Creating a Floor-Ready Nurse

Instructor Resources—Redefined!

INTRODUCING
Pearson Nursing Class Preparation Resources

- **New and Unique!** Correlation to Today's Nursing Standards!
  - Correlation guides link book and supplement content to nursing standards such as the *2010 ANA Scope and Standards of Practice*, *QSEN, National Patient Safety Goals, AACN Essentials of Baccalaureate Education* and more!

- **New and Unique! Pearson Nursing Lecture Series**
  - Highly visual, fully narrated and animated, these short lectures focus on topics that are traditionally difficult to teach and difficult for students to grasp
  - All lectures accompanied by case studies and classroom response questions for greater interactivity within even the largest classroom
  - Useful as lecture tools, remediation material, homework assignments and more!

- **Additional instructor resources!**
  - Find assets such as **videos, animations, lecture starters, classroom and clinical activities** and more!
  - **Add selected resources** to presentations that can be shown online or exported to PowerPoint™ or HTML pages
  - Organized by topic and **fully searchable** by type and keyword
  - **Upload your own resources** to keep everything in one place
  - **Rate resources** and view other instructor ratings!

- **Pearson** Nursing Question Bank
  - Even **more** accessible with both pencil and paper and online delivery options
  - **All NCLEX®-style** questions
  - **All New!** Approximately 30% of questions now in alternate-item format!
  - **Complete rationales** for both correct and incorrect answers mapped to learning outcomes

Book-specific resources also available to instructors including:

- Instructor's Manual and Resource Guide organized by learning outcome
- Comprehensive PowerPoint™ presentations integrating lecture notes and images
- Image library
- Classroom Response Questions
- Online course management systems complete with instructor tools and student activities

mynursinglab

- Saves instructor time by providing quality feedback, ongoing formative assessments, and customized remediation for students
- **New and Unique!** *ECG: The Art and Science of Interpretation.* A special ECG module prepares students for the important skill of interpreting ECGs. Includes:
  - Mini-lectures, quizzes, animations, and hundreds of practice strips
- **New!** Select *Real Nursing Simulation* scenarios
- Includes select set of *Real Nursing Skill 2.0* videos
- Available with *Pearson's Interactive e-Text*
  - Integrated media and website links
  - Full search capability and note-taking functionality
  - Customizable organization

REAL NURSING SIMULATIONS

- 25 simulation scenarios that span the nursing curriculum
- Consistent format includes learning objectives, case flow, set-up instructions, debriefing questions and more!

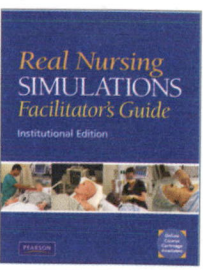

- Companion online course cartridge with student pre- and post-simulation activities, videos, skill checklists and reflective discussion questions

Brief Contents

Medical-Surgical
NURSING
Critical Thinking in Client Care
Volume One

FIFTH EDITION

Priscilla LeMone, RN, DSN, FAAN
Associate Professor Emeritus
Sinclair School of Nursing
University of Missouri
Columbia, Missouri

Karen Burke, RN, MS
Education Consultant
Astoria, Oregon

Gerene Bauldoff, RN, PhD, FAAN
Associate Professor of Clinical Nursing
The Ohio State University
Columbus, Ohio

Pearson

Boston   Columbus   Indianapolis   New York   San Francisco   Upper Saddle River
Amsterdam   Cape Town   Dubai   London   Madrid   Milan   Munich   Paris   Montreal   Toronto
Delhi   Mexico City   Sao Paulo   Sydney   Hong Kong   Seoul   Singapore   Taipei   Tokyo

Library of Congress Cataloging-in-Publication Data

LeMone, Priscilla.
  Medical-surgical nursing : critical thinking in client care / Priscilla LeMone, Karen Burke, Gerene
Bauldoff. -- 5th ed.
     p. ; cm.
  Rev. ed. of: Medical-surgical nursing. 4th ed. c2008.
  Includes bibliographical references and index.
  ISBN-13: 978-0-13-507594-4
  ISBN-10: 0-13-507594-7
  1. Nursing. 2. Surgical nursing. 3. Critical thinking. I. Burke, Karen M. II. Bauldoff, Gerene. III.
Medical-surgical nursing. IV. Title.
  [DNLM: 1. Nursing Process. 2. Nursing Care. 3. Patient Care Planning. 4. Perioperative Nursing.
WY 100.1]
  RT41.M493 2011
  617'.0231--dc22

                              2010042914

Publisher: Julie Levin Alexander
Assistant to Publisher: Regina Bruno
Executive Acquisitions Editor: Pamela Fuller
Editorial Assistant: Lisa Pierce/Cynthia Gates
Development Editor: Barbara Price
Director of Marketing: David Gesell
Marketing Manager: Phoenix Harvey
Marketing Specialist: Michael Sirinides
Managing Editor, Production: Patrick Walsh
Production Editor: GEX Publishing Services
Production Liaison: Cathy O'Connell
Digital Media Product Manager: Travis Moses-Westphal
Media Project Manager: Rachel Collett
Manufacturing Manager: Ilene Sanford
Senior Art Director: Mary Siener
Art Editor: Patricia Gutierrez
Assistant Editor for Media: Sarah Wrocklage
Interior Design: GEX Publishing Services
Cover and Interior Design: Mary Siener
Manager, Image Rights and Permissions: Annette Linder
Composition: GEX Publishing Services
Printer/Binder: Courier Kendallville
Cover Printer: Lehigh-Phoenix Color/Hagerstown
Cover Photograph: Rick Brady

Notice: Care has been taken to confirm the accuracy of information presented in this book. The authors, editors, and the publisher, however, cannot accept any responsibility for errors or omissions or for consequences from application of the information in this book and make no warranty, express or implied, with respect to its contents.

   The authors and publisher have exerted every effort to ensure that drug selections and dosages set forth in this text are in accord with current recommendations and practice at time of publication. However, in view of ongoing research, changes in government regulations, and the constant flow of information relating to drug therapy and reactions, the reader is urged to check the package inserts of all drugs for any change in indications or dosage and for added warning and precautions. This is particularly important when the recommended agent is a new and/or infrequently employed drug.

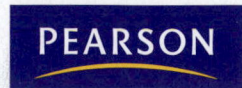

www.pearsonhighered.com

10 9 8 7 6 5 4 3 2

ISBN-13: 978-0-13-254180-0
ISBN-10: 0-13-254180-7

About the Authors

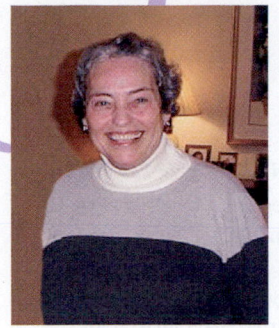

Priscilla LeMone, RN, DSN, FAAN

Associate Professor Emeritus, Sinclair School of Nursing, University of Missouri; Adjunct Associate Professor of Nursing, College of Nursing, The Ohio State University

Priscilla LeMone spent most of her career as a nurse educator, teaching medical-surgical nursing and pathophysiology at all levels from diploma to doctoral students. She has a diploma in nursing from Deaconess College of Nursing (St. Louis, Missouri), baccalaureate and master's degrees from Southeast Missouri State University, and a doctorate in nursing from the University of Alabama–Birmingham. She is retired as an Associate Professor Emeritus, Sinclair School of Nursing, University of Missouri, but continues to keep up to date in nursing both as an Adjunct Associate Professor at The Ohio State University, College of Nursing and as an author of nursing textbooks.

Dr. LeMone had numerous awards for scholarship and teaching during her more than 30 years as a nurse educator. She is most honored for receiving the Kemper Fellowship for Teaching Excellence from the University of Missouri, the Unique Contribution Award from the North American Nursing Diagnosis Association, and for being selected as a Fellow in the American Academy of Nursing

Dr. LeMone currently lives in Ohio. She enjoys traveling, gardening, knitting, and reading fiction.

She believes that her education gave her solid and everlasting roots in nursing. Her work with students has given her the wings that have allowed her love of nursing and teaching to continue through the years.

I dedicate this book to all the students who will become the caregivers. The following quote provides a solid base for your professional future:

How far you go in life depends on your being tender with the young, compassionate with the aged, sympathetic with the striving and tolerant of the weak and the strong, because someday in your life you will have been all of these. (George Washington Carver)

Priscilla LeMone

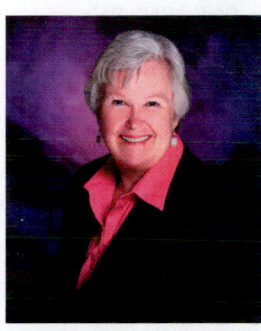

Karen M. Burke, RN, MS

Karen Burke has been a nurse educator for much of her career, teaching basic and advanced medical-surgical nursing and pathophysiology. She retired as director of the nursing and health occupations programs at Clatsop Community College in Astoria, Oregon, subsequently serving as nursing education consultant and program manager for the Oregon State Board of Nursing. She currently provides consulting services for nursing and higher education.

Ms. Burke earned her diploma in nursing from Emanuel Hospital School of Nursing in Portland, Oregon, later completing baccalaureate studies at Oregon Health & Science University, and a master's degree in nursing at the University of Portland. She has been actively involved in nursing education and clinical nursing education reform, as well as in initiatives to address the nursing faculty shortage. Ms. Burke is coauthor of another text, *Medical-Surgical Nursing Care* (3rd edition) with Elaine Mohn-Brown and Linda Eby.

Ms. Burke strongly values the nursing profession and the importance of providing a strong education in the art and science of nursing for students preparing to enter the profession, no matter which educational path is being pursued.

I dedicate this book to Brad, Faith, Max, and Aliya – who will carry our family into the future – and to all the nursing students who carry our profession into the future.

Karen Burke

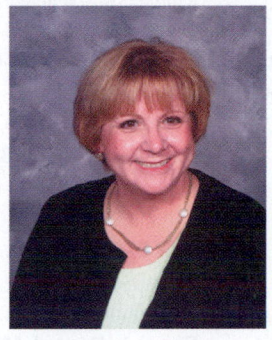

Gerene Bauldoff, RN, PhD, FAAN

Gerene Bauldoff is an Associate Professor of Clinical Nursing at The Ohio State University College of Nursing in Columbus, Ohio. She has been a nurse educator for ten years, teaching medical-surgical nursing, clinical specialist role and translational science courses at the baccalaureate, master's and doctoral levels. Prior to her nursing educator role, her clinical background includes home health nurse, lung transplant coordinator and pulmonary rehabilitation coordinator. Dr. Bauldoff has a diploma from the Western Pennsylvania Hospital School of Nursing, Pittsburgh, PA, and a BSN from LaRoche College in Pittsburgh. Her graduate education is from the University of Pittsburgh, with a MSN in medical-surgical nursing (Cardiopulmonary clinical nurse specialist) and PhD in nursing in 2001, training under Leslie Hoffman, PhD, RN, FAAN.

Dr. Bauldoff is an active member in multiple professional organizations including Sigma Theta Tau International Honor Society of Nursing, the American Association of Cardiovascular and Pulmonary Rehabilitation (AACVPR), the American Thoracic Society Nursing Assembly and the American College of Chest Physicians (ACCP). She is a recognized expert in medical-surgical nursing, focusing on the care of the patient with chronic pulmonary disease and served as the nursing representative on the ACCP/AACVPR Evidence-based Guidelines for Pulmonary Rehabilitation published in 2007. She has been honored with fellowship in AACVPR and ACCP. She currently serves on the Board of Directors of the American Association of Cardiovascular and Pulmonary Rehabilitation and has been appointed to the Community-Based Care board of the Ohio Council of Home Care and Hospice.

Dr. Bauldoff feels nursing is the best profession, using scientific evidence to provide the highest quality of care while maintaining the personal relationship with the patient and their family. Her experiences provide her with insights and lessons learned that she shares with her students.

Dr. Bauldoff resides in central Ohio. She enjoys reading, walking, bicycling, golf, and spending time with her family and friends. She is learning the intricacies of social networking and keeps up to date with technology to be able to interface with her students, family, and friends.

I dedicate this book to my parents, Melvin and the late Frieda Bauldoff, who taught me and my sisters that education is the springboard to a life of great joy and adventure. I also dedicate this book to Dr. Leslie Hoffman, my mentor and role model—she remains who I would like to be when I grow up!

Gerene Bauldoff

Thank You

Contributors

We extend a heartfelt thanks to our contributors, who gave their time, effort, and expertise so tirelessly to the development and writing of chapters and resources that helped foster our goal of preparing student nurses for evidence-based practice.

Textbook Contributors

Jane E. Bostick, PhD, RN, PMHCNS-BC

Associate Teaching Professor, University of Missouri Sinclair School of Nursing, Columbia, Missouri
Chapters 3 and 6

Renae L. Dougal, MSN, RN, CLNC, CCRP

Nurse Educator Specialist, Clinical Education & Research Department , Saint Alphonsus Regional Medical Center, Boise, Idaho,
Research Feature

Mei R. Fu, PhD, RN, ACNS-BC

Assistant Professor, College of Nursing, New York University, New York, New York
Chapter 14

Gina Dahlby, MSN, RN

Assistant Professor, MedCentral College of Nursing, Mansfield, Ohio, *Chapter 7*

Bonnie L. Kirkpatrick RN, MS, CNS, CNL

Clinical Instructor, The Ohio State University College of Nursing, Columbus, Ohio
Chapter 10

Kimberly R. Regis, RN, MS,CPNP

Nurse Practitioner, Section of Molecular and Human Genetics, Nationwide Children's Hospital, Columbus, Ohio, *Chapter 8*

Mary Ann Towle, BSN, MSN, MEd

Senior Instructor, Boise State University, Boise, Idaho, *Clinical competencies/End of unit features*

Marjorie Whitman RN, MSN, AOCN

Nursing Consultant, University of Missouri Hospital & Clinics (retired), Columbia, Missouri, *Chapters 4, 12, 13, 19, 20*

Janice Wilcox, MSN, RN

Nursing Educator, The Ohio State Medical Center, Columbus, Ohio
Chapters 48 and 49

Student and Instructional Resource Contributors

Tracy Blanc, RN, BSN

Nursing Instructor, Ivy Tech Community College, Terre Haute, Indiana

Wanda Bonnel, PhD, RN, ANEF

Associate Professor, University of Kansas, Kansas City, Kansas

Jane Bostick, PhD, RN, PMHCNS-BC

Associate Teaching Professor, University of Missouri-Columbia, Columbia, Missouri

Donna Bowles, RN, EdD, CNE

Associate Professor, Indiana University Southeast, New Albany, Indiana

Janet Brown, PhD, RN, CNE

Associate Professor, The University of Tennessee, Knoxville, Knoxville, Tennessee

Janet E. Burton, MSN, RN, CMSRN

Medical-Surgical Nursing Instructor, Ivy Tech Community College, Columbus, Indiana

Emily Cannon, RN, MSN

Associate Professor, Ivy Tech Community College, Terre Haute, Indiana

Kathleen A. Clark, BSN, MSN

Assistant Professor, College of Saint Mary, Omaha, Nebraska

Kim D. Cooper, RN, MSN

Nursing Department Chair, Ivy Tech Community College, Terre Haute, Indiana

Renae L. Dougal, MSN, RN, CLNC, CCRP

Nurse Educator Specialist, Clinical Education & Research Department , Saint Alphonsus Regional Medical Center, Boise, Idaho

Daniel B. Flores Jr., MSN, RN

Faculty, Baptist Health System School of Health Professions, San Antonio, Texas

Pam Fowler, MS, RN

Retired, Rogers State University, Claremore, Oklahoma

Kathy Garza, MS, BSN, RN

Associate Professor, Hocking College, Nelsonville, Ohio

Caushauana Harvey, MSN, RN

Nursing Faculty, Fortis College-Columbus, Westerville, Ohio

Tiffany Johnson, MSN, RN

Instructor, West Georgia Technical College, Waco, Georgia

Christina D. Keller, RN, MSN

Assistant Professor, Virginia Western Community College, Roanoke, Virginia

Cynthia J. Larsen, MSN, RN, CNE

Nursing Instructor, Southwest Wisconsin Technical College, Fennimore, Wisconsin

Anne M Larson PhD, RN, CNE, BC

Professor, Midland Lutheran College, Fremont, Nebraska

Wanda Lawrence, PhD, RNC, MSN

Assistant Professor, Winston-Salem State University, Winston-Salem, North Carolina

Dawna Martich, RN, MSN

Nursing Education Consultant, Pittsburgh, Pennsylvania

Joni Meeker, RN, MSN, FNP-BC

Professor, Hondros College, Westerville, Ohio

Dona Molyneaux, PhD

Associate Professor, Gwynedd Mercy College, Gwynedd Valley, Pennsylvania

Leigh Moore, MSN, RN, CNOR, CNE

Associate Professor, Southside Virginia Community College, Alberta, Virginia

Traci Moxley, RN, MSN

Nursing Faculty, Harrisburg Area Community College, Lancaster, Pennsylvania

Christina C. Olson, RN, MSN

Program Coordinator of Nursing, San Antonio College, San Antonio, Texas

Felicia Vergara Omick, MSN, RN, CNE

Assistant Professor, Southside Virginia Community College, Alberta, Virginia

Jill Price, MSN, RN, CCRN

Online Services, DeVry Inc., Faculty Manager, Chamberlain College of Nursing, Senior Faculty, Chamberlain College of Nursing, US Virgin Islands

Sharon R. Redding, MN, RN, CNE

Associate Professor of Nursing, College of Saint Mary, Omaha, Nebraska

Margaret Reneau, RN, MSN

Online Faculty Manager and Operations Liaison, Chamberlain College of Nursing, Jacksonville, Florida

Elizabeth Schneider, RN, MSN, CNS

Program Director, Keiser University, Ft. Lauderdale Campus, Florida

Caryn A. Sheehan, DNP, ARNP, RN

Associate Professor, Saint Anselm College, Manchester, New Hampshire

Judy K. Smith, MSN, RN, BC

Assistant Professor, Lamar University, Beaumont, Texas

Betsy Swinny, MSN, RN, CCRN

Faculty II, BHS School of Health Professions, San Antonio, Texas

Jeri Taylor, BS, RN

Associate Professor, Ivy Tech Community College, Terre Haute, Indiana

Charlotte A. Wisnewski, PhD, RN, BC, CDE, CNE

Associate Professor, University of Texas Medical Branch, Galveston, Texas

Reviewers

Our heartfelt thanks go out to our colleagues from schools of nursing across the country who have given their time generously to help create this exciting new edition of our medical–surgical nursing textbook. These individuals helped us plan and shape our book and resources by reviewing chapters, art, design, and more. *Medical–Surgical Nursing: Critical Thinking in Patient Care* has reaped the benefits of your collective knowledge and experience as nurses and teachers, and we have improved the materials due to your efforts, suggestions, objections, endorsements, and inspiration. Among those who gave their time generously to help us are the following:

Academic Reviewers

Julie Baldwin, RN, MSN, BC

Assistant Professor, Missouri Western State University, St. Joseph, Missouri

Michael Beach DNP, ACNP-BC, PNP

Assistant Professor, University of Pittsburgh, Pittsburgh, Pennsylvania

Sophia Beydoun RN MSN

Nursing Instructor, Henry Ford Community College, Dearborn, Michigan

Tracy Blanc, RN, BSN

Nursing Instructor, Ivy Tech Community College, Terre Haute, Indiana

Jill Brennan-Cook, DNP, RN, CEN

Associate Professor of Nursing, Mount Saint Mary College, Newburgh, New York

Janet E. Burton, MSN, RN, CMSRN

Medical-Surgical Nursing Instructor, Ivy Tech Community College, Columbus, Indiana

Theresa Delahoyde, EdD, RN

Associate Professor, BryanLGH College of Health Sciences, Waverly, Nebraska

Deborah Ellis RN, MSN, NP-C

Assistant Professor, Missouri Western State University, St. Joseph, Missouri

Maria Farber, MSN, RN, BC, OCN

Instructor, Middlesex County College, Edison, New Jersey

Karlynne Galczyk MPH, MSN, RN

Lecturer, Widener University, Chester, Pennsylvania

Carman Godfrey, MSN, RN

Nursing Instructor, Faulkner State Community College, Bay Minette, Alabama

Janet Riga Goeldner, RN, MSN, AOCN

Professor, University of Cincinnati, Cincinnati, Ohio

Claudia Haile, RN, MSN

Instructor, Corning Community College, Corning, New York

Jackie Harris, MNSc, RN

Assistant Professor, Harding University, Searcy, Arkansas

Caushauana Harvey, MSN, RN

Nursing Faculty, Fortis College-Columbus, Westerville, Ohio

Roseann Kaminsky, RN, BSN, BSEd, MSN

Associate Professor, Lorain County Community College, Elyria, Ohio

Cheryl Lantz, RN, MS, PhDc

Assistant Professor, Dickinson State University, Dickinson, North Dakota

Anne M Larson PhD, RN, CNE, BC

Professor, Midland Lutheran College, Fremont, Nebraska

Karla Larson, MSN, RN, GNP

Assistant Professor, Indiana Wesleyan University, Marion, Indiana

Virginia Lester, RN MSN

Assistant Professor, Department of Nursing, Angelo State University, San Angelo, Texas

Margie Lovett-Scott, FNP

Associate Professor, The College at Brockport, Brockport, New York

Ann Marie E. McSwain, RN, MSN, CCNS, CCRN, APRN, BC

Assistant Professor, Lincoln University, Jefferson City, Missouri

Dianne Murphy, DNP, RN, CCRN

Associate Professor, Mount Saint Mary College, Newburgh, New York

Donna Molyneaux, PhD

Associate Professor, Gwynedd-Mercy College, Gwynedd Valley, Pennsylvania

Karen Sheffield O'Brien, RN PhD, ACNP-BC

Assistant Professor, University of Texas Medical Branch, Galveston, Texas

Stefani O'Connor, MS, RN, CCM

Clinical Instructor, The Ohio State University, Columbus, Ohio

Mia Toles-Pickard, MSN, MHA

Instructor, University of Phoenix/Axia College, Phoenix, Arizona

Sharon R. Redding, MN, RN, CNE

Associate Professor of Nursing, College of Saint Mary, Omaha, Nebraska

Stacy Rose, MSN, RN, CRNP

Assistant Professor, Kent State University, Ashtabula, Ohio

Sonia Rudolph, RN, MSN, ARNP, FNP-BC

Associate Professor, Jefferson Community & Technical College, Louisville, Kentucky

Joanne Farley Serembus, EdD, RN, CCRN, CNE

Clinical Associate Professor, Drexel University, Philadelphia, Pennsylvania

Marianne F. Swihart, RN, BSN, MEd, MSN

Associate Professor, Pasco Hernando Community College, New Port Richey, Florida

Shirley Van Zandt, MS, MPH, CRNP

Instructor, Johns Hopkins University, Baltimore, Maryland

Denyce Watties-Daniels, RN, MSN

Assistant Professor, Coppin State University, Baltimore, Maryland

Charlotte A. Wisnewski, PhD, RN, BC, CDE, CNE

Associate Professor, University of Texas Medical Branch, Galveston, Texas

Denise York, RNC, CNS, MS, MEd

Professor, Columbus State Community College, Columbus, Ohio

Preface

Why We Wrote this Book

Medical-Surgical Nursing: Critical Thinking in Patient Care is based on our philosophy that nursing care is provided for the whole person, and not just for a malfunction of one or more body systems. Therefore, our text is structured by functional health patterns. Functional health patterns, as defined by Dr. Marjorie Gordon, include several important components: patterns of behavior, nursing assessment, and nursing diagnoses. Patterns indicate a sequence of recurring behavior and are interrelated, interactive, and interdependent. Health behaviors may be functional or dysfunctional. Dysfunctional patterns of health are indicated by manifestations of an illness or trauma, or may be risk factors for illness or injury. Both functional and dysfunctional patterns of health are identified by assessment and are given labels (nursing diagnoses) to direct care within the nursing process.

We revised and updated the fifth edition of *Medical-Surgical Nursing: Critical Thinking in Patient Care* to provide the knowledge and skills needed to care for adult patients to promote health, facilitate recovery from illness and injury, and provide support when coping with disability or loss. Throughout the text, we make every effort to communicate that both nurses and patients may be male or female; and that patients require holistic, individualized care regardless of their age, gender, or racial, cultural, or socioeconomic background. Our goal is to provide the knowledge and resources that ensure a solid base for critical thinking and clinical judgment and that can be applied to provide safe, individualized, and competent clinical nursing care. We use understandable language and a consistent format, and students overwhelmingly report that they actually like reading our text. We have developed multiple learning strategies to facilitate success—audio, illustrations, teaching tips, and video and animation media.

Starting with the first edition, we have held fast to our vision that this textbook

- maintains a strong focus on nursing care as the essential element in learning and doing nursing, regardless of the gender, age, race, culture, or socioeconomic background of the patient or the setting for care.

- provides a balance of pathophysiology, pharmacology, and interdisciplinary care to support dependent, interdependent, and independent nursing interventions.

- emphasizes the nurse's role as a caregiver, educator, advocate, leader and manager, and as an essential member of the interdisciplinary healthcare team.

- uses functional health patterns and the nursing process as the structure for providing nursing care in today's world by prioritizing nursing diagnoses and interventions specific to altered responses to illness.

- fosters critical thinking and decision-making skills as the basis for safe, knowledgeable, individualized clinical practice.

ORGANIZATION

The book is organized into 50 chapters in six major parts, organized by functional health patterns. Each part opens with a concept map illustrating the relationship of a specific functional health pattern to possible nursing diagnoses. The parts are then divided into units based on alterations in human structure and function. Each unit with a focus on altered health states opens with an assessment chapter. This chapter draws upon the student's prerequisite knowledge, and serves to reinforce basic principles of anatomy and physiology as applied to assessment in both health and illness. To increase student learning, each chapter in the book includes key terms, learning outcomes and clinical competencies, chapter highlights (not included in the assessment chapters), test yourself NCLEX-type questions, and a bibliography that provides additional reading.

Following the assessment chapter in each unit, the nursing care chapters provide information about major illnesses and traumatic injuries. Each of the nursing care chapters follows a consistent format, including three key components:

PATHOPHYSIOLOGY The discussion of each *major* illness or injury begins with incidence and prevalence, risk factors, and an overview of pathophysiology, followed by manifestations (signs and symptoms) and complications. Selected *Focus on Cultural Diversity* boxes demonstrate how race, age, and gender affect differences in incidence, prevalence, and mortality. *Pathophysiology Linkage* tables provide the pathophysiologic basis for manifestations. Throughout, *Pathophysiology Illustrated* and *Multisystem Effects of Illness* art brings changes in physiologic processes to life. *Manifestation* boxes summarize specific subjective and objective manifestations.

INTERDISCIPLINARY CARE Interdisciplinary care considers diagnosis and treatment by the healthcare team. The section includes information, as appropriate, about specific tests necessary for diagnosis, medications, surgery and other treatments, fluid management, dietary management, and complementary and alternative therapies. Specific information with related nursing care is highlighted in *Medication Administration* boxes, *Nursing Care of Patients (such as those having a specific treatment or surgery)* boxes, and Procedure boxes describing care for advanced procedures.

NURSING CARE Because illness prevention is critical in health care today, health promotion information introduces the nursing care discussion of major illnesses or injuries. Selected major illnesses also include *Evidence for Nursing Care* boxes with resources for additional review in applying evidence to practice. We discuss nursing assessment and care within a context of priority nursing diagnoses and interventions, with rationales provided for each intervention. Boxes throughout each illness discussion section present information essential to patient care. These features include *Nursing Care*, *Nursing Care of the Older Adult*, *Meeting Individualized Needs*, *Practice Alerts*, *Safety Alerts*, *Moving Evidence into Action* (a summary of a nursing study with critical thinking questions), and *NANDA, NIC, and NOC Linkages*. Last, for 80 major disorders or trauma, we provide a narrative *Case Study & Nursing Care Plan*. Critical thinking questions specific to the care plan conclude with a section called *Evaluate Your Response* that provides additional guidance for critical thinking (with suggestions for decisions provided in the appendix). The nursing care section ends with information about community-based care with suggestions for referrals and additional patient resources.

CHAPTER REVIEW This end-of-chapter section concludes with ten or more multiple-choice NCLEX-type review questions to reinforce comprehension of the chapter content. (The correct answers with rationales are found in Appendix C.) Students can log on to the student resources website to apply what they have learned from the textbook through critical thinking and interactive exercises.

What's New in the Fifth Edition

■ We are delighted to welcome Gerene Bauldoff as a co-author of this book. Information about Dr. Bauldoff is included in a separate section.

All the chapters of the fifth edition of this book were extensively reviewed, and reviewer comments were used to make this revision. New features of the fifth edition include the following:

■ Using the term *patient* to describe the recipient of nursing care; this change reflects current language used by major nursing organizations.

■ A reorganization of some units as follows:

• ***Responses to Altered Nutrition*** (unit 6) includes chapters on assessment and care of patients with nutritional disorders, upper gastrointestinal disorders, bowel disorders, and disorders of the gallbladder, liver, and pancreas.

• ***Responses to Altered Cardiovascular Function*** (unit 8) includes chapters on assessment and care of patients with coronary heart disease, cardiac disorders, vascular and lymphatic disorders, and hematologic disorders.

• ***Responses to Altered Neurologic Function*** includes chapters on assessment and care of patients with intracranial disorders, spinal cord disorders, and neurologic disorders.

■ The diagnostic tables in each assessment chapter have been expanded and are listed alphabetically, and a question about spirituality was added to the functional health pattern interview guide.

■ Memory cues provide methods of remembering important information.

■ Pathophysiology Linkage tables illustrate the way in which a specific disease pathophysiology results in patient manifestations.

Features

PATHOPHYSIOLOGY ILLUSTRATED

The 3-D art brings the content to life—visual illustrations of disease processes make processes easy to visualize.

PATHOPHYSIOLOGY ILLUSTRATED
Acute Renal Failure

The initial kidney injury is usually associated with an acute condition such as sepsis, trauma, and hypotension, or the result of treatment for an acute condition with a nephrotoxic medication. Injury to the kidney can occur because of glomerular injury, vasoconstriction of capillaries, or tubular injury. All consequences of injury lead to decreased glomerular filtration and oliguria.

PATHOPHYSIOLOGY LINKAGE Fluid Volume Excess

MANIFESTATIONS	RELATED PATHOPHYSIOLOGY
Peripheral edema, or if severe, anasarca (severe, generalized edema)	Excess fluid in the interstitial spaces, usually resulting from conditions that cause retention of both sodium and water (heart failure, cirrhosis of the liver, renal failure, adrenal gland disorders, corticosteroid administration, and stress conditions causing the release of ADH and aldosterone, such as surgery)
Full bounding pulse, distended neck and peripheral veins, increased central venous pressure (>11–12 cm of water), cough, dyspnea (labored or difficult breathing), **orthopnea** (difficult breathing when supine)	Circulatory overload from increased water and sodium retention
Dyspnea at rest	Impaired gas exchange from pulmonary interstitial edema
Tachycardia and hypertension	Increased circulatory fluid volume
Reduced oxygen saturation	As fluid increases in the interstitial spaces and alveoli, gas exchange is impaired, leading to hypoxia and hypercapnia
Moist crackles on auscultation of the lungs, pulmonary edema	Excess fluid in pulmonary interstitial spaces and alveoli
Increased urine output (polyuria)	Increased sodium and water retention resulting in increased circulatory volume and increased perfusion of the renal arteries
Ascites (excess fluid in the peritoneal cavity)	Sodium and water retention
Decreased hematocrit and BUN	Dilutional effect of increased circulatory volume
Altered mental status and anxiety	Pressure on the cerebral cortex from an increase in cerebral contents and cerebral hypertension causes decreased oxygenation (hypoxia) of neurons
Pulmonary edema	Elevation of left-sided filling pressures resulting from increased circulatory volume and heart failure

PATHOPHYSIOLOGY LINKAGE

Pathophysiology linkages are tables that show the relationships between specific disease pathophysiologies and resulting clinical manifestations.

Features

DIAGNOSTIC TESTS

The three-column tables summarize information about key diagnostic tests for each body system.

MOVING EVIDENCE INTO ACTION

These boxes focus on research into specific topics and how the research relates to current nursing care. Critical-thinking questions help students understand the material.

MOVING EVIDENCE INTO ACTION — Preventing Pressure Ulcers in Acute Care and Home Care Settings

Despite advances in health care to extend life and improve functional status, older adults with chronic illnesses are at increased risk of developing pressure ulcers. The older adult, with age-related compromised cellular activity is especially vulnerable to impaired healing of injured tissue such as pressure ulcers. This article (Frantz, 2004) describes an evidence-based protocol designed to enhance the healing of pressure ulcers in older patients by using evidence-based interventions. The following interventions are recommended:

- Assess all individuals admitted to a healthcare facility with a pressure ulcer for the risk of developing additional pressure ulcers by using a standardized risk assessment scale.
- Perform a complete history and physical examination, combined with a detailed assessment of the ulcer characteristics (location, stage, type of tissue, presence of tunneling or tracts, exudate, odor, and condition of skin around the ulcer).
- Remove necrotic tissue and debris from the ulcer to decrease the growth of bacteria and remove foreign materials, such as exudates and metabolic wastes.
- Provide a moist wound environment to promote reepithelialization and healing.
- Control bacterial levels in the wound by using cleansing and debridment, as well as systemic and topical antibiotics.
- Supply essential substrates for tissue repair, including protein, calories, vitamins, and minerals. Maintain a positive nitrogen balance.
- Manage tissue loads by positioning to avoid external force on the ulcer.

IMPLICATIONS FOR NURSING
The design and implementation of a pressure ulcer prevention and treatment plan is essential for any person at risk, including older adults, those with debilitating or multiple illnesses, and those with health problems limiting mobility. To effectively implement a plan, it is important to prepare providers to use a standard protocol through educational programs, and to monitor indicators of improvement or deterioration in the ulcer and presence or absence of new ulcers. These outcomes should be assessed and recorded on a weekly basis.

CRITICAL THINKING IN PATIENT CARE
1. Describe the differences and similarities in a pressure ulcer prevention plan of care you would develop for two patients: a 76-year-old man in a nursing home who has had a stroke that paralyzed his left side, and a 36-year-old man with a spinal cord injury from a motorcycle accident who cannot walk and lives at home.
2. Consider the activities to treat pressure ulcers, and answer the following:
   a. What level of healthcare provider would you delegate to care for the patient?
   b. How much time in an 8-hour period would be needed for nursing care?
3. What would you teach family caregivers about providing care at home?

EVIDENCE FOR NURSING CARE

Evidence for Nursing Care boxes provide resources for additional review in applying evidence to practice.

EVIDENCE FOR NURSING CARE — The Patient with Bacterial Infection of the Skin

Selected resources that nurses may find helpful when planning evidence-based nursing care follow.

- Casey, M. L., & Chasens, E. R. (2009). Community-associated methicillin-resistant staphylococcus aureus: Implications for emergency department nursing. *Journal of Emergency Nursing, 35*(3), 224–229.
- Haas, J. P., & Larson, E. L. (2008). Compliance with hand hygiene. *The American Journal of Nursing, 108*(8), 40–44.
- Hodgkinson, B., Agnew, J., Godfrey, C., Goldie, B., Kenner, C., González, R. L., Ramirez, B. A., Maria, E. G., McInerney, P., & Robertson-Malt, S. (2007). Topical skin care in aged care facilities. *Best Practice, The Joanna Briggs Institute, 11*(3), 1–4. Retrieved from http://www.joannabriggs.edu.au/pdf/BPISEng_11_3.pdf
- Johnson, D., Lineweaver, L., & Maze, L. M. (2009). Patients' bath basins as potential sources of infection: A multicenter sampling study. *American Journal of Critical Care, 18*(1), 31–38.

FUNCTIONAL HEALTH PATTERN ASSESSMENT

Health history questions are described for the functional health patterns related to each unit.

GENETIC CONSIDERATIONS

For each unit, this feature lists genetic issues related to the body system.

GENETIC CONSIDERATIONS — Examples of Integumentary Disorders

- Oculocutaneous albinism, an autosomal recessive inheritance disorder, causes hypopigmentation (albinism or absence of color) of the skin, hair, and eyes as a result of an inability to synthesize melanin.
- Keloids, which are elevated scars, have a familial tendency and are more commonly found in Blacks.
- Vitiligo, the sudden appearance of white patches on the skin, has a familial tendency.
- Male pattern baldness (the most common cause of baldness in men) is genetically predetermined.
- Hirsutism (excessive hair in women) may be genetically predetermined.
- Blacks may have very dry scalps and dry, fragile hair of genetic origin.
- A family history of skin cancer is a risk factor for skin cancer

DIAGNOSTIC TESTS of the Integumentary System

NAME OF TEST	PURPOSE & DESCRIPTION	RELATED NURSING INTERVENTIONS
Biopsy	A punch biopsy is done to differentiate benign lesions from skin cancers. An instrument is used to remove a small section of dermis and subcutaneous fat. Depending on size, the incision may be sutured with a single suture. An incisional biopsy is done to differentiate benign lesions from skin cancers. An incision is made and the skin lesion or tumor is removed for analysis. The incision is closed with sutures.	Apply dressing and provide information about self-care and when to return for suture removal.
Culture	A culture of scrapings from a lesion, from drainage, or of exudate is done to identify fungal, bacterial, or viral skin infections.	Obtain the culture with a sterile Culturette swab and culture tubes. Maintain strict asepsis while obtaining the culture.
Immunofluorescent Slides	Immunofluorescent studies of samples from skin and/or serum may be done to identify IgG antibodies (present in pemphigus vulgaris) and to identify varicella in skin cells (for herpes zoster). Skin or blood samples are placed on a slide and examined microscopically.	No special preparation is necessary.
Oil Slides	Oil slides are used to determine the type of skin infestation present. Scrapings of the lesion are placed on a slide with mineral oil and examined microscopically.	No special preparation is necessary.
	These tests are used to determine a specific allergen. In a patch test, a small amount of the suspected material is placed on the skin under an occlusive bandage. In a scratch test, a needle is used to "scratch" small amounts of potentially allergic materials on the skin surface.	Explain to the patient the need to return in 48 hours to have the patched area or scratched areas evaluated.
	A specimen from hair or nails is examined for a fungal infection. The specimen is obtained by placing material from a scraping on a slide, adding a potassium hydroxide solution, and examining it microscopically.	No special preparation is necessary.
	This test is used to diagnose herpes infections, but it does not differentiate herpes simplex from herpes zoster. Fluid and cells from the vesicles are obtained, put on a slide, stained, and examined microscopically.	
	This test uses an ultraviolet light that causes certain organisms to fluoresce (such as *Pseudomonas* organisms and fungi). The skin is examined under a special lamp.	

FUNCTIONAL HEALTH PATTERN INTERVIEW   Integumentary System

Functional Health Pattern	Interview Questions and Leading Statements
Health Perception-Health Management	- Describe any health problems, injuries, or surgeries you have had. How were these treated? - Describe medications, herbs, and vitamins you currently are taking. - Describe your current problem. How long has it lasted? What have you done to treat it? - Do you have allergies to foods, plants, pets? Explain how the allergy affects you. - Describe what you do each day to care for your skin, hair, and nails.
Nutritional-Metabolic	- Describe what you eat and how much and type of fluids you drink in a 24-hour period. - Do you have a history of food allergies? If so, describe what you are allergic to and how you respond. - Have you recently eaten any new foods? - Do you take any nutritional supplements, herbs, or vitamins? If so, what are they? - How well do your cuts and scratches heal?
Elimination	- Is your skin and scalp dry or oily? - Have you noticed swelling around your eyes or ankles? - Do you perspire a lot?
Activity-Exercise	- Describe your physical activities in a typical day. - Do you bruise easily? - Do you use a sunscreen when you are outside? If so, what SPF? - Do you visit tanning salons?
Sleep-Rest	- How many hours do you sleep each night? - Do you have trouble sleeping because of itching or sweating?
Cognitive-Perceptual	- Do you have any of the following: pain, discomfort, itching, tingling, burning, tenderness, or numbness? If so, where?
Self-Perception-Self-Concept	- How does this condition make you feel about yourself?
Role-Relationships	- How does this condition affect your relationships with others? - Is there anything in your work environment that may have caused this condition?
Sexuality-Reproductive	- Has this condition interfered with your usual sexual activities?
Coping-Stress-Tolerance	- Have you experienced any type of stress that may have worsened this condition? - Has this condition created stress for you? - Describe what you do when you feel stressed.
Value-Belief	- Tell me how specific relationships or activities help you cope with this condition. - Describe specific cultural beliefs or practices that affect how you care for and feel about this condition. - Is there anything interfering with your spiritual beliefs, needs, or practices as a result of this condition? What can I or another caregiver do to help you with your spiritual needs? - Are there any specific treatments that you would not use to treat this condition?

MEDICATION ADMINISTRATION

Drugs appropriate for the chapter disorders are featured, as well as the related nursing responsibilities and patient/family teaching.

MEDICATION ADMINISTRATION Therapeutic Baths

AGENTS USED IN THERAPEUTIC BATHS

Saline or tap water

Antibacterial agents: potassium permanganate, acetic acid, hexachlorophene

Colloid substances: oatmeal (Aveeno), cornstarch, sodium bicarbonate

Coal tar derivatives: Balnetar, Zetar, Polytar

Emollients: Alpha Keri, Lubath, mineral oil

Therapeutic baths have a variety of uses in treating skin disorders. Depending on the agent used, therapeutic baths soothe the skin, lower the skin bacteria count, clean and hydrate the skin, loosen scales, and relieve itching.

Nursing Responsibilities
- Ensure that the bath water is at a comfortable temperature that is neither too hot nor too cool, usually 110°F to 115°F (45°C to 46°C).
- Fill the tub one-third to one-half full.
- Mix the agent well with the water.

- Assist the patient into and out of the tub to prevent falls.
- Dry the patient's skin by blotting with the towel.

Health Education for the Patient and Family
- Use a bath mat in the tub because the medications may cause the tub to become slippery.
- Keep the bathroom warm but adequately ventilated.
- Follow directions carefully for the amount of medication to use in the bath.
- Fill the bath one-third to o... comfortable temperature.
- Stay in the bath for 20 to ... areas to be treated.
- Do not get the bathwater ...
- Dry by blotting (not rubbi...
- If the medications cause s...
- If the itching is not relieve... dry, call your healthcare ...

NURSING CARE OF THE OLDER ADULT

This feature provides essential guidelines for caring for older adults.

NURSING CARE OF THE OLDER ADULT Age-Related Skin Changes

AGE-RELATED CHANGE	SIGNIFICANCE
Epidermis: ↓ thickness and miotic activity	▪ Skin is more fragile and at greater risk for tears or injury ▪ Delayed wound healing ▪ Hyperkeratoses and skin cancers in sun-exposed areas are more evident
Epidermis: ↑ permeability, ↓ Langerhans cells	▪ Increased risk of reactions to irritants ▪ Decreased inflammatory response
Epidermis: ↓ number of active melanocytes	▪ Increased susceptibility to sun exposure
Epidermis: hyperplasia of melanocytes, especially in sun-exposed areas	▪ Small areas of hyperpigmentation ("liver spots") and hypopigmentation ("age spots"), especially on the hands
Epidermis: ↓ vitamin D production	▪ Increased risk of osteomalacia, osteoporosis
...on flattens	▪ Increased risk of skin tears, purpura, and pressure ulcers
	▪ More susceptible to dry skin ▪ Decreased sensation (pain, touch, temperature, and peripheral vibration) ▪ Increased risk of injury
	▪ Greater risk of hyperthermia and hypothermia
	▪ Decreased tone and elasticity, with wrinkle formation
	▪ Cherry hemangiomas are common
	▪ Greater risk of hypothermia ▪ Increased risk of pressure ulcers
...tissue is redistributed	▪ Cellulite forms ▪ Bags over and under the eyes ▪ Double chin forms ▪ Abdominal fat increases ▪ Breasts sag ▪ Skin returns to normal more slowly when pinched (also called tenting)
...tivity	▪ Dry skin is common ▪ Absent perspiration

CASE STUDY & NURSING CARE PLAN A Patient with Herpes Zoster

Jesus Rivera is a 34-year-old migrant farm worker who currently lives in temporary housing in a rural area of the southwestern United States. His family includes his wife, Marta, who is 3 months pregnant, and two children, ages 3 and 5. He takes his wife to a medical clinic staffed by volunteer nurses, physicians, and students from a nearby university for a prenatal checkup. The clinic is open only on Saturday and provides care on a sliding fee scale or for free if the family is unable to pay. While Mrs. Rivera is being examined, Mr. Rivera asks the nurse to have someone look at some very painful blisters on his chest that developed about a week ago. He is afraid that exposure to pesticides has caused the sores.

ASSESSMENT

Mr. Rivera speaks Spanish and is able to communicate only slightly in English. The initial assessment of Mr. Rivera is performed by Anita Mendez, a student nurse fluent in Spanish. Mr. Rivera's history reveals problems with lower back pain but no significant past medical illnesses. He is not aware of any allergies and cannot remember having had chickenpox as a child. Two years ago, both children were sick and had blisters on their bodies, and a friend told them it was chickenpox. Mrs. Rivera thinks she had chickenpox as a child.

Because Mr. Rivera has not had any medical care for several years, baseline laboratory tests are ordered to screen for any other illnesses. The complete blood count (CBC), blood chemistry, and urinalysis are all within normal limits.

Mr. Rivera says that he did not feel well for several days before the blisters appeared, having experienced chills and general achiness. He had not taken his temperature because the family does not own a thermometer. Current vital signs are as follows: T 99°F (37.2°C), P 74, R 22, and BP 148/88.

Physical examination of the trunk reveals a bandlike pattern of lesions across the left thorax. Some of the lesions are vesicles filled with serous fluid; others are darker in color and are oozing a light yellow drainage. The skin around the lesions is red and inflamed. Mr. Rivera complains of a severe, burning pain with itching across his chest. He is diagnosed with herpes zoster.

DIAGNOSES
- *Risk for Infection* related to open oozing areas on the left thorax
- *Acute Pain* related to the presence of lesions and pruritus
- *Deficient Knowledge* of the cause of the skin disorder and recommended treatment
- *Anxiety* related to need to work in areas of pesticide application
- *Ineffective Health Maintenance* related to limited access to health care due to transitory work conditions and cultural and language barriers

EXPECTED OUTCOMES
- Skin lesions will heal without evidence of a secondary infection.
- Limit exposure (as much as possible) to his wife and children and to persons with debilitating illnesses to prevent the spread of the virus.
- Obtain relief of pain and pruritus with the proper use of medications.

- Verbalize an understanding of the disease process and participate in the treatment plan.
- Obtain follow-up care.
- Make an appointment for a referral for information about occupational hazards.

PLANNING AND IMPLEMENTATION
- Provide verbal and written instructions (in Spanish) for self-care:
  - Wear a clean cotton undershirt each day.
  - Trim the fingernails short, and keep the hands clean.
  - Wash the hands each time the infected area is touched.
  - Wash any soiled clothes or linens in hot water and soap.
  - Do not allow other family members to use your towels.
  - Take medications as prescribed for itching and pain.
  - Take the medicine for your sores every 4 hours, even during nighttime hours, for 7 days.
  - As much as possible, do not touch your wife and children until the sores are covered with scabs. Do not have sex with your wife while you have these sores.
- Teach how to take care of skin lesions:
  - Wear disposable gloves every time you do this treatment.
  - Wash the sores and the skin around them very gently with a soft washcloth and a mild soap.
  - Using your fingers, carefully rub the cream on the sores. Do this once every morning after breakfast and once every evening after supper.
  - Wash your hands carefully before and after each treatment.
- Make a follow-up appointment for the next week.
- Provide Mr. Rivera with the name and phone number of the Occupational Safety and Health Administration (OSHA) and recommend he call for an appointment to discuss his concerns about pesticides.

EVALUATION

Mrs. Rivera explains how she has taken care of her husband, and Mr. Rivera is careful to describe how he has followed the nurse's instructions. The skin lesions are dry and crusty, with no new blister formation. Mr. Rivera says he has not called OSHA and is not sure that he will, but he thanks Miss Mendez for the phone number. The nurses make an appointment in 1 month for a prenatal checkup for Mrs. Rivera and for follow-up of Mr. Rivera's herpes zoster. Mr. Rivera promises to return if they are still living close enough to keep the appointment.

CRITICAL THINKING IN THE NURSING PROCESS
1. Identify barriers to care present in this case study. How may nursing interventions promote healthcare delivery to disadvantaged populations?
2. Although most cases of herpes zoster are self-limiting, what further assessments and interventions might have been indicated had the lesions shown little improvement over time and/or the pain remained severe?
3. If Mr. Rivera is advised not to work until his lesions heal, the family may face economic and sociocultural hardships. Develop a plan of care for Mr. Rivera for the nursing diagnosis *Ineffective Role Performance*.

See Evaluating Your Response in Appendix C.

CASE STUDY & NURSING CARE PLAN

The two-column Case Study & Nursing Care Plan includes Assessment, Diagnoses, Expected Outcomes, Planning and Implementation, Evaluation, and Critical Thinking in the Nursing Process.

NURSING CARE OF THE PATIENT
Receiving Intraspinal Analgesia

Intraspinal analgesia is used to manage chronic intractable malignant pain and postoperative pain, particularly after orthopedic and abdominal surgeries. The intraspinal route may be either intrathecal (into the subarachnoid space) or epidural (into the epidural space). Infusion of an opioid into these spaces provides for a direct effect on the opiate receptors in the dorsal horn of the spinal cord. The opioid analgesic is also absorbed systemically, affecting pain responses in the brain. This method can provide complete pain relief but has some potentially dangerous adverse effects.

PROCEDURE

The physician places a catheter into the epidural space. The catheter is connected to infusion tubing and an infusion pump, and the prescribed medication is administered. A portable or implantable pump may be used for longer term opioid analgesic administration.

NURSING CARE
- Monitor vital signs every 15 minutes for the first 2–3 hours and every hour for the first 24 hours; the patient is at risk for respiratory depression and hypotension. These adverse responses may not develop immediately, becoming evident only after several hours.

NURSING CARE OF THE PATIENT

Essential information needed for nursing care of various disorders is described—detailed illustrations help students understand the steps of the nursing process.

Features

END OF CHAPTER TEST YOURSELF NCLEX-RN® REVIEW

At the end of each chapter, NCLEX-style review questions reinforce comprehension of the chapter content.

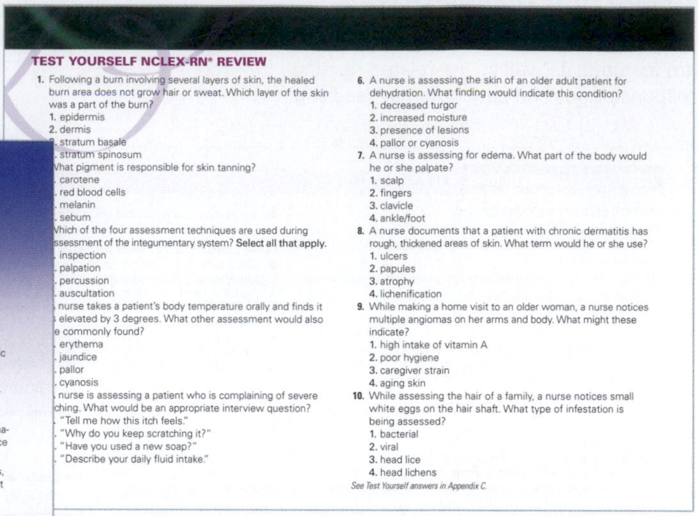
TEST YOURSELF NCLEX-RN® REVIEW

1. Following a burn involving several layers of skin, the healed burn area does not grow hair or sweat. Which layer of the skin was a part of the burn?
   1. epidermis
   2. dermis
   3. stratum basale
   4. stratum spinosum
2. What pigment is responsible for skin tanning?
   1. carotene
   2. red blood cells
   3. melanin
   4. sebum
3. Which of the four assessment techniques are used during assessment of the integumentary system? Select all that apply.
   1. inspection
   2. palpation
   3. percussion
   4. auscultation
4. A nurse takes a patient's body temperature orally and finds it elevated by 3 degrees. What other assessment would also be commonly found?
   1. erythema
   2. jaundice
   3. pallor
   4. cyanosis
5. A nurse is assessing a patient who is complaining of severe itching. What would be an appropriate interview question?
   1. "Tell me how this itch feels."
   2. "Why do you keep scratching it?"
   3. "Have you used a new soap?"
   4. "Describe your daily fluid intake."
6. A nurse is assessing the skin of an older adult patient for dehydration. What finding would indicate this condition?
   1. decreased turgor
   2. increased moisture
   3. presence of lesions
   4. pallor or cyanosis
7. A nurse is assessing for edema. What part of the body would he or she palpate?
   1. scalp
   2. fingers
   3. clavicle
   4. ankle/foot
8. A nurse documents that a patient with chronic dermatitis has rough, thickened areas of skin. What term would he or she use?
   1. ulcers
   2. papules
   3. atrophy
   4. lichenification
9. While making a home visit to an older woman, a nurse notices multiple angiomas on her arms and body. What might these indicate?
   1. high intake of vitamin A
   2. poor hygiene
   3. caregiver strain
   4. aging skin
10. While assessing the hair of a family, a nurse notices small white eggs on the hair shaft. What type of infestation is being assessed?
    1. bacterial
    2. viral
    3. head lice
    4. head lichens

See Test Yourself answers in Appendix C.

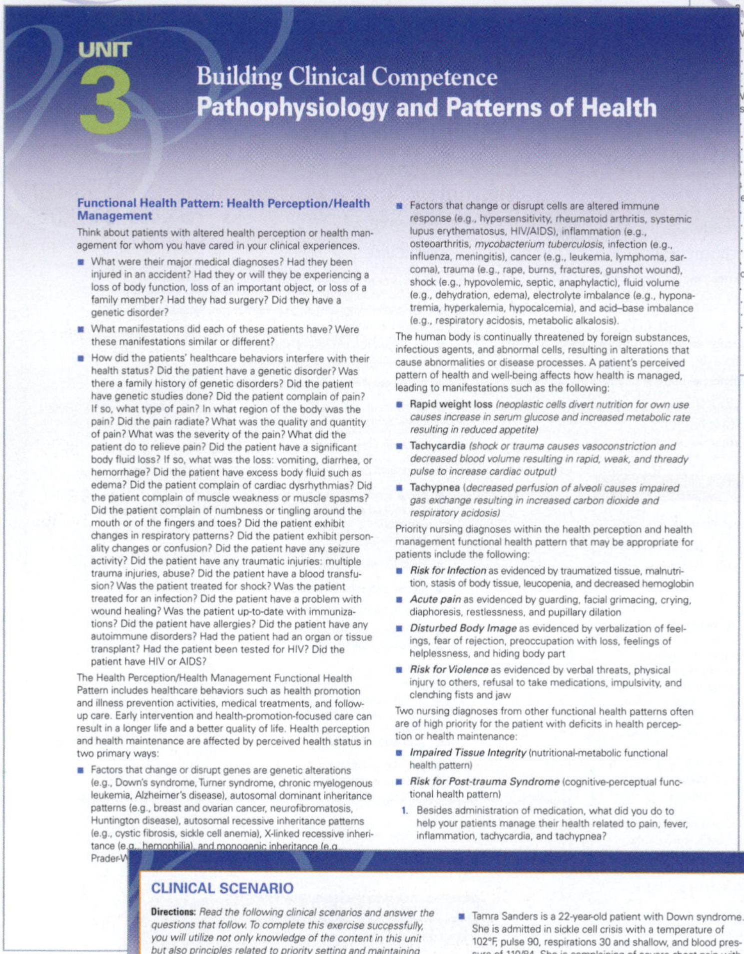
UNIT 3

Building Clinical Competence

Pathophysiology and Patterns of Health

Functional Health Pattern: Health Perception/Health Management

Think about patients with altered health perception or health management for whom you have cared in your clinical experiences.

- What were their major medical diagnoses? Had they been injured in an accident? Had they or will they be experiencing a loss of body function, loss of an important object, or loss of a family member? Had they had surgery? Did they have a genetic disorder?
- What manifestations did each of these patients have? Were these manifestations similar or different?
- How did the patients' healthcare behaviors interfere with their health status? Did the patient have a genetic disorder? Was there a family history of genetic disorders? Did the patient have genetic studies done? Did the patient complain of pain? If so, what type of pain? In what region of the body was the pain? Did the pain radiate? What was the quality and quantity of pain? What was the severity of the pain? What did the patient do to relieve pain? Did the patient have a significant body fluid loss? If so, what was the loss: vomiting, diarrhea, or hemorrhage? Did the patient have excess body fluid such as edema? Did the patient complain of cardiac dysrhythmias? Did the patient complain of muscle weakness or muscle spasms? Did the patient complain of numbness or tingling around the mouth or of the fingers and toes? Did the patient exhibit changes in respiratory patterns? Did the patient exhibit personality changes or confusion? Did the patient have any seizure activity? Did the patient have any traumatic injuries: multiple trauma injuries, abuse? Did the patient have a blood transfusion? Was the patient treated for shock? Was the patient treated for an infection? Did the patient have a problem with wound healing? Was the patient up-to-date with immunizations? Did the patient have allergies? Did the patient have any autoimmune disorders? Had the patient had an organ or tissue transplant? Had the patient been tested for HIV? Did the patient have HIV or AIDS?

The Health Perception/Health Management Functional Health Pattern includes healthcare behaviors such as health promotion and illness prevention activities, medical treatments, and follow-up care. Early intervention and health-promotion-focused care can result in a longer life and a better quality of life. Health perception and health maintenance are affected by perceived health status in two primary ways:

- Factors that change or disrupt genes are genetic alterations (e.g., Down's syndrome, Turner syndrome, chronic myelogenous leukemia, Alzheimer's disease), autosomal dominant inheritance patterns (e.g., breast and ovarian cancer, neurofibromatosis, Huntington disease), autosomal recessive inheritance patterns (e.g., cystic fibrosis, sickle cell anemia), X-linked recessive inheritance (e.g., hemophilia), and monogenic inheritance (e.g., Prader-W...
- Factors that change or disrupt cells are altered immune response (e.g., hypersensitivity, rheumatoid arthritis, systemic lupus erythematosus, HIV/AIDS), inflammation (e.g., osteoarthritis, *mycobacterium tuberculosis*, infection (e.g., influenza, meningitis), cancer (e.g., leukemia, lymphoma, sarcoma), trauma (e.g., rape, burns, fractures, gunshot wound), shock (e.g., hypovolemic, septic, anaphylactic), fluid volume (e.g., dehydration, edema), electrolyte imbalance (e.g., hyponatremia, hyperkalemia, hypocalcemia), and acid–base imbalance (e.g., respiratory acidosis, metabolic alkalosis).

The human body is continually threatened by foreign substances, infectious agents, and abnormal cells, resulting in alterations that cause abnormalities or disease processes. A patient's perceived pattern of health and well-being affects how health is managed, leading to manifestations such as the following:

- **Rapid weight loss** *(neoplastic cells divert nutrition for own use causes increase in serum glucose and increased metabolic rate resulting in reduced appetite)*
- **Tachycardia** *(shock or trauma causes vasoconstriction and decreased blood volume resulting in rapid, weak, and thready pulse to increase cardiac output)*
- **Tachypnea** *(decreased perfusion of alveoli causes impaired gas exchange resulting in increased carbon dioxide and respiratory acidosis)*

Priority nursing diagnoses within the health perception and health management functional health pattern that may be appropriate for patients include the following:

- ***Risk for Infection*** as evidenced by traumatized tissue, malnutrition, stasis of body tissue, leucopenia, and decreased hemoglobin
- ***Acute pain*** as evidenced by guarding, facial grimacing, crying, diaphoresis, restlessness, and pupillary dilation
- ***Disturbed Body Image*** as evidenced by verbalization of feelings, fear of rejection, preoccupation with loss, feelings of helplessness, and hiding body part
- ***Risk for Violence*** as evidenced by verbal threats, physical injury to others, refusal to take medications, impulsivity, and clenching fists and jaw

Two nursing diagnoses from other functional health patterns often are of high priority for the patient with deficits in health perception or health maintenance:

- ***Impaired Tissue Integrity*** (nutritional-metabolic functional health pattern)
- ***Risk for Post-trauma Syndrome*** (cognitive-perceptual functional health pattern)

1. Besides administration of medication, what did you do to help your patients manage their health related to pain, fever, inflammation, tachycardia, and tachypnea?

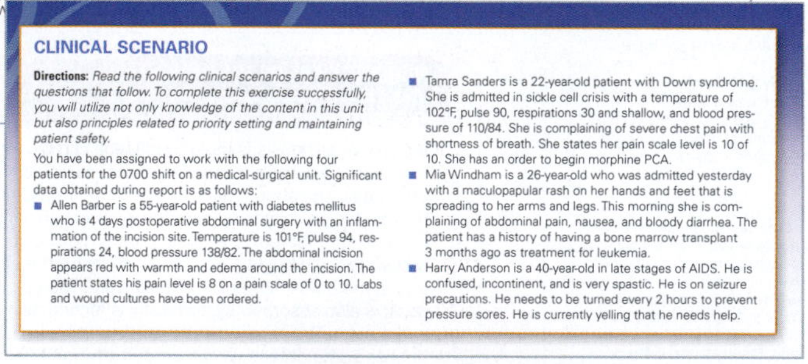
CLINICAL SCENARIO

Directions: *Read the following clinical scenarios and answer the questions that follow. To complete this exercise successfully, you will utilize not only knowledge of the content in this unit but also principles related to priority setting and maintaining patient safety.*

You have been assigned to work with the following four patients for the 0700 shift on a medical-surgical unit. Significant data obtained during report is as follows:

- Allen Barber is a 55-year-old patient with diabetes mellitus who is 4 days postoperative abdominal surgery with an inflammation of the incision site. Temperature is 101°F, pulse 94, respirations 24, blood pressure 138/82. The abdominal incision appears red with warmth and edema around the incision. The patient states his pain level is 8 on a pain scale of 0 to 10. Labs and wound cultures have been ordered.
- Tamra Sanders is a 22-year-old patient with Down syndrome. She is admitted in sickle cell crisis with a temperature of 102°F, pulse 90, respirations 30 and shallow, and blood pressure of 110/84. She is complaining of severe chest pain with shortness of breath. She states her pain scale level is 10 of 10. She has an order to begin morphine PCA.
- Mia Windham is a 26-year-old who was admitted yesterday with a maculopapular rash on her hands and feet that is spreading to her arms and legs. This morning she is complaining of abdominal pain, nausea, and bloody diarrhea. The patient has a history of having a bone marrow transplant 3 months ago as treatment for leukemia.
- Harry Anderson is a 40-year-old in late stages of AIDS. He is confused, incontinent, and is very spastic. He is on seizure precautions. He needs to be turned every 2 hours to prevent pressure sores. He is currently yelling that he needs help.

BUILDING CLINICAL COMPETENCE

Appearing at the end of each unit, this feature integrates information from the unit chapters and gives readers opportunities to apply what they have learned to simulated clinical situations. "Building Clinical Competence" is made up of three separate assignments, which focus on the essential skills of critical thinking, prioritization, and delegation.

FUNCTIONAL HEALTH PATTERN ACTIVITY

This feature provides more detail about how the disorders discussed in the unit impact patients' functional health status. The Functional Health Patterns are described in further detail. Priority nursing diagnoses are described and critical thinking questions focus on applying the most important content.

CLINICAL SCENARIO

This activity presents the reader with multiple patients, and the associated questions focus on setting priorities while managing multiple patients. This activity is particularly good preparation for NCLEX questions that test prioritization, delegation, and safe nursing care.

CASE STUDY WITH CONCEPT MAP

This activity offers readers opportunities to apply specific patient information to the process of concept mapping. Critical-thinking questions prepare the groundwork for creating the concept map, and readers have the opportunity to create a concept map of their own in the Student Resources section of the student website.

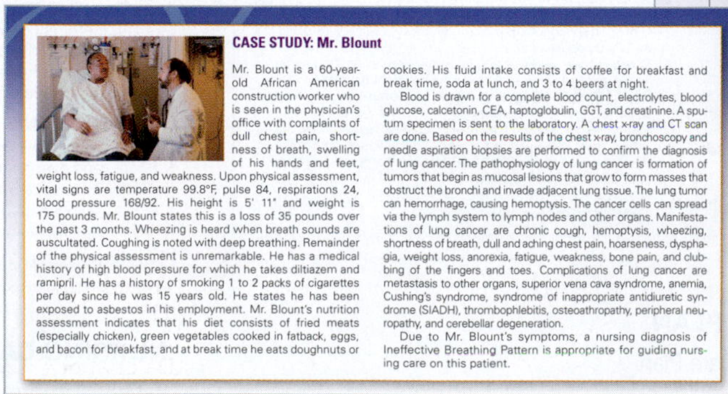
CASE STUDY: Mr. Blount

Mr. Blount is a 60-year-old African American construction worker who is seen in the physician's office with complaints of dull chest pain, shortness of breath, swelling of his hands and feet, weight loss, fatigue, and weakness. Upon physical assessment, vital signs are temperature 99.8°F, pulse 84, respirations 24, blood pressure 168/92. His height is 5' 11" and weight is 175 pounds. Mr. Blount states this is a loss of 35 pounds over the past 3 months. Wheezing is heard when breath sounds are auscultated. Coughing is noted with deep breathing. Remainder of the physical assessment is unremarkable. He has a medical history of high blood pressure for which he takes diltiazem and ramipril. He has a history of smoking 1 to 2 packs of cigarettes per day since he was 15 years old. He states he has been exposed to asbestos in his employment. Mr. Blount's nutrition assessment indicates that his diet consists of fried meats (especially chicken), green vegetables cooked in fatback, eggs, and bacon for breakfast, and at break time he eats doughnuts or cookies. His fluid intake consists of coffee for breakfast and break time, soda at lunch, and 3 to 4 beers at night.

Blood is drawn for a complete blood count, electrolytes, blood glucose, calcetonin, CEA, haptoglobulin, GGT, and creatinine. A sputum specimen is sent to the laboratory. A chest x-ray and CT scan are done. Based on the results of the chest x-ray, bronchoscopy and needle aspiration biopsies are performed to confirm the diagnosis of lung cancer. The pathophysiology of lung cancer is formation of tumors that begin as mucosal lesions that grow to form masses that obstruct the bronchi and invade adjacent lung tissue. The lung tumor can hemorrhage, causing hemoptysis. The cancer cells can spread via the lymph system to lymph nodes and other organs. Manifestations of lung cancer are chronic cough, hemoptysis, wheezing, shortness of breath, dull and aching chest pain, hoarseness, dysphagia, weight loss, anorexia, fatigue, weakness, bone pain, and clubbing of the fingers and toes. Complications of lung cancer are metastasis to other organs, superior vena cava syndrome, anemia, Cushing's syndrome, syndrome of inappropriate antidiuretic syndrome (SIADH), thrombophlebitis, osteoathropathy, peripheral neuropathy, and cerebellar degeneration.

Due to Mr. Blount's symptoms, a nursing diagnosis of Ineffective Breathing Pattern is appropriate for guiding nursing care on this patient.

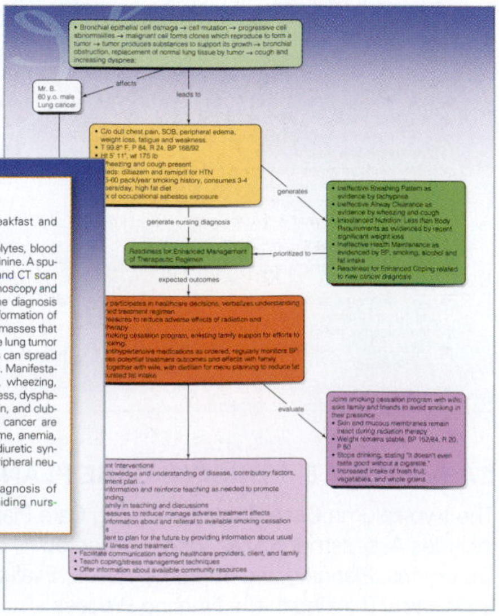

Contents

Contents **xix**

Medical-Surgical Nursing Practice

PART I

Functional Health Patterns with Related Nursing Diagnoses

HEALTH PERCEPTION HEALTH MANAGEMENT

- Perceived health status
- Perceived health management
- Health care behaviors: health promotion and illness prevention activities, medical treatments, follow-up care

VALUE-BELIEF

- Values, goals, or beliefs (including spirituality) that guide choices or decisions
- Perceived conflicts in values, beliefs, or expectations that are health related

COPING-STRESS-TOLERANCE

- Capacity to resist challenges to self-integrity
- Methods of handling stress
- Support systems
- Perceived ability to control and manage situations

NUTRITIONAL-METABOLIC

- Daily consumption of food and fluids
- Favorite foods
- Use of dietary supplements
- Skin lesions and ability to heal
- Condition of the integument
- Weight, height, temperature

PART I
Medical Surgical Nursing Practice: Practical Examples Related NANDA Nursing Diagnoses

- Anxiety
- Caregiver Role Strain
- Chronic Pain
- Compromised Family Coping
- Death Anxiety
- Decisional Conflict
- Deficient Knowledge
- Fatigue
- Fear
- Fluid Volume Excess
- Health Promoting Behavior
- Infection
- Latex Allergy Response
- Nausea
- Powerlessness
- Risk for Bleeding
- Risk for Electrolyte Imbalance
- Risk for Injury
- Risk for Shock
- Risk Prone Health Behavior
- Self-Care Deficit
- Situational Low Self-Esteem

Functional Health Patterns with Related Nursing Diagnoses
Adapted from Gordon, M., (1994). *Nursing diagnosis: Process and application* (3rd ed.), St. Louis: Mosby-Year Book, pp. 80–96.
Copyright © 1994, with permission from Elsevier Science.

SEXUALITY-REPRODUCTIVE

- Satisfaction with sexuality or sexual relationships
- Reproductive pattern
- Female menstrual and perimeno-pausal history

ELIMINATION

- Patterns of bowel and urinary excretion
- Perceived regularity or irregularity of elimination
- Use of laxatives or routines
- Changes in time, modes, quality or quantity of excretions
- Use of devices for control

ROLE-RELATIONSHIP

- Perception of major roles, relationships, and responsibilities in current life situation
- Satisfaction with or disturbances in roles and relationships

ACTIVITY-EXERCISE

- Patterns of personally relevant exercise, activity, leisure, and recreation
- ADLs which require energy expenditure
- Factors that interfere with the desired pattern (e.g., illness or injury)

SELF-PERCEPTION– SELF-CONCEPT

- Attitudes about self
- Perceived abilities, worth, self-image, emotions
- Body posture and movement, eye contact, voice and speech patterns

SLEEP-REST

- Patterns of sleep and rest/relaxation in a 24-hr period
- Perceptions of quality and quantity of sleep and rest
- Use of sleep aids and routines

COGNITIVE-PERCEPTUAL

- Adequacy of vision, hearing, taste, touch, smell
- Pain perception and management
- Language, judgment, memory, decisions

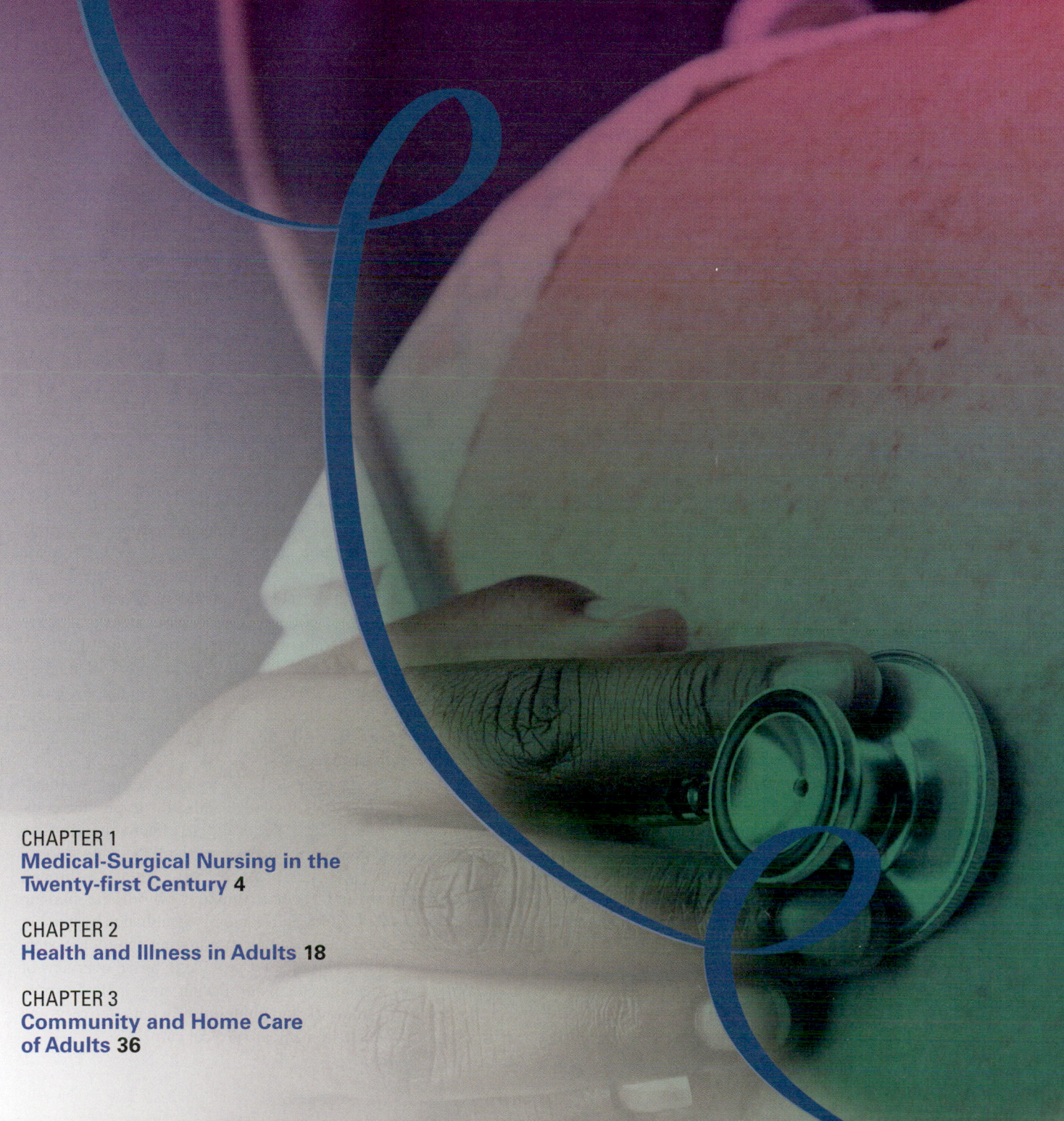

Dimensions of Medical-Surgical Nursing

1 Medical-Surgical Nursing in the Twenty-first Century

LEARNING OUTCOMES

1. Describe the core competencies for healthcare professionals: patient-centered care, interdisciplinary teams, evidence-based practice, quality improvement, safety, and informatics.
2. Apply the attitudes, mental habits, and skills necessary for critical thinking when using the nursing process in patient care.
3. Explain the importance of nursing codes and standards as guidelines for clinical nursing practice.
4. Explain the activities and characteristics of the nurse as caregiver, educator, advocate, leader and manager, and researcher.

CLINICAL COMPETENCIES

1. Demonstrate critical thinking when using the nursing process to provide knowledgeable, safe, and patient-centered care.
2. Provide clinical care within a framework that integrates, as appropriate, the medical-surgical nursing roles of caregiver, educator, advocate, leader/manager, and researcher.

KEY TERMS

code of ethics, 11	delegation, 14	nursing process, 6
core competencies, 5	dilemma, 12	patient, 4
critical pathway, 9	ethics, 11	professional boundaries, 11
critical thinking, 5	medical-surgical nursing, 4	standard, 11

Nursing, as defined by the American Nurses Association (ANA) (2004a), "is the protection, promotion, and optimization of health and abilities, prevention of illness and injury, alleviation of suffering through the diagnosis and treatment of human response, and advocacy in the care of individuals, families, communities, and populations" (p. 7). **Medical-surgical nursing** is the health promotion, health care, and illness care of adults based on knowledge derived from the arts and sciences and shaped by knowledge (the science) of nursing. The adult **patient**—the person with whom and for whom nursing care is designed and implemented—ranges in age from the late teens to the early 100s. Medical-surgical nursing focuses on the adult patient's response to actual or potential alterations in health. Medical-surgical nurses must be knowledgeable about all body systems, the disorders that affect them, and the interrelatedness of body systems and health problems. Medical-surgical nurses need to be strong communicators, able to effectively communicate with other members of the healthcare team, patients, and their families. Medical-surgical nurses need to be able to safely perform often complex nursing care skills and tasks. Delegation to and management and supervision of nursing assistive personnel is an ever-increasing component of effective medical-surgical nursing care.

The wide range of ages and the variety of healthcare needs specific to individual patients make medical-surgical nursing an ever-changing and challenging area of nursing practice. It also is important to remember that individual patients are part of families and live in communities. In some instances, nursing care is directed toward the family (for example, supporting the family of a dying person) or even the community (for example, immunizing people to prevent an outbreak of hepatitis A).

In this textbook, discussions of the human responses are structured within the framework of functional health patterns, and nursing care is presented within the context of nursing diagnoses. Throughout the text, nursing care planning is based on a philosophy that individuals, their families, and communities are active participants in health and illness as well as consumers of healthcare services.

No matter the type of healthcare service or setting, medical-surgical nurses must use knowledge and skills to provide competent and safe patient care. The ability to effectively prioritize activities and patient care needs is critical. Nursing care is structured by the activities planned and carried out through clinical reasoning and critical thinking within the nursing process, is based on ethics and standards established by nursing organizations, and is focused on returning the patient to a state of functional health. This chapter provides a broad overview of the clinical practice of medical-surgical nursing, including core competencies, framework and guidelines for care delivery, and the roles of the nurse in medical-surgical care.

Core Competencies for Safe and Effective Health Care

The healthcare system in North America faces numerous challenges, including an increasingly older patient population, changing consumer desires and expectations, rapidly expanding information and technologies, and a focus on improving quality and safety of care. After examining a number of studies about these challenges, the Institute of Medicine (IOM) (2001) found that although misuse of services and injuries resulting from errors are becoming more common, the safety and quality problems exist largely because of problems within the system and not through fault of highly dedicated healthcare professionals.

To meet the challenges, the National Academy of Sciences (2003) proposed a set of five **core competencies** that all healthcare professionals should possess, regardless of their discipline, to meet the needs of the twenty-first-century health system. The competencies are based on using communication, knowledge, technical skills, clinical reasoning, critical thinking, and values in clinical practice. The Quality and Safety Education for Nurses (QSEN) initiative (Cronenwett et al., 2007) followed, with a major goal of preparing nurses with the necessary knowledge, skills, and attitudes to continuously improve the quality and safety of care in healthcare systems (Sullivan, 2010, p. 37). The core competencies with a description of related activities are outlined in Table 1–1.

Framework for Practice: Critical Thinking in the Nursing Process

As nurses care for patients, they use nursing knowledge, critical thinking, clinical reasoning, and the nursing process as they care for patients. It is these mental activities and their application that differentiate nursing from other helping professions.

Critical Thinking

Critical thinking is goal-oriented, purposeful, and reflective thinking. It is self-directed thinking that is focused on what to believe or do in a specific situation. It involves attitudes and skills. The nurse uses critical thinking to collect and interpret information, consider the patient's needs, and determine appropriate interventions.

As you practice critical thinking, you will use the following:

- Knowledge gained though classroom studies, textbooks and current resources, and by interacting with experienced nurses
- Experience gained by working with patients experiencing similar problems or disorders
- An understanding of the patient as an individual who presents with both current and previous illness experiences
- Personal values and beliefs, including recognition of prejudices that may influence thinking (e.g., believing that all homeless people are dirty, or that aged people cannot learn to care for themselves)

TABLE 1–1 Core Competencies for Healthcare Professionals

COMPETENCY	DESCRIPTION OF ACTIVITIES
Provide patient-centered care	■ Identify, respect, and communicate patient's differences, values, preferences, and expressed needs. ■ Relieve pain and suffering, considering patient values, preferences, and needs. ■ Coordinate care, promoting active patient and family involvement in health care. ■ Listen to, communicate with, and educate patients. ■ Facilitate informed patient consent for care. ■ Communicate care needs and provide them at each transition in care.
Work in interdisciplinary teams	■ Effectively communicate with team members to develop and achieve patient goals. ■ Clarify roles and responsibilities of team members, collaborating and integrating care. ■ Use communication practices that minimize risks associated with care transitions.
Use evidence-based practice	■ Integrate research and evidence with clinical expertise and patient values for optimum care. ■ Participate in learning and research activities to the extent possible.
Apply quality improvement	■ Identify actual and potential errors and hazards in care. ■ Understand and implement basic safety principles and tools. ■ Understand and measure quality of care in terms of structure, process, and outcomes in relation to patient and community needs. ■ Design and test interventions to change processes and systems of care, with the objective of improving quality.
Promote safety	■ Effectively use technology and practices that support safety and quality. ■ Effectively use strategies to reduce the risk of harm to self or others. ■ Communicate recognized hazards or concerns to patients, families, and the healthcare team. ■ Use organizational systems to report near misses and errors. ■ Participate in root cause analysis of errors and near misses to identify and design system improvements.
Use informatics	■ Communicate, manage knowledge, decrease error, and support decision making [critical thinking] using information technology.

Source: Data from National Academy of Sciences. (2003). Health professions education: A bridge to quality, pp. 1–15. Available at http://www.nap.edu, and from Quality and safety education for nurses (2007). Nursing Outlook, 55(3), pp. 122–131.

- An ability to identify other possible options, evaluate the alternatives, and reach a conclusion

It takes practice to make critical thinking an integral component of a nurse's clinical reasoning. The beginning nurse uses a deliberate process of assessing, considering possible alternative causes and action options, and choosing the most appropriate of the alternatives considered. With knowledge and experience, the nurse recognizes expected patterns of response, deviations from the expected, and the probable meaning of the deviation. Clinical reasoning and critical thinking gradually become more internalized; the nurse begins "thinking like a nurse." Critical-thinking exercises are included throughout this book to provide practice in clinical reasoning.

Attitudes and Mental Habits Necessary for Critical Thinking

Thinking critically involves more than just cognitive (knowledge) skills. It is strongly influenced by one's attitudes and mental habits. To think critically, you must be aware of your attitudes and how they affect your thinking. These attitudes and mental habits are the following:

- Being able to think independently so that you make clinical decisions based on sound thinking and judgment. This means, for example, that you are not influenced by negative comments from other healthcare providers about a patient.
- Being willing to listen to and be fair in your evaluation of others' ideas and beliefs. This involves listening carefully to other ideas and thoughts, and making a decision based on what you learn instead of how you feel.
- Having empathy by being able to put yourself in the place of another to better understand that other person. For example, if you put yourself in the place of the person with severe pain, you are better able to understand why he or she is so upset when pain medications are late.
- Being fair-minded and considering all viewpoints before making a decision through a sense of justice and being humble. This means you consider the viewpoints of others that may be different from yours before reaching a conclusion. You also realize that you are constantly learning from others. You are not afraid to say, "I don't know the answer to that question, but I will find out and let you know."
- Being disciplined so that you do not stop at easy answers, but continue to consider alternatives.
- Being creative and self-confident. Nurses often need to consider different ways of providing care and constantly look for better, more cost-effective methods. Confidence in one's decisions is gained through critical thinking.

Critical Thinking Skills

The major critical thinking skills used by nurses are divergent thinking, reasoning, clarifying, and reflection. A description of each follows:

Divergent thinking is the ability to weigh the importance of information. This means that when you collect data from a patient, you can sort out the data that are relevant for care from the data that are not relevant, and explore alternatives to draw a conclusion. Abnormal data are usually considered relevant; normal data are helpful but may not change the care you provide.

Reasoning is the ability to discriminate between facts and guesses. By using known facts, problems are solved and decisions are made in a systematic, logical way. For example, when you take a pulse you must know the facts of normal pulse rate for a person of this age, types of medications the patient is taking that may alter the pulse rate, and the emotional and physical state of the patient. Based on these facts, you are able to decide if the pulse rate is normal or abnormal.

Clarifying involves noting similarities and differences to sort information to help focus on the present situation. For example, when caring for a patient with chronic pain, you must know the definition of chronic pain and the similarities and differences between acute pain and chronic pain.

Reflection occurs when you take time to think about something, comparing different situations with similar solutions. It cannot take place in an emergency situation. As you reflect on your experiences in nursing, many of those experiences may in turn become alternatives when caring for a different patient.

All nurses are expected to think critically, making reasoned clinical judgments. Using critical thinking to provide care that is structured by the nursing process allows the nurse to provide safe, effective, holistic, and individualized care.

The Nursing Process

The **nursing process** is the series of critical-thinking and clinical-reasoning activities nurses use as they provide care to patients. As nurses gain increasing autonomy in their practice, the nursing process helps them identify their independent practice domain. The nursing process provides a common reference system and a common terminology to serve as a base for improving clinical practice through research. In addition, the nursing process can serve as a framework for the evaluation of quality care.

The nursing process can be used in any setting. The purpose of care may be to promote wellness, maintain health, restore health, or provide comfort and facilitate coping with disability or death. Regardless of the purpose of care, the planned process of nursing allows for the inclusion of specific, individualized, and holistic activities.

The nursing process also benefits the patient receiving care and the agency or institution providing that care. The patient receives planned, individualized interventions; participates in all steps of the process; and is assured continuity of care through the written care plan. The nursing process benefits the healthcare institution through better resource utilization, increased patient satisfaction, and improved documentation of care.

The five phases in the nursing process are assessment, diagnosis, planning, implementation, and evaluation. These phases are interrelated and interdependent. They are often used cyclically, with the patient central to all phases, as illustrated in Figure 1–1 ■. The steps have been legitimized by the ANA Standards of Practice, state nursing practice acts, and licensing examinations that are structured on a nursing model of care based on the nursing process.

This textbook assumes that the student already has a basic understanding of the nursing process and is now ready to expand and apply that knowledge to adult patients with medical-surgical health problems. The following discussion is intended to serve only as a review; for more information, consult books specifically

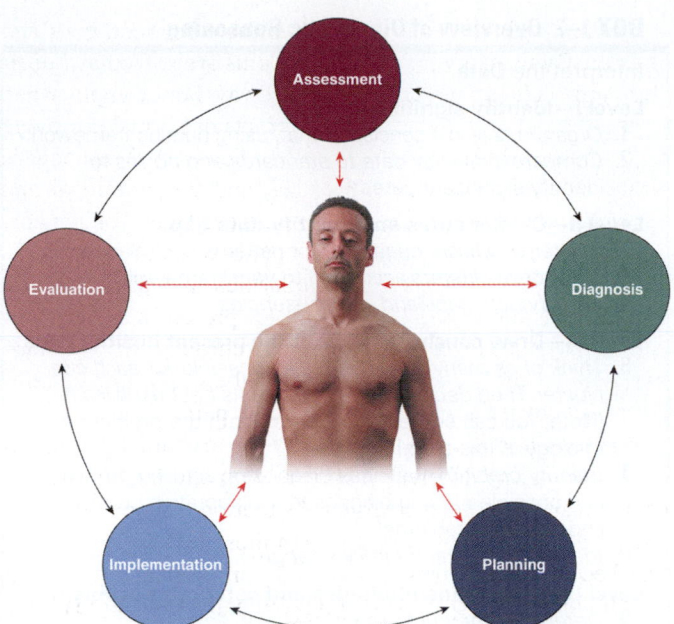

Figure 1–1 ■ Steps of the nursing process. Notice that the steps are interrelated and interdependent. For example, evaluation of the patient might reveal the need for further assessment, additional nursing diagnoses, and/or a revision of the plan of care.

focused on the use of the nursing process, and read the case studies in the nursing care chapters throughout this textbook.

In addition to nursing care plans based on a patient care situation that describe each step of the process, charts are included throughout the text that illustrate the relationship of nursing diagnoses (NANDA), nursing interventions (NIC), and nursing outcomes (NOC). Categorized as the NNN Alliance, the links between and among NANDA, NIC, and NOC represent the collaborative relationship between the North American Nursing Diagnosis Association (NANDA) and the Center for Nursing Classification and Clinical Effectiveness (Nursing Interventions Classification [NIC] and Nursing Outcomes Classification [NOC]) at the University of Iowa.

Assessment

Assessment is a critical element in each phase of the nursing process. It begins with the patient's first encounter with the healthcare system and continues as long as the patient requires care. During assessment, data (pieces of information) about health status are collected, validated, organized, clustered into patterns, and communicated either verbally or in written form. Assessment serves as the basis for deriving accurate nursing diagnoses, for planning and implementing both initial and ongoing individualized care, and for evaluating care.

The nurse collects holistic assessment data, considering all dimensions of the patient. The data collected are both objective and subjective. Information that the nurse perceives by the senses is *objective data*; it is seen, heard, touched, or smelled, and can be verified by another person (e.g., blood pressure, temperature, pulse, or the presence of infected drainage). Information that is perceived only by the person experiencing it (e.g., pain, dizziness, or anxiety) is *subjective data*.

Nurses conduct both initial and ongoing assessments. The initial assessment, conducted through a nursing history and physical assessment, is obtained to provide a comprehensive

picture of the patient's health status. It is necessary to provide comprehensive data about the individual's health responses, identify specific factors that contribute to these responses, and facilitate mutually established goals and outcomes of care.

Focused assessments are ongoing and continuous, occurring whenever the nurse interacts with the patient. In a focused assessment, data is gathered about an identified or potential problem. This data is used to evaluate nursing actions and make decisions about whether to continue or change interventions to meet outcomes. Assessments also provide structure for documenting nursing care. In addition, focused assessments enable the nurse to identify responses to a disease process or treatment modality not present during the initial assessment, and to identify new problems (Alfaro-LeFevre, 2009).

To make accurate and holistic assessments, nurses must have and use a wide variety of knowledge and skills. The ability to assess the physical status of the patient is essential, as is the ability to communicate effectively. Nurses must know and understand pathophysiology and pharmacology and be able to identify abnormal laboratory and diagnostic test data. Finally, nurses need a solid foundation of nursing knowledge and skill to interpret assessment data and to use that interpretation as the basis for individualized care.

Nurses use a number of critical thinking skills when assessing. An attitude of inquiry is used during data gathering. The nurse must distinguish data that is relevant from that which is irrelevant, as well as important data from unimportant data. In addition, the nurse identifies missing data and seeks additional information to fill in gaps (Wilkinson, 2007).

> **MEMORY CUE**
> Remember that assessment is collecting and interpreting the meaning of data; it is *not* forming judgments. "Patient is angry and out-of-control" is a judgment; "Pacing, talking loudly and with a rapid cadence" is an assessment.

Diagnosis

The ANA defines nursing as "the protection, promotion, and optimization of health and abilities, prevention of illness and injury alleviation of suffering through the diagnosis and treatment of human response" (2004a, p. 7). In the diagnosis phase of the nursing process, the nurse uses assessed data, knowledge of expected responses, intuition, and prior experience to analyze data and draw conclusions about its meaning. The nurse then labels each identified health problem with a nursing diagnosis, a statement that describes the patient's current health status. Nursing diagnoses describe actual or potential health problems that can legally be diagnosed by the nurse, for which the nurse can prescribe the primary interventions, and for which the nurse is accountable (Wilkinson, 2007).

The nurse analyzes assessment data to support appropriate nursing diagnoses. During analysis, the nurse organizes or categorizes data so that it can be used to identify actual or potential health problems. Data can be organized within a variety of frameworks. Methods commonly used are basic human needs (Maslow, 1970), body systems, human response patterns, and functional health patterns (Gordon, 1982). The broad organizational structure used to categorize information in this book is based on functional health patterns, outlined in Box 1–1.

Identifying health problems or needs and making a diagnosis is a complex process that always involves uncertainty. Therefore, the nurse uses diagnostic reasoning to choose nursing diagnoses that best define the individual patient's health problems. Diagnostic reasoning is a form of clinical judgment used to make decisions about which label (or diagnosis) best describes the patterns of data. Box 1–2 outlines the steps and processes the nurse uses in diagnostic reasoning.

Diagnoses made by nurses generally fall within three categories:

1. Actual nursing diagnoses: A health problem identified during assessment that can be relieved or resolved through nursing interventions
2. Potential (or risk) nursing diagnoses: A health problem that is likely to develop unless the nurse intervenes
3. Collaborative problems: A health problem that requires both medical and nursing interventions; nurses monitor for and intervene to reduce complications (Wilkinson, 2007)

NANDA Although there is no universal list of diagnoses used in nursing, the ongoing work of NANDA is widely accepted. The diagnoses are classified by a taxonomy; that is, they are grouped into classes and subclasses based on patterns and relationships. The NANDA system was accepted in 1988 by the ANA as the official system of nursing diagnosis for the United States. Nursing diagnoses within the NANDA taxonomy are used in this book. Where appropriate, collaborative problems also are identified. A complete list of current NANDA nursing diagnoses can be found in ∞ Appendix B.

BOX 1–1 Functional Health Patterns

1. *Health perception–health management pattern.* Describes client's perceived pattern of health and well-being and how health is managed.
2. *Nutritional-metabolic pattern.* Describes pattern of food and fluid consumption relative to metabolic need and pattern indicators of local nutrient supply.
3. *Elimination pattern.* Describes pattern of excretory function (bowel, bladder, and skin).
4. *Activity-exercise pattern.* Describes pattern of exercise, activity, leisure, and recreation.
5. *Cognitive-perceptual pattern.* Describes sensory-perceptual and cognitive patterns.
6. *Sleep-rest pattern.* Describes patterns of sleep, rest, and relaxation.
7. *Self-perception–self-concept pattern.* Describes self-concept pattern and perceptions of self (e.g., body comfort, body image, feeling state).
8. *Role-relationship pattern.* Describes patterns of role engagements and relationships.
9. *Sexuality-reproductive pattern.* Describes client's patterns of satisfaction and dissatisfaction with sexuality; describes reproductive patterns.
10. *Coping–stress tolerance pattern.* Describes general coping pattern and effectiveness of the pattern in terms of stress tolerance.
11. *Value-belief pattern.* Describes patterns of values, beliefs (including spiritual), or goals that guide choices or decisions.

Source: Adapted from Gordon, M., (1994). *Nursing diagnosis: Process and application* (3rd ed.), St. Louis: Mosby-Year Book. Used with permission.

BOX 1–2 Overview of Diagnostic Reasoning

Interpret the Data

Level I—Identify significant cues
1. *Organize data* in a concise format, using nursing framework
2. *Compare individual data to standards and norms* to identify significant cures

Level II—Cluster cures and identify data gaps
3. *Cluster significant cues*; look for patterns and relationships
4. *Categorize clusters* according to your framework
5. *Identify data gaps and inconsistencies*

Level III—Draw conclusions about the present health status
6. *Think of as many explanations as possible for each cue cluster. Then decide which hypothesis best explains it.* (Note: You can sometimes identify both the problem and etiology in this step.)
7. *Identify problem* (wellness diagnoses; actual, potential, and possible nursing diagnoses; collaborative problems; and medical problems)
8. *Identify patient and family strengths.*

Level IV—Determine etiologies and categorize problems
9. *Determine the etiologies of the problems*
10. *Categorize problems according to your framework*

Verify the Diagnoses
11. *Verify the diagnoses and strengths* with the patient, family, other professionals, and references

Label the Diagnoses
12. *Choose standardized problem label.* Write formal health status statements: nursing and wellness diagnoses, collaborative problems, and strengths
13. *Prioritize the problems*

Record the Data
14. *Record the problem statements* on the appropriate documents: patent care plan, chart, etc.

Source: From Wilkinson, Judith M., *Nursing Process and Critical Thinking*, 4th, © 2007. Reproduced by permission of Pearson Education, Inc., Upper Saddle River, New Jersey.

WRITING DIAGNOSES A diagnosis is written in two parts joined by the phrase "related to." The first part of the statement describes the patient's health status. It identifies what needs to change in a specific patient as a result of nursing interventions, and suggests the patient outcomes that measure the change. The part of the statement that follows the "related to" phrase identifies the physical, psychosocial, cultural, spiritual, and/or environmental factors (etiologies) that cause or contribute to the occurrence of the response.

Many nurses write nursing diagnoses using a method known as PES (Gordon, 1994). Diagnoses written with this method have three components:

1. The problem (P), which is the NANDA label.
2. The etiology (E) of the problem, which names the related factors and is indicated by the phrase "related to."
3. The signs and symptoms (S), which are the defining characteristics and are indicated by the phrase "as manifested by."

Examples of nursing diagnoses written with the PES method are as follows:

- *Anxiety* related to hospitalization as manifested by statements of nervousness and by crying
- *Bowel incontinence* related to loss of sphincter control as manifested by involuntary passage of stool

- *Fatigue* related to the side effects of chemotherapy as manifested by the inability to carry out normal daily routines and statements of overwhelming exhaustion

Planning

During the planning step, the nurse identifies the desired patient outcomes of care and nursing interventions to achieve those outcomes. *Outcomes*, which are mutually established by the patient and nurse, describe the expected patient responses that will occur as a result of the nursing interventions. Nursing interventions (actions) are specifically planned to achieve the desired outcomes. Both outcomes and nursing interventions are documented in a written plan of care that directs nursing activities and documentation and provides a tool for evaluation (Alfaro-LeFevre, 2009).

Nurses plan interventions for problems that require nursing management (stated as nursing diagnoses) and for collaborative or clinical problems. Nursing diagnoses provide the basis for selecting nurse-initiated interventions to achieve outcomes for which the nurse is accountable. Collaborative problems are often based on medical diagnoses (such as hemorrhage) that nurses monitor to detect onset or changes in status.

Outcome criteria for nursing diagnoses are patient centered, time specific, and measurable. They are classified into three domains: cognitive (knowing), affective (feeling), and psychomotor (doing). The nurse considers all three domains to ensure holistic care.

The Nursing Outcomes Classification (NOC) provides standardized outcome labels and measurable indicators that can be used to evaluate patient status and nursing care.

Outcome criteria for collaborative problems follow the same pattern. For example, "Respiratory complications will not occur as evidenced by clear lung sounds, pulse, respiratory rate, and temperature in normal range for patient throughout recovery period."

Planned nursing interventions must be specific and individualized. If, for example, the nurse identifies that a patient is at risk for fluid volume deficit, it is not enough that the nurse simply encourage the patient to drink increased amounts of fluid. The nurse and the patient together must identify those liquids the patient prefers, the times that will be best for drinking them, and the amount of fluid (in ounces or milliliters); this information is documented as a nursing order on the written care plan. Only then does care truly become a part of the plan of care.

EVIDENCE-BASED PRACTICE GUIDELINES Whenever possible, planned nursing interventions are based on evidence, that is, nursing research and nursing practice guidelines. Currently, significant work is being done to develop evidence-based nursing practice guidelines. Guidelines are collections of practical information used to help guide decisions related to specific circumstances (Hanson et al., 2008). Nurses use guidelines to help identify appropriate interventions for a given nursing care problem or diagnosis. Evidence-based nursing care guidelines also show the strength of the evidence (research) used, allowing nurses to evaluate the appropriateness of a given guideline for the individual circumstance. Evidence-based nursing guidelines are available through specialty nursing organizations, healthcare systems, on the web, and in published resources. See the accompanying Moving Evidence into Action feature for more information about nurses' use of evidence for nursing practice.

Using research and evidence for planning nursing care is a relatively new skill for many nurses. Brief features such as the accompanying box will be found throughout this book. These boxes identify potential resources for planning evidence-based nursing care.

NURSING INTERVENTIONS CLASSIFICATION Just as NANDA has provided standardized language for nursing diagnoses and NOC provides standardized outcome labels and criteria, the NIC provides standardized nursing intervention labels and nursing activities to carry out the intervention.

CRITICAL PATHWAYS A **critical pathway** (also called a clinical path or pathway) is a healthcare plan designed to provide care with a multidisciplinary, managed action focus. Such pathways are generally developed for specific diagnoses—usually

---

MOVING EVIDENCE INTO ACTION | **Nursing Practice**

Recognition of the need to base nursing practice on the best available evidence has significantly increased in recent years. Despite this recognition and the increased availability of published nursing research, current nursing practice often is based on experience, tradition and intuition—not on science. Koehn & Lehman (2008) surveyed registered nurses in a large medical center to identify their knowledge and skills, attitudes, and current use of evidence-based practice (EBP). Overall, nurses rated their knowledge and skills lower than their attitudes and use of EBP. Lack of time was identified by nurses as the major barrier to implementing EBP; nurses identified limited knowledge of research as a significant barrier as well.

IMPLICATIONS FOR NURSING

With increasing emphasis on and recognition of the importance of EBP, it is clear that practicing nurses need support to effectively implement it. Many nurses in the current workforce were educated at a time when EBP was not taught or emphasized. In addition to administrative leadership and support for implementing evidence-based nursing practice, nurses need support for developing the knowledge and skills to find and critically evaluate the research to support EBP.

CRITICAL THINKING IN PATIENT CARE

1. In this study, less than half of the nurses responding to the survey reported reading or subscribing to a professional journal. What implications do you think this finding has for the use of evidence-based nursing practice? What do you think nurse managers and administrators could do to encourage more nurses to stay up-to-date on current nursing practice?
2. Lack of time was identified in this study as a major barrier to implementing EBP. How could you, as a staff nurse, support your peers in developing and implementing EBP?
3. Nurses are responsible for not only using evidence in their nursing practice, but also for contributing to nursing research and the evidence for nursing practice. What steps might you take to identify a research question that could provide evidence for practicing nurses to use?

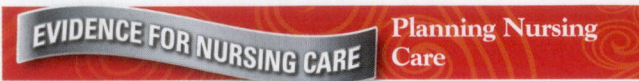

EVIDENCE FOR NURSING CARE   Planning Nursing Care

Selected resources that nurses may find helpful when planning evidence-based nursing care follow.

- Carlson, C. (2009, December). Use of three evidence-based postoperative pain assessment practices by registered nurses. *Pain Management Nursing, 10*(4), 174–187.
- D'Arcy, Y. (2009). Putting pain research into practice. *Nursing 2009, 39*(8), 58.
- Rauen, C. A., Makic, M. B. F., & Bridges, E. (2009). Evidence-based practice habits: Transforming research into bedside practice. *Critical Care Nurse, 29*(2), 46–59.
- Scott, K., & McSherry, R. (2009). Evidence-based nursing: Clarifying the concepts for nurses in practice. *Journal of Clinical Nursing, 18*(8), 1085–1095.
- Sund-Levander, M., & Grodzinsky, E. (2010, January 12–18). What is the evidence base for the assessment and evaluation of body temperature? *Nursing Times, 106*(1), 10–13.

high volume, high risk, and high cost case types—with the collaboration of members of the healthcare team. Critical pathways are outcome driven and provide a time line to achieve specified goals. They also establish the sequence of multidisciplinary interventions, including education, discharge planning, consultations, medication administration, diagnostics, therapeutics, and treatments.

The overall goal is to design pathways that facilitate a reproducible standard of care for specific patient populations and improve the quality and proficiency of that care.

When patients do not achieve expected outcomes, variances (deviations from the established plan) from the critical pathways are recorded and studied by the multidisciplinary team. In many agencies, critical pathways are designed so that interventions and variances can be easily documented. Most documentation systems require a check off when interventions are performed or variances occur.

Implementation

The implementation step is the action or "doing" phase of the nursing process, during which the nurse carries out planned interventions. In some instances, the nurse assigns and supervises nursing assistive personnel in carrying out planned interventions. Ongoing assessment of the patient before, during, and after the intervention is an essential component of implementation in either case. Although the plan may be appropriate, many variables can modify or negate any planned intervention, making a change in the plan necessary. For example, the nurse would not be able to force fluids if the patient were nauseated or vomiting.

When implementing the planned interventions, the nurse follows several important principles:

- Set daily priorities, based on initial assessments and on the patient's condition as reported during the change of shift report and/or documented in the patient's chart. Ensure that critical assessments (such as status of invasive lines, fluids infusing, or changes in health status during the preceding shift) take first priority.
- Be aware of the interrelated nature of nursing interventions. For example, while giving a bath the nurse can also assess

physical and psychologic status, use therapeutic communication, teach the patient, do range-of-motion exercises, and provide skin care.
- Determine the most appropriate interventions for each patient, based on health status and illness treatment. Examples of appropriate interventions include the following:
  - Directly performing the activity for the patient.
  - Assisting the patient to perform the activity.
  - Supervising the patient/family while they are performing the activity.
  - Assigning and supervising nursing assistive personnel to perform the activity.
  - Teaching the patient/family about health care.
  - Monitoring the patient at risk for potential complications or problems.
- Use available resources to provide interventions that are realistic for the situation and practical in terms of equipment available, financial status of the patient, and resources available (including staff, agency, family, and community resources).

Documenting interventions is the final component of implementation, and it is a legal requirement. There are many different ways of documenting care. Narrative source-oriented and problem-oriented charting methods are used, as are focused charting, charting by exception, and computer-assisted documentation.

Evaluation

The evaluation step allows the nurse to determine whether the plan was effective and either to continue the plan, to revise the plan, or to terminate the plan. The outcome criteria that were established during the planning step provide the basis for evaluation. Evaluation takes place continuously throughout patient care, as illustrated in Figure 1–1.

To evaluate a plan, the nurse collects data from the patient and the patient's chart. The nurse then compares the status of the patient with the written outcomes. If the outcomes have been accomplished, the nurse may either continue or terminate the plan. If the outcomes have not been accomplished, the nurse must modify the nursing diagnoses, outcomes, or plan.

The Nursing Process in Clinical Practice

With experience, the nurse does not consciously stop and consider each step. Rather, using the process as a framework, care is based on the patient's specific, individualized needs. For example, when caring for a patient who is hemorrhaging, the nurse uses all five steps simultaneously to meet critical, life-threatening needs. In contrast, when considering long-term needs for a patient with a chronic illness or disability, the nurse makes in-depth assessments, mutually determines goals with the patient, and documents a written plan of care that is developed and revised as necessary by all nurses providing care. As a nurse becomes an expert practitioner, the nursing process becomes so much a part of the nurse that he or she may not even consciously consider it while providing care; the practice is the process (Benner, 1984).

Guidelines for Nursing Practice

Nursing practice is structured by codes of ethics and standards that guide nursing practice and protect the public. Individual nursing practice is held to these standards in a court of law. The guidelines are especially important because nurses encounter legal and ethical problems almost daily.

Codes for Nurses

An established **code of ethics** is one criterion that defines a profession. **Ethics** are principles of conduct. Ethical behavior is concerned with moral duty, values, obligations, and the distinction between right and wrong. Codes of ethics for nurses provide a frame of reference for "professionally valued and ideal nursing behaviors that are congruent with the principles expressed in the Code for Nurses" (Ketefian, 1987, p. 13).

The large number of ethical issues facing nurses in clinical practice makes the established codes for nurses critical to moral and ethical decision making. The codes also help to define the roles of nurses. The codes of ethics presented here were developed by and for members of the International Council of Nurses (ICN) and the ANA.

The ICN Code

The ICN Code of Ethics for Nurses (2006) helps guide nurses in setting priorities, making judgments, and taking action when they face ethical dilemmas in clinical practice. The ICN Code specifies what nurses are accountable for in terms of people, practice, society, coworkers, and the profession. The philosophical base for the ICN code is that nurses are responsible to promote health, to prevent illness, and to alleviate suffering.

The ANA Code

The ANA Code for Nurses (2001) states principles of ethical concern, guiding the behavior of nurses and also defining nursing for the general public (Box 1–3).

Standards of Nursing Practice

A **standard** is a statement or criterion that can be used by a profession and by the general public to measure quality of practice. Established standards of nursing practice make each individual nurse accountable for practice. This means that each nurse providing care has the responsibility or obligation to account for his or her own behaviors within that role. Professional nursing organizations develop and implement standards of practice to identify clearly the nurse's responsibilities to society.

The ANA standards of nursing practice (2004) are outlined in Box 1–4. These standards allow objective evaluation of nursing licensure and certification, institutional accreditation, quality assurance, and public policy.

Health Information Privacy Rules

Although the right to privacy of health and other personal information is an accepted ethical principle of nurses and other healthcare providers, federal rules also govern what can be shared and with whom. The Health Insurance Portability and Accountability Act and the Standards for Privacy of Individually Identifiable Health Information, commonly referred to together as HIPAA, are designed to protect individuals' health information while allowing such information to be shared as needed for effective care. The rules apply to those who transmit health information electronically—including nurses and others employed in hospitals, clinics, and other settings.

While often misinterpreted, HIPAA rules allow disclosure of health information for treatment purposes, even without the

BOX 1–3 The American Nurses Association Code of Ethics for Nurses

- The nurse, in all professional relationships, practices with compassion and respect for the inherent dignity, worth, and uniqueness of every individual, unrestricted by considerations of social or economic status, personal attributes, or the nature of health problems.
- The nurse's primary commitment is to the patient, whether an individual, family, group, or community.
- The nurse promotes, advocates for, and strives to protect the health, safety, and rights of the patient.
- The nurse is responsible and accountable for individual nursing practice and determines the appropriate delegation of tasks consistent with the nurse's obligation to provide optimum patient care.
- The nurse owes the same duties to self as to others, including the responsibility to preserve integrity and safety, to maintain competence, and to continue personal and professional growth.
- The nurse participates in establishing, maintaining, and improving health care environments and conditions of employment conducive to the provision of quality health care and consistent with the values of the profession through individual and collective action.
- The nurse participates in the advancement of the profession through contributions in practice, education, administration, and knowledge development.
- The nurse collaborates with other health professionals and the public in promoting community, national, and international efforts to meet health needs.
- The profession of nursing, as represented by associations and their members, is responsible for articulating nursing values, for maintaining the integrity of the profession and its practice, and for shaping social policy.

Source: ©2001 From *Code of Ethics for Nurses with Interpretive Statements.* By American Nurses Association. Reprinted with permission. All Rights Reserved.

patient's explicit consent. Although the patient's privacy is to be protected, safety protections such as posting the patient's name outside his or her room are allowed to help ensure that care is provided to the correct patient (Anderson, 2007). Unless the patient specifically objects, health information also can be shared with family members who are involved in the patient's care. Other state or federal laws may override the patient's right to privacy of health information, for example, laws that require nurses and other healthcare providers to report evidence of child, elder, or spousal abuse.

Professional Boundaries

Nurses are expected to act in the best interests of the patient, avoiding use of their position for personal gain or to become involved in the patient's personal relationships. **Professional boundaries** are the borders between the vulnerability of the patient and the power of the nurse. The nurse's position as care provider and knowledge of private information about the patient places the nurse in a position of power. It is vital that nurses recognize this relationship, and establish boundaries to safely and effectively meet the patient's needs. Confusion between the needs of the nurse and those of the patient can result in boundary violations (National Council of State Boards of Nursing, 1996). It is the nurse's responsibility to establish and maintain professional boundaries, maintaining an appropriate level of involvement for effective care.

BOX 1–4 ANA Standards of Practice

Standards of Practice	Standards of Professional Practice

Standards of Practice

- Assessment: The registered nurse collects comprehensive data pertinent to the patient's health or the situation.
- Diagnosis: The registered nurse analyzes the assessment data to determine the diagnoses or issues.
- Outcomes Identification: The registered nurse identifies expected outcomes for a plan individualized to the patient or the situation.
- Planning: The registered nurse develops a plan that prescribes strategies and alternatives to attain expected outcomes.
- Implementation: The registered nurse implements the identified plan, coordinates care delivery, and employs strategies to promote health and a safe environment. The advanced practice registered nurse also provides consultation and uses prescriptive authority, procedures, referrals, treatments and therapies.
- Evaluation: The registered nurse evaluates progress toward attainment of outcomes.

Standards of Professional Practice

- Quality of Practice: The registered nurse systematically enhances the quality and effectiveness of nursing practice.
- Education: The registered nurse attains knowledge and competency that reflects current nursing practice.
- Professional Practice Evaluation: The registered nurse evaluates one's own nursing practice in relation to professional practice standards and guidelines, relevant statutes, rules, and regulations.
- Collegiality: The registered nurse interacts with and contributes to the professional development of peers and colleagues.
- Collaboration: The registered nurse collaborates with patient, family, and others in the conduct of nursing practice.
- Ethics: The registered nurse integrates ethical provisions in all areas of practice.
- Research: The registered nurse integrates research findings into practice.
- Resource Utilization: The registered nurse considers factors related to safety, effectiveness, cost, and impact on practice in the planning and delivery of nursing services.
- Leadership: The registered nurse provides leadership in the professional practice setting and the profession.

Source: ©2004 From *Nursing Scope and Standards of Practice.* By American Nurses Association. Reprinted with permission. All Rights Reserved.

Legal and Ethical Dilemmas in Nursing

A **dilemma** is a choice between two unpleasant, ethically troubling alternatives. Nurses who provide medical-surgical nursing care face dilemmas almost daily. Many commonly experienced dilemmas involve confidentiality, patient rights, and issues of dying and death. The nurse must use ethical and legal guidelines to make decisions about moral actions when providing care in these and in many other situations.

Nurses respect the right to confidentiality of patient information found in the patient's record or secured during interviews. However, an individual's right to privacy and confidentiality creates a dilemma when it conflicts with the nurse's right to information that may affect personal safety. The law in most states mandates that HIV test results can be given to another person only with the patient's written consent. Many healthcare providers believe that this law violates their own right to personal safety.

The right to refuse treatment (including surgery, medication, medical therapy, and nourishment) also raises nursing dilemmas. The situation, the alternatives, and the potential harm from refusal must be carefully explained. The nurse is faced with the dilemma of respecting the patient's autonomy or following the ethical principle of beneficence, doing what is best for the patient.

Issues surrounding dying and death have become increasingly pressing as advances in technology extend the lives of people with chronic, debilitating illness and major trauma. These changes have altered concepts of living and dying, resulting in ethical conflicts regarding quality of life and death with dignity versus technologic methods of preserving life in any form.

Even if the patient is competent and requests that no heroic measures be used to maintain life, many questions arise in nursing care. What constitutes a heroic measure? Should nursing interventions to provide comfort include administering narcotics at a level known to depress respirations? These and other questions are being debated not only within the healthcare system but also in the courts.

Roles of the Nurse in Medical-Surgical Nursing Practice

Health care today is a vast and complex system. It reflects changes in society, changes in the populations requiring nursing care, and a philosophical shift toward health promotion rather than illness care. Roles of the medical-surgical nurse have broadened and expanded in response to these changes. Medical-surgical nurses are increasingly expected to be care managers, educators, advocates, leaders, and researchers. The nurse assumes these various roles to promote and maintain health, to prevent illness, and to facilitate coping with disability or death for the adult patient (a person requiring healthcare services) in any setting.

The Nurse as Caregiver

Nurses have always been caregivers. However, the activities carried out within the caregiver role have changed tremendously in the twenty-first century. From 1900 to the 1960s, the nurse was regarded primarily as the person who gave personal care and carried out physicians' orders. This dependent role has changed as a result of the increased education of nurses, research in and the development of nursing knowledge, and the recognition that nurses are autonomous and informed professionals.

The caregiver role for the nurse today is both independent and collaborative. Nurses independently make assessments and plan and implement patient care based on nursing knowledge and skills. Nurses also collaborate with other members of the healthcare team to implement and evaluate care (Figure 1–2 ■).

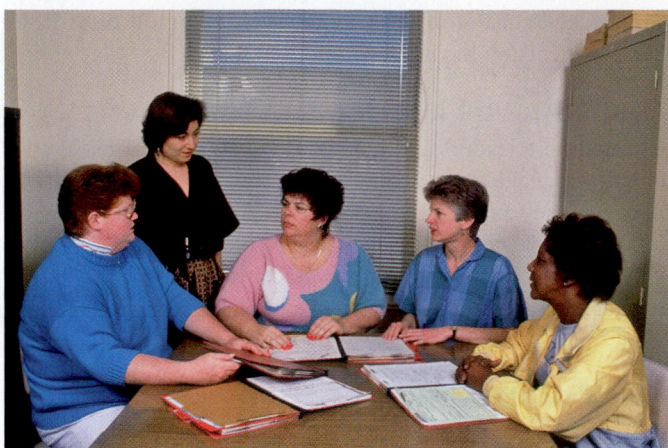

Figure 1–2 ■ The healthcare team discusses the individualized plan of care and outcomes.

As a caregiver, the nurse practices both the science and the art of nursing. In medical-surgical nursing, the science requires a deep understanding of normal physiology and the pathophysiology underlying disease processes commonly affecting adults. Just as the pediatric nurse must understand the physical and psychosocial development of children, the medical-surgical nurse must understand the physical, psychosocial, economic and developmental differences among adults spanning a range of more than 60 years. Using critical

thinking in the nursing process as the framework for care, the nurse provides interventions to meet not only the physical needs but also the psychosocial, cultural, spiritual, and environmental needs of patients and families. See Box 1–5 for a discussion of culturally sensitive nursing care. Considering all aspects of the patient ensures a holistic approach to nursing. Holistic nursing care is based on a philosophical view that interacting wholes are greater than the sum of their parts. A holistic approach also emphasizes the uniqueness of the individual.

In providing comprehensive, individualized care, the nurse uses critical thinking skills to analyze and synthesize knowledge from the arts, the sciences, and nursing research and theory. The science (knowledge base) of nursing is translated into the art of nursing through caring. Caring is the means by which the nurse is connected with and concerned for the patient (Benner & Wrubel, 1989). Thus, the nurse as caregiver is knowledgeable, skilled, empathic, and caring.

The Nurse as Educator

The nurse's role as educator is increasingly important for several reasons. Healthcare providers and consumers as well as local, state, and federal governments are placing greater emphasis on health promotion and illness prevention, hospital stays are shorter, and the number of chronically ill in our society is increasing. Early discharge of patients from the hospital setting or rehabilitation facility to home care means that family

BOX 1–5 Culturally Sensitive Nursing

The primary focus of nursing care is the patient, as the patient relates to the environment and experiences events or situations related to health or illness. These experiences are given shape and personal meaning by culture—the socially inherited characteristics of a human group. These characteristics include the beliefs, practices, habits, likes, dislikes, customs, and rituals people learn from their families and pass on to their children. Cultural background is an essential component of a person's ethnic identity. A person's ethnic identity includes belonging to a social group within a culture and a social system and sharing a common religion, language, ancestry, and physical characteristics.

The healthcare system encompasses patients who are culturally diverse. This diversity includes differences in country of origin, health beliefs, sexual orientation, race, socioeconomic level, and age. Despite increasing diversity, nursing has been slow to address the need for culturally sensitive care. Many different factors account for this inattention, including ethnocentrism (people's belief that their own cultural group's beliefs and values are the only acceptable ones) and prejudice. The healthcare system is itself a culture, composed primarily of white middle-class people, and it often serves as a barrier to culturally sensitive care.

The 1992 American Academy of Nursing Expert Panel on Culturally Competent Nursing Care identified several reasons why it has become increasingly important that nurses plan culturally sensitive care:

■ The demographic and ethnic composition of the population of the world in general, and the United States in particular, has changed markedly, and there is a lack of ethnic representation in healthcare professionals in the healthcare system. Information on and knowledge about values, beliefs, experiences, and healthcare needs of various populations is limited.

■ There is a growing awareness and acceptance of diversity and an increased willingness to maintain and support ethnic and cultural heritage.

■ People of color and immigrants are facing increasing unemployment, decreasing opportunity, and limited access to health care. These conditions may contribute to the establishment of new minorities, such as the homeless.

■ The international focus on providing health care for all people (within the context of inequity, barriers, and lack of access) may have raised the consciousness of healthcare professionals to some of the inequities inherent in healthcare systems in both developing countries and developed countries.

■ Nurses comprise the largest force in the delivery of health care and therefore have the potential to contribute to the changing inequities in and inaccessibility to health care.

■ Consumers are becoming increasingly aware of what is competent and sensitive health care.

This same panel of experts proposed general principles for nurses for becoming sensitive to cultural diversity and providing culturally sensitive care. For example,

■ nurses must learn to appreciate intergroup and intragroup cultural diversity and commonalties in racial/ethnic minority populations.

■ nurses must understand how social structure factors shape health behaviors and practices among members of racial/ethnic minorities.

■ nurses must confront their own ethnocentrism and racism.

■ nurses must begin rehearsing, practicing, and evaluating services provided to cross-cultural populations.

People of every culture have the right to have their cultural values known, respected, and addressed appropriately in nursing and other healthcare services (Leininger, 1991). To provide nursing care that is culturally sensitive, nurses must develop a sensitivity to personal fundamental values about health and illness; must accept the existence of differing values; and must be respectful of, interested in, and understanding of other cultures without being judgmental.

caregivers must learn how to perform complex skills. All these factors make the educator role essential to maintaining the health and well-being of patients.

The framework for the role of educator is the teaching–learning process. Within this framework, the nurse assesses learning needs, plans and implements teaching methods to meet those needs, and evaluates the effectiveness of the teaching. To be an effective educator, the nurse must have effective interpersonal skills and be familiar with adult learning principles (Figure 1–3 ■).

A major component of the educator role today is discharge planning. Discharge planning, which begins on admission to a healthcare setting, is a systematic method of preparing the patient and family for exit from the healthcare agency and for maintaining continuity of care after the patient leaves the setting. Discharge planning also involves making referrals, identifying community and personal resources, and arranging for necessary equipment and supplies for home care.

The Nurse as Advocate

The patient entering the healthcare system may be unprepared to make independent decisions. However, today's healthcare consumer is better educated about options for care, and may have very definite opinions. The nurse as patient advocate actively promotes the patient's rights to autonomy and free choice. The nurse as advocate speaks for the patient, mediates between the patient and other persons, and/or protects the patient's right to self-determination (Ellis & Hartley, 2007). The goals of the nurse as advocate are to do the following:

- Assess the need for advocacy.
- Communicate with other healthcare team members.
- Provide patient and family teaching.
- Assist and support patient decision making.
- Serve as a change agent in the healthcare system.
- Participate in health policy formulation.

The nurse must practice advocacy based on the belief that patients have the right to choose treatment options, based on information about the results of accepting or rejecting the treatment, without coercion. The nurse must also accept and respect the decision of the patient, even though it may differ from the decision the nurse would make.

The Nurse as Leader and Manager

All nurses are leaders and managers. They practice leadership and they manage time, people, resources, and the environment in which they provide care. Nurses carry out these roles by directing, delegating, supervising and coordinating nursing activities. Nurses must be knowledgeable of how and when to delegate, as well as the legal requirements of delegation. Nurses also evaluate the quality of care provided.

Models of Care Delivery

Nurses are leaders and managers of patient care within a variety of models of care delivery. Examples are primary nursing, team nursing, and case management. The nursing shortage made the combination of primary and team nursing more economically feasible.

PRIMARY NURSING Primary nursing allows the nurse to provide individualized direct care to a small number of patients during their entire inpatient stay. This model was developed to reduce the fragmentation of care experienced by the patient and to facilitate family-centered continuity of care. In primary nursing, the nurse provides and coordinates care; communicates with patients, families, and other healthcare providers; and carries out discharge planning.

TEAM NURSING Team nursing is practiced by teams of variously educated healthcare providers. For example, a team may consist of a registered nurse, a licensed practical nurse, and two unlicensed assistive personnel (UAPs). The registered nurse is the team leader. The team leader is responsible for making assignments and has overall responsibility for patient care by team members. All team members work together, each performing the activities for which he or she is best prepared.

CASE MANAGEMENT Case management focuses on management of a caseload (group) of patients and the members of the healthcare team caring for those patients. The purpose of case management is to maximize positive outcomes and contain costs. The nurse who is case manager is usually a clinical specialist, and the caseload consists of patients with similar healthcare needs. As case manager, the nurse makes appropriate referrals to other healthcare providers and manages the quality of care provided, including accuracy, timeliness, and cost. The case manager also is in contact with patients after discharge, ensuring continuity of care and health maintenance.

Delegation

Delegation is carried out when the nurse assigns appropriate and effective work activities to other members of the healthcare team. When the nurse delegates nursing care activities to another person, that person is authorized to act in the place of the nurse, while the nurse retains the accountability for the activities performed. Delegation skills are becoming increasingly important in healthcare as agencies restructure and implement cost containment measures. More categories of healthcare workers with often minimal nursing education and experience

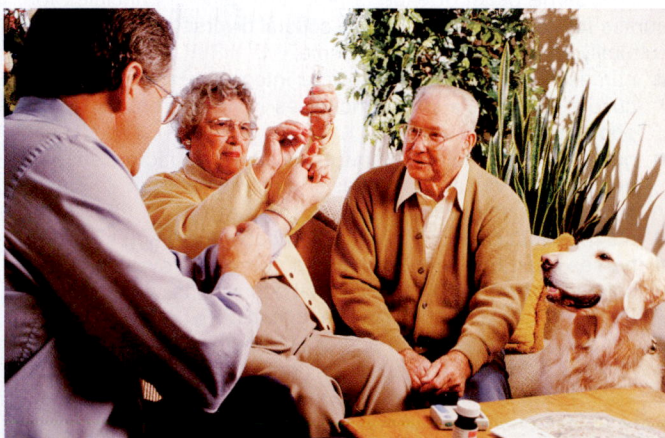

Figure 1–3 ■ The nurse's role as educator is an essential component of care. As part of the discharge planning process, the nurse is responsible for teaching for self-care at home.

are being hired to assist the registered nurse as *nurse extenders*, or *UAPs*. Guidelines for delegation include the following:

- Consider the training, experience, and competence of each member of the healthcare team, the complexity of the task to be assigned, and the amount of time available to supervise the tasks.
- Determine the level of nursing judgment and evaluation required for the task.
- Consider the patient's condition and the potential harm and difficulty of performing the task.
- Know the state's nurse practice act and any practice limitations that may exist.
- Delegate only tasks that are within the scope of practice or authorized duties for each category of worker.
- Assign the right job to the right person. Tasks that are routine and standard are the best to assign to others.
- Know when it is appropriate to retain direct responsibility for care activities. Tasks that are complex or require a high level of nursing judgment should be performed by the nurse.
- Give clear and complete directions for assignments. Ask questions to be sure directions have been understood.
- Give the team member the authority to complete the task while remaining accountable for the outcomes of care.
- Monitor the care provided and give constructive evaluation if necessary.

Quality and Safety

As a major sector within the healthcare workforce, nurses have a significant responsibility for ensuring the quality and safety of care patients receive. This responsibility goes beyond ensuring that individual patients receive safe and effective patient-centered nursing care to recognizing healthcare system issues that impact quality of care. The current focus of safety initiatives is on minimizing the risk of harm to patients and providers by improving the performance and effectiveness of both individuals and healthcare systems (Cronenwett et al., 2007). All nurses must be prepared to understand, take seriously, and participate in quality and safety improvement strategies.

As a leader and manager, the nurse encourages the use of strategies such as standardized practices, checklists, and technology to improve safety and quality. When an error or near miss occurs, the nurse's focus is on reporting the incident to promote analysis of the factors and systems leading up to it, not on blaming the individuals involved.

In the role of leader and manager, the nurse is responsible for the quality of patient care through a process of quality improvement. Quality improvement uses data to monitor the outcomes of care and the processes used to deliver that care. Changes to improve the quality and safety of healthcare systems are continuously designed and tested through quality improvement strategies and initiatives (Cronenwett et al., 2007).

Quality improvement methods also are used to evaluate patient care. They commonly evaluate actual care against an established set of standards of care. Nurses and other healthcare providers make this evaluation by reviewing documentation, by conducting patient surveys and nurse interviews, and/or by direct observation of nurse or patient performance. The data are then used to identify differences between actual practice and established standards and to develop a plan of action to resolve the differences. The actions are then assessed through internal peer review or by an external medical review organization, called a utilization and quality control peer review organization (PRO), to determine whether they were effective in improving practice.

The Nurse as Researcher

Nurses have always identified problems in patient care. Early nurse researchers showed the link between effective preoperative patient education and shorter postoperative hospital stays with fewer complications. Today, nurse researchers are studying a broad variety of questions and issues. To develop the science of nursing, nursing knowledge must be established through clinical research and then published so that the findings can be used by all nurses to provide evidence-based patient care.

To be relevant, nursing research must have a goal to improve the care that nurses provide patients. This means that all nurses must consider the researcher role to be integral to nursing practice. Summaries of relevant nursing research are included in almost all the nursing care chapters of this textbook. After the summary and discussion of each study, a critical-thinking section specifically related to the findings of the study encourages the student to apply the findings to the clinical setting.

CHAPTER HIGHLIGHTS

- Recommended core competencies for all healthcare professionals include providing patient-centered care, working in interdisciplinary teams, using evidence-based practice, applying quality improvement, promoting safe healthcare systems, and using informatics.
- The nursing process is the cyclical series of critical-thinking activities used by nurses to provide patient care to promote wellness, maintain health, restore health, or facilitate coping with disability or death. The five inter-related phases of the nursing process are assessment, diagnosis, planning, implementation, and evaluation.

- The clinical practice of nursing is guided by codes for nurses and standards of practice.
- The human responses that nurses must consider when planning and implementing care result from changes in the structure and/or function of all body systems, as well as the effects of those changes on the psychosocial, cultural, spiritual, economic, and personal life of the patient.
- Nurses function as caregivers, educators, advocates, leaders and managers, and researchers to promote and maintain health, prevent illness, improve health care delivery and systems, and facilitate coping with disability or death for the adult patient.

TEST YOURSELF NCLEX-RN® REVIEW

1. The National Academy of Sciences has proposed a set of core competencies for healthcare professionals. What is the primary purpose of these competencies?
   1. to make all healthcare professionals equal
   2. to improve safety and quality of care
   3. to reduce the number of medical law suits
   4. to maintain public faith in physicians

2. What does the nurse use in the practice setting to make clinical judgments and decisions?
   1. nursing process
   2. standards of care
   3. nursing ethics
   4. critical thinking

3. Which of the following statements is true of outcomes developed during the planning phase of the nursing process?
   1. Outcomes are mutually established by the patient and the nurse.
   2. Outcomes are mutually established by the nurse and the physician.
   3. Outcomes are mandated by institutional policies and standards.
   4. Outcomes are written by patients and family members.

4. The phases of the nursing process are used when providing care to patients. From the following list, choose the order in which these phases are most often used.
   1. outcomes
   2. assessment
   3. evaluation
   4. implementation
   5. planning

5. When nurses discuss the "science of nursing," what does this phrase mean?
   1. clinical competency
   2. holistic care
   3. knowledge base
   4. practice component

6. What role does the nurse demonstrate when developing and providing health information?
   1. advocate
   2. caregiver
   3. researcher
   4. educator

7. What goal is a component of the nurse's role as advocate?
   1. assisting and supporting patient decision making
   2. conducting research about the effects of exercise
   3. delegating responsibilities for patient care to others
   4. performing range-of-motion exercises

8. A nurse assigns appropriate work activities to other members of his or her team. What role is being illustrated?
   1. advocate
   2. leader/manager
   3. researcher
   4. caregiver

9. A method of establishing a standard of care and evaluating outcomes of that standard involves which of the following?
   1. writing a dress code policy for a healthcare agency
   2. creating a critical pathway for a specific type of patient
   3. establishing quality assurance regulations
   4. implementing a new procedure to change dressings

10. A nurse delegates vital sign assessment to a UAP. Who is accountable for the assessment findings?
    1. the UAP
    2. the patient
    3. the nurse
    4. the physician

See Test Yourself answers in Appendix C.

Pearson Nursing Student Resources

Find additional review materials at
nursing.pearsonhighered.com

Prepare for success with additional NCLEX®-style practice questions, interactive assignments and activities, Web links, animations and videos, and more!

BIBLIOGRAPHY

Alfaro-LeFevre, R. (2009). *Applying nursing process: A tool for critical thinking* (7th ed.). Philadelphia: Lippincott.

American Nurses Association. (2001). *Code of ethics for nurses.* Silver Spring, MD: Author.

American Nurses Association. (2003). *Nursing's social policy statement* (2nd ed.). Washington, DC: Author.

American Nurses Association. (2004a). Managed care: Challenges & opportunities for nursing. Retrieved from http://nursingworld.org/readroom/fsmgdcar.htm

American Nurses Association. (2004b). *Nursing: Scope and standards of practice.* Silver Spring, MD: Author.

American Nurses Association. (2005). *ANA's health care agenda 2005.* Washington, DC: Author.

Anderson, F. (2007). Finding HIPAA in your soup: Decoding the privacy rule. *American Journal of Nursing, 107*(2), 66–71.

Andrews, M. M., & Boyle, J. S. (2008). *Transcultural concepts in nursing care* (5th ed.). Philadelphia, PA: Lippincott.

Banning, M. (2008, May). Clinical reasoning and its application to nursing: concepts and research studies. *Nurse Education in Practice, 8*(3), 177–183.

Benner, P. (1984). *From novice to expert: Excellence and power in clinical nursing practice.* Redwood City, CA: Addison-Wesley Nursing.

Benner, P., & Wrubel, J. (1989). The primacy of caring: Stress and coping in clinical nursing practice. Redwood City, CA: Addison-Wesley Nursing.

Bulechek, G. M., Butcher, H. K., & Dochterman, J. M. (2008). *Nursing Interventions Classification (NIC)* (5th ed.). St. Louis: Mosby.

Chitty, K., & Black, B. P. (2007). *Professional nursing: Concepts & challenges* (5th ed.). Philadelphia: Saunders.

Cronenwett, L., Sherwood, G., Barnsteiner, J., Disch, J., Johnson, J., Mitchell, P., et al. (2007). Quality and safety education for nurses. *Nursing Outlook, 55*(3), 122–131.

Ellis, J., & Hartley, C. (2008). *Managing and coordinating nursing care* (5th ed.). Philadelphia: Lippincott.

Esterhuizen, P. (2006). Is the professional code still the cornerstone of clinical nursing practice? *Journal of Advanced Nursing, 53*(1), 104–110.

Foust, J. (2007, May). Discharge planning as part of daily nursing practice. *Applied Nursing Research, 20*(2), 72–77.

Giger, J. N., & Davidhizar, R. E. (2008). *Transcultural nursing: Assessment and intervention* (5th ed.). St. Louis, MO: Mosby.

Greggs-McQuilkin, D. (2003). The specialty of medical-surgical nursing: The solid rock, not the stepping stone. *MEDSURG Nursing, 12*(1), 5, 26.

Hanks, R. (2008, July). The lived experience of nursing advocacy. *Nursing Ethics, 15*(4), 468–477.

Hanson, D., Hoss, B., & Wesorick, B. (2008, August). Evaluating the evidence: Guidelines. *AORN Journal, 88*(2), 184, 186, 188–196.

International Council of Nurses. (2006). *The ICN Code of ethics for nurses.* Geneva: Imprimerie Fornara.

Institute of Medicine. Committee on Quality of Health Care in America. (2001). *Crossing the quality chasm: A new health system for the 21st century.* Washington, DC: National Academy Press.

Johnson, K., Hallsey, D., Meredith, R., & Warden, E. (2006, April). A nurse-driven system for improving patient quality outcomes. *Journal of Nursing Care Quality, 21*(2), 168–175.

Klenner, S. (2000). Mapping out a clinical pathway. *RN, 63*(6), 33–36.

Koehn, M., & Lehman, K. (2008). Nurses' perceptions of evidence-based nursing practice. *Journal of Advanced Nursing, 62*(2), 209–215.

Lachman, V. D. (2007). Ethics, law, and policy. Moral courage in action: Case studies. *Medsurg Nursing, 16*(4), 275–277.

Lachman, V. (2008, October). Making ethical choices: weighing obligations & virtues. *Nursing, 38*(10), 42–46.

Leininger, M. (1991). Transcultural care principles, human rights, and ethical considerations. *Journal of Transcultural Nursing, 3*(1), 21–23.

Mathes, M. (2005). Ethics, law, and policy. On nursing, moral autonomy, and moral responsibility. *Medsurg Nursing, 14*(6), 395–398.

Matter, S. (2006, December). Empower nurses with evidence-based knowledge. *Nursing Management.* Retrieved from www.nursingmanagement.com

National Academy of Sciences. (2003). Executive summary. *Health professions education: A bridge to quality,* pp. 1–18. Retrieved from http://www.nap.edu

National Council of State Boards of Nursing, Inc. (1996). Professional boundaries: A nurse's guide to the importance of appropriate professional boundaries. Chicago, IL: National Council of State Boards of Nursing, Inc.

Olson, D. P. (2007). Ethical issues. Unwanted treatment: What are the ethical implications? *American Journal of Nursing, 107*(9), 51–53.

Radwin, L. (1990). Research on diagnostic reasoning in nursing. *Nursing Diagnosis, 1*(2), 70–77.

Riddell, T. (2007, March). Critical assumptions: thinking critically about critical thinking. *Journal of Nursing Education, 46*(3), 121–126.

Spector, R. (2009). *Cultural diversity in health and illness* (7th ed.). Upper Saddle River, NJ: Prentice Hall.

Spotlight on medical-surgical nursing. (2003). *Nursing, 33*(4), 88–R2.

Sullivan, D. (2010). Connecting nursing education and practice: A focus on shared goals for quality and safety. *Creative Nursing, 16*(1), 37–43.

Tanner, C. A. (2006). Thinking like a nurse: A research-based model of clinical judgment in nursing. *Journal of Nursing Education, 45*(6), 204–211.

Uhrenfeldt, L., & Hall, E. (2007, May). Clinical wisdom among proficient nurses. *Nursing Ethics, 14*(3), 387–398.

Wallace, C., Bigelow, S., Xu, X., & Elstein, L. (2007, January–February). Collaborative practice: usability of text-based, electronic patient care guidelines. *CIN: Computers, Informatics, Nursing, 25*(1), 39–44.

Wilkinson, J. M. (2007). *Nursing process and critical thinking* (4th ed.). Upper Saddle River, NJ: Prentice Hall.

World Health Organization. (1974). *Constitution of the World Health Organization: Chronicle of the World Health Organization.* Geneva: World Health Organization.

Health and Illness in Adults

LEARNING OUTCOMES

1. Define health, incorporating the health–illness continuum and the concept of high-level wellness.
2. Explain factors affecting functional health status.
3. Discuss the nurse's role in health promotion.
4. Describe characteristics of health, disease, and illness.
5. Describe illness behaviors and needs of the patient with acute illness and chronic illness.
6. Describe the primary, secondary, and tertiary levels of illness prevention.
7. Compare and contrast the physical status, risks for alterations in health, assessment guidelines, and healthy behaviors of the young adult, middle adult, and older adult.
8. Explain the definitions, functions, and developmental stages and tasks of the family.

CLINICAL COMPETENCIES

1. Use knowledge of developmental levels and of activities to promote, restore, and maintain health when planning and implementing patient-centered care for adults.
2. Engage patients and family members in active partnerships to promote and maintain health of the adult.

KEY TERMS

acute illness, *22*
chronic illness, *23*
disease, *22*
exacerbation, *23*

family, *31*
health, *18*
health–illness continuum, *18*
holistic health care, *19*

illness, *22*
manifestations, *22*
remission, *23*
wellness, *18*

The human responses that nurses must consider when planning and implementing care result from changes in the structure and/or function of all body systems, as well as the interrelated effects of those changes on the psychosocial, cultural, spiritual, economic, and personal life of the patient.

In 1948, the World Health Organization (WHO) defined **health** as "a state of complete physical, mental, and social well-being, and not merely the absence of disease or infirmity." This definition, which WHO maintains to date, addresses the importance of physical, mental, emotional, and social components of health, but fails to take into account the various levels of health a person may experience. Health is not just a state of being, but the resources (e.g., physical, personal, social) used by each person in dealing with the challenges of living. These factors, which greatly influence nursing care, include the health–illness continuum and high-level wellness.

The Health–Illness Continuum and High-Level Wellness

The **health–illness continuum** represents health as a dynamic process, with high-level **wellness** at one extreme of the continuum and death at the opposite extreme (Figure 2–1 ■).

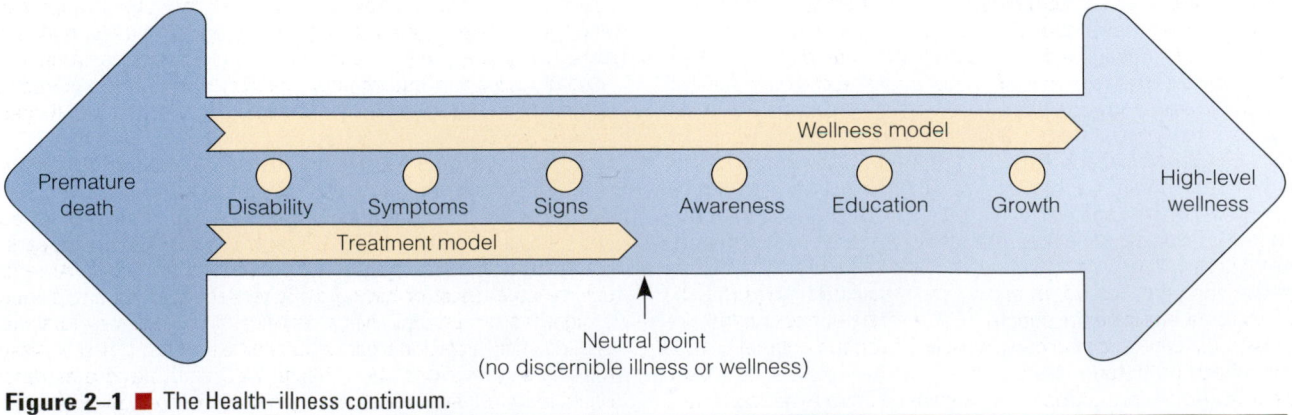

Figure 2–1 ■ The Health–illness continuum.

Source: From Travis, J. W., & Ryan, R. S. (1998). *Wellness Workbook.* Berkeley, CA: Ten Speed Press. Used with permission.

Individuals place themselves at different locations on the continuum at specific points in time.

Dunn (1959) expanded the concept of a continuum of health and illness in his description of high-level wellness. Dunn conceptualized wellness as an active process influenced by the environment. He differentiated good health from wellness:

> Good health can exist as a relatively passive state. . . . Wellness is an integrated method of functioning. . . oriented toward maximizing the potential of which the individual is capable, within the environment where he is functioning. (1959, p. 4)

A variety of factors influence wellness, including self-concept, environment, culture, and spiritual values. Providing care based on a framework of wellness facilitates active involvement by both the nurse and the patient in promoting, maintaining, or restoring health. It also supports the philosophy of **holistic health care**, in which all aspects of a person (physical, psychosocial, cultural, spiritual, and intellectual) are considered as essential components of individualized care.

Factors Affecting Health

Many different factors affect a person's health or level of wellness. These factors often interact to promote health or to become risk factors for alterations in health.

Genetic Makeup

Each person's genetic makeup influences health status throughout life. Genetic makeup affects personality, temperament, body structure, intellectual potential, and susceptibility to the development of hereditary alterations in health. Examples of chronic illnesses that are associated with genetic makeup include sickle cell disease, hemophilia, diabetes mellitus, and cancer.

Cognitive Abilities and Educational Level

Although cognitive abilities are determined prior to adulthood, cognitive development affects whether people view themselves as healthy or ill; cognitive levels also may affect health practices. Injuries to and illnesses affecting the brain may alter cognitive abilities. Educational level affects the ability to understand and follow guidelines for health. For example, if an individual is functionally illiterate, written information about healthy behaviors and health resources is worthless.

Race, Ethnicity, and Cultural Background

Certain diseases occur at a higher rate of incidence in some races and ethnic groups than in others. For example, in the United States hypertension is more common in African Americans, diabetes mellitus and chronic liver disease are among the leading causes of illness in Native Americans, and eye disorders are more prevalent in Chinese Americans. See the accompanying Cultural Diversity feature. The ethnic and cultural background of an individual also influences health values and behaviors, lifestyle, and illness behaviors. Every culture defines health and illness in a way that is unique; in addition, each culture has its own health beliefs and illness treatment practices.

Age, Gender, and Developmental Level

Age, gender, and developmental level are factors in health and illness. Cardiovascular disorders are uncommon in young adults, but the incidence increases after the age of 40. Myocardial infarctions are more common in men than women until women are postmenopausal. Some diseases occur only in one gender or the other (e.g., prostate cancer in men and cervical cancer in women). The older adult often has increased incidence of chronic illness and increased potential for serious illness or death from infectious illnesses such as influenza and pneumonia.

Lifestyle and Environment

The components of a person's lifestyle that affect health status include patterns of eating, use of chemical substances (alcohol, nicotine, caffeine, legal and illegal drugs), exercise and rest patterns, and coping methods. Examples of altered responses are the relationship of obesity to hypertension, cigarette smoking to chronic obstructive pulmonary disease, a sedentary lifestyle to heart disease, and a high-stress career to alcoholism. The environment has a major influence on health. Occupational exposure to toxic substances (such as asbestos and coal dust) increases the risk of pulmonary disorders. Air, water, and food pollution increase the risk of respiratory disorders, infectious diseases, and cancer. Environmental temperature variations can result in hypothermia or hyperthermia, especially in the older adult.

FOCUS ON CULTURAL DIVERSITY
Biologic Variations Among Cultures

As genetic science and our understanding of disease causes and pathology have advanced, there is increasing recognition that differences between peoples of the world are more than skin deep. Certain diseases and conditions are much more likely to develop in some groups than in others; for example, sickle cell anemia occurs more frequently in people whose ancestors are from central Africa, the Near East, the Mediterranean region, and parts of India; Caucasian women of small stature and of Scandinavian heritage have a higher risk of developing osteoporosis. Biological variations also may affect the way the body metabolizes drugs, leading to an effect that is either less than or greater than anticipated. In other cases, selected drugs may be found to be effective for people of one race but not another.

Biologic differences among people of various cultural groups also affect both food preferences and food tolerance. Most Mexican Americans, African Americans, Native Americans, and Asians are lactose intolerant; that is, they do not produce enough lactose to tolerate large amounts of milk and milk products. If too much milk (or yogurt or milk chocolate) is eaten, undigested lactose in the intestine causes manifestations such as cramping, flatulence, abdominal bloating, and diarrhea (Giger & Davidhizar, 2008).

Although known biologic variables among people of different races and cultures can be helpful in providing individualized health education, it is important to avoid stereotyping based on racial and cultural differences. For example, a person who appears to be African American may actually identify with Native American culture as a result of having a Native American parent; a recent emigrant from Ethiopia has a significantly different cultural background than a black person who is a descendent of U.S. slaves. Making assumptions about health risk factors and preferences could lead to inappropriate care planning for these individuals.

Socioeconomic Background

Both lifestyle and environmental influences are affected by one's income level. The culture of poverty, which crosses all racial and ethnic boundaries, negatively influences health status. Living at or below the poverty level may result in crowded, unsanitary living conditions or homelessness. Housing often is overcrowded, lacks adequate heating or cooling, and is infested with insects and rats. Crowded living conditions increase the risk of transferring communicable diseases. Other problems include lack of infant and child care, lack of medical care for injuries or illness, inadequate nutrition, use of addictive substances, and violence.

Geographic Area

The geographic area in which one lives influences health status. Such illnesses as malaria are more common in tropical areas of North America, whereas multiple sclerosis occurs with greater frequency in the northern United States and Canada. Other geographic influences are seen in the number of skin cancers in people living in sunny, hot areas and sinus infections in people living in areas of high humidity.

Health Promotion and Maintenance

For many years, the emphasis in nursing was on care of the acutely ill patient in the hospital setting. With changes in society and in health care, this emphasis is shifting toward preventive, community-based care, including managing chronic illness. Although the focus of this textbook is not community health nursing, the importance of teaching health-promoting behaviors is an essential component of medical-surgical nursing.

Healthy Living

Practices that are known to promote health and wellness include the following:

- Eat three balanced meals a day, following the guidelines developed jointly by the U.S. Department of Agriculture

---

BOX 2–1 Dietary Guidelines for Health

- Eat a variety of foods to get the energy, proteins, vitamins, minerals, and fiber needed for good health.
- Balance intake of food with physical activity. Maintain or improve body weight to reduce the risks of high blood pressure, heart disease, stroke, certain cancers, and type 2 diabetes mellitus.
- Choose a diet with plenty of grain products, vegetables, and fruits, which provide needed fiber and complex carbohydrates and can help lower intake of fat.
- Choose a diet low in fat, saturated fat, and cholesterol to reduce the risk of heart attack and certain types of cancer, and to help maintain a healthy weight.
- Choose a diet moderate in sugars. Increased sugar intake can increase weight, decrease nutrient intake, and contribute to tooth decay.
- Choose a diet moderate in salt and sodium to help reduce the risk of high blood pressure.
- Drink alcoholic beverages, if at all, in moderation. Alcohol provides non-nutrient calories, may be addicting, and causes many health problems.

(USDA) and the U.S. Department of Health and Human Services (HHS) (Box 2–1). It is also helpful to follow a general guideline of what to eat each day, such as with the Food Guide Pyramid illustrated in Figure 2–2 ■. The food pyramid was revised in 2005, with recommendations for a greater emphasis on monounsaturated and polyunsaturated fats, the inclusion of whole-grain foods with each meal, and increased intake of fish and vegetables. The goal of the revision is to reduce obesity and cardiovascular disease. A website is available to individualize the plan by helping consumers choose foods and amounts. After entering their age, gender, and activity level, consumers get their own plan at an appropriate calorie level, and can print out a miniposter and worksheet to track progress.

(vertical text, left margin) Health Promotion for Young Adults Video

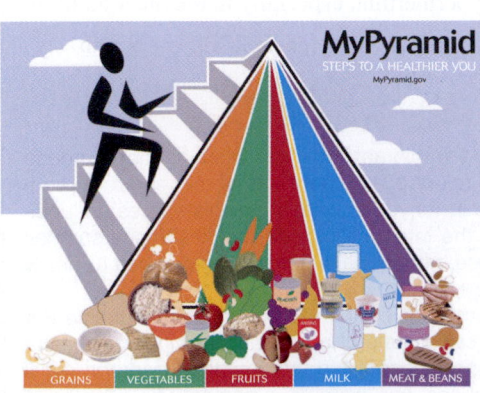
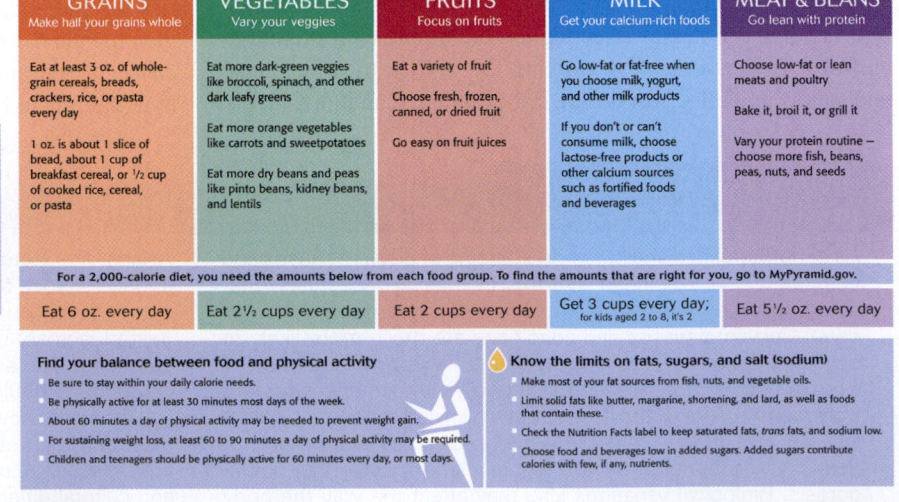
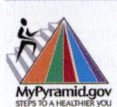
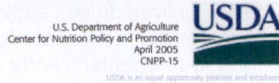

Figure 2–2 ■ The USDA Food Guide Pyramid is designed to be used as a method of helping Americans make healthy food choices and be active every day.

Source: U.S. Department of Agriculture and U.S. Department of Health and Human Services. (2005). Retrieved from http://www.mypyramid.gov/downloads/miniposter.pdf

- Exercise moderately and regularly, engaging in at least 20 minutes of continuous activity (such as walking) five or more days per week.
- Sleep 7 to 8 hours each day.
- Limit alcohol consumption to a moderate amount (no more than two drinks per day for men or one drink daily for women), and favor red wine.
- Eliminate smoking and use of other tobacco products such as smokeless tobacco.
- Keep sun exposure to a minimum.
- Maintain recommended immunizations (Table 2–1).

The nurse promotes health by teaching the activities that maintain wellness, by providing information about the characteristics and consequences of diseases when risk factors have been identified, and by supplying specific information about decreasing risk factors (Pender, Parsons, & Murdaugh, 2006). The nurse also promotes health by following healthy practices and serving as a role model.

NATIONAL HEALTH PROMOTION The U.S. Department of Health and Human Services (HHS) has published national public health objectives each decade since 1980. Overarching goals for the current decade are described in Box 2–2.

BOX 2–2 *Healthy People 2020:* Overarching Goals

With the overall mission of improving the nation's health, *Healthy People 2020* has four overarching major goals. These goals address factors that contribute to the health status of individuals or populations, and include social and physical determinants of health.

Overarching Goals
- Eliminate preventable disease, disability, injury, and premature death.
- Achieve health equity, eliminate disparities, and improve the health of all groups.
- Create social and physical environments that promote good health for all.
- Promote healthy development and healthy behaviors across every stage of life.

Objectives to achieve these overarching goals fall under such diverse topics as the following:
- Access to health services
- Chronic disease conditions
- Educational and community-based programs
- Food safety
- Global health
- Injury and violence prevention
- Nutrition and weight status, and
- Social determinants of health

Source: U.S. Department of Health and Human Services. (2010). *Healthy People 2020.* Washington, DC: Author.

TABLE 2–1 Recommended Immunizations for Adults

VACCINE	INDICATIONS	DO NOT GIVE TO
Measles-mumps-rubella	Anyone born after 1956 and never infected, or those likely to be exposed, such as those entering college or the military and healthcare personnel.	Pregnant women, immunocompromised people, or anyone with a history of anaphylactic reaction to egg protein or neomycin.
Tetanus, diphtheria, pertussis (Td, Tdap)	Anyone who has never been vaccinated should have the primary tetanus and diphtheria toxoid series, followed by booster every 10 years. Adults younger than 65 years should receive one dose of Tdap.	People with a history of anaphylactic reaction to the vaccine. People with a history of encephalopathy following pertussis vaccine should not receive Tdap.
Hepatitis A	Anyone who wishes protection and those traveling to countries in which hepatitis A infection is endemic.	People with a history of hypersensitivity to aluminum hydroxide or phenoxyethanol.
Hepatitis B	Anyone likely to have repeated exposure (such as healthcare providers or sex partners of a known carrier) or who have had exposure (such as a needle-stick injury to a healthcare worker).	People with a history of anaphylactic reaction to common baker's yeast.
Human papillomavirus (HPV)	All previously unvaccinated women through age 26 years.	People with a history of anaphylactic reaction to the vaccine or its components.
Influenza	Anyone at high risk for complications, healthcare providers, and those wanting immunity.	Those with a high fever, or a history of anaphylactic reaction to egg protein.
Pneumococcal pneumonia	Anyone at high risk for pneumococcal disease, those over 65 years of age.	Pregnant women.
Varicella	Anyone never infected, especially healthcare providers and child care workers.	Pregnant women, immunocompromised people, those who have received an immune globulin or a blood transfusion within 5 months, or those with a history of anaphylactic reactions to neomycin or gelatin.
Zoster (shingles)	Persons age 60 years and older.	Pregnant women, immunocompromised people, and those with a history of anaphylactic reactions to neomycin or gelatin.

Disease and Illness

Disease and *illness* are terms that are often used interchangeably, but in fact they have different meanings. In general, nursing is concerned with illness, whereas medicine is concerned with disease.

Disease

Disease (literally meaning "without ease") is a medical term describing alterations in structure and function of the body or mind. Diseases may have mechanical, biologic, or normative causes. Mechanical causes of disease result in damage to the structure of the body and are the result of trauma or extremes of temperature. Biologic causes of disease affect body function and are the result of genetic defects, the effects of aging, infestation and infection, alterations in the immune system, and alterations in normal organ secretions. Normative causes are psychologic but involve a mind–body interaction, so that physical manifestations occur in response to the psychologic disturbance.

The cause of many diseases is still unknown. The following are generally accepted as common causes of disease:

- Genetic defects
- Developmental defects resulting from exposure to viruses, chemicals, or drugs that affect the developing fetus
- Biologic agents or toxins (including viruses, bacteria, rickettsia, fungi, protozoa, and helminths)
- Physical agents such as temperature extremes, radiation, and electricity
- Chemical agents such as alcohol, drugs, strong acids or bases, and heavy metals
- Generalized response of tissues to injury or irritation
- Alterations in the production of antibodies, resulting in allergies or hypersensitivities
- Faulty metabolic processes (e.g., a production of hormones or enzymes above or below normal)
- Continued, unabated stress

Diseases may be classified as acute or chronic, communicable, congenital, degenerative, functional, malignant, psychosomatic, idiopathic, or iatrogenic. These classifications are defined in Table 2–2. In all types of disease, alterations in structure or function cause signs and symptoms (**manifestations**) that prompt a person to seek treatment from a physician or traditional healer. Although both subjective symptoms and objective signs commonly appear with disease, objective signs often predominate. Subjective symptoms may include such manifestations as nausea, general malaise, or fatigue. Examples of objective signs include bleeding, vomiting, diarrhea, limitation of movement, swelling, visual disturbances, and changes in elimination. However, pain (a subjective symptom) is often the primary reason that prompts a person to seek health care.

Illness

Illness is the response a person has to a disease. This response is highly individualized because the person responds not only to his or her own perceptions of the disease but also to the perceptions of others. Illness integrates pathophysiologic alterations; psychologic effects of those alterations; effects on roles, relationships, and values; and cultural and spiritual beliefs. A person may have a disease and not categorize him- or herself as ill, or may validate feelings of illness through the comments of others ("You don't look as though you feel well today").

ACUTE ILLNESS An **acute illness** occurs rapidly, lasts for a relatively short time, and is self-limiting. The condition responds to self-treatment or to medical-surgical intervention. Patients with uncomplicated acute illnesses usually have full recovery and return to normal pre-illness functioning.

Illness behaviors are the way people cope with the alterations in health and function caused by a disease. Illness behaviors are highly individualized and are influenced by age, gender, family values, socioeconomic status, culture, educational level, and mental status. The commonly recognized sequence of illness behaviors follows:

1. *Experiencing symptoms.* In the first stage of an acute illness, a person experiences one or more manifestations that prompt awareness of a change in normal health. Examples of symptoms that signal an illness are pain, bleeding, swelling, fever, or difficulty with breathing. If the manifestations are mild or are familiar (such as symptoms of the common cold or influenza), the person usually uses over-the-counter medications or a traditional remedy for self-treatment. If the symptoms are relieved, no further action is taken; however, if the symptoms are severe or become worse, the person moves to the next stage.

2. *Assuming the sick role.* In the second stage of illness behavior, the person assumes the sick role. This signals acceptance of the symptoms as indicative of an illness. The person usually validates this belief with others and seeks support for seeking professional treatment or remaining

TABLE 2–2 Disease Classifications and Definitions

CLASSIFICATION	DEFINITION
Acute	A disease that has a rapid onset, lasts a relatively short time, and is self-limiting
Chronic	A disease that requires continuing management over a long period—years or even decades
Communicable	A disease that can spread from one person to another
Congenital	A disease or disorder that exists at or before birth
Degenerative	A disease that results from deterioration or impairment of organs or tissues
Functional	A disease that affects function or performance but does not have manifestations of organic illness
Malignant	A disease that tends to become worse and cause death
Psychosomatic	A psychologic disease that is manifested by physiologic symptoms
Idiopathic	A disease that has an unknown cause
Iatrogenic	A disease that is caused by medical therapy

home from school or work. Self-preoccupation is characteristic of this stage, and the person focuses on alterations in function resulting from the illness. If the illness is resolved, the person validates a return to health with others and resumes normal activities; however, if manifestations remain or increase in severity and others agree that no improvement has occurred, the person moves to the next stage by seeking medical care.

3. *Seeking medical care.* In our society, a physician or other healthcare provider usually provides validation of illness. People who believe themselves to be ill (and who are encouraged by others to contact a healthcare provider) make the medical contact for diagnosis, prognosis, and treatment of the illness. If the medical diagnosis is of an illness, the person moves to the next stage. If the medical diagnosis does not support illness, the patient may return to normal functioning or may seek validation from a different healthcare provider.

4. *Assuming a dependent role.* The stage of assuming a dependent role begins when a person accepts the diagnosis and planned treatment of the illness. As the severity of the illness increases, so does the dependent role. It is during this stage that the person may enter the hospital for treatment and care. The responses of the person to care depend on many different variables: the severity of the illness, the degree of anxiety or fear about the outcome, the loss of roles, the support systems available, individualized reactions to stress, and previous experiences with illness care. The severity of the illness and the individual's resources affect whether the person moves to the next stage, recovery and rehabilitation, or to chronic illness or even death.

5. *Achieving recovery and rehabilitation.* The final stage of an acute illness is recovery and rehabilitation. The person now gives up the dependent role and resumes normal roles and responsibilities. As a result of education during treatment and care, the person may be at a higher level of wellness after recovery is complete. There is no set timetable for recovery from an illness. The severity of the illness and the method of treatment affect the length of time required, as does the person's compliance with treatment plans and motivation to return to normal health.

CHRONIC ILLNESS **Chronic illness** is a term that encompasses many different long-term pathologic and psychologic alterations in health. It is the leading health problem in the world today, accounting for 70% of all deaths in the United States (CDC, 2009). The incidence and prevalence of chronic illness is increasing, a trend that is predicted to continue. Current trends contributing to an increased incidence of chronic illnesses include an aging population, diseases of lifestyle and behavior (e.g., obesity, smoking), and environmental factors.

Chronic illness is defined as a condition that requires continuing management over a long period—years or even decades. Chronic conditions may be caused by noncommunicable disease (e.g. cancer, heart disease); persistent illnesses such as asthma or diabetes; long-term mental health disorders such as schizophrenia; or physical, sensory, or structural impairments (e.g. arthritis, visual impairment).

Chronic illness is often also characterized by impaired function in more than one body system; responses to this impaired function may occur in sensory perception, self-care abilities, mobility, cognition, and social skills. The demands on the individual and family as a result of these responses are often lifelong (Crumbie et al., 2004; Lee, 2009).

The intensity of a chronic illness and its related manifestations range from mild to severe. Chronic illness may be characterized by periods of remission and exacerbation. During periods of **remission**, the person does not experience symptoms, even though the disease is still clinically present. During periods of **exacerbation**, the symptoms reappear. These periods of change in symptoms do not appear in all chronic diseases.

Each person with a chronic illness has a unique set of responses and needs. The response of the person to the illness is influenced by the following factors:

- The point in the life cycle at which the illness develops
- The type and degree of limitations imposed by the illness
- The visibility of impairment or disfigurement
- The pathophysiology causing the illness
- The relationship between the impairment and functioning in social roles
- Pain and fear

These factors are highly complex. They are interrelated within each person, resulting in individualized illness behaviors and needs. Because there are so many different chronic diseases and because the experience of each person with the illness is a composite of individualized responses, it is difficult to generalize about needs. However, almost all people with a chronic illness will need to do the following:

- Live as normally as possible, despite symptoms and treatment that may make the person with a chronic illness feel alienated, lonely, and different from others without the illness.
- Learn to adapt activities of daily living and self-care activities.
- Grieve the loss of physical function and, in some cases, life roles, structure, income, status, and dignity.
- Learn to manage an ongoing treatment plan.
- Maintain a positive self-concept and a sense of hope.
- Maintain a feeling of being in control.
- Confront the inevitability of death (Miller, 2000).

Many people with chronic illness successfully meet health-related needs, whereas others do not. Research indicates that adaptation is influenced by variables such as anger, depression, denial, self-concept, locus of control, hardiness, and disability. Nursing interventions for the person with a chronic illness focus on education to promote independent functioning, reduce healthcare costs, and improve well-being and quality of life.

ILLNESS PREVENTION Activities to prevent illness include any measures that limit the progression of an illness at any point of its course. Three levels of illness prevention have been defined (Leavell & Clark, 1965). Each level of prevention occurs at a distinct point in the development of a disease process and requires specific nursing interventions (Edelman & Mandle, 2006). The levels are as follows:

1. *Primary level of prevention.* This level includes generalized health promotion activities as well as specific actions

that prevent or delay the occurrence of a disease. Following are examples of primary prevention activities:

- Reducing exposure to environmental risks, such as air and water pollution
- Eating nutritious foods
- Protecting oneself against industrial hazards
- Obeying seat belt and helmet laws
- Obtaining sex counseling and practicing safer sex
- Obtaining immunizations
- Undergoing genetic screenings
- Eliminating the use of alcohol and cigarettes

2. *Secondary level of prevention.* This level involves activities that emphasize early diagnosis and treatment of an illness to stop the pathologic process and enable the person to return to his or her former state of health as soon as possible. Following are examples of secondary prevention activities:

- Being screened for diseases such as hypertension, diabetes mellitus, and glaucoma
- Obtaining physical examinations and diagnostic tests for cancer
- Performing self-examination for breast and/or testicular cancer
- Obtaining tuberculosis skin tests
- Obtaining specific treatment for illness (e.g., treatment of streptococcal infections of the throat helps prevent secondary disorders involving the heart and/or kidneys)

3. *Tertiary level of prevention.* This level focuses on stopping the disease process and returning the affected individual to a useful place in society within the constraints of any disability. The activities primarily revolve around rehabilitation. Following are examples of tertiary prevention measures:

- Obtaining medical or surgical treatment for an illness
- Enrolling in specific rehabilitation programs for cardiovascular problems, head injuries, and strokes
- Joining work training programs following illness or injury
- Educating the public to employ rehabilitated people to the fullest possible extent

Meeting Health Needs of Adults

The adult years commonly are divided into three stages: the young adult (ages 18 to 40), the middle adult (ages 40 to 65), and the older adult (over age 65). Although developmental markers are not as clearly delineated in the adult as in the infant or child, specific changes do occur with aging in intellectual, psychosocial, and spiritual development, as well as in physical structures and functions.

The developmental theories specific to the adult, with related stages and tasks, are listed in Table 2–3. Applying a variety of developmental theories is important to the holistic care of the adult as nurses assess, plan and implement care, and provide teaching.

The Young Adult

From ages 18 to 25, the healthy young adult is at the peak of physical development (Figure 2–3 ■). All body systems are functioning at maximum efficiency. Then, during the 30s, some

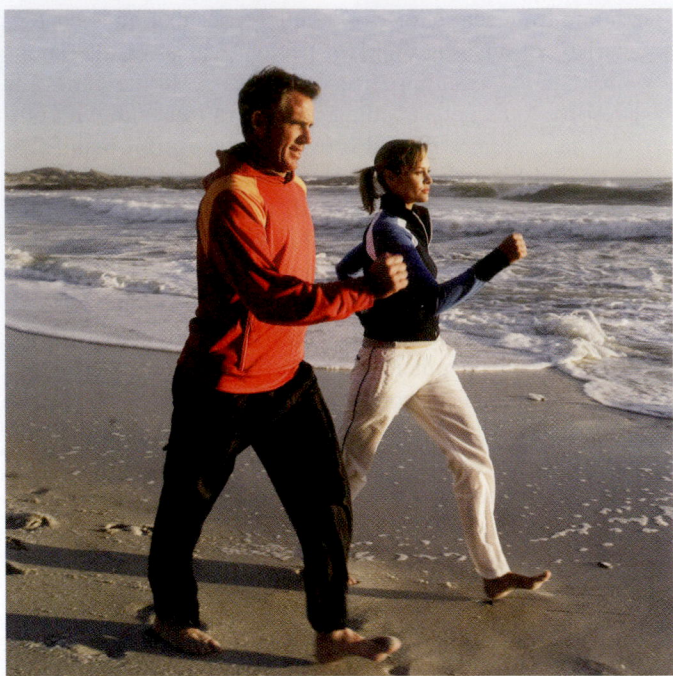

Figure 2–3 ■ Regular exercise is a key healthy behavior for the young adult.

normal physiologic changes begin to occur. A comparison of physical status for young adults during their 20s and 30s is shown in Table 2–4.

Risks for Alterations in Health

The young adult is at risk for alterations in health from accidents, sexually transmitted infections, substance abuse, and physical or psychosocial stressors. These risk factors may be interrelated (see the Moving Evidence into Action Moving Evidence into Action).

INJURIES Unintentional injuries are the leading cause of injury and death in people between ages 15 and 24 (National Center for Health Statistics [NCHS], 2007). Most injuries and fatalities occur as the result of motor vehicle crashes, but injuries and death also result from assaults (homicide), drowning, fire, guns, occupational accidents, and exposure to environmental hazards. Accidental injury or death is often associated with the use of alcohol or other chemical substances, or with psychologic stress. Intentional self-harm (suicide) is the third leading cause of death in young adults of both genders.

SEXUALLY TRANSMITTED INFECTIONS Sexually transmitted infections include genital herpes, chlamydia, gonorrhea, syphilis, and HIV/AIDS. The young adult who is sexually active with a variety of partners and who does not use condoms is at greatest risk for development of these diseases. Nursing care of patients with sexually transmitted infections is discussed in ∞ Chapter 50.

SUBSTANCE ABUSE Substance abuse is a major cause for concern in the young adult population. Although alcohol abuse occurs at all ages, it is greater in the 20s than during any other decade of the life span. Alcohol contributes to motor vehicle crashes and physical violence, and it is damaging to the developing fetus in pregnant women. It can also cause liver disease and nutritional deficits.

TABLE 2–3 Theories of Adult Development

	THEORIST	AGE	TASK
Psychosocial Development	Erikson	18–25	Identity versus role confusion ■ Establishing an intimate relationship with another person ■ Committing oneself to work and to relationships
		25–65	Generativity versus stagnation ■ Accepting one's own life as creative and productive ■ Having concern for others
		65–death	Integrity versus despair ■ Accepting worth of one's own life ■ Accepting inevitability of death
Spiritual Development	Fowler	After 18	■ Having a high degree of self-consciousness ■ Constructing one's own spiritual system
		After 30	■ Being aware of truth from a variety of viewpoints
	Westerhoff	Young adult	Searching faith ■ Acquiring a cognitive and an affective faith through questioning one's own faith
		Middle–older adult	Owned faith ■ Putting faith into action and standing up for beliefs
Moral Development	Kohlberg	Adult	Postconventional level Social contract/legalistic orientation ■ Defining morality in terms of personal principles ■ Adhering to laws that protect the welfare and rights of others Universal-ethical principles ■ Internalizing universal moral principles ■ Respecting others; believing that relationships are based on mutual trust
Developmental Tasks	Havighurst	18–35	■ Selecting and learning to live with a mate ■ Starting a family and rearing children ■ Managing a home ■ Starting an occupation ■ Taking on civic responsibility ■ Finding a congenial social group
		35–60	■ Achieving civic and social responsibility ■ Establishing and maintaining an economic standard of living ■ Assisting teenage children in becoming responsible and happy adults ■ Developing leisure-time activities ■ Relating to one's spouse as a person ■ Accepting and adjusting to the physiologic changes of middle age ■ Adjusting to aging parents
		60 and over	■ Meeting civic and social obligations ■ Establishing an affiliation with one's own age group ■ Establishing satisfactory physical living arrangements ■ Adjusting to decreasing physical strength, health, retirement, reduced income, death of spouse

Source: Data from Erickson, E. (1963). *Childhood and Society* (2nd ed.). New York: Norton; Fowler, W. (1981). *Stages of Faith: The Psychology of Human Development and the Quest for Meaning*. New York: Harper & Row; Havighurst, R. J. (1972). *Human Development and Education* (3rd ed.). New York: Longman; Kohlberg, L. (1979). *The Meaning and Measurement of Moral Development*. New York: Clark University; and Westerhoff, J. (1976). *Will Our Children Have Faith?* New York: Seabury Press.

Other substances that are commonly abused include nicotine, marijuana, amphetamines (including methamphetamine), cocaine, and crack. Smoking increases the risk of respiratory and cardiovascular diseases. Marijuana can affect memory and learning for days to weeks after its use. Methamphetamine, a highly addictive substance, can lead to structural and functional changes in the areas of the brain associated with emotion and memory. Cocaine and crack can cause death from cardiovascular effects (increased heart rate and ventricular dysrhythmias), and can lead to addiction and health problems in the baby born to an addicted mother. Nursing care of patients with problems of substance abuse is discussed in ∞ Chapter 6.

TABLE 2–4 Physical Status and Changes in the Young Adult Years

ASSESSMENT	STATUS DURING THE 20S	STATUS DURING THE 30S
Skin	Smooth, even temperature	Wrinkles begin to appear
Hair	Slightly oily, shiny	Graying may begin
	Balding may begin	Balding may begin
Vision	Snellen 20/20	Some loss of visual acuity and accommodation
Musculoskeletal	Strong, coordinated	Some loss of strength and muscle mass
Cardiovascular	Maximum cardiac output	Slight decline in cardiac output
	60–90 beats/minute	60–90 beats/minute
	Mean BP: 120/80	Mean BP: 120/80
Respiratory	Rate: 12–20	Rate: 12–20
	Full vital capacity	Slight decline in vital capacity

PHYSICAL AND PSYCHOSOCIAL STRESSORS Physical stressors that increase the risk of illness include environmental pollutants and work-related risks (e.g., electrical hazards, mechanical injuries, or exposure to toxins or infectious agents). Other physical stressors include exposure to the sun, participation in high-risk activities (e.g., contact sports, driving too fast), ingestion of chemical substances (e.g., caffeine, alcohol, nicotine), and pregnancy. Young adults have the highest rate of injury-related visits to emergency departments (NCHS, 2009).

Many different and individualized psychosocial stressors may affect the young adult. Choices must be made about education, occupation, relationships, independence, and lifestyle. These choices indirectly affect future health. The young adult without adequate education or job skills may face unemployment, poverty, homelessness, and limited access to health care. Nearly half of all marriages end in divorce, usually within the first 10 years. People who are divorced have more health problems than those who remain married (NCHS, 2002). Divorce often results in loneliness, feelings of failure, financial difficulties, domestic violence, and child abuse. The inability of the young adult to cope with these stressors may result in suicide, which ranks close to accidents as a major cause of death in this age group. Although difficult to prove, it is believed that some accidental deaths, especially when associated with substance abuse, are actually suicides.

Assessment Guidelines

The following guidelines are useful in assessing the achievement of significant developmental tasks in the young adult. Does the young adult

- feel independent from parents?
- have a realistic self-concept?
- like oneself and the direction in which life is going?
- interact well with family?
- cope with the stresses of constant change and growth?
- have well-established bonds with significant others, such as marriage partners or close friends?
- have a meaningful social life?
- have a career or occupation?
- demonstrate emotional, social, and economic responsibility for his or her own life?
- have a set of values that guide behavior?
- have a healthy lifestyle?

Physical assessment of the young adult includes height and weight, blood pressure, and vision. During the health history, the nurse should ask specific questions about substance use, sexual activity and concerns, exercise, eating habits, menstrual history and patterns, coping mechanisms, any familial chronic illnesses, and family changes. See Table 2–5 for health screening recommendations for young and middle adults.

MOVING EVIDENCE INTO ACTION **Health Promotion for Young Adults**

Traditional college students who fall into the young adult age group (ages 18 to 24) often engage in risky behaviors that increase their health risks. Students responding to a 2008 survey by the American College Health Association reported the following:

- stress that interfered with academic performance (34%)
- sleep difficulties (26%)
- consuming one to four drinks while partying (38%)
- engaging in behaviors they regretted after drinking (36%)
- feeling depressed (18.4%)
- being in an emotionally abusive relationship (13.6%)

These behaviors have major implications for the health of this segment of young adults. This survey also found that students identify health educators and health center staff as credible sources of health-related information.

IMPLICATIONS FOR NURSING

Nurses in college-based health centers and primary care settings are in position to provide resources and education for college-age students. Interventions that focus on wellness, health promotion, and coping strategies can have a positive impact on student outcomes (Ahern, 2009). Nurses should reach out to young, college-age adults to provide support and education to promote healthy behaviors.

CRITICAL THINKING IN PATIENT CARE

1. Considering the current preferred methods of communicating among adolescents and young adults, develop potential strategies for outreach to and health and wellness education for students on a traditional, residential college campus.
2. How might you modify these planned strategies to reach students enrolled in a college where the primary student population is commuters?
3. Would your strategies and focus change if your goal was health promotion for nontraditional college students (ages 25 and older)?

TABLE 2–5 Recommended Health Screening for Healthy Adults (without specific risk factors)

EXAMINATION	RECOMMENDED FREQUENCY		
	YOUNG ADULTS (18–40)	MIDDLE ADULTS (40–65)	OLDER ADULTS (65 AND OLDER)
Health maintenance examination: ■ Height, weight, body mass index ■ Risk evaluation & counseling ■ Safety ■ Behavioral assessment	Every 1 to 5 years	Every 1 to 3 years	Every 1 to 2 years
Blood pressure	Every 2 years; more frequently if 120/80 or higher	Every 2 years; more frequently if 120/80 or higher	Every 2 years; more frequently if 120/80 or higher
Breast cancer: ■ Clinical breast exam ■ Mammography	Every 3 years	Annually Annually	Annually Annually to age 75
Cervical cancer (Pap test)	Annually until age 30, then every 2 to 3 years after three normal results	Every 2 to 3 years if normal	May discontinue; resume if has new sexual partner
Cholesterol and lipid profile	Every 5 years	Every 5 years	Every 5 years
Chlamydia	All sexually active women under age 26		
Colorectal cancer: ■ Fecal occult blood test (FOBT) or fecal immunochemical test (FIT) ■ Flexible sigmoidoscopy or double contrast barium enema ■ Colonoscopy		Annually beginning at age 50 Every 5 years beginning at age 50 Every 10 years beginning at age 50	Annually Every 5 years Every 10 years to age 80
Diabetes mellitus		Fasting plasma glucose every 3 years	Fasting plasma glucose every 3 years
Glaucoma			Every 2 years
Osteoporosis			Bone mineral density; repeat every 2 years for those at risk
Prostate cancer		Digital rectal exam (DRE) and prostate-specific antigen (PSA) annually beginning at age 50 (age 45 for black males and men with strong family history of prostate cancer)	DRE and PSA annually

Sources: Cokkinides, V., Bandi, P., Siegel, R., Ward, E. M., & Thun, M. J. (2007). *Cancer prevention & early detection facts & figures 2008.* Atlanta, GA: American Cancer Society; National Guideline Clearinghouse. (2006). Adult preventive services (ages 18–49). Southfield, MI: Michigan Quality Improvement Consortium; National Guideline Clearinghouse. (2006). Adult preventive services (ages 50–65+). Southfield, MI: Michigan Quality Improvement Consortium.

Promoting Healthy Behaviors in the Young Adult

The nurse promotes health in the young adult by teaching the behaviors listed in Box 2–3. Health information for the young adult is primarily provided in community settings. Examples are as follows:

■ Health-related courses and seminars at colleges and universities include information on the use of sports and exercise facilities, alcohol and drug abuse, smoking cessation, mental health, and sexual health.
■ Workplace programs include blood pressure monitoring, exercise, smoking cessation, cafeteria nutrition guidelines, and stress reduction activities.
■ Community programs include media information, health fairs, support groups, and information about risk factors for disease and injury.

The Middle Adult

The middle adult, ages 40 to 65, has physical status and function similar to that of the young adult. However, many changes take place between ages 40 and 65. Table 2–6 lists the physical changes that normally occur in the middle years.

Risks for Alterations in Health

The middle adult is at risk for alterations in health from obesity, cardiovascular disease, cancer, substance abuse, and physical and psychosocial stressors. These factors may be interrelated.

OBESITY   The middle adult often has a problem maintaining a healthy weight. Weight gain in middle adulthood is usually the result of continuing to consume the same number of calories while decreasing physical activity and experiencing a

BOX 2–3 Healthy Behaviors in the Young Adult

- Choose foods from all food groups, and eat a variety of foods.
- Choose a diet low in fat (30% or less of total calories), saturated fat (less than 10% of calories), and cholesterol (less than 300 mg daily).
- Choose a diet that each day includes at least seven servings of fruits and vegetables, and six servings of grains.
- Use sugar, salt, and sodium in moderation.
- For females, increase to or maintain 18 mg of iron daily in the diet, 1000 mg of calcium, and 400 mg of folic acid per day through diet or supplements.
- Have regular dental examinations and cleanings.
- Make exercise a regular part of life, carrying out activities that increase the heart rate to a set target, and maintain that rate for 30–60 minutes five or more days a week.
- Include exercise as part of any weight reduction program.
- Maintain immunizations.

decrease in basal metabolic rate. Obesity affects all of the major organ systems of the body, increasing the risk of atherosclerosis, hypertension, elevated cholesterol and triglyceride levels, and diabetes. Obesity is also associated with heart disease, cancer, osteoarthritis, and gallbladder disease.

TABLE 2–6 Physical Changes in the Middle Adult Years

ASSESSMENT	CHANGES
Skin	■ Decreased turgor, moisture, and subcutaneous fat result in wrinkles. ■ Fat is deposited in the abdominal and hip areas.
Hair	■ Loss of melanin in hair shaft causes graying. ■ Hairline recedes in males.
Sensory	■ Visual acuity for near vision decreases (presbyopia) during the 40s. ■ Auditory acuity for high-frequency sounds decreases (presbycusis); more common in men. ■ Sense of taste diminishes.
Musculoskeletal	■ Skeletal muscle mass decreases by about age 60. ■ Thinning of intervertebral discs results in loss of height (about 2.5 cm [1 inch]). ■ Postmenopausal women may develop low bone density or osteoporosis.
Cardiovascular	■ Blood vessels lose elasticity. ■ Systolic blood pressure may increase.
Respiratory	■ Loss of vital capacity (about 1 L from age 20 to 60) occurs.
Gastrointestinal	■ Large intestine gradually loses muscle tone; constipation may result. ■ Gastric secretions are decreased.
Genitourinary	■ Hormonal changes occur: menopause, women ($\downarrow$ estrogen); andropause, men ($\downarrow$ testosterone).
Endocrine	■ Gradual decrease in glucose tolerance occurs.

CARDIOVASCULAR DISEASE   The major risk factors, especially for coronary heart disease, include age, male gender, family history, physical inactivity, cigarette smoking, hypertension, elevated blood cholesterol levels, and diabetes. Other contributing factors include obesity, stress, and lack of exercise. The middle adult is at risk for peripheral vascular, cerebrovascular, and cardiovascular disease.

CANCER   Cancer is the third leading cause of death in adults between ages 25 and 64 in the United States, with one-third of cases occurring between ages 35 and 64. Cancers of the breast, colon, lung, and reproductive system are common in the middle years. Prolonged exposure to environmental carcinogens and use of alcohol and nicotine are significant cancer risk factors for the middle adult. Nursing care of the patient with cancer is discussed in ∞ Chapter 14.

SUBSTANCE ABUSE   Although the middle adult may abuse a variety of substances, the most commonly abused are alcohol, nicotine, and prescription drugs. Excess alcohol use in the middle adult contributes to an increased risk of liver cancer, cirrhosis, pancreatitis, hyperlipidemia, and anemia. Alcoholism also increases the risk of accidental injury or death and disrupts careers and relationships. Cigarette smoking increases the risk of cancer of the larynx, lung, mouth, pharynx, bladder, pancreas, esophagus, and kidney; of chronic obstructive pulmonary disorders; and of cardiovascular disease.

PHYSICAL AND PSYCHOSOCIAL STRESSORS   The middle adult years are ones of change and transition, frequently resulting in stress. Both men and women must adapt to changes in physical appearance and function and accept their own mortality. Children may leave home or choose to remain at home longer than they are welcome. Parents are aging, with illness probable and death inevitable. The middle adult thus becomes part of what has been called "the sandwich generation," caught between the need to care for both children and aging parents. Both men and women may make career changes, and approaching retirement becomes a reality. Divorce in the middle years is a major emotional, social, and financial stressor.

Assessment Guidelines

The following guidelines are useful in assessing the achievement of significant developmental tasks in the middle adult. Does the middle adult

- accept the aging body?
- feel comfortable with and respect him- or herself?
- enjoy some new freedom to be independent?
- accept changes in family roles?
- enjoy success and satisfaction from work and/or family roles?
- interact well and share companionable activities with a partner?
- expand or renew previous interests?
- pursue charitable and altruistic activities?
- consider plans for retirement?
- have a meaningful philosophy of life?
- follow preventive healthcare practices?

EVIDENCE FOR NURSING CARE Health Promotion for Middle Adults

Selected resources that nurses may find helpful when planning evidence-based nursing care follow.
- O'Rourke, J. (2009). Blazing the trail into boomer wellness and prevention. *Rehab Management, 22*(6), 10, 12–13.
- Zender, R., & Olshansky, E. (2009). Promoting wellness in women across the life span. *The Nursing Clinics of North America, 44*(3), 281–291.

Physical assessment of the middle adult includes all body systems, including blood pressure, vision, and hearing. Monitoring for risks and onset of cancer symptoms is essential (see Table 2–5). During the health history, the nurse should ask specific questions about food intake and exercise habits, substance abuse, sexual concerns, changes in the reproductive system, coping mechanisms, and family history of chronic illnesses.

Promoting Healthy Behaviors in the Middle Adult

The nurse promotes health in the middle adult by teaching the behaviors listed in Box 2–4. Information about health for the middle adult may be provided in a variety of community settings, including outpatient clinics, occupational health clinics, and private practice. Examples are as follows:

- Specific programs emphasize accepting responsibility for one's own health. This type of teaching can be in a seminar or on a one-to-one basis, and includes information specific to a group of individuals with an identified need, such as smokers, women who have just entered the workforce, or men nearing retirement.
- The community and industries provide information about safety hazards in the home and workplace, as well as during leisure activities.
- Literature about community resources is available for health promotion, including programs offered at alcohol/drug abuse treatment centers, clinics and health centers, counseling services, crisis intervention centers, spouse abuse programs, and health education and promotion agencies (e.g., American Red Cross, American Cancer Society, American Heart Association, YWCA, YMCA).

BOX 2–4 Healthy Behaviors in the Middle Adult

- Choose foods from all food groups, and eat a variety of foods.
- Choose a diet low in fat (30% or less of total calories), saturated fat (less than 10% of calories), and cholesterol (less than 300 mg daily). Adjust daily calorie intake to maintain healthy weight.
- Choose a diet that each day includes at least seven servings of fruits and vegetables, and six servings of grains.
- Use sugar, salt, and sodium in moderation.
- Increase calcium intake (in perimenopausal women) to 1200 mg daily.
- Consume high-fiber foods.
- Have regular dental examinations and cleanings.
- Make exercise a part of life, carrying out regular exercise that is moderately strenuous, is consistent, and avoids overexertion; exercise for 30 minutes five or more days a week.
- Include exercise as part of any weight reduction program.

The Older Adult

The older adult period begins at age 65, but it can be further divided into three periods: the young-old (ages 65 to 74), the middle-old (ages 75 to 84), and the old-old (age 85 and over). With increasing age, a number of normal physiologic changes occur, as listed in Table 2–7.

The older adult population is increasing more rapidly than any other age group. In the last century, the number of adults in the United States living to age 65 or older increased from 4% in 1900 to 12.4% in 2006. There will be 71.5 million older adults by the year 2030, almost twice the number in 2005. The average life expectancy in the United States is 75.2 years for men and 80.4 years for women (Administration on Aging, 2007; NCHS, 2009).

FAST FACTS
Diversity in Older Adults
- Currently, minority older adults comprise over 19% of all older Americans.
- By 2030, the minority older adult population is projected to increase by 183%, compared with 74% for the older adult white population.
- Minority elders will increase as follows: African Americans = 147%, Asians = 208%, Hispanic Americans = 254%, American Indians and Alaska Natives = 143%.

Source: Data from Administration on Aging. (2007). *A profile of older Americans: 2007.* Retrieved from www.aoa.gov/prof/Statistics/profile/profiles.aspx

The increasing numbers of older adults have important implications for nursing. Patients in all healthcare settings will be older, with nursing care and teaching needs that differ from those of young and middle adults. Although gerontologic nursing (care of the older adult) is a nursing specialty area, it is also an integral component of medical-surgical nursing (Figure 2–4 ■).

Risks for Alterations in Health

The older adult is at risk for alterations in health from a variety of causes. Most older adults have one or more chronic health problems; many have multiple illnesses. The most frequently

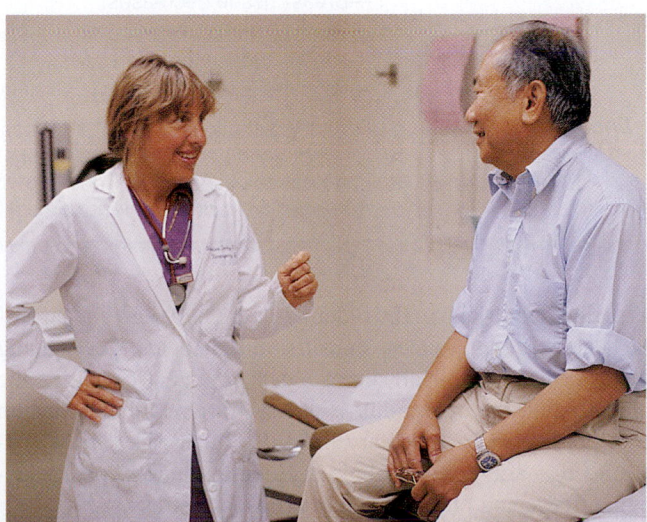

Figure 2–4 ■ The older adult population is increasing more rapidly than any other age group, making gerontologic nursing an integral component of medical-surgical nursing practice.

TABLE 2–7 Physical Changes in the Older Adult Years

ASSESSMENT	CHANGES
Skin	■ Decreased turgor and sebaceous gland activity result in dry, wrinkled skin. Melanocytes cluster, causing "age spots" or "liver spots."
Hair and nails	■ Scalp, axillary, and pubic hair thins; nose and ear hair thickens. Women may develop facial hair. ■ Nails grow more slowly; may become thick and brittle.
Sensory	■ Visual field narrows, and depth perception is distorted. ■ Pupils are smaller, reducing night vision. ■ Lenses yellow and become opaque, resulting in distortion of green, blue, and violet tones and increased sensitivity to glare. ■ Production of tears decreases. ■ Sense of smell decreases. ■ Age-related hearing loss progresses, involving middle- and low-frequency sounds. ■ Threshold for pain and touch increases. ■ Proprioception (sense of physical position) may be altered, increasing risk for falls.
Musculoskeletal	■ Loss of overall mass, strength, and movement of muscles occurs; tremors may occur. ■ Loss of bone structure and deterioration of joint cartilage results in kyphosis, increased risk of fractures, and restricted range of motion.
Cardiovascular	■ Systolic blood pressure rises. ■ Cardiac output decreases. ■ Peripheral resistance increases, and capillary walls thicken.
Respiratory	■ Continued loss of vital capacity occurs as the lungs become less elastic and more rigid. ■ Anteroposterior chest diameter and residual volume increase. ■ Although blood carbon dioxide levels remain relatively constant, blood oxygen levels decrease by 10%–15%.
Gastrointestinal	■ Decreased saliva production and loss of taste buds decrease ability to taste salt and sweet. ■ Gag reflex is decreased, stomach motility reduced, and gastric emptying is delayed. ■ Both large and small intestines have some atrophy, with decreased peristalsis. ■ The liver decreases in weight and storage capacity; gallstones increase; pancreatic enzymes decrease.

Genitourinary	■ Kidneys lose mass, and the glomerular filtration rate is reduced (by nearly 50% from young adulthood to old age).
	■ Bladder capacity decreases, and the micturition reflex is delayed. Urinary retention is more common.
	■ Women may have stress incontinence; men may have an enlarged prostate gland.
	■ Reproductive changes in men occur:
	  —Testosterone decreases.
	  —Sperm count decreases.
	  —Testes become smaller.
	  —Length of time to achieve an erection increases; erection is less full.
	■ Reproductive changes in women occur:
	  —Estrogen levels decrease.
	  —Breast tissue decreases.
	  —Vagina, uterus, ovaries, and urethra atrophy.
	  —Vaginal lubrication decreases.
	  —Vaginal secretions become alkaline.

Endocrine	■ Pituitary gland loses weight and vascularity. ■ Thyroid gland becomes more fibrous, and plasma T_3 levels decrease. ■ Pancreas releases insulin more slowly; increased blood glucose levels are common. ■ Adrenal glands produce less cortisol.

occurring conditions in the older adult are hypertension, arthritis, heart diseases, cancer, sinusitis, and diabetes. The leading causes of death are heart disease, cancer, and stroke. Like the middle adult, the older adult is at risk for alterations in health from obesity and a sedentary lifestyle. Other risk factors specific to this age group include accidental injuries, pharmacologic effects, and physical and psychosocial stress.

INJURIES Injuries in the older adult cause many different problems: illness, financial burdens, hospitalization, self-care deficits, loss of independence, and even death. The risk of injury is increased by normal physiologic changes that accompany aging, pathophysiologic alterations in health, environmental hazards, and lack of support systems. The three major causes of injury in the older adult are falls, fires, and motor vehicle crashes. Of these, falls with resultant hip fractures are the most significant in terms of long-term disability and death.

PHARMACOLOGIC EFFECTS A number of risk factors predispose the older adult to toxic drug effects. Age-related changes in tissue and organ structure and function alter the absorption of both oral and parenteral medications. Low nutritional levels and decreased liver function may alter drug metabolism. The aging kidney may not excrete drugs at the normal clearance rate. Self-administration of both prescribed and over-the-counter medications presents risks for error resulting from confusion, forgetfulness, or misreading the directions. The older adult may take several drugs at once, increasing the risk for adverse drug interactions. In addition, the older adult living on a fixed income may have to make a choice between buying medications or food, resulting in undermedication and ineffective treatment of an illness.

PHYSICAL AND PSYCHOSOCIAL STRESSORS The older adult is exposed to the same environmental hazards as the young and middle adult, but the effects of an accumulation of years of exposure may now appear. For example, exposure to the sun in earlier years may be manifested by skin cancer, and the long-term effects of exposure to noise pollution can result in impaired hearing. The older adult is at increased risk for respiratory disorders as a result of years of smoking, or from such pollutants as coal or asbestos dust. Living conditions and economic constraints may prevent the older adult from having necessary heating and cooling, contributing to thermal-related illnesses and even death. Elder abuse and neglect further increase the risk of injury or illness.

Psychosocial stressors for the older adult include the illness or death of a spouse, decreased or limited income, retirement, isolation from friends and family because of lack of transportation or distance, return to the home of a child, or relocation to a long-term healthcare facility. A further stressor may be role loss or reversal—for example, when the wife becomes the caretaker of her chronically ill husband.

Assessment Guidelines

The following guidelines are useful in assessing the achievement of significant developmental tasks in the older adult. Does the older adult

- adjust to the physiologic changes related to aging?
- manage retirement years in a satisfying manner?
- have satisfactory living arrangements and income to meet changing needs?
- participate in social and leisure activities?
- have a social network of friends and support persons?
- view life as worthwhile?
- have high self-esteem?
- have the abilities to care for self or to secure appropriate help?
- gain support from a value system or spiritual philosophy?
- adapt lifestyle to diminishing energy and ability?
- accept and adjust to the death of significant others?

Physical assessment of the older adult includes a careful examination of all body systems. During the health history, the nurse should ask specific questions about usual dietary patterns; elimination; exercise and rest; use of alcohol, nicotine, over-the-counter medications and prescription drugs; sexual concerns; financial concerns; and support systems.

Promoting Healthy Behaviors in the Older Adult

The nurse promotes health in the older adult by teaching the behaviors listed in Box 2–5 and encouraging screening examinations as outlined in Table 2–5. Medicare covers the cost of

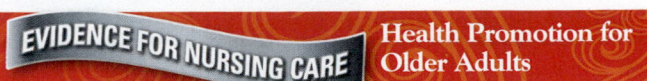

EVIDENCE FOR NURSING CARE **Health Promotion for Older Adults**

Selected resources that nurses may find helpful when planning evidence-based nursing care follow.

- Kennedy, R. D., & Cullamar, K. (2007). Try this: Best practices in nursing care to older adults. Immunizations for older adults. The Hartford Institute for Geriatric Nursing, Division of Nursing, New York University. Available at www.hartfordign.org.
- Lee, C. (2009). A comparison of health promotion behaviors in rural and urban community-dwelling spousal caregivers. *Journal of Gerontological Nursing, 35*(5), 34–40.

most regular screening examinations, based on recommended frequency of the exam. Older adults may be concerned about the cost of undergoing health promotion and screening exams; providing information about Medicare coverage can relieve concerns and promote compliance with recommended schedules.

Older adults get the same benefits from health teaching as young adults and middle adults; they should never be viewed as being "too old" for healthy living practices. However, nurses should structure teaching activities to meet age-related physiologic changes, such as using charts and literature with large print. Health education for the older adult is provided in hospitals, long-term care facilities, retirement centers, outpatient clinics, senior citizen centers, and other community settings. Examples are as follows:

- Educational seminars teach about accident prevention in the home, in automobiles, and when taking public transportation.
- Health screenings and information from health fairs can specifically aid the older adult.
- Community programs provide immunization for influenza and pneumonia.
- Literature is available about financial assistance for health care, crisis hot lines, community services and resources (as described earlier for the middle adult), transportation, and nutrition (such as the Meals on Wheels program).

The Family of the Adult Patient

Although some patients are totally alone in the world, most have one or more people who are significant in their lives. These significant others may be related or bonded to the patient by birth, adoption, marriage, or friendship. Although not always meeting traditional definitions, people (or even pets) significant to the patient are the patient's family. The nurse includes the family as an integral component of care in all healthcare settings.

Definitions and Functions of the Family

What is a **family**? The definitions of family vary by culture and change as society changes. According to one definition, a family is a unit of people related by marriage, birth, or adoption (Duvall, 1977). A more comprehensive definition is that a family is a social unit composed of two or more people who are emotionally involved with each other.

Although every family is unique, all families have certain structural and functional features in common. Family structure (family roles and relationships) and family function

BOX 2–5 Healthy Behaviors in the Older Adult

- Eat a variety of nutrient-dense foods and beverages within and among the basic food groups while choosing foods that limit the intake of saturated and trans fats, cholesterol, added sugars, salt, and alcohol.
- Choose a diet low in fat (30% or less of total calories), saturated fat (less than 10% of calories), and cholesterol (less than 300 mg daily). Choose foods high in fiber, low in sodium, and high in potassium.
- People with dark skin and those with little sunlight exposure should consume extra vitamin D from fortified foods or supplements.
- Individuals with hypertension and African Americans should consume no more than 1500 mg of sodium each day.
- If weight loss is needed, aim for a slow, steady loss by decreasing caloric intake while maintaining an adequate nutrient intake and increasing physical activity.
- Increase calcium intake to 1200 mg daily.
- Make exercise a part of life, carrying out regular exercise that is moderately strenuous, is consistent, and avoids overexertion; exercise for 30 to 60 minutes every day, if possible.
- Practice good oral hygiene with teeth brushing and flossing and have a dental checkup one to two times a year.
- Use sunscreen and avoid sunburn.
- Obtain an annual influenza immunization and have the pneumonia vaccine at age 65. *(Medicare pays for an annual influenza immunization once a year in the fall or winter and covers the cost of the pneumococcal vaccine, which most people only need once.)*

(interactions among family members and with the community) provide the following:

- *Interdependence.* The behaviors and developmental level of individual family members constantly influence and are influenced by the behaviors and developmental level of all other members of the family.
- *Maintaining boundaries.* The family creates boundaries that guide its members, providing a distinct and unique family culture. This culture, in turn, provides values.
- *Adapting to change.* The family changes as new members are added, current members leave, and the development of each member progresses.
- *Performing family tasks.* Essential tasks maintain the stability and continuity of the family. These tasks include physical maintenance of the home and the people in the home, the production and socialization of family members, and the maintenance of the psychologic well-being of members.

Family Developmental Stages and Tasks

The family, like the individual, has developmental stages and tasks. Each stage brings change, requiring adaptation; each new stage also brings family-related risk factors for alterations in health. The nurse must consider the needs of the patient both at a specific developmental stage and within a family with specific developmental tasks. Family developmental stages and developmental tasks are described next; related risk factors and health problems for each stage are listed in Table 2–8.

Couple

Two people living together with or without being married are in a period of establishing themselves as a couple. The developmental tasks of the couple include adjusting to living together as a couple, establishing a mutually satisfying relationship, relating to kin, and deciding whether to have children (in those of child-bearing age).

Family with Infants and Preschoolers

The family with infants or preschoolers must adjust to having and supporting the needs of more than two members. Other developmental tasks of the family at this stage are developing an attachment between parents and children, adjusting to the economic costs of having more members, coping with energy depletion and lack of privacy, and carrying out activities that enhance growth and development of the children.

Family with School-Age Children

The family with school-age children has the developmental tasks of adjusting to the expanded world of children in school and encouraging educational achievement. A further task is promoting joint decision making between children and parents.

Family with Adolescents and Young Adults

The developmental tasks of the family with adolescents and young adults focus on transition. While providing a supportive home base and maintaining open communications, parents must balance freedom with responsibility and release adult children as they seek independence.

Family with Middle Adults

The family with middle adults (in which the parents are middle aged and children are no longer at home) has the developmental tasks of maintaining ties with older and younger generations and planning for retirement. If the family consists of just the middle-aged couple, they have the developmental task of reestablishing the relationship and (if necessary) acquiring the role of grandparents.

Family with Older Adults

The older adult family has the developmental tasks of adjusting to retirement, adjusting to aging, and coping with the loss of a spouse. If a spouse dies, further tasks include adjusting to living alone or closing the family home.

The Family of the Patient with a Chronic Illness

The patient with a chronic illness may be hospitalized for diagnosis and treatment of acute exacerbations, but the care of the patient is primarily provided at home. Chronic illness in a family member is a major stressor that may cause changes in family structure and function, as well as changes in performing family developmental tasks.

Many different factors affect family responses to chronic illness; family responses in turn affect the patient's response to and perception of the illness. Factors influencing response to chronic illness include personal, social, and economic resources; the nature and course of the disease; and demands of the illness as perceived by family members.

Support for the family is essential. The following information should be considered when performing any family assessment and developing a patient's plan of care:

- Cohesiveness and communication patterns within the family
- Family interactions that support self-care

TABLE 2–8 Family-Related Risk Factors for Alterations in Health

STAGE	RISK FACTORS	HEALTH PROBLEMS
Couple or Family with Infants and Preschoolers	■ Lack of knowledge about family planning, contraception, sexual and marital roles ■ Inadequate prenatal care ■ Altered nutrition: inadequate nutrition, overweight, underweight ■ Smoking, alcohol/drug abuse ■ First pregnancy before age 16 or after age 35 ■ Low socioeconomic status ■ Lack of knowledge about child health and safety	Sexually transmitted infection Premature pregnancy Infertility Low-birth-weight infant Birth defects Poisoning Injury to infant or child Accidents Psychologic stress Family violence (child or spousal abuse)
Family with School-Age Children	■ Unsafe home environment ■ Working parents with inappropriate or inadequate resources for child care ■ Low socioeconomic status ■ Child abuse or neglect ■ Multiple, closely spaced children ■ Repeated infections, accidents, and hospitalizations ■ Unrecognized and unattended health problems ■ Poor or inappropriate nutrition ■ Toxic substances in the home	Behavior problems Speech and vision problems Learning disabilities Communicable diseases Physical abuse Cancer Developmental delay Obesity, underweight
Family with Adolescents and Young Adults	■ Family values of aggressiveness and competition ■ Lifestyle and behavior leading to chronic illness (substance abuse, inadequate diet) ■ Lack of problem-solving skills ■ Conflicts between parent and children	Violent death and injury Alcohol/drug abuse Unwanted pregnancy Suicide Sexually transmitted infections Domestic abuse
Family with Middle Adults	■ High-fat, high-cholesterol diet ■ Overweight ■ Hypertension ■ Smoking, alcohol abuse ■ Physical inactivity ■ Personality patterns related to stress ■ Exposure to environment: sunlight, radiation, asbestos, water or air pollution ■ Depression	Cardiovascular disease (coronary heart disease and cerebral vascular disease) Cancer Diabetes mellitus Accidents Suicide Mental illness
Family with Older Adults	■ Depression ■ Drug interactions ■ Chronic illness ■ Death of spouse ■ Reduced income ■ Poor nutrition ■ Lack of exercise ■ Past environment and lifestyle	Impaired vision and hearing Hypertension Acute illness Chronic illness Infectious diseases (influenza, pneumonia) Injuries from burns and falls Depression, suicide Alcohol abuse

■ Number of friends, relatives, and social support systems (e.g., church members) available
■ Family values and beliefs about health and illness
■ Cultural and spiritual beliefs
■ Developmental level of the patient and family

It is important to remember that standardized teaching plans may not be effective. Rather, patients with chronic illnesses and their families should be given the freedom to choose appropriate literature, self-help or support groups, and interactions with others who have the same illness.

CHAPTER HIGHLIGHTS

- Health, an ever-changing state, is affected by genetic makeup; cognitive abilities and educational level; race, ethnicity, and cultural background; age, gender, and developmental level; lifestyle and environment; socioeconomic background; and geographic area.
- The emphasis of nursing has shifted from acute illness care in the hospital setting to preventive community-based care. An essential component of medical-surgical nursing is teaching health-promoting behaviors to promote and maintain functional health status.
- Illnesses may be acute or chronic, with behaviors of illness individualized within a fairly predictable sequence of experiencing symptoms, assuming the sick role, seeking medical help, assuming a dependent role, and achieving recovery and rehabilitation.

- Young adults are at risk for alterations in health from injuries, sexually transmitted infections, substance abuse, workplace exposure to pollutants, sun exposure, and psychologic stressors.
- Middle adults are at risk for alterations in health from obesity, cardiovascular disease, cancer, substance abuse, and the stresses of change and transition.
- Older adults are at risk for alterations in health from chronic illnesses (including hypertension, heart disease, cancer, and stroke), injuries, drug toxicities, and changes in income and marital status.
- The family is an integral component in planning and implementing nursing care for the adult patient.

TEST YOURSELF NCLEX-RN® REVIEW

1. Which definition best describes wellness?
   1. a complete absence of disease
   2. presence of no more than one chronic illness
   3. never having to take medications
   4. actively practicing healthy behaviors
2. Many different factors affect the health of an individual. Which of the following are included? **Select all that apply.**
   1. genetic makeup
   2. cognitive abilities
   3. height
   4. age
   5. race
3. Which of the following diseases has a genetic basis?
   1. tuberculosis
   2. sickle cell disease
   3. appendicitis
   4. indigestion
4. Primary levels of prevention are general health promotion actions that prevent or delay the occurrence of a disease. Which of the following is a primary preventive activity?
   1. practicing safer sex
   2. having a screening for hypertension
   3. doing a self-breast examination
   4. having surgery
5. You call your instructor to say you have the "flu" and will not be in class. What level of illness behavior are you demonstrating?
   1. experiencing symptoms
   2. assuming the sick role
   3. seeking medical care
   4. assuming a dependent role

6. Your nephew was born with a heart defect. How would this disorder be classified?
   1. an acute illness
   2. a malignant illness
   3. an iatrogenic illness
   4. a congenital illness
7. Of the following descriptors, which is specific to a chronic illness?
   1. occurs rapidly
   2. lasts for a lifetime
   3. self-limiting
   4. lasts for a short time
8. Mr. Jones, aged 50, is 30 pounds overweight, smokes, and rarely exercises. As a middle adult, these factors increase his risk for disorders of which body system?
   1. cardiovascular
   2. renal
   3. gastrointestinal
   4. nervous
9. You have been asked to present a health-related program at the local senior center. What would be an appropriate topic?
   1. the hazards of substance abuse
   2. accident prevention in the home
   3. family roles and tasks
   4. treating acute illness
10. Which of the following developmental tasks are a part of the life of a family with older adults if a spouse dies? **Select all that apply.**
    1. coping with lack of privacy
    2. planning for retirement
    3. adjusting to aging
    4. coping with loss
    5. relating to kin

See Test Yourself answers in Appendix C.

Pearson Nursing Student Resources

Find additional review materials at
nursing.pearsonhighered.com

Prepare for success with additional NCLEX®-style practice questions, interactive assignments and activities, Web links, animations and videos, and more!

BIBLIOGRAPHY

Administration on Aging, U.S. Department of Health and Human Services. (2007). *A profile of older Americans: 2007.* Retrieved from www.aoa.gov/prof/Statistics/profile/profiles.aspx

Administration on Aging, U.S. Department of Health and Human Services. (2008). *A statistical profile of older Americans aged 65+.* Retrieved from www.aoa.gov

Amella, E. J. (2004). Presentation of illness in older adults. *American Journal of Nursing, 104*(10), 40–51.

Brooks, Y., Black, D., Coster, D., Blue, C., Abood, D., & Gretebeck, R. (2007, November). Body mass index and percentage body fat as health indicators for young adults. *American Journal of Health Behavior, 31*(6), 687–700. Retrieved from Health Source: Nursing/Academic Edition database.

Byrne, S. (2008, September). Healthcare avoidance: a critical review. *Holistic Nursing Practice, 22*(5), 280–292. Retrieved from CINAHL database.

Centers for Disease Control and Prevention. (2007). Recommended adult immunization schedule—United States, October 2007–September 2008. Atlanta, GA: MMWR.

Centers for Disease Control and Prevention and The Merck Company Foundation. (2007). The state of aging and health in America 2007. Retrieved from www.cdc.gov/aging

Cokkinides, V., Bandi, P., Siegel, R., Ward, E. M., & Thun, M. J. (2007). *Cancer prevention & early detection facts & figures 2008.* Atlanta, GA: American Cancer Society.

Cumbie, S., Conley, V., & Burman, M. (2004 January–March). Advanced practice nursing model for comprehensive care with chronic illness. *Advances in Nursing Science, 27*(1), 70–80.

D'Cruz, P. (2003). Family-focused interventions in health and illness. *Journal of Health Management, 5*(1), 37–56.

Dunn, H. (1959). High-level wellness for man and society. *American Journal of Public Health, 49,* 786–972.

Duvall, E. (1977). *Marriage and family development.* Philadelphia: Lippincott.

Edelman, C., & Mandle, C. (2006). *Health promotion throughout the lifespan* (6th ed.). St. Louis, MO: Mosby.

Erikson, E. (1963). *Childhood and society* (2nd ed.). New York: Norton.

Federal Citizen Information Center. (2004). *The food guide pyramid.* Retrieved from http://www.pueblo.gsa.gov/cic_text/food/food-pyramid/main.htm

Fowler, J. (1981). *Stages of faith: The psychology of human development and the quest for meaning.* New York: Harper & Row.

Freidman, M., Bowden, V., & Jones, E. (2003). *Family nursing: Research, theory and practice.* Upper Saddle River, NJ: Prentice Hall.

Grossman, S. & Lange, J. (2006). Theories of aging as a basis for assessment. *MEDSURG Nursing, 15*(2), 77–83.

Havighurst, R. (1972). *Human development and education* (3rd ed.). New York: Longman.

Kennedy, R. D., & Cullamar, K. (2007). Try this: Best practices in nursing care to older adults. Immunizations for older adults. The Hartford Institute for Geriatric Nursing, Division of Nursing, New York University. Retrieved from www.hartfordign.org

Kohlberg, L. (1979). *The meaning and measurement of moral development.* New York: clark University.

Langer, N. (2008, May). Integrating Compliance, communication, and culture: Delivering health care to an aging population. *Educational Gerontology, 34*(5), 385–396.

Leavell, H., & Clark, A. (1965). *Preventive medicine for doctors in the community.* New York: McGraw-Hill.

Lee, C. (2009). A comparison of health promotion behaviors in rural and urban community-dwelling spousal caregivers. *Journal of Gerontological Nursing, 35*(5), 34–40.

Lubkin, I., & Larsen, P. (2006). *Chronic illness: Impact and interventions* (6th ed.). Boston: Jones & Bartlett.

Miller, C. (2003). Safe medication practices: Nursing assessment of medications in older adults. *Geriatric Nursing, 24*(5), 314–315, 317.

Miller, C. (2008). *Nursing for wellness in older adults: Theory and practice* (5th ed.). Philadelphia: Lippincott.

Miller, J. (2000). *Coping with chronic illness: Overcoming powerlessness* (3rd ed.). Philadelphia: F. A. Davis.

National Center for Health Statistics. (2009). *Health, United States, 2008.* Hyattsville, MD: U. S. Department of Health and Human Services, Centers for Disease Control and Prevention.

National Guideline Clearinghouse. (2006). Adult preventive services (ages 18–49). Southfield, MI: Michigan Quality Improvement Consortium. Retrieved from www.guideline.gov

National Guideline Clearinghouse. (2006). Adult preventive services (ages 50– 65+). Southfield, MI: Michigan Quality Improvement Consortium. Retrieved from www.guideline.gov

Pender, N., Parsons, M., & Murdaugh, C. (2006). *Health promotion in nursing practice* (5th ed.). Upper Saddle River, NJ: Prentice Hall.

Senior Site. (2004). *Learning to cope with chronic illness.* Retrieved from http://seniors-site.com/coping/chronic.html

Strandberg, T., & Pitkälä, K. (2007, April 21). Frailty in elderly people. *Lancet,* pp. 1328, 1329. Retrieved from Health Source: Nursing/Academic Edition database.

Strauss, A., et al. (1984). *Chronic illness and the quality of life.* St. Louis, MO: Mosby.

Suchman, E. (1972). Stages of illness and medical care. In E. Jaco (Ed.), *Patients, physicians and illness.* New York: Free Press.

Tabloski, P. A. (2006). *Gerontological nursing.* Upper Saddle River, NJ: Pearson/Prentice Hall.

U.S. Department of Health and Human Services. (2010). *Healthy people 2020.* Washington, DC: Author.

Westerhoff, J. (1976). *Will our children have faith?* New York: Seabury Press.

World Health Organization. (1974). *Constitution of the World Health Organization: Chronicle of the World Health Organization.* Geneva: Author.

3 Community and Home Care of Adults

LEARNING OUTCOMES

1. Differentiate community-based care from community health care.
2. Discuss selected factors affecting health in the community.
3. Describe services and settings for healthcare consumers receiving community-based and home care.
4. Describe the components of the home healthcare system, including agencies, patients, referrals, nursing care, physicians, reimbursement, and legal considerations.
5. Compare and contrast the roles of the nurse providing home care with the roles of the nurse in medical-surgical nursing discussed in ∞ Chapter 1.
6. Discuss nursing interventions to deliver safe and competent care to patients in their homes.
7. Explain the purpose of rehabilitation in health care.

CLINICAL COMPETENCIES

1. Assess factors affecting the health of individuals in the community.
2. Provide patient care in community-based settings and the home.
3. Apply the nursing process to care of the patient in the home.

KEY TERMS

community-based care, *36*
contracting, *42*
disability, *47*
faith community nursing, *38*

handicap, *47*
home care, *38*
hospice care, *39*
impairment, *47*

referral source, *39*
rehabilitation, *47*
respite care, *39*

Healthcare is provided by medical-surgical nurses in a variety of settings. Currently, only patients requiring complex surgery, who are acutely ill or seriously injured, or who are having babies are hospitalized and then only for a minimum period of time. As a result, most healthcare services are provided in settings outside the hospital. Those settings include clinics, schools, prisons, day-care centers for children and seniors, offices, and homes. The discussion in this chapter focuses on selected community services and settings and home care.

People requiring healthcare services may access and use the system through a variety of providers and settings, including hospital-based outpatient care, community-based offices and clinics, and home care. In the healthcare system of the twenty-first century, hospitals are primarily acute care providers with services focused on high-technology care for severely ill or injured people or for people having major surgery. Even those patients rarely remain in the hospital for long. They are moved as rapidly as possible to less acute care settings within the hospital and then to community-based and home care. Health care has become a managed care, community-based system. Although many nurses are still employed in hospitals, they are increasingly providing nursing care outside of the acute care, in-hospital setting.

Community-Based Nursing Care

A community may be a small neighborhood in a major urban city or a large area of rural residents. Communities are formed by the characteristics of people, area, social interaction, and common ties. Each community, however, is unique. People who live in a community may share a culture, history, or heritage. Although a community is where people live, have homes, raise families, and carry on daily activities, its members often cross community boundaries to work or to seek health care. Nurses who provide care within a community must know the composition and characteristics of the patients with whom they will work.

In contrast to community health nursing, which focuses on the health of the community, **community-based care** centers on individual and family healthcare needs. The nurse practicing community-based care provides direct services to individuals to manage acute or chronic health problems and to promote self-care. The care is provided in the local community, is culturally competent, and is family centered. The philosophy of community-based nursing directs nursing care for patients wherever they are, including where they live, work, play, worship, and go to school.

Nurses provide community-based care in many different ways and locations, ranging from leading support groups in a hospital (for individuals and family members diagnosed with such illnesses as cancer or diabetes) to managing a freestanding clinic to providing care at the patient's home. Box 3–1 illustrates the varied settings within the community in which a nurse may provide care.

Factors Affecting Health in the Community

Many factors can affect the health of individuals in a community. These factors include social support systems, the community healthcare structure, environmental factors, and economic resources.

Social Support Systems

A person's social support system consists of the people who lend assistance to meet financial, personal, physical, or emotional needs. In most instances, family, friends, and neighbors provide the best social support within the community. To understand the community social structure, the nurse needs to know what support is available for health care for the patient and family, including neighbors, friends, their church, organizations, self-help groups, and professional providers. The nurse also must know and respect the cultural and ethnic background of the community.

Community Healthcare Structure

The healthcare structure of a community has a direct effect on the health of the people living and working within it. The size of the community often determines the type of services provided as well as the access to the services. For example, urban residents have various means of transportation to a variety of community healthcare providers, whereas rural residents must often travel long distances for any type of care. The financial base of the community is also important, in many cases determining state and county funding of services.

Nurses who provide community-based care must know about public health services, the number and kind of health screenings offered, the location and specialty of healthcare professionals within the community, and the availability and accessibility of services and supplies. Other factors to consider include facilities (e.g., day care and long-term care), housing, and the number and kind of support agencies providing assistance (e.g., for housing, shelter, and food).

Environmental Factors

The environment within which a person lives and works may have both helpful and harmful effects on health. Air and water quality differ across communities. Air pollution may occur across a large area, or may be limited to the home. Within the home, pollution may occur from such sources as molds, pesticides, and fumes from new carpet. The water source also varies, with water supplies coming from rivers, lakes, reservoirs, or wells. No matter the source, chemical runoff or bacteria may contaminate water. It is critical to determine whether patients have a safe supply of running water.

Household and community safety and health resource accessibility are also important. Nurses must consider lighting, street and sidewalk or road upkeep and conditions, effects of ice and snow, condition of stairs and floors, and usefulness and availability of bathroom facilities. Physical barriers to residents accessing community resources include lack of transportation, distance to services, and location of services.

Economic Resources

Economic resources encompass the financial and insurance coverage necessary to provide the means for health care within the community. As private medical insurance becomes more and more expensive, fewer citizens have it, and many U.S. citizens have no insurance at all. Most unskilled and semi-skilled jobs do not provide healthcare benefits, resulting in a substantial percentage of what might be labeled "the working poor," those who have no financial assistance for illness care or healthcare screenings from an employer. However, the healthcare bill of 2010 mandates healthcare insurance for all citizens, with provisions made requiring employers to provide insurance and Medicaid expanded to assist low-income people. Older adults with fixed or limited incomes often find their monthly income consumed by medicines and medical supplies.

Medicare and Medicaid are health assistance programs created by 1965 Social Security amendments. Medicare is a federal health insurance plan for acute care needs of the disabled and those over 65 years. This plan covers some services provided in hospitals, long-term facilities, and the home; however, many necessary healthcare components are not covered fully or at all, including prescribed and over-the-counter medications and adaptive equipment for safety, such as shower seats or raised toilet seats. Coverage for care at home continues only as long as skilled providers are needed, and the person is not considered homebound even if he or she needs a wheelchair and assistance from others to leave the home. Medicaid is a state-run health insurance program for people with limited incomes. Each state has different benefits and criteria for coverage.

Community-Based Healthcare Services

Community-based healthcare services have many forms. Selected examples are discussed in the following sections.

Community Centers and Clinics

Community centers and clinics may be directed by physicians, advanced practice nurses in collaboration with physicians, or advanced practice nurses working independently (depending on state regulations). These healthcare settings may be located within a hospital, be part of a hospital but located in another area, or be independent of a hospital base. Healthcare centers and clinics provide a wide range of services and often meet the health needs of patients who are unable to access care elsewhere. This group includes the homeless, the poor, those with substance abuse problems, those with sexually transmitted diseases, and the victims of violent or abusive behavior.

Day Care Programs

Day care programs, such as senior centers, are usually located where people gather for social, nutritional, and recreational purposes. They may provide care for older adults with physical

BOX 3–1 Community-Based Nursing Care Settings

- Hospitals
    - Outpatient (ambulatory) surgery
    - Outpatient diagnostics and treatments
    - Cardiac rehabilitation
    - Support groups
    - Education groups
- County health departments
- Senior centers
- Long-term care
- Parish nursing
- Adult day care centers
- Homeless shelters
- Mobile vans
- Mental health centers
- Schools
- Crisis intervention centers
- Ambulatory surgery centers
- Alcohol/drug rehabilitation
- Healthcare provider offices
- Healthcare clinics
- Free clinics
- Urgent care centers
- Rural health centers
- Home care
- Hospice care
- Industry
- Jails and prisons

Hospice (NAHC) (2009) defines **home care** as services for recovering, disabled, or chronically ill people who are in need of treatment or support to function effectively in the home environment. The U.S. Department of Health and Human Services places home care along a continuum of health care. Home care is provided in the patient's place of residence for the purpose of promoting, maintaining, or restoring health or of maximizing the level of independence while minimizing the effects of disability and illness, including terminal illness.

Home care encompasses both health and social services provided to the chronically ill, disabled, or recovering person in his or her own home. Home care is usually provided when a person needs help that cannot be provided by a family member or friend. Among patients who benefit from home care services are those who

- cannot live independently at home because of age, illness, or disability.
- have chronic, debilitating illnesses such as congestive heart failure, heart disease, kidney disease, respiratory diseases, diabetes mellitus, or muscle-nerve disorders.
- are terminally ill and want to die with comfort and dignity at home.
- do not need in-patient hospital or nursing home care but require additional assistance.
- need short-term help at home for postoperative care.

The services provided in the home may include professional nursing care, care provided by home care aides, physical therapy, speech therapy, occupational therapy, medical social worker services, and nutritional services. Patients receiving home care services are usually under the care of a physician, with the focus of care being treatment or rehabilitation. Registered nurses or licensed practical nurses provide nursing care based on physician orders. These nurses give direct care, supervise other care providers, coordinate patient care with the physician, advocate for the patient and family, and teach family members and friends how to care for the patient when professional services are no longer necessary.

Home care is both professional and technical. Professional home care is provided by people who are practice driven, licensed, certified, and/or have special qualifications. Nurses, therapists, social workers, and home aides are considered professional providers. Durable medical equipment companies (businesses that deliver medical equipment to homes) are technical providers. Technical home care providers are business and product driven. Customer satisfaction, field service, reimbursement, and profits are their primary concerns.

disabilities or mild Alzheimer's disease while family caregivers are at work. These programs vary among communities. Meals may be provided at low cost.

Faith Community Nursing

Faith community nursing, also known as parish nursing, is a nontraditional, community-based way of providing health promotion and health restoration nursing interventions to specific groups of people. It meets the needs of people who are often underserved by the traditional healthcare system.

A nurse who practices faith community nursing works with the pastor and staff of a faith community to promote health and healing through counseling, referrals, teaching, and assessment of healthcare needs. A faith community nurse may be employed by a hospital and contracted by a church, be employed directly by a church, or work as a volunteer with the congregation of a church. The faith community nurse helps bridge gaps between members of the church and the healthcare system (American Nurses Association [ANA], 2005).

Meals on Wheels

Many communities have a food service, usually called Meals on Wheels, for older people who do not have assistance in the home for food preparation. A hot, nutritionally balanced meal is delivered once a day, usually at noon. Volunteers often deliver the meals, providing not only nutrition but also a friendly, caring visit each day.

Home Care

Home care is not easily defined. It is not simply illness care at home, nor is it the act of setting up a hospital room in someone's house. The National Association for Home Care and

Brief History of Home Care

Many milestones marked the growth and development of home care in the United States. The passage of Medicare in 1965, Medicaid in 1970, the addition of hospice benefits in 1973, and the introduction of diagnosis-related groups (DRGs) in 1983 dramatically affected home care. Medicare legislation entitled the nation's older adult to home care services, primarily skilled nursing, and other curative or restorative therapies. This same benefit was extended to certain disabled younger Americans in 1973.

The introduction of DRGs to help control healthcare costs greatly increased home care. DRGs are categories for reimbursement of inpatient services. The DRG system pays the same predetermined amount of money for the care of different persons with the same medical diagnosis. Many changes in the healthcare system have been attributed to the introduction of DRGs, including earlier discharge from hospitals and the increased need for home care services.

Hospice and Respite Care

Hospice care is a special component of home care, designed to provide medical, nursing, social, psychological, and spiritual care for terminally ill patients and their families. Hospice care relies on a philosophy of relieving pain and suffering and allowing the patient to die with dignity in a comfortable environment. Licensed nurses, medical social workers, physicians, occupational and physical therapists, and volunteers provide care. Hospice care is discussed in ∞ Chapter 5.

Respite care provides short-term or intermittent home care, often using volunteers. These services exist primarily to give the family member or friend who is the primary caregiver some time away from care. Respite care does much to relieve the burden of full-time caregiving.

The Home Care System

Nurses who practice home care do so within a system that includes home healthcare agencies, patients, referral sources, physicians, reimbursement sources, and legal considerations. The system is interactive and functions best when its members communicate, cooperate, and collaborate with one another.

Types of Home Health Agencies

Home care agencies are either public or private organizations engaged in providing skilled nursing and other therapeutic services in the patient's home. The several different types of home care agencies differ only in the way their programs are organized and administered. All home care agencies are similar in that they must meet uniform standards for licensing, certification, and accreditation. Home care agencies include the following:

- *Official or public agencies.* State or local governments operate these agencies, which are financed primarily by tax funds. Most official agencies offer home care, health education, and disease-prevention programs in the community.
- *Voluntary or private not-for-profit agencies.* Donations, endowments, charities such as the United Way, and third-party (insurance company) reimbursement support these agencies. They are governed by a volunteer board of directors, which usually represents the community they serve.
- *Private, proprietary agencies.* Most of these agencies are for-profit organizations governed by either individual owners or national corporations. Although some participate in third-party reimbursement, others rely on patients paying their own bills (often called out-of-pocket expenses).
- *Institution-based agencies.* These agencies operate under a parent organization, such as a hospital. The home care agency is governed by the sponsoring organization, and the mission of both is similar. Often, the majority of home care referrals come from the parent organization.

Home care agency personnel typically include administrators, managers, care providers (these may be experienced in areas such as social work, medical-surgical care, mental health care, or infusion services) and business office staff. Depending on the agency and geographic location, professional providers may include registered nurses, practical nurses, nurse practitioners, enterostomal therapists, physical therapists, occupational therapists, speech therapists, respiratory therapists, social workers, a chaplain or pastoral minister, dietitians, and home care aides. It is not unusual for patients to require the services of several professionals simultaneously. No matter how many providers are in the home, the responsibility for case coordination (also called case management) remains with the registered nurse.

Patients

The patients in home care are the person receiving care and the person's family. The recognition that the family is also a patient acknowledges the powerful influence that families exert on health. A patient's family is not limited to persons related by birth, adoption, or marriage. In the home, family members may include partners, friends, colleagues, other significant people, and even animals that hold the potential of greatly affecting the health care environment.

Age and functional disability are the primary predictors of need for home care services. Information from a national survey conducted by the Agency for Health Care Policy and Research found that about half of all home care patients are over the age of 65 and that the number of home care services that patients need seems to increase with age.

The old adage that discharge plans begin at admission makes more sense today than ever before. With shortened lengths of hospital stay, it is imperative for nurses to evaluate all patients for their ability to manage at home. Nurses preparing to send patients home must consider many of the questions outlined in the Meeting Individualized Needs box on page 40.

Referrals

A **referral source** is a person recommending home care services and supplying the agency with details about the patient's needs. The source may be a physician, nurse, social worker, therapist, or discharge planner. Families sometimes generate their own referrals, either by approaching one of the sources already mentioned or by calling a home care agency directly to make an inquiry. When the family seeks a referral and the agency believes that the patient qualifies for services, usually the agency contacts the patient's physician and requests a referral on the patient's behalf.

The nurse may make a referral to a home care agency, a hospice, or a community resource if the patient seems to need formal follow-up beyond the present clinical setting. Hospital discharge planners, social workers, organizations for older adults, and local nonprofit agencies usually have a good command of the services and support groups available in their communities.

The nurse must talk to patients and their caregivers about concerns related to home management. It is not unusual for one family member to think that no additional help is necessary and

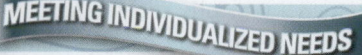

MEETING INDIVIDUALIZED NEEDS The Patient Being Discharged from Acute Care to Home Care

QUESTIONS FOR CONSIDERATION
- Does the patient need follow-up therapy, treatments, or additional education?
- What equipment, supplies, or information about community resources is necessary?
- What teaching materials can be sent home? Are they written at an acceptable reading level? Do they come in other languages?
- What cognitive abilities do the patient and the caregiver seem to have? Are there any sensory deprivations that impede learning?
- Who will be the principal caregiver in the home? Is there one? Are all caregivers comfortable in doing what needs to be done? If not, what support do they need to become comfortable?
- Was the caregiver present during and included in instruction? How have the patient and caregiver responded to health teaching thus far? Have they comprehended what has been taught? Was their stress level such that they could not listen?
- Has a devastating diagnosis and/or prognosis just been determined?
- Is high-technology intervention necessary?

for another to feel differently. The nurse can facilitate an informal family meeting in which everyone shares concerns and can make inquiries about the family's insurance coverage for home care. Suggesting services that families cannot afford only adds to the problem. For patients with limited means, the nurse can consult with staff in the institution who are most knowledgeable about funding. In every instance, it is important that the nurse avoid making assumptions: Well-educated and financially secure patients can be just as overwhelmed by illness as patients who are poor and less learned. Everyone is a referral candidate.

If the family believes that no help is necessary and the nurse believes otherwise, then the nurse may ask the family to consider an evaluation visit, explaining how the situation may look different once the patient is home. If family members continue to refuse, the nurse can let them know that the door is never closed and give them contacts in the community that they can access independently should their needs change.

Physicians

Home care cannot begin without a physician's order, nor can it proceed without a physician-approved treatment plan. This is a legal and reimbursement requirement. Only after a referral is made and an initial set of physician orders is obtained can a nursing assessment visit be scheduled to identify the patient's needs. If the input of another provider, such as a physical therapist, is necessary to complete the initial assessment, then the nurse arranges for this visit.

At the nursing assessment visit, the nurse begins to formulate the plan of care. Box 3–2 lists Medicare's required data for the nursing plan of care. Once formulated, the nurse sends the plan of care back to the physician for review and approval. The physician's signature on the plan of care authorizes the home care agency's providers to continue with services and also serves as a contract indicating agreement to participate in the care of the patient on an ongoing basis. The plan is reviewed as necessary, but at least once every 60 days.

Reimbursement for Services

A reimbursement source pays for home care services. Medicare is home care's largest single reimbursement source, although other sources exist (Medicaid, other public funding, private insurance, and public donation). The reimbursement source evaluates each treatment plan to determine if the goals and plans set forth by the professional providers match the needs assessed. Only interventions identified on the treatment plan

are covered. Periodically the reimbursement source may ask for the home care provider's notes to substantiate what is being done in the home. This is one reason why accurate documentation is critical.

Medicare does not reimburse visits made to support general health maintenance, health promotion, or patients' emotional or socioeconomic needs. Both patient and nurse must meet specific criteria to secure Medicare reimbursement. The patient must meet all of the following criteria:

- The physician must decide that the patient needs care at home and make a plan for home care.
- The patient must need at least one of the following: intermittent (not full time) skilled nursing care, physical therapy, speech language pathology services, or occupational therapy.
- The patient must be homebound. This means leaving the home is a major effort. When leaving the home, it must be infrequent, for a short time, to get medical care, or to attend religious services.
- The home care agency must be Medicare approved.

Medicare will reimburse only when the skilled provider performs at least one of the following tasks:

- Teaching about a new or acute situation.
- Assessing an acute process or a change in the patient's condition.
- Performing a skilled procedure or a hands-on service requiring the professional skill, knowledge, ability, and judgment of a licensed nurse (Figure 3–1 ■).

BOX 3–2 Medicare's Required Data for the Plan of Care

1. All pertinent diagnoses
2. A notation of the beneficiary's mental status
3. Types of services, supplies, and equipment ordered
4. Frequency of visits to be made
5. Patient's prognosis
6. Patient's rehabilitation potential
7. Patient's functional limitations
8. Activities permitted
9. Patient's nutritional requirements
10. Patient's medications and treatments
11. Safety measures to protect against injuries
12. Discharge plans
13. Any other items the home health agency or physician wishes to include

Source: Data from Medicare Health Insurance Manual-11, Section 204.2.

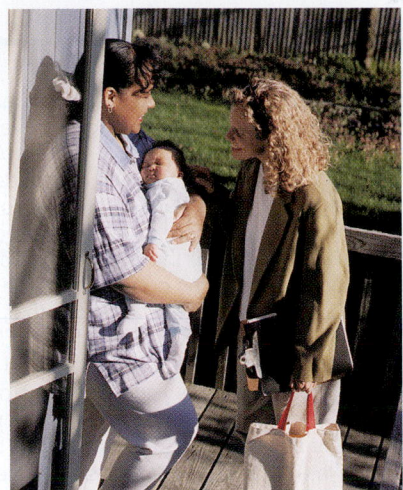

Figure 3–1 ■ The nurse is arriving for a home visit.

The reimbursement guidelines present problems because they are not sensitive to the full scope of nursing practice. Many of the patient and family needs that nurses encounter during home visits are complex and time consuming, reflecting both intense psychosocial and economic concerns. This situation presents a profound dilemma. How are nurses to reconcile spending time on issues for which their agency will receive no payment? How are they to meet agency home visit productivity standards when each home they enter requires more and more from them? How are they to document activities and interventions that are not considered "skilled"? There are no easy answers to these questions.

Legal Considerations

The legal considerations in home care center around issues of privacy and confidentiality, the patient's access to health information, the patient's freedom from unreasonable restraint, witnessing of documents, informed consent, and matters of negligence and/or malpractice. Numerous sources suggest that nurses can best avoid lawsuits by familiarizing themselves with the standards of practice, providing care that is consistent with both the standards and their agency's policies, and documenting all care fully and accurately according to agency guidelines.

Home care nurses are responsible for adhering to the same codes and standards that guide all other nurses. These codes and standards guide nursing practice and protect the public. In addition to these guidelines, other codes and statements give specific guidance on issues that affect care in the home.

The ANA Scope and Standards of Practice for Home Health Nursing (2007a) and Public Health Nursing (2007b) are used in conjunction as a basis for the practice of nursing in the home. These standards address the nursing process, interdisciplinary collaboration, quality assurance, professional development, and research. The standards speak to two levels of practitioners (generalist, who is prepared on the baccalaureate level, and specialist, who is prepared on the graduate level) and outline what achievements are expected of the professional nurse in the home.

Another source of guidance regarding home care is the National Association of Home Care (NAHC) Bill of Rights. Its use is a federal requirement for all home care agencies. Although they are permitted to make additions to the NAHC's original bill of rights, home care agencies are required by law to address the concepts in the NAHC Bill of Rights with all home care patients on the initial visit. The bill of rights is listed in Box 3–3.

The Nursing Process in Home Care

The nursing process used in home care is no different from that practiced in any other setting. The unique challenges of home care present themselves chiefly in the implementation step. Generally, the differences lie in assessing how the home's unique environment affects the need or problem and using outcome criteria and mutual participation to plan goals and interventions.

Assessment

In home care, nursing assessment and data collection center chiefly around the first home visit. This is not to say that nurses do not collect information on an ongoing basis, but because most agencies require the submission of a plan of care within 48 hours of the initial evaluation, the first visit carries tremendous weight. Under ideal circumstances, a preliminary review of background information initiates the assessment process; the reality in home care, however, is that few patients are referred with copies of either their medical records or their discharge summaries. If the patient has received home care services in the past, records may be available, but often all the nurse has prior to initiating care is the referral form describing the present problem, some notations about past medical history, and a projection of the skilled interventions needed. Therefore, it falls to the nurse to try to obtain as complete a clinical picture as possible when meeting the patient.

Assessment begins when the nurse calls the patient to arrange a visit. This initial telephone call can yield much information to the nurse who pays close attention. For example,

- How alert, oriented, and stressed does the patient (and/or family) seem to be?
- Does the patient know the reason for the home care referral?
- How open to intervention do the patient and family seem to be?
- Have they encountered any difficulties since discharge from the prior setting?
- Do they need any supplies on the first visit?

During the visit, much of the assessment process centers on collecting the information requested on the tools and forms contained in the agency's admission packet. These packets usually include a physical and psychosocial database; a medication sheet; forms for pain assessment, spiritual assessment, financial assessment; and a family roster. It is extremely important that the data collected be as complete and accurate as possible and reflect subjective, objective, current, and historical information. Through interviewing, direct observation, and physical assessment, the nurse can achieve the goal of the initial visit, namely, to gain as clear and accurate a clinical picture of the patient as possible.

Diagnosis

After completing the initial assessment, the nurse identifies the real and/or potential patient problems that emerge from the data. Nursing diagnoses describing the patient's health problems and needs, based on data collection, must be part of the home care record both to organize care and to justify reimbursement.

In almost all home care situations, *Deficient Knowledge* is an appropriate nursing diagnosis. Nursing interventions for this diagnosis specific to a patient with Alzheimer's disease and the patient's family can be found in the Meeting Individualized Needs box on page 43.

BOX 3–3 Example of a Home Health Agency's Bill of Rights

The agency acknowledges the patient's rights and encourages the patient and family to participate in their plan of care through informed decision making. In accordance with this belief, each patient/family member will receive, prior to admission, the following bill of rights and responsibilities.

1. The patient and the patient's property will be treated with respect by the program's staff.
2. The patient will receive care without regard to race, color, creed, age, sex, religion, national origin, or mental or physical handicap.
3. The patient has the right to be free from mental and physical abuse.
4. The patient's medical record and related information is maintained in a confidential manner by the program.
5. The patient will receive a written statement of the program's objectives, scope of services, and grievance process prior to admission.
6. The patient, family, or guardian has the right to file a complaint regarding the services provided by the program without fear of disruption of service, coercion, or discrimination.
7. The patient will be advised of the following in advance of service:
   a. Description of services and proposed visit frequency
   b. Overview of the anticipated plan of care and its likely outcome
   c. Options that may be available
8. The patient/family is encouraged to participate in the plan of care. The patient will receive the necessary information concerning the patient's condition and will be encouraged to participate in changes that may arise in care.
9. The program shall provide for the right of the patient to refuse any portion of planned treatment to the extent permitted by law without relinquishing other portions of the treatment plan, except where medical contraindications exist. The patient will be informed of the expected consequences of such action.

10. The patient has a right to continuity of care:
    a. Services provided within a reasonable time frame
    b. A program that is capable of providing the level of care required by the patient
    c. Timely referral to alternative services, as needed
    d. Information regarding impending discharge, continuing care requirements, and other services, as needed
11. The patient will be informed of the extent to which payment will be expected for items or services to be furnished to patients by Medicare, Medicaid, and any other program that is funded partially or fully with federal funds. Upon admission, the patient will be informed orally and in writing of any charges for items and services that the program expects will not be covered upon admission. The patient will be informed of any change in this amount as soon as possible, but no later than within 25 days after the program is made aware of the change.
12. Upon request, the patient may obtain:
    a. An itemized bill
    b. The program's policy for uncompensated care
    c. The program's policy for disclosure of the medical record
    d. Identity of healthcare providers with which the program has contractual agreements, insofar as the patient's care is concerned
    e. The name of the responsible person supervising the patient's care and how to contact this person during regular business hours
13. The patient has the right to obtain medical equipment and other health-related items from the company of the patient's choice and assumes financial responsibility for such. The program's staff will assist in obtaining supplies and physician approvals as needed.
14. The patient/family is responsible for:
    a. Giving the program accurate, necessary information
    b. Being available and cooperative during scheduled visits
    c. Assisting, as much as possible, in the plan of care
    d. Alerting the staff to any problems as soon as possible

Planning

Planning in home care includes setting priorities, establishing goals, and deciding on interventions designed to meet the needs of the patient. The greatest level of success is achieved when patients feel an ownership of the suggested plan. For this reason, planned interventions and outcome criteria should be patient centered, realistic, achievable, and mutually accepted. The nurse works with the patient to do the following:

- Identify significant issues and needs.
- Set mutually agreed-upon goals (outcome criteria).
- Make and initiate acceptable plans to meet the goals.

Outcome criteria should be verbally stated to patients and documented clearly and concisely, in timed, measurable, and observable terms. These measures help patients and care providers better focus their work together and evaluate the effectiveness of care. In addition, outcome criteria provide the reimbursement source a measurable standard from which to judge the appropriateness of the plan of care.

Implementation

The home care nurse implements most of the planned interventions, although some may be carried out by another agency provider, a paraprofessional introduced into the setting by the nurse case manager, or the patient.

Nurses and patients reach an agreement about the implementation of care through a process called **contracting**, the negotiation of a cooperative working agreement between the nurse and patient that is continuously renegotiated. Contracting is a concept used often in, but not exclusive to, many home and community health settings. Contracting can occur both formally and informally. It involves exploring a need, establishing goals, evaluating resources, developing a plan, assigning responsibilities, agreeing on a time frame, and evaluating or terminating. Contracting requires the nurse to relinquish control as the expert and consider the patient as an equal partner in the process.

Contracting is not appropriate with all patients. It is certainly inadvisable if the nurse–patient relationship is to be no more than two visits or if the patient has limited cognitive abilities. However, contracting is useful for patients who demonstrate a willingness to be active participants in their health care. It is empowering, can save time, and keeps the nursing goals directed and focused.

Evaluation

Evaluation in home care is both formative and summative. Formative evaluation is the systematic, ongoing comparison of the plan of care with the goals actually being achieved from visit to

MEETING INDIVIDUALIZED NEEDS Family Home Care for the Older Adult with a Dementing Disorder

NURSING DIAGNOSIS
Deficient Knowledge related to lack of information about Alzheimer's disease process and care

OUTCOME CRITERIA
Short term: Adequate knowledge, as evidenced by family's stating of disease progression and treatment (expected within 1 week)
Long term: Adequate knowledge, as evidenced by family's following of the recommended interventions throughout illness course (within 1 month) or by discharge from home health

INTERVENTIONS
- Alert the family to both environmental hazards and patient habits that could threaten safety. (first visit)
- Provide the family with specific recommendations for keeping the patient safe, for example, serving foods warm, not hot; allowing the patient to eat with fingers; cutting food in small pieces; wearing an ID bracelet; discouraging daytime sleep. (first visit)
- Discuss the disease course (degenerative), the prognosis (incurable), typical issues of concern (promoting adequate nutrition, activity, rest, safety, and independence); supporting cognitive function; communication, socialization, and family caregiving; the supportive care available; and the ultimate need for long-term placement with disease progression. (first visit)
- Discuss local resources, including adult day care, support groups, and Alzheimer's Disease Association. Give family a list of these resources. (first visit)
- Include all family members or significant persons in teaching and planning care. (each visit)
- Prepare the family for typical types of Alzheimer's disease behaviors: forgetfulness, disorientation, agitation, screaming, crying, physical or verbal abuse, accusations of infidelity. (subsequent visits)
- Teach the family specific interventions for dealing with these behaviors: calm, unhurried manner, music, stroking, rocking, structuring the environment, distracting the patient. (subsequent visits)
- Stress the importance of both exercise and recreation in terms of quality of life and decreasing nighttime restlessness. (subsequent visits)
- Reinforce the patient's continued needs for socialization and intimacy. (subsequent visits)
- Suggest specific interventions for meeting socialization needs: limiting visitors to one or two at a time, pet therapy, use of the phone. (subsequent visits)
- Suggest useful interventions that are described in the literature and/or that are utilized in more formal Alzheimer's disease settings and may also be helpful in the home. (subsequent visits)
- Keep the environment safe for the patient.
- Use reality orientation with patient several times a day, and post clocks, calendars, and telephone numbers within easy sight of the patient.
- Give patient simple directions, using simple sentences and a quiet, monotone voice so as not to excite the patient.
- Allow the use of the telephone, because calls will help orient the patient.

visit. In summative evaluation, the nurse reviews the total plan of care and the patient's progress toward goals to determine the patient's eligibility for discharge.

Reimbursement guidelines may be helpful in driving the evaluation process. Because reimbursement sources require that all skilled services be justified, many home care agencies have designed their clinical notes to include areas for evaluation of the patient's response to the visit's interventions and documentation of a plan of care for the next scheduled visit.

Roles of the Home Care Nurse

The role expectations of the home care nurse are similar to those of the professional nurse in any setting. On behalf of patients in the home, the nurse serves as an advocate, a provider of direct care, an educator, and a coordinator of services.

Advocate

As patient advocate, the nurse explores, informs, supports, and affirms the choices of patients. Advocacy begins on the first visit, when the nurse discusses advanced directives, living wills, and durable power of attorney for health care. The home care agency's bill of rights also needs to be discussed. During the course of care, patients may need help negotiating the complex medical system (especially in regard to healthcare insurance), accessing community resources, recognizing and coping with required changes in lifestyle, and making informed decisions. When the family's desires differ from the patient's, advocacy can be a challenge. If a conflict arises, the nurse must remain the patient's primary advocate.

In the home there are no colleagues present to consult, to assist, or to rely on for support. The home is a practice setting where nurses learn to trust their theoretical and intuitive knowledge and to be totally accountable.

Provider of Direct Care

Home care nurses usually are not involved in providing personal care for patients (such as bathing and changing linens). The families often provide routine personal care, or the nurse may arrange for a home care aide. If a personal care need arises during the course of the skilled visit (e.g., if a patient has an incontinent episode), the nurse typically either bathes and changes the patient or assists the caregiver to do so before moving on to the skilled activities planned for the visit.

As a provider of direct care, the nurse uses the nursing process to assess, diagnose, plan care, intervene, and evaluate patient needs. During the course of this process, home care nurses frequently are involved in performing specific procedures and treatments such as physical assessments, care of intravenous lines, ostomy care, wound care, and pain management.

Personal health habits, living conditions, resources, and support systems may leave much to be desired. It is not unusual for home care nurses to face unchanged dressings, undertreated infections, off-and-on self-medication, poor nutrition, filthy conditions, and unreliable caregivers. No matter how vigilant nurses may be, practice settings like these work against their best efforts. If the conditions cannot be changed, the nurse may withdraw from the situation, or continue to practice within the environment and report substandard care by caregivers.

Educator

Most of the home care nurse's time is spent teaching. Many nurses believe that their role as teacher is the crux of their nursing practice and that nurses in the home are always teaching (Figure 3–2 ■). For this reason, it is important that home care nurses develop expertise in the theory and principles of patient education.

The greatest educational challenge may be motivating the patient. Discovering what it takes to make the patient want to learn and focusing the patient on what is most important can tax the ingenuity of even the most dedicated nurse. Despite the work involved, nurses are rewarded by the knowledge that through their efforts, patients have learned to manage independently. Because the nurse's role as educator is becoming increasingly important, guidelines for community-based care are included in the discussion of each major disorder addressed in this textbook.

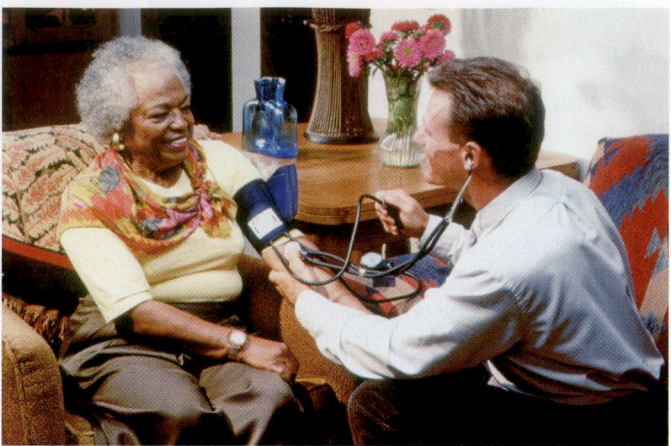

Figure 3–2 ■ Home visits offer opportunities to carry out health promotion activities. This nurse takes a patient's blood pressure while visiting for an unrelated condition.

SAFETY ALERT
Promoting Safety in Home Care

When preparing patients for discharge to home, the nurse focuses on safety and survival first. Even if health education is to continue with home care, a day or two may elapse before the nurse arrives, and patients must be able to manage by themselves until then. The nurse must not discharge patients without giving them the correct information and supplies to get them through the first few days at home. Additionally, patients should not be discharged without phone numbers and complete written information about their medications and the manifestations of complications they should report to their doctor or the nurse that discharged them. Finally, all patients should be able to at least minimally manage any necessary treatments. Management includes not only performing procedures safely but also knowing how to obtain necessary supplies in the community.

Patients need help understanding their situations, making healthcare decisions, and changing health behaviors. It is unrealistic, however, to believe that patients can be taught everything they need to know during today's shortened hospital stays. The nurse should therefore recommend a home care referral for anyone in need of follow-up teaching. Prioritized teaching is essential: Even under the best of circumstances, patients generally forget about one-third of what is said to them and their recall of specific instructions and advice is less than 50%. Comprehensive information related to patient and family teaching is included in most of the following chapters in this textbook. This can be used as a guide in planning teaching.

Coordinator of Services

As coordinator of services, the home care nurse is the main contact with the patient's physician and all other providers involved in the treatment plan. It is the responsibility of the registered nurse case coordinator (or clinical case manager) to report patient changes, discuss responses, and develop and secure treatment plan revisions on an ongoing basis. This is accomplished formally, through scheduled case and team conferences, and informally (often over the phone) with concerned providers. Documentation of all coordination activities is legally required.

Special Considerations in Home Care Nursing

Nursing practice in the home is a unique experience that differs in many ways from nursing practice in a hospital setting. The word "home" generates strong feelings of ownership, control, security, family history, independence, comfort, protection, and conflict. Family members perceive a sharing of self when they consistently allow entry to a stranger. Because patients and nurses most often meet during periods of vulnerability and crisis, and because socializing is such an integral part of the home visit process, nurse providers are often perceived as friends or extended family members, blurring the boundaries of practice.

Nurses are invited into homes, meaning they are guests and cannot assume entry as they do in formal clinical settings. The environment belongs to the patient, who retains control. Every nursing action must communicate respect for these boundaries. To negotiate both repeated entry and a share of power in the patient's domain, the nurse must establish trust and rapport quickly. This is often difficult because most home care nurses are with each patient for only 1 hour a few times a week.

During the course of establishing rapport and getting to know each other as people, the nurse–patient relationship often becomes something more. Nurses and patients end up giving to each other and learning from each other. By connecting as human beings, they touch each other's spirits in profound ways (Taylor, 2008). In home health, it is not unusual for nurses to realize suddenly not only that they do things to create a healing environment but also that their very presence has become the healing environment. Over time, as the nurse becomes a familiar presence and the family's behavior relaxes, the nurse can gain a clearer and more complete picture of family relationships, dynamics, lifestyle choices, and coping patterns.

Caregiver burden is not easily hidden in the home. In nearly one out of four American households (23%), people are taking care of disabled relatives and friends (USDHHS, 2008). Many

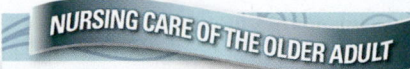

Special Needs of Older Adults Living Alone

Many older adults live alone. Some may have current or potential caregivers nearby, whereas others, for various reasons, have no one. These people often require considerable nursing support to remain strong, independent, and resourceful. Caring for "families of one" can take a toll on even the strongest home care nurse. Some nurses have reported calling between visits, keeping in touch after discharge, and driving by on days off because they have such difficulty "letting go" their concerns about these

patients. Transitioning between healthcare settings is especially problematic for those with chronic illness or long-term health problems. Older adults are at high risk for "falling through the gap" and frequently need assistance to navigate the complex healthcare system. High quality transitional care can reduce adverse events and re-hospitalization rates while improving patient satisfaction with care (Naylor & Keating, 2008).

of these caregivers are themselves older adults. Healthcare planners visualize the home as a place where all kinds of medical services can occur but may give little thought to how people manage. Few ever ask whether families can cope with the level of care they are expected to assume. Caregiving has only recently been acknowledged as a complex activity, requiring adjustment in family living patterns, relationships, and finances. Early hospital discharge of family members with chronic conditions places enormous emotional, physical, and financial burdens on family caregivers (Toofany, 2008). For some families, the crisis of caregiving is short lived, but for others it lasts for years. As a result, caregivers are at great risk for both physical and emotional illness. Because the success of home care heavily depends on the supports in place, addressing the needs of the support network is imperative.

Nursing Interventions to Ensure Competent Home Care

Despite differences in the setting, nursing care for patients in their homes is a highly rewarding clinical practice. The following discussion provides practical information for competent care with successful outcomes.

Establish Trust and Rapport

To establish trust and rapport in the patient's home, nurses must try to find common ground and let go of ethnocentric ("my culture's way is the best way") views. Nurses must be sure everything they say and do communicates an understanding that they are guests—offering suggestions in a way that acknowledges the patient's right to say no, sensing and honoring "where people are in their situation," maintaining a respectful distance, and noticing and honoring family customs ("I see that no one wears shoes in your house; I'll take mine off, too."). Nurses should try to negotiate their schedules around the family's needs; nursing should enhance family coping, not complicate it. Above all, nurses should validate patients' illness experiences, remembering that everyone needs someone who is willing to listen and say, "I hear what you are saying, and I think I have a sense of how you feel."

Proceed Slowly

The nurse must enter the home with awareness that the first contact is important. On the first nursing visit, the nurse can suggest to patients that they have someone else present "to help them listen." To avoid overwhelming patients with too much information, the nurse stresses the essential information and

repeats it on subsequent visits. When making suggestions, the nurse offers patients the pluses and minuses of each alternative. Informed decisions are difficult to make if people are too overwhelmed to think of their options. The nurse speaks slowly, directly, and within the patient's range of vision (the patient may have to lip-read) and refrains from shouting at patients who are hearing-impaired. The nurse must also allow time for families to process new information.

Set Goals and Boundaries

The nurse explores patients' expectations of home care. In particular, the nurse explains the primary goal (to achieve self-care), defines nurse and patient roles within this framework, and discusses limitations. The nurse may make statements such as, "No, a home care nurse is not the same as a private duty nurse" and "Home care nurses do not routinely do that, but today I will make an exception." It is important that the nurse stresses mutual accountability, choice, and negotiation as part of the process.

Assess the Home Environment

The nurse surveys the overall home environment, using common sense, intuition, and imagination. Among the variables to note are sights, sounds, smells, dress, tone of voice, body language, and the use of touch; visiting patterns among family members; significant relationships; what is sacred and what is not; the appearance of the house, yard, sidewalk, and neighborhood; and the effect of illness on the family. The nurse asks questions and listens carefully to stories and offhand remarks.

Set Priorities

It is important that nurses are flexible and realize they cannot tackle everything. Although it is necessary to enter the home with a plan in mind, nurses must be prepared to modify the plan according to conditions they encounter once inside. Safety, issues that are of concern to patients, and those problems that can most easily be solved should be addressed first. Alternatively, the nurse can focus on safety first, then short-term and long-term goals. If the priorities that are set are primarily the nurse's and not the patient's, then they may not be met.

Promote Learning

Instead of just teaching the patient, the nurse tries actively to promote the patient's ability to learn by, for example, identifying what is most important to the patient and teaching that. Survival takes first priority; the nurse teaches the information people need to ensure their safety until the next visit. The nurse prioritizes material on a needs-to-know, wants-to-know, ought-to-know basis, assessing and responding to learner readiness.

Timing is important; people who are not ready to listen cannot be taught. In addition, the nurse must allow a sufficient amount of time to teach, ask patients how and when they learn best, use appropriate methods and materials when possible, and capitalize on patients' frustrations and desires to regain control of self-care. When possible, the nurse teaches while providing care.

The nurse can empower patients to learn by talking them through learning tasks, encouraging them to listen to their own bodies and to ask questions, and urging them to write thoughts and questions about their care and bring them to the next visit or doctor's appointment.

Limit Distractions

Homes are full of events or circumstances that may divert attention from the job at hand. Such distractions as children, animals, noise, clutter, and mannerisms that are controlling, manipulative, or aggressive can try even the most experienced nurse. However, environmental and behavioral distractions can yield useful information about people, their relationships, and their values. For example, a dirty house could indicate a lack of interest in housekeeping, outright neglect and abuse, depression, or increased disability.

Distractions should be limited as much as possible. For example, the nurse might ask a patient, "May I please turn off your television while we visit?" or "I would like to schedule my next visit for a time when the children are in school. Is that all right with you?" The nurse must be truthful about allergies, fear of a patient's pet, or difficulty hearing in a particular room, but should not debate the priority of the visit over the distraction (such as a favorite television show). The nurse may not change the patient's views and may also risk losing the patient's trust and rapport. If all efforts at limiting distractions fail, the nurse should leave the home and return on another day: "I can see this is not going to work for us today. I will need to leave."

If any distraction originates with the nurse, such as fear of harm, reaction to the patient's lifestyle, preoccupation with role or a feeling of being overwhelmed by the situation in the home, the nurse should seek out a colleague to discuss the problem. Often, another perspective helps when dealing with the issue.

Put Safety First

Safety assessment in the home is a nursing responsibility and a legal requirement. Nurses cannot close their eyes to an unsafe environment. Upon entering the home and on a continuing basis, it is imperative that the nurse alert the family to unsafe and hazardous conditions, suggest remedies, and document in the clinical record the family's response to the nurse's suggestions. See Box 3–4 for a sample home safety assessment list. In particular, nurses must remain alert to the following:

- How patients handle stairs.
- How patients manage their own care if they are alone.
- The presence of a smoke detector in the home.
- The presence of bathroom safety equipment.
- Electrical hazards.
- Slippery throw rugs, clutter, or a furniture arrangement that may cause a fall.
- A supply of expired medications.
- Inappropriate clothing or shoes.
- Cooking habits that may precipitate a fire.

BOX 3–4 Home Safety Assessment Checklist

General Household Safety
1. Do stairwells and halls have good lighting?
2. Do staircases have handrails on both sides?
3. Are rugs securely tacked down?
4. Is the telephone readily accessible? Is the dial easy to read?
5. Are electrical cords in good condition and out of the way?
6. Is furniture sturdy?
7. Is the temperature of the home comfortable?
8. Are protective screens in front of fireplaces or heating devices?
9. Are smoke detectors and carbon monoxide detectors present and working?

Bathroom
1. Are grab bars present in the tub and/or shower? Around the toilet?
2. Are toilet seats high enough?
3. Are nonskid materials (rugs, mats) on the floor, tub/shower?
4. Are medications stored safely? Out of the reach of children?
5. Is the water temperature safe?
6. Are electrical outlets and appliances a safe distance from the tub?

Kitchen
1. Are floors slippery? Are nonskid rugs used?
2. Is the stove in good working order?
3. Is the refrigerator in good working order? Clean?
4. Are electrical outlets overloaded with appliance cords?
5. Are sharp objects kept in a special container or safe area?
6. Is food storage adequate? Clean?
7. Are cleaning materials stored safely?

- An inadequate food supply.
- Poorly functioning utilities.
- Chipping paint.
- Signs of abusive behavior.

Nurses cannot go into homes and change the family's living space and lifestyle, but they can register their concern and react appropriately if the situation suggests that an injury is about to occur or if they suspect abuse or neglect. In the home and community setting, ignoring an unsafe environment is considered nursing negligence.

The disposal of toxic medications and sharp objects (such as needles used for injections) is also a safety issue in the home, especially if young children are present. Once again, it is imperative that the nurse address this with the patient, demonstrate safe disposal, and provide the necessary equipment to accomplish that end. Documentation should address what information the nurse has covered, the family's response to the teaching, and assessment of the family's ongoing practice of safety precautions.

Nurses must focus on safety and survival first, for themselves as well as their patients, in all that they do. When traveling in the community, the nurse takes such precautions as keeping car doors locked, having a cellular phone, keeping supplies out of sight, and staying inside the car in potentially dangerous situations. Colleagues, families, and community members can offer useful guidelines for maintaining safety and self-protection.

It is important to avoid overwhelming families with numerous healthcare providers in the home. Most people dislike having strangers in their home, no matter how helpful they may seem to be. The nurse can help families manage moments of crisis by staying as close as possible. If abuse is suspected, the nurse must notify authorities and/or remove patients from potentially dangerous situations.

Make Do

Nurses must learn to be resourceful and cost conscious with equipment, supplies, and services in the home. When needing to make do or improvise, they should do so in a low-key manner to avoid causing the family additional anxiety. The nurse must make every effort to convey the message that the situation is under control; after leaving the home, the nurse can react as necessary.

Control Infection

Infection control in the home centers on protecting patients, caregivers, and the community from the spread of disease. Within the home, nurses may encounter patients with infectious or communicable diseases, patients who are immuno-compromised, and/or patients having multiple access devices, drainage tubes, or draining wounds. The home presents a challenging environment in which to practice infection control for several reasons: Families typically are set in their own ways of doing things; caregivers often lack any formal education on the subject; the setting itself may not be conducive; and the facilities for even the most basic of aseptic practices (hand hygiene) may be lacking. Without a doubt, the single most important nursing intervention in controlling infection is health teaching. Patients and caregivers need to know the importance of effective hand hygiene, the use of gloves, the disposal of wastes and soiled dressings, the handling of linens, and the practice of standard precautions. Unfortunately, the imparting of important information does not always bring about a change in behavior. Trying to change a family's values frequently demands a great deal of ingenuity from the nurse.

Rehabilitation

Rehabilitation is the process of learning to live to one's maximum potential with a chronic impairment and its resultant functional disability. Rehabilitation nursing is based on a philosophy that each person has a unique set of strengths and abilities that can enable that person to live with dignity, self-worth, and independence. Nursing care to promote rehabilitation primarily focuses on patients with chronic illnesses or impairments. Rehabilitation most often begins in the acute phase of an illness or injury.

The terms *impairment*, *disability*, and *handicap* are often used as synonyms, but they have different meanings. **Impairment** is a disturbance in structure or function resulting from physiologic or psychologic abnormalities. A **disability** is the degree of observable and measurable impairment. A **handicap** is the total adjustment to disability that limits functioning at a normal level (Stanhope & Lancaster, 2006). For example, following a motorcycle accident, a patient had damage to her left leg that led to impairment in the ability to flex her knee. This resulted in a 50% disability of that leg and caused a handicap because the patient was a school bus driver and could no longer operate the bus safely.

Rehabilitation promotes reintegration into the patient's family and community through a team approach. Many different aspects of the patient's life are included in the plan of care, including physical function, mental health, interpersonal relationships, social interactions, family support, and vocational status. This comprehensive consideration of the patient requires the expertise of a team of healthcare providers who usually meet weekly to discuss the achievement of patient goals.

Assessment of the patient and family includes functional health level and self-care abilities, educational needs, psychosocial needs, and the home environment. It is critical to determine the priorities of needs from the patient and family perspective before establishing any plan of care. The nurse assesses the patient's level of physical function, goals, concerns, stage of loss, home environment, and available resources.

Interventions to facilitate rehabilitation are revised to meet patient and family needs as the patient progresses toward reintegration. In general, interventions are planned and implemented to prevent complications, assist in achieving a realistic level of independence, educate the patient and family about home care, and make referrals to community agencies (for nursing care, special equipment or supplies, support groups, counseling, physical therapy, occupational therapy, respiratory therapy, vocational guidance, house cleaning, and meals).

CHAPTER HIGHLIGHTS

- In contrast to community health, which focuses on health of a population, community-based care focuses on individual and family healthcare needs. Services are provided in many different settings, including community centers and clinics, day care programs, faith community nursing, and Meals on Wheels.
- Factors affecting health in the community include social support systems, community healthcare structures, environment, and economic resources.
- Home care is defined as services for recovering, disabled, or chronically ill people who are in need of treatment or support to function effectively in the home environment.
- Two special components of home care are hospice care and respite care.

- The home care system includes agencies, patients, referral sources, physicians, reimbursement sources, and legal considerations.
- The roles of the home care nurse include advocate, provider of direct care, educator, and coordinator of services.
- Nursing interventions to ensure competent care include those used to establish trust and rapport, proceed slowly, set goals and boundaries, assess the home environment, set priorities, promote learning, limit distractions, put safety first, and control infection.
- Rehabilitation is the process of learning to live to one's maximum potential with a chronic health impairment and its resultant disability.

TEST YOURSELF NCLEX-RN® REVIEW

1. What is the focus of community-based nursing care?
   1. the function of the community
   2. the health of the community
   3. individual and family health
   4. older adult needs and services

2. What is one way in which urban and rural residents may differ?
   1. access to healthcare services
   2. age and gender of residents
   3. family tasks and values
   4. ability to follow directions

3. As part of the initial assessment of a disabled older adult receiving community-based care, the nurse asks, "Who takes you to your doctor's appointments and picks up your prescriptions or groceries for you?" Which of the following factors is the nurse assessing?
   1. social support systems
   2. community healthcare structure
   3. environmental factors
   4. economic resources

4. Which of the following services helps relieve the stress of full-time caregiving?
   1. faith community nursing
   2. block nursing
   3. day care
   4. respite care

5. Home health nurses provide care to patients with a wide variety of healthcare needs. Which of the following patients would benefit from home care? **Select all that apply.**
   1. an older adult recently discharged from the hospital after a total hip replacement
   2. a teenager recently discharged from the hospital following an appendectomy
   3. a middle-aged patient with a terminal illness who wants to die at home
   4. a single mother of toddlers recently discharged following major abdominal surgery
   5. a frail older adult experiencing weakness and impaired mobility from osteoarthritis

6. While making the first home health visit, the nurse discusses advance directives, living wills, and durable power of attorney for health care. These topics are part of which nursing role?
   1. provider of direct care
   2. coordinator of services
   3. educator
   4. advocate

7. The nurse is assessing the safety of a patient's home environment. Which of the following outcomes indicate an unsafe environment? **Select all that apply.**
   1. the presence of overloaded extension cords
   2. the presence of a smoke detector in the home
   3. the presence of several throw rugs and a cluttered floor space
   4. a supply of expired medications
   5. a supply of frozen dinners and canned goods

8. Which of the following factors should have the highest priority when planning rehabilitative care for the patient?
   1. physician and nurse perspective of needs
   2. patient and family perspective of needs
   3. patient and family insurance coverage
   4. physician and nurse goals and concerns

9. Nurses practicing in the home provide teaching for a variety of topics. Which of the following areas is essential to maintaining infection control?
   1. fire and smoke detectors
   2. hand hygiene
   3. uncluttered floors and stairs
   4. medications

10. What element of home care is a requirement for reimbursement?
    1. family member approval
    2. completion of agency forms
    3. physician's order
    4. treatment plan

See Test Yourself answers in Appendix C.

Pearson Nursing Student Resources

Find additional review materials at
nursing.pearsonhighered.com

Prepare for success with additional NCLEX®-style practice questions, interactive assignments and activities, Web links, animations and videos, and more!

BIBLIOGRAPHY

American Nurses Association. (2005). *Faith community nursing scope and standards of practice.* Washington, DC: Author.

American Nurses Association. (2007a). *Home health nursing scope and standards of practice.* Washington, DC: Author.

American Nurses Association. (2007b). *Public health nursing scope and standards of practice.* Washington, DC: Author.

Carter, A. (2009). Home healthcare nurses and clinicians can bring significant savings to the table. *Home Healthcare Nurse, 27*(1), 64–65.

Eddy, T., Kilburn, E., Chang, C., Bullock, L., & Sharps, B. (2008). Facilitators and barriers for implementing home visit interventions to address intimate partner violence. *Nursing Clinics of North America, 43*(3), 419–435.

Grafova, I., Freedman, V., Kumar, K., & Ropgowski, J. (2008). Neighborhoods and obesity in later life. *American Journal of Public Health, 98*(11), 2065–2071.

Hoare, K. (2004). Care home placement: Can admission direct from acute hospital be justified? *Nursing Older People, 16*(6), 14–17.

Medicare. (2007). Types of long-term care. Retrieved from http://www.medicare.gov/LongTermCare/Static/TypesOverview.asp

National Association for Home Care and Hospice. (2009). *What are my rights as a patient?* Retrieved from http://www.nahc.org/consumer/rights.html

Naylor, M., & Keating, S. (2008). Transitional care. *American Journal of Nursing, 108*(9 supplement), 58–63.

North American Nursing Diagnosis Association International. (2009). *Nursing diagnoses: Definitions & classification 2009–2011.* Oxford, UK: Wiley-Blackwell.

Schneider, J., Barkauskas, V., & Keenan, G. (2008). Evaluating home health care nursing outcomes with OASIS and NOC. *Journal of Nursing Scholarship, 40*(1), 76–42.

Spotlight on home health nursing. (2007). *Nursing, 37*(12), 56–R2.

Stanhope, M., & Lancaster, J. (2006). Foundations of nursing in the community (2nd ed.). St. Louis: Mosby.

Taylor, E. J. (2008). Promoting spiritual health in home healthcare. *Home Healthcare Nurse 26*(6), 367–374.

Toofany, S. (2008). Hospital at home: A resurgence. *Primary Health Care, 18*(7), 20–23.

US Department of Health and Human Services (USDHHS), Administration on Aging (AOA). (2007). *Hospice care: A guide for families*. Retrieved from http://www.aoa.gov/press/prodsmats/fact/pdf/fs_hospice.pdf

US Department of Health and Human Services (USDHHS), Administration on Aging (AOA). (2008). *National family caregiver support program*. Retrieved from http://www.aoa.gov/prof/aoaprog/caregiver/caregiver.aspx

US Department of Health and Human Services (USDHHS), Centers for Medicare & Medicaid Services (CMS). (2007). *Medicare and home health care.* (Pub. No. CMS-10969). Baltimore, MD: CMS. Retrieved from http://www.medicare.gov/Publications/Pubs/pdf/10969.pdf

US Department of Health and Human Services (USDHHS), Centers for Medicare & Medicaid Services (CMS). (2008). *Medicare & You 2009.* (Pub. No. CMS-10050). Baltimore, MD: CMS. Retrieved from http://www.medicare.gov/Publications/Pubs/pdf/10050.pdf

Wilkinson, J. & Ahern, N. (2008). *Prentice Hall nursing diagnosis handbook with NIC interventions and NOC outcomes,* (9th ed.). Upper Saddle River, NJ: Prentice Hall.

Building Clinical Competence
Dimensions of Medical-Surgical Nursing

Functional Health Pattern: Health Perception-Health Management

Think about patients with altered health perception or health management for whom you have cared in your clinical experiences.

- What were the patient's major medical diagnoses (e.g. hypertension, diabetes mellitus, cancer, chronic obstructive pulmonary disease, stroke and alcoholism)?

- What kinds of manifestations did each of these patients have? Were these manifestations similar or very different?

- How did the patients' healthcare behaviors interfere with their health status? Did they have yearly physical examinations and routine eye examinations? Did they obtain recommended immunizations? Did they use preventative measures, such as breast self-examinations or testicular examinations, sunscreen, dietary changes, decreasing alcohol intake, stopping smoking, beginning exercising regularly, practicing safe sex, and using stress reduction activities? Did they achieve developmental tasks appropriate for their age? Did they interact well with family, friends, and coworkers?

The Health Perception-Health Management Functional Health Pattern include healthcare behaviors, such as health promotion and illness prevention activities, medical treatments, and follow-up care. Individuals are at different locations on the illness-wellness continuum at specific points in time. Health perception and health maintenance are affected by factors that influence the individual's health status or level of wellness in two primary ways:

- Factors affecting health that can be altered to possibly prevent disease processes are diet (e.g., osteoporosis), substance abuse (e.g., alcoholism), smoking (e.g., chronic obstructive pulmonary disease, lung cancer), socioeconomic status (e.g., communicable disease, violence or abuse) or occupational exposure (e.g., pulmonary disease due to asbestos, tuberculosis).

- Factors affecting health that cannot be altered and that may result in disease processes are genetics (e.g., sickle cell disease, hemophilia), age (e.g., type II diabetes mellitus, myocardial infarction), or race (e.g., hypertension).

A patient's perceived pattern of health and well-being affects how health is managed. Improper health management affects the body's ability to maintain itself, leading to manifestations such as the following:

- **Vomiting** (*unpleasant, wave-like sensations in the stomach with sweating and pulse rate changes result in sudden, forceful expulsion of stomach contents through the mouth*)

- **Bleeding** (*trauma, decreased platelets or deficient clotting factors result in the delay of or inability of the activation of the clotting pathway cause leakage of blood*)

- **Pain** (*swollen tissue, changes in pH and inflammatory changes cause tissue damage stimulate pain receptors transmit pain impulses to the brain*)

Priority nursing diagnoses within the health perception and health management functional health pattern that may be appropriate for patients include the following:

- *Health-Seeking Behaviors* as evidenced by dietary changes as prescribed, decreasing alcohol intake, stopping smoking, and joining a health club to participate in an exercise program.

- *Deficient Knowledge* as evidenced by lack of interest in learning about health care, inability to understand healthcare teaching (developmental level), and misinterpretation of healthcare teaching completed.

- *Ineffective Health Maintenance* as evidenced by smoking, drinking alcohol or other substance abuse, sedentary lifestyle, and not seeking routine health care.

- *Risk for Injury* as evidenced by poor hygiene habits, self treatment of illnesses, not taking prescribed medications, and participation in risk-seeking behaviors.

Two nursing diagnoses from other functional health patterns often are of high priority for the patient with deficits in health perception or health management:

- *Self-Care Deficit* (Activity-Exercise Functional Health Pattern)

- *Low Self-Esteem* (Self-Perception–Self-concept Functional health pattern)

Question

1. What questions will you ask your patients to determine his or her perceived pattern of health and well-being?

CLINICAL SCENARIO

Directions: *Read the following clinical scenario and answer the related questions. To complete this exercise successfully you will not only use knowledge of the content in this unit, but also principles related to setting priorities and maintaining patient safety.*

You have been assigned to work with the following home health care patients on the day shift. You receive a report at 0800. Significant data obtained during report is as follows:

- Mrs. Cora Swank, a 76-year-old female, had surgery 10 days ago for an obstructed colon that resulted in a permanent transverse colostomy. She was discharged from the acute care hospital yesterday. She lives with her 78-year-old husband. You need to evaluate her care of the colostomy and how well she can care for herself at home.
- Tom Smith is a 24-year-old who is at home due to osteomyelitis in the left leg from a previous leg fracture obtained when the motorcycle he was riding was involved in an accident. You need to change his left leg dressing and administer IV vancomycin (Vancocin) that is to be given every 12 hours. The next dose is due at 0930.
- Marguerite Garcia is an 86-year-old Hispanic who lives alone. She has hypertension, type II diabetes mellitus, and congestive heart failure. She is to have her blood pressure taken and a glucometer check for her blood sugar level. You will need to make sure she is taking her prescribed medications and set up her medications for the week.
- Sebastian Huian is a 56-year-old Asian who had a stroke which left him with left-sided weakness and some speech difficulties in addition to speaking little English. He smokes a half a pack of cigarettes daily. He is being discharged from the rehabilitation unit this morning. You will be doing an intake as the first home health visit to determine what his needs will be and how much assistance he will need from home health.

Questions

Priority Setting

1. What factors will you consider when deciding in which order you will visit these patients after report?
   A. _____
   B. _____
   C. _____

Health Promotion

1. An important part of primary prevention is to provide patient teaching related to the primary diagnosis. What primary prevention interventions will you talk to each patient about?
   A. _____
   B. _____
   C. _____
   D. _____

2. Tertiary level of prevention focuses on stopping the disease process and returning the affected patient to a useful place in society. Which is an example of a tertiary level of prevention for Mr. Huian?
   A. Eating a nutritious diet to promote healing and gain more strength.
   B. Having screenings for other disease processes, such as hypertension.
   C. Enrolling in a work training program for individuals with extremity weakness.
   D. Eliminating the use of smoking and alcohol.

Nursing Process

1. Besides obtaining vital signs, what diagnosis-specific assessment data should be collected for each patient?
   A. _____
   B. _____
   C. _____
   D. _____

2. Identify one nursing diagnoses for each of the patients presented earlier. What is the rationale for your choices?

	Nursing Diagnosis	Rationale
Cora Swank		
Tom Smith		
Marguerite Garcia		
Sebastian Huian		

3. Nursing interventions to ensure competent home care for Mr. Huian include which of the following? Select all that apply.
   A. Establish trust and rapport.
   B. Have his 14-year-old son translate for him.
   C. Assess the home environment for safety.
   D. Discuss having family members feed him due to his left arm weakness.
   E. Set goals for home health care and rehabilitation.

4. The nurse explains a diet of low sodium foods to Mrs. Garcia. What is the best way to evaluate Mrs. Garcia's understanding of the low sodium diet?

Communication

1. What information will you report to the next home health nurse who will be caring for Mr. Huian?

Delegation

1. What care or data collection for each patient can be delegated to a home health certified nursing assistant?

Nursing Ethics

1. During your initial visit to Tom Smith, he states, "When my leg is better, let's go dancing." How will you respond?

CASE STUDY: Betty Jo Moore

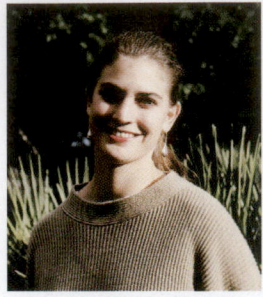

Betty Jo Moore is a 20-year-old who is admitted to the women's health unit for treatment of lower abdominal pain and tenderness, chills, and foul-smelling vaginal discharge. During the admission assessment she states that she is unmarried and has been sexually active for the past three years with multiple sexual partners. Vital signs are as follows: temperature 100.4°F, pulse 92, respirations 22, blood pressure 118/76. Lab studies drawn in the emergency department indicate a WBC count of 25,000 mm³, an erythrocyte sedimentation rate of 22mm/h, and a positive c-reactive protein. She is to begin IV antibiotic therapy and is in need of being educated about safe sex practices.

Ms. Moore is diagnosed with pelvic inflammatory disease. The pathophysiology of pelvic inflammatory disease (PID) is that pathogenic microorganisms enter the vagina during intercourse or other sexual activity and alter the cervical mucosa, allowing the microorganisms to travel to the uterus. The microorganisms can travel to the fallopian tubes and ovaries also. Multiplication of the microorganisms results in infection and possibly abscess formation. Manifestations of pelvic inflammatory disease include fever, chills, purulent vaginal discharge, vaginal bleeding, severe lower abdominal pain, pain on movement of the cervix, and dysuria. Complications that can occur from pelvic inflammatory disease are pelvic abscess, infertility, ectopic pregnancy, chronic pelvic pain, pelvic adhesions, and dyspareunia. Due to her medical diagnosis and history of unsafe sexual practices, the nursing diagnosis of Deficient Knowledge is appropriate for guiding nursing care.

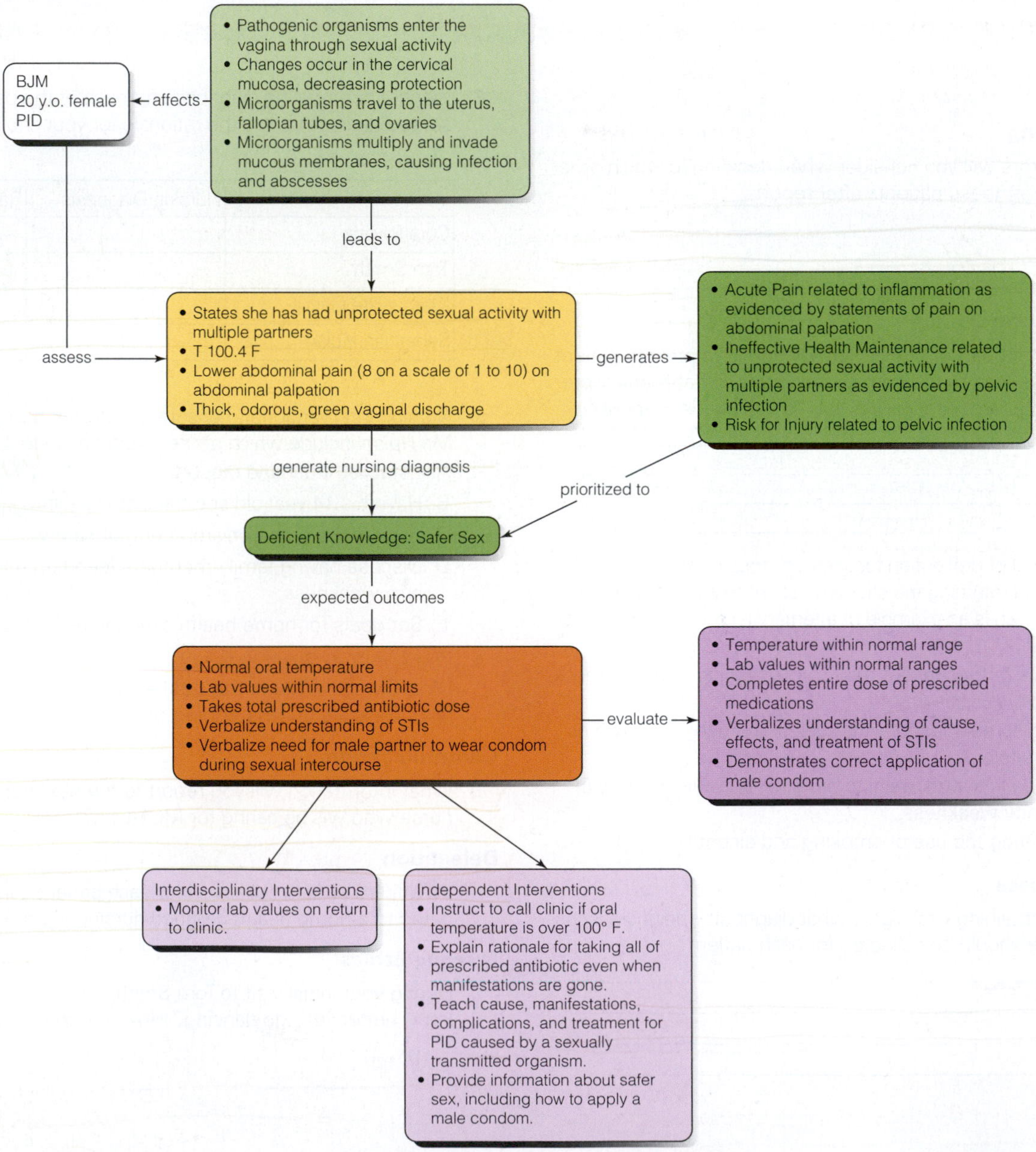

BJM
20 y.o. female
PID

← affects —

- Pathogenic organisms enter the vagina through sexual activity
- Changes occur in the cervical mucosa, decreasing protection
- Microorganisms travel to the uterus, fallopian tubes, and ovaries
- Microorganisms multiply and invade mucous membranes, causing infection and abscesses

leads to

assess →

- States she has had unprotected sexual activity with multiple partners
- T 100.4 F
- Lower abdominal pain (8 on a scale of 1 to 10) on abdominal palpation
- Thick, odorous, green vaginal discharge

— generates →

- Acute Pain related to inflammation as evidenced by statements of pain on abdominal palpation
- Ineffective Health Maintenance related to unprotected sexual activity with multiple partners as evidenced by pelvic infection
- Risk for Injury related to pelvic infection

generate nursing diagnosis

prioritized to

Deficient Knowledge: Safer Sex

expected outcomes

- Normal oral temperature
- Lab values within normal limits
- Takes total prescribed antibiotic dose
- Verbalize understanding of STIs
- Verbalize need for male partner to wear condom during sexual intercourse

— evaluate →

- Temperature within normal range
- Lab values within normal ranges
- Completes entire dose of prescribed medications
- Verbalizes understanding of cause, effects, and treatment of STIs
- Demonstrates correct application of male condom

Interdisciplinary Interventions
- Monitor lab values on return to clinic.

Independent Interventions
- Instruct to call clinic if oral temperature is over 100° F.
- Explain rationale for taking all of prescribed antibiotic even when manifestations are gone.
- Teach cause, manifestations, complications, and treatment for PID caused by a sexually transmitted organism.
- Provide information about safer sex, including how to apply a male condom.

Activity:

1. After reviewing the concept map, go to the Pearson Nursing Student Resources for this book at www.nursing.pearsonhighered.com to write a concept map based on the nursing diagnosis *Risk-Prone Health Behavior* as evidenced by multiple sexual partners. See answers and hints in Appendix C.

Alterations in Patterns of Health

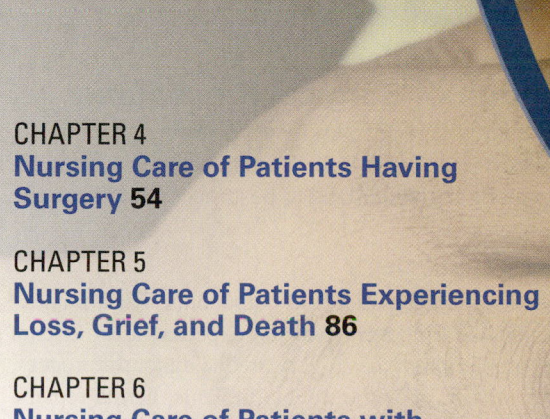

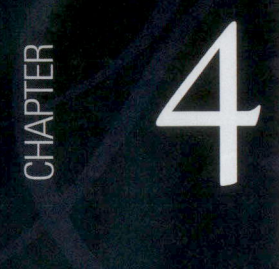
4 Nursing Care of Patients Having Surgery

LEARNING OUTCOMES

1. Compare the differences and similarities between outpatient and inpatient surgery.
2. Identify the three phases of perioperative care.
3. Interpret the significance of diagnostic tests used in the perioperative period.
4. Explain nursing implications for medications prescribed for the surgical patient.
5. Identify variations in perioperative care for the older adult.
6. Describe principles of pain management specific to acute postoperative pain control.

CLINICAL COMPETENCIES

1. Assess the physiologic and psychosocial health status of patients for surgery to determine their ability to tolerate surgery and identify risks for complications.
2. Participate in patient and family teaching prior to anesthesia, during postoperative care, and prior to discharge from the facility.
3. Use appropriate communication techniques to minimize risks associated with handoffs among healthcare team members during transitions between phases of the perioperative experience.
4. Observe and participate as appropriate with nursing responsibilities and interventions to promote patient safety and integrity and to prevent hazards in the operating room.
5. Use the nursing process to provide safe and effective nursing care for the patient in the preoperative, intraoperative, and postoperative phases of surgery.

KEY TERMS

anesthesia, 64	evisceration, 79	postoperative phase, 54
circulating nurse, 67	general anesthesia, 64	preoperative phase, 54
conscious sedation, 65	informed consent, 55	regional anesthesia, 64
dehiscence, 79	intraoperative phase, 54	scrub person, 67
equianalgesia, 80	perioperative nursing, 54	surgery, 54

Perioperative nursing is a specialized area of practice. It incorporates the three phases of the surgical experience: preoperative, intraoperative, and postoperative. The **preoperative phase** begins when the decision for surgery is made and ends when the patient is transferred to the operating room. The **intraoperative phase** begins with the patient's entry into the operating room and ends with admittance to the postanesthesia care unit (PACU), or recovery room. The **postoperative phase** begins with the patient's admittance to the PACU and ends with the patient's complete recovery from the surgical intervention. Although the perioperative nurse works in collaboration with other healthcare professionals to identify and meet the patient's needs, the perioperative nurse has the primary responsibility and accountability for nursing care of the patient undergoing surgery.

Surgery

Surgery is an invasive medical procedure performed to diagnose or treat illness, injury, or deformity. Although surgery is a medical treatment, the nurse assumes an active role in caring for the patient before, during, and after surgery. Interdisciplinary care and independent nursing care together prevent complications and promote the surgical patient's optimal recovery

Classification of Surgical Procedures

Surgical procedures can be classified according to purpose, risk, and urgency (see Table 4–1). Based on this information, nursing care can be individualized to best meet patient needs.

Settings for Surgery

Surgical patients may be inpatients or outpatients. The complexity of the surgery and recovery and the expected level of care needed upon completion of the surgery are the major differences. Cataract removal with or without lens implants, hernia repairs, tubal ligations, vasectomies, dilation and curettage (D&C), hemorrhoidectomies, diagnostic procedures, and biopsies are commonly performed as outpatient (same-day) surgeries.

Inpatient and outpatient surgeries are performed in the same operating suites in most hospitals. Outpatient surgery is also performed in freestanding surgical facilities and in physician's

TABLE 4–1 Classification of Surgical Procedures

	CLASSIFICATION	FUNCTION	EXAMPLES
Purpose	Diagnostic	Determine or confirm a diagnosis	Breast biopsy, bronchoscopy
	Ablative	Remove diseased tissue, organ, or extremity	Appendectomy, amputation
	Constructive	Build tissue/organs that are absent (congenital anomalies)	Repair of cleft palate
	Reconstructive	Rebuild tissue/organ that has been damaged	Skin graft after a burn, total joint replacement
	Palliative	Alleviate symptoms of a disease (not curative)	Bowel resection in patient with terminal cancer
	Transplant	Replace organs/tissue to restore function	Heart, lung, liver, kidney transplant
Risk	Minor	Minimal physical assault with minimal risk	Removal of skin lesions, dilation and curettage (D&C), cataract extraction
	Major	Extensive physical assault and/or serious risk	Transplant, total joint replacement, thoracotomy, colostomy, nephrectomy
Urgency	Elective	Suggested, though no foreseen ill effects if postponed	Cosmetic surgery, cataract surgery, bunionectomy
	Urgent	Necessary to be performed within 1 to 2 days	Heart bypass surgery, amputation resulting from gangrene, fractured hip
	Emergency	Performed immediately	Obstetric emergencies, bowel obstruction, ruptured aneurysm, life-threatening trauma

offices. The number of outpatient surgeries has grown rapidly in the past decade as part of the effort to contain the high costs of surgery. Moreover, increasingly complex surgeries on patients with complicated medical problems are now commonly performed on an outpatient basis. This increase in number of procedures and acuity level of the patients has presented a challenge to the perioperative nurse, the patient, and the family.

Outpatient surgery potentially offers several advantages:

- Decreased cost to the patient, hospital, and insuring agency
- Reduced risk of hospital-acquired infection
- Less interruption in the patient's and family's routine
- Possible reduction in time lost from work and/or other responsibilities
- Less physiologic stress to the patient and family

Many similarities exist between nursing care of inpatient and outpatient surgical patients. Physical care is provided in much the same manner in the preoperative, intraoperative, and postoperative phases of surgery. The major differences lie in the degree of teaching and emotional support that are necessary for outpatient surgical patients and their families. In addition to the physiologic insult of surgery, the outpatient surgical patient must cope with the additional stress of needing to learn a great deal of information in a short span of time. The nurse teaches the patient and family in both the preoperative and postoperative periods to enable the patient to perform self-care following discharge. More extensive teaching and emotional support is essential as patients requiring more complex surgical procedures and experiencing more complicated health problems undergo outpatient surgery.

PRACTICE ALERT
Patients having outpatient surgery should wear or bring clothing that will be easy to put on after surgery and will accommodate any dressings or appliances. Patients must also bring any medications, including herbal preparations, they regularly use.

Following outpatient surgery, the patient is discharged after meeting the institution's criteria, which are typically as follows:

- Vital signs are stable.
- Patient is able to stand and begin to walk without dizziness or nausea.
- Pain is controlled or alleviated.
- Patient is able to urinate.
- Patient is oriented.
- Patient and/or significant other demonstrates understanding of postoperative instructions.

Legal Requirements

It is the responsibility of the surgeon who performs the procedure to obtain the patient's consent for care. The surgeon should discuss the procedure with the patient and family in language they can understand. **Informed consent** is disclosure of risks associated with the intended procedure or operation to the patient, and is usually obtained by means of a legal document required for certain diagnostic procedures or therapeutic measures, including surgery. The language of the document varies according to statutory and common law of each state. This legal document protects the patient, nurse, physician, and healthcare facility. Informed consent includes the following information:

- Need for the procedure in relation to the diagnoses
- Description and purpose of the proposed procedure
- Possible benefits and potential risks
- Likelihood of a successful outcome
- Alternative treatments or procedures available
- Anticipated risks should the procedure not be performed
- Physician's advice as to what is needed
- Right to refuse treatment or withdraw consent

Ideally, the nurse should be present when the preceding information is provided. Later, the nurse can discuss the information with the patient and family, if necessary. If the patient has questions or concerns that were not discussed or made clear, or if the nurse questions the patient's understanding, the surgeon is responsible for supplying further information. If these situations arise, the nurse should contact the surgeon before having the patient sign a consent for the operation or special procedures. Following a thorough discussion of the consent, the nurse witnesses the patient's voluntary signature on the form (Figure 4–1 ■). The nurse also signs the form, indicating that the correct patient (or legal designee) is signing the form and that the patient was alert and aware of what was being signed.

Risk Factors

An independent national organization called the Institute for Healthcare Improvement (IHI) launched a campaign in 2004 to prevent an alleged 100,000 avoidable deaths in U.S. hospitals by 2006. Guided by these goals, hospitals implemented changes that spared more than 122,000 lives (Daniels, 2007). A 2006 initiative by IHI to further reduce medical harm was joined by a coalition of healthcare organizations called the Surgical Care Improve Project (SCIP). SCIP focuses on evidence-based interventions to reduce surgical complications including surgical site infections (SSIs), adverse cardiac events, and blood clots. Perioperative nursing should support and follow guidelines that will achieve these goals.

Prior to planning and implementing care for the surgical patient, the nurse must first assess the patient's needs and the factors that may increase the risks associated with surgery. The type of surgical procedure determines the assessment and interventions planned by the nurse. However, a complete assessment is also necessary to identify *risk factors* and to determine the patient's overall health status. Table 4–2 lists common risk factors for the patient undergoing surgery, and the related nursing interventions and implications. For example, when a patient is admitted for surgery on the right knee, it should be of concern to the nurse if this patient has diabetes, smokes 1.5 packs of cigarettes per day, has numbness in the right foot, and takes insulin. This information should be incorporated into a care plan, using appropriate nursing diagnoses and interventions to meet the patient's needs and assist the patient toward full postoperative recovery.

Risks are associated with all phases of surgery. For example, transporting the patient to and from the operating room (OR) requires assessment of the needs of the patient for supplemental oxygen, intravenous therapy, cardiac monitoring, and safety issues pertaining to the means of transport. Many patients enter

the operating suite highly anxious and may benefit from medication to help them relax prior to administration of anesthesia. This can be discussed with the anesthetist. Chemicals, electrical equipment, and environmental hazards in the surgical area have the potential for harm and must be monitored and maintained carefully. Also read about risks for the older patient in the Nursing Care of the Older Adult box on page 69.

Patient and Procedure Identification

The 2009 Patient Safety Goals issued by the Joint Commission specifically address patient and procedure identification prior to any treatment or procedure. The patient must be actively involved in identification procedures, and if the patient is not able to participate or reliability is questioned, the family or designated caregiver is responsible for verifying identification. Hence any patient whose reliability is questionable must be accompanied by the caregiver into the surgical area for the "time out" procedure (AORN, 2010).

Unfortunately, there is a risk of performing the wrong surgery on the wrong patient: wrong site, wrong procedure, wrong person (Gibbs, 2005). In 2004, the Joint Commission issued the Universal Protocol (Box 4–1) mandating preoperatively (1) verifying the procedure, (2) physically marking and initialing the site, and (3) taking a "time out" before starting any procedure. A time out is an intentional stoppage of the preparation for the operation in the operating suite before the patient is anesthetized. The goal of the time out is to ensure the right procedure will be performed on the right patient on the correct site with the necessary and correct healthcare providers in attendance. All participants are introduced, including the patient, and encouraged to ask any questions or express any concerns before the surgery is commenced.

BOX 4–1 The Universal Protocol

The Universal Protocol to reduce surgical errors calls for three specific actions by the healthcare team:

1. *Conduct a pre-procedure verification process* when the procedure is scheduled, during pre-admission testing, on admission to the facility, before entering the procedure room, and whenever the patient is transferred to another caregiver during the procedure. This process includes verifying the availability of the following:
   - ✓ Relevant documents such as the history and physical, pre-anesthesia assessment
   - ✓ Accurate, complete, and signed procedure consent form
   - ✓ Correct and accurately labeled diagnostic test results including x-rays
   - ✓ Any required blood products, implants, devices, or special equipment
2. *Mark the procedure site* for any procedure that involves incisions, punctures, or insertion of instruments. The site is to be marked by the healthcare provider performing the procedure or by an individual who will be directly involved and present during the procedure and while the patient is awake.
3. *"Time out" before starting the procedure* to conduct a final verification that the correct patient, site, positioning, and procedure are identified, and that all relevant documents, information, and equipment are available.

M.R. # _____

Informed Consent to Operation, Administration of Anesthetics, and to the Rendering of Other Medical Services

Saint
Francis
Medical
Center

1. I do hereby authorize and direct _____ M.D./D.O./D.D.S., my physician, and/or such associates or assistants of his choice, to perform the following operation or procedure:

_____

_____

upon _____ (patient's name). I understand that the above named physician and his associates or assistants are employed by me and will be occupied solely with performing such operation or procedure.

2. The nature of the operation or procedure has been explained to me and no warranty or guarantee has been made as to result or cure. I have been advised that additional surgical and/or medical procedures or treatment may be deemed necessary during the course of the operation or procedure consented hereto, and I fully consent to such additional procedures and treatment which, in the opinion of my physician, are deemed necessary or desirable for the well-being of the patient. The possible risks and complications of the operation or procedure have been explained to me. The physician has explained to me the above medical terminology and I satisfactorily understand the type of operation/procedure.

3. I hereby authorize and direct the above named physician and/or his associates or assistants or those working under his direction to provide for _____ (patient's name) such additional services as he or they may deem reasonable and necessary, including, but not limited to, the administration and maintenance of anesthesia, blood or blood derivatives, and the performance of services involving pathology and radiology and I hereby consent thereto. The possible risks and complications of blood transfusions and the administration of anesthetics have also been explained to me.

4. I understand also that the persons in attendance at such operation or procedure for the purpose of administering anesthesia, and the radiologists in attendance at such operation or procedure for the purpose of performing radiological (X-ray) service are not the agents, servants, or employees of St. Francis Medical Center nor of any physician, but are independent healthcare providers who are employed by me in the same way that my surgeon and physician are employed by me.

5. I hereby authorize the Medical Center pathologist or personnel to use their discretion in the disposal of any severed tissue or member.

6. I hereby grant permission for St. Francis Medical Center to obtain clinical photographs for educational purposes or for my patient record as deemed necessary by my physician.

7. The **exception to this consent:** (If none, write "none".) _____ _____ and I assume full responsibility for these exceptions.

_____   _____
PATIENT'S SIGNATURE   DATE

If the patient is a minor or incompetent or is unable to sign, the following must be completed:

I hereby certify that I am the (relationship) _____ of the above named patient who is unable to sign because _____ ,

and I am fully authorized to give the consent herein granted.

_____   _____
SIGNATURE   DATE

_____   _____
WITNESSED BY/date   **WITNESSED BY/date**

If signed in the physician's office, the following   **MUST be completed by the Medical Center.**

_____   _____
REVIEWED BY (patient name) **/date**   **WITNESSED BY /date**

Figure 4–1 ■ Informed consent form.

TABLE 4–2 Nursing Implications for Surgical Risk Factors

FACTOR	ASSOCIATED RISK	NURSING IMPLICATIONS
Adolescence *[handwritten: Developmental]*	Diversity in age and physical, cognitive, and psychologic maturation makes preparation for surgery vary in content and inclusion of significant others. Increased need for control, privacy, and peer interaction poses special challenges in the acute care setting.	Adapt assessment and interventions to the development level of individual patients, involving them in preparation and care to the extent possible. Allow for regressive and independent behavior including rejection of adult support.
Advanced age *[handwritten: Developmental]*	Older adults have age-related changes that affect physiologic, cognitive, and psychosocial responses to the stress of surgery; decreased tolerance of general anesthesia and postoperative medications; and delayed wound healing.	Selected nursing interventions are summarized in Table 4–6.
Malnutrition	Reserves may not be sufficient to allow the body to respond satisfactorily to the physical assault of surgery; organ failure and shock may result. Increased metabolic demands may result in poor wound healing and infection.	With the physician and dietitian, promote weight gain by providing a well-balanced diet high in calories, protein, and vitamin C. Administer parenteral nutrition, nutritional supplements, and enteral feedings as prescribed. Daily weights and calorie counts also may be ordered.
Obesity *[handwritten: psycho-sociocultural]*	The obese patient is at increased risk for delayed wound healing, wound dehiscence, infection, pneumonia, atelectasis, thrombophlebitis, dysrhythmias, and heart failure.	Promote weight reduction if time permits. Monitor closely for wound, pulmonary, and cardiovascular complications postoperatively. Encourage coughing, turning, and diaphragmatic breathing exercises and early ambulation.
Poverty *[handwritten: Psychosociocultural]*	Because of limited access to health care, pathology may be more advanced at diagnosis. Greater risk of exposure to hazardous waste and emotional stress, poor nutrition, lack of exercise, and poor social support systems.	Assess for undiagnosed chronic conditions, assess nutritional status, and involve a social worker for help with resources. Unattended children may accompany the patient and need assistance.
Chronic Conditions		
Alcoholism *[handwritten: Chemical]*	The patient may be malnourished and experience delirium tremens (acute withdrawal symptoms). More general anesthesia may be required. Hemorrhage and delayed wound healing can result from liver damage and poor nutritional status.	Monitor closely for signs of delirium tremens. Encourage well-balanced diet. Monitor for wound complications. Administer supplemental nutrients parenterally as ordered.
Arthritis *[handwritten: physiological]*	Inflammation or degenerative changes in joints limits mobility and comfort.	Position and pad arthritic joints including the spine. Handle joints gently to avoid strain on ligaments and tendons.
Cardiovascular disorders *[handwritten: physiological]*	Presence of cardiovascular disease increases the risk of heart failure, hemorrhage and shock, hypotension, venous thrombosis, pulmonary embolism, stroke (especially in the older patient), and fluid volume overload.	Diligently monitor vital signs, especially pulse rate, regularity, and rhythm, and general condition of the patient. Closely monitor fluid intake (oral and parenteral) to prevent circulatory overload. Assess skin color. Assess for chest pain, lung congestion, and peripheral edema. Observe for signs of hypoxia, and administer oxygen as ordered. Early postoperative ambulation and leg exercises reduce the risk of vascular problems, such as venous thrombosis and pulmonary embolism. Determine that prescribed beta-blockers are given preoperatively.
Diabetes mellitus *[handwritten: physiological]*	Diabetes causes an increased risk for fluctuating blood glucose levels, which can lead to life-threatening hypoglycemia or ketoacidosis. Diabetes also increases the risk for cardiovascular disease, delayed wound healing, and wound infection.	Monitor the patient closely for manifestations of hypoglycemia and hyperglycemia. Monitor blood glucose levels every 4 hours or as ordered. Administer insulin as prescribed. Encourage intake of food at the designated meal and snack times.
Immune suppression	Suppressed immunity impairs ability to resist infection and promote tissue repair. Advanced age, HIV, autoimmune diseases, chronic pain, immune deficiency diseases, malnutrition, splenectomy, and alcohol abuse compromise immunity.	Prevent hypothermia, maintain sterile fields, consistently prevent infection. Nourishment and normoglycemia promote wound healing.

TABLE 4–2 Nursing Implications for Surgical Risk Factors (continued)

FACTOR	ASSOCIATED RISK	NURSING IMPLICATIONS
Nicotine use *chemical*	Cigarette smokers are at increased risk for respiratory complications such as pneumonia, atelectasis, and bronchitis because of increased mucous secretions and a decreased ability to expel them.	Ideally, the patient should quit smoking. Be supportive of the patient, and monitor closely for respiratory difficulties. Coughing, turning, and diaphragmatic breathing exercises with early ambulation are very important. Increase daily fluid intake to 2500–3000 mL (unless contraindicated) to help liquefy respiratory secretions to aid expectoration. A nicotine patch may help the patient tolerate withdrawal during the postoperative period.
Renal and liver disorders *physiological*	The patient with renal or liver dysfunction may poorly tolerate general anesthesia, have fluid/electrolyte and acid–base imbalances, decreased metabolism and excretion of drugs, increased risk for hemorrhage, and delayed wound healing.	Monitor for fluid volume overload, intake and output (I&O), and response to medication. Evaluate closely for drug side effects and evidence of acidosis or alkalosis.
Respiratory disorders *physiological*	Respiratory complications such as bronchitis, atelectasis, and pneumonia are some of the most common and serious postoperative complications. Respiratory depression from general anesthesia and acid–base imbalance may also occur. Patients with pulmonary disease are more at risk for developing these complications.	Closely monitor respirations, pulse, and breath sounds. Also assess for hypoxia, dyspnea, lung congestion, and chest pain. Encourage coughing, turning, and diaphragmatic breathing exercises and early postoperative ambulation. Encourage the patient to quit smoking or at least to reduce the number of cigarettes smoked.
Medical Therapies		
Medications *chemical*	Anesthesia interaction with some medications can cause respiratory difficulties, hypotension, and circulatory collapse. Other medications can produce side effects that may increase surgical risk.	Inform the anesthesiologist of all prescribed and over-the-counter medications, as well as any herbal preparations.
Anticoagulants	May cause intraoperative and postoperative hemorrhage.	Monitor for bleeding. Assess PT/PTT values.
Antidepressants (particularly monoamine oxidase inhibitors)	Increase the hypotensive effects of anesthesia.	Closely monitor blood pressure.
Antihypertensives	Increase the hypotensive effects of anesthesia.	Closely monitor blood pressure.
Antibiotics (particularly the "mycin" group)	May cause apnea and respiratory paralysis.	Monitor respirations.
Diuretics	May lead to fluid and electrolyte imbalances, producing altered cardiovascular response and respiratory depression.	Monitor I&O and electrolytes. Assess cardiovascular and respiratory status.
Herbal supplements	Some may prolong the effects of anesthesia. Others may increase the risks of bleeding or raise blood pressure.	Inquire about the use of herbs or other dietary supplements. These should be discontinued at least 2 weeks before surgery.
Immunosuppressants	Steroids, drugs to treat cancer, and transplant rejection drugs suppress the immune system and increase the risk of infection and hypothermia (Neil, 2007).	Monitor CBC with differential for leukopenia. Document current dosage of medications and time of last dose. Administer prescribed steroids in the perioperative period to prevent adrenal crisis. Prevent hypothermia and maintain sterile fields. Monitor wound and protect from infection.
Treatments	Radiation therapy	Tissue integrity may be compromised in targeted fields.
In the OR		
Fluid/electrolyte imbalance	Depending on the degree of dehydration and/or the type of electrolyte imbalance, cardiac dysrhythmias or heart failure may occur. Liver and renal failure may also result.	Administer intravenous fluids as ordered. Monitor I&O. Monitor patient for evidence of electrolyte imbalance (∞ see Chapter 10).
Hypothermia/hyperthermia	Deviations from normothermia, either hypothermia or hyperthermia, may cause infection, cardiac morbidity, myocardial ischemia, surgical bleeding, skin damage, or patient discomfort.	Monitor core temperatures and prevent chilling or overheating. Remove wet drapes and test the temperature of fluids used.

(continued)

TABLE 4–2 Nursing Implications for Surgical Risk Factors (continued)

FACTOR	ASSOCIATED RISK	NURSING IMPLICATIONS
Surgical site infections	Contamination of sterile fields as well as opening body organs containing pathogens leads to infection.	Administer antibiotics prior to incision as ordered. Carefully maintain sterile fields. Monitor and sustain core body temperature between 36°C and 38°C.
Venous stasis	Lower limbs, especially when tourniquets are applied, are susceptible to blood clotting. Patients with cancer have higher risks of blood clots.	Promote venous circulation with intermittent pneumatic compression devices as ordered. Monitor circulation in arms and legs during surgery.

SAFETY ALERT

It is very important to establish the right and duty of all members of the surgical team to advocate for the safety of the patient. Important processes such as counting of sponges and equipment are time-consuming and may seem less important when urged by team members with less "power" (Jackson & Brady, 2008).

Retainment of Foreign Objects

Another potential error is retained foreign bodies such as instruments, needles, or sponges. To prevent accidental retention the American College of Surgeons recommends

- consistent application and adherence to standardized procedures for the counting of objects used in the surgery,
- methodical wound exploration before closing the site,
- using x-ray detectable materials in the wound,
- maintenance of optimal OR environments to allow focused surgical performance (minimizing distractions such as change of personnel, telephone calls, beepers, and pages),
- employing technological methods to ensure no unintended item remains, and
- suspension of these measures as needed in life-threatening situations (Gibbs, 2005; Jackson & Brady, 2008).

While not all surgeries have equal risk for retainment of items, those that do must include a careful count procedure with appropriate action if the count is incorrect. Stopping a closing procedure to recount and search for missing items increases anesthesia and wound exposure, but leaving items contributes to serious infections and other potential liabilities (Jackson & Brady, 2008).

Medication Reconciliation

A complete history of medications the patient has been taking regularly is vital information at every transition point in the care continuum. Over-the-counter medicines and herbal preparations as well as prescription medications may interact with drugs given during surgery, putting a patient at increased risk (Saber, 2006). As part of the preoperative planning and teaching, early consideration of all medications including complementary and alternative medicine is important. This information should be obtained in a matter-of-fact and nonjudgmental manner, because a judgmental attitude could cause the patient to withhold information. This process needs to be repeated at

every transition: admission to the hospital, preoperatively, in postoperative reports, and at discharge.

Medications may interact with anesthesia drugs during surgery, augmenting hemodynamic effects such as hypertension or hypotension. Some categories of medication require special consideration in regard to surgery (Saber, 2006). These include drugs that alter blood clotting, replace adrenal hormones, prevent seizures, antiparkinsonian drugs, antipsychotics, anxiolytics, bronchodilators, cardiovascular drugs, glaucoma drugs, immunosuppressants, and thyroid or antithyroid drugs. Patients with diabetes or HIV infection who are being treated with antivirals require expert advice (Rahman & Beattie, 2008). Anticoagulant medications should be discontinued prior to surgery to prevent excessive blood loss during surgery. These include aspirin and nonsteroidal anti-inflammatory drugs. If laboratory tests of bleeding time, prothrombin time (PT), partial thromboplastin time (PTT), and international normalized ratio (INR) are elevated, the surgery may be cancelled. Guidelines for discontinuing use vary according to the particular medication; it is generally recommended that aspirin or products containing aspirin be discontinued 5 days or longer before surgery. Similarly, herbs or nutritional supplements that impair clotting should be discontinued 2 weeks prior to surgery (Saper, 2005). The most common self-prescribed medicines that may inhibit coagulation are vitamin E, garlic, ginkgo, ginseng, fish oil, and chamomile. Many plants contain coumarins with the potential to interact with warfarin and inhibit coagulation. Others inhibit platelet aggregation or prevent the conversion of fibrinogen to fibrin. Patients taking warfarin for the risk of blood clots due to atrial fibrillation will be counseled about the appropriate time to withdraw warfarin. If surgery is urgent due to trauma or sudden onset of morbidity, the impact of anticoagulants needs to be evaluated with PT, PTT, and INR before the operation and appropriate support for clotting administered.

In addition to clotting impairment, excessive consumption of herbal medicines or dietary supplements can produce levels of chemicals that interact with conventional medications, exacerbating or impairing the intended effect. Anesthesia drugs often decrease hepatic blood flow and interfere with metabolism and elimination of medications (Bressler, 2005). This increases the risk of adverse drug–herbal supplement interactions during surgery. Cardiovascular instability, impaired glucose control, increased metabolism of perioperative medication, and unpredictable response to anesthesia are categories of adverse reactions of perioperative herbal use (Saper, 2005).

Thromboembolism

The risk of bleeding has to be balanced against the risk of postoperative deep venous thrombosis (DVT) and thromboembolism. Prophylactic anticoagulation with low-dose unfractionated heparin, low-molecular-weight heparin, factor Xa, or warfarin may be used for this purpose. Aspirin-only therapy is not considered adequate protection from DVT formation (Daniels, 2007). In addition, use of intermittent pneumatic compression devices (IPCDs) and graduated compression stockings is recommended. DVTs can lead to pulmonary embolism (PE) and to significant patient morbidity, mortality, and increased healthcare cost. Each patient's risk for developing DVT and PE needs to be assessed and appropriate prophylaxis initiated when indicated.

Hypothermia

Hypothermia is a risk in the perioperative period. The anesthetized patient loses heat intraoperatively and is unable to restore temperature through the normal mechanisms of shivering or muscle contractions. Typically, surgical suites are maintained quite cold for the comfort of the personnel gowned in several layers of protective clothing and wearing masks. Lowering environmental temperature is common in surgical suites, but research shows that normothermia (core body temperature in the range of 36.0°C to 37.5°C [Porth, 2007]) in the patient provides less risk to the patient for infection, cardiac morbidity, myocardial ischemia, surgical bleeding, and patient discomfort. Methods to minimize the risk of hypothermia include applying warm blankets, limiting the amount of skin exposed, warming intravenous fluids, and monitoring the patient's temperature.

Hyperthermia should also be avoided. Heating of fluids or use of heating units necessitates accurate measurement of the temperature and assessment of the patient's skin integrity. Body temperature is best evaluated through core temperature monitoring, which includes esophageal or tympanic assessment (AORN, 2010; Weirich, 2008).

Surgical Site Infections (SSIs)

Despite the carefully clean OR environment and use of sterile equipment, gloves, and gowns, a significant percentage of patients develop wound infections. Patients suffer increased morbidity and mortality, and healthcare costs increase dramatically as a result of SSIs. Four strategies are recommended by SCIP guidelines: prophylactic antibiotics in select procedures, appropriate hair removal, glucose control in patients having major cardiac surgery, and normothermia in patients undergoing colon surgery. Prophylactic antibiotic administration immediately before the surgical incision is indicated for hip and knee arthroplasty, cardiac surgery including coronary artery bypass graft, hysterectomy, and some colon and vascular procedures (Daniels, 2007).

Adverse Cardiac Events

Myocardial infarction is a risk following major surgery, especially among elderly patients. The circulatory system is stressed during surgery, increasing the risk for cardiac ischemia. Beta-blocker medications slow nerve conduction to the myocardium and reduce oxygen demand, thereby reducing the risk for infarction. Any patient who is taking beta-blocker medication regularly needs to take the usual dose prior to any type of surgery.

Interpreting and responding to identified risk factors require nursing judgment. It is important to bring information to the attention of the surgeons and anesthesiologists prior to surgery so necessary modifications can be made for the patient.

Interdisciplinary Care

The patient undergoing surgery receives care from a number of healthcare providers. Surgeons, nurses, scrub technicians, anesthetists, phlebotomists, x-ray technicians, registration clerks, and transporters are often involved in securing the safety and health of patients. Case managers, social workers, and spiritual care providers are available based on patient need and desire. This interdisciplinary approach focuses on placing the patient in the best possible health status before, during, and after surgery.

Diagnostic Tests

Diagnostic tests performed prior to surgery provide baseline data or reveal problems that may place the patient at additional risk during and after surgery. Because of the trend toward shortened hospital stays, many diagnostic studies and procedures are performed in a preadmission clinic within a week prior to elective surgery.

Complete blood counts, electrolyte studies, coagulation studies, and urinalysis are the most commonly performed preoperative laboratory tests. Table 4–3 discusses the significance and nursing implications of abnormal findings for these common tests. Additional diagnostic tests may be performed as the history and physical findings indicate. For example, if the patient has a low hemoglobin and hematocrit, and significant blood loss during surgery is anticipated, the surgeon may order a type and crossmatch of the patient's blood for a possible transfusion.

In addition to laboratory tests, older patients or those with risk factors related to heart and lung function typically have a chest x-ray. This radiologic procedure provides baseline information about the size, shape, and condition of the heart and lungs. Pulmonary complications such as lung disease, tuberculosis, calcification, infiltration, or pneumonia may require that surgery be postponed to allow the patient to undergo further evaluation or treatment. If findings are abnormal and the surgery cannot be postponed, information from the chest x-ray study can be used to determine the safest form of anesthesia.

Another commonly performed preoperative diagnostic procedure is the electrocardiogram (ECG). This test is ordered routinely on patients undergoing general anesthesia when they are over 40 years of age or have cardiovascular disease. The ECG provides data for evaluation about either new or preexisting cardiac conditions. The patient's surgery may be cancelled or postponed if a life-threatening cardiac condition is discovered.

In addition to the chest x-ray study and ECG, other diagnostic tests may be performed preoperatively to gather further assessment data. For example, for patients who have chronic

TABLE 4–3 Laboratory Tests for Perioperative Assessment

TEST	SIGNIFICANCE OF INCREASED VALUES	SIGNIFICANCE OF DECREASED VALUES	NURSING IMPLICATIONS
Hemoglobin (Hgb) and hematocrit (Hct)	Dehydration, excessive fluid plasma loss, polycythemia vera	Fluid overload, excessive blood loss, anemia	Monitor oxygenation, and vital signs; assess for bleeding.
Glucose and hemoglobin-A1c	Impaired glucose metabolism, stress, or infection	Inadequate glucose intake in relation to insulin	If decreased, monitor for manifestations of hypoglycemia. Notify surgeon of glucose <70 mg/dL or >180 mg/dL.
White blood cell (WBC) count	Infectious/inflammatory processes, leukemia	Immune deficiencies	Monitor for manifestations of inflammation; monitor drainage, temperature, and pulse. Use strict standard precautions.
Platelet count	Malignancies, polycythemia vera	Clotting deficiency disorders, chemotherapy	If decreased, assess for bleeding at incision sites and drainage tubes, and assess for hematomas.
Carbon dioxide (CO_2)	Emphysema, chronic bronchitis, asthma, pneumonia, respiratory acidosis, vomiting, nasogastric suctioning	Metabolic acidosis, hyperventilation	Monitor respiratory status and arterial blood gases (ABGs).
Electrolytes			
Potassium (K^+)	Kidney dysfunction, dehydration, suctioning	Side effects of diuretics, vomiting, NG suctioning	Monitor K^+ level, cardiac and neurologic function, and preoperative diuretic therapy.
Sodium (Na^+)	Kidney dysfunction, dehydration, normal saline-containing intravenous fluids	Side effects of diuretics, vomiting, NG suctioning, fluid volume excess	Monitor Na^+ level and I&O; assess for peripheral edema and effects of perioperative diuretic therapy.
Chloride (Cl^-)	Kidney dysfunction, dehydration, alkalosis	Side effects of diuretics, vomiting, NG suctioning	Monitor Cl^- level and I&O; assess for peripheral edema and perioperative diuretic therapy.
Prothrombin time (protime, or PT) and partial thromboplastin time (PTT)	Defect in mechanism for blood clotting, anticoagulant therapy (aspirin, heparin, warfarin), side effect of other drugs affecting clotting time	Hypercoagulability of the blood may lead to thrombus formation in the veins	If clotting time is elevated, monitor PT/PTT values. Assess for bleeding at incision site and drainage tubes and for hematomas. If clotting time is decreased, monitor for thrombus formation (pulmonary emboli, venous thrombosis), and evaluate PT and PTT values.
Urinalysis	Varied	Varied	Used to detect abnormal substances (e.g., protein, glucose, red blood cells, or bacteria) in the urine. Notify surgeon if abnormalities are detected.
Serum creatinine, BUN	Renal dysfunction	Malnutrition, musculoskeletal wasting	Monitor urinary output, wound healing.

obstructive pulmonary disease, pulmonary function studies often are performed to determine the extent of respiratory dysfunction. This information guides the anesthesiologist before and during surgery in choosing the type of anesthetic to be used, and it guides the surgeon and nursing staff in the recovery phase.

Renal function is evaluated on the basis of glomerular filtration rate (GFR) which is estimated by using serum creatinine (reported as the eGFR) or by measuring urinary creatine. Creatinine is a stable product of muscle mass; it is filtered by the kidneys or secreted by the kidney tubules. In kidney failure, serum creatinine rises and the GFR is low. The best indicator of GFR is the creatinine clearance, a comparison of both serum and urinary creatinine levels. In older adults with decreased muscle mass and low dietary meat intake, serum creatinine may be falsely low. Older adults are especially susceptible to renal insufficiency, which puts them at risk for fluid volume overload in the perioperative period and for accumulation of metabolic by-products and medications dependent on renal clearance (Loran et al., 2005; Giannelli, 2007).

Medications

The patient having surgery receives medications before, during, and after surgery to achieve specific therapeutic outcomes. Traditionally, all medication orders are cancelled when the patient goes to surgery and must be rewritten by the physician when the patient returns to the postsurgical care unit. Following surgery it is very important that medications are re-ordered so that chronic as well as acute conditions will be treated.

PREOPERATIVE MEDICATIONS A combination of preoperative drugs may be ordered to achieve a multitude of desired outcomes with minimal side effects. Such outcomes include sedation, reducing anxiety, inducing amnesia to minimize unpleasant surgical memories, increasing comfort during preoperative procedures, reducing gastric acidity and volume, increasing gastric emptying, decreasing nausea and vomiting, and reducing the incidence of aspiration by drying oral and respiratory secretions.

The surgical patient usually is given preoperative medications 45 to 70 minutes before the scheduled surgery. Any delay in administration should be reported promptly to the surgical department. Preoperative medications are often given in the surgical holding area.

TABLE 4–4 Examples of Commonly Used Preoperative Medications

GENERIC	TRADE	ACTION BY CATEGORY	NURSING IMPLICATIONS
Antibiotics			
Cefazolin	Ancef	Prevents surgical site infections in orthopedic and general surgeries and is associated with lower risk of mortality in elderly patients	Patients with beta-lactam allergies receive vancomycin or clindamycin.
Benzodiazepines			
Midazolam	Versed	Decreases anxiety and produces sedation to some extent	Monitor for respiratory depression, hypotension, drowsiness, and lack of coordination.
Diazepam	Valium	Induces amnesia	
Lorazepam	Ativan	May induce substantial amnesia	
Opioid Analgesics			
Morphine	Morphine	Decreases anxiety, provides analgesia	Monitor for respiratory depression and safety if ambulating. ∞ See Chapter 9 for nursing implications of specific opioid analgesics.
Fentanyl	Sublimaze	Allows reduced anesthetic dose	
Oxycodone	Roxicodone		
Hydrocodone	Vicodin		
Tramadol	Ultram		
Codeine	Tylenol with Codeine		
Antacids			
Sodium citrate	Bicitra	Increases the pH and reduces volume of gastric fluid; used in patients with GERD and/or trauma	No significant factors in this setting.
H₂ Receptor Antagonists			
Cimetidine	Tagamet	Reduces gastric acid volume and concentration	Monitor for confusion and dizziness in older adults.
Famotidine	Pepcid		
Nizatidine	Axid		
Ranitidine	Zantac		
Gastric Acid (Proton) Pump Inhibitors			
Lansoprazole	Prevacid	Suppresses gastric acid secretion	Monitor for dizziness and headache, rash, or thirst.
Omeprazole	Prilosec		
Pantoprazole	Protonix		
Antiemetics			
Metoclopramide	Reglan	Enhances gastric emptying	Monitor for sedation and extrapyramidal symptoms (involuntary movement, muscle tone changes, and abnormal posture).
Droperidol	Inapsine	Tranquilizer	
Anticholinergics			
Atropine sulfate	Atropine sulfate	Reduces oral and respiratory secretions to decrease risk of aspiration; decreases vomiting and laryngospasm	Monitor for confusion, restlessness, and tachycardia. Prepare patient to expect a dry mouth.
Glycopyrrolate	Robinul		
Scopolamine	Scopolamine		

Preoperative antibiotic prophylaxis is effective in the prevention of postoperative complications in many surgeries (Andersen et al., 2005; Daniels, 2007). Table 4–4 outlines commonly prescribed preoperative medications.

An increasingly common and controversial strategy to prevent intense or lingering pain is the use of *preemptive analgesia* (D'Arcy, 2008). The goal of preemptive analgesia is to prevent sensitization of the central and peripheral nervous system from painful stimuli by blocking the pain pathways with local, regional, or epidural analgesia prior to incision. Sensitization to pain is believed to prolong the painful experience; blocking the sensitization throughout the perioperative period should result in decreased pain in the postoperative period, shortened hospital stay, quicker return to self-care, and decreased residual pain (Polomano et al., 2008; Ong et al., 2005). To date, the best combination of methods and medications for the great variety of surgical interventions has not been identified. The best method to improve postoperative pain scores, reduce total analgesic consumption, and extend the time to first rescue dose following anesthesia seems to be a combination of epidural, local wound infiltration, and nonsteroidal anti-inflammatory drugs (NSAIDs). Opioids given preoperatively do not enhance comfort in the postoperative period (Ong et al, 2005).

Decisions about which of the patient's routine medications to administer prior to surgery when the patient is NPO require careful analysis. The best guideline is to confer with the surgeon and anesthetist about specific medications. The reason for caution has to do with potential interactions between anesthesia and medications and the effect on the patient if drugs such as steroids, antiseizure medications, and tranquilizers are discontinued abruptly. Generally, insulin is withheld when the patient is NPO, but depending on the anticipated length of the surgery, the dosage may be adjusted for the previous evening as well as the morning of surgery. Under anesthesia the manifestations of hypoglycemia (insulin reaction) are absent, so withholding insulin the morning of surgery when the patient is NPO is advisable. Plasma glucose is monitored intermittently during surgery with the goal of maintaining normal blood sugar level (see Table 4–2). Patients who ordinarily manage their diabetes mellitus with oral medications often are placed on sliding scale insulin to manage blood glucose during the perioperative experience. Evidence-based practice supports subcutaneous basal insulin administration for hyperglycemic patients to maintain glycemia below 180 mg/dL throughout the perioperative period. This practice is associated with better healing, fewer infections, and shorter hospital stays (Odom-Forren, 2006).

INTRAOPERATIVE MEDICATIONS

Anesthesia is used to produce unconsciousness, analgesia, reflex loss, and muscle relaxation during a surgical procedure. **General anesthesia** produces all of these effects, whereas **regional anesthesia** results in analgesia, reflex loss, and muscle relaxation but does not cause the patient to lose consciousness. An anesthesiologist (physician) or certified registered nurse anesthetist (CRNA) administers anesthetics during the intraoperative phase of surgery.

General Anesthesia General anesthesia is most commonly administered by inhalation and, to a lesser extent, by the intravenous route. It produces central nervous system depression. As a result, the patient loses consciousness and does not perceive pain, the skeletal muscles relax, and reflexes diminish.

Advantages to general anesthesia include rapid excretion of the anesthetic agent and prompt reversal of its effects when desired. Additionally, general anesthesia can be used with all age groups and any type of surgical procedure. It produces amnesia.

Disadvantages of general anesthesia include risks associated with circulatory, respiratory, hepatic, and renal side effects. Patients with serious respiratory or circulatory diseases, such as emphysema or congestive heart failure, are at greater risk for complications. Patients with renal or hepatic disease cannot metabolize and eliminate anesthetics safely. Inhalation agents are avoided in patients with a history of malignant hyperthermia (MH) because they can trigger MH (Box 4–1). With the increase in ambulatory and minimally invasive surgeries, anesthetics are used that enable shorter recovery phases. Drugs with a very short half-life have a rapid recovery phase, allowing *fast-tracking*, often bypassing the post anesthesia care unit (PACU) (Hassan & Fahy, 2005).

The phases of general anesthesia are divided into three distinct categories: induction, maintenance, and emergence. During the induction phase, the patient receives the anesthetic agent intravenously or by inhalation. During this phase, airway

---

BOX 4–2 Malignant Hyperthermia (MH)

Malignant hyperthermia (MH) is a rare autosomal dominant disorder that can be triggered by inhalational anesthetic gases and succinylcholine, a depolarizing neuromuscular blocker. The initial manifestations are an unexplained rise in end-tidal carbon dioxide that does not respond to ventilation and sustained skeletal muscle contraction (Carter-Templeton, 2005). The temperature rises rapidly as high as 43°C as result of sustained hypermetabolism. Cardiac dysrhythmias develop and oxygen and ATP are rapidly consumed. Lactate and carbon dioxide, byproducts of metabolism, are produced in excess (Porth & Matfin, 2009). If unchecked the condition will progress to hyperkalemia, myoglobinuria, disseminated intravascular coagulation, congestive heart failure, bowel ischemia, and compartment syndrome in the limbs.

MH can develop during surgery or when the patient returns to the PACU. If the early symptoms of MH (e.g., escalating temperature, increased carbon dioxide production) are identified, suspected triggering agents are immediately discontinued. Oxygen is immediately administered with a nonrebreather mask. The patient should not be unattended, good IV access should be maintained, and the anesthesia provider should be summoned. Dantrolene, a muscle relaxant, is administered and measures to decrease core body temperature should be started at once and continued until core temperature is 36.0°C. A urinary catheter should be placed to monitor urine output and blood drawn for testing. Blood gases should be drawn to measure pH; sodium bicarbonate is given to correct metabolic acidosis. Insulin may be ordered to decrease serum potassium. This patient may be transferred to the ICU for continued monitoring and doses of dantrolene every 4–6 hours.

patency is achieved and maintained with either endotracheal intubation or newer devices including the laryngeal mask airway (LMA) esophageal-tracheal Combitube, or lighted stylet or wand (Hassan & Fahy, 2005). These newer methods of airway maintenance do not require direct visualization of the vocal cords for placement. They allow effective ventilation and can prevent the need for surgical tracheostomy in patients who are difficult to intubate.

The next phase of general anesthesia is maintenance. During this period, the patient is positioned, the skin is prepared, and surgery is performed. The anesthesiologist maintains the proper depth of anesthesia while constantly monitoring physiologic parameters such as heart rate, blood pressure, respiratory rate, temperature, and oxygen and carbon dioxide levels.

The final phase of anesthesia is the patient's emergence from this altered physiologic state. As the anesthetic agents are withdrawn or the effects reversed pharmacologically, the patient begins to awaken. The endotracheal tube or laryngeal mask is removed (extubated) once the patient is able to reestablish voluntary breathing. It is critical to ensure airway patency during this period, because extubation may cause bronchospasm or laryngospasm.

Regional Anesthesia

Regional anesthesia is a type of anesthesia in which medication instilled around the nerves blocks transmission of nerve impulses in a particular area. Regional anesthesia produces analgesia, relaxation, and reduced reflexes. The patient is awake and conscious during the surgical procedure but does not perceive pain. Regional anesthesia may be classified in several ways:

- **Local nerve infiltration** is achieved by injecting lidocaine, bupivacaine, or tetracaine around a local nerve to suppress sensation over a limited area of the body. This technique may be used when a skin or muscle biopsy is obtained or when a small wound is sutured.
- **Nerve blocks** are accomplished by injecting an anesthetic agent at the nerve trunk to produce a lack of sensation over a specific larger area, such as an extremity.
- **Epidural blocks** are local anesthetic agents injected into the epidural space, outside the dura mater of the spinal cord. This type of intraspinal anesthesia provides safe and effective pain relief for patients of all ages with less risk of adverse effects than general anesthesia. It is indicated for surgeries of the arms and shoulders, thorax, abdomen, pelvis, and lower extremities (Schwartz, 2006). The epidural catheter is often left in place for pain relief in the postoperative period; it can also be used for chronic pain management.

Spinal anesthesia is administered similarly to epidural except the anesthetic medication is infused in a single injection. Spinal anesthesia is effective for approximately 90 minutes. Surgeries of the lower abdomen, perineum, and lower extremities are likely to use this type of regional anesthesia. Leakage of cerebrospinal fluid (CSF) into the epidural space can cause reduced CSF pressure and postoperative headaches. Treatment may include hydration, caffeine, analgesics, or administration of an epidural blood patch (Schwartz, 2006). Hypotension is common with epidural and spinal anesthesia. Blood pressure should be monitored and, if critical hypotension occurs, the anesthesia provider should be alerted and expected to increase intravenous fluids and administer vasoactive medications.

Conscious Sedation

An increasing number of surgical and diagnostic procedures are being performed using **conscious sedation**. This type of anesthesia provides analgesia, amnesia, and moderate sedation. The pharmacologic effects are produced by administering a combination of intravenous medications with opioids (such as morphine sulfate or fentanyl [Sublimaze]) or sedatives (such as diazepam [Valium] and midazolam [Versed]). During conscious sedation the patient is able to independently maintain an open airway. This allows the patient to respond to verbal and physical stimulation. Physician supervision is always required and a registered nurse must be prepared to initiate rescue if sedation becomes too deep. Institutions base their policies defining the qualifications of those who care for patients undergoing conscious sedation on professional organization guidelines, regulatory agency requirements, and state law.

Assessment prior to conscious sedation includes evaluating the appropriateness of the patient based on physical status. Patients with compromised circulation or airway, a history of sleep apnea or snoring, a history of problems with anesthesia or analgesia, or medications that would potentially interact with conscious analgesia medications may require the anesthesiologist to manage conscious sedation procedures. Patients need to be appropriately fasting, and baseline vital signs must be taken prior to giving the sedative. A consent form must be signed by the patient, and a patent IV line must be in place. Equipment to rescue the patient should be available if sedation becomes too deep. Oxygen saturation, pulse, breathing, and level of consciousness must be monitored throughout the procedure.

Common adverse side effects include venous thrombosis, phlebitis, local irritation, confusion, drowsiness, hypotension, and apnea. Reversal agents (naloxone hydrochloride [Narcan] and flumazenil [Romazicon]) are used as needed to enhance the safety of conscious sedation.

POSTOPERATIVE MEDICATIONS Management of acute postoperative pain by medication improves with greater understanding of pain physiology and the development of better methods to deliver adequate pain medication. For more information on pain management, ∞ see Chapter 9.

Established, persistent, severe pain is more difficult to treat than pain that is at its onset. Therefore, postoperative analgesics should be administered at regular intervals around the clock (ATC) to maintain a therapeutic blood level. Administering analgesics as needed (prn) lowers this therapeutic level; delays in medication administration further increase pain intensity. Therefore, prn administration of analgesics is not recommended in the first 36 to 48 hours postoperatively. Patients using patient-controlled analgesia (PCA) or patient-controlled epidural analgesia (PCEA) in the postoperative period need to be taught the importance of using the allowed dosages regularly to prevent increasing pain levels.

In the immediate postoperative period, older adult patients benefit from the same protocol for morphine titration as do younger patients. Intravenous morphine may be initiated at a slightly reduced dose and then titrated to the same protocol as for younger patients. Morphine-related adverse effects such as nausea, vomiting, respiratory depression, constipation, urinary retention, pruritus, and allergy or sedation are similar among varying age groups. However, older adult patients require fewer opioids than younger patients in the later postoperative period. PCEA may be more effective for older adult patients and is associated with earlier improved mental status and bowel activity (Loran et al., 2005).

PRACTICE ALERT
Nurses are responsible for assessing patients' pain level and administering pain medication. They must work collaboratively with surgeons to schedule postoperative analgesics rather than rely on prn administration orders.

NSAIDs treat mild to moderate postoperative pain. This category of drugs should be given soon after surgery (orally, parenterally, or rectally) along with opioids unless contraindicated. Although NSAIDs may not be sufficient to control pain completely, they allow lower doses of opioid analgesics and therefore fewer side effects. NSAIDs can be given safely to older patients, but they should be observed closely for side effects, particularly gastric and renal toxicity.

Opioid analgesics, such as morphine, are considered the foundation for managing moderate to severe postoperative pain. Opioid dosage requirements vary greatly from one patient to another, so the dosage must be individually tailored. Later in the postoperative recovery period, opioid analgesics (oral or parenteral) may be given prn. In this way, pain relief can be maintained, while the potential for drug side effects is decreased.

Contrary to the belief of many healthcare providers (including nurses), physical dependence and tolerance to opioid analgesics is extremely uncommon in short-term postoperative use. Additionally, opioid analgesics, when used to treat acute pain, rarely lead to psychologic dependence and addiction. According to the World Health Organization pain ladder, acute pain is appropriately treated with opioids, tapering to acetaminophen as healing progresses. Chronic pain, in contrast, is treated with analgesics that increase from acetaminophen to opioids as tolerance develops or the condition worsens.

Analgesic options continue to develop, especially methods of delivery. Relatively new is the Q-ball, which provides wound infiltration with analgesia. Using combinations of analgesics and simultaneous methods of delivery, the patient can appreciate better pain control and experience fewer analgesic gaps (periods of ineffective pain control). Among the newest methods to achieve control are transdermal fentanyl by iontophoresis and extended-release epidural morphine. Iontophoresis is the delivery of "charged molecules across intact skin using a small electric current" (Polomano et al., 2008, p. S48). By providing combinations of opioids via multiple routes preemptively as well as intraopertively and postoperatively, the doses of each can be reduced and pain control enhanced.

Older patients tend to be more sensitive to the analgesic effects of opioids, experiencing a higher peak effect with a longer duration of pain control. The Moving Evidence into Action box on page 67 provides additional information.

PRACTICE ALERT
Oral analgesia requires a significantly greater dose than parenteral for most analgesics. Teach patients who are being discharged and their caregivers the relative strength of oral analgesics. (Caution them to not rely on trade names to gauge effectiveness.) Two acetaminophen with codeine (30 mg) is *equianalgesia* to 10 mg parenteral morphine; however, oral meperidine 100 mg does not provide equianalgesia with 10 mg parenteral morphine. (∞ See Chapter 9 for details about equianalgesia.)

Surgical Environment

MEMBERS OF THE SURGICAL TEAM   Because of the complexity of the intraoperative environment, members of the surgical team must function as a coordinated unit. The surgeon, surgical assistant(s), anesthesiologist or CRNA, circulating nurse, and scrub person or operating room technician (Figure 4–2 ■) constitute the surgical team. Each member provides specialized skills and is essential to the successful outcome of the surgery. Risks to members of the surgical team

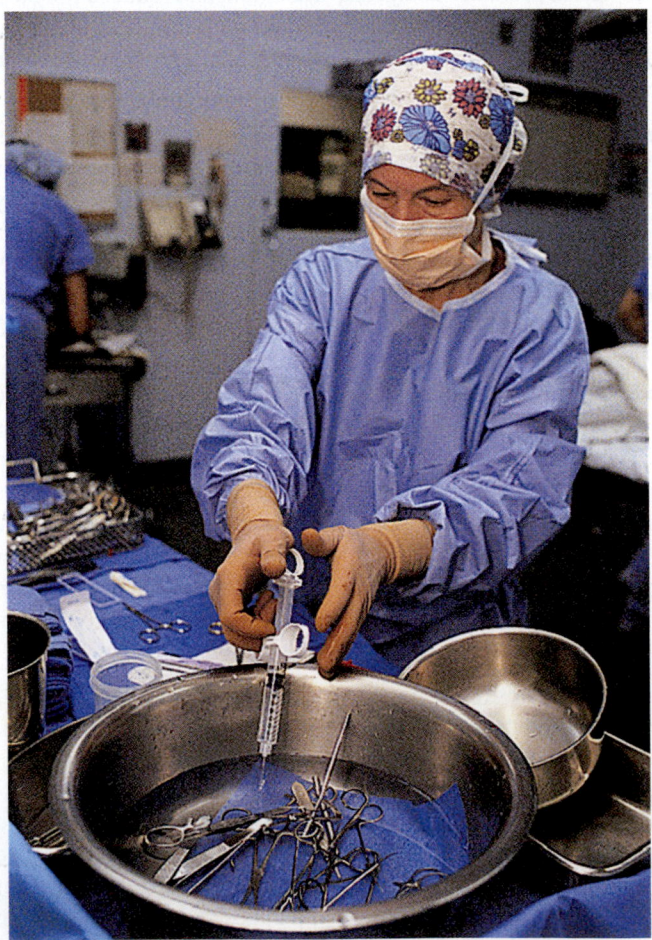

Figure 4–2 ■ A scrub nurse in the operating room.

MOVING EVIDENCE INTO ACTION | Assisting Older Adults to Communicate Postoperative Pain

Pain is a subjective experience. Nurses rely heavily on patients' assessments of the pain they are experiencing. Rating of pain intensity by the patient is the gold standard for knowing when to provide an intervention to decrease pain, and it is considered more accurate than nurses' evaluations of behavioral manifestations of pain. Older patients who believe that healthcare providers know best how to manage their pain are at risk for inadequately treated pain.

McDonald and colleagues (2005) used a program for coaching older adults about postoperative pain communication and management. In this study, older adults preparing for single-knee replacement surgery attended a preoperative joint replacement class where they learned about recovering from the surgery and pain management. Forty subjects greater than age 65 were randomly assigned either to the regular class, which included pain management information, or an intervention class, which included both information on pain management and skills to effectively communicate about pain. Pain severity scores were similar for both groups on postoperative days 1 and 2. There was no significant difference between the two groups in the postdischarge measures (day 7) of any pain dimension.

IMPLICATIONS FOR NURSING

Findings from this study highlight the importance of coaching older adults to report their pain experience candidly, particularly in the immediate postoperative period. Establishing trust within

the nurse–patient relationship is critical to relieving pain. Coaching older patients to describe their pain location, intensity, and sensation gives them permission to communicate in a manner with which they may feel uncomfortable at first. Coaching is necessary to dispel myths about professional expertise and to allow patients control and independence so that they are willing to ask for pain medications. Exploring with older patients their perception of pain, as well as the significance it has for recovery from illness, are necessary elements in providing adequate pain relief and restoring health.

CRITICAL THINKING IN PATIENT CARE

1. Your older patient says, "I deserved this pain, so I don't want to take anything to make it better." What would be your response and why?
2. A man of Native American descent, aged 76, replies that "something doesn't feel right" when asked to rate his pain on a scale of 0 to 10. His pulse is increased and he is protective of his abdominal incision. What could you ask or do to accurately assess his pain?
3. An independent, 85-year-old woman has a PCA pump for analgesia following major surgery. She continuously presses the pump button, but continues to complain of severe pain. What do you do now?

---

from bloodborne pathogens or injury are minimized when the surgical team is well organized and prepared.

The surgeon is the physician performing the procedure. As head of the surgical team, the surgeon is responsible for all medical actions and judgments.

The surgical assistant works closely with the surgeon in performing the operation. The number of assistants varies according to the complexity of the procedure. The assistant may be another physician, a nurse, a physician assistant, or other trained person. The assistant performs such duties as exposing the operative site, retracting nearby tissue, sponging and/or suctioning the wound, ligating bleeding vessels, and suturing or helping suture the surgical wound.

The anesthesiologist (medical doctor) or CRNA relieves the surgeon of the responsibility for the patient's general well-being, thus allowing the surgeon to focus on the technical aspects of the procedure. The anesthesiologist or CRNA evaluates the patient preoperatively, administers the anesthesia and other required medications, transfuses blood or other blood products, infuses intravenous fluids, continuously monitors the patient's physiologic status, alerts the surgeon to developing problems and treats them as they arise, and supervises the patient's recovery in the PACU.

The **circulating nurse** is a highly experienced registered nurse who coordinates and manages a wide range of activities before, during, and after the surgical procedure. The circulating nurse oversees the physical aspects of the operating room itself, including the equipment, assists with transferring and positioning the patient, prepares the patient's skin, ensures that no break in aseptic technique occurs, and counts all sponges

and instruments. The circulating nurse assists all other team members, including the anesthesiologist or CRNA. Thorough documentation of the case in the surgical area is essential, and the circulating nurse is responsible for documenting intraoperative nursing activities, medications, blood administration, placement of drains and catheters, and length of the procedure. The circulating nurse also formulates a care plan based on physiologic and psychosocial assessments of the patient. Finally, the circulating nurse is at all times an advocate for the safety and well-being of the patient.

The role of the **scrub person** primarily involves technical skills, manual dexterity, and in-depth knowledge of the anatomic and mechanical aspects of a particular surgery. The scrub person handles sutures, instruments, and other equipment immediately adjacent to the sterile field. The role of the scrub person may be assumed by a registered nurse or an operating room technician (ORT), depending on hospital policy and the complexity of the surgery. Registered nurses are responsible for patient outcomes including the performance of the person functioning in the role of scrub person. The Association of Operating Room Nurses (AORN) believes that registered nurses should maintain an active presence in the role of scrub person to ensure appropriate delegation and supervision of scrub duties and to maintain an integral link between scrub and circulating responsibilities (AORN, 2010).

The role of nurses in surgery continues to evolve to improve patient care. Although not participating in the surgical procedure, PACU nurses are part of the surgical team. In recent years, nurses have begun to specialize within the already specialized field of perioperative nursing. Specialty surgical teams are developing in response to the demands of increasingly complex technical surgeries. For example, a designated open heart surgical team may be responsible for all open heart cases and ordinarily not be involved with other procedures. The use of specialty surgical teams allows nurses to become highly skilled in a particular range of procedures.

Safety in the surgical environment is important for surgical team members as well as patients. Team members need to be aware of and strictly comply with guidelines to prevent exposure to scatter radiation when fluoroscopy is used in surgical procedures. Fluoroscopy is a real time continuous image of the internal structures of a patient. This technique is used in many types of surgeries including cardiac catheterization, orthopedic placement of metalwork, urologic cases, cardiovascular cases, and digestive system cases. The facility's radiation safety officer assures that protective equipment such as lead aprons, protective eye-glasses, and thyroid shields are available to all personnel at risk for exposure. In the surgical setting, the risk of scatter radiation is small with each event, but the cumulative dose may exceed safe limits. Therefore, personnel need to be informed about protection and limit their exposure (AORN, 2010).

SURGICAL METHODS Open invasive surgical procedures have traditionally been the gold standard for successful outcomes. This approach was necessary in order to see and protect vital structures surrounding a target organ. Today, miniaturization and technology allow minimally invasive surgeries carried out through small incisions with the aid of cameras and remotely controlled tools and instruments for incising and suturing. While laparoscopic surgeries have been available since 1985, a newer method of minimally invasive surgery is robot-assisted surgery. Robotic technology offers three-dimensional views, while laparoscopic technology offers only two-dimensional views. Instruments are easier for the surgeon to manipulate with the robotic systems. Robotic, computer-aided surgical systems are not independent, preprogrammed systems. Two surgeons perform the procedures—the primary surgeon at the robotic controls and the other at the patient's side to exchange sterile instruments, retract patient tissues, and manipulate nonrobotic sterile instruments used to assist the procedure (Francis & Winifield, 2006). Nurses must be familiar with the equipment and the procedures and ready to assist at all times.

Minimally invasive surgery, whether performed robotically or laparoscopically, has advantages for patients. There is less operative trauma, leading to improved postoperative comfort and decreased pain. While these procedures may take longer than similar open surgeries, they result in decreased hospital stays and fewer complications such as adhesions. General anesthesia is required for most minimally invasive surgeries and the risk for some complications similar to open surgeries remains.

SURGICAL ATTIRE Strict dress codes are necessary in the surgical department to provide infection control within the operating room suites, reduce cross-contamination between the surgery department and other hospital units or departments, and promote both personnel and patient health and safety. While based on research and recommendations by hospital infection

control authorities, guidelines for attire differ among surgical facilities. Following institutional guidelines, all personnel in the surgical department must be in proper surgical attire. The design and composition of the surgical attire minimize bacterial shedding, thus reducing wound contamination. The area in the surgical department is divided into *unrestricted*, *semirestricted*, and *restricted* zones. The unrestricted zones permit access by those in hospital uniforms or street clothes. These areas facilitate communication with operating room personnel.

The semirestricted zones require scrub attire, including a scrub suit, shoe covers, and a cap or hood (Figure 4–3 ■). Hallways, work areas, and storage areas are considered semirestricted. New guidelines exist for attire in the semirestricted and restricted areas of the OR. Previously, each person had to disrobe and don hospital-laundered scrubs. Today, home-laundered scrubs are accepted by many institutions based on data comparing hospital and home-laundered apparel. Only woven or disposable fabrics that will not harbor bacteria are allowed, and all items of apparel must be covered by appropriate fabric. No fabric other than the approved scrub uniform fabric can be exposed to the environment. AORN guidelines (2010) suggest that home-laundered scrubs be brought to the OR in a clean covering and donned at the facility, not worn into the hospital from home. Institutions vary in their interpretation of these guidelines. Artificial nails are discouraged in surgery and anywhere the nurse will have direct contact with high-risk patients. These nails are associated with glove tears and even after careful hand hygiene can harbor potential pathogens (Ogg & Peterson, 2007).

Restricted zones are within operating rooms. Personnel wear masks, sterile gowns, and gloves in addition to appropriate scrub attire if they are participating at the operating table.

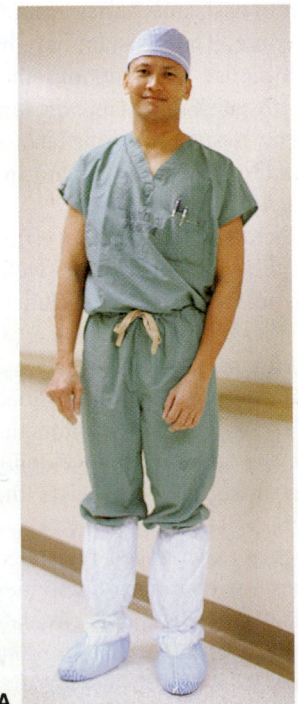 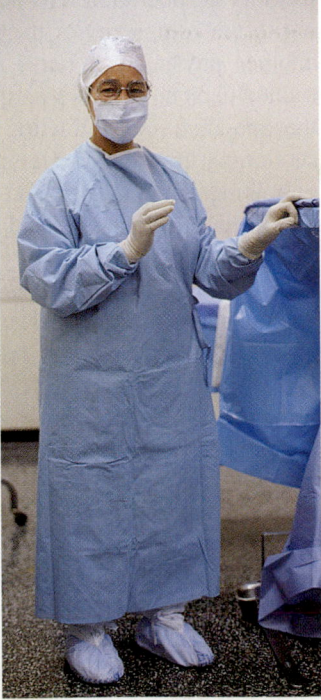

Figure 4–3 ■ Surgical attire. *A*, Scrub attire includes scrub suit, shoe covers, and cap or hood to cover hair. *B*, Sterile attire includes scrub suit, shoe covers, and cap or hood, plus gown, gloves, and mask.

Because of cardiovascular and tissue changes that result from aging, long, complicated surgeries (especially of the thorax and abdomen) place the older adult at increased risk for complications The older adult is more prone to hypotension, hypothermia, and hypoxemia resulting from anesthesia and the cool temperature in the operating room

Positioning may cause complications in the older adult. Intraoperative positioning of arthritic joints can cause postoperative joint pain unrelated to the operative site. Also, the longer the surgery, the greater the chance of decubitus ulcer formation. The older patient is at increased risk for developing decubitus ulcers because of decreased subcutaneous fat tissue and reduced peripheral circulation.

Infections are a particular problem in the older adult because of increased susceptibility from potential immune system decline and unusual manifestations such as confusion, lethargy, and anorexia. The classic signs of infection, fever, redness, pain, and swelling may be diminished in the elderly patient especially if there is immune system decline. The focus of care needs to be strongly on prevention.

Finally, the older adult often has some degree of hearing and/or visual impairment. These impairments coupled with a strange environment can make the operating room a frightening, disorienting place. By effectively communicating with the patient, the nurse can provide support and reassurance to minimize these factors. To decrease confusion and assist in communication, hearing aids and glasses should be used when appropriate and possible.

Factors that contribute to successful surgical outcomes for older adults include stabilizing nutrition and hydration, controlling concurrent chronic conditions with appropriate medication reconciliation, and providing information for realistic expectations about the surgery and the recovery (Clayton, 2008). Advanced age alone is not a contra-indication for surgery.

The outer sterile covering is changed between procedures and when it becomes soiled or wet. These practices are designed to protect the patient and the practitioner, especially from blood-borne pathogens. Continual evaluation by the hospital's infection control team is the source for guiding these practices. Strict adherence to proper usage of gowns, gloves, and masks is vital for protection (Belkin, 2006).

THE SURGICAL SCRUB The surgical scrub is performed to render hands and arms as clean as possible in preparation for a procedure. All personnel who participate directly in the procedure must perform a surgical scrub with a brush and antimicrobial soap. Skin cannot be rendered sterile, but it can be considered "surgically clean" following the scrub. The purposes of the surgical scrub are to do the following:

- Remove dirt, skin oils, and transient microorganisms from hands and forearms.
- Increase patient safety by reducing microorganisms on surgical personnel.
- Leave an antimicrobial residue on the skin to inhibit growth of microbes for several hours.

Following the 5- to 10-minute surgical scrub, hands and arms are dried with sterile towels.

Patient Preparation

Although much preparation has taken place prior to the patient's transfer to the surgical department, additional activities such as hair removal and positioning may be performed there. The skin preparation, which usually includes cleansing the area with a prescribed antimicrobial agent, may have been performed either by the patient or by nursing personnel before the transfer to the surgical department. Additional skin cleansing is performed in the surgical department to further decrease microorganisms on the skin and thereby reduce the possibility of wound infection.

Shaving as part of skin preparation is associated with increased risk for infection secondary to nicks in the skin. Hair removal by clippers or by depilatory solutions is preferable (Daniels, 2007). The surgeon may order hair removed in and around the proposed incision area. This is more often performed in the holding area of the surgical department. Generally, the prepared area is wider than the planned incision because of the possibility of unexpected extension of the incision. Hospital policy and surgeon preference should be followed.

Preparing the patient for surgery also includes positioning the patient on the operating table. Table 4–5 shows frequently used positions and describes corresponding surgical procedures and possible adverse effects. Positioning exposes the operative site and provides access for anesthesia administration.

> **SAFETY ALERT**
> Proper positioning is imperative to prevent injury to the patient. Pressure, rubbing, and/or shearing forces can cause injury to the tissue over bony prominences. If positioning causes normal joint range of motion to be exceeded, injury to muscles and joints can occur.

Improper positioning also can lead to sensory and motor dysfunction, resulting in nerve damage. Pressure on peripheral blood vessels can decrease venous return to the heart and negatively affect the patient's blood pressure. Additionally, oxygenation of the blood can be decreased if the patient is not properly positioned to promote lung expansion.

Because the anesthetized patient cannot respond to discomfort, it is the surgical team's responsibility to position the patient not only for the best surgical advantage but also for patient safety and comfort. The circulating nurse refers to hospital policy, the surgeon's preference, and the patient's history to ensure optimal positioning, and continuously assesses the patient. Be aware that tendons and ligaments can be overstretched by improper positioning (Clayton, 2008).

INTRAOPERATIVE AWARENESS Prior to induction of anesthesia, the circulating nurse establishes rapport with the patient to assess the patient's psychologic status. This assessment is continued throughout the surgical procedure. After anesthetic medications have been given, the patient may appear oblivious to the surroundings; however, anesthesiologists are concerned

TABLE 4–5 Common Surgical Positions

POSITION AND USE	POSSIBLE ADVERSE EFFECTS AND NURSING INTERVENTIONS
(a) The *dorsal recumbent* (or *supine*) *position* is used for many abdominal surgeries (e.g., colostomy and herniorrhaphy) as well as for some thoracic surgeries (e.g., open heart surgery) and some surgeries on the extremities. 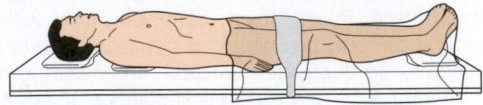	This position may cause excessive pressure on posterior bony prominences, such as the back of the head, scapulae, sacrum, and heels. Pad these areas with soft materials. To avoid compression of blood vessels and sluggish circulation, ensure that the knees are not flexed. Use trochanter rolls or other padding to avoid internal or external rotation of the hips and shoulders.
(b) The *semisitting position* is used for surgeries on the thyroid and neck areas. 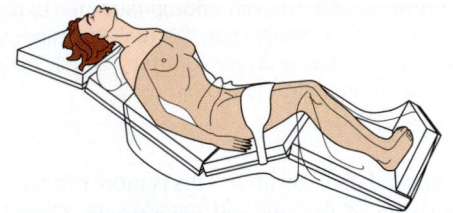	This position can lead to postural hypotension and venous pooling in the legs. It may promote skin breakdown on the buttocks. Sciatic nerve injury is possible. Assess for hypotension. Ensure that knees are not sharply flexed. Use soft padding to prevent nerve compression.
(c) The *prone position* is used for spinal fusions and removal of hemorrhoids. 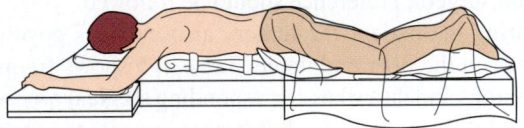	This position causes pressure on the face, knees, thighs, anterior ankles, and toes. Pad bony prominences, and support the feet under the ankles. To promote optimum respiratory function, raise the patient's chest and abdomen, and support with padding. Corneal abrasion could occur if the eyes are not closed or are insufficiently padded.
(d) The *lateral chest position* is used for some thoracic surgeries, as well as hip replacements. 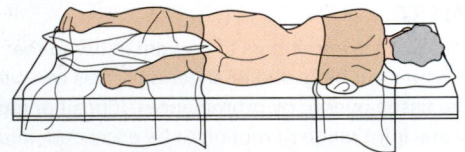	This may cause excessive pressure on the bony prominences on the side on which the patient is positioned. Ensure adequate padding and support, especially of the downside arm. The weight of the upper leg may cause peroneal nerve injury on the downside leg. Both legs must therefore be padded.
(e) The *lithotomy position* is used for gynecologic, perineal, or rectal surgeries. 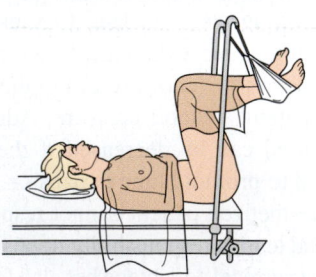	This position causes an 18% decrease (from a standing position) in vital capacity of the lungs. Monitor respirations, and assess for hypoxia and dyspnea. The lithotomy position can lead to joint damage, peroneal nerve damage, and damage to peripheral blood vessels. To avoid injury, ensure adequate padding, and manipulate both legs into the stirrups simultaneously.
(f) The *jackknife position* is used for proctologic surgeries, such as removal of hemorrhoids, and for some spinal surgeries. 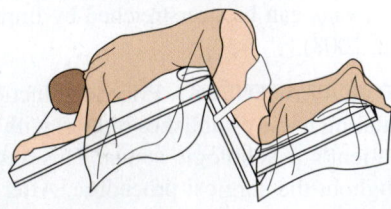	This position causes a 12% decrease (from a standing position) in vital capacity of the lungs. Monitor respirations, and assess for hypoxia and dyspnea. In this position, the greatest pressure is felt at the bends in the table. Therefore, the patient is supported with pads at the groin and knees, as well as at the ankles. Padding of the chest and knees helps prevent skin breakdown. Padding and proper positioning help prevent pressure on the ear, the neck, and the nerves of the upper arm.

about patient awareness with recall of intraoperative events (Hassan & Fahy, 2005). Intraoperative awareness is the patient's subconscious awareness of what is being said and done during surgery. Although most patients do not consciously remember what happened or what was said, psychologic trauma can result. Because loss of consciousness is gradual, conversations during surgery should be professional.

> **PRACTICE ALERT**
> Do not say anything while the patient is unconscious that would be inappropriate if the patient were awake. Maintain a respectful, professional demeanor throughout the operative period.

Nutrition

Wound healing after surgery depends on adequate nutritional intake. During the immediate postoperative phase, dietary intake is withheld until evidence of peristalsis (either audible bowel sounds or passage of flatus) is found and the patient can tolerate liquids without nausea and vomiting. While intravenous fluids maintain hydration and electrolyte balance, they do not provide nutrition. Unless balanced nutrition through gastrointestinal intake can be reestablished within 3 to 4 days, parenteral nutrition is critical for homeostasis and wound healing.

- Protein, calories, and vitamins are needed for wound healing and recovery from surgery.
- Low-fat, high-fiber diets are important for chronic cardiovascular fitness, but are contraindicated in the wound healing phase following surgery.
- Failure to use the gastrointestinal tract for more than 4 or 5 days allows the intestinal mucosa to atrophy, putting the patient at risk for infection.

Fluid administered through peripheral veins must be isotonic or only moderately hypertonic to prevent injury to the small peripheral veins. Solutions of 10% dextrose are tolerable peripherally for a short time but do not provide adequate calories for healing and maintenance. To provide adequate nutrition, central vein access must be established and solutions must be prepared with protein, carbohydrates, lipids, vitamins, and minerals. This is important for patients who have extended recovery periods without eating after surgery.

Parenteral nutrition has serious risks. Central vein access may cause infection and sepsis. Normal stimulation to the intestinal tract is lost when the parenteral approach is used alone. Using the gut is better than using the vein because it (1) prevents intestinal atrophy, which results in a very thin bowel wall poorly suited to absorb nutrients; (2) prevents bacteria and inert particles from translocating across the bowel lining into the bloodstream; (3) introduces fats and other large particles into the lymphatic circulation and stimulates the immune system; and (4) is safer and far less expensive than parenteral nutritional support (Heimburger & Weinsier, 1997; Lindgren & Ames, 2005). Education and counseling to support adequate nutritional intake should be ongoing throughout the preoperative and postoperative period.

✿ Nursing Care

The following section discusses nursing care in each of the three phases of surgery. The Case Study & Nursing Care Plan at the end of the section follows one patient through the postoperative experience, bringing this information together.

Preoperative Nursing Care

The patient's response to planned surgery varies greatly. When planning and implementing nursing care, consider individual psychologic and physical differences, the type of surgery, and the circumstances surrounding the need for surgery. A thorough nursing assessment is needed to determine the most appropriate care for each patient undergoing surgery.

Before planning and implementing care for the surgical patient, gather assessment information by taking a nursing history and performing a physical examination. Use this information to establish baseline data, identify physical needs, determine teaching needs and psychologic support for the patient and family, and prioritize nursing care. The type of surgical procedure directs the assessment and intervention planned by the nurse.

> **PRACTICE ALERT**
> Be sure to assess information about use of over-the-counter medications including herbal supplements. These drugs can interact with medications administered in the perioperative period.

Surgery is a significant and stressful event. Regardless of the nature of the surgery (whether major or minor), the patient and family will be anxious. Some patients and their families seek care from a spiritual provider during this time. The degree of anxiety they will feel is not necessarily proportional to the magnitude of the surgical procedure. For example, a patient scheduled to have a biopsy to rule out cancer, which is considered minor surgery, may be more anxious than a patient undergoing gallbladder removal, which is considered major surgery.

The nurse's ability to listen actively to both verbal and nonverbal messages is imperative to establishing a trusting relationship with the patient and family (Majasaari et al., 2005). Therapeutic communication can help the patient and family identify fears and concerns. The nurse can then plan nursing interventions and supportive care to reduce the patient's anxiety level and assist the patient to cope successfully with the stressors encountered during the perioperative period.

Preoperative Patient and Family Teaching

Patient teaching is an essential nursing responsibility in the preoperative period. Patient education and emotional support have a positive effect on the patient's physical and psychologic well-being, and on family members, both before and after surgery. Majasaari et al. (2005) surveyed 100 patients who underwent general, orthopedic, or gynecologic surgery as outpatients and their family members. Results of the survey showed the greatest dissatisfaction with outpatient surgery was lack or inadequacy of information. Because outpatient surgical stays are

BOX 4–3 Preoperative Patient Teaching

Diaphragmatic Breathing Exercise

Diaphragmatic (abdominal) breathing exercises are taught to the patient who is at risk for developing pulmonary complications, such as atelectasis or pneumonia. Risk factors for pulmonary complications include general anesthesia, abdominal or thoracic surgery, history of smoking, chronic lung disease, obesity, and advanced age.

In diaphragmatic breathing, the patient inspires deeply while allowing the abdomen to expand outward. On expiration, the abdomen contracts inward as air from the lungs is expelled.

1. Explain to the patient that the diaphragm is a muscle that makes up the floor of the abdominal cavity and assists in breathing. The purpose of diaphragmatic breathing is to promote lung expansion and ventilation and enhance blood oxygenation.
2. Position the patient in a high or semi-Fowler's position.
3. Ask the patient to place the hands lightly on the abdomen (see the following figure).
4. Instruct the patient to breathe in deeply through the nose, allowing the chest and abdomen to expand.
5. Have the patient hold the breath for a count of 5.
6. Tell the patient to exhale completely through pursed (puckered) lips, allowing the chest and abdomen to deflate.
7. Have the patient repeat the exercise five times consecutively.

Encourage the patient to perform diaphragmatic breathing exercises every 1 to 2 waking hours, depending on the patient's needs and institutional protocol.

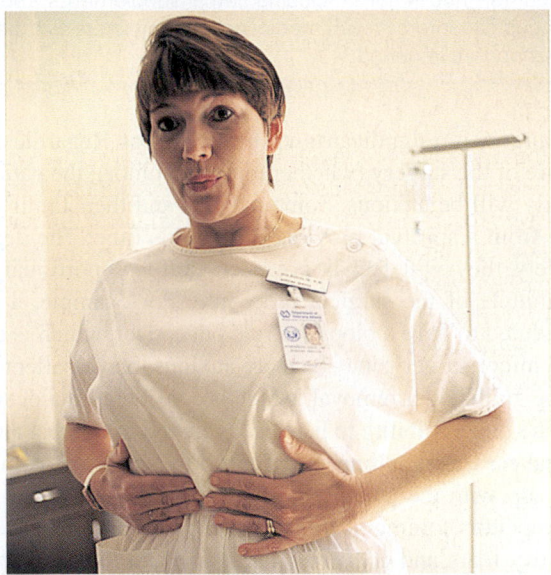

Diaphragmatic breathing exercise.

Coughing Exercise

Coughing exercises are also taught to the patient who is at risk for developing pulmonary complications. The purpose of coughing is to loosen, mobilize, and remove pulmonary secretions. Splinting the incision decreases the physical and psychologic discomfort associated with coughing.

1. Assist the patient in following steps 1 through 4 for diaphragmatic breathing.
2. Ask the patient to splint the incision with interlocked hands or a pillow (see the following figure).
3. Tell the patient to take three deep breaths and then cough while contracting abdominal muscles.
4. Have the patient repeat the exercise five times consecutively every 2 hours while awake, taking short rest periods between coughs if necessary.

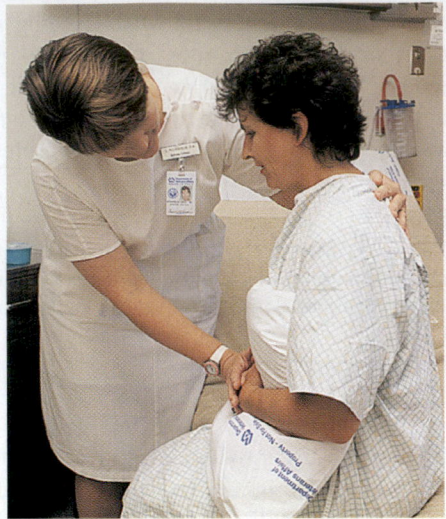

Splinting abdomen while coughing.

Leg, Ankle, and Foot Exercises

Leg exercises are taught to the patient who is at risk for developing venous thrombosis (formation of blood clots in a vein, often accompanied by inflammation). Risk factors for developing venous thrombosis include decreased mobility preoperatively and/or postoperatively; a history of difficulties with peripheral circulation; and cardiovascular, pelvic, or lower extremity surgeries.

The purpose of leg exercises is to promote venous blood return from the extremities. As the leg muscles contract and relax, blood is pumped back to the heart, promoting cardiac output and reducing venous stasis. These exercises also maintain muscle tone and range of motion, which facilitate early ambulation.

Teach the patient to perform the following exercises while lying in bed:

1. Muscle pumping exercise: Contract and relax calf and thigh muscles at least 10 times consecutively.
2. Leg exercises:
   a. Bend the knee and raise it toward the chest (see the following figure).
   b. Straighten out leg and hold for a few seconds before lowering the leg back to the bed.
   c. Repeat exercise five times consecutively prior to alternating to the other foot.

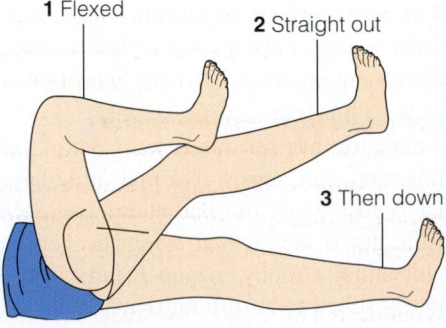

1 Flexed   **2** Straight out   **3** Then down

Leg exercises.

3. Ankle and foot exercises:
   a. Rotate both ankles by making complete circles, first to the right and then to the left (see the following figure).
   b. Repeat five times and then relax.
   c. With feet together, point toes toward the head and then to the foot of the bed (see the following figure).
   d. Repeat this pumping action 10 times, and then relax.

(continued)

BOX 4–3 Preoperative Patient Teaching (continued)

Encourage the patient to perform leg, ankle, and foot exercises every 1 to 2 hours while awake, depending on the patient's needs and ambulatory status, the physician's preference, and institutional protocol.

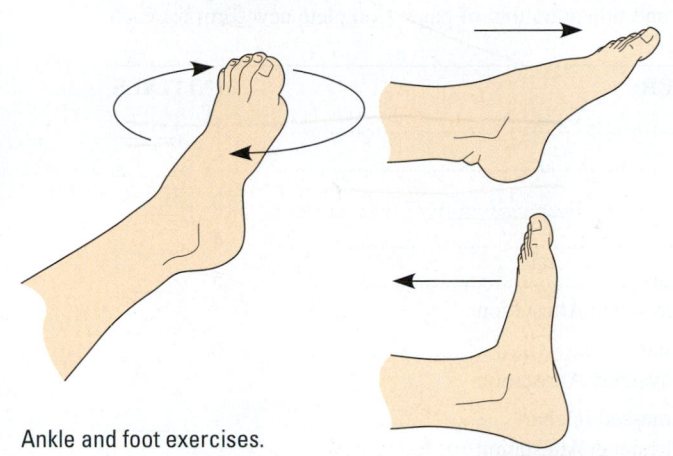

Ankle and foot exercises.

Turning in Bed

The patient who is at risk for circulatory, respiratory, or gastrointestinal dysfunction following surgery is taught to turn in bed. Although this may be a simple task prior to surgery, after surgery (particularly after abdominal surgery) the patient may find it a difficult procedure. To make the procedure more comfortable, the patient may need to splint the incision by using the hand placed on a small pillow or blanket. Additionally, the patient should be taught that analgesics can be given to ease postoperative discomfort involved with turning. Encourage the patient to turn every 2 hours while awake.

1. Tell the patient to grasp the side rail toward the direction to be turned, to rest the opposite foot on the mattress, and to bend the knee.
2. Instruct the patient to roll over in one smooth motion by pulling on the side rail while pushing off with the bent knee.
3. Pillows may need to be positioned behind the patient's back to help the patient maintain a side-lying position. The older patient may also need padding over pressure points between the knees and ankles to decrease the chance of decubitus ulcer formation from pressure.

---

brief, it is valuable for nurses to be sensitive, perceptive, and able to listen to and identify the patient as an individual within a unique family.

Patient teaching should begin as soon as the patient learns of the upcoming surgery. Teaching may begin as early as in the physician's office or at the time of preadmission testing. Although education continues during postoperative care, most teaching is done before surgery because pain and the effects of anesthesia can greatly diminish the patient's ability to learn.

The amount of information desired varies from patient to patient. Therefore, assess the patient's need for and readiness to accept information. The teaching will be directed in part by the particular surgical procedure that is being performed and by the type of anesthesia. The information in Box 4–3 is relevant to most patients undergoing major surgery.

In addition to teaching the patient and family about measures that will decrease the risk of complications, provide other preoperative information to prepare the patient and family for surgery. This information should include the following:

- Diagnostic tests—reasons and preparations
- Arrival time if surgery is scheduled the day of admission
- Preparations for surgery, including fasting prior to surgery, skin preparation, indwelling catheter or bladder elimination, start of intravenous infusion, preoperative medication, handling of valuables (rings, watch, money)
- Sedative/hypnotic medication to be taken the night before surgery to promote rest and sleep
- Counseling on whether to take significant medications the morning of surgery
- Informed consent
- Expected timetable for surgery and the recovery room
- Method to inform family of progress throughout surgery
- Transfer to the surgery department
- Location of the surgical waiting room
- Transfer to recovery room

- Anticipated postoperative routine and devices or equipment (drains, tubes, equipment for IV infusions, oxygen or humidifying mask, dressings, splints, casts)
- Plans for postoperative pain control
- Appropriate clothing for dressing prior to discharge from outpatient surgery

The American Society of Anesthesiologists provides guidelines for preoperative fasting in healthy patients undergoing elective procedures; they are available online. Withdrawal from caffeine in beverages such as coffee or colas may cause headaches and irritability. Dehydration, hypovolemia, and hypoglycemia are other recognized side effects. Thirst, worry, and hunger are reported by patients to be related to fasting. Fasting does not ensure that the stomach will be empty or that the gastric contents will be less acidic.

Preoperative Patient Preparation

A preoperative surgical checklist (Figure 4–4 ■) serves as an outline for finalizing preparation of the patient for surgery in most institutions. Complete the checklist before the patient is transported to surgery. Nursing responsibilities the day of surgery are as follows:

- Assist with bathing, grooming, and changing into operating room gown.
- Ensure that the patient takes nothing by mouth (NPO). Provide additional teaching, and reinforce prior teaching.
- Remove nail polish, lipstick, and makeup to facilitate circulatory assessment during and after surgery. Artificial nails worn by the patient should not be altered.
- Ensure that identification, blood, and allergy bands are correct, legible, and secure.
- Remove hair pins and jewelry; a wedding ring may be worn if it is removed from the finger, covered with gauze, replaced, and then taped to the finger.
- Complete skin or bowel preparation as ordered.

To be completed 24 hours prior to surgery

DATE:

* CALL REPORT AT 4474 (6 AM - 6 PM)
CALL REPORT AT 6171 (6 PM - 6 AM & weekends & holidays)

INSTRUCTIONS: Indicate that the task has been completed or the proper form is on the chart by initializing the item. Place NA in the column if item does not apply. Sign full name and title at bottom of page. Complete new form for each surgery procedure date.

REVIEW MEDICAL RECORD AND PHYSICIAN'S ORDER: **INITIALS**

1. History and Physical completed and in chart .... 1. _____

2. Laboratory studies/Reports in chart .... 2. _____

3. EKG report in chart .... 3. _____

4. Chest X-ray report in chart .... 4. _____

5. Operative Permit completed, signed, & witnessed in chart .... 5. _____
   ☐ Patient Affirmation   ☐ Witness Affirmation   ☐ Physician Attestation

6. Anesthesia Permit completed, signed, & witnessed in chart .... 6. _____
   ☐ Patient Affirmation   ☐ Witness Affirmation   ☐ Physician Attestation

7. Consent for blood transfusion completed, signed, & witnessed in chart .... 7. _____
   ☐ Patient Affirmation   ☐ Witness Affirmation   ☐ Physician Attestation

8. Medication Reconciliation Form Completed & Signed .... 8. _____

9. 4 pages of labels .... 9. _____

PREOPERATIVE PREPARATION: **INITIALS**

1. Identification bracelet accurate and affixed to wrist or ankle prior to transport .... 1. _____

2. Allergies checked, allergies bracelet on and allergy sticker on chart .... 2. _____

3. Isolation label on chart .... 3. _____

4. Jewelry, hairpieces, hairpins, contact lenses, glasses, prosthesis, underwear, money removed .. 4. _____

5. Vital signs taken and recorded .... 5. _____
   Time taken_____ BP_____ Temp_____ HR_____ Resp_____ FS_____ 6. _____

6. Dentures: ☐ Full: ☐ Upper ☐ Lower   ☐ Partial: ☐ Upper ☐ Lower
   ☐ Other:_____
   ☐ **Removed:** ☐ Sent Home ☐ Left at bedside
   ☐ **Left in place as requested by:** ☐ Anesthesiologist ☐ Patient

7. Patient NPO ☐ yes since _____ ☐ no .... 7. _____
   If no: O.R. notified (Time) _____ (Whom)..

8. Medication sheets on chart... 8. _____

9. Most recent nursing assessment attached... 9. _____

10. Report called to _____ at_____ (time) .... 10. _____

INITIALS	SIGNATURE AND TITLE	INITIALS	SIGNATURE AND TITLE

THE GEORGE WASHINGTON UNIVERSITY HOSPITAL

UHS
Universal Health

Patient Label

NURSING PREOPERATIVE CHECKLIST

OP0070

75-041 (12/06)

Figure 4–4 ■ The preoperative checklist helps ensure consistent completion of preoperative care activities.

- Insert an indwelling catheter, intravenous line, or nasogastric tube as ordered.
- Remove dentures, artificial eye, and contact lenses, and store them in a safe place.
- Leave a hearing aid in place if the patient cannot hear without it, and notify the operating room nurse.
- Verify that the informed consent has been signed prior to administering preoperative medications.
- Weigh the patient and record height and weight in the chart (for dosage of anesthesia).
- Verify that all ordered diagnostic test reports are in the chart.
- Have the patient empty the bladder immediately before the preoperative medication is administered (unless an indwelling catheter is in place).
- Administer preoperative medication as scheduled (refer to the Medications section earlier in the chapter and Table 4–4).
- Ensure the safety of the patient once the medication has been given by placing the patient on bed rest with raised side rails and by placing the call light within reach.
- Obtain and record vital signs.
- Provide ongoing supportive care to the patient and the patient's family.
- Document all preoperative care in the appropriate location, such as the preoperative surgical checklist, the medication record, and the narrative preoperative nursing notes.
- Verify with the surgical personnel the patient's identity, and verify that all patient information is documented appropriately.
- Help the surgical personnel transfer the patient from the bed to the stretcher.
- Prepare the patient's room for postoperative care, including making the surgical bed and ensuring that the anticipated supplies and equipment are in the room.

Having completed the preoperative check list and upon "call" from the OR, the patient enters the operating suite via stretcher and resides in a "holding area" prior to entry into the designated operating room. Additional preparations are made here and may include hair removal and intravenous access. Surgery nurses rotate their staffing assignments among holding areas, operating room, and postanesthesia care units. Preoperative care is completed in this setting. Some hospitals allow a family member or significant other to accompany the patient in the holding area while awaiting transfer to the operating room.

Intraoperative Nursing Care

The intraoperative phase of surgery begins when the patient enters the operating room and ends when the patient is transferred to the postanesthesia care unit. Nursing care in this phase focuses on keeping the patient and the environment safe and providing physiologic monitoring and psychologic support. Circulating nurses and scrub nurses, according to specific role definitions, support and care for the patient and assist the surgeons.

On entry into the surgical suite, the nurse verifies the patient's identity, the type and site of surgery, and previously obtained assessment data. The nurse participates in the Universal Protocol, calling for a "time out" before the procedure to conduct final verification of the correct patient, site,

positioning, and procedure, and that all relevant documents, information, and equipment are available.

The patient is appropriately positioned, using safety belts to secure him or her while assuring distal circulation remains unimpaired. Bone prominences are padded to reduce the risk of tissue breakdown. During surgery, the nurse observes for and informs the team if any breaks or potential breaks in sterile technique are noted.

> **PRACTICE ALERT**
> Objects on the sterile drape are considered sterile. Remain a minimum of 12 inches away from draped tables and sterile fields to avoid contamination if you are not attired in sterile gown and gloves.

Postoperative Nursing Care

Immediate Postoperative Care

Immediate postoperative care begins when the patient has been transferred from the operating room to the PACU. The PACU nurse immediately assesses the patient's airway and breathing and monitors vital signs and the surgical site to determine the response to the surgical procedure and to detect significant changes. Assessing mental status and level of consciousness is another ongoing nursing responsibility, and the patient may require repeated orientation to time, place, and person. Emotional support also is essential, because the patient is in a vulnerable and dependent position. Assessing and evaluating hydration status by monitoring intake and output is crucial to detecting cardiovascular or renal complications. In addition, the PACU nurse assesses the patient's pain level. Careful administration of analgesics provides comfort without compounding the potential side effects from the anesthesia.

Care When the Patient Is Stable

When awake and after being stabilized, the patient is transferred to his or her room. The PACU nurse communicates information about the patient's condition and postoperative orders to the floor nurse prior to the patient's arrival. This prepares the floor nurse for additional problems or needed equipment.

Immediate and continuing assessment is essential to detect and/or prevent complications. In documenting assessment findings, the nurse completes a flow record of the individual patient's situation. Baseline data are obtained and compared with preoperative data. A postoperative head-to-toe assessment includes but may not be limited to the following:

- General appearance
- Vital signs
- Level of consciousness
- Emotional status
- Quantity of respirations
- Skin color and temperature
- Discomfort/pain
- Nausea/vomiting
- Type of intravenous fluids and flow rate
- Dressing site

- Drainage on the dressing and/or bed linen
- Urinary output (catheter or ability to urinate)
- Ability to move all extremities

The hospital policy or physician's orders dictate the frequency of follow-up assessments. After major surgery, the nurse generally assesses the patient every 15 minutes during the first hour and, if the patient is stable, every 30 minutes for the next 2 hours, and then every hour during the subsequent 4 hours. Assessments are then carried out every 4 hours, subject to change according to the patient's condition and protocol for the particular surgical procedure. It is critically important to inform the surgeon immediately if the assessment reveals any signs of impending shock or other life-threatening changes.

After carrying out the initial assessment and ensuring the patient's safety by lowering the bed, raising the side rails, and placing the call light within reach, the nurse notes the physician's postoperative orders. These orders guide the nurse in the care of the postoperative patient. For example, the orders specify activity level, diet, medications for pain and nausea, antibiotics, continuation of preoperative medications, frequency of vital sign assessments, administration of intravenous fluids, and laboratory tests such as hemoglobin and potassium level. In most institutions, orders written prior to surgery must be reordered following surgery because the patient's condition is presumed to have changed.

Nursing Care of Common Postoperative Complications

Several factors place the patient at risk for postoperative complications. Nursing care before, during, and after surgery is aimed at preventing and/or minimizing the effects of these complications.

Preoperative care and teaching to decrease postoperative complications have been discussed. The following section addresses postoperative cardiovascular, respiratory, and wound complications, and problems associated with elimination.

Cardiovascular Complications

Common postoperative cardiovascular complications include shock, hemorrhage, deep venous thrombosis, and pulmonary embolism.

SHOCK   Shock is a life-threatening postoperative complication. It results from an insufficient blood flow to vital organs, an inability to use oxygen and nutrients, or the inability to rid tissues of waste material. Hypovolemic shock, the most common type in the postoperative patient, results from a decrease in circulating fluid volume. Decreased fluid volume develops with blood or plasma loss or, less commonly, from severe prolonged vomiting or diarrhea. Symptoms vary according to the severity of the shock; the greater the loss of fluid volume, the more severe the symptoms. ∞ Chapter 11 provides a detailed discussion of nursing care of the patient with various types of shock.

HEMORRHAGE   Hemorrhage is an excessive loss of blood. A concealed hemorrhage occurs internally from a blood vessel that is no longer sutured or cauterized or from a drainage tube that has eroded a blood vessel. An obvious hemorrhage occurs externally from a dislodged or ill-formed clot at the wound. Hemorrhage also may result from abnormalities in the blood's ability to clot; these abnormalities may result from a pathologic condition, or they may be a side effect of medications.

Hemorrhage from a venous source oozes out quickly and is dark red, whereas an arterial hemorrhage is characterized by bright red spurts of blood pulsating with each heartbeat. Whether the hemorrhage is from a venous or an arterial source, hypovolemic shock will occur if sufficient blood is lost from the circulation.

Assessment findings with hemorrhage depend on the amount and rate of blood loss. Restlessness and anxiety are observed in the early stage of hemorrhage. Frank bleeding will be present if the hemorrhage is external. The patient will have symptoms characteristic of shock.

Care of the patient who is hemorrhaging centers around stopping the bleeding and replenishing the circulating blood volume. Nursing care includes providing care for shock and one or more of the following:

- Applying one or more sterile gauze pads and a snug pressure dressing to the area
- Applying pressure with gloved hands (may be necessary for severe external bleeding)
- Preparing patient and family for emergency surgery (in severe situations when bleeding cannot be stopped)

DEEP VENOUS THROMBOSIS   Deep venous thrombosis (DVT) is the formation of a thrombus (blood clot) in association with inflammation in deep veins. This complication most often occurs in the lower extremities of the postoperative patient. It may result from the combination of several factors, including trauma during surgery, pressure applied under the knees, and sluggish blood flow during and after surgery. Patients particularly at risk for developing DVT include those who are over age 40 and who

- have experienced trauma or undergone orthopedic surgery to lower extremities; urologic, gynecologic, or obstetric surgeries; or neurosurgery.
- are pregnant or have recently given birth, have varicose veins, are undergoing hormone replacement therapy, or are using birth control pills.
- have a history of venous thrombosis, pulmonary emboli, or atrial fibrillation.
- are obese, smoke, have prolonged travel time in plane or car, or are immobilized.
- have an infection or sepsis.
- have a malignancy.

Prevention of venous stasis is an important nursing responsibility; it reduces adverse patient outcomes and decreases healthcare costs. Early ambulation is the key to preventing venous stasis but when patients are immobilized there is risk for blood clots. Anticoagulant medications such as low molecular weight heparin are used in high risk populations. Use of mechanical prophylactic devices (intermittent pneumatic compression devices [IPCDs]) on the foot, entire leg, or calf only is documented as effective prevention. Given the frequency and seriousness of the development of DVT and pulmonary embolism, attention to prevention is very important.

Common assessment findings reveal pain or cramping in the involved calf or thigh. Redness and edema of the entire extremity may occur along with a slightly elevated temperature. The patient may have a positive Homans' sign (pain in the calf on dorsiflexion of the affected foot).

Nursing care of the patient with DVT focuses on preventing a portion of the clot from dislodging and becoming an embolus (traveling blood clot) circulating to the heart, brain, or lungs; preventing other clots from forming; and supporting the patient's own physiologic mechanism for dissolving clots. Nursing care includes the following measures:

- Administer anticoagulants and analgesics as prescribed.
- Monitor laboratory values for clotting times. PT, PTT
- Maintain bed rest and keep affected extremity at or above heart level.
- Apply thigh-high antiemboli stockings or IPCDs to stimulate venous return.
- Ensure that the affected area is not rubbed or massaged.
- Apply heat as prescribed.
- Record bilateral calf or thigh circumferences every shift.
- Teach and support the patient and family.
- Assess color and temperature of involved extremity every shift.

PULMONARY EMBOLISM A pulmonary embolism is a dislodged blood clot or other substance that lodges in a pulmonary artery. For the postoperative patient with DVT, the threat that a portion of the thrombus may break off or dislodge from the vein wall and travel to the lung is a constant concern. Early detection of this potentially life-threatening complication depends on the nurse's astute, continuing assessment of the postoperative patient.

Common assessment findings of the patient experiencing a pulmonary embolism include mild to moderate dyspnea, chest pain, diaphoresis, anxiety, restlessness, rapid respirations and pulse, dysrhythmias, cough, and cyanosis. The severity of the symptoms is determined by the degree of pulmonary vascular blockage. Sudden death can occur if a major pulmonary artery becomes completely blocked.

Stabilizing respiratory and cardiovascular functioning while preventing the formation of additional emboli is of utmost importance in the care of the patient with a pulmonary embolism. Nursing care includes the following measures:

- Immediately notify the physician and nursing supervisor.
- Frequently assess and record general condition and vital signs.
- Maintain the patient on bed rest, and keep the head of the bed elevated.
- Provide oxygen as ordered and monitor pulse oximetry.
- Administer prescribed intravenous fluids to maintain fluid balance while preventing fluid overload.
- Administer prescribed anticoagulants.
- Maintain comfort by administering analgesics and sedatives (use caution to prevent respiratory depression).
- Provide supportive measures for the patient and family.

Refer to ∞ Chapter 37 for a detailed discussion of pulmonary embolism.

Respiratory Complications

Common postoperative respiratory complications include pneumonia and atelectasis.

PNEUMONIA Pneumonia is an inflammation of lung tissue. Inflammation is caused either by a microbial infection or by a foreign substance in the lung, which leads to inflammation. Numerous factors may be involved in the development of pneumonia, including aspiration of gastric contents, retained pulmonary secretions, failure to cough deeply, and impaired cough reflex and decreased mobility.

Common assessment findings of the postoperative patient with pneumonia are as follows:

- High fever
- Rapid pulse and respirations
- Chills (may be present initially)
- Productive cough (may be present depending on the type of pneumonia)
- Dyspnea
- Chest pain
- Crackles and wheezes

Treating the pulmonary infection, supporting the patient's respiratory efforts, promoting lung expansion, and preventing the organisms' spread are the goals in the care of the patient with pneumonia. Nursing care includes the following measures:

- Obtain sputum specimens for culture and sensitivity testing.
- Position patient with the head of the bed elevated.
- Encourage the patient to turn, cough, and perform deep-breathing exercises at least every 2 hours.
- Assist with incentive spirometry, intermittent positive pressure breathing (IPPB), and/or nebulizer treatments as ordered.
- Ambulate patient as condition permits and as prescribed.
- Administer oxygen as ordered.
- Assess vital signs, breath sounds, oxygen saturation, and general condition.
- Maintain hydration to help liquefy pulmonary secretions.
- Administer antibiotics, expectorants, antipyretics, and analgesics as ordered.
- Provide or assist with frequent oral hygiene.
- Prevent the spread of microorganisms by teaching proper disposal of tissues, covering mouth when coughing, and good hand hygiene technique.
- Provide supportive measures for the patient and family.
  ∞ Chapter 36 provides a detailed discussion of pneumonia.

ATELECTASIS Atelectasis is an incomplete expansion or collapse of lung tissue resulting in inadequate ventilation and retention of pulmonary secretions. Common assessment findings include dyspnea, diminished breath sounds over the affected area, anxiety, restlessness, crackles, and cyanosis.

Promoting lung expansion and systemic oxygenation of tissues is a goal in the care of the patient with atelectasis. Nursing care includes these tasks:

- Position the patient with the head of the bed elevated.

- Administer oxygen as prescribed.
- Encourage coughing, turning, and deep breathing every 2 hours.
- Ambulate the patient as condition permits and as prescribed.
- Assist with incentive spirometry or other pulmonary exercises, such as inflating a balloon, as ordered.
- Administer analgesics as prescribed.
- Promote hydration.
- Provide supportive measures to the patient and family.

Wound Complications

Discussion of the complications associated with surgical wounds follows an overview of wound healing, wound drainage, and nursing care of wounds.

Wounds heal by either *primary*, *secondary*, or *tertiary intention* (Figure 4–5 ■). Healing by primary intention takes place when the wound is uncomplicated and clean and has sustained little tissue loss. The edges of the incision are well approximated (have come together well) with sutures, staples, or superglue for drain holes or superficial wounds (Zide, 2005). This type of surgical incision heals quickly, and very little scarring is expected.

Secondary intention refers to the healing that occurs when the wound is large, gaping, and irregular. Tissue loss prevents wound edges from approximating; therefore, granulation tissue fills in the wound. This type of wound takes longer to heal, is more prone to infection, and develops more scar tissue.

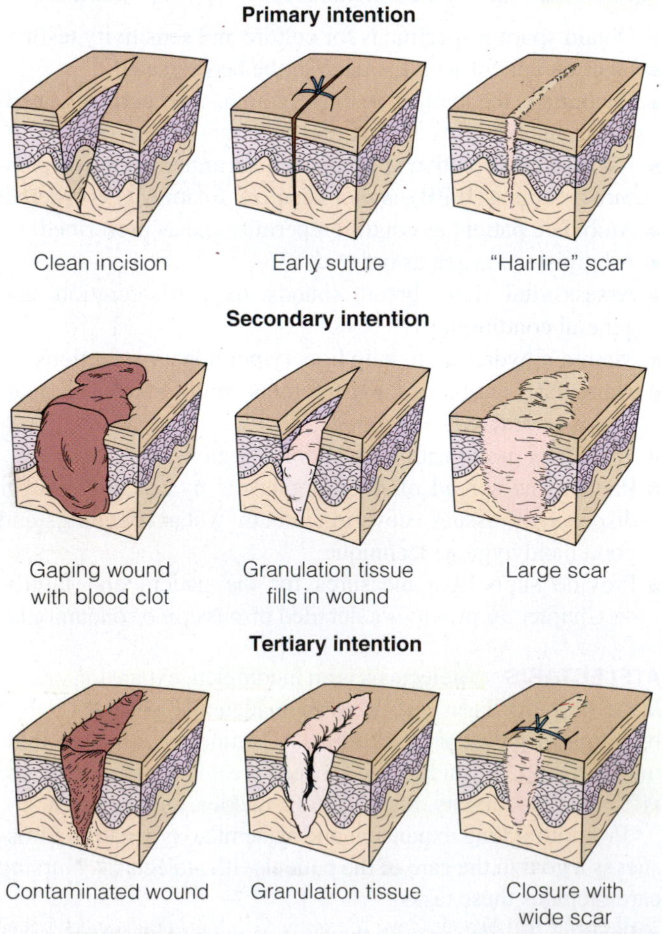

Primary intention

Clean incision   Early suture   "Hairline" scar

Secondary intention

Gaping wound with blood clot   Granulation tissue fills in wound   Large scar

Tertiary intention

Contaminated wound   Granulation tissue   Closure with wide scar

Figure 4–5 ■ Wound healing by primary, secondary, and tertiary intention.

If enough time passes before a wound is sutured, healing by tertiary intention occurs. Infection is more likely to take place. Because the wound edges are not approximated, tissue is regenerated by the granulation process. Closure of the wound results in a wide scar.

From the time the surgical incision is made until the wound is completely healed, all wounds progress through four stages of healing. However, healing time varies according to many factors, such as age, nutritional status, general health, and the type and location of the wound. Figure 4–5 provides a summary of the stages of wound healing.

Wound drainage (exudate) results from the inflammatory process in the first two stages of wound healing. The drainage is from the rich blood supply that surrounds the wound tissue and is composed of escaped fluid and cells. The drainage is described as serous, sanguineous, or purulent.

- Serous drainage contains mostly the clear serous portion of the blood. The drainage appears clear or slightly yellow and is thin in consistency.
- Sanguineous drainage contains a combination of serum and red blood cells and has a thick, reddish appearance. This is the most common type of drainage from a noncomplicated surgical wound.
- Purulent drainage is composed of white blood cells, tissue debris, and bacteria. Purulent drainage is the result of infection and tends to be of a thicker consistency, with various colors specific to the type of organism. It also may have an unpleasant odor.

Box 4–4 describes and illustrates various types of wound drainage devices. These devices decrease pressure in the wound area by removing excess fluid, which promotes healing and decreases complications.

Nursing care of the postoperative patient with a surgical wound focuses on preventing and monitoring for wound complications. The nurse assumes a leading role in supporting the wound healing process, providing emotional support to the patient and teaching wound care to the patient.

Common assessment findings of an infected wound include pain; purulent, odorous discharge and redness; warmth; tenderness; and edema around the edges of the incision. Additionally, the patient may have a fever, chills, and increased respiratory and pulse rates. Nursing care includes the following measures:

- Maintain medical asepsis (e.g., by using good hand hygiene technique).
- Follow Centers for Disease Control and Prevention guidelines for wound care.
- Observe aseptic technique during dressing changes and handling of tubes and drains.
- Assess vital signs, especially temperature.
- Evaluate the characteristics of wound discharge (color, odor, and amount).
- Assess the condition of the incision (approximation of the edges, sutures, staples, or drains).
- Clean, irrigate, and pack the wound in the prescribed manner. Sterile normal saline is often prescribed; povidone-iodine (Betadine) is no longer recommended for wound care.

BOX 4–4 Wound Drainage Devices

A Penrose drain, used for passive wound drainage, promotes healing from the inside to the outside (see figure A). The use of the drain decreases the chance of abscess formation. The safety pin in the Penrose drain prevents the exposed end from slipping down into the wound. Wound care focuses on cleaning around the drain with a prescribed solution, such as sterile normal saline, and replacing the precut gauze dressing as necessary to keep the surrounding skin dry and encourage further drainage. An absorbent dressing is placed over the drain and gauze (not shown).

Wound suction devices promote drainage of fluid from the incision site, decreasing pressure on healing tissues and reducing abscess formation. Shown are the Jackson-Pratt and Hemovac wound suction devices (see figures B and C).

The frequency with which the nurse empties the device depends on the time elapsed since surgery, type of surgery, amount of drainage, and hospital policy. For example, immediately after surgery the nurse may empty the device every 15 to 60 minutes. With time, as drainage decreases, the device is emptied every 2 to 4 hours (per hospital policy). Care is taken to maintain asepsis when emptying suction devices, avoiding contamination of the drain or the drain plug. Amount, color, consistency, and odor of drainage are documented. Usually, the drain is removed on the second to fourth day after surgery. Removal causes minor patient discomfort. The drain site is cleaned, superglue may be applied to the hole, and a sterile dressing is applied.

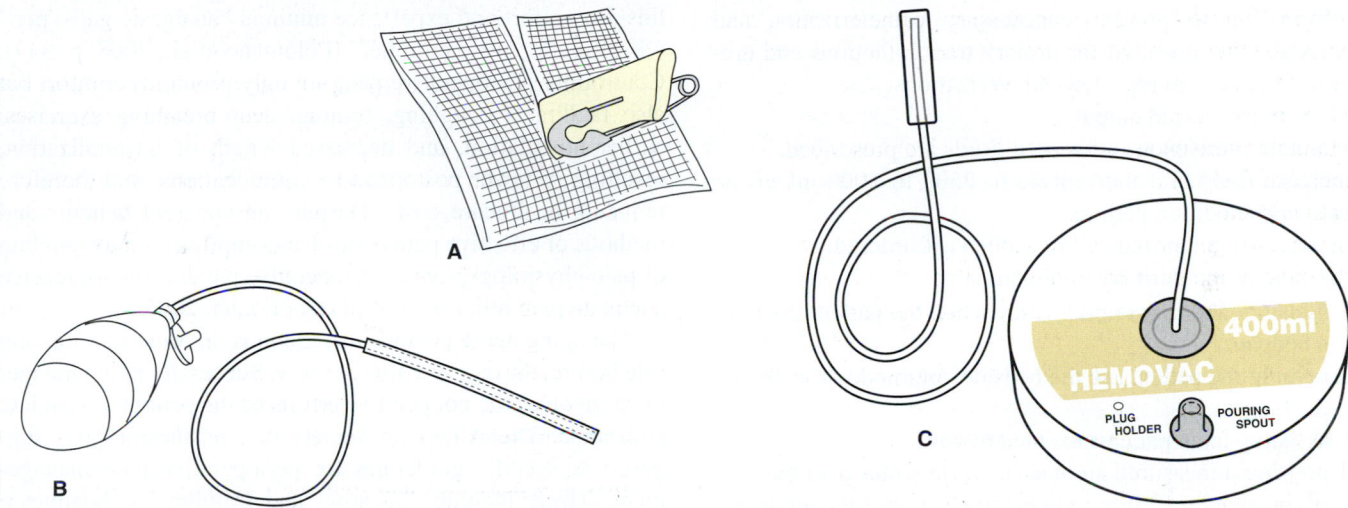

Wound drainage devices. *A*, Penrose passive wound drainage device. *B*, Jackson-Pratt wound suction device. *C*, Hemovac wound suction device.

- Maintain the patient's hydration and nutritional status.
- Culture the wound prior to beginning antibiotic therapy.
- Administer antibiotics and antipyretics as prescribed.
- Provide supportive measures to patient and family.

Dehiscence is a separation in the layers of the incisional wound (Figure 4–6A ■). Treatment depends on the extent of wound disruption. If the dehiscence is extensive, the incision must be resutured in surgery. **Evisceration** is the protrusion of body organs from a wound dehiscence (Figure 4–6B). These serious complications may result from delayed wound healing or may occur immediately following surgery. They also may occur after forceful straining (coughing, sneezing, or vomiting). When dehiscence occurs, immediately cover the wound with a sterile dressing moistened with normal saline. Emergency surgery is performed to repair these conditions.

Either the nurse, physician, physician assistant (PA), or nurse practitioner (NP) removes sutures or staples after the wound has healed sufficiently (usually 5 to 10 days after surgery). Removal is performed using medical aseptic technique. Additional support may be provided to the incision by applying strips of tape (or Steri-Strips) as directed by institutional policy or by the physician.

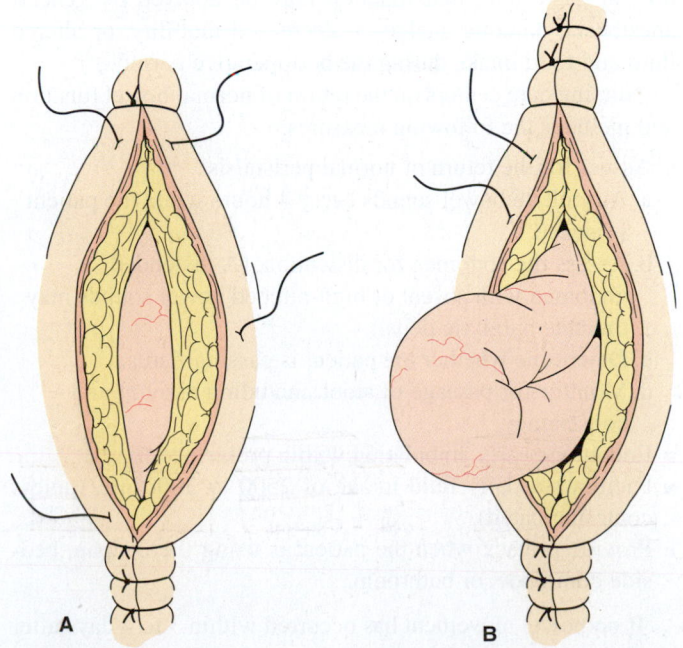

Figure 4–6 ■ Wound complications. *A*, Dehiscence is a disruption in the incision resulting in a separation of the layers of the wound. *B*, Evisceration is a protrusion of a body organ through a surgical incision.

Complications Associated with Elimination

Common postoperative complications associated with elimination include urinary retention and altered bowel elimination. The inability to urinate with urinary retention may occur postoperatively as a result of the recumbent position, effects of anesthesia and narcotics, inactivity, altered fluid balance, nervous tension, or surgical manipulation in the pelvic area. Nursing care centers on promoting normal urinary elimination and includes the following measures:

- Assess for bladder distention if the patient has not voided within 7 to 8 hours after surgery or if the patient is urinating small amounts frequently.
- Assess the amount of urine in the bladder with a portable ultrasound scanner. This noninvasive procedure provides information to prevent unnecessary catheterization and decreases the potential for urinary tract infections and urethral trauma from repeated catheterizations.
- Monitor intake and output.
- Maintain intravenous infusion if fluids are prescribed.
- Increase daily oral fluid intake to 2500 to 3000 mL if the patient's condition permits.
- Insert a straight or indwelling catheter if ordered.
- Promote normal urinary elimination by
  a. assisting and providing privacy when the patient uses a bedpan.
  b. helping the patient use the bedside commode or walk to the bathroom.
  c. assisting male patients to stand to void.
  d. pouring a measured amount of warm water over the perineal area. (If urination occurs, subtract the amount of water from the total amount for an accurate output measurement.)

Bowel elimination frequently is altered after abdominal or pelvic surgery and sometimes after other surgeries. Return to normal gastrointestinal function may be delayed by general anesthesia, narcotic analgesia, decreased mobility, or altered fluid and food intake during the perioperative period.

Nursing care centers on the return of normal bowel function and includes the following measures:

- Assess for the return of normal peristalsis:
  a. Auscultate bowel sounds every 4 hours while the patient is awake.
  b. Assess the abdomen for distention. (A distended abdomen with absent or high-pitched bowel sounds may indicate paralytic ileus.)
  c. Determine whether the patient is passing flatus.
  d. Monitor for passage of stool, including amount and consistency.
- Encourage early ambulation within prescribed limits.
- Facilitate a daily fluid intake of 2500 to 3000 mL (unless contraindicated).
- Provide privacy when the patient is using the bedpan, bedside commode, or bathroom.

If no bowel movement has occurred within 3 to 4 days after surgery, a suppository or an enema may be ordered.

Special Considerations for Older Adults

Physiologic, cognitive, and psychosocial changes associated with the aging process place the older adult at increased risk for postoperative complications. These age-related changes with selected nursing interventions are summarized in Table 4–6. With an ever-increasing population of older adults, particularly the very old, the nurse must be aware of these normal changes and modify nursing care accordingly in an effort to provide safe, supportive care.

Managing Acute Postoperative Pain

Pain is expected after surgery. It is neither realistic nor practical to eliminate postoperative pain completely. Nevertheless, the patient should receive substantial relief from and control of this discomfort and experience minimal "analgesic gaps: periods of ineffective pain relief" (Polomano et al., 2008, p. S44). Controlling postoperative pain not only promotes comfort but also facilitates coughing, turning, deep-breathing exercises, earlier ambulation, and decreased length of hospitalization, resulting in fewer postoperative complications, and therefore reducing healthcare costs. Despite the apparent benefits and methods of effective pain control and improved understanding of pain physiology, many postoperative patients do not receive adequate pain relief or control (MacLellan, 2004).

Managing acute postoperative pain is an important nursing role before, during, and after surgery. Successful pain management involves the cooperative efforts of the patient, physician, and nurse. The American Society of Anesthesiologists suggests six specific guidelines for perioperative pain management. These include education and training for healthcare providers, monitoring of patient outcomes, 24-hour availability of anesthesiologists providing perioperative pain management, and use of a dedicated acute pain service. Preoperatively, the patient should learn how much pain to anticipate and what methods are available to control pain. After discussing options with the patient, healthcare providers must respect the patient's personal preferences.

Postoperative medications were discussed earlier in the chapter. Various nonpharmacologic approaches to pain management are used alone or in combination to control acute postoperative pain. Relaxation, music, distraction, and imagery techniques can decrease mild pain and anxiety. Massage and the application of heat or cold can also relieve postoperative pain. Transcutaneous electrical nerve stimulation (TENS) has been used successfully to decrease postoperative incisional pain. Other approaches include acupuncture, acupressure, and therapeutic touch. Additional information on pain management techniques is found in ∞ Chapter 9.

Opioid dosage requirements vary greatly from one patient to another and by the route they are taken. Remember that oral doses of analgesics are not equal to parenteral doses. Oral doses need to be higher to provide **equianalgesia**. (See Table 9–3 for equianalgesic doses.)

The patient's input and participation in assessing pain and pain relief is essential to a successful pain control regime. For example, the patient can rate the pain on a scale of 0 to 10

TABLE 4–6 Nursing Interventions for Older Surgical Patients

SYSTEM	AGE-RELATED CHANGES	NURSING INTERVENTIONS
General appearance	Change in height, weight, and fat distribution	Assess physical parameters. Provide for warmth. Turn frequently.
Integument	Diminished integrity secondary to loss of subcutaneous fat and decreased oil production, elasticity, and hydration	Provide careful preoperative preparation to avoid trauma. Avoid shaving. Assess oxygenation and hydration by evaluation of mucous membranes, laboratory studies, and urine output.
Sensory-perceptual	Decline in vision and hearing ability; dryness of mouth	Compensate for sensory deficits: speak low, not loud; minimize noise in environment; provide adequate room light; stay within patient's field of vision when speaking; encourage patient to wear hearing aid to the operating room. Whenever possible, do not remove dentures or glasses. Provide comfort measures when NPO.
Respiratory	Decreased efficiency of cough reflex and decreased aeration of lung fields	Teach and encourage coughing and diaphragmatic breathing exercises. Assess baseline parameters. Constantly monitor lung sounds and respiratory status.
Cardiovascular	Less efficient, decreased adaptation to stress	Monitor for hypotension and shock. Assess for thrombus formation, cardiac dysrhythmias, peripheral pulses, and edema.
Gastrointestinal	Decline in gastric motility	Encourage intake of adequate fluids, nutritious meals, soft diet. Assist with feeding; monitor bowel function.
Genitourinary	Decreased efficiency of kidney; loss of bladder control	Monitor I&O and electrolyte levels. Assess for drug side effects. Assist with voiding as needed.
Musculoskeletal	Stiffness of joints; decrease in strength; brittleness of bones	Carefully position on OR table. Move carefully and gently. Prevent pressure sores.
Cognitive-psychosocial	Decreased reaction time; stable intellectual ability; proneness to delirium and altered mental status while in hospital	Provide ample time for making decisions. Implement safety measures. Talk to patient as adult, not as child. Unique to older adults, fear of increasing dependency on others. Orient frequently.

Reprinted from *AORN Journal*, Vol. 83, No. 3, Judith L. Clayton, "Special Needs of Older Adults Undergoing Surgery," p 557–574, © 2008, Association of periOperative Registered Nurses, with permission from Elsevier.

(where 0 signifies no pain and 10 signifies unbearable pain). Assess and document pain at scheduled intervals to determine the degree of pain control, to observe for drug side effects, and to assess the need for changes in the dosage and/or frequency of medication administration. When a range of dosage is ordered, carefully titrate opioid dosages based on individual assessments of need and response to therapy.

Using NANDA, NIC, and NOC

Linkages between a selected NANDA nursing diagnosis, NIC, and NOC for the postoperative patient are shown in the chart that follows.

Community-Based Care

Because the postoperative phase does not end until the patient has recovered completely from the surgical intervention, the nurse plays a vital role as the patient nears discharge. As the patient prepares to recuperate at home, provide information and support to help the patient successfully meet self-care demands. All aspects of teaching should be accompanied by written guidelines, directions, and information. This is

NANDA, NIC, AND NOC LINKAGES
The Postoperative Patient

NANDA   Acute Pain

↓

NIC   Medication Administration
Patient-Controlled Analgesia (PCA) Assistance
Pain Management
Postanesthesia Care

↓

NOC   Pain Level
Pain Control
Symptom Control

Data from NANDA International. (2009). *Nursing diagnoses: Definitions & classification 2009–2011.* Oxford, UK: Wiley-Blackwell; Bulechek, G. M., Butcher, H. K., & Dochterman, J. M. (Eds.). (2008). *Nursing Interventions Classification (NIC)* (5th ed.). St. Louis, MO: Mosby; and Moorhead, S., Johnson, M., Maas, M., & Swanson, E. (Eds.). (2008). *Nursing Outcomes Classification (NOC)* (4th ed.). St. Louis, MO: Mosby.

CASE STUDY & NURSING CARE PLAN A Patient Having Surgery

Martha Overbeck is a 74-year-old widow of German descent who lives alone in a senior citizens' housing complex. She is active there, as well as in the Lutheran Church. She has been in good health and is independent, but she has become progressively less active as a result of arthritic pain and stiffness. Mrs. Overbeck has degenerative joint changes that have particularly affected her right hip. On the recommendation of her physician and following a discussion with her friends, Mrs. Overbeck has been admitted to the hospital for an elective right total hip replacement. Her surgery has been scheduled for 8:00 AM the following day.

Mrs. Eva Jackson, a close friend and neighbor, accompanies Mrs. Overbeck to the hospital. Mrs. Overbeck explains that her friend will help in her home and assist her with the wound care and prescribed exercises.

ASSESSMENT

Gloria Nobis, RN, is assigned to Mrs. Overbeck's care on return to her room. Ms. Nobis performs a complete head-to-toe assessment and determines that Mrs. Overbeck is drowsy but oriented. Her skin is pale and slightly cool. Mrs. Overbeck states she is cold and requests additional covers. Ms. Nobis places a warmed cotton blanket next to Mrs. Overbeck's body, adds another blanket to her covers, and adjusts the room's thermostat to increase the room temperature. Mrs. Overbeck states that she is in no pain and would like to sleep. She has even, unlabored respirations and stable vital signs as compared to preoperative readings.

Mrs. Overbeck is NPO. An intravenous solution of dextrose and water is infusing at 100 mL/h per infusion pump. No redness or edema is noted at the infusion site. Ms. Nobis notes that the antibiotic ciprofloxacin hydrochloride (Cipro) is to be administered by mouth when the patient is able to tolerate fluids. Mrs. Overbeck has a large gauze dressing over her right upper lateral thigh and hip with no indications of drainage from the wound. Tubing protrudes from the distal end of the dressing and is attached to a passive suctioning device (Hemovac). Ms. Nobis empties 50 mL of dark red drainage from the suctioning device and records the amount and characteristics on a flow record. Mrs. Overbeck has a Foley catheter in place with 250 mL of clear, light amber urine in the dependent gravity drainage bag.

When assessing Mrs. Overbeck's lower extremities, Ms. Nobis finds her feet slightly cool and pale with rapid capillary refill time bilaterally. Dorsalis pedis and posterior tibial pulses are strong and equal bilaterally. Ms. Nobis notes slight pitting edema in the right foot and ankle as compared with the left extremity. She also notes sensation and ability to move both feet and toes, without numbness or tingling (paresthesia).

Ms. Nobis records these findings on a postoperative flowsheet. After ensuring that Mrs. Overbeck is safely positioned and can reach her call light, Ms. Nobis gives Mrs. Overbeck's friend, Mrs. Jackson, a progress report. They then go into Mrs. Overbeck's room.

DIAGNOSES

Ms. Nobis makes the following postoperative nursing diagnoses for Mrs. Overbeck:

- *Risk for Infection* of right hip wound related to disruption of normal skin integrity by the surgical incision
- *Risk for Injury* related to potential dislocation of right hip prosthesis secondary to total hip replacement
- *Pain* related to right hip incision and positioning of arthritic joints during surgery
- *Risk for Impaired Physical Mobility* related to right hip wound

EXPECTED OUTCOMES

The expected outcomes established in the plan of care specify that Mrs. Overbeck will

- regain skin integrity of the right hip incision without experiencing signs or symptoms of infection.

- demonstrate (along with Mrs. Jackson) proper aseptic technique while performing the dressing change.
- verbalize signs and symptoms of infection to be reported to her physician.
- describe measures to be taken to prevent dislocation of right hip prosthesis.
- report control of pain at incision and in arthritic joints.
- remain afebrile.
- remain free of complications related to immobility such as respiratory obstruction, muscle weakness, urinary retention, constipation, and disorientation.

PLANNING AND IMPLEMENTATION

Ms. Nobis develops a care plan that includes the following interventions to assist Mrs. Overbeck during her postoperative recovery:

- Use aseptic technique while changing dressing.
- Monitor temperature and pulse every 4 hours to assess for elevation.
- Assist to change positions frequently (q2h) and cough and deep breathe. Assist with early ambulation.
- Assess wound every 8 hours for purulent drainage and odor. Assess edges of wound for approximation, edema, redness, or inflammation in excess of expected inflammatory response.
- Teach Mrs. Overbeck and Mrs. Jackson how to use aseptic technique while assessing the wound and performing the dressing change.
- Teach Mrs. Overbeck and Mrs. Jackson the signs and symptoms of infection and when to report findings to the physician.
- Review and discuss with Mrs. Overbeck the written materials on total hip replacement.
- Convey empathetic understanding of Mrs. Overbeck's incisional and arthritic joint pain.
- Medicate Mrs. Overbeck every 4 hours (or as ordered) to maintain a therapeutic analgesic blood level.

EVALUATION

Throughout Mrs. Overbeck's hospitalization, Ms. Nobis works with Mrs. Overbeck and Mrs. Jackson to ensure that Mrs. Overbeck can care for herself after discharge from the hospital. Five days after her surgery, Mrs. Overbeck is discharged with a well-approximated incision with no indications of an infection. Prior to discharge, Ms. Nobis is confident that with Mrs. Jackson's help Mrs. Overbeck can properly assess the incision. With minimal help, Mrs. Overbeck is able to replace the dressing using aseptic technique. She can cite the signs and symptoms of an infection, take her own oral temperature, and describe preventive measures to decrease the chances of dislocating her prosthetic hip. Because of her reduced mobility the past 5 days, Mrs. Overbeck says she can tell the arthritis in her "old bones" is "acting up." She reports less pain in her right hip than before the surgery. Mrs. Overbeck tells Ms. Nobis she will be back the following winter to have her left hip replaced.

CRITICAL THINKING IN THE NURSING PROCESS

1. Describe risk factors for Mrs. Overbeck's safety. What changes in her home environment would you suggest to promote safety until she recovers more fully?
2. Why is Mrs. Overbeck placed on the antibiotic Cipro although she has no indications of an infection? What teaching would you do?
3. Mrs. Overbeck's clotting time is slightly elevated as a result of an ordered anticoagulant. Why would this medication be ordered? Consider the patient's age and the area of surgery.
4. Mrs. Overbeck is 30 pounds above her ideal weight and has osteoarthritis. Develop a care plan for the nursing diagnosis *Ineffective Health Maintenance* related to intake in excess of metabolic requirements.

See Evaluating Your Response in Appendix C.

particularly helpful when a large amount of unfamiliar, detailed information is presented. Because the hospital stay is often brief, make an organized, coordinated effort to educate the patient and family. Teaching needs vary, but the most common needs include the following:

- How to perform wound care. Teaching is more effective if the nurse first demonstrates and explains the procedure for the patient and family or other caregiver. The patient and family should then participate in the care. To evaluate the effectiveness of the teaching, ask the patient or caregiver to demonstrate the procedure in return. Ideally, teaching is carried out over several days, evaluated, and periodically reinforced.

- Signs and symptoms of a wound infection. The patient should be able to determine what is normal and what should be reported to the physician.
- Method and the frequency of taking one's temperature.
- Limitations or restrictions that may be imposed on such activities as lifting, driving, bathing, sexual activity, and other physical activities.
- Control of pain. If analgesics are prescribed, instruct the patient in the dosage, frequency, purpose, common side effects, and other side effects to report to the physician. Reinforce the use of relaxation, distraction, imagery, or other pain control techniques that the patient has found useful in controlling postoperative pain.

CHAPTER HIGHLIGHTS

- Surgeries take place in traditional and nontraditional settings with increasing use of minimally invasive procedures that expedite discharge, facilitate healing, and increase patient satisfaction.
- Surgery is an invasive procedure and legal guidelines must be followed to protect the patient and the healthcare providers. The surgical team includes surgeons, anesthetists, nurses, and technicians; all are responsible for the safety of the patient and the progression of the surgery.
- The focus on safety during surgery continues to increase with attention directed to preventing wrong site and wrong patient surgeries (using the Universal Protocol), surgical site infections, DVT and PE, and adverse cardiac events. A team approach to safety works best; each member of the team must feel accountable for the results of the surgery and entitled to share observations and concerns as the procedure progresses.
- Inpatients have relatively short stays. Providing information for self-care is challenging with the shortened stays and rate of admissions and discharges. From the time of entry to the surgical setting, the patient's discharge must be planned and prepared.
- Patient teaching prior to and following surgery empowers patients to achieve successful recovery, discharge, and rehabilitation. Most of the care patients receive during healing is either provided by self or a caregiver outside the healthcare environment. Patients and their families need to know appropriate

assessments and interventions to monitor the healing process and contact information for additional help.
- Pain management is offered prior to, during, and after surgery with methods designed to give the best therapeutic response. While acute pain occurs related to the surgery, many patients also experience chronic pain that affects their response to pain management therapies.
- Behaviors characteristic of older adult patients and ethnically diverse populations increase the need for individualized care. Assessment of physical and emotional status can be more difficult when patients have hearing or visual impairments or when individuals speak and understand a foreign language. Surgery can be frightening to patients and their families and they need reassurance and interventions to decrease pain, relieve anxiety, and promote healing.
- Operating room and postanesthesia care nursing are professional specialties that require unique orientation and education. These professionals make careful assessments of the risks each patient faces and make plans to ensure safe, successful surgical outcomes. Special attention is focused on early recognition and treatment of postoperative complications associated with cardiopulmonary function, respiratory function, wound healing, elimination, and pain.

TEST YOURSELF NCLEX-RN® REVIEW

1. The nurse's primary responsibility related to informed consent is which of the following?
   1. defining the risks and benefits of the surgery
   2. witnessing the patient's signature on the consent form
   3. explaining the right to refuse treatment or withdraw consent
   4. advising the patient and family about what is needed for the diagnosis
2. Given shorter hospital stays for outpatient surgery, patients require which of the following?
   1. increased opioid doses
   2. increased information about complications
   3. increased attention to nutrition
   4. increased parenteral hydration

3. Nonsteroidal anti-inflammatory drugs are given in the postoperative period to do which of the following?
   1. stimulate appetite
   2. increase amnesia
   3. potentiate analgesia
   4. improve renal function
4. When reviewing a preoperative patient's chart, the nurse notes some abnormal findings. Which abnormal finding may indicate renal impairment?
   1. decreased hemoglobin
   2. increased chloride
   3. decreased glucose
   4. increased creatinine

5. In the immediate postoperative period for knee surgery, neurovascular concern is raised if which of the following is found distal to the site?
   1. bounding pedal pulse
   2. muscle cramps in the foot
   3. redness or swelling in the calf
   4. skin that is cool to the touch
6. What would the nurse do postoperatively about medications prescribed prior to surgery?
   1. continue after surgery
   2. decrease by half for 36 hours
   3. order anew prior to administration
   4. withhold until evidence of anesthesia is absent
7. A nurse is preparing a patient with diabetes mellitus for surgery. The patient is NPO prior to surgery. What would the nurse consider about this patient?
   1. has no risk for hyperglycemia
   2. should receive sliding-scale insulin prescriptions
   3. will benefit from hypoglycemia during anesthesia
   4. will fail to manifest signs of hypoglycemia under anesthesia

8. Acute pain management medications in the immediate post-operative period generally do which of the following?
   1. progress from NSAIDs to opioids
   2. progress from oral to parenteral routes
   3. are scheduled rather than prn to promote control
   4. induce a strong sedative effect to decrease the risk of nausea
9. What risks for the older adult patient are posed from lengthy operative procedures?
   1. memory loss due to blood loss
   2. hearing loss due to extended anesthesia
   3. weight loss due to lack of nutritional intake
   4. pressure sores and joint pain from operative positioning
10. A nurse working in the PACU would know that hypothermia in the perioperative period has what effect?
    1. decreases cardiac ischemia
    2. reduces the risk for wound infection
    3. increases patient comfort and analgesia
    4. is associated with cardiac morbidity and surgical bleeding

See Test Yourself answers in Appendix C.

Pearson Nursing Student Resources

Find additional review materials at
nursing.pearsonhighered.com

Prepare for success with additional NCLEX®-style practice questions, interactive assignments and activities, Web links, animations and videos, and more!

BIBLIOGRAPHY

American Society for Pain Management Nursing and the American Pain Society. (2010). Consensus statement: The use of "as needed" range orders for opioid analgesics in the management of acute pain. Retrieved from http://www.ampainsoc.org/advocacy/opioids2.htm

Andersen, B. R., Kallehave, F. L., & Andersen, H. K. (2005). Antibiotics versus placebo for prevention of postoperative infection after appendectomy (Review). *The Cochrane Database of Systematic Reviews, 4.*

AORN. (2010). *Perioperative standards and recommended practices.* Denver, CO: AORN, Inc.

AORN Journal. (2007). AORN Guidelines for prevention of venous stasis. *AORN Journal, 85,* 607–614; 616–624.

Asher, M. E. (2004). Surgical considerations in the elderly. *Journal of Perianesthesia Nursing, 19*(6), 406–414.

Belkin, N. L. (2006). Masks, barriers, laundering, and gloving: Where is the evidence? *AORN, 84*(4), 655–657; 660–664.

Berry, D., Wick, C., & Magons, P. (2008). A Clinical Evaluation of the cost and time effectiveness of the ASPAN Hypothermia Guideline. *Journal of PeriAnesthesia Nursing 23*(1), 24–35.

Bhattacharyya, T., Yeon, H., & Harris, M. B. (2005). The medical-legal aspects of informed consent in orthopaedic surgery. *The Journal of Bone and Joint Surgery, 87A*(11), 2395–2400.

Brandom, B. W. (2005). The genetics of malignant hyperthermia. *Anesthesiology Clinics of North America, 23,* 615–619.

Bratzler, D. W., & Houck, P. M. (2005). Surgical Infection Prevention Guideline Writers Workgroup. Antimicrobial prophylaxis for surgery: An advisory statement from the National Surgical Infection Prevention Project. *American Journal of Surgery, 189*(4), 395–404.

Brendle, T. A. (2007). Surgical Care Improvement Project and the perioperative nurse's role. *AORN Journal, 86*(1), 94–95; 97–101.

Bressler, R. (2005). Herb-drug interactions: Interactions between Kava and prescription medications. *Geriatrics, 60*(9), 24–25.

Byme, M. (2006). Special needs populations: Patients in poverty. *AORN, 84*(5), 837–839.

Carter-Templeton, H. (2005). Malignant hyperthermia. *Nursing, 35*(6), 88.

Cawley, Y. (2008). Mechanical thromboprophylaxis in the perioperative setting. *MedSurg Nursing 17*(3), 177–182.

Clayton, J. L. (2008). Special needs of older adults undergoing surgery. *AORN, 87*(3), 557–570.

Cohen, M. J., & Schecter, W. P. (2005). Perioperative pain control: A strategy for management. *Surgical Clinics of North America, 85,* 1243–1257.

Daniels, S. M. (2007). Protecting patients from harm: Improving hospital care for surgical patients. *Nursing 2007, 37*(8), 36–42.

D'Arcy, Y. (2008). First strike: Does preemptive analgesia work? *Nursing, 38*(4), 52–55.

Fanning, J., Fenton, B, & Purohit, M. (2008). Robotic radical hysterectomy. *American Journal of Obstetrics & Gynecology, 198,* 649.e1–649e1.

Francis, P, & Winifield, H.N. Medical robotics: The impact on perioperative nursing practice. *Urology Nursing, 26*(2), 99–108.

Giannelli, S. V., Patel, K. V., Windham, B. G., Pizzarelli, F., Ferrucci, L., & Guralnik, J. M. (2007). Magnitude of underascertainment of impaired kidney function in older adults with normal serum creatinine. *Journal of the American Geriatrics Society, 55*(6), 816–823.

Gibbs, V. C. (2005). Patient safety practices in the operating room: Correct-site surgery and nothing left behind. *Surgical Clinics of North America, 85,* 1207–1319.

Hassan, Z., & Fahy, B. G. (2005). Anesthetic choices in surgery. *Surgical Clinics of North America, 85,* 1075–1089.

Jackson, S., & Brady, S. (2008). Counting difficulties: Retained instruments, sponges, and needles. *AORN, 87*(2), 315–321.

Lindgren, V. A., & Ames, N. (2005). Caring for patients on mechanical ventilation: What research indicates is best practice. *American Journal of Nursing, 105*(5), 50–60.

Loran, D. B., Hyde, B. R., & Zwischenberger, J. B. (2005). Perioperative management of special populations: The geriatric patient. *Surgical Clinics of North America, 85,* 1259–1266.

MacLellan, K. (2004). Postoperative pain: Strategy for improving patient experiences. *Journal of Advanced Nursing, 46*(2), 179–193.

Majasaari, H., Sarajärvi, A., Koskinen, H., Autere, S., & Paavilainen, E. (2005). Patients' perceptions of emotional support and information provided to family members. *AORN Journal, 81*(5), 1030–1039.

McDonald, D. D., Thomas, G. J., Livingston, K. E., & Severson, J. S. (2005). Assisting older adults to communicate their postoperative pain. *Clinical Nursing Research, 14*(2), 109–126.

Neil, J. A. (2007). Perioperative care of the immunocompromised patient. *AORN Journal, 85*(3), 544–560.

Odom-Forren, J. (2006). Preventing surgical site infections. *Nursing, 36*(6), 58–63.

Ogg, M., & Petersen, C. (2007). Clinical issues: surgical hand antisepsis; hand lotions and creams, gel overlays as artificial nails; benchmarking. *AORN Journal, 85*(4), 815–818.

Pagana, K. D., & Pagana, T. J. (2009). *Mosby's manual of diagnostic and laboratory tests* (9th. ed.). St. Louis, MO: Mosby.

Phillips, N. (2007). *Berry & Kohn's operating room technique* (11th ed.). St. Louis, MO: Mosby.

Polomano, R. C., Rathmell, J. P., Krenzischek, D. A., & Dunwoody, C. J. (2008). Emerging trends and new approaches to acute pain management. *Journal of PeriAnesthesia Nursing (23)*1a, 843–853.

Porth, C. M. (2007). Essentials of *Pathophysiology: Concepts of altered health states* (2nd ed.). Philadelphia: Lippincott Williams & Wilkins.

Porth, C. M., & Matfin, G. (2009). *Pathophysiology: Concepts of altered health states.* (8th ed.). Philadelphia: Lippincott Williams & Wilkins.

Rahman, M. H., & Beattie, J. (2004). Medication in the perioperative period. *The Pharmaceutical Journal, 272,* 287–289.

Saber, W. (2006). Perioperative medication management: a case-based review of general principles. *Cleveland Clinic Journal of Medicine, 73,* S1, S82–S87.

Saper, R. B. (2005). *Overview of herbal medicine.* UpToDate online. Retrieved January 9, 2006, from http://www.uptodate.com

Schwartz, A. J. (2006). Learning the essentials of epidural anesthesia. *Nursing, 36*(1), 44–50.

Silber, J. H., Rosenbaum, P. R., Trudeau, M. E., Chen, W., Zhang, X., Lorch, S. A., et al. (2005). Preoperative antibiotics and mortality in the elderly. *Annals of Surgery, 242*(1), 107–114.

The Joint Commission (2009). The Universal Protocol. Retrieved from www.jointcommission.org/PatientSafety/UniversalProtocol/

The Joint Commission. (2008). 2009 National Patient Safety Goals. Accreditation Program: Hospital, 01.01.01. Retrieved September, 6 2008, from http://www.jointcommission.org/NR/rdonlyres/31666E86-E7F4-423E-9BE8-F05BD1CB0AA8/0/HAP_NPSG.pdf

Washington, G. T., & Matney, J. L. (2007). Comparison of temperature measurement devices in post anesthesia patients. *Journal of PeriAnesthesia Nursing, 23*(1), 36–348.

Weirich, T. L. (2008). Hypothermia/warming protocols: Why are they not widely used in the OR? *AORN, 87*(2), 333–344.

Zide, B. M. (2005). Seven more tips for the operating room. *Plastic & Reconstructive Surgery, 115*(3), 973–975.

Nursing Care of Patients Experiencing Loss, Grief, and Death

LEARNING OUTCOMES

1. Compare and contrast theories of loss and grief.
2. Explain factors affecting responses to loss.
3. Explain the physiologic basis for manifestations associated with the end of life.

4. Discuss legal and ethical issues in end-of-life care.
5. Describe the philosophy and activities of hospice and palliative care.

CLINICAL COMPETENCIES

1. Identify physiological changes in the dying patient.
2. Use assessments, patient values, and evidence to provide nursing interventions to promote a comfortable and dignified death.

3. Effectively communicate with and function within the interdisciplinary team to plan and provide individualized care for patients and families experiencing loss, grief, or death.
4. Adapt individual and cultural values and variations, as well as expressed needs and preferences, into the plan of care for patients and families experiencing loss, grief, or death.

KEY TERMS

advance directives, 92	durable power of attorney, 92	hospice, 92
bereavement, 93	end-of-life, 91	living will, 92
chronic sorrow, 98	euthanasia, 92	loss, 86
death, 87	grief, 86	mourning, 86
death anxiety, 98	grieving, 86	palliative care, 93
do-not-resuscitate order, 92	healthcare surrogate, 92	

Loss may be defined as an actual or potential situation in which a valued object, person, body part, or emotion that was formerly present is lost or changed and can no longer be seen, felt, heard, known, or experienced. A loss may be temporary or permanent, complete or partial, objectively verifiable or perceived, physical or symbolic. Only the person who experiences the loss can determine the meaning of the loss. Although the order of importance varies with the person, people most commonly fear the losses listed in Box 5–1.

Loss always results in change. The stress associated with the loss may be the precipitating factor leading to physiologic or psychologic change in the person or family. The effective or ineffective resolution of feelings surrounding the loss determines the person's ability to deal with the resulting changes.

BOX 5–1 Types of Losses

- Death
- Health
- Body part
- Social status
- Lifestyle
- Marital relationship (i.e., through divorce)
- Reproductive function
- Sexual function

There are many different types of loss, with responses to the loss individualized within each person. This chapter considers loss from both a general and from a specific focus. There is, within the chapter, a greater emphasis on loss from death, as this is often a difficult situation because nurses care for the person who is dying and also for the people who are left to experience the loss. Some of the terms that are used throughout the chapter are introduced in the following paragraphs.

Grief is the emotional response to loss and its accompanying changes. Grief as a response to loss is an inevitable dimension of the human experience. The loss of a job, a role (e.g., the loss of the role of spouse, as occurs in divorce), a goal, body integrity, a loved one, or the impending loss of one's own life or a loved one's life may trigger grief. Although death is the ultimate loss, losses that occur in any phase of the life cycle may produce grief responses as intensely painful as those observed in the death experience.

Grieving may be thought of as the internal process the person uses to work through the response to loss. **Mourning** describes the actions or expressions of the bereaved, including the symbols, clothing, and ceremonies that make up the outward manifestations of grief. Both grieving and mourning are healthy responses to loss because they ultimately lead the person to invest energy in new relationships and to develop positive self-regard.

Death is defined in many ways. One commonly used definition of death is an irreversible cessation of circulatory and respiratory functions or irreversible cessation of all functions of the entire brain, including the brainstem. With the current life-support systems available, the most often used criterion for determining death is whole-brain death (permanent irreversible cessation of the functioning of all areas of the brain). The criteria for whole-brain death are listed in ∞ Chapter 11.

Although death is an inevitable part of life, it is often an immensely difficult loss for the person who is dying and for his or her loved ones. Death may be accidental (for example, from trauma), purposeful (from suicide), occur suddenly or at the end of a long and painful struggle with a terminal illness such as cancer or AIDS, or be the natural end of the aging process.

Theories of Loss, Grief, and Dying

Medical-surgical nurses often care for patients exhibiting responses typical of various stages of the grieving process. Highly individual in quality and duration, the grief process may range from discomforting to debilitating, and it may last a day or a lifetime, depending on what the loss means to the person experiencing it. Although each person experiences loss in a different manner, knowledge of some of the major theories of loss, grief, and dying can give the nurse a framework for holistic care of the patient and family anticipating or experiencing a loss. Table 5–1 summarizes these theories.

Freud: Psychoanalytic Theory

Freud (1917, 1957) wrote about grief and mourning as reactions to loss. Freud described the process of mourning as one in which the person gradually withdraws attachment from the lost object or person. He observed that with normal grieving, this withdrawal of attachment is followed by a readiness to make new attachments. In comparing melancholia (prolonged gloominess, depression) with the "normal" emotions of grief and its expression in mourning, Freud observed that the "work of mourning" is a nonpathologic condition that reaches a state of completion after a period of inner labor.

Bowlby: Attachment Theory

Bowlby (1973, 1980) believed that the grieving process initiated by a loss or separation from a loved object or person successfully ends when the grieving person experiences feelings of emancipation from the lost object or person. He divided the grieving process into three phases and identified behaviors characteristic of each phase.

- *Protest.* The protest phase is marked by a lack of acceptance of the loss. All energy is directed toward protesting the loss. The person experiences feelings of anger toward self and others, and feelings of ambivalence toward the lost object or person. Crying and angry behaviors characterize this phase.
- *Despair.* The person's behavior becomes disorganized. Despair mounts as efforts to deny the loss compete with acceptance of permanent loss. Crying and sadness, coupled with a desire for the lost object or person to return, result in disorganized thoughts as the patient recognizes the reality of the loss.
- *Detachment.* As the person realizes the permanence of the loss and gradually relinquishes attachment to the lost object, a reinvestment of energy occurs. Both the positive and negative aspects of the relationship are remembered. Expressions of hopefulness and readiness to move forward are characteristic of this phase.

Bolby's theory was used as a base for a "continuing bonds" theory, developed by Field, Gao, and Paderna (2005). This theory poses the belief that mourners of loved ones lost by death continue to have memories of the deceased, feel their presence, and save meaningful belongings. These actions bring comfort to the bereaved, and allow a new relationship to form with those lost by death. As a result the mourners resolve their grief and accept the loss.

Engel: Acute Grief, Restitution, and Long-Term Grief

Engel (1964) related the grief process to other methods of coping with stress: After the person perceives and evaluates the loss (the stressful event), the person adapts to it. Engel's recognition of the effect of cognitive factors on the grieving process was an important contribution to the understanding of grieving. The acute stage is initiated by shock and disbelief and may be manifested by denial, which in turn may help the person to cope with the overwhelming pain. As the shock and disbelief begin to fade the loss becomes a reality, and pain, anguish, anger, guilt, and blame surface. Culturally patterned behaviors, such as maintaining a stoic pose in public or weeping openly, characterize this phase. During restitution friends and family gather to support the grieving person through rituals dictated by their culture. The mourner continues to feel a painful void and is preoccupied with thoughts of the loss. The mourner may join

TABLE 5–1 Summary of Selected Theories of Loss

THEORIST	DYNAMICS
Freud	Grief and mourning are reactions to loss. Grieving is the inner labor of mourning a loss. Inability to grieve a loss results in depression.
Bowlby	The successful grieving process initiated by a loss or separation during childhood ends with feelings of emancipation from the lost person or object.
Engel	After the person perceives and evaluates the loss, the person adapts to it. Shock and disbelief, developing awareness, and restitution occur during the first year following the loss; in the months following, the person puts the lost relationship into perspective.
Lindemann	A sequence of responses is experienced following a catastrophic event; concepts of anticipatory grieving and morbid grief reactions are defined.
Caplan	Periods of psychologic crisis are precipitated by hazardous circumstances; successful resolution of grief involves feelings of hope and engaging in activities of ordinary living.
Kübler-Ross	Five stages define the response to loss: denial, anger, bargaining, depression, and acceptance. Stages are not necessarily sequential.

a support group or seek other social support for coping with the loss. This stage lasts about one year, after which the mourner begins to come to terms with the loss and interests in people and activities are renewed.

Lindemann: Categories of Symptoms

Lindemann (1944) interviewed people who had lost a loved one during the course of medical treatment, disaster victims, and relatives of members of the armed forces who had died. Lindemann's research led him to describe normal grief, anticipatory grieving, and morbid grief reactions. He described symptoms characteristic of normal grief into categories of somatic (physical symptoms without an organic cause) distress, preoccupation with the image of the deceased, feelings of guilt, hostile reactions, and loss of patterns of conduct.

Anticipatory grieving was defined as a cluster of predictable responses to an anticipated loss. These responses include the range of feelings experienced by the person or family preoccupied with an anticipated loss. The term *morbid grief reaction* described delayed and dysfunctional reactions to loss; a variety of debilitating health problems were seen in people who displayed excessive or delayed responses to loss.

Caplan: Stress and Loss

Caplan's (1990) theory of stress and its relationship to loss is useful in understanding the grief process. He expanded the focus of the grief process to include not only bereavement but also other episodes of stress that people experience, such as may result from surgery or childbirth. Caplan described three factors that influence the person's ability to deal with a loss. He believed these factors might cause distress for a year or more following the loss.

■ The psychic pain of the broken bond and the agony of coming to terms with the loss
■ Living without the assets and guidance of the lost person or resource
■ The reduced cognitive and problem-solving effectiveness associated with the distressing emotional arousal

Caplan described the process of building new attachments to replace those that have been lost as involving two elements: a feeling of hope and the assumption of regular activity as a form of participating in ordinary living.

Kübler-Ross: Stages of Coping with Loss

Kübler-Ross's (1969, 1978) research on death and dying provided a framework for gaining insight about the stages of coping with an impending or actual loss. According to Kübler-Ross, not all people dealing with a loss go through these stages, and those who do may not experience the stages in the sequence described. In identifying the stages of death and dying, Kübler-Ross stressed the danger of prematurely labeling a "stage" and emphasized that her goal was to describe her observations of how people come to terms with situations of loss.

Some or all of the following reactions may occur during the grieving process and may reappear as the person experiences the loss:

■ *Denial.* A person may react with shock and disbelief after receiving word of an actual or potential loss. After receiving a terminal diagnosis, notification of a death, or other serious loss, people may make such statements as "This can't be happening to me" or "This can't be true."
■ *Anger.* In the anger stage, the person resists the loss. The anger is often directed toward family and healthcare providers.
■ *Bargaining.* The bargaining stage serves as an attempt to postpone the reality of the loss. The person makes a secret bargain with God, expressing a willingness to do anything to postpone the loss or change the prognosis.
■ *Depression.* The person enters a stage of depression as the full impact of the actual or perceived loss is realized. The person prepares for the impending loss by working through the struggle of separation. While grieving over "what cannot be," the person may either talk freely about the loss or withdraw from others.
■ *Acceptance.* The person begins to come to terms with the loss and resumes activities with hopefulness for the future. Some dying people reach a stage of acceptance in which they may appear to be almost devoid of emotion. The struggle is past, and the emotional pain is gone.

Factors Affecting Responses to Loss

A variety of factors affect a person's responses to loss. These include age, social support, families, culture and spiritual practices, and rituals of mourning.

Age

The understanding of and reaction to loss is influenced by the age of the person experiencing the loss. In general, as people experience life transitions, their ability to understand and accept the losses associated with the transitions increases. From the age of 3 years, the development of the concept of death as a loss proceeds rapidly. Table 5–2 outlines the development of the concept of death throughout the life span.

Social Support

Grieving is painful and lonely. One's social support system is important because of its potentially positive influence on the successful resolution of grief. Some losses may lead to social isolation, placing affected people at high risk for dysfunctional grief reactions. For example, partners of people who die with AIDS often report feeling excluded by the deceased person's family and by healthcare providers. Characteristic factors that can interfere with successful grieving include the following:

■ Perceived inability to share the loss
■ Lack of social recognition of the loss
■ Ambivalent relationships prior to the loss
■ Traumatic circumstances of the loss

A move, a divorce, or even the death of a pet can cause a person to feel extremely isolated, yet the person experiencing these types of loss does not ordinarily receive the same social support offered to the person mourning the death of a loved one. A woman having an abortion or giving up a child for adoption seldom receives the same social support as the mother of a child who died at birth. It is therefore especially important that

TABLE 5–2 Development of the Concept of Death

AGE	BELIEFS/ATTITUDES ABOUT DEATH
3	Fears separation; lacks comprehension of permanent separation.
3 to 5	Believes death is like sleeping and is reversible.
	Expresses curiosity about what happens to the body.
6 to 10	Understands finality of death.
	Views own death as avoidable.
	Associates death with violence.
	Believes wishes can be responsible for death.
11 to 12	Reflects views of death expressed by parents. Expresses interest in afterlife as an understanding of mortality develops. Recognizes death as irreversible and inevitable.
13 to 21	Usually has a religious and philosophic view of death but seldom thinks about it.
	Views own death as distant or a challenge, acting out defiance through reckless behavior.
	Previously held developmental awareness of death may still be present.
22 to 45	Does not think about death unless confronted with it.
	Emotionally distances self from death.
	Attitude toward death influenced by religious and cultural beliefs.
46 to 65	Experiences the death of parents or friends.
	Accepts own mortality.
	Experiences waves of death anxiety.
	Puts life in order to prepare for death and decrease anxiety.
66 and older	Fears lingering, incapacitating illness. Views death as inevitable but from a philosophical viewpoint, that is, as freedom from pain and illness or as a spiritual reunion with deceased friends and loved ones.

the nurse does not place a value on the patient's loss when assessing the need for support.

The painful nature of grief can cause the patient to withdraw from a previously established social support system, thereby increasing the feelings of loneliness caused by the loss. A recently widowed woman, for example, may refuse invitations involving married couples with whom she had socialized while her husband was alive, even though her needs for social interaction remain similar to those established before the loss.

Families

A well-functioning family usually rallies after the initial shock and disbelief and provides support for each other during all phases of the grieving process. After a loss, the functional family is able to shift roles, levels of responsibility, and ways of communicating. See the Moving Evidence into Action box for research about factors that affect a family member's ability to care for a dying family member at home.

The family may have negative as well as positive effects. For example, the dying patient may request that someone the family perceives as an outsider be near, and the family may respond with anger to the perceived "intrusion." Similarly, certain family members may express hurt feelings or anger if the patient is unresponsive to other family members. Well-meaning family members also may try to shield the patient from the pain of grieving. It is rare for the family and the patient to experience anger, denial, and acceptance in unison. While one member is in denial, another may be angry because "not enough is being done."

Culture and Spiritual Practices

The influence of culture and ethnic identity on communication, family values, and beliefs about and practices related to illness and death are important considerations when providing nursing care. There are countless ethnocultural and religious differences in the way people observe dying, death, and mourning. For example, differences in the way death is expressed in the United States include "passed away," "died peacefully," "departed this life," "went home to be with God," and "passed from this life." Objects, too, express death and death rituals, such as masks, statues, and candles. Examples of religious traditions in mourning and end-of-life rituals (Spector, 2009) include the following:

- *Catholicism:* An obligation to take ordinary, not extraordinary, measures to prolong life. Autopsy and organ donation are acceptable.
- *Islam:* Euthanasia is prohibited. Medical help to prolong life is not sought. The body is washed only by Muslims of the same gender.
- *Judaism:* Neither autopsy nor organ donation is acceptable. The body is ritually washed and burial is as soon as possible. There is a 7-day mourning period.
- *Protestantism:* Organ donation, autopsy, burial, or cremation are individual decisions. Prolonging life many have restrictions.

Spiritual Beliefs

Patients who are dying often ask questions of themselves and others as to what their life has meant, why this illness has affected them, and what will happen to them when they die. They may feel abandoned by God, or worry that their behavior caused the illness resulting in death. These questions and concerns lead to spiritual distress, which if unresolved may lead to hopelessness, anxiety, and depression. When spiritual distress is resolved, the patient can die more peacefully.

The principles, values, personal philosophy, and meaning of life by which the patient has pursued goals and self-actualization may be called into question when the patient responds to an actual or perceived loss. Because of a fear of intruding on the personal spiritual beliefs and practices of the patient, the nurse often feels uncertain about implementing interventions that would be helpful to the patient responding to a loss. The following questions (using the mnemonic device FICA) may be used to assess a patient's spiritual or religious practices (AACN, 2002):

- *Faith:* What is your faith or belief? Do you consider yourself a spiritual or a religious person? Does religious faith or spirituality play an important part in your life? What do you believe gives your life meaning?

Patients who are terminally ill often choose to die at home and are supported in this choice by many healthcare providers as a way to enhance the dying experience for the patient and for his or her family members. This shift to the setting for healthcare as a patient nears the end of life is contingent upon the availability and readiness of members of the family to assume care of the patient at home. Family caregivers become responsible for providing most of the physical and emotional care of the patient, for managing complex care in the home, and for organizing and coordinating health services on behalf of the dying person. Stajduhar, Martin, Barwidh, & Fykes (2008) collected data from family caregivers of home-care patients who were diagnosed with advanced cancer and had a life expectancy of 6 months or less. The themes identified were (1) the caregiver's approach to life (having a "just do it" positive attitude), (2) the patient's illness experience (caregivers coped best when the patient was "doing well"), (3) the patient's recognition of the caregivers' contribution to his or her care (coping was facilitated by patient's recognition and appreciation of caregiving efforts), (4) the quality of the relationship between the caregiver and dying person (caregiving was easier when the relationship was based on mutual love and respect), and (5) the caregiver's sense of security (security in the caregiving role was enhanced by having family and friends to listen and provide hands-on help, access to relevant and timely information, and support from the healthcare system when it was needed).

IMPLICATIONS FOR NURSING

Although this study focused on patients with terminal cancer, the findings are applicable to family caregivers of all patients who require end-of-life care at home. As the population of older

adults increases, so too will the number of people who wish to die at home. Nurses must be able to teach the skills of physical care and the importance of maintaining comfort. It is also important for nurses to know how to help family members learn to talk with the patient about dying and what the patient wants to facilitate a good death. The family caregiver must know that other family members and friends support what is being done and that it is often a difficult and lonely responsibility. Nurses can provide emotional support through referrals for hospice care and spiritual support, and by being available to provide information throughout end-of-life care. Caring for the caregiver of a dying patient is an important nursing role.

CRITICAL THINKING IN PATIENT CARE

1. An older man, dying of advanced lung caner, says, "I just want to go home to die." He has no family living near him. How would you respond?
2. Make a list of teaching topics needed by the daughter of an 83-year-old woman who has had three major strokes and also has Alzheimer's disease. The daughter wants to care for her mother at home during the last days of her life.
3. The wife of a man dying of kidney failure says, "I just can't leave him. I don't need time for myself." What could you say to convince her that she does need time for herself?

Data from Stajduhar, K., Martin, W., Barwidh, D., & Fyles, G. (2008). Factors influencing family caregivers' ability to cope with providing end-of-life cancer care at home. *Cancer Nursing, 31*(1), 77–85.

- *Influence:* How does your religious faith or spirituality influence your thoughts about health? How does it affect the way that you take care of yourself?
- *Community:* Do you consider yourself part of a spiritual or religious community or congregation? How is that community or congregation a source of support for you?
- *Address:* Do you have any special religious or spiritual issues or concerns that you would like me to address with you? Is there someone else you would like to speak to about these matters?

It is often difficult for patients with an incurable illness to maintain hope and a sense that their lives have had meaning. To meet spiritual needs, nurses can help patients accept the uncertainty that comes with their illness and future death, and respect the spiritual beliefs and practices of patients and their families. Patients who are religious need opportunities for prayer, devotions, and religious rituals. Other resources for spirituality include meditation, guided imagery, music, and art. Privacy and space for these activities should be provided without question.

Rituals of Mourning

Through participation in religious ceremonies such as baptism, confirmation, and bat or bar mitzvah, people joyously celebrate progression to a new stage of life and loss of a former way of being. The funeral ceremony serves many of the same purposes in meeting the needs of the bereaved as people gather to share loss. Through the ceremony, people symbolically express

triumph over death and deny the fear of death. Culture is the primary factor that dictates the rituals of mourning. See the Focus on Cultural Diversity feature on page 91, which provides examples of values and rituals for death in selected groups of people.

Nurses' Response to Patients' Loss

Nurses care for patients and families at various stages of the grief process and may feel that crisis situations are not the time for self-reflection. However, because the nurse's conscious or unconscious reactions to the patient's responses to the loss will influence the outcome of any intervention, nurses need to take time to analyze their own feelings and values related to loss and the expression of grief. The nurse can promote self-awareness by reflecting on the following questions:

- What are my personal feelings about how grief should be expressed?
- Am I making judgments about the meaning of this loss to the patient?
- Are unresolved losses in my own life preventing me from relating therapeutically to the patient?

The following Internet resources may be useful in helping nurses provide care to dying patients:

- Dying Well
- National Hospice and Palliative Care Organization
- AARP Grief and Loss Program
- GriefNet
- National Resource Center on Diversity at End-of-Life Care

FOCUS ON CULTURAL DIVERSITY
Cultural Aspects of Terminal Illness Care

Culture/Ethnicity	Nursing Considerations
American Indian	Some tribes prefer not to openly discuss terminal prognosis and do-not-resuscitate (DNR) decisions, because negative thoughts may make inevitable loss occur sooner. Suggest a family meeting to discuss care and end-of-life issues. If the family feels comfortable, all members of the family and close friends may remain 24 hours a day (eating, joking, singing). Mourning is done in private, away from the dying person. After death, the family may hug, touch, sing, and stay close to the deceased.
Black/African American	Suggest that the family have a family meeting or talk with a minister or family elder. Patients may decide to have older family member disclose a poor prognosis. Care for the dying family member is often done at home until death is imminent.
Chinese American	Ensure the head of the family is present when terminal illness is discussed. The patient may not want to discuss approaching death. Special amulets or cloths may be brought from home. Family members may prefer to bathe the body after death.
Iranian	Information about a terminal illness should be presented by a trusted member of the healthcare team to the family, and never to the patient when he or she is alone. Most Iranians believe in tagdir (will of God) in life and death as a predestined journey. When death occurs, notify the head of the family first. DNR decisions are often made by the family. The family may want to bathe the body.
Mexican American	Based on the belief that worry may make health worse, the family may want to protect the patient from the seriousness of illness. The information is often handled by an older daughter or son. Extended family members are obligated to pay respects to the sick and dying, although pregnant women do not care for dying persons or attend funerals. The family may prefer the patient die at home. Prayers, amulets, and rosary beads are used, and the priest should be notified. Death is seen as an important spiritual event. The family may bathe the body and spend time with the body.
Vietnamese	Consult head of family before telling patient about a terminal illness. The entire family will make DNR decision, often with assistance from a priest or monk. Patients often prefer to die at home. Family should have extra time with the body, and may cry loudly and uncontrollably. Spiritual/religious rites are often conducted in the room.

Source: Adapted from Lipson, J. G., Dibble, S. L., & Minarik, P. A. (Eds.). (1996). *Culture & nursing care: A pocket guide.* San Francisco: UCSF Nursing Press; Spector, R. E. (2009). *Cultural diversity in health & illness* (7th ed.). Upper Saddle River, N.J.: Prentice Hall Health.

End-of-Life Care

End of Life Care or Grieving Video

End-of-life (the final weeks of life when death is imminent) nursing care that ensures a peaceful death was mandated by the International Council of Nurses (1997) and further supported by the American Association of Colleges of Nursing (AACN) (1999). Following are selected competencies necessary for nurses to provide high-quality end-of-life care as defined by the AACN (2004).

- Promote the provision of comfort care to the dying as an active, desirable, and important skill, and an integral component of nursing care (Figure 5–1 ■).
- Communicate effectively and compassionately with the patient, family, and healthcare team members about end-of-life issues.
- Recognize one's own attitudes, feelings, values, and expectations about death and the individual, cultural, and spiritual diversity existing in those beliefs and customs.
- Demonstrate respect for the patient's views and wishes during end-of-life care.
- Use scientifically based standardized tools to assess manifestations (e.g., pain, dyspnea, constipation, anxiety, fatigue, nausea/vomiting, and altered cognition) experienced by patients at the end of life.
- Use data from assessment to plan and intervene in symptom management using state-of-the-art traditional and complementary approaches.

- Assist the patient, family, colleagues, and one's self to cope with suffering, grief, loss, and bereavement in end-of-life care.

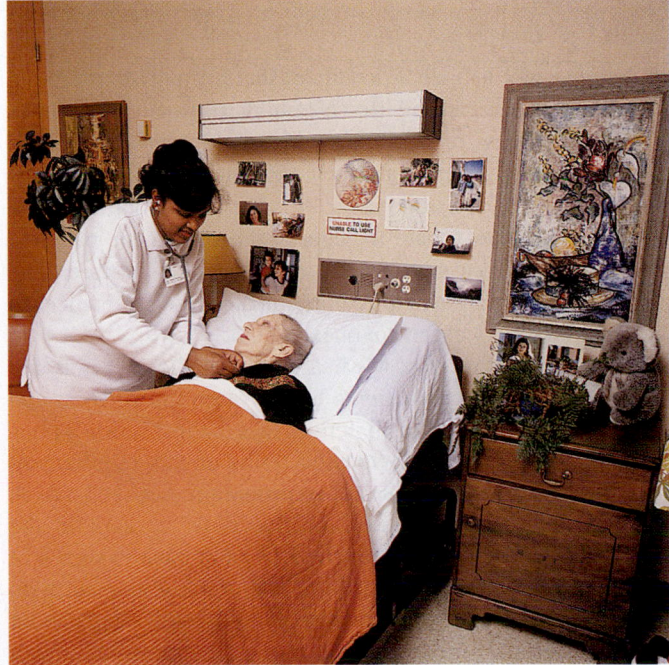

Figure 5–1 ■ The nurse helps the patient visualize the hospital room as a safe, comfortable place to die by surrounding the patient with familiar pictures and objects.

Nursing Considerations for End-of-Life Care

Nurses care for the dying patient in critical care units, emergency rooms, hospital units, long-term care facilities, and the home. Regardless of the setting, the patient's wishes about death should be respected. The Dying Person's Bill of Rights states that each person has "the right to be cared for by caring, sensitive, knowledgeable people who will attempt to understand my needs and will be able to gain some satisfaction in helping me face my death" (Barbus, 1975).

Legal and Ethical Issues

Issues such as those involved in advance directives and living wills, euthanasia, and quality of life are especially important to nurses in upholding the specific care requests of their patients.

Advance Directives

Advance directives are legal documents that allow a person to plan for health care and/or financial affairs in the event of incapacity. They include living wills, healthcare surrogates, and durable power of attorney.

FAST FACTS

Types of Advance Directives

- **Living will**: A document that provides written directions about life-prolonging procedures to provide instructions when a person can no longer communicate in a life-threatening situation.
- **Healthcare surrogate**: An individual selected to make medical decisions when a person is no longer able to make them for him- or herself.
- **Durable power of attorney**: A document that can delegate the authority to make health, financial, and/or legal decisions on a person's behalf. It must be in writing and must state that the designated person is authorized to make healthcare decisions.

A living will is a legal document that formally expresses a person's wishes regarding life-sustaining treatment in the event of terminal illness or permanent unconsciousness. It is not a type of durable power of attorney and usually does not designate a substitute decision maker. It is the responsibility of the nurse as patient advocate to request and record the patient's preference for care and include it in the plan of care. The nurse's documentation helps communicate these preferences to the other members of the healthcare team.

Facilities that receive Medicare and Medicaid funds are required to provide all patients with written information and counseling about advance directives and the institution's policies governing them. The specific terms of this requirement are found in the Patient Self-Determination Act (PSDA). A copy of the signed advance directive must be kept in the patient's medical record, but patients do not have to sign it in order to be treated. Nurses are the ones in close contact with patients, so they are often left with unresolved feelings about the moral, ethical, and legal aspects of their actions. Although advance directives do not ease the pain of seeing patients die, they do help nurses provide patients with the care that the patients have chosen.

Do-Not-Resuscitate Orders

A **do-not-resuscitate order** (DNR, or "no-code") is written by the physician for the patient who has a terminal illness or is near death. This order is based on the wishes of the patient and family that no cardiopulmonary resuscitation be performed for respiratory or cardiac arrest. A "comfort measures only" order indicates that no further life-sustaining interventions are necessary and that the goal of care is a comfortable, dignified death. Agency protocols should be established defining "comfort care" for consistency in nursing care. Confusing or conflicting DNR orders create dilemmas because nurses are involved in resuscitation and either begin CPR or ensure that unwanted attempts do not occur. The American Nurses' Association (ANA) (2004) recommends that the DNR order should be directed by what the informed patient wants or wanted. The ANA further recommends that guidelines and policies be developed to help resolve conflicts between patients and their families, between patients and healthcare professionals, and among healthcare professionals.

Euthanasia

Euthanasia (from the Greek for "painless," "easy," "gentle," or "good death") is now commonly used to signify a killing prompted by some humanitarian motive. There are many arguments for and against euthanasia, and nurses have often found themselves at the center of the debate. As a result, nurses have pushed for the development of appropriate guidelines and procedures for DNR orders. When no such orders exist, the nurse faces a dilemma. Certainly, there are situations in which the nurse's role is clear. For example, it is considered malpractice to participate in "slow codes" (in which the nurse does not hurry to alert the emergency team when a terminally ill patient who does not have a DNR order stops breathing).

The natural death laws seek to preserve the notion of voluntary versus involuntary euthanasia. In voluntary euthanasia, the competent adult patient and a physician, nurse, or adult friend or relative make the decision to terminate life. Involuntary euthanasia ("mercy killing") is performed without the patient's consent. Because care settings offer many complex and technologic interventions, it is not likely that the ethical aspects of euthanasia will soon be resolved. However, advance directives do give patients a much more active role in decisions about their own care.

Settings and Services for End-of-Life Care

Settings and services for end-of-life care range from the critical care unit in a hospital to the patient's own home. Two methods of providing end-of-life care—hospice and palliative care—are described in this section.

Hospice

Hospice is a philosophy of care rather than a program of care. It is comprehensive and coordinated care for patients with limited life expectancy, provided at home, hospitals, and long-term care facilities, that reaffirms the right of every patient and family to fully participate in the final stages of life. Provided by hospice agency nurses and other members of a healthcare team (including social workers, ministers, home health aides, and volunteers), it is based on a philosophy of death with comfort and dignity, encompassing biomedical, psychosocial, and spiritual aspects of the dying experience. Although most hospice care is provided in the home, it may also be provided in hospitals, long-term care facilities, or other community-based settings.

There are more than 3250 hospice agencies in the United States, with services and care reimbursed by private insurance or a Medicare hospice benefit. Services are reimbursed by Medicare for an initial 90-day period, followed by a subsequent 90-day period, and an unlimited number of 60-day periods as long as the patient continues to meet eligibility requirements. The average length of service is 71 days (Hospice Association of America, 2008). Hospice services usually begin when the patient has 6 months or less to live and ends with the family 1 year after the death of the patient. This continuation of care for the family is called bereavement care (**bereavement** is the time of mourning experienced after a loss).

To be eligible for hospice benefits from Medicare or Medicaid, the patient must have a serious, progressive illness with a limited life expectancy. In most cases, a family (or other) caregiver must be continuously in the home with the patient. The patient must have Medicare, waive traditional Medicare benefits for the terminal illness, have physician certification of a terminal illness with a life expectancy of 6 months or less, and care must be provided by a Medicare-certified hospice agency or program. Hospice care under Medicare includes home care, inpatient care when needed, and a variety of services not otherwise covered by Medicare (US Department of Health & Human Services, 2008). The focus is on care, not cure.

Palliative Care

Palliative care is an area of care that has evolved out of the hospice experience, but exists outside of hospice programs, is not restricted to the end of life, and is used earlier in the disease experience. Palliative care, which can be used in all types of healthcare settings, is focused on the relief of physical, mental, and spiritual distress for individuals who have an incurable illness. The goal of palliative care is to prevent and relieve suffering by early assessment and treatment of pain and other physical, psychosocial, and spiritual needs to improve the patient's quality of life.

Although palliative care may be provided by a single person, it usually involves the combined efforts of an interdisciplinary team, including physicians, nurses, social workers, chaplains, home health aides, and volunteers. Care is provided in the patient's home (or long-term care facility, senior living facility, or hospital). The expected outcomes of care are directed by interventions to manage current manifestations of the illness and to prevent new manifestations from occurring.

Physiological Changes in the Dying Patient

Death is a highly individualized process, and may occur rapidly or slowly. Physiological changes are a part of the dying process. These changes result in any or all of the manifestations listed in the accompanying box as death nears. Although each person responds differently, there are certain manifestations common in the dying process, regardless of the trauma or disease process that is causing death. The discussion that follows includes treatments and related nursing care.

MANIFESTATIONS of Impending Death

- Difficulty talking or swallowing
- Nausea, flatus, abdominal distention
- Urinary and/or bowel incontinence, constipation
- Decreased sensation, taste, and smell
- Weak, slow, and/or irregular pulse
- Decreasing blood pressure
- Decreased, irregular, or Cheyne-Stokes respirations
- Changes in level of consciousness
- Restlessness, agitation
- Coolness, mottling, and cyanosis of the extremities

Pain

A common problem for patients at the end of life, pain is what people often say they fear the most. Pain, a subjective experience, is influenced by the patient's emotions, previous experiences with pain, and family and culture. Unfortunately, pain is often undertreated at the end of life because physicians and nurses fear they will cause addiction or cause harm from the high does of opioids necessary to control pain. However, nearly all pain at the end of life can be managed without causing addiction or hastening death through respiratory depression. It is of utmost importance to keep the patient comfortable through general comfort measures (Box 5–2) and by administering ordered medications for pain, neuropathic pain (which is rarely relieved by opioids), seizures, and/or anxiety. The pathophysiology, treatment, and nursing care of patients experiencing pain are fully described in ∞ Chapter 9.

PRACTICE ALERT

There is no maximum allowable dose for full agonist opioids such as morphine sulfate; the dose should be increased to whatever is necessary to relieve pain. Meperidine (Demerol) is not useful for chronic pain as it has a short half-life and a toxic metabolite that can caused irritability and seizures (McPhee, Papadakis, & Tierney, 2008, p. 69).

Dyspnea

Respiratory changes, including dyspnea, are normal as death nears. Dyspnea is a subjective experience, and the patient often reports having a feeling of suffocation, shortness of breath, or

---

BOX 5–2 Providing Comfort for the Patient Nearing Death

- Maintain clean skin and bed linens.
- Use a draw sheet to turn the patient as often as possible so the patient is comfortable.
- Position the patient to promote comfort and protect bony areas with padding. Reposition the patient and raise the head of the bed if fluids accumulate in the upper airways and back of the throat.
- Use bed pads or insert a Foley catheter (if ordered) for urinary incontinence.
- Use gentle massage to improve circulation and shift edema.
- Provide small, frequent sips of fluids, ice chips, or Popsicles.
- Provide oral care, using a soft moist brush or glycerin swab.
- Clean secretions from the eyes and nose.
- Administer ordered pain medications as needed to maintain comfort.
- Administer oxygen as prescribed to relieve dyspnea.

tightness in the chest. Up to 50% of dying patients have severe dyspnea, especially those with lung tumors (primary or metastatic), restrictive lung disease, or pleural effusion (Tierney et al. 2008). Regardless of the terminal illness or fatal injury, the final cause of death is a lack of oxygen to the brain.

As death nears, respirations often become fast or slow, shallow, and labored. The patient may have apnea or Cheyne-Stokes respirations (regular periods of deep, rapid breathing following by no breaths for 5 to 30 seconds). Fluid may accumulate in the lungs, causing crackles, especially in patients who are well hydrated, and in those who are having difficulty swallowing or coughing. These sounds are not painful for the patient, but they may be treated with oxygen, opioids (to improve respirations and decrease anxiety), and medications to decrease secretions (atropine, scopolamine, hyoscyamine, or glycopyrrolate). It should be noted that oxygen and suctioning are only temporary measures, and (especially with suctioning) may even be traumatic for the patient. Nursing care to improve respirations include keeping the head of the bed elevated. Keeping the room cool and providing a breeze from a fan often makes the patient more comfortable.

> **PRACTICE ALERT**
> Morphine is the medication of choice for palliative treatment of dyspnea. Nebulized morphine may be used, and is often more effective than that given by other routes, but it increases the risk of bronchospasm. Nebulized morphine is contraindicated in patients with chronic obstructive pulmonary disease because of the risk of respiratory depression and increasing hypercapnia.

Anorexia, Nausea, and Dehydration

Although anorexia and a decrease in food and fluid intake are normal in the dying patient, the family often views this as "giving up." Anorexia may be a protective mechanism; the breakdown of body fats results in ketosis, which leads to a sense of well-being and helps decrease pain. Parenteral or enteral feedings do not improve manifestations or prolong life and may actually cause discomfort. As weakness and difficulty swallowing progress, the gag reflex is decreased and patients are at increased risk for aspiration if oral foods are given.

Nausea, with or without vomiting, is a common problem in dying patients. Nausea and vomiting may be caused by reduced gastric emptying, constipation, bowel obstruction (a side effect of morphine), uremia, or hypercalcemia. If the patient is conscious and complains of nausea, antiemetics such as prochlorperazine (Compazine) or ondansetron (Zofran) should be administered.

Dehydration is less of a problem than overhydration. Forcing fluids or initiating intravenous fluids for hydration may in turn increase fluid in the lungs, peripheral edema, ascites, and vomiting. Dehydration in the patient nearing death primarily causes discomfort from dry mouth and thirst. The patient should be given small sips of water or an atomizer can be used to spray the inside of the mouth. Oral care should be given at least every 2 hours, and more often if the patient is breathing through his or her mouth. Glycerine swabs may be used to moisten the lips.

Altered Levels of Consciousness

Neurologic dysfunction results from any or all of the following: decreased cerebral perfusion, hypoxemia, metabolic acidosis, sepsis, an accumulation of toxins from liver and renal failure, the effects of medications, and disease-related factors. These changes may result in decreased level of consciousness or agitated delirium. Patients with terminal delirium may be confused, restless, or agitated. Moaning, groaning, and grimacing often accompany the agitation and may be misinterpreted as pain. Level of consciousness often decreases to the point where the patient cannot be aroused. Although decreased consciousness and agitation are both normal states at the end of life, they are very distressing to the patient's family.

If possible, confusion or agitation is treated based on its cause, for example, by relieving pain or dyspnea. Other medications include low doses of neuroleptics, tranquilizers, or anti-anxiety medications. A patient near death often has altered cerebral function, so the nurse must stand near the bedside and speak clearly. Hearing is thought to be the last sense a dying patient loses; the nurse should never whisper or engage in conversation with the family as if the patient were not there. Nursing care for the comatose patient includes the following:

- Using artificial tears if the patient does not blink
- Keeping lights at a low level
- Keeping skin clean and dry
- Covering the patient only with a light blanket
- Using adult incontinence pads or pants for incontinence
- Turning every 2 hours and maintaining joints in position of comfort

Hypotension

As death nears, the cardiac output decreases, as does intravascular blood volume. As a result, blood pressure gradually decreases and the pulse is often rapid and irregular. The extremities are cooler, and cyanosis is present in nailbeds, skin, and lips. The skin on the legs and in dependent areas may become mottled in color. Renal perfusion decreases and the kidneys cease to function. Urinary output is scanty. The patient will have tachycardia, hypotension, cool extremities, and cyanosis with skin mottling.

Support for the Patient and Family

As the patient's condition deteriorates, the nurse's knowledge of the patient and family guides the care provided. It may be necessary to provide opportunities for patients to express personal preferences about where they want to die and about funeral and burial arrangements. If the family feels that this is morbid, the nurse explains that it helps patients to keep a sense of control as they approach death.

The patient needs the opportunity to say goodbye to others. The nurse encourages and supports the patient and family as they terminate relationships as a necessary part of the grief process. The nurse acknowledges that termination is painful and, if the patient or family desires, stays with them during this time. Family members are often afraid to be present at the moment of death, yet dying alone is the greatest fear expressed by patients.

Death

The manifestations listed below are seen after death occurs, and are the basis for pronouncing death. They appear gradually and not in any special order. Pronouncement of death is legally required by a physician or other healthcare provider to confirm death. The time of death, with any related data, is documented in the patient's chart.

The nurse may also fear being present at the moment of the patient's death. In fact, Kübler-Ross (1969) noted that the nurse's fear of death frequently interferes with the ability to provide support for the dying patient and family. Thoughts such as, "Please, God, don't let him die on my shift," are common, and they express the nurse's emotional turmoil in dealing with the task. Nurses who have worked through their own feelings about death and dying are more at ease in assisting the dying patient toward a peaceful death.

After the death, the family is encouraged to acknowledge the pain of loss. The nurse's presence and support as the bereaved express their sorrow, anger, or guilt can help them resolve their grief. It is important for the bereaved not to suppress the pain of grieving with drugs. By accepting variations in the expression of grief, the nurse supports the family's grief reactions.

Resolution of grief begins with acceptance of the loss. The nurse can encourage this acceptance by maintaining open, honest dialogue and by providing the family with the opportunity to view, touch, hold, and kiss the person's body. As family members realize the finality of the death, they are often comforted by the presence of the nurse who cared for the patient during the final days.

Postmortem Care

The nurse documents the time of death (required for the death certificate and all official records), notifies the physician, and assists the family (if needed) in choice of a funeral home. If the patient dies at home, death must be pronounced before the body is removed. In some states and in some situations, nurses can pronounce death; for specifics, consult state practice acts, laws, and agency policy. All jewelry is removed and given to the family unless the request is made that it be left on. The body is kept in place until the family is ready and gives permission for it to be moved. If an autopsy is required or requested, the body must be left undisturbed (e.g., do not remove any tubes) for transportation to the medical examiner.

Documentation of the death is completed by sending a completed death certificate to the funeral home (for a death in the home), or by completing the required paperwork and sending the body to the morgue or funeral home (for a death in the hospital or long-term care setting).

MANIFESTATIONS of Death

- Absence of respirations, pulse, and heartbeat
- Fixed and dilated pupils; eyes may stay open
- Release of stool and urine
- Waxen color (pallor) as blood settles to dependent areas
- Body temperature drops
- Lack of reflexes
- Flat encephalogram

Nurses' Grief

The nurse who has developed a close relationship with the patient who has died may experience strong feelings of grief. Sharing grief with the family after the death of a loved one helps both the nurse and family to cope with their feelings about the loss. Taking time to grieve after the death of a patient provides a release that can help prevent "blunting" of feelings, a problem often experienced by nurses who care for patients who are terminally ill.

> **PRACTICE ALERT**
> Crying with families, at one time considered unprofessional, is now recognized as an expression of empathy and caring.

Nurses working with critically or terminally ill patients should be aware that witnessing a patient's death and the family's grief may reactivate feelings about some unresolved grief in their own lives. In these cases, nurses may need to reflect on their responses to their own losses. Also, nurses who work with dying patients need support from peers and other professionals to work through the often overwhelming feelings that result from dealing with death, grief, and loss (Figure 5–2 ■).

Interdisciplinary Care

Interventions for loss and grief may be planned and implemented by any or all members of the healthcare team. Nurses and social workers provide interventions to help patients or families adapt to a loss. They also make referrals to mental health professionals (grief counselors, social services), support groups, chaplains, or legal or financial assistance agencies.

Grieving patients frequently enter the healthcare system with significant somatic symptoms. In some cases, the symptoms of

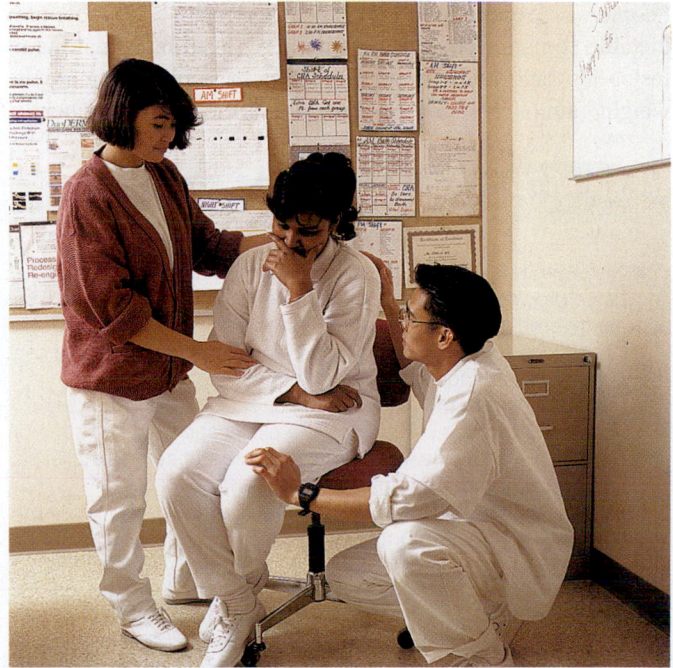

Figure 5–2 ■ Nurses who work with dying patients need support from their colleagues to work through their often overwhelming feelings of grief.

grief and loss are overlooked until the patient reaches a crisis state requiring psychiatric medical intervention. Collaborative care by the physician and the nurse early in the normal grieving process can help the patient achieve an early and effective resolution of grief and avoid physical or psychiatric health problems.

∽ Nursing Care

Nurses practicing in all types of settings care for patients who are in various stages of the grieving process. Grief is highly individual. The grief process may range from uncomfortable to debilitating, and it may last for a day or a lifetime, depending on what the loss means to the person experiencing it. A case study and care plan for a patient who is grieving is included at the end of this section.

Health Promotion

In planning and implementing nursing care for the patient experiencing a loss, the nurse considers the individual responses, which may vary greatly. In an era of short acute care stays for patients, nurses may feel that an elaborate grief assessment is impossible or, at the least, impractical. But research and clinical experience suggest that patients who delay the grieving process after a loss are prone to have health problems that may last a lifetime. See below for an end-of-life checklist for older adults.

Assessment

Knowledge of the expected physical reactions to loss provides the nurse with a basis for identifying reactions requiring further assessment. To assess the extent of physical distress, the nurse observes for changes in sensory processes and asks questions about the patient's sleeping and eating patterns, activities of daily living, general health status, and pain.

Physical Assessment

People who experience a loss may experience one or more predictable somatic (physical) symptoms. Gastrointestinal manifestations such as indigestion, nausea or vomiting, anorexia, weight gain or loss, constipation, or diarrhea occur frequently.

The shock and disbelief that accompany a loss may cause shortness of breath, a choking sensation, hyperventilation, or weakness. Some people also report insomnia, preoccupation with sleep, fatigue, and decreased or increased activity level.

Crying and sadness are observed during normal grief states. Crying may make the individual feel exhausted and interfere with carrying out activities of daily living. However, a person who is unable to cry may have difficulty completing the mourning process. If the person does not express feelings of grief, somatic symptoms may increase.

Reactions to loss are not always obvious. For example, in patients who experience an illness following a serious loss, assessment may reveal somatic complaints related to the grief state as well as the illness. When a person who has been healthy begins to develop patterns of increased illness, the nurse should be aware that this may signal dysfunctional grieving. This is especially common in the loss and grieving associated with a change in body image. In addition to making a physical assessment, assess the patient's perception of the alteration in body image. The loss of a body part, weight gain or loss, and scars from surgery or trauma can be difficult for the patient to accept. Some patients may grieve hair loss that accompanies chemotherapy used in cancer treatment.

It is imperative that the dying patient's concerns about pain be assessed, especially if the patient has cancer or another painful illness. Knowledge of pain theories and pain assessment can help the nurse assess the need for pain medication (∞ see Chapter 9). During the last stages of dying, the patient usually becomes very weak, and sensations and reflexes decrease; these changes call for careful assessment of the patient's physical needs.

Spiritual Assessment

Because spiritual beliefs and practices greatly influence people's reaction to loss, it is important to explore them with the patient when assessing a loss. The spiritually healthy patient has inner resources that help work through the grief process. Faith, prayer, trust in God or a superior being, perception of a purpose in life, or belief in immortality are examples of the inner resources that may sustain the patient during an actual or

---

NURSING CARE OF THE OLDER ADULT   **End-of-Life Checklist**

- Take time a day or so before appointments with your healthcare provider to think about the questions you need answered and concerns you want to discuss. It is often a good idea to keep a pad of paper and a pen handy so you can write down things as they come to you.
- Do not hesitate to have your doctor explain your diagnosis again if you didn't understand the explanation the first time or if you missed some key points. The same goes for details about using medications and possible side effects.
- You may wish to have a friend or family member go with you to medical appointments.
- When you visit the doctor, take an up-to-date list of all the medications (prescribed and over-the-counter) you are currently taking.
- If you have physical pain, tell your healthcare provider. You will probably be asked to rate your pain on a scale of 1 (no pain) to 10 (severe pain). Your rating helps determine what pain relief measures are appropriate.

- It is a good idea to ask your healthcare provider about hospice services well before you are likely to need them.
- Your family and close friends should be aware of your treatment preferences (such as the existence of a DNR order). You might consider documenting your wishes in a living will.
- Think about asking and appointing someone you trust to make your healthcare decisions in case the moment comes when you can no longer make them yourself.
- If you are feeling depressed or anxious or need emotional support, consider talking to a pastor, chaplain, rabbi, or other trusted person in your faith community. If necessary, ask your healthcare provider to recommend someone to help you sort out your feelings.
- Avoid withdrawing from social activities. Keep communicating with your family, friends, and the people who help care for you. If you are open with them you are more likely to get the care you need.

perceived loss. Patients who had not considered themselves religious before the actual or perceived loss often turn to religion to seek comfort or to cope with feelings of despair, helplessness, hopelessness, or guilt.

Assessing the dying patient's spiritual life and its significance to the patient and family helps identify spiritual support systems. Some nurses are uncomfortable with assessing the patient's spiritual needs; the following questions may be helpful.

- What are the spiritual aspects of the patient's philosophy about life? Death?
- Are the values and beliefs about life and death congruent with those of people who are important to the patient?
- Which spiritual resources and rituals have significance for the patient?

Belief systems that are incompatible with those of family members can be an additional source of stress for patients dealing with a loss. The anger and resentment often observed among families faced with decisions concerning dying members may be avoided if the nurse assesses the potential effect of differing beliefs.

Patients coping with a loss often perceive that it is a punishment from God for their wrongdoing or for their failure to remain faithful to their religious practices. Therefore, it is important to assess the level of guilt the patient or family expresses. Assessing the patient's comments regarding feelings of responsibility for the loss helps determine whether these feelings are an expected phase of grieving or indicate dysfunctional grieving.

Psychosocial Assessment

When working through the grief process, patients can be overwhelmed by the fears associated with the loss and the changes it will produce. The patient responding to an actual or perceived loss commonly expresses anxiety (fear of the unknown). An extreme level of anxiety can threaten the patient's well-being. Assessment includes helping patients openly acknowledge their fears. Some patients may fear the feelings they experience while proceeding through the grief process more than the loss itself. The most common fear expressed by patients facing a loss is that of losing self-control.

Talking with dying patients is often difficult. The following suggestions by Roncour (personal communication) provide assistance.

- Often, when patients initiate conversations about dying, you may feel unprepared for their questions. They can take you by surprise, and can often lead you to believe that the patient expects a crystal ball response. Remember that the purpose of all such discussions is to keep the lines of communication open with the patient. The idea is to make the subject of dying discussible, and to communicate to the patient that it does not make you afraid to do so. An open-ended statement, such as "Tell me what concerns you the most" provide a means of encouraging communication.
- Some patients may be too fearful to ask physicians such questions. They often approach staff who they perceive as less intimidating or more approachable. The question often comes in the middle of the night, when there are no distractions, when anxiety or pain may keep the patient awake, and when the patient may feel most alone with psycho-spiritual

distress. In any case, it is often on the nurse's watch when questions about dying may arise.

- Because of the surprising nature of such questions, you may feel tempted to escape ("I've got to go take that patient's vital signs right now"), or pass the buck ("That sounds like a question for your doctor"). Be vigilant about such impulsive behavior and realize that it only serves your own need to reduce your anxiety, but does nothing to assist the patient with his or her own. It is well within the scope of your professional practice as a competent nurse to provide counseling and death education, especially when the patient asks you for it or indicates an unmet need for such information and support. *When in doubt, ask a question in response, such as "Tell me how you feel about that" or "What have you been told already?"* This will accomplish several things. First, it will help you to regain your composure. The second point of asking a question is that it will give you more information about what is on the patient's mind so that your intervention can be as specific and responsive to that patient as possible.
- Do not provide false reassurance. It is important to remember that avoiding discussions about death robs the patient of precious time to accomplish goals that produce hope. Dying people hope for many things even when they cannot hope for a cure, such as hope for freedom from pain, to be surrounded by loved ones, and for the rest of their allotted time to be spent in meaningful pursuits.

Awareness of the altered sensorium observed during the stage of shock and disbelief provides parameters for assessment. The nurse may note in the patient feelings of numbness, unreality, emotional distance, intense preoccupation with the lost object, helplessness, loneliness, and disorganization. As awareness of the loss begins to develop, preoccupation with the lost person or object may increase, and self-accusation and ambivalence toward the lost person or object may follow.

Nursing Diagnoses and Interventions

A variety of nursing diagnoses may be appropriate for the patient experiencing loss and grief, as well as for the patient who is nearing death. Nurses practicing medical-surgical nursing will most often provide interventions for grieving, chronic sorrow, and death anxiety.

Grieving

Grieving is a combination of intellectual and emotional responses and behaviors by which people adjust their self-concept in the face of an actual or potential loss. Grieving may be a response to one's own future death; to loss of body parts or functions; to loss of a significant person, animal, or possession; or to loss of a social role. Nursing interventions are designed to assist with grief resolution.

- Assess for factors causing or contributing to the grief. Ask about support systems, how many losses have occurred, relationship with the lost person, significance of the body part, and previous experiences with loss and grief. *Grief and mourning occur when a person experiences any type of loss.*
- Use open-ended questions to encourage the person to share concerns and the possible effect on the family. *Grief resolution cannot occur until the patient acknowledges the loss.*

- Promote a trusting nurse–patient relationship: Allow enough time for communications; speak clearly, simply, and concisely; listen; be honest in responses to questions; do not give unrealistic hope; offer support; and demonstrate respect for the person's age, culture, religion, race, and values. *An effective nurse–patient relationship begins with acceptance of the patient's feelings, attitudes, and values related to the loss. If the patient is ready to talk, listening and being present are the most appropriate interventions.*
- Ask about strengths and weakness in coping with the other losses. *Current responses are influenced by past experiences with loss, illness, and death. Socioeconomic and cultural background, as well as cultural and spiritual beliefs and values, affect a person's ability to adapt to loss.*
- Teach the patient and family the stages of grief. *This helps them to be aware of their emotions in each stage and reassures them that their reactions are normal.*
- Provide time for decision making. *In periods of stress, people may need extra time to make informed decisions.*
- Provide information about appropriate resources, including support from family, friends, support groups, community resources, and legal/financial aides. *Support from others decreases feelings of loneliness and isolation and facilitates grief work.*

Chronic Sorrow

Chronic sorrow is a "cyclical, recurring, and potentially progressive pattern of pervasive sadness experienced in response to continual loss, throughout the trajectory of an illness or disability" (Nanda International, 2009, p. 276). It is triggered by situations that bring to mind the person's losses, disappointments, or fears. It may be experienced by a patient, parent or caregiver, or person with chronic illness or disability.

- Explain the difference between chronic sorrow and chronic grieving. *Grieving is time-limited and ends in adaptation to the loss. Chronic sorrow may vary in intensity, but it persists as long as the person with the disability or chronic sorrow condition lives.*
- Encourage verbalization of feelings about the loss, and about the personal relevance of the changes to hopes for the future. *Expressing feelings is normal and necessary to decrease the emotional pain.*
- Help identify triggers that intensify the sorrow, such as birthdays, anniversaries, and holidays. *When triggers have been identified, role-playing may make the events less painful.*
- Refer to appropriate community support groups. *Participating in support groups with others experiencing grief is helpful in coping with loss.*
- Encourage use of personal, family, significant other, and spiritual support systems *to facilitate coping with loss.*

Death Anxiety

Death anxiety is worry or fear related to death or dying. It may be present in patients who have an acute life-threatening illness, who have a terminal illness, who have experienced the death of a family member or friend, or who have experienced multiple deaths in the same family.

- Explore the patient's knowledge of the situation. For example, ask, "What has your doctor told you about your condition?" *This provides information about the patient's*

knowledge base about the condition and about his or her ability to make informed decisions.

- Ask the patient to identify specific fears about death. *This provides data about any unrealistic expectations or misperceptions.*
- Determine the patient's perceptions of strengths and weakness in coping with death. *Identifying past strengths can help the patient cope with loss, illness, and death.*
- Ask the patient to identify needed help. *This determines whether available resources are adequate.*
- Encourage independence and control in decisions about treatment and care. *This promotes self-esteem, decreases feelings of powerlessness, and allows the patient to retain dignity in dying.*
- Facilitate access to culturally appropriate spiritual rituals and practices. *This provides spiritual comfort.*
- Explain advance directives and assist with them if necessary. *Advance directives help ensure that the patient's wishes for end-of-life care are carried out.*
- Encourage life review and reminiscence. *Life review is self-affirming.*
- Encourage activities such as listening to music, aromatherapy, massage, or relaxation exercises. *These activities decrease anxiety.*
- Suggest keeping a journal or leaving a written legacy. *A written document provides continuing support to others after death.*

Using NANDA, NIC, and NOC

Linkages between a selected NANDA nursing diagnosis, NIC, and NOC for the patient experiencing death anxiety are shown in the chart that follows.

Community-Based Care

In addition to teaching patients and families to carry out the physical skills that are necessary to the patient's care, nurses also provide information on identifying signs of deterioration

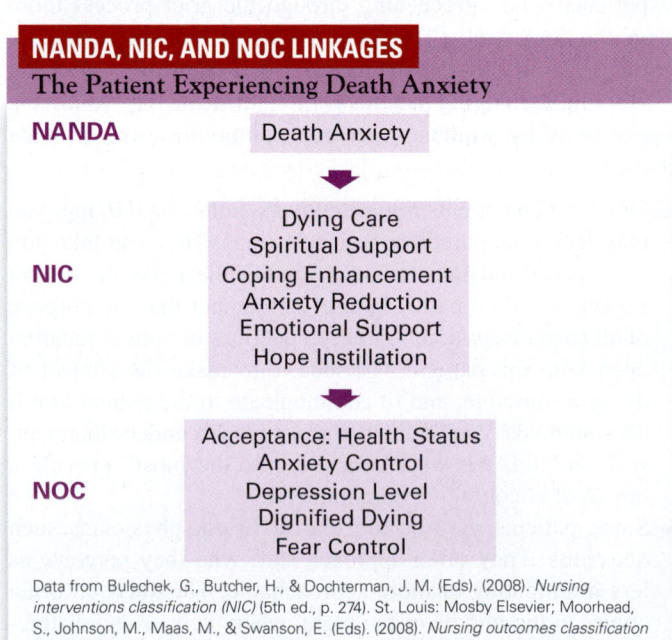

NANDA, NIC, AND NOC LINKAGES
The Patient Experiencing Death Anxiety

NANDA   Death Anxiety

NIC
Dying Care
Spiritual Support
Coping Enhancement
Anxiety Reduction
Emotional Support
Hope Instillation

NOC
Acceptance: Health Status
Anxiety Control
Depression Level
Dignified Dying
Fear Control

Data from Bulechek, G., Butcher, H., & Dochterman, J. M. (Eds). (2008). *Nursing interventions classification (NIC)* (5th ed., p. 274). St. Louis: Mosby Elsevier; Moorhead, S., Johnson, M., Maas, M., & Swanson, E. (Eds). (2008). *Nursing outcomes classification (NOC)* (4th ed., p. 761). St. Louis: Mosby Elsevier; NANDA International. (2009). *Nursing diagnoses: Definitions & classification 2009–20011.* Oxford, UK: Wiley-Blackwell.

CASE STUDY & NURSING CARE PLAN   Loss and Grief

Pearl Rogers is a 79-year-old woman who is admitted to the Methodist Home Nursing Center. Mrs. Rogers lived with her husband of 58 years until his death 9 months ago. She had one son who died in an auto crash 2 years ago, and she has one daughter who lives nearby. After her husband's death, Mrs. Rogers lived with her daughter until her admission to the nursing center. Mrs. Rogers has become increasingly agitated and helpless, complaining constantly of pain. Her daughter states that Mrs. Rogers is chronically constipated, has difficulty sleeping, and has stopped engaging in all social activities, including weekly church services. She cries frequently. Extensive medical testing prior to her admission to the nursing center revealed Mrs. Rogers has arthritis but no other pathologic disorder.

ASSESSMENT

On admission to the nursing center, Mrs. Rogers says, "I'm a sick woman, and no one will listen to me! I can't walk, I'm so weak. My head hurts, and I'm always sick at my stomach. I haven't had a bowel movement in a week, and I never sleep more than 3 hours a night." Physical assessment findings include swollen knees and ankles, with limited mobility of the lower extremities.

DIAGNOSES

- Grieving related to stress of husband's death
- Disturbed Sleep Pattern related to grieving
- Constipation related to inactivity

EXPECTED OUTCOMES

- Engage in normal grief work: Work through grief process, discuss reality of losses, use nondestructive coping mechanisms, and discuss positive and negative aspects of the loss.
- Experience adequate and restful sleep: Fall asleep 20 to 30 minutes after retiring and awaken feeling rested after 7 to 8 hours of sleep.
- Have a bowel movement with soft, formed stools at least every other day.

PLANNING AND IMPLEMENTATION

- Promote trust: Show empathy and caring, demonstrate respect for Mrs. Roger's culture and values, offer support and reassurance, be honest, engage in active listening.

- Assist in labeling Mrs. Roger's feelings: anger, fear, loneliness, guilt, isolation.
- Explore previous losses and the ways in which the patient has coped.
- Encourage review of Mrs. Roger's relationship with her dead husband.
- Reinforce expressions of behaviors associated with normal grieving.
- Encourage participation in usual spiritual practices.
- Encourage participation in a grief group that meets at the facility.
- Consult with the physical and recreational therapist to help the nursing staff provide afternoon activities.
- Provide measures that assist in bowel evacuation: Encourage exercise as tolerated, including walks and rocking in a rocking chair. Offer foods that stimulate bowel movements. Offer privacy: Close the door, ensuring that the emergency call bell is within reach, and do not interrupt.
- Administer a mild laxative and/or stool softener, if necessary, but discontinue as soon as possible.

EVALUATION

After 4 weeks at the nursing center, Mrs. Rogers states, "I don't feel any better, but I know I have to accept my situation." Although Mrs. Rogers states that she doesn't feel better, she is walking the length of the hall, sleeping better, and having regular bowel movements. Mrs. Rogers is also less withdrawn and has openly discussed her feelings related to her husband's death, including her anger at the loss of her son and her husband less than 2 years apart. She has attended the grief group once and has attended chapel services on Sunday for the past 2 weeks. Her daughter visits her each Saturday and takes her in a wheelchair to the shopping mall.

CRITICAL THINKING IN THE NURSING PROCESS

1. What common physical manifestations of grief did Mrs. Rogers experience?
2. How might Mrs. Rogers's daughter be more involved in developing and implementing her mother's plan of care?
3. Suppose Mrs. Rogers says that she does not want any help, that she just wants to be left alone to die. How would you respond?

See Evaluating Your Response in Appendix C.

---

and additional sources of support. General guidelines for teaching patients and families about grief include those suggested in the accompanying Meeting Individualized Needs feature that appears below. In addition, suggest the following resources:

- Hospice
- Home healthcare agencies
- Support groups
- Public health departments
- Church, synagogue, or mosque
- Pastoral counseling centers
- Mental health agencies

MEETING INDIVIDUALIZED NEEDS   Teaching for Patients Experiencing a Loss

- Encourage both children and adults to discuss expected or impending loss and to express feelings.
- Teach problem-solving skills: Define what the possible changes and problems are related to the predicted loss, develop potential strategies for dealing with problems, list pros and cons of each strategy, and decide which strategies might be most useful to try first to solve potential problems associated with loss.
- Teach individuals and families how to support a person who is dealing with an impending loss.

- Explain what to expect with a loss: sadness, fear, rejection, anger, guilt, loneliness.
- Teach signs of grief resolution:
  - No longer living in the past, becoming future oriented
  - Breaking ties with the lost object or person (acute stage often shows signs of resolving in 6 to 12 months)
  - The possibility of having painful "waves" of grief years after the loss, especially on the anniversary of the loss and in response to "triggers" such as pictures, events, songs, or memories

CHAPTER HIGHLIGHTS

- Grief is the emotional response to a loss, experienced by a person as grieving. Bereavement, a form of depression accompanied by anxiety, is a common response to loss of a loved one by death. Death, although inevitable, is an immensely difficult loss.
- There are many different theories of how people respond to loss, grief, and death. These theories are useful when providing nursing care to patients and families.
- A person's response to loss is influenced by age, culture, social support, family members, spiritual beliefs, and rituals of mourning. Nurses need to assess the way in which they respond to loss to better care for patients.
- Legal and ethical issues involved in end-of-life care include advance directives (living wills, healthcare surrogate, and durable power of attorney), do-not-resuscitate orders, and euthanasia.

- Hospice, a model of care for patients and their families when faced with limited life expectancy, supports a dignified and peaceful death. Palliative care is focused on the relief of physical, mental, and spiritual distress for people with an incurable illness.
- To provide knowledgeable and compassionate care at the end of life, nurses must recognize physiological changes as the patient nears death, support the patient and family, provide postmortem care, and resolve their own grief.
- Nursing care of patients experiencing an actual or potential loss includes accurate physical, spiritual, and psychosocial assessment, and interventions for the human responses of grieving, chronic sorrow, and/or death anxiety.

TEST YOURSELF NCLEX-RN® REVIEW

1. Which of the following statements best describes loss?
   1. It is determined by one's cultural values.
   2. It is largely dependent on support of family and friends.
   3. It can be determined only by the person who experiences it.
   4. It is the same as grief and mourning.
2. A newly diagnosed patient states, "I hate this cancer." According to Kübler-Ross, what stage of loss is being verbalized?
   1. anger
   2. bargaining
   3. depression
   4. denial
3. What is an important factor in the successful resolution of grief?
   1. social isolation
   2. support systems
   3. triggers of grief
   4. loss acknowledgement
4. What element is the primary factor that dictates the rituals of mourning?
   1. culture
   2. age
   3. gender
   4. religion
5. A patient says, "I don't want anything heroic done if I die. Just let me go." What document expresses a person's wishes for life-sustaining treatment in the event of terminal illness or permanent unconsciousness?
   1. durable power of attorney
   2. living will
   3. no-code order
   4. healthcare surrogate
6. A patient has been referred to hospice and asks what it means. The nurse's response is based on what knowledge about hospice?
   1. Hospice is a special place of care.
   2. Hospice care is a life-long type of care.
   3. Hospice is a model of care rather than a place of care.
   4. Hospice is designed for patients with serious chronic illness.

7. A patient nearing death requests that no medication be given that would cause a loss of consciousness, including pain medication. What would a nurse do to provide the best end-of-life care in this situation?
   1. Give the medication; comfort is the highest priority.
   2. Give half the ordered dose to provide compassionate care.
   3. Discuss this with family members and follow their wishes.
   4. Respect the patient's wishes and withhold pain medications.
8. Which of the senses is believed to be the last one lost as a person nears death?
   1. hearing
   2. vision
   3. touch
   4. smell
9. Which of the following statements best describes the treatment of pain at the end of life?
   1. As patient nears death, no pain is perceived and no medications are necessary.
   2. It is important to withhold pain medications if the patient has respiratory changes.
   3. There is no maximum allowable dose for opioids during end-of-life care.
   4. Nurses should not administer opioids to the dying patient.
10. A woman, recently widowed, tells the nurse, "I just can't even get out of bed in the mornings anymore." What response by the nurse would be most helpful in resolving the patient's grief?
    1. "I don't know why you feel that way."
    2. "This must be a difficult time for you."
    3. "Why do you think you feel this way?"
    4. "After you get up, you will feel better."

See Test Yourself answers in Appendix C.

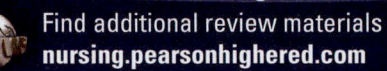

Pearson Nursing Student Resources

Find additional review materials at
nursing.pearsonhighered.com

Prepare for success with additional NCLEX®-style practice questions,
interactive assignments and activities, Web links, animations and
videos, and more!

BIBLIOGRAPHY

American Association of Colleges of Nursing (AACN). (2004). *Peaceful death: Recommended competencies and curricular guidelines for end-of-life nursing care.* Washington, DC: AACN.

American Association of Retired Persons (AARP). (2010). *End of life: Beginning the conversation.* Retrieved from http://www.aarp.org

American Geriatrics Society. (2007). *Position statement: The care of dying patients.* Retrieved from http://americangeriatrics.org/products/positionpapers/careofd

American Nurses Association. (2003). *Position statements: Pain management and control of distressing symptoms in dying patients.* Retrieved from http://www.nursingworld.org/readroom/position/ethics/etpain.htm

Bialk, J. (2004). Ethical guidelines for assisting patients with end-of-life decision making. *MEDSURG Nursing, 13*(2), 87–90.

Bowlby, J. (1973). *Attachment and loss, Separation, anxiety, and anger* (Vol. 2). New York: Basic Books.

Bowlby, J. (1980). *Attachment and loss, loss, sadness, and depression* (Vol. 3). New York: Basic Books.

Bulechek, G., Butcher, H., & Dochterman, J. M. (Eds.) (2008). *Nursing interventions classification (NIC)* (5th ed). St. Louis: Mosby Elsevier.

Caplan, G. (1990). Loss, stress, and mental health. *Community Mental Health Journal, 26*(1), 27–48.

Chart Smart: Documenting a patient's death. (2008). *Nursing, 38* (7), 19.

Emanuel, L., Ferris, F., von Guten, C., & Von Rooenn, J. (2006). *The last hours of living: Practical advice for clinicians.* Medscape. Retrieved from http://cme.medscape.com/viewprogram/5808?src=top10

Engel, G. (1964). Grief and grieving. *American Journal of Nursing, 64*, 93.

Field, N., Gao, B., & Paderna, L. (2005). Continued bonds in bereavement: An attachment theory based perspective. *Death Studies, 29*(4), 277–299.

Fields, L. (2007). DNR does not mean no care. *Journal of Neuroscience Nursing, 39*(5), 294–296

Florida Department of Elder Affairs and the Florida Partnership for End-of-life Care. (2005). *Making choices: A guide to plan for end-of-life planning.* Retrieved from http://elderaffairs.state.fl.us

Freud, S. (1917/1957). Mourning and melancholia. In J. Strachey & A. Tyson (Eds.), *The complete psychological works of Sigmund Freud* (Vol. 14). London: Hogarth Press.

Henneman, E., & Karras, G. (2004). Determining brain death in adults: A guideline for use in critical care. *Critical Care Nurse, 24*, 50–56. Retrieved from http://ccn.aacnjournals.org/cgi/contents/full/24/5/50

Holtslander, L. (2008). Ways of knowing hope: Carper's fundamental patterns as a guide for hope research with bereaved palliative caregivers. *Nursing Outlook, 56*(1), 25–30.

Hospice Foundation of America. (2005). *The dying process: A guide for caregivers.* Washington, DC: Hospice Foundation of America.

Hospice Foundation of America. (2008). *HFA grief resource page. What is grief?* Retrieved from http://www.hospicefoundation.org/griefAndLoss/

Huggins, M., & Brooks, L. (2007). Discussing end-of-life care with older patients: What are you waiting for? *Geriatrics Aging, 10*(7), 461–464.

International Council of Nurses. (2005). *The ICN definition of nursing.* Geneva: The International Council of Nurses.

Jonhson, J., & Johnson, M. (1995). *Grief. What it is and what you can do.* Omaha, NE: Centering Corporation.

Kantor, D. (2008). Caring for the dying patient. *American Journal of Nursing, 108*(11), 72CCC.

Kübler-Ross, E. (1969). *On death and dying.* New York: Macmillan.

Kübler-Ross, E. (1978). *To live until we say goodbye.* Englewood Cliffs, NJ: Prentice Hall.

Kübler-Ross, E. (1997). *On death and dying: What the dying have to teach doctors, nurses, clergy, and their own families.* New York: Simon & Schuster.

Living wills and health care proxies. (2004). *Harvard Women's Health Watch, 11*(5), 6–7.

Mananec, P., & Tyler, M. (2003). Cultural considerations in end-of-life care. *American Journal of Nursing, 103*(3), 50–58.

McPhee, S. J., Papadakis, M. A., & Tierney, L. M. (2008). *Current medical diagnosis & treatment* (47th ed.). New York: McGraw Hill.

Moorhead, S., Johnson, M., Maas, M., & Swanson, E. (Eds.). (2008). *Nursing outcomes classification (NOC)* (4th ed.). St. Louis: Mosby Elsevier.

NANDA International. (2009). *Nursing diagnoses: Definitions & classification 2009–2011.* Oxford, UK: Wiley-Blackwell.

National Association for Home Care & Hospice. (2008). *Hospice facts & statistics.* Washington, DC: National Association for Home Care & Hospice.

Norlander, L. (2008). *To comfort always: A nurse's guide to end-of-life care.* Indianapolis: Sigma Theta Tau International.

Pomeranz, J., & Brustman, M. (2005). When's the time right to enter hospice care? *Nursing, 55*(8), 43.

Rancour, P. (2008). *Personal communications.* Columbus, OH.

Rancour, P. (2008). *Tales from the pager chronicles.* Indianapolis: Sigma Theta Tau International.

Rushton, C., Roshi, J., & Dossey, B. (2007). Being with dying: Contemporary practices for compassionate end-of-life care. *American Nurse Today, 2*(9), 16–18.

Spector, R. (2009). *Cultural diversity in health and illness* (7th ed.). Upper Saddle River, NJ: Pearson Prentice Hall.

Springhouse (Eds.). (2006). *End of life: A nurse's guide to compassionate care.* Philadelphia: Lippincott Williams & Wilkins.

Stajduhar, K., Martin, W., Barwich, D., & Fyles, G. (2008). Factors influencing family caregivers' ability to cope with providing end-of-life cancer care at home. *Cancer Nursing, 31*(1), 77–85.

Ufema, J. (2007). *Insights on death & dying.* Philadelphia: Lippincott Williams & Wilkins.

U.S. Department of Health & Human Services. (2008). *Medicare hospice benefits.* Baltimore: Centers for Medicare & Medicaid Services.

Wilkinson, J., & Ahern, N. (2009). *Prentice Hall nursing diagnosis handbook* (9th ed.). Upper Saddle River, NJ: Pearson Prentice Hall.

6 Nursing Care of Patients with Problems of Substance Abuse

LEARNING OUTCOMES

1. Discuss risk factors associated with substance abuse.
2. Recognize the manifestations of potential substance abuse in coworkers.
3. Describe common characteristics of substance abusers.

4. Explain the effects of addictive substances on physiological, cognitive, psychological, and social well-being.
5. Support interdisciplinary care for the patient with substance abuse problems, including diagnostic tests, emergency care for overdose, and treatment of withdrawal.

CLINICAL COMPETENCIES

1. Assess functional health status of patients with substance abuse or dependence.
2. Monitor for signs of withdrawal and life-threatening conditions.
3. Provide skilled nursing care during the detoxification period.
4. Collaborate with other disciplines when caring for patients with substance abuse problems.

5. Educate patients about stress management, coping skills, nutrition, relapse prevention, and healthy lifestyle choices.
6. Use the nursing process to provide individualized nursing care for patients experiencing problems with substance abuse.
7. Revise plan of care as needed to promote, maintain, or restore functional health status to patients with substance abuse problems.

KEY TERMS

alcohol, *107*
amphetamine, *108*
caffeine, *105*
cannabis sativa, *106*
central nervous system depressants, *108*
cocaine, *108*
co-occurring disorders, *103*
delirium tremens (DT), *108*

hallucinogens, *109*
inhalants, *110*
kindling, *103*
Korsakoff's psychosis, *108*
nicotine, *106*
opiates, *109*
polysubstance abuse, *115*

psychostimulants, *108*
substance abuse, *102*
substance dependence, *102*
tolerance, *102*
Wernicke's encephalopathy, *108*
withdrawal, *102*
withdrawal symptoms, *102*

Disease Process: The Patient with Substance Abuse Problems

Substance abuse refers to the use of any chemical in a fashion inconsistent with medical or culturally defined social norms despite physical, psychological, or social adverse effects. Anxiety and depressive disorders frequently occur with substance abuse. More than 90% of people who commit suicide have a depressive or substance abuse disorder (National Institute of Mental Health [NIMH], 2008). In 2007, over 22 million Americans, or 9% of the population, were classified with substance dependence or abuse (Substance Abuse and Mental Health Services Administration [SAMHSA], 2008a).

The *Diagnostic and Statistical Manual of Mental Disorders* (*DSM-IV-TR*) (American Psychiatric Association [APA], 2000) includes a classification scheme for distinguishing between substance abuse and substance dependence. **Substance dependence** refers to a severe condition occurring when the use of the chemical substance is no longer under an individual's control for at least 3 months. Continued use of the substance usually persists despite adverse effects on the

person's physical condition, psychological health, and interpersonal relationships. The *DSM-IV-TR* criteria deal with the behavioral aspects and the maladaptive patterns of substance use, emphasizing the physical symptoms of **tolerance** and **withdrawal**. Tolerance is a cumulative state in which a particular dose of the chemical elicits a smaller response than before. With increased tolerance, the individual needs higher and higher doses to obtain the desired effect. When a person is physically addicted to the drug and stops taking it, **withdrawal symptoms** can occur within hours. Withdrawal is an uncomfortable state lasting several days, manifested by tremors, diaphoresis, anxiety, high blood pressure, tachycardia, and possibly convulsions. An overview of the *DSM-IV-TR* diagnostic criteria for substance abuse and substance dependence is shown in Box 6–1.

Pathophysiology and Manifestations

The human tendency to seek pleasure and avoid stress and pain is partially responsible for substance abuse. Although far from definite, evidence implicates the endogenous opioid system in

BOX 6–1 Substance Abuse versus Substance Dependence

Substance Abuse

Maladaptive pattern of substance use leading to clinically significant impairment or distress, manifested by **one or more** of the following within a 12-month period:

1. Failure to fulfill major role obligations at work, school, and home.
2. Involvement in physically hazardous situations while impaired (driving while intoxicated, operating a machine, exacerbation of physical symptoms such as ulcers).
3. Recurrent legal or interpersonal problems.
4. Continued use despite recurrent social and interpersonal problems.

Substance Dependence

Maladaptive pattern of substance use leading to clinically significant impairment or distress, manifested by **three or more** of the following within a 12-month period:

1. Presence of tolerance to the drug.
2. Presence of withdrawal symptoms.
3. Substance is taken in larger amounts or for longer periods than is intended.
4. Unsuccessful or persistent desire to cut down or control substance use.
5. More time spent in getting, taking, and recovering from the substance. May withdraw from family or friends and spend more time using substance in private.
6. Decline in or absence of important social, occupational, or recreational activities.
7. Continued use of substance despite knowledge of adverse effects.

Adapted from American Psychiatric Association. (2000). *Diagnostic and Statistical Manual of Mental Disorders* (4th ed., text rev.). Washington, DC: APA.

the development and maintenance of addictive behaviors. Current data suggest that alcohol increases opioid neurotransmission and that this activation is partly responsible for its reinforcing effect. Dopamine has been identified as the primary neurotransmitter responsible for sustaining the addictive quality of drugs as well as increasing drug-seeking behavior. The reinforcing properties of drugs can create a pleasurable experience and reduce the intensity of unpleasant experiences.

The craving one has for a particular substance may also be heightened by a phenomenon known as the "kindling" effect. **Kindling** refers to long-term changes in brain neurotransmission that occur after repeated detoxifications. Recurrent detoxifications increase neuron sensitivity and are thought to intensify obsessive thoughts or cravings for a substance. Eventually the brain responds spontaneously in a dysfunctional manner even when the substance is no longer being used (Stuart, 2009). This phenomenon may explain why subsequent episodes of withdrawal from a substance tend to progressively worsen.

Although there is no greater prevalence of psychiatric illness in substance abusers than in the general population, co-occurring disorders are often present. **Co-occurring disorders** (previously called dual diagnosis and dual disorders) refer to the coexistence of substance abuse or dependence and a psychiatric disorder in one individual. One disorder can be an indication of another, such as the relationship between alcoholism and depression. Alcohol dependence and major depression commonly occur together, posing a significant risk for the development of the other disorder. A depressed person may use self-medication in the form of alcohol to treat the depression, or the alcoholic person may become depressed. The most commonly co-occurring mental disorders in adults are alcohol abuse or alcohol dependence with depression or psychoses. Patients with co-occurring disorders are more likely to be unemployed younger males living in unstable conditions with more than one psychiatric diagnosis and a personality disorder. The combination of these factors results in more crises and a greater risk to the person and others. Box 6–2 lists terminology associated with substance abuse.

Risk Factors

Various risk factors help explain why one person becomes addicted while another does not. Genetic, biological, psychological, and sociocultural factors shed light on how a person may abuse or become dependent on a substance.

- *Genetic factors* include an apparent hereditary factor, especially with alcohol use and dependence. Most of the related genetic research has focused on alcoholism. Evidence supports the D2 dopamine receptor gene (DRD2 A1 allele) as a genetic marker in adolescent males with increased risk for developing substance use problems (Conner et al., 2005). The discovery that the DRD2 A1 allele gene appeared to be associated with alcoholism has led to a growing body of genetic research into substance abuse disorders (Stuart, 2009).

GENETIC CONSIDERATIONS
Alcoholic Fathers and Their Sons

Genetic research has also identified that children of alcoholics (COAs) are at higher risk for developing substance use problems (Conner et al., 2005). This is primarily true with male relatives. One type of alcoholism seen mostly in the sons of alcoholic fathers is associated with an early onset, inability to abstain, and an antisocial personality (Stuart, 2009). Results of one study revealed that adolescent boys of alcoholics with the D2 dopamine receptor gene (DRD2 A1 allele) tried and got intoxicated on alcohol more often than boys without this genetic marker. In addition, they tried more, and used more substances overall. Boys with the allele developed a tobacco habit more and experienced a marijuana high at an earlier age than boys without the allele (Conner et al., 2005).

Critical Thinking in Patient Care

1. Why is it important to ask your patients if they have a family history of substance abuse?
2. What questions should you ask when assessing for increased risk of substance abuse?
3. Does having a positive family history of substance abuse indicate that a person will develop a substance abuse problem? Why or why not?

BOX 6–2 Terminology Associated with Substance Abuse

Term	Definition
Abstinence	Voluntarily going without drugs or alcohol.
Addiction	A disease process characterized by the continued use of a specific chemical substance despite physical, psychological, or social harm (used interchangeably with substance dependence).
Codependence	A cluster of maladaptive behaviors exhibited by significant others of a substance abusing individual that serves to enable and protect the abuse at the expense of living a full and satisfying life.
Co-occurring disorders	Concurrent diagnosis of a substance use disorder and a psychiatric disorder. One disorder can precede and cause the other, such as the relationship between alcoholism and depression.
Cross-tolerance	Tolerance to one drug confers tolerance to another.
Delirium tremens	A medical emergency usually occurring 3 to 5 days following alcohol withdrawal and lasting 2 to 3 days. Characterized by paranoia, disorientation, delusions, visual hallucinations, elevated vital signs, vomiting, diarrhea, and diaphoresis.
Detoxification	The process of helping an addicted individual safely through withdrawal.
Dual diagnosis	The coexistence of substance abuse/dependence and a psychiatric disorder in one individual (used interchangeably with dual disorder and co-occurring disorders).
Kindling	Brain sensitization to events such as stress, trauma, or the effects of substance use.
Korsakoff's psychosis	Secondary dementia caused by thiamine (B_1) deficiency that may be associated with chronic alcoholism; characterized by progressive cognitive deterioration, confabulation, peripheral neuropathy, and myopathy.
Physical dependence	A state in which withdrawal syndrome will occur if drug use is discontinued.
Polysubstance abuse	The simultaneous use of many substances.
Psychologic dependence	An intensive subjective need for a particular psychoactive drug.
Substance abuse	Continued use of a chemical substance in a fashion inconsistent with medical or social norms, for at least 1 month, despite related problems.
Substance dependence	A severe condition occurring when the use of the chemical substance is no longer under control, for at least 3 months; continued use persists despite adverse effects (used interchangeably with addiction).
Tolerance	State in which a particular dose elicits a smaller response than it formerly did. With increased tolerance the individual needs higher and higher doses to obtain the desired response.
Wernicke's encephalopathy	Caused by thiamine (B_1) deficiency, characterized by nystagmus, ptosis, ataxia, confusion, coma, and possible death. Thiamine deficiency is common in chronic alcoholism.
Withdrawal syndrome	Constellation of signs and symptoms that occurs in physically dependent individuals when they discontinue drug use.

Women drink less alcohol and have fewer alcohol-related problems than men. In addition, women are less likely to have characteristics associated with heavy drinking including aggressiveness, drinking to reduce distress, and antisocial tendencies. See the Genetics Consideration box on page 103.

■ *Biological factors* were first identified by Jellinek in his Disease Model of Alcoholism. He hypothesized that addiction to alcohol may have a biochemical basis and identified specific phases of the disease (Jellinek, 1946). Expanding on Jellinek's early work, researchers have implicated low levels of dopamine and serotonin in the development of alcohol dependence. Dopamine and dopamine receptor sites are intricately involved in the complex workings between the nervous system and abusive substances. Any drug's ability to have an impact on the biochemical mechanism of the brain must be able to do so at a receptor site or at a number of receptor sites (Figure 6–1 ■). Most abused substances either mimic or block the brain's most important neurotransmitters at their respective receptor sites. For example, heroin and other opiates mimic natural opiate-like neurotransmitters such as endorphin, enkephalin, and dynorphin. In contrast, cocaine and other stimulants block the reuptake of dopamine, serotonin, and norepinephrine (Stuart, 2009).

■ *Psychological factors* attempt to explain substance abuse through a combination of psychoanalytic, behavioral, and family system theories. Psychoanalytic theorists view substance abuse as a fixation at the oral stage of development, while behavioral theorists see addiction as a learned, maladaptive behavior. Family system theory focuses on the pattern of family relationships throughout several generations. No addictive personality type has been identified; however, several common factors seem to exist among alcoholics and drug users. Another type of alcoholism may be more environmentally influenced and is linked with onset after the age of 25, inability to stop after one drink, and a passive-dependent personality (Stuart, 2009). Many substance abusers have experienced sexual or physical abuse in their childhood and as a result have low self-esteem and difficulty expressing emotions. A link also exists between substance abuse and psychiatric disorders such as depression, anxiety, and antisocial and dependent personalities. The habit of using a substance becomes a form of self-medication to cope with day-to-day problems, and over time develops into an addiction.

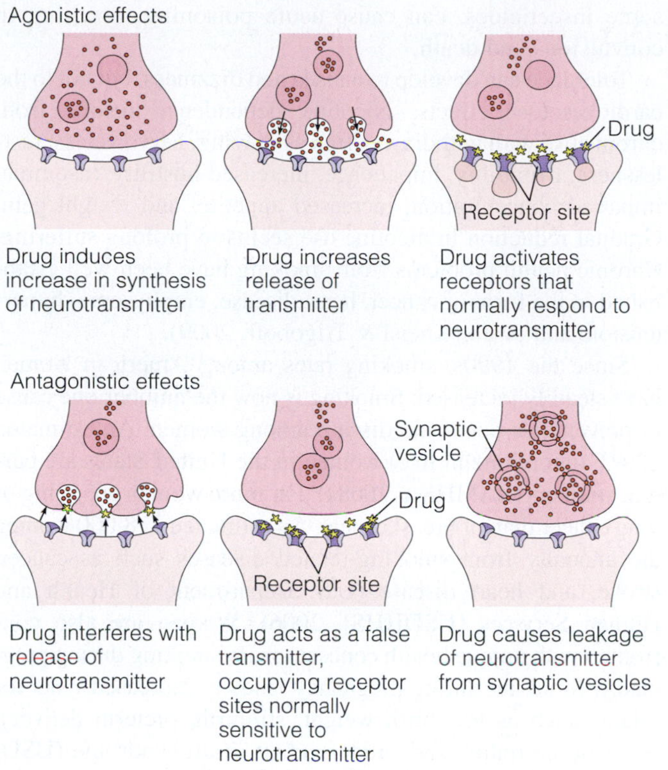

Agonistic effects

Drug induces increase in synthesis of neurotransmitter

Drug increases release of transmitter

Drug activates receptors that normally respond to neurotransmitter

Drug

Receptor site

Antagonistic effects

Drug interferes with release of neurotransmitter

Drug acts as a false transmitter, occupying receptor sites normally sensitive to neurotransmitter

Drug causes leakage of neurotransmitter from synaptic vesicles

Synaptic vesicle

Drug

Receptor site

Figure 6–1 ■ Action of abusive substances at brain receptor sites.

■ *Sociocultural factors* often influence individuals' decisions as to when, what, and how they use substances. Ethnic differences in the way alcohol is metabolized may explain why some individuals choose not to drink. Compared to other ethnic groups, Asian Americans report the lowest prevalence of family history of alcoholism. It is hypothesized that the Asian population has a deficiency of aldehyde dehydrogenase (ADH), the chemical in the brain that breaks down alcohol acetaldehyde (Cook et al., 2005). A buildup of acetaldehyde in the brain causes toxic symptoms characterized by vomiting, flushing and tachycardia. Caucasians, Hispanics, and African Americans, on the other hand, have sufficient ADH for metabolizing alcohol and report higher alcoholism rates (Bersamin, Paschall, & Flewelling, 2005).

Religious background may also correlate with the likelihood that a person will abuse alcohol. Among major religions, people of Jewish faith have the lowest rate of alcoholism while Roman Catholics have the highest rate. See the accompanying Focus on Diversity feature.

Many factors place a person at risk for substance use, abuse, and dependence. No single cause can explain why one individual develops a pattern of drug use and another person does not. Thorough assessment of these factors is necessary to understand the whole person and plan appropriate interventions.

Characteristics of Abusers

As mentioned, no addictive personality type exists; however, many abusers have several characteristics in common. Addictive behavior associated with alcoholism and other substances is characterized by compulsive preoccupation with obtaining the substance, loss of control over consumption, and development of tolerance and dependence as well as impaired social and occupational functioning. There is a tendency for drug users to indulge in impulsive, risk-taking behaviors. Abusers often have a low tolerance for frustration and pain. Often, drug users are rebellious against social norms and engage in various antisocial and risky behaviors such as stealing, promiscuity, driving while intoxicated, and violence against others. There is also a tendency toward anxiety, anger, and low self-esteem in substance abusers. Many people have a desire for social acceptance and initiate drug use to "fit in" with a peer group. Others may suffer from social anxiety and need drugs or alcohol to feel less inhibited while interacting with others.

Addictive Substances and Their Effects
Caffeine

Caffeine is a stimulant that increases the heart rate and acts as a diuretic. Although commonly consumed daily in soft drinks, coffee, tea, chocolate, and some pain relievers, an excessive amount of caffeine can cause negative physiologic effects, especially cardiac related risks. Approximately 300 mg per day

FOCUS ON CULTURAL DIVERSITY
Substance Use and Ethnicity

Ethnic identity plays a unique role in drug use behavior. Patterns of substance use are influenced by cultural norms and practices, in addition to other environmental and biological factors. Adolescents in particular are influenced by ethnic and cultural practices. Positive ethnic identity (i.e., strong ethnic affiliation, attachment, and pride) may "protect" adolescents against drug use and help them form resistant behaviors to substance abuse (Marsiglia, Kulis, Hecht, & Sills, 2004). A higher number of Black and Hispanic children are exposed to alcohol problems in the home than white children (Ramisetty-Mikler & Caetano, 2004). Use of tobacco, alcohol, and illicit drugs are reportedly different in racial and ethnic groups. American Indians and Alaska Natives have higher levels of tobacco, alcohol, and illicit drug use when compared to other racial groups (SAMHSA, 2008a). Substance abuse and Type 2 diabetes are serious health problems among

American Indians (Leonardson et al., 2005). Asian Americans have the lowest rates of tobacco, alcohol, and illicit drug usage (SAMHSA).

CRITICAL THINKING IN PATIENT CARE

1. You are a school nurse with a large population of American Indians, Latin Americans, and African Americans in the community. An increasing problem with alcohol use and binge drinking among the high school students has become evident. The school superintendent has asked you for ideas to address this problem. How would you respond?

2. You are caring for a 23-year-old Asian American female brought to the emergency room by her boyfriend who tells you they were at a college party where she had alcohol for the first time. She is weak, her face is flushed, and she is vomiting violently. What would you do?

is safe for most people, but over 600 mg is considered excessive and not recommended (Kneisl & Trigoboff, 2009). Individuals with a history of cardiac disease are advised to cut down or eliminate caffeine intake altogether. Caffeine, if consumed in large quantities, can also cause higher total cholesterol levels and insomnia.

Many people in today's society recognize the adverse effects of too much caffeine in the system and voluntarily cut down on caffeine by drinking decaffeinated beverages. A caffeine-addicted person who abruptly withdraws from caffeine often experiences headaches and irritability. A rising number of adolescents are developing caffeine dependence by consuming sizeable quantities of soft drinks and coffee.

Nicotine

Nicotine is found in tobacco and enters the system via the lungs (cigarettes and cigars) and oral mucous membranes (chewing tobacco as well as smoking). In low doses, nicotine stimulates nicotinic receptors in the brain to release norepinephrine and epinephrine, causing vasoconstriction. As a result, the heart rate accelerates and the force of ventricular contractions increases. Gastrointestinal (GI) effects include an increase in gastric acid secretion, tone and motility of GI smooth muscle, and promotion of vomiting. Nicotine acts on the central nervous system (CNS) as a stimulant, binding to acetylcholine receptors in the brain and causing the release of dopamine and norepinephrine. Quitting smoking is thought to be more difficult because of dopamine release, which in turn reinforces the addictive craving for more. Smoking cessation can pose a problem for hospitalized patients. See Moving Evidence into Action: Smoking Cessation in Hospitalized Patients.

Initially, nicotine increases respiration, mental alertness, and cognitive ability, but eventually depresses these responses (Kneisl & Trigoboff, 2009). Moderate doses of nicotine can cause tremors. High doses of nicotine, found in

some insecticides, can cause acute poisoning, resulting in convulsions and death.

Tolerance can develop to nausea and dizziness, but not to the cardiovascular effects. Nicotine dependence results from chronic use with withdrawal seen as craving, nervousness, restlessness, irritability, impatience, increased hostility, insomnia, impaired concentration, increased appetite, and weight gain. Gradual reduction in nicotine use seems to prolong suffering. Chronic health problems from smoking have been well established in the form of cancer, heart disease, emphysema, hypertension, and death (Kneisl & Trigoboff, 2009).

Since the 1990s, smoking rates among American women have steadily increased. Smoking is now the number one cause of preventable death and disease among women. An estimated 22.4% (about one in five) women in the United States are current smokers (SAMHSA, 2008a). Far more women are dying of lung cancer than of breast cancer. An estimated 178,000 women die annually from smoking-related diseases such as cancer, stroke, and heart disease (U.S. Department of Health and Human Services [USDHHS], 2006). Women are also confronted with unique health concerns from smoking during pregnancy. Smoking during pregnancy leads to increased risks for infants such as low birth weight, stillbirth, preterm delivery, perinatal mortality, and sudden infant death syndrome (USDHHS). Secondhand effects from smoking have been demonstrated, especially to fetuses during pregnancy. Smoking also increases the risk for infertility. Postmenopausal women who smoke have lower bone density and increased risk for hip fracture than women who have never smoked (USDHHS).

Cannabis

Cannabis sativa is the source of marijuana. According to 2007 NSDUH data, marijuana is the most commonly used illicit drug (14.4 million users) (SAMHSA, 2008a). A majority of illicit drug users (56.2%) reported that their first drug was marijuana,

---

MOVING EVIDENCE INTO ACTION — Smoking Cessation in Hospitalized Patients

Despite the well-publicized deleterious health effects posed by cigarette smoking and the legally restricted access to cigarettes, it still remains a persistent problem. Smoking has been banned in stores, malls, hospitals, office buildings, and even a number of restaurants. Admission to the hospital provides an excellent opportunity for nurses to assist patients to quit smoking. Patients in hospitals may find it easier to quit in an environment where smoking is restricted or prohibited. In addition, individuals may be more open to cessation efforts when faced with the risks associated with surgery. In a review of the literature, researchers found that high intensity behavioral interventions that include at least 1 month of follow-up contact were effective in helping hospitalized patients quit smoking (Rigotti, Munafo, Murphy, & Stead, 2005). Healthcare professionals, especially nurses, can be very instrumental in smoking cessation efforts. Another literature review provided evidence that nursing interventions for smoking cessation has potential benefits (Rice & Stead, 2005). Nicotine replacement therapy (NRT) also increases quit rates with or without additional counseling (Rice & Stead, 2005; Silagy et al., 2005). NRT aims to reduce withdrawal from tobacco products by replacing nicotine in the blood. All forms of NRT, available as chewing gum, skin

patches, nose spray, inhalers, and tablets, increases the likelihood that a person will succeed in quitting smoking (Silagy et al., 2005). Effective nursing strategies include asking patients about their tobacco use, counseling those who want to quit, reinforcing cessation efforts, and early follow-up with those who quit smoking. This evidence points to the important role nurses possess to encourage their patients to quit smoking and the need for nurses to incorporate smoking cessation interventions as part of their standard practice.

CRITICAL THINKING IN PATIENT CARE

1. You are caring for a 55-year-old man recently hospitalized for acute angina who asks you what is the best way to stop smoking. What would you do?
2. Why do you think nurses and other healthcare professionals should (or should not) quit smoking?
3. You are caring for a 12-year-old girl who tells you she has smoked cigarettes occasionally and believes it makes her more popular with her older friends. She admits that she knows that smoking is supposed to be bad for you but doesn't see the harm in smoking a few cigarettes every day. How would you respond?

supporting the notion that marijuana is a "gateway" drug. The greatest psychoactive substances are in the flowering tops of the cannabis plant. Marijuana (also know as grass, weed, pot, dope, joint, and reefer) and hashish are the most common derivatives. The psychoactive component of marijuana is an oily chemical known as delta-9-tetrahydrocannabinol (THC). THC activates specific cannabinoid receptors in the brain. Evidence suggests that marijuana may act like opioids and cocaine in producing a pleasurable sensation, probably by causing release of endogenous opioids and then dopamine (Kneisl & Trigoboff, 2009). Marijuana use can trigger psychosis in schizophrenic patients and according to recent research cannabis use may be a risk factor in developing future psychotic symptoms (Ferdinand et al., 2005).

Physiologic effects of cannabis are dose related and can cause an increase in heart rate and bronchodilation in short-term use. Chronic long-term use can lead to airway constriction, bronchitis, sinusitis, asthma, and increased risk for respiratory cancer. The reproductive system is also affected by marijuana; it causes decreased spermatogenesis and testosterone levels in males and suppresses follicle-stimulating, luteinizing, and prolactin hormones in females, making breast feeding for new mothers impossible. Birth defects may also be associated with cannabis use. Marijuana crosses the placental barrier and is spread to fetal tissues. When a pregnant woman smokes marijuana she increases the risk of abnormalities in the fetus such as CNS disturbances, low birth weight, decreased length, smaller head circumference, and fetal death (Kneisl & Trigoboff, 2009). Subjective effects of marijuana include euphoria, sedation, and hallucinations. In addition, chronic use of marijuana can result in amotivational behaviors such as apathy, dullness, poor grooming, reduced interest in achievement, and disinterest. At extremely high doses, tolerance and physical dependence result.

Alcohol

Alcohol is the most commonly used and abused legal substance in the United States. Alcohol and other CNS depressants act on other neurotransmitters in the brain such as gamma-aminobutyric acid (GABA). GABA is the most prevalent inhibitory neurotransmitter in the brain and has a major role in decreasing neuronal excitability. Alcohol creates an additive effect with GABA, further inhibiting arousal and depressing the autonomic nervous system. This may explain why cross-tolerance effects occur when alcohol and other CNS depressants are used in combination. When taken together, alcohol and other CNS depressants such as benzodiazepines and barbiturates can lead to respiratory depression and death.

Slightly more than half, or 126.8 million, of the nation's population over age 12 report current alcohol use (SAMHSA, 2008a). Of this number, an estimated 17 million, or 1 in every 7, report heavy drinking (defined as binge drinking on at least 5 days in the past 30 days) (SAMHSA). Although the legal drinking age in all 50 states is 21, many underage people use alcohol. Of the 14 million adults in America who abuse alcohol, 95% report drinking before the age of 21 (SAMHSA, 2008b). Alcohol use increases with increasing age among underage persons and, unfortunately, this pattern has remained stable since 2002. In 2007, slightly more

than half (50.7%) of 18 to 20 year olds drank alcohol during the month before they were surveyed (SAMHSA, 2008a). Alcohol is considered a "gateway" drug, leading to the use of "harder" substances like cocaine, heroin, or methamphetamine. During 2006, over 130,000 alcohol-related emergency department (ED) visits were made by patients under the age of 21 (SAMSHA, 2008b). Almost one-third (31%) of those alcohol-related ED visits for minors involved other substances as well. Table 6–1 lists the drugs most frequently reported with alcohol in ED visits.

> **FAST FACTS**
> **Underage Drinking**
> - The rate of underage drinking remains consistently high. In 2007, approximately 10.7 million persons aged 12 to 20 reported drinking alcohol in the past month (27.9% of this age group).
> - Of these, nearly 18.6% were binge drinkers, and 6% were heavy drinkers.
> - Among persons aged 12 to 20 in 2007, past month alcohol use rates were lowest among Asians (16.8%) and highest among whites (32%).
> - The highest prevalence of binge and heavy drinking in 2007 was for young adults aged 18 to 20 (50.7%).
> - In 2007, over 26% of teens (16 to 20 years) reported driving under the influence at least once in the past year.
>
> *Source: SAMHSA, 2008a NSDUH.*

Alcohol is absorbed in the mouth, stomach, and digestive tract. The liver metabolizes approximately 95% of the ingested alcohol and the rest is excreted via the skin, kidney, and lungs. Generally, an individual can break down approximately 1 ounce of whiskey every 90 minutes. Factors such as body mass, food intake, and liver function can affect the rate of alcohol absorption.

When used in moderation, certain types of alcohol can have positive physiological effects by decreasing coronary artery disease and protecting against stroke. However, when consumed in excess, alcohol can severely diminish one's ability to function and will ultimately lead to life-threatening conditions. Chronic use of alcohol can cause severe neurological and psychiatric disorders. Severe damage to the liver occurs with chronic alcohol abuse, and can progress from fatty liver to other

TABLE 6–1 Drugs Most Frequently Reported with Alcohol-Related ED Visits

RANK	DRUG	ESTIMATED VISITS
1	No other drug	126,704
2	Cocaine only	101,588
3	Marijuana only	41,653
4	Cocaine and marijuana	21,241
5	Heroin only	14,958
6	Stimulants only	7,895
7	Alprazolam only	8,007
8	Cocaine and heroin	10,628

Source: SAMHSA, Office of Applied Studies, Drug Abuse Warning Network, 2008b.

liver diseases such as hepatitis or cirrhosis. Chronic alcoholism is the major cause of fatal cirrhosis. Alcohol causes damaging effects to many other systems; its effects include myocardial disease, erosive gastritis, acute and chronic pancreatitis, sexual dysfunction, and an increased risk of breast cancer.

Malnutrition is another serious complication of chronic alcoholism, especially thiamine (B_1) deficiency that can result in neurological impairments. Thiamine depletion is thought to cause the Wernicke-Korsakoff syndrome observed in chronic alcoholics (Stuart, 2009). Severe cognitive impairment is a principal feature of **Wernicke's encephalopathy** and **Korsakoff's psychosis**. Although these are sometimes considered to be two distinctive disorders, they are actually different phases of the same disease, commonly called Wernicke-Korsakoff syndrome. Wernicke's encephalopathy indicates the acute stage of the illness, and Korsakoff's psychosis indicates the chronic stage.

Although alcohol is a CNS depressant, it actually disrupts sleep, thus altering the sleep cycle, decreasing the quality of sleep, intensifying obstructive sleep apnea, and reducing total sleeping time. Heavy drinkers have a higher mortality rate and many fatalities occur from alcohol-related accidents. Blood alcohol levels (BALs) are highly predictive of CNS effects. Euphoria, reduced inhibitions, impaired judgment, and increased confidence are seen at 0.05% (Kneisl & Trigoboff, 2009). The legal level of intoxication in many states is 0.08%. Toxic levels in excess of 0.5% can cause coma, respiratory depression, peripheral collapse, and death (Kneisl & Trigoboff, 2009). Chronic consumption of alcohol produces tolerance and creates cross-tolerance to general anesthetics, barbiturates, benzodiazepines, and other CNS depressants. If alcohol is withdrawn abruptly, the brain becomes overly excited because receptors previously inhibited are no longer inhibited. This hyperexcitability manifests clinically as anxiety, tachycardia, hypertension, diaphoresis, nausea, vomiting, tremors, sleeplessness, and irritability (Llussier et al., 2007). Severe manifestations of alcohol withdrawal include seizures, convulsions, and **delirium tremens (DT)**. Episodes of delirium tremens have a mortality rate of 1% to 5%.

CNS Depressants

Central nervous system depressants, including barbiturates, benzodiazepines, paraldehyde, meprobamate, and chloral hydrate are also subject to abuse. Cross dependence exists among all CNS depressants and cross-tolerance can develop to alcohol and general anesthetics. Chronic users of barbiturates require progressively higher doses to achieve subjective effects as tolerance develops, but they develop little tolerance to respiratory depression. The depressant effects related to barbiturates are dose dependent and range from mild sedation to sleep to coma to death. With larger doses over time and a combination of alcohol and barbiturates, the risk of death increases greatly. The risk of accidental overdose and death resulting from barbiturates has resulted in decreased use, yet barbiturates are still clinically useful for seizure disorders and alcohol withdrawal. Benzodiazepines have replaced barbiturates as the drugs of choice for anxiety-related disorders. Benzodiazepines alone are safer than barbiturates, because an overdose of oral benzodiazepines rarely results in death. However, CNS depressants when taken together (for example alcohol and benzodiazepines) can result in death.

Psychostimulants

Psychostimulants such as cocaine and amphetamines have a high potential for abuse. Euphoria is the main subjective effect associated with cocaine and amphetamines, leading to addiction. **Cocaine** powder has been "snorted" (inhaled through the nostrils) for thousands of years, but a more dangerous method now is called freebasing. Cocaine base (freebased cocaine, or "crack") is heat stable and is usually "cooked" in a baking soda solution and smoked (freebasing). Cocaine hydrochloride (HCl) is diluted or cut before sale and the pure form ("rocks") is administered intranasally (snorted) or injected intravenously. "Skin popping," a subcutaneous method many substance abusers are using to administer drugs, may lead to the formation of abscesses under the skin. Mild overdose of cocaine produces agitation, dizziness, tremor, and blurred vision. Severe overdose produces anxiety, hyperpyrexia, convulsions, ventricular dysrhythmias, severe hypertension, and hemorrhagic stroke with possible angina or myocardial infarction (MI). The use of cocaine during pregnancy is especially problematic because the drug crosses the placenta and enters the fetal bloodstream. Spontaneous abortion, premature delivery, retardation of intrauterine growth, congenital abnormalities, and fetal addiction can result. Long-term intranasal use of cocaine can cause atrophy of the nasal mucosa, necrosis and perforation of the nasal septum, and lung damage. The growing practice of crack cocaine injection requires serious attention, as this new drug use behavior is associated with increased rates of high risk behaviors. Recent research indicates that injection drug users (IDUs) exhibit significantly higher rates of risky health behaviors. High risk sexual behaviors were especially prevalent among female crack cocaine injectors. Higher self-reported rates of adverse health outcomes, such as sexually transmitted infections (STIs), Hepatitis C, and abscesses among crack injectors were found, although no differences in rates of HIV infection were self-reported (Buchanan et al., 2006).

Amphetamine use is on the rise and poses a severe health risk to society due to its devastating physical and neurological consequences, including amphetamine-induced mental disorders. Methamphetamine is illegally manufactured, distributed, and abused and is currently the most widespread amphetamine used in the United States (SAMHSA, 2008a). In 2007, there were an estimated 529,000 current users of methamphetamine aged 12 or older (SAMHSA). Methamphetamine is a powerful stimulant drug commonly referred to as "speed," "crystal," "crank," "go," and, most recently, "ice," a smokable form of methamphetamine. The manufacture of methamphetamine is a relatively simple process and can be carried out by individuals without special knowledge or expertise in chemistry. Methamphetamine is often taken in combination with other drugs such as cocaine and marijuana and, like heroin and cocaine, can be inhaled, injected, ingested, or smoked.

It appears that methamphetamine is an "equal-opportunity" drug for addiction without regard to gender, age, race, or sexual preferences. In regard to race or ethnicity, the highest percentage rates of methamphetamine use were found among Native Hawaiians or other Pacific Islanders and the lowest rates of methamphetamine use were among Caucasians, Hispanics, Asians, and African Americans (SAMHSA, 2008a).

Methamphetamine use has been linked with human immunodeficiency virus (HIV) infection and high rates of sexually transmitted infections (STIs) in homosexual, heterosexual, and bisexual men and women all over the United States (Brown, Domier, & Rawson, 2005; Semple Grant, & Patterson, 2004; Shoptaw et al., 2005). Heterosexual men and women displayed severe to moderate depressive symptoms due to perceived stigma associated with methamphetamine use, emphasizing the importance of identifying and treating depression in this population (Semple, Patterson, & Rant, 2005).

Amphetamines cause arousal and an elevation of mood with a sense of increased strength, mental capacity, self-confidence, and a decreased need for food and sleep. Methamphetamine users experience numerous physical symptoms including weight loss, tachycardia, tachypnea, hyperthermia, insomnia, and muscular tremors. The behavioral and psychiatric symptoms reported most often include violent behavior, repetitive activity, memory loss, paranoia, delusions of reference, auditory hallucinations, and confusion or fright. A psychotic state with hallucinations and paranoia is common with long-term use, requiring treatment similar to other psychotic disorders. The cardiovascular effects of amphetamines are comparable to those of cocaine, including vasoconstriction, tachycardia, hypertension, angina, and dysrhythmias. Tolerance to mood elevation, appetite suppression, and cardiovascular effects develops with amphetamines; however, dependence is more psychological than physical.

Withdrawal from amphetamines produces dysphoria and craving with fatigue, prolonged sleep, excessive eating, and depression. Although a large number of people cope with amphetamine dependence worldwide, limited evidence exists for effective treatment (Srisuraponont, Jarusuraisin, & Kittirattanapalboon, 2005). In a systematic review of treatment measures for amphetamine dependence and abuse, antidepressants provided little benefit concerning amphetamine use. Both biological and psychosocial treatments should be further investigated (Srisuraponont, Jarusuraisin, & Kitirattanapalboon, 2005).

Opiates

Opiates such as morphine, meperidine, codeine, hydrocodone, and oxycodone are narcotic analgesics. Examples of some common brand names include Vicodin®, Percocet®, OxyContin®, and Darvon®. Narcotic analgesics are a type of pain reliever derived from natural or synthetic opiates. A small percentage of individuals are originally exposed to opiates in the context of prescription pain management; however, most people use opiates under social or illicit circumstances. The urban poor constitute the majority of abusers, although opiates are used and abused by people of all socioeconomic statuses. The problem of abuse of and addiction to prescribed narcotics has resurfaced as a major issue for the United States in the past decade and has worsened over the past few years (Compton & Volkow, 2006). Approximately 6.9 million Americans over the age of 12 reported nonmedical use of prescription pain relievers (SAMHSA, 2008a). According to the 2007 NSDUH, the number of new nonmedical users of OxyContin® was 554,000, with an average age at first use of 24 years (SAMHSA). A steady increase in opiate abuse seems to reflect, in part, changes in

medication prescribing practices, changes in drug formulations, and fairly easy access via the Internet or from family and friends. Over 56% of persons abusing pain relievers reported that the source of the drug was from a friend or relative for free.

Although the use of narcotic analgesics for acute pain management looks benign, long-term use has been associated with significant rates of abuse or addiction. OxyContin® is a controlled-released form of oxycodone prescribed for the management of moderate to severe pain. OxyContin® diversion and abuse has become a major problem in certain areas of the United States, particularly rural areas and Appalachia. A retrospective review of 534 medical records revealed that 27% of patients admitted and discharged from an addiction detoxification unit were dependent on prescription opiate medications (Miller & Greenfeld, 2004). The most frequently mentioned medication was Vicodin® (hydrocodone) followed by OxyContin® (oxycodone). Almost 0.75 million ED visits in 2006 involved illicit use of prescription or over-the-counter (OTC) pharmaceuticals (SAMHSA, 2008b). The most frequent opiates included methadone, oxycodone, and combination forms (e.g., hydrocodone with acetaminophen).

Heroin has been abused for many centuries and is usually administered intravenously. It induces a "rush" or "kick" that lasts less than a minute, followed by a sense of euphoria lasting several hours. Tolerance develops to the euphoria, respiratory depression, and nausea but not to constipation and miosis. Physical dependence occurs with long-term use of opiates. Initial withdrawal symptoms such as drug craving, lacrimation, rhinorrhea, yawning, and diaphoresis usually take 10 days to run their course, with the second phase of opiate withdrawal lasting for months with insomnia, irritability, fatigue, and potential GI hyperactivity and premature ejaculation as problems. Methadone is a synthetic opiate used to treat chronic pain and addiction to other opiates. Methadone does not hinder one's ability to function productively as other narcotics do and is a viable support for withdrawal (Stuart, 2009).

Hallucinogens

Hallucinogens are also called psychedelics and include phencyclidine (PCP), 3,4-methylenediosy-methamphetamine (MDMA), d-lysergic acid diethylamide (LSD), mescaline, dimethyltryptamine (DMT), and psilocin. Psychedelics bring on the same types of thoughts, perceptions, and feelings that occur in dreams. PCP (also called angel dust and peace pill) was developed in the 1950s as an anesthetic similar to ketamine, but due to its severe side effects its development for human use was discontinued. PCP is known for inducing violent behavior and for inducing negative physical reactions such as seizures, coma, and death. The most common route of administration is smoking tobacco, marijuana, or herbal cigarettes laced with PCP powder or the liquid form of PCP.

MDMA, commonly known as Ecstasy, had high use in the 1980s as a popular recreational "club drug" associated with dance clubs or "raves" and has reappeared in recent years as a date or rape drug. According to 2007 NSDUH data, approximately 0.5 million persons aged 12 or older (0.2%) used Ecstasy during the past year (SAMHSA, 2008a). Ecstasy use peaked in 2002, but has shown a steady decline in recent years, possibly due to a heightened awareness and vigilance. Parties where other drugs such as marijuana or alcohol are present may lead to easier access or availability of Ecstasy, thereby increasing the chances for first-time Ecstasy use. One study suggests that cannabis use is a powerful risk factor for subsequent first onset of Ecstasy use (Zimmerman et al., 2005). Another study reported approximately 20% of youths aged 16 to 23 admitted to using one or more of the following drugs: methamphetamine, MDMA (Ecstasy), LSD, ketamine, GHB (gamma-hydroxybutyrate), and flunitrazepam (Rohypnol) (Wu, Schlenger, & Galvin, 2006). Females were more likely than males to report using multiple club drugs. Staying in school and getting married were associated with decreased odds of club drug use. On the other hand, use of club drugs was increased by criminal behaviors and recent alcohol abuse or dependence.

LSD was first used to simulate psychosis. It affects serotonin receptors at multiple sites in the brain and spinal cord. LSD is usually taken orally but can be injected or smoked, as in tobacco- or marijuana-laced cigarettes. The individual's response to a "trip," the experience of being high on LSD, cannot be predicted and psychological effects and "flashbacks" are common. Serotonin imbalance is thought to affect impulse control and may be responsible for uninhibited sexual responses in women who have been given the drug without their knowledge. Other hallucinogens are similar to LSD but with different potency and course of action. Because physical dependence to hallucinogens does not appear to occur, withdrawal symptoms are not present.

Inhalants

Inhalants are categorized into three types: anesthetics, volatile nitrites, and organic solvents. Nitrous oxide (laughing gas) and ether are the most abused anesthetics. Amyl nitrite, butyl nitrite, and isobutyl nitrite are volatile nitrites used especially by homosexual males to induce venodilation and anal sphincter relaxation. Amyl nitrite is manufactured for medical use, but butyl and isobutyl nitrites are sold for recreational use. Other names for butyl and isobutyl nitrites are climax, rush, and locker room. Street names for amyl nitrite are "poppers" or "snappers" (Box 6–3). Brain damage or sudden death can occur the first, tenth, or hundredth time an individual uses an inhalant, resulting in "sudden sniffing death." This danger makes the use of inhalants more hazardous than some other substances.

Another danger is the wide assortment of organic solvents that are available to and inhaled by young children. Organic solvents are ingested in three different methods: bagging, huffing, or sniffing. *Bagging* involves pouring the solvent in a plastic bag and inhaling the vapor. *Huffing* refers to pouring the solvent on a rag and inhaling. *Sniffing* refers to inhaling the solvent directly from the container. Common organic solvents are toluene, gasoline, lighter fluid, paint thinner, nail polish remover, benzene, acetone, chloroform, and model airplane glue. The effects from inhaling organic solvents are similar to alcohol, with prolonged use leading to multiple toxicities and an increased risk for abusing other substances. Children who used inhalants before the age of 14 were twice as likely to initiate opiate use, as compared to those who had never tried opiates (Storr, Westergaard, & Anthony, 2005). There are no antidotes for these inhalants; therefore, management of overdose is supportive.

BOX 6–3 Common Street Names for Abused Substances

Substance	Street Name
Alcohol	Booze, brew, spirits, juice, hootch
Amphetamines	Bennies, crystal, crystal meth, crank, dexies, diet pills, dolls, eye-openers, ice, lid poppers, pep pills, purple hearts, speed, uppers
Barbiturates	Barbs, beans, black beauties, blue angels, candy, downers, goof balls, ludes, nebbies, reds, sleepers, tranks, yellow jackets, yellows
Benzodiazepines	Bennies, blues, rainbows, reds, sopors, yellows
Cocaine	Bernice, bernies, big C, blow, Charlie, coke, dust, girl, heaven, jay, lady, nose candy, nose powder, snow, sugar, white lady
	Crack: conan, freebase, rock, toke, white cloud, white tornado
Heroin, morphine	H, horse, harry, boy, M, Miss Emma, scag, "shit," smack, stuff, white junk, white stuff
Opiates	Meperidine (Demerol), hydrocodone (Vicodin®), Percocet®, oxycodone (OxyContin®), and Darvon®
Marijuana	Acapulco gold, Aunt Mary, broccoli, dope, grass, grunt, hay, hemp, herb, J, joint, joy stick, killer weed, Mary Jane, pot, ragweed, reefer, smoke, weed, "shit"
Hallucinogens	Acid, big D, blotter, blue heaven, cap D, deeda, flash, L, mellow yellows, microdots, paper acid, sugar, ticket, yello, Ecstasy

Interdisciplinary Care

Effective treatment of substance abuse and dependence results from the efforts of an interdisciplinary team specializing in the treatment of psychiatric and substance abuse disorders. Therapies may include detoxification, aversion therapy to maintain abstinence, group and/or individual psychotherapy, psychotropic medications, cognitive-behavioral strategies, family counseling, and self-help groups. Patients suffering from substance abuse can be treated in either inpatient or outpatient settings. A substance overdose is a life-threatening condition that requires emergency hospitalization to stabilize the patient medically before implementing any of these interventions. Several diagnostic tests can provide valuable information about the patient's physical condition and set the course for treatment.

Diagnostic Tests

The body fluids most often tested for drug content are blood and urine, although saliva, perspiration, and even hair can be tested. The simplest method of detecting blood alcohol content is by using a Breathalyzer. More invasive procedures such as serum drug levels are useful in the ED and other hospital settings to treat drug overdoses or complications. Urine drug screens (UDS) and/or blood alcohol levels (BAL) are the main biological measures for assessment purposes. Urine drug screening is noninvasive and the preferred method for detecting substances in the body. Companies often require a UDS of prospective employees before hiring them. In addition, professional and college athletes are now required to submit to random drug testing. Results of UDS are also used within the court system to determine drug use in relation to criminal activity. The length of time that drugs can be found in blood and urine varies according to dosage and metabolic properties of the drug. All traces of the drug may disappear within 24 hours or may still be detectable 30 days later. The psychoactive substance found in marijuana, delta 6-3, 4-tetrahydrocannabinol (THC) is stored in fatty tissues (especially the brain and reproductive system) and can be detected in the body for up to 6 weeks (Kneisl & Trigoboff, 2009).

Knowledge of the BAL is helpful in ascertaining the level of intoxication, the level of tolerance, and whether the person accurately reported recent drinking. At 0.10% (after 5 to 6 drinks in 1 to 2 hours), voluntary motor action becomes clumsy and reaction time is impaired. The degree of impairment varies with gender, weight, and food ingestion. Small women who drink alcohol on an empty stomach will experience intoxication more rapidly than large males who have eaten a full meal. At 0.20% (after 10 to 12 drinks in 2 to 4 hours), function of the motor area in the brain is depressed, causing staggering and ataxia (Kneisl & Trigoboff, 2009). A level above 0.10% without associated behavioral symptoms indicates the presence of tolerance. A BAL greater than 0.08% is considered legal intoxication in most states. High tolerance is a sign of physical dependence. Assessing for withdrawal symptoms is important when the BAL is high.

> **PRACTICE ALERT**
> Medications given for treatment of withdrawal from alcohol are usually not started until the BAL is below a set norm (usually below 0.10%) unless withdrawal symptoms become severe. The BAL may be repeated several times, several hours apart, to determine the body's metabolism of alcohol and when it is safe to give the patient medication to minimize the withdrawal symptoms.

High Acuity Care

Emergency Care for Overdose

The care of a patient who has overdosed on any substance is a serious medical emergency. Respiratory depression may require mechanical ventilation. The patient may become severely sedated and difficult to arouse. Every effort must be made to keep the patient awake; however, stupor and coma may often result. A seizure is another serious complication that requires emergency treatment. If the overdose was intentional, the patient must be constantly monitored for further signs of suicidal ideation. Never leave an actively suicidal patient alone. Signs of overdose and withdrawal from major substances are summarized in Table 6–2 along with recommended treatments.

Treatment of Withdrawal

All CNS depressants, including alcohol, benzodiazepines, and barbiturates, have a potentially dangerous progression of withdrawal. Alcohol and the entire class of CNS depressants share the same withdrawal syndrome. Early signs of withdrawal appear within a few hours following cessation of the drug, peak after 24 to 48 hours, and then rapidly disappear unless the withdrawal progresses to delirium tremens. Severe withdrawal or delirium tremens is a medical emergency that usually occurs 2 to 5 days following alcohol withdrawal and persists 2 to

3 days. The symptoms of severe withdrawal include disorientation, paranoid delusions, visual hallucinations, and marked withdrawal symptoms. Seizures may also occur, requiring the use of emergency equipment. Treatment of severe withdrawal during detoxification is mostly symptomatic through acetaminophen, vitamins, and medications to minimize discomfort.

In managing alcohol withdrawal, the goal is to minimize adverse outcomes, such as patient discomfort, seizures, delirium and mortality, and to avoid the adverse effects of withdrawal medications, such as excess sedation. Close monitoring is essential to assure protection of the patient. Critical care monitoring may be indicated to manage alcohol withdrawal delirium, particularly when very high doses of benzodiazepines are needed, or when there are significant concurrent medical conditions. Medications such as benzodiazepines are effectively used to minimize the discomfort associated with alcohol withdrawal and prevent serious adverse effects, in particular seizures. A symptom-triggered approach to the administration of benzodiazepines during alcohol withdrawal results in less total medication use and requires a shorter duration of treatment.

> **PRACTICE ALERT**
> The Clinical Institute Withdrawal Assessment for Alcohol (CIWA-Ar) is recommended to manage the symptoms of acute alcohol withdrawal. Benzodiazepines such as lorazepam (Ativan) are commonly administered according to a sliding scale based on the CIWA-Ar score. Medication is given only when the CIWA-Ar score is higher than 8 points.

Medications used to treat alcoholism are disulfiram (Antabuse), naltrexone (ReVia, Depade), and acamprosate (Campral). Disulfiram is a form of aversion therapy that prevents the breakdown of alcohol, causing physical illness (intense vomiting) if taken while drinking alcohol. All forms of alcohol, including OTC cough and cold preparations, must be avoided.

Naltrexone can help reduce the craving for alcohol by blocking the pathways to the brain that trigger a feeling of pleasure when alcohol and other narcotics are used. Because naltrexone blocks opiate receptors, patients should avoid taking any narcotics, such as codeine, morphine, or heroin, while on naltrexone. Patients should also discontinue all narcotics 7 to 10 days before starting on naltrexone. It is also recommended that patients wear a medical alert bracelet stating they are on naltrexone, in case of emergency medical treatment. While on disulfiram or naltrexone, psychosocial treatments such as Alcoholics Anonymous meetings, individual counseling, or group therapy are important, as the desire to "take a break" from treatment can overcome the patient's motivation to continue taking the medication.

Acamprosate is another medication prescribed for patients wanting to abstain from alcohol. The chemical structure of acamprosate is similar to gamma amino butyric acid (GABA) and glutamate neurotransmitters. Acamprosate is thought to block glutamate receptors while simultaneously activating GABA receptors in the brain; thus stabilizing the chemical imbalance that is disrupted by alcoholism. Evidence suggests that acamprosate is fairly effective in reducing cravings of alcohol-dependent patients when used in combination with psychosocial interventions (Snyder & Bowers, 2008).

TABLE 6–2 Signs and Treatment of Overdose and Withdrawal

	OVERDOSE		WITHDRAWAL	
DRUG	**SIGNS**	**TREATMENT**	**SIGNS**	**TREATMENT**
CNS Depressants: Alcohol Barbiturates Benzodiazepines	Cardiovascular or respiratory depression or arrest (mostly with barbiturates) Coma Shock Convulsions Death	*If awake:* Keep awake Induce vomiting Activated charcoal to absorb drug VS q 15 minutes *Coma:* Clear airway, intubate IV fluids Gastric lavage Seizure precautions Possible hemo or peritoneal dialysis Frequent VS Assess for shock and cardiac arrest	Nausea and vomiting Tachycardia Diaphoresis Anxiety or agitation Tremors Marked insomnia Grand mal seizures Delirium (after 5–15 years of heavy use)	Carefully titrated detoxification with similar drug *NOTE:* Abrupt withdrawal can lead to death.
Stimulants: Cocaine-crack Amphetamines	Respiratory distress Ataxia Hyperpyrexia Convulsions Coma Stroke Myocardial infarction (MI) Death	Antipsychotics Management for 1. Hyperpyrexia 2. Convulsions 3. Respiratory distress 4. Cardiovascular shock 5. Acidify urine (ammonium Cl for amphetamine)	Fatigue Depression Agitation Apathy Anxiety Sleepiness Disorientation Lethargy Craving	Antidepressants (desipramine) Dopamine agonist Bromocriptine
Opiates: Heroin Meperidine Morphine Methadone	Pupil dilation due to anoxia Respiratory depression-arrest Coma Shock Convulsions Death	Narcotic antagonist, (Narcan) quickly reverses CNS depression	Yawning, insomnia Irritability Rhinorrhea Panic Diaphoresis Cramps Nausea and vomiting Muscle aches Chills and fever Lacrimation Diarrhea	Methadone tapering Clonidine-naltrexone detoxification Buprenorphine substitution
Hallucinogens:		Low stimuli with minimal light, sound, activity	No pattern of withdrawal	
Lysergic acid diethylamide (LSD)	Psychosis Brain damage Death	Have one person "talk down patient," reassure Speak slowly and clearly Diazepam or chloral hydrate for anxiety		
Phencyclidine piperidine (PCP)	Possible hypertensive crisis Respiratory arrest Hyperthermia Seizures	Acidify urine to help excrete drug (cranberry juice, ascorbic acid); in acute stage use ammonium chloride Minimal stimulus Do NOT attempt to talk down, speak slowly in low voice Diazepam or Haldol		

TABLE 6–2 Signs and Treatment of Overdose and Withdrawal (continued)

	OVERDOSE		WITHDRAWAL	
DRUG	SIGNS	TREATMENT	SIGNS	TREATMENT
Inhalants: Volatile solvents such as butane, paint thinner, airplane glue, or nail polish remover	Intoxication: Excitation Drowsiness Disinhibition Staggering Lightheadedness Agitation Side Effects: Damage to nervous system Death	Support affected systems	No pattern of withdrawal	
Nitrates	Enhance sexual pleasure	Neurological symptoms may respond to vitamin B$_{12}$ and folate		
Anesthetics such as nitrous oxide	Giggling, laughter Euphoria	Chronic users may experience polyneuropathy and myelopathy		

MEMORY CUE

Alcohol abuse is a disease with definite genetic propensity, passed down from generation to generation through family members' DNA. The three main medications currently available to help alcohol-dependent patients maintain sobriety can be easily remembered by using the acronym DNA: Disulfiram, Naltrexone, and Acamprosate. Disulfiram interacts with alcohol to cause adverse effects, while naltrexone and acamprosate help to reduce the craving for alcohol.

Withdrawal symptoms from opiates and stimulants can be very unpleasant but are generally not life threatening. The patient experiencing an acute phase of cocaine withdrawal may become suicidal. Common drugs used in the treatment of substance abuse and withdrawal are presented in Table 6–3.

TABLE 6–3 Drugs Used in the Treatment of Substance Withdrawal/Abuse

DRUG	DOSE	PURPOSE
Benzodiazepines		
Clordiazepoxide (Librium)	15–100 mg	Diminishes anxiety and has anticonvulsant qualities to provide safe withdrawal. May be ordered q4h or prn to manage adverse effects from withdrawal; then dose is tapered to zero.
Diazepam (Valium)	4–40 mg	
Oxazepam (Serax)	30–120 mg	
Lorazepam (Ativan)	2–6 mg	
Vitamins		
Thiamine (Vitamin B$_1$)	100 mg/day	Prevents Wernicke's encephalopathy.
Folic acid	1 mg/day	Corrects vitamin deficiency caused by heavy long-term alcohol abuse.
Multivitamins	1 tab/cap daily	
Anticonvulsants		
Phenobarbital	30–320 mg	For seizure control and sedation.
Magnesium sulfate	1 g q6h	Reduces postwithdrawal seizures.
Abstinence medications		
Disulfiram (Antabuse)	250 mg/day	Prevents breakdown of alcohol.
Naltrexone (ReVia)	50 mg/day	Diminishes cravings for alcohol and opioids.
Acamprosate (Campral)	300 mg/TID	Diminishes cravings for alcohol.
Methadone	40 mg/day	Blocks craving for heroin.
Antidepressants		
Fluoxetine (Prozac)	20–80 mg/day	Enhances and stabilizes mood and diminishes anxiety.
Sertraline (Zoloft)	50–200 mg/day	

NURSING CARE OF THE OLDER ADULT   **Substance Abuse in the Older Adult**

Substance abuse in older adults is likely to increase over subsequent decades as baby boomers reach retirement age. People of any age can have substance abuse problems, but the consequences in older adults can be more critical (Lewis, 2008). Falls and accidents can rob older adults of their independence, and substance abuse increases the risk of falls by affecting alertness, judgment, coordination, and reaction time. In addition, older adults (especially older women) are more likely than younger people to use prescription or OTC medicines, which can be harmful when mixed with alcohol and/or illicit drugs (Lantz, 2005). Alcohol and drug abuse can also make certain medical problems hard to diagnose, for example, by dulling a pain sensation that might warn of a heart attack.

While substance abuse and dependence is not as common in older adults, it is less likely to be recognized. Unfortunately, a substance abuse problem in an older adult can be difficult to detect because many of the symptoms of abuse (e.g., insomnia, depression, loss of memory, anxiety, musculoskeletal pain) may be confused with conditions commonly seen in older patients (Lantz, 2005). Healthcare professionals frequently attribute these symptoms to the aging process and fail to address the misuse and abuse of substances in the elderly. Often, the *symptoms* of substance abuse are treated rather than confronting the abuse itself. Older adults are also at greater risk for numerous physical problems and premature death because alcohol negatively interacts with the natural aging process to increase risks for injuries, hypertension, cardiac dysrhythmias, cancers, gastrointestinal problems, cognitive deficits, bone loss, and emotional challenges, most notably depression (Stevenson, 2005). Because depression and alcohol abuse are the most frequently found disorders in completed suicides, nurses should routinely screen older adults for both substance abuse and mental disorders.

✎ Nursing Care

Substance Abuse Video

Nurses may interact with patients experiencing substance abuse or substance dependence in a variety of settings. The most common setting is an alcohol and drug abuse (ADA) treatment program where patients are hospitalized for 20 to 30 days for detoxification and in-patient therapy. These patients may be voluntarily admitted but most are court-ordered to undergo treatment after charges of driving under the influence (DUI) or driving while intoxicated (DWI). Patients with substance abuse or dependence have impaired senses and risk-taking behaviors that lead to injuries from falls and accidents requiring medical attention. Therefore, hospital EDs as well as medical and surgical units are places where nurses will frequently encounter these patients. Box 6–4 summarizes key safety considerations for hospitalized patients with substance abuse problems. Occupational nurses and community health nurses will also interact with substance abusing patients in employee assistance programs and community health departments. Urgent care, pain clinics, and ambulatory care centers are other settings in which patients with substance abuse disorders will frequently appear for minor health problems associated with chronic disorders related to substance abuse or dependence.

Health Promotion

Nursing care of the patient with substance abuse or dependence is challenging and requires a nonjudgmental atmosphere promoting trust and respect. Health promotion efforts are aimed at preventing drug use among children and adolescents and reducing the risks among adults. Adolescence is the most common phase for the first experience with drugs (Stuart, 2009); therefore, teenagers are a vulnerable population, often succumbing to peer pressure. Healthy lifestyles, parental support, stress management, good nutrition, and information about ways to steer clear of peer pressure are important topics for the nurse to provide in school programs.

Nurses should provide adults with information on healthy coping mechanisms, relaxation, and stress reduction techniques to decrease the risks of substance abuse. Nurses have a responsibility to educate their patients about the physiological effects of substances on the body as well as ways to manage stress and anxiety. Nurses must encourage and support periods of abstinence while assisting patients to make major changes in lifestyles, habits, relationships, and coping methods. See Nursing Care of the Older Adult for meeting the individualized needs of older patients with substance abuse problems.

Assessment

A comprehensive approach to the assessment of substance use is essential to ensure adequate and appropriate intervention. Three important areas to assess are a history of the patient's past substance use, medical and psychiatric history, and the presence of psychosocial concerns. Questions should be asked in a nonthreatening, matter-of-fact manner, phrased as to not imply wrongdoing (Savage, 2008). For instance, a nonthreatening question such as "How much alcohol do you drink?" is preferable to the judgmental question "You don't drink too much alcohol, do you?" Open-ended questions that elicit more than a simple yes or no answer help to determine the direction of future counseling. Examples of open-ended questions are

---

BOX 6–4   Safety Considerations for Hospitalized Patients with Substance Abuse

- Closely monitor patients admitted for a drug overdose for signs of suicidal ideation.
- Never leave an actively suicidal patient alone.
- During acute alcohol withdrawal (first 72 hours), assess for withdrawal symptoms and administer benzodiazepines as ordered.
- Monitor unconscious patients closely for possibility of aspiration. Never place an intoxicated, unconscious patient in a supine position.
- Seizure precautions are indicated for patients experiencing acute withdrawal symptoms.
- Expect signs of delirium tremens to occur after 72 hours of abstinence from alcohol.
- Monitor patient for signs of hallucinations, delusions, or altered sensory perceptions that may lead to injuries.
- Assess for fall and choking risk. Provide one-to-one assistance as needed.
- Maintain fluid and electrolyte balance.

provided in Box 6–5. Use therapeutic communication techniques to establish trust prior to the assessment process.

History of Past Substance Use

A thorough history of the patient's past substance use is important to ascertain the possibility of tolerance, physical dependence, or withdrawal syndrome. The following questions are helpful in eliciting a pattern of substance use behavior.

■ How many substances has the patient used simultaneously (**polysubstance abuse** or simultaneous use of many substances) in the past?
■ How often, how much, and when did the patient first use the substance(s)?
■ Is there a history of blackouts, delirium, or seizures?
■ Is there a history of withdrawal syndrome, overdoses, and complications from previous substance use?
■ Has the patient ever been treated in an alcohol or drug abuse clinic?
■ Has the patient ever been arrested for DUI or charged with any criminal offense while using drugs or alcohol?
■ Is there a family history of drug or alcohol use?

Medical and Psychiatric History

The patient's medical history is another important area for assessment and should include the existence of any concomitant physical or mental condition (e.g., HIV, hepatitis, cirrhosis, esophageal varices, pancreatitis, gastritis, Wernicke-Korsakoff syndrome, depression, schizophrenia, anxiety, or personality disorder). Ask about prescribed and OTC medications as well as any allergies or sensitivity to drugs. A brief overview of the patient's current mental status is also significant.

■ Is there a history of abuse (physical or sexual) or family violence?
■ Has the patient ever tried to commit suicide?
■ Is the patient currently having suicidal or homicidal ideation?

Psychosocial Issues

Information about the patient's level of stress and other psychosocial concerns can help in the assessment of substance use problems.

■ Has the patient's substance use affected his or her ability to hold a job?
■ Has the patient's substance use affected relationships with spouse, family, friends, or coworkers?
■ How does the patient usually cope with stress?

BOX 6–5 Examples of Open-Ended Questions for Assessment

■ On average, how many days per week do you drink alcohol or use drugs?
■ On a typical day when you use drugs or alcohol, how many hits or drinks do you have?
■ What is the greatest number of drinks you have had at any one time during the past month?
■ What drug(s) did you take before coming to the hospital or clinic?
■ How long have you been using the substances?
■ How often and how much do you usually use?
■ What kinds of problems has substance use caused for you, your family, friends, finances, and health?

■ Does the patient have a support system that helps in times of need?
■ How does the patient spend his or her leisure time?

Screening Tools

Several screening tools such as the Michigan Alcohol Screening Test (MAST) (Pokorny, Miller, & Kaplan, 1972), Brief Drug Abuse Screening Test (B-DAST) (Skinner, 1982), and the CAGE questionnaire (Ewing, 1984) may help the nurse determine the degree of severity of substance abuse or dependence (Figure 6–2 ■). These screening tools provide a nonjudgmental, brief, and easy method to ascertain patterns of substance abuse behaviors.

■ *Michigan Alcohol Screening Test (MAST) Brief Version* is a 10-question, dichotomous, self-administered questionnaire that takes 10 to 15 minutes to complete. An answer of yes to 3 or more questions indicates a potentially dangerous pattern of alcohol abuse.
■ *CAGE questionnaire* is more useful when the patient may not recognize he or she has an alcohol problem or is uncomfortable acknowledging it. This questionnaire is designed to be a self-report of drinking behavior or may be administered by a professional. One affirmative response indicates the need for further discussion and follow-up. Two or more yes answers signify a problem with alcohol that may require treatment.
  ■ Have you ever felt you should *Cut* down on your drinking?
  ■ Have people *Annoyed* you by criticizing your drinking?
  ■ Have you ever felt bad or *Guilty* about your drinking?
  ■ Have you ever had a drink first thing in the morning (an "*Eye-opener*") to steady your nerves or to get rid of a hangover?
■ *Brief Drug Abuse Screening Test (B-DAST)* is a yes/no self-administered questionnaire that is useful in identifying people who are possibly addicted to drugs other than alcohol. A positive response to one or more questions suggests significant drug abuse problems and warrants further evaluation. Because self-report tools are not always answered truthfully, all patients who screen positive for drug addiction should be evaluated according to other diagnostic criteria.

Withdrawal Assessment Tools

Nurses working in medical-surgical units, psychiatric units, and special substance abuse units routinely care for patients experiencing acute alcohol or opiate withdrawal. Several assessment tools are available to determine the severity of withdrawal symptoms and indicate the need for pharmacological treatment to manage withdrawal symptoms. Examples of withdrawal assessment tools are the revised *Clinical Institute Withdrawal Assessment (CIWA-Ar)* (Sullivan et al., 1989) and the *Clinical Opiate Withdrawal Scale (COWS)* (Wesson & Ling, 2003).

■ The *Clinical Institute Withdrawal Assessment of Alcohol-Revised (CIWA-Ar)* (Sullivan et al., 1989) (Figure 6–3 ■) is used widely in clinical and research settings for initial assessment and ongoing monitoring of alcohol withdrawal signs and symptoms. The CIWA-Ar scale is a validated 10-item assessment tool that can be used to monitor and medicate patients going through alcohol withdrawal. The CIWA-Ar assesses for several alcohol withdrawal symptoms (e.g. high blood pressure, rapid pulse

Brief MAST   Scoring Yes to 3 or more indicates alcoholism

1. Do you feel you are a normal drinker?
2. Do friends or relatives think you are a normal drinker?
3. Have you ever attended a meeting of Alcoholics Anonymous?
4. Have you ever gotten in trouble at work because of drinking?
5. Have you ever lost friends or girlfriends/boyfriends because of drinking?
6. Have you ever neglected your obligations, your family, or your work for 2 or more days in a row because of your drinking?
7. Have you ever had delirium tremens (DTs), severe shaking, or heard voices or seen things that were not there after heavy drinking?
8. Have you ever gone to anyone for help about your drinking?
9. Have you ever been in a hospital because of your drinking?
10. Have you ever been arrested for drunken driving or other drunken behavior?

B-DAST   The following questions concern information about your involvement with drugs *not including alcoholic beverages* during the past 12 months.

In the statements, "drug abuse" refers to (1) the use of prescribed or OTC drugs in excess of the directions and (2) any nonmedical use of drugs. The various classes of drugs may include cannabis, solvents, antianxiety drugs, sedative-hypnotics, cocaine, stimulants, hallucinogens, and narcotics. Remember *do not include alcoholic beverages*.

Have you used drugs other than those required for medical purposes?	Yes ___	No ___
Do you abuse more than one drug at a time?	Yes ___	No ___
Are you always able to stop using drugs when you want to?	Yes ___	No ___
Have you had "blackouts" or "flashbacks" as a result of drug use?	Yes ___	No ___
Do you ever feel bad about your drug abuse?	Yes ___	No ___
Does your spouse (or parents) ever complain about your involvement with drugs?	Yes ___	No ___
Have you neglected your family because of your use of drugs?	Yes ___	No ___
Have you engaged in illegal activities in order to obtain drugs?	Yes ___	No ___
Have you ever experienced withdrawal symptoms (felt sick) when you stopped taking drugs?	Yes ___	No ___
Have you had medical problems as a result of your drug use (e.g., memory loss, hepatitis, convulsions, bleeding, etc.)?	Yes ___	No ___

Scoring: one positive response warrants further evaluation

Figure 6–2 ■ Screening Tools for Alcohol and Drug Abuse.

Source: Brief MAST adapted from "The Brief MAST: A Shortened Version of the Michigan Alcohol Screening Test" by A. D. Porkorny, B. A. Miller, and H. B. Kaplan, 1972, *American Journal of Psychiatry,* September 1972, Vol. 129, pp. 342–345, Table 3. Used with permission from the American Journal of Psychiatry, © 1972 American Psychiatric Association. *Source:* Reprinted from Addictive Behaviors, Vol. 7, No. 4, H. A. Skinner, "Brief Drug Abuse Screening Test (B-DAST)", p. 363, © 1982, with permission from Elsevier.

and respirations, tremors, insomnia, irritability, sweating, and convulsions) and results in a score that is used to direct the administration of benzodiazepines or other drugs to relieve associated symptoms of withdrawal and prevent seizures. A score of 8 points or fewer corresponds to mild withdrawal symptoms. Scores of 9–15 points indicate moderate withdrawal, while a score of 15 or greater denotes severe withdrawal and an increased risk of delirium tremens and seizures.

■ *Clinical Opiate Withdrawal Scale (COWS)* (Wesson & Ling, 2003) rates eleven common signs or symptoms of opiate withdrawal. The summed total score of the 11 items can be used to assess the intensity of opiate withdrawal and determine the extent of a patient's physical dependence on opioids. A score of less than 12 on the COWS indicates mild or no opiate withdrawal symptoms while a score of 13 or more indicates moderate to severe withdrawal symptoms (Figure 6–4 ■).

Nursing Diagnoses and Interventions

The primary nursing diagnoses and interventions for patients with substance abuse problems are listed in this section. Implications for nursing care in acute and home care settings are combined in this discussion. See the Case Study & Nursing Care Plan on page 119 for the patient experiencing withdrawal from alcohol.

Injury, Risk for; Violence, Risk for

■ Assess patient's level of disorientation to determine specific risks to safety. *Knowledge of the patient's level of cognitive functioning is essential to the development of an appropriate plan of care.*

■ Obtain a drug history as well as urine and blood samples for laboratory analysis of substance content. *Subjective history is often not accurate and knowledge regarding substance use is important for accurate assessment.*

■ Place patient in a quiet, private room to decrease excessive stimuli, but do not leave patient alone if excessive hyperactivity or suicidal ideation is present. *Excessive stimuli increase patient's agitation.*

■ Frequently orient patient to reality and the environment, ensuring that potentially harmful objects are stored outside the patient's access. *Patient may harm self or others if disoriented and confused.*

■ Monitor vital signs every 15 minutes until stable and assess for signs of intoxication or withdrawal. *The most reliable information about withdrawal symptoms are vital signs; they provide information about the need for medication during detoxification.*

Clinical Institute Withdrawal Assessment of Alcohol Scale, Revised (CIWA-Ar)

Patient:_____ Date: _____ Time: _____ (24 hour clock, midnight = 00:00)

Pulse or heart rate, taken for one minute:_____ Blood pressure:_____

NAUSEA AND VOMITING -- Ask "Do you feel sick to your stomach? Have you vomited?" Observation.
0 no nausea and no vomiting
1 mild nausea with no vomiting
2
3
4 intermittent nausea with dry heaves
5
6
7 constant nausea, frequent dry heaves and vomiting

TREMOR -- Arms extended and fingers spread apart. Observation.
0 no tremor
1 not visible, but can be felt fingertip to fingertip
2
3
4 moderate, with patient's arms extended
5
6
7 severe, even with arms not extended

PAROXYSMAL SWEATS -- Observation.
0 no sweat visible
1 barely perceptible sweating, palms moist
2
3
4 beads of sweat obvious on forehead
5
6
7 drenching sweats

ANXIETY -- Ask "Do you feel nervous?" Observation.
0 no anxiety, at ease
1 mild anxious
2
3
4 moderately anxious, or guarded, so anxiety is inferred
5
6
7 equivalent to acute panic states as seen in severe delirium or acute schizophrenic reactions

AGITATION -- Observation.
0 normal activity
1 somewhat more than normal activity
2
3
4 moderately fidgety and restless
5
6
7 paces back and forth during most of the interview, or constantly thrashes about

TACTILE DISTURBANCES -- Ask "Have you any itching, pins and needles sensations, any burning, any numbness, or do you feel bugs crawling on or under your skin?" Observation.
0 none
1 very mild itching, pins and needles, burning or numbness
2 mild itching, pins and needles, burning or numbness
3 moderate itching, pins and needles, burning or numbness
4 moderately severe hallucinations
5 severe hallucinations
6 extremely severe hallucinations
7 continuous hallucinations

AUDITORY DISTURBANCES -- Ask "Are you more aware of sounds around you? Are they harsh? Do they frighten you? Are you hearing anything that is disturbing to you? Are you hearing things you know are not there?" Observation.
0 not present
1 very mild harshness or ability to frighten
2 mild harshness or ability to frighten
3 moderate harshness or ability to frighten
4 moderately severe hallucinations
5 severe hallucinations
6 extremely severe hallucinations
7 continuous hallucinations

VISUAL DISTURBANCES -- Ask "Does the light appear to be too bright? Is its color different? Does it hurt your eyes? Are you seeing anything that is disturbing to you? Are you seeing things you know are not there?" Observation.
0 not present
1 very mild sensitivity
2 mild sensitivity
3 moderate sensitivity
4 moderately severe hallucinations
5 severe hallucinations
6 extremely severe hallucinations
7 continuous hallucinations

HEADACHE, FULLNESS IN HEAD -- Ask "Does your head feel different? Does it feel like there is a band around your head?" Do not rate for dizziness or lightheadedness. Otherwise, rate severity.
0 not present
1 very mild
2 mild
3 moderate
4 moderately severe
5 severe
6 very severe
7 extremely severe

ORIENTATION AND CLOUDING OF SENSORIUM -- Ask "What day is this? Where are you? Who am I?"
0 oriented and can do serial additions
1 cannot do serial additions or is uncertain about date
2 disoriented for date by no more than 2 calendar days
3 disoriented for date by more than 2 calendar days
4 disoriented for place/or person

Total **CIWA-Ar** Score _____
Rater's Initials _____
Maximum Possible Score 67

The **CIWA-Ar** is not copyrighted and may be reproduced freely. This assessment for monitoring withdrawal symptoms requires approximately 5 minutes to administer. The maximum score is 67 (see instrument). Patients scoring less than 10 do not usually need additional medication for withdrawal.

Sullivan, J.T.; Sykora, K.; Schneiderman, J.; Naranjo, C.A.; and Sellers, E.M. Assessment of alcohol withdrawal: The revised Clinical Institute Withdrawal Assessment for Alcohol scale (**CIWA-Ar**). *British Journal of Addiction* 84:1353-1357, 1989.

Figure 6–3 ■ Assessment Tool for Alcohol Withdrawal.

Source: Clinical Institute Withdrawal Assessment of Alcohol Scale, Revised (CIWA-Ar) from "The Revised Clinical Institute Withdrawal Assessment for Alcohol scale (CIWA-Ar)" by J. T. Sullivan, K. Sykora, J. Schneiderman, C. A. Naranjo, & E. M. Sellers, 1989, *British Journal of Addictions*, 84, 1353–1357. Used by permission of Wiley-Blackwell.

Clinical Opiate Withdrawal Scale

For each item, circle the number that best describes the patient's signs or symptom. Rate on just the apparent relationship to opiate withdrawal. For example, if heart rate is increased because the patient was jogging just prior to assessment, the increase pulse rate would not add to the score.

Patient's Name:_____   Date and Time ____/____/____:_____

Reason for this assessment:_____

Resting Pulse Rate: _____ beats/minute *Measured after patient is sitting or lying for one minute* 0 pulse rate 80 or below 1 pulse rate 81-100 2 pulse rate 101-120 4 pulse rate greater than 120	**GI Upset**: *over last ½ hour* 0 no GI symptoms 1 stomach cramps 2 nausea or loose stool 3 vomiting or diarrhea 5 Multiple episodes of diarrhea or vomiting
Sweating: *over past ½ hour not accounted for by room temperature or patient activity.* 0 no report of chills or flushing 1 subjective report of chills or flushing 2 flushed or observable moistness on face 3 beads of sweat on brow or face 4 sweat streaming off face	**Tremor** *observation of outstretched hands* 0 No tremor 1 tremor can be felt, but not observed 2 slight tremor observable 4 gross tremor or muscle twitching
Restlessness *Observation during assessment* 0 able to sit still 1 reports difficulty sitting still, but is able to do so 3 frequent shifting or extraneous movements of legs/arms 5 Unable to sit still for more than a few seconds	**Yawning** *Observation during assessment* 0 no yawning 1 yawning once or twice during assessment 2 yawning three or more times during assessment 4 yawning several times/minute
Pupil size 0 pupils pinned or normal size for room light 1 pupils possibly larger than normal for room light 2 pupils moderately dilated 5 pupils so dilated that only the rim of the iris is visible	**Anxiety or Irritability** 0 none 1 patient reports increasing irritability or anxiousness 2 patient obviously irritable anxious 4 patient so irritable or anxious that participation in the assessment is difficult
Bone or Joint aches *If patient was having pain previously, only the additional component attributed to opiates withdrawal is scored* 0 not present 1 mild diffuse discomfort 2 patient reports severe diffuse aching of joints/ muscles 4 patient is rubbing joints or muscles and is unable to sit still because of discomfort	**Gooseflesh skin** 0 skin is smooth 3 piloerrection of skin can be felt or hairs standing up on arms 5 prominent piloerrection
Runny nose or tearing *Not accounted for by cold symptoms or allergies* 0 not present 1 nasal stuffiness or unusually moist eyes 2 nose running or tearing 4 nose constantly running or tears streaming down cheeks	Total Score _____ The total score is the sum of all 11 items Initials of person completing Assessment: _____

Score: 5-12 = mild; 13-24 = moderate; 25-36 = moderately severe; more than 36 = severe withdrawal

Provided by: Physician Clinical Support System, (877) 630-8812; PCSSproject@asam.org; www.PCSSmentor.org

Figure 6–4 ■ Assessment Tool for Opiate Withdrawal.

Source: Excerpted from Wesson & Ling "The Clinical Opiate Withdrawal Scale (COWS)," Vol. 35, No. 2, of the Journal of Psychoactive Drugs. Reprinted with permission of Haight Ashbury Publications (www.hajpd.com).

George Russell, aged 58, fell at home and broke his arm. His wife took him to the ER and an open reduction internal fixation (ORIF) of his right wrist was performed under general anesthesia in the operating room. He was admitted to the postoperative unit for observation following surgery because he required large amounts of anesthesia during the procedure.

Mr. Russell has a ruddy complexion and looks older than his stated age. He discloses that he was laid off from his factory job 2 years ago and has been working odd jobs until last week when he was hired by a local assembly plant. His father was a recovering alcoholic and his 30-year-old son has been treated for alcohol abuse in the past. Mr. Russell states that he knows alcoholism runs in the family, but he feels that he has his drinking under control. However, he cannot remember the events that led up to his fall and how he might have broken his arm.

ASSESSMENT

During the nursing assessment, Mr. Russell is hesitant to provide information and refuses to make eye contact. Prior to his operation, a BAL was drawn because the ER nurse detected alcohol on his breath. His BAL was 0.40 %, which is 5 times the legal limit for intoxication in many states. His vital signs are within the upper limits of normal, but he is confused and disoriented with slurred speech and a slight tremor of the hands. He is 6 feet tall and weighs 140 pounds. His total albumin is 2.9 mg and he has elevated liver enzymes. His wife states that he rarely eats the meals she prepares because he is usually drinking and has no appetite for food.

DIAGNOSES

- *Ineffective Coping* related to possible hereditary factor and personal vulnerability
- *Risk for Injury* related to aggressive behavior, unsteady gait and impaired motor responses
- *Ineffective Denial* related to inability to recognize maladaptive behaviors caused by substance use
- *Imbalanced Nutrition: Less than Body Requirements* related to anorexia manifested by decreased weight and low serum protein levels

EXPECTED OUTCOMES

- Patient will express his true feelings associated with using alcohol as a method of coping with stressful situations.
- Patient will identify three adaptive coping mechanisms he can use as alternatives to alcohol in response to stress.
- Patient will verbalize the negative effects of alcohol and agree to seek professional help with his drinking.

- Patient will be free of injury as evidenced by steady gait and absence of subsequent falls.
- Patient will gain 1 lb (0.45 kg) per week without evidence of increased fluid retention. Serum albumin levels will return to normal range.

PLANNING AND IMPLEMENTATION

- Establish trusting relationship with patient and spend time with him discussing his feelings, fears, and anxieties.
- Consult with a physician regarding a schedule for medications during detoxification and observe for signs of withdrawal syndrome.
- Explain the effects of alcohol abuse on the body and emphasize that prognosis is closely associated with abstinence.
- Teach a relaxation technique that is useful in the patient's opinion.
- Provide community resource information about self-help groups and, if patient is receptive, a list of meeting times and phone numbers.
- Consult with a dietitian to determine number of calories needed to provide adequate nutrition and realistic weight gain. Document intake, output, and calorie count.
- Consult with physician to begin vitamin B_1 (Thiamine) and dietary supplements.

EVALUATION

Mr. Russell was discharged from the postoperative unit without complications. He successfully underwent detoxification and contacted the Employee Assistance Program (EAP) at his new place of employment. He was on medical leave while his arm completely healed and now attends Alcoholics Anonymous meetings 5 days a week. He reports that he enjoys taking long walks with his wife in the warm weather and that his appetite has returned. He has gained 10 pounds in the past 6 weeks and feels physically better than he has in many years.

CRITICAL THINKING IN THE NURSING PROCESS

1. Explain why it would be important to include questions about Mr. Russell's medication history and his use of other medications during the initial nursing assessment.
2. Mr. Russell asks you to explain the risks of taking disulfiram (Antabuse). What should you tell him?
3. Develop a care plan for Mr. Russell for the nursing diagnosis of *Alteration in Nutrition: Less than Body Requirements*. Why is this necessary?

See Evaluating Your Response in Appendix C.

Denial, Ineffective

- Be genuine, honest, and respectful of the patient. Keep all promises and convey an attitude of acceptance of the patient. *The development of a nonjudgmental, therapeutic nurse–patient relationship is essential to gain the patient's trust.*
- Identify maladaptive behaviors or situations that have occurred in the patient's life and discuss how the use of substances may have been a contributing factor. *The first step in combating denial is for the patient to recognize the relationship between substance use and personal problems.*
- Do not accept the use of defense mechanisms such as rationalization or projection as the patient attempts to blame others or make excuses for his or her behavior. Use confrontation with caring to avoid placing the patient on the defensive. *Confrontation interferes with the patient's ability to use denial.*

- Encourage patient participation in therapeutic group activities such as co-occurring disorder or Alcoholics Anonymous (AA) meetings with other people who are experiencing or have experienced similar problems. *Peer feedback is often more accepted than feedback from authority figures.*

Coping, Ineffective

- Establish trusting relationship. *Trust is essential to the nurse–patient relationship.*
- Set limits on manipulative behavior and maintain consistency in responses. *Patient is unable to set own limits and must begin to accept responsibility without being manipulative.*
- Encourage patient to verbalize feelings, fears, or anxieties. Use attentive listening and validate patient's feelings with observations or statements that acknowledge feelings.

Verbalization of feelings helps patient to develop insight into behaviors and long-standing problems.

- Explore methods of dealing with stressful situations other than resorting to substance use. Provide encouragement for changing to a healthier lifestyle. Teach healthy coping mechanisms (e.g., physical exercise, progressive muscle relaxation, deep breathing exercises, meditation, and imagery). *Patient needs knowledge about how to adapt to stress without resorting to drug use.*

Nutrition, Imbalanced: Less than Body Requirements

- Administer vitamins and dietary supplements as ordered by physician. *Vitamin B$_1$ is necessary to prevent complications from chronic alcoholism such as Wernicke's syndrome.*
- Monitor lab work (e.g., total albumin, complete blood count, urinalysis, electrolytes, and liver enzymes) and report significant changes to physician. *Objective laboratory tests provide necessary information to determine the extent of malnourishment.*
- Collaborate with dietitian to determine number of calories needed to provide adequate nutrition and realistic weight gain. Document intake, output, and calorie count. Weigh daily if condition warrants. *Weight loss or gain is important assessment information so that an appropriate plan of care can be developed.*
- Teach the importance of adequate nutrition by explaining the food guide pyramid and relating the physical effects of malnutrition on body systems. *Patient may have inadequate knowledge of proper nutritional habits.*

Self-Esteem, Chronic or Situational Low

- Spend time with the patient and convey an attitude of acceptance. Encourage the patient to accept responsibility for his or her own behaviors and feelings. *An attitude of acceptance enhances self-worth.*
- Encourage the patient to focus on strengths and accomplishments rather than weaknesses and failures. *Minimize attention to negative ruminations.*
- Encourage participation in therapeutic group activities. Offer recognition and positive feedback for actual achievements. *Success and recognition increase self-esteem.*
- Teach assertiveness techniques and effective communication techniques such as the use of "I feel" rather than "You make me feel" statements. *Previous patterns of communication may have been aggressive and accusatory, causing barriers to interpersonal relationships.*

Deficient Knowledge

- Assess the patient's level of knowledge and readiness to learn the effects of drugs and alcohol on the body. *Baseline assessment is required to develop appropriate teaching material.*
- Develop a teaching plan that includes measurable objectives. Include significant others, if possible. *Lifestyle changes often affect all family members.*
- Begin with simple concepts and progress to more complex issues. Use interactive teaching strategies and written materials appropriate to the patient's educational level. Include information on physiological effects of substances, the propensity for physical and psychological dependence, and the risks to a

fetus if the patient is pregnant. *Active participation and handouts enhance retention of important concepts.*

Sensory Perception, Disturbed

- Observe for withdrawal symptoms. Monitor vital signs. Provide adequate nutrition and hydration. Place on seizure precautions. *These actions provide supportive physical care during detoxification.*
- Assess level of orientation frequently. Orient and reassure the patient of safety in presence of hallucinations, delusions, or illusions. *Patient may be frightened.*
- Explain all interventions before approaching the patient. Avoid loud noises and talk softly to the patient. Decrease external stimuli by dimming lights. *Excessive stimuli increase agitation.*
- Administer prn medications according to detoxification schedule. *Benzodiazepines help to minimize the discomfort of withdrawal symptoms.*

Thought Processes, Disturbed

- Give positive reinforcement when thinking and behavior are appropriate or when the patient recognizes that delusions are not based in reality. *Drugs and alcohol can interfere with the patient's perception of reality.*
- Use simple, step-by-step instructions and face-to-face interaction when communicating with the patient. *Patient may be confused or disoriented.*
- Express reasonable doubt if the patient relays suspicious or paranoid beliefs. Reinforce accurate perception of people or situations. *It is important to communicate that you do not share that false belief as reality.*
- Do not argue with delusions or hallucinations. Convey acceptance that the patient believes a situation to be true, but that the nurse does not see or hear what is not there. *Arguing with the patient or denying the belief serves no useful purpose, because delusions are not eliminated.*
- Talk to the patient about real events and real people. Respond to feelings and reassure the patient that he or she is safe from harm. *Discussions that focus on the delusions may aggravate the condition. Verbalization of feelings in a nonthreatening environment may help the patient develop insight.*

Using NANDA, NIC, and NOC

Linkages between a selected NANDA nursing diagnosis, NIC, and NOC for the patient with a substance abuse problem are shown in the chart that follows.

Community-Based Care

The community provides many options for treating substance abuse including a mixture of individual, group, and family therapy. Medical detoxification can occur in hospitals, psychiatric units, special substance abuse units, methadone clinics, or outpatient settings. Less restrictive environments include residential rehabilitation programs, halfway houses, and partial hospitalization programs. These programs provide structured environments for the recovering substance abuser while maintaining a viable presence in the community. In addition, patients can obtain vocational counseling, become involved in self-help groups such as Alcoholics Anonymous or Narcotics Anonymous, and receive drug and health education.

The Patient with a Substance Abuse Problem

Nursing Diagnoses	Nursing Interventions	Nursing Outcomes
■ Defensive Coping	■ Patient Contracting ■ Anxiety Reduction ■ Coping Enhancement ■ Counseling ■ Decision-Making Support ■ Self-Awareness Enhancement	■ Risk Control: Alcohol Use, Drug Use, Tobacco Use ■ Anxiety Control ■ Coping ■ Symptom Control Behavior ■ Self-Esteem

Note: Data from Moorhead, S., Johnson, M., Maas, M., & Swanson, E. (Eds.). (2008). *Nursing outcomes classification (NOC)* (4th ed.). St. Louis: Mosby; North American Nursing Diagnosis Association. (2009). *Nursing diagnoses: Definitions & classification 2009–2011*. Philadelphia: Wiley-Blackwell; Bulechek, G. M., Butcher, H. K., & Dochterman, J. (2008). *Nursing interventions classification (NIC)* (4th ed.). St. Louis: Mosby. Reprinted by permission.

Teaching the patient and family includes the following:

■ The negative effects of substance abuse, including physical and psychological complications of substance abuse
■ The signs of relapse and the importance of after care programs and self-help groups to prevent relapse
■ Information about specific medications that help to reduce the craving for alcohol (naltrexone [ReVia] and acamprosate [Campral]) and maintain abstinence (disulfiram [Antabuse]), including the potential side effects, possible drug interactions, and any special precautions to be taken (e.g., avoiding OTC medications such as cough syrup that may have alcohol content)
■ Ways to manage stress including techniques such as progressive muscle relaxation, abdominal breathing techniques, imagery, meditation, and effective coping skills

In addition, suggest the following resources:

■ Alcoholics Anonymous, Narcotics Anonymous, and other self-help groups
■ Employee assistance programs
■ Individual, group, and/or family counseling
■ Community rehabilitation programs
■ National Alliance for the Mentally Ill

MEMORY CUE

Patients are at highest risk for relapse within the first few months after stopping the abused substance. An acronym that can assist the patient in recognizing behaviors that lead to relapse is **HALT**: **h**ungry, **a**ngry, **l**onely, and **t**ired. Nurses should emphasize the importance of a balanced diet, adequate sleep, healthy recreation activities, and a caring support system to prevent relapse.

Impaired Nurses

Healthcare providers are as susceptible as anyone else for developing substance abuse. By nature of their roles, dentists, pharmacists, physicians, and nurses are in frequent contact with drugs and are at high risk for substance abuse problems. One study exploring family history of alcohol and drug use in healthcare professionals found that nurses reported a higher prevalence of alcoholism in their families than dentists and physicians (Kenna & Wood, 2005). However, no significant differences were found in healthcare professionals' drinking levels. As a rule, nurses experience many pressures in the workplace and have easy access to drugs. This temptation may result in greater vulnerability for substance abuse and dependence and can lead to impaired professional practice. Nurses must act responsibly when coworkers display signs of substance use. Healthcare professionals have a higher risk for opiate abuse than other professionals due to the high accessibility of opiates in their line of work. If colleagues are showing signs of a substance abuse problem, information about impaired nurse programs is available through most state boards of nursing to help individual nurses. Nurses convicted of working or driving under the influence of alcohol, illegal substances, or nonmedical use of prescription drugs are subject to disciplinary action by their state board of nursing. A disciplinary hearing is held and may result in censure, probation, or suspension of a professional license. The loss of professional licensure is the most severe form of disciplinary action and may prevent an individual from ever practicing nursing again. Warning signs of impaired nurses in the workplace are listed in Table 6–4.

TABLE 6–4 Warning Signs of Impaired Nurses in the Workplace

AT-RISK SITUATIONS	OBSERVABLE WARNING SIGNS
Easy access to prescription drugs	Inaccurate narcotic counts or frequent missing drugs
	Patients complain of ineffective pain control, deny receiving pain meds
	Excessive "wasting" of drugs
	Volunteering to give medications to patients
	Frequent trips to the bathroom
Role strain	Frequent tardiness or absenteeism, especially before and after scheduled days off
	Haphazard, shoddy charting
	Patient care judgment errors
	Unorganized, erratic behavior, unkempt appearance
Depression	Irritability, unable to focus or concentrate
	Abrupt mood swings
	Isolating self, taking long breaks
	Apathetic, depressed, lethargic
	Unexplained absences from assigned unit
Signs of alcohol or drug use	Smell of alcohol on breath
	Excessive use of perfumes, mouthwash, or mints
	Slurred speech, flushed face, reddened eyes, unsteady gait
	Wearing long sleeves in hot weather to cover up arms
Signs of withdrawal	Tremors, restlessness, sweating
	Watery eyes, runny nose, stomach aches

CHAPTER HIGHLIGHTS

- Substance abuse is the unsanctioned use of any chemical despite adverse effects on the individual's physical, psychological, interpersonal, or social health.
- Substance dependence occurs when control over the chemical substance is lost and the individual must use increasing amounts to produce the desired effect (tolerance) and must use the substance to avoid or relieve uncomfortable symptoms (withdrawal).
- Combinations of genetic, biologic, psychological, and sociocultural factors contribute to substance abuse or dependence. Addictive behavior has been linked to biochemical changes in dopamine and serotonin brain levels as well as heredity, ethnic differences, and peer pressure. Thorough assessment of individual risk factors is necessary to plan and deliver appropriate nursing interventions.
- Adolescents are particularly influenced by society and peers to use substances, predominantly tobacco, alcohol, and illicit drugs. A positive ethnic identity and family environment act as "protective" deterrents for substance use.
- Substance abusers have common characteristics including risk-taking behavior, low tolerance for frustration or pain, compulsive preoccupation with the substance, anxiety, anger, and low self-esteem. Stress management, anger control, social support, and counseling are helpful strategies to avoid substance abuse and dependence.
- Alcohol is the most commonly used and abused legal substance in America; however, polysubstance abuse is frequent in many individuals. Marijuana is the most commonly used illicit drug. Both alcohol and marijuana are considered "gateway" drugs to harder substance abuse. Substances such as cocaine and methamphetamine are often used in conjunction with alcohol. Prescription anti-anxiety agents have been abused in the past, and there is a growing trend in prescription narcotic analgesic abuse.
- Nursing care of patients experiencing substance abuse problems includes health promotion efforts to prevent substance abuse; comprehensive physical, spiritual, and psychosocial assessment; and interventions for the human responses of ineffective coping and denial, imbalanced nutrition, low self-esteem, disturbed thought processes, disturbed sensory perception, and risk for injury or violence.
- Severe alcohol withdrawal or delirium tremens is a medical emergency that usually occurs 2 to 5 days following cessation of use. A symptom-triggered approach to the administration of benzodiazepines during alcohol withdrawal results in less total medication use and requires a shorter duration of treatment.
- The community provides many options for treating substance abuse including a mixture of individual, group, and family therapy. A successful after-care program includes resources to help manage stress and prevent relapse.
- Nurses are susceptible to substance abuse due to pressures in the workplace and easy access to drugs. Nurses need to assess their response to stress and seek early treatment for depressive symptoms to avoid impaired professional practice.

TEST YOURSELF NCLEX-RN® REVIEW

1. What is the minimum level of alcohol in the blood for an individual to be considered intoxicated?
   1. 0.05%
   2. 0.08%
   3. 0.50%
   4. 1.00%
2. Which of the following questions is *most* appropriate when interviewing the patient who is suspected of alcohol abuse problems?
   1. "Typically, how many days per week do you drink alcoholic beverages?"
   2. "Have you been drinking lately?"
   3. "You don't drink much alcohol, do you?"
   4. "Has your drinking caused a lot of problems between you and your spouse?"
3. What is the rationale behind ordering thiamine (vitamin B_1) for a person with a history of chronic alcoholism?
   1. to prevent acute pancreatitis
   2. to prevent cirrhosis of the liver
   3. to prevent hepatic encephalopathy
   4. to prevent Wernicke's encephalopathy
4. Which of the following substances present the highest medical danger during withdrawal?
   1. CNS stimulants and amphetamines
   2. opiates and marijuana
   3. alcohol and CNS depressants
   4. amphetamines and hallucinogens
5. What is the rationale for prescribing disulfiram (Antabuse) for a person who suffers from alcohol abuse?
   1. to decrease the discomfort of withdrawal symptoms
   2. to decrease the pleasant, reinforcing effects of alcohol
   3. to prevent the breakdown of alcohol, thereby inhibiting impulsive drinking
   4. to block the signs and symptoms of alcohol withdrawal
6. Which is NOT a warning sign of substance abuse in the nurse?
   1. impaired motor coordination, slurred speech, bloodshot eyes
   2. unkempt appearance, disorganized, erratic behavior
   3. patients consistently report effective pain control
   4. frequent absenteeism or tardiness, unexplained absences from the unit
7. Which of the following statements is false?
   1. Smoking is the leading known cause of preventable death and disease among women.
   2. The smoking rates for women have steadily declined since the 1950s.
   3. Women who smoke during pregnancy have a higher risk for spontaneous abortions.
   4. Women who smoke have an increased risk for stroke and heart disease.
8. Which statement by the patient illustrates an understanding of your teaching regarding naltrexone (ReVia)?
   1. "I should read labels of OTC cold medicines to make sure they don't have alcohol."
   2. "I should stop taking all pain medications before starting on naltrexone."
   3. "I should go to my Narcotics Anonymous meetings for 1 month, then I can stop going."
   4. "I should wear a medical alert bracelet that states I'm taking naltrexone."

9. Which of the following is a realistic goal for a patient with substance abuse?
   1. The patient will identify ways to deal with stressful situations instead of resorting to substance use.
   2. The patient will refrain from using substances until craving for the substance has been eliminated.
   3. The patient will focus on negative aspects of past behaviors and interpersonal relationships.
   4. The patient be able to use alcohol or drugs in moderation.

10. An appropriate nursing diagnosis for a patient with substance abuse problems is which of the following.
    1. *Imbalanced Nutrition: Greater than Body Requirements* related to food intake in excess of energy expenditure
    2. *Excess Fluid Volume* related to increased intake of vitamins and dietary supplements
    3. *Ineffective Denial* related to inability to recognize maladaptive behaviors related to substance use
    4. *Disturbed Thought Processes* related to infectious process and pain

See Test Yourself answers in Appendix C.

Pearson Nursing Student Resources

Find additional review materials at
nursing.pearsonhighered.com
Prepare for success with additional NCLEX®-style practice questions, interactive assignments and activities, Web links, animations and videos, and more!

BIBLIOGRAPHY

American Psychiatric Association (2000). *Diagnostic and statistical manual of mental disorders (DSM-IV-TR)* (4th ed., text revision). Washington, DC: Author.

Bersamin, M., Paschall, M. F., & Flewelling, R. L. (2005). Ethnic differences in relationships between risk factors and adolescent binge drinking: A national study. *Prevention Science, 6*(2), 127–137.

Brown, A. H., Domier, C. P., & Rawson, R. A. (2005). Stimulants, sex, and gender. *Sexual Addiction & Compulsivity, 12*(2-3), 169–180.

Buchanan, D., Tooze, J. A., Shaw, S., Kinzly, M., Heimer, R., & Singer, M. (2006). Demographic, HIV risk behavior, and health status characteristics of "crack" cocaine injectors compared to other injection drug users in three New England cities. *Drug and Alcohol Dependence, 81*(3), 221–229.

Bulechek, G. M., Butcher, H. K. & Dochterman, J. M. (Eds.). (2008). *Nursing interventions classification (NIC)* (5th ed.). St. Louis: Mosby.

Compton, W. M. & Volkow, N. D. (2006). Major increases in opioid analgesic abuse in the United States: Concerns and strategies. *Drug and Alcohol Dependence, 81*(2), 103–107.

Conner, B. T., Noble, E. P., Berman, S. M., Ozkaragoz, T., Ritchie, T., Antolin, T., & Sheen, C. (2005). DRD2 genotypes and substance use in adolescent children of alcoholics. *Drug and Alcohol Dependence, 79*(3), 379–387.

Cook, T. A., Luczak, S. E., Shea, S. H., Ehlers, C. L., Carr, L. G., & Wall, T. L. (2005). Associations of ALDH2 and ADH1B genotypes with response to alcohol in Asian Americans. *Journal of Studies on Alcohol, 66*(2), 196–204.

Ewing, J. A. (1984). Detecting alcoholism: The CAGE questionnaire. *Journal of the American Medical Association, 252*(14), 1905–1907.

Ferdinand, R. F., Sondeijker, F., van der Ende, J., Selten, J., Huizink, A., & Verhulst, F. C. (2005). Cannabis use predicts future psychotic symptoms, and vice versa. *Addiction, 100*(5), 612–618.

Jellinek, E. (1946). *Phases in the drinking history of alcoholics.* New Haven, CT: Hillhouse Press.

Kenna, G. A., & Wood, M. D. (2005). Family history of alcohol and drug use in healthcare professionals. *Journal of Substance Use, 10*(4), 225–238.

Kneisl, C. R., & Trigoboff, E. (2009). *Contemporary psychiatric–mental health nursing* (2nd ed.). Upper Saddle River, NJ: Prentice Hall.

Lantz, M. S. (2005). Prescription drug and alcohol abuse in an older woman. *Clinical Geriatrics, 12*(1), 39–43.

Leonardson, G. R., Kemper, E., Ness, F. K., Koplin, B. A., Daniels, M. C., & Leonardson, G. A. (2005). Validity and reliability of the audit and CAGE-AID in Northern Plains American Indians. *Psychological Reports, 97*(1), 161–166.

Lewis, T. (2008). Assessing an older adult for alcohol use disorders. *Nursing, 32*(8), 60–61.

Llussier-Cushing, M., Repper-DeLisi, J., Mitchell, M., Lakatos, B., Mahmoud, F., & Lipkos-Orlando. (2007). Is your medical-surgical patient withdrawing from alcohol? *Nursing2007, 37*(10), 50–55.

Miller, N. S., & Greenfeld, A. (2004). Patient characteristics and risk factors for development of dependence on hydrocodone and oxycodone. *American Journal of Therapeutics, 11*(1), 26–32.

Moorhead, S., Johnson, M., & Maas, M. & Swanson, E. (Eds.). (2008). *Nursing outcomes classification (NOC)* (4th ed.). St. Louis: Mosby.

National Institute of Mental Health. (2008). *The numbers count: Mental disorders in America.* NIH Publication No. 01-4584. Bethesda, MD: NIMH. Retrieved from http://www.nimh.nih.gov/publicat/numbers.cfm

North American Nursing Diagnosis Association International. (2009). *Nursing diagnoses: Definitions & classification 2009–2011.* Philadelphia: Wiley-Blackwell.

Pokorny, A. D., Miller, B. A., & Kaplan, H. B. (1972). The brief MAST: A shortened version of the Michigan Alcohol Screening Test. *American Journal of Psychiatry, 129,* 342–345.

Rice, V. H., & Stead, L. F. (2005). Nursing interventions for smoking cessation. *The Cochrane Database of Systematic Reviews,* Issue 4, The Cochrane Collaboration: John Wiley & Sons.

Rigotti, N. A., Munafo, M. R., Murphy, M. F. G., Stead, L. F. (2005). Interventions for smoking cessation in hospitalized patients. *The Cochrane Database of Systematic Reviews,* Issue 4, The Cochrane Collaboration: John Wiley & Sons.

Savage, C. (2008). How to screen patients for alcohol use disorders. *American Nurse Today, 3*(12), 7–9.

Semple, S. J., Patterson, T. L., & Rant, I. (2005). Methamphetamine use and depressive symptoms among heterosexual men and women. *Journal of Substance Use, 10*(1), 31–47.

Shoptaw, S., Reback, C. J., Peck, J. A., Yang, X., Rotheram-Fuller, E., Larkins, S., Veniegas, R. C., Freese, T. E., & Hucks-Ortiz, C. (2005). Behavioral treatment approaches for methamphetamine dependence and HIV-related sexual risk behaviors among urban gay and bisexual men. *Drug and Alcohol Dependence, 78*(2), 125–134.

Silagy, C. Lancaster, T., Stead, M., & Fowler, G. (2005). Nicotine replacement therapy for smoking cessation. *The Cochrane Database of Systematic Reviews,* Issue 4, The Cochrane Collaboration: John Wiley & Sons.

Skinner, H. A. (1982). *Drug Abuse Screening Test (DAST)* (p. 363). Langford Lance, England: Elsevier Science Ltd.

Snyder, J. L., & Bowers, T. G. (2008). The efficacy of acamprosate and naltrexone in the treatment of alcohol dependence: a relative benefits analysis of randomized controlled trials. *Journal of Drug and Alcohol Abuse, 34*(4), 449–461.

Srisurapanont, M., Jarusuraisin, N., & Kittirattanapalboon, P. (2005). Treatment for amphetamine dependence and abuse. *The Cochrane Database of Systematic Reviews,* (4): ID #CD003022.

Stevenson, J. S. (2005). Alcohol use, misuse, abuse, and dependence in later adulthood. *Annual Review of Nursing Research, 23,* 245–280.

Storr, C. L., Westergaard, R., & Anthony, J. C. (2005). Early onset inhalant use and risk for opiate initiation by young adulthood. *Drug and Alcohol Dependence, 78*(3), 253–261.

Stuart, G. W. (2009). *Principles and practice of psychiatric nursing* (9th ed.). St. Louis: Mosby.

Substance Abuse and Mental Health Services Administration (SAMHSA), Office of Applied Studies. (2008a). *Results from the 2007 National Survey on Drug Use and Health: National findings* (NSDUH Series H-34, DHHS Publication No. SMA 08-4343). Rockville, MD.

Substance Abuse and Mental Health Services Administration (SAMHSA), Office of Applied Studies. (2008b). *Drug abuse warning network, 2006: National estimates of drug-related emergency department visits* (DAWN Series D-30, DHHS Publication No. (SMA) 08-4339). Rockville, MD: Author.

Sullivan, J. T., Sykora, K., Schneiderman, J., Naranjo, C. A., & Sellers, E. M. (1989). Assessment of alcohol withdrawal: the revised Clinical Institute Withdrawal Assessment for Alcohol scale (CIWA-Ar). *British Journal of Addictions, 84,* 1353–1357.

U.S. Department of Health and Human Services (USDHHS), Centers for Disease Control and Prevention. (2007). *Fact sheet: Women and tobacco.* National Center for Chronic Disease Prevention and Health Promotion, Office on Smoking and Health. Retrieved January 12, 2009, from http://www.cdc.gov/tobacco/data_statistics/fact_sheets/populations/women_tobacco.htm

Wesson, D. R., & Ling, W. (2003). The clinical opiate withdrawal scale (COWS). *Journal of Psychoactive Drugs, 35*(2), 253–259.

Wu, L. T., Schlenger, W. E. & Gavin, D. M. (2006). Concurrent use of methamphetamine, MDMA, LSD, ketamine, GHB, and flunitrazepam among American youths. *Drug and Alcohol Dependence, 84*(1), 102–113.

Zimmerman, P., Wittchen, H., Waszak, F., Nocon, A., Hofler, M., & Lieb, R. (2005). Pathways into Ecstasy use: the role of prior cannabis use and Ecstasy availability. *Drug and Alcohol Dependence, 79*(3), 331–341.

7 Nursing Care of Patients Experiencing Disasters

LEARNING OUTCOMES

1. Distinguish the difference between an emergency and a disaster.
2. Describe the types of injuries and manifestations associated with biologic, chemical, or radiologic terrorism.
3. Discuss nursing interventions for the treatment of injuries related to biologic, chemical, or radiologic terrorism.
4. Explain the rationale for reverse triage in disasters versus conventional triage in emergencies.
5. Discuss situations requiring the need for patient isolation or patient decontamination.
6. Discuss the role of the nurse in disaster planning, response, and mitigation.

CLINICAL COMPETENCIES

1. Assess health status of patients who have experienced a disaster and monitor, document, and triage to the appropriate level of care.
2. Use evidence-based interventions to plan and implement nursing care for patients with injuries suffered as a result of a disaster.
3. Using assessment skills, implement and evaluate individualized nursing interventions for patients who are victims of disasters.
4. Provide safe and knowledgeable nursing care to treat disaster-related injuries.
5. Evaluate and revise plan of care to restore functional health status to patients who have sustained injuries due to a disaster.
6. Provide education to promote prevention of disaster-related injuries.

KEY TERMS

bioterrorism, *126*
cold zone, *133*
conventional weapons, *125*
disasters, *124*
emergency, *125*
hot zone, *133*
man-made disasters, *125*
mass casualty incidents, *125*

mitigation, *131*
multiple casualty incidents, *125*
natural disasters, *124*
nonconventional terrorist weapons, *125*
personal protective equipment (PPE), *133*
preparedness, *131*

radiation sickness, *129*
recovery, *131*
reverse triage, *132*
surge capacity, *131*
terrorism, *125*
triage, *132*
warm zone, *133*

All nurses will be expected to know how to provide care for victims of disasters whether they work in acute care settings, ambulatory sites, long-term care facilities, or at home in their communities. There is no way to know where or when disasters may strike. Because of this, nurses must be prepared to assist patients, families, friends, healthcare workers, first responders, and communities in their recovery from disastrous events. There are a number of basic competencies that nurses should be cognizant of related to disaster preparedness. The International Nursing Coalition for Mass Casualty Education (INCMCE) was founded to ensure a competent nurse workforce to respond to mass casualty incidents (MCIs) by facilitating the development of policies related to mass casualty events as they influence the public health infrastructure and affect nursing practice, education, research, and regulation (International Nursing Coalition for Mass Casualty Education [INCMCE], 2003).

The purpose of the *Educational Competencies for Registered Nurses Responding to Mass Casualty Incidents* publication (2003) is to provide registered nurses with the awareness of critical competencies necessary to respond effectively to mass casualty events (Box 7–1). Nurses are expected to have sufficient knowledge to recognize the potential for a disaster event; when such an event has occurred; and what nurses can do to protect themselves, family members, and community members from harm or from potential exacerbation of conditions. Nurses must be aware of their role in disaster planning, response, and mitigation. Equally important, nurses must be aware of professional limitations and be able to respond to MCIs appropriately within the scope of nursing practice.

Disasters and Emergencies

Noji (1997) defined disasters as "events that require extraordinary efforts beyond those needed to respond to everyday emergencies." **Disasters** may be natural or man-made. **Natural disasters** are caused by acts of nature or emerging diseases. They may be predictable through advanced meteorologic technologies or unexpected. For example, Hurricane Katrina hit landfall on August 29, 2005, along the Central Gulf Coast. The hurricane caused vast devastation as its storm surge breached the levee system that protected New Orleans from Lake Ponchartrain and the Mississippi River. Most of the New Orleans area was flooded, and heavy damage was also inflicted on the coasts of Mississippi and Alabama. Katrina is considered one of the most destructive and costliest natural disasters in the history of the United States (U.S. Department of Homeland Security, 2008). **Man-made disasters** are either accidental or intentional. They include complex emergencies, technologic disasters, material shortages, and other disasters not caused by natural hazards. Examples of man-made or human-generated disasters include war; chemical, biologic, radiologic, and nuclear terrorism; transportation accidents; group violence; food or water contamination; deforestation; and building collapses. Contamination of large amounts of vegetables at a grocery store is an example of a deliberate or *intentional* man-made disaster. A campfire that has been left unattended such that the embers are carried by high winds to the dry trees and brush nearby, creating a massive forest fire is an example of a man-made *accidental* disaster.

An **emergency** is distinguished from a disaster in that an emergency encompasses an unforeseen combination of circumstances calling for immediate action for a range of victims from one to many. For example, a motor vehicle crash may call for emergency assistance for a small number of individuals whose injuries are minor to very severe or fatal. Emergencies are generally accommodated within the emergency management system. Disasters seldom involve a single victim. Instead, disasters are complex emergencies that significantly overwhelm available hospitals, emergency medical services, facilities, and resources. Disasters are typically labeled as **multiple casualty incidents** with more than 2 but fewer than 100 persons injured or **mass casualty incidents** in which 100 or more casualties are involved (Beachley, 2005). An example of a mass casualty incident is that of an entire community affected by the release of a hazardous material such as a chemical as a result of a train derailment. With human fatalities of approximately 200,000 and 1,300 in Banda Aceh and the Gulf

Coast, respectively, the tsunami in Indonesia and Hurricane Katrina are prime examples of mass casualty incidents (American Red Cross, 2006). In summary, the key difference between an emergency and a disaster is that an emergency can be handled by the usual emergency management systems already in place, while a disaster overwhelms general emergency systems and requires additional resources.

Causes of Disasters

Disasters may result from a variety of causes, including hazardous materials and terrorism.

Hazardous Materials

Hazardous materials pose a potential risk to life, health, or property if they are released because of their chemical, biologic, or physical nature. The hazard exists during any stage of use, from the production and storage of these substances to their transportation, use, or disposal. Hazardous materials accidents range from the unintentional release of household hazardous materials, to chemical spills on highways, to groundwater contamination by naturally occurring methane gas (Langan & James, 2005).

Terrorism

Terrorism is defined by the U.S. Department of Defense as the "calculated use of violence or the threat of violence to inculcate fear; intended to coerce or to intimidate governments or societies in the pursuit of goals that are generally political, religious or ideological." One of the goals of terrorism is to cause psychologic effects that reach a much wider audience than the immediate victims or object of an attack. High-profile acts draw attention to the terrorists and their cause. It is thought that terrorists seek to obtain leverage, influence, and power through the publicity generated by their violence (Hoffman, 2008).

The weapons terrorists use are often described as conventional and nonconventional. **Conventional weapons** include bombs and guns. Car and truck bombs have become powerful weapons in suicide attacks such as the Oklahoma City bombing of the Alfred P. Murrah Federal Building on April 19, 1995. Terrorists use explosive bombs such as letter, parcel, pipe, barometric, and fertilizer truckbombs, as well as incendiary bombs such as Molotov cocktails. Other types of conventional terrorist weapons include handguns, rifles, semiautomatic weapons, hand grenades, rocket-propelled devices, and even surface-to-air, shoulder-fired missiles that can bring down helicopters, fighter aircraft, and civilian airliners (Through The Eyes of Terror, n.d.).

Nonconventional terrorist weapons include those in the chemical, biologic, and nuclear categories. Chemical terrorism attacks may manifest as the release of a toxin into highly populated areas, bodies of water, and unventilated areas. Another type of chemical terrorism is a specific attack on a particular product, especially a food product. This is accomplished by introducing a toxic chemical substance directly into the product. The anthrax attacks against U.S. public officials after 9/11 illustrate how these small amounts of "white powder" can encourage mass panic and hysteria in the public (Simonsen & Spindlove, 2007) (See Box 7–2).

BOX 7–1 Educational Competencies for Registered Nurses Responding to Mass Casualty Incidents

Core Competencies
1. Critical thinking
2. Assessment
3. Technical skills
4. Communication

Core Knowledge Areas
1. Health promotion, risk reduction, and disease prevention
2. Healthcare systems and policy
3. Illness and disease management
4. Information and healthcare technologies
5. Ethics
6. Human diversity

Professional Role Development
1. A description of nursing roles in MCIs
2. Identification of the most appropriate or most likely healthcare role for oneself during an MCI

Source: INCMCE (2003).

Bioterrorism

Another name for biologic terrorism is **bioterrorism**. Biologic terrorism is the "use of etiological agents (disease) to cause harm or kill a population, food, and/or livestock. Biological terrorism includes the use of organisms such as bacteria, viruses, and rickettsia and the use of products of organisms—toxins. The main purpose of biologic weapon use is mass devastation. Unfortunately, it is not uncommon for the results of a biologic attack not to be known for several hours or days after the attack because aerosolized biologic particles are odorless, colorless, and tasteless. Unless the terrorists announce the biologic attack, it may remain unknown until patients begin to present at emergency departments or physicians' offices a few days or weeks after the release of the agent. Detection is difficult because of the numerous different healthcare facilities available for patient treatment. Surveillance is essential to detect such an event. The goal of the surveillance system is to determine the status of the public's health and detect any sudden change in that status. Fortunately, biologic weapons are not as common, accessible, or available as chemical weapons.

Healthcare providers must be alert to the recognition, reporting, and treatment of high-priority biologic agents. A disaster preparedness plan should be established in every healthcare facility that outlines the protocol and procedures to be taken with a suspected bioterrorism attack. Hospital staff will alert the infection control nurse when subtle changes or trends in symptoms among patients are seen. The public health department is also given this data. When an unusual disease pattern presents itself, laboratories perform tests on cultures that would normally be discarded as contaminants. Laboratory personnel report unusual clusters of laboratory results. Special laboratories have been established to perform a battery of tests on suspicious specimens of rarely seen bacteria, toxins, viruses, or increased numbers of a particular strain or specimen. The Centers for Disease Control and Prevention (CDC) have created detailed "Fact Sheets" about bioterrorism agents and diseases for healthcare providers.

Nuclear/Radiologic Terrorism

The nuclear category of nonconventional terrorist weapons encompasses the use of a nuclear device to cause mass murder and devastation. This category of terrorism includes the use or threat of the use of fissionable radioactive materials in an attack. An explosion at a nuclear power plant is an example of this type of terrorism. Using conventional weapons against one of the many nuclear reactors in the world could cause an explosion that would cause extensive and possibly irreversible environmental damage. Damage to the reactors could cause radioactive matter to be released into the atmosphere, potentially endangering large population centers (U.S. Department of State, 2009).

The radiologic dispersion bomb is probably the most accessible nuclear device to be used by terrorists. Another name for this device is dirty bomb because it consists of a conventional explosive and radioactive waste by-products from nuclear reactors. The dirty bomb discharges deadly radioactive particles into the environment. It is cheaper to make than a nuclear bomb

---

BOX 7–2 Biologic Threat Infections

Following the terrorist attacks on September 11, 2001, and the development of anthrax cases in the United States, concern has arisen about the possible use of biologic weapons. The most likely pathogens to be used for this purpose include anthrax, smallpox, botulism, pneumonic plague, and viral hemorrhagic fevers.

Anthrax is an acute bacterial infection caused by *Bacillus anthracis*, a gram-positive, spore-producing organism that occurs in inhaled, cutaneous, and gastrointestinal forms. The spores are impervious to temperature and sunlight, and remain viable for years.

Inhalation anthrax carries the highest mortality rate because spores of one to five microns are easily inhaled and deposited in the alveoli. The patient initially exhibits influenza-like symptoms such as fever, nonproductive cough, headache, and malaise that advances to respiratory distress, mediastinal widening, and hemodynamic collapse in 3 to 5 days. Death may occur shortly thereafter. Untreated patients die in 2 to 3 days. The characteristic lesion of cutaneous anthrax progresses from an itching papule to a painless, serosanguineous-filled vesicle that forms a black necrotic center. Patients who ingest the anthrax bacillus develop nausea, vomiting, severe abdominal pain, and bloody diarrhea. Diagnosis is confirmed by a positive blood culture, polymerase chain reaction, and serology. On confirmation of anthrax exposure, prophylaxis is initiated with oral ciprofloxacin (Cipro) or doxycycline (Doxycin) for 60 days; people with confirmed systemic anthrax cases must receive anti-infectives intravenously (CDC, 2006).

Healthcare workers risk exposure to anthrax through direct contact with a contaminated surface, exposed persons' contaminated clothes, or direct unprotected contact with the open lesions of cutaneous anthrax. Guidelines for decontamination of extensively exposed persons include removal of clothing and storage in a sealed plastic bag, and showering with soap and water. If gross contamination with the agent occurs and soap and water decontamination is ineffective, use a bleach solution (1:10 dilution of household bleach/final hypochlorite concentration 0.5%) and rinse after 10 to 15 minutes (Heymann, 2004).

In 1980, the World Health Organization certified that *smallpox* was eradicated. Routine smallpox vaccination was discontinued in 1972, leaving people under the age of 39 at risk for this disease if it reappears or is used as a weapon. Smallpox spreads by direct contact or by inhalation of respiratory droplets. Symptoms include a high fever, headache, and malaise, followed by a vesicular/pustular rash appearing simultaneously on the face and extremities. Once the lesions break open and spread large amounts of the virus into the mouth and throat, people are highly contagious and should be placed in negative-pressure rooms. Anyone exposed to the patient should be vaccinated and monitored closely. Vaccination up to 4 days after exposure and before a rash appears provides almost complete protection (World Health Organization (WHO), 2009). Healthcare providers should be alert to illness patterns that could indicate an unusual infectious disease outbreak. Indicators of a biologic agent release include increased disease incidence among people in the same geographic area (e.g., people who attended the same event); the disease pattern is inconsistent with patient age, such as chickenpox among adults; and a patient presents with symptoms of a rare disease. The presence of one or more of these indicators should be reported to public health authorities to determine the infectious disease source and to prevent further exposure (WHO, 2009).

and radioactive waste material is relatively easy to obtain. Radioactive waste is found throughout the world and is typically not as well guarded as nuclear weapons.

Types of Disasters with Common Injuries

This section describes a variety of disasters with the injuries that are common to each specific disaster. Table 7–1 outlines types of disasters with related injuries and nursing implications.

Hurricanes, Tornados, and Tsunamis

A hurricane is a type of tropical cyclone. It is a low-pressure system that generally forms in the tropics. Hurricanes can wreak havoc on coastlines as well as several hundred miles inland. Hurricanes and tropical storms can also spawn tornadoes, create storm surges along the coast, and cause extensive damage from heavy rainfall. Floods are deadly and destructive. Excessive rain can trigger landslides or mudslides, especially in mountainous regions. Flooding on rivers and streams may persist for several days or more after the storm (Federal Emergency Management Agency, 2008).

Common physical effects include asphyxia due to drowning; wounds; bone, joint, and muscle injuries; aggravation of chronic illnesses; stress-related symptoms; upper respiratory infections; gastrointestinal illnesses; clean-up injuries; animal, snake, and insect bites; skin irritations and infections; obstetrical complications; and waterborne and insect-borne diseases from contaminated water supplies and insect breeding grounds (Clark, 2008; Smith & Maurer, 2005).

As a result of Hurricane Katrina, many people lost their homes, family members, friends, and the environment that supported their daily routines. Many basic physical needs in the aftermath of the hurricane could not be met, which put survivors at risk of dehydration, starvation or malnutrition, heat-related illnesses, and diseases and injuries related to lack of sanitation and safe housing (Myers-Walls, 2005). The CDC offers a number of specific strategies to promote health and safety after a hurricane.

A tsunami, a seismic sea wave, is a series of ocean waves characterized by having a long period and wavelength and the ability to travel at speeds greater than 500 miles per hour. As the tsunami encounters shallow water, its height increases drastically, resulting in a sudden increase in sea level, thereby flooding low-lying coastal areas. Injuries are similar to those seen with hurricanes.

Thunderstorms

Risk of a lightning strike is possible during a thunderstorm. The short duration of a lightning strike results in a very short flow of current internally, despite the high voltage of lightning. Additionally, the almost immediate flashover of current around the body usually results in very little, if any, skin breakdown or burning of tissues (Daley et al., 2008).

High electrolyte and water content in the body conduct the greatest electrical current. Hence, the greatest conductors of

electrical current in the body are the nerves, muscle, and blood vessels. High resistors to electric current are bone, tendon, and fat, due to their tendency to heat up and coagulate instead of transmitting current. Much of the energy current may be dissipated at the skin surface. This results in significant surface burns, especially in calloused areas (Daley et al., 2008).

Tornados

Flying debris causes most fatalities and injuries in tornadoes. The physical effects include bone, muscle, and joint injuries; fractures; aggravation of chronic illnesses, obstetrical complications, stress-related symptoms; upper respiratory infections and those associated with fiberglass; eye injuries (see Box 7–3 for first aid); clean-up wounds; and gastrointestinal illnesses (Smith & Maurer, 2005).

Earthquakes

Earthquakes have a high incidence of mortality and morbidity. The most common health effects experienced by victims of earthquakes include stress-related symptoms; wounds; bone, joint, and muscle injuries; burns from explosions; clean-up injuries; gastrointestinal and respiratory problems; aggravation of chronic illnesses; obstetrical complications; and death (Smith & Maurer, 2005).

Snowstorms

Overexertion and exhaustion are major problems during the snow shoveling that is done following a snowstorm. The exertion required to shovel heavy snow in the extreme cold may cause a myocardial infarction.

BOX 7–3 First Aid for Eye Injuries

Specks in the Eye
- Do not rub the eye.
- Flush the eye with large amounts of water.
- Seek medical attention if the speck does not wash out.

Cuts, Punctures, and Foreign Objects in the Eye
- Do NOT wash out the eye.
- Do NOT try to remove a foreign object stuck in the eye.
- Seek immediate medical attention.

Chemical Burns
- Immediately flush the eye with water or any drinkable fluid. Open the eye as wide as possible. Continue flushing for at least 15 minutes. For caustic or basic solutions, continue flushing while on the way to medical care.
- If a contact lens is in the eye, begin flushing over the lens immediately. Flushing may dislodge the lens.
- Seek immediate medical attention.

Blows to the Eye
- Apply a cold compress without pressure, or tape crushed iced in a plastic bag to the forehead and allow it to rest gently on the injured eye.
- Seek immediate medical attention if pain continues, if vision is reduced, or if blood or discoloration appears in the eye.

Source: National Institute for Occupational Safety and Health (NIOSH). (2009). Available at http://www.cdd.gov/niosh/topics/eye/eyesafe.html

TABLE 7–1 Types of Disasters and Common Injuries

TYPE OF DISASTER	COMMON INJURIES	NURSING IMPLICATIONS
Hurricane-Related Injuries	Drowning; clean-up injuries; aggravation of chronic illnesses; stress-related symptoms; upper respiratory infections; gastrointestinal illnesses; animal, snake, and insect bites; obstetrical complications; contaminated water supplies and insect-breeding grounds; heat-related illnesses; lack of sanitation and safe housing	Asphyxia; wounds; bone, joint, and muscle injuries; infections; skin irritations; waterborne and insect-borne diseases; dehydration; starvation or malnutrition; diseases.
Tsunami-Related Injuries	"Tsunami lung," a severe infection caused by swallowing muddy, bacteria-laden water	Requires aggressive respiratory and ventilator management, blood transfusions, antibiotics, and other medical support.
Thunderstorm-Related Injuries	Resistance of body tissues to electrical current *Least resistance:* nerves, blood, mucous membranes, muscle *Intermediate resistance:* dry skin *Most resistance:* tendon, fat, bone	Potential for tissue destruction with longer duration of contact with high-voltage current; if energy current is dissipated at the skin surface, significant surface burns result, especially in calloused areas.
Tornado-Related Injuries	Flying debris; injuries similar to hurricane-related injuries	Injuries and fatalities can occur.
Earthquake-Related Injuries	High incidence of mortality and morbidity; explosions	May result in stress-related symptoms; wounds; bone, joint, and muscle injuries; clean-up injuries; gastrointestinal and respiratory problems; aggravation of chronic illnesses; obstetrical complications; burns.
Snowstorm-Related Injuries	Overexertion and exhaustion	Myocardial infarction can occur.
Disaster-Related Eye Injuries	"Specks" of dust or debris; cuts, punctures, or stuck objects; blows to the eye	Administer eyewash or flushing versus rubbing; stabilize eye with rigid shield. Apply cold compress, no pressure; patient should visit healthcare professional to rule out serious injury or internal eye damage.
Blast Injuries	Auditory	Tympanic membrane rupture, ossicular disruption, and cochlear damage occur; damage from foreign body can occur.
	Eye, orbit, face	Perforated globe, air embolisms, fractures are common; damage from foreign body can occur.
	Respiratory	May result in blast lung, hemothorax, pneumothorax, pulmonary contusion and hemorrhage, atrioventricular fistulas (source of air embolism), airway epithelial damage, aspiration pneumonitis, sepsis.
	Digestive	May result in bowel perforation, hemorrhage, ruptured liver or spleen, sepsis, mesenteric ischemia from air embolism.
	Circulatory	Cardiac contusion, myocardial infarction from air embolism, shock, vasovagal hypotension, peripheral vascular injury, and air embolism-induced injury can occur.
	Central nervous system injury	Concussion, closed and open brain injury, stroke, spinal cord injury, air embolism-induced injury can occur.
	Renal injury	May result in renal contusion, laceration, acute renal failure due to rhabdomyolysis, hypotension, and hypovolemia.
	Extremity injury	Traumatic amputation, fractures, crush injuries, compartment syndrome, burns, cuts, lacerations, acute arterial occlusion, air embolism-induced injury can occur.
Blunt Trauma	Head and torso blunt trauma, penetrating trauma	Fractured limbs and spinal injury can occur.
Pressure Trauma	Lungs	Tearing of the alveoli cause swelling, fluid accumulation, possible pulmonary emboli, eventual hypoxia.
	Ear injury: ear pain, hearing loss	Keep auditory canal clean.

TABLE 7–1 Types of Disasters and Common Injuries (continued)

TYPE OF DISASTER	COMMON INJURIES	NURSING IMPLICATIONS
	Bowel injury	Make the patient comfortable.
Radiological Dispersion Bomb (Dirty Bomb) Blast	Radiation sickness	Get rid of contaminated clothes, shower, and evacuate the area within a day of a small or medium blast. Those close to the blast could suffer radiation sickness and require hospital care.
Nuclear Detonation	Thermal burns	May involve only the epidermis and upper layers of dermis with short duration of heat exposure.
Bright Light Flash of Nuclear Detonation	Eye burn injuries	May blind the patient momentarily, effects will disappear with time, can impair a patient's ability to perform self-care and other ADLs.
Radiation Exposure Injury	Bone marrow and blood cell damage	A reduction in the blood's oxygen-carrying capacity results in nausea, fatigue, and a general feeling of malaise. Reduced platelet production causes clotting disorders and possibly hemorrhage. When the body's white blood cells are destroyed, it is important to reduce the patient's exposure to infection. Infection at the time of reduced WBC production can be severe and even fatal.
	Bowel	Cells that reproduce the bowel lining are damaged, resulting in nausea, loss of appetite, vomiting, diarrhea, fluid loss, and malaise in the acute stage; later, dehydration, malnutrition, bowel hemorrhage, and perforation may occur; if radiation exposure is not exacerbated by other injury or pathology, patients will generally survive.
	Integument	Erythema or generalized reddening of the skin occurs when skin cells are damaged, with the appearance of a sunburn; more serious burns may occur with persistent exposure or extremely high radiation doses.
	Nervous and cardiovascular systems	With acute radiation exposure, blood vessel and nerve cells are damaged and the patient is incapacitated and experiences cardiovascular collapse, confusion, and even an "on fire" sensation throughout the body; symptoms this severe generally do not permit survival.
Chemical Burns	Range from minor to life-threatening injuries	Remove clothing from injury site as well as any jewelry; flush chemical from skin with thorough decontamination; cover wounds loosely with a dry, sterile, or clean cloth.

Source: Adapted from *Centers for Disease Control and Prevention* (2003a), Daley, Aycinena, & Mallat (2008), DeLorenzo & Porter (2000), and Harris (2002).

Explosives

Blast injuries are the result of explosive munitions, often involving car or package bombs. Care for persons injured by blast injuries typically focuses on abdominal and lung injuries, penetrating wounds, traumatic amputations, and burns (Scott, Vanderploeg, Belanger & Scholten, 2005).

Radiologic Dispersion Bomb (Dirty Bomb) Blast

A dirty bomb consists of a conventional explosive such as trinitrotoluene (TNT) packed with radioactive waste by-products from nuclear reactors. When the dirty bomb explodes, the radioactive material spreads in the wind like a dust cloud. In this way, it reaches far wider areas than the initial explosion (Harris, 2005). The long-term destructive force of the dirty bomb is caused by the ionizing radiation from the radioactive material. In a person's body, an ion's electrical charge may lead to unnatural chemical reactions inside the cells. The charge can break DNA chains. Cells with broken DNA strands either die or the DNA develops a mutation. Diseases develop as the result of widespread cell death. If the DNA mutates, a cell may become cancerous. The cancer may spread and the cells may malfunction. This series of events may result in a wide variety of symptoms collectively referred to as **radiation sickness**. While this condition can be deadly, it is survivable with bone marrow transplantation.

People are exposed to ionizing radiation frequently, but in small doses, with little if any ill effects. Some of the sources of this everyday exposure are outer space, the stars, sun, natural radioactive isotopes, and x-ray machines. The risk of cancer and radiation sickness is increased by exposure to a dirty bomb and the subsequent rise in radiation levels above normal. The fatal effects of the dirty bomb may not be apparent in the short term after exposure, but could kill people years later.

Nuclear Detonations

A thermal burn is the most common mechanism resulting in injury and death associated with nuclear detonation. A tremendous amount of thermal energy is created by a nuclear reaction. This energy travels unimpeded through the air. The energy is absorbed by the contact surface. It may create burns or ignite combustibles. The burns may involve only the epidermis and upper layers of dermis because of the short duration of heat exposure. Thermal burn injuries can be severe and are treated as any other burn. Radiation exposure results in injury from ionizing radiation altering some cell structures. Cells are damaged from the changes in DNA in bone marrow, blood, bowel, skin, and nervous and cardiovascular systems. Radiation suppresses the immune system, so special care must be taken to reduce the potential infection often associated with full-thickness burns. More information on burn care can be found in ∞ Chapter 17.

The major activities performed for patients who have suffered a nuclear casualty are triage, evacuation or sheltering, search and rescue, radioactive monitoring, decontamination, and direct patient care. The patient will be assessed for injuries such as burns or blunt trauma. Pressure injuries such as lung injury, difficult breathing, or minor stroke-like symptoms (air emboli) must be assessed quickly. There may be some early complaints of radiation exposure such as nausea or fatigue. The manifestations of serious radiation exposure may not occur for several hours and do not suggest imminent death. Since radiation has a cumulative danger, shorter exposure times are less damaging. Flash blindness to the eyes caused by a detonation blast lasts only a few minutes during daylight and up to 30 minutes at night. Reassure patients that their eyesight will return and have someone remain with them until their sight is restored.

The victim should be evacuated from the exposure area, along with the healthcare provider and first responders. Wind shifts are monitored continuously to minimize exposure. Triage is done to classify the patients into categories of immediate, delayed, and minimal. Comfort measures, such as psychologic support and empathy, are given to patients.

Disaster Planning, Response, and Mitigation

In the United States, disaster preparedness has been a priority issue for government and military agencies. These efforts have been expanded to public and private healthcare sectors. Healthcare professionals are among the essential personnel in addressing disaster preparations and in dealing with the consequences of a disaster. Nurses comprise the largest group of healthcare professionals, and will play key roles in disaster relief whether they work in hospitals, residential facilities, ambulatory care, schools, or simply at home in their communities. The general public looks to nurses for information and trusts that what nurses advise is true and accurate. Nurses have a responsibility to be educated and to assimilate the new skills and demands necessary to assist patients, families, and communities in preparing for and responding to disastrous situations effectively.

Numerous disaster agencies are involved in disaster planning, response, and mitigation depending on the severity of the disaster and the resultant necessary response:

- A Level I disaster is dealt with effectively by local emergency response personnel and organizations.
- A Level II disaster requires mutual aid from surrounding communities and regional efforts.
- A Level III disaster overwhelms local and regional assets and statewide or federal assistance is required (Goolsby & Mothershead, 2008).

Agencies that may become involved include the Federal Emergency Management Agency (FEMA), the U.S. Army Corps of Engineers, the U.S. Department of Health and Human Services (DHHS), the American Red Cross (an international disaster relief agency), United Nations Headquarters of the Disaster Relief Organization, Pan American Health Organization (PAHO), International Reserve Committee, and local volunteer organizations such as the Boy Scouts of America, Goodwill Industries, and Volunteers of America. National agencies have state and local offices that respond to disasters. However, the most immediate response is from the local groups and organizations. Individual states may request aid from neighboring states or the federal government if the disaster exceeds local and state resources. The local disaster response organizations include fire departments, police departments, public health departments, public works, emergency services, and the local branch of the American Red Cross.

Local disaster response plans include action plans for various types of disaster situations, designation of the overall incident commander, and identification of community resources. The local emergency management agency is also represented in the state management planning efforts.

Hospitals and other healthcare agencies develop their own disaster plans. However, it is very important that each agency understands its role within the larger community disaster plan. When disasters occur, competing healthcare systems must put the competition aside and work collaboratively in the response effort to ensure favorable outcomes following the impact of the disaster.

Stages of Disaster Preparedness

The five stages of disaster preparedness are the *nondisaster* or *interdisaster* stage, the *predisaster* stage, the *impact* stage, the *emergency* stage, and the *reconstruction* or *rehabilitation* stage (see Figure 7–1 ■). The nondisaster stage is the time for planning and preparation as the threat of a disaster is still in the future. It is a time for prevention, preparedness, and mitigation activities. The predisaster stage occurs when there is knowledge about an impending disaster that has not yet occurred. Activities during this stage include warning, preimpact mobilization, and evacuation if appropriate. The impact stage is a time when the disaster event has occurred and the community experiences the immediate effects. The emergency stage involves the immediate response to the effects of the disaster. The community relies on local assistance or aid because outside sources of aid have not yet arrived. In the reconstruction or recovery stage, restoration, reconstitution, and mitigation take

STAGES AND PHASES OF A DISASTER

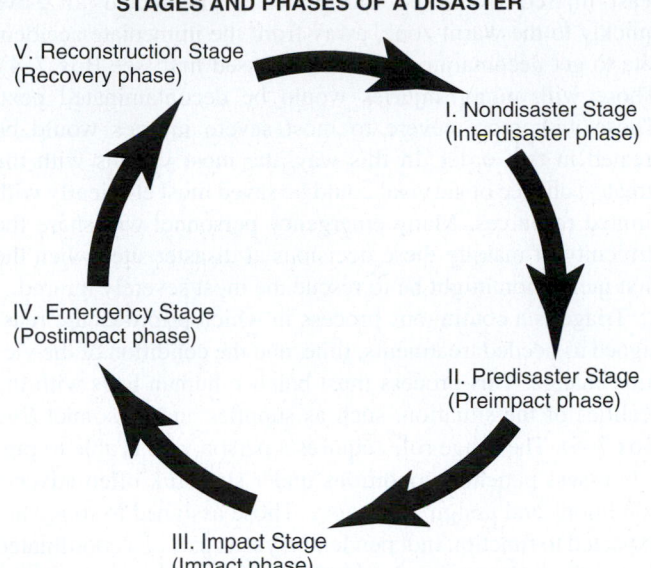

Figure 7–1 ■ The stages of a disaster are cyclical. After a disaster, the planning cycle begins again, with evaluation of the current disaster plan and community response, debriefing with all disaster response agencies and personnel, and modifying disaster plans based on lessons learned.

Source: From Langan, Joanne C.; James, Dotti C., *Preparing Nurses for Disasters Management*, 1st, © 2005. Reproduced by permission of Pearson Education, Inc., Upper Saddle River, New Jersey.

place. This stage involves rebuilding and returning to some semblance of "normalcy" but also includes mitigation activities or planning to prevent subsequent disasters or to minimize the effects of future disasters (Langan & James, 2005b).

The key to effective disaster management is predisaster planning and preparation. Clark (2008) stated that the two purposes of disaster planning are to reduce the community's vulnerability to the disaster and to prevent it, if possible, and to ensure that resources are available for effective response in the event of a disaster. A comprehensive emergency management plan addresses four major areas: mitigation, preparedness, response, and recovery.

Mitigation is the action taken to prevent or reduce the harmful effects of a disaster on human health or property. It involves future-oriented activities to prevent subsequent disasters or to minimize their effects. Mitigation may take the form of reinforcing highway over-passes and levees, sandbagging, developing communication strategies as backup systems to what is currently in place, and educating professionals and the public regarding preparation and response to disasters. A key nursing activity related to mitigation is the active participation in learning about the major aspects of disasters to remain current in their knowledge base and be able to teach the general public. Another mitigation activity is the anticipation of needed resources and policies to assist nurses and other professionals in implementing an effective disaster response.

Preparedness is having a comprehensive disaster plan in place that coordinates efforts among many people, agencies, and levels of government. The plan will be based on familiarity with possible disaster agents based on previous experiences, as well as experiences of others from various regions and countries. It is

imperative that all persons and agencies who may be involved in the disaster response be involved in the planning. In this way, information is shared and representatives from each agency explain and offer their respective resources and expertise and note deficiencies in the plan. Planning committees will exist on all levels—federal, regional, state, local, and individual agency. Nurses participate in this facet of disaster planning by having a nurse representative on the planning committee at least at the agency level.

Response to disasters happens in the emergency stage, after the disaster event has occurred. The community has been rapidly assessed for damage, and the types and extent of injuries suffered as well as the immediate needs of the community have been determined. Hospital disaster planners must plan for the possibility that the next disaster may involve the hospital. The hospital's response may include the evacuation of patients as well as relocating and operating from an independent facility. **Surge capacity** is the healthcare system's ability to rapidly expand beyond normal services to meet the increased demand for qualified personnel, medical care, and public health in the event of a large-scale disaster. The Agency for Healthcare Research and Quality (2005) has published a report discussing the use of former "shuttered" hospitals to expand surge capacity during mass casualty events. Hospitals must be constantly aware of the number of beds available, which patients may be discharged, staffing, equipment, other resources, and their overall ability to manage casualties quickly.

The local community provides assistance or aid initially, because outside sources of aid have not yet arrived. Assistance from outside of the affected area arrives later and search and rescue operations commence as well as first aid, emergency medical assistance, establishment or restoration of communication and transportation, assessment of infectious diseases and mental health problems, and evacuation of residents, if necessary. Nurses should follow the disaster plan of their agencies, communities, and the local emergency management agency. This includes having a disaster plan for the nurse's immediate family. In this way, the nurse will feel secure in the fact that the immediate family is situated safely and the nurse can respond to the staging area to await instructions. Nurses use their expertise in infectious disease control and in assessing physical as well as psychosocial needs. In a disaster, mental health issues are extremely significant for victims, families, friends, first responders, and all healthcare workers. Nurses will ensure that patients receive follow-up care for both physical wounds and mental health concerns. Advanced practice nurses may take on significantly greater responsibilities especially if they are competent and prepared in emergency and trauma care. Protocols and standards of care are in place to guide the practice of all nurses. It is imperative that nurses determine the boundaries of their practice in times of emergencies when mass numbers of victims must be treated without the luxury of an on-site physician.

The **recovery** aspect of disaster response is also called *reconstruction*. During this stage, restoration, reconstitution, and mitigation take place. Restoration includes rebuilding, replacing lost or damaged property, returning to school and work, and continuing life without those who were killed in the disaster. Reconstitution occurs when the life of the community returns to a new normal. The final stage of recovery is mitigation, which is also an activity in the preparation and planning aspects of the nondisaster stage. This illustrates the cyclical nature of planning and disaster response. The work is never complete. Future-oriented activities take place to prevent subsequent disasters or to minimize their effects. Some of these activities may include increased security and surveillance measures. Nurses may suggest ideas for responding to the victims of disasters more effectively and efficiently. For example, nurses may communicate the need for carts stocked with specific items that will assist them in treating patients faster. They may also suggest a more efficient method of tracking patients as they enter the healthcare system and move from area to area based on the patients' acuity and condition. Nurses will participate in mock disasters, read updated protocols, and practice their skills repeatedly to maintain competence. Mock disasters or disaster drills can take the form of tabletop exercises/discussions or simulated drills with mock victims. Mock disaster drills allow the participants to become familiar with the plan, and the areas that need strengthening in the plan will become evident (Langan & James, 2005b).

Casualty Management

During a disaster, nurses may be expected to perform triage. Nurses perform triage every day in every emergency department. **Triage** means sorting. A very basic triage system is to categorize or label victims needing the most support and emergency care as "red." Those less critical but still in need of transport to emergency centers for care are classified as "yellow." Victims who have minor injuries and do not warrant transport to an emergency center are categorized as "green." Victims who are least likely to survive or are already deceased are color coded as "black" (see Table 7–2). These are the triage levels given to patients under normal circumstances or when there are only a few victims. However, when there is a mass casualty event with greater than 100 victims, **reverse triage** may be instituted. Reverse triage works on the principle of the greatest good for the greatest number. For example, if there were a collision between a train full of railroad cars filled with toxic chemicals and a full tour bus in a highly populated area, this disaster would likely be called a mass casualty event. In this case, those persons who were the most ambulatory and

least injured would be transported or instructed to move quickly to the warm zone, away from the immediate accident site to get decontaminated and processed first (see Box 7–4). Those with minor injuries would be decontaminated next. Those with more severe to most severe injuries would be treated in that order. In this way, the most victims with the greatest chance of survival could be saved most efficiently with limited resources. Many emergency personnel will share the difficulty of making these decisions at disaster sites when the first inclination might be to rescue the most severely injured.

Triage is a continuous process in which priorities are reassigned as needed treatments, time, and the condition of the victims change. This process must balance human lives with the realities of the situation, such as supplies and personnel (see Box 7–5). The triage role requires a person who is able to rapidly assess patients' conditions under stressful, often adverse conditions and assign a category. Those assigned to triage are expected to function independently, yet as part of a coordinated team effort (James et al., 2005). It has been suggested that emergency personnel should triage/categorize the victims so that physicians and nurses can be best utilized in the treatment area, performing patient care. Advanced practice personnel will continue to triage and perform more complete assessments.

Isolation and Personal Protective Equipment

Persons suspected of having smallpox or some other highly contagious disease will need to be isolated from other patients, visitors, or healthcare personnel. For example, persons with pulmonary tuberculosis and a severe illness requiring hospitalization should be placed in a private room with negative-pressure ventilation. Patients are taught to cover their nose and mouth when coughing or sneezing. All persons entering the room should wear personal respiratory protective devices capable of filtering submicron particles. Decontamination of the air may be achieved through ventilation and supplemented by ultraviolet light.

Gas masks are used in a broad range of military, industrial, and emergency situations to protect the user from hazardous dust, gas, or other aerosols. Biologic contaminants that are spread through aerosolized droplets create a threat to those not wearing PPE. A gas mask may be considered a high-performance respirator and is

---

TABLE 7–2 Simple Triage and Rapid Transport (START) System

Red (Immediate)	Critically injured, with problems that will require immediate intervention to correct. (Patients with a respiratory rate above 30 are tagged "red." If their respirations are below 30, assess their circulatory status. If capillary refill takes more than 2 seconds, tag them "red." If it is below 2 seconds, assess mental status.)
Yellow (Delayed)	Injured, and will require some medical attention, but they will not die if care is delayed while you care for other patients; not ambulatory and will require a stretcher for transportation. (Patients who can follow simple commands such as hand grips are tagged as "yellow." Patients who cannot follow simple commands are tagged "red.")
Green (Ambulatory)	Not critically injured, and can walk and care for themselves. (Have them walk to a safe place, but do not lose track of them; every patient triaged at an incident is tracked to the best of the responder's ability.)
Black (Expectant)	Deceased, or have such catastrophic injuries that they are not expected to survive to be transported. (If the patient is not breathing, open the airway manually. If they remain apneic, tag them "black"; if they begin breathing, they are tagged "red.")

Source: Start.(n.d.) Managing the scene. Retrieved January 10, 2009, from http://www.citmt.org/start/rpm.htm

BOX 7–4 Hot, Warm, and Cold Zones

The site of the disaster where a weapon was released or where the contamination occurred is called the **hot zone**. It is considered contaminated and only those persons in the appropriate **personal protective equipment (PPE)** may enter it. PPE is equipment used for the protection of personnel and includes gloves, masks, goggles, gowns, and biologic disposal bags. Typically, fire, police, and military personnel will collect evidence and begin their investigation in this zone. The **warm zone** is adjacent to the hot zone. Another name for this area is the *control zone*. This area is where decontamination of victims or triage and emergency treatment take place. The level of PPE required is based on the dynamic risk assessment of the threat and agent involved. The **cold zone** is considered to be the safe zone. It is adjacent to the warm zone and is the area where a more in-depth triage of victims would occur. Survivors may find shelter in this area, and the command and control vehicles would be found here as well as the emergency transport vehicles.

usually equipped with both eye protection and air supply protection or treatment. A hood, helmet, or headgear is generally worn to protect the skin, eyes, airways, and respiratory systems. Protective clothing is made to guard against mild irritants and even serious lethal materials. Some protective suits are disposable, intended for one use only. Others are durable, multilayered fabrics that are completely impermeable and are reusable. The Occupational Safety and Health Administration (OSHA) (2005) has issued guidelines to inform healthcare workers and first responders about the correct level of PPE for various situations. The Chemical, Biological, Radiological, and Nuclear (CBRN) Personal Protection Equipment Selection Matrix for Emergency Responders and other information specific to PPE can be located online at the OSHA website. In addition to the isolation of patients, special air handling systems are used in the isolation

BOX 7–5 Key Triage Points to Remember

1. Use a triage system that is easy to learn, easy to implement in stressful conditions, and does not require advanced diagnostic skills yet allows for basic patient interventions.
2. Use the Incident Management System (defined by each facility, and based on the area's civilian and military authorities) for every incident and wear personnel identification vests. Incident management systems use logical management structure, defined responsibilities, clear reporting channels, and a common language (Langan & James, 2005).
3. Get accurate preliminary and final patient counts and relay this information to the incident commander.
4. Use some type of visual color-coded identification system to indicate patient priority.
5. Do not fall into the trap of using your time providing one-to-one patient care.
6. Retriage patients frequently, at the incident, on arrival at the treatment area, and periodically thereafter.
7. Make certain the walking-wounded are gathered and treated.
8. Preplan for potential incidents that may occur.
9. Be aware that emergency responders may be potential targets.
10. Practice, practice, practice.

rooms to prevent the spread of the contaminated droplets into the general hospital air vents. Many hospitals also have the capability to shut off airflow in contaminated areas to prevent the spread of contaminants to other "clean" areas of the hospital. The heating, ventilation, air conditioning, and refrigeration (HVAC) systems are closely monitored and can be shut down in designated areas to avoid air intake from the outside as well, especially in cases of outdoor environmental contamination.

Recording Victim Data

The CDC has created a Mass Trauma Data Instrument (available on the CDC website: Mass Casualty Event Preparedness and Response) to record data about victims of disasters. The categories on the data sheet include demographics, circumstances of the injury, injury conditions, and disposition and details of the conditions. The completion of this form is initiated by the triage nurse and completed by the nurse who implements the treatment or transfers the patient to another unit/department.

Crowd Control

When a disaster occurs, many people converge on the site. Those who come are the curious and those who truly mean to assist in the rescue and recovery of victims. However, this crowd of people needs to be controlled by authorities in charge of the site and rescue and recovery. Similarly, crowds may arrive at the hospital or healthcare delivery sites when injured or even when they just think they may be injured or contaminated in some way. The job of crowd control is not under the auspices of nurses or other healthcare personnel. The agency's security personnel and/or the local police force must control these crowds. If control is not maintained, chaos ensues and those in greatest need of medical assistance may be unable to reach healthcare providers in order to avoid further declines in their health status. In fact, nurses, physicians, and other healthcare workers should not enter an area that has not been secured. To put one's safety at risk jeopardizes the potential treatment of many. Additionally, social services personnel or psychiatric service providers should be available to assist the "worried well" cope with the trauma they have experienced or witnessed or simply heard about through the news media.

Psychosocial Needs

The importance of mental health services for victims, the public, first responders, and healthcare workers cannot be overstated. Both those persons directly affected by the disaster as well as those indirectly affected will seek medical care and advice. Many who seek medical attention are simply anxious about the threat of injury. At times, reassurance is all that is necessary. However, with large numbers of people seeking health care, the system is quickly overwhelmed. Mental health experts may quickly assess individual needs, offer immediate advice, and refer for follow-up care if deemed appropriate.

People react to disasters in a variety of ways, both physically and behaviorally. Their reactions depend on the severity of the threat and their proximity to the area of direct impact. The closer the person is to the area of impact and the longer the exposure, the greater the likelihood of a more severe reaction to the event. Table 7–3 summarizes the normal initial responses aimed at survival (Ganong, 2005; Murray, Zentner & Yakimo, 2009; Selye, 1965, 1980).

Most people exhibit great coping mechanisms and resilience in the aftermath of a disaster. However, mechanisms should be developed for identifying and referring those who need psychologic counseling. After the September 2001 terrorist attacks on the World Trade Center and the Pentagon, it was reported that 71% of the persons surveyed felt depressed, 49% had difficulty concentrating, and 33% had trouble sleeping at night. Most (92%) felt sad when watching news coverage of the event, yet 63% stated a compulsion to continue to watch the news (Pew Research Center for the People and the Press, 2001). Reactions to terrorist events and disasters in general are influenced by developmental level and maturity, prior experiences with disasters, and cultural background (McLaughlin et al., 2005).

✍ Nursing Care

The Role of the Nurse in Disaster Relief

Because nurses have an obligation to keep current in new and emerging trends in health care and threats to society, learning about the prevention and mitigation of disasters is essential. Nurses must be aware of the roles they play in all aspects of disaster preparedness and response (Box 7–6.) It is imperative that nurses first know how to take care of themselves in order to assist others. By educating oneself and being proactive in regular drills and practice of skills, nurses take an active role in helping others to save lives and fulfill an important obligation to society.

Applying basic first aid skills can be very helpful in immediate disaster relief efforts until emergency help can be obtained. The American Red Cross invites nurse volunteers and will provide the necessary training. Many nurses have taken advantage of online disaster certificate programs, and efforts are being made to integrate disaster preparedness content into nursing courses.

BOX 7–6   Roles of Nurses in Disasters

1. Prepare selves, families, friends, and communities for disasters in conjunction with the local disaster preparedness plan.
2. Continue educating self on various types of disasters and appropriate response.
3. Provide emergency services with consideration of victims' abilities, deficits, culture, language, or special needs.
4. Assist in the mobilization of healthcare personnel, food, water, shelter, medication, clothing, and other assistive devices.
5. Collaborate with agencies in authority including local, state, and federal representatives to deploy resources based on the greatest good for the greatest number.
6. Consider needs of victims including shelter both temporary and permanent, as well as psychologic, economic, legal, and spiritual factors.
7. Become involved with local, state, and national disaster planning agencies to schedule regular meetings to continually review and modify disaster plans.

In many different practice settings, nurses serve on disaster preparedness and response planning committees. Nurses are receiving in-service education on biologic, chemical, and radiologic threats to patient health as well as surveillance and reporting of suspicious activities. Although nursing professionals may not be asked to don decontamination gear to decontaminate victims, nurses should be aware of decontamination basics so that they will remain safe from exposure and be able to direct others when threatened with contamination. Some nurses choose to be actively involved with disaster medical assistance teams as part of the National Disaster Medical System (NDMS). The NDMS is a program, coordinated by the federal government, that supplements an integrated national medical response to assisting states and local authorities in dealing with the medical aspects of peacetime disasters.

In a true mass casualty event, it is impossible to have physicians present at every station where they are needed. Nurses may have to assume expanded roles in making decisions for the most appropriate treatment of casualties. Discussions should

TABLE 7–3   Responses to Stress: General Adaptation Syndrome (GAS) and Levels of Anxiety

GAS STAGE	PHYSICAL RESPONSE	BEHAVIORS RELATED TO ANXIETY
Alarm Stage	Pupils dilate; blurred vision. Hearing sharper or diminished.	Misinterpretation of stimuli. Confusion. Poor concentration. Selective inattention. Need for assistance.
Severe Anxiety or Panic	Stronger, faster heart rate and respirations. Palpitations, arrhythmias, elevated blood pressure.	Feeling of impending doom. Terror. Fear. Agitation. Irritability. Increased demands. Impulsivity. Paresthesias.
	Muscle tone increased. Headaches.	Muscle tension. Excitability, restless movements. Tremors. Rigidity. Weakness.
	Basal metabolism rate increased. Body temperature. Perspiration. Altered glucose, protein, and lipid metabolism. Increased startle response.	Insomnia. Urgency of speech and movement. Fatigue. Dehydration. Weight loss. Appetite changes. Smooth muscle of gastrointestinal and urinary tracts less motile, interfering with digestion and elimination of wastes.
	Hypoglycemia from glycogenolysis due to high energy demands.	Blood glucose increase. Appetite changes. Dehydration. Fatigue. Poor concentration.
	Increased blood clotting and suppressed immune response if stage persists.	Blood stasis; thrombus formation. Resistance to infection and disease reduced.

take place among physicians, nurses, and policy makers regarding the necessity of the nurses' expanded roles in crisis situations. As noted earlier in the chapter, these agency policies must be documented in the agency-wide plan. Additionally, all healthcare personnel must receive any specialized training required to be safe and competent practitioners of the expanded duties. This training must be practiced and updated and those participating in the training must be tracked and notified of additional requirements as necessary. See the Moving Evidence into Action box on page 135.

Roles of Nurses Working with Victims of Disasters

The role of the nurse in a disaster depends greatly on a number of variables including the nature of the disaster, the number of victims and severity of injuries, the location of the disaster as well as the location of the nurse, the availability of supplies, rescue and command personnel, and other necessary resources. The nurse must be able to perform under stressful conditions but will not be expected to endanger self, other nurses, or other rescuers.

If it is safe to do so, the nurse begins by triaging and assessing the victims for the best care and best use of available resources. Very quick, direct treatment may be given, or the nurse may be involved in extended periods of time with a mobile surgical unit. Local authorities such as the police, fire, and emergency medical services will guide the nurse in securing the area and determining the safe zone for the nurse and others to work. The National Disaster Medical System is the agency responsible for coordinating disaster relief with local fire, police, and emergency medical services to provide overall disaster assistance. Victim assistance may be offered in the field in mobile shelters, in local clinics, in hospitals, or in makeshift buildings.

Nurses take on a variety of roles based on their expertise and the needs of the victims. Nurses will be expected to follow the emergency preparedness plans outlined in their communities and in their agencies of employment. When a disaster occurs, it is not a time for individual creativity. However, individual nurses should be the leaders in their communities in discussing emergency preparedness and contingency plans.

Considerations for Patients with Special Needs

Older Adults

It is not appropriate to generalize needs to all older adults. Many are quite independent and active into their 90s. However, some older persons lack the physical stamina to recover quickly from disastrous events. The nurse must assess the individual's ability to cope with and recover from unexpected events, socioeconomic factors, support systems, potential healthcare needs, and resources. See the accompanying Case Study & Nursing Care Plan.

Teaching about disaster preparedness is important in all communities. Older adults need to determine the appropriateness of "sheltering in place" should there be an environmental event outside of their homes, or of being evacuated if they are unable to care for themselves for extended periods of time. This becomes a very real issue when roads become impassable or usual modes of transportation and communication are disrupted.

MOVING EVIDENCE INTO ACTION **Disaster Education**

The nursing profession has recognized the need to develop resources to teach practicing and future nurses to improve their response to victims of radiologic, biologic, and chemical terrorism. However, nursing students may have different perceptions about working with disaster victims. The purpose of this descriptive study (Young & Persell, 2004) was to identify student nurses' major concerns and learning needs in working with victims of terrorism. Ninety-five junior and senior baccalaureate nursing students participated in the study by completing an anonymous questionnaire regarding their concerns about terrorism and how their lives had changed following September 11, 2001 ("9/11"). The students' main concern was for the safety of themselves and their families. The students indicated they would not be willing to care for victims if there was a lack of protection for all types of terrorist agents for themselves and their families. The students did not demonstrate an accurate understanding of the pathogenic nature of many terrorist agents even though the nursing faculty members had provided self-education articles for the students. The students' concerns for specific infectious agents appeared to be based on unnecessary fear or inappropriate confidence.

IMPLICATIONS FOR NURSING

If nurses do not believe that a terrorist event is a real threat in their communities, they may not be motivated to become more prepared for terrorist events. The nation's emergency healthcare planners and trauma nurses will have a major challenge preparing more nurses for disasters, especially mass casualty events. During a terrorist attack, the general public will seek information about the event from all healthcare providers. The public will also expect nurses to deliver safe and competent care to the victims of terrorism. Disaster care information should be a part of the curriculum in all basic nursing education schools. Continuing education and elective courses should continue to be planned. Basic disaster preparedness competencies should be required for all new graduate nurses so that they have a solid foundation on which to build.

CRITICAL THINKING IN PATIENT CARE

1. Make a list of all the barriers that nurses might express as reasons they do not need or value disaster/terrorism education and preparation.
2. Discuss the rationale for including basic disaster preparedness content in all basic nursing education programs.
3. Consider the results of this study. What could have been done differently to assist nursing students in learning facts and the pathogenic nature of the terrorist agents presented in the articles?

Source: Young, C. F., & Persell, D. (2004). Biological, chemical, and nuclear terrorism readiness: Major concerns and preparedness of future nurses. *Disaster Management & Response, 2*(4), 109–114.

A current list of medications, doses, and times of administration should be kept in an easily accessible, secure place. The names and phone numbers of significant persons, relatives, those with power of attorney, healthcare providers, or any others to be notified in case of emergency should also be kept in an easily accessible place. Additionally, the following materials should be considered essential in keeping with the person should evacuation to a shelter be necessary: eyeglasses and eyeglass prescriptions, style and serial numbers of medical devices such as pacemakers, healthcare policies and numbers, identification, list of allergies, blood type, checkbook, credit cards, insurance agent's name and number, driver's license, 72-hour supply of medications, dentures, list of special dietary needs, sturdy shoes, warm clothing, blankets, incontinence briefs, prostheses, hearing aids, hearing aid batteries, extra wheelchair batteries, oxygen, and other assistive devices.

Immunocompromised Patients

Patients who are immunocompromised pose special problems to the healthcare community especially if these persons are unable to access health care quickly in a disaster situation. A compromised immune system may be due to treatments such as chemotherapy or immunosuppressants or from an underlying disease such as HIV. The immunocompromised population would be at greater risk for complications and death than the general population should a bioterrorist attack occur. For example, a potential complication following smallpox vaccination is generalized vaccinia. It is believed to result from a vaccinia viremia with skin manifestations. In noncompromised persons, generalized vaccinia consists of vesicles or pustules appearing on normal skin distant from the vaccination site. The rash is generally self-limited and usually requires only supportive therapy. However, immunocompromised patients may have a toxic course and require vaccinia immune globulin (VIG), available only from the CDC (Center for Disease Control (CDC), 2008).

An additional issue the nurse should discuss with this population is the patients' preparation for disaster events related to infection control. Patients should carry treatment calendars with them at all times so that any healthcare provider can determine where they are in their treatment program and disease process. Patients should plan a backup location to visit for chemotherapy if their usual office is inaccessible. Nurses should also assess their patients' knowledge level regarding the avoidance of raw seafood or possibly contaminated water. Bottled water should be ready so the patient can avoid drinking water of questionable purity. Bone marrow transplant patients are instructed not to eat fresh fruits and vegetables due to the risk of contamination and subsequent infection. It is safest for this population of patients to consume processed or canned foods if they can be heated to the proper temperatures.

Patients with Sensory, Speech, or Literacy Deficits

Persons who have sensory deficits, speech or language impairments, or who are illiterate must be assessed for the most effective means of communicating steps to be taken in the case of a disaster. One cannot generalize that all people with hearing impairments or speech impairments will choose a particular means of communication. This may be an individual preference. A multitude of communication means are available through technological support systems as well as written and visual cue boards. Public service announcements may inform the general public about impending natural disasters and about proper steps to be taken to be safely rescued or sheltered. Nurses are in the position of alerting community leaders about special needs of members of their communities. Public service personnel, including fire, police, and emergency services, should be alerted to extenuating circumstances and needs of specific individuals in the community. The collaborative planning efforts of the individual, family members, caregivers, and emergency service personnel will help alleviate any undue pain and suffering caused by the lack of understanding of emergency messages and directives.

Patients with Mobility and Sensory Deficits

The U.S. Department of Health and Human Services (2005) has estimated that 13% of the U.S. population experiences some form of activity limitation due to a chronic condition. Many persons require the use of assistive technology devices (ATDs) to accommodate mobility and other impairments. Careful planning must be in place in order to provide necessary support during and after a disaster. Arrangements must be made in advance to provide adequate numbers of volunteers or staff to assist when this group must be relocated or regrouped in a safe room or shelter. These individuals or their caregivers must provide input to service personnel to determine what kind of support services would be necessary in an emergency or disaster. Emergency personnel or rescue teams may need to learn a few basic phrases in American Sign Language. Something as simple as carrying a notepad and pencil or directions in large print may be just what is necessary to share information with people who have hearing impairments or visual impairments, respectively.

Non-English-Speaking Patients

The literacy of non-English-speaking patients should be assessed in both their own language and in English. One cannot assume that individuals are literate in their own language. It is ideal to obtain the assistance of an interpreter, preferably an interpreter with whom the patient is familiar, to assist in translating information for the patient. Communication aids can be prepared in advance of disasters to be used during emergencies. The communication aids or disaster preparedness and response procedures should be practiced on a regular basis prior to an emergency. The use of visual aids is very helpful. Do not use children as interpreters if adults are available. The stress of interpretation can be overwhelming to the children and place an unnecessary burden on them.

Spiritual Considerations

Religion tends to be a source of comfort for those who are experiencing the threat of loss of life, property, or way of living. Churches, synagogues, and clergy become active in supporting

CASE STUDY & NURSING CARE PLAN   A Patient with Injuries from a Natural Disaster

Mr. Ed Jones, a 84-year-old widower, is retired from his job as a cabinetmaker. He continues to work with wood as a hobby in the basement of his home located on the banks of the Deep River. He sells small toys at craft fairs and flea markets in nearby communities. His daughter lives approximately 20 minutes away and checks in on him at least every weekend. Mr. Jones is independent and sees his primary care physician occasionally for monitoring of his blood pressure, which is controlled with antihypertensive medications. Following a week of heavy rainstorms, flash flooding occurred in the area and Mr. Jones's basement sustained much water damage and ruined most of his stored wood, wooden toy products, and the woodworking machinery. Mr. Jones waded through the waist-deep water to get to the rescue boat rather than wait for the boat to get to him. He is subsequently admitted to the medical/surgical unit due to concerns from the EMTs who triaged him at the fire station 5 miles inland from Mr. Jones's neighborhood.

ASSESSMENT

Lisa Smith, RN, obtains a nursing assessment. Mr. Jones states that he has been on antihypertensive medications for "a few years" but only takes his medication "once in awhile" since it has been some time since his last office visit and he wants his remaining pills "to last" until he can get back to the doctor. He has had numerous cuts to his hands from his woodworking and has had a big ulcer on his right foot "for a few weeks" caused by a tool that fell on his foot. He did not seek medical care because he believed it would get better on its own. "It looks worse than it is. It really doesn't even hurt."

When asked about his home he stated, "Everything is gone. My wife is gone, my wood, my tools...it's all over."

Physical assessment findings include T 100.7°F PO, P 96, R 20, and BP 178/100. Skin cool and dry with multiple lesions on both hands and a Stage II ulcer on his right dorsal foot with yellow-green exudate. Pain rated at a 2 on a 10 scale with 10 being the worst pain there could be. Lungs are clear, heart rate regular. No edema noted. Abdominal assessment is normal. Neurologically intact. Weight is normal for height and frame. A culture is ordered and taken of the yellow-green exudate of the right foot.

Preliminary blood work results show WBCs at 15,000/mm³. A peripheral IV is initiated with continuous fluids and IV antibiotics are ordered every 6 hours. An antihypertensive medication is ordered on a regular schedule plus a prn antihypertensive for systolic >180 and diastolic >90.

DIAGNOSES

- *Impaired Skin Integrity* of the right foot and hands related to lesions (cuts) on the hands and Stage II ulcer with exudates on the right foot
- *Powerlessness* related to perceived loss of control over life situation
- *Ineffective Thermoregulation* related to trauma
- *Acute Pain* related to expression of pain secondary to skin lesions

EXPECTED OUTCOMES

- Regain skin integrity—ulcer on right foot and lesions on hands will heal.
- Identify aspects of his life still under his control.
- Maintain body temperature at normothermic levels.
- Express feeling of comfort and relief from pain.

PLANNING AND IMPLEMENTATION

- Assess skin every shift; describe and document skin condition; report changes.
- Clean lesions on hands and right foot every 8 hours and assess healing.
- Administer prescribed antibiotics and assess for effectiveness in treating infection.
- Arrange psychosocial consult(s).
- Guide Mr. Jones through a life review. Encourage reflection on past achievements.
- Help Mr. Jones identify the aspects of his life that are still under his control.
- Monitor temperature every 4 hours, more often if indicated.
- Monitor and record patient's heart rate and rhythm, blood pressure, and respiratory rate every 4 hours.
- Administer analgesics, antipyretics, and medications as indicated.
- Maintain hydration; monitor intake and output.
- Assess level of pain and administer pain medication as prescribed.

EVALUATION

Mr. Jones was hospitalized for 3 days, receiving intravenous antibiotic therapy, analgesics, an antidepressant, monitoring of his cardiac response to a new antihypertensive medication, wound care, and sessions with the social services representative and his daughter. His hand lesions are healed, the foot ulcer has developed new granulation tissue with no signs of infection, he is afebrile, and his blood pressure is maintained within normal limits. He will be discharged to his daughter's home until his home can be assessed for the extent of the water damage and feasibility of repair. He has agreed to visit a therapist to work through his feelings of grief and loss. He has expressed an interest in attending monthly support group meetings with his neighbors who also experienced losses in this disaster.

CRITICAL THINKING IN THE NURSING PROCESS

1. What action did Mr. Jones take that probably exacerbated his skin lesions?
2. What other testing might you anticipate related to Mr. Jones's delayed healing?
3. What were the contributing factors to Mr. Jones's fever?
4. What life situations contributed to Mr. Jones's attitude about life?

See Evaluating Your Response in Appendix C.

---

their congregations in times of disaster. Religious leaders should be actively involved in community planning for disaster preparedness especially if certain religious considerations should be strictly followed. For example, in some religions, the human body and all of its parts are considered sacred. To be sensitive to this religious belief, all tissues and blood would be collected at the site of a disaster by those trained to collect such material versus washing this matter away from the scene. In general, rescue personnel would need to be informed of specific religious obligations or rights to be able to be sensitive to the individual's religious beliefs and practices.

CHAPTER HIGHLIGHTS

- Disasters require extraordinary efforts beyond those needed to respond to everyday emergencies.
- Nurses have an obligation to keep current in new and emerging trends in health care and threats to society.
- Learning about the prevention and mitigation of bioterrorism and disasters in general is essential.
- Reverse triage is used in mass casualty events instead of traditional triage in order to do the greatest good for the greatest number.

- Nurses will be actively engaged in assessing the physical as well as the mental needs of victims, their families, first responders, and other healthcare personnel.
- Nurses need to have their own family disaster plans in place to be able to assist others in times of disasters.
- Nurses are actively involved in disaster mitigation, planning, and response efforts by learning and practicing their communities' and agencies' disaster preparedness systems.

TEST YOURSELF NCLEX-RN® REVIEW

1. What is the key difference between emergencies and disasters?
   1. Emergencies are controlled.
   2. Disasters result from man-made errors.
   3. Emergencies can typically be handled by available emergency services.
   4. Disasters typically involve the local emergency services and no other agencies.
2. Which of the following is NOT true regarding nurses' responsibilities in disaster preparedness?
   1. Nurses have a responsibility to the public to be knowledgeable about disaster preparedness and response.
   2. Nurses must have a personal and family plan as a part of their disaster preparedness and response plan.
   3. Nurses will be the leaders in the incident command structure set up at the site of the disaster.
   4. Nurses who are prepared for disasters will be better able to help themselves, their families, and their communities in a disaster situation.
3. What is the purpose of reverse triage?
   1. Save scarce resources for future use.
   2. Test first responders on their triage classification categories.
   3. Save those persons who are in the most critical condition.
   4. Do the greatest good for the greatest number with limited resources.
4. Why is important for nurses to assess patients' literacy in their primary language?
   1. They are most comfortable speaking in their primary language.
   2. They are most comfortable reading in their primary language.
   3. They may not be able to read and comprehend in their primary language.
   4. They may be too shy to communicate in English if it is not their primary language.
5. Which of the following is true about personal protective equipment (PPE)?
   1. PPE protects by creating a barrier against hazards.
   2. Eye, face, head, foot, and hand protection are addressed in PPE programs.
   3. PPE should reduce the likelihood of occupational injury and/or illness.
   4. Healthcare workers do not need to wear PPE if they follow strict hand hygiene protocol and universal precautions.

6. Which of the following is NOT true about decontamination?
   1. Decontamination corridors should be set up in an area downwind from the hospital entrance.
   2. Decontamination begins in the hot zone, closest to the site of the disaster.
   3. Decontamination must take place before the patient enters the hospital.
   4. Decontaminating a person should be done by sweeping strokes away from you and the patient.
7. What is another name for a radiological dispersion bomb?
   1. a dirty bomb
   2. an ionization radiation bomb
   3. a nonfiltered bomb
   4. a radio-controlled remote bomb
8. One of the results of DNA mutation inside cells exposed to ionizing radiation that can be deadly, but is survivable with bone marrow transplantation, is a description of which of the following?
   1. ionizing sickness
   2. radiation sickness
   3. TNT sickness
   4. compromised immune sickness
9. Why should a nurses assess the special needs of older adults as part of the emergency preparedness plan?
   1. All older adults will need some kind of special support.
   2. Some older adults will take the lead in evacuation efforts in nursing homes.
   3. Not all older adults need the same level of support in emergencies and disasters.
   4. Some older adults will be unable to evacuate even with multiple support agencies.
10. Why would nurses need the assistance of a mental health worker following a disaster?
    1. All nurses need the help of a mental health worker at one point or another in their nursing careers.
    2. Nurses are trained to provide care, regardless of the situation encountered.
    3. Nurses maintain good mental health and rarely require mental health assistance.
    4. The nurse may feel as overwhelmed and traumatized as the population for whom he or she is caring.

See Test Yourself answers in Appendix C.

Pearson Nursing Student Resources

Find additional review materials at
nursing.pearsonhighered.com

Prepare for success with additional NCLEX®-style practice questions, interactive assignments and activities, Web links, animations and videos, and more!

BIBLIOGRAPHY

Agency for Healthcare Research and Quality. (2005, September). *Use of former ("shuttered") hospitals to expand surge capacity*. Retrieved from http://www.ahrq.gov/research/shuttered/American Red Cross

American Red Cross. (n.d.). *Disaster preparedness for seniors by seniors*. Retrieved from http://www.redcross.org/services/disaster/beprepared/seniors.html

American Red Cross. (n.d.). *Your evacuation plan*. Retrieved from http://www.redcross.org/services/disaster/0,1082,0_6_,00.html

American Red Cross and IOM open new homes in Indonesia. (2006). Retrieved from http://www.redcross.org/article/0,1072,0_332_5110,00.html

Beachley, M. (2005). Nursing in a disaster. In C. M. Smith & F. A. Maurer (Eds.), *Community public/health nursing practice* (pp. 496–514). Philadelphia: Elsevier Health Sciences.

Centers for Disease Control and Prevention. (2006a). *Explosions and blast injuries: A primer for clinicians*. Retrieved from http://www.bt.cdc.gov/masstrauma/explosions.asp

Centers for Disease Control and Prevention. (2006b). *Fact sheet: Anthrax information for health care providers*. Retrieved from http://www.bt.cdc.gov/agent/anthrax/anthrax-hcp-factsheet.asp#cutaneous

Centers for Disease Control and Prevention. (2008a). *Key facts about hurricane recovery: Protect your health and safety after a hurricane*. Retrieved from http://www.bt.cdc.gov/disasters/hurricanes/pdf/recovery.pdf

Centers for Disease Control and Prevention. (2008b) *Blast injuries: Fact sheets for professionals*. Retrieved from http://www.bt.cdc.gov/masscasualties/blastinjuryfacts.asp

Centers for Disease Control and Prevention. (2008c). *Smallpox fact sheet—Adverse reactions following smallpox vaccination*. Retrieved from http://www.bt.cdc.gov/agent/smallpox/vaccination/reactions-vacc-clinic.asp

Clark, M. J. (2008). Care of client patients in disaster settings. In M. J. Clark, *Community health nursing: Advocacy for population health* (5th ed.) (Chapter 27). Upper Saddle River, NJ: Pearson/Prentice Hall.

Clark, M. J. (2008). Communicable diseases. In M. J. Clark, *Community health nursing: Advocacy for population health* (5th ed.) (Chapter 28). Upper Saddle River, NJ: Pearson/Prentice Hall.

County of Henrico (n.d.). *Community disaster preparedness manual*. Retrieved from http://www.co.henrico.va.us/fire/pdfs/cpm_man.pdf

Daley, B. J., Aycinena, J. F., & Mallat, A. F. (2008). *Electrical Injuries*. Retrieved from http://emedicine.medscape.com/article/433682-overview

Federal Emergency Management Agency. (2008). *Are you ready? Hurricanes*. Retrieved from http://www.fema.gov/areyouready/hurricanes.shtm

Ganong, W. (2005). *Review of medical physiology* (22nd ed.). New York: McGraw-Hill.

Goolsby, C., & Mothershead, J. L. (2008). *Disaster planning*. Retrieved from http://www.emedicine.com/emerg/topic718.htm

Hoffman, B. (2008). Terrorism. *In Microsoft Encarta Online Encyclopedia 2008*. Retrieved from http://encarta.msn.com/encyclopedia_761564344/Terrorism.html#s3

International Nursing Coalition for Mass Casualty Education. (2003). *Educational competencies for registered nurses related to mass casualty incidents*. Retrieved from http://www.aacn.nche.edu/Education/pdf/INCMCECompetencies.pdf

James, D. C., Langan, J. C., Sandkuhl, H., & Benbenishty, J. (2005). Preparing staff and inactive registered nurses to manage casualties. In J. C. Langan & D. C. James (Eds.), *Preparing nurses for disaster management* (pp. 95–123). Upper Saddle River, NJ: Pearson/Prentice Hall.

Laditka, S., Laditka, J., Zirasagar, S., Cornman, C., Davis, C., & Richter, J. (2008). Providing shelter to nursing home evacuees in disasters: Lessons learned from hurricane Katrina. *American Journal of Public Health, 98*(7), 1288–1293.

Langan, J. C. & James, D. C. (2005). *Preparing nurses for disaster management*. Upper Saddle River, NJ: Pearson/Prentice Hall.

McLaughlin, D. E., Murray, R. B., & Benbenishty, J. (2005). Promoting mental health: Predisaster and postdisaster. In J. C. Langan & D. C. James (Eds.), *Preparing nurses for disaster management* (pp. 55–77). Upper Saddle River, NJ: Pearson/Prentice Hall.

Murray, R. B., Zentner, J., & Yakimo, R. (2009). *Health promotion strategies through the life span* (8th ed.). Upper Saddle River, NJ: Pearson/Prentice Hall.

National Institute of Mental Health. (2002). *Mental health and mass violence: Evidence-based early psychological interventions for victims/survivors of mass violence. A workshop to reach consensus on best practices* (NIH Publication No. 02-5138). Washington, DC: U.S. Government Printing Office.

National Institute for Occupational Safety and Health. (2009). *Eye safety for emergency response and disaster recovery*. Retrieved from http://www.cdc.gov/niosh/topics/eye/eyesafe.html

Noji, E. K. (1997). The nature of disaster: General characteristics and public health effects. In E. K. Noji (Ed.), *The public health consequences of disasters* (pp. 3–20). New York: Oxford University Press.

North Carolina Department of Health and Human Services. (2007). *After the storm: Injury prevention*. Retrieved from http://www.dhhs.state.nc.us/docs/hurricanepreventinjury.htm

Occupational Safety and Health Administration. (2005). *CBRN personal protective equipment selection matrix for emergency responders*. Retrieved from http://www.osha.gov/SLTC/emergencypreparedness/cbrnmatrix/index.html

Pacific Tsunami Museum. (2007). *Tsunami glossary*. Retrieved from http://www.tsunami.org/definitions.html

Pew Research Center for the People and the Press. (2001). *American psyche reeling from terror attacks*. Retrieved from http://people-press.org/reports/display.php3?ReportID=3

Pryor, T. (2005). Remembering the tsunami: Story of hope. *Reflections on Nursing Leadership*, 4th Quarter, pp. 26–27.

Scott, S. G., Vanderploeg, R. D., Belanger, H. G., & Scholten, J. D. (2005). Blast injuries: Evaluating and treating the postacute sequelace. *Federal Practitioner*, 67–75.

Selye, H. (1965). Stress syndrome. *American Journal of Nursing, 65*(3), 97–99.

Simonsen, C. E., & Spindlove, J. R. (2007). *Terrorism today: The past, the players, the future* (3rd ed.). Upper Saddle River, NJ: Pearson/Prentice Hall.

Smith, C. M., & Maurer, F. A. (2005). *Community/public health nursing practice: Health for families and populations* (3rd ed.). Philadelphia: Saunders.

Start. (n.d.). Managing the scene. Retrieved from http://www.citmt.org/start/rpm.htm

Stevens, S., & Slone, L. (2005). *Tsunami and mental health: What can we expect?* Retrieved from http://www.ncptsd.va.gov/ncmain/ncdocs/fact_shts/fs_tsunami_mental_health.html

Through The Eyes of Terrorism. (n.d.). *Weapons*. Retrieved from http://library.thinkquest.org/CR0212088/terweap.htm

U. S. Department of Homeland Security. (2008, October 16). *The first year after Hurricane Katrina: What the federal government did*. Retrieved from http://www.dhs.gov/xprepresp/programs/gc_1157649340100.shtm

U.S. Department of State. (2009). *Fact sheet: Guidance for responding to radiological and nuclear incidents*. Retrieved from http://travel.state.gov/travel/tips/health/health_1184.html

World Health Organization. (2009). *Smallpox*. Retrieved from http://www.who.int/mediacentre/factsheets/smallpox/en/index.html

Functional Health Pattern: Health Perception-Health Management

Think about patients with altered health perception or health management for whom you have cared in your clinical experiences.

- What were their major medical diagnoses (e.g., surgery, terminal illness, impending death, alcoholism or other substance abuse, or victim of multiple or mass casualty incident)?

- What kinds of manifestations did each of these patients have? Were these manifestations similar or different?

- How did the each patient's healthcare behaviors interfere with his or her health status? Had the patient had surgery before? Did the patient experience any complications due to having surgery? Did the patient have any problems with anesthesia? What medications was the patient taking? Did the patient take medications as prescribed? Did the patient use any substances other than prescribed medications and over-the-counter medications? If so, what substances and how much were used? How much alcohol did the patient drink? What kind of problems had substance abuse caused for the patient, family, friends, finances, and health? Was the patient exposed to environmental hazards? Did the patient have sensory deficits or sight or speech impairments? Did the patient speak English? What religious considerations did the patient verbalize? Did the patient have a living will, do-not-resuscitate orders, or power of attorney? Had end-of-life issues been discussed with the family?

The Health Perception-Health Management Functional Health Pattern includes healthcare behaviors such as health promotion and illness prevention activities, medical treatments, and follow-up care. Individuals may or may not have the ability to change their healthcare practices. Health perception and health maintenance are affected by perceived health status in two primary ways:

- Factors that interfere with health care are lack of understanding basic health practices (e.g., altered cognition, altered coping), inability to take responsibility for meeting health needs (e.g., alcoholism, substance abuse), or lack of communication skills (e.g., non-English-speaking, illiterate).

- Factors that interfere with the desire to seek higher level of wellness are inability to change declining health status (e.g., cancer, kidney failure, impending death), need for treatment (e.g., surgery), catastrophic events (e.g., motor vehicle accidents injuries, weather-related event injuries, thermal or chemical burns).

A patient's perceived pattern of health and well-being affects how health is managed. Unexpected events can alter the patient's health status, leading to manifestations such as the following:

- **Anxiety** *(uneasy feeling of the unknown → resulting in sympathetic nervous system responses)*

- **Grief** *(physical and emotional responses → due to loss or impending loss → resulting in withdrawal of attachment)*

- **Death** *(irreversible condition → resulting from cessation of circulatory and respiratory functions or irreversible cessation of all functions of the brain)*

Priority nursing diagnoses within the health perception and health management functional health pattern that may be appropriate for patients include the following:

- *Impaired Skin Integrity* as evidenced by surgical incisions, injuries due to accidents or falls, physical immobility, and skin changes in the elderly

- *Risk for Injury* as evidenced by misuse of drugs and alcohol, environmental hazards, intraoperative complications, and inadequate postoperative care

- *Ineffective Therapeutic Regimen Management* as evidenced by ineffective patterns of health care, lack of knowledge of health care, and mistrust of healthcare personnel

- *Powerlessness* as evidenced by loss of privacy, loss of control due to chronic or debilitating conditions, and dependency on others

Two nursing diagnoses from other functional health patterns often are of high priority for the patient with alterations in patterns of health perception or health maintenance:

- *Impaired Verbal Communication* (Cognitive-Perceptual Functional Health Pattern)

- *Ineffective Individual Coping* (Coping-Stress-Tolerance Functional Health Pattern)

Question

1. How did you decrease your patient's anxiety, thus altering his or her health status?

Questions

Refer to the Clinical Scenario on the next page in order to answer the following questions.

Priority Setting

1. In what order would you visit these patients after report? What is your rationale for your choice?
   A. _____
   B. _____
   C. _____
   D. _____

Health Promotion

1. Diet is important for wound healing. What nutrients will you encourage Mary Black to eat in order to ensure proper healing of her fractured ankle?

2. Mary Black understands her diet when she picks which meal plan?
   A. hamburger, french fries, and a cola beverage
   B. tossed salad, chocolate pudding, and iced tea
   C. baked chicken, broccoli and cheese, and lemonade
   D. salmon patty, baked potato, and milk

CLINICAL SCENARIO

Directions: *Read the following clinical scenario and answer the questions that follow. To complete this exercise successfully you will not only use knowledge of the content in this unit, but also principles related to setting priorities and maintaining patient safety.*

You have been assigned to work with the following four patients for the 0700 shift on a medical-surgical unit. Significant data obtained during report is as follows:

■ Peter Black is a 46-year-old who was admitted from the emergency room 2 hours ago for observation after being thrown 50 yards during a tornado. His vital signs on admission were stable: T 99.8°F, P 86, R 24, and BP 140/86. He had multiple abrasions and lacerations that were sutured in the emergency room. He is now complaining of numbness in both legs.

■ Mary Black is a 44-year-old wife of Peter Black who was admitted 1 hour ago with multiple abrasions and ecchymotic areas. She is scheduled to go to surgery at 0900 for an open reduction of a left ankle fracture. Current vital signs are T 99°F, P 90, R 26, BP 134/88. She is requesting pain medication and wants to see her children, who were admitted to the pediatric unit, before going to surgery.

■ John Linzer, aged 67, was admitted one week ago in the terminal stages of colon cancer. Vital signs are T 96.8°F, P 54, R 10, BP 88/68. The family is requesting that a nurse check on Mr. Linzer as they feel that death is imminent. There is a do-not-resuscitate order.

■ Paul Goetz, aged 47, was admitted three days ago due to being found unconscious in his car. On admission his alcohol level was 0.45. Current vital signs are T 100°F, P 110, R 30, BP 168/94. He is diaphoretic, disoriented, and complaining of nausea and seeing spiders on the wall.

Nursing Process

1. Besides obtaining vital signs, what diagnosis-specific assessment data should be collected for each patient?
   A. _____
   B. _____
   C. _____
   D. _____

2. Identify one priority nursing diagnosis for each patient presented earlier. What is the rationale for your choices?

	Nursing Diagnosis	Rationale
Peter Black		
Mary Black		
John Linzer		
Paul Goetz		

3. Identify five nursing interventions for John Linzer as he progresses through the dying process.

4. With history of alcoholism for 5 years, which is a priority nursing intervention in the plan of care for Mr. Goetz?
   A. Identify maladaptive behaviors that may contribute to the alcoholism.
   B. Encourage patient participation in therapeutic group activities.
   C. Teach the patient the effects of alcohol use on his body.
   D. Use a respectful, nonjudgmental approach to gain the patient's trust.

5. Paul Goetz is given Ativan (lorazepam) to prevent symptoms of alcohol withdrawal. How would you evaluate the effectiveness of this medication?

6. Mrs. Black understands the postoperative teaching done by the nurse when she states which of the following?
   A. "Since my surgery is on my ankle, I will need to stay still in the bed to prevent pain."
   B. "I will need to cough frequently to remove fluids from my lungs."
   C. "Since I will have a PCA machine for pain medication, I will not have to ask for pain medication."
   D. "I will be able to eat and drink as soon as I return from surgery."

Communication

1. What information will you report to Peter Black's doctor regarding his new symptom of numbness in both legs?

2. What information should be communicated with the pediatric unit nurses prior to Mary Black's being allowed to visit her children before she has surgery on her ankle?

Delegation

1. What nursing interventions for each patient can be delegated to a certified nursing assistant (CNA)?
   A. _____
   B. _____
   C. _____
   D. _____

Nursing Ethics

1. Paul Goetz asks you to bring him some beer. He says, "You can smuggle it in and no one will know." How will you respond?

2. When preparing for the role the nurse will play in disaster relief, the nurse must first do which of the following?
   A. Be able to apply basic first aid skills.
   B. Be aware of decontamination procedures.
   C. Serve on disaster preparedness committees.
   D. Know how to take care of him- or herself.

CASE STUDY: Maria Rodriguez

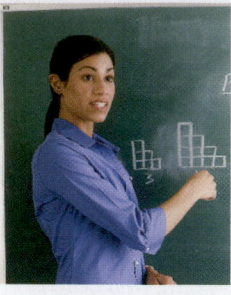

Mrs. Maria Rodriguez is admitted to the emergency room with an open left leg fracture, left upper quadrant pain, and reddened areas across the left shoulder, neck, and chest. According to the paramedics, she was involved in a multiple car accident on an icy highway. Upon assessment she is found to be a non-English-speaking Hispanic, 28 years of age, 5' 4'' in height, and weighing 115 pounds. Her vital signs are T 100°F, P 100, R 28 and shallow, BP 150/86. She indicates that her pain scale level is at 9 out of 10, even after being medicated with Morphine in the ambulance.

After chest, abdominal, and leg x-rays, Mrs. Rodriguez is diagnosed with a severe comminuted left leg fracture; a lacerated spleen; and bruising across the shoulder, neck, and chest due to the seat belt. With the use of a translator, the physician explains to the patient that due to the seriousness of the left leg fracture, the left leg may need to be amputated during surgery. Mrs. Rodriguez begins crying and wringing her hands after speaking with the physician.

Blood is drawn for the following laboratory studies: complete blood count with differential, electrolytes, prothrombin time (PT), partial thromboplastin time (PTT), and blood gases. A urine specimen is sent to the laboratory for a urinalysis. Preoperative preparation is completed. Through the use of a translator, the nurse explains postoperative teaching to the patient to prevent the following complications of surgery: shock, hemorrhage, deep vein thrombosis, pulmonary embolism, pneumonia, infection, urinary retention, and delayed bowel elimination. The nurse tries to calm the patient and answer any questions she has regarding the surgery and what will happen in the postoperative period. The nurse attempts to contact family members and a priest to see the patient before she goes to surgery. At the ordered time, the nurse administers preoperative medication as ordered and the patient is sent to the operating room.

Due to difficulty understanding the English language, the need for surgery, and the possibility of leg amputation, the patient is very anxious. The nursing diagnosis of Anxiety is appropriate for guiding nursing care. Anxiety is an uneasy feeling of not knowing what is going to happen. The pathophysiology of anxiety is anticipation of danger or a threat to health status that leads to a "fight or flight" response from the sympathetic nervous system. Manifestations of anxiety are restlessness, tachycardia, rapid breathing, facial flushing, increased perspiration, weakness, tremors, and impaired attention and concentration. Complications of anxiety are nausea, vomiting, diarrhea, loss of appetite, insomnia, immobility, and powerlessness that can lead to panic or phobias.

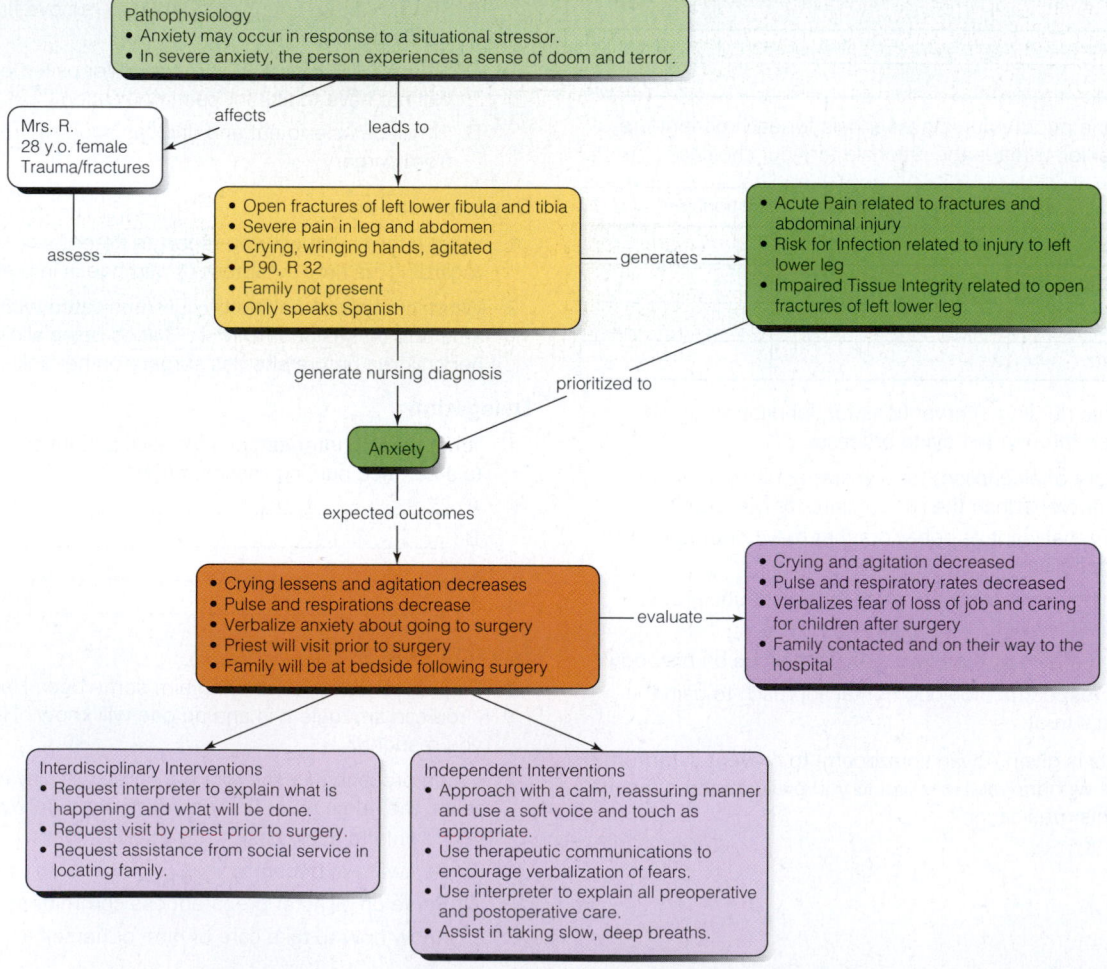

Activity:

1. After reviewing the concept map, go to the Pearson Nursing Student Resources for this book at www.nursing. pearsonhighered.com to write a concept map based on the nursing diagnosis Grieving related to potential amputation of left leg. In your concept map, be sure to include consideration of Mrs. Rodriguez's communication barriers and culture. See answers and hints in Appendix C.

2. Write another concept map using another appropriate nursing diagnosis.

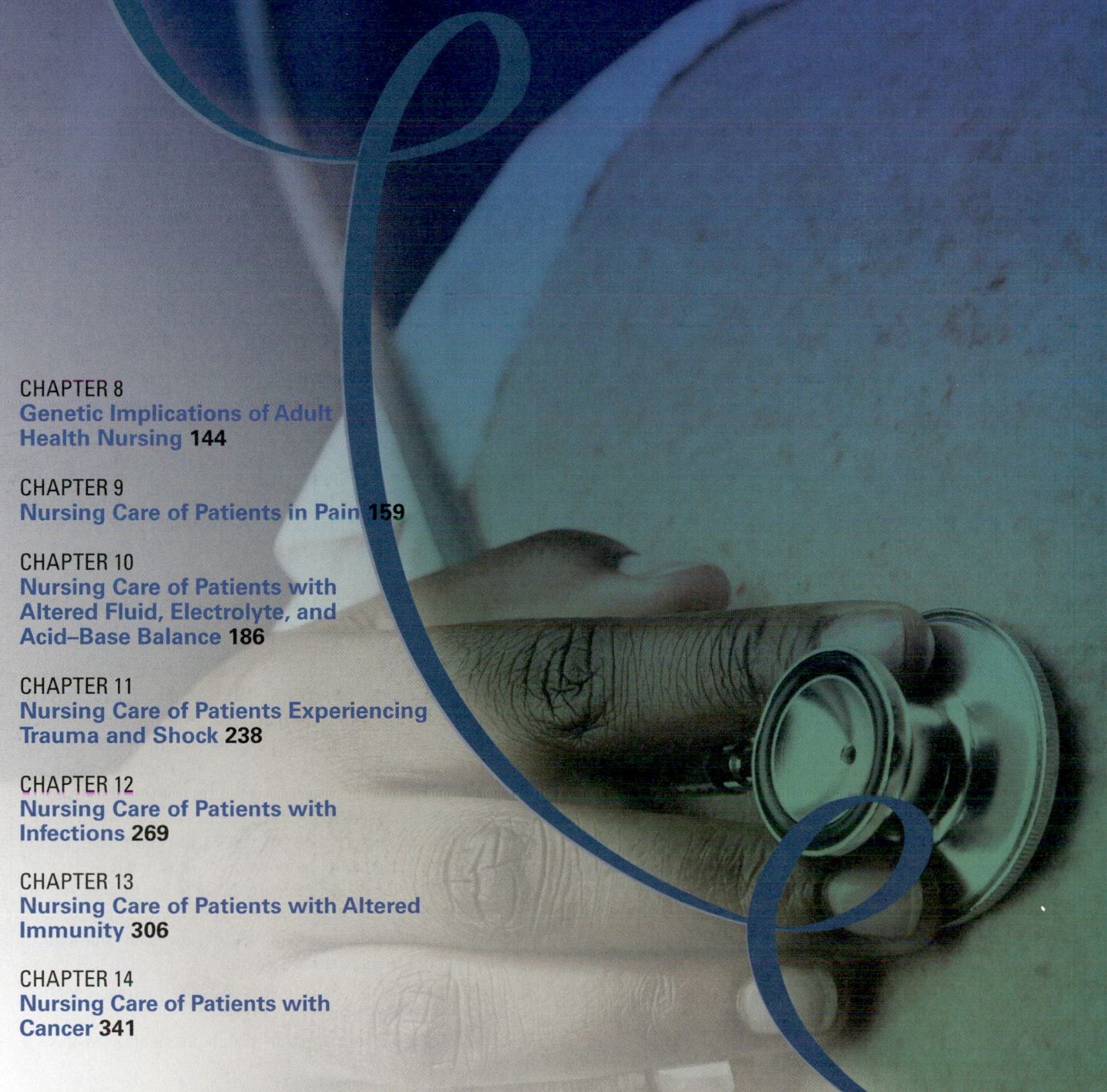

Pathophysiology and Patterns of Health

UNIT 3

Genetic Implications of Adult Health Nursing

LEARNING OUTCOMES

1. Discuss the role of genetic concepts in health promotion and health maintenance.
2. Apply knowledge of the principles of genetic transmission and risk factors for genetic disorders.
3. Describe the significance of delivering genetic education and counseling follow-up in a professional manner.
4. Explain the implications of genetic advances on the role of nurses with particular attention to spiritual, cultural, ethical, legal, and social issues.
5. Identify the significance of recent advances in human genetics and the effect on healthcare delivery.

CLINICAL COMPETENCIES

1. Integrate genetic physical assessment and the use of a pedigree family history into delivery of nursing care.
2. Identify patients or families with actual or potential genetic conditions and initiate referrals to a genetics professional.
3. Prepare patients and their families for a genetic evaluation and facilitate the genetic counseling process.
4. Integrate basic genetic concepts into patient and family education and the reinforcement of information provided to patients by genetic professionals.

KEY TERMS

alleles, *147*
autosomes, *145*
biological markers, *148*
chromosomes, *145*
gene, *147*
genotype, *147*
heterozygous, *147*

homozygous, *147*
human genome, *144*
meiosis, *146*
mitosis, *146*
penetrance, *149*
phenotype, *147*
polymorphisms, *148*

sex chromosomes, *146*
somatic cell, *146*
translocation, *147*
trisomy 21, *146*
X-linked dominant, *148*
X-linked recessive, *148*

Ongoing research in genetics has enhanced our understanding of the causes and natural course for disease, and our understanding of the factors that increase risk for the development of many diseases. Genetics research is not only focused on traditional genetic disorders, but also common complex diseases such as heart disease, stroke, diabetes, and several kinds of cancer. The knowledge gained from the Human Genome Project (Box 8–1) and the continued efforts of scientists and clinicians has and will continue to have a profound impact on the prevention, diagnosis, and treatment of genetic disorders and complex diseases (Figure 8–1 ■).

Integrating Genetics into Nursing Practice

Genetic knowledge will continue to revolutionize how persons perceive themselves, their health status, and their health potential. Therefore, it is expected that nurses must integrate genetics into nursing practice. The *Statement on the Scope and Standards of Genetics Clinical Nursing Practice* from the American Nurses Association and the International Society of Nurses in Genetics (ANA/ISONG) defines the role of all nurses regardless of practice setting (Box 8–2), thus emphasizing the importance of genetics in every arena of health care.

Nurses must have basic genetic knowledge to care for the needs of patients and their families with known or suspected genetic disease. Basic interventions that meet the standard of genetic nursing include the following:

■ Identifying simple risk factors by completing genetics-focused family history
■ Performing an accurate and thorough physical assessment

BOX 8–1 Human Genome Project

In 1986, the U.S. Department of Energy (USDOE) announced the Human Genome initiative, and in 1990 the USDOE joined with the National Institutes of Health (NIH) to develop the Human Genome Project (HGP). The ultimate goal was to sequence the **human genome** and to identify all human genes. The completion of a high-quality reference sequence was announced in April 2003. Information obtained through the sequencing of the human genome has had a tremendous impact on finding the genes associated with human disease. Future research will now be directed toward understanding the complex functions of cellular regulation, human variation, and the interplay of genes and environment and how all the cell organelles, genes, and proteins work together in life's functions (USDOE Genome Programs, 2008).

Source: From Ball, Jane W.; Bindler, Ruth McGillis W.; Cowen, Kay J., *Child Health Nursing: Partnering with Children and Families*, 2nd, © 2010. Reproduced by permission of Pearson Education, Inc., Upper Saddle River, New Jersey.

Nursing Role in Genetic Testing Video

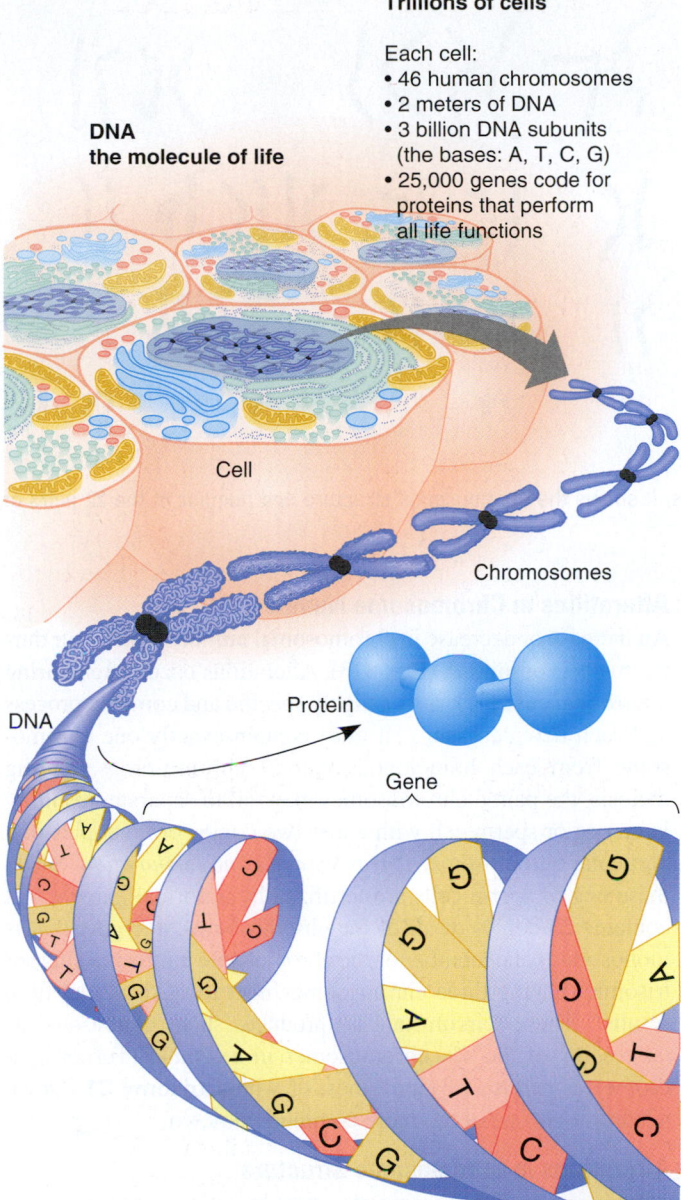

Trillions of cells

Each cell:
- 46 human chromosomes
- 2 meters of DNA
- 3 billion DNA subunits
  (the bases: A, T, C, G)
- 25,000 genes code for
  proteins that perform
  all life functions

DNA
the molecule of life

Cell

Chromosomes

DNA

Protein

Gene

Figure 8–1 ■ Each cell nucleus throughout the body contains the genes, DNA, and chromosomes that make up the majority of an individual's genome. The remaining portion of the human genome is in the mitochondria.

Source: From Ball, Jane W., Bindler, Ruth McGillis W., and Cowen, Kay J., *Child Health Nursing: Partnering with Children and Families,* 2nd, p. 89, © 2009 Pearson Prentice Hall. Reproduced by permission of Pearson Education, Inc., Upper Saddle River, New Jersey.

- Applying concepts of health promotion and health maintenance to assist the patient and family in making informed decisions about their health and lifestyle choices while facilitating autonomy
- Being a patient advocate and providing patients with information about available resources and services
- Providing patient education and making referrals when appropriate
- Completing an evaluation of the plan of care for the patient
- Applying knowledge of the ethical, legal, and social implications of genetic information

Nurses can improve the nursing care provided to patients by applying fundamental genetic concepts to their practice.

Genetic Basics

Life starts as a single cell, but the developed human body is made up of many cells. These cells share common features such as a nucleus that contains 46 chromosomes, and organelles such as mitochondria. There are many different types of specialized cells that function differently depending on their location. For example, pancreatic cells have a very different function than that of nerve cells.

All human cells, except mature red blood cells, contain a complete set of deoxyribonucleic acid (DNA) molecules. DNA molecules consist of long sequences of nucleotides or bases represented by the letters A, T, G, and C. The order of these bases gives the exact instructions for the functioning of that particular cell. Writing the correct order of the bases using the abbreviations represents the sequence of the bases in DNA. Together, the total sum of DNA in a human cell is referred to as the human *genome*, or the complete set of inheritance for an individual. The human genome includes the DNA in the cell nucleus as well as the DNA found in the mitochondria, which will be discussed later in this section. Each person's genome is unique. Identical (monozygotic) twins are the exception because they develop from only one fertilized ovum and share identical DNA.

The cell nucleus contains about 6 feet of DNA that is tightly wound and packaged into 23 pairs of chromosomes, making a complete set of 46 **chromosomes**. The structure and number of chromosomes can be shown by a karyotype, or picture, of an individual's chromosomes (Figure 8–2 ■) There are two copies of each chromosome. One copy, or half of the complete set of these 46 chromosomes, is inherited from the mother and the other copy, or the other half of the 46 chromosomes, is inherited from the father. For example, an individual will have two copies of chromosome 1, one inherited from his or her mother and one inherited from his or her father. These two copies or pairs of inherited chromosomes are called homologous (the same) chromosomes. Chromosomes are numbered according to size (largest to smallest), with chromosome 1 being the largest. The first 22 pairs of chromosomes, known as **autosomes**, are alike

Nursing Role in Genetic Testing Animation

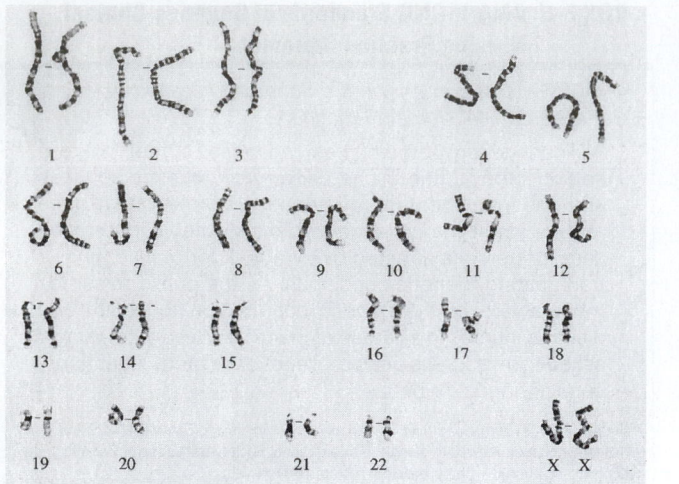
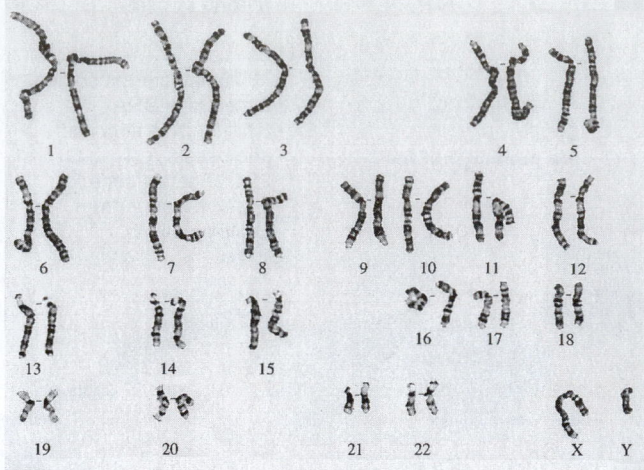

Figure 8–2 ■ A karyotype is a picture of an individual's chromosomes. It shows the chromosomal structure and number of the 22 pairs of autosomes and the sex chromosomes.

in males and females. The 23rd pair, the **sex chromosomes**, determines an individual's gender. A female has two copies of the X chromosome (one copy inherited from each parent) and a male has one X chromosome (inherited from his mother) and a Y chromosome (inherited from his father).

Cell Division

Mitosis and meiosis are the two types of cell division in human cells. **Mitosis** is the process of making new cells and it takes place in the **somatic**, or tissue, **cells** of the body. Cell division through mitosis heals wounds and replaces cells lost daily on skin surfaces and in the lining of gastrointestinal and respiratory tracts. In addition, mitosis is responsible for human development. The mitotic activity of the zygote and its daughter cells is the foundation for a human's growth and development. The zygote undergoes mitosis to form a multicellular embryo, then fetus, then infant. Cell division through mitosis results in two cells called *daughter cells* that are genetically identical to the original cell, or *mother cell*, and each other.

Meiosis is also known as the reduction division of the cell. Meiosis occurs only in the sex cells of the testes and ovaries and results in the formation of the sperm and oocyte (gametes). Meiosis is very similar to mitosis in that it is a form of cell division; however, through a series of complex mechanisms, the amount of genetic material is reduced in half (23 chromosomes). This is very important because when the two sex cells combine during fertilization, the total number of chromosomes (46) is present in the offspring's cells. There are three purposes of meiosis: (1) to produce gametes, (2) to reduce the number of chromosomes by half, and (3) to make new combinations of genetic material from crossing over and independent assortment processes, which allows diversity in the human population.

Chromosomal Alterations

Alterations in chromosomes often occur during cell division and are classified as either alterations in the number of chromosomes or structural alterations. They involve either part of or the whole chromosome. The clinical consequences of number and structural changes in the chromosomes in an individual vary depending on the amount and type of DNA affected by the alterations.

Alterations in Chromosome Number

An increase or decrease in chromosomal numbers can occur during meiosis or mitosis (Box 8–3). Alterations occur often during meiosis because meiosis is a highly specific and complex process and each new daughter cell must contain exactly one chromosome from each homologous pair of chromosomes. During meiosis, the paired chromosomes may fail to separate, resulting in an egg or sperm cell with either two copies or no copies of a particular chromosome. This is known as *nondisjunction*. When these egg or sperm cells are fertilized by a normal gamete that contains 23 copies of all of the chromosomes, a zygote that is monosomic (one member of the chromosome pair is missing) or trisomic (having three chromosomes instead of the usual two) results. These circumstances produce such conditions as *monosomy* of the sex chromosomes in a female (Turner syndrome) or *trisomy* of autosomes, of which **trisomy 21** (Down syndrome) is one of the more commonly known.

Alterations in Chromosome Structure

Alterations in chromosome structure include inversions, deletions, duplications, and translocations. In a chromosomal inversion a segment of a chromosome is reversed, changing the DNA sequence for that portion of the chromosome. It occurs when a chromosome breaks in two places and the piece between the breaks turns upside down and reattaches within the same chromosome. The clinical consequences of an inversion

---

BOX 8–3 Variations in Chromosomal Number

Aneuploidy—the condition when extra or missing chromosomes exist; in affected living individuals, physical abnormalities and/or mental retardation are common

Monosomy—the loss of a single chromosome from a pair, i.e., Turner syndrome (45,XO)

Trisomy—the gain of a single chromosome, making a total of three copies of a certain chromosome, i.e., trisomy 21 or Down syndrome

Euploidy—the presence of the normal number of 46 chromosomes

Polyploidy—the condition when more than two pairs of all the chromosomes are present

depend on how much chromosomal material is involved, where the inversion occurs, and what type of inversion is present.

A chromosomal alteration that includes a missing (deletion) or additional (duplication) whole chromosome or segment of a chromosome is an unbalanced rearrangement. An unbalanced rearrangement can result in missing genes, confusing directions from the genes, or too much gene product, which often results in a condition that is not compatible with life or altered physical and/or mental development. An example is *cri du chat* syndrome (mental retardation, crying that sounds like a cat mewing, and low-set ears), which results from a large deletion on 5p (the short arm of chromosome 5).

Translocation (chromosomal reshuffling) occurs when a segment of a chromosome transfers or moves and attaches itself to another chromosome. An example is the reciprocal translocation that is found in 95% of patients with chronic myelogenous leukemia (CML) (Wang et al., 2006). The contributing translocation occurs between chromosomes 9 and 22 and is known as the Philadelphia chromosome. The translocation that occurs between chromosomes 9 and 22 is not inheritable. However, this is not true for all translocations. About 4% of trisomy 21 cases are caused by a translocation; of these, half can be attributed to a translocation inherited from a parent (Mayo Clinic, 2008). The parent remains unaffected because although he or she has extra material his or hers is a balanced chromosomal rearrangement.

Genes

A **gene** is a small portion (segment) of the nucleotide (base) sequence of a chromosome DNA molecule that can be identified as having specific directions for a particular function or characteristic. The specific sequence of nucleotides (the genes and the variations therein) is referred to as the individual's **genotype**. Each chromosome contains numerous genes arranged in a linear order. Researchers currently believe there are about 20,000 to 25,000 genes in the human genome (USDOE Human Genome Programs, 2008).

All genes come in pairs because chromosomes come in pairs. The only exception to all genes being paired are the genes on the sex chromosomes (X and Y) present in males. All genes have a specific location on a specific chromosome. This is known as the *genetic locus*. For example, one of the many genes located on chromosome 19 is a gene for eye color. There may be slight variations or different forms of a gene, for instance, green versus blue eye color, and these different forms or versions of genes are called **alleles**. When an individual has two identical forms (alleles) of a gene they are said to be **homozygous** (homo = same). If an individual has two different forms (alleles) of the gene, they are said to be **heterozygous** (hetero = different). Genes can be described as *altered* or *mutated* when a change has taken place, or *expressed* when the gene has an impact on the outward appearance of an individual and/or the functioning of cells. The observable, outward expression of an individual's entire physical, biochemical, and physiologic makeup, as determined by his or her genotype (alleles) and environmental factors, is referred to as **phenotype**.

Function and Distribution of Genes

One function of genes is to provide directions for how to make proteins. These protein-directing genes are very important to life and functioning as a human and are responsible for transmitting messages between cells, fighting infection, directing genes to turn "on" or "off," forming structures, as well as sensing light, taste, and smell (U.S. National Library of Medicine, 2008). Some gene activities change from moment to moment in response to tens of thousands of intra- and extracellular environmental signals (USDOE Genome Programs, 2008). An example of this is the feedback mechanism that stimulates a cell to produce insulin after eating a candy bar. After eating, a gene on chromosome 11 directs pancreatic cells to produce, modify, and secrete insulin. Although the gene for producing insulin is present in all nucleated cells of the body, it is only functional in insulin-secreting pancreatic cells.

Mitochondrial Genes

Chromosomes in the cell nucleus are not the only site where genes reside. Several dozen that are involved in energy metabolism are located in the cell mitochondria (the "powerhouse" of the cell). *Mitochondria* are concerned with energy production and metabolism. Some cells contain more mitochondria than others, but each mitochondrion contains its own copies of DNA identified as mitochondrial DNA (mtDNA). Because ova have many mitochondria and sperm do not (most mitochondria are located in the tail of the sperm that detaches after fertilization), mtDNA is primarily inherited from the mother. Therefore, mitochondrial genes and any diseases due to DNA alterations on those genes are transmitted through the mother in a matrilineal pattern. This pattern of inheritance is very different from the pattern of inheritance of genes found in the nucleus of the cell. Thus, an affected female will pass the mtDNA mutation to all of her children; however, an affected male will not pass the mtDNA mutation to any of his children (Nussbaum et al., 2007). Manifestations of conditions as a result of mitochondrial gene alterations are primarily involved in high-energy tissues and organs such as skeletal muscle, heart muscle, the liver, kidney, brain, and nerve cells. The ears, eyes, and endocrine system are also affected. Symptoms develop over years as unhealthy or dying cells are not replaced. Hypertrophic cardiomyopathy, heart block, seizures, and deafness are also associated with mtDNA gene alterations (Nussbaum et al., 2007).

Gene Alterations and Disease

Today, we know that gene alterations are responsible for approximately 6000 hereditary diseases (Winkleman, 2004). However, different gene alterations within a particular gene can result in a wide variety of signs and symptoms. For example, the *CFTR* gene for cystic fibrosis is a very large gene located on chromosome 7. More than 1100 different mutations of the CFTR gene have been reported to be associated with disease (Giusti et al., 2007). The area of the *CFTR* gene that controls mucous production can have more than 300 different gene alterations resulting in a variety of symptoms ranging from mild, to severe, or no symptoms at all (U.S. National Library of Medicine, 2008). Gene alterations, not the genes themselves, cause genetic diseases and conditions.

Gene Alterations That Decrease Risk of Disease

Although it is common to associate gene mutations with disease, it is important to remember that gene mutations can also be helpful to decrease the risk of disease. Gene alterations and genetic variations may also have a protective role in the expression of diseases. A common example is the protective value of the gene alteration that causes sickle cell disease. Those individuals with this gene alteration have protection against malaria. Another example is the APOE gene. The APOE gene provides instructions for making a protein called apolipoprotein E. This protein combines with fats (lipids) in the body to form molecules called lipoproteins that are responsible for packaging cholesterol and other fats and carrying them through the bloodstream. There are at least three slightly different versions (alleles) of the APOE gene. The major alleles are called e2, e3, and e4. Research has shown that a person who inherits at least one e4 allele will have a greater chance of developing Alzheimer's disease. However, inheriting the e2 allele seems to indicate that a person is less likely to develop Alzheimer's (Genetics Home Reference, 2008).

Single Nucleotide Polymorphisms

Greater than 99% of human DNA sequences are the same (HGP, 2008c). **Polymorphisms** are DNA sequences that are natural variations in a gene in which each possible sequence is present in at least 1% of people, but usually have no adverse effect on the individual. *Single nucleotide polymorphisms* (SNPs, or "snips") are the most common type of genetic variation among humans and are one-letter (base pair) variations in the DNA sequence and serve as biological markers. **Biological markers** are important for the construction of chromosome maps and are easily tracked, stable segments of DNA. Scientists are hopeful that information gained from SNPs will provide information on how subtle differences in humans impact their response to drugs and the environment, thus making medical treatment and pharmacologic management more individualized.

Principles of Inheritance

Knowledge of inheritance allows the nurse to provide genetic information to patients and their families to assist them in managing their care and in making reproductive decisions. The basic underlying principles of inheritance that nurses can apply to inheritance risk assessment and teaching include (1) all genes are paired, (2) only one gene of each pair is transmitted (passed on) to an offspring, and (3) one copy of each gene in the offspring comes from the mother and the other copy comes from the father. Understanding the Mendelian patterns of inheritance is made easier by relating these principles.

Mendelian Pattern of Inheritance

Conditions that are caused by a mutation or alteration of a single gene are known as *monogenic* or *single-gene disorders*. The most common gene alterations that result in genetic disorders are categorized into Mendelian inheritance patterns because they are predictably passed on from generation to generation following Mendel's laws of inheritance. These single-gene mutations follow an autosomal dominant, autosomal recessive, **X-linked recessive**, or **X-linked dominant** inheritance pattern. The first three of these patterns are the most common. Modes of transmission or inheritance for thousands of conditions resulting from monogenic alterations have been identified (U.S. National Library of Medicine, 2008).

Autosomal Dominant

Autosomal dominant (AD) conditions are the result of an altered gene on any of the 22 autosomes or non–sex chromosomes (Figure 8–3 ■). More than half of the known Mendelian

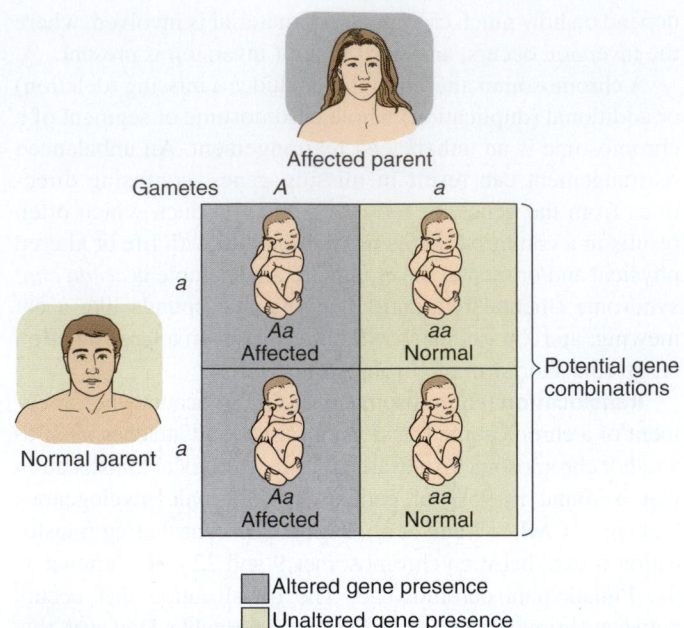

Figure 8–3 ■ This Punnett square shows potential gene combinations (genotypes) and resulting phenotypes of children from parent genotypes with an autosomal dominant altered gene. Phenotypes are expressed (affected) when a male *or* female has one copy of the gene alteration.

Source: From Ball, Jane W.; Bindler, Ruth McGillis W.; Cowen, Kay J., Child Health Nursing: Partnering with Children and Families, 2nd, © 2010. Reproduced by permission of Pearson Education, Inc., Upper Saddle River, New Jersey.

conditions are autosomal dominant. In AD conditions, disease occurs in spite of the fact that there exists one unaltered or normal gene. Also, homozygous dominant conditions are generally much more severe than heterozygous dominant conditions and are often lethal. Because homozygous dominant conditions are usually lethal and would result from both parents being affected, the nurse should consider an individual exhibiting an autosomal dominant condition as heterozygous. See Box 8–4 for characteristics of an AD pattern of inheritance.

Autosomal Recessive

A gene or genetic condition is considered recessive when two copies of altered genes are needed to express the condition. Autosomal recessive (AR) conditions are the result of an

BOX 8–4 Autosomal Dominant Mendelian Inheritance Characteristics

(Examples: neurofibromatosis, breast and ovarian cancer, autosomal dominant polycystic kidney disease, Marfan syndrome, Huntington disease, familial hypercholesterolemia)

When the nurse gathers a family history, the nurse should assess for any of the following characteristics of autosomal dominant inheritance:

1. Both males and females are affected.
2. Males and females are usually affected in equal numbers.
3. An affected child will have an affected parent and/or all generations will have an affected individual (appearing as a vertical pattern of affected individuals on the family pedigree).
4. Unaffected children of an affected parent will have unaffected offspring.
5. A significant proportion of isolated cases are due to a new mutation.

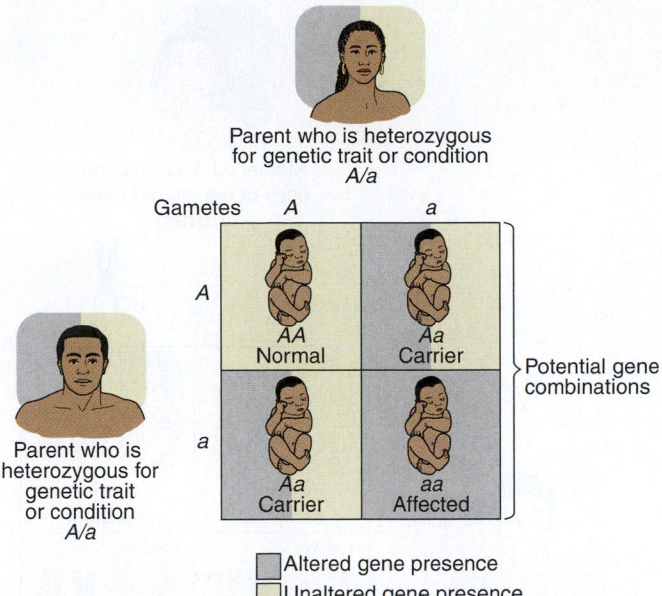

Parent who is heterozygous for genetic trait or condition *A/a*

Gametes

Parent who is heterozygous for genetic trait or condition *A/a*

Potential gene combinations

AA Normal
Aa Carrier
Aa Carrier
aa Affected

Altered gene presence
Unaltered gene presence

Figure 8–4 ■ This Punnett square shows potential gene combinations (genotypes) and resulting phenotypes of children from parent genotypes with an autosomal recessive altered gene. Phenotypes are expressed (affected) when a male *or* female has two copies of the gene alteration.

Source: From Ball, Jane W.; Bindler, Ruth McGillis W.; Cowen, Kay J., Child Health Nursing: Partnering with Children and Families, 2nd, © 2010. Reproduced by permission of Pearson Education, Inc., Upper Saddle River, New Jersey.

altered gene on any of the 22 autosomes or non–sex chromosomes (Figure 8–4 ■). An individual with a recessive condition has inherited one altered gene from his mother and one from his father. In most cases, neither of the parents is affected and, therefore, each of the parents must have a single gene alteration on one chromosome of a pair and the normal, wild-type or unaltered form of the gene on the other chromosome. These parents would be known as *carriers* of the condition and they do not usually exhibit any signs and symptoms of the condition. Because the gene alteration occurs on a non–sex chromosome, both males and females have an equal chance of inheriting the altered gene from their parent. See Box 8–5 for characteristics of an AR pattern of inheritance.

X-Linked Recessive

X-linked conditions are the result of an altered gene on the X chromosome. Unlike the autosomes, the sex chromosome, X, is unevenly distributed to males and females. The female has two X chromosomes and the male has only one. Thus, the family history and pattern of inheritance has a characteristic distribution pattern among the males and females in the family (Figure 8–5 ■). Because the male has only one copy of any gene on the X chromosome, it becomes the only copy available to give direction for those particular functions of these genes regardless of whether it is considered dominant or recessive in the female. Thus, if any of these genes are altered, an unaltered counterpart is not present to "override" the altered functioning gene.

The consequences of the altered gene on an X chromosome will be expressed in all males. Females, on the other hand, will have two copies and the unaltered gene generally compensates for the altered gene, making the female a carrier. The male

receives his X chromosome from his mother and his Y chromosome from his father. The female offspring receives an X chromosome from each of her parents. Thus, all affected males will pass on the altered X chromosome to all of his daughters who will be carriers of the altered gene. A male can never transmit an altered gene on the X chromosome to his sons because the male will transmit only the Y chromosome to his sons. Because of these transmission patterns, the most commonly occurring transmission of an X-linked condition is through a female who is a carrier of an altered gene. See Box 8–6 for characteristics of an X-linked recessive pattern of inheritance.

X-Linked Dominant

X-linked dominant conditions also exist but these conditions are very rare. If a male is affected, the condition is severe and often lethal. A family history of multiple male miscarriages may be a sign of an X-linked dominant condition. An example of a viable X-linked dominant condition is vitamin-D resistant rickets, also known as hypophosphatemic rickets.

Variability in Classic Mendelian Patterns of Inheritance

Along with understanding the classic Mendelian inheritance patterns, several other concepts are also important for families to understand when the nurse is assisting patients with or at risk for inheriting a genetic disorder. These include the following exceptions or variations to the traditional Mendelian patterns of inheritance.

Penetrance

Penetrance is the probability that a gene will be expressed phenotypically. It is an "all or none" concept in that either the gene will be expressed (even if mildly expressed) or it will not be expressed at all. Penetrance can be measured in the following way. In a certain group of individuals with the same genotype, what percentage of them will exhibit at least some signs and/or symptoms of the condition? If the number is less than 100%, then that condition is said to show reduced penetrance. For example, the gene alterations that cause achondroplasia (dwarfism) exhibit 100% penetrance and all individuals with

BOX 8–5 Autosomal Recessive Mendelian Inheritance Characteristics

(Examples: hemochromatosis type 1, cystic fibrosis, phenylketonuria, sickle cell anemia)

When the nurse gathers a family history, the nurse should assess for any of the following characteristics of autosomal recessive inheritance:
1. Both males and females are affected.
2. Males and females are usually affected in equal numbers.
3. An affected child will have an unaffected parent but may have affected siblings (appearing as a horizontal pattern of affected individuals on the family pedigree).
4. The condition may appear to skip a generation.
5. The parents of the affected child may be consanguineous (close blood relatives).
6. The family may be descendants of a certain ethnic group that is known to have a more frequent occurrence of a certain genetic condition.

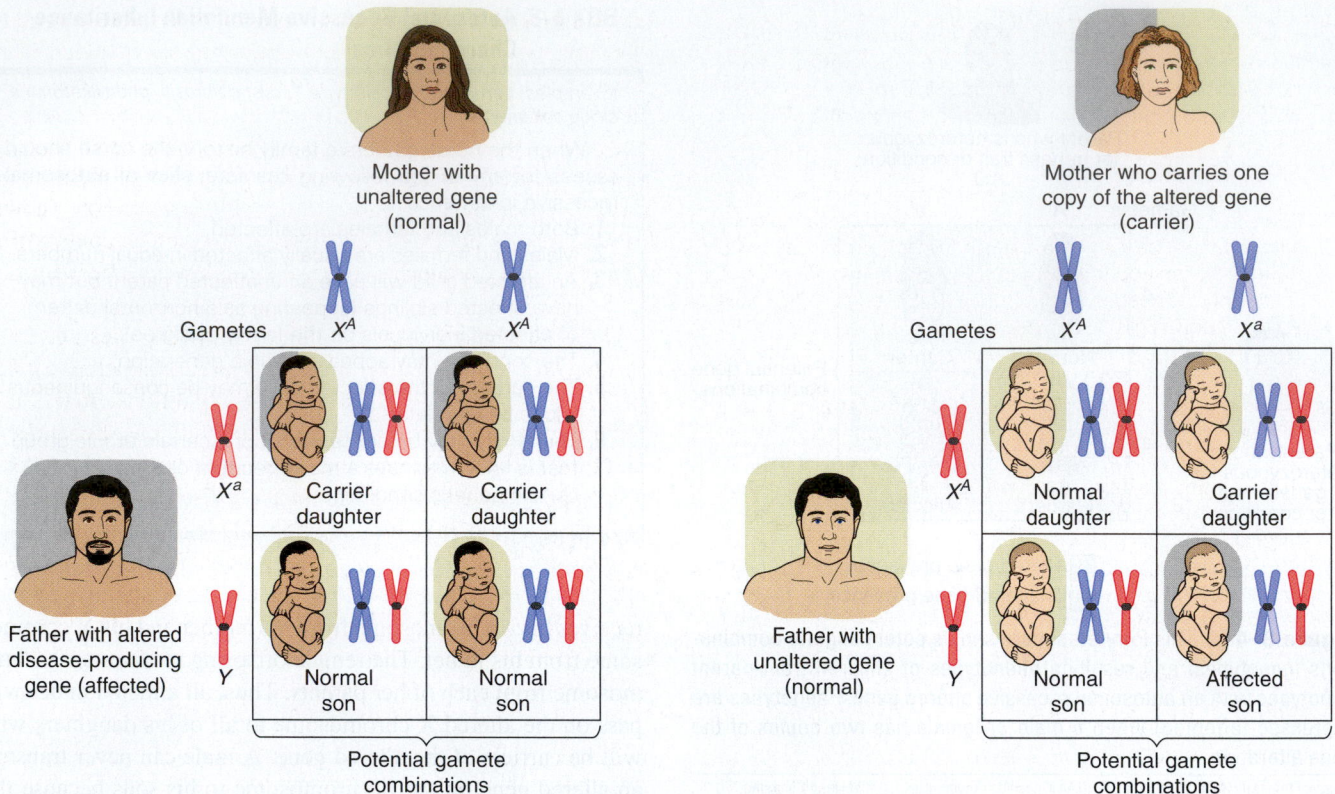

Figure 8–5 ■ These Punnett squares show potential gene combinations (genotypes) and resulting phenotypes of children from different parent genotypes with an X-linked recessive altered gene. Phenotypes are expressed (affected) in a male with only one copy of the gene alteration and in a female with two copies of the altered gene.

Source: From Ball, Jane W.; Bindler, Ruth McGillis W.; Cowen, Kay J., Child Health Nursing: Partnering with Children and Families, 2nd, © 2010. Reproduced by permission of Pearson Education, Inc., Upper Saddle River, New Jersey.

one copy of the gene alteration will exhibit signs and symptoms of the disease (Nussbaum et al., 2007).

New Mutation

When there is no previous history of a condition including even subtle signs and symptoms of the disease in any other immediate or distant family member, the disease may be caused by a spontaneous new mutation. This case is usually called a *de novo* mutation. New mutations of a gene are most frequently seen in autosomal dominant conditions because one copy of an altered gene is all that is necessary to elicit a state of altered health. Autosomal dominant diseases known to have high mutation rates include neurofibromatosis, achondroplasia, and

---

BOX 8–6 X-Linked Recessive Mendelian Inheritance Characteristics

(Examples: hemophilia A; Duchenne muscular dystrophy)

When the nurse gathers a family history, he or she should assess for any of the following characteristics of X-linked recessive inheritance:

1. More males will be affected than females; rarely seen in females.
2. An affected male will have all carrier daughters.
3. There is no male-to-male inheritance.
4. Affected males are related by carrier females.
5. Females may report varying milder symptoms of the condition.
6. A new sporadic case could be due to a new mutation.

Marfan syndrome. New mutations are also possible in autosomal recessive diseases although rarely expressed because two altered genes are necessary for signs and symptoms to appear. Finally, new mutations are often seen in X-linked recessive disorders, such as hemophilia A, as the male with just one altered gene will express the disease phenotype.

Anticipation

Anticipation occurs when successive generations of a family exhibit more severe signs and symptoms of certain diseases and the disease often has an earlier onset. An example of a condition where this occurs is fragile X. Fragile X is the most common cause of inherited mental impairment, caused by a mutation in a gene known as FMR-1, which is located on the X chromosome. The mutation is a "genetic stutter" in which a small section within the gene is repeated too many times. A person who does not have fragile X has between 6 and 45 repeats (trinucleotide repeats). Individuals with 55 to 200 repeats have a pre-mutation that can possibly expand when passed on to offspring. When this mutation is greater than 200 repeats an individual has a full mutation. See Box 8–7 for more information about fragile X.

Variable Expressivity

Expressivity is used to describe the severity of the *gene expression* of the phenotype. When people with the same genetic makeup (genotype) exhibit signs and/or symptoms with varying degrees of severity the phenotype is described as

BOX 8–7 Fragile X and Anticipation

- **Normal number of repeats.** Individuals with a normal number of repeats (6 to 45) cannot pass fragile X syndrome on to their offspring. The number of repeats in the offspring generally does not change.
- **Intermediate number of repeats or "gray zone":** When an individual has more than about 45 repeats but fewer than 55 repeats, the number of repeats can sometimes expand slightly when passed from parent to child. Individuals who have between about 45 and 55 repeats are considered in a "gray zone." These individuals have not been found to have a child with fragile X syndrome. However, the number of repeats can grow with each generation, so their grandchildren could be at risk.
- **Pre-mutation.** Individuals with between about 55 and 200 repeats have what is called a pre-mutation. Both men and women can be carriers of the pre-mutation. About 1 in 250 women and 1 in 800 men carries the pre-mutation. However, only women who carry the pre-mutation are at risk for having a child with fragile X syndrome.

  A pre-mutation carrier mother has a 50 percent chance of passing along the abnormal gene to her baby during each pregnancy. Some children who inherit the abnormal gene have a pre-mutation and no symptoms of fragile X syndrome. However, the number of repeats is likely to expand when the gene is passed from mother to child. As a result, some children of carrier mothers inherit the full mutation (more than 200 repeats) and show symptoms of fragile X syndrome.

  A male pre-mutation carrier passes on the pre-mutation to all of his daughters but to none of his sons. The daughters generally have no symptoms of fragile X syndrome, but they are carriers of a pre-mutation that may be passed on to their children. Unlike in females, in males the pre-mutation does not usually expand in size when passed on to their daughters. Sons of men with the pre-mutation do not inherit it because they do not get an X chromosome from their father.
- **Full mutation.** Individuals with more than 200 repeats have the full mutation. A woman with a full fragile X mutation has a 50 percent chance of passing along the full mutation in each pregnancy. If a man with a full mutation has children, he will pass the pre-mutation on to all of his daughters. For reasons that are not understood, the full mutation shrinks back to a pre-mutation in sperm. His sons are not at risk because they do not inherit the X chromosome from their father.

Source: Copyright 2007 March of Dimes. Used by permission.

variable expression (Nussbaum et al., 2007). Variable expression is common in the autosomal dominant condition, neurofibromatosis. Although neurofibromatosis has 100% penetrance, variable expressivity can occur within family members with each family member exhibiting a variety of signs and/or symptoms.

Multifactorial (Polygenic or Complex) Disorders

Many birth defects such as cleft lip and palate, as well as many adult-onset conditions such as cancer, mental illness, asthma, diabetes, obesity, heart disease, and Alzheimer's disease have a multifactorial cause. *Multifactorial conditions* occur as a result of several gene (polygenic) variations, lifestyle, and

environmental influences that work together. The polygenic concept is illustrated with the multiple genes involved in an individual's susceptibility for breast cancer. These genes have been identified on chromosomes 6, 11, 13, 14, 15, 17, and 22. Exactly which genes interrelate and how many environmental influences are enough to cause the presentation of many of the common complex diseases or conditions is not known. However, it is believed that by 2010, the major contributing genes for many common complex conditions will be identified (HGP, 2008a).

Multifactorial conditions accumulate in families but these conditions do not follow the characteristic Mendelian pattern of inheritance seen with single-gene conditions. Inheritable recurrence risks vary in multifactorial conditions. Scheuner et al. (1997) developed a method of risk stratification that allows risk to be quantified for common adult diseases. For example, premature death in a first-degree relative, two affected first-degree relatives, and two second-degree maternal or paternal relatives with at least one individual having premature onset of the disease are all considered high inheritance risks. A patient considered as high risk for an inheritable condition should be referred for genetics consultation.

Interdisciplinary Care

Many health professionals work together in screening, diagnosis, identification, and treatment of genetic disorders. The goals of interdisciplinary care are early diagnosis through testing and assessment and development of an effective treatment plan, combined with psychosocial support to enhance coping and referral to a genetic specialist when needed.

Genetic Testing

Genetic testing involves the analysis of DNA, RNA, chromosomes, and serum levels of specific enzymes or metabolites. Genetic tests can be classified into two categories: screening and diagnostic. A positive screening genetic test result indicates an increased risk or probability but must always be confirmed by diagnostic testing. Screening genetic tests are most commonly completed in prenatal, newborn, and carrier circumstances. In contrast, a diagnostic test can definitively validate or eliminate a genetic disorder in the symptomatic patient and then guide clinical management. Box 8–8 lists some of the benefits and negative outcomes of genetic testing. Several categories of genetic tests follow:

- *Newborn screening* provides a means to identify children who have an increased risk for having a genetic disease such as phenylketonuria, sickle cell disease, or maple syrup urine disease. Several states now screen for more than 30 conditions (expanded newborn screen) as part of routine newborn care.
- *Carrier testing* is completed on asymptomatic individuals who may be carriers of one copy of a gene alteration that can be transmitted to future children in an autosomal recessive or X-linked pattern of inheritance. This may be part of a couple's premarriage or preconception planning if they belong to a particular ethnic group with known incidence to genetic disorders such as sickle cell anemia and Tay-Sachs disease.

BOX 8–8 Outcomes Related to Genetic Testing

Benefits of Genetic Testing
Provide for:
- Early screening and preventive measures
- Future planning and life preparation
- Lifestyle adaptations
- Decreased confusion and anxiety
- Psychologic stress relief
- Reproductive choices
- Informed immediate/extended family members
- Early medical and/or surgical intervention
- Cost of medical follow-up reduced (if negative result)

Possible Negative Outcomes of Genetic Testing
- Survivor guilt
- Loss of identity
- No treatment may exist
- Employability and insurability affected
- Confusion about accessing health care and resources
- Risk for invasion of confidentiality and privacy
- Social stigmatization

Source: Data from Secretary's Advisory Committee on Genetic Testing (SACGT), National Institutes of Health, 2000.

It may be necessary to determine the exact gene mutation from an affected family member prior to carrier testing. This is often completed through lineage analysis.

- *Preimplantation genetic diagnosis (PGD)* involves the detection of disease-causing gene alterations in human embryos just after *in vitro* fertilization and before implantation in the uterus, thus providing an opportunity for preselection of unaffected embryos for implantation. This type of genetic testing is most often used by parents who are both carriers of a single-gene recessive disorder and who wish to implant into the uterus only the embryo(s) without the disease-causing gene alteration. It has also been used to determine tissue type for donation of tissue such as bone marrow to a sibling or parent PGD is usually not covered by insurance, is very costly, and is available at only a small number of centers and for only a small number of disorders (U.S. National Library of Medicine, 2008).

- *Predictive genetic testing* is usually made available to the asymptomatic individual and includes both predispositional and presymptomatic testing. A positive predispositional testing result will indicate there is an increased risk that the individual might eventually develop the disease. Common examples include breast cancer and hereditary nonpolyposis colorectal cancer. A presymptomatic test is performed when development of the disease is certain if the gene alteration is present. These tests are medically indicated when the seriousness and mortality of the disease can be reduced with knowledge of the gene alteration. An example of this would be hereditary hemochromatosis or familial hypercholesterolemia. Life planning and lifestyle choices can be influenced by predictive testing.

- Other uses of genetic testing include organ transplantation tissue typing and pharmacogenetic testing, which involves predicting or studying the patient's response to particular

medications. For example, pharmacogenetic testing has shown that 20% of Caucasians have a polymorphism on the cytochrome P450 CYP2C9 gene and consequently metabolize Warfarin more slowly and take longer to achieve therapeutic dosing (Ryan, Byrne, & O'Shea, 2008). These patients require significantly less Warfarin and are two to three times more likely to have a hemorrhagic adverse event. Controversy remains as to whether genetic testing should be undertaken for every patient prior to initiating Warfarin therapy; however, the United States Food and Drug Administration has revised the product label for Warfarin to include information on the benefits of genetic testing to guide Warfarin treatment (2008).

DIAGNOSING CHROMOSOMAL ALTERATIONS
Chromosomal diagnostic examination can be accomplished with a blood, skin, or buccal cell sampling. A karyotype is completed in a cytogenetics laboratory. Chromosomes can be identified by their size and unique light and dark banding patterns. The pairs of autosomal chromosomes are arranged from 1 to 22 according to each chromosome's size, unique banding patterns, and *centromere* position. The sex chromosomes complete the picture, with the X chromosome(s) first, then the Y chromosome (if present). The karyotype shows all of the chromosome pairs lined up and positioned on a piece of paper allowing for visual chromosomal analysis. (See Figure 8–2 earlier in this chapter.) The final report contains numerical data that includes the total number of chromosomes present. Guidelines for writing results of karyotyping are determined by the International System of Human Cytogenetic Nomenclature (ISCN). The guidelines established by this organization allow for a standardized universal language that is utilized by cytogenetic laboratories and in medical publications. For example, a normal female karyotype is written as 46, XX, whereas a karyotype of a female with trisomy 21 is written as 47, XX, +21. In the second example, the (+) symbol signifies an additional copy of chromosome 21, whereas a (−) would signify a deletion (ISCN, 2005).

DIAGNOSING GENE ALTERATIONS More than 1000 tests are available from several laboratories, with some tests only available by a small number of sites. *DNA-based tests* involve sophisticated technology that permits the examination of the DNA itself. Genetic testing that is DNA based can be obtained from blood, bone marrow, amniotic fluid, fibroblast cells of the skin, or buccal cells from the mouth. These tests can be focused looking for common mutation(s) for a specific disorder or a mutation already identified in a previous family member. Several of the conditions screened for on newborn screening such as galactosemia are biochemical tests that look at enzyme levels. Genotyping must be done to confirm the diagnosis and specific type of galactosemia the patient has and to provide more accurate genetic counseling for family planning. A third type of DNA-based test is a complete gene sequence that may be utilized when only one mutation can be found in a symptomatic patient or when none of the common mutations were found (U.S. National Library of Medicine, 2008).

✍ Nursing Care

The Role of the Nurse in Genetic Testing

Although confidentiality and privacy are integral parts of delivery of care for all nurses, this issue is of even more concern as it relates to genetic information. Results of genetic tests can affect employment and insurance options. Will the results affect the patient's ability to obtain and/or maintain insurance coverage? Can an employer refuse to hire or promote an individual because of genetic testing results? Can genetic information be released to the courts, military, schools, or adoption agencies? Would a patient with a known gene alteration for Huntington disease be offered a college scholarship to the best law school? There is debate over whether genetic privacy is different from medical privacy. The nurse should inform patients of their rights and responsibility to know who will have access to the genetic test results. Those providing the genetic tests must provide the patient with assurance that the results will be handled confidentially, and that there will be no access to the genetic information by a third party without written permission of the individual being tested. All genetic testing should be voluntary and it is the nurse's responsibility to ensure that the informed consent process includes discussion of the risks and benefits of the test, including any physical harm as well as potential psychologic and societal injury by stigmatization, discrimination, and emotional stress. Healthcare providers are legally liable to maintain that confidence. Exceptions to the individual's privacy may be made only when the individual refuses to inform extended family members when a very high probability of irreversible harm exists for an extended family member and informing the family member can prevent harm from occurring (National Human Genome Research Institute, 2005).

Psychosocial Issues

Although family and individual anxiety may be decreased with a negative test result, potential problems do exist and the nurse must be prepared to address them. Concerns about carrier status may interfere with development of intimacy and interpersonal relationships. Nonpaternity may be revealed through genetic testing. For example, the parents of a child born with an autosomal recessive condition will be considered carriers of the altered gene the majority of the time. To counsel the parents about future pregnancies, the parents would be tested to confirm their genotype, and nonpaternity may become an issue. A positive test result may lead to feelings of unworthiness, confusion, anger, depression, and self-image disturbance. Survivor guilt may affect adults with negative results if their siblings are positive. The individual carrying a gene alteration for a late-onset disease may have an increased tendency for risky behaviors and may choose not to be a positive member of society. Relatives of an individual affected with a genetic disorder may be very frightened when they realize what their own future might be. The individual who has inherited an altered disease-producing gene may foster deep resentment toward the parent who carries the altered gene. Parents and older generations may feel tremendous guilt for passing the altered gene to their children and grandchildren.

Economic Issues

The nurse should consider the cost of genetic tests, which can range from hundreds to thousands of dollars, depending on the size of the gene being tested. Most insurance companies do not cover genetic tests, but if there is insurance coverage the individual must weigh the cost of allowing the insurance company to have access to the genetic information (HGPb, 2008). Additionally, depending on the information that will be gained from obtaining the test, the family may wish to defer testing if it does not provide better outcomes or change in treatment strategy for the patient.

Assessment

Health Promotion and Health Maintenance

Health promotion and health maintenance of the patient are viewed as goals of nursing care.

With knowledge of genetic conditions, the nurse can ensure health teaching and early detection of complications from genetic conditions with emphasis on primary and secondary care interventions. For example,

- a woman with a strong family history and/or mutations in the *BRCA1* and *BRCA2* tumor suppressor genes should have screening clinical breast exams and mammographies at an earlier age than the general population.
- a man with a strong family history and/or mutations in the *BRCA1* and *BRCA2* tumor suppressor genes should report any mass, tenderness, or swelling in the breast tissue and maintain early screening for prostate cancer.
- colonoscopy screening every 1 to 2 years beginning at age 25 is important for the individual with a positive family history and/or mutations in the *MLH1/MSH2* gene, which increases the risk for hereditary nonpolyposis colorectal cancer.

Patients receiving early intervention and health-promotion-focused care can live longer and with a much better quality of life that those who do not. The nurse must be able to identify both community-based and genetic-based resources that are available to assist the patient in strategies to support both health promotion and health maintenance activities.

Patient Intake and History

Family history has long been a part of nursing assessment, but the relative importance of obtaining a family history has recently increased as our knowledge of the interaction of genes and the environment has expanded. In fact, it is an inexpensive first "genetic screen," often underused by healthcare professionals. Yet, with the number of genetics professionals being less than the projected need, professionals in primary care and other specialties will have to share some of the responsibility in obtaining this information and making appropriate referrals.

Pedigrees

A pedigree is a pictorial representation or diagram of the medical history of a family (typically three generations). Multiple symbols are utilized to present this picture (Figure 8–6 ■) and the finished pedigree presents a family's medical data and biologic

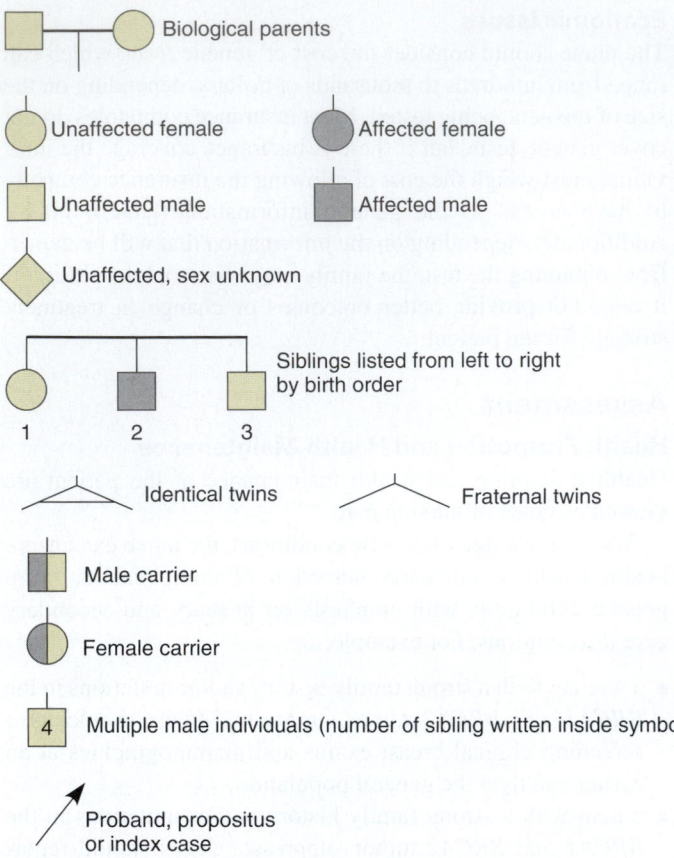

Figure 8–6 ■ Selected standardized symbols for use in drawing a pedigree.

Source: From Ball, Jane W.; Bindler, Ruth McGillis W.; Cowen, Kay J., *Child Health Nursing: Partnering with Children and Families*, 2nd, © 2010. Reproduced by permission of Pearson Education, Inc., Upper Saddle River, New Jersey.

relationship information at a glance (Figure 8–7 ■). A pedigree provides the nurse, genetic counselor, or geneticist with a clear, visual representation of relationships of affected individuals to the immediate and extended family. It can identify other individuals in the family who might benefit from a genetic consultation. It also can identify a single-gene alteration pattern of inheritance or a cluster of multifactorial conditions, and a referral and/or reproductive risk teaching for the individual and family can result. A family's learning can be enhanced by the visual teaching contribution a pedigree can provide and also clarify any inheritance misunderstandings or misconceptions.

By simply integrating into practice the genetic aspects of assessment, observation, and history gathering, the nurse can improve the standard of care delivered and have a positive effect on the patient. The nurse does not need to be a genetic expert, but with heightened awareness, appropriate inquiries and referrals to genetic specialists can be completed.

Nursing Diagnosis and Interventions

Nurses are responsible for comprehensively delivering the correct standard of care to patients, but at the same time being aware of the limitations of their own knowledge and expertise. In addition to the continuous integration of genetic aspects into nurses' assessments of family history and physical assessment, nurses are also responsible for carrying out interventions that include initiating referrals to genetic specialists and delivering

care to the individual or family in any of the following ways. Nursing diagnoses to consider include the following:

- *Grieving*
- *Anxiety*
- *Disturbed Body Image*
- *Ineffective Coping*
- *Decisional Conflict*
- *Interrupted Family Processes*
- *Ineffective Health Maintenance*
- *Deficient Knowledge*
- *Powerlessness*
- *Spiritual Distress*

Genetic Referrals and Counseling

Referral of a patient with a suspected genetic problem to a geneticist, genetic clinical nurse specialist, or genetic clinic is an expected nursing responsibility in the same way as referrals to a dietitian or a social worker. After gathering assessment data that incorporates genetic concepts, the nurse is able to initiate a referral to genetic specialists if there are indicators for a genetic referral (Box 8–9). The nurse should provide the patient with information about the advantages of a referral to genetic specialists, the disadvantages of not following through with the referral, and provide anticipatory guidance as to what to expect from his or her visit (Box 8–10).

Usually before the first genetic evaluation visit, the patient will be contacted to provide a detailed medical and family history and to make an appointment for genetic consultation. The patient should be prepared to give as exact a family history as possible so that a detailed three-generation pedigree can be constructed. The patient should be informed that a genetic consultation usually lasts several hours. During the appointment, a genetic clinical nurse, genetic counselor, and/or a physician will perform an initial interview with the patient. A geneticist will examine the patient in order to establish an accurate diagnosis. Tests may be ordered. These may include chromosome (cytogenetic) analysis, DNA-based testing, x-rays, biopsy, biochemical tests, and linkage studies (Lashley, 2005). After the exam and the completion of any applicable testing, the geneticist and/or genetic counselor will discuss the findings with the patient and make recommendations. The discussion will include the natural history of the condition, the inheritance patterns, the current preventive or treatment options, and the risks to the patient and/or family. The visit will also include opportunities for questions and answers as well as the assessment and evaluation of the patients' understanding. It is typical for the retention of information for a patient facing a new genetic diagnosis to be very low. This makes it imperative for the nurse to take advantage of opportunities to reinforce genetic concepts at a later time when the patient is ready.

As the visit concludes, the patient can expect appropriate referrals to be made, discussion of available services or research studies, and possible scheduling of a follow-up visit. A summary of the information is usually sent to the patient and the patient's healthcare provider will receive a report if requested by the patient.

Genetic healthcare providers present the patient with information to promote informed decisions. They are also sensitive to the importance of protecting the individual's autonomy. A challenge during any visit to a genetic specialist is providing

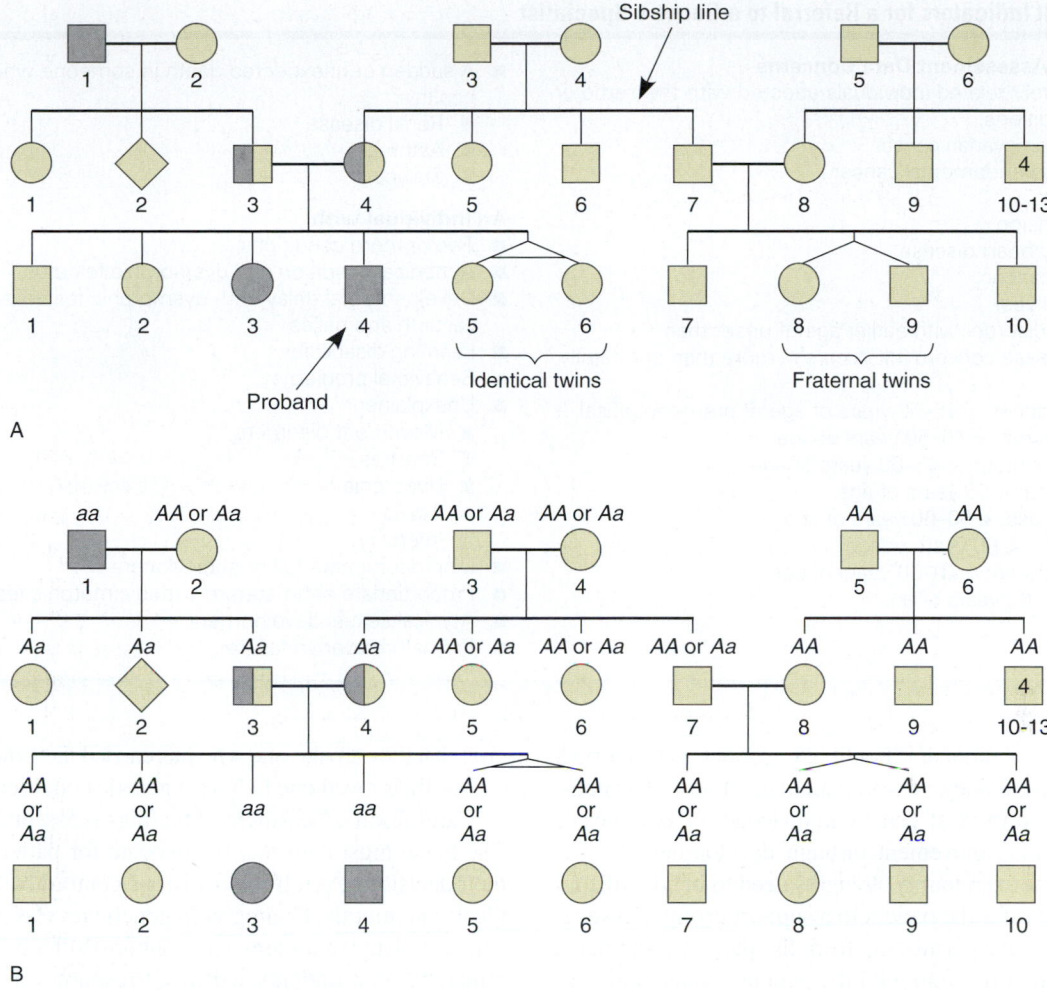

(A) A representative pedigree for a single character or genetic condition through three generations.
(B) The most probable genotypes of each individual in the pedigree for an autosomal recessive condition, represented by AA, Aa, or aa.

Figure 8–7 ■ Sample three-generation pedigree.

Source: Fig. 3.13, p. 63 from *Concepts of Genetics*, 7th ed. by William S. Klug and Michael R. Cummings. Copyright © 2003 by William S. Klug and Michael R. Cummings. Reproduced by permission of Pearson Education, Inc..

nondirective counseling. Patients should be permitted to make decisions that are not influenced by any biases or values from the nurse, counselor, or geneticist. Many patients are accustomed to practitioners and nurses providing direction and guidance in their decision making, and patients may be very uncomfortable with the nondirectional approach of the nurse. They may believe that the nurse or healthcare provider is withholding very bad news. The nurse should discuss the positives and negatives of each decision and present as many options as possible through the use of therapeutic listening and communication skills.

Patient Teaching and Support

The nurse must be aware of available genetic resources and participate in the education of genetic disorders as well as health promotion and prevention. The cultural and religious beliefs and values of the patient must be assessed prior to teaching. Are the gene alterations viewed as uncontrollable and believed to be occurring secondary to cultural belief such as a stranger looking at the patient? Or, are the gene alterations considered a "punishment"? Obtaining educational materials in the native language of the patient will also help facilitate the

teaching–learning experience. Also, identifying and dealing with barriers to learning, such as denial, anxiety, or guilt, will enable teaching to be more useful and effective for the patient and family.

Nurses should encourage open discussions and the expression of fears and concerns. Reinforce to patients that genetic alterations are caused by changes within a gene and not by superstitions related to sin or other cultural beliefs. However, it is important to remember that everyone has superstitions or beliefs and the nurse must remain nonjudgmental. The nurse is responsible for assessing the patient's coping mechanisms as well as available family, spiritual, cultural, and community support systems. Genetic conditions can cause a permanent strain on family dynamics and relationships. The nurse may need to help the patient reaffirm his or her self-worth and value (Lashley, 2005).

Growth and development and meeting adult developmental milestones can be altered by actual or potential genetic disorders. Especially unique is the potential or actual inheritance of a late-onset condition such as Huntington disease. The patient with this altered gene may not meet any of the developmental tasks in

BOX 8–9 Adult Indicators for a Referral to a Genetic Specialist

Adult History Assessment Data Concerns
- Several closely related individuals affected with the same or related conditions:
  - Breast and ovarian cancer
  - Colon and endometrial cancer
  - Diabetes
  - Hypertension
  - Coronary heart disease
  - Thyroid cancer
  - Colon polyps
- A common disorder with earlier age of onset than typical (increase concern if it occurs in more than one family member):
  - Breast cancer: < 45–50 years of age or premenopausal
  - Colon cancer: < 45–50 years of age
  - Prostate cancer: < 45–60 years of age
  - Vision loss: < 55 years of age
  - Hearing loss: < 50–60 years of age
  - Dementia: < 60 years of age
  - Heart disease: < 40–60 years of age
  - Stroke: < 60 years of age

- A sudden or unexpected death in someone who seemed healthy:
  - Renal disease
  - Asthma
  - Suicide

An Individual with:
- Two or more conditions
- A medical condition and dysmorphic features
- Developmental delay with dysmorphic features and/or physical birth anomalies
- Learning disabilities
- Behavioral problems
- Unexplained:
  - Movement disorders
  - Seizures
  - Hypotonia
  - Ataxia
  - Infertility
- Disproportionate tall or short stature
- Proportionate short stature with dysmorphic features
- Atypical sexual development
- Premature ovarian failure

moving through adulthood. Should the patient get married, attend college, save money, or worry about the future? The nurse must identify the impact of genetic knowledge on activities of daily living but also movement through developmental milestones. Both patient and family strengths need to be identified.

The nurse can refer the patient to a support group. However it is important to have permission from the patient if the nurse is providing a support group with the patient's name and contact information.

Another key role for the nurse is to help patients with the often difficult task of communicating genetic information such as inheritance patterns to extended family members. Cultural values of autonomy and privacy are affected when a patient must consider whether to communicate genetic information to extended family members who may also carry the altered gene. The history of a genetic alteration that may or may not cause disease can be extensive within a family, affecting multiple family members. Family members often have difficulty understanding that some genetic conditions have variable expressivity. Members of the extended family often are shocked and feel a profound sense of

guilt that they are the one who has carried the gene alteration that caused their loved one to have a genetic condition.

Careful self-assessment of feelings is essential for the nurse. The nurse must continually advocate for patients and support their decisions even if the decisions contradict the nurse's own ideals and morals. Coping with genetic revelations and making genetic-related treatment decisions are difficult. The nurse must remember that patients will need resources and support, and also help in gathering information about reproductive options.

Evaluation

Expected outcomes of delivering nursing care with a genetic focus include the following:

- The patient will make informed and voluntary decisions related to genetic health issues.
- The patient will accurately identify the following:
  - Basic genetic concepts and simple inheritance risk probabilities
  - What to expect from a genetic referral
  - The influence of genetic factors in health promotion and health maintenance
  - Differences between medical and genetic tests
  - Social, legal, and ethical issues related to genetic testing

BOX 8–10 Genetic Information Nondiscrimination Act of 2008 (GINA)

After 13 years of debate, on May 21, 2008, President George W. Bush signed into law the Genetic Information Nondiscrimination Act of 2008 (GINA). The purpose of this federal law is to protect consumers from discrimination by employers and health insurance companies based on genetic information. Examples of protected tests are BRCA1/BRCA2 (breast cancer); Huntington's disease; and carrier screening for cystic fibrosis, sickle cell anemia, and cystic fibrosis. The health insurance regulations will take place 1 year after legislation was signed, while employment regulations are effective 6 months after signing. Some of the things not covered under GINA are life, disability, or long-term care insurance, and members of the military.

Visions for the Future

Nurses are often the primary caregivers to whom patients turn for information, guidance, and clarification of ideas. This nursing role is essential not only in providing direct nursing care but as a member of the community. As more information about the genetic revolution becomes available to consumers—in areas such as pharmacogenomics, gene transfer, ethics, genetic engineering, and stem cell research—the role of nurses remains not only vital but grows enormously. Nurses should remain educated, informed, knowledgeable, and ready to discuss trends and changes with patients and their families.

CHAPTER HIGHLIGHTS

■ Nurses are responsible for basic genetic knowledge and delivering the expected standard of genetic nursing care. The nurse must be aware of the social, ethical, cultural, and spiritual issues related to the delivery of genetic nursing care.

■ When cell division does not occur as expected, chromosomal alterations on the autosomes or sex chromosomes can result. Chromosomal alterations can be seen in a human karyotype.

■ An individual may be identified as heterozygous or homozygous for a single gene. Some gene alterations cause disease and some are protective from disease. Multifactorial inheritance does not follow Mendelian inheritance patterns.

■ Many types of genetic tests are available. All genetic tests have special considerations related to social, financial, ethical, and legal implications. Genetic healthcare providers are obligated to present the individual and his or her family with information to promote informed decisions.

■ Basic genetic nursing care involves family risk assessment through a detailed family history, integrating genetic concepts into a physical assessment, and initiating a referral to a genetic specialist.

■ Genetic concepts can be applied to health promotion and health maintenance. Knowledge of the principles of inheritance allows the nurse to not only offer and reinforce genetic information to patients and their families but also to assist them in managing their care and in making reproductive decisions.

TEST YOURSELF NCLEX-RN® REVIEW

1. The patient is discussing the inheritance of an autosomal dominant trait. The patient has the condition and the patient's wife does not. They have one child without the condition. The nurse would be correct in explaining to the patient that he is most likely which genotype?
   1. FF
   2. Ff
   3. ff
   4. X_fY

2. A male patient diagnosed with Fabry disease is admitted to the unit. Which statement made by the patient would indicate to the nurse that the patient understands Mendelian inheritance concepts? "I have the disease because... **Select all that apply.**
   1. my mother had Fabry and my father did not."
   2. my father's mother had Fabry disease."
   3. my grandmother's brother had Fabry disease."
   4. my father has Fabry disease."

3. The nurse is providing information regarding genetic testing to a couple who believe they are carriers of an autosomal recessive gene alteration. Which statement by the nurse is appropriate?
   1. "If both of you are carriers, all of your sons will be affected and all of your daughters will be carriers."
   2. "Chromosomal studies will reveal if you are actually a carrier."
   3. "Newborn screening will reveal if your child is affected."
   4. "During the genetic evaluation, you will be asked to provide at least a three-generation family history."

4. When analyzing a family pedigree, the nurse notes the pedigree demonstrates that successive generations contain affected individuals, both males and females are affected, and there is no father-to-offspring inheritance. What is the most likely pattern of inheritance?
   1. autosomal dominant
   2. autosomal recessive
   3. x-linked recessive
   4. mitochondrial

5. When the nurse is developing a teaching plan, which statement is a correct rationale regarding the health promotion and health maintenance benefits from an assessment of family history?
   1. Clinical treatment options can be more focused.
   2. Prophylactic treatments can be started early.
   3. Specific diet, exercise regimen, and genotype can be determined.
   4. Single-gene alteration can be diagnosed.

6. When developing a teaching plan for a patient with a newly diagnosed genetic disorder, what is the rationale for including time for questions and answers?
   1. genetic disorders frequently are accompanied by learning difficulty
   2. retention of information is typically low at this time
   3. the information is complex and high-level
   4. many patients do not want to know this information

7. The patient asks the nurse if a genetic referral is necessary. Which information would be appropriate for the nurse to provide? Most likely genetic specialists will do which of the following? **Select all that apply.**
   1. Provide direction for important decision making.
   2. Complete chromosomal studies.
   3. Ask to see photographs of relatives.
   4. Provide information about the natural history of the condition.

8. The nurse would consider which assessment finding(s) as minor anomalies? **Select all that apply.**
   1. café au lait spots
   2. ear pits
   3. atrial septal defect (ASD)
   4. hypertelorism

9. A young man has a positive family history for mutations of the MLH/MLH2 gene. What would the nurse recommend?
   1. clinical breast examinations annually
   2. self-testing of blood glucose daily
   3. colonoscopy screening every 1 to 2 years
   4. hematocrit levels every 3 months

10. What was one purpose of the Genetic Information Nondiscrimination Act (GINA), signed into law in 2008?
    1. protection against gender bias in the workplace
    2. guidelines for specific sexual harassment activities
    3. mandated genetic testing for all government employees and their children
    4. protection against discrimination by employers based on genetic information

See Test Yourself answers in Appendix C.

Pearson Nursing Student Resources

Find additional review materials at
nursing.pearsonhighered.com

Prepare for success with additional NCLEX®-style practice questions, interactive assignments and activities, Web links, animations and videos, and more!

BIBLIOGRAPHY

American Nurses Association and International Society of Nurses in Genetics, Inc. (2007). *Statement on the scope and standards of genetics clinical nursing practice.* Washington, DC: American Nurses Publishing.

Bradley, A. (2005). Utility and limitations of genetic testing information. *Nursing Standard, 20*(5), 52–55.

Burke, W. (2004). Genetic testing in primary care. *Annual Review Genomics: Human Genetics, 5*, 1–14.

Chinnery, P. F. (2005, April 12). Leber hereditary optic neuropathy. In *GeneReviews at GeneTests: Medical Genetics Information Resource* [Online database]. University of Washington, Seattle, 1997–2005. Retrieved from http://www.genetests.org

Dietz, H. C. (2005, October 26). Marfan syndrome. In *GeneReviews at GeneTests: Medical Genetics Information Resource* [Online database]. University of Washington, Seattle, 1997–2005. Retrieved from http://www.genetests.org

Duncan, R., Savulescu, J., & Gillam, L. et al., (2005). An international survey of predictive genetic testing in children for adult onset conditions. *Genetics in Medicine, 7*(6), 390–396.

Gene reviews. In *GeneTests: Medical Genetics Information Resource* [Online database]. University of Washington, Seattle, 1993–2005. Retrieved from http://www.genetests.org

Genetics Home Reference (2008). *Genes: APOE.* Retrieved from http://ghr.nlm.nih.gov/gene=apoe

Giusti, R., Badgwell, A., Iglesias, A. D., & New York State Cystic Fibrosis Newborn Screening Consortium. (2007). New York State Cystic Fibrosis Consortium: The first 2.5 years of experience with cystic fibrosis newborn screening in an ethnically diverse population. *Pediatrics, 119*, e460–e467.

Guttmacher, A. E., Collins, F. S., & Carmona, R. H. (2004). The family history—more important than ever. *New England Journal of Medicine, 35*(22), 2333–2336.

Hudson, K., Holohan, M., & Collins, F. (2008). Keeping pace with the times – the genetic information nondiscrimination act of 2008. *The New England Journal of Medicine, 358*(25), 2661–2663.

Human Genome Project. (2008a). *From genome to the proteome.* Retrieved from http://www.ornl.gov/sci/techresources/Human_Genome/project/info.shtml

Human Genome Project. (2008b). *Gene testing.* Retrieved from http://www.ornl.gov/sci/techresources/Human_Genome/medicine/genetest.shtml

Human Genome Project. (2008c). *SNP fact sheet.* Retrieved from http://www.ornl.gov/techresources/Human_Genome/faq/snps.shtml

International Society of Nurses in Genetics. (2005). *Position statement: Informed decision-making consent: The role of the nurse.* Retrieved from http://www.isong.org/about/position_statements/index.html

Jones, K. L. (2005). *Smith's recognizable patterns of human malformations* (6th ed.). Philadelphia: Saunders.

Klug, W. S., Cummings, M. R., Spencer, C., & Palladino, M. A. (2009). *Concepts of genetics* (8th ed.). Upper Saddle River, NJ: Pearson/Prentice Hall.

Klug, W. S., Cummings, M. R., Spencer, C., & Palladino, M. A. (2010). *Essentials of genetics.* (7th ed.). Upper Saddle River, NJ: Pearson/Prentice Hall.

Lashley, F. R. (2005). *Clinical genetics in nursing practice.* (3rd ed.). New York: Springer.

Lea, D. (2008, January). Genetic and genomic healthcare: Ethical issues of importance to nurses. *The Online Journal of Issues in Nursing*, Vol. 13, No. 1.

Levy, H. P. (2007, May 1). Ehlers-Danlos Syndrome, Hypermoblity Type I. *Gene reviews.* In *GeneTests: Medical Genetics Information Resource.* Retrieved from http://www.ncbi.nlm.nih.gov/sites/GeneTests/?db=GeneTests [Online database].

Mayo Clinic. (2008). *Children's Health: Down Syndrome.* Retrieved from www.mayoclinic.com

National Cancer Institute. (2009). *Chronic myelogenous leukemia.* Retrieved from http://www.cancer.gov

National Coalition for Health Professional Education in Genetics. (2005). *Core competencies in genetics essential for all health-care professionals.* Retrieved from http://www.nchpeg.org

National Human Genome Research Institute. (2008). *FISH Fact Sheet.* Retrieved from http://www.genome.gov/10000206

Nussbaum, R. L., McInnes, R. R., Willard, H. F., & Boerkoel, C. F. (2007). *Thompson & Thompson genetics in medicine* (6th ed.). Philadelphia: Saunders.

Online Mendelian Inheritance in Man. (2003). McKusick-Nathans Institute for Genetics Medicine, Johns Hopkins University (Baltimore, MD) and National Center for Biotechnology Information Library of Medicine (Bethesda, MD). Retrieved from http://www.ncbi.nlm.nih.gov/omim/

Ryan, F., Byrne, S., & O'Shea, S. (2008). Managing oral anticoagulation therapy: Improving clinical outcomes: A review. *Journal of Clinical Pharmacy and Therapeutics. 33*, 581–590.

Theos, A., &, Korf, B. (2006). Pathophysiology of neurofibromatosis type 1. *Annals of Internal Medicine, 144*(11), 842–849.

U.S. Department of Energy Biological and Environmental Research Source. (2008). *Gene gateway—Exploring genes and genetic disorders.* Retrieved from http://www.ornl.gov/TechResources/Human_Genome/posters/chromosome/

U.S. Department of Energy Genome Programs. (2008). *Genomics and its impact on science and society: The human genome project and beyond.* Retrieved from http://www.ornl.gov/hgmis/publicat/primer/

U.S. National Library of Medicine (2008). *Genetics home reference.* Retrieved from http://ghr.nlm.nih.gov/

Winkleman, C. (2004). Genomics: What every critical care nurse needs to know about the genetic contribution to critical illness. *Critical Care Nurse, 24*(3), 34–35.

Nursing Care of Patients in **Pain**

LEARNING OUTCOMES

1. Describe the neurophysiology of pain.
2. Compare and contrast definitions and characteristics of acute, chronic, central, malignant, phantom, and psychogenic pain.
3. Discuss factors affecting individualized responses to pain.
4. Discuss interdisciplinary care for the patient in pain, including medications, surgery, transcutaneous electrical nerve stimulation, and complementary therapies.
5. Use the nursing process as a framework for providing individualized nursing care for patients experiencing pain.

CLINICAL COMPETENCIES

1. Assess patients' pain intensity, quality, location, pattern, intensifiers, relievers; side effects of analgesics; and effect on function and mood.
2. Determine patient's expressed desire, values, preference, and support for pain management.
3. In collaboration with the healthcare team, intervene with appropriate evidence-based pharmacologic and nonpharmacologic methodologies. Revise plan of care according to patient's response to interventions and need for control.
4. Use equianalgesia tables to select and transition between opioid analgesics.
5. Teach patients about safe and effective self-management of pain.
6. Evaluate effectiveness of interventions to relieve pain and promote comfort; re-treat or adjust doses of medication and interventions as necessary.

KEY TERMS

acute pain, *163*
addiction, *166*
analgesic, *167*
breakthrough pain, *165*

chronic pain, *164*
equianalgesic, *168*
neuropathic pain, *165*
nociceptive pain, *165*

nociceptors, *161*
pain, *159*
titrate, *172*

Pain is a subjective response to both physical and psychologic stressors. All people experience pain at some point during their lives. An estimated 50 million Americans live with chronic pain; low back pain is one of the most common types of chronic pain, along with migraine or severe headache and joint pain. Another 25 million experience acute pain related to surgery or trauma (American Academy of Pain Management, 2009; Centers for Disease Control and Prevention [CDC], 2006). Although pain as a health condition falls within the cognitive-perceptual health pattern, its effects have the potential to cause dysfunction in all functional health patterns, whether the pain is acute, chronic, severe, or mild to moderate.

FAST FACTS

- More than 25% of adults report low back pain within the past 3 months.
- Approximately 15% of adults, most between age 18 and 44, experience recurrent migraine or severe headache.
- Pain is common among older adults, with 20% reporting pain lasting more than 24 hours within the past month (CDC, 2006).

Although pain usually is experienced as uncomfortable and unwelcome, it also serves a protective role, warning of potentially health-threatening conditions. For this reason, pain is increasingly referred to as the *fifth vital sign*, with recommendations to assess pain with each vital sign assessment. The Joint Commission (2001) established pain standards that identify the relief of pain as a patient right. Joint Commission standards require healthcare facilities to implement specific procedures for, and provider education on, pain assessment and management.

Pain is a distinct and personal experience influenced by physiologic, psychologic, cognitive, sociocultural, and spiritual factors. It is the symptom most associated with describing oneself as ill, and it is the most common reason for seeking health care. The International Association for the Study of Pain (IASP) defines pain as an unpleasant sensory and emotional experience associated with actual or potential tissue damage, or described in terms of such damage. Although there are many definitions and descriptors of pain, the one most relevant for nurses is that pain is "whatever the person experiencing it says it is, and existing whenever the person says it does" (McCaffery, 1979, p. 11). This definition acknowledges the patient as the only person who can accurately define and describe his or her own pain and serves as the basis for nursing assessment and care of patients in pain. It also supports the values and beliefs about pain necessary for holistic nursing care, including the following:

- Only the person affected can experience pain; that is, pain has a personal meaning.
- If the patient says he or she has pain, the patient is in pain. All pain is real.
- Pain has physical, emotional, cognitive, sociocultural, and spiritual dimensions.
- Pain affects the whole body, usually negatively.
- Pain may serve as both a response to and a warning of actual or potential trauma.

Myths and Misconceptions about Pain

Myths and misconceptions about pain and its management are common in both healthcare providers and patients. Some of the most common of these myths are included here.

- *Pain is a result, not a cause.*   According to the traditional view of pain, pain is a symptom, not a condition. Pain is now recognized to have both immediate and long-term effects, such as immobility, anger, and anxiety; pain may also delay healing and rehabilitation.
- *Chronic pain is really a masked form of depression.* Serotonin plays a chemical role in pain transmission and is also the major modulator of depression. Therefore, pain and depression are chemically related, not mutually exclusive. It is common to find them coexisting.
- *Narcotic medication is too risky to be used in chronic pain.*   This common misconception often deprives patients of the most effective source of pain relief. Opioid (narcotic) analgesics are now recognized as an appropriate strategy for managing chronic pain unrelieved by other strategies.
- *It is best to wait until a patient has pain before giving medication.*   Relieving pain before it escalates is widely accepted as having a noticeable effect on the amount of pain a patient experiences.
- *Many patients lie about the existence or severity of their pain.*   Very few patients lie about their pain.
- *Pain relief interferes with diagnosis.*   Effective pain management with analgesics in the emergency department (ED) has been shown to have no impact on physical assessment findings or diagnosis (Pasero, 2003).

Neurophysiology of Pain

The peripheral nervous system has two types of neurons: sensory and motor. The pain experience involves both sensory stimulation and perception. Pain stimuli are generated and transmitted through the sensory neurons, perceived within the central nervous system, and responded to through the motor neurons. Connections or synapses occur within the spinal cord and again within the brain, where interpretation of the painful stimulus leads to a response. A pain stimulus may prompt an immediate reflex response that precedes awareness of the pain.

Pain Theories

Several theories explain the response to pain and the diversity of human experiences with pain. The meaning or perception of pain can be modified by past experiences, motivation, attention, suggestion, personality, and culture. *Specificity* and *pattern* theories describe nerve impulses of varying intensity terminating in pain centers in the forebrain. These theories provide explanations of the neurophysiologic basis of pain. Later, in 1965, Melzack and Wall postulated the *gate-control theory* (Helms & Barone, 2008). According to this theory, activation of large-diameter, faster-propagating fibers by a tactile stimulus (e.g., massaging the elbow after hitting it on a sharp object) activates a gating mechanism that then blocks impulses from smaller pain fibers (Porth & Matfin, 2009). This mechanism was thought to exist at the segmental spinal cord level (Figure 9–1 ■).

Ongoing research demonstrates that the control and modulation of pain is much more complex than the description in the gate-control theory, which served as a base for further research about pain-modulating systems Tactile information is now known to be transmitted by both large- and small-diameter fibers, and interaction between sensory neurons is known to occur at multiple levels of the central nervous system. Melzack subsequently developed the *neuromatrix* theory of pain to integrate cultural and genetic factors with basic neurophysiologic function. This theory is consistent with but more complex than the gate-control theory. According to the neuromatrix theory, the brain contains a *body-self neuromatrix*, a widely distributed network of neurons that is affected by both genetic factors and sensory experiences. The neuromatrix integrates multiple sources of input in addition to the stimuli of pain and touch. The pain experience for the individual is affected by inputs from other sensory systems that help interpret the stimuli (e.g., seeing

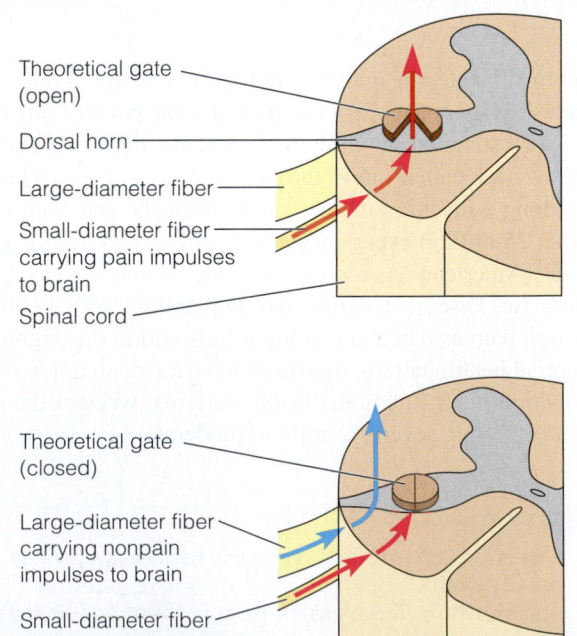

Theoretical gate (open)

Dorsal horn

Large-diameter fiber

Small-diameter fiber carrying pain impulses to brain

Spinal cord

Theoretical gate (closed)

Large-diameter fiber carrying nonpain impulses to brain

Small-diameter fiber carrying pain impulses

Figure 9–1 ■ The spinal cord component of the gate-control theory. Pain transmission by small-diameter fibers is blocked when large-diameter fibers carrying touch impulses dominate, closing the gate in the dorsal horn of the spinal cord.

a wound); factors such as attention, expectation, personality, and culture; innate pain modulation systems; and components of stress-regulation systems (Porth & Matfin, 2009).

One pain theory that is quite significant in clinical terms describes the effect of sensitizing the central and peripheral nervous system to painful stimuli. According to this theory, painful signals create a cascade of changes in the nervous system that increase the responsiveness of the peripheral and central neurons. These changes, in turn, increase the response to future signals and amplify pain. Studies of infants undergoing painful procedures show that those who received analgesia experienced reduced sensitivity to future painful events, while those who did not receive analgesia experienced greater sensitivity (Taddio & Katz, 2005). Sensitization occurs from nociceptive barrage as well as inflammation that follows the injury or incision. In adults this theory indicates the value of preventing sensitization as well as treating perceived pain with multimodal pain therapy. Local and regional anesthesia used in combination with central anesthesia prior to incision to diminish sensitization of these pathways results in significantly reduced consumption of intravenous morphine by PCA in the 5 days following surgery (Hartrick, 2004).

Physiology

Nerve receptors for pain are called **nociceptors** (Figure 9–2 ■). These free nerve endings are woven throughout all the tissues of the body except the brain. Nociceptors are especially numerous in the skin and muscles. Pain occurs when the tissue containing nociceptors is subjected to a noxious insult. The intensity and duration of the stimuli determine the sensation. Long-lasting, intense stimulation produces greater pain than brief, mild stimulation.

Nociceptors respond to several different types of noxious stimuli: mechanical, chemical, or thermal. Some nociceptors respond to only a single type of stimulus, whereas others respond to all three types of stimuli (Table 9–1). The perception of pain in different parts of the body is affected by this variation in sensitivity to type of stimulus and the distribution of nociceptors in various tissues.

Tissue trauma, inflammation, and ischemia prompt the release of a number of biochemicals. These biochemicals have several effects. Chemicals such as bradykinin, histamine, serotonin, and potassium ion directly stimulate nociceptors, producing pain. These chemicals and others (such as ATP and prostaglandins) also sensitize nociceptors, intensifying the pain response and causing normally innocuous stimuli (such as touch) to be perceived as pain. Chemical mediators also act to perpetuate inflammation, which, in turn, causes release of additional chemicals that stimulate pain receptors. Furthermore, so-called *silent nociceptors* (e.g., sensory receptors in the gut that normally do not respond to mechanical or thermal stimuli) can become sensitive to mechanical stimuli in the presence of inflammatory mediators, leading to severe and debilitating pain and tenderness (Fauci et al., 2008).

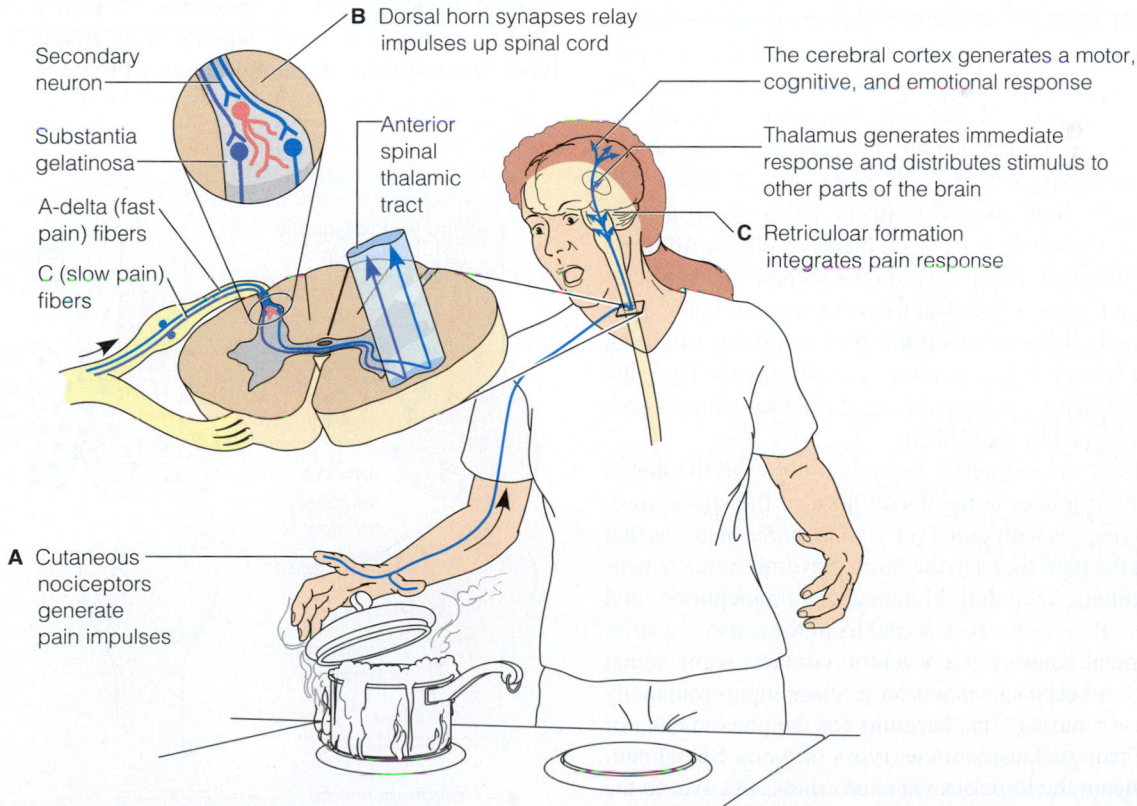

Figure 9–2 ■ *A,* Touching the hot lid activates nociceptors in the skin, generating pain impulses that travel via fast Aδ and slower C fibers to the spinal cord. *B,* Secondary neurons in the dorsal horn pass impulses across the spinal cord to the anterior spinothalamic tract. *C,* Pain impulses ascend to the thalamus and, from there, to the cerebral cortex and the reticular and limbic systems in the brainstem, which integrate the emotional, cognitive, and autonomic responses to pain.

TABLE 9–1 Painful Stimuli

STIMULUS	EXAMPLES
Chemical	■ Ischemia (e.g., angina, bowel infarct) ■ Tissue trauma ■ Inflammation, inflammatory mediators such as histamine, prostaglandins
Mechanical	■ Spasm (ureteral colic, gallstones) ■ Compression (e.g., mechanical or by a tumor, carpal tunnel syndrome, or compartment syndrome) ■ Extreme muscle stretch or contraction (e.g., following a fracture)
Thermal	■ Contact with extreme heat or cold

Pain Pathways

The neural pathways of pain are illustrated in Figure 9–1 and can be summarized as follows:

1. A noxious stimulus is translated by nociceptors into an action potential that then is transmitted through small A-delta (Aδ) and even smaller C nerve fibers to the spinal cord. Aδ fibers are myelinated and transmit impulses rapidly. They produce what is called *fast pain* or first pain—sharp, well-defined pain sensations, such as those that result from cuts, electric shocks, or the impact of a blow. Aδ fibers are associated with acute pain from mechanical or thermal injury. C fibers are not myelinated and thus transmit pain impulses more slowly. Pain transmitted by C fibers may be described as *slow-wave pain* or second pain because it is slower to develop and lasts longer. This pain is more often prompted by chemical stimuli or persistent mechanical or thermal stimuli (Porth & Matfin, 2009). The pain from deep body structures (such as muscles and viscera) is primarily transmitted by C fibers, producing diffuse burning or aching sensations. C fibers are associated with chronic pain. Both Aδ and C fibers are involved in most injuries. For example, if a person bangs an elbow, Aδ fibers transmit this pain stimulus within 0.1 second, and can actually prompt reflex withdrawal from the stimulus before pain is perceived. The person feels this pain as a sharp, localized, smarting sensation. One or more seconds after the blow, the person experiences a duller, aching, diffuse sensation of pain impulses carried by the C fibers.

2. The sensory neuron enters the spinal cord via the dorsal root and terminates in the dorsal horn of the spinal cord. Here it synapses with spinal (or *second-order*) neurons that transmit the pain signal to the brain. Several chemical neurotransmitters, including glutamate, norepinephrine, and substance P, carry the pain signal from the sensory neuron to the spinal neurons. Each neuron contacts many spinal neurons, and each spinal neuron receives input from many peripheral neurons. This accounts for the phenomenon of referred pain (discussed under types of pain). Spinal neurons transmit the impulses via axons that cross over to the spinothalamic tract.

3. The impulses ascend the spinothalamic tracts and pass through the medulla and midbrain to the thalamus.

4. From the thalamus, the pain signal is distributed via third-order neurons to several areas of the cerebral cortex. The somatosensory area of the cerebral cortex localizes the pain and interprets its intensity and quality. Other thalamic neurons reach areas of the frontal lobe, generating an emotional or affective response to pain. Connections to the reticular and limbic systems of the brain also are involved in the emotional and autonomic responses to painful stimuli. Pain signals to these areas can activate the "fight or flight" response, stress responses, and cardiovascular changes. A noxious impulse becomes pain when the sensation reaches conscious levels and is perceived and evaluated by the person experiencing the sensation.

Pain Modulation

No two people experience pain from an identical stimulus in the same way or at the same intensity; furthermore, the same person may perceive pain from the same stimulus differently on different occasions. A number of neural and chemical responses explain some of these differences.

Neural circuits that are thought to arise in the cerebral cortex link with the hypothalamus, midbrain, and medulla. These circuits interact with peripheral sensory axon terminals in the dorsal horn of the spinal cord to selectively control neurons that transmit pain signals. As a result, that pain response can be modified, that is, changed, increased, or dampened. Neurons within this circuit produce *endogenous opioids*, naturally occurring morphine-like neuropeptides. They also contain opioid receptors sensitive to endorphins and opioid drugs. Four types of endogenous opioids have been identified: enkephalins, endorphins, dynorphins, and endomorphins. They are hormones that act like neurotransmitters, binding with opioid receptors to block transmission of painful stimuli (Figure 9–3 ■). These

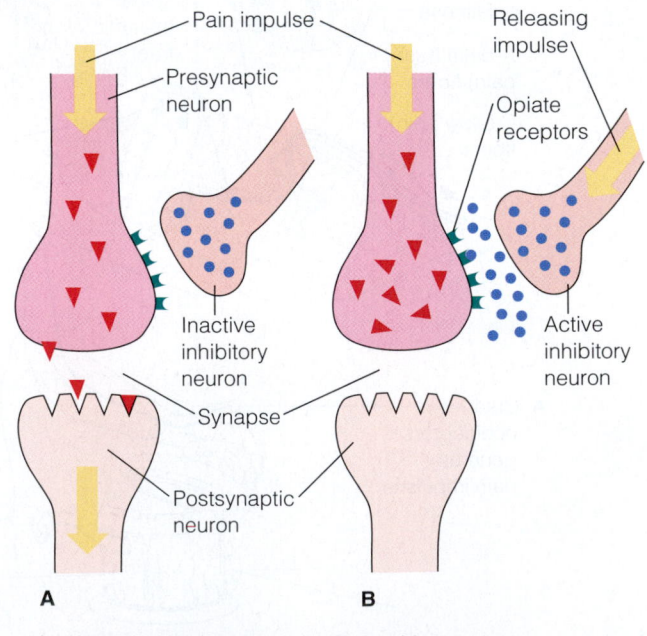

▲ = Neurotransmitters   • = Endorphins

Figure 9–3 ■ *A,* Pain impulse causes presynaptic neuron to release burst of neurotransmitters across synapse. These bind to postsynaptic neuron and propagate impulse. *B,* Inhibitory neuron releases endorphins, which bind to presynaptic opiate receptors. Neurotransmitter release is inhibited, and pain impulse interrupted.

substances also have been linked to a general sense of well-being (McCance & Huether, 2010).

Chemicals such as peptides and neurotransmitters also affect responses to pain stimuli. Locally, inflammatory mediators (e.g., prostaglandins, nitric oxide, histamine) lower the threshold for pain perception and tend to augment pain. ATP, substance P, and other peptides promote the local spread of pain and contribute to vasodilation and vascular permeability, increasing discomfort (McCance & Huether, 2010). In contrast, substances such as serotonin, norepinephrine, and others inhibit pain impulse transmission in the spinal cord and brain.

Types and Characteristics of Pain

Pain typically is described and characterized in several ways: by its duration (acute or chronic), its source or location, and referral.

Acute Pain

Acute pain has a sudden onset, is usually self-limited, and is localized. The cause of acute pain generally can be identified ("I tripped and twisted my ankle; now it really hurts"). The onset is usually sudden, most often resulting from tissue injury from trauma, surgery, or inflammation. The pain is usually sharp and localized, although it may radiate. Tissue healing relieves the pain. The three major types of acute pain are the following:

- *Cutaneous and deep somatic pain*, which arises from nerve receptors originating in the skin (e.g., from a laceration), subcutaneous tissues, or deep body structures such as periosteum, muscles, tendons, joints, and blood vessels (acute pain

from a fracture or sprain, for example). Somatic pain may be either sharp and well localized, or dull and diffuse.

- *Visceral pain*, which arises from body organs. Visceral pain is dull and poorly localized because of the low number of nociceptors. The viscera are sensitive to stretching, inflammation, and ischemia but relatively insensitive to cutting and temperature extremes. Visceral pain often radiates or is referred. It may be described as deep cramping, splitting or stabbing pain, intermittent pain, or colicky pain. A kidney stone passing through the ureter to the bladder causes severe, acute visceral pain.

- *Referred pain* is pain that is perceived in an area distant from the site of the stimuli. It commonly occurs with pain that originates in thoracic or abdominal viscera. Visceral sensory fibers synapse at the level of the spinal cord, close to fibers innervating other subcutaneous tissue areas of the body (Figure 9–4 ■). For example, the phrenic nerve, which innervates the central part of the diaphragm enters the spinal cord at the C3 to C5 level; pain originating in the diaphragm or the parietal peritoneum lining it (e.g., peritonitis) may be perceived as shoulder pain. Sites of referred pain are determined during embryologic development.

Acute pain warns of actual or potential injury to tissues. As a stressor, it initiates the fight-or-flight autonomic stress response. Characteristic physical responses include tachycardia, rapid and shallow respirations, increased blood pressure, dilated pupils, sweating, and pallor. The pain may be accompanied by nausea and vomiting. Secondary reflex muscle spasms may develop, intensifying the pain. The person experiencing acute pain responds to this threat with anxiety and fear. This psychologic

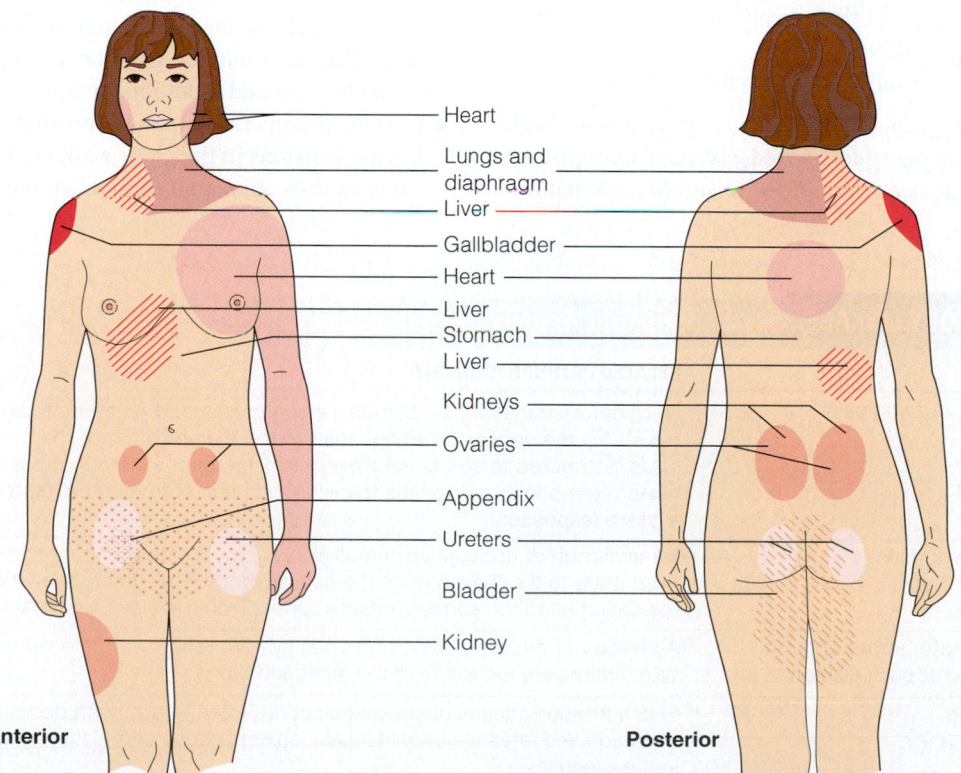

Heart
Lungs and diaphragm
Liver
Gallbladder
Heart
Liver
Stomach
Liver
Kidneys
Ovaries
Appendix
Ureters
Bladder
Kidney

Anterior

Posterior

Figure 9–4 ■ Referred pain results of the convergence of sensory nerves from certain areas of the body within the spinal cord. For example, a toothache may be felt in the ear, pain from inflammation of the diaphragm may be felt in the shoulder, and pain from ischemia of the heart muscle (angina) may be felt in the left arm.

response may further increase the physical responses to acute pain. The accompanying Pathophysiology Linkage box describes manifestations of pain with an abbreviated explanation of the pathophysiology underlying the manifestation.

Chronic Pain

Chronic pain is prolonged pain, or pain that persists after the condition causing it has resolved. Although the cause may be identifiable (e.g., arthritis, cancer, migraine headache, diabetic neuropathy), chronic pain does not always have an identifiable cause. In some cases, pain may be perpetuated by disease-caused damage that persists after the disease has resolved (e.g., sensory nerve damage or reflex muscle contraction). In others, an imbalance of pain modulation mechanisms is thought to cause the persistent pain. This imbalance may relate to changes in the peripheral nervous system such as increased neuronal sensitivity to stimuli (a lower pain threshold) or spontaneous impulse generation by damaged neurons. Changes in the dorsal root, spinal cord, and brain also affect pain modulation. Repeated stimulation of peripheral nerves leads to a progressive buildup of electrical response in the central nervous system (CNS), leading to more intense and prolonged pain.

Unlike acute pain, chronic pain has much more complex and poorly understood neurophysiology and purpose. Persistent chronic pain often serves no useful function. The pain itself becomes the problem, creating physical, psychosocial, and economic stresses on the affected individual and his or her family. Furthermore, emotional and psychologic factors can cause the pain itself or make it worse. There is a clear association between chronic pain and depression. Depletion of serotonin (a neurotransmitter) and endorphins, found in both chronic pain and in depression, suggest common physiology in these disorders (Porth & Matlin, 2009).

Chronic pain can be subdivided into three categories:

- *Recurrent acute pain*, characterized by relatively well-defined episodes of pain interspersed with pain-free episodes. Migraine headache is an example of recurrent acute pain.
- *Chronic malignant pain*, caused by advance of a life-threatening disease or associated with treatment. Cancer pain is a type of chronic malignant pain.
- *Chronic nonmalignant pain*, non-life-threatening pain that nevertheless persists beyond the expected time for healing. Chronic lower back pain, a major cause of suffering and lost work time, falls into this category.

Patients with chronic pain often do not have the same physiologic responses to pain as are seen in acute pain. The heart and respiratory rates and blood pressure may remain within the normal range. Other autonomic nervous system responses such as nausea, vomiting, pallor, or sweating may not occur with persistent pain. The patient with chronic pain often is depressed, may have difficulty sleeping, and may be preoccupied with the pain. Table 9–2 compares acute and chronic pain.

The most common chronic pain condition is lower back pain. Other common chronic pain conditions include the following (McCance & Huether, 2010):

- *Myofascial pain syndromes* are marked by injury to or disease of muscle and fascia. They include myositis, fibrositis, myofibrositis, myalgia, and muscle strain. Pain results from muscle spasm, stiffness, and collection of lactic acid in the muscle. The pain leads to *guarding* (a defensive tensing of the muscle) and limited motion, which, in turn, leads to weakness, stiffness, and spasm—and more pain.
- Cancer often produces chronic pain, usually due to factors such as tumor growth that presses on nerves or other structures, stretching of viscera, obstruction of ducts, or metastasis to bones. The malignant tumor also may mechanically stimulate pain or the production of biochemicals that cause pain. Pain also may be associated with treatments such as chemotherapy and radiation therapy.
- Chronic postoperative pain is uncommon, but may occur following incisions in the chest wall, radical mastectomy, radical neck dissection, and surgical amputation.

PATHOPHYSIOLOGY LINKAGE	Acute Pain and Associated Manifestations
MANIFESTATION	**RELATED PATHOPHYSIOLOGY**
Localized, sharp, burning pain	Nociceptors transmit pain stimulus along myelinated Aδ fibers to spinal cord, where it travels via the neospinothalamic tract to the thalamus. From the thalamus, the stimulus is distributed to somatosensory cortex (perception and interpretation), the limbic system (emotional responses to pain), and brain stem centers (autonomic nervous system responses).
Diffuse, dull, aching pain	Transmission of nociceptive stimuli along unmyelinated C fibers to the spinal cord, and from there to the thalamus via the paleospinothalamic tract. Stimuli are distributed from the thalamus to the somatosensory cortex, limbic system, and brain stem centers.
Increased heart rate, stroke volume, and blood pressure; pupil dilation	Activation of the sympathetic nervous system (SNS) with release of catecholamines, which stimulate receptors in the heart and blood vessels.
Nausea, vomiting	SNS activation causes decreased blood flow to the gut, with decreased gastric acid secretion and intestinal motility; pain, anxiety cause stimulation of the vomiting center in the medulla.
Muscle tension	Protective responses initiated by higher brain centers to reduce nociceptive stimuli.
Anxiety, fear	Emotional responses to pain stimuli generated by limbic system.

TABLE 9–2 Characteristics of Acute and Chronic Pain

CHARACTERISTIC	ACUTE PAIN	CHRONIC PAIN
Purpose	Signals actual or potential tissue damage	May serve no useful function
Onset and duration	Sudden; relieved by healing	Persists after acute problem is resolved
Cause	Actual or potential tissue damage	May not be readily identifiable May result from nerve damage or pain modulation mechanism imbalance
Associated symptoms	Sympathetic nervous system responses (increased pulse and respiratory rates, increased blood pressure, sweating, nausea) Muscle spasms Anxiety, fear	Depression common Insomnia Possible preoccupation with pain

Breakthrough Pain

Breakthrough pain is pain that exceeds baseline chronic or persistent pain. It is often described as a sudden flare that exceeds the analgesic effect of long-acting pain medications. Whether the pain is malignant or non-malignant in origin, treated or untreated, breakthrough pain is temporary and can be debilitating. The onset and intensity of breakthrough pain vary; its unpredictability and inconsistency are distressing to the patient and can make it difficult to manage.

Incident pain is a subtype of breakthrough pain. Incident or *episodic pain* is predictable, precipitated by an event or activity such as coughing, changing position, or being touched. Pain associated with a fractured bone is a good example of incident pain. When the patient remains still and the fracture is aligned and supported, little pain is experienced. Movement of the affected part, however, can precipitate sharp, intense pain.

Nociceptive Pain

Nociceptive pain is pain caused by stimulation of peripheral or visceral pain receptors. It generally is localized and responsive to treatment. Nociceptive pain may be either acute or chronic, resulting from disease processes (e.g., arthritis), tissue trauma, and medical treatment (e.g., surgery).

Neuropathic Pain

Neuropathic pain results from injury to the peripheral nerves that leads to abnormal impulse processing by the peripheral and central nervous systems. Although neuropathic pain may be acute (e.g., the pain associated with shingles [herpes zoster]), usually it is chronic, associated with conditions such as diabetic neuropathy or postherpetic neuralgia. Neuropathic pain is thought to result from hyperactivity of neurons in the spinal cord and thalamus. The hyperactive neurons generate *ectopic* (arising from an abnormal site) impulses, leading to spontaneous paresthesias, numbness, pain, and tenderness, despite peripheral nerve damage. The pain may be described as gnawing, electric shock-like, burning, shooting, or tingling. Pain may occur with a stimulus such as touch that normally does not produce pain (*allodynia*), or its intensity may be disproportionate to the stimulus (*hyperalgesia*) (Helms & Barone, 2008; McCance & Huether, 2010).

Central Pain

Central pain is caused by a lesion or damage in the brain or spinal cord. This damage leads to spontaneous generation of impulses that are perceived as pain. An infarction, tumor, trauma, or disorder such as multiple sclerosis or epilepsy may cause central pain. Central pain is constant, of moderate to severe intensity, and difficult to treat. The location of the pain depends on the area of the CNS affected. The pain may be described as burning, pressing, lacerating, or aching. "Pins and needles" sensations may be experienced along with the underlying pain. Affected areas may have decreased sensation (numbness). Thalamic pain, a type of central pain, may cause hyperesthesia (an abnormal sensitivity to touch, pain, or other sensory stimuli) on the side of the body opposite to the thalamic lesion.

Complex Regional Pain Syndromes

Complex regional pain syndromes (CRPS) cause extremity pain that is severe, diffuse, and burning. The pain is accompanied by vasomotor changes that affect skin color and temperature. Initially the affected extremity has typical inflammatory symptoms, with redness, warmth, and swelling. Later, it is cool, cyanotic, and edematous; skin and nail changes may be seen (McCance & Huether, 2010). The cause of CRPS is unclear; there may, in fact, be several causes, including damage to the central or peripheral nervous system, or a disrupted healing or immune process. In CRPS, pain receptors in the affected part of the body become sensitized to catecholamines, neurotransmitters associated with sympathetic nervous system activity.

Phantom Limb Pain

Phantom limb pain is a pain syndrome that occurs following amputation of a body part. The patient experiences pain in the missing body part that may be described as burning, cramping, or shooting. Phantom limb pain more frequently affects people who had pain in the amputated limb prior to its removal than those who did not. Several theories for phantom limb pain have been developed. These include regeneration of severed peripheral nerves and abnormal impulses generated by spinal cord neurons that no longer receive normal sensory input from the body (Porth & Matfin, 2009).

Adverse Effects of Pain

Acute pain has a defined purpose: to warn of injury to body tissues. Although often attributable to a defined disorder (such as arthritis, migraine, or cancer), chronic pain often serves no useful purpose, becoming instead part of the problem. Physiologic responses to pain extend beyond the muscle spasm and fight-or-flight response (increased blood pressure, heart rate, and cardiac output, decreased gastric and intestinal motility), and can have adverse effects on the patient's health. Pain interferes with sleep quantity and quality, leading to exhaustion and possible disorientation. Metabolism and myocardial oxygen demand are increased. Catabolism (breakdown of body tissues) increases, and healing is impaired. Immune function is suppressed, increasing the risk for infection. Research shows a clear link between chronic pain and depression.

Factors Affecting Responses to Pain

Responses to pain stimuli are as individualized as the person experiencing the stimulus. The previous discussion focused on types of pain and physiologic responses to pain stimuli. The individualized response to pain is shaped not only by physiologic responses, but by multiple and interacting factors, including age, gender, sociocultural influences, emotional state, past experiences with pain, the source and meaning of the pain, and knowledge base.

The *pain threshold* is the point at which a stimulus elicits a response. Although the pain threshold is relatively consistent, meaning that a given pain stimulus will elicit pain perception among most people, it can be affected by factors such as the presence of chronic pain (which tends to lower the threshold) or more intense pain at another site (which tends to raise the threshold).

Pain tolerance is the amount (duration, intensity) of pain a person can endure before outwardly responding to it (McCance & Huether, 2010). Pain tolerance varies significantly among individuals and within an individual over time. It is influenced by culture, expectations, emotions, and psychosocial factors. The ability to tolerate pain may be decreased by repeated episodes of pain, fatigue, anger, anxiety, and sleep deprivation. Medications, alcohol, hypnosis, warmth, distraction, and spiritual practices may increase pain tolerance.

Age

Age influences a person's perception and expression of pain. There is, however, no evidence that nociception is altered by age. When compared with younger adults, pain stimulus transmission relies more on C fibers in older adults than on $A\delta$ fibers. As a result, pain stimulus transmission is slower, and pain more frequently may be described as burning, dull, or aching. Central processing often is slowed, resulting in a slower response time

to pain. Referred pain is less typical in older adults, and visceral pain may present as less severe than in younger adults. The older adult may report vague complaints of pain, or may present with manifestations such as delirium rather than subjective reports of pain (Helms & Barone, 2008; Tabloski, 2006).

Many older adults experience both acute and chronic pain related to disorders such as arthritis or peripheral neuropathy. While peripheral vascular disease or diabetes may lead to neuropathy and interfere with normal nerve impulse transmission, neuropathy can manifest as hyperesthesias as well as hypoesthesias. Both of these manifestations cause discomfort. Pain tolerance decreases with aging, perhaps related to the prevalence of chronic pain in this population. Studies of elderly nursing home residents found daily, persistent pain among them, with 40% of those who reported pain on the first assessment still in pain 60 to 180 days later (Teno, 2002).

Effective assessment and management of pain in the elderly can be challenging. Patients and healthcare professionals (including nurses) may believe that pain and discomfort are unavoidable aspects of aging. Individuals in this age group may fail to acknowledge pain, believing that pain is inevitable or fearing dependency if they alarm their loved ones. Patients and healthcare professionals may have misconceptions about the use of analgesics, including opioid medications, fearing adverse effects (such as respiratory depression) or **addiction**. Sensory impairments (e.g., impaired hearing) or cognitive impairments can interfere with the patient's ability to report pain and the healthcare professional's ability to assess pain. The Nursing Care of the Older Adult table lists some age-related changes and their effects on pain.

Gender

Clinical and animal studies show that women have a lower pain threshold and experience higher intensity of pain than men (Toomey, 2008; Wilson, 2006). It has long been held that sociocultural factors account for these recognized differences in the pain experience. Research has recently provided evidence of physiologic differences in pain responses and the analgesic effect of opioid medications. Positron emission tomography (PET) demonstrates greater activation of areas of the brain associated with emotions in women experiencing a painful stimulus than in men (Toomey, 2008). These physiologic responses appear to be genetically encoded, involving the sex

NURSING CARE OF THE OLDER ADULT   **Age-Related Changes in Pain Perception and Response**

AGE-RELATED FACTOR	EFFECTS
Decreased $A\delta$ fiber transmission, greater reliance on C fiber transmission	Pain perceived as dull, aching, more diffuse rather than sharp, localized
Slowed central processing	Slower motor or avoidance responses
Reduced norepinephrine levels	Reduced sympathetic nervous system responses to pain (pulse, blood pressure, papillary dilation)
Decreased referred pain	May not exhibit "classic" manifestations of such disorders as myocardial infarction, acute abdomen
Reduced neurotransmitter levels	Increased risk of depression related to chronic pain

hormones and the activity of opioid receptors in the brain. Fluctuating estrogen levels associated with the menstrual cycle affect perceived pain intensity. The circuits that mediate the pain response differ in men and women, the opioid pain modulatory system in particular. Because of these differences, women and men may respond differently to opioid analgesics such as morphine (Wilson, 2006).

Sociocultural Influences

Each person's response to pain is strongly influenced by the family, community, and culture. Sociocultural influences affect pain behavior, dictating appropriate and inappropriate expressions of pain. In general, cultural responses to pain fall into two categories: stoic and emotive (Andrews & Boyle, 2008). For example, if the patient's culture teaches that people should tolerate pain stoically, the patient may appear withdrawn and refuse (or not request) pain medication. If the cultural norm encourages open and intense emotional expression, the patient may cry freely and appear comfortable requesting pain medication.

Cultural standards also teach an individual how much pain to tolerate, what types of pain to report, to whom to report the pain, and what kind of treatment to seek. For example, patients of northern European ancestry may value "being a good patient," which may cause them to avoid "complaining" about their pain, whereas patients of Jewish ancestry may value seeking information about their pain, which may cause them to discuss their pain often and in detail. Note, however, that behaviors vary greatly within a culture and from generation to generation. The nurse should approach each patient as an individual, observing the patient carefully, taking the time to ask questions, and avoiding assumptions.

The nurse also has a set of sociocultural values and beliefs about pain. If these values and beliefs differ from those of the patient, the assessment and management of pain may be based on the values of the nurse rather than on the needs of the patient. The nurse must be familiar with ethnic and cultural diversity in pain expression and management and respect cultural differences. It is particularly important to remember that pain behaviors are not an objective indicator of the amount of pain present for any individual. Finally, most experts agree that cultural differences in the expression of, response to, and interpretation of the meaning of pain need further research.

Psychological Influences

The intensity of perceived pain has been shown to be affected by psychological variables such as attention, expectation, and suggestion. The sensation of pain may be blocked by intense concentration (during sports activities, for example) or may be increased by anxiety or fear. Pain often is increased when it occurs in conjunction with other illnesses or physical discomforts such as nausea or vomiting. The presence or absence of support people or caregivers that genuinely care about pain management also may alter emotional status and the perception of pain. The placebo effect, a positive patient response to an inactive substance, has been demonstrated through both observational studies and brain MRI studies (Fauci et al., 2008).

Anxiety may increase the perception of pain, and pain in turn may cause anxiety. In addition, the muscle tension common with anxiety can create its own source of pain. This association explains why nonpharmacologic interventions such as relaxation or guided imagery are helpful in relieving or decreasing pain.

Fatigue, lack of sleep, and depression also are related to pain experiences. Pain interferes with a person's ability to fall asleep and stay asleep and thus induces fatigue. In turn, fatigue can lower pain tolerance. Depression is clearly linked to pain: Serotonin, a neurotransmitter, is involved in the modulation of pain in the CNS. In clinically depressed people, serotonin is decreased, leading to an increase in pain sensations. The reverse is also true: In the presence of pain, depression is common.

The meaning associated with the pain influences the experience of pain. For example, the pain of labor to deliver a baby is experienced differently from the pain following removal of a major organ for cancer. Because pain is the major signal for health problems, it is strongly linked to all associated meanings of health problems, such as disability, loss of role, and death. A lack of understanding of the source, outcome, and meaning of the pain can contribute negatively to the pain experience. For this reason, it is important to explain to patients the etiology and prognosis for the pain assessed.

If the patient perceives the pain as deserved (e.g., "just punishment for sins"), the patient may actually feel relief that the "punishment" has commenced. If the patient believes that the pain will relieve him or her from an unrewarding job, dangerous military service, or even stressful social obligations, there may similarly be a feeling of relief. In contrast, pain that is perceived as meaningless—for example, chronic low back pain or the unrelieved pain of arthritis—can cause anxiety and depression.

Interdisciplinary Care

Effective pain relief results from collaboration among patient and all members of the healthcare team. Acute pain management may be straightforward, accomplished though short-term analgesia and management of the underlying problem. Chronic pain, on the other hand, frequently requires a multidisciplinary approach. Pain clinics are centers staffed by a team of healthcare professionals who use traditional pharmacologic agents as well as herbs, vitamins, and other dietary supplements; nutritional counseling; psychotherapy; biofeedback; hypnosis; acupuncture; massage; and other treatments. Hospices for dying patients also provide a multifaceted approach to pain management. Chapter 5 provides information about pain management during end-of-life care.

Medications

Medication is the most common approach to pain management. Management of acute pain often is relatively straightforward, relying on **analgesic** (pain-relieving) drugs such as acetaminophen, nonsteroidal anti-inflammatory drugs (NSAIDs), and opioid analgesics. Chronic pain presents additional challenges; a broader range of drug classes may be employed, including antidepressant medications, anticonvulsants, and chronic opioid medication use.

In addition to administering the prescribed medications, the nurse may act interdependently in selecting the appropriate dosage and timing. The nurse is also responsible for assessing the side effects of the medications, evaluating the medication's effectiveness, and providing patient teaching. The nurse's role in pain relief is patient advocate as well as direct caregiver.

The World Health Organization (WHO) "ladder of analgesia" effectively guides the use of medications for patients with malignant pain (WHO, 2009) (Figure 9–5 ■). Aspirin and NSAIDs are initially used, followed by the addition of mild opioid analgesics and then strong opioids until pain is relieved, reflecting the interactive nature of these two types of analgesics. Adjuvant drugs are used to manage fear and anxiety. This approach also emphasizes administering analgesics by the clock, rather than on-demand, to maintain comfort.

ASPIRIN, ACETAMINOPHEN, AND NSAIDS Nonopioid analgesics such as acetaminophen (Tylenol), aspirin and NSAIDs produce analgesia and reduce fever. They are used to treat mild to moderate pain, and are particularly effective for treating headache and musculoskeletal pain.

Acetaminophen appears to act on the CNS to relieve pain. Its exact mechanism of action is unknown, but it is believed to raise the pain threshold by acting on receptors in pain pathways. Acetaminophen is considered to be a very safe drug, and often is combined with opioid analgesics to allow effective pain relief with a lower opioid dose (e.g., Percocet, Tylenol #3, Vicodin). It is important to remember, however, that acetaminophen is toxic to the liver. Hepatotoxicity is a particular risk in patients who are malnourished or who have a history of alcohol abuse (DiPiro et al., 2008). It also is a consideration when given in combination with an opioid analgesic. As the patient develops tolerance to the opioid, increasing doses may be required to achieve effective analgesia, resulting in acetaminophen doses that increase the risk for hepatotoxicity.

Aspirin and NSAIDs act on peripheral nerve endings and minimize pain by interfering with two enzymes necessary for prostaglandin synthesis, cyclooxygenase type 1 (COX-1) and cyclooxygenase type 2 (COX-2). Examples include ibuprofen, indomethacin (Indocin), and ketorolac (Toradol). The NSAIDs have anti-inflammatory, analgesic, and antipyretic actions. NSAIDs are the treatment of choice for mild to moderate pain and continue to be effective when combined with narcotics for moderate to severe pain. NSAIDs are increasingly used in a *multimodal* approach to analgesic therapy; that is, in combination with opioid and adjunctive pain relief measures.

As a class, aspirin and NSAIDs are associated with gastric irritation. As cyclooxygenase (COX) inhibitors, they interfere with prostaglandin production. While this accounts for their anti-inflammatory effects, prostaglandins are necessary to maintain the gastric mucosal barrier. The gastric mucosal barrier (composed of mucus and bicarbonate) protects gastric mucosa from the irritating effects of ingested substances. NSAIDS, therefore, are not only irritating to gastric mucosa, they interfere with its protection as well. The risk for resultant gastrointestinal bleeding is greatest with aspirin, because it also interferes with platelets and blood clotting (Lehne, 2007).

NSAIDs also increase blood pressure in many patients, and, with long-term use, may be toxic to the kidneys. With the exception of aspirin, NSAIDs have been shown to have an associated increased cardiovascular risk (DiPiro, 2008). They are not recommended for use in people with kidney or liver disease, bleeding disorders, peptic ulcer disease, pregnancy, or a history of hypersensitivity to aspirin or other NSAIDs. Nursing implications for NSAIDs are found in the Medication Administration box on page 169. For more information about doses and precautions for specific NSAIDs, see Table 40–5 on page 1368.

OPIOID ANALGESICS *Opioid* (also called *narcotic*) analgesics are derivatives of the opium plant. These drugs (and their synthetic forms) are the most potent pain relieving drugs available, and are the treatment of choice for acute moderate-to-severe pain. Examples are morphine, codeine, and fentanyl (Duragesic, Actiq). Opioid analgesics produce analgesia by binding to opioid receptors both within and outside the CNS. They differ from one another in potency, speed of onset, duration of action, and preferred route of administration. Opioid *agonists* such as morphine produce their effect by stimulating the receptor they bind with. Drugs with a mixed *agonist-antagonist* effect block the activity of some receptors (mu receptors), while activating others (kappa receptors). This mixed agonist-antagonist activity can actually intensify pain responses in some patients. Buprenorphine (Buprenex), butorphanol (Stadol), nalbuphine (Nubain), and pentazocine (Talwin) are examples of opioids with mixed agonist-antagonist effects.

A summary of **equianalgesic** or approximate equivalent doses of selected opioid analgesics used to treat moderate to severe pain, their peak effect and duration, and nursing implications is provided in Table 9–3.

Opioid analgesics tend to have similar unintended effects. They are CNS and respiratory depressants. They commonly produce sedation, drowsiness, and dizziness. All should be

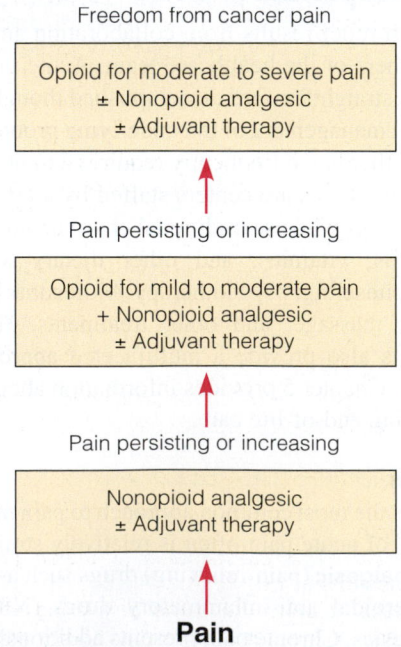

Freedom from cancer pain

Opioid for moderate to severe pain
± Nonopioid analgesic
± Adjuvant therapy

↑

Pain persisting or increasing

Opioid for mild to moderate pain
+ Nonopioid analgesic
± Adjuvant therapy

↑

Pain persisting or increasing

Nonopioid analgesic
± Adjuvant therapy

↑

Pain

Figure 9–5 ■ The WHO analgesic ladder illustrates the process for selection of analgesic medications for pain management.

Source: The WHO Analgesic Ladder from Cancer Pain Relief and Palliative Care, Technical Report Series, No. 804, The World Health Organization, Geneva, Switzerland. Reprinted by permission.

MEDICATION ADMINISTRATION Nonsteroidal Anti-Inflammatory Drugs

EXAMPLES OF NSAIDS ARE THE FOLLOWING:

aspirin (acetylsalicylic acid)

celecoxib (Celebrex)

diflunisal (Dolobid)

fenoprofen calcium (Nalfon)

ibuprofen (Advil, Motrin)

indomethacin (Indocin)

ketoprofen (Actron, Orudis)

ketorolac tromethamine (Toradol)

nabumetone (Relafen)

naproxen (Aleve, Naprosyn)

piroxicam (Feldene)

sulindac (Clinoril)

tolmetin (Tolectin)

The NSAIDs have anti-inflammatory, analgesic, and antipyretic effects. It is believed that they inhibit the enzyme COX, thereby decreasing synthesis of prostaglandins. These drugs provide analgesic effects by reducing inflammation and by perhaps blocking the generation of noxious impulses.

Nursing Responsibilities
- Do not administer aspirin with other NSAIDs.
- Assess and document if the patient is taking a hypoglycemic agent or insulin; the NSAIDs may increase the hypoglycemic effect.
- Administer with meals, milk, or a full glass of water to decrease gastric irritation.
- Assess patients who are also taking anticoagulants for bleeding; the NSAIDs increase this risk.

Health Education for the Patient and Family
- Drugs may cause gastrointestinal bleeding (report nausea, vomiting of blood, dark stools), visual disturbances (report blurred or diminished vision), increased blood pressure, hearing problems, dizziness, skin rash, and kidney problems (report weight gain or edema).
- Take medications with meals to decrease gastric irritation.
- Avoid drinking alcohol or taking any over-the-counter drug unless approved by the healthcare provider.
- The desired effects may not appear for 3–5 days, and the full effects may not appear for 2–4 weeks.
- Maintain regular healthcare appointments.

avoided or used with caution in patients with chronic obstructive lung disease (COPD) or who are experiencing an acute asthma attack because they can suppress respirations. Nausea and vomiting are common adverse effects, as is constipation. All opioid analgesics have the potential to cause physical and psychologic dependence, particularly when taken at high doses for an extended time (Adams, Holland, & Bostwick, 2008).

A common myth among healthcare professionals is that using opioids for pain treatment poses a real threat of addiction.

Actually, when the medications are used as recommended, there is little to no risk of addiction. Rather, if pain is not adequately treated, the patient may seek more and more analgesic relief, thus increasing the risk of an adversarial relationship with the provider and a weakening of the trust relationship between patient and provider (Trame, 2002) (Box 9–1).

Opioid analgesics commonly are used to treat chronic malignant pain (see Figure 9–5). Because of their potency and efficacy, they also may be used to treat chronic nonmalignant

BOX 9–1 Pain Management, Addiction, and Regulation

The goals of pain control are to minimize discomfort and promote normal functioning. While these goals often can be achieved through use of nonpharmacologic strategies and nonnarcotic analgesics, opioid medications currently provide the only effective option for pain associated with acute trauma, surgery, cancer, and some chronic conditions.

Crude opium has been available for thousands of years. Abuse of opium and its derivatives (e.g., heroin, morphine) increased dramatically with development of the hypodermic syringe. International efforts to control narcotic trafficking and abuse while ensuring availability for medical and scientific purposes began in the early twentieth century. And yet today, while much of the world's population still lacks access to these effective and inexpensive analgesics, illicit narcotic trafficking accounts for $400–$500 billion per year; nearly 10% of world trade (Taylor, 2007).

The WHO estimates than 80% of people with severe pain are inadequately treated (Taylor, 2007). Despite significant data showing very little *addiction* as the result of treating pain with adequate analgesia, prescribers still tend to undertreat chronic nonmalignant pain (American Pain Society, 2009). Cook et al. (2004) found that physicians prescribe significantly more nonopioid analgesics for a patient addicted to heroin than for a nonaddicted patient with identical injuries. The authors observe that analgesics may be rationed to addicted persons in an effort to wean them from their addiction. Addiction is a neurophysiologic disease, separate and distinct from *physical dependence* and tolerance. See the following list for definitions of relevant terms.

The development of highly effective oral opioid analgesics such as oxycodone (OxyContin) and hydrocodone (Vicodin) has resulted in increased illegal trafficking of legally manufactured opioids. This has led to calls for legislation to limit the use and availability of these drugs, an option that concerns palliative care specialists.

Opioid analgesics are among the most effective, highly regulated, and significantly abused drugs available today. Clearly, there are no simple answers to the problems associated with drug trafficking, abuse, and addiction.
- *Addiction:* A primary, chronic neurobiologic disease characterized by compulsive use of a substance despite negative consequences, such as health threats or legal problems.
- *Drug abuse:* The use of any chemical substance for other than a medical purpose.
- *Physical drug dependence:* A biologic need for a substance. If the substance is not supplied, physical withdrawal symptoms occur.
- *Psychologic drug dependence:* A psychologic need for a substance. If the substance is not supplied, psychologic withdrawal symptoms occur.
- *Drug tolerance:* Physical adaptation to the drug resulting in its diminished effects over time.
- *Equianalgesic:* Having the same pain-killing effect when administered to the same individual. Drug dosages are equianalgesic if they have the same effect as morphine sulfate 10 mg administered parenterally.
- *Pseudoaddiction:* Behavior involving drug seeking; a result of receiving inadequate pain relief.

TABLE 9–3 Equianalgesic Drug Chart

ANALGESIC	DOSAGE(MG)	PEAK(MIN)	DURATION(H)	NURSING CONSIDERATIONS
Morphine sulfate	10 SC, IV 30–60 PO	30–60 min 60–120 min	4–5 h 4–5 h	PO dose is 3–6 times the IM dose. A lower dose may be appropriate for older patients with chronic pain. Smaller doses (e.g., 2 to 5 mg) may be administered more frequently when using IV route.
Codeine	130 IM, SC 200 PO	30–60 min 60–120 min	4 h 4 h	PO dose is about 1.5 times the parenteral dose. IM absorption unpredictable. Analgesic potency about one-sixth that of morphine. Often given in combination with aspirin or acetaminophen for mild to moderate pain. Also used for its antitussive (cough suppressant) effect.
Fentanyl (Duragesic, Sublimaze)	0.1(100 mcg)/h IV or transdermal	1 min	5–7 min IV	100 mcg/hr parenteral or transdermal is equivalent to 4 mg/hr of parenteral morphine. Rapid onset and short half-life; tissue storage can prolong half-life and effect with longer-term use. Transdermal fentanyl not recommended for acute pain management. Available by oral transmucosal route (lozenge on a stick).
Hydromorphone HCl (Dilaudid)	1.5 IM, SC, IV 7.5 PO	15–30 min 30 min	4 h 4 h	PO dose is 5 times IM dose. Shorter acting than morphine.
Levorphanol (Levo-Dromoran)	2 IM, SC, IV 4 PO	60 min 90–120 min	4–5 h 4–5 h	Longer acting than morphine when given in repeated, regular doses. Accumulates, so analgesic effect may increase over time.
Meperidine (Demerol)	75 IM, SC, IV 300 PO	30–50 min 60–90 min	2–4 h 2–4 h	Not recommended as first-line opioid for acute or chronic pain. Metabolized to normeperidine, which is toxic to the CNS. Not recommended for older adults, patients with impaired kidney function, or for administration by continuous IV infusion.
Methadone HCl (Dolophine)	10 IM, SC, IV 20 PO	60–120 min 90–120 min	4–6 h 4–6 h	Initial PO dose is twice IM dose. Accumulates, so analgesic effect may increase over time. Initial doses lower in opioid-tolerant patients. Also used for heroin detoxification and temporary maintenance.
Oxycodone (Percocet, OxyContin)	30 PO (NA parenteral)	60 min	3–6 h	Used in combination with nonopioid analgesic (Percocet, Tylox) for moderate pain. Available as a single-entity product in immediate- or controlled-release forms (OxyContin) for severe pain. Has faster onset and higher peak effect than most PO narcotics, equivalent to oral morphine.
Oxymorphone (Numorphan)	1–1.5 IM, SC, IV 10 PO or PR	30–60 min 30–60 min	3–6 h 4–6 h	Also available as rectal suppository (10 mg equianalgesic). Used for moderate to severe pain.
Tramadol (Ultram, Zydol)	100 PO	120–180 min	3–6 h	Used for moderate to moderately severe pain. Causes less respiratory depression than morphine.

Note: Morphine sulfate 10 mg IM is the analgesic dose to which all other parenteral and PO doses in this table are considered equianalgesic.

pain. Oral preparations of a fixed combination of an opioid and acetaminophen are used with caution. Tolerance can lead to higher required doses of the opioid, increasing the risk for hepatoxicity due to the increasing dose of acetaminophen. Nursing implications for opioid analgesics are found in the Medication Administration box on page 171.

Certain opioid analgesics, while still available, are not recommended for use because of toxic effects or their potential for abuse. As previously noted, the metabolite of meperidine (Demerol) is toxic to the CNS. While a single dose of meperidine may be used to relieve acute pain (e.g., migraine), it is not recommended for continued use (DiPiro, 2008). Propoxyphene (Darvon, Darvocet, Balacet), a synthetic opioid analgesic for mild to moderate pain has a high potential for abuse, with significant risk for psychologic dependence. The risk of fatal overdose is significant with propoxyphene (FDA, 2009), and it

MEDICATION ADMINISTRATION Opioid Analgesics

EXAMPLES OF OPIOID ANALGESICS ARE THE FOLLOWING:
buprenorphine HCl (Buprenex)

codeine

fentanyl (Duragesic)

hydrocodone (Hycodan, Vicodin)

hydromorphone HCl (Dilaudid)

levorphanol (Levo-Dromoran)

morphine sulfate

nalbuphine HCl (Nubain)

oxycodone (OxyContin)

oxymorphone HCl (Numorphan)

pentazocine (Talwin)

Opioid analgesics are used to treat severe pain. The drugs in this category include morphine, codeine, opium derivatives, and synthetic substances with activity similar to natural opioids. Morphine and codeine are pure chemical substances isolated from opium. These drugs decrease the awareness of the sensation of pain by binding to opiate receptors in the brain and spinal cord. It is also believed that they diminish the transmission of pain impulses by altering cell membrane permeability to sodium and by affecting the release of neurotransmitters for efferent nerves sensitive to noxious stimuli. Opioid analgesics affect the central nervous system, causing analgesia, euphoria, drowsiness, mental clouding, and lethargy. They also have various other effects: Depending on the drug used, they can depress respirations, stimulate the vomiting center, suppress the cough reflex, induce peripheral vasodilatation (resulting in hypotension), constrict the pupils, and decrease intestinal peristalsis (DiPiro, 2008). Opioid analgesics have the potential to cause tolerance and psychologic and physical dependence.

Nursing Responsibilities
■ Opioids are regulated by federal law; the nurse must record the date, time, patient name, type and amount of the drug used, and sign the entry in a narcotic inventory sheet. If the drug must be wasted after it is signed out, the act must be witnessed and the narcotic sheet signed by the nurse and the witness. Computerized narcotic documentation methods are also available.
■ Keep an opioid antagonist, such as naloxone, immediately available to treat respiratory depression.
■ Assess allergies or adverse effects from opioids previously experienced by the patient.

■ Assess for respiratory disorders (e.g., asthma or COPD), neuromuscular disorders (e.g. multiple sclerosis), and other conditions that might increase the risk associated with respiratory depression.
■ Assess the characteristics of the pain and the effectiveness of drugs that have been previously used to treat the pain.
■ Take and record baseline vital signs before administering the drug.
■ Administer the drugs, following established guidelines.
■ Monitor vital signs and respiratory status, level of consciousness, papillary response, nausea, bowel function, urinary function, and effectiveness of pain management at regular intervals and as indicated.
■ Provide for patient safety.
■ Report adverse effects such as continued nausea, vomiting, or itching.
■ Employ protocols or prn orders as needed to promote bowel function and prevent constipation.
■ Meperidine (Demerol) is associated with CNS toxicity and thus involves significant patient risk (DiPiro, 2008). Monitor any patient who is receiving more than one dose for nervousness, restlessness, tremors, twitching, shakiness, myoclonic jerks, diaphoresis, changes in level of awareness, agitation, disorientation, confusion, delirium, hallucinations, violent shivering, and/or seizures. Toxicity can occur with any route of administration or any dosing regimen. The risk is increased in patients with decreased renal function (including normal changes with aging). Report these manifestations to the physician. Oral administration is not recommended.
■ Teach noninvasive methods of pain management for use in conjunction with opioid analgesics.

Health Education for the Patient and Family
■ The use of opioid analgesics to treat severe pain is unlikely to cause addiction (American Pain Society, 2009).
■ Do not drink alcohol while taking these drugs.
■ Do not take over-the-counter medications unless approved by the healthcare provider.
■ Increase intake of fluids and fiber in the diet to prevent constipation. Contact your provider if additional measures (such as laxatives) are needed to manage constipation.
■ The drugs often cause dizziness, drowsiness, and impaired thinking; use caution when driving or making decisions.
■ Report adverse effects or decreasing effectiveness to the physician.

should not be taken concurrently with any other CNS depressant such as alcohol. Furthermore, clinical studies have shown propoxyphene to be no more effective as an analgesic than acetaminophen.

ANTIDEPRESSANTS Antidepressants, particularly those within the tricyclic and related chemical groups, are useful for treating chronic pain. Tricyclic antidepressants act on the production and retention of serotonin in the CNS, thus inhibiting pain sensation. The dose to provide analgesia is lower than that required to treat depression. These drugs also potentiate the effects of opioid analgesics, and may be used to help manage severe persistent or malignant pain. They also promote normal sleeping patterns, further alleviating the suffering of the patient in pain. They are particularly useful in treating neuropathic pain. Tricyclic antidepressants are not without adverse

effects, however. They may cause orthostatic hypotension, drowsiness, urinary retention, constipation, and impaired memory. These effects can limit their usefulness in older adults in particular. Antidepressants from other classes such as serotonin norepinephrine reuptake inhibitors (venlafaxine [Effexor], duloxetine [Cymbalta]) appear to have an analgesic effect similar to that of tricyclic antidepressants with fewer adverse effects (Fauci et al., 2008).

ANTICONVULSANTS Similar to antidepressants, some seizure medications such as gabapentin (Neurontin), pregabalin (Lyrica), and carbamazepine (Tegretol) are useful with neuropathic pain, including shingles (herpes zoster), migraine headaches, and diabetic neuropathy. These drugs reduce pain and sleep disruption. Drugs that are primarily used to treat epilepsy (seizures) have been used to treat nerve pain conditions and migraine headache for several decades. Many anticonvulsant drugs have been shown in clinical studies to be effective in managing chronic pain (DiPiro, 2008).

LOCAL ANESTHETICS Drugs such as benzocaine and lidocaine are part of a large group of substances that block the initiation and transmission of nerve impulses in a local area, thus blocking pain as well. Local anesthetics can be delivered by a variety of methods, including via transdermal patch to treat focal neuropathic pain (DiPiro, 2008). They are sometimes used to enable a patient to begin moving and using a painful area to diminish long-term pain.

Local anesthetics can be delivered directly to the sheath of a nerve through a peripheral nerve catheter. During surgery, a soaker type catheter can be inserted along a surgical incision to deliver local relief; this method may decrease the need for opioids and allow the patient to resume activity sooner (D'Arcy, 2005).

Analgesic Administration

The ideal drug, route of administration, and dosing schedule to provide optimal pain relief varies, depending on such factors as the type of pain, its intensity and duration, and the individual patient. Each drug has a unique absorption and duration of action. The nurse must understand that no drug will have a totally predictable effect, because each person absorbs, metabolizes, and excretes medications at different dosage levels. The only way to obtain reliable data about the effectiveness of the medication for the individual is to assess how that patient responds. Therefore, the best choice is to individualize the drug, route, and schedule.

Giving analgesics before the pain occurs or increases prevents some of the untoward effects of pain. This holds true for both acute and chronic pain: Poorly managed acute pain is one of the leading causes of persistent pain syndrome. Additional benefits of a preventive approach to pain can be summarized as follows:

- The patient may spend less time in pain. Pain has been shown to have a negative effect on healing; poorly relieved pain is associated with longer hospital stays.
- Inadequate relief of acute pain has been shown to be a significant contributing factor to chronic pain (Barclay, Lee, & Martin, 2008).
- Frequent analgesic administration may allow for smaller doses and less analgesic administration.
- Smaller doses will in turn mean fewer side effects.
- The patient's fear and anxiety about the return of pain will decrease.
- Pain relief allows the patient to be more physically active and avoid complications of immobility.

Analgesics may be given either around-the-clock (ATC) or as necessary (PRN, meaning *pro re nata*, Latin for "as circumstances may require"). ATC administration is recommended for the first 48 hours for acute pain related to surgery or traumatic injury. It also is appropriate for pain that has a predictable intensity and pattern. PRN administration is appropriate for pain that is not predictable or constant. PRN medication should be given as soon as the pain begins. Breakthrough pain occurs to patients receiving long-acting analgesics for chronic pain. It

is a transitory experience of moderate to severe pain often precipitated by coughing or movement but that may occur spontaneously. Breakthrough pain is managed using short-acting opioid analgesics in addition to ATC medications.

Maintaining effective pain relief while minimizing adverse effects of the medication can be challenging. Within a prescribed range, the nurse can choose the correct dose according to the patient's response. It is also the role of the nurse to notify the physician if the prescribed dosage does not meet the patient's needs or causes excessive drowsiness, unsteadiness, or significant adverse effects.

Routes of Administration

The route of administration significantly affects how much of the medication is needed to relieve pain. For example, because of differences in absorption and distribution, oral doses of some opioids must be up to five times greater than parenteral doses to achieve the same degree of pain relief. In addition, the potency of opioid analgesics vary. Consulting an equianalgesic chart when converting from one route of administration to another or from one drug to another helps ensure an equivalent effect for the patient. The analgesic effect of 10 mg of parenteral morphine is used as the base to which other opioids and routes of administration are compared. Table 9–3 is an example of an equianalgesic chart.

ORAL The simplest route for both patient and nurse is the oral (PO) route. Unless contraindicated, the oral route is preferred for most patients. Special nursing care is still required, because some medications must be given with food, some are irritating to the gastrointestinal system, and some patients have trouble swallowing pills. Liquid and timed-release forms are available for special applications.

Some analgesics, such as fentanyl, are available in alternative forms, including a buccal tablet, a lozenge, or a lollipop. The buccal route provides a rapid onset of action, as the medication is absorbed directly into the circulation, bypassing the gastrointestinal tract and first-pass liver metabolism. These delivery systems are particularly helpful for managing breakthrough pain. Special precautions must be taken in storing the lozenge and lollipop, as these may be mistaken for candy by children and pets (Cranwell-Bruce, 2007).

RECTAL The rectal route is helpful for patients who are unable to swallow or who are experiencing nausea and vomiting. Acetaminophen, aspirin, and some NSAIDs and opioid analgesics are available in this form. The rectal route is effective and simple, but the patient and family may not accept it. To be effective, any rectal medication must be placed above the rectal sphincter.

TRANSDERMAL The transdermal, or "patch," form of medication is increasingly being used because it is simple, painless, and delivers a continuous level of medication (Figure 9–6 ■). Transdermal medications are easy to store and apply. Reapplication every 72 hours enhances compliance. Additional short-acting medication may be needed for breakthrough pain. As with any route of administration, overdosage can occur. It is important to start with a low dose and **titrate** (which means to increase or decrease dose in small increments) to the effective

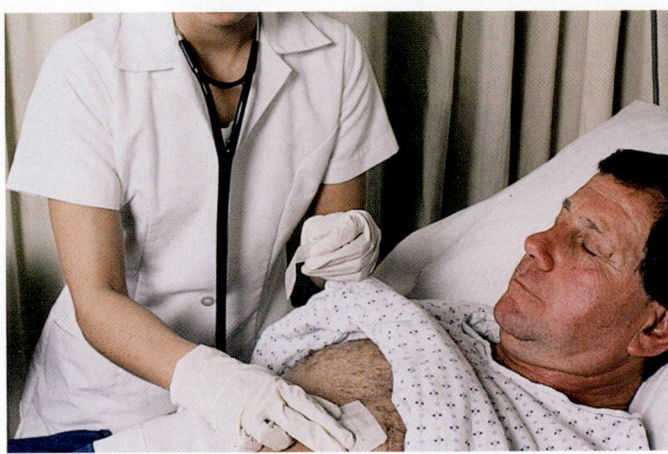

Figure 9–6 ■ The transdermal patch administers medication in predictable doses.

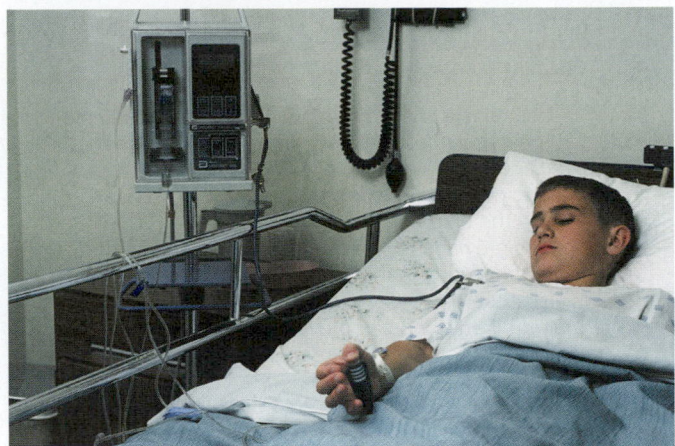

Figure 9–7 ■ PCA units allow the patient to self-manage acute pain. The units may be portable or mounted on intravenous poles.

level. Medication administered transdermally is in a lipid-soluble form, and may be stored in fat cells longer than expected. Monitor level of sedation and respiratory effort.

A transdermal patch is applied to a clean, dry area on the upper torso. If hair is present, it should be clipped before applying the patch. Apply the patch immediately after opening the package, ensuring complete contact with the skin, especially around the edges. The patch is effective for about 72 hours. When replaced, the new patch should be applied on a different site. When transdermal therapy is initiated, approximately 12–24 hours is necessary until therapeutic level is absorbed; similarly, when discontinuing, expect a gradual decline in level because of medication reservoir in the skin. Absorption is enhanced by fever or inflammation of the skin, exercise, and use of electric blankets or heating pads.

PARENTERAL Once the most popular route for pain medication administration, the intramuscular (IM) route is no longer preferred. Its disadvantages include uneven absorption from the muscle, discomfort on administration, and time consumed to prepare and administer the medication. Subcutaneous administration may be used, primarily when continuous analgesic administration via a parenteral route is required.

INTRAVENOUS The intravenous (IV) route provides the most rapid onset of effect, usually ranging from 1 to 15 minutes. Medication can be given by drip, bolus, or patient-controlled analgesia (PCA). PCA uses a pump with a control mechanism that allows the patient to self-manage pain (Figure 9–7 ■). The advantages of PCA are dose precision, timeliness, and convenience. The patient does not have to wait for a nurse to assess the need for pain medication, then procure and deliver the analgesia. Respiratory depression and sedation is minimized when plasma levels of opioids are steady. PCA, especially with basal dosing (continuous infusion of a very small dose), facilitates frequent small dosing. Several drugs can be administered by this route. The disadvantages are the nursing care needed for any intravenous line, the potential for infection, and the cost of disposable supplies. In addition, the risk for serious medication error requiring interventions in response has been shown to be greater with PCA than when other methods of analgesic delivery are used. Adverse events associated with PCA errors include

depressed respirations, inadequate pain relief, and even patient death (Sheehan, 2008). This increased risk is attributed to the complexity of the systems involved when PCA is used to provide analgesia. The PCA method of administration requires close attention by the physician, pharmacist, and nurse, as well as careful patient teaching and monitoring.

INTRASPINAL The intraspinal (intrathecal or epidural) route is invasive and requires more extensive nursing care but may provide better analgesia and postoperative recovery than intravenous delivery for some patients. When a combination of local anesthetics and opioids are infused by the epidural route, many patients experience better pain relief, earlier bowel recovery, and earlier mobility. The risk for respiratory depression and failure is lower with epidural analgesia than with administration by other parenteral routes. Other complications can occur, however, including hypotension, development of an epidural hematoma or abscess, and neurologic damage. Some patients achieve little or no pain relief with epidural analgesia, another potential complication (Gendall, Kennedy, Watson, & Frizell, 2007). See page 174 for nursing implications for patients receiving epidural analgesia.

NERVE BLOCKS In a nerve block, a local anesthetic, sometimes in combination with steroidal anti-inflammatory drugs, is injected by a physician or nurse anesthetist into or near a nerve, usually in an area between the nociceptor and the dorsal root. The procedure may be performed to determine the precise location of the source of the pain: Pain relief indicates that the injection site is the site of the source of the pain.

Temporary (local) nerve blocks may give the patient enough relief to (1) develop a more hopeful attitude that pain relief is possible, (2) allow local procedures to be performed without causing discomfort, or (3) exercise and move the affected part. A temporary nerve block may be particularly useful for such painful conditions as fractured ribs, allowing the patient to deep breathe, cough, and move with more ease during healing. Nerve blocks may also be performed to predict the results of neurosurgery. For long-term pain relief, a permanent neurolytic agent is used. Neurolytic blocks usually are reserved for terminally ill patients because of the risks of weakness, paralysis, and bowel and bladder dysfunction.

Receiving Intraspinal Analgesia

Intraspinal analgesia is used to manage chronic intractable malignant pain and postoperative pain, particularly after orthopedic and abdominal surgeries. The intraspinal route may be either intrathecal (into the subarachnoid space) or epidural (into the epidural space). Infusion of an opioid into these spaces provides for a direct effect on the opiate receptors in the dorsal horn of the spinal cord. The opioid analgesic is also absorbed systemically, affecting pain responses in the brain. This method can provide complete pain relief but has some potentially dangerous adverse effects.

PROCEDURE

The physician places a catheter into the epidural space. The catheter is connected to infusion tubing and an infusion pump, and the prescribed medication is administered. A portable or implantable pump may be used for longer term opioid analgesic administration.

NURSING CARE

- Monitor vital signs every 15 minutes for the first 2–3 hours and every hour for the first 24 hours; the patient is at risk for respiratory depression and hypotension. These adverse responses may not develop immediately, becoming evident only after several hours.

SAFETY ALERT

Ensure that naloxone, an opioid antagonist, is immediately available to reverse respiratory depression if necessary.
- Monitor the effectiveness of the pain management. Administer supplemental analgesics as ordered, and notify the physician if analgesia is inadequate (patient rates pain at 4 or higher on a scale of 0 to 10).
- Monitor intake and output. Intraspinal narcotics may block the micturition reflex, causing urinary retention and necessitating intermittent catheterization or placement of an indwelling urinary catheter.
- Use sterile technique to care for the intraspinal catheter.

Surgery

As a pain-relief measure, surgery usually is considered only after all other methods have failed. Surgical intervention typically is reserved for patients experiencing nerve pain, for example, the pain of trigeminal neuralgia, complex regional pain syndrome, or pain associated with spinal nerve or spinal cord injury. Patients need thorough knowledge of the implications of the use of surgery for pain relief. For example, motor function loss is an unwelcome side effect of some surgeries. Surgical procedures used to relieve pain are shown in Figure 9–8 ■. Some surgical procedures can be accomplished through minimally invasive techniques (e.g., percutaneously); others require an open surgical procedure. Surgical approaches to pain relief may include the following:

CORDOTOMY A *cordotomy* is an incision into the anterolateral tracts of the spinal cord to interrupt the transmission of pain. Because it is difficult to isolate the nerves responsible for upper body pain, this surgery is most often performed for pain in the abdominal region and legs, including severe pain from terminal cancer. A percutaneous cordotomy produces lesions of the anterolateral surface of the spinal cord by means of a radio frequency current.

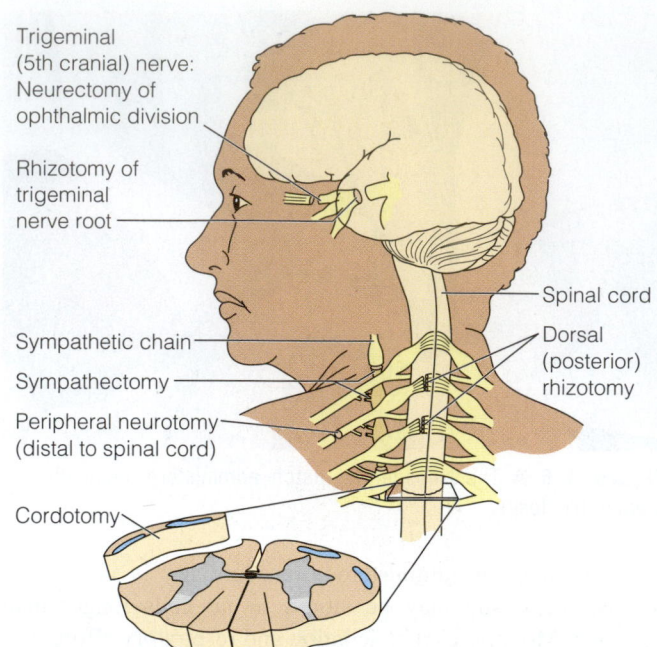

Figure 9–8 ■ Surgical procedures may be used to treat severe pain that does not respond to other types of management. They include cordotomy, neurectomy, sympathectomy, and rhizotomy.

NEURECTOMY A *neurectomy* is the removal or destruction of a nerve. It is sometimes used for pain relief, for example, to relieve the pain of trigeminal neuralgia. The nerve may be destroyed through several different methods, including injection of glycerol into the nerve, using radiofrequency-generated heat, or by compressing the nerve using a balloon. When an open approach is used, the nerve is exposed and severed. A peripheral neurectomy is the severing of a nerve at any point distal to the spinal cord.

SYMPATHECTOMY The sympathetic nerves play an important role in producing and transmitting the sensation of pain. A *sympathectomy* involves destruction by injection or incision of the ganglia of sympathetic nerves, usually in the lumbar region or the cervicodorsal region at the base of the neck.

RHIZOTOMY *Rhizotomy* is surgical severing of the dorsal spinal roots. It is most often performed to relieve the pain of cancer of the head, neck, or lungs. A rhizotomy may be performed by surgically cutting the nerve fibers, by injecting a chemical such as alcohol or phenol into the subarachnoid space, or by using a radio frequency current to selectively destroy pain fibers.

Transcutaneous Electrical Nerve Stimulation (TENS)

Transcutaneous electrical nerve stimulation (TENS) is the application of electrical current through the skin to control acute or chronic pain. A TENS unit consists of a battery-operated low-voltage transmitter connected to the skin using two or more electrodes (Figure 9–9 ■). Electrodes may be placed by the patient or by the physical therapist. The TENS unit generates a high-frequency or a low-frequency electrical pulse. With high-frequency application, pulse intensity is low and does not cause muscle contraction; low-frequency applications produce an intensity that does produce muscle contraction. The patient experiences a gentle tapping or vibrating sensation over the electrodes. He or she can adjust the voltage to achieve maximum pain relief.

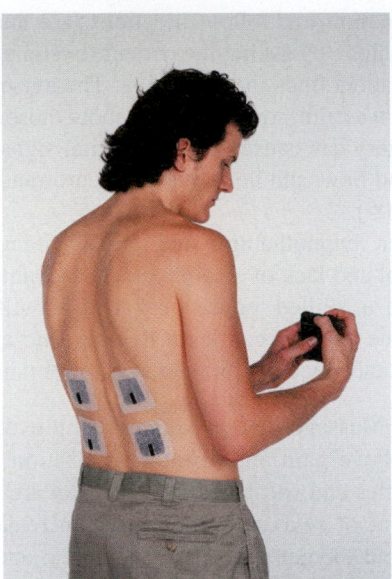

Figure 9–9 ■ The TENS unit is used to assist in acute and chronic in pain management. Electrodes deliver low-voltage electrical stimuli through the skin to block transmission of pain stimuli.

TENS controls pain in several ways. It activates opioid receptors in the spinal cord and medulla. It also affects release of both excitatory and inhibitory neurotransmitters, reducing the transmission of pain signals within the CNS. Furthermore, TENS stimulates large-diameter A-beta touch fibers to close the gate controlling pain transmission within the spinal cord. Low frequency TENS stimulates serotonin release and activates serotonin receptors, as well as prompting endorphin release.

A TENS unit is most commonly used to relieve chronic benign pain, neuropathic pain, and acute postoperative pain. Their use during obstetric care (labor in particular) is increasing, as is their use in treating orthopedic conditions. In any case, thorough patient teaching is essential, including an explanation of manufacturer's directions, instructions on where to place the electrodes, and the importance of placing the electrodes on clean, unbroken skin. The patient should assess the skin daily for signs of irritation. Patients who have a cardiac pacemaker or implanted cardioverter-defibrillator should not use TENS.

TENS offers several advantages: avoidance of drug side effects, patient control, and good interaction with other therapies. Disadvantages are its cost and the need for expert training for initiation. It also should be noted that TENS is not effective in relieving all types of pain or for all patients.

Complementary Therapies

The benefit of complementary and adjunctive therapies (or *CAM*—complementary and alternative medicine) as part of a comprehensive pain management strategy is increasingly recognized. According to a report issued in December 2008 by the National Center for Complementary and Alternative Medicine (NCCAM) and National Center for Health Statistics (part of the Centers for Disease Control and Prevention), about 38% of adults in the United States are using some form of CAM. See the accompanying Focus on Cultural Diversity box for the prevalence of CAM use among people of various cultures.

Pain—back, neck, or joint pain—and arthritis are the most common conditions that prompt adults to use CAM. A number of CAM therapies are used to treat pain, including acupuncture, chiropractic and osteopathic medicine, massage, and relaxation. Some of the more commonly used therapies follow.

ACUPUNCTURE Acupuncture is an ancient Chinese system involving the stimulation of certain specific points on the body to enhance the flow of vital energy (chi) along pathways called meridians. Acupuncture points can be stimulated by inserting and withdrawing needles, applying heat, massage, laser, electrical stimulation, or a combination of these methods. Only care providers with training in acupuncture techniques can use this method. Acupuncture is becoming a more widely accepted therapy, although evidence of its effectiveness in treating pain is mixed. Acupuncture has been shown to enhance traditional analgesia when used after abdominal surgery. The effectiveness of acupuncture in relieving chronic musculoskeletal pain has been extensively studied, with a beneficial effect shown in relieving chronic pain in the neck, lower back, or shoulder. Numerous studies also have shown that acupuncture may increase the pain threshold and promote well-being in patients with fibromyalgia (Spencer & Jacobs, 2003).

BIOFEEDBACK Biofeedback is method for learning to control physiologic responses of the body. Physiologic responses such as brain waves, muscle contraction, and skin temperature are measured electronically, "feeding" this information back to the patient. Biofeedback units use electrodes placed on the skin to transform data into visual cues, such as colored lights. The patient thus learns to recognize stress-related responses and to replace them with relaxation responses. Eventually, the patient learns to repeat independently those actions that produce the desired brain wave effect.

Biofeedback gives the patient a measure of control over the response to pain. It has been studied as a CAM therapy for migraine, fibromyalgia, traumatic brain injury, and temporomandibular disorder (TMD). In all studies, a beneficial effect was found, for example, reduced frequency of migraine headache or reduced intensity of pain associated with fibromyalgia and TMD (Fontaine, 2005; Spencer & Jacobs, 2003).

CHIROPRACTIC Chiropractic uses on hands-on therapy, focusing on the relationship between body structure and function. This relationship between structure (primarily that of the

---

FOCUS ON CULTURAL DIVERSTY
Use of CAM Therapies

Although about 38% of adults in the United States use CAM therapies, the number of people using CAM varies among different cultural groups. The National Center for Complementary and Alternative Medicine estimates that in 2007 CAM was used by the following:

50.3% of American Indian/Alaska Natives

43.1% of non-Hispanic White Americans

39.9% of Asian Americans

25.5% of Black Americans

23.7% of Hispanic Americans

spine) and function and its affect on health is a key concept of chiropractic medicine. Chiropractic therapy is directed at normalizing the relationship between structure and function to promote the body's innate ability to self-heal (NCCAM, 2008). The practice of chiropractic in the United States is limited to those who earn a doctor of chiropractic degree from an accredited college. Chiropractic is among the 10 most commonly used CAM procedures, with an estimated 20% of Americans receiving chiropractic care at some point during their lives. Most often, it is used in conjunction with conventional medical services.

Spinal manipulation has been demonstrated to be as effective for relieving mild-to-moderate low back pain as conventional treatments (NCCAM, 2008). Chiropractic generally is safe, with discomfort of the treated area, headache, and fatigue the most common adverse effects. Chiropractors may combine treatments such as application of heat or ice, electrical stimulation, exercise prescriptions, counseling, and dietary supplements with spinal manipulation.

DISTRACTION Distraction involves redirecting attention away from the pain and onto something that the patient finds more pleasant. Examples of distracting activities are practicing focused breathing, listening to music, or doing some form of rhythmic activity to music. For example, the patient using recorded music for distraction may sing along with the song, tap out the rhythm with the fingers or foot, clap to the music, conduct the music, or add harmony.

Participating in an activity that promotes laughter, such as reading a joke book or viewing a comedy, has been found to be highly effective in pain relief. Laughing for 20 minutes or more is known to produce an increase in endorphins that may continue pain relief even after the patient stops laughing.

HYPNOTHERAPY AND GUIDED IMAGERY Hypnotherapy is the use of hypnosis, a trance state in which the mind becomes extremely responsive to suggestion, to address a specific problem such as pain. Guided imagery is similar, helping patients achieve a state of focused attention. During hypnotherapy or guided imagery, the patient enters a trance state in which he or she is aware of the surroundings without focusing on them. The patient may go through three trance levels: superficial trance, in which awareness of the surroundings is maintained; alpha trance, a deeper trance state during which the heart rate, blood pressure, and respirations fall; and somnambulism, the level believed to be most beneficial. The patient's muscles relax, alpha brain waves predominate, and the patient experiences a sense of well-being and the ability to accept new ideas. During this state, the therapist may make suggestions to encourage pain relief. It is possible to achieve complete anesthesia or to modify pain in a variety of ways through hypnotism. For the technique to work, however, the patient must be fully relaxed and must want to be hypnotized.

Guided imagery, also called creative visualization, is use of the mind to create a scene or sensory experience that relaxes the muscles and moves the attention of the mind away from the pain experience. Images may be created by the therapist to help the patient modify physical responses to stressors such as pain. To use guided imagery, the patient must be able to concentrate,

use the imagination, and follow directions. The nurse can facilitate this technique by asking the patient for some descriptions of what the patient finds most relaxing. The nurse then speaks to the patient in a calm, soothing voice about those places or situations. Imagery can cause changes in vital signs, brain wave patterns, blood flow, and hormone and neurotransmitter levels (Fontaine, 2005).

Advantages hypnotherapy and guided imagery include patient control and lack of side effects. Disadvantages include the need for a skilled practitioner and a willing patient. However, some patients can learn to enter into a trance state without assistance by a practitioner to achieve pain relief.

MASSAGE Massage therapy often is employed as a CAM therapy to relieve pain and promote relaxation. In massage therapy, muscles and soft tissues of the body are manipulated with the intent of relaxing soft tissues; increasing warmth, blood flow, and oxygen delivery to the area; and decreasing pain. There are over 80 different types of massage therapy. Among the most common are Swedish massage, deep tissue massage, trigger point massage, and shiatsu massage. Massage therapy carries very little risk, but should be used appropriately and performed by a licensed or certified massage professional.

NATURAL PRODUCTS Natural products are the most frequently employed CAM therapy overall, used by nearly 20% of adults. A number of products, including herbals, natural oils, and other natural substances are available. Glucosamine, a natural substance that is found in cartilage, is among the most commonly used natural products. When combined with chondroitin, another natural substance found in cartilage, glucosamine has been found to have a beneficial effect on moderate to severe pain associated with osteoarthritis of the knee (NCCAM, 2006). Other natural products have been studied for the relief of pain associated with migraine and other musculoskeletal conditions such as fibromyalgia and rheumatoid arthritis with mixed results (Spencer & Jacobs, 2003).

RELAXATION Relaxation involves learning activities that deeply relax the body and mind. Relaxation distracts the patient's focus from the pain, lessens the effects of stress from pain, increases pain tolerance, increases the effectiveness of other pain relief measures, and increases perception of pain control. Some examples of relaxation activities are the following:

- *Diaphragmatic breathing* can relax muscles, improve oxygen levels, and provide a feeling of release from tension. This technique is more effective when the patient either lies down or sits comfortably, remains in a quiet environment, and keeps the eyelids closed. Inhaling and exhaling slowly and regularly is also helpful. The technique for diaphragmatic breathing is described and illustrated in ∞ Chapter 4.
- *Progressive muscle relaxation* may be used alone or in conjunction with deep breathing to help manage pain. The patient is taught to tighten one group of muscles (such as those of the face), hold the tension for a few seconds, and then relax the muscle group completely, repeating these actions for all parts of the body. This method is also more effective when the patient lies or sits comfortably, is in a quiet environment, and

keeps the eyelids closed. There are tapes available to help the patient with this relaxation process.

- *Meditation* is a process whereby the patient empties the mind of all sensory data and, typically, concentrates on a single object, word, or idea. This activity produces a deeply relaxed state in which oxygen consumption decreases, muscles relax, and endorphins are produced. At its deepest level, the meditative state may resemble a trance state. A variety of exercises can induce the meditative state, and all are relatively easy to learn. Many books and tapes are available commercially.

- *Music therapy* uses music and the therapeutic relationship to reduce pain, anxiety, and depression. Music provides a familiar sensory stimulus that can provoke favorable responses such as muscle relaxation and reduced heart rate and blood pressure. Studies on the efficacy of music therapy to reduce pain perception in an acute care setting have been mixed; however, patients rated music therapy as a positive experience even when its effect on pain perception was statistically insignificant (Richards, Johnson, Sparks, & Emerson, 2007).

Nursing Care

Nursing care of the patient with pain presents perhaps more of a challenge than almost any other type of illness or injury. Regardless of the type of pain, the goal of nursing care is to assist the patient to achieve optimal control of the pain. See the accompanying Case Study & Nursing Care Plan: A Patient Experiencing Chronic Pain.

Health Promotion

Health promotion activities related to pain focus on providing effective relief of acute pain to avoid the negative consequences of inadequately managed pain. Evidence points to the existence of pain circuits established when acute pain is inadequately treated that perpetuate pain and contribute to chronic pain. Furthermore, pain has a negative effect on quality of life, resulting in decreased job performance, exercise, socialization, and activity-of-daily-living (ADL) performance. Longer-term effects include depression, isolation, and loss of self-esteem (American Academy of Pain Management, 2009).

CASE STUDY & NURSING CARE PLAN   A Patient Experiencing Chronic Pain

Susan Akers, aged 37, is currently being seen at an outpatient clinic for chronic nonmalignant pain. She works at a local paper factory. She has a 3-year history of neck and shoulder pain that usually is accompanied by headaches. She believes the pain is related to lifting objects at work, but it is now precipitated by activities of daily living. Susan is absent from work approximately three times a month and states that the absences are due to her pain and headaches. She has been seeking care in the local emergency department on the average of twice monthly for injections for pain. She does not regularly use medications but does take Percocet-5 as needed (usually two to three times a day). Ms. Akers is divorced and has two children. She states that she has several friends in the area, but her parents and siblings live in another part of the United States.

ASSESSMENT

During the nursing history, Ms. Akers rates her pain during an acute episode as a 7 on a scale of 1 to 10. She states that lifting objects and moving her hands and arms above shoulder level precipitate sharp pain. The pain never really goes away, but it does decrease with upper extremity rest. She says that when she lifts a lot at work, she has difficulty sleeping that night. She takes two Percocet-5 tablets every 6 hours when the pain is severe, but does not get complete relief.

DIAGNOSIS

- *Chronic Pain* related to muscle inflammation

EXPECTED OUTCOMES

Ms. Akers will:
- Return for follow-up visits with a journal of activities and pain experiences.
- After 3 to 5 days on regularly scheduled doses of pain medication, report a decrease in the level of pain from 7 to 3 or 4 on a scale of 1 to 10.
- Decrease number of absences from work.
- Modify activities at work and at home, especially when pain is intense.

PLANNING AND IMPLEMENTATION

- Encourage discussion of pain, and acknowledge belief in Ms. Akers's report of pain.
- Consult with a physician for an appropriate nonsteroidal anti-inflammatory analgesic with a minimum of side effects, and instruct in maintaining regular dosing schedules.
- For episodes of acute pain, take opioid analgesic as soon as the pain begins and every 6 hours while continuing the dosage of NSAID analgesic.
- Teach one relaxation technique that is personally useful.
- Explore distraction techniques such as listening to music, watching comedies, or reading.
- Provide clinic phone number and instruct to call if pain is unrelieved with opioid and NSAID analgesics.

EVALUATION

Ms. Akers returns for scheduled follow-up visits with a completed journal of her activities and associated pain. She reports that taking oral opioid analgesics has relieved her pain and that within 3 weeks regular use, NSAID analgesics brought her pain under control. She also reports that her supervisor has reassigned her to a position that requires no lifting. She now rates her pain at 2 or 3 on a scale of 1 to 10. She has missed only 1 day of work in the last 3 months and reports that her children and friends have helped with her household tasks when she has requested they do so.

CRITICAL THINKING IN THE NURSING PROCESS

1. Describe three factors that support the statement "Pain is a personal experience."
2. Ms. Akers asks you how often she should take her pain medications. You tell her to (a) take them on a regular basis or (b) wait until she experiences pain. Which action would you choose, and why?
3. Develop a care plan for Ms. Akers for the nursing diagnosis of *Risk for Constipation*. Why is this necessary?

See Evaluating Your Response in Appendix C.

Assessment

Pain assessment varies by the acuity of the pain and circumstances surrounding the patient's entry into the healthcare setting. Identifying the location, intensity, and triggering event may be the most appropriate initial assessment for a patient experiencing acute pain related to trauma. The approach to a patient experiencing acute pain without known trauma (e.g., acute chest, flank, or abdominal pain) may still be very focused due to the acuity of the situation. Additional information regarding the quality and timing of the pain, as well as the patient's health history often provide valuable clues about the underlying cause. When pain is chronic, a comprehensive approach to pain assessment is essential to ensure adequate and appropriate interventions. The four essential areas to assess are patient perceptions, physiologic responses, behavioral responses, the patient's attempts to manage the pain, and the effectiveness of these pain-management strategies.

Patient Perceptions

The most reliable indicator of the presence and degree of pain is the patient's own statement about the pain.

> **MEMORY CUE**
>
> The PQRST mnemonic provides a useful tool for conducting a focused pain assessment:
>
> P = What precipitated (triggered, stimulated) the pain? Has anything relieved the pain? What is the pattern of the pain (constant, episodic)?
>
> Q = What are the qualities of the pain? How would you describe the pain (sharp, stabbing, aching, burning, stinging, deep, crushing, viselike, gnawing)?
>
> R = What is the region (location) of the pain? Can you put your finger on where the pain is? Does the pain radiate to other areas of the body?
>
> S = What is the severity or intensity of the pain?
>
> T = What is the timing of the pain? When does it begin, how long does it last, and how is it related to other events in the patient's life?

The McGill Pain Questionnaire is a useful tool in assessing the subjective pain experience. It asks the patient to locate the pain and to describe its quality and intensity using terms to describe its sensory, affective, evaluative, and miscellaneous

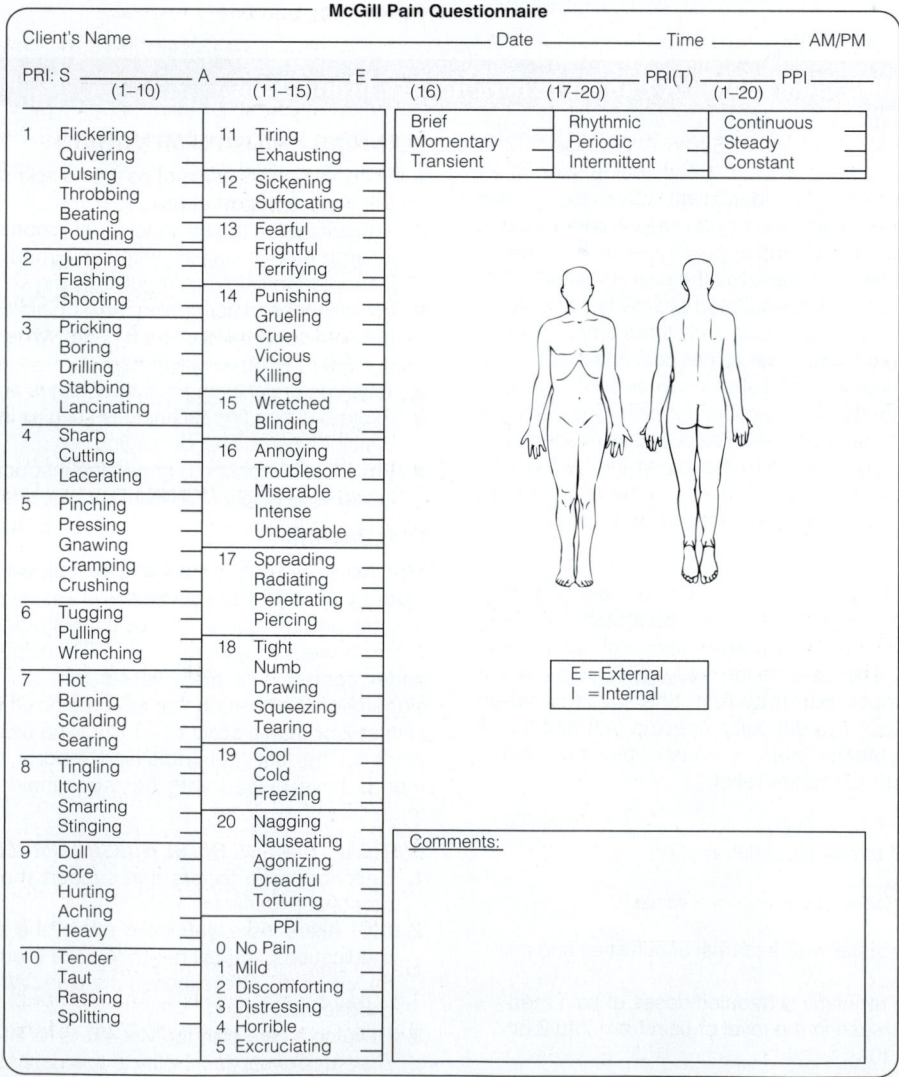

Figure 9–10 ■ The McGill Pain Questionnaire. The descriptors fall into four major groups: sensory (1–10), affective (11–15), evaluative (16), and miscellaneous (17–20). The rank value for each descriptor is based on its position in the word set; the sum of the rank values is the pain rating index (PRI). The present pain intensity (PPI) is based on a scale of 0 to 5.

components. Additional components of the questionnaire address the pattern and timing of the pain (Figure 9–10 ■).

The most common method to assess the severity of pain is a pain rating scale. Pain rating scales can be used even in the most emergent situations. Several scales are illustrated in Figure 9–11 ■. For patients who do not understand English or numerals, a scale using colors (e.g., light blue for no pain through bright red for worst possible pain) or the Faces Pain Scale-Revised (FPS-R) may be helpful. The following guidelines will help the nurse effectively use a pain rating scale:

- To ensure consistent communication, explain the specific pain rating scale being used. If a word descriptor scale is used, verify that the patient can read the language being used. If a numerical scale is used, be sure the patient can count to 10. Discuss the definition of the word "pain" to ensure that the patient and the provider are communicating on the same level. It is often helpful to use the patient's own words when describing the pain.
- Explain that the report of pain is important for promoting recovery, not just for achieving temporary comfort.
- Ask the patient to establish a comfort-function goal. This is a level of pain that does not interfere with or prevent the performance of essential activities of recovery or living. Often, pain assessment is made while a patient is sedentary. In this state the patient may experience less pain than when active and falsely estimate tolerable pain ratings. Provide guidelines for setting goals. Researchers found that pain ratings higher than 3 (scale of 0–10) interfered significantly with patients' activities, and scores of 6 and 7 decrease quality of life (Slaughter, Pasero, & Manworren, 2002).

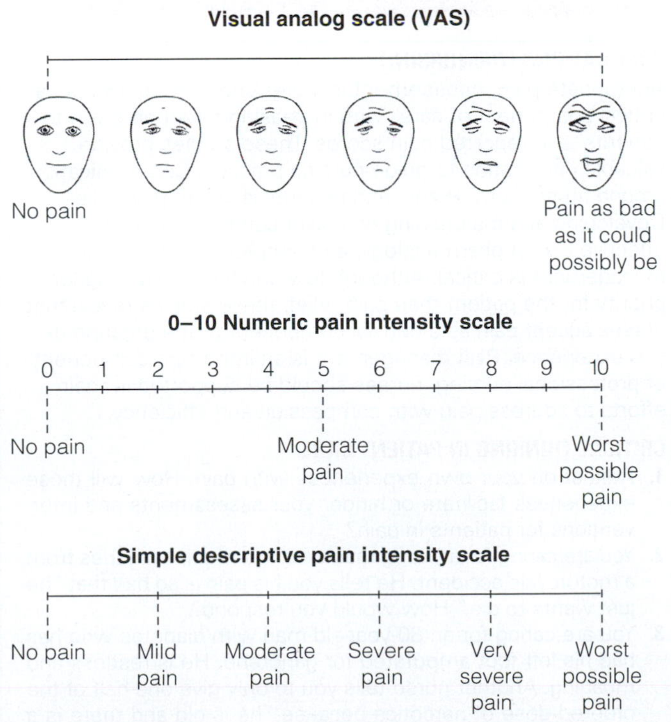

Figure 9–11 ■ Examples of commonly used pain scales.

Commonly Used Pain Scale from FPS-R. This figure has been reproduced with permission of the International Association for the Study of Pain® (IASP®). The figure may not be reproduced for any other purpose without permission.

Research has shown the numeric rating, verbal descriptor, and faces rating scales to be effective with young, middle, and older adults. These scales also are effective in cognitively impaired older adults, although the faces scale was the preferred tool. Additionally, the faces scale was preferred by African Americans and Hispanics (Flaherty, 2007).

Physiologic Responses
Predictable physiologic changes occur in the presence of acute pain. These may include muscle tension; tachycardia; rapid, shallow respirations; increased blood pressure; dilated pupils; sweating; and pallor. Over time, however, the pain stimulus triggers less of a sympathetic nervous system response, and these physiologic changes may be extinguished in patients with chronic pain.

Behavioral Responses
Some behaviors are so typical of people in pain that the behaviors are referred to as *pain behaviors*. They include bracing or guarding the painful part, taking medication, crying, moaning, grimacing, withdrawing from activity and socialization, becoming immobile, talking about pain, holding the painful area, breathing with increased effort, exhibiting a sad facial expression, and being restless.

Behavioral responses to pain may or may not coincide with the patient's report of pain and are not always reliable cues to the pain experience. Discrepancies between the patient's report of pain and behavioral responses may be the result of cultural factors, coping skills, fear, denial, or the utilization of relaxation or distraction techniques.

Patients may deny pain for a variety of reasons, including fear of injections, fear of drug/narcotic addiction, misinterpretation of terms (the patient may not think that aching, soreness, or discomfort qualify as pain), or the misconception that healthcare providers know when patients experience pain. Some patients may deny pain as part of an attempt to deny that there is something wrong with them. Other patients, by contrast, may think that "as needed" medications will be given only if their pain rating is high. Patients may also use pain as a mechanism to gain attention from family and healthcare providers.

Patients with Advanced Dementia
Behavior cues are critical for assessing pain intensity in patients with advanced dementia (unable to respond to simple yes or no questions) or who are nonverbal. The Pain Assessment in Advanced Dementia (PAINAD) scale uses five behavioral indicators of pain. Once trained, the nurse can use the scale by observing patient behaviors related to breathing (normal, labored, hyperventilation), vocalization (moaning, calling out, crying), facial expression (smiling or without expression, sad, frowning, grimacing), body language (relaxed, tense, rigid or striking out), and consolability (distractible, reassured, or unable to console) (Horgas & Miller, 2008).

Self-Management of Pain
The patient's attempts to manage pain are useful additions to the assessment database. This information is individualized and patient specific, including many factors such as culture, age, and patient knowledge. Get detailed descriptions of actions the patient or significant others took, when and how these measures were applied, and how well they worked.

Nursing Diagnoses and Interventions

The primary nursing diagnoses for patients in pain are acute pain and chronic pain.

Acute Pain

Assess the characteristics of the pain by asking the patient to do the following:

- Point to the pain location or mark the pain location on a figure drawing. *Pain location provides information about the etiology of the pain and the type of pain being experienced.*
- Rate the intensity of the pain by using an evidence-based pain scale (see Figure 9–11). Use the same scale with each assessment. *Pain and its intensity is a subjective experience. Consistently using the same scale to rate pain intensity allows evaluation of intervention effectiveness.*

PRACTICE ALERT
Do not assume that the older patient or the cognitively-impaired patient is not having pain or is unable to identify its intensity. Many cognitively impaired patients are able to use a pain scale such as faces, numeric rating, or verbal descriptor (Flaherty, 2007).

- Describe the quality of the pain, saying, for example, "Describe what your pain feels like." If necessary, suggest word descriptors for the patient to select. *Descriptive terms provide insight into the nature and cause of the pain.*
- Describe the pattern of the pain, including time of onset, duration, persistence, and times without pain. Ask whether the pain is worse at regular times of the day and about its relationship to activity. *The pattern of pain provides clues about cause and location.*
- Describe any precipitating or relieving factors. *Precipitating factors provide clues to any underlying pathophysiology of the pain; relieving factors provide information that can be used when planning nursing interventions for pain management.*
- Monitor manifestations of pain by taking vital signs; assessing skin temperature and moisture; observing pupils; observing facial expressions, position in bed, guarding of body parts; and noting restlessness. *Autonomic responses to pain may result in an increased blood pressure, tachycardia, rapid respirations, perspiration, and dilated pupils. Other responses to pain include grimacing, clenching the hands, muscle rigidity, guarding, restlessness, and nausea.*

PRACTICE ALERT
Consider pain the fifth vital sign and assess patients for pain every time you check temperature, pulse, respirations, and blood pressure.

- Communicate belief in the patient's pain. *Verbally acknowledge the presence of the pain, listen carefully to the description of pain, and act to help the patient manage the pain. Because pain is a personal, subjective experience, the nurse must convey belief in the patient's pain. By conveying belief in the patient's pain, the nurse reduces anxiety and thereby lessens pain.* See the accompanying Moving Evidence into Action box.
- Administer prescribed analgesics, determining the preferred route of administration. Provide pain-relieving measures for

MOVING EVIDENCE INTO ACTION   The Patient Experiencing Pain

Pain that is not adequately managed is the focus of regulatory agencies, professional healthcare organizations, and consumer groups. Despite well-defined guidelines for pain management, there is a gap between guideline standards of care and implementation of care. A number of studies have compared nurses' perceptions of pain management with the experience related by patients. In a study by Manias et al. (2005) nurses were observed for 2-hour periods of high environmental, patient, and nursing activity, revealing varied responses to patients' pain. The pain was (1) responded to effectively; (2) prioritized as less important than other nursing tasks; (3) ignored because cues were missed; (4) treated as part of the medication administration regimen, with medication given or withheld according to schedule; (5) prevented through comfort measures, pre-medicating, and teaching the importance of early communication about pain; and (6) only addressed reactively, after the painful experience. A later study by Gunningberg and Idvall (2007) compared patient and nurse assessments of the pain management of postoperative patients on two surgery units. This study found areas for improvements in pain management related to communication, action, trust, and environment. Patients who experienced more pain than expected were less satisfied with their care and reported higher levels of pain intensity. The study also pointed to the importance of considering patients' previous pain experience and goals for pain relief in accurately assessing pain.

IMPLICATIONS FOR NURSING

Appropriate pain management is increasingly recognized as a critical component of care, with increasing attention given to patients' self-reported pain scores. These studies provide valuable information to guide nursing practice. Communication among nurses, physicians, and patients is key to pain relief. Developing and maintaining caregiver competence in the effective use of pharmacologic and nonpharmacologic pain management is critical. Although few conditions have higher priority for the patient than pain relief, these studies reveal that nurses accept pain as a normal component of the postoperative experience. Pain management is an important component of professional nursing; nurses should be supported in their efforts to address pain with compassion and efficiency.

CRITICAL THINKING IN PATIENT CARE

1. Reflect on your own experiences with pain. How will those experiences facilitate or hinder your assessments and interventions for patients in pain?
2. You are caring for a young man who has multiple injuries from a motorcycle accident. He tells you his pain is so bad that "he just wants to die." How would you respond?
3. You are caring for an 80-year-old man with diabetes who has had his left foot amputated for gangrene. He is restless and moaning. Another nurse tells you to only give one-half of the ordered dose of narcotics because "he is old and there is a danger of respiratory depression." What would you do?
4. Why do you think nurses tend to underestimate and under-medicate pain?

severe pain on a regular around-the-clock basis or by self-administration (such as with a PCA pump). *The patient is a part of the decision-making process and can exert some control over the situation by choosing the administration route. Analgesics are usually most effective when they are administered before pain occurs or becomes severe. Around-the-clock administration has been proven to provide better pain management for both acute and chronic pain.*

> **SAFETY ALERT**
> Use extreme care to ensure the correct patient, medication, and dose when setting up and monitoring PCA for analgesia. Patient harm resulting from medication errors with PCA often is greater than harm resulting from other types of medication errors.

- To reduce the risk of medication error associated with PCA, work with administration to develop the following strategies:
  - Use a single brand or type of pump within a facility to reduce programming and use complexity for caregivers.
  - Use bar codes and electronic medical records to reduce errors that involve the wrong medication.
  - Develop and use easily understood and standardized forms for PCA.
    The complexity of activities required to safely program PCA pumps, the use of different medications and concentrations, confusion of medical orders, and variations in documentation related to PCA are identified as contributing factors to PCA medication errors (Sheehan, 2008).
- Evaluate and monitor the effects of analgesics and other pain-relieving measures. Teach family members or significant others to be alert for adverse reactions to pain medications. Sedation, constipation, nausea and dizziness are common side effects of opioid analgesics. *Opioid analgesics stimulate mu receptors, leading to common adverse effects such as respiratory depression, nausea, and constipation.*
- Provide for safety of the patient receiving opioid analgesics:
  - Check respiratory rate and oxygen saturation every 2 hours at the beginning of opioid therapy and after increasing dosage. Reduce the dose and notify the physician if the respiratory rate falls to eight per minute or lower or if the oxygen saturation falls. *Excessive sedation can progress to significant respiratory depression.*

- Prevent falls that may result from sedation or dizziness. *Opioid analgesics can affect balance and judgment, increasing the risk for falls, particularly in the elderly.*
- Administer an opioid antagonist such as naloxone (Narcan) if the patient develops symptoms of excessive opioid dosage. Administer prescribed dose (0.4–2 mg) by direct intravenous push over 10 to 15 seconds or by intravenous infusion. Titrate infusion or repeat direct IV push every 2–3 minutes (up to a total of 10 mg) to reverse respiratory depression or excessive sedation. Continue to monitor respiratory status and sedation, repeating naloxone as necessary. *The opioid agonist causing excessive sedation and respiratory depression may have a longer half-life than naloxone, leading to a fall in respiratory rate and decreased LOC after the initial dose of naloxone has been substantially eliminated. Administration of excessive naloxone may cause acute withdrawal and failure of pain relief. It may take considerable time to re-establish a therapeutic comfort level.*
- Teach the patient and family nonpharmacologic methods of pain management, such as relaxation, distraction, and cutaneous stimulation. *These techniques are especially useful when used in conjunction with pain medications. They can be beneficial for patients experiencing either acute or chronic pain.*
- Provide comfort measures, such as changing positions, back massage, oral care, skin care, and changing bed linens. *Basic comfort measures for personal cleanliness, skin care, and mobility promote physical and psychosocial well-being, lessening the perception of pain.*
- Provide patient and family teaching, and make referrals if necessary to assist with coping, financial resources, and home care. *The patient (and family) with pain requires information about medications, noninvasive techniques for pain management, and sources of assistance with home-based care. The patient with acute pain requires information about the expected course of pain resolution.*

Chronic Pain

The patient who has chronic pain may not demonstrate the same physiologic and behavioral responses to pain as are seen in the patient with acute pain. The intensity of the pain, however, may be as high or even higher than acute pain. Furthermore, chronic pain, whether of malignant or nonmalignant origin, has a negative

Chronic Pain Video

NURSING CARE OF THE OLDER ADULT   **Pain Management for the Older Adult**

Older adults often have medical conditions associated with pain, such as arthritis, peripheral vascular disease, and diabetes. Many older adults have multiple health disorders causing them to experience both acute and chronic pain.

The nursing standard of care calls for older adults to be pain free or have their pain controlled to an acceptable level that allows the highest possible level of functioning (Horgas & Yoon, 2008). Achieving this standard requires comprehensive assessment of the patient, including the patient's history, subjective reports of pain, nonverbal and behavioral responses, and information from family members about the patient's pain experiences.

In addition to frequent and ongoing assessment, nursing care guidelines call for the nurse to anticipate and treat pain before, during, and after painful procedures and treatments. The nurse should educate the patient, family, and other clinicians about prophylactic analgesic use, using analgesics on a regular basis, and how to avoid allowing pain to escalate. Teaching must include information about the medications themselves, their side and adverse effects, and issues about addiction, dependence, and tolerance. Finally, the nurse teaches the patient, family, and other healthcare providers about nonpharmacologic pain management strategies such as relaxation, massage, and application of heat or cold (Horgas & Yoon, 2008).

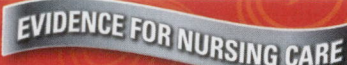

EVIDENCE FOR NURSING CARE — The Patient with Acute Pain

Selected resources that nurses may find helpful when planning evidence-based nursing care follow.

- Herr, K., Bjoro, K., Steffensmeier, J., & Rakel, B. (2006, July). *Acute pain management in older adults.* Iowa City, IA: University of Iowa Gerontological Nursing Interventions Research Center, Research Translation and Dissemination Core.
- Institute for Clinical Systems Improvement. (2008). *Health care guideline: Assessment and management of acute pain* (6th ed., pp. 1–58). Retrieved from http://www.icsi.org/pain_acute/pain__acute__assessment_and_management_of__3.html
- Registered Nurses Association of Ontario (RNAO). (2007 February 27). *Assessment and management of pain: supplement.* Toronto, ON: Author.

effect on the patient's physical, psychosocial, emotional, and functional status. In addition to the nursing assessments and interventions identified for acute pain, consider the following interventions for the patient experiencing chronic pain.

- Ask the patient to describe the pain and its meaning, including its effects on life style, self-concept, roles, and relationships. *Pain is a stressor that may affect the patient's coping ability. Chronic pain often interferes with sleep quality, job performance, personal relationships, and social interactions. The patient may have concerns about addiction to pain medication and costs as well.*
- Assess for depression using an accepted depression screening tool. *Chronic pain and depression commonly occur concurrently (Fauci et al., 2008).*
- If the underlying cause of chronic pain has not been identified, advocate for consultations, diagnostic testing, or other means of establishing an accurate diagnosis. *Guidelines for chronic pain management call for treatment of the underlying cause whenever it can be identified (WHO, 2008).*

EVIDENCE FOR NURSING CARE — The Patient with Chronic Pain

Selected resources that nurses may find helpful when planning evidence-based nursing care follow.

- D'Arcy, Y. (2009). Chronic opioid therapy clinical guidelines. *The Nurse Practitioner: The American Journal of Primary Health Care, 34*(10), 13–15. Retrieved from http://www.nursingcenter.com/library/JournalArticle.asp?Article_ID=935533
- D'Arcy, Y. (2009). Overturning barriers to pain relief in older adults. *Nursing2009, 39*(10), 32–39. Retrieved from www.nursing2009.com
- Institute for Clinical Systems Improvement (ICSI). (2008, July). *Assessment and management of chronic pain.* Bloomington, MN: Institute for Clinical Systems Improvement.
- University of Michigan Health System. (2009, March). *Managing chronic non-terminal pain including prescribing controlled substances.* Ann Arbor, MI: University of Michigan Health System.

- Administer prescribed NSAIDs, opioid and nonopioid analgesics, and other medications around the clock and as ordered. Whenever possible, the oral or transdermal routes should be used. *Around-the-clock analgesic administration helps maintain pain within an acceptable range within which the patient remains comfortable and functional. As needed medications may be required for breakthrough pain.*
- Do not crush or break or allow patients to chew controlled-release oral preparations. *Crushing, breaking or chewing controlled release oral preparations may lead to overdose. Capsules containing controlled-release pellets can be opened and sprinkled over soft food. See the accompanying box for more information about standards of pain management in the older adult.*
- Teach the patient, family, and caregivers how to manage side and adverse effects of prescribed medications. Advise about the importance of taking NSAIDs with food to reduce the risk of gastrointestinal irritation and bleeding. Provide information about appropriate laxatives for the patient taking opioid analgesics. Instruct when to contact the prescribing care provider should adverse effects become problematic. *Many analgesics, while effective, have adverse effects that may limit the patient's willingness to continue therapy. In most cases, appropriate management of these effects allows continued use of the medication.*
- Encourage and advocate for a multimodal approach to pain management, teaching about the use of heat, cold, and CAM therapies, providing for referrals to healthcare providers (e.g. physical therapists, chiropractic physicians, massage therapists, acupuncturists) and chronic pain clinics as appropriate. *Using a multimodal approach to management of chronic pain improves the patient's perception of control over the pain and its effect on lifestyle. This also may allow less dependence on opioid and nonopioid analgesics.*

Using NANDA, NIC, and NOC

Linkages between a selected NANDA nursing diagnosis, NIC, and NOC for the patient with chronic pain are shown in the chart that follows.

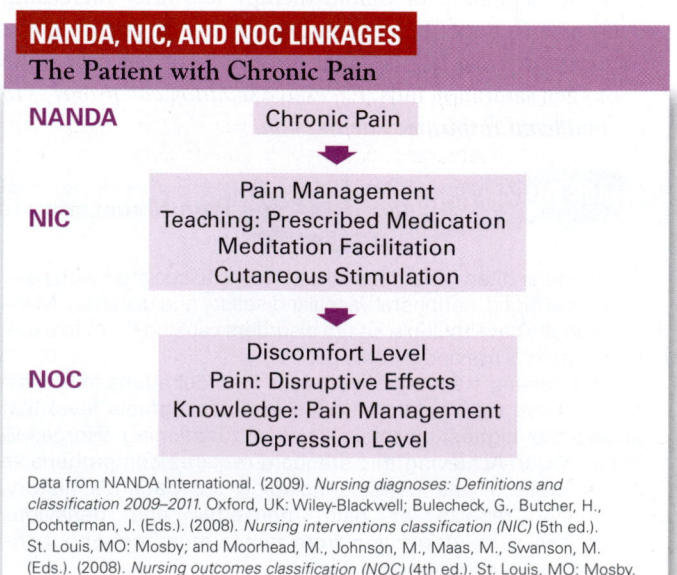

NANDA, NIC, AND NOC LINKAGES
The Patient with Chronic Pain

NANDA
Chronic Pain

NIC
Pain Management
Teaching: Prescribed Medication
Meditation Facilitation
Cutaneous Stimulation

NOC
Discomfort Level
Pain: Disruptive Effects
Knowledge: Pain Management
Depression Level

Data from NANDA International. (2009). *Nursing diagnoses: Definitions and classification 2009–2011.* Oxford, UK: Wiley-Blackwell; Bulecheck, G., Butcher, H., Dochterman, J. (Eds.). (2008). *Nursing interventions classification (NIC)* (5th ed.). St. Louis, MO: Mosby; and Moorhead, M., Johnson, M., Maas, M., Swanson, M. (Eds.). (2008). *Nursing outcomes classification (NOC)* (4th ed.). St. Louis, MO: Mosby.

Community-Based Care

Teaching the patient and family includes the following:

- Specific drugs to be taken, including the frequency, potential side effects, possible drug interactions, and any special precautions to be taken (such as taking with food or avoiding alcohol).
- How to take or administer the drugs ordered for managing chronic malignant or nonmalignant pain (Box 9–2).
- The importance of taking pain medications before the pain becomes severe.
- An explanation that the risk of addiction to pain medications is very small when they are used for pain relief and management.
- Discussion about physical tolerance and the importance of contacting the prescriber should medications become less effective.
- The importance of scheduling periods of rest and sleep.
- Use of CAM therapies to supplement or enhance traditional approaches to pain management.
- In addition, suggest the following resources:
  - Pain clinics
  - Community support groups
  - American Cancer Society
  - American Pain Society

BOX 9–2 Opioids for Long-Term Analgesia for Chronic Pain

Drug	Route	Nursing Implications
Oxycodone (OxyContin)	Oral	Available in a timed-release formulation for 12-hour dosing and as fast-acting formulations (OxyIR, OxyFAST) for breakthrough pain.
Morphine (Kadian)	Oral	Formulated of timed-release particles in a capsule. If patient can't swallow the capsule, may be sprinkled over food or given by nasogastric or gastric tube.
Fentanyl (Duragesic)	Transdermal	Absorbed slowly through the skin; allows 72-hour dose schedule. Up to 14 ours to achieve therapeutic level; when discontinued therapeutic effect will decay slowly.
Fentanyl citrate (Actiq)	Transmucosal	A lozenge formulation used to treat breakthrough cancer pain in opioid-tolerant patients.

CHAPTER HIGHLIGHTS

- Pain is transmitted by the peripheral and central nervous systems and perceived in the CNS. Opioids and other analgesics block the perception of pain; NSAIDs and most nonpharmacological interventions block or decrease the transmission of pain from the periphery to the CNS. Measures to block the sensitization of pain-transmitting fibers can help prevent chronic pain.
- There are many types of pain and treatment varies according to the type and combination of types. Acute pain, which may be cutaneous or deep somatic, visceral, or referred, usually decreases as healing progresses. Chronic pain may be episodic, experienced as recurrent acute pain, or may be persistent pain of either malignant or nonmalignant origin. Breakthrough pain is that which exceeds the baseline or persistent level of pain. Phantom limb pain is a type of neuropathic pain that occurs after amputations. Central pain and complex regional pain syndrome also are types of neuropathic pain.
- Culture and gender impact pain perception and behavior. A patient's emotional state, past experiences with pain, and the underlying cause and meaning of the painful experience also affect responses to pain. A mnemonic such as PQRST or a tool such as the McGill Pain Questionnaire may be used when assessing pain. Important components of the assessment include the location, intensity, and character (quality) of the pain; its onset, duration, and timing; factors that aggravate or relieve the pain; associated symptoms; and measures taken to treat the pain or its cause. When rating pain intensity, one pain scale should be consistently used with the individual patient.
- Behavioral assessment of pain intensity is less accurate than a patient's report of pain intensity, particularly when pain is chronic. Behavioral responses may be used to assess pain in patients who are significantly cognitively impaired, however. Older adults perceive pain as intensely as younger adults, but may hesitate to report pain for fear of losing independence or being considered a bother. Physical tolerance develops with long-term opioid use, necessitating dose increases to achieve the same effect. Although patients who are addicted to opioids need greater doses of opioid analgesics to control pain because of tolerance, treating physicians and nurses providing care often withhold or use lower doses of opioid analgesics, leading to inadequate pain relief.
- Pain management includes assessment, intervention, and evaluation. It is important to verify that interventions have been effective. If not, interventions must be identified that bring pain down to a level of intensity with which the patient feels satisfied.

TEST YOURSELF NCLEX-RN® REVIEW

1. During your assessment, a patient tells you he has had lower back pain for 9 months. When planning nursing care, you recognize this type of pain as which of the following?
   1. neuropathic pain
   2. chronic pain
   3. visceral pain
   4. somatic pain

2. A patient presents to the ED after smashing her finger in the car door. She relates that her pain initially was sharp and so intense she thought she would faint, but now it is dull and throbbing. The nurse appropriately recognizes this as which of the following?
   1. indicative that the injury is less severe than initially perceived
   2. the result of interpretation of the pain stimulus by the thalamus
   3. an example of the gate theory of pain transmission
   4. transmission of pain stimuli via unmyelinated C fibers

3. You are taking a health history for a patient who has taken an NSAID for several years. Which of the following questions should you ask? **Select all that apply.**
   1. "Tell me how and when you take this drug."
   2. "Have you ever vomited blood or had very dark stools?"
   3. "Do you know that you may become addicted to this drug?"
   4. "Have you noticed any problems with your breathing?"
   5. "Do you have your blood pressure checked regularly?"

4. Which of the following would you include when teaching a patient about a transdermal pain medication?
   1. Contact your physician if this medication makes you excessively sleepy.
   2. Replace this patch every 24 hours, applying it to clean, dry skin.
   3. When reapplying the patch, place it on the anterior thigh.
   4. This medication should be effective within 2 to 4 hours; contact your physician if your pain is not at an acceptable level after that.

5. Which of the following statements would be most useful in determining the quality of a patient's pain?
   1. "Tell me where you hurt."
   2. "Rate your pain on a scale of 0–10."
   3. "Describe what your pain feels like."
   4. "Tell me how this pain affects your sleep."

6. When assessing a postoperative patient's pain, you note that he is relaxed, smiling, and visiting with friends. He rates his pain as a 7 on a scale of 0–10. The most appropriate response is to do which of the following?
   1. Reassess the patient's pain after his friends have left.
   2. Document your assessment but take no further action.
   3. Administer the prescribed analgesic dose.
   4. Note that the patient is developing tolerance to the prescribed opioid analgesic.

7. When teaching a patient with chronic malignant pain about using opioid analgesics, you would include which of the following instructions?
   1. "This drug may interfere with urination; contact your physician if that becomes a problem."
   2. "Increase fluid and fiber intake; you may need a stool softener or laxative to prevent constipation."
   3. "This drug may cause itching and rash; take Benadryl (diphenhydramine) as needed."
   4. "There is a risk of addiction with this drug; stop the drug if you find that it no longer provides the degree of pain relief necessary."

8. When assessing pain in a patient who is moderately cognitively impaired due to dementia, the nurse should do which of the following?
   1. Ask the patient to rate his pain using the faces pain scale.
   2. Use only behavioral cues such as grimacing, pacing, or agitation.
   3. Have the family evaluate the intensity of the patient's pain.
   4. Administer the prescribed analgesic on an around-the-clock basis.

9. A patient asks the nurse if she should take glucosamine for her knee pain. The nurse bases her response on the knowledge of which of the following?
   1. There is no evidence that natural products such as glucosamine are effective for treating any type of pain.
   2. Chronic pain such as that associated with osteoarthritis is best treated with NSAIDs and acetaminophen.
   3. When combined with chondroitin, glucosamine has been effective in relieving moderate to severe knee pain in some patients.
   4. Although no studies have shown a benefit from taking glucosamine, other CAM therapies such as acupuncture are effective for treating pain.

10. A patient who recently took up running to lose weight asks why she feels better after running when she should be tired and sore. The most accurate response would be which of the following?
    1. Natural narcotic-like substances are released during physical activities like running.
    2. Activities such as running activate a natural "gate" in the spinal cord, blocking pain signals.
    3. Engaging in activities that actively use large muscle groups changes pain circuits in the brain, reducing the perception of pain.
    4. With repeated stimulation through activities such as running, nociceptors in deep tissues become less sensitive to stimuli.

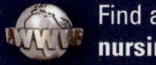

BIBLIOGRAPHY

Adams, M., P., Holland, L. N., Jr., & Bostwick, P. M. (2008). *Pharmacology for nurses: A pathophysiologic approach* (2nd ed.). Upper Saddle River, NJ: Pearson Prentice Hall.

American Academy of Pain Management. (2009). Pain is an epidemic – A message from the director. Retrieved from www.aapainmanage.org

American Music Therapy Association, Inc. Music therapy in the treatment and management of pain. Retrieved from www.musictherapy.org

Andrews, M. M., & Boyle, J. S. (2008). *Transcultural concepts in nursing care* (5th ed.). Philadelphia, PA: Lippincott Williams & Wilkins.

Ashley, J. L. (2008). Pain management: Nurses in jeopardy. *Oncology Nursing Forum, 35*(5), E70–E75.

ASPAN pain and comfort clinical guideline. (2008). Retrieved from www.guideline.gov

Barclay, L., Lee, D., & Martin, B., N. (2008). Patients may need better pain interventions after traumatic injury. *Medscape Medical News, 2008 March 25.*

Barnes, P. M., Bloom, B., Nahin, R. (2008 December). Complementary and alternative medicine use among adults and children: United States, 2007. *CDC National Health Statistics Report #12.* Retrieved from www.nccam.nih.gov

Breivik, H., Borchgrevink, P. C., Allen, S. M., Rosseland, L. A., Romundstad, L., Breivik Hals, E. K., et al. (2008). Assessment of pain. *British Journal of Anaesthesia, 101*(1), 17–24. Retrieved from www.medscape.com

Centers for Disease Control and Prevention (CDC). (2006). New report finds pain affects millions of Americans. Retrieved from www.cdc.gov

Comptom, P., & Athanasos, P. (2003). Chronic pain, substance abuse and addiction. *The Nursing Clinics of North America, 38*; 525–537.

Cranwell-Bruce, L. (2007 October). Update on pain management: New methods of opiate delivery. *Medsurg Nursing, 16*(5), 333–335.

DiPiro, J., Talbert, R., Yee, G., Matzke, G., Wells, B., & Posey, L. (2008). *Pharmacotherapy: A pathophysiologic approach* (7th ed.). New York, NY: McGraw Hill.

Doyle, S. (2008). Fentanyl buccal tablets safe, well tolerated in cancer patients. *Medscape Medical News, 2008.* Retrieved from www.medscape.com

Fauci, A. S., Braunwald, E., Kasper, D. L., Hauser, S. L., Longo, D. L., Jameson, J. L., et al. (2008). *Harrison's principles of internal medicine* (17th ed.). New York, NY: McGraw Hill.

Flaherty, E. (2007). Pain assessment for older adults. *Try This: Best Practices in Nursing Care to Older Adults.* New York, NY: The Hartford Institute for Geriatric Nursing, College of Nursing, New York University.

Flaherty, E. (2008). How to try this. Using pain-rating scales with older adults. *American Journal of Nursing, 108*(6), 40–47.

Fontaine, K. L. (2005). *Complementary & alternative therapies for nursing practice* (2nd ed.). Upper Saddle River, NJ: Pearson Prentice Hall.

Galvagno, S. M., Jr., Correll, D. J., & Narang, S. (2007 April). Safe oral equianalgesic opioid dosing for patients with moderate-to-severe pain. *Resident & Staff Physician, 2007-04.* Retrieved from www.residentandstaff.com

Gendall, K. A., Kennedy, R. R., Watson, A. J. M., & Frizelle, F. A. (2007 March). The effect of epidural analgesia on postoperative outcome after colorectal surgery. *Colorectal Disease, 9,* 584–600.

Gunningberb, L., & Idvall, E. (2007). The quality of postoperative pain management from the perspectives of patients, nurses and patient records. *Journal of Nursing Management, 15,* 756–766.

Hartrick, C. T. (2004). Multimodal postoperative pain management. *American Journal of Health-System Pharmacology, 61,* S1, S4–S10.

Helms, J. E., & Barone, C. P. (2008 December). Physiology and treatment of pain. *Critical Care Nurse, 28*(6), 38–49.

Horgas, A., & Miller, L. (2008 July). How to try this. Pain assessment in people with dementia. *American Journal of Nursing, 108*(7), 62–70.

Horgas, A. L., & Yoon, S. L. (2008 January). Want to know more: Pain. Nursing Standard of Practice Protocol: Pain management in older adults. New York, NY: The Harford Institute for Geriatric Nursing, New York University. Retrieved from www.consultgerirn.org

International Association for the Study of Pain (IASP). (2008). What's new: IASP pain terminology. Retrieved from www.iasp-pain.org

Joint Commission on Accreditation of Healthcare Organizations. (2004). *Joint Commission on Accreditation of Healthcare Organizations pain standards for 2004.* Retrieved from www.jcaho.org

Lehne, R. A. (2007). Pharmacology for Nursing Care (6th ed.). St. Louis, MO: W.B. Saunders.

Low, J., Johnston, N., & Morris, C. (2008). Editorial. Epidural analgesia: First do no harm. *Anaesthesia, 63,* 1–3.

McCaffery, M. (1979). *Nursing management of the patient with pain.* Philadelphia: Lippincott.

McCaffery, M., Pasero, C., & Ferrell, B. R. (2007 December). Pain control. Nurses' decisions about opioid dose. *American Journal of Nursing, 107*(12), 35–39.

McCance, K., & Huether, S. (2010). *Pathophysiology: The biologic basis for disease in adults and children* (6th ed.). St. Louis: Mosby.

McCarberg, B. H. (2008). What are we afraid of? Barriers to providing adequate pain relief. *Medscape Neurology & Neurosurgery, 2008.* Retrieved from www.medscape.com

McCarberg, B., & D'Arcy, Y. (2007 July). Target pain with topical peripheral analgesics. *The Nurse Practitioner, 32*(7), 44–49.

Melzack, R. (1975). The McGill Pain Questionnaire: Major properties and scoring methods. Pain, 1, 277.

Miaskowski, C., Cleary, J., Burney, R., Coyne, P, Finley, R., Foster, R., et al. (2008). Guideline for the treatment of cancer pain in adults and children. Glenview, IL: American Pain Society (APS). Retrieved from www.guideline.gov

NANDA International. (2009). *Nursing diagnoses: Definitions and classification 2009–2011.* Oxford, UK: Wiley-Blackwell.

National Center for Complementary and Alternative Medicine (NCCAM). (2008). CAM use by race/ethnicity among adults—2007. Retrieved from www.nccam.nih.gov

NCCAM. (2006). Efficacy of glucosamine and chondroitin sulfate may depend on level of osteoarthritis pain. Retrieved from www.nccam.nih.gov

NCCAM. (2008). Spinal manipulation for low-back pain. Retrieved from www.nccam.nih.gov

National Comprehensive Cancer Network. (2008). NCCN practice guidelines in oncology: Adult cancer pain. Retrieved from www.nccn.org

National Institute of Neurological Disorders and Stroke. (2008). NINDS central pain syndrome information page. Retrieved from www.ninds.nih.gov

National Institute of Neurological Disorders and Stroke. (2009). Complex regional pain syndrome fact sheet. Retrieved from www.ninds.nih.gov

Pasero, C. (2003). Pain in the emergency department. Withholding pain medication is not justified. *American Journal of Nursing, 103*(7), 73–74.

Porth, C., & Matfin, G. (2009). Pathophysiology: Concepts of altered health states (8th ed.). Philadelphia: Lippincott.

Richards, T., Johnson, J., Sparks, A., & Emerson, H. (2007 February). The effect of music therapy on patients' perception and manifestation of pain, anxiety, and patient satisfaction. *MEDSURG Nursing, 16*(1), 7–14.

Sheehan, S. (2008). Study: Patient harm more common with patient-controlled pain medication. Joint Commission Resources. Retrieved from www.jcrinc.com

Slatkin, N. E., & Rhiner, M. I. (2008). Breakthrough pain: Improving recognition and management to enhance quality of life. Retrieved from www.medscape.com

Spencer, J. W., & Jacobs, J. J. (2003). *Complementary and alternative medicine: An evidence-based approach* (2nd ed.). St. Louis, MO: Mosby.

Tabloski, P. (2006). *Gerontological Nursing.* Upper Saddle River, NJ: Pearson Prentice Hall.

Taddio, A., & Katz, J. (2005). The effects of early pain experience in neonates on pain responses in infancy and childhood. *Pediatric Drugs, 7*(4), 245–257.

Taylor, A. (2007 Winter). Addressing the global tragedy of needless pain: Rethinking the United Nations Single Convention on Narcotic Drugs. *Journal of Law, Medicine & Ethics, Winter 2007,* 556–570.

Toomey, M. (2008, October). Gender differences in pain: Does X = Y? *AANA Journal, 76*(5), 355–359.

World Health Organization (WHO). (2008). *Scoping document for WHO treatment guidelines on chronic non-malignant pain in adults.* Geneva: WHO.

WHO. (2008). *Scoping document for WHO treatment guidelines on pain related to cancer, HIV and other progressive life-threatening illnesses in adults.* Geneva: WHO.

WHO. (2009). *WHO's pain ladder.* Geneva: WHO.

Wilkinson, J. M., & Ahern, N. R. (2009). *Nursing diagnosis handbook* (9th ed.). Upper Saddle River, NJ: Pearson Prentice Hall.

Wilson, B. A., Shannon, M. T., Shields, K. M., & Stang, C. L. (2008). *Nurse's drug guide 2008.* Upper Saddle River, NJ: Pearson Prentice Hall.

10 Nursing Care of Patients with Altered Fluid, Electrolyte, and Acid–Base Balance

LEARNING OUTCOMES

1. Describe the functions and regulatory mechanisms that maintain water and electrolyte balance in the body.
2. Compare and contrast the causes, effects, and care of the patient with fluid volume or electrolyte imbalance.
3. Explain the pathophysiology and manifestations of imbalances of sodium, potassium, calcium, magnesium, and phosphorus.
4. Describe the causes and effects of acid–base imbalances.

CLINICAL COMPETENCIES

1. Assess and monitor fluid, electrolyte, and acid–base balance.
2. Administer fluids and medications knowledgeably and safely.
3. Determine priority nursing diagnoses, based on assessment data, to select and implement individualized nursing interventions.
4. Use assessed data, patient values, and evidence to provide patient and family teaching about diet and medications used to promote, restore, and maintain fluid, electrolyte, and acid–base balance.
5. Effectively communicate and function within the interdisciplinary team to plan and provide care to patients with altered fluid, electrolyte, and acid–base balance.
6. Adapt individual cultural values and variations and expressed needs and preferences into the plan of care to provide knowledgeable and safe care to patients with fluid and electrolyte imbalances.

KEY TERMS

acidosis, 222	base excess (BE), 223	Kussmaul's respirations, 227
alkalis, 222	dehydration, 193	orthopnea, 198
alkalosis, 222	fluid volume deficit (FVD), 193	serum bicarbonate, 223
arterial blood gases (ABGs), 201	fluid volume excess, 198	tetany, 214
atrial natriuretic peptide (ANP), 192	homeostasis, 186	third spacing, 193

Normal physiologic processes depend on **homeostasis** (the ability to maintain internal equilibrium by adjusting physiological processes) in the internal environment of the body. The fluid volume, electrolyte composition, and pH of both intracellular and extracellular spaces must remain constant within a relatively narrow range to maintain health and life. Changes in the normal distribution and composition of body fluids often occur in response to illness and trauma. These changes affect fluid balance of the intracellular and extracellular compartments of the body, the concentration of electrolytes within fluid compartments, and the body's hydrogen ion concentration (pH). Fluid and electrolyte imbalances occur in all adult age groups, and in all healthcare settings.

Changes in the normal volume of fluids, their composition, distribution, and relative acidity or alkalinity have the potential to disrupt most functional health patterns. Imbalances of fluids, electrolytes, and pH affect the ability to maintain activities of daily living (activity-exercise), think clearly (cognitive-perceptual), and engage in self-care (health perception-health management). Conversely, alterations in a number of health patterns affect the ability to maintain homeostasis. Alterations in the nutritional-metabolic pattern affect the ability to consume adequate food and fluids. Disruptions of the elimination pattern may lead to retention or loss of excess amounts of fluids and electrolytes. Disrupted heart or respiratory function, which falls within the activity-exercise pattern, has the potential to affect fluid, electrolyte, and acid–base balance.

The goal in managing fluid, electrolyte, and acid–base imbalances is to reestablish and maintain homeostasis. Nursing care includes identifying and assessing patients who are likely to develop imbalances, monitoring patients for early manifestations, and implementing interdisciplinary and nursing interventions to prevent or correct imbalances. Effective nursing interventions require an understanding of the multiple processes that maintain fluid, electrolyte, and acid–base balance and an understanding of the causes and treatment of imbalances that occur. This chapter contains many references to disease processes that are discussed throughout the book and is most useful as a reference when learning about those disorders.

Overview of Fluid and Electrolyte Balance

Fluid and electrolyte balance in the body involves regulatory mechanisms that maintain the composition, distribution, and movement of fluids and electrolytes.

Body Fluid Composition

Body fluid is composed of water and various dissolved substances (solutes).

Water

Water is the primary component of body fluids and functions in several ways to maintain normal cellular function. Water provides a medium for the transport and exchange of nutrients and other substances such as oxygen, carbon dioxide, and metabolic wastes to and from cells; provides a medium for metabolic reactions within cells; and assists in regulating body temperature through the evaporation of perspiration.

Total body water constitutes about 60% of the total body weight, but this amount varies with age, gender, and the amount of body fat. Total body water decreases from 45% to 50% of total body weight with obesity and with aging (Porth & Matfin, 2009). Fat cells contain comparatively little water: In the person who is obese, the proportion of water to total body weight is less than in the person of average weight; in a person who is very thin, the proportion of water to total body weight is greater than in the person of average weight. Adult females have a greater ratio of fat to lean tissue mass than adult males; therefore, they have a lower percentage of total body water.

To maintain normal fluid balance, body water intake and output should be approximately equal. The average fluid intake and output is about 2500 mL over a 24-hour period. Most water gain is from the intake of foods and fluids; carbohydrate metabolism and other metabolic processes produce an additional small amount. Urine production and excretion account for most water loss. The average daily urine output is 1500 mL in adults. About 300 mL to 400 mL of urine per day is required to excrete metabolic wastes produced by the body (Porth & Matfin, 2009). Insensible water loss occurs through the skin, lungs, and feces. These losses, while normally small, can increase significantly during exercise, when environmental temperatures are high, and during illness that increases the respiratory rate, perspiration, or gastrointestinal (GI) losses (particularly diarrhea). Table 10–1 shows the sources of fluid gain and loss (Porth & Matfin, 2009).

Electrolytes

Body fluids contain both water molecules and chemical compounds. These chemical compounds can either remain intact in solution or dissociate into discrete particles. Electrolytes are substances that dissociate in solution to form charged particles called ions. Cations are positively charged electrolytes; anions are negatively charged electrolytes. Electrolytes have many functions, including assisting with the regulation of water balance, regulating and maintaining acid–base balance, and contributing to enzyme reactions. They are also essential for neuromuscular activity.

Body Fluid Distribution

Body fluid is classified by its location inside or outside of cells. Intracellular fluid (ICF) is found within cells (Figure 10–1 ■). ICF is essential for normal cell function, providing a medium for metabolic processes. Extracellular fluid (ECF) is located outside of cells and is further classified by location:

- Interstitial fluid is located in the spaces between most of the cells of the body.
- Intravascular fluid, called *plasma*, is contained within the arteries, veins, and capillaries.
- Transcellular fluid includes urine; digestive secretions; perspiration; and cerebrospinal, pleural, synovial, intraocular, gonadal, and pericardial fluids.

Solutes. Although the overall concentration of solutes in ICF and ECF is nearly identical, the concentration of specific electrolytes differs significantly between these compartments, as shown in Figure 10–2 ■. ICF contains high concentrations of

TABLE 10–1 24-Hour Fluid Gain and Loss for an Adult

	SOURCE	AMOUNT (mL)
Gain	Fluids taken orally	1000
	Water in food	1300
	Water as by-product of food metabolism	200
		↓
	Total	2500
		↑
Loss	Urine	1500
	Feces	200
	Perspiration	500
	Respiration	300

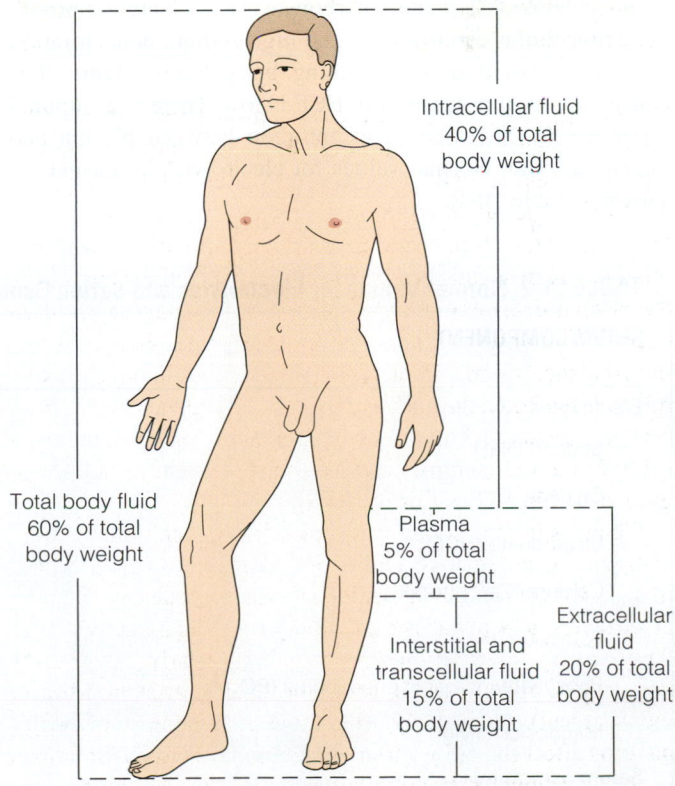

Intracellular fluid
40% of total
body weight

Total body fluid
60% of total
body weight

Plasma
5% of total
body weight

Interstitial and
transcellular fluid
15% of total
body weight

Extracellular
fluid
20% of total
body weight

Figure 10–1 ■ The major fluid compartments of the body.

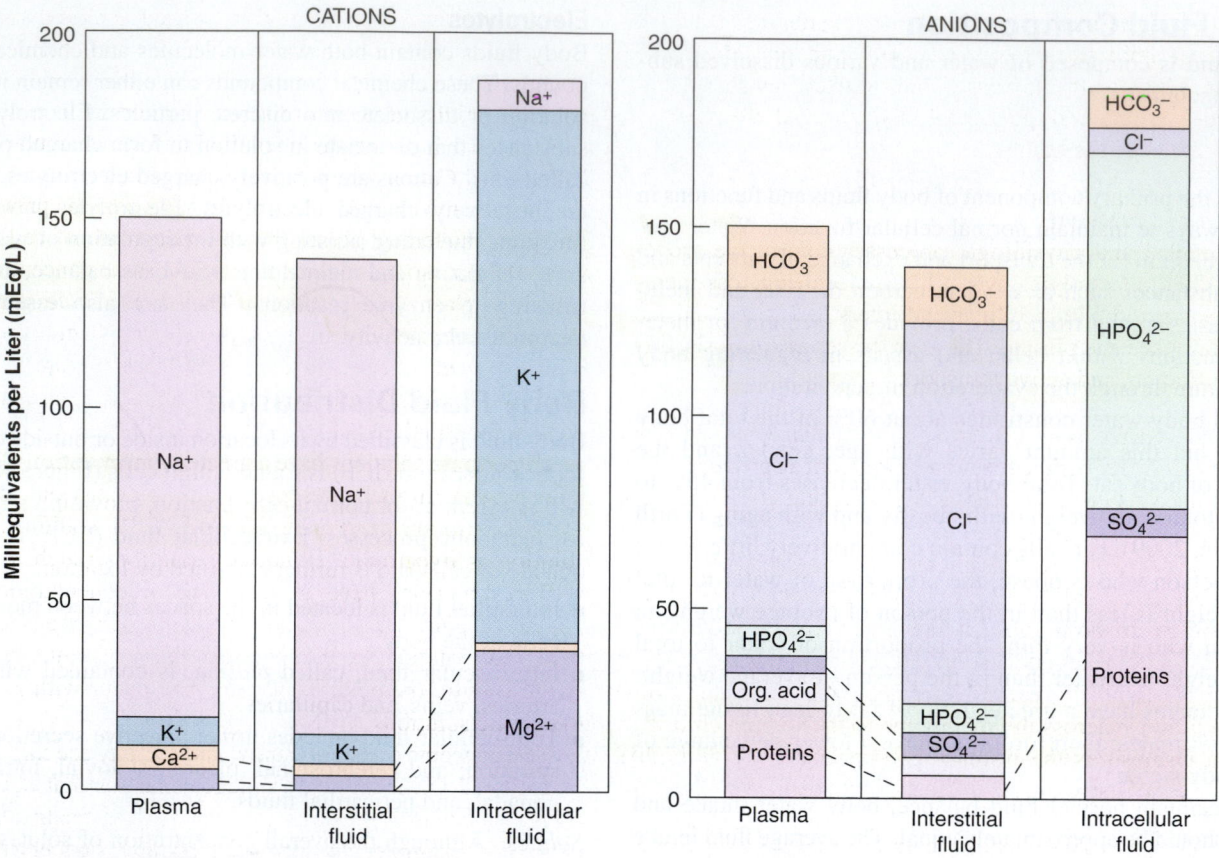

Figure 10–2 ■ Electrolyte composition (cations and anions) of body fluid compartments.

Source: Fig. 27.2, p. 1009 from *Fundamentals of Anatomy and Physiology*, 4th ed. by Frederic H. Martini. Copyright © 1998 by Frederic H. Martini, Inc. Reproduced by permission of Pearson Education, Inc.

potassium (K^+), magnesium (Mg^{2+}), and phosphate (PO_4^{2-}), as well as other solutes such as glucose and oxygen. Sodium (Na^+), chloride (Cl^-), and bicarbonate (HCO_3^-) are the principal extracellular electrolytes. The high sodium concentration in ECF is essential to regulating body fluid volume. The concentration of potassium in ECF is low. There is a minimal difference in electrolyte concentration between plasma and interstitial fluid. Normal values for electrolytes in plasma are shown in Table 10–2.

The body fluid compartments are separated by cell membranes and epithelial membranes. The cell membrane is selectively permeable; that is, it allows the passage of water, oxygen, carbon dioxide, and small water-soluble molecules, but bars proteins and other intracellular colloids. Capillary membranes separate plasma from interstitial fluid. The capillary membrane separating the plasma from the interstitial space is made of squamous epithelial cells. Pores in the membrane allow solute molecules (such as glucose and sodium), dissolved gases, and

TABLE 10–2 Normal Values for Electrolytes and Serum Osmolality

SERUM COMPONENT	VALUES	
	CONVENTIONAL	SI
Electrolytes		
Sodium (Na^+)	135–145 mEq/L	135–145 mmol/L
Chloride (Cl^-)	98–106 mEq/L	98–106 mmol/L
Bicarbonate (HCO_3^-)	22–26 mEq/L	22–26 mmol/L
Calcium (Ca^{2+}) (total)	8.5–10.0 mg/dL	2.1–2.6 mmol/L
Potassium (K^+)	3.5–5.0 mEq/L	3.5–5.0 mmol/L
Phosphate/inorganic phosphorus (PO_4^{-2})	1.7–2.6 mEq/L (2.5–4.5 mg/dL)	0.8–1.5 mmol/L
Magnesium (Mg^{2+})	1.6–2.6 mg/dL (1.3–2.1 mEq/L)	0.8–1.3 mmol/L
Serum osmolality	275–295 mOsm/kg	275–295 mmol/kg

water to cross the membrane. Epithelial membranes separate transcellular fluid from interstitial fluid and plasma. These membranes include the mucosa of the stomach, intestines, and gallbladder; the pleural, peritoneal, and synovial membranes; and the tubules of the kidney.

Body Fluid Movement

Four chemical and physiologic processes control the movement of fluid, electrolytes, and other molecules across membranes between the intracellular and interstitial space and the interstitial space and plasma. These processes are osmosis, diffusion, filtration, and active transport.

OSMOSIS Osmosis is the process by which water moves across a selectively permeable membrane from an area of lower solute concentration to an area of higher solute concentration (Figure 10–3 ■). A selectively permeable membrane allows water molecules to cross but is relatively impermeable to dissolved substances (solutes). Osmosis continues until the solute concentration on both sides of the membrane is equal. For example, if pure water and a sodium chloride solution are separated by a selectively permeable membrane, then water molecules will move across the membrane to the sodium chloride solution. Osmosis is the primary process that controls body fluid movement between the ICF and ECF compartments.

Osmolality   Osmolality, or concentration of a solution, refers to the number of solutes per kilogram of water (by weight); it is reported in milliosmoles per kilogram (mOsm/kg). The osmolality of the ECF depends chiefly on sodium concentration. Serum osmolality may be estimated by doubling the serum sodium concentration (approximately 142 mEq/L). Glucose and urea contribute to the osmolality of ECF, although to a lesser extent than sodium.

Osmotic Pressure and Tonicity   The power of a solution to draw water across a membrane is known as the osmotic pressure of the solution. The composition of interstitial fluid and intravascular plasma is essentially the same except for a higher concentration of proteins in the plasma. These proteins (especially albumin) exert colloid osmotic pressure (also called

oncotic pressure), pulling fluid from the interstitial space into the intravascular compartment. Because the osmolality of intravascular and interstitial fluid is essentially identical, the osmotic activity of plasma proteins is important in maintaining fluid balance between the interstitial and intravascular spaces, helping hold water within the vascular system.

Tonicity refers to the effect a solution's osmotic pressure has on water movement across the cell membrane of cells within that solution. Isotonic solutions have the same concentration of solutes as plasma. Cells placed in an isotonic solution will neither shrink nor swell because there is no net gain or loss of water within the cell, and no change in cell volume (Figure 10–4A ■). Normal saline (0.9% sodium chloride solution) is an example of an isotonic solution.

Hypertonic solutions have a greater concentration of solutes than plasma. In their presence, water is drawn out of a cell, causing it to shrink (Figure 10–4B). A 3% sodium chloride solution is hypertonic. Hypotonic solutions (such as 0.45% sodium chloride) have a lower solute concentration than plasma (Figure 10–4C). When red blood cells are placed in a hypotonic solution, water moves into the cells, causing them to swell; rupture (hemolysis) of cells may occur with extremely hypotonic solutions.

The concepts of osmotic draw and tonicity are important in understanding the pathophysiologic changes that occur with fluid and electrolyte imbalances, as well as treatment measures. For example, an increased sodium concentration of extracellular fluid pulls water from the ICF compartment into the ECF compartment, causing cells to shrink. In this case, administering a hypotonic IV solution to reduce the sodium concentration and osmolality of ECF will facilitate water movement back into the cells.

DIFFUSION Diffusion is the process by which solute molecules move from an area of high solute concentration to an area of low solute concentration to become evenly distributed (Figure 10–5 ■). The two types of diffusion are simple and facilitated diffusion. Simple diffusion occurs by the random movement of particles through a solution. Water, carbon dioxide, oxygen, and solutes move between plasma and the interstitial space by simple diffusion through the capillary membrane. Water and solutes move into the cell by passing through protein channels or by dissolving in the lipid cell membrane. Facilitated diffusion, also called carrier-mediated diffusion, allows large water-soluble molecules, such as glucose and amino acids, to diffuse across cell membranes. Proteins embedded in the cell membrane function as carriers, helping large molecules cross the membrane. The rate of diffusion is influenced by a number of factors, such as the concentration of solute and the availability of carrier proteins in the cell membrane. The effect of both simple and facilitated diffusion is to establish equal concentrations of the molecules on both sides of a membrane.

FILTRATION Filtration is the process by which water and dissolved substances (solutes) move from an area of high hydrostatic pressure to an area of low hydrostatic pressure. This usually occurs across capillary membranes. Hydrostatic pressure

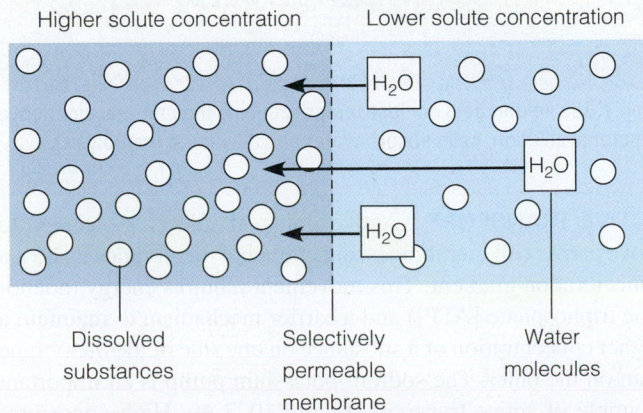

Higher solute concentration   Lower solute concentration

Dissolved substances   Selectively permeable membrane   Water molecules

Figure 10–3 ■ Osmosis. Water molecules move through a selectively permeable membrane from an area of low solute concentration to an area of high solute concentration.

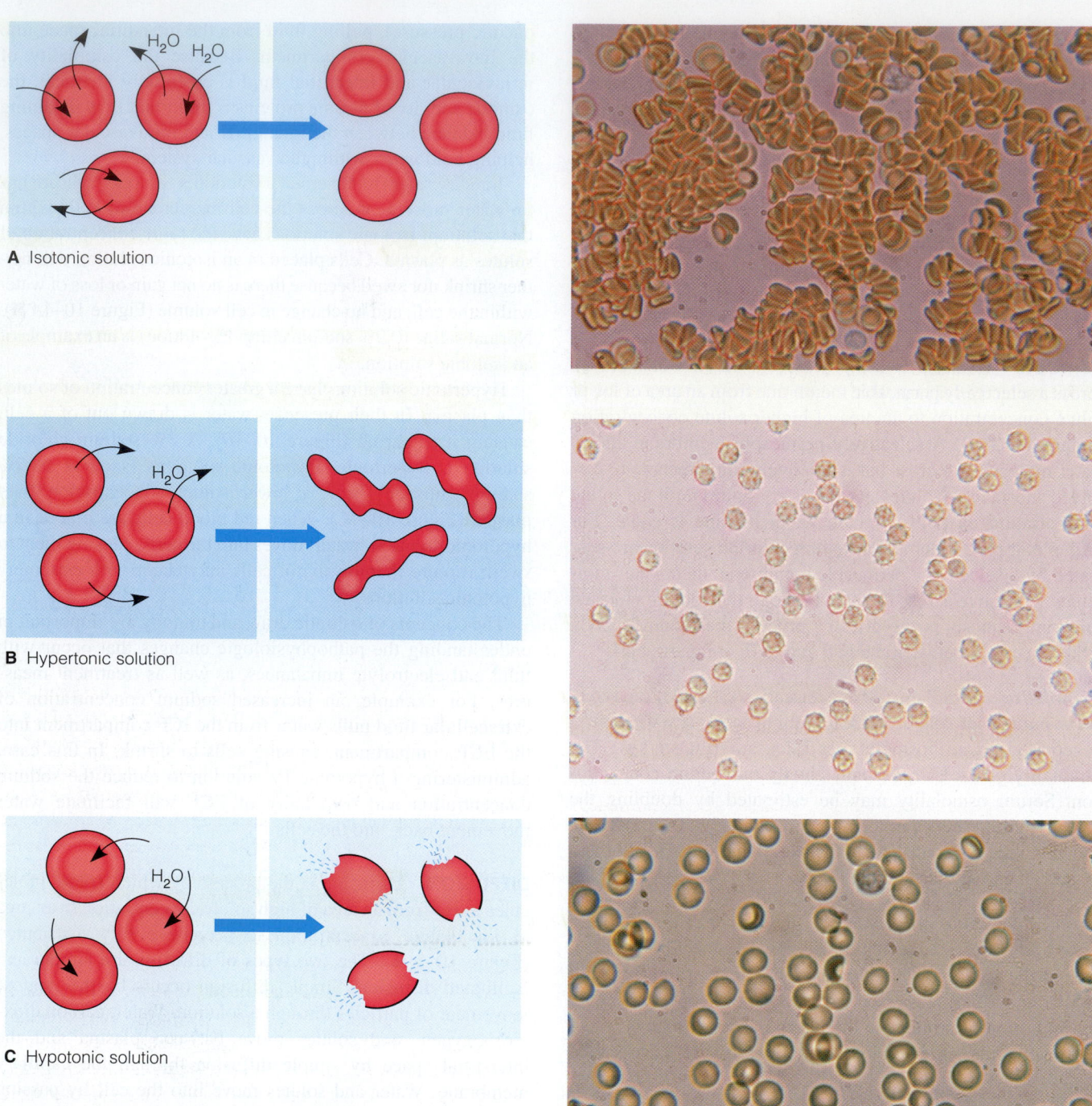

Figure 10–4 ■ The effect of tonicity on red blood cells. *A,* In an isotonic solution, RBCs neither gain nor lose water, retaining their normal biconcave shape. *B,* In a hypertonic solution, cells lose water and shrink in size. *C,* In a hypotonic solution, cells absorb water and may burst (hemolysis).

is created by the pumping action of the heart and gravity against the capillary wall. Filtration occurs in the glomerulus of the kidneys, as well as at the arterial end of capillaries.

A balance of hydrostatic (filtration) pressure and osmotic pressure regulates the movement of water between the intravascular and interstitial spaces in the capillary beds of the body. Hydrostatic pressure within the arterial end of the capillary pushes water into the interstitial space. At the venous end of the capillary, the osmotic force of plasma proteins draws fluid back into the capillary (Figure 10–6 ■).

ACTIVE TRANSPORT Active transport allows molecules to move across cell membranes and epithelial membranes against a concentration gradient. This movement requires energy (adenosine triphosphate [ATP]) and a carrier mechanism to maintain a higher concentration of a substance on one side of the membrane than on the other. The sodium-potassium pump is an important example of active transport (Figure 10–7 ■). High concentrations of potassium in intracellular fluids and of sodium in extracellular fluids are maintained because cells actively transport potassium from interstitial fluid into intracellular fluid.

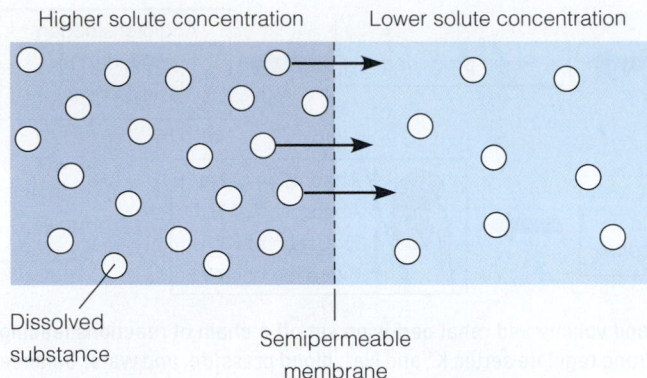

Figure 10–5 ■ Diffusion. Solute molecules move through a semipermeable membrane from an area of high solute concentration to an area of low solute concentration.

Body Fluid Regulation

Homeostasis requires several regulatory mechanisms and processes to maintain the balance between fluid intake and excretion. These include thirst, the kidneys, the renin–angiotensin–aldosterone mechanism, antidiuretic hormone, and atrial natriuretic peptide. These mechanisms affect the volume, distribution, and composition of body fluids.

Thirst

Thirst is the primary regulator of water intake. Thirst plays an important role in maintaining fluid balance and preventing dehydration. The thirst center, located in the hypothalamus, is stimulated when the blood volume drops because of water losses or when serum osmolality increases. The thirst mechanism is highly effective in regulating extracellular sodium levels. Increased sodium in ECF increases serum osmolality, stimulating the thirst center. Fluid intake in turn reduces the sodium concentration of ECF and lowers serum osmolality. Conversely, a drop in serum sodium and low serum osmolality inhibit the thirst center.

> **PRACTICE ALERT**
> The thirst mechanism declines with aging, making older adults more vulnerable to dehydration and hyperosmolality. Patients with an altered level of consciousness or who are unable to respond to thirst, such as intubated patients and artificially fed patients, are also at risk.

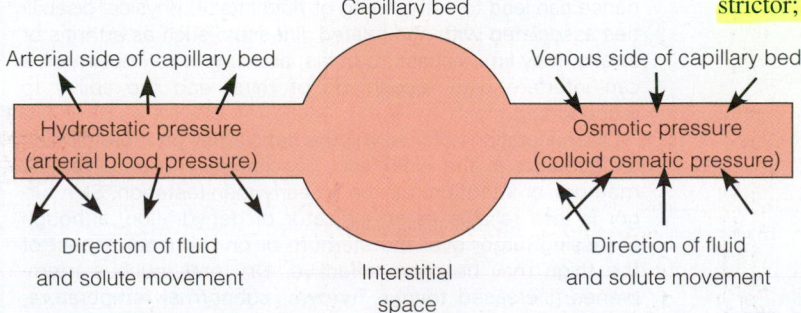

Figure 10–6 ■ Fluid balance between the intravascular and interstitial spaces is maintained in the capillary beds by a balance of filtration at the arterial end and osmotic draw at the venous end.

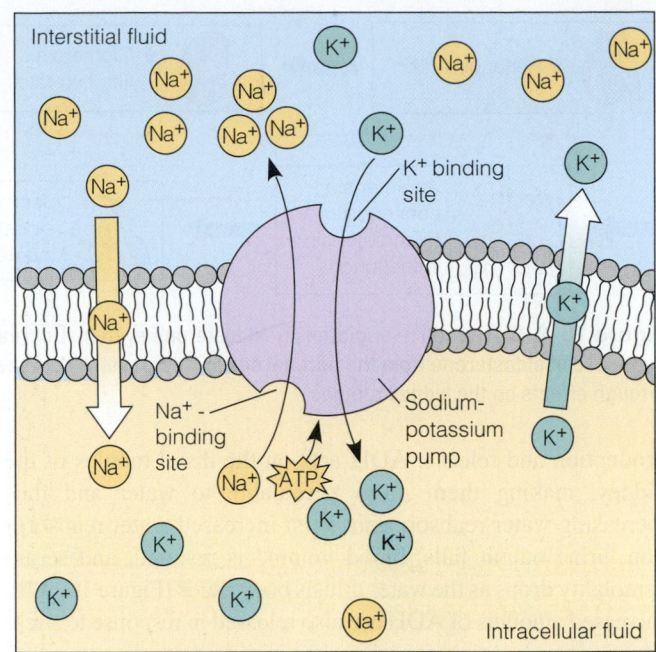

Figure 10–7 ■ The sodium-potassium pump. Sodium and potassium ions are moved across the cell membranes against their concentration gradients. This active transport process is fueled by energy from ATP.

Kidneys

The kidneys are primarily responsible for regulating fluid volume and electrolyte balance in the body. They regulate the volume and osmolality of body fluids by controlling the excretion of water and electrolytes. In adults, about 170 L of plasma are filtered through the glomeruli every day. By selectively reabsorbing water and electrolytes, the kidneys maintain the volume and osmolality of body fluids. About 99% of the glomerular filtrate is reabsorbed, and only about 1500 mL of urine is produced over a 24-hour period (Porth & Matfin, 2009).

Renin–Angiotensin–Aldosterone System

The renin–angiotensin–aldosterone system helps to maintain intravascular fluid balance and blood pressure. A decrease in blood flow or blood pressure to the kidneys stimulates specialized receptors in the juxtaglomerular cells of the nephrons to produce renin, an enzyme. Renin converts angiotensinogen (a plasma protein) in the circulating blood into angiotensin I. Angiotensin I travels through the bloodstream to the lungs where it is converted to angiotensin II by angiotensin-converting enzyme (ACE). Angiotensin II is a potent vasoconstrictor; it raises the blood pressure. It also stimulates the thirst mechanism to promote fluid intake and acts directly on the kidneys, causing them to retain sodium and water. Angiotensin II stimulates the adrenal cortex to release aldosterone. Aldosterone promotes sodium and water retention in the distal nephron of the kidney, restoring blood volume (Figure 10–8 ■).

Antidiuretic Hormone

Antidiuretic hormone (ADH), released by the posterior pituitary gland, regulates water excretion from the kidneys. Osmoreceptors in the hypothalamus respond to increases in serum osmolality and decreases in blood volume, stimulating ADH

Respiratory Acidosis Animation

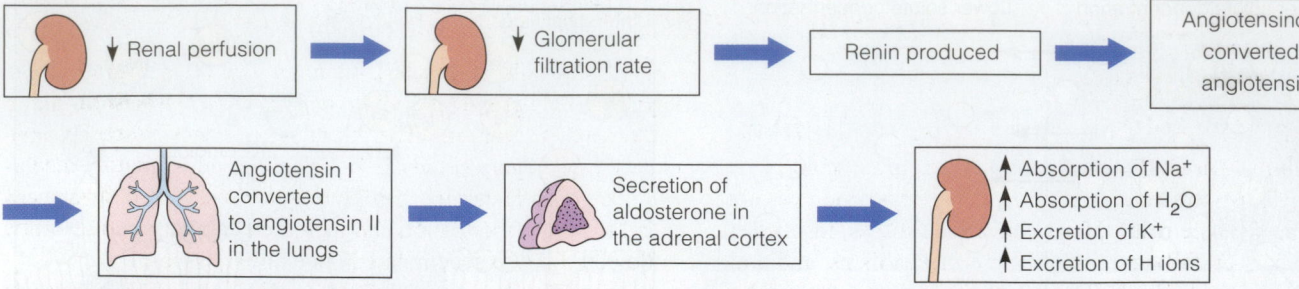

Figure 10–8 ■ The renin–angiotensin–aldosterone system. Decreased blood volume and renal perfusion set off a chain of reactions leading to release of aldosterone from the adrenal cortex. Increased levels of aldosterone regulate serum K+ and Na+, blood pressure, and water balance through effects on the kidney tubules.

production and release. ADH acts on the distal tubules of the kidney, making them more permeable to water and thus increasing water reabsorption. With increased water reabsorption, urine output falls, blood volume is restored, and serum osmolality drops as the water dilutes body fluids (Figure 10–9 ■). Increased amounts of ADH are also released in response to stress situations such as nausea, pain, surgery and anesthesia, narcotics, and nicotine. Its release is inhibited by alcohol and medications such as phenytoin, as well as by increased blood volume and decreased serum osmolality (Porth, 2007).

Atrial Natriuretic Peptide

Atrial natriuretic peptide (ANP) is a hormone released by atrial muscle cells in response to distention from fluid overload. ANP affects several body systems, including the cardiovascular, renal, neural, GI, and endocrine systems, but it primarily opposes the renin–angiotensin–aldosterone system by inhibiting renin secretion and blocking the secretion and sodium-retaining effects of aldosterone. As a result, ANP promotes sodium wasting and increased urine output.

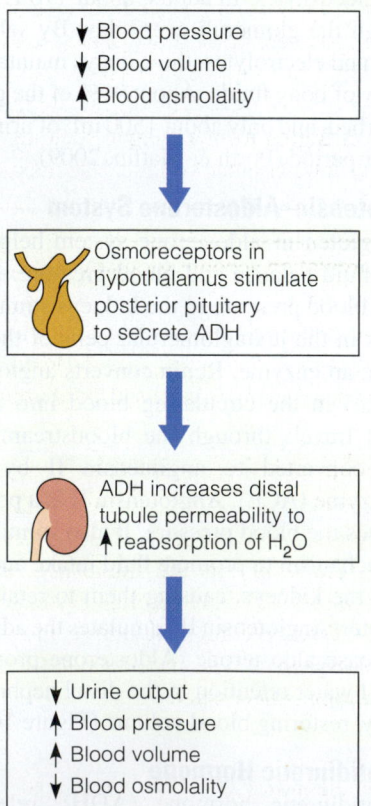

Figure 10–9 ■ Antidiuretic hormone (ADH) release and effect. Increased serum osmolality or a fall in blood volume stimulates the release of ADH from the posterior pituitary. ADH increases the permeability of distal tubules, promoting water reabsorption.

NURSING CARE OF THE OLDER ADULT   **Fluid Volume Deficit**

Changes in the normal aging process affect homeostasis in several ways. In older adults, the percentage of total body water is about 10% lower than in younger or middle-aged adults, and thus they have less body reserve. Lean muscle mass is lower in older adults, and the percentage of body fat is higher; as a result water accounts for about 50% of the total body weight (TBW) of an older man and about 45% TBW of an older woman (Porth & Matfin, 2009). Sodium and water regulation become less efficient with aging. Renal blood flow and glomerular filtration decline with aging; the kidneys are less able to effectively concentrate the urine and conserve sodium and water. The perception of thirst decreases, interfering with the thirst mechanism. Consequently, the older adult may become dehydrated without being aware of the need to increase fluid intake.

Undetected fever in older adults can increase the total body need for water with every degree of temperature. Dehydration can cause a fever and further compound dehydration in the older adult. Older adults who have self-care deficits, or who are confused, depressed, tube fed, on bed rest, or taking medications (such as sedatives, tranquilizers, diuretics, and laxatives) are at greatest risk for fluid volume imbalance. Older adults without air conditioning are at risk during extremely hot weather. In addition, functional changes and illnesses can affect fluid balance. For example, fear of incontinence can lead to self-limiting of fluid intake; physical disabilities associated with age-related illnesses, such as arthritis or stroke, may limit access to fluids; and cognitive impairments can interfere with recognition of thirst and the ability to respond to it.

Manifestations of fluid volume deficit may be more difficult to recognize in the older adult. A change in mental status, memory, or attention may be an early manifestation. Skin turgor is less reliable as an indicator of dehydration, although assessing turgor over the sternum or on the inner aspect of the thigh may be more effective. Dry oral mucous membranes, increased tongue furrows, subnormal temperature, tachycardia, and a pinched facial expression are also indicative of dehydration. Orthostatic vital signs may not demonstrate typical changes in the dehydrated older adult.

Fluid and Electrolyte Imbalances

Fluid Imbalance

The Patient with a Fluid Volume Deficit

Fluid volume deficit (FVD) is a decrease in intravascular, interstitial, and/or intracellular fluid in the body. Fluid volume deficits may be the result of excessive fluid losses, insufficient fluid intake, or failure of regulatory mechanisms and fluid shifts within the body. FVD is a relatively common problem that may exist alone or in combination with other electrolyte or acid–base imbalances. The term **dehydration** refers to loss of water alone, even though it often is used interchangeably with fluid volume deficit.

Pathophysiology

The most common cause of fluid volume deficit is excessive loss of GI fluids from vomiting, diarrhea, GI suctioning, intestinal fistulas, and intestinal drainage. Other causes of fluid losses include diuretics, renal disorders, endocrine disorders, excessive exercise, hot environment, hemorrhage, and chronic abuse of laxatives and/or enemas. Other factors involved in inadequate fluid intake include inability to access fluids, inability to request or to swallow fluids, oral trauma, or altered thirst mechanisms. Older adults are at particular risk for fluid volume deficit (see the Nursing Care of the Older Adult box on page 192).

Fluid volume deficit can develop slowly or rapidly, depending on the type of fluid loss. Loss of extracellular fluid volume can lead to hypovolemia, decreased circulating blood volume. Electrolytes often are lost along with fluid, resulting in an isotonic fluid volume deficit. When both water and electrolytes are lost, the serum sodium level remains normal, although levels of other electrolytes such as potassium may fall. Fluid is drawn into the vascular compartment from the interstitial spaces as the body attempts to maintain tissue perfusion. This eventually depletes fluid in the intracellular compartment as well.

Hypovolemia stimulates regulatory mechanisms to maintain circulation. The sympathetic nervous system is stimulated, as is the thirst mechanism. ADH and aldosterone are released, prompting sodium and water retention by the kidneys. Severe fluid loss, as in hemorrhage, can lead to shock and cardiovascular collapse.

THIRD SPACING **Third spacing** is a shift of fluid from the vascular space into an area where it is not available to support normal physiologic processes. Fluid may be sequestered in the abdomen or bowel, or in other actual or potential body spaces as the pleural or peritoneal space. Fluid may also become trapped within soft tissues following trauma or burns. The trapped fluid represents a volume loss and is unavailable for normal physiologic processes.

In many cases, fluid is sequestered in interstitial tissues and is unavailable to support cardiovascular function. As an example, surgery triggers adaptive stress responses and the release of stress hormones (ACTH, cortisol, and catecholamines). These hormones increase blood glucose levels to provide increased fuel for metabolic processes and promote vasoconstriction that redistributes blood to vital organs (the heart and brain). Renal blood flow falls, stimulating the renin–angiotensin–aldosterone system. This promotes sodium and water retention to maintain intravascular volume. The blood vessel and tissue damage caused by surgery stimulate the release of inflammatory mediators such as histamine and prostaglandins. These substances lead to local vasodilation and increased capillary permeability, allowing fluid to accumulate in interstitial tissues.

Assessing the extent of FVD resulting from third spacing is difficult. It may not be reflected in weight or intake and output records, and it may not become apparent until after organ malfunction occurs. Daily weights may be helpful in uncovering third spaced fluids; however, due to fluid or weight loss due to disease processes, these gains may be obscured. Delays in recognition and treatment can lead to irreversible shock and multiorgan system failure (Perrin, 2009).

Manifestations

With a rapid fluid loss (such as hemorrhage or uncontrolled vomiting), manifestations of hypovolemia develop rapidly. When the loss of fluid occurs more gradually, the patient's fluid volume may be very low before manifestations develop. See the Multisystem Effects of Fluid Volume Deficit feature on page 194.

Rapid weight loss is a good indicator of fluid volume deficit. Each liter of body fluid weighs about 1 kg (2.2 lb). The severity of the fluid volume deficit can be estimated by the percentage of rapid weight loss: A loss of 2% of body weight represents a mild FVD; 5%, moderate FVD; and 8% or greater, severe FVD (Metheny, 2000). Loss of interstitial fluid causes skin turgor to diminish. When pinched, the skin of a patient with FVD remains elevated. Postural or orthostatic hypotension is a sign of hypovolemia. A drop of more than 15 mmHg in systolic blood pressure when changing from a lying to standing position often indicates loss of intravascular volume. Venous pressure falls as well, causing flat neck veins, even when the patient is recumbent. Compensatory mechanisms to conserve water and sodium and maintain circulation account for many of the manifestations of fluid volume deficit, such as tachycardia; pale, cool skin (vasoconstriction); and decreased urine output. The specific gravity of urine increases as water is reabsorbed in the tubules. Table 10–3 compares manifestations of fluid imbalances.

Interdisciplinary Care

The primary goals of care are to prevent deficits in patients at risk and to correct deficits and their underlying causes. Depending on the acuity of the imbalance, treatment may include replacement of fluids and electrolytes by the IV, oral, or enteral route. When possible, the oral or enteral route is preferred for administering fluids. In acute situations, however, IV fluid administration is necessary.

Diagnosis

Laboratory and diagnostic tests may be ordered when fluid volume deficit is suspected. Such tests measure the following:

- *Serum electrolytes.* In an isotonic fluid deficit, sodium levels are within normal limits; when the loss is water only, sodium levels are high. Decreases in potassium are common.

MULTISYSTEM EFFECTS OF
Fluid Volume Deficit

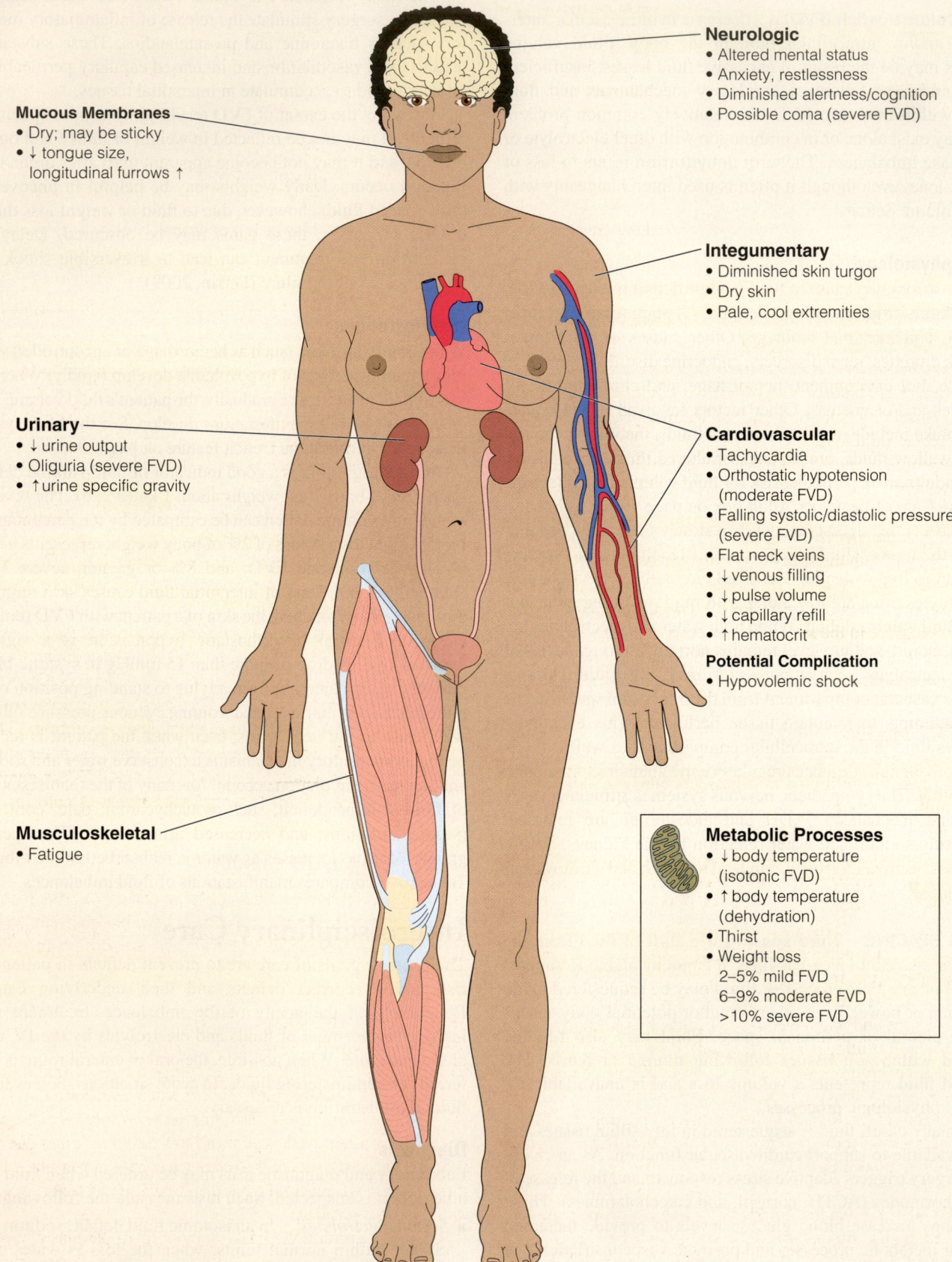

Neurologic
- Altered mental status
- Anxiety, restlessness
- Diminished alertness/cognition
- Possible coma (severe FVD)

Mucous Membranes
- Dry; may be sticky
- ↓ tongue size, longitudinal furrows ↑

Integumentary
- Diminished skin turgor
- Dry skin
- Pale, cool extremities

Urinary
- ↓ urine output
- Oliguria (severe FVD)
- ↑urine specific gravity

Cardiovascular
- Tachycardia
- Orthostatic hypotension (moderate FVD)
- Falling systolic/diastolic pressure (severe FVD)
- Flat neck veins
- ↓ venous filling
- ↓ pulse volume
- ↓ capillary refill
- ↑ hematocrit

Potential Complication
- Hypovolemic shock

Musculoskeletal
- Fatigue

Metabolic Processes
- ↓ body temperature (isotonic FVD)
- ↑ body temperature (dehydration)
- Thirst
- Weight loss
  2–5% mild FVD
  6–9% moderate FVD
  >10% severe FVD

TABLE 10–3 Comparison of the Manifestations of Fluid Imbalance

ASSESSMENT	FLUID DEFICIT	FLUID EXCESS
Blood pressure	Decreased systolic	Increased
	Postural hypotension	
Heart rate	Increased	Increased
Pulse amplitude	Decreased	Increased
Respirations	Normal	Moist crackles
		Wheezes
Jugular vein	Flat	Distended
Edema	Rare	Dependent
Skin turgor	Loose, poor turgor	Taut
Output	Low, concentrated	May be low or normal
Urine specific gravity	High	Low
Weight	Loss	Gain

- *Serum osmolality.* Measurement of serum osmolality helps to differentiate isotonic fluid loss from water loss. With water loss, osmolality is high; it may be within normal limits with an isotonic fluid loss.
- *Hemoglobin and hematocrit.* The hematocrit often is elevated due to loss of intravascular volume and hemoconcentration.
- *Urine specific gravity and osmolality.* As the kidneys conserve water, both the specific gravity and osmolality of urine increase.
- *Central venous pressure (CVP).* The CVP measures the mean pressure in the superior vena cava or right atrium, providing an accurate assessment of fluid volume status. The technique for measuring CVP is described in ∞ Chapter 31.

Fluid Management

Oral rehydration is the safest and most effective treatment for fluid volume deficit in alert patients who are able to take oral fluids. Adults require a minimum of 1500 mL of fluid per day or approximately 30 mL per kg of body weight (ideal body weight is used to calculate fluid requirements for obese patients) for maintenance. Fluids are replaced gradually, particularly in older adults, to prevent rapid rehydration of the cells.

For mild fluid deficits in which a loss of electrolytes has been minimal (e.g., moderate exercise in warm weather), water alone may be used for fluid replacement. When the fluid deficit is more severe and when electrolytes have also been lost (e.g., FVD due to vomiting and/or diarrhea, strenuous exercise for longer than an hour or two), a carbohydrate/electrolyte solution such as a sports drink, ginger ale, or a rehydrating solution (e.g., Pedialyte or Rehydralyte) is more appropriate. These solutions provide sodium, potassium, chloride, and calories to help meet metabolic needs.

IV THERAPY   When the fluid deficit is severe or the patient is unable to ingest fluids, the IV route is used to administer replacement fluids. Table 10–4 describes commonly administered IV fluids with nursing implications. Isotonic electrolyte solutions (0.9% NaCl or Ringer's solution) are used to expand plasma volume in hypotensive patients or to replace abnormal losses, which are usually isotonic in nature. Normal saline (0.9% NaCl) tends to remain in the vascular compartment, increasing blood volume. When administered rapidly, however, this solution can precipitate acid–base imbalances, so balanced electrolyte solutions such as Lactated Ringer's solution are preferred to expand plasma volume.

Five percent dextrose in 0.45% saline (D_5 1/2; NS) or 0.45% NaCl (one-half normal saline or 1/2 NS) are given to provide water to treat total body water deficits. D_5W, although isotonic in the bag, is not used for fluid resuscitation as the dextrose is rapidly metabolized and the subsequent fluid is hypotonic (David, 2007). Saline solution (0.45% NaCl with or without added electrolytes) or 5% dextrose in 0.45% sodium chloride (D_5 1/2 NS) are used as maintenance solutions. These solutions provide additional electrolytes such as potassium, a buffer (lactate or acetate) as needed, and water. When dextrose is added, they also provide a minimal number of calories.

∞ Nursing Care

Nurses are responsible for identifying patients at risk for fluid volume deficit, initiating and carrying out interventions to prevent and treat fluid volume deficit, and monitoring the effects of therapy.

Health Promotion

Health promotion activities focus on teaching to prevent fluid volume deficit. Discuss the importance of maintaining adequate fluid intake, particularly when exercising and during hot weather. Advise patients to use commercial sports drinks to replace both water and electrolytes when exercising during warm weather. Instruct patients to maintain fluid intake when ill, particularly during periods of fever or when diarrhea is a problem.

Carefully monitor the intake and output of patients at risk for abnormal fluid losses through vomiting, diarrhea, nasogastric suction, increased urine output, fever, or draining wounds. Monitor

TABLE 10–4 Commonly Administered IV Fluids with Nursing Implications

I. Isotonic Solutions

0.9% Saline
Lactated Ringer's solution

- Monitor for fluid overload; if manifestations occur, discontinue fluids and notify the healthcare provider.
- Do not administer lactated Ringer's solution to patients with severe liver disease as the liver may be unable to convert the lactate to bicarbonate and the patient may become acidotic. Do not administer if the patient has a blood pH of > 7.50.
- If administering lactated Ringer's solution, monitor potassium levels and cardiac rhythm; if abnormals are present, notify the healthcare provider.

II. Hypotonic Solutions

0.45% saline or 0.25% saline
D_5W

- Monitor for inflammation and infiltration at IV insertion site as hypotonic solutions may cause cells to swell and burst, including those at the insertions site; this narrows the lumen of the vein.
- Monitor blood sodium levels.
- Do not administer to patients at risk for increased intracranial pressure (e.g., head trauma, stroke, neurosurgery).
- Do not administer to patients at risk for third-space shifts (burns, trauma, liver disease, malnutrition).

III. Hypertonic Solutions

Hypertonic fluids have a tonicity > 350 mEq/L and include the following:

Fluids containing medications

D_5W sodium chloride

D_5W in lactated Ringer's solution

Total parenteral solutions

- Monitor for inflammation and infiltration at IV insertion site as hypertonic solutions cause cells to shrink, exposing the basement membrane of the vein.
- Monitor blood sodium levels.
- Monitor for circulatory overload.
- Do not administer to patients with diabetic ketoacidosis or impaired cardiac or kidney function.

Clinical alert: The Infusion Nurses Society mandates that all fluids with a tonicity exceeding 500 mEq/L be infused through a central venous access device; this includes $D_{10}W$, 5% protein hydrolysate, or a high electrolyte solution.

Adapted from David, K. (2007). *IV fluids: Do you know what's hanging and why?* RN Web and AHA Media LLC; Hogan, M., Gringrich, M., Overby, P., & Ricci, M. (2007). *Fluids, electrolytes, & acid–base balance* (2nd ed). Upper Saddle River, NJ: Pearson Prentice Hall; and Rosenthal, K., (2009). *Tonicity and IV fluids.* Resource Nurse.com.

---

fluid intake in patients with decreased level of consciousness, disorientation, nausea, anorexia, and physical limitations.

Assessment

Collect assessment data through the health history interview and physical examination.

- *Health history:* Risk factors such as medications, acute or chronic renal or endocrine disease; precipitating factors such as hot weather, extensive exercise, lack of access to fluids, recent illness (especially if accompanied by fever, vomiting, and/or diarrhea); onset and duration of manifestations.
- *Physical assessment:* Weight; vital signs including orthostatic blood pressure and pulse; peripheral pulses and capillary refill; jugular neck vein distention; skin color, temperature, turgor; level of consciousness and mentation; urine output. Allow the older adult to stand quietly for a full minute before rechecking blood pressure and pulse when measuring orthostatic vital signs.

Nursing Diagnoses and Interventions

Nursing diagnoses and interventions for the patient with fluid volume deficit focus on managing the effects of the deficit and preventing complications.

Deficient Fluid Volume

Patients with a fluid volume deficit due to abnormal losses, inadequate intake, or impaired fluid regulation require close monitoring as well as immediate and ongoing fluid replacement.

- Assess intake and output accurately, monitoring fluid balance. In acute situations, hourly intake and output may be indicated. *Urine output should normally be 30 to 60 mL per hour. Urine output of less than 30 mL per hour in adults indicates inadequate renal perfusion and an increased risk for acute renal failure and inadequate tissue perfusion (Perrin, 2009).*

> **PRACTICE ALERT**
> Report a urine output of less than 30 mL per hour to the patient's healthcare provider.

- Assess vital signs, CVP, and peripheral pulse volume at least every 4 hours. *Hypotension, tachycardia, low CVP, and weak, easily obliterated peripheral pulses indicate hypovolemia.*
- Weigh daily under standard conditions (time of day, clothing, and scale). *In most instances (except third spacing), changes in weight accurately reflect fluid balance.*

- Administer and monitor the intake of oral fluids as prescribed. Identify beverage preferences and provide these on a schedule. *Oral fluid replacement is preferred when the patient is able to drink and retain fluids.*
- Administer IV fluids as prescribed using an infusion pump. Monitor for indicators of fluid overload if rapid fluid replacement is ordered: dyspnea, tachypnea, tachycardia, increased CVP, jugular vein distention, and edema. *Rapid fluid replacement may lead to hypervolemia, resulting in pulmonary edema and cardiac failure, particularly in patients with compromised cardiac and renal function.*
- Monitor laboratory values: electrolytes, serum osmolality, blood urea nitrogen (BUN), and hematocrit. *Rehydration may lead to changes in serum electrolytes, osmolality, BUN, and hematocrit. In some cases, electrolyte replacement may be necessary during rehydration.*

Ineffective Tissue Perfusion

A fluid volume deficit can lead to decreased perfusion of renal, cerebral, and peripheral tissues. Inadequate renal perfusion can lead to acute renal failure. Decreased cerebral perfusion leads to changes in mental status and cognitive function, causing restlessness, anxiety, agitation, excitability, confusion, vertigo, fainting, and weakness.

- Monitor for changes in level of consciousness and mental status. *Restlessness, anxiety, confusion, and agitation may indicate inadequate cerebral blood flow and circulatory collapse.*
- Monitor serum creatinine, BUN, and cardiac enzymes, reporting elevated levels to the physician. *Elevated levels may indicate impaired renal function or cardiac perfusion related to circulatory failure.*
- Turn at least every 2 hours. Provide good skin care and monitor for evidence of skin or tissue breakdown. *Impaired circulation to peripheral tissues increases the risk of skin breakdown. Turn frequently to relieve pressure over bony prominences. Keep skin clean, dry, and moisturized to help maintain integrity.*

Risk for Injury

The patient with fluid volume deficit is at risk for injury because of dizziness and loss of balance resulting from decreased cerebral perfusion secondary to hypovolemia.

- Institute safety precautions, including keeping the bed in a low position, using side rails as needed, and slowly raising the patient from supine to sitting or sitting to standing position. *Using safety precautions and allowing time for the blood pressure to adjust to position changes reduce the risk of injury.*
- Teach patient and family members how to reduce orthostatic hypotension:
  a. Move from one position to another in stages; for example, raise the head of the bed before sitting up, and sit for a few minutes before standing.
  b. Avoid prolonged standing.
  c. Rest in a recliner rather than in bed during the day.
  d. Use assistive devices to pick up objects from the floor rather than stooping.

Teaching measures to reduce orthostatic hypotension reduces the patient's risk for injury. Prolonged bed rest increases skeletal muscle weakness and decreases venous tone, contributing to postural hypotension. Prolonged standing allows blood to pool in the legs, reducing venous return and cardiac output.

Using NANDA, NIC, and NOC

Linkages between a selected NANDA nursing diagnosis, NIC, and NOC for the patient with fluid volume deficit are shown in the chart that follows.

Community-Based Care

Depending on the severity of the fluid volume deficit, the patient may be managed in the home or long-term care facility, or may be admitted as a hospital inpatient. Assess the patient's understanding of the cause of the deficit and the fluids necessary for providing replacement. Address the following topics when preparing the patient and family for home care:

- The importance of maintaining adequate fluid intake (at least 1500 mL per day; more if extra fluid is being lost through perspiration, fever, or diarrhea)
- Manifestations of fluid imbalance, and how to monitor fluid balance
- How to prevent fluid deficit:
  - Avoid exercising during extreme heat.
  - Increase fluid intake during hot weather.
  - If vomiting, take small frequent amounts of ice chips or clear liquids, such as weak tea, flat cola, or ginger ale.
  - Reduce intake of coffee, tea, and alcohol, which increase urine output and can cause fluid loss.
- Replacement of fluids lost through diarrhea with fruit juices or bouillon, rather than large amounts of tap water
- Alternate sources of fluid (such as gelatin, frozen juices, or ice cream) for effective replacement of lost fluids.

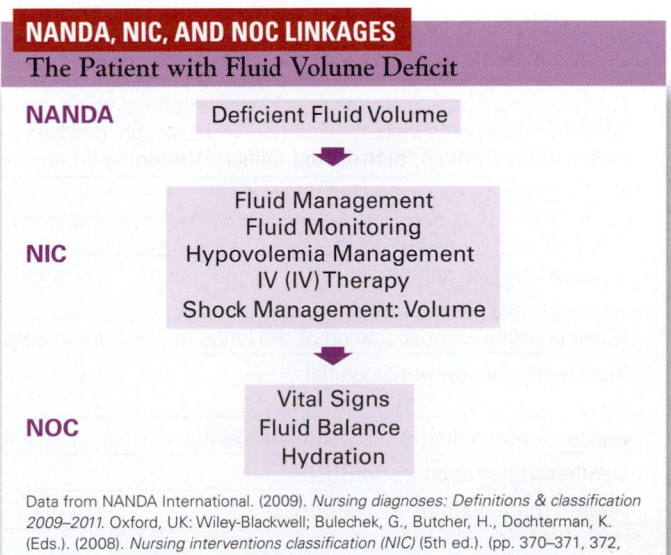

NANDA, NIC, AND NOC LINKAGES
The Patient with Fluid Volume Deficit

NANDA	Deficient Fluid Volume
NIC	Fluid Management Fluid Monitoring Hypovolemia Management IV (IV) Therapy Shock Management: Volume
NOC	Vital Signs Fluid Balance Hydration

Data from NANDA International. (2009). *Nursing diagnoses: Definitions & classification 2009–2011.* Oxford, UK: Wiley-Blackwell; Bulechek, G., Butcher, H., Dochterman, K. (Eds.). (2008). *Nursing interventions classification (NIC)* (5th ed.). (pp. 370–371, 372, 420–421, 441, 655), St. Louis: Elsevier Mosby; and Moorhead, M., Johnson, M., Maas, M., and Swanson, E. (Eds.). (2008). *Nursing outcomes classification (NOC)* (4th ed.) (p. 771). St. Louis: Elsevier Mosby.

The Patient with Fluid Volume Excess

Fluid volume excess results when both water and sodium are retained in the body. Fluid volume excess may be caused by fluid overload (excess water and sodium intake) or by impairment of the mechanisms that maintain homeostasis. The excess fluid can lead to excess intravascular fluid (hypervolemia) and excess interstitial fluid (edema).

Pathophysiology

Fluid volume excess usually results from conditions that cause retention of both sodium and water. These conditions include heart failure, cirrhosis of the liver, renal failure, adrenal gland disorders, corticosteroid administration, and stress conditions causing the release of ADH and aldosterone. Other causes include an excessive intake of sodium-containing foods, drugs that cause sodium retention, and the administration of excess amounts of sodium-containing IV fluids (such as 0.9% NaCl or Ringer's solution). This *iatrogenic* (induced by the effects of treatment) cause of fluid volume excess primarily affects patients with impaired regulatory mechanisms.

In fluid volume excess, both water and sodium are gained in about the same proportions as normally exists in extracellular fluid. The total body sodium content is increased, which in turn causes an increase in total body water. Because the increase in sodium and water is isotonic, the serum sodium and osmolality remain normal, and the excess fluid remains in the extracellular space.

Stress responses activated before, during, and immediately after surgery commonly lead to increased ADH and aldosterone levels, leading to sodium and water retention. In the immediate postoperative period, however, this additional fluid tends to be sequestered in interstitial tissues and unavailable to support cardiovascular and renal function (see the earlier Third Spacing section in this chapter). This sequestered fluid is reabsorbed into the circulation within about 48 to 72 hours after surgery. Although it is then normally eliminated through a process of diuresis, patients with heart or kidney failure are at risk for developing fluid overload.

Manifestations

Excess extracellular fluid leads to hypervolemia and circulatory overload. Excess fluid in the interstitial space causes peripheral or generalized edema. The manifestations of fluid volume excess relate to both the excess fluid and its effects on circulation. Manifestations of fluid volume excess with related pathophysiology are described in the table below.

Complications

Congestive heart failure (CHF) is not only a potential cause of fluid volume excess, but it is also a potential complication of the condition if the heart is unable to increase its workload to handle the excess blood volume. Severe fluid overload and CHF can lead to pulmonary edema, a medical emergency. ∞ See Chapter 31 for information about CHF and pulmonary edema.

Interdisciplinary Care

Managing fluid volume excess focuses on prevention in patients at risk, treating its manifestations, and correcting the underlying cause. Management includes limiting sodium and water intake and administering diuretics.

PATHOPHYSIOLOGY LINKAGE   Fluid Volume Excess

MANIFESTATIONS	RELATED PATHOPHYSIOLOGY
Peripheral edema, or if severe, anasarca (severe, generalized edema)	Excess fluid in the interstitial spaces, usually resulting from conditions that cause retention of both sodium and water (heart failure, cirrhosis of the liver, renal failure, adrenal gland disorders, corticosteroid administration, and stress conditions causing the release of ADH and aldosterone, such as surgery)
Full bounding pulse, distended neck and peripheral veins, increased central venous pressure (>11–12 cm of water), cough, dyspnea (labored or difficult breathing), **orthopnea** (difficult breathing when supine)	Circulatory overload from increased water and sodium retention
Dyspnea at rest	Impaired gas exchange from pulmonary interstitial edema
Tachycardia and hypertension	Increased circulatory fluid volume
Reduced oxygen saturation	As fluid increases in the interstitial spaces and alveoli, gas exchange is impaired, leading to hypoxia and hypercapnia
Moist crackles on auscultation of the lungs, pulmonary edema	Excess fluid in pulmonary interstitial spaces and alveoli
Increased urine output (polyuria)	Increased sodium and water retention resulting in increased circulatory volume and increased perfusion of the renal arteries
Ascites (excess fluid in the peritoneal cavity)	Sodium and water retention
Decreased hematocrit and BUN	Dilutional effect of increased circulatory volume
Altered mental status and anxiety	Pressure on the cerebral cortex from an increase in cerebral contents and cerebral hypertension causes decreased oxygenation (hypoxia) of neurons
Pulmonary edema	Elevation of left-sided filling pressures resulting from increased circulatory volume and heart failure

Diagnosis

The following laboratory tests may be ordered.

- *Serum electrolytes* and *serum osmolality* are measured, but usually remain within normal limits.
- *Serum hematocrit* and *hemoglobin* often are decreased due to plasma dilution from excess extracellular fluid.

Additional tests of *renal* and *liver function* (such as serum creatinine, BUN, and liver enzymes) may be ordered to help determine the cause of fluid volume excess.

Medications

Diuretics are commonly used to treat fluid volume excess. They inhibit sodium and water reabsorption, increasing urine output. The three major classes of diuretics, each of which acts on a different part of the kidney tubule, are as follows:

- Loop diuretics act in the ascending loop of Henle.
- Thiazide-type diuretics act on the distal convoluted tubule.
- Potassium-sparing diuretics affect the distal nephron.

The nursing implications for diuretics are outlined in the following Medication Administration box.

Treatments

FLUID MANAGEMENT   Fluid intake may be restricted in patients who have fluid volume excess. The amount of fluid allowed per day is prescribed by the primary care provider. All fluid intake must be calculated, including meals and that used to administer medications orally or IV. Box 10–1 provides guidelines for hospitalized patients with a fluid restriction.

DIETARY MANAGEMENT   Because sodium retention is a primary cause of fluid volume excess, a sodium-restricted diet often is prescribed. The primary dietary sources of sodium are the salt shaker, processed foods, and foods themselves.

A mild sodium restriction can be achieved by instructing the patient and primary food preparer in the household to reduce the amount of salt in recipes by half, avoid using the salt shaker during meals, and avoid foods that contain high levels of sodium (either naturally or because of processing). In moderate and severely sodium-restricted diets, salt is avoided altogether, as are all foods containing significant amounts of sodium.

MEDICATION ADMINISTRATION   **Diuretics for Fluid Volume Excess**

Diuretics increase urinary excretion of water and sodium. They are categorized into three major groups: loop diuretics, thiazide and thiazide-like diuretics, and potassium-sparing diuretics. Diuretics are used to enhance renal function and to treat vascular fluid overload and edema. Common side effects include orthostatic hypotension, dehydration, electrolyte imbalance, and possible hyperglycemia. Diuretics should be used with caution in the older adult. Examples of each major type follow.

LOOP DIURETICS

Furosemide (Lasix)

Ethacrynic Acid (Edecrin)

Bumetanide (Bumex)

Torsemide (Demadex)

Loop diuretics inhibit sodium and chloride reabsorption in the ascending loop of Henle (∞ see Chapter 26 for the anatomy of the kidneys). As a result, loop diuretics promote the excretion of sodium, chloride, potassium, and water.

THIAZIDE AND THIAZIDE-LIKE DIURETICS

Bendroflumethiazide (Naturetin)

Chlorothiazide (Diuril)

Hydrochlorothiazide (HydroDIURIL, Oretic)

Metolazone (Zaroxolyn)

Polythiazide (Renese)

Chlorthalidone (Hygroton)

Trichlormethiazide (Naqua)

Indapamide (Lozol)

xipamid (Xipamide)

Thiazide and thiazide-like diuretics promote the excretion of sodium, chloride, potassium, and water by decreasing absorption in the distal tubule.

POTASSIUM-SPARING DIURETICS

Spironolactone (Aldactone)

Amiloride HCl (Midamor)

Triamterene (Dyrenium)

Potassium-sparing diuretics promote excretion of sodium and water by inhibiting sodium-potassium exchange in the distal tubule.

NATRIURETIC PEPTIDE FAMILY

The natriuretic peptide family consists of atrial natriuretic peptide, brain natriuretic peptide, and C-type natriuretic peptide. Although the primary action of the natriuretic peptides is vasodilation, it has multiple effects on the kidneys including diuresis from renal hemodynamics and direct renal tubular effects.

Health Education for the Patient and Family

- The drug will increase the amount and frequency of urination.
- The drugs must be taken even when you feel well.
- Take the drugs in the morning and afternoon to avoid having to get up at night to urinate.
- Change position slowly to avoid dizziness.
- Report the following to your primary healthcare provider: dizziness; trouble breathing; or swelling of face, hands, or feet.
- Weigh yourself every day, and report sudden gains or losses.
- Avoid using the salt shaker when eating.
- If the drug increases potassium loss, consume foods high in potassium, such as orange juice and bananas.
- Do not use salt substitute if you are taking a potassium sparing diuretic.

BOX 10–1 Fluid Restriction Guidelines

- Subtract required fluids (e.g., ordered IV fluids, fluid used to dilute IV medications) from total daily allowance.
- Divide remaining fluid allowance—Day shift: 50% of total; Evening shift: 25% to 33% of total; Night shift: Remainder.
- Explain the fluid restriction to the patient and family members.
- Identify preferred fluids and intake pattern of patient.
- Place allowed amounts of fluid in small glasses (gives perception of a full glass).
- Offer ice chips (when melted, ice chips are approximately half the frozen volume).
- Provide frequent oral care.
- Provide sugarless chewing gum (if allowed) to reduce thirst sensation.

Examples of food high in sodium include lunch meat, bacon, cheese, dry cereal, canned soup, popcorn, ketchup, pickles, and seafood.

Nursing Care

Nursing care focuses on preventing fluid volume excess in patients at risk and on managing problems resulting from its effects.

Health Promotion

Health promotion related to fluid volume excess focuses on teaching preventive measures to patients who are at risk (e.g., patients who have heart disease or kidney failure). Discuss the relationship between sodium intake and water retention. Provide guidelines for a low-sodium diet, and teach patients to carefully read food labels to identify sodium in processed foods. Instruct patients at risk to weigh themselves on a regular basis, using the same scale, and to notify their primary care provider if they gain more than 5 lb in a week or less.

Assessment

Collect assessment data through the health history interview and physical examination.

- *Health history:* Risk factors such as medications, heart failure, acute or chronic renal or endocrine disease; precipitating factors such as a recent illness, change in diet, or change in medications. Recent weight gain; complaints of persistent cough, shortness of breath, swelling of feet and ankles, or difficulty sleeping when lying down.
- *Physical assessment:* Weight; vital signs; peripheral pulses and capillary refill; jugular neck vein distention; edema; lung sounds (crackles or wheezes), dyspnea, cough, and sputum; urine output; mental status.

Nursing Diagnoses and Interventions

Nursing diagnoses and interventions for the patient with fluid volume excess focus on the multisystem effects of the fluid overload.

Fluid Volume Excess

Nursing care for the patient with excess fluid volume includes collaborative interventions such as administering diuretics and maintaining a fluid restriction, as well as monitoring the status

and effects of the excess fluid volume. This is particularly critical in older patients because of the age-related decline in cardiac and renal compensatory responses.

- Assess vital signs, heart sounds, and volume of peripheral arteries. *Hypervolemia can cause hypertension, bounding peripheral pulses, and a third heart sound (S_3) due to the volume of blood flow through the hearts.*
- Assess for the presence and extent of edema, particularly in the lower extremities and the back, sacral, and periorbital areas. *Initially, edema affects the dependent portions of the body—the lower extremities of ambulatory patients and the sacrum in bedridden patients. Periorbital edema indicates more generalized edema.*

PRACTICE ALERT
Assess urine output hourly. Maintain accurate intake and output records. Note urine output of less than 30 mL per hour or a positive fluid balance on 24-hour total intake and output calculations. Congestive heart failure and inadequate renal perfusion may result in decreased urine output and fluid retention.

- Obtain daily weights at the same time of day, using approximately the same clothing and a balanced scale. *Daily weights are one of the most important gauges of fluid balance. Acute weight gain or loss represents fluid gain or loss. Weight gain of 2.2 lbs is equivalent to 1 L of fluid gain.*
- Administer oral fluids cautiously, adhering to any prescribed fluid restriction. Discuss the restriction with the patient and significant others, including the total volume allowed, the rationale, and the importance of reporting all fluid taken. *All sources of fluid intake, including ice chips, are recorded to avoid excess fluid intake.*
- Provide oral hygiene at least every 2 hours. *Oral hygiene contributes to patient comfort and keeps mucous membranes intact; it also helps relieve thirst if fluids are restricted.*
- Teach patient and significant others about the sodium-restricted diet (see Box 10–2), and emphasize the importance of checking before bringing foods to the patient. *Excess sodium promotes water retention; a sodium-restricted diet is ordered to reduce water gain.*
- Administer prescribed diuretics as ordered, monitoring the patient's response to therapy. *Loop or high-ceiling diuretics such as furosemide can lead to rapid fluid loss and manifestations of hypovolemia and electrolyte imbalance.*
- Promptly report significant changes in serum electrolytes or osmolality or abnormal results of tests done to determine contributing factors to the fluid volume excess. *Gradual correction of serum electrolytes and osmolality is expected; however, aggressive diuretic therapy can lead to overcorrection.*

Risk for Impaired Skin Integrity

Tissue edema decreases oxygen and nutrient delivery to the skin and subcutaneous tissues, increasing the risk of injury.

- Frequently assess skin, particularly in pressure areas and over bony prominences. *Skin breakdown can progress rapidly when circulation is impaired.*
- Reposition the patient at least every 2 hours. Provide skin care with each position change. *Frequent position changes minimize tissue pressure and promote blood flow to tissues.*

- Provide an egg-crate mattress or alternating pressure mattress, foot cradle, heel protectors, and other devices to reduce pressure on tissues. *These devices, which distribute pressure away from bony prominences, reduce the risk of skin breakdown.*

Impaired Gas Exchange

With fluid volume excess, gas exchange may be impaired by edema of pulmonary interstitial tissues. Acute pulmonary edema is a serious and potentially life-threatening complication of pulmonary congestion.

- Auscultate lungs for presence or worsening of crackles and wheezes; auscultate heart for extra heart sounds. *Crackles and wheezes indicate pulmonary congestion and edema. A gallop rhythm (S_3) may indicate diastolic overloading of the ventricles secondary to fluid volume excess.*
- Place in Fowler's position if dyspnea or orthopnea is present. *Fowler's position improves lung expansion by decreasing the pressure of abdominal contents on the diaphragm.*
- Monitor oxygen saturation levels and **arterial blood gases (ABGs)** for evidence of impaired gas exchange ($SaO_2 < 92\%$ to 95%; $PaO_2 < 80$ mmHg). Administer oxygen as indicated. *Edema of interstitial lung tissues can interfere with gas exchange and delivery to body tissues. Supplemental oxygen promotes gas exchange across the alveolar-capillary membrane, improving tissue oxygenation.*

Community-Based Care

Teaching for home care focuses on managing the underlying cause of fluid volume excess and preventing future episodes of excess fluid volume. Address the following topics when preparing the patient and family for home care:

- Manifestations of excess fluid and when to contact the care provider
- Prescribed medications: when and how to take, intended and adverse effects, what to report to care provider

BOX 10–2 Patient Teaching: Low-Sodium Diet

Low-Sodium Diet
- Reducing sodium intake will help the body excrete excess sodium and water.
- The body needs less than one-tenth of a teaspoon of salt per day.
- Approximately one-third of sodium intake comes from salt added to foods during cooking and at the table; one-fourth to one-third comes from processed foods; and the rest comes from food and water naturally high in sodium.
- Sodium compounds are used in foods as preservatives, leavening agents, and flavor enhancers.
- Many nonprescription drugs (such as analgesics, cough medicine, laxatives, and antacids) as well as toothpastes and mouthwashes contain high amounts of sodium.
- Low-sodium salt substitutes are not really sodium free and may contain half as much sodium as regular salt.
- Use salt substitutes sparingly; larger amounts often taste bitter instead of salty.
- The preference for salt will eventually diminish.
- Salt, monosodium glutamate, baking soda, and baking powder contain substantial amounts of sodium.
- Read labels.
- In place of salt or salt substitutes, use herbs, spices, lemon juice, vinegar, and wine as flavoring when cooking.

- Recommended or prescribed diet; ways to reduce sodium intake; how to read food labels for salt and sodium content; use of salt substitutes, if allowed
- If restricted, the amount and type of fluids to take each day; how to balance intake over 24 hours
- Monitoring weight; changes reported to care provider
- Ways to decrease dependent edema:
  a. Change position frequently.
  b. Avoid restrictive clothing.
  c. Avoid crossing the legs when sitting.
  d. Wear support stockings or hose.
  e. Elevate feet and legs when sitting.
- How to protect edematous skin from injury:
  a. Do not walk barefoot.
  b. Buy good-fitting shoes; shop in the afternoon when feet are more likely to be swollen.
- Using additional pillows or a recliner to sleep, to relieve orthopnea

Sodium Imbalance

Sodium is the most plentiful electrolyte in ECF, with normal serum sodium levels ranging from 135 to 145 mEq/L. Sodium is the primary regulator of the volume, osmolality, and distribution of ECF. It also is important in maintaining neuromuscular activity. Because of the close interrelationship between sodium and water balance, disorders of fluid volume and sodium balance often occur together. Sodium imbalances affect the osmolality of ECF and water distribution between the fluid compartments. When sodium levels are low (hyponatremia), water is drawn into the cells of the body, causing them to swell. In contrast, high levels of sodium in ECF (hypernatremia) draw water out of body cells, causing them to shrink.

Most of the body's sodium comes from dietary intake. Although a sodium intake of 500 mg per day is usually sufficient to meet the body's needs, and the CDC suggests that two-thirds of Americans should limit their intake to 1500 mg per day (about 3/4 teaspoon), the average intake of sodium by adults in the United States is about 3500 mg per day (CDC, 2009). Other sources of sodium include prescription drugs and some self-prescribed remedies.

The kidney is the primary regulator of sodium balance in the body. The kidney excretes or conserves sodium in response to changes in vascular volume. A fall in blood volume prompts several mechanisms that lead to sodium and water retention:

- The renin–angiotensin–aldosterone system (see Figure 10–8) is stimulated. Angiotensin II prompts the renal tubules to reabsorb sodium. It also causes vasoconstriction, slowing blood flow through the kidney and reducing glomerular filtration. This further reduces the amount of sodium excreted. Angiotensin II promotes the release of aldosterone from the adrenal cortex. In the presence of aldosterone, more sodium is reabsorbed in the cortical collecting tubules of the kidney, and more potassium is eliminated in the urine.
- ADH is released from the posterior pituitary (see Figure 10–9). ADH promotes sodium and water reabsorption in the distal tubules of the kidney, reducing urine output and expanding blood volume.

In contrast, when blood volume expands, sodium and water elimination by the kidneys increases.

- The glomerular filtration rate increases, allowing more water and sodium to be filtered and excreted.
- The hormone ANP is released by cells in the atria of the heart. ANP increases renal blood flow and glomerular filtration rate and also inhibits the aldosterone secretion to increase sodium excretion by the kidneys.
- ADH release from the pituitary gland is inhibited by ANP. In the absence of ADH, the distal tubule is relatively impermeable to water, allowing more to be excreted in the urine. Table 10–5 summarizes the manifestations of sodium imbalances.

The Patient with Hyponatremia

Hyponatremia is a serum sodium of less than 135 mEq/L. Hyponatremia usually results from a loss of sodium from the body, but it may also be caused by water gains that dilute ECF.

Pathophysiology

Excess sodium loss can occur through the kidneys, GI tract, or skin. Diuretics, kidney diseases, or adrenal insufficiency with impaired aldosterone and cortisol production can lead to excessive sodium excretion in urine. Vomiting, diarrhea, and GI suction are common causes of excess sodium loss through the GI tract. Sodium may also be lost when GI tubes are irrigated with water instead of saline, or when repeated tap water enemas are administered (Porth & Matfin, 2009). Excessive sweating, loss of skin surface (as with an extensive burn), and third spacing can also cause excessive sodium loss.

Hyponatremia causes a decrease in serum osmolality. Water shifts from ECF into the intracellular space, causing cells to swell and reducing the osmolality of intracellular fluid. Many of the manifestations of hyponatremia can be attributed to cellular edema and hypo-osmolality. Water gains that can lead to hyponatremia may occur with systemic diseases such as heart failure, renal failure, or cirrhosis of the liver; syndrome of inappropriate secretion of antidiuretic hormone (SIADH); excessive administration of hypotonic IV fluids; and self-induced water intoxication.

TABLE 10–5 Manifestations of Sodium Imbalances

HYPONATREMIA	HYPERNATREMIA
- Plasma sodium <135 mEq/L	- Plasma sodium >145 mEq/L
- Decreased serum osmolality	- Increased serum osmolality
- Decreased hematocrit and BUN	- Increased hematocrit and BUN
- Weight loss	- Weight gain
- Muscle cramps, weakness	- Increased thirst, oliguria, increased urine output and specific gravity
- Headache	- Dry skin and mucous membranes, decreased skin turgor, furrowed tongue, dry mouth
- Anxiety	
- Lethargy, stupor, coma	
- Anorexia, nausea, vomiting, diarrhea	- Headache, restlessness
- Hypotension, shock	- Seizures, coma
	- Tachycardia, hypotension, vascular collapse

Manifestations

The manifestations of hyponatremia depend on the rapidity of onset, the severity, and the cause of the imbalance. If the condition develops slowly, manifestations are usually not experienced until the serum sodium levels reach 125 mEq/L. In addition, the manifestations of hyponatremia vary, depending on extracellular fluid volume. Early manifestations of hyponatremia include muscle cramps, weakness, and fatigue from its effects on muscle cells. Gastrointestinal function is affected, causing anorexia, nausea and vomiting, abdominal cramping, and diarrhea.

As sodium levels continue to decrease, the brain and nervous system are affected by cellular edema. Neurologic manifestations progress rapidly when the serum sodium level falls below 120 mEq/L and include headache, depression, dulled sensorium, personality changes, irritability, lethargy, hyperreflexia, muscle twitching, and tremors. If serum sodium falls to very low levels, coma is likely to occur. When hyponatremia is associated with decreased ECF volume, the manifestations are those of hypovolemia (*hypotonic dehydration*). In hyponatremia associated with fluid volume excess, manifestations include those of hypervolemia.

Interdisciplinary Care

Interdisciplinary management of hyponatremia focuses on restoring normal blood volume and serum sodium levels.

Diagnosis

The following laboratory tests may be ordered.

- *Serum sodium* and *osmolality* are decreased in hyponatremia.
- A *24-hour urine specimen* is obtained to evaluate sodium excretion. In conditions associated with normal or increased extracellular volume (such as SIADH), urinary sodium is increased; in conditions resulting from losses of isotonic fluids (e.g., sweating, diarrhea, vomiting, and third-space fluid accumulation), by contrast, urinary sodium is decreased.

Medications

When both sodium and water have been lost (hyponatremia with hypovolemia), sodium-containing fluids are given to replace both water and sodium. Isotonic Ringer's solution or isotonic saline (0.9% NaCl) solution may be administered. Cautious administration of IV 3% or 5% NaCl solution may be necessary in patients who have very low plasma sodium levels (110 to 115 mEq/L).

Loop diuretics are administered to patients who have hyponatremia with normal or excess ECF volume. Loop diuretics promote an isotonic diuresis and fluid volume loss without hyponatremia. Thiazide diuretics are avoided because they cause a relatively greater sodium loss in relation to water loss. In addition, drugs to treat the underlying cause of hyponatremia may be administered.

Fluid and Dietary Management

If hyponatremia is mild, increasing the intake of foods high in sodium may restore normal sodium balance. Fluids often are restricted to help reduce ECF volume and correct hyponatremia (see Box 10–1 for fluid restriction guidelines).

⚘ Nursing Care

Nursing care of the patient with hyponatremia focuses on identifying patients at risk and managing problems resulting from the systemic effects of the disorder.

Health Promotion

People at risk for mild hyponatremia include those who participate in activities that increase fluid loss through excessive perspiration (diaphoresis) and then replace those losses by drinking large amounts of water or drinks with high sugar content. This includes athletes, people who do heavy labor in high environmental temperatures, and older adults living in non-air-conditioned settings during hot weather. Teach the following to patients who are at risk:

- Manifestations of mild hyponatremia, including nausea, abdominal cramps, and muscle weakness
- The importance of drinking liquids containing sodium and other electrolytes at frequent intervals when perspiring heavily, when environmental temperatures are high, and/or if watery diarrhea persists for several days

Assessment

Assessment data related to hyponatremia include the following:
- *Health history:* Current manifestations, including nausea and vomiting, abdominal discomfort, muscle weakness, headache, other manifestations; duration of manifestations and any precipitating factors such as heavy perspiration, vomiting, or diarrhea; chronic diseases such as heart or renal failure, cirrhosis of the liver, or endocrine disorders; current medications.
- *Physical assessment:* Mental status and level of consciousness; vital signs including orthostatic vital signs and peripheral pulses; presence of edema or weight gain.

Nursing Diagnoses and Interventions

Risk for Imbalanced Fluid Volume

Because of its role in maintaining fluid balance, sodium imbalances often are accompanied by water imbalances. In addition, treatment of hyponatremia can affect the patient's fluid balance.

- Monitor intake and output, weigh daily, and calculate 24-hour fluid balance. *Fluid excess or deficit may occur with hyponatremia.*

> **PRACTICE ALERT**
> Carefully monitor patients receiving sodium-containing IV solutions for manifestations of hypervolemia (increased blood pressure and CVP, tachypnea, tachycardia, gallop rhythm [S_3 and/or S_4 heart sounds], shortness of breath, crackles). Hypertonic saline solutions can lead to hypervolemia, particularly in patients with cardiovascular or renal disease.

- Use an infusion pump to administer hypertonic saline (3% and 5% NaCl) solutions; carefully monitor flow rate and response. *Hypertonic solutions can increase the risk of pulmonary and cerebral edema due to water retention. Careful monitoring is vital to prevent these complications and possible permanent damage.*

- If fluids are restricted, explain the reason for the restriction, the amount of fluid allowed, and how to calculate fluid intake. *Teaching increases the patient's sense of control and compliance.*

For additional nursing interventions that may apply to the patient with hyponatremia, review the discussions of fluid volume deficit and fluid volume excess.

Risk for Ineffective Cerebral Tissue Perfusion

The patient with severe hyponatremia experiences fluid shifts that cause an increase in intracellular fluid volume. This can cause brain cells to swell, increasing pressure within the cranial vault.

- Monitor serum electrolytes and serum osmolality. Report abnormal results to the healthcare provider. *As serum sodium and osmolality levels fall, the manifestations and neurologic effects of hyponatremia become increasingly severe.*
- Assess for neurologic changes, such as lethargy, altered level of consciousness, confusion, and convulsions. Monitor mental status and orientation. Compare baseline data with continuing assessments. *If serum sodium levels continue to fall, the patient may become increasingly less responsive.*
- Assess muscle strength and tone, and deep tendon reflexes. *Increasing muscle weakness and decreased deep tendon reflexes are manifestations of increasing hyponatremia.*

Community-Based Care

Teaching for home care focuses on the underlying cause of the sodium deficit and prevention. Teach patients about the following:

- Manifestations of mild and more severe hyponatremia to report to the primary care provider
- The importance of regular serum electrolyte monitoring if taking a potent diuretic or on a low-sodium diet
- Types of foods and fluids to replace sodium orally if dietary sodium is not restricted
- Older adults' increased risk for hyponatremia from the effects of medications and potential fluid imbalances

The Patient with Hypernatremia

Hypernatremia is a serum sodium level greater than 145 mEq/L. It may develop when sodium is gained in excess of water, or when water is lost in excess of sodium. Either fluid volume deficit or fluid volume excess often accompany hypernatremia.

Pathophysiology

Two regulatory mechanisms protect the body from hypernatremia: Excess sodium in ECF stimulates the release of ADH so more water is retained by the kidneys, and the thirst mechanism is stimulated to increase the intake of water. These two factors increase extracellular water, diluting the excess sodium and restoring normal levels.

Hypernatremia (also known as *hypertonic dehydration*) causes hyperosmolality of the ECF. As a result, water is drawn out of cells, leading to cellular dehydration. The most serious effects of cellular dehydration are seen in the brain. As brain cells contract, neurologic manifestations develop. The brain itself shrinks, causing mechanical traction on cerebral vessels. These vessels may tear and bleed. Although the brain rapidly adapts to hyperosmolality to minimize the water loss, acute hypernatremia can cause coma and seizures (Porth & Matfin, 2009).

Water deprivation is a cause of hypernatremia in patients who are unable to respond to thirst due to altered mental status or physical disability. Excess water loss may also occur with watery diarrhea or increased water losses from fever, hyperventilation, excessive perspiration, or massive burns. Unless water is adequately replaced, patients with diabetes insipidus (∞ see Chapter 19) also may develop hypernatremia. Excess sodium intake can result from ingestion of excess salt or hypertonic IV solutions. Patients who experience near-drowning in seawater are at risk for hypernatremia, as are patients with heatstroke.

Manifestations

Thirst is the first manifestation of hypernatremia. If thirst is not relieved, the primary manifestations relate to altered neurologic function (see Table 10–5). Initial lethargy, weakness, and irritability can progress to seizures, coma, and death in severe hypernatremia. Both the severity of the sodium excess and the rapidity of its onset affect the manifestations of hypernatremia.

Interdisciplinary Care

Treatment of hypernatremia depends on its cause. Hypernatremia is corrected slowly (over a 48-hour period) to avoid development of cerebral edema secondary to a shift of water into the brain cells.

Diagnosis

The following laboratory and diagnostic tests may be ordered:

- *Serum sodium levels* are greater than 145 mEq/L in hypernatremia.
- *Serum osmolality* is greater than 295 mOsm/kg in hypernatremia.

Medications

The principal treatment for hypernatremia is oral or IV water replacement. Hypotonic IV fluids such as 0.45% NaCl solution or 5% dextrose in water (which is isotonic when administered, but becomes hypotonic and provides pure water when the glucose is metabolized) may be administered to correct the water deficit. Diuretics may also be given to increase sodium excretion.

∞ Nursing Care

The primary focus of nursing care related to hypernatremia is prevention. Measures to prevent hypernatremia include identifying risk factors, teaching patients and caregivers, monitoring laboratory test results, and collaborating with the interdisciplinary team to reduce the potential for hypernatremia.

Health Promotion

Patients at risk for hypernatremia, as well as their caregivers, need teaching to prevent this electrolyte disorder. Instruct caregivers of debilitated patients who are unable to perceive thirst or unable to respond to it to offer fluids at regular intervals. If the patient is unable to maintain adequate fluid intake, contact the healthcare provider about an alternate route for fluid intake (e.g., a feeding tube). Teach caregivers the importance of

providing adequate water for patients receiving tube feedings (many of which are hypertonic).

Assessment

Assessment data related to hypernatremia include the following:
- *Health history:* Duration of manifestations and any precipitating factors such as water deprivation, increased water loss due to heavy perspiration, temperature or rapid breathing, diarrhea, excess salt intake, or diabetes insipidus; current medications; perception of thirst.
- *Physical assessment:* Vital signs, mucous membranes; mental status or level of consciousness; manifestations of fluid volume excess or fluid volume deficit.

Nursing Diagnoses and Interventions

Risk for Injury

Mental status and brain function may be affected by hypernatremia itself or by rapid correction of the condition that leads to cerebral edema. In either case, closely monitor the patient and take precautions to reduce risk of injury.

- Monitor and maintain fluid replacement to within the prescribed limits. Monitor serum sodium levels and osmolality; report rapid changes to the care provider. *Rapid water replacement or rapid changes in serum sodium or osmolality can increase the risk of bleeding or cerebral edema.*
- Monitor neurologic function, including mental status, level of consciousness, and other manifestations such as headache, nausea, vomiting, hypertension, and bradycardia. *Both hypernatremia and rapid correction of hypernatremia affect cerebral function. Careful monitoring is vital to detect changes in mental status that may indicate cerebral bleeding or edema.*
- Institute safety precautions as necessary: Keep the bed in its lowest position, side rails up and padded, and an airway at bedside. *Patients with sodium disorders are at risk for injury due to seizure activity and changes in mental status.*
- Keep clocks, calendars, and familiar objects at bedside. Orient to time, place, and circumstances as needed. Allow significant others to remain with the patient as much as possible. *An unfamiliar environment and altered thought processes can further increase the patient's risk for injury. Significant others provide a sense of security and reduce the patient's anxiety.*

Community-Based Care

When preparing the patient who has experienced hypernatremia for home care, discuss the following topics:

- The importance of responding to thirst and consuming adequate fluids (If the patient is dependent on a caregiver, stress to the caregiver the importance of regularly offering fluids.)
- If prescribed, guidelines for following a low-sodium diet (see Box 10–2)
- Use and effects of any prescribed diuretic
- The importance of following a schedule for regular monitoring of serum electrolyte levels and reporting manifestations of imbalance to healthcare provider

Potassium Imbalance

Potassium, the primary intracellular cation, plays a vital role in cell metabolism and cardiac and neuromuscular function. The normal serum (ECF) potassium level is 3.5 to 5.0 mEq/L. To maintain balance, potassium must be replaced daily through diet. Virtually all foods contain potassium, although some foods and fluids are richer sources of this element than others.

Most potassium in the body is found within the ICF, which has a concentration of 140 to 150 mEq/L. This significant difference in the potassium concentrations of ICF and ECF helps maintain the resting membrane potential of nerve and muscle cells. Potassium imbalances affect transmission and conduction of nerve impulses, maintenance of normal cardiac rhythms, and contraction of skeletal and smooth muscle. The higher intracellular potassium concentration is maintained by the sodium-potassium pump. Potassium constantly shifts into and out of the cells. This movement between ICF and ECF can significantly affect the serum potassium level. For example, potassium shifts into or out of the cells in response to changes in hydrogen ion concentration (pH, discussed later in this chapter) as the body strives to maintain a stable acid–base balance.

Aldosterone helps regulate potassium elimination by the kidneys. An increased potassium concentration in ECF stimulates aldosterone production by the adrenal gland. The kidneys respond to aldosterone by increasing potassium excretion. Changes in aldosterone secretion can profoundly affect the serum potassium level.

The Patient with Hypokalemia

Hypokalemia is an abnormally low serum potassium level (less than 3.5 mEq/L). It usually results from excess potassium loss, although hospitalized patients may be at risk for hypokalemia because of inadequate potassium intake.

Pathophysiology

Hypokalemia may result from inadequate intake of potassium; excessive renal, intestinal, or skin losses; or redistribution between the ICF and ECF. An intake of a minimum of 40 to 50 mEq/day is needed to compensate for urinary losses (Porth & Matfin, 2009). The kidneys are the main source of potassium loss. Normally only small amounts of potassium are lost in the feces, but substantial amounts may be lost from the GI tract with diarrhea or through drainage from an ileostomy (a permanent opening into the small bowel). Excessive sweating may also cause potassium loss.

These losses deplete total potassium stores in the body.

- Excess potassium loss through the kidneys often is secondary to drugs such as potassium-wasting diuretics, corticosteroids, amphotericin B, and large doses of some antibiotics. Hyperaldosteronism, a condition in which the adrenal glands secrete excess aldosterone, also causes excess elimination of potassium through the kidneys. Renal losses of potassium also occur from stress, trauma, metabolic acidosis, and a magnesium deficit.
- Gastrointestinal losses of potassium result from severe vomiting, gastric suction, or loss of intestinal fluids through diarrhea or ileostomy drainage.
- Transcellular shifts (from the ECF to the ICF) occur in conditions such as treatment of diabetic ketoacidosis with insulin (insulin increases the movement of potassium into the cells) and the use of beta2-adrenergic decongestants and bronchodilators (these drugs have the same effect as insulin).

Potassium intake may be inadequate in patients who are unable or unwilling to eat for prolonged periods. Hospitalized patients are at risk, especially those on extended parenteral fluid therapy with solutions that do not contain potassium. Patients with anorexia nervosa or alcoholism may develop hypokalemia due to both inadequate intake and loss of potassium through vomiting, diarrhea, or laxative or diuretic use.

PATHOPHYSIOLOGY LINKAGE   Hypokalemia

MANIFESTATIONS	RELATED PATHOPHYSIOLOGY
Characteristic electrocardiogram (ECG) changes of hypokalemia include flattened or inverted T waves, the development of U waves, and a depressed ST segment (Figure 10–10).	Low levels of potassium interfere with the contractility of cardiac muscle and the regulation and transmission of cardiac impulses, which maintain normal cardiac rhythms.
Nausea and vomiting, anorexia, decreased bowel sounds, ileus	Loss of potassium from severe vomiting, gastric suctioning, diarrhea, or ileostomy drainage affects the resting membrane potential and intracellular enzymes in smooth muscle cells, slowing peristalsis of the GI tract.
Decreased cardiac output, dysrhythmias (abnormal rhythms)	Decreased strength of cardiac contractions and dysrhythmias in turn cause a decrease in cardiac output. The most serious cardiac effect is an increased risk of atrial and ventricular dysrhythmias. Hypokalemia increases the risk for digitalis toxicity in patients receiving this drug used to treat heart failure (∞ see Chapter 31).
Muscle weakness and leg cramps	Low potassium levels affect the resting membrane potential and intracellular enzymes in skeletal muscle cells. Muscles of the lower extremities are affected first, then the trunk and upper extremities. This effect of hypokalemia is magnified when serum calcium levels are above normal.
	Severe hypokalemia can lead to rhabdomyolysis, a condition in which muscle fibers disintegrate, releasing myoglobin to be excreted in the urine.
Altered kidney function	Inability to concentrate urine due to decreased collecting tubule responsiveness to antidiuretic hormone.

Manifestations

Hypokalemia affects the transmission of nerve impulses, interfering with the contractility of smooth, skeletal, and cardiac muscle, as well as the regulation and transmission of cardiac impulses. Carbohydrate metabolism is affected by hypokalemia. Insulin secretion is suppressed, as is the synthesis of glycogen in skeletal muscle and the liver.

See the Pathophysiology Linkages box for manifestations of hypokalemia.

Manifestations of hypokalemia are more pronounced when potassium losses occur acutely. When hypokalemia develops gradually, potassium shifts out of the cells, helping maintain the ratio of intracellular to extracellular potassium. As a result, the neuromuscular manifestations of hypokalemia are less severe. See the Multisystem Effects of Hypokalemia feature on the following page.

Interdisciplinary Care

The management of hypokalemia focuses on prevention and treatment of a deficiency.

Diagnosis

The following laboratory and diagnostic tests may be ordered:

- *Serum potassium* (K^+) is used to monitor potassium levels in patients who are at risk for or who are being treated for hypokalemia.
- *Arterial blood gases (ABGs)* are measured to determine acid–base status. An increased pH (alkalosis) often is associated with hypokalemia. (See Table 10–10 later in this chapter for normal ABG values.)
- *Renal function studies*, such as *serum creatinine* and *blood urea nitrogen (BUN)*, may be ordered to evaluate for potential causes or effects of hypokalemia.

- *ECG recordings* are obtained to evaluate the effects of hypokalemia on the cardiac conduction system.

Medications

Oral and/or parenteral potassium supplements are given to prevent and, as needed, treat hypokalemia. To prevent hypokalemia in the patient taking nothing by mouth, potassium chloride is added to IV fluids. The dose used to treat hypokalemia includes the daily maintenance requirement, replacement of ongoing losses (e.g., gastric suction), and additional potassium to correct the existing deficit. Several days of therapy may be required. Commonly prescribed potassium supplements, their actions, and nursing implications are described in the following Medication Administration box.

Nutrition

A diet high in potassium-rich foods is recommended for patients at risk for developing hypokalemia or to supplement drug therapy. Examples of foods high in potassium include bananas, oranges, avocados, spinach, potatoes, tomatoes, meat, seafood, milk, and yogurt.

✎ Nursing Care

See the Case Study & Nursing Care Plan on page 209.

Health Promotion

When providing general health education, discuss using balanced electrolyte solutions (e.g., Pedialyte or sports drinks) to replace abnormal fluid losses (excess perspiration, vomiting, or severe diarrhea). Discuss the necessity of preventing hypokalemia with patients at risk. Provide diet teaching and refer patients with anorexia nervosa for counseling. Stress the potassium-losing effects of diuretics. Encourage a diet rich in high-potassium foods, as well as regular monitoring of serum potassium levels.

MEDICATION ADMINISTRATION Hypokalemia

POTASSIUM SOURCES

Potassium acetate (Tri-K)

Potassium bicarbonate (K + Care ET)

Potassium citrate (K-Lyte)

Potassium chloride (K-Lease, Micro-K 10, Apo-K)

Potassium gluconate (Kaon Elixir, Royonate)

Potassium is rapidly absorbed from the GI tract; potassium chloride is the agent of choice, because low chloride often accompanies low potassium. Potassium is used to prevent and/or treat hypokalemia (e.g., with parenteral nutrition and potassium-wasting diuretics, and prophylactically after major surgery).

Nursing Responsibilities

- When giving oral forms of potassium
  a. dilute or dissolve effervescent, soluble, or liquid potassium in fruit or vegetable juice or cold water.
  b. chill to increase palatability.
  c. give with food to minimize GI effects.
- When giving parenteral forms of potassium (KCl)
  a. do not administer IV push, do not add to fluids already hanging, and infuse at rate not to exceed 10 mEq/hour.
  b. do **NOT** administer undiluted.

  c. assess injection site frequently for manifestations of pain and inflammation. Discontinue and restart in another vein at first sign of infiltration.
  d. use an infusion pump.
  e. use cardiac monitoring if high or rapid doses are administered.
- Assess for abdominal pain, distention, GI bleeding; if present, do not administer medication. Notify healthcare provider.
- Monitor fluid intake and output.
- Assess for manifestations of hyperkalemia: weakness, feeling of heaviness in legs, mental confusion, hypotension, cardiac dysrhythmias, changes in ECG, increased serum potassium levels.

Health Education for the Patient and Family

- Do not take potassium supplements if you are also taking a potassium-sparing diuretic.
- When parenteral potassium is discontinued, eat potassium-rich foods.
- Do not chew enteric-coated tablets or allow them to dissolve in the mouth; this may affect the potency and action of the medications.
- Take potassium supplements with meals.
- Do not use salt substitutes when taking potassium (most salt substitutes are potassium based).

MULTISYSTEM EFFECTS OF
Hypokalemia

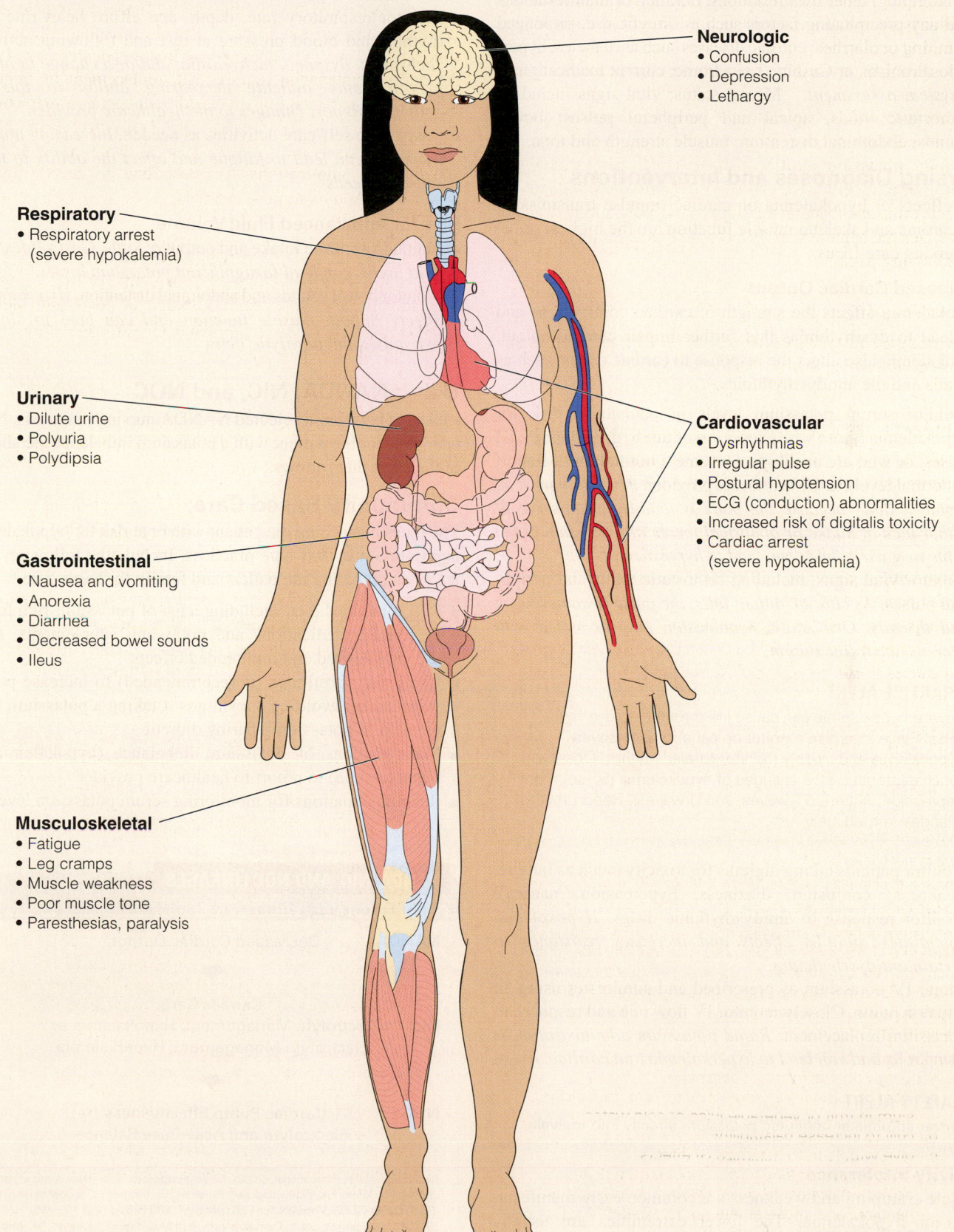

Neurologic
- Confusion
- Depression
- Lethargy

Respiratory
- Respiratory arrest
  (severe hypokalemia)

Urinary
- Dilute urine
- Polyuria
- Polydipsia

Cardiovascular
- Dysrhythmias
- Irregular pulse
- Postural hypotension
- ECG (conduction) abnormalities
- Increased risk of digitalis toxicity
- Cardiac arrest
  (severe hypokalemia)

Gastrointestinal
- Nausea and vomiting
- Anorexia
- Diarrhea
- Decreased bowel sounds
- Ileus

Musculoskeletal
- Fatigue
- Leg cramps
- Muscle weakness
- Poor muscle tone
- Paresthesias, paralysis

Assessment

Assessment data related to hypokalemia include the following:

- *Health history:* Current manifestations, including anorexia, nausea and vomiting, abdominal discomfort, muscle weakness or cramping, other manifestations; duration of manifestations and any precipitating factors such as diuretic use, prolonged vomiting or diarrhea; chronic diseases such as diabetes, hyperaldosteronism, or Cushing's syndrome; current medications.
- *Physical assessment:* Mental status; vital signs including orthostatic vitals, apical and peripheral pulses; bowel sounds, abdominal distention; muscle strength and tone.

Nursing Diagnoses and Interventions

The effects of hypokalemia on cardiac impulse transmission and cardiac and skeletal muscle function are the highest priority nursing care focus.

Decreased Cardiac Output

Hypokalemia affects the strength of cardiac contractions and can lead to dysrhythmias that further impair cardiac output. Hypokalemia also alters the response to cardiac drugs, such as digitalis and the antidysrhythmics.

- Monitor serum potassium levels in patients at risk for hypokalemia (those with excess losses due to drug therapy, GI losses, or who are unable to consume a normal diet). Report abnormal levels to the healthcare provider. *Potassium must be replaced daily because the body is unable to conserve it. Either lack of intake or abnormal losses of potassium in the urine or gastric fluids can lead to hypokalemia.*
- Monitor vital signs, including orthostatic vitals and peripheral pulses. *As cardiac output falls, the pulse becomes weak and thready. Orthostatic hypotension may be noted with decreased cardiac output.*

> **PRACTICE ALERT**
> Severe hypokalemia can cause life-threatening dysrhythmias. Place a cardiac monitor on patients with severe hypokalemia and closely monitor cardiac rhythm. Observe for characteristic ECG changes of hypokalemia (ST segment depression, flattened T waves, and U waves). Report rhythm changes immediately.

- Monitor patients taking digitalis for toxicity (such as fatigue, weakness, confusion, dizziness, hypotension, nausea). Monitor response to antidysrhythmic drugs. *Hypokalemia potentiates digitalis effects and increases resistance to certain antidysrhythmics.*
- Dilute IV potassium as prescribed and administer using an infusion pump. Closely monitor IV flow rate and response to potassium replacement. *Rapid potassium administration is dangerous and can lead to hyperkalemia and cardiac arrest.*

> **SAFETY ALERT**
> Never administer undiluted potassium directly into the vein.

Activity Intolerance

Muscle cramping and weakness are common early manifestations of hypokalemia. The lower extremities are usually affected first. This muscle weakness can cause the patient to fatigue easily, particularly with activity.

- Monitor skeletal muscle strength and tone, which are affected by moderate hypokalemia. *Increasing weakness, paresthesias, or paralysis of muscles or progression of affected muscles to include the upper extremities or trunk can indicate a further drop in serum potassium levels.*
- Monitor respiratory rate, depth, and effort; heart rate and rhythm; and blood pressure at rest and following activity. *Tachypnea, dyspnea, tachycardia, and/or a change in blood pressure may indicate decreasing ability to tolerate activities. Report changes to the healthcare provider.*
- Assist with self-care activities as needed. *Increasing muscle weakness can lead to fatigue and affect the ability to meet self-care needs.*

Risk for Imbalanced Fluid Volume

- Maintain accurate intake and output records. *Gastrointestinal fluid losses can lead to significant potassium losses.*
- Monitor bowel sounds and abdominal distention. *Hypokalemia affects smooth muscle function and can lead to slowed peristalsis and paralytic ileus.*

Using NANDA, NIC, and NOC

Linkages between a selected NANDA nursing diagnosis, NIC, and NOC for the patient with a potassium imbalance are shown in the chart that follows.

Community-Based Care

The focus in teaching the patient with or at risk for hypokalemia is prevention by self-care practices. Include the following topics when preparing the patient and family for home care.

- Recommended diet, including a list of potassium-rich foods
- Prescribed medications and potassium supplements, their use, and desired and unintended effects
- Using salt substitutes (if recommended) to increase potassium intake; avoiding substitutes if taking a potassium supplement or potassium-sparing diuretic
- Manifestations of potassium imbalance (hypokalemia or hyperkalemia) to report to healthcare provider
- Recommendations for monitoring serum potassium levels

NANDA, NIC, AND NOC LINKAGES
The Patient with Potassium Imbalance

NANDA	Decreased Cardiac Output
NIC	Cardiac Care
Electrolyte Management: Hypokalemia *or*
Electrolyte Management: Hyperkalemia
NOC	Cardiac Pump Effectiveness
Electrolyte and Acid–Base Balance

Data from NANDA International. (2009). *Nursing diagnoses: Definitions & classification 2009–2011*. Oxford, UK: Wiley-Blackwell; Bulechek, G., Butcher, H., & Dochterman, K. (Eds.). (2008). *Nursing interventions classification (NIC)* (5th ed.) (pp. 195–196, 286–287, 294–295). St. Louis, Elsevier Mosby; and Moorhead, S., Johnson, M., Maas, M., & Swanson, E. (Eds.). (2008). *Nursing outcomes classification (NOC)* (4th ed.) (pp.211–212, 340–341). St. Louis: Elsevier Mosby.

CASE STUDY & NURSING CARE PLAN · Hypokalemia

Rose Ortiz is a 72-year-old widow who lives alone, although close to her daughter's home. Ms. Ortiz has mild heart failure and is being treated with digoxin (Lanoxin) 0.125 mg, furosemide (Lasix) 40 mg PO daily, and a mildly restricted sodium diet (2 g daily). For the last several weeks, Ms. Ortiz has complained that she feels weak and sometimes faint, light-headed, and dizzy. Serum electrolyte tests ordered by her physician reveal a potassium level of 2.4 mEq/L. Potassium chloride solution (Kaochlor 10%, 20 mEq/15 mL) PO twice daily is prescribed, and Ms. Ortiz is referred to Nancy Walters, RN, for follow-up care.

ASSESSMENT

Ms. Ortiz's health history reveals that she has adhered to her sodium-restricted diet and has been compliant in taking her prescribed medications, with the exception of occasionally taking an additional "water pill" when her ankles swell. She takes a laxative every evening to ensure a daily bowel movement. She states that she is reluctant to take the potassium chloride the doctor has ordered because her neighbor complains that his potassium supplement upsets his stomach. Physical assessment findings included T 98.4, P 70, R 20, and BP 138/84. Muscle strength in her upper extremities is normal and equal; lower extremity strength is weak but equal. Sensation is normal.

DIAGNOSES

- *Risk for Injury* related to muscle weakness
- *Risk for Ineffective Health Maintenance* related to lack of knowledge about how diuretic therapy and laxative use affect potassium levels

EXPECTED OUTCOMES

- Maintain potassium level within normal limits (3.5 to 5.0 mEq/L).
- Regain normal muscle strength.
- Remain free of injury.
- Verbalize understanding of the effects of diuretic therapy and laxatives on potassium levels.

- Identify measures to avoid GI irritation when taking oral potassium.
- Identify potassium-rich foods.

PLANNING AND IMPLEMENTATION

- Explain need to use caution when ambulating, particularly when going up and down stairs.
- Discuss side effects of furosemide, and explain how taking additional tablets may have contributed to hypokalemia.
- Discuss alternative measures to prevent constipation without using laxatives on a regular basis (e.g., high-fiber diet, adequate fluid intake).
- Explain purpose of the prescribed potassium and its role in reversing muscle weakness.
- Teach to take potassium supplement after breakfast and supper, diluted in 4 oz of juice or water, and to sip it slowly over a 5- to 10-minute period. Advise to call if gastric irritation occurs.
- Discuss dietary sources of potassium; provide a list of potassium-rich foods.

EVALUATION

On a follow-up visit 1 week later, Ms. Ortiz states that her muscle weakness, dizziness, and other manifestations have resolved. She is taking the prescribed drugs as directed and is using laxatives only two or three times a week. Ms. Ortiz reports that she has increased her intake of potassium-rich foods and fluids and of high-fiber foods. Her potassium level is within normal limits.

CRITICAL THINKING IN THE NURSING PROCESS

1. What is the pathophysiologic basis for Ms. Ortiz's muscle weakness and dizziness?
2. How might the chronic overuse of laxatives contribute to hypokalemia?
3. Describe the interaction of digitalis, diuretics, and potassium.
4. Develop a plan of care for Ms. Ortiz for the nursing diagnosis of *Perceived Constipation.*

See Evaluating Your Response in Appendix C.

- If taking digitalis, manifestations of digitalis toxicity to report to healthcare provider
- Managing GI disorders that cause potassium loss (vomiting, diarrhea, ileostomy drainage) to prevent hypokalemia

The Patient with Hyperkalemia

Hyperkalemia is an abnormally high serum potassium (greater than 5 mEq/L). Hyperkalemia can result from inadequate excretion of potassium, excessively high intake of potassium, or a shift of potassium from the ICF to the ECF. Hyperkalemia affects neuromuscular and cardiac function.

Pathophysiology

Impaired renal excretion of potassium is a primary cause of hyperkalemia. Untreated renal failure, adrenal insufficiency (e.g., Addison's disease or inadequate aldosterone production), and medications (such as potassium-sparing diuretics, the antimicrobial drug trimethoprim [Trimpex], and some NSAIDs) impair potassium excretion by the kidneys. Rapid IV administration of potassium or transfusion of aged blood can lead to hyperkalemia. A shift of potassium ions from the ICF can occur in acidosis, with severe tissue trauma, during chemotherapy, and due to starvation. In acidosis, excess hydrogen ions enter the cells, displacing potassium and causing it to shift into the extracellular space. The extent of this shift is greater with metabolic acidosis than with respiratory acidosis (see the Acid–Base Disorders section later in this chapter).

Hyperkalemia alters the cell membrane potential, affecting the heart, skeletal muscle function, and the GI tract. The most harmful consequence of hyperkalemia is its effect on cardiac function. The cardiac conduction system is affected first, with slowing of the heart rate, possible heart blocks, and prolonged depolarization. ECG changes include peaked T waves, a prolonged PR interval, and widening of the QRS complex (see Figure 10–10 ■). Ventricular dysrhythmias develop, and cardiac arrest may occur. Severe hyperkalemia decreases the strength of myocardial contractions.

Manifestations

The manifestations of hyperkalemia result from its effects on the heart, skeletal, and smooth muscles. Early manifestations include diarrhea, colic (abdominal cramping), anxiety, paresthesias, irritability, and muscle tremors and twitching. As serum potassium levels increase, muscle weakness develops,

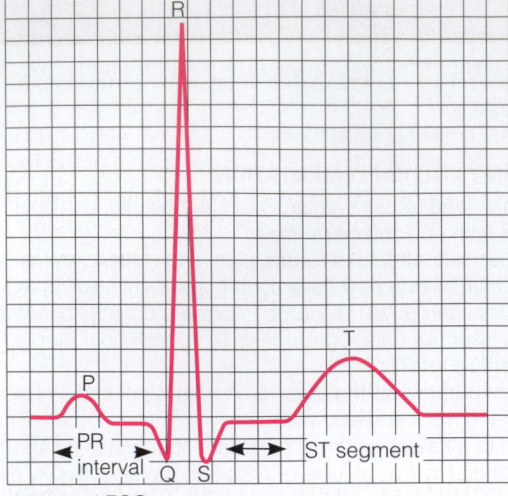

A Normal ECG

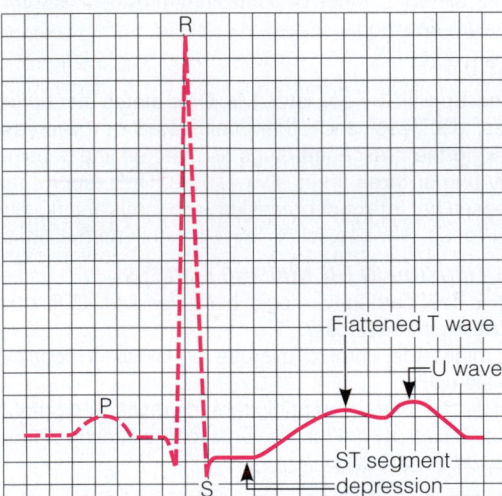

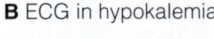

B ECG in hypokalemia

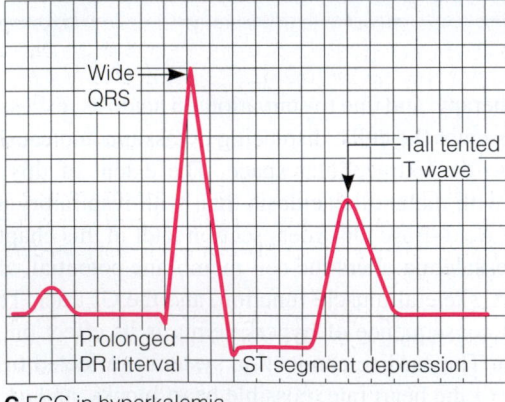

C ECG in hyperkalemia

Figure 10–10 ■ The effects of changes in potassium levels on the electrocardiogram (ECG). *A,* Normal ECG; *B,* ECG in hypokalemia; *C,* ECG in hyperkalemia.

TABLE 10–6 Pathophysiologic Indicators and Manifestations of Hyperkalemia

PATHOPHYSIOLOGIC INDICATOR	MANIFESTATIONS
Changes in laboratory values	■ Serum sodium level >145 mEq/L ■ Increased serum osmolality ■ Increased hematocrit and BUN
Increased ADH	■ Thirst ■ Decreased urine output ■ Increased urine specific gravity
Intracellular dehydration	■ Dry skin, dry mucous membranes ■ Increased tongue furrows ■ Decreased salivation
Hyperosmolality of ECF = Dehydration of brain neurons	■ Headache ■ Restlessness ■ Seizures ■ Coma
Decreased vascular volume	■ Tachycardia ■ Pulse weak and thready ■ Decreased blood pressure ■ Vascular collapse ■ ECG changes (see Figure 10–10)

Interdisciplinary Care

The management of hyperkalemia focuses on returning the serum potassium level to normal by treating the underlying cause and avoiding additional potassium intake. The choice of therapy for existing hyperkalemia is based on the severity of the hyperkalemia.

Diagnosis

The following laboratory and diagnostic tests may be ordered:

■ *Serum electrolytes* show a serum potassium level greater than 5.0 mEq/L. Low calcium and sodium levels may increase the effects of hyperkalemia; therefore, these electrolytes are usually measured as well.
■ *ABGs* are measured to determine if acidosis is present.
■ An *ECG* is obtained and *continuous ECG monitoring* is instituted to evaluate the effects of hyperkalemia on cardiac conduction and rhythm.

Medications

Medications are administered to lower the serum potassium and to stabilize the conduction system of the heart. For moderate to severe hyperkalemia, calcium gluconate is given IV to counter the effects of hyperkalemia on the cardiac conduction system. While the effect of calcium gluconate lasts only for 1 hour, it allows time to initiate measures to lower serum potassium levels. To rapidly lower these levels, regular insulin and 50 g of glucose are administered. Insulin and glucose promote potassium uptake by the cells, shifting potassium out of ECF. In some cases, a ß₂-agonist such as albuterol may be given by nebulizer to temporarily push potassium into the cells. Sodium bicarbonate may be given to treat acidosis. As the pH returns toward normal, hydrogen ions are released from the cells and potassium returns into the cells.

progressing to flaccid paralysis. The lower extremities are affected first, progressing to the trunk and upper extremities. The heart rate may be slow (bradycardia) and irregular. Table 10–6 summarizes the pathophysiologic indicators and manifestations of hyperkalemia.

To remove potassium from the body, sodium polystyrene sulfonate (Kayexalate), a resin that binds potassium in the GI tract, may be administered orally or rectally. If renal function is normal, diuretics such as furosemide are given to promote potassium excretion. Commonly prescribed drugs, their actions, and nursing implications are listed in the accompanying Medication Administration box.

Dialysis

When renal function is severely limited, either peritoneal dialysis or hemodialysis may be implemented to remove excess potassium. These measures are invasive and typically used only when other measures are ineffective. ∞ See Chapter 28 for more information about dialysis.

✍ Nursing Care

Nursing care interventions related to hyperkalemia include identifying patients at risk, preventing hyperkalemia, and addressing problems resulting from the systemic effects of hyperkalemia. A Case Study & Nursing Care Plan for a patient with hyperkalemia is found on page 212.

Health Promotion

Patients at the greatest risk for developing hyperkalemia include those taking potassium supplements (prescribed or over-the-counter), using potassium-sparing diuretics or salt substitutes, and experiencing renal failure. Athletes participating in competition sports such as body building and those using anabolic steroids, muscle-building compounds, or "energy drinks" also may be at risk for hyperkalemia.

Teach all patients to carefully read food and dietary supplement labels. Discuss the importance of taking prescribed potassium supplements as ordered, and not increasing the dose unless prescribed by the care provider. Advise patients taking a potassium supplement or potassium-sparing diuretic to avoid salt substitutes, which usually contain potassium. Discuss the importance of maintaining an adequate fluid intake (unless a fluid restriction has been prescribed) to maintain renal function to eliminate potassium from the body.

Assessment

Assessment data related to hyperkalemia include the following:
- *Health history:* Current manifestations, including numbness and tingling, nausea and vomiting, abdominal cramping, muscle weakness, palpitations; duration of manifestations and any precipitating factors such as use of salt substitutes, potassium supplements, or reduced urine output; chronic diseases such as renal failure or endocrine disorders; current medications.
- *Physical assessment:* Apical and peripheral pulses; bowel sounds; muscle strength in upper and lower extremities; ECG pattern.

MEDICATION ADMINISTRATION | Hyperkalemia

DIURETICS
Potassium-wasting diuretics, such as furosemide (Lasix), may be used to enhance renal excretion of potassium.

Nursing Responsibilities
- Monitor serum electrolytes.
- Monitor and record weight at regular intervals under standard conditions (same time of day, balanced scale, same clothing).
- Monitor intake and output.

INSULIN, HYPERTONIC DEXTROSE, AND SODIUM BICARBONATE
Insulin, hypertonic dextrose (10% to 50%), and sodium bicarbonate are used in the emergency treatment of moderate to severe hyperkalemia. Insulin promotes the movement of potassium into the cell, and glucose prevents hypoglycemia. The onset of action of insulin and hypertonic dextrose occurs within 30 minutes and is effective for approximately 4 to 6 hours.

Sodium bicarbonate elevates the serum pH; potassium is moved into the cell in exchange for hydrogen ion. Sodium bicarbonate is particularly useful in the patient with metabolic acidosis (Perrin, 2009). Onset of effects occurs within 15 to 30 minutes and is effective for approximately 2 hours.

Nursing Responsibilities
- Administer IV insulin and dextrose over prescribed interval of time using an infusion pump.
- Administer sodium bicarbonate as prescribed. It may be administered as an IV bolus or added to a dextrose-in-water solution and given by infusion.
- In patients receiving sodium bicarbonate, monitor for sodium overload, particularly in patients with hypernatremia, heart failure, and renal failure.

- Monitor the ECG pattern closely.
- Monitor serum electrolytes (K^+, Na^+, Ca^{2+}, Mg^{2+}) frequently during treatment.

CALCIUM GLUCONATE AND CALCIUM CHLORIDE
IV calcium gluconate or calcium chloride is used as a temporary emergency measure to counteract the toxic effects of potassium on myocardial conduction and function.

Nursing Responsibilities
- Closely monitor the ECG of the patient receiving IV calcium, particularly for bradycardia.
- Calcium should be used cautiously in patients receiving digitalis, because calcium increases the cardiotonic effects of digitalis and may precipitate digitalis toxicity, leading to dysrhythmias.

SODIUM POLYSTYRENE SULFONATE (KAYEXALATE) AND SORBITOL
Sodium polystyrene sulfonate (Kayexalate) is used to treat moderate or severe hyperkalemia. Categorized as a cation exchange resin, Kayexalate exchanges sodium or calcium for potassium in the large intestine. Sorbitol is given with Kayexalate to promote bowel elimination. Kayexalate and sorbitol may be administered orally, through a nasogastric tube, or rectally as a retention enema.

Nursing Responsibilities
- Because Kayexalate contains sodium, monitor patients with heart failure and edema closely for water retention.
- Monitor serum electrolytes (K^+, Na^+, Ca^{2+}, Mg^{2+}) frequently during therapy.
- Restrict sodium intake in patients who are unable to tolerate increased sodium load (e.g., those with CHF or hypertension).

CASE STUDY & NURSING CARE PLAN   Hyperkalemia

Montigue Longacre, a 51-year-old African American male, has end-stage renal failure. He arrives at the emergency clinic complaining of shortness of breath on exertion and extreme weakness.

ASSESSMENT

Mr. Longacre tells the nurse, Janet Allen, RN, that he normally receives dialysis three times a week. He missed his last treatment, however, to attend his father's funeral. During the last several days, he has eaten a number of fresh oranges he received as a gift. Physical assessment findings include T 99.2, P 100, R 28, BP 168/96, 2+ pretibial edema, and a 6-lb (3.6-kg) weight gain since his last hemodialysis treatment 4 days ago. Laboratory and diagnostic tests show the following abnormal results:

- K^+ 6.5 mEq/L (normal 3.5 to 5 mEq/L)
- BUN 118 mg/dL (normal 7 to 18 mg/dL)
- Creatinine 14 mg/dL (normal 0.7 to 1.3 mg/dL)
- HCO_3^- 17 mEq/L (normal 22 to 26 mEq/L)
- Peaked T wave noted on ECG

Mr. Longacre is placed on continuous ECG monitoring, and the physician prescribes hemodialysis. As an interim measure to lower the serum potassium, the physician prescribes D50W (25 g of dextrose), one ampule, to be administered IV with 10 units of regular insulin over 30 minutes.

DIAGNOSES

- *Activity Intolerance* related to skeletal muscle weakness
- *Risk for Decreased Cardiac Output* related to hyperkalemia
- *Risk for Ineffective Health Maintenance* related to inadequate knowledge of recommended diet
- *Fluid Volume Excess* related to renal failure

EXPECTED OUTCOMES

- Gradually resume usual physical activities.
- Maintain serum potassium level within normal range.
- Verbalize causes of hyperkalemia, the importance of hemodialysis treatments as scheduled, and the role of diet in preventing hyperkalemia.

PLANNING AND IMPLEMENTATION

- Monitor intake and output.
- Monitor serum potassium and ECG closely during treatment.
- Teach causes of hyperkalemia and the relationship between hemodialysis and hyperkalemia.
- Discuss the importance of avoiding foods high in potassium to prevent or control hyperkalemia.

EVALUATION

Following emergency treatment and hemodialysis, Mr. Longacre's ECG and serum potassium level have returned to normal. His muscle strength has returned to near normal, and he verbalizes an understanding of his prescribed hemodialysis regimen. Janet Allen provides verbal and written information about hyperkalemia, the importance of complying with the hemodialysis regimen, and the importance of limiting intake of dietary sources of potassium in renal failure. She also furnishes a list of foods high in potassium and cautions against using potassium-containing salt substitutes and nonprescription drugs.

CRITICAL THINKING IN THE NURSING PROCESS

1. What information given by Mr. Longacre indicated that he might be experiencing hyperkalemia?
2. Why was continuous ECG monitoring instituted as an emergency measure?
3. What additional emergency measures might have been instituted if Mr. Longacre's serum potassium level had been 8.5 mEq/L and his ECG had showed changes in impulse conduction?
4. Develop a care plan for Mr. Longacre for the nursing diagnosis of *Anxiety*.

See Evaluating Your Response in Appendix C.

Nursing Diagnoses and Interventions

The effects of excess potassium on the electrical conduction and contractility of the heart are the highest priority for nursing care, particularly when the serum potassium level is 6.5 mEq/L or higher.

Risk for Decreased Cardiac Output

Hyperkalemia affects depolarization of the atria and ventricles of the heart. Severe hyperkalemia can cause dysrhythmias with ventricular fibrillation and cardiac arrest. The cardiac effects of hyperkalemia are more pronounced when the serum potassium level rises rapidly. Low serum sodium and calcium levels, high serum magnesium levels, and acidosis contribute to the adverse effects of hyperkalemia on the heart muscle.

> **PRACTICE ALERT**
> Monitor the ECG pattern for development of peaked, narrow T waves, prolongation of the PR interval, depression of the ST segment, widened QRS interval, and loss of the P wave (see Figure 10–10). Notify the physician of changes. Progressive ECG changes from a peaked T wave to loss of the P wave and widening of the QRS complex indicate an increasing risk of dysrhythmias and cardiac arrest.

- Closely monitor the response to IV calcium gluconate, particularly in patients taking digitalis. *Calcium increases the risk of digitalis toxicity.*

Risk for Activity Intolerance

Both hypokalemia (low serum potassium levels) and hyperkalemia (high serum potassium levels) affect neuromuscular activity and the function of cardiac, smooth, and skeletal muscles. Hyperkalemia can cause muscle weakness and even paralysis.

- Monitor skeletal muscle strength and tone. *Increasing weakness, muscle paralysis, or progression of affected muscles to affect the upper extremities or trunk can indicate increasing serum potassium levels.*
- Monitor respiratory rate and depth. Regularly assess lung sounds. *Muscle weakness due to hyperkalemia can impair ventilation. In addition, medications such as sodium bicarbonate or sodium polystyrene sulfonate can cause fluid retention and pulmonary edema in patients with preexisting cardiovascular disease.*
- Assist with self-care activities as needed. *Increasing muscle weakness can lead to fatigue and affect the ability to meet self-care needs.*

Community-Based Care

Preventing future episodes of hyperkalemia is the focus when preparing the patient for home care. Include the family, a significant other, or a caregiver when teaching the following topics:

- Recommended diet and any restrictions including salt substitutes and foods high in potassium
- Medications to be avoided, including over-the-counter and fitness supplements

Calcium Imbalance

Calcium is one of the most abundant ions in the body. The normal adult total serum calcium concentration is 8.5 to 10.0 mg/dL. Calcium is obtained from dietary sources, although only about 20% of the calcium ingested is absorbed into the blood. The remainder is excreted in feces. Extracellular calcium is excreted by the kidneys. Approximately 99% of the total calcium in the body is bound to phosphorus to form the minerals in bones and teeth. The remaining 1% is in extracellular fluid. About half of this extracellular calcium is ionized (free); it is this ionized calcium that is physiologically active. The remaining extracellular calcium is bound to protein or other ions. Ionized calcium is essential to a number of processes: stabilizing cell membranes, regulating muscle contraction and relaxation, maintaining cardiac function, and blood clotting.

Serum calcium levels are regulated by the interaction of three hormones: parathyroid hormone (PTH), calcitonin, and calcitriol (a metabolite of vitamin D). When serum calcium levels fall, the parathyroid glands secrete PTH, which mobilizes skeletal calcium stores, increases calcium absorption in the intestines, and promotes calcium reabsorption by the kidneys (Figure 10–11 ■). Calcitriol facilitates this process by stimulating calcium release from the bones, absorption in the intestines, and reabsorption by the kidneys. Calcitonin is secreted by the thyroid gland in response to high serum calcium levels. Its effect on serum calcium levels is the opposite of PTH: It inhibits the movement of calcium out of bone, reduces intestinal absorption of calcium, and promotes calcium excretion by the kidneys.

Serum calcium levels are also affected by acid–base balance. When hydrogen ion concentration falls and the pH rises (alkalosis), more calcium is bound to protein. While the total serum calcium remains unchanged, less calcium is available in the ionized, active form. Conversely, when hydrogen ion concentration increases and the pH falls (acidosis), calcium is released from protein, making more ionized calcium available.

Finally, the total amount of calcium in blood plasma fluctuates with plasma protein levels, particularly the albumin level. As the albumin level falls, the total amount of plasma calcium declines. Table 10–7 summarizes the manifestations of calcium imbalances.

The Patient with Hypocalcemia

Hypocalcemia is a total serum calcium level of less than 8.5 mg/dL. Hypocalcemia can result from decreased total body calcium stores or low levels of extracellular calcium with normal amounts of calcium stored in bone. The systemic effects of hypocalcemia are caused by decreased levels of ionized calcium in extracellular fluid.

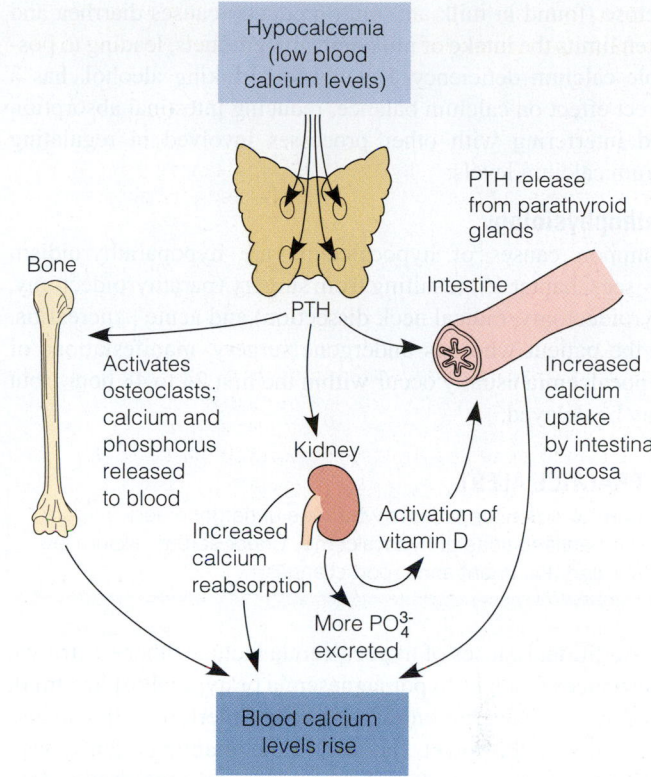

Figure 10–11 ■ Low calcium levels (hypocalcemia) trigger the release of parathyroid hormone (PTH), increasing calcium ion levels through stimulation of bones, kidneys, and intestines.

Risk Factors

Certain people are at greater risk for hypocalcemia: those who have had a parathyroidectomy (removal of the parathyroid glands), older adults (especially women), people with lactose intolerance, and those who have alcoholism. Older adults often consume less milk and milk products (good sources of calcium) and may have decreased exposure to the sun (a source of vitamin D). Older adults also may be less active, promoting calcium loss from bones. They are more likely to be taking drugs that interfere with calcium absorption or promote calcium excretion (e.g., furosemide). Older women are at particular risk after menopause because of reduced estrogen levels. Intolerance to

TABLE 10–7 Manifestations of Calcium Imbalances

HYPOCALCEMIA	HYPERCALCEMIA
■ Serum calcium level <8.5 mg/dL	■ Serum calcium level >10.0 mg/dL
■ Numbness and tingling	■ Increased thirst and urine output
■ Muscle cramping	■ Anorexia
■ Hyperactive reflexes	■ Nausea, vomiting
■ Tetany	■ Constipation
■ Carpopedal and laryngeal spasms	■ Muscle weakness
■ Positive Chvostek and Trousseau signs (see Figure 10–12)	■ Increased blood pressure
	■ AV block
■ Decreased blood pressure	■ Lethargy
■ Ventricular dysrhythmias	■ Coma
■ Bone pain, fractures (chronic form)	

lactose (found in milk and milk products) causes diarrhea and often limits the intake of milk and milk products, leading to possible calcium deficiency. Ethanol, or drinking alcohol, has a direct effect on calcium balance, reducing intestinal absorption and interfering with other processes involved in regulating serum calcium levels.

Pathophysiology

Common causes of hypocalcemia are hypoparathyroidism (∞ see Chapter 19) resulting from surgery (parathyroidectomy, thyroidectomy, radical neck dissection) and acute pancreatitis. In the patient who has undergone surgery, manifestations of hypocalcemia usually occur within the first 24 to 48 hours, but may be delayed.

> **PRACTICE ALERT**
> Carefully monitor patients who have undergone neck surgery for manifestations of hypocalcemia. Check serum calcium levels, and document and report changes.

Additional causes of hypocalcemia include other electrolyte imbalances (such as hypomagnesemia or hyperphosphatemia), alkalosis, malabsorption disorders that interfere with calcium absorption in the bowel, and inadequate vitamin D (due to lack of sun exposure or malabsorption). Hyperphosphatemia often occurs in acute renal failure, with reciprocal hypocalcemia. Massive transfusion of banked blood can lead to hypocalcemia. Citrate is added to blood to prevent clotting and as a preservative. When blood is administered faster than the liver can metabolize the citrate, it can bind with calcium, temporarily removing ionized calcium from circulation. Many drugs increase the risk for hypocalcemia, including loop diuretics (such as furosemide [Lasix]), anticonvulsants (such as phenytoin [Dilantin] and phenobarbital), phosphates (including phosphate enemas), and drugs that lower serum magnesium levels (such as cisplatin [Platinol]).

Extracellular calcium acts to stabilize neuromuscular cell membranes. This effect is reduced in hypocalcemia, increasing neuromuscular irritability. The threshold of excitation of sensory nerve fibers is lowered as well, leading to paresthesias (altered sensation). The nervous system becomes more excitable, and muscle spasms develop. In the heart, this change in cell membranes can lead to dysrhythmias such as ventricular tachycardia and cardiac arrest. Hypocalcemia decreases the contractility of cardiac muscle fibers, leading to decreased cardiac output.

Manifestations and Complications

The most serious manifestations of hypocalcemia are **tetany** (tonic muscular spasms) and convulsions. Numbness and tingling around the mouth (circumoral) and in the hands and feet develop. Muscle spasms of the face and extremities occur, and deep tendon reflexes become hyperactive. Chvostek's sign, contraction of the facial muscles produced by tapping the facial nerve in front of the ear (Figure 10–12A ■), and Trousseau's sign, carpal spasm induced by inflating a blood pressure cuff on the upper arm to above systolic blood pressure for 2 to 5 minutes (Figure 10–12B), indicate increased neuromuscular excitability in patients without obvious manifestations. Tetany can also cause bronchial muscle spasms, simulating an asthma attack,

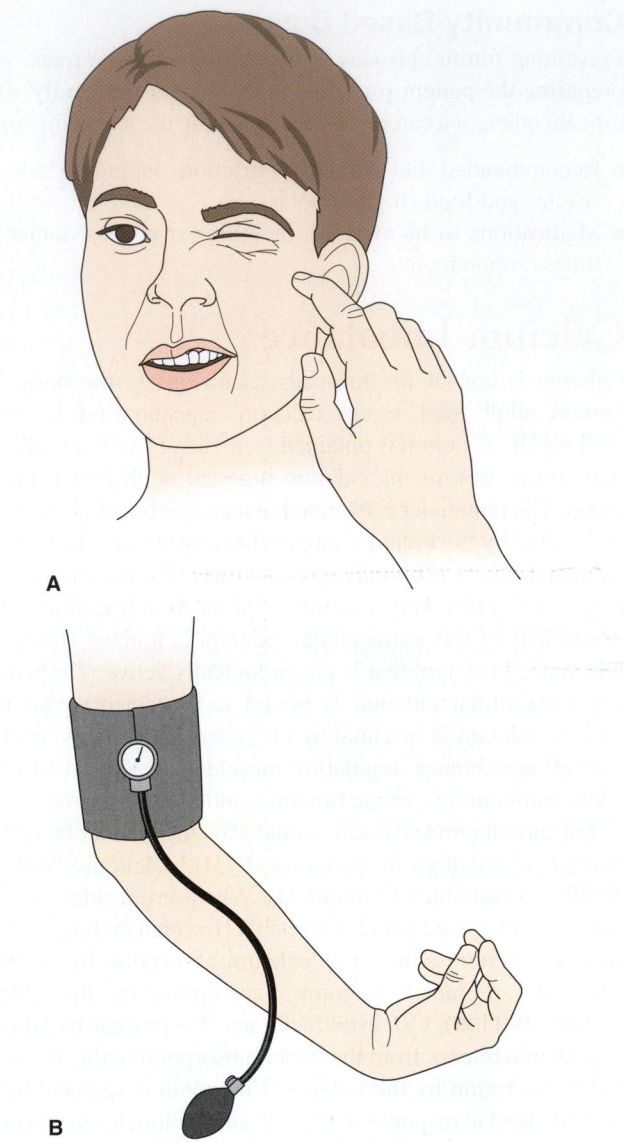

Figure 10–12 ■ *A*, Positive Chvostek's sign. *B*, Positive Trousseau's sign.

and visceral muscle spasms, producing acute abdominal pain. Cardiovascular manifestations include hypotension, possible bradycardia (slow heart rate), and ventricular dysrhythmias.

Serious complications of hypocalcemia include airway obstruction and possible respiratory arrest from laryngospasm, ventricular dysrhythmias, prolonged QT intervals, cardiac arrest, heart failure, and convulsions.

Interdisciplinary Care

Management of hypocalcemia is directed toward restoring normal calcium balance and correcting the underlying cause.

Diagnosis

The following laboratory and diagnostic tests may be ordered when hypocalcemia is known or suspected:

■ *Total serum calcium*, the amount of ionized (active) calcium available, usually is estimated. In critically ill patients, however, *ionized calcium* may be directly measured using ion-selective electrodes. Direct measurement of ionized calcium requires special handling of the blood specimen, including placing the specimen on ice and analyzing it immediately.

- *Serum albumin*, because the albumin level affects serum calcium results. When the albumin level is low (hypoalbuminemia), the amount of ionized calcium may remain normal even though the total calcium level is low.
- *Serum magnesium*, because hypocalcemia is often associated with hypomagnesemia (serum magnesium < 1.6 mg/dL). In this case, normal magnesium levels must be restored to correct the hypocalcemia.
- *Serum phosphate*, because hyperphosphatemia (serum phosphate > 4.5 mg/dL) can lead to hypocalcemia due to the inverse relationship between phosphorus and calcium (as phosphate levels rise, calcium levels fall).
- *Parathyroid hormone (PTH)*, to identify the possible diagnoses of hyperparathyroidism.
- An *ECG*, to evaluate the effects of hypocalcemia on the heart, such as a prolonged ST segment.

Medications

Hypocalcemia is treated with oral or IV calcium. The patient with severe hypocalcemia is treated with IV calcium to prevent life-threatening problems such as airway obstruction. The most common IV calcium preparations include calcium chloride and calcium gluconate. Although calcium chloride contains more elemental calcium than calcium gluconate, it also is more irritating to the veins and may cause venous sclerosis (hardening of the vein walls) if given into a peripheral vein. IV calcium preparations can cause necrosis and sloughing of tissue if they infiltrate into subcutaneous tissue. Rapid drug administration can lead to bradycardia and possible cardiac arrest due to overcorrection of hypocalcemia with resulting hypercalcemia. See the accompanying Medication Administration box for further information about calcium administration.

Oral calcium preparations (calcium carbonate, calcium gluconate, or calcium lactate) are used to treat chronic, asymptomatic hypocalcemia. Calcium supplements may be combined with vitamin D, or vitamin D may be given alone to increase GI absorption of calcium.

Nutrition

A diet high in calcium-rich foods may be recommended for patients with chronic hypocalcemia or with low total body stores of calcium. Foods high in calcium include dairy products, canned salmon, broccoli, spinach, and tofu.

℘ Nursing Care

Health Promotion

Because of the large stores of calcium in bones, most healthy adults have a very low risk of developing hypocalcemia. However, a deficit of total body calcium is often associated with aging, increasing the risk of osteoporosis, fractures, and disability. Women have a higher risk for developing osteoporosis than men due to lower bone density and hormonal influences. Teach women of all ages the importance of maintaining adequate calcium intake through diet and, as needed, calcium supplements. Stress the relationship between weight-bearing exercise and bone density, and encourage women to engage in a regular aerobic and weight-training exercise regime. Recommend screening for bone density in older women. ∞ See Chapter 40 for more information about osteoporosis.

Assessment

Assessment data related to hypocalcemia include the following:
- *Health history:* Current manifestations, including numbness and tingling around mouth and of hands and feet, abdominal pain, shortness of breath; acute or chronic diseases such as pancreatitis, liver or kidney disease; current medications.

MEDICATION ADMINISTRATION Calcium Salts

CALCIUM SALTS
Calcium carbonate (BioCal, Calsam, Caltrate, OsCal, Tums, others)
Calcium chloride
Calcium citrate (Citracal)
Calcium glubionate
Calcium gluceptate
Calcium gluconate (Kalcinate)
Calcium lactate

Calcium salts are given to increase calcium levels when there is a deficit (a total body deficit or inadequate levels of extracellular calcium). Calcium is necessary to maintain bone structure and for multiple physiologic processes including neuromuscular and cardiac function as well as blood coagulation. In the presence of vitamin D, calcium is well absorbed from the GI tract. Severe hypocalcemia is treated with IV calcium preparations.

Nursing Responsibilities
Oral calcium salts:
- Administer 1 to 1.5 hours after meals and at bedtime.
- Give calcium tablets with a full glass of water.
IV calcium salts:
- Assess IV site for patency. Do not administer calcium if there is a risk of leakage into the tissues.

- May be given by slow IV push (dilute with sterile normal saline for injection prior to administering) or added to compatible parenteral fluids such as NS, lactated Ringer's solution, or D_5W.
- Administer into the largest available vein; use a central line if available.
- Do not administer with bicarbonate or phosphate.
- Continuously monitor ECG when administering IV calcium to patients taking digitalis due to increased risk of digitalis toxicity.
- Frequently monitor serum calcium levels and response to therapy.

Health Education for the Patient and Family
- Take calcium tablets with a full glass of water 1 to 2 hours after meals. Do not take with food or milk. If possible, do not take within 1 to 2 hours of other medications.
- Maintain adequate vitamin D intake through diet or exposure to the sun to promote calcium absorption.
- Calcium carbonate can cause constipation. Eat a high-fiber diet and maintain a generous fluid intake to prevent constipation.

■ *Physical assessment:* Muscle spasms; deep tendon reflexes; Chvostek's sign and Trousseau's sign; vital signs and apical pulse; presence of convulsions.

Nursing Diagnoses and Interventions

The effect of hypocalcemia on neuromuscular irritability, with the risk for muscle spasm and convulsions, is the highest priority for nursing care of the patient.

Risk for Injury

The patient with hypocalcemia is at risk for injury from possible laryngospasm, cardiac dysrhythmias, or convulsions. In addition, too rapid administration of IV calcium or infiltration of the medication into subcutaneous tissues can lead to injury.

■ Frequently monitor airway and respiratory status. Report changes such as respiratory stridor (a high-pitched, harsh inspiratory sound indicative of upper airway obstruction) or increased respiratory rate or effort to the physician. *These changes may indicate laryngeal spasm due to tetany.*

> **PRACTICE ALERT**
> Laryngeal spasm is a respiratory emergency, requiring immediate intervention to maintain ventilation and gas exchange.

■ Monitor cardiovascular status including heart rate and rhythm, blood pressure, and peripheral pulses. *Hypocalcemia decreases myocardial contractility, causing reduced cardiac output and hypotension. It also can cause bradycardia or ventricular dysrhythmias. Cardiac arrest may occur in severe hypocalcemia.*

■ Continuously monitor ECG in patients receiving IV calcium preparations, especially if the patient also is taking digitalis. *Rapid administration of calcium salts can lead to hypercalcemia and cardiac dysrhythmias. Calcium administration increases the risk of digitalis toxicity and resultant dysrhythmias.*

■ If the patient has tetany, provide a quiet environment and institute seizure precautions such as raising the side rails and keeping an airway at bedside. *A quiet environment reduces central nervous system stimuli and the risk of convulsions in the patient with tetany.*

Community-Based Care

In preparing the patient with hypocalcemia for home care, consider the circumstances leading to low serum calcium levels. Discuss risk factors for hypocalcemia specific to the patient, and provide information about managing these risk factors to avoid future episodes of hypocalcemia. Teach about prescribed medications, including calcium supplements. Provide a list of foods high in calcium, as well as sources of vitamin D if recommended. Discuss manifestations to report to the healthcare provider, and stress the importance of follow-up care as scheduled.

The Patient with Hypercalcemia

Hypercalcemia is a serum calcium value greater than 10.0 mg/dL. Excess ionized calcium in ECF can have serious widespread effects.

Pathophysiology

Hypercalcemia usually results from increased resorption of calcium from the bones. The two most common causes of bone resorption are hyperparathyroidism and malignancies. In hyperparathyroidism, excess PTH is produced. This causes calcium to be released from bones, as well as increased calcium absorption in the intestines and retention of calcium by the kidneys. Hypercalcemia is a common complication of malignancies. It may develop as a result of bone destruction by the tumor or due to hormone-like substances produced by the tumor itself. Prolonged immobility and lack of weight bearing also cause increased resorption of bone with calcium release into extracellular fluids. Self-limiting hypercalcemia may follow successful kidney transplant. Levels of parathyroid hormone may be altered in chronic renal failure, leading to increased serum calcium levels.

Increased intestinal absorption of calcium also can lead to hypercalcemia. This may result from excess vitamin D, overuse of calcium-containing antacids, or excessive milk ingestion. Renal failure and some drugs such as thiazide diuretics and lithium can interfere with elimination of calcium by the kidneys, causing high serum calcium levels.

The effects of hypercalcemia largely depend on the degree of serum calcium elevation and the length of time over which it develops. In general, higher serum calcium levels are associated with more serious effects. Calcium has a stabilizing effect on the neuromuscular junction; hypercalcemia decreases neuromuscular excitability, leading to muscle weakness and depressed deep tendon reflexes. Gastrointestinal motility is reduced as well. In the heart, calcium exerts an effect similar to digitalis (∞ see Chapter 30), strengthening contractions and reducing the heart rate. Hypercalcemia affects the conduction system of the heart, leading to bradycardia and heart blocks. The ability of the kidneys to concentrate urine is impaired by hypercalcemia, causing excess sodium and water loss and increased thirst.

Extremely high serum calcium levels affect mental status. This is thought to be due to increased calcium in cerebrospinal fluid. Behavioral effects range from personality changes to confusion, impaired memory, and acute psychoses.

Manifestations and Complications

Manifestations of hypercalcemia relate to its effects on neuromuscular activity, the central nervous system, the cardiovascular system, and the kidneys. Decreased neuromuscular excitability causes muscle weakness and fatigue, as well as GI manifestations such as anorexia, nausea, vomiting, and constipation. Central nervous system (CNS) effects may include confusion, lethargy, behavior or personality changes, and coma. Cardiovascular effects include dysrhythmias, ECG changes, and possible hypertension. Hypercalcemia causes polyuria and, as a result, increased thirst (see Table 10–7).

Complications of hypercalcemia can affect several different organ systems. Peptic ulcer disease may develop due to increased gastric acid secretion. Pancreatitis can occur as a result of calcium deposits in pancreatic ducts. Excess calcium can precipitate out of urine to form kidney stones. Hypercalcemic crisis, an acute increase in the serum calcium level, can lead to cardiac arrest.

Interdisciplinary Care

The management of hypercalcemia focuses on correcting the underlying cause and reducing the serum calcium level. Treatment is particularly important in patients who have one or more of the following: serum calcium levels greater than 12 mg/dL, overt manifestations of hypercalcemia, compromised renal function, and inability to maintain an adequate fluid intake.

Diagnosis

The laboratory and diagnostic tests that may be ordered are as follows:

- *Serum electrolytes* show a total serum calcium greater than 10.0 mg/dL.
- *Serum PTH levels* are measured to identify or rule out hyperparathyroidism as the cause of hypercalcemia.
- *ECG* changes in hypercalcemia include a shortened QT interval, shortened and depressed ST segment, and widened T wave. Bradycardia or heart block may be identified on the ECG.
- *Bone density scans* may be done to monitor bone resorption and the effects of treatment measures on mineralization of bone.

Medications

Measures to promote calcium elimination by the kidneys and reduce calcium resorption from bone are used to treat hypercalcemia. In acute hypercalcemia, IV fluids are given with a loop diuretic such as furosemide [Lasix] to promote elimination of excess calcium. Calcitonin, which promotes the uptake of calcium into bones, also may be used to rapidly lower serum calcium levels.

A number of drugs that inhibit bone resorption are available. The bisphosphonates (pamidronate and etidronate) are commonly used to treat hypercalcemia associated with malignancies. These drugs also are used to prevent and treat osteoporosis. Nursing implications for calcitonin and bisphosphonate drugs are presented in the Medication Administration boxes in ∞ Chapter 40. When a bisphosphonate drug is ineffective to correct hypercalcemia, mithramycin, a chemotherapeutic agent, may be used.

Rapid reversal of hypercalcemia in emergency situations may be accomplished by IV administration of sodium phosphate or potassium phosphate. Calcium binds to phosphate, thus decreasing serum calcium levels. Paradoxically, complications of this therapy can include fatal hypocalcemia resulting from binding of the ionized calcium and soft tissue calcifications.

Other drug therapies include the use of IV plicamycin (Mithramycin) to inhibit bone resorption. Glucocorticoids (cortisone), which compete with vitamin D, and a low-calcium diet may be prescribed to decrease GI absorption of calcium, inhibit bone resorption, and to increase urinary calcium excretion. Also, calcitonin may be prescribed to decrease skeletal mobilization of calcium and phosphorus and to increase renal output of calcium and phosphorus. ∞ See Chapter 19 for more information about and nursing implications of glucocorticoid therapy.

Fluid Management

IV fluids, usually isotonic saline, are administered to patients with severe hypercalcemia to restore vascular volume and promote renal excretion of calcium. Isotonic saline is used because sodium excretion is accompanied by calcium excretion. Careful assessment of cardiovascular and renal function is done prior to fluid therapy; the patient is carefully monitored for evidence of fluid overload during treatment.

ℳ Nursing Care

Health Promotion

Identify and monitor patients at risk for hypercalcemia. Promote mobility in patients when possible. Assist hospitalized patients to ambulate as soon as possible. In the home setting, discuss the benefits of regular weight-bearing activity with patients, families, and caregivers. Encourage a generous fluid intake of up to 3 to 4 quarts per day. Encourage patients at risk to limit their intake of milk and milk products, as well as calcium-containing antacids and supplements. In addition, patients with prolonged immobility or hypercalcemia are encouraged to consume fluids that increase the acidity of urine (which inhibits calcium stone formation), such as cranberry or prune juice.

Assessment

Assessment data related to hypercalcemia include the following:

- *Health history:* Current manifestations, including weakness or fatigue, abdominal discomfort, nausea or vomiting, increased urination and thirst; changes in memory or thinking; duration of manifestations and any risk factors such as excess intake of milk or calcium products, prolonged immobility, malignancy, renal failure, or endocrine disorders; current medications.
- *Physical assessment:* Mental status and level of consciousness; vital signs including apical pulse; bowel sounds; muscle strength of upper and lower extremities; deep tendon reflexes.

> **MEMORY CUE**
> Remember, calcium has a stabilizing or sedative effect on neuromuscular transmission. Therefore,
> Hypocalcemia → Increased neuromuscular excitability, muscle twitching, spasms, and possible tetany
> Hypercalcemia → Decreased neuromuscular excitability, muscle weakness, and fatigue

Nursing Diagnoses and Interventions

Risk for Injury

Patients with hypercalcemia are at risk for injury due to changes in mental status, the effects of hypercalcemia on muscle strength, and loss of calcium from bones.

- Institute safety precautions if confusion or other changes in mental status are noted. *Changes in mental status may impair judgment and the patient's ability to maintain his or her own safety.*

■ Observe for manifestations of digitalis toxicity (if administered), including vision changes, anorexia, and changes in heart rate and rhythm. Monitor serum digitalis levels. *Hypercalcemia increases the risk of digitalis toxicity.*

■ Promote fluid intake to keep the patient well hydrated and maintain dilute urine. Encourage fluids such as prune or cranberry juice to help maintain acidic urine. *Acidic, dilute urine reduces the risk of calcium salts precipitating out to form kidney stones.*

■ If excess bone reabsorption has occurred, use caution when turning, positioning, transferring, or ambulating. *Bones that have lost excess calcium may fracture with minimal stress or trauma (pathologic fractures).*

Risk for Fluid Volume Excess

Large amounts of isotonic IV fluid often are administered to help correct acute hypercalcemia, leading to a risk for hypervolemia. Patients with preexisting cardiac or renal disease are at particular risk. Loop diuretics may be prescribed to help eliminate excess fluid and calcium.

■ Closely monitor intake and output. *A loop diuretic such as furosemide may be necessary if urinary output does not keep up with fluid administration.*

■ Frequently assess vital signs, respiratory status, and heart sounds. *Increasing pulse rate, dyspnea, adventitious lung sounds, and an S_3 on auscultation of the heart may indicate excess fluid volume and potential heart failure.*

■ Place in semi-Fowler's to Fowler's position. *Elevating the head of the bed improves lung expansion and reduces the work of breathing.*

Community-Based Care

Discuss the following topics when preparing the patient for discharge:

■ Avoid excess intake of calcium-rich foods and antacids.

■ Use prescribed drugs to prevent excess calcium resorption. Discuss their dose, use, and desired and possible adverse effects.

■ Increase fluid intake to 3 to 4 quarts per day; increase the intake of acid ash foods (meats, fish, poultry, eggs, cranberries, plums, prunes); increase dietary fiber and fluid intake to prevent constipation.

■ Maintain weight-bearing physical activity to prevent hypercalcemia.

Magnesium Imbalance

Only about 1% of the magnesium in the body is in extracellular fluid; the rest is found within the cells and in bone. The normal serum concentration of magnesium ranges from 1.6 to 2.6 mg/dL (1.3 to 2.1 mEq/L).

Magnesium is obtained through the diet (it is plentiful in green vegetables, grains, nuts, meats, and seafood) and excreted by the kidneys. Magnesium is vital to many intracellular processes, including enzyme reactions and synthesis of proteins and nucleic acids. Magnesium exerts a sedative effect on the neuromuscular junction, decreasing acetylcholine release. It is an essential ion for neuromuscular transmission and cardiovascular function. The physiologic effects of magnesium are affected by both potassium and calcium levels.

The Patient with Hypomagnesemia

Hypomagnesemia is a magnesium level of less than 1.6 mg/dL. It is a common problem in critically ill patients. Hypomagnesemia may be caused by deficient magnesium intake, excessive losses, or a shift between the intracellular and extracellular compartments.

Risk Factors

Loss of GI fluids, particularly from diarrhea, an ileostomy, or intestinal fistula is a major risk factor for hypomagnesemia. Disruption of nutrient absorption in the small intestine also increases the risk. Multiple factors associated with alcoholism contribute to hypomagnesemia: deficient nutrient intake, increased GI losses, impaired absorption, and increased renal excretion. Other risk factors for hypomagnesemia include protein-calorie malnutrition or starvation; diabetic ketoacidosis; kidney disease; drugs such as loop or thiazide diuretics, aminoglycoside antibiotics, amphotericin B, and cyclosporine; and rapid administration of citrated blood.

Pathophysiology

Magnesium deficiency usually occurs along with low serum potassium and calcium levels. The effects of hypomagnesemia relate not only to the magnesium deficiency but also to hypokalemia and hypocalcemia.

Hypomagnesemia causes increased neuromuscular excitability, with muscle weakness and tremors. The accompanying hypocalcemia contributes to this effect. In the central nervous system, this increased neural excitability can lead to seizures and changes in mental status. Deficient intracellular magnesium in the myocardium increases the risk of cardiac dysrhythmias and sudden death. Hypokalemia increases this risk. Hypomagnesemia also increases the risk of digitalis toxicity. Chronic hypomagnesemia may contribute to hypertension, probably due to increased vasoconstriction. Severe hypomagnesia is strongly linked to low serum calcium levels because both are associated with renal and GI losses.

Manifestations and Complications

Neuromuscular manifestations of hypomagnesemia include tremors, hyperreactive reflexes, positive Chvostek's and Trousseau's signs (see Figure 10–12), tetany, paresthesias, and seizures. CNS effects include confusion, mood changes (apathy, depression, agitation), hallucinations, and possible psychoses. An increased heart rate and ventricular dysrhythmias are common, especially when hypokalemia is present or the patient is taking digitalis. Cardiac arrest and sudden death may occur. Table 10–8 summarizes manifestations of magnesium imbalances.

TABLE 10–8 Manifestations of Magnesium Disorders	
HYPOMAGNESEMIA	**HYPERMAGNESEMIA**
■ Serum magnesium level < 1.6 mg/dL	■ Serum magnesium level > 2.6 mg/dL
■ Changes in personality	■ Confusion and lethargy
■ Nystagmus (lateral twitching of eyeballs)	■ Hypotension
■ Positive Babinski, Chvostek, and Trousseau signs	■ Cardiac dysrhythmias
■ Hypertension	■ Coma
■ Tachycardia	■ Cardiac arrest
■ Cardiac dysrhythmias	

Interdisciplinary Care

Hypomagnesemia is diagnosed by measuring serum electrolyte levels. The ECG shows a prolonged PR interval, widened QRS complex, and depression of the ST segment with T-wave inversion. Treatment is directed toward prevention and identification of an existing deficiency. Magnesium is added to IV total parenteral nutrition solutions to prevent hypomagnesemia.

In patients able to eat, a mild deficiency may be corrected by increasing the intake of foods rich in magnesium (such as green leafy vegetables, seafood, milk, bananas, citrus fruits, and chocolate), or with oral magnesium supplements. Oral magnesium supplements may cause diarrhea, however, limiting their use.

Patients with manifestations of hypomagnesemia are treated with parenteral magnesium sulfate. Treatment is continued for several days to restore intracellular magnesium levels. Magnesium may be given IV or by deep IM injection. Renal function is evaluated prior to administration, and serum magnesium levels are monitored during treatment. The IV route is used for severe magnesium deficiency or if neurologic changes or cardiac dysrhythmias are present. See the Medication Administration box below for the nursing implications of parenteral magnesium sulfate.

∾ Nursing Care

Health Promotion

Discuss the importance of maintaining adequate magnesium intake through a well-balanced diet, particularly with patients at risk (people with alcoholism, malabsorption, or bowel surgery). Many hospitalized patients are at risk for hypomagnesemia due to protein-calorie malnutrition and other disorders.

Monitor serum magnesium levels, reporting changes to the healthcare provider.

Assessment

In addition to asking questions related to risk factors for hypomagnesemia, assess for manifestations of hypokalemia and hypocalcemia. Monitor diagnostic studies such as serum electrolytes, serum albumin levels, and the ECG.

Nursing Diagnoses and Interventions

Nursing care for patients with hypomagnesemia focuses on careful monitoring of manifestations and responses to treatment, promoting safety, patient and family teaching, and administering prescribed medications.

Risk for Injury

■ Monitor serum electrolytes, including magnesium, potassium, and calcium. *Magnesium deficiency often is accompanied by deficiencies of potassium and calcium.*

■ Monitor GI function, including bowel sounds and abdominal distention. *Hypomagnesemia reduces GI motility.*

■ Initiate cardiac monitoring, reporting and treating (as prescribed) ECG changes and dysrhythmias. In patients receiving digitalis, monitor for digitalis toxicity. *Low magnesium levels can precipitate ventricular dysrhythmias, including lethal dysrhythmias such as ventricular fibrillation.*

■ Assess deep tendon reflexes frequently during IV magnesium infusions and prior to each IM dose. *Depressed tendon reflexes indicate a high serum magnesium level.*

■ Maintain a quiet, darkened environment. Institute seizure precautions. *Increased neuromuscular and CNS irritability can lead to seizures. A quiet, dark environment reduces stimuli.*

Community-Based Care

Prior to discharge, instruct the patient to increase dietary intake of foods high in magnesium and provide information about magnesium supplements. In addition, if alcohol abuse has precipitated a magnesium deficit, discuss alcohol treatment options, including support groups such as Alcoholics Anonymous, Al-Anon, and/or Alateen.

The Patient with Hypermagnesemia

Hypermagnesemia is a serum magnesium level greater than 2.6 mg/dL. It is much less common than hypomagnesemia. Hypermagnesemia can develop in renal failure, particularly if

---

MEDICATION ADMINISTRATION Magnesium Sulfate

Magnesium sulfate is used to prevent or treat hypomagnesemia. It may be given IV or by IM injection.

Nursing Responsibilities
■ Assess serum magnesium levels and renal function tests (BUN and serum creatinine) prior to administering. Notify the care provider if magnesium levels are above normal limits or renal function is impaired.
■ Frequently monitor neurologic status and deep tendon reflexes during therapy. Withhold magnesium and notify the care provider if deep tendon reflexes are hypoactive or absent.

■ Monitor intake and output.
■ Administer IM doses deep into the ventral or dorsal gluteal sites.
■ IV magnesium sulfate may be given by direct IV push or by continuous infusion.

Health Education for the Patient and Family
Explain purpose and duration of treatment. Discuss reason for frequent neurologic and reflex assessments.

magnesium is administered parenterally or orally (e.g., magnesium-containing antacids or laxatives). Older adults are at risk for hypermagnesemia as renal function declines with aging and they may be more likely to use over-the-counter laxatives and other preparations that contain magnesium.

Pathophysiology and Manifestations

Elevated serum magnesium levels interfere with neuromuscular transmission and depress the central nervous system. Hypermagnesemia also affects the cardiovascular system, potentially causing hypotension, flushing, sweating, and bradydysrhythmias.

Predictable manifestations occur with increasing serum magnesium levels. With lower levels, nausea and vomiting, hypotension, facial flushing, sweating, and a feeling of warmth occur. As levels increase, manifestations of CNS depression appear (weakness, lethargy, drowsiness, weak or absent deep tendon reflexes). Marked elevations cause respiratory depression, coma, and compromised cardiac function (ECG changes, bradycardia, heart block, and cardiac arrest).

Interdisciplinary Care

The management of hypermagnesemia focuses on identifying and treating the underlying cause. All medications or compounds containing magnesium (such as antacids, IV solutions, or enemas) are withheld. In the patient with renal failure, hemodialysis or peritoneal dialysis is instituted to remove the excess magnesium.

Calcium gluconate is administered IV to reverse the neuromuscular and cardiac effects of hypermagnesemia. The patient may require mechanical ventilation to support respiratory function, and a pacemaker to maintain adequate cardiac output.

∾ Nursing Care

Nursing care includes instituting measures to prevent and identify hypermagnesemia in patients at risk, monitoring for critical effects of hypermagnesemia, and providing measures to ensure the patient's safety. Consider the following nursing diagnoses for the patient with hypermagnesemia:

- *Decreased Cardiac Output* related to altered myocardial conduction
- *Ineffective Breathing Pattern* related to respiratory depression
- *Risk for Injury* related to muscle weakness and altered level of consciousness
- *Risk for Ineffective Health Maintenance* related to lack of knowledge about use of magnesium-containing supplements, antacids, laxatives, and enemas.

Phosphate Imbalance

Although most phosphate (85%) is found in bones, it is the primary intracellular anion. About 14% is in intracellular fluid, and the remainder (1%) is in extracellular fluid. The normal serum phosphate (or phosphorus) level in adults is 2.5 to 4.5 mg/dL. Phosphorus levels vary with age, gender, and diet.

Overview of Normal Phosphate Balance

Phosphate is essential to intracellular processes such as the production of ATP, the fuel that supports muscle contraction, nerve cell transmission, and electrolyte transport. Phosphate is vital for red blood cell function and oxygen delivery to tissues; nervous system and muscle function; and the metabolism of fats, carbohydrates, and protein. It also assists in maintaining acid–base balance.

Phosphorus is ingested in the diet, absorbed in the jejunum, and primarily excreted by the kidneys. When phosphate intake is low, the kidneys conserve phosphorus, excreting less. An inverse relationship exists between phosphate and calcium levels: When one increases, the other decreases. Regulatory mechanisms for calcium levels (parathyroid hormone, calcitonin, and vitamin D) also influence phosphate levels. The manifestations of phosphate imbalances are summarized in Table 10–9.

The Patient with Hypophosphatemia

Hypophosphatemia is a serum phosphorus of less than 2.5 mg/dL. Low serum phosphate levels may indicate a total body deficit of phosphate or a shift of phosphate into the intracellular space, the most common cause of hypophosphatemia. Decreased GI absorption of phosphate or increased renal excretion of phosphate also can cause low phosphate levels. Hypophosphatemia often is iatrogenic (related to treatment). Selected causes of hypophosphatemia include the following:

- Refeeding syndrome can develop when malnourished patients are started on enteral or total parenteral nutrition. Glucose in the formula or solution stimulates insulin release, which promotes the entry of glucose and phosphate into the cells, depleting extracellular phosphate levels.
- Medications frequently contribute to hypophosphatemia, including IV glucose solutions, antacids (aluminum- or magnesium-based antacids bind with phosphate), anabolic steroids, and diuretics.
- Alcoholism affects both the intake and absorption of phosphate.
- Hyperventilation and respiratory alkalosis cause phosphate to shift out of extracellular fluids into the intracellular space.
- Other causes include diabetic ketoacidosis with excess phosphate loss in the urine, stress responses, and extensive burns.

TABLE 10–9 Manifestations of Phosphate Imbalances

HYPOPHOSPHATEMIA	HYPERPHOSPHATEMIA
■ Serum phosphate level < 2.5 mg/dL	■ Serum phosphate level > 4.5 mg/dL
■ Intention tremor, paresthesias	■ Paresthesias
■ Confusion, stuporous	■ Muscle weakness
■ Bone pain	■ Nausea and vomiting
■ Joint stiffness	■ Dysphagia
■ Bleeding disorders (platelet dysfunction)	■ Tetany
■ Impaired white blood cell function	■ Decreased blood pressure
■ Seizures	■ Cardiac dysrhythmias

Pathophysiology and Manifestations

Most effects of hypophosphatemia result from depletion of ATP and impaired oxygen delivery to the cells due to a deficiency of the red blood cell enzyme 2,3-DPG. Severe hypophosphatemia affects virtually every major organ system:

- *Central nervous system:* Reduced oxygen and ATP synthesis in the brain causes neurologic manifestations such as irritability, apprehension, weakness, paresthesias, lack of coordination, confusion, seizures, and coma.
- *Hematologic:* Oxygen delivery to the cells is reduced. Hemolytic anemia (excessive RBC destruction) may develop due to lack of ATP in red blood cells.
- *Musculoskeletal:* Decreased ATP causes muscle weakness and release of creatinine phosphokinase (CPK, a muscle enzyme); acute rhabdomyolysis (muscle cell breakdown) can develop. Muscle cell destruction, in turn, can lead to acute renal failure as myoglobin, a muscle cell protein, exerts a toxic effect on the kidney tubule.
- *Cardiovascular:* Hypophosphatemia decreases myocardial contractility; decreased oxygenation of the heart muscle can cause chest pain and dysrhythmias.
- *Gastrointestinal:* Anorexia can occur, as well as dysphagia (difficulty swallowing), nausea and vomiting, decreased bowel sounds, and possible ileus due to reduced GI motility.

Interdisciplinary Care

Treatment for hypophosphatemia is directed at prevention, treating the underlying cause of the disorder, and replacing phosphate. An improved diet and oral phosphate supplement (such as Neutra-Phos or Neutra-Phos K capsules) may restore normal phosphate levels in patients with a mild to moderate deficiency. IV phosphate (sodium phosphate or potassium phosphate) is given when serum phosphate levels are less than 1 mg/dL.

∽ Nursing Care

Nurses can be instrumental in identifying patients at risk for phosphate deficiency and preventing it from developing. Nurses should closely monitor serum electrolyte values in patients at risk, including those who are malnourished, receiving IV glucose solutions or total parenteral nutrition, or being treated with diuretic therapy or antacids that bind with phosphate. Nursing diagnoses that may be appropriate for the patient with hypophosphatemia include the following:

- *Impaired Physical Mobility* related to muscle weakness and poor coordination
- *Decreased Cardiac Output* related to reduced myocardial contractility
- *Risk for Injury* related to muscle weakness and altered mental status

Community-Based Care

In preparing for discharge, teach the patient and family about the causes and manifestations of hypophosphatemia. Discuss the importance of avoiding phosphorus-binding antacids, unless prescribed. Stress a well-balanced diet to maintain an adequate intake of phosphate.

The Patient with Hyperphosphatemia

Hyperphosphatemia is a serum phosphate level greater than 4.5 mg/dL. As with other electrolyte imbalances, it may be the result of impaired phosphate excretion, excess intake, or a shift of phosphate from the intracellular space into extracellular fluids.

- Acute or chronic renal failure is the primary cause of impaired phosphate excretion.
- Rapid administration of phosphate-containing solutions, including phosphate enemas, can increase serum phosphate levels. In addition, excess vitamin D increases phosphate absorption and can lead to hyperphosphatemia in patients with impaired renal function.
- A shift of phosphate from the intracellular to extracellular space can occur during chemotherapy, from sepsis or hypothermia, or because of extensive trauma or heat stroke.
- Because phosphate levels are affected by serum calcium concentrations, disruption of the mechanisms that regulate calcium levels (e.g., hypoparathyroidism, hyperthyroidism, or vitamin D intoxication) can lead to hyperphosphatemia.

Pathophysiology and Manifestations

Excessive serum phosphate levels cause few specific manifestations. The effects of high serum phosphate levels on nerves and muscles (muscle cramps and pain, paresthesias, tingling around the mouth, muscle spasms, tetany) are more the result of hypocalcemia that develops secondary to an elevated serum phosphorus level. The phosphate in the serum combines with ionized calcium, and the ionized serum calcium level falls.

Interdisciplinary Care

Treatment of the underlying disorder often corrects hyperphosphatemia. When this is not feasible, phosphate-containing drugs are eliminated and intake of phosphate-rich foods such as organ meats and milk and milk products is restricted. Agents that bind with phosphate in the GI tract (such as calcium-containing antacids) may be prescribed. If renal function is adequate, IV normal saline may be given to promote renal excretion of phosphate. Dialysis may be necessary to reduce phosphate levels in patients with renal failure.

∽ Nursing Care

When providing nursing care for the patient with hyperphosphatemia, monitor the laboratory data for an excess of phosphorus and a deficit of calcium, as well as the manifestations of hypocalcemia.

Community-Based Care

Discuss the risk of hyperphosphatemia related to using phosphate preparations as laxatives or enemas, particularly with patients who have other risk factors for the disorder. When preparing the patient for discharge, teach about the use of phosphate-binding preparations as ordered and dietary phosphate restrictions.

Acid–Base Disorders

Homeostasis and optimal cellular function require maintenance of the hydrogen ion (H^+) concentration of body fluids within a relatively narrow range. Hydrogen ions determine the relative acidity of body fluids. Acids release hydrogen ions in solution; bases (or **alkalis**) accept hydrogen ions in solution. The hydrogen ion concentration of a solution is measured as its pH. The relationship between hydrogen ion concentration and pH is inverse; that is, as hydrogen ion concentration increases, the pH falls, and the solution becomes more acidic. As hydrogen ion concentration falls, the pH rises, and the solution becomes more alkaline or basic. The pH of body fluids is slightly basic, with the normal pH ranging from 7.35 to 7.45 (a pH of 7 is neutral).

Regulation of Acid–Base Balance

A number of mechanisms work together to maintain the pH of the body within normal range. Metabolic processes in the body continuously produce acids, which fall into two categories: volatile acids and nonvolatile acids. Volatile acids can be eliminated from the body as a gas. Carbonic acid (H_2CO_3) is the only volatile acid produced in the body. It dissociates into carbon dioxide (CO_2) and water (H_2O); the carbon dioxide is then eliminated from the body through the lungs. All other acids produced in the body are nonvolatile acids that must be metabolized or excreted from the body in fluid. Lactic acid, hydrochloric acid, phosphoric acid, and sulfuric acid are examples of nonvolatile acids. Most acids and bases in the body are weak; that is, they neither release nor accept a significant amount of hydrogen ion.

Three systems work together in the body to maintain the pH despite continuous acid production: buffers, the respiratory system, and the renal system.

Buffer Systems

Buffers are substances that prevent major changes in pH by removing or releasing hydrogen ions. When excess acid is present in body fluid, buffers bind with hydrogen ions to minimize the change in pH. If body fluids become too basic or alkaline, buffers release hydrogen ions, restoring the pH. Although buffers act within a fraction of a second, their capacity to maintain pH is limited. The major buffer systems of the body are the bicarbonate-carbonic acid buffer system, phosphate buffer system, and protein buffers.

The bicarbonate-carbonic acid buffer system can be illustrated by the following equation:

$$CO_2 + H_2O \rightleftarrows H_2CO_3 \rightleftarrows H^+ + HCO_3^-$$

Bicarbonate (HCO_3^-) is a weak base; when an acid is added to the system, the hydrogen ion in the acid combines with bicarbonate, and the pH changes only slightly. Carbonic acid (H_2CO_3) is a weak acid produced when carbon dioxide dissolves in water. If a base is added to the system, it combines with carbonic acid, and the pH remains within the normal range. Although the amounts of bicarbonate and carbonic acid in the body vary to a certain extent, as long as a ratio of 20 parts

bicarbonate (HCO_3^-) to 1 part carbonic acid (H_2CO_3) is maintained, the pH remains within the 7.35 to 7.45 range (Figure 10–13 ■).

The normal serum bicarbonate level is 24 mEq/L, and that of carbonic acid is 1.2 mEq/L. Thus, the ratio of bicarbonate to carbonic acid is 20:1. It is this ratio that maintains the pH within the normal range. Adding a strong acid to extracellular fluid depletes bicarbonate, changing the 20:1 ratio and causing the pH to drop below 7.35. This is known as **acidosis**. Addition of a strong base depletes carbonic acid as it combines with the base. The 20:1 ratio again is disrupted and the pH rises above 7.45, a condition known as **alkalosis**.

Intracellular and plasma proteins also serve as buffers. Plasma proteins contribute to buffering of extracellular fluids. Proteins in intracellular fluid provide extensive buffering for organic acids produced by cellular metabolism. In red blood cells, hemoglobin acts as a buffer for hydrogen ion when carbonic acid dissociates. Inorganic phosphates also serve as extracellular buffers, although their roles are not as important as the bicarbonate-carbonic acid buffer system. Phosphates are, however, important intracellular buffers, helping to maintain a stable pH within the cells.

Respiratory System

The respiratory system (and the cerebral respiratory center) regulates carbonic acid in the body by eliminating or retaining carbon dioxide. Carbon dioxide is a potential acid; when combined with water, it forms carbonic acid (see the previous equation), a volatile acid. Acute increases in either carbon dioxide or hydrogen ions in the blood stimulate the respiratory center in the brain. As a result, both the rate and depth of respiration increase. The increased rate and depth of lung ventilation eliminate carbon dioxide from the body, and carbonic acid levels fall, bringing the pH to a more normal range. Although this compensation for increased hydrogen ion concentration occurs

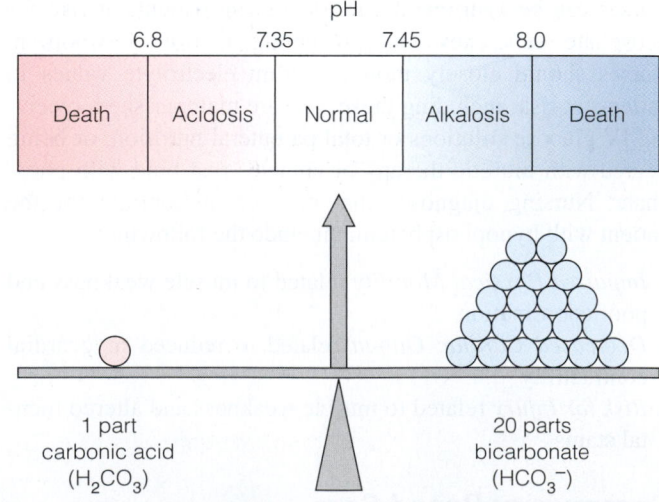

Figure 10–13 ■ The normal ratio of bicarbonate to carbonic acid is 20:1. As long as this ratio is maintained, the pH remains within the normal range of 7.35 to 7.45.

within minutes, it becomes less effective over time. Patients with chronic lung disease may have consistently high carbon dioxide levels in their blood.

Alkalosis, by contrast, depresses the respiratory center. Both the rate and depth of respiration decrease, and carbon dioxide is retained. The retained carbon dioxide then combines with water to restore carbonic acid levels and bring the pH back within the normal range.

Renal System

The renal system is responsible for the long-term regulation of acid–base balance in the body. Excess nonvolatile acids produced during metabolism normally are eliminated by the kidneys. The kidneys also regulate bicarbonate levels in extracellular fluid by regenerating bicarbonate ions as well as reabsorbing them in the renal tubules. Although the kidneys respond more slowly to changes in pH (over hours to days), they can generate bicarbonate and selectively excrete or retain hydrogen ions as needed. In acidosis, when excess hydrogen ion is present and the pH falls, the kidneys excrete hydrogen ions and retain bicarbonate. In alkalosis, the kidneys retain hydrogen ions and excrete bicarbonate to restore acid–base balance.

Assessing Acid–Base Balance

Acid–base balance is evaluated primarily by measuring arterial blood gases. Arterial blood is used because it reflects acid–base balance throughout the entire body better than venous blood. Arterial blood also provides information about the effectiveness of the lungs in oxygenating blood. The elements measured are pH, the $PaCO_2$, the PaO_2, and bicarbonate level.

The abbreviations $PaCO_2$ and PaO_2 are used interchangeably with PCO_2 and PO_2. The P stands for partial pressure, the pressure exerted by the gas dissolved in the blood. The *a* indicates that the sample is arterial blood. Because these measurements rarely are done on venous blood, the *a* often is deleted from the abbreviation.

The $PaCO_2$ measures the pressure exerted by dissolved carbon dioxide in the blood. It reflects the respiratory component of acid–base regulation and balance, and is regulated by the lungs. The normal value is 35–45 mmHg. A $PaCO_2$ of less than

35 mmHg is known as *hypocapnia*; a $PaCO_2$ greater than 45 mmHg is *hypercapnia*.

The PaO_2 is a measure of the pressure exerted by oxygen that is dissolved in the plasma. Only about 3% of oxygen in the blood is transported in solution; most is combined with hemoglobin. However, it is the dissolved oxygen that is available to the cells for metabolism. As dissolved oxygen diffuses out of plasma into the tissues, more is released from hemoglobin. The normal value for PaO_2 is 80 to 100 mmHg. A PaO_2 of less than 80 mmHg is indicative of hypoxemia. The PaO_2 is valuable for evaluating respiratory function, but is not used as a primary measurement in determining acid–base status.

The **serum bicarbonate** (HCO_3^-) reflects the renal regulation of acid–base balance. It is often called the metabolic component of arterial blood gases. The normal HCO_3^- value is 22 to 26 mEq/L.

The **base excess (BE)** is a calculated value also known as *buffer base capacity*. The base excess measures substances that can accept or combine with hydrogen ion. It reflects the degree of acid–base imbalance by indicating the status of the body's total buffering capacity. It represents the amount of acid or base that must be added to a blood sample to achieve a pH of 7.4. This is essentially a measure of increased or decreased bicarbonate. The normal value for base excess for arterial blood is –3.0 to +3.0. Normal ABG values are summarized in Table 10–10.

ABGs are analyzed to identify acid–base disorders and their probable cause, to determine the extent of the imbalance, and to monitor treatment. When analyzing ABG results, it is important to use a systematic approach. First evaluate each individual measurement, then look at the interrelationships to determine the patient's acid–base status (see Box 10–3).

Acid–Base Imbalance

Acid–base imbalances fall into two major categories: acidosis and alkalosis. Acidosis occurs when the hydrogen ion concentration increases above normal (pH below 7.35). Alkalosis occurs when the hydrogen ion concentration falls below normal (pH above 7.45).

Acid–base imbalances are further classified as metabolic or respiratory disorders. In metabolic disorders, the primary

TABLE 10–10 Normal Arterial Blood Gas Values

VALUE	NORMAL RANGE	SIGNIFICANCE
pH	7.35 to 7.45	Reflects hydrogen ion (H$^+$) concentration ■ < 7.35 = acidosis ■ > 7.45 = alkalosis
$PaCO_2$	35 to 45 mmHg	Partial pressure of carbon dioxide (CO_2) in arterial blood ■ < 35 mmHg = hypocapnia ■ > 45 mmHg = hypercapnia
PaO_2	80 to 100 mmHg	Partial pressure of oxygen (O_2) in arterial blood ■ < 80 mmHg = hypoxemia
HCO_3^-	22 to 26 mEq/L	Bicarbonate concentration in plasma
BE	–3 to +3	Base excess; a measure of buffering capacity

BOX 10–3 Interpreting Arterial Blood Gases

1. Look at the pH.
   - pH < 7.35 = acidosis
   - pH > 7.45 = alkalosis
2. Look at the $PaCO_2$.
   - $PaCO_2$ < 35 mmHg = hypocapnia; more carbon dioxide is being exhaled than normal
   - $PaCO_2$ > 45 mmHg = hypercapnia; carbon dioxide is being retained
3. Evaluate the pH–$PaCO_2$ relationship for a possible respiratory problem.
   - If the pH is < 7.35 (acidosis) and the $PaCO_2$ is > 45 mmHg (hypercapnia), retained carbon dioxide is causing increased H^+ concentration and *respiratory acidosis*.
   - If the pH is > 7.45 (alkalosis) and the $PaCO_2$ is < 35 mmHg (hypocapnia), low carbon dioxide levels and decreased H^+ concentration are causing *respiratory alkalosis*.
4. Look at the bicarbonate.
   - If the HCO_3^- is < 22 mEq/L, bicarbonate levels are lower than normal.
   - If the HCO_3^- is > 26 mEq/L, bicarbonate levels are higher than normal.
5. Evaluate the pH, HCO_3^-, and BE for a possible metabolic problem.
   - If the pH is < 7.35 (acidosis), the HCO_3^- is < 22 mEq/L, and the BE is < –3 mEq/L, then low bicarbonate levels and high H^+ concentrations are causing *metabolic acidosis*.
   - If the pH is > 7.45 (alkalosis), the HCO_3^- is > 26 mEq/L, and the BE is > +3 mEq/L, then high bicarbonate levels are causing *metabolic alkalosis*.
6. Look for compensation.
   - *Renal compensation:*
     - In respiratory acidosis (pH < 7.35, $PaCO_2$ > 45 mmHg), the kidneys retain HCO_3^- to buffer the excess acid, so the HCO_3^- is > 26 mEq/L.
     - In respiratory alkalosis (pH > 7.45, $PaCO_2$ < 35 mmHg), the kidneys excrete HO_3^- to minimize the alkalosis, so the HCO_3^- is < 22 mEq/L.
   - *Respiratory compensation*
     - In metabolic acidosis (pH < 7.35, HCO_3^- < 22 mEq/L), the rate and depth of respirations increase, increasing carbon dioxide elimination, so the $PaCO_2$ is < 35 mmHg.
     - In metabolic alkalosis (pH > 7.45, HCO_3^- > 26 mEq/L), respirations slow, carbon dioxide is retained, so the $PaCO_2$ is > 45 mmHg.
7. Evaluate oxygenation.
   - PaO_2 < 80 mmHg = hypoxemia; possible hypoventilation
   - PaO_2 > 100 mmHg = hyperventilation

change is in the concentration of bicarbonate. In metabolic acidosis, the amount of bicarbonate is decreased in relation to the amount of acid in the body (Figure 10–14A ■). It can develop as a result of abnormal bicarbonate losses or because of excess nonvolatile acids in the body. The pH falls below 7.35 and the bicarbonate concentration is less than 22 mEq/L. Metabolic alkalosis, by contrast, occurs when there is an excess of bicarbonate in relation to the amount of hydrogen ion (Figure 10–14B). The pH is above 7.45 and the bicarbonate concentration is greater than 26 mEq/L.

In respiratory disorders, the primary change is in the concentration of carbonic acid. Respiratory acidosis occurs when carbon dioxide is retained, increasing the amount of carbonic acid in the body (Figure 10–15A ■). As a result, the pH falls to less than 7.35, and the $PaCO_2$ is greater than 45 mmHg. When too much carbon dioxide is "blown off," carbonic acid levels fall and respiratory alkalosis develops (Figure 10–15B). The pH rises to above 7.45 and the $PaCO_2$ is less than 35 mmHg.

Acid–base disorders are further defined as *primary* (simple) and *mixed*. Primary disorders usually are due to one cause. For example, respiratory failure often causes respiratory acidosis due to retained carbon dioxide; renal failure usually causes metabolic acidosis due to retained hydrogen ion

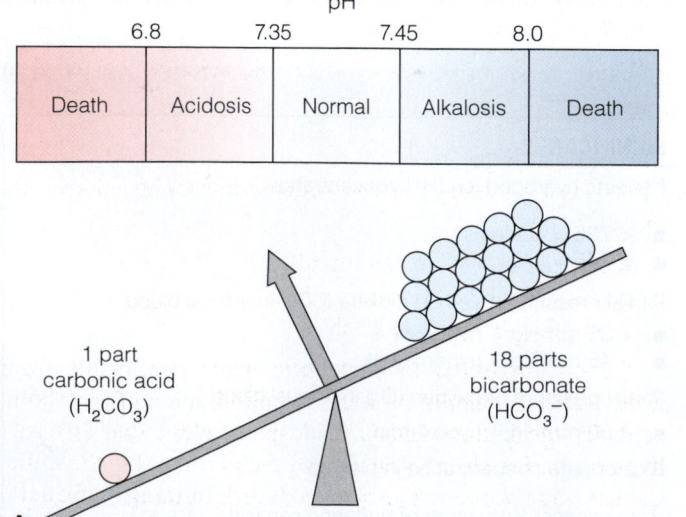

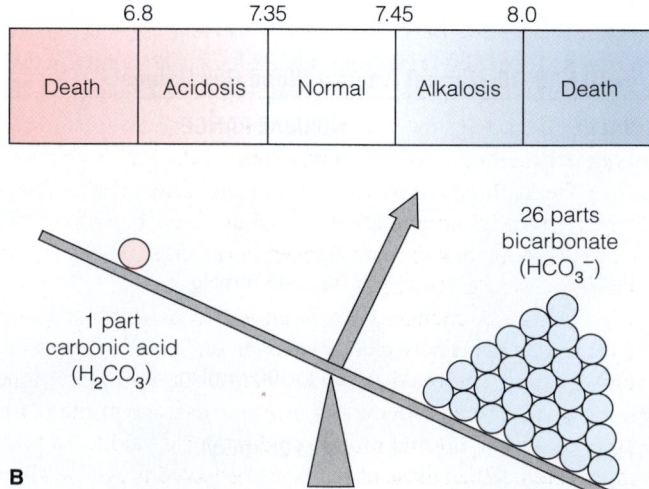

Figure 10–14 ■ Metabolic acid–base imbalances. *A,* Metabolic acidosis. *B,* Metabolic alkalosis.

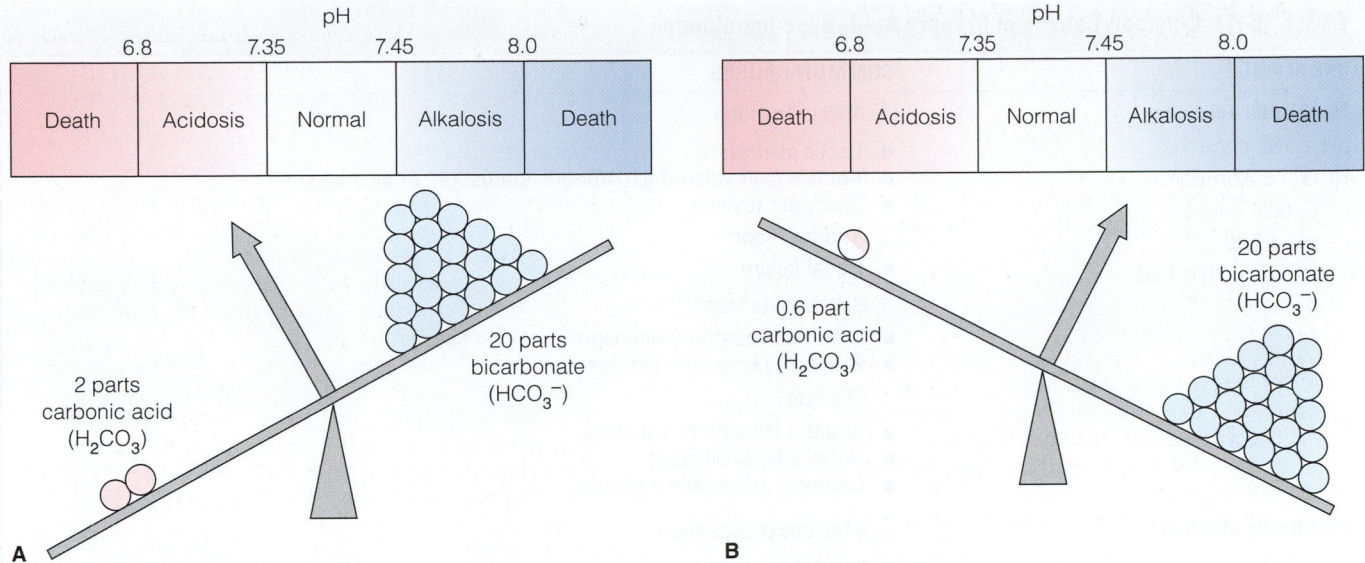

Figure 10–15 ■ Respiratory acid–base imbalances. *A,* Respiratory acidosis. *B,* Respiratory alkalosis.

and impaired bicarbonate production. Table 10–11 summarizes primary acid–base imbalances with common causes of each. Mixed disorders occur from combinations of respiratory and metabolic disturbances. For example, a patient in cardiac arrest develops a mixed respiratory and metabolic acidosis due to lack of ventilation (and retained CO_2) and hypoxia of body tissues that leads to anaerobic metabolism and acid by-products (excess nonvolatile acids).

FAST FACTS
- Simple acid–base imbalances are more commonly seen than mixed imbalances. Common causes of simple acid–base imbalances include the following:
  - Diabetic ketoacidosis (metabolic acidosis)
  - Chronic obstructive lung disease (respiratory acidosis)
  - Anxiety-related (psychogenic) hyperventilation (respiratory alkalosis)
- Critically ill patients are at higher risk for mixed acid–base imbalances.

Compensation

With primary acid–base disorders, compensatory changes in the other part of the regulatory system occur to restore a normal pH and homeostasis. In metabolic acid–base disorders, the change in pH affects the rate and depth of respirations. This, in turn, affects carbon dioxide elimination and the $PaCO_2$, helping restore the carbonic acid to bicarbonate ratio. The kidneys compensate for simple respiratory imbalances. The change in pH affects both bicarbonate conservation and hydrogen ion elimination (Table 10–12).

Compensatory changes in respirations occur within minutes of a change in pH. These changes, however, become less effective over time. The renal response takes longer to restore the pH, but is a more effective long-term mechanism. If the pH is restored to within normal limits, the disorder is said to be fully compensated. When these changes are reflected in ABG values but the pH remains outside normal limits, the disorder is said to be partially compensated.

The Patient with Metabolic Acidosis

Metabolic acidosis (bicarbonate deficit) is characterized by a low pH (< 7.35) and a low bicarbonate (< 22 mEq/L). It may be caused by excess acid in the body or loss of bicarbonate from the body. When metabolic acidosis develops, the respiratory system attempts to return the pH to normal by increasing the rate and depth of respirations. Carbon dioxide elimination increases, and the $PaCO_2$ falls (< 35 mmHg).

Risk Factors

Metabolic acidosis rarely is a primary disorder; it usually develops during the course of another disease:

- Acute lactic acidosis usually results from tissue hypoxia due to shock or cardiac arrest.
- Patients with type 1 diabetes mellitus are at risk for developing diabetic ketoacidosis. (∞ See Chapter 20 for more information about diabetes and its complications.)
- Acute or chronic renal failure impairs the excretion of metabolic acids.
- Diarrhea, intestinal suction, or abdominal fistulas increase the risk for excess bicarbonate loss.

Other common causes of metabolic acidosis are listed in Table 10–11.

Pathophysiology

Three basic mechanisms that can cause metabolic acidosis are the following:

- Accumulation of metabolic acids
- Excess loss of bicarbonate
- An increase in chloride levels

An accumulation of metabolic acids can result from excess acid production or impaired elimination of metabolic acids by the kidney. Lactic acidosis develops due to tissue hypoxia and a shift to anaerobic metabolism by the cells. Lactate and hydrogen ions are produced, forming lactic acid. Both oxygen and glucose are necessary for normal cell metabolism. When intracellular glucose is inadequate due to

TABLE 10–11 Common Causes of Primary Acid–Base Imbalances

IMBALANCE	COMMON CAUSES

Metabolic acidosis
 	
pH < 7.35
HCO_3^- < 22 mEq/L
   Critical values
   pH < 7.20
   HCO_3^- < 10 mEq/L
	↑ Acid production
	■ Lactic acidosis
	■ Ketoacidosis related to diabetes, starvation, or alcoholism
	■ Salicylate toxicity
	↓ Acid excretion
	■ Renal failure
	
	↑ Bicarbonate loss
	■ Diarrhea, ileostomy drainage, intestinal fistula
	■ Biliary or pancreatic fistulas
	↑ Chloride
	■ Sodium chloride IV solutions
	■ Renal tubular acidosis
	■ Carbonic anhydrase inhibitors

Metabolic alkalosis
 	
pH > 7.45
HCO_3^- > 26 mEq/L
   Critical values
   pH > 7.60
   HCO_3^- > 40 mEq/L
	↑ Acid loss or excretion
	■ Vomiting, gastric suction
	■ Hypokalemia
	↑ Bicarbonate
	■ Alkali ingestion (bicarbonate of soda)
	■ Excess bicarbonate administration

Respiratory acidosis
 	
pH < 7.35
$PaCO_2$ >45 mm Hg
   Critical values
   pH < 7.2
   $PaCO_2$ > 77 mmHg
	Acute respiratory acidosis
	■ Acute respiratory conditions (pulmonary edema, pneumonia, acute asthma)
	■ Opiate overdose
	■ Foreign body aspiration
	■ Chest trauma
	Chronic respiratory acidosis
	■ Chronic respiratory conditions (COPD, cystic fibrosis)
	■ Multiple sclerosis, other neuromuscular diseases
	■ Stroke

Respiratory alkalosis
 	
pH > 7.45
$PaCO_2$ < 35 mm Hg
 	
   Critical values
   pH > 7.60
   $PaCO_2$ < 20 mmHg
	■ Anxiety-induced hyperventilation (e.g., anxiety)
	■ Fever
	■ Early salicylate intoxication
	■ Hyperventilation with mechanical ventilator

starvation or a lack of insulin to move it into cells, the body breaks down fatty tissue to meet its metabolic needs. In this process, fatty acids are released, which are converted to ketones; ketoacidosis develops. Substances such as aspirin, methanol (wood alcohol), and ethylene (contained in antifreeze and solvents) cause a toxic increase in body acids by either breaking down into acid products (salicylic acid) or stimulating metabolic acid production (Porth & Matfin, 2009). Renal failure impairs the body's ability to excrete excess hydrogen ions and form bicarbonate.

Excess metabolic acids increase the hydrogen ion concentration of body fluids. The excess acid is buffered by bicarbonate, leading to what is known as a high anion gap acidosis (see Box 10–4).

The pancreas secretes bicarbonate-rich fluid into the small intestine. Intestinal suction, severe diarrhea, ileostomy drainage,

or fistulas can lead to excess losses of bicarbonate. Hyperchloremic acidosis can develop when excess chloride solutions (such as NaCl or ammonium chloride) are infused, causing a rise in chloride concentrations. It also may be related to renal disease or administration of carbonic anhydrate inhibitor diuretics. The anion gap remains normal in metabolic acidosis due to bicarbonate loss or excess chloride.

Acidosis depresses cell membrane excitability, affecting neuromuscular function. It also increases the amount of free calcium in ECF by interfering with protein binding. Severe acidosis (pH of 7.0 or less) depresses myocardial contractility, leading to a fall in cardiac output. If kidney function is normal, acid excretion and ammonia production increase to eliminate excess hydrogen ions.

Acid–base imbalances also affect electrolyte balance. In acidosis, potassium is retained as the kidney excretes excess

TABLE 10–12 Compensation for Simple Acid–Base Imbalances

PRIMARY DISORDER	CAUSE	COMPENSATION	EFFECT ON ABGS
Metabolic acidosis	Excess nonvolatile acids; bicarbonate deficiency	Rate and depth of respirations increase, eliminating additional CO_2.	↓ pH ↓ HCO_3^- ↓ $PaCO_2$
Metabolic alkalosis	Bicarbonate excess	Rate and depth of respirations decrease, retaining CO_2.	↑ pH ↑ HCO_3^- ↑ $PaCO_2$
Respiratory acidosis	Retained CO_2 and excess carbonic acid	Kidneys conserve bicarbonate to restore carbonic acid: bicarbonate ratio of 1:20.	↓ pH ↑ $PaCO_2$ ↑ HCO_3^-
Respiratory alkalosis	Loss of CO_2 and deficient carbonic acid	Kidneys excrete bicarbonate and conserve H^+ to restore carbonic acid:bicarbonate ratio.	↑ pH ↓ $PaCO_2$ ↓ HCO_3^-

hydrogen ions. Excess hydrogen ions also enter the cells, displacing potassium from the intracellular space to maintain the balance of cations and anions within the cells. The effect of both processes is to increase serum potassium levels. Also in acidosis, calcium is released from its bonds with plasma proteins, increasing the amount of ionized (free) calcium in the blood. Magnesium levels may fall in acidosis.

Manifestations

Metabolic acidosis affects the function of many body systems. Its general manifestations include weakness and fatigue, headache, and general malaise. Gastrointestinal function is affected, causing anorexia, nausea, vomiting, and abdominal pain. The level of consciousness declines, leading to stupor and coma. Cardiac dysrhythmias develop, and cardiac arrest may occur. The skin is often warm and flushed. Skeletal problems may develop in chronic acidosis, as calcium and phosphate are released from the bones.

Manifestations of compensatory mechanisms are seen. The respirations are labored, deep and rapid, known as **Kussmaul's respirations**. The patient may complain of shortness of breath or dyspnea. See the Manifestations box on page 228.

Interdisciplinary Care

Management of metabolic acidosis focuses on treating the underlying cause of the disorder and correcting the acid–base imbalance.

Diagnosis

The following laboratory and diagnostic tests may be ordered.

■ *ABGs* generally show a pH of less than 7.35 and a bicarbonate level of less than 22 mEq/L. A compensatory decrease in $PaCO_2$ to less than 35 mmHg is usually present.

BOX 10–4 Unraveling the Anion Gap

Calculation of the anion gap can help identify the underlying mechanism in metabolic acidosis if it is unclear.

The number of cations (positively charged ions) and anions (negatively charged ions) in ECF normally is equal (refer to Figure 10–2). Not all of these ions, however, are measured in laboratory testing (e.g., organic acids and proteins). The anion gap is calculated by subtracting the sum of two measured anions, chloride and bicarbonate, from the concentration of the major cation, sodium (see the following figure). The normal anion gap is 8 to 12 mEq/L.

Excess acids in ECF are buffered by bicarbonate, reducing serum bicarbonate levels and the total measured concentration of anions. This increases the anion gap (B in figure). When bicarbonate is lost from the body or chloride levels increase, however, the anion gap remains within normal limits (C in figure). This occurs because an increase or decrease in one of these negatively charged ions causes a corresponding change in the other to maintain balance (e.g., ↓ HCO_3^- ↔ ↑ Cl^-), and there is no change in the amount of unmeasured anions.

Illustration of the anion gap in metabolic acidosis. *A,* Normal anion gap. *B,* High anion gap caused by excess acids. *C,* Normal anion gap with hyperchloremia.

- *Serum electrolytes* demonstrate elevated serum potassium levels and possible low magnesium levels. The total calcium may remain unchanged, although more physiologically active ionized calcium is available. Sodium, chloride, and bicarbonate levels are used to calculate the anion gap.
- The *ECG* may show changes that reflect both the acidosis (particularly when severe) and the accompanying hyperkalemia.
- Other diagnostic studies such as the blood glucose and renal function studies may be ordered to identify the underlying cause of metabolic acidosis.

Medications

An alkalinizing solution such as bicarbonate may be given if the pH is less than 7.2 to reduce the effects of the acidosis on cardiac function. Sodium bicarbonate is the most commonly used alkalinizing solution; others include lactate, citrate, and acetate solutions (which are metabolized to bicarbonate). Alkalinizing solutions are given IV for severe acute metabolic acidosis. In chronic metabolic acidosis, the oral route is used.

The patient treated with bicarbonate must be carefully monitored. Rapid correction of the acidosis may lead to metabolic alkalosis and hypokalemia. Hypernatremia and hyperosmolality may develop as well, leading to water retention and fluid overload.

> **PRACTICE ALERT**
> As metabolic acidosis is corrected, potassium shifts back into the intracellular space. This can lead to hypokalemia and cardiac dysrhythmias. Carefully monitor serum potassium levels during treatment.

Treatment for diabetic ketoacidosis includes IV insulin and fluid replacement (∞ see Chapter 20 for the treatment of diabetic ketoacidosis). Alcoholic ketoacidosis is treated with saline solutions and glucose. Treatment for lactic acidosis from decreased tissue perfusion (e.g., shock or cardiac arrest) focuses on correcting the underlying problem and improving tissue perfusion. Patients with chronic renal failure and mild or moderate metabolic acidosis may or may not require treatment, depending on the pH and bicarbonate levels. When metabolic acidosis is due to diarrhea, treatment includes correcting the underlying cause and providing fluid and electrolyte replacement.

MANIFESTATIONS of Metabolic Acidosis

- Anorexia
- Nausea and vomiting
- Abdominal pain
- Weakness
- Fatigue
- General malaise
- Decreasing levels of consciousness
- Dysrhythmias
- Bradycardia
- Warm, flushed skin
- Hyperventilation (Kussmaul's respirations)

Nursing Care

Nurses frequently provide care for patients with metabolic acidosis, although the focus of care often is the disorder underlying the acidosis (e.g., diabetes mellitus, renal failure) rather than the acidosis itself. For this reason, it is vital for the nurse to be aware of the effects of the acidosis and its implications for nursing care.

Health Promotion

To promote health in patients at risk for metabolic acidosis, discuss management of their underlying disease process (e.g., type 1 diabetes or renal failure) to prevent complications such as diabetic ketoacidosis and metabolic acidosis. Because early manifestations of metabolic acidosis (e.g., fatigue, general malaise, anorexia, nausea, abdominal pain) resemble those of common viral disorders such as "the flu," stress the importance of promptly seeking treatment if these manifestations develop.

Assessment

Assessment data related to metabolic acidosis include the following:

- *Health history:* Current manifestations, including anorexia, nausea, vomiting, abdominal discomfort, fatigue, lethargy, other manifestations; duration of manifestations and any precipitating factors such as diarrhea, ingestion of a toxin such as aspirin, methanol, or ethylene; chronic diseases such as diabetes or renal failure, cirrhosis of the liver, or endocrine disorders; current medications.
- *Physical assessment:* Mental status and level of consciousness; vital signs; apical and peripheral pulses; skin color and temperature; abdominal contour and distention; bowel sounds; urine output.

> **PRACTICE ALERT**
> Apply firm pressure to the puncture site for 2–5 minutes after the needle is withdrawn following aspiration of arterial blood to measure ABGs to prevent bleeding into the surrounding tissues. Pressure may need to be applied longer for patients receiving anticoagulation medications.

Nursing Diagnoses and Interventions

Nursing management of patients with metabolic acidosis often focuses on the primary disorder (e.g., diabetic ketoacidosis or renal failure); however, the acidosis itself has effects that must be attended to when providing care.

Decreased Cardiac Output

Metabolic acidosis affects cardiac output by decreasing myocardial contractility, slowing the heart rate, and increasing the risk for dysrhythmias. The accompanying hyperkalemia increases the risk for decreased cardiac output as well (see the earlier discussion about hyperkalemia).

- Monitor vital signs, including peripheral pulses and capillary refill. *Hypotension, diminished pulse strength, and slowed capillary refill may indicate decreased cardiac output and impaired tissue perfusion. Poor tissue perfusion can increase the risk for lactic acidosis.*

- Monitor the ECG pattern for dysrhythmias and changes characteristic of hyperkalemia. Notify the physician of changes. *Progressive ECG changes such as widening of the QRS complex indicate an increasing risk of dysrhythmias and cardiac arrest. Dysrhythmias further decrease cardiac output, possibly intensifying the degree of acidosis.*
- Monitor laboratory values, including ABGs, serum electrolytes, and renal function studies (serum creatinine and BUN). *Frequent monitoring of laboratory values allows evaluation of the effectiveness of treatment as well as early identification of potential problems.*

Risk for Fluid Volume Excess

Administering bicarbonate to correct acidosis increases the risk for hypernatremia, hyperosmolality, and fluid volume excess.

- Monitor and maintain fluid replacement as ordered. Monitor serum sodium levels and osmolality. *Bicarbonate administration can cause hypernatremia and hyperosmolality, leading to water retention.*
- Monitor heart and lung sounds, CVP, and respiratory status. *Increasing dyspnea, adventitious lung sounds and a high CVP reading, and a third heart sound (S_3) due to the volume of blood flow through the heart are indicative of hypervolemia and should be reported to the healthcare provider.*
- Assess for edema, particularly in the back, sacral, and periorbital areas. *Initially, edema affects dependent tissues—the back and sacrum in patients who are bedridden. Periorbital edema indicates more generalized edema.*
- Assess urine output hourly. Maintain accurate intake and output records. Note urine output less than 30 mL/hour or a positive fluid balance on 24-hour total intake and output calculations. *Heart failure and inadequate renal perfusion may lead to decreased urine output.*
- Obtain daily weights using consistent conditions. *Daily weights are an accurate indicator of fluid balance.*
- Administer prescribed diuretics as ordered, monitoring the patient's response to therapy. *Loop or high-ceiling diuretics such as furosemide [Lasix] can lead to further electrolyte imbalances, especially hypokalemia. This is a significant risk like that seen during correction of metabolic acidosis.*

Risk for Injury

Mental status and brain function are affected by acidosis, increasing the risk for injury.

- Monitor neurologic function, including mental status, level of consciousness, and muscle strength. *As the pH falls, mental functioning declines, leading to confusion, stupor, and a decreasing level of consciousness.*
- Institute safety precautions as necessary: Keep the bed in its lowest position, side rails raised. *These measures help protect the patient from injury resulting from confusion or disorientation.*
- Keep clocks, calendars, and familiar objects at bedside. Orient to time, place, and circumstances as needed. Allow significant others to remain with the patient as much as possible. *An unfamiliar environment and altered thought*

processes can further increase the risk for injury. Significant others provide a sense of security and reduce anxiety.

Nursing care also includes measures to treat the underlying disorder, such as diabetic ketoacidosis. Refer to the chapters on diabetes (∞ Chapter 20) and renal failure (∞ Chapter 28) for specific interventions.

Community-Based Care

Discharge planning and teaching focus on the underlying cause of the imbalance. The patient who has developed ketoacidosis as a result of diabetes mellitus, starvation, or alcoholism needs interventions and teaching to prevent future episodes of acidosis. Diet, medication management, and alcohol dependency treatment are vital teaching areas. When metabolic acidosis is related to renal failure, the patient should be referred for management of the renal failure itself. Patients who have experienced diarrhea or excess ileostomy drainage leading to bicarbonate loss need information about appropriate diarrhea treatment strategies and when to call their primary care provider.

The Patient with Metabolic Alkalosis

Metabolic alkalosis (bicarbonate excess) is characterized by a high pH (> 7.45) and a high bicarbonate (> 26 mEq/L). It may be caused by loss of acid or excess bicarbonate in the body. When metabolic alkalosis develops, the respiratory system attempts to return the pH to normal by slowing the respiratory rate. Carbon dioxide is retained, and the $PaCO_2$ increases (> 45 mmHg).

Risk Factors

As is the case with other acid–base imbalances, metabolic alkalosis rarely occurs as a primary disorder. Risk factors include hospitalization, hypokalemia, and treatment with alkalinizing solutions (e.g., bicarbonate).

Pathophysiology

Hydrogen ions may be lost via gastric secretions through the kidneys, or because of a shift of H^+ into the cells. Metabolic alkalosis due to loss of hydrogen ions usually occurs because of vomiting or gastric suction. Gastric secretions are highly acidic (pH 1 to 3). When these are lost through vomiting or gastric suction, the alkalinity of body fluids increases. This increased alkalinity results both from the loss of acid and selective retention of bicarbonate by the kidneys as chloride is depleted. (Chloride is the major anion in ECF; when it is lost, bicarbonate is retained as a replacement anion.)

Increased renal excretion of hydrogen ions can be prompted by hypokalemia as the kidneys try to conserve potassium, excreting hydrogen ion instead. Hypokalemia contributes to metabolic alkalosis in another way as well. When potassium shifts out of cells to maintain extracellular potassium levels, hydrogen ions shift into the cells to maintain the balance between cations and anions within the cell.

Excess bicarbonate usually occurs as a result of ingesting antacids that contain bicarbonate (such as soda bicarbonate or Alka-Seltzer) or overzealous administration of bicarbonate to treat metabolic acidosis. Common causes of metabolic alkalosis are summarized in Table 10–11.

In alkalosis, more calcium combines with serum proteins, reducing the amount of ionized (physiologically active) calcium in the blood. This accounts for many of the common manifestations of metabolic alkalosis. Alkalosis also affects potassium balance: Hypokalemia not only can cause metabolic alkalosis (see the earlier discussion), but it also can result from metabolic alkalosis. Hydrogen ions shift out of the intracellular space to help restore the pH, prompting more potassium to enter the cells and depleting ECF potassium. The high pH depresses the respiratory system as the body retains carbon dioxide to restore the carbonic acid to bicarbonate ratio.

Manifestations and Complications

Manifestations of metabolic alkalosis (see the following box) occur as a result of decreased calcium ionization and are similar to those of hypocalcemia, including numbness and tingling around the mouth, fingers, and toes; dizziness; Trousseau's sign; and muscle spasm. As the respiratory system compensates for metabolic alkalosis, respirations are depressed and respiratory failure with hypoxemia and respiratory acidosis may develop.

Interdisciplinary Care

Interdisciplinary management of metabolic alkalosis focuses on diagnosing and correcting the underlying cause.

Diagnosis

The following laboratory and diagnostic tests may be ordered.

- *ABGs* show a pH greater than 7.45 and bicarbonate level greater than 26 mEq/L. With compensatory hypoventilation, carbon dioxide is retained, and the $PaCO_2$ is greater than 45 mmHg.
- *Serum electrolytes* often demonstrate decreased serum potassium (< 3.5 mEq/L) and decreased chloride (< 95 mEq/L) levels. The serum bicarbonate level is high. Although the total serum calcium may be normal, the ionized fraction of calcium is low.
- *Urine pH* may be low (pH 1 to 3) if metabolic acidosis is caused by hypokalemia. The kidneys selectively retain potassium and excrete hydrogen ion to restore ECF potassium levels. Urinary chloride levels may be normal or greater than 250 mEq/24 hours.
- The *ECG pattern* shows changes similar to those seen with hypokalemia. These changes may be due to hypokalemia or to the alkalosis.

MANIFESTATIONS of Metabolic Alkalosis

- Confusion
- Decreasing level of consciousness
- Hyperreflexia
- Tetany
- Dysrhythmias
- Hypotension
- Seizures
- Respiratory failure

Medications

Treatment of metabolic alkalosis includes restoring normal fluid volume and administering potassium chloride and sodium chloride solution. The potassium restores serum and intracellular potassium levels, allowing the kidneys to more effectively conserve hydrogen ions. Chloride promotes renal excretion of bicarbonate. Sodium chloride solutions restore fluid volume deficits that can contribute to metabolic alkalosis. In severe alkalosis, an acidifying solution such as dilute hydrochloric acid or ammonium chloride may be administered. In addition, drugs may be used to treat the underlying cause of the alkalosis.

✑ Nursing Care

Health Promotion

Health promotion activities focus on teaching patients the risks of using sodium bicarbonate as an antacid to relieve heartburn or gastric distress. Stress the availability of other effective antacid preparations and the need to seek medical evaluation for persistent gastric manifestations. In the hospital setting, carefully monitor laboratory values for patients at risk for developing metabolic alkalosis, particularly patients undergoing continuous gastric suction.

Assessment

Focused assessment data related to metabolic alkalosis include the following:

- *Health history:*   Current manifestations, such as numbness and tingling, muscle spasms, dizziness, other manifestations; duration of manifestations and any precipitating factors such as bicarbonate ingestion, vomiting, diuretic therapy, or endocrine disorders; current medications.
- *Physical assessment:*   Vital signs including apical pulse and rate and depth of respirations; muscle strength; deep tendon reflexes.

Nursing Diagnoses and Interventions

As with metabolic acidosis, nursing care of the patient with metabolic alkalosis often focuses on intervening for patient responses to the primary problem, rather than the alkalosis itself. However, the risk for impaired gas exchange is a priority problem, especially with severe metabolic alkalosis.

Risk for Impaired Gas Exchange

Respiratory compensation for metabolic alkalosis depresses the respiratory rate and reduces the depth of breathing to promote carbon dioxide retention. As a result, the patient is at risk for impaired gas exchange, especially in the presence of underlying lung disease.

- Monitor respiratory rate, depth, and effort. Monitor oxygen saturation continuously, reporting an oxygen saturation level of less than 95% (or as ordered). *The depressed respiratory drive associated with metabolic alkalosis can lead to hypoxemia and impaired oxygenation of tissues. Oxygen saturation levels of less than 90% indicate significant oxygenation problems.*
- Assess skin color; note and report cyanosis around the mouth. *Central cyanosis, seen around the mouth and oral mucous membranes, indicates significant hypoxia.*

- Monitor mental status and level of consciousness (LOC). Report decreasing LOC or behavior changes such as restlessness, agitation, or confusion. *Changes in mental status or behavior may be early manifestations of hypoxia.*
- Place in semi-Fowler's or Fowler's position as tolerated. *Elevating the head of the bed facilitates alveolar ventilation and gas exchange.*
- Schedule nursing care activities to allow rest periods. *The patient who is hypoxemic has limited energy reserves, necessitating frequent rest and limited activities.*
- Administer oxygen as ordered or necessary to maintain oxygen saturation levels. *Supplemental oxygen can help maintain blood and tissue oxygenation despite depressed respirations.*

Fluid Volume Deficit

Patients with metabolic alkalosis often have an accompanying fluid volume deficit.

- Assess vital signs, CVP, and peripheral pulse volume at least every 4 hours. *Hypotension, tachycardia, a low CVP, and weak, easily obliterated peripheral pulses indicate hypovolemia.*
- Weigh daily under standard conditions (time of day, clothing, and scale). *Rapid weight changes accurately reflect fluid balance.*
- Administer IV fluids as prescribed using an infusion pump. Monitor for indicators of fluid overload if rapid fluid replacement is ordered: dyspnea, tachypnea, tachycardia, increased CVP, jugular vein distension, and edema. *Rapid fluid replacement may lead to hypervolemia, resulting in pulmonary edema and cardiac failure, particularly in patients with compromised cardiac and renal function.*
- Monitor serum electrolytes, osmolality, and ABG values. *Rehydration and administration of potassium chloride will affect both acid–base and fluid and electrolyte balance. Careful monitoring is important to identify changes.*

Community-Based Care

When preparing the patient with metabolic alkalosis for discharge, consider the cause of the alkalosis and any underlying factors. For example, provide teaching about the following:

- Using appropriate antacids for heartburn and gastric distress
- Using potassium supplements as ordered or eating high-potassium foods to avoid hypokalemia if taking a potassium-wasting diuretic or if aldosterone production is impaired
- Contacting the primary care provider if uncontrolled or extended vomiting develops

The Patient with Respiratory Acidosis

Respiratory acidosis is caused by an excess of dissolved carbon dioxide, or carbonic acid. It is characterized by a pH less than 7.35 and a $PaCO_2$ greater than 45 mmHg. Respiratory acidosis may be either acute or chronic. In chronic respiratory acidosis, the bicarbonate is higher than 26 mEq/L as the kidneys compensate by retaining bicarbonate.

Risk Factors

Acute or chronic lung disease (e.g., pneumonia or chronic obstructive pulmonary disease [COPD]) is the primary risk factor for respiratory acidosis. Other conditions that depress or interfere with ventilation, such as excess narcotic analgesics, airway obstruction, or neuromuscular disease, also are risk factors for respiratory acidosis. Selected causes of respiratory acidosis are listed in Table 10–11.

Pathophysiology

Both acute and chronic respiratory acidosis result from carbon dioxide retention caused by alveolar hypoventilation. Hypoxemia (low oxygen in the arterial blood) frequently accompanies respiratory acidosis.

ACUTE RESPIRATORY ACIDOSIS Acute respiratory acidosis occurs as the result of a sudden failure of ventilation. Chest trauma, aspiration of a foreign body, acute pneumonia, and overdoses of narcotic or sedative medications can lead to this condition. Because acute respiratory acidosis occurs with the sudden onset of hypoventilation—for example, with cardiac arrest—the $PaCO_2$ rises rapidly and the pH falls markedly. A pH of 7 or lower can occur within minutes (Metheny, 2000). The serum bicarbonate level initially is unchanged because the compensatory response of the kidneys occurs over hours to days.

Hypercapnia (increased carbon dioxide levels) affects neurologic function and the cardiovascular system. Carbon dioxide rapidly crosses the blood–brain barrier. Cerebral blood vessels dilate and, if the condition continues, intracranial pressure increases and papilledema (swelling and inflammation of the optic nerve where it enters the retina) develops (Porth & Matfin, 2009). Peripheral vasodilation also occurs, and the pulse rate increases to maintain cardiac output.

CHRONIC RESPIRATORY ACIDOSIS Chronic respiratory acidosis is associated with chronic respiratory or neuromuscular conditions such as COPD, asthma, cystic fibrosis, or multiple sclerosis. These conditions affect alveolar ventilation because of airway obstruction, structural changes in the lung, or limited chest wall expansion. Most patients with chronic respiratory acidosis have COPD with chronic bronchitis and emphysema. (∞ See Chapter 37 for more information about COPD.) In chronic respiratory acidosis, the $PaCO_2$ increases over time and remains elevated. The kidneys retain bicarbonate, increasing bicarbonate levels, and the pH often remains close to the normal range.

The acute effects of hypercapnia may not develop because carbon dioxide levels rise gradually, allowing compensatory changes to occur. When carbon dioxide levels are chronically elevated, the respiratory center becomes less sensitive to the gas as a stimulant of the respiratory drive. The PaO_2 provides the primary stimulus for respirations. Patients with chronic respiratory acidosis are at risk for developing carbon dioxide narcosis, with manifestations of acute respiratory acidosis, if the respiratory center is suppressed by administering excess supplemental oxygen.

> **PRACTICE ALERT**
> Carefully monitor neurologic and respiratory status in patients with chronic respiratory acidosis who are receiving oxygen therapy. Immediately report a decreasing LOC or depressed respirations.

Manifestations

The manifestations of acute and chronic respiratory acidosis differ. In acute respiratory acidosis, the rapid rise in $PaCO_2$ levels causes manifestations of hypercapnia. Cerebral vasodilation causes manifestations such as headache, blurred vision, irritability, and mental cloudiness. If the condition continues, the level of consciousness progressively decreases. Rapid and dramatic changes in ABGs can lead to unconsciousness and ventricular fibrillation, a potentially lethal cardiac dysrhythmia. The skin of the patient with acute respiratory acidosis may be warm and flushed, and the pulse rate is elevated.

The manifestations of chronic respiratory acidosis include weakness and a dull headache. Sleep disturbances, daytime sleepiness, impaired memory, and personality changes also may be manifestations of chronic respiratory acidosis (see the following box).

Interdisciplinary Care

Patients with acute respiratory failure usually require treatment in the emergency department or intensive care unit. The focus is on restoring adequate ventilation and gas exchange. Hypoxemia often accompanies acute respiratory acidosis, so oxygen is administered as well. Supplemental oxygen is administered with caution to patients with chronic respiratory acidosis.

Diagnosis

The following laboratory and diagnostic tests may be ordered.

- *ABGs* show a pH of less than 7.35 and a $PaCO_2$ of more than 45 mmHg. In acute respiratory acidosis, the bicarbonate level is initially within normal range but increases to greater than 26 mEq/L if the condition persists. In chronic respiratory acidosis, both the $PaCO_2$ and the HCO_3^- may be significantly elevated.
- *Serum electrolytes* may show hypochloremia (chloride level < 98 mEq/L) in chronic respiratory acidosis.
- *Pulmonary function tests* may be done to determine if chronic lung disease is the cause of the respiratory acidosis. These studies would not be done during the acute period, however.

Additional diagnostic tests may be done to identify the underlying cause of the respiratory acidosis. *Chest x-ray* and *sputum studies* (cytology and culture) may be ordered to identify an acute or chronic lung disorder. If drug overdose is suspected, serum levels of the drug may be obtained.

Medications

Bronchodilator drugs may be administered to open the airways and antibiotics prescribed to treat respiratory infections. If excess narcotics or anesthetic has caused acute respiratory acidosis, drugs to reverse their effects (such as naloxone) may be given.

Respiratory Support

Treatment of respiratory acidosis, either acute or chronic, focuses on improving alveolar ventilation and gas exchange. Patients with severe respiratory acidosis and hypoxemia may require intubation and mechanical ventilation (∞ see Chapter 37 for more information about these procedures). The $PaCO_2$ level is lowered slowly to avoid complications such as cardiac dysrhythmias and decreased cerebral perfusion. In patients with chronic respiratory acidosis, oxygen is administered cautiously to avoid carbon dioxide narcosis.

Pulmonary hygiene measures, such as breathing treatments or percussion and drainage, may be instituted. Adequate hydration is important to promote removal of respiratory secretions.

∞ Nursing Care

See the Case Study & Nursing Care Plan: Acute Respiratory Acidosis on page 234.

Health Promotion

Health promotion activities related to respiratory acidosis focus on identifying, monitoring, and teaching patients at risk. Carefully monitor patients receiving anesthesia, narcotic analgesics, or sedatives for manifestations of respiratory depression. Monitor the response of patients with a history of chronic lung disease to oxygen therapy. Teach patients who have an identified risk for respiratory acidosis (such as people using narcotic analgesia for cancer pain and people with chronic lung disease) and their families about early manifestations of respiratory depression and acidosis, and instruct them to immediately contact their care provider if manifestations develop.

Assessment

Assessment data related to respiratory acidosis include the following:

- *Health history:* Current manifestations, including headache, irritability or lethargy, difficulty thinking, blurred vision, and other manifestations; duration of manifestations and any precipitating factors such as drug use or respiratory infection; chronic diseases such as cystic fibrosis or COPD; current medications.
- *Physical assessment:* Mental status and level of consciousness; vital signs; skin color and temperature; rate and depth of respirations, pulmonary excursion, lung sounds; examination of optic fundus for possible papilledema.

Nursing Diagnoses and Interventions

Restoring effective alveolar ventilation and gas exchange is the priority of interdisciplinary and nursing care for patients with respiratory acidosis.

MANIFESTATIONS of Respiratory Acidosis

ACUTE RESPIRATORY ACIDOSIS
- Headache
- Warm, flushed skin
- Blurred vision
- Irritability, altered mental status
- Decreasing level of consciousness
- Cardiac arrest

CHRONIC RESPIRATORY ACIDOSIS
- Weakness
- Dull headache
- Sleep disturbances with daytime sleepiness
- Impaired memory
- Personality changes

Impaired Gas Exchange

- Frequently assess respiratory status, including rate, depth, effort, and oxygen saturation levels. *Decreasing respiratory rate and effort along with decreasing oxygen saturation levels may signal worsening respiratory failure and respiratory acidosis.*
- Frequently assess level of consciousness. *A decline in LOC may indicate increasing hypercapnia and the need for increasing ventilatory support (such as intubation and mechanical ventilation).*
- Promptly evaluate and report ABG results to the physician and respiratory therapist. *Rapid changes in carbon dioxide or oxygen levels may necessitate modification of the treatment plan to prevent complications of overcorrection of respiratory acidosis.*
- Place in semi-Fowler's to Fowler's position as tolerated. *Elevating the head of the bed promotes lung expansion and gas exchange.*
- Administer oxygen as ordered. Carefully monitor response. Reduce the oxygen flow rate or percentage and immediately report increasing somnolence. *Supplemental oxygen can suppress the respiratory drive in patients with chronic respiratory acidosis.*

Ineffective Airway Clearance

- Frequently auscultate breath sounds (whether on or off a mechanical ventilator). *Increasing adventitious sounds or decreasing breath sounds (faint or absent) may indicate worsening airway clearance due to obstruction or fatigue.*
- Encourage the patient with chronic respiratory acidosis to use pursed-lip breathing. *Pursed-lip breathing helps maintain open airways throughout exhalation, promoting carbon dioxide elimination.*
- Frequently reposition and encourage ambulation as tolerated. *Repositioning, sitting at the bedside, and ambulation promote airway clearance and lung expansion.*
- Encourage fluid intake of up to 3000 mL per day as tolerated or allowed. *Fluids help liquefy secretions and hydrate respiratory mucous membranes, promoting airway clearance.*
- Administer medications such as inhaled bronchodilators as ordered. *Inhaled bronchodilators help relieve bronchial spasm, dilating airways.*
- Provide percussion, vibration, and postural drainage as ordered. *Pulmonary hygiene measures such as these help loosen respiratory secretions so they can be coughed out of airways.*

Using NANDA, NIC, and NOC

Linkages between a selected NANDA nursing diagnosis, NIC, and NOC for the patient with respiratory acidosis are shown in the chart that follows.

Community-Based Care

Planning and teaching for home care focuses on the health problem that caused the patient to develop respiratory acidosis. The patient who developed acute respiratory acidosis as a result of acute pneumonia or chest trauma may only require teaching to prevent future problems. If acute respiratory acidosis occurred secondarily to a narcotic overdose, determine if the drug was prescribed for pain or if it was an illicit street drug.

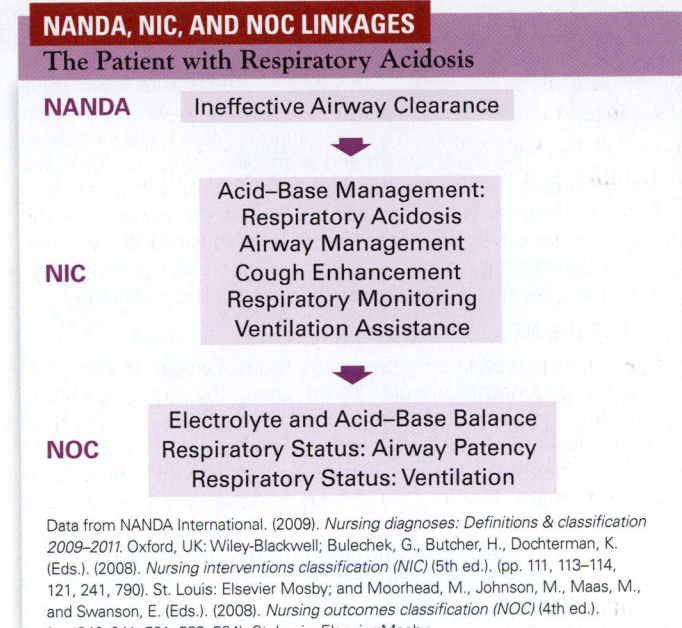

NANDA, NIC, AND NOC LINKAGES
The Patient with Respiratory Acidosis

NANDA — Ineffective Airway Clearance

NIC — Acid–Base Management: Respiratory Acidosis
Airway Management
Cough Enhancement
Respiratory Monitoring
Ventilation Assistance

NOC — Electrolyte and Acid–Base Balance
Respiratory Status: Airway Patency
Respiratory Status: Ventilation

Data from NANDA International. (2009). *Nursing diagnoses: Definitions & classification 2009–2011.* Oxford, UK: Wiley-Blackwell; Bulechek, G., Butcher, H., Dochterman, K. (Eds.). (2008). *Nursing interventions classification (NIC)* (5th ed.). (pp. 111, 113–114, 121, 241, 790). St. Louis: Elsevier Mosby; and Moorhead, M., Johnson, M., Maas, M., and Swanson, E. (Eds.). (2008). *Nursing outcomes classification (NOC)* (4th ed.). (pp. 340–341, 581, 583–584). St. Louis: Elsevier Mosby.

Provide teaching to the patient who requires narcotic medication on a continuing basis. Refer the patient using illicit drugs to a substance abuse counselor, treatment center, or Narcotics Anonymous as appropriate.

For patients with chronic lung disease, discuss ways to avoid future episodes of acute respiratory failure. Encourage the patient to be immunized against pneumococcal pneumonia and influenza. Discuss ways to avoid acute respiratory infections and measures to take when respiratory status is further compromised.

The Patient with Respiratory Alkalosis

Respiratory alkalosis is characterized by a pH greater than 7.45 and a $PaCO_2$ of less than 35 mmHg. It is always caused by hyperventilation leading to a carbon dioxide deficit.

Risk Factors

Anxiety with hyperventilation is the most common cause of respiratory alkalosis; therefore, anxiety disorders increase the risk for this acid–base imbalance. In the patient who is critically ill, mechanical ventilation is a risk factor for respiratory alkalosis.

Pathophysiology

In acute respiratory alkalosis, the pH rises rapidly as the $PaCO_2$ falls. Because the kidneys are unable to rapidly adapt to the change in pH, the bicarbonate level remains within normal limits. Anxiety-based hyperventilation is the most common cause of acute respiratory alkalosis. Other physiologic causes of hyperventilation include high fever, hypoxia, gram-negative bacteremia, and thyrotoxicosis. Early salicylate intoxication (aspirin overdose), encephalitis, and high progesterone levels in pregnancy directly stimulate the respiratory center, potentially leading to hyperventilation and respiratory alkalosis. Hyperventilation also can occur during anesthesia or mechanical ventilation if the rate and tidal volume (depth) of ventilations is excessive.

If hyperventilation continues, the kidneys compensate by eliminating bicarbonate to restore the bicarbonate to carbonic

CASE STUDY & NURSING CARE PLAN   Acute Respiratory Acidosis

Marlene Hitz, aged 76, is eating lunch with her friends when she suddenly begins to choke and is unable to breathe. After several minutes of trying, an attendant at the senior center successfully dislodges some meat caught in Ms. Hitz's throat by using the Heimlich maneuver. Ms. Hitz is taken by ambulance to the emergency department for follow-up because she was apneic for 3 to 4 minutes, her respirations are shallow, and she is disoriented.

ASSESSMENT

Ms. Hitz is placed in an observation room. Oxygen is started at 4 L/min per nasal cannula. David Love, the nurse admitting Ms. Hitz, makes the following assessments: T 98.2, P 102, R 36 and shallow, BP 146/92. Skin is warm and dry. Alert but restless and not oriented to time or place; responds slowly to questions. Stat ABGs are drawn, a chest x-ray is done, and D5 1/2 NS is started IV at 50 mL/h.

The chest x-ray shows no abnormality. ABG results are pH 7.38 (normal: 7.35 to 7.45), $PaCO_2$ 48 mmHg (normal: 35 to 45 mmHg), PaO_2 92 mmHg (normal: 80 to 100 mmHg), and HCO_3^- 24 mEq/L (normal: 22 to 26 mEq/L).

DIAGNOSES

- *Impaired Gas Exchange* related to temporary airway obstruction
- *Anxiety* related to emergency hospital admission
- *Risk for Injury* related to confusion

EXPECTED OUTCOMES

- Regain normal gas exchange and ABG values.
- Be oriented to time, place, and person.
- Regain appropriate mental status.
- Remain free of injury.

PLANNING AND IMPLEMENTATION

- Monitor ABGs, to be redrawn in 2 hours.
- Monitor vital signs and respiratory status (including oxygen saturation) every 15 minutes for the first hour, then every hour.
- Assess color of skin, nail beds, and oral mucous membranes every hour.
- Assess mental status and orientation every hour.
- Monitor anxiety level as evidenced by restlessness and agitation.
- Maintain a calm, quiet environment.
- Provide reorientation and explain all activities.
- Keep side rails in place, and place call bell within reach.

EVALUATION

Ms. Hitz remains in the emergency department for 6 hours. Her ABGs are still abnormal, and David now notes the presence of respiratory crackles and wheezes. She is less anxious and responds appropriately when asked who and where she is. Because she has not regained normal gas exchange, Ms. Hitz is admitted to the hospital for continued observation and treatment.

CRITICAL THINKING IN THE NURSING PROCESS

1. Describe the pathophysiologic process that leads to acute respiratory acidosis in Ms. Hitz.
2. Describe the effect of acidosis on mental function.
3. What teaching would you provide to Ms. Hitz to prevent future episodes of choking?

See Evaluating Your Response in Appendix C.

---

acid ratio. The bicarbonate level is lower than normal in chronic respiratory alkalosis, and the pH may be close to the normal range.

Alkalosis increases binding of extracellular calcium to albumin, reducing ionized calcium levels. As a result, neuromuscular excitability increases and manifestations similar to hypocalcemia develop. Low carbon dioxide levels in the blood cause vasoconstriction of cerebral vessels, increasing the neurologic manifestations of the disorder.

Manifestations

The manifestations of respiratory alkalosis include lightheadedness, a feeling of panic and difficulty concentrating, circumoral and distal extremity paresthesias, tremors, and positive Chvostek's and Trousseau's signs. The patient also may experience tinnitus, a sensation of chest tightness, and palpitations (cardiac dysrhythmias). Seizures and loss of consciousness may occur. (See the following Manifestations box.)

Interdisciplinary Care

Management of respiratory alkalosis focuses on correcting the imbalance and treating the underlying cause.

Diagnosis

ABGs generally show a pH greater than 7.45 and a $PaCO_2$ of less than 35 mmHg. In chronic hyperventilation, there is a compensatory decrease in serum bicarbonate to less than 22 mEq/L and the pH may be near normal.

Medications

A sedative or antianxiety agent may be necessary to relieve anxiety and restore a normal breathing pattern. Additional drugs to correct underlying problems other than anxiety-induced hyperventilation may be ordered.

Respiratory Therapy

The usual treatment for anxiety-related respiratory alkalosis involves instructing the patient to breathe more slowly and having the patient breathe into a paper bag or rebreather mask. This allows rebreathing of exhaled carbon dioxide, increasing $PaCO_2$ levels, and reducing the pH. If excessive ventilation by a mechanical ventilator is the cause of respiratory alkalosis, ventilator settings are adjusted to reduce the respiratory rate and tidal volume as indicated. When hypoxia is the underlying cause of hyperventilation, oxygen is administered.

MANIFESTATIONS of Respiratory Alkalosis

- Dizziness
- Numbness and tingling around mouth, hands, and feet
- Palpitations
- Dyspnea
- Chest tightness
- Anxiety/panic
- Tremors
- Tetany
- Seizures, loss of consciousness

∾ Nursing Care

Health Promotion

Identify patients at risk in the hospital (e.g., patients on mechanical ventilation or who have a fever or infection), and monitor assessment data and ABGs to identify early manifestations of hyperventilation and respiratory alkalosis.

Assessment, Diagnoses, and Interventions

Ineffective Breathing Pattern

The usual cause of hyperventilation and respiratory alkalosis is psychologic, although physiologic disorders also can lead to hyperventilation. It is important to not only address the hyperventilation, but also to identify the underlying cause.

- Assess respiratory rate, depth, and ease. Monitor vital signs (including temperature) and skin color. *Assessment data can help identify the underlying cause, such as a fever or hypoxia.*
- Obtain subjective assessment data such as circumstances leading up to the current situation, current health and recent illnesses or medication use, and current manifestations. *Subjective data provide cues to the cause and circumstances of the hyperventilation response.*
- Reassure the patient that he or she is not experiencing a heart attack and that manifestations will resolve when breathing

returns to normal. *Manifestations of hyperventilation and respiratory alkalosis such as dyspnea, chest tightness or pain, and palpitations can mimic those of a heart attack.*

- Instruct the patient to maintain eye contact and breathe with you to slow the respiratory rate. *These measures help to make the patient aware of respirations and provide a sense of support and control (Ackley & Ladwig, 2006).*
- Have the patient breathe into a paper bag. *This allows the patient to rebreathe exhaled carbon dioxide, increasing the $PaCO_2$ and decreasing the pH.*
- Protect the patient from injury. *If hyperventilation continues to the point at which the patient loses consciousness, respirations will return to normal, as will acid–base balance.*
- If the patient has experienced repeated episodes of hyperventilation or has a chronic anxiety disorder, refer for counseling. *Counseling can help the patient develop alternative strategies for dealing with anxiety.*

Community-Based Care

Planning and teaching for home care is directed toward the underlying cause of hyperventilation. If anxiety precipitated the episode, discuss anxiety management strategies with the patient. Refer the patient and family to a counselor if appropriate. Teach the patient to identify a hyperventilation reaction, and how to breathe into a paper bag to manage it at home.

CHAPTER HIGHLIGHTS

- The volume and composition of body fluid is normally maintained by a balance of fluid and electrolyte intake; elimination of water, electrolytes, and acids by the kidneys; and hormonal influences. Change in any of these factors can lead to a fluid, electrolyte, or acid–base imbalance that adversely affects health.
- Fluid, electrolyte, and acid–base imbalances can affect all body systems, especially the cardiovascular system, the central nervous system, and the transmission of nerve impulses. Conversely, primary disorders of the respiratory, renal, cardiovascular, endocrine, or other body systems can lead to an imbalance of fluids, electrolytes, or acid–base status.
- Fluid and sodium imbalances are related; both affect serum osmolality.
- Potassium imbalances are commonly seen in patients with acute or chronic illnesses. Both hypokalemia and hyperkalemia affect cardiac conduction and function. Carefully monitor cardiac rhythm and status in patients with very low or very high potassium levels.
- Calcium imbalances primarily affect neuromuscular transmission: Hypocalcemia increases neuromuscular irritability; hypercalcemia

depresses neuromuscular transmission. Magnesium imbalances have a similar effect.

- Acid–base imbalances may be caused by either metabolic or respiratory health problems. Simple acid–base imbalances (respiratory or metabolic acidosis or alkalosis) are more commonly seen than mixed imbalances.
- Buffers, lungs, and kidneys work together to maintain acid–base balance in the body. Buffers respond to changes almost immediately; the lungs respond within minutes; the kidneys, require hours to days to restore normal acid–base balance.
- The lungs compensate for metabolic acid–base imbalances by excreting or retaining carbon dioxide. This is accomplished by increasing or decreasing the rate and depth of respirations.
- The kidneys compensate for respiratory acid–base imbalances by producing and retaining or excreting bicarbonate, and by retaining or excreting hydrogen ions.
- Careful monitoring of respiratory and cardiovascular status, mental status, neuromuscular function, and laboratory values is an important nursing responsibility for all patients with fluid, electrolyte, or acid–base imbalances.

TEST YOURSELF NCLEX-RN® REVIEW

1. A patient is admitted to the emergency department with hypovolemia. Which IV solution would the nurse anticipate administering?
   1. lactated Ringer's solution
   2. 10% dextrose in water
   3. 3% sodium chloride
   4. 0.45% sodium chloride

2. When assessing a patient with fluid volume deficit, what would the nurse expect to find?
   1. increased pulse rate and blood pressure
   2. dyspnea and respiratory crackles
   3. headache and muscle cramps
   4. orthostatic hypotension and flat neck veins

3. The nurse caring for a patient with acute hypernatremia includes which of the following in the plan of care? **Select all that apply.**
   1. Conduct frequent neurologic checks.
   2. Restrict fluids to 1500 mL per day.
   3. Orient to time, place, and person frequently.
   4. Maintain IV access.
   5. Limit length of visits.
4. Laboratory results for a patient show a serum potassium level of 2.2 mEq/L. Which of the following nursing actions is of highest priority for this patient?
   1. Keep the patient on bed rest.
   2. Initiate cardiac monitoring.
   3. Start oxygen at 2 L/min.
   4. Initiate seizure precautions.
5. The nurse evaluates teaching about calcium supplement therapy as effective when the patient states that she will take her calcium tablets how?
   1. all at one time in the morning
   2. with meals
   3. as needed for tremulousness
   4. with a full glass of water
6. A patient who is known to be an alcoholic presents with confusion, hallucinations, and a positive Chvostek's sign. Which medication(s) should the nurse anticipate administering?
   1. magnesium sulfate
   2. calcium chloride
   3. insulin and glucose
   4. sodium bicarbonate

7. Arterial blood gas results for a patient show pH 7.21, PaO_2 98 mmHg, $PaCO_2$ 32 mmHg, and HCO_3^- 17 mEq/L. The nurse correctly interprets these values as indicative of which of the following acid–base imbalances?
   1. metabolic acidosis
   2. metabolic alkalosis
   3. respiratory acidosis
   4. respiratory alkalosis
8. A patient is admitted with a suspected heroin overdose and a respiratory rate of 5 to 6 per minute. Which of the following assessment data would the nurse anticipate? **Select all that apply.**
   1. pH 7.29
   2. alert and oriented
   3. $PaCO_2$ 54 mmHg
   4. HCO_3^- 32 mEq/L
   5. skin warm and flushed
9. The nurse caring for a patient undergoing several days of gastric decompression recognizes that the patient is at risk for which of the following acid–base imbalances?
   1. metabolic acidosis
   2. metabolic alkalosis
   3. respiratory acidosis
   4. respiratory alkalosis
10. A patient undergoing mechanical ventilation following a severe chest wall injury and flail chest complains of chest tightness, anxiety, and feeling as though she cannot get enough air. She is afraid she is having a heart attack. The nurse should first do which of the following?
    1. Administer prescribed analgesic.
    2. Contact respiratory therapy to evaluate ventilator settings.
    3. Obtain arterial blood gases.
    4. Notify the physician.

See Test Yourself answers in Appendix C.

Pearson Nursing Student Resources
Find additional review materials at **nursing.pearsonhighered.com**
Prepare for success with additional NCLEX®-style practice questions, interactive assignments and activities, Web links, animations and videos, and more!

BIBLIOGRAPHY

American Association of Critical Care Nurses. (2007). Practice alert: Oral care in the critically ill. Retrieved from http://www.aacn.org

Astle, S. M. (2005). Restoring electrolyte balance. *RN, 68*(5), 34–40.

Beer, M. H., Porter, R., & Jones, T. V. (Eds.). (2008). *The Merck manual of diagnosis and therapy* (18th ed.). Merck & Co., Inc. Internet edition provided by Medical Services, USMEDSA, USHH.

Blackmer, S. (2010). Cerebral salt wasting: An overlooked cause of hyponatremia. *American Nurse Today, 5*(3), 34, 36.

Bulechek, G., Butcher, H., & Dochterman, J. (Eds.). (2008). *Nursing interventions classification (NIC)* (5th ed.). Mosby Elsevier.

Centers for Disease Control. (2009). Application of lower sodium intake recommendations to adults—United States, 1999–2006. *MMWR Weekly*, March 27, 2009/ *58*(11).

David, K. (2007). *IV fluids: Do you know what's hanging and why?* RN Web. Available RN/AHC Home Study Program.

Dougherty, L. (2008). Back to basics in IV therapy: An unfortunate necessity. *British Journal of Nursing, 17*(19), S3.

Edwards, S. L. (2005). Maintaining calcium balance: Physiology and implications. *Nursing Times, 101*(19), 58–61.

Fauci, A. S., Braunwald, E., Kasper, D., Hauser, S. L., Longo, D. L., Jameson, J. L., & Loscalzo (Eds.). (2008). *Harrison's principles of internal medicine* (17th ed.). New York: McGraw-Hill.

Fournier, M. (2009). Perfecting your acid-base balancing act. How to detect and correct acid-base disorders. *American Nurse Today, 4*(1), 17–22.

Gobbi, M., Cowen, M., & Ugboma, D. (2006). Fluid and electrolyte balance. In M. Alexander, J. Fawcett, & P. Runciman (Eds) *Nursing practice: Hospital and home: The adult* (3rd ed., pp. 763–785). Philadelphia: Churchill Livingstone.

Hayes, D. (2007). How to respond to abnormal serum sodium levels. *Nursing, 37*(12), 56hn1–2, 56hn4.

Hogan, M., Gingrich, M., Overby, P., & Ricci, M. (2007). *Fluids, electrolytes, & acid-base balance* (2nd ed). Pearson Prentice Hall.

Holman, C., Roberts, S., & Nicol, M. (2005). Promoting adequate hydration in older people. *Nursing Older People, 17*(4), 31–32.

Kee, J. L. (2008). *Prentice Hall handbook of laboratory and diagnostic tests with nursing implications* (6th ed). Pearson Prentice Hall.

Lawes, R. (2009). Body out of balance: Understanding metabolic acidosis and alkalosis. *Nursing, 39*(11), 50–54.

Macafee, D., Allison, S., & Lobo, D. (2005). Some interactions between GI function and fluid and electrolyte homeostasis. *Current Opinion in Clinical Nutrition and Metabolic Care, 8*(2), 197–203.

McPhee, S., Papadakis, M., & Tierney, L. (2008). *Current medical diagnosis and treatment* (47th ed.). New York: Lange /McGraw-Hill.

Mentes, J. (2008). *Hydration management: Nursing standard of practice protocol: Oral hydration management.* Hartford Institute for Geriatric Nursing. Retrieved from http://www.consultgerirn.org/topics

Metheny, N. M. (2000). *Fluid and electrolyte balance: Nursing considerations* (4th ed.). Philadelphia: Lippincott.

Moorhead, S., Johnson, M., Maas, M., & Swanson, E. (Eds). (2008). *Nursing outcomes classification (NOC)* (4th ed.). St. Louis: Mosby Elsevier.

ROME

NANDA International. (2009). *Nursing diagnoses: Definitions and classification 2009–2011*. Oxford, UK: Wiley-Blackwell.

Nemec, K., Kopelent-Frank, H., & Greif, R. (2008). Standardization of infusion solutions to reduce the risk of incompatibility. *American Journal of Health-System Pharmacy, 65*(17), 1648–1654.

Oh, H., & Seo, W. (2007). Alterations in fluid, electrolytes and other serum chemistry values and their relations with enteral tube feeding in acute brain infarction patients. *Journal of Clinical Nursing, 16*(2), 298–307.

Oh, H., Suh, Y., Hwang, S., & Seo, W. (2005). Effects of nasogastric tube feeding on serum sodium, potassium and glucose levels. *Journal of Nursing Scholarship, 37*(2), 141–147.

O'Keeffe, S. (2005). Clinician's guide to interpreting arterial blood gases (ABG's). *Clinical Times, 2*(3), 3.

O'Neill, P. (2007). Helping your patient to restrict potassium: Teach him how to modify his diet to maintain optimum levels of this vital electrolyte. *Nursing, 37*(4), 64hn6, 64hn8.

Perrin, K. O. (2009). *Understanding the essentials of critical care nursing*. Upper Saddle River: Pearson Prentice Hall.

Porth, C. M. (2007). *Essentials of pathophysiology: Concepts of altered health states* (2nd ed.). Philadelphia: Lippincott Williams & Wilkins.

Porth, C. M., & Matfin, G. (2009). *Pathophysiology: Concepts of altered health states*. (8th ed.). Philadelphia: Lippincott Williams & Wilkins.

Pruitt, W. C., & Jacobs, M. (2004). Interpreting arterial blood gases: Easy as ABC. *Nursing, 34*(8), 50–53.

Rosenthal, K. (2009). *Tonicity and IV fluids*. Resource Nurse. Retrieved from http://www.resourcenurse.com/feature_tonicity_fluids.html

Scroggs, J. (2008). Improving patient safety using clinical needs assessment in IV therapy. *British Journal of Nursing, 17*(19), S22–S28.

Stanner, S. (2005). Preventing undernutrition and dehydration in older people. *Nursing & Residential Care, 7*(1), 17–19.

Sweeney, J. (2005a). What causes hyponatremia? *Nursing, 35*(6), 18.

Sweeney, J. (2005b). What causes sudden hypokalemia? *Nursing, 35*(4), 12.

Ulrich, S., & McCutcheon, H. (2008). Nursing practice and oral fluid intake of older people with dementia. *Journal of Clinical Nursing, 17*(21), 2910–2919.

Urden, L. D., Stacy, K. M., & Lough, M. E. (2006). *Thelan's critical care nursing: Diagnosis and management* (5th ed.). St. Louis, MO: Mosby.

Wilson, B., Shannon, M., & Shields, K. (2009). *Prentice Hall Nurses Drug Guide 2009*. Pearson Prentice Hall.

Young, E., Shrrard-Jacob, A., Knapp, K., et al., (2009). Perioperative fluid management. *AORN Journal, 39*(1), 167–182.

CHAPTER 11

Nursing Care of Patients Experiencing Trauma and Shock

LEARNING OUTCOMES

1. Define the word *trauma*.
2. Define the components and types of trauma.
3. Describe the result of energy transfer to the human body.
4. Discuss causes, effects, and initial management of trauma.
5. Discuss diagnostic tests used in assessing patients experiencing trauma and shock.
6. Describe collaborative interventions for patients experiencing trauma and shock, including medications, blood transfusion, and intravenous fluids.
7. Discuss organ donation and forensic implications of traumatic injury or death.
8. Discuss cellular homeostasis and basic hemodynamics.
9. Discuss the risk factors, etiologies, and pathophysiologies of hypovolemic shock, cardiogenic shock, obstructive shock, and distributive shock.
10. Use the nursing process as a framework for providing individualized care to patients experiencing trauma and shock.

CLINICAL COMPETENCIES

1. Describe steps of the primary survey to diagnose and manage life-threatening injuries.
2. Obtain initial subjective and objective data of the trauma patient to include history taking, assessment, review of past medical history, and communication with pre-hospital and other healthcare providers and family members.
3. Evaluate patient response to medical and surgical interventions for patients sustaining multiple trauma and shock.
4. Provide essential ongoing written communication for patient care and continuity of the trauma patient.
5. Describe the role of the nurse in trauma prevention education and develop a plan of care to restore the functional health status of trauma patients.
6. Communicate significant data and changes in the condition of the patient who has sustained trauma.
7. Identify nursing diagnoses based on signs and symptoms recognized during the nursing assessment.
8. Develop a plan of care for the trauma patient based on scientific knowledge and patient diversity that addresses the nursing diagnosis.
9. Document quality of care issues associated with the trauma patient.
10. Advocate for the patient's rights as indicated by documents that address end-of-life issues.
11. Comply with guidelines related to the Uniform Anatomical Gift Act.

KEY TERMS

abrasion, *242*
brain death criteria, *248*
contusion, *242*
laceration, *242*

pneumothorax, *241*
puncture wound, *242*
shock, *253*

tension pneumothorax, *241*
transfusion, *245*
trauma, *238*

The Patient Experiencing Trauma

Trauma is defined as injury to human tissues and organs resulting from the transfer of energy from the environment. In the past the term *trauma* has been associated with the word *accident*. *Accident* means that the injury occurred without intent, a result of random chance. We now know that a considerable number of injuries are preventable and not of random chance. Intentional and nonintentional trauma encompasses a variety of injuries resulting from motor vehicle crashes, pedestrian injuries, gunshot wounds, falls, violence toward others, or self-inflicted violence. The injuries, disabilities, and deaths resulting from these acts constitute a major healthcare challenge.

FAST FACTS
- Trauma kills more people between the ages of 1 and 44 than any other disease or illness.
- Forty-three percent of all deaths from ages 1 to 4 are due to trauma.
- Forty-eight percent of all deaths from ages 5 to 14 are due to trauma.
- Sixty-two percent of all deaths from ages 15 to 24 are due to trauma.

Trauma usually occurs suddenly, leaving the patient and family with little time to prepare for its consequences. Nurses provide a vital link in both the physical and psychosocial care for the injured patient and family. In caring for the patient who has experienced trauma, nurses must consider not only the initial physical injury, but also its long-term consequences, including rehabilitation. Trauma may alter the patient's previous way of life, potentially effecting independence, mobility, cognitive thinking, and appearance.

Components of Trauma

Trauma results from an abnormal exchange of energy between a host and a mechanism in a predisposing environment. The *host* is the person or group at risk of injury. Multiple factors influence the host's potential for injury: age, sex, race, economic status, preexisting illnesses, and use of substances such as street drugs and alcohol.

The *mechanism* is the source of the energy transmitted to the host. The energy exchanged can be mechanical, gravitational, thermal, electrical, physical, or chemical. Table 11–1 lists the most common mechanisms for each type of energy. Mechanical energy is the most common type of energy transferred to a host in trauma. The most common mechanical source of injury in all adult age groups is the motor vehicle.

Guns are another common mechanical source of injury. Trauma from gunshot wounds has steadily increased over the past 20 years and remains a major reason for emergency department and trauma center admissions, especially in large cities.

When describing a traumatic injury, *intention* is included as a component. Most gunshot and stab wounds are examples of intentional injuries. It is important to remember, however, that some gunshot wounds are unintentional, such as those that occur when children play with their parents' guns. Other common unintentional injuries result from motor vehicle crashes, falls, drowning, fires, and hunting accidents.

The final component of trauma is the *environment*. For example, a road that has become slippery after a snowstorm is a physical environment that may contribute to an injury.

TABLE 11–1 Common Mechanisms of Injury by Energy Source

ENERGY SOURCE	COMMON MECHANISMS OF INJURY
Mechanical	Motor vehicles
	Firearms
	Machines
Gravitational	Falls
Thermal	Heating appliances
	Fire
	Freezing temperatures
Electrical	Wires, sockets, and other electrical objects
	Lightning
Physical	Fists, feet, and other body parts (as in physical assault)
	Sharp objects, such as knives
	Ultraviolet radiation
	Ionizing radiation
	Water (drowning)
	Other submersion agents (e.g., grain)
	Explosions
Chemical	Drugs
	Poisons
	Industrial chemicals

Occupation is an important environmental factor to consider. Those in certain occupations face a high risk of trauma; examples include police officers, firefighters, professional athletes, racecar drivers, and taxi cab drivers. One's social environment also influences risk for injury, such as the presence of gangs and neighborhood violence. (See the following box for one example, intimate partner violence.)

MEETING INDIVIDUALIZED NEEDS   Assessing Intimate Partner Violence (IPV)

Most IPV incidents are not reported, thus it is believed that the available data greatly underestimates the true magnitude of the problem. It is estimated that more than 5.3 million women are beaten by male partners every year, resulting in 1300 deaths annually. Among men, 3.2 million IPV episodes occur annually, accounting for approximately 800,000 men raped or physically assaulted by an intimate partner. IPV is the single largest cause of injury to women in the United States. This is a widespread problem that occurs regardless of age, sex, race, socioeconomic status, or education. IPV is also referred to as partner abuse or spousal abuse (CDC, 2003). In 2001, intimate partner violence made up 20% of violent crime against women. The same year, intimate partners committed 3% of all violent crimes against men.

Note: From Bureau of Justice Statistics Crime Data. *Intimate Partner Violence, 1993–2001.* February 2003.

VIOLENCE IN THE ELDERLY
Elder abuse is defined as anything that endangers the life of an elderly person. This can range from physical or emotional assault to intimidation, neglect, or financial exploitation. In addition, willful deprivation of food or medical care is included. The National Elder Abuse Incidence study found that approximately 551,000 persons

aged 60 or older were abused or neglected in a 1-year period. Persons 80 years of age and older experienced abuse and neglect two to three times their proportion of the older population. The perpetrator is a family member in 90% of the cases.

The general approach to diagnosis in abuse situations is challenging and many times hidden. As with spousal, elder, or child abuse, the task of identification is complex. The following are clues to identify violence-related injuries:

- Injuries that do not correlate with the history
- Injuries that suggest a defensive posture
- Injuries during pregnancy
- Pattern injuries
- Pattern burns
- Sexual abuse/rape
- Unusual or unexplained fractures
- Signs of confinement
- Unusual interaction between patient and caregiver
- Lack of medical attention; immunizations not up to date, poor dental health
- Unexplained dehydration or malnutrition

Types of Trauma

Minor trauma causes injury to a single part or system of the body and is usually treated in a physician's office or in the hospital emergency department. A fracture of the clavicle, a small second-degree burn, and a laceration requiring sutures are examples of minor trauma. Major or multiple trauma involves serious single-system injury (such as the traumatic amputation of a leg) or multiple-system injuries. Multiple trauma is most often the result of a motor vehicle crash.

Trauma is further classified as either blunt or penetrating. Blunt trauma occurs when there is no communication between the damaged tissues and the outside environment. It is caused by various forces including *deceleration* (a decrease in the speed of a moving object), *acceleration* (an increase in the speed of a moving object), *shearing* (forces occurring across a plane, with structures slipping across each other), *compression* (acute tissue pressure resulting in increased density), and *crushing* (high force that results in tissue destruction). Blunt forces often cause multiple injuries that may affect the head, spinal cord, bones, thorax, and abdomen. Blunt trauma is frequently caused by motor vehicle crashes, falls, assaults, and sports activities.

Penetrating trauma occurs when a foreign object enters the body, causing damage to body structures. Structures commonly affected include the brain, lungs, heart, liver, spleen, the intestines, and the vascular system. Examples of penetrating trauma are gunshot or stab wounds and impalement.

Other types of trauma include inhalation injuries from gases, smoke, or steam, burn or freezing injuries, and blast injuries from explosions. Blast injuries result from the temperature and velocity of air movement and the force of projectiles from the explosion. Blast injuries are more severe in water than in air since blast waves travel farther and faster in water. Trauma from blast injuries includes pulmonary edema and hemorrhage, damage to abdominal organs, burns, penetrating injuries, and ruptured tympanic membranes.

Outcome studies show a correlation between survival rates of multiple trauma victims and rapid response times by pre-hospital providers, coupled with appropriate decision making with regards to transporting victims to a facility capable of treating their injuries. As a result, a system was devised to assist pre-hospital providers to make the appropriate decisions. Trauma patients are classified as Class 1, 2, or 3 based on factors including mechanism of injury, vehicle speed, height of falls, and location of penetrating injuries. Class 3 trauma is the least severe. An example would be a same level fall without loss of consciousness or significant injury. Class 1 trauma involves life-threatening injuries likely to require medical specialists or immediate surgical intervention. While any hospital emergency department should be capable of caring for Class 3 trauma patients, patients meeting Class 1 or 2 criteria should be transported to a designated trauma center when possible. Facilities designated as trauma centers have medical specialists and surgical coverage available or on call 24 hours a day.

Effects of Traumatic Injury

Death is a common result of serious traumatic injury, and may be immediate, early, or late. Immediate death happens within minutes at the scene from such injuries as a torn thoracic aorta or decapitation. Early death occurs during the "golden hour" (the first hour following the injury) from major abdominal or thoracic injuries or progression of intracranial hemorrhage. Appropriate care during this time has been shown to improve survival. Late death generally occurs days or weeks after the injury and results from multiple organ failure, sepsis, and coagulopathies.

Because of the serious consequences of trauma, it is important to rapidly identify the patient's injuries and institute appropriate interventions quickly. Following are common results of trauma and interventions necessary for good outcomes.

Head and Neck Effects—Airway Obstruction

Maintenance of the airway and cervical spine are the highest priority in the trauma patient. Other distracting injuries may take the inexperienced practitioner away from the airway, but if the airway is not patent and the patient is unable to deliver oxygen to vital organs, all other interventions are futile.

Assessment includes determining airway patency. If the patient is unresponsive, manual opening of the airway using a jaw thrust maneuver is necessary. The jaw thrust is recommended in patients with actual and potential C-spine injury. Once the airway is opened, the practitioner must identify any potential obstruction from the tongue, loose teeth, foreign bodies, bleeding, secretions, vomitus, or edema. If the patient is responsive and can vocalize, that is a good indication that the airway is clear.

Any time the nurse performs an intervention it is important that you reassess the effectiveness of the intervention. For example, if you suction the airway to remove vomitus, you would reassess the airway after suctioning to determine if that intervention was successful or if you have to re-suction the airway a second time.

All trauma patients should receive high flow oxygen until stabilized. Assessment of breathing effectiveness is paramount. Assessment should include if the patient has spontaneous breathing, good rise and fall of the chest, determination of skin color, general rate and depth of respirations, abdominal or accessory muscle use, position of the trachea, observation of chest wall integrity and presence of jugular vein distention, bilateral breath sounds, as well as the presence of any surface trauma.

In addition to suctioning, other airway adjuncts available include oral or nasal pharyngeal airways, oxygen delivery devices, laryngeal mask airway, Combitube, and endotracheal intubation (Figure 11–1 ■). Intubation is the preferred method of airway management if the patient is unable to maintain oxygenation or an open airway.

Trauma patients may exhibit several aspects of airway management that are unique and require special preparation and precautions, as discussed next.

CLOSED HEAD INJURY Changes in hemodynamics, oxygenation, and ventilation should be minimized in order to maintain adequate cerebral perfusion pressure. Laryngoscopy causes a marked increase in intracranial pressure (ICP).

The goal is to maintain a $PaCO_2$ of 30–35 mmHg. Lidocaine administered 3–5 minutes prior to intubation can blunt an increase in ICP that is secondary to laryngeal stimulation. In a normotensive patient, beta blockers are given 2–3 minutes prior to intubation to attenuate the sympathetic response. Effective induction agents such as Etomidate or thiopental have not been shown to increase ICP.

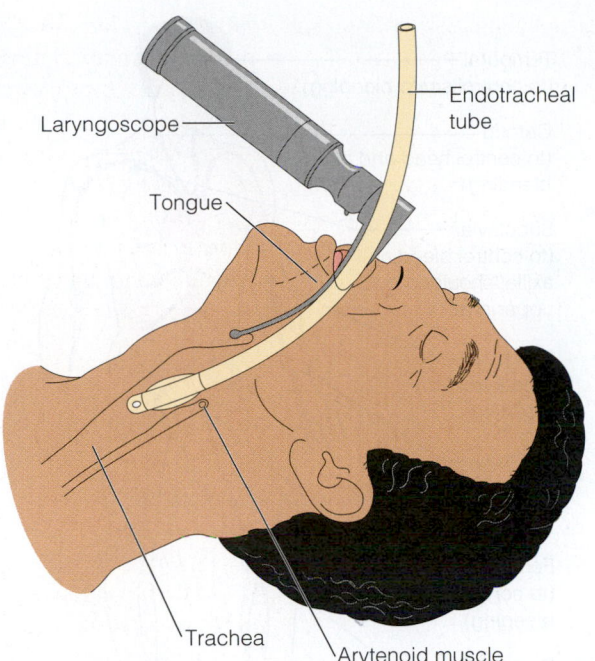

Figure 11–1 ■ Placement of an oral endotracheal tube (ETT) for intubation. When the ETT is in place, air or oxygen can be blown into the external opening of the tube and enter the trachea.

MAXILLOFACIAL TRAUMA   Significant distortion of normal anatomy in facial trauma and respiratory compromise is not uncommon. Even in patients who present with mild respiratory compromise rapid deterioration from edema or hemorrhage can occur. A surgical airway may be the only alternative.

DIRECT AIRWAY TRAUMA   Penetrating trauma to the neck is associated with a high degree of morbidity and mortality. Airway involvement includes dyspnea, cyanosis, subcutaneous emphysema, hoarseness, or air bubbling from the wound. Orotracheal intubation with rapid sequence intubation is the technique of choice. The key is early identification of the need for intubation before the patient has no airway at all. Tracheobronchial injury occurs in approximately 10%–20% of patients with penetrating neck injuries.

CERVICAL SPINE INJURY   Precautions for securing an airway in the presence of a presumed C-spine injury is not unusual. Approximately 3%–6% of major trauma victims have clinically significant C-spine injuries. Oral intubation with manual in-line axial head and neck stabilization (MIAS) is a safe method. There is a decreased probability of C-spine injury if the following criteria are met:

■ Absence of midline cervical spine tenderness
■ Normal alertness
■ Absence of intoxication
■ Absence of a painful distracting injury
■ No focal neurological defects

BURNS   Burn patients with airway compromise require aggressive management. Upper airway edema associated with inhalation or enclosed space fires can progress during the post burn phase. Securing an airway sooner than later is the goal. ∞ See Chapter 17 for nursing care of the patient with burns.

Thoracic Effects

TENSION PNEUMOTHORAX   A **pneumothorax** results when air enters the potential space between the parietal and visceral pleura. The thorax is completely filled by the lungs. Surface tension between the pleural surfaces hold the lungs to the chest wall. Air present in the pleural space will eventually collapse the lungs. A **tension pneumothorax** is life threatening and requires immediate intervention. On inspiration air enters the pleural space, does not escape on expiration, and increases the intrapleural pressure. This pressure collapses the injured lung, shifts the mediastinal contents, compressing the heart, great vessels, trachea, and eventually the uninjured lung. In turn, this causes the following signs and symptoms:

■ Severe respiratory distress
■ Hypotension
■ Jugular vein distension
■ Tracheal deviation toward the uninjured side
■ Cyanosis

The immediate short-term life-saving intervention is a needle thoracostomy, inserting a large bore over the needle catheter into the second intercostal space at the mid-clavicular line (MCL). See Figure 11–2 ■.

FLAIL CHEST   Flail chest is the fracture of two or more ribs in two or more separate locations, leading to an unstable thoracic wall segment. Paradoxical movement of the chest wall is

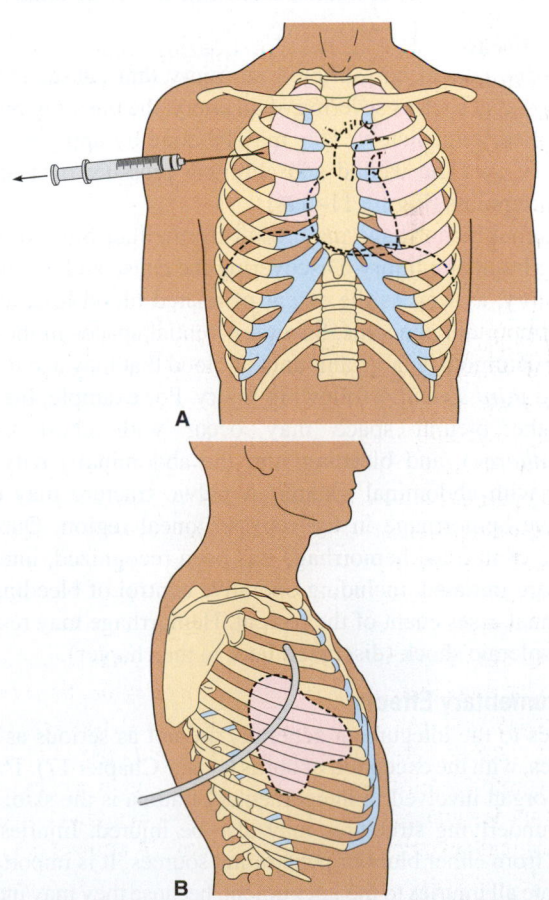

Figure 11–2 ■ A needle thoracostomy may be used in the emergency treatment of a tension pneumothorax. *A,* A large-gauge needle is introduced, and air and fluid are aspirated. *B,* Alternatively, a chest tube may be inserted and connected to a chest drainage system.

Hemo/Pneumothorax Animation

seen with the area sinking into the chest cavity with inspiration and protrusion with expiration. The area must be supported quickly to re-establish the thoracic bellows effect.

THORACIC CONTUSION AND RUPTURE Bruising of thoracic tissue is referred to as contusion. Pulmonary contusion is the most common traumatic chest injury. As a shock wave of force travels through the parenchyma, diffuse hemorrhage and alveolar edema develops, impairing gas exchange. Motor vehicle accidents are the most common cause of pulmonary contusions. Diaphragmatic rupture is a rare traumatic injury but can result in herniation of abdominal contents into the thoracic cavity, causing respiratory compromise.

Myocardial contusion results in extravasation of red blood cells into myocardial fibers. As myocardial cells are injured, it is believed that cardiac output diminishes due to reductions in contractile strength. Myocardial rupture is an acute traumatic tear of any structures of the heart. While rare, myocardial rupture is usually fatal with atrial rupture having the best chance for survival.

Cardiac tamponade occurs when blood or fluid collects in the pericardial sac. Resulting in myocardial compression, this condition is potentially life threatening and should be addressed immediately with pericardiocentesis.

Aortic rupture (transection) can result in acceleration-deceleration injury or blunt chest trauma. This injury is commonly fatal due to profuse bleeding. Aortic rupture is the second most common cause of trauma death after traumatic brain injury.

Hemorrhage

When the patient has suffered an injury that causes external hemorrhage, such as severing of an artery, the bleeding must be controlled immediately. This may be done by applying direct pressure over the wound and applying pressure over arterial pressure points (Figure 11–3 ■).

Internal hemorrhage may result from either blunt or penetrating traumatic injury. Discovering the cause and location of the injury, as well as the extent of related blood loss, are the most important concerns. Several potential spaces in the body can accommodate large amounts of blood that may accumulate (called *third spacing*) following injury. For example, bleeding into the pleural space may occur with chest trauma (*hemothorax*), and bleeding into the abdominal cavity may occur with abdominal trauma. A pelvic fracture may cause massive hemorrhage in the retroperitoneal region. Once the source of internal hemorrhage has been recognized, interventions are initiated, including operative control of bleeding and continual assessment of the patient. Hemorrhage may result in hypovolemic shock (discussed later in the chapter).

Integumentary Effects

Injuries to the integument generally are not as serious as other injuries, with the exception of burns (∞ see Chapter 17). The primary organ involved in integumentary trauma is the skin; however, underlying structures may also be injured. Injuries may result from either blunt or penetrating sources. It is important to evaluate all injuries to the integument, because they may indicate a more serious injury such as an open fracture. Additionally, large wounds may contribute to significant blood loss.

Five specific injuries to the integument are contusions, abrasions, puncture wounds, lacerations, and full thickness avulsion

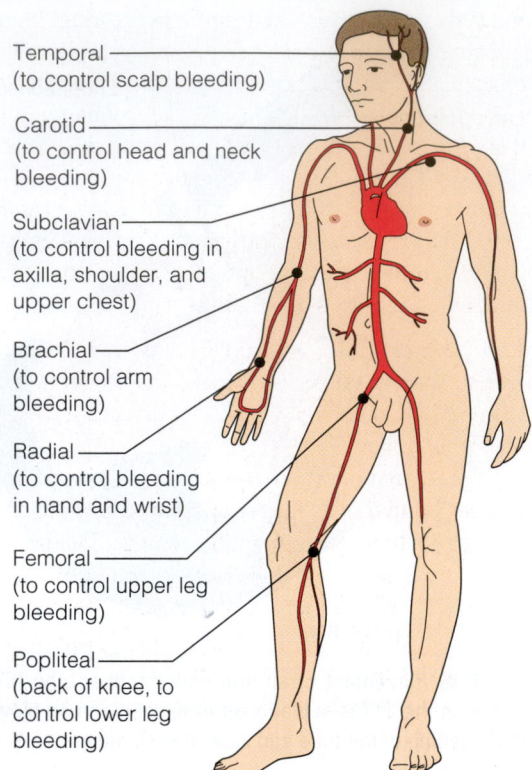

Temporal (to control scalp bleeding)

Carotid (to control head and neck bleeding)

Subclavian (to control bleeding in axilla, shoulder, and upper chest)

Brachial (to control arm bleeding)

Radial (to control bleeding in hand and wrist)

Femoral (to control upper leg bleeding)

Popliteal (back of knee, to control lower leg bleeding)

Figure 11–3 ■ The major pressure points used for the control of bleeding.

injuries (Figure 11–4 ■). **Contusions**, or superficial tissue injuries, result from blunt trauma that causes the breakage of small blood vessels and bleeding into the surrounding tissue. **Abrasions**, or partial-thickness denudations of an area of integument, generally result from falls or scrapes. **Puncture wounds** occur when a sharp or blunt object penetrates the integument. **Lacerations** are

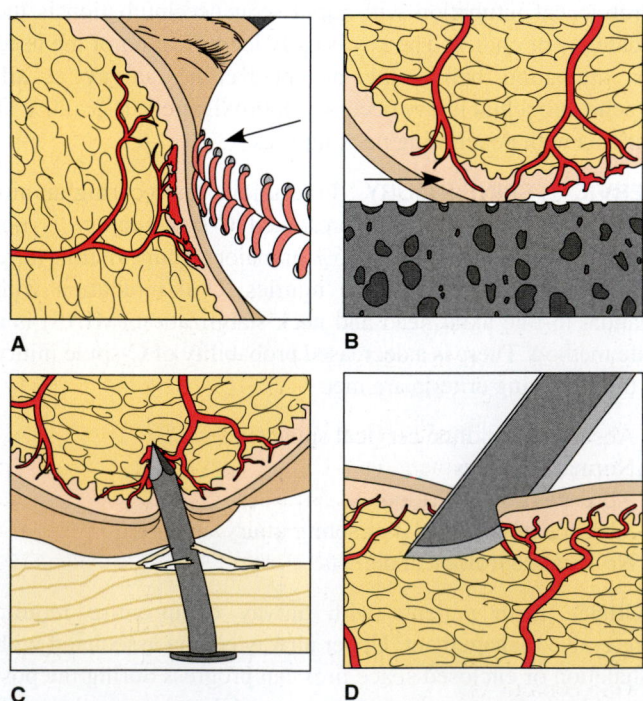

Figure 11–4 ■ Traumatic injuries to the skin include *A*, contusion; *B*, abrasion; *C*, puncture wound; and *D*, laceration.

open wounds that result from sharp cutting or tearing. Injuries to the integument are at risk for contamination from dirt, debris, or foreign objects. Infection may cause further physical stress to the patient with multiple injuries. Full thickness avulsion injuries are injuries that result in loss of all of the layers of the skin, causing fat and muscle to be exposed. The size of the wound impacts both the length of time necessary for healing to take place as well as the risk for infection. These types of injuries are treated by allowing new skin to grow from the edges, stitching the wound together, reattaching avulsed skin, or by skin grafting.

Abdominal Effects

The abdomen contains both solid organs (liver, spleen, and pancreas) and hollow organs (stomach and intestines). Direct trauma to the abdomen can lacerate and compress the solid organs and cause burst injuries to the hollow organs. Blood vessels may be torn and organs may be displaced from their blood supply, producing life-threatening hemorrhage. Damage to the mesenteric vessels supplying the bowel can result in bowel ischemia and infarction. Injury to the stomach, pancreas, and small bowel may allow digestive enzymes to leak out into the abdominal cavity. Rupture of the large bowel results in escape of feces, which causes peritonitis. The immediate threat following abdominal trauma is hemorrhage; the later threat is peritonitis.

Musculoskeletal Effects

Musculoskeletal injuries may occur alone or with multiple injuries as the result of blunt or penetrating trauma. Musculoskeletal injuries usually are not considered a high priority in the care of the patient with multiple injuries. Exceptions are the life- or limb-threatening musculoskeletal injury, such as a dislocated hip, pulseless extremity, or significant blood loss such as from a femur or pelvic fracture. Other exceptions include fractures or dislocations with neurovascular compromise, open fractures, or compartment syndromes. Musculoskeletal injuries may provide clues to the presence of other serious injuries; for example, a fractured clavicle may indicate an associated thoracic injury. Care of the patient who has suffered a musculoskeletal injury is discussed in ∞ Chapter 38.

Neurologic Effects

Head injuries are a common type of injury sustained as the result of trauma. Injuries to the spinal cord, resulting in loss of neurologic function, are devastating outcomes of trauma, but they are much less common than head injuries. Most head and spinal cord injuries result from blunt trauma and are sustained in motor vehicle crashes. Falls, sports injuries, and assault are other sources of neurologic injury. Care of the patient with a neurologic injury is discussed in ∞ Chapters 41 and 42.

Multiple Organ Dysfunction Syndromes (MODS)

Multiple organ dysfunction syndrome (MODS) is a common complication of severe injury and a frequent cause of death in intensive care units. It is a progressive impairment of two or more organ systems. This is the result of an uncontrolled inflammatory response to severe injury or illness.

Patients at risk for MODS are those with a disturbance in homeostasis resulting from one or a combination of the following conditions:

- infection
- injury
- inflammation
- ischemia
- immune response
- intoxication of substances
- iatrogenic factors

The primary organ systems involved in MODS are the respiratory, renal, hepatic, hematologic, cardiovascular, gastrointestinal, and neurological. Supportive therapy depends on the identification of correctable causes. It may be one or a combination of several therapies. Surgical intervention, antibiotic administration, corticosteroid administration, or correction coagulopathies are some therapies used for this condition. MODS following injuries produces more than half of the late mortality following trauma.

Effects on the Family

Trauma usually occurs suddenly and with little warning. It may result in death or cause injury serious enough to alter both the patient's and the family's lives. The suddenness and seriousness of the event are precipitating factors in the development of a psychologic crisis. Over the past decade, some emergency departments have instituted care plans that allow families to be present during resuscitation. This type of care is not without controversy, but it should be considered when appropriate.

Interdisciplinary Care

Interdisciplinary care of the trauma patient depends on a team approach. Providing trauma care with a team focus helps each team member know his or her role. Prompt delegation of tasks and responsibilities improves the patient's chances for survival and decreases the morbidity that may result from traumatic injuries.

Pre-hospital Care

The major functions of pre-hospital care include injury identification, critical interventions, and rapid transport.

INJURY IDENTIFICATION Emergency care of the patient experiencing trauma is based on rapid assessment to identify injuries and begin appropriate interventions. Injuries that indicate the need for trauma center care include the following:

- Penetrating injuries to the abdomen, pelvis, chest, neck, or head
- Spinal cord injuries with deficit
- Crushing injuries to the abdomen, chest, or head
- Major burns
- Injuries leading to airway compromise or obstruction

Many methods help healthcare providers determine the seriousness of the patient's injuries and the potential for survival. Scoring systems such as the Champion Revised Trauma Scoring System can be helpful (Table 11–2). A primary trauma assessment follows an alphabet mnemonic:

- **A** is airway assessment (with C-spine immobilization) to determine if the airway is patent, maintainable, or nonmaintainable.
- **B** is breathing evaluation for spontaneous respirations or ventilatory impedance such as by rib fractures or a collapsed lung.
- **C** is circulatory assessment to palpate peripheral and central pulses; to assess capillary refill, skin color, and temperature; and to identify any external sources of bleeding.
- **D** is disability and refers to the neurovascular status. Assessment includes level of consciousness, pupillary function, and response to verbal or painful stimuli.

TABLE 11–2 Champion Revised Trauma Scoring System

TEST	SCORE	CODED VALUE
Glasgow Coma Scale*	13 to 15	4
	9 to 12	3
	6 to 8	2
	4 to 5	1
	3	0
Systolic blood pressure	> 89	4
	76 to 89	3
	50 to 75	2
	1 to 49	1
	0	0
Respiratory rate	10 to 29	4
	> 29	3
	6 to 9	2
	1 to 5	1
	0	0
Total score:		_____

The highest possible total score is 12. The lowest possible score is 0. The higher the total score, the greater the chance of survival.

*∞ See Chapter 41 for instructions for using the Glasgow Coma Scale.

Note: From "A Revision of the Trauma Score" by H. Champion et al., 1989, **Journal of Trauma**, Vol 29, No 5, p. 624, with permission from Wolters Kluwer Health.

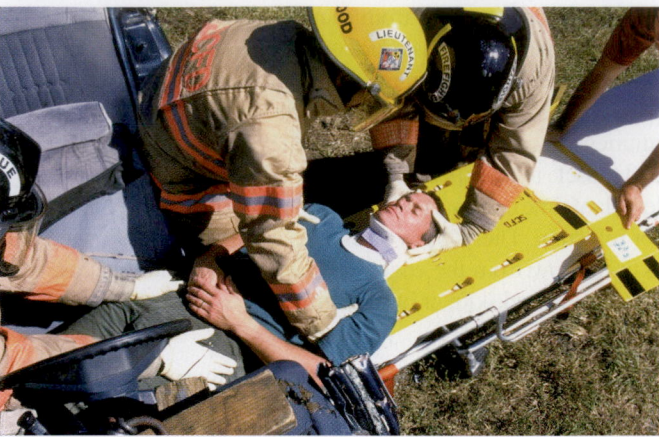

Figure 11–5 ■ Immobilization of the cervical spine at the scene of the accident is essential to preventing further injury to the spinal cord. The combined use of a hard cervical collar, head blocks, and tape best restricts flexion, extension, rotation, and lateral bending of the neck.
Source: Spencer Grant/Photo Researchers, Inc.

- **E** is expose/environment where a whole body assessment is completed while assuring that hypothermia doesn't occur (i.e., heated blankets, warmed intravenous fluids).

Secondary assessment usually begins while the primary assessment is underway. This assessment extends the alphabetical mnemonic:

- **F** is "full set of vital signs." F can also stand for having family members present during treatment.
- **G** is giving comfort measures for both physical and emotional comfort for the patient and family.
- **H** is head-to-toe assessment and medical history that includes visual and manual assessment as well as appropriate auscultation.
- **I** is inspection of posterior surfaces for any injuries.

The Glasgow Coma Scale is another scoring system that is used to quantify the level of consciousness following traumatic brain injury. ∞ See Chapters 41 and 45.

CRITICAL INTERVENTIONS As life-threatening problems are identified during the primary assessment, appropriate on-the-scene interventions must be performed immediately. These include providing life support, immobilizing the cervical spine, managing the airway, and treating hemorrhage and shock.

Immobilization of the patient's cervical spine is a primary intervention. The patient is placed on a spine board, and a cervical collar and a head immobilizer are applied (Figure 11–5 ■). The cervical spine may also be immobilized by logrolling the patient onto a board, placing towel rolls or a head immobilizer along the sides of the patient's head, and securing the patient to the board. If

the patient was wearing a helmet at the time of injury, the helmet should remain on until the patient arrives at the hospital, unless the patient's airway is at risk. If necessary, healthcare personnel at the scene will remove the helmet by manipulating it over the patient's nose and ears while holding the patient's head and neck immobile; safe removal requires at least two people. Improper removal risks injury or additional injury to the spinal cord.

If the patient's airway is patent, oxygen is administered. Ventilations may be assisted with a bag-valve-mask resuscitator until airway management is achieved. Active external bleeding is controlled by direct pressure. Measures to reverse shock (discussed later in the chapter) are initiated.

RAPID TRANSPORT Patients who have multiple injuries must be transported as soon as possible to a regional trauma center. The most common modes of rapid transport are ground ambulance and air ambulance, which includes helicopters specially staffed and equipped to care for trauma victims. Figure 11–6 ■ shows a flight nurse assessing a patient. Stable patients within access of a ground ambulance are best transported by ground. Unstable patients and those injured in the wilderness or other areas in which ground access is difficult may best be transported by air. When these transport systems are unavailable, the patient is transported by any possible means.

Emergency Department Care

DIAGNOSIS The diagnostic tests ordered once the patient reaches the hospital depend on the type of injury the patient has sustained. Tests that may be ordered for victims of trauma include the following:

- *Blood type and crossmatch* involves typing the patient's blood for ABO antigens and Rh factor, screening the blood for antibodies, and crossmatching the patient's serum and donor red blood cells.
- *Complete blood count* evaluates the components of blood including red blood cell count and white blood cell count.
- *Arterial blood gas* evaluates oxygenation, acid–base balance, presence of metabolic or respiratory compensatory mechanisms.

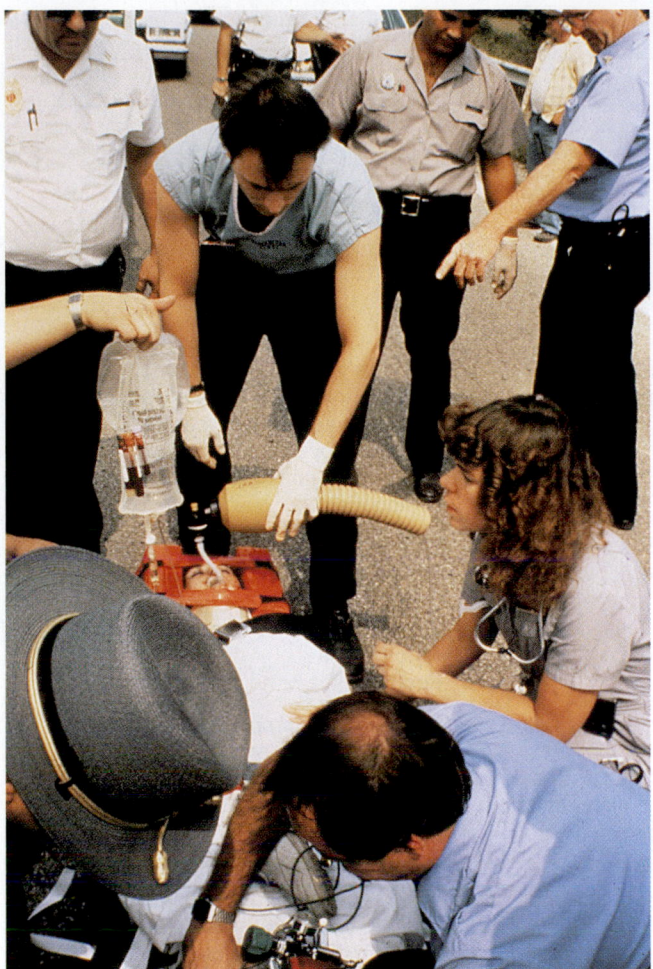

Figure 11–6 ■ Flight nurses provide initial assessment, stabilization, and support for patients with trauma.

Courtesy of University Air Care/University of Cincinnati Hospital.

- *Blood alcohol level* measures the amount of alcohol in a patient's blood. It has been found that between 20% and 50% of people who are injured may be intoxicated. Alcohol alters the patient's level of consciousness and response to pain.
- *Urine drug screen* may also be ordered. Like alcohol, such drugs as cocaine alter the patient's level of consciousness and overall response to the primary survey.
- *Pregnancy test* for any woman of childbearing age rules out the potential for pregnancy and fetal injury.
- *Focused assessment by sonography in trauma (FAST)* primarily focuses on evaluating the identification of blood in body cavities where it is not supposed to be. Primary focus is on the peritoneum. It is also helpful in identification of blood in the pleura and pericardium.
- *Diagnostic peritoneal lavage* determines the presence of blood in the peritoneal cavity, which may indicate abdominal injury. The test is generally done in the emergency department. A local anesthetic (such as lidocaine) is injected subcutaneously, and a small incision is made in the lower abdomen. A catheter is placed into the peritoneal cavity, and any free blood is aspirated. If 10 mL of blood is found, the patient is taken to the operating room for exploratory surgery. If no free blood is aspirated, 1 L of a warm isotonic solution (Ringer's solution or normal saline) is rapidly infused into

the peritoneal cavity and then allowed to drain by gravity. If the solution returns pink and is found to have a red blood cell count of 100,000 mm^3; a white blood cell count of $\geq$ 500; or bile, food, or feces, the test is considered positive and the patient is taken to the operating room for exploratory surgery. This procedure is used less with the inception of the FAST exam. This test does not detect retroperitoneal injuries (injuries of the kidneys, pancreas, great vessels, duodenum, or portions of the ascending or descending colon).
- *Computerized tomography (CT) scans* can discover injuries to the brain, skull, spine, spinal cord, chest, and abdomen.
- *Magnetic resonance imaging (MRI) scans* can discover injuries to the brain and spinal cord.

Medications

Medications used to treat the patient who has experienced trauma depend on the type and severity of the injuries, as well as the degree of traumatic shock that is present. The following general categories of medications may be used. (Fluid administration and the drugs listed are covered later in the chapter in discussion of the collaborative care of the patient in shock.)

- Blood components and crystalloids are administered intravenously in the initial treatment of traumatic shock to replace intravascular volume.
- Inotropic drugs (drugs that increase myocardial contractility) are given to increase cardiac output and improve tissue perfusion. These drugs, administered only after fluid volume restoration, include dopamine (Dopastat, Intropin), dobutamine (Dobutrex), and isoproterenol (Isuprel).
- Vasopressors may be administered in conjunction with fluid replacement to treat neurogenic, septic, or anaphylactic shock. Examples of vasopressors include dopamine (Dopastat), epinephrine (Adrenalin), norepinephrine (Levophed), and phenylephrine (Neo-synephrine).
- Opioids, administered by bolus or continuous infusion, are used to treat pain as soon as possible. However, the effects of the pain medications may alter patient responses to injury, cause hypotension and respiratory depression, and mask potential injuries. If pain medications are administered, they must be carefully regulated, and the patient must be closely monitored.
- Immunization: If the patient has penetrating and open wounds, tetanus immunization status must be determined. If the patient is unable to remember when the last tetanus immunization was given, is unable to answer, or has not received a tetanus immunization within the past 5 years, then tetanus prophylaxis is given.

Blood Transfusions

Blood and blood components are initially produced in the body and then donated for use by another person through a **transfusion** (an infusion of blood or blood components). A patient may be given whole blood, packed red blood cells (RBCs), platelets, plasma, albumin, clotting factors, prothrombin, or cryoprecipitate (Table 11–3). Blood and blood components increase the amount of hemoglobin available to carry oxygen to the cells, improve hemoglobin and hematocrit levels during active bleeding, increase intravascular volume, and replace deficient substances such as platelets and clotting factors.

TABLE 11–3 Volume Resuscitation Therapies

COMPONENT	INDICATIONS	ADVANTAGES	DISADVANTAGES
Ringer's lactate	■ Restoration of circulating volume ■ Replacement of electrolyte deficits	■ Good availability ■ Safe to use ■ Low cost ■ Aids in buffering acidosis	■ Rapid movement from the intravascular to the extravascular space, leading to three or more times requirement for replacement
Normal saline	■ Restoration of circulating volume ■ Vehicle compatible with administration of blood	■ Good availability ■ Low cost ■ Safe to use	■ Hyperchloremic acidosis associated with prolonged use of sodium solutions
Whole blood	■ Replaces blood volume and oxygen carrying capacity in hemorrhage and shock	■ Contains RBCs, plasma proteins, clotting factors, and plasma	■ Contains few platelets or granulocytes; deficient in clotting factors V and VII ■ Greatest risks are for incompatibility or circulatory overload ■ Risk of transmitting blood-borne pathogens
Packed red blood cells (RBCs)	■ Restoration of intravascular volume ■ Replacement of oxygen carrying capacity	■ One unit of RBCs should increase the hemoglobin of a 70 kg adult by approximately 1 gm/dl in the absence of volume overload or continuing blood loss.	■ Red cells require compatibility testing ■ Risk of transmitting blood borne pathogens ■ Should be warmed to prevent hypothermia ■ Contains little or no clotting factors
Platelets	■ Significant thrombocytopenia (platelet count less than 20,000–50,000 per mm^3) ■ Continued hemorrhage	■ Compatibility testing is not required ■ Typical platelet transfusion should raise the platelets of a 70 kg adult approximately 30,000–50,000/UL	■ Post exposure prophylaxis with anti-Rh immune globulin should be considered following Rh+ platelet transfusion to an Rh– woman ■ Risk of transmitting blood-borne pathogens
Albumin	■ Expends blood volume in shock and trauma	■ Good availability	■ Is not a substitute for whole blood ■ Risk of hypersensitivity reactions ■ Risk of transmitting blood-borne pathogens
Fresh frozen plasma (FFP)	■ Documented coagulopathy ■ Restoration of clotting factors ■ Supplies plasma proteins	■ Cross matching and Rh compatibility is not required	■ Must be thawed in a 37°C water bath for approximately 30 minutes ■ Should be ABO compatible ■ Risk of transmitting blood-borne pathogens
Cryoprecipitate	■ Coagulopathy with low fibrinogen ■ Restoration of fibrinogen	■ Rh type not important	■ Risk of transmitting blood-borne pathogens ■ Contains hemagglutinins ■ If large volume of ABO incompatible cryoprecipitate are administered intravascular hemolysis can occur

Each person has one of four blood types: A, B, AB, or O. The blood group antigens A and B, present on RBC membranes, form the basis for the ABO blood categorization. The presence or absence of these inherited antigens determines one's blood type. People with blood type A have A antigens, those with type B have B antigens, those with type AB have both antigens, and those with neither antigen have blood type O (called a universal donor).

> ### FAST FACTS
> ■ Type AB blood is the "universal receiver."
> ■ Type O blood is the "universal donor."

ABO antibodies develop in the serum of people whose RBCs lack the corresponding antigen; these antibodies are called anti-A and anti-B. The person with blood type B has A antibodies, the person with type A has B antibodies, the person with type O has both types of antibodies, and the person with blood type AB has no antibodies (called a universal recipient).

A third antigen on the RBC membrane is D. People who are Rh positive have the D antigen, whereas people who are Rh negative do not. These antigens and antibodies may cause ABO and Rh incompatibilities.

A transfusion of incompatible blood causes hemolysis (breakdown) of the RBCs and agglutination of erythrocytes. (Agglutination is the clumping of cells that results from their interaction with specific antibodies.) The ABO blood group names and compatibilities are listed in Table 11–4.

TABLE 11–4 Blood Group Types and Compatibilities

BLOOD GROUP	RBC AGGLUTINOGENS	SERUM AGGLUTINOGENS	COMPATIBLE DONOR BLOOD GROUPS	INCOMPATIBLE DONOR BLOOD GROUPS
A	A	Anti-B	A, O	B, AB
B	B	Anti-A	B, O	A, AB
AB	A, B	None	A, B, AB, O	None
O	None	Anti-A, Anti-B	O	A, B, AB

Before RBCs or whole blood can be administered, a series of procedures determine donor and recipient ABO types and Rh groups. These procedures, called a type and crossmatch, are performed by mixing the donor cells with the recipient's serum and watching for agglutination. If none occurs, the blood is considered compatible.

Despite meticulous procedures for matching blood types and antigens, blood transfusion reactions may still occur. The most common is a *febrile reaction*. Antibodies within the patient receiving the blood are directed against the donor's white blood cells, causing fever and chills. Febrile reactions typically begin during the first 15 minutes of the transfusion. Using leukocyte-poor blood avoids future febrile reactions.

Hypersensitivity reactions result when antibodies in the patient's blood react against proteins, such as immunoglobulin A, in the donor blood. Hypersensitivity reactions may appear during or after the transfusion. The manifestations of hypersensitivity reaction include *urticaria* (the appearance of reddened wheals of various sizes on the skin) and itching.

Hemolytic reactions, the most dangerous transfusion reactions, usually result from an ABO incompatibility. Clumping RBCs block capillaries, decreasing blood flow to vital organs. In addition, macrophages engulf the clumped RBCs, releasing free hemoglobin into the circulating blood; the hemoglobin is then filtered by the kidneys and may block the renal tubules, causing renal failure. Hemolytic reactions usually begin after infusion of 100 to 200 mL of the incompatible blood. Manifestations of a hemolytic reaction include flushing of the face, a burning sensation along the vein, headache, urticaria, chills, fever, lumbar pain, abdominal pain, chest pain, nausea and vomiting, tachycardia, hypotension, and dyspnea. If any of these manifestations appear, the blood transfusion must be immediately discontinued.

Other risks to patients receiving blood include circulatory overload, electrolyte imbalances, and infectious diseases such as hepatitis or cytomegalovirus.

Patients who have experienced trauma of any severity have had substantial blood loss and are usually in hypovolemic shock. Blood replacement is the treatment of choice to restore oxygen-carrying capacity. Patients in severe shock with active bleeding are given universal, type O red blood cells immediately. Patients with less severe injuries or bleeding may be stabilized with other types of fluids until type-specific or crossmatched blood is available.

Some emergency departments and trauma centers use autotransfusion to provide blood for transfusions for the patient with multiple injuries and/or severe shock. Autotransfusion is a method of blood administration in which special equipment collects and returns the patient's own blood. The chest cavity is the typical source of blood to be autotransfused.

Nursing considerations for blood transfusion therapy are described in the following Medication Administration box.

Emergency Surgery

Immediate surgical intervention is indicated when the patient remains in shock despite resuscitation and there is no obvious external sign of blood loss. Abdominal and chest x-rays, ultrasound studies, diagnostic peritoneal lavage, or CT scan may be performed to help identify the potential source of the blood loss. It is important that the emergency or trauma nurse speak with the family as soon as possible and keep everyone informed about what is happening to his or her family member. Unfortunately, the need for emergency surgery may not allow time for family members or significant others to see their loved one before transfer to the operating room.

Organ Donation

The Uniform Anatomical Gift Act (1968, 1987) requires that people be informed about their options for organ donation. Under this act, consent for organ donation may be given not only by the donor but also by a spouse, adult children, parents, adult siblings, guardian, or any adult authorized to do so. The act also encourages people to carry donor cards.

The increased success of organ transplant has made it a more common and valuable method of prolonging and improving life; however, many people are still waiting for organs, and many people who may be suitable organ donors die each year from trauma. Organs and tissues that may be transplanted include bones, eyes, liver, lungs, skin, muscles and tendons, pancreas, intestines, kidneys, heart, and heart valves.

The organ donation process begins with identification of the potential organ donor. Most people are potential organ donors. Exceptions include those who

- currently abuse intravenous drugs.
- have preexisting untreated infections, such as septicemia.
- have any malignancy other than a primary brain tumor.
- have active tuberculosis.

In the past HIV positive patients were excluded as donors. A recent legislative change now allows HIV positive patients to donate to HIV positive recipients.

The family needs to be made aware of the patient's prognosis and presented with the option of donating the patient's organs. Both the family's and the patient's feelings about

MEDICATION ADMINISTRATION Blood Transfusion

The risk for and seriousness of blood transfusion reactions require that extreme caution be taken when blood is administered. Most fatal transfusion reactions are the result of human error. Although general guidelines are provided here, each institution has specific policies and procedures that must be followed. Prior to beginning the transfusion, the nurse must determine that typed and crossmatched blood is available and collect the needed equipment: a Y-tubing blood administration set with a filter, a large-bore intravenous catheter (usually 18 or 19 gauge), and normal saline solution. Only normal saline is used with a blood transfusion. Dextrose causes clumping of RBCs, and distilled water causes hemolysis.

Nursing Responsibilities
■ Obtain patient consent.
■ Assess for any previous reactions to blood.
■ Explain the procedure to the patient, and answer any questions.
■ Prepare the intravenous equipment. Shut off one side of the Y tubing, and attach the other side to the saline solution. Flush the tubing and filter with the saline.
■ If venous access is not already in place, insert the intravenous needle (following body substance precautions), and begin administering the saline.
■ Using institutional procedure, obtain the blood from the blood bank or laboratory. Administer the blood immediately; if this is not possible, return it to the blood bank or laboratory.
■ Check and document that the donor and recipient blood have been tested and are compatible. This usually involves two nurses, each verifying the following:
   a. an order for blood has been written
   b. type and crossmatch have been done
   c. the name of the patient and the name on the blood bag are identical
   d. the number assigned to the unit of blood is identical to the one on the requisition for the blood
   e. blood type and Rh factor are compatible
   f. the blood has not exceeded its expiration date
   g. the unit of blood is intact and has no bubbles or discoloration
■ Identify the patient by reading the arm band and asking the patient to tell you his or her name. Check the arm band against the unit of blood.
■ Gently invert the blood bag several times to mix the plasma and RBCs.
■ Take and record vital signs as a baseline.
■ Attach the open side of the Y tubing to the blood unit, and begin the transfusion at a slow rate of about 2 mL per minute. (Some trauma patients may have blood infused at a rapid rate. If blood is infused rapidly, it may need to be warmed prior to administration to prevent hypothermia.)

■ Stay with the patient for at least the first 15 minutes of the transfusion, monitoring for manifestations of a reaction and taking the patient's vital signs.
■ Continue to monitor the patient during the transfusion, assessing for manifestations of hypersensitivity or hemolytic reactions and taking and recording vital signs as directed by institutional policy.
■ After the first 15 minutes, the rate of infusion is increased. If there is no danger of fluid volume overload, most patients can tolerate an infusion of a unit of blood (ranging from 250 to 500 mL, depending on the blood component administered) in 2 hours. The unit of blood should be administered in 3 to 4 hours; after this time, it has warmed and begins to deteriorate.
■ Take the following actions if manifestations of a reaction occur:
   a. Stop the infusion of blood immediately, and notify the physician. Continue to infuse the saline.
   b. Take vital signs and assess manifestations.
   c. Compare the blood slip with the unit of blood to ensure that an identification error was not made.
   d. Save the blood bag and any remaining blood for return to the laboratory for further tests to determine the cause of the reaction.
   e. Follow institutional policy for collecting urine and venous blood samples.
   f. Continue to monitor the patient and provide prescribed interventions to treat hypersensitivity or hemolytic manifestations.

Health Education for the Patient and Family
■ The possible risks of blood transfusions include infectious diseases and acquired immune deficiency syndrome (AIDS). However, because of careful handling and storage of blood, bacterial contamination is rare. Although hepatitis may be transmitted by contaminated blood, new tests for hepatitis antibodies in the donor blood are reducing this risk. Many people are afraid of contracting AIDS from blood; however, donor screening and HIV-antibody testing of donor blood has virtually eliminated the transmission of HIV by blood transfusion. A new risk that has been identified is the transmission of West Nile Virus through blood transfusions. Screening for this risk is asking potential donors about the presence of symptoms indicative of West Nile Virus.
■ During the transfusion, immediately report any warm feelings, chills, itching, feelings of weakness or fainting, or difficulty breathing.
■ Report any signs of a delayed transfusion reaction: chills, fever, cough, difficulty breathing, hives, itching, or changes in circulation, and seek medical care immediately.
■ Discuss any religious or cultural considerations related to blood transfusions.

---

organ donation must be explored. Even if the patient carries an organ donation card, many institutions will not remove any organs without a signature from a family member or other authorized person. The nurse must always respect the family's concerns and feelings in this process. Organ procurement agencies employ specially trained personnel who oversee organ donor identification and procurement. These professionals are trained to approach families regarding potential organ donation. Box 11–1 lists **brain death criteria**. Once brain death has been confirmed, the family must also

understand the diagnosis and be allowed time to accept the patient's death.

When caring for an adult patient who is an organ donor, the nurse carries out the following:

■ Maintain systolic blood pressure of 90 mmHg to keep the patient's organs perfused until removal.
■ Maintain urine output at more than 30 mL per hour. This is usually accomplished by administering fluids and/or inotropic agents such as dopamine.
■ Maintain oxygen saturation at 90% or greater.

BOX 11–1 Brain Death Criteria

Clinical Signs
- Irreversible condition
- Apnea with a $PaCO_2$ greater than 60 mmHg
- No response to deep stimuli
- No spontaneous movement (some spinal cord reflexes may be present)
- No gag or corneal reflex
- No oculocephalic or oculovestibular reflex
- Absence of toxic or metabolic disorders

Confirmatory Tests
- Cerebral blood flow study
- Electroencephalogram

Forensic Considerations

Injuries often happen under circumstances that require legal investigation. Many injuries, particularly penetrating trauma, may involve criminal activity. Therefore, the nurse must recognize the need to identify, store, and properly transfer potential evidence for medical–legal investigations.

Each item of clothing removed from the patient must be placed in a breathable container, such as a paper bag, and documented appropriately. Bullets or knives should be labeled, with their source specified, and given to the proper authorities. Holes found in clothing should not be disturbed. When it is necessary to cut off clothing, these areas should be avoided and never cut through if at all possible.

The patient's hands may yield important evidence, such as powder burns or residue on the skin, or tissue or hair samples beneath the fingernails. In the case of death, it is recommended that paper bags be placed over the patient's hands if the presence of evidence is suspected; otherwise, the evidence should be collected by nail clippings.

Identify all wounds and document these findings with pictures, diagrams, or written descriptions. Once the evidence has been collected, identified, and properly stored, ensure that it is given to the appropriate authorities. A chain of custody needs to be maintained throughout the entire process. All evidence must be identified and labeled, and documentation procedures must chronicle where and in whose possession the evidence has been. For the chain of custody to remain intact, the evidence must remain in the continuous possession of identified people and be marked and sealed in tamper-proof containers.

∞ Nursing Care

Nursing care of the patient who has been injured begins with a primary assessment and the initiation of collaborative interventions for any life-threatening injuries. Nursing care is directed toward the patient's specific responses to trauma.

Health Promotion

Prevention efforts can reduce the incidence and severity of trauma. Areas of health promotion and trauma prevention interventions for individuals and communities include the following:

- Motor vehicle safety: seatbelts, airbags, helmets, driving under the influence of alcohol or drugs, reckless driving,

visual or cognitive deficits in the older adult, cell phone use, driver fatigue
- Home safety: snow and ice removal, electrical wiring, falls, burns, drowning
- Farm safety: operating heavy equipment, safe storage of chemicals such as fertilizers
- Work safety: operating work equipment, wearing safety equipment, removal of jewelry
- Relationships: domestic violence, child abuse, elder abuse, or neglect
- Communities: gun control, gangs, condition of streets, neighborhood safety

(In providing information about trauma prevention to members of the community, the nurse serves as a healthcare educator, political activist, and safety advocate.)

Assessment

See Interdisciplinary Care for assessment of the patient experiencing trauma.

Nursing Diagnoses and Interventions

The trauma patient has many complex and interrelated actual or potential alterations in health. The nursing care in this section focuses on patient and family problems with respirations, infection, immobility, and spirituality. Nursing interventions for decreased cardiac output and altered perfusion are discussed in the section of the chapter on nursing care of the patient in shock. See the accompanying Case Study & Nursing Care Plan on page 252.

EVIDENCE FOR NURSING CARE — The Patient with Brain Death

Selected resources that nurses may find helpful when planning evidence-based nursing care follow.

- Arbour, R. (2009). Cardiogenic oscillation and ventilator autotriggering in brain-dead patients: A case series. *American Journal of Critical Care, 18*(5), 496, 488–495.
- Catlin, A. J. & Volat, D. (2009). When the fetus is alive but the mother is not: Critical care somatic support as an accepted model of care in the twenty-first century? *Critical Care Nursing Clinics of North America, 21*(2), 267–276.
- Greer, D. M., Varelas, P. N., Haque, S., & Wijdicks, E. F. M. (2008). Variability of brain death determination guidelines in leading US neurologic institutions. *Neurology, 70*(4), 284–289.
- Linde, E. B. (2009). Speaking up for organ donors. *Nursing2009, 39*(1), 29–31.
- Recommendations for end-of-life care in the intensive care unit: A consensus statement by the American Academy of Critical Care Medicine. (2008). National Guideline Clearinghouse. Retrieved from http://www.guideline.gov/summary/summary.aspx?doc_id=12655&nbr=006550&string=brain+AND+death
- Wijdicks, E. F. M., Rabinstein, A. A., Manno, E. M. & Atkinson, J. D. (2008). Pronouncing brain death: Contemporary practice and safety of the apnea test. *Neurology, 71*(16), 1240–1244.

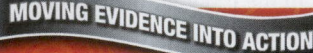

MOVING EVIDENCE INTO ACTION | The Care of ICU Patients

SUSTAINING MULTIPLE TRAUMA

Ventilator-associated pneumonia (VAP) is an important patient safety issue in critically injured patients. The purpose of this study (Dodek, 2004) was to develop an evidenced-based guideline for prevention of ventilator-assisted pneumonia.

Data extraction consisted of gathering physical, positional, and pharmacologic interventions that may influence the development of VAP. The authors searched for pertinent randomized trails and case reviews that involved patients on mechanical ventilation. The study was isolated to include only adults and only studies published before 1 April 2003 were considered.

Physical strategies included the following:
- Route of endotracheal intubations
- Systematic search for maxillary sinusitis
- Frequency of ventilator circuit changes
- Airway humidification
- Endotracheal suctioning system
- Sublette secretion drainage
- Chest physiology
- Timing of tracheotomy

Positional strategies included the following:
- Kinetic bed therapy
- Semi-recumbent positioning
- Prone positioning

Pharmacologic strategies include the following:
- Stress ulcer prophylaxis
- Prophylactic antibiotics, including selective decontamination of the digestive track

IMPLICATIONS FOR NURSING

The following section identifies pertinent findings to support the conclusion that effectively implemented guidelines may decrease the morbidity, mortality, and costs of VAP in mechanically ventilated patients.

Based on direct evidence the following recommendations are encouraged:
- Alternatively, orotracheal intubations should be used when intubation is necessary.
- Recommend that new circuits for each patient be instituted and changed if the circuits become soiled.
- Recommend weekly changes of heat and moisture exchangers on equipment providing mechanical ventilation.
- Recommend the use of closed endotracheal suction systems that are changed for each new patient and as clinically indicated.
- Recommend that clinicians consider the use of subglottic secretion drainage.
- Recommend that clinicians consider the use of kinetic beds.
- Recommend the use of semi-recumbent positioning, with a goal of 45 degrees, in patients without contraindications.

The pharmacologic strategies that were studied were unfounded and not recommended for the VAP guideline.

CRITICAL THINKING IN PATIENT CARE

1. Considering the information from this study, how would you communicate the recommendations to the medical staff for the patient with mechanical ventilation?
2. What is the rationale behind the preceding recommendations?

Ineffective Airway Clearance

The patient with multiple injuries is at great risk for developing airway obstruction and apnea. Facial injuries, loose teeth, blood, and vomitus increase the risk for aspiration and obstruction. Neurologic injuries and cerebral edema alter the patient's respiratory drive and ability to keep the airway clear.

- Assess if airway is patent, maintainable, or nonmaintainable. Assess for manifestations of airway obstruction: stridor, tachypnea, bradypnea, cough, cyanosis, dyspnea, decreased or absent breath sounds, changes in oxygen levels, and changes in level of consciousness. *Assessing the airway and initiating interventions are the first steps in managing the patient with multiple injuries.*
- Monitor oxygen saturation by applying a pulse oximeter. Adjust oxygen flow to maintain oxygen saturation from 94% to 100%. *Changes in oxygen saturation as measured by the pulse oximeter indicate the effectiveness of the patient's airway. Pulse oximetry in patients who have been exposed to carbon monoxide (i.e., house fires) is unreliable since it cannot differentiate carboxyhemoglobin from oxyhemoglobin.*
- Monitor level of consciousness. *An early sign of an ineffective airway is change in the patient's behavior. If the patient becomes restless, anxious, combative, or unresponsive, the effectiveness of the airway needs to be immediately evaluated and appropriate interventions initiated.*

Risk for Infection

Traumatic injuries are considered dirty wounds. Projectiles enter the body through dirty surfaces and clothing, carrying dirt and debris into the wound. Open fractures provide a portal for the entry of bacteria and dirt. Even with surgical intervention, the wounds often remain contaminated.

- Use careful hand hygiene practices. *Hand hygiene remains the single most important factor in preventing the spread of infection.*
- Use strict standard precautions and aseptic technique when caring for wounds. *Standard precautions are essential to protect the patient and the nurse from infection.* In addition,
  - monitor wounds for odor, redness, heat, swelling, and copious or purulent drainage.
  - monitor hidden wounds, such as those under casts, by asking the patient whether the pain has increased and observing for increased drainage and heat over the area of the wound.
  - ensure that cross-contamination between wounds does not occur. Collect drainage in ostomy bags if it is copious. *The skin is the first line of defense against infection. Wounds provide a portal of entry for organisms. Risk factors for wound infection include contamination, inadequate wound care, and the condition of the wound at the time of closure. Aseptic techniques used in applying and changing dressings reduce the entry of organisms.*

- Take and record vital signs, including temperature, every 2 to 4 hours. *Vital signs, particularly an elevated body temperature, indicate the presence of an infection.*
- Provide adequate fluids and nutrition. *Adequate fluids, calories, and protein are essential to wound healing.*
- Assess for manifestations of gas gangrene: fever, pain, and swelling in traumatized tissues; drainage with a foul odor. *Gas gangrene is usually caused by the organism* Clostridium perfringens. *This bacterium is found in the soil and can be introduced into the body during a traumatic injury. The organism grows in the tissues, causing necrosis; hydrogen and carbon dioxide are released, with resultant swelling of tissues. If the infection continues, tissues are progressively destroyed, and sepsis and death may result.*
- Assess for development of potentially life-threatening conditions such as necrotizing fasciitis where flesh-eating bacteria infect subcutaneous and dermal layers, spreading to the fascial plane. *Many types of bacteria can cause necrotizing fasciitis; however, the methicillin-resistant* Staphylococcus aureus *is occurring with increasing frequency.*
- Assess the status of tetanus immunization and administer tetanus toxoid or human toxin-antitoxin (TAT) as prescribed. *Tetanus is caused by an exotoxin produced by* Clostridium tetani, *usually introduced through an open wound. The organism is commonly found in the soil.*
- Use strict aseptic technique when inserting catheters, suctioning, administering parenteral medications, or performing any other invasive procedure. *Using aseptic technique during invasive procedures reduces the risk of entry of organisms.*

Impaired Physical Mobility

The patient with trauma injuries is often unable to change positions independently and is at risk for complications of the integumentary, cardiovascular, gastrointestinal, respiratory, musculoskeletal, and renal systems. Patients at greatest risk are those who have had multiple injuries, spinal cord injuries, peripheral nerve injuries, and traumatic amputations. Collaborate with the physical therapist and occupational therapist (if available) to determine the most effective types and schedule of exercises and assistive devices.

- If active bleeding or edema is not present, provide active or passive exercises to affected and unaffected extremities at least once every 8 hours. *Exercise improves muscle tone, maintains joint mobility, improves circulation, and prevents contractures.*
- Help the patient turn, cough, and deep breathe and use the incentive spirometer at least every 2 hours. *Changing positions, coughing, deep breathing, and incentive spirometry reduce the risk of integumentary and respiratory complications.*
- If the patient is unable to be moved and positioned, consider a specialty bed, such as the kinetic continuous rotation bed (Figure 11–7 ■). *The kinetic continuous rotation bed allows continuous turning of the patient; the motion decreases pulmonary complications, venous stasis, postural hypotension, urinary stasis, muscle wasting, and bone demineralization.*
- Monitor the lower extremities each day for manifestations of deep vein thrombosis: heat, swelling, and pain. Measure and record the circumference of the thigh and calf each day. If antiemboli stockings or intermittent compression stockings

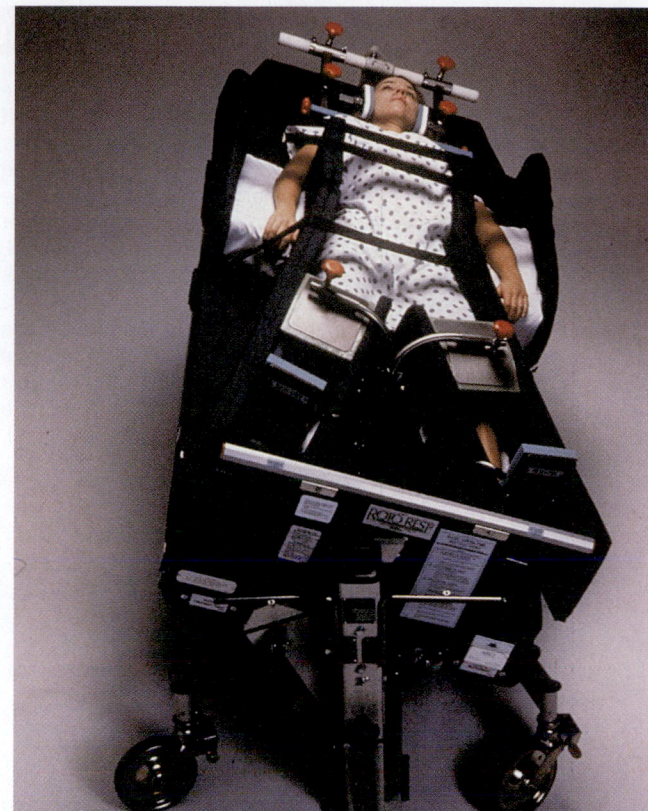

Figure 11–7 ■ A kinetic continuous rotation bed provides a means of turning the patient with multiple injuries to decrease the hazards of immobility.
Courtesy of Kinetic Concepts, Inc.

are used, remove them for 1 hour during each shift and assess the skin. *Venous stasis results when surrounding muscles are unable to contract and help move the blood through the veins. Thrombus (clot) formation in deep veins is a major risk for pulmonary embolism.*

Spiritual Distress

Trauma generally strikes without warning and carries potentially devastating consequences, including severe alterations in the lives of the victim and family, and death. The traumatic death of a loved one may be the most difficult event a family may ever experience. The decision to cease life support systems or to donate organs challenges the family's belief systems and psychologic stability. Nursing care of the family (or patient) experiencing spiritual distress includes the following:

- Offer referral to spiritual advisor if needed. *Most hospitals have chaplain programs.*
- Give the family information about the option to donate the patient's organs. *The decision to donate organs needs to be based on information about the patient's condition, prognosis, and criteria by which brain death is determined. It is important to convey to family members that organ donation is only an option and that they should not feel they are obligated to consent or are doing something wrong if they do not consent.*
- Encourage the family to ask questions and express any feelings about the traumatic event and/or organ donation. *Allowing families to express their feelings may help prevent long-term consequences such as guilt.*

CASE STUDY & NURSING CARE PLAN   A Patient with Multiple Injuries

Jane Souza is a 25-year-old married woman with two children who provides day care for preschool children in her home. As she is driving the interstate at 65 miles per hour, a car crosses the median and strikes her vehicle head-on. Mrs. Souza, who is not wearing a seat belt, is thrown forward against the steering wheel. The front of her car is pushed up against her by the car that struck her, entrapping her lower extremities.

After extensive efforts to extricate her from the car, Jane is transported to the local trauma center. She is still conscious, is receiving high-flow oxygen by mask, and has one intravenous line in place. Her vital signs are a palpable systolic blood pressure of 80, a pulse rate of 120, and a respiratory rate of 36. On arrival, she states that she is having difficulty breathing.

ASSESSMENT

- Airway: Maintainable with high-flow oxygen in place.
- Breathing: Respiratory rate of 36, multiple bruising and abrasions on right side of her chest, decreased breath sounds on the right side.
- Circulation: No palpable radial pulses; palpable brachial pulses. Monitor shows sinus tachycardia. No active external bleeding noted. Skin color pale, cool to the touch, and diaphoretic. One intravenous line already established.
- Neurologic: Moved her fingers when asked; complains of difficulty breathing; denies that she is hurt. Pupils 4 mm, equal, and react to light. Has a broken right arm and an open fracture of the left ankle; because of these injuries, extremity movement is limited.

Because of Mrs. Souza's respiratory distress, she is intubated and ventilated with 100% oxygen. Another intravenous line is inserted and O-negative blood administered. It is determined that Jane has sustained a pneumothorax in the right side and a chest tube is inserted.

DIAGNOSES

- *Ineffective Breathing Pattern* related to multiple bruises and abrasions on the right side of the chest, and respiratory difficulty

- *Deficient Fluid Volume* related to acute internal blood loss (presumed because no active bleeding can be found)
- *Risk for Injury* related to trauma resuscitation

EXPECTED OUTCOMES

- Maintain adequate oxygenation.
- Maintain adequate circulating blood volume.

PLANNING AND IMPLEMENTATION

- Monitor airway and assist in any needed airway management.
- Explain all procedures.
- Monitor the effects of fluid and blood administration, including any changes in blood pressure and pulse.
- Prepare for transfer to the operating room for emergency surgery.
- Keep family informed about her condition.

EVALUATION

Mrs. Souza is transferred to the operating room, where it is determined that she has a ruptured spleen and a serious pelvic fracture. Her treatment continues in the operating room.

CRITICAL THINKING IN THE NURSING PROCESS

1. Is the nursing diagnosis Deficient Fluid Volume appropriate for Jane Souza? Why or why not?
2. The assessment of a patient who has experienced trauma is, in order, A = airway, B = breathing, and C = circulation. What is the rationale for this sequence?
3. Following surgery, Mrs. Souza is moved to the surgical intensive care unit. She is very anxious and restless. What methods of assessments would help you identify the cause of her restlessness?
4. Infection is a common complication for the trauma patient. Describe five risks for infection that are present from the time of injury to the time of hospital discharge.

See Evaluating Your Response in Appendix C.

- Refer the family for follow-up care. Long-term follow-up is important for the family facing the sudden death of a loved one. *Grieving is not an overnight process, and providing the family with resources that may be used in the future may help prevent future crises and dysfunction.* (For more information, ∞ see Chapter 5.)

Post-traumatic Stress Disorder

Post-traumatic stress disorder is an intense, sustained emotional response to a disastrous event. It is also referred to as post-trauma syndrome. It is characterized by emotions that range from anger to fear and by flashbacks or psychic numbing. In the initial stage, the patient may be calm or may express feelings of anger, disbelief, terror, and shock. In the long-term phase, which begins anywhere from a few days to several months after the event, the patient often experiences flashbacks and nightmares of the traumatic event. The patient may call on ineffective coping mechanisms, such as alcohol or drugs, and withdraw from relationships.

- Assess emotional responses while providing physical care. Observe for crying, sleep problems, suspiciousness, and fear

during the initial phase of treatment. If the patient is unconscious, encourage family members and friends to express their feelings. *These assessments provide valuable information about the patient's ability to cope with the trauma.*

- Be available if the patient wishes to talk about the trauma, and encourage expression of feelings. *The patient may initially deny negative feelings; this denial is a coping mechanism in the initial phase of recovery.*
- Teach relaxation techniques, such as deep breathing, progressive muscle relaxation, or imagery (∞ see Chapter 4). *These techniques are often useful in coping when thoughts of the trauma recur.*
- Refer the patient and family members for counseling, psychotherapy, or support groups as appropriate. *Continued therapy may be necessary in assisting the patient and family to resolve the acute and long-term effects of trauma.*

Using NANDA, NIC, and NOC

Linkages between a selected NANDA nursing diagnosis, NIC, and NOC for the patient experiencing trauma are shown in the chart that follows.

Community-based Care

Address the following topics to prepare the patient and family for home care:

- The type of home environment to which the patient will be returning, including any changes that will be required to let the patient function in that environment
- Medications, dressings, wound care, equipment, and supplies
- Special diet, if needed
- Rehabilitation plan and its effect on the patient's family
- Follow-up appointments with the physician or at the trauma clinic
- Emotional changes that the patient may undergo as a result of the trauma
- Helpful resources:
  - Home health care
  - Community support groups
  - National Institute of Neurological Disorders and Stroke

The Patient Experiencing Shock

Shock is a clinical syndrome characterized by a systemic imbalance between oxygen supply and demand. This imbalance results in a state of inadequate blood flow to body organs and tissues, causing life-threatening cellular dysfunction.

Overview of Cellular Homeostasis and Hemodynamics

To maintain cellular metabolism, cells of all body organs and tissues require a regular and consistent supply of oxygen and the removal of metabolic wastes. This homeostatic regulation is maintained primarily by the cardiovascular system and depends on four physiologic components.

1. A cardiac output sufficient to meet bodily requirements
2. An uncompromised vascular system, in which the vessels have a diameter sufficient to allow unimpeded blood flow and have good tone (the ability to constrict or dilate to maintain normal pressure)

3. A volume of blood sufficient to fill the circulatory system, and a blood pressure adequate to maintain blood flow
4. Tissues that are able to extract and use the oxygen delivered through the capillaries

In a healthy person, these components function as a system to maintain tissue perfusion.

During shock, however, one or more of these components are disrupted. An understanding of basic hemodynamics is necessary to understand the pathophysiology of shock.

- Stroke volume (SV) is the amount of blood pumped into the aorta with each contraction of the left ventricle.
- Cardiac output (CO) is the amount of blood pumped per minute into the aorta by the left ventricle. CO is determined by multiplying the SV by the heart rate (HR): CO = SV × HR.
- Systemic vascular resistance (SVR) is the resistance offered by the peripheral circulation.

> **PRACTICE ALERT**
> Cardiac Output (CO) = Stroke Volume (SV) × Heart Rate (HR).

- Mean arterial pressure (MAP) is the product of cardiac output and SVR: MAP = CO × SVR. It can also be calculated as MAP = [(2x diastolic BP) + systolic BP] / 3. When CO, SVR, or total blood volume rises, MAP and tissue perfusion increase. Conversely, when CO, SVR, or total blood volume falls, MAP and tissue perfusion decrease. A MAP of 70 to 110 is normal. A MAP of 60 mmHg is required to maintain adequate perfusion to the brain, heart, and kidneys.
- The sympathetic nervous system maintains the smooth muscle surrounding the arteries and arterioles in a state of partial contraction called sympathetic tone. Increased sympathetic stimulation increases vasoconstriction and SVR; decreased sympathetic stimulation allows vasodilatation, which decreases SVR.

Pathophysiology

When one or more cardiovascular components do not function properly, the body's hemodynamic properties are altered. Consequently, tissue perfusion may be inadequate to sustain normal cellular metabolism. The result is the clinical syndrome known as shock. The manifestations of shock result from the body's attempts to maintain vital organs (heart and brain) and to preserve life following a drop in cellular perfusion. However, if the injury or condition triggering shock is severe enough or of long enough duration, cellular hypoxia and cellular death occur.

Shock is triggered by a sustained drop in mean arterial pressure. This drop can occur after a decrease in cardiac output, a decrease in the circulating blood volume, or an increase in the size of the vascular bed due to peripheral vasodilatation. If intervention is timely and effective, the physiologic events that characterize shock may be stopped; if not, shock may lead to death.

Stage I: Early, Reversible, and Compensatory Shock

The initial stage of shock begins when baroreceptors in the aortic arch and the carotid sinus detect a sustained drop in MAP of less than 10 mmHg from normal levels. The circulating blood volume may decrease (usually to less then 500 mL), but not enough to cause serious effects.

The body reacts to the decrease in arterial pressure. The cerebral integration center initiates the body's response systems, causing the sympathetic nervous system to increase the heart rate and the force of cardiac contraction, thus increasing cardiac output. Sympathetic stimulation also causes peripheral vasoconstriction, resulting in increased systemic vascular resistance and a rise in arterial pressure. The net result is that the perfusion of cells, tissues, and organs is maintained. Symptoms are almost imperceptible during the early stage of shock. The pulse rate may be slightly elevated. If the injury is minor or of short duration, arterial pressure is usually maintained, and no further symptoms occur.

Compensatory shock begins after the MAP falls 10 to 15 mmHg below normal levels. The circulating blood volume is reduced by 25% to 35% (1000 mL or more), but compensatory mechanisms are able to maintain blood pressure and tissue perfusion to vital organs, thereby preventing cell damage.

- Stimulation of the sympathetic nervous system results in the release of epinephrine from the adrenal medulla and the release of norepinephrine from the adrenal medulla and the sympathetic fibers. Both hormones rapidly stimulate the alpha- and beta-adrenergic fibers. Stimulated alpha-adrenergic fibers cause vasoconstriction in the blood vessels supplying the skin and most of the abdominal viscera. Perfusion of these areas decreases. Stimulated beta-adrenergic fibers cause vasodilatation in vessels supplying the heart and skeletal muscles (beta one response), and increase the heart rate and force of cardiac contraction (beta two response). Further, blood vessels in the respiratory system dilate, and the respiratory rate increases (beta two response). Thus, stimulation of the sympathetic nervous system results in increased cardiac output and oxygenation of these tissues.
- The renin-angiotensin response occurs as the blood flow to the kidneys decreases. Renin released from the kidneys acts on angiotensinogen to form angiotensin I. This is converted by angiotensin converting enzyme in the lungs to angiotensin II, which causes vasoconstriction and stimulates the adrenal cortex to release aldosterone. Aldosterone causes the kidneys to reabsorb water and sodium and to lose potassium. The absorption of water maintains circulating blood volume while increased vasoconstriction increases SVR, maintaining central vascular volume and raising blood pressure.
- The hypothalamus releases adrenocorticotropic hormone (ACTH), causing the adrenal glands to secrete aldosterone. Aldosterone promotes the reabsorption of water and sodium by the kidneys, preserving blood volume and pressure.
- The posterior pituitary gland releases antidiuretic hormone (ADH), which increases renal reabsorption of water to increase intravascular volume. The combined effects of hormones released by the hypothalamus and posterior pituitary glands work to conserve central vascular volume.
- As MAP falls in the compensatory stage of shock, decreased capillary hydrostatic pressure causes a fluid shift from the interstitial space into the capillaries. The net gain of fluid raises the blood volume.

Working together, these compensatory mechanisms can maintain MAP for only a short period of time. During this period, the perfusion and oxygenation of the heart and brain are adequate. If effective treatment is provided, the process is arrested, and no permanent damage occurs. However, unless the underlying cause of shock is reversed, these compensatory mechanisms soon become harmful, and shock perpetuates shock.

Stage II: Intermediate or Progressive Shock

The progressive stage of shock occurs after a sustained decrease in MAP of 20 mmHg or more below normal levels and a fluid loss of 35% to 50% (1800 to 2500 mL of fluid). Although the compensatory mechanisms in the previous state remain activated, they are no longer able to maintain MAP at a level sufficient to ensure perfusion of vital organs.

The vasoconstriction response that first helped sustain MAP eventually limits blood flow to the point that cells become oxygen deficient. To remain alive, the affected cells switch from aerobic to anaerobic metabolism. The lactic acid formed as a by-product of anaerobic metabolism contributes to an acidotic state at the cellular level. As a result, adenosine triphosphate (ATP), the source of cellular energy, is produced inefficiently. Lacking energy, the sodium-potassium pump fails. Potassium moves out of the cell, while sodium and water move inward. As this process continues, the cell swells, cell membrane integrity is lost, and cell organelles are damaged. Lysosomes within the cell spill out their digestive enzymes, which disintegrate any remaining organelles. Some enzymes spread to adjacent cells, where they erode and rupture cell membranes.

The acid by-products of anaerobic metabolism dilate the precapillary arterioles and constrict the postcapillary venules. This causes increased hydrostatic pressure within the capillary, and fluid shifts back into the interstitial space. The capillaries also become increasingly permeable, allowing serum proteins to shift from the vascular space into the interstitium. The buildup of plasma proteins increases the osmotic pressure in the interstitium, further accelerating the fluid shift out of the capillaries.

Throughout this period, the heart rate and vasoconstriction increase; however, perfusion of the skin, skeletal muscles, kidneys, and gastrointestinal organs is greatly diminished. Cells in the heart and brain become hypoxic while other body cells and tissues become ischemic and anoxic. A generalized state of acidosis and hyperkalemia ensues (∞ see Chapter 10). Unless this stage of shock is treated rapidly, the patient's chances of survival are poor.

Stage III: Refractory or Irreversible Shock

If shock progresses to the irreversible stage, tissue anoxia becomes so generalized and cellular death so widespread that no treatment can reverse the damage. Even if MAP is temporarily restored, too much cellular damage has occurred to maintain life. Death of cells is followed by death of tissues, which results in death of organs. Death of vital organs contributes to subsequent death of the body.

Effects of Shock on Body Systems

Whatever its causes, shock produces predictable effects on the body's organ systems. (See the Multisystem Effects of Shock feature on page 255.)

CARDIOVASCULAR SYSTEM The perfusion and oxygenation of the heart are adequate in the early stages of shock. As shock progresses, myocardial cells become hypoxic, and myocardial

MULTISYSTEM EFFECTS OF
Shock

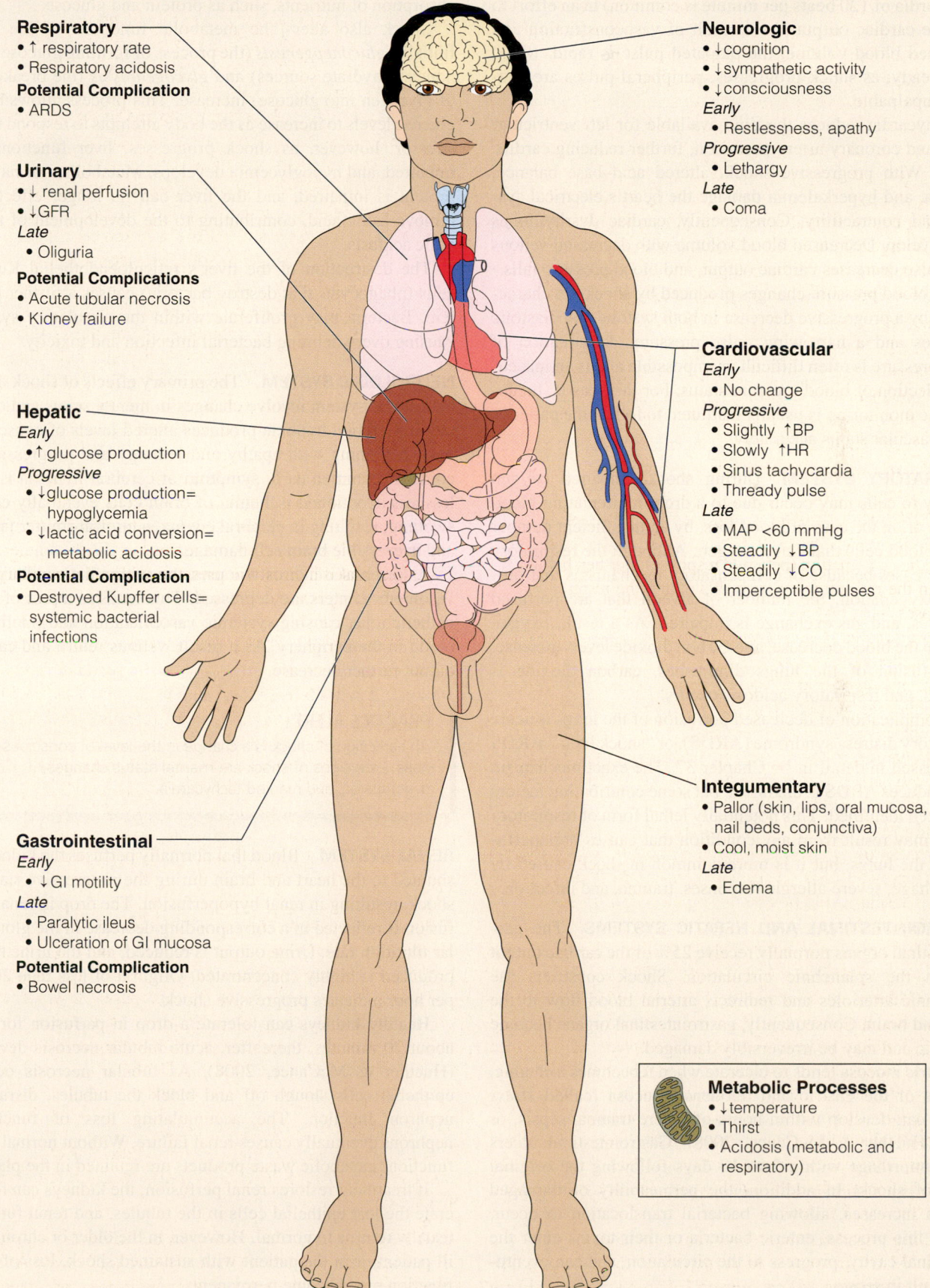

Respiratory
- ↑ respiratory rate
- Respiratory acidosis

Potential Complication
- ARDS

Urinary
- ↓ renal perfusion
- ↓GFR

Late
- Oliguria

Potential Complications
- Acute tubular necrosis
- Kidney failure

Hepatic
Early
- ↑ glucose production

Progressive
- ↓glucose production=
  hypoglycemia
- ↓lactic acid conversion=
  metabolic acidosis

Potential Complication
- Destroyed Kupffer cells=
  systemic bacterial
  infections

Gastrointestinal
Early
- ↓GI motility

Late
- Paralytic ileus
- Ulceration of GI mucosa

Potential Complication
- Bowel necrosis

Neurologic
- ↓cognition
- ↓sympathetic activity
- ↓consciousness

Early
- Restlessness, apathy

Progressive
- Lethargy

Late
- Coma

Cardiovascular
Early
- No change

Progressive
- Slightly ↑BP
- Slowly ↑HR
- Sinus tachycardia
- Thready pulse

Late
- MAP <60 mmHg
- Steadily ↓BP
- Steadily ↓CO
- Imperceptible pulses

Integumentary
- Pallor (skin, lips, oral mucosa,
  nail beds, conjunctiva)
- Cool, moist skin

Late
- Edema

Metabolic Processes
- ↓temperature
- Thirst
- Acidosis (metabolic and
  respiratory)

muscle function diminishes. Initially, the blood pressure may be normal or even slightly elevated (as a result of compensatory mechanisms) and the heart rate only slightly increased. Sympathetic stimulation increases the heart rate (a sinus tachycardia of 120 beats per minute is common) in an effort to increase cardiac output. As a result of vasoconstriction and decreased blood volume, the palpated pulse is rapid, weak, and thready; as shock progresses, peripheral pulses are usually nonpalpable.

Tachycardia reduces the time available for left ventricular filling and coronary artery perfusion, further reducing cardiac output. With progressive shock, altered acid–base balance, hypoxia, and hyperkalemia damage the heart's electrical systems and contractility. Consequently, cardiac dysrhythmias may develop. Decreased blood volume with decreased venous return also decreases cardiac output, and blood pressure falls.

The blood pressure changes produced by shock are characterized by a progressive decrease in both systolic and diastolic pressures and a narrowing pulse pressure. Auscultation of blood pressure is often difficult or impossible and is an inaccurate reflection of blood pressure status. For this reason, hemodynamic monitoring is usually instituted to follow the patient's cardiovascular status accurately.

RESPIRATORY SYSTEM   During shock, impaired oxygen delivery to cells may occur due to a drop in circulating blood volume or, in the case of blood loss, by an insufficient number of red blood cells that carry oxygen. Although the respiratory rate increases because of compensatory mechanisms that promote oxygenation, the number of alveoli that are perfused decreases, and gas exchange is impaired. As a result, oxygen levels in the blood decrease, and carbon dioxide levels increase. As perfusion of the lungs diminishes, carbon dioxide is retained, and respiratory acidosis occurs.

A complication of decreased perfusion of the lungs is acute respiratory distress syndrome (ARDS), or "shock lung." ARDS is discussed in detail in ∞ Chapter 37. The exact mechanism that produces ARDS is unknown, but some contributing factors have been identified. This potentially lethal form of respiratory failure may result from any condition that causes hypoperfusion of the lungs, but it is more common in shock caused by hemorrhage, severe allergic responses, trauma, and infection.

GASTROINTESTINAL AND HEPATIC SYSTEMS   The gastrointestinal organs normally receive 25% of the cardiac output through the splanchnic circulation. Shock constricts the splanchnic arterioles and redirects arterial blood flow to the heart and brain. Consequently, gastrointestinal organs become ischemic and may be irreversibly damaged.

Gastric mucosa tends to ulcerate when it becomes ischemic. Lesions of the gastric and duodenal mucosa (called *stress ulcers*) can develop within hours of severe trauma, sepsis, or burns (Huether & McCance, 2008). Gastrointestinal ulcers may hemorrhage within 2 to 10 days following the original cause of shock. In addition, the permeability of damaged mucosa increases, allowing bacterial translocation to occur. During this process, enteric bacteria or their toxins enter the abdominal cavity, progress to the circulation, and can eventually result in sepsis.

Gastric and intestinal motility is impaired during shock, and paralytic ileus may result. If the episode of shock is prolonged, necrosis of the bowel may occur. In many cases, alterations in the structure and function of the gastrointestinal tract impair absorption of nutrients, such as protein and glucose.

Shock also alters the metabolic functions of the liver. Initially, *gluconeogenesis* (the process of forming glucose from noncarbohydrate sources) and *glycogenolysis* (the breakdown of glycogen into glucose) increase. This process allows blood glucose levels to increase as the body attempts to respond to the stressor; however, as shock progresses, liver functions are impaired, and hypoglycemia develops. Metabolism of fats and protein is impaired, and the liver can no longer effectively remove lactic acid, contributing to the development of metabolic acidosis.

The destruction of the liver's reticuloendothelial Kupffer cells (phagocytes that destroy bacteria) causes a further problem. Bacteria may proliferate within the circulatory system, causing overwhelming bacterial infection and toxicity.

NEUROLOGIC SYSTEM   The primary effects of shock on the neurologic system involve changes in mental status and orientation. Cerebral hypoxia produces altered levels of consciousness, beginning with apathy and lethargy and progressing to coma. A common early symptom of cerebral hypoxia is restlessness. Continued ischemia of brain cells eventually causes swelling, resulting in cerebral edema, neurotransmitter failure, and irreversible brain cell damage.

As cerebral ischemia worsens, the sympathetic activity and vasomotor centers are depressed. This leads to a loss of sympathetic tone, causing systemic vasodilatation and pooling of blood in the periphery. As a result, venous return and cardiac output further decrease.

> **PRACTICE ALERT**
> An early sign of shock is a change in the level of consciousness. Late signs of shock are mental status changes, hypotension, and marked tachycardia.

RENAL SYSTEM   Blood that normally perfuses the kidneys is shunted to the heart and brain during the progressive stage of shock, resulting in renal hypoperfusion. The drop in renal perfusion is reflected in a corresponding decrease in the glomerular filtration rate. Urine output is reduced, and the urine that is produced is highly concentrated. Oliguria of less than 20 mL per hour indicates progressive shock.

Healthy kidneys can tolerate a drop in perfusion for only about 20 minutes; thereafter, acute tubular necrosis develops (Huether & McCance, 2008). As tubular necrosis occurs, epithelial cells slough off and block the tubules, disrupting nephron function. The accumulating loss of functional nephrons eventually causes renal failure. Without normal renal function, metabolic waste products are retained in the plasma.

If treatment restores renal perfusion, the kidneys can regenerate the lost epithelial cells in the tubules, and renal function usually returns to normal. However, in the older or chronically ill patient or in the patient with sustained shock, loss of renal function may become permanent.

EFFECTS ON SKIN, TEMPERATURE, AND THIRST In most types of shock, blood vessels supplying the skin are vasoconstricted, and the sweat glands are activated. As a result, changes in skin color occur. The skin of Caucasian patients becomes pale. In people with darker skin (such as those of African, Hispanic, or Mediterranean descent), shock-related skin color changes may be assessed as paleness of the lips, oral mucous membranes, nail beds, and conjunctiva. The skin is usually cool and moist and, in the later stages of shock, often edematous.

The body temperature decreases as shock progresses, the result of a decrease in overall body metabolism. Some people in shock become thirsty, probably a response to decreased blood volume and increased serum osmolality (Huether & McCance, 2008).

Types of Shock

Shock is identified according to its underlying cause. All types of shock progress through the same stages and exert similar effects on body systems. Any differences are noted in the following discussion.

Hypovolemic Shock

Hypovolemic Shock Video

Hypovolemic shock is caused by a decrease in intravascular volume of 15% or more (Huether & McCance, 2008). In hypovolemic shock, the venous blood returning to the heart decreases, and ventricular filling drops. As a result, stroke volume, cardiac output, and blood pressure decrease. Hypovolemic shock is the most common type of shock, and it often occurs simultaneously with other types.

The decrease in circulating blood volume that triggers hypovolemic shock may result from the following:

- Loss of blood volume from hemorrhage (from surgery, trauma, gastrointestinal bleeding, blood coagulation disorders, ruptured esophageal varices)
- Loss of intravascular fluid from the skin due to injuries such as burns (see Chapter 17)
- Loss of intravascular volume from severe dehydration
- Loss of body fluid from the gastrointestinal system due to persistent and severe vomiting or diarrhea, or continuous nasogastric suctioning
- Renal losses of fluid due to the use of diuretics or to endocrine disorders such as diabetes insipidus
- Conditions causing fluid shifts from the intravascular compartment to the interstitial space
- Third spacing due to such disorders as liver diseases with ascites, pleural effusion, or intestinal obstruction

Hypovolemic shock affects all body systems. Its effects vary depending on the patient's age, general state of health, extent of injury or severity of illness, length of time before treatment is provided, and the rate of volume loss.

The manifestations of hypovolemic shock result directly from the decrease in circulating blood volume and the initiation of compensatory mechanisms (Figure 11–8 ■). The loss of circulating blood volume reduces cardiac output by decreasing venous return to the heart. As a result, blood pressure drops. The carotid and cardiac baroreceptors sense the decrease in blood pressure and communicate it to the vasomotor centers in the brainstem. The vasomotor centers then induce the sympathetic compensatory responses. If the fluid loss is less than 500 mL, activation of the sympathetic response is generally adequate to restore cardiac output and blood pressure to near normal, although the heart rate may remain elevated.

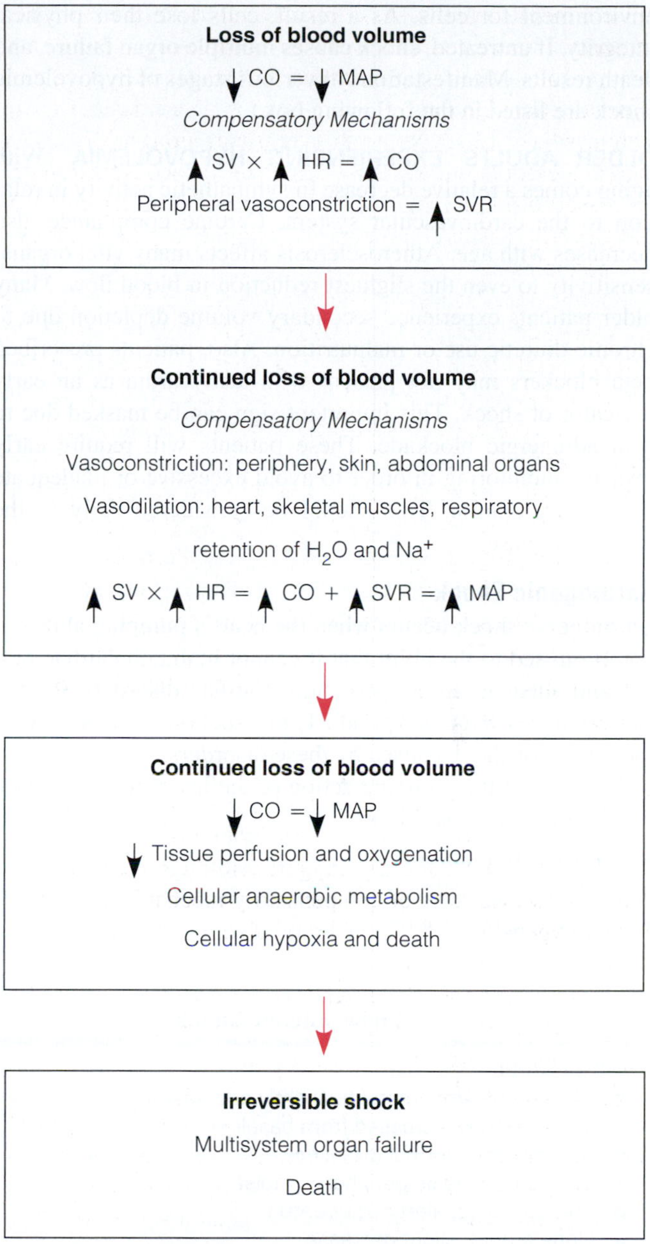
Loss of blood volume
↓ CO = ↓ MAP
Compensatory Mechanisms
↑ SV × ↑ HR = ↑ CO
Peripheral vasoconstriction = ↑ SVR
Continued loss of blood volume
Compensatory Mechanisms
Vasoconstriction: periphery, skin, abdominal organs
Vasodilation: heart, skeletal muscles, respiratory
retention of H2O and Na+
↑ SV × ↑ HR = ↑ CO + ↑ SVR = ↑ MAP
Continued loss of blood volume
↓ CO = ↓ MAP
↓ Tissue perfusion and oxygenation
Cellular anaerobic metabolism
Cellular hypoxia and death
Irreversible shock
Multisystem organ failure
Death

Key CO: Cardiac output
HR: Heart rate
MAP: Mean arterial pressure
SV: Stroke volume
SVR: Systemic vascular resistance

Figure 11–8 ■ The stages of hypovolemic shock.

With a sustained loss of blood volume (1000 mL or more), the shock stage progresses. Heart rate and vasoconstriction increase, and blood flow to the skin, skeletal muscles, kidneys, and abdominal organs decreases. Several renal mechanisms and a decline in capillary pressure help conserve blood volume. Eventually, the amount of blood flowing to cells is too low to oxygenate them and sustain production of cellular energy. Anaerobic metabolism begins, producing an acidotic environment for cells. As a result, cells lose their physical integrity. If untreated, shock causes multiple organ failure, and death results. Manifestations of various stages of hypovolemic shock are listed in the following box.

OLDER ADULTS EXPERIENCING HYPOVOLEMIA With aging comes a relative decrease in sympathetic activity in relation to the cardiovascular system. Cardiac compliance also decreases with age. Atherosclerosis affects many vital organs' sensitivity to even the slightest reduction in blood flow. Many older patients experience secondary volume depletion due to chronic diuretic use or malnutrition. Also, patients prescribed beta blockers may not present with tachycardia as an early indicator of shock. This important sign can be masked due to beta adrenergic blockade. These patients will require early invasive monitoring in order to avoid excessive or inadequate volume restoration. This should be considered early in the treatment phase.

Cardiogenic Shock

Cardiogenic shock occurs when the heart's pumping ability is compromised to the point that it cannot maintain cardiac output and adequate tissue perfusion. Cardiac disorders are discussed in ∞ Chapters 30 and 31; this section focuses only on the effects of shock caused by these disorders.

The loss of the pumping action of the heart may be caused by the following conditions:

- Myocardial infarction
- Cardiac tamponade
- Restrictive pericarditis

MANIFESTATIONS of Hypovolemic Shock

INITIAL STAGE
- Blood pressure: normal to slightly decreased
- Pulse: slightly increased from baseline
- Respirations: normal (baseline)
- Skin: cool, pale (in periphery), moist
- Mental status: alert and oriented
- Urine output: slight decrease
- Other: thirst, decreased capillary refill time

COMPENSATORY AND PROGRESSIVE STAGES
- Blood pressure: hypotension
- Pulse: rapid, thready
- Respirations: increased
- Skin: cool, pale (includes trunk); poor turgor with fluid loss, edematous with fluid shift
- Mental status: restless, anxious, confused, agitated
- Urine output: oliguria (less than 30 mL/hour)
- Other: marked thirst, acidosis, hyperkalemia, decreased capillary refill time, decreased or absent peripheral pulses

IRREVERSIBLE STAGE
- Blood pressure: severe hypotension (often, systolic pressure is below 80 mmHg)
- Pulse: very rapid, weak
- Respirations: rapid, shallow; crackles and wheezes
- Skin: cool, pale, mottled with cyanosis
- Mental status: disoriented, lethargic, comatose
- Urine output: anuria
- Other: loss of reflexes, decreased or absent peripheral pulses

- Cardiac arrest
- Dysrhythmias, such as fibrillation or ventricular tachycardia
- Pathologic changes in the valves
- Cardiomyopathies from hypertension, alcohol, bacterial or viral infections, or ischemia
- Complications of cardiac surgery
- Electrolyte imbalances (especially changes in normal potassium and calcium levels)
- Drugs affecting cardiac muscle contractility
- Head injuries causing damage to the cardioregulatory center

Myocardial infarction is the most common cause of cardiogenic shock. Patients admitted to the hospital for treatment of myocardial infarction or cardiac surgery are at risk for cardiogenic shock. The severity and progression of shock are related to the amount of myocardial damage.

Whatever the cardiogenic cause, the decrease in cardiac output causes a decrease in MAP. Heart rate may increase in response to compensatory mechanisms. However, tachycardia increases myocardial oxygen consumption and decreases coronary perfusion. The myocardium becomes progressively depleted of oxygen, causing further myocardial ischemia and necrosis. The typical sequence of shock is essentially unchanged in cardiogenic shock.

Cyanosis, however, is more common in cardiogenic shock because stagnating blood increases extraction of oxygen from the hemoglobin at the capillary beds. As a result, the skin, lips, and nail beds may appear cyanotic. As cardiac failure (and cardiogenic shock) progresses, left ventricular end-diastolic pressure increases. The increase is transmitted to the pulmonary capillary bed, and pulmonary edema may occur. Retention of blood in the right side of the heart increases right atrial pressure, which leads to jugular venous distention as a result of backflow through the vena cava. Manifestations of cardiogenic shock are listed in the following box.

Obstructive Shock

Obstructive shock is caused by an obstruction in the heart or great vessels that either impedes venous return or prevents effective cardiac pumping action. The causes of obstructive shock are impaired diastolic filling (e.g., pericardial tamponade or pneumothorax), increased right ventricular afterload (e.g., pulmonary emboli), and increased left ventricular afterload (e.g., aortic stenosis, abdominal distention). The manifestations are the result of decreased cardiac output and blood pressure, with reduced tissue perfusion and cellular metabolism.

MANIFESTATIONS of Cardiogenic Shock

- Blood pressure: hypotension, possible narrowing pulse pressures
- Pulse: rapid, thready; distention of veins of hands and neck
- Respirations: increased, labored; crackles and wheezes; pulmonary edema
- Skin: pale, cyanotic, cold, moist
- Mental status: restless, anxious, lethargic progressing to comatose
- Urine output: oliguria to anuria
- Other: dependent edema; elevated CVP; elevated pulmonary capillary wedge pressure; arrhythmias

Distributive Shock

Distributive shock (also called vasogenic shock) includes several types of shock that result from widespread vasodilatation and decreased peripheral resistance. As the blood volume does not change, relative hypovolemia results. Examples of distributive shock include septic, neurogenic, and anaphylactic shock. Treatment is based on the underlying pathogenesis.

Septic Shock

Septic shock, the leading cause of death for patients in intensive care units, is one part of a progressive syndrome called systemic inflammatory response syndrome (SIRS). This condition is most often the result of gram-negative bacterial infections (i.e., *Pseudomonas*, *E. coli*, *Klebsiella*), but may also follow gram-positive infections from *Staphylococcus* and *Streptococcus* bacteria. Gram-negative sepsis has greatly increased in the past 10 years, with a 60% mortality rate despite treatment. The pathophysiology of septic shock is complex and not completely understood.

Patients at risk for developing infections leading to septic shock include those who are hospitalized, have debilitating chronic illnesses, or have poor nutritional status. The risk is heightened after invasive procedures or surgery. Other patients at risk of septic shock include older adults and those who are immunocompromised. Portals of entry for infection that may lead to septic shock are as follows:

- Urinary system: catheterizations, suprapubic tubes, cystoscopy
- Respiratory system: suctioning, aspiration, tracheostomy, endotracheal tubes, respiratory therapy, mechanical ventilators
- Gastrointestinal system: peptic ulcers, ruptured appendix, peritonitis
- Integumentary system: surgical wounds, intravenous catheters, intra-arterial catheters, invasive monitoring, decubitus ulcers, burns, trauma
- Female reproductive system: elective surgical abortion, ascending infections from transmission of bacteria during the intrapartal and postpartal periods, tampon use, sexually transmitted diseases

Septic shock begins with *septicemia* (the presence of pathogens and their toxins in the blood). As pathogens are destroyed, their ruptured cell membranes allow endotoxins to leak into the plasma. The endotoxins disrupt the vascular system, coagulation mechanism, and immune system and trigger an immune and inflammatory response (∞ see Chapter 13 for more information). For this reason, the initial effects of septic shock differ from those of hypovolemic and cardiogenic shock; cardiac output is high and systemic vascular resistance is low.

Endotoxins directly damage the endothelial lining of small blood vessels first; the small blood vessels of the kidneys and lungs are most susceptible. Cellular damage stimulates the release of vasoactive proteins and activates coagulation factor XII. The vasoactive proteins stimulate peripheral vasodilatation and increase capillary permeability; the activation of coagulation factors results in the production of multiple intravascular blood clots.

As a result of the increased capillary permeability and vasodilatation, fluid shifts from the intravascular space to the interstitial space. Hypovolemia results as fluid volume is lost from the circulating blood. Hypovolemia and intravascular coagulation alter oxygenation and cellular metabolism, leading to anaerobic metabolism, lactic acidosis, and cellular death.

Septic shock has an early phase and a late phase. In early septic shock (sometimes called the *warm* phase), vasodilatation results in weakness and warm, flushed skin, and the septicemia often causes high fever and chills. In late septic shock (sometimes called the *cold* phase), hypovolemia and activity of the compensatory mechanisms result in typical shock manifestations, including cold, moist skin; oliguria; and changes in mental status. Death may result from respiratory failure, cardiac failure, or renal failure. Manifestations of septic shock are listed in the following box.

Toxic shock syndrome is an especially virulent form of septic shock, occurring most frequently in menstruating women who use tampons. It is thought that bacterial toxins diffuse from the site of infection in the vagina into the circulation. The toxins then trigger a widespread inflammatory response and septic shock. The manifestations of toxic shock syndrome include extreme hypotension, hyperpyrexia, headache, myalgia, confusion, skin rash, vomiting, and diarrhea (Huether & McCance, 2008).

Disseminated intravascular coagulation (DIC), a generalized response to injury, is a potential risk in septic shock. This condition is characterized by simultaneous bleeding and clotting throughout the vasculature. Sepsis injures blood cells, causing platelet aggregation and decreased blood flow. As a result, blood clots form throughout the microcirculation. The clotting slows circulation further while stimulating excess fibrinolysis. As the body's stores of clotting factors are depleted, generalized bleeding begins. DIC is further discussed in ∞ Chapter 33.

Neurogenic Shock

Neurogenic shock is the result of an imbalance between parasympathetic and sympathetic stimulation of vascular smooth muscle. If parasympathetic overstimulation or sympathetic understimulation persists, sustained vasodilatation occurs, and blood pools in the venous and capillary beds.

MANIFESTATIONS of Septic Shock

EARLY (WARM) SEPTIC SHOCK
- Blood pressure: normal to hypotension
- Pulse: increased, thready
- Respirations: rapid and deep
- Skin: warm, flushed
- Mental status: alert, oriented, anxious
- Urine output: normal
- Other: increased body temperature; chills; weakness; nausea, vomiting, diarrhea; decreased CVP

LATE (COLD) SEPTIC SHOCK
- Blood pressure: hypotension
- Pulse: tachycardia, arrhythmias
- Respirations: rapid, shallow, dyspneic
- Skin: cool, pale, edematous
- Mental status: lethargic to comatose
- Urine output: oliguria to anuria
- Other: normal to decreased body temperature; decreased CVP

Neurogenic shock causes dramatic reduction in systemic vascular resistance as the size of the vascular compartment increases. As systemic vascular resistance decreases, pressure in the blood vessels becomes too low to drive nutrients across capillary membranes, and cellular metabolism is impaired.

The following conditions can cause neurogenic shock by increasing parasympathetic stimulation or inhibiting sympathetic stimulation of the smooth muscle of blood vessels:

- Head injury
- Trauma to the spinal cord (spinal shock, a form of neurogenic shock, is described in ∞ Chapter 43)
- Insulin reactions (which cause hypoglycemia, decreasing glucose to the medulla)
- Central nervous system depressant drugs (such as sedatives, barbiturates, or narcotics)
- Anesthesia (spinal and general)
- Severe pain
- Prolonged exposure to heat

Bradycardia occurs early, but tachycardia begins as compensatory mechanisms are initiated. Central venous pressure drops as veins dilate, venous return to the heart decreases, stroke volume decreases, and MAP falls. In early stages, the extremities are warm and pink (from the pooling of blood), but as shock progresses, the skin becomes pale and cool. Manifestations of neurogenic shock are listed in the following box.

Anaphylactic Shock

Anaphylactic shock is the result of a widespread humorally mediated hypersensitivity reaction (called *anaphylaxis*). The pathophysiology in this type of shock includes vasodilatation, pooling of blood in the periphery, and hypovolemia with altered cellular metabolism. These physiologic alterations occur when a sensitized person has contact with an *allergen* (a foreign substance to which an individual is hypersensitive). Many different allergens can cause anaphylactic shock, including medications, blood administration, latex, foods, snake venom, and insect stings.

Anaphylactic shock does not occur with the first exposure to an allergen. With the first exposure to a foreign substance (the *antigen*), the body produces specific immunoglobulin E (IgE) antibodies against this antigen. The person is thus sensitized to that specific antigen. With subsequent exposure, the antigen reacts with the already formed IgE antibodies, disrupting cellular integrity. In addition, large amounts of histamine and other vasoactive amines are released and distributed through the circulatory system. These substances cause increased capillary permeability and massive vasodilatation, resulting in profound hypotension and eventual vascular collapse.

MANIFESTATIONS of Neurogenic Shock

- Blood pressure: hypotension
- Pulse: slow and bounding
- Respirations: vary
- Skin: warm, dry
- Mental status: anxious, restless, lethargic progressing to comatose
- Urine output: oliguria to anuria
- Other: lowered body temperature

MANIFESTATIONS of Anaphylactic Shock

- Blood pressure: hypotension
- Pulse: increased, dysrhythmias
- Respirations: dyspnea, stridor, wheezes, laryngospasm, bronchospasm, pulmonary edema
- Skin: warm, edematous (lips, eyelids, tongue, hands, feet, genitals)
- Mental status: restless, anxious, lethargic to comatose
- Urine output: oliguria to anuria
- Other: paresthesias; urticaria; pruritus; abdominal cramps, vomiting, diarrhea

Histamine also causes constriction of smooth muscles in the bladder, uterus, intestines, and bronchioles. Respiratory distress, bronchospasm, laryngospasm, and severe abdominal cramping result. Serotonin (a neurotransmitter with vasoconstrictive properties) is released, further affecting respiratory status by increasing capillary permeability in the lungs. As a result, plasma leaks into the alveoli, gas exchange is impaired, and pulmonary edema may occur.

Anaphylactic shock begins and progresses rapidly. Manifestations may begin within 20 minutes of contact with an antigen. Unless appropriate intervention is provided, death can occur within a matter of minutes. Because anaphylaxis is rapid and potentially lethal, people with known allergies should carry some form of warning (such as a MedicAlert bracelet) informing others of their susceptibility. Some patients carry an *Epi-pen* (epinephrine) to halt anaphylaxis. Healthcare providers should be extremely careful to assess and document allergies or previous drug reactions. Manifestations of anaphylactic shock are listed in the following box. Similar, but not related, are anaphylactoid reactions that are not humorally mediated and do not require prior exposure to a trigger. These can have similar symptoms and are treated in a similar manner.

Interdisciplinary Care

Medical care for the patient in shock focuses on treating the underlying cause, increasing arterial oxygenation, and improving tissue perfusion. Depending on the cause and type of shock, interventions include emergency care measures, oxygen therapy, fluid replacement, and medications. Emergency care is often the first course of collaborative action taken to arrest shock, as discussed earlier in this chapter. A *central venous catheter* may be used to aid in the differential diagnosis of shock and to provide information about the preload of the heart. A pulmonary artery catheter may be inserted to monitor cardiac dynamics, fluid balance, and the effects of vasoactive medications.

Diagnosis

The following diagnostic tests can help identify the type of shock and assess the patient's physical status. Measurements include the following:

- *Blood hemoglobin* and *hematocrit*, to detect the concentration that usually occurs in hypovolemic shock. These changes reflect the underlying etiology. In hypovolemic shock resulting from hemorrhage, the hemoglobin and hematocrit concentrations are lower than normal; in hypovolemic shock resulting from intravascular fluid loss, by contrast, the hemoglobin and hematocrit concentrations are higher than normal.

- *Arterial blood gases (ABGs)*, to determine oxygen and carbon dioxide levels and pH. The effects of shock and of the body's compensatory mechanisms cause a decrease in pH (indicating acidosis), a decrease in the partial pressure of oxygen (PaO_2) and in total oxygen saturation, and an increase in the partial pressure of carbon dioxide ($PaCO_2$).
- *Serum electrolytes*, to monitor the severity and progression of shock. As shock progresses, glucose levels decrease, sodium levels decrease, and potassium levels increase.
- *Blood urea nitrogen (BUN), serum creatinine levels, urine specific gravity*, and *osmolality*, to check renal function. As perfusion of the kidneys is decreased and renal function is reduced, the BUN and creatinine levels increase as does urine specific gravity and osmolality.
- *Blood cultures*, to identify the causative organism in septic shock.
- *White blood cell count* and *differential*, in the patient with septic or anaphylactic shock. The total WBC count is increased in septic shock. Elevated neutrophils indicate acute infection, increased monocytes indicate a bacterial infection, and increased eosinophils indicate an allergic response.
- *Serum cardiac enzymes*, which are elevated in cardiogenic shock: creatine kinase (CK), myoglobin, and c-reactive protein. Troponin can be elevated if the cause of cardiogenic shock is acute MI.

Other diagnostic tests may be ordered to determine the extent of injury or damage or to locate the site of internal hemorrhage. These tests might include x-ray studies, computerized tomography (CT) scans, magnetic resonance imaging (MRI), endoscopic examinations, and echocardiograms. Newer diagnostic methods for hypoperfusion include gastric tonometry and sublingual PCO_2. Gastric tonometry measures the partial pressure of carbon dioxide in the gastric lumen. The measurement of sublingual carbon dioxide correlates well with decreased MAP (Sole, Lamborn, & Hartshorn, 2001).

Medications

When fluid replacement alone is not sufficient to reverse shock, vasoactive drugs (drugs causing vasoconstriction or vasodilatation) and inotropic drugs (drugs improving cardiac contractility) may be administered. When used to treat shock, these drugs increase venous return through vasoconstriction of peripheral vessels; they also improve the pumping ability of the heart by facilitating myocardial contractility and by dilating coronary arteries to increase perfusion of the myocardium.

Drugs used to treat shock are discussed in the Medication Administration box on page 262. Other drugs that may be administered to the patient in shock include the following:

- Diuretics to increase urine output after fluid replacement has been initiated
- Sodium bicarbonate to treat acidosis
- Calcium to replace calcium lost as a result of blood transfusions
- Antiarrhythmic agents to stabilize heart rhythm
- Broad spectrum antibiotics to suppress organisms responsible for septic shock

- Epinephrine, antihistamines, and inhaled beta-2 agonists to treat anaphylactic shock
- Morphine to dilate veins and decrease anxiety

Oxygen Therapy

Establishing and maintaining a patent airway and ensuring adequate oxygenation are critical interventions in reversing shock. All patients in shock (even those with adequate respirations) should receive oxygen therapy (usually by mask or nasal cannula) to maintain the PaO_2 at greater than 80 mmHg during the first 4 to 6 hours of care. If the patient's unassisted respiration cannot maintain PaO_2 at this level, ventilatory assistance may be necessary. Care of the patient requiring ventilatory assistance is discussed in ∞ Chapter 37.

Fluid Resuscitation

The most effective treatment for the patient in hypovolemic shock is the administration of intravenous fluids or blood. Fluids also treat septic and, more judiciously, neurogenic shock. However, the patient with cardiogenic shock may require either fluid replacement or restriction, depending on pulmonary artery pressure.

Various fluids may be administered alone or in combination as part of fluid replacement therapy in treating shock. Fluid replacements are administered in massive amounts through two large-bore peripheral lines or through a central line. Current fluid resuscitation protocols include rapid crystalloid infusion followed by blood transfusion. Fluid replacements, such as crystalloid and colloid solutions, increase circulating blood volume and tissue perfusion. Whole blood or blood products increase the oxygen-carrying capacity of the blood and thus increase oxygenation of cells. However, these resuscitation fluids are not thought to minimize inflammation. Studies are underway to evaluate alternative resuscitation fluids such as a alternative colloid (hydroxyethyl starch [Hextend Biotime, Inc./Berkley, CA]), alternative crystalloid (Ringer's ethyl pyruvate), and hypertonic saline with dextran and polymerized hemoglobin.

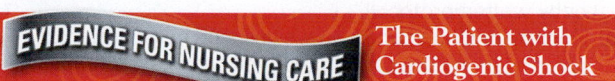

EVIDENCE FOR NURSING CARE — The Patient with Cardiogenic Shock

Selected current resources that nurses may find helpful when planning evidence-based nursing care follow.

- Acute Coronary Syndromes. A National Clinical Guideline. (2008). *National Guideline Clearinghouse*. Retrieved November 3, 2009, from http://www.guideline.gov/summary/summary.aspx?doc_id=10585&nbr=005527&string=cardiogenic+AND+shock
- Cooper, B. E. (2008). Review and update on inotropes and vasopressors. *AACN Advanced Critical Care, 19*(1), 5–15.
- Ellender, T. J., & Skinner, J. C. (2008). The use of vasopressors and inotropes in the emergency medical treatment of shock. *Emergency Medicine Clinics of North America, 26*(3), 759–786.
- Gorman, D., Calhoun, K., Carassco, M., Niclaus, D., Neron, M., McNally, L., & Thompson, P. (2008). Take a rapid treatment approach to cardiogenic shock. *Nursing2008, 3*(4), 18–27.
- Spaniol, J. R., Knight, A. R., Zebley, J. L. Anderson, D., & Pierce, J. D. (2007). Fluid resuscitation therapy for hemorrhagic shock. *Journal of Trauma Nursing, 14*(3), 152–160.

MEDICATION ADMINISTRATION   The Patient in Shock

ADRENERGICS (SYMPATHOMIMETICS)

Vasoconstrictors

    Epinephrine (Adrenalin)

    Norepinephrine (Levophed)

    Metaraminol (Aramine)

    Vasopressin (Pitressin)

Inotropes

    Dopamine (Inotropin)

    Dobutamine (Dobutrex)

    Isoproterenol (Isuprel)

Adrenergic drugs (also called sympathomimetics) mimic the fight-or-flight response of the sympathetic nervous system, selectively stimulating alpha-adrenergic and beta-adrenergic receptors. Many of these drugs have both vasopressor (vaso-constricting) effects and positive inotropic effects. Stimulation of alpha-adrenergic receptors results in vasoconstriction and increased systemic blood pressure. Stimulation of beta-adrenergic receptors increases the force and rate of myo-cardial contraction.

The physiologic effect of these drugs includes improved perfusion and oxygenation of the heart, with increased stroke volume and heart rate, and increased cardiac output. Increased cardiac output in turn increases tissue perfusion and oxygenation. The major disadvantage is that increases in stroke volume and heart rate also increase the oxygen require-ments of the myocardium. These drugs may be used in the early stages of shock, especially in types of shock character-ized by vasodilation.

Nursing Responsibilities

- Carefully monitor responses in the older adult, who may be especially sensitive to sympathomimetics and require lower doses.
- When administering these drugs by the subcutaneous route, carefully aspirate the injection site to avoid injecting the drug directly into a blood vessel.
- Use the intravenous route only with continuous infusion pumps. Carefully adjust the dose to accommodate the patient's cardiovascular status (as ordered by the physician or by written protocol).
- Document lung sounds, vital signs, and hemodynamic parameters before starting the medication, and then accord-ing to institutional policy (usually every 5 to 15 minutes).
- Record and monitor urine output. Report output of less than 30 mL per hour.
- Be aware that the sympathomimetics are incompatible with sodium bicarbonate or alkaline solutions.
- When administering drugs that cause vasoconstriction, such as norepinephrine (Levophed) and metaraminol (Aramine), monitor the intravenous insertion site for

infiltration. If infiltration does occur, stop the infusion and notify the physician immediately. (Infiltration may cause ischemia and necrosis of tissue.)

Patient Teaching

- Because these drugs mimic a physiologic reaction to stress, they may cause feelings of anxiety.
- Close monitoring to adjust the dose will be carried out by qualified nurses using written protocols.
- Report heart palpitations or chest pain immediately.

Vasodilators

    Amrinone (Inocor)

    Nitroglycerin (Tridil)

    Nitroprusside (Nipride)

Drugs that cause vasodilation act directly on smooth muscle, affecting both arterioles and veins. Peripheral resistance, cardiac output, and pulmonary wedge pressure are all reduced as a result of the vasodilation. These effects decrease the oxygen need of the heart and decrease pulmonary congestion. Vasodilators are used primarily in the treatment of cardiogenic shock and may be com-bined with a sympathomimetic (e.g., dopamine).

Nursing Responsibilities

- Mix with D_5W or 0.9% saline.
- IV nitroglycerin must be mixed in glass bottles and infused through special, non-PVC tubing. Up to 40% to 80% of nitroglycerin can be absorbed by PVC bags or tubing.
- Infuse with an infusion pump, and use within 4 hours of reconstitution.
- Do not add other medications to the solution.
- Use cautiously in patients with increased intracranial pressure.
- Assess mental status, blood pressure, and pulse prior to ini-tiating medication. Thereafter, assess blood pressure and pulse according to institutional policy (usually every 5 min-utes initially, then every 15 minutes until stable, and then every hour).
- Monitor for confusion, dizziness, tachycardia, arrhythmias, hypotension, and adventitious breath sounds. Report these immediately if they occur, and slow infusion to a keep-open rate.
- Monitor patients receiving nitroprusside for signs of thio-cyanate poisoning (nausea, disorientation, muscle spasms, decreased or absent reflexes) if infusion lasts longer than 72 hours.
- Keep patient in bed with side rails up.

Health Education for the Patient and Family

- It is important to stay in bed and change positions slowly to avoid dizziness.
- The blood pressure and pulse are taken frequently to adjust the dose of medication.
- Headache is a common side effect.

CRYSTALLOID SOLUTIONS Crystalloid solutions contain dextrose or electrolytes dissolved in water; they are hypertonic, isotonic, or hypotonic. Hypertonic solutions include 3% saline. Isotonic solutions include normal saline (0.9%), lactated Ringer's solution, and Ringer's solution. Hypotonic solutions include one-half normal saline (0.45%) and 5% dextrose in water (D5W).

Hypertonic crystalloid solutions pull fluid into the vascular space to promote excretion. Isotonic and hypotonic crystalloid solutions increase fluid volume in both the intravascular and the interstitial space. Of the total amount infused, only about 25% remains in the intravascular system; the remaining 75% moves into the interstitial space. Consequently, fluid volume is only minimally expanded and the potential for peripheral edema is increased when crystalloid solutions are used. However, Ringer's lactate (an electrolyte solution) and 0.9% saline are the fluids of choice in treating hypovolemic shock, especially in the emergency phase of care while blood is being typed and crossmatched. Large amounts of these solutions may be infused rapidly, increasing blood volume and tissue perfusion.

COLLOID SOLUTIONS Colloid solutions contain substances (colloids) that should not diffuse through capillary walls. Hence, colloids tend to remain in the vascular system and increase the osmotic pressure of the serum, causing fluid to move into the vascular compartment from the interstitial space. As a result, plasma volume expands. Colloid solutions used to treat shock include 5% albumin, 25% albumin, hetastarch, plasma protein fraction, and dextran.

Colloid products reduce platelet adhesiveness and have been associated with reductions in blood coagulation. Consequently, the patient's prothrombin time (PT), INR, platelet count, and activated partial thromboplastin time (PTT) should be monitored when these solutions are administered. Normal values are as follows:

PT	10–15 seconds
INR	1–1.2 seconds
Platelets	150,000–400,000
APTT	< 35 seconds

See the following Medication Administration box for further information about colloid solutions and associated nursing responsibilities and patient teaching.

BLOOD AND BLOOD PRODUCTS If hypovolemic shock is due to hemorrhage, the infusion of blood and blood products may be indicated. The goal of blood administration is to keep the hematocrit at 30% to 35% and the hemoglobin level between 12.5 and 14.5 g/100 mL. Available blood and blood products include fresh whole blood, stored whole blood, packed red blood cells, platelet concentrate, fresh-frozen plasma, and cryoprecipitate. Often, packed red blood cells are given to provide hemoglobin concentration and are supplemented with crystalloids to maintain an adequate circulatory volume (see the discussion of blood administration earlier in the chapter).

∂ Nursing Care

Nursing assessments and interventions to prevent shock are an essential part of the nursing care of every patient. The primary nursing interventions to prevent shock are assessment and monitoring.

Health Promotion and Assessment

Nursing assessments are critical in preventing shock. Identifying patients at risk and making focused assessments are essential. Although shock may occur at any age, physiologic changes with aging make the older adult a high-risk population (see the following box).

- *Hypovolemic shock:* Patients who have undergone surgery, have sustained multiple traumatic injuries, or have been seriously burned are most likely to develop hypovolemic shock. Monitoring fluid status is essential in preventing shock and includes daily assessments of weight, fluid intake by all routes, measurable fluid loss (e.g., urine, vomitus, wound drainage, gastric drainage, and chest tube drainage), and fluid loss that must be estimated, such as profuse perspiration and wound drainage. Assessments for the critically ill patient

---

MEDICATION ADMINISTRATION Colloid Solutions (Plasma Expanders)

Albumin 5% (Albuminar-5, Buminate 5%)

Albumin 25% (Albuminar-25, Buminate 25%)

Dextran 40 (Gentran 40)

Dextran 70 (Gentran 70, Macrodex)

Dextran 75 (Gentran 75)

Hetastarch (Hespan [HES])

Plasma protein fraction (Plasmanate, Plasma-Plex, Plasmatein, Protenate)

These solutions are blood volume expanders and are used to treat hypovolemic shock due to surgery, hemorrhage, burns, or other trauma. Albumin and plasma protein fraction are prepared from healthy blood donors. Dextran and hetastarch are synthetically prepared large molecules. The solutions promote circulatory volume and tissue perfusion by rapidly expanding plasma volume. Dextran solutions are infrequently used.

Nursing Responsibilities
- Before infusion begins, establish baseline of vital signs, lung sounds, heart sounds, and (if possible) CVP and pulmonary artery wedge pressure.
- Start administration of ordered intravenous fluids, using a large-gauge (18-gauge or larger) infusion needle.
- Obtain and record vital signs as required by institutional policy (usually every 15 to 60 minutes) and patient status.
- Obtain and record intake and output every 1 to 2 hours.

- Monitor for manifestations of congestive heart failure or pulmonary edema (dyspnea, cyanosis, cough, crackles, wheezes). If these manifestations appear, stop the fluids and notify the physician immediately.
- Monitor for bleeding from new sites; an increase in blood pressure may cause bleeding in severed vessels that did not bleed with decreased blood pressure.
- Monitor for manifestations of dehydration (dry lips; scant, dark-colored urine; loss of skin turgor). Increased intravenous fluids are usually ordered if the patient becomes dehydrated.
- Monitor for manifestations of circulatory overload (jugular vein distention, increase in CVP, increase in pulmonary capillary wedge pressure). If these manifestations occur, slow rate of infusion and notify physician.
- Monitor prothrombin time, partial thromboplastin time, and platelet counts.
- If administering dextran or plasma protein fraction, have epinephrine and antihistamines readily available for any manifestations of a hypersensitivity reaction (fever, chills, rash, headache, wheezing, flushing).
- Maintain patient on bed rest with side rails elevated.

Health Education for the Patient and Family
- The solutions are given to replace lost serum protein, which helps maintain the volume of blood.
- The vital signs are taken frequently to ensure the safety of the patient.

are ongoing and include fluid balance, hemodynamic values, and vital signs.

- *Cardiogenic shock:* Patients with left anterior wall myocardial infarctions are at risk for developing cardiogenic shock. Nursing care to prevent the development of cardiogenic shock focuses on maintaining or improving myocardial oxygen supply by providing immediate pain relief, maintaining rest, and administering supplemental oxygen.
- *Neurogenic shock:* The risk of neurogenic shock is increased in patients who have spinal cord injuries and those who have received spinal anesthesia. Preventive nursing care includes maintaining immobility of patients with spinal cord trauma and elevating the head of the bed 15 to 20 degrees following spinal anesthesia. Elevations of more than 20 degrees, however, can potentiate headaches following spinal anesthesia and should be avoided.
- *Anaphylactic shock:* Prevent anaphylactic shock by collecting information about allergies and drug reactions during the health history. Note these allergies clearly on all documents and place a special armband on the patient. Careful and frequent assessments during blood administration may prevent serious reactions to blood or blood products.
- *Septic shock:* Patients who are hospitalized, are debilitated, are chronically ill, or have undergone invasive procedures or tube insertions are at high risk for septic shock. Nursing care to prevent septic shock includes careful and consistent hand hygiene, the use of aseptic techniques for procedures (e.g., catheterizations, suctioning, changing dressings, starting and maintaining intravenous fluids or medications), and monitoring for local and systemic manifestations (e.g., white blood cell and differential counts) of infection.

Nursing Diagnoses and Interventions

Nursing care for the patient in shock focuses on assessing and monitoring overall tissue perfusion and on meeting psychosocial needs of the patient and the family. This section discusses nursing diagnoses that are appropriate for the patient with hypovolemic shock. See the accompanying Case Study & Nursing Care Plan on page 265.

EVIDENCE FOR NURSING CARE — **The Patient with Pneumothorax**

Selected resources that nurses may find helpful when planning evidence-based nursing care follow.

- Farrington, M., Lang, S., Cullen, L., & Stewart, S. (2009). Nasogastric tube placement verification in pediatric and neonatal patients. *Pediatric Nursing, 35*(1), 17–24.
- Global strategy for the diagnosis, management, and prevention of chronic obstructive pulmonary disease. (2008). National Guideline Clearinghouse. Retrieved from http://www.goldcopd.com
- Robinson, P. D., Cooper, P., & Ranganathan, S. C. (2009). Evidence-based management of paediatric primary spontaneous pneumothorax. *Paediatric Respiratory Reviews, 10*(3), 110–117.

Decreased Cardiac Output

Decreased cardiac output is the primary problem for the patient in shock. Although much of the care related to this diagnosis is collaborative, many independent nursing interventions are critical to the care of the patient in shock.

- *Assess and monitor cardiovascular function via the following:*
  - Blood pressure
  - Heart rate and rhythm
  - Pulse oximetry
  - Peripheral pulses
  - Hemodynamic monitoring of arterial pressures, pulmonary artery pressures, and central venous pressures (CVPs). *A baseline assessment is necessary to establish the stage of shock. If palpable peripheral pulses and audible (to auscultation) blood pressure are lost, inserting central arterial, venous, and pulmonary artery catheters is essential to establish progression of shock accurately and to evaluate the patient's response to therapy.*
- Measure and record intake and output (total output and urinary output) hourly. *A decrease in circulating blood volume with hypotension and the effect of the compensatory mechanisms associated with shock can cause renal failure. Urinary output of less than 30 mL per hour in an acutely ill adult indicates reduced renal blood flow.*
- Monitor bowel sounds, abdominal distention, and abdominal pain. *Decreased splanchnic blood flow reduces bowel motility and peristalsis; paralytic ileus may result.*
- Monitor for sudden sharp chest pain, dyspnea, cyanosis, anxiety, and restlessness. *Hemoconcentration and increased platelet aggregation may result in pulmonary emboli.*
  - Maintain bed rest and provide (to the extent possible) a calm, quiet environment. Place in a supine position with the legs elevated to about 20 degrees, trunk flat, and head and shoulders elevated higher than the chest (semi-fowler's can also be used with mechanically-ventilated patients) (Figure 11–9 ■). *Limiting activity and ensuring rest decreases the workload of the heart. The supine position with legs elevated increases venous return; however, this position should not be used for patients in cardiogenic shock. The Trendelenburg position is no longer recommended, because it causes the abdominal organs to press against the diaphragm (limiting respirations), decreases filling of the coronary arteries, and initiates aortic and carotid sinus reflexes.*

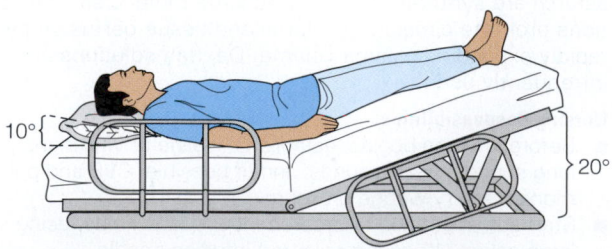

Figure 11–9 ■ The patient in shock should be positioned with the lower extremities elevated approximately 20 degrees (knees straight), trunk horizontal, and the head elevated about 10 degrees.

CASE STUDY & NURSING CARE PLAN   A Patient with Septic Shock

Huang Mei Lan is a 43-year-old unmarried female who lives alone in a major West Coast city. Ms. Huang came to America 15 years ago from China and now speaks English well. Her family still lives in China. She worked in a neighborhood sewing shop until 3 years ago, when she was diagnosed with breast cancer. Her treatment included mastectomy of the affected breast and follow-up chemotherapy.

Last month, Ms. Huang experienced a recurrence of cancer in the lymph glands of the affected side. Surgery to remove the glands was performed and chemotherapy started. Ms. Huang has a central line, a urinary catheter, and a surgical incision. She is underweight, weak, and depressed. Although she has multiple physical problems, she never complains or asks for any kind of medication.

ASSESSMENT

Ms. Huang's primary nurse, Robert O'Brien, enters her room early in the morning to make an initial assessment. He finds Ms. Huang huddled in the middle of the bed, shivering violently. Her vital signs are T 104° F, P 110, R 30, and BP 106/66. Her skin is hot, dry, and flushed with poor turgor. She is alert and oriented, but is restless and appears anxious. Ms. Huang states she is nauseated and suddenly begins vomiting and is incontinent of liquid stool. Laboratory data indicate leukocytosis, respiratory alkalosis, and reduced platelet count. Blood cultures, as well as cultures of Ms. Huang's sputum, urine, and wound drainage, are conducted. She is diagnosed as having septic shock.

Hetastarch is ordered per intravenous line, and intravenous broad-spectrum antibiotics are begun until the organism and its portal of entry can be determined. Despite treatment, Ms. Huang's condition worsens. Her blood pressure continues to drop, her skin becomes cool and cyanotic, and she begins to have periods of disorientation. She is transferred to the critical care unit. As she is being prepared for the transfer, she begins to cry and asks, "Am I going to die?"

DIAGNOSES

- *Ineffective Breathing Pattern* related to rapid respirations and progression of septic shock
- *Ineffective Tissue Perfusion* related to progression of septic shock with decreased cardiac output, hypotension, and massive vasodilatation
- *Deficient Fluid Volume* related to vomiting, diarrhea, high fever, and shift of intravascular volume to interstitial spaces

- *Anxiety* related to feelings that illness is worsening and is potentially life threatening, and the transfer to the critical care unit

EXPECTED OUTCOMES

- Regain and maintain blood gas parameters within normal limits.
- Maintain adequate circulating blood volume.
- Regain and maintain stable hemodynamic levels.
- Verbalize increased ability to cope with stressors.

PLANNING AND IMPLEMENTATION

- Monitor results of arterial blood gases, blood counts, clotting times, and platelet counts.
- Monitor respiratory status, including respiratory rate, rhythm, and breath sounds.
- Monitor neurologic status, including mental status and level of consciousness.
- Monitor cardiovascular status, including arterial blood pressure; rate, rhythm, and quality of pulses; central venous pressure; pulmonary artery pressure; and cardiac output.
- Monitor body temperature every 2 hours.
- Monitor urinary output hourly, reporting any output of less than 30 mL per hour.
- Monitor color and character of skin.
- Explain procedures and provide comfort measures (oral care, skin care, turning, positioning).

EVALUATION

Despite intensive nursing and medical care, Ms. Huang's condition remains critical. The interventions are continued.

CRITICAL THINKING IN THE NURSING PROCESS

1. Vasopressors may be used in the treatment of septic shock. Explain the rationale for their use.
2. While monitoring Ms. Huang's arterial blood gases, the nurse notes that her PaO_2 is < 60 mmHg and her $PaCO_2$ is > 50. What do these findings indicate, and why have they occurred?
3. Ms. Huang has been given large amounts of colloids intravenously. Hemodynamic monitoring indicates a higher than normal CVP and pulmonary artery pressure. What do these findings indicate? What physical assessments would you make to confirm the changes?

See Evaluating Your Response in Appendix C.

NURSING CARE OF THE OLDER ADULT   Variations in Assessment Findings—Shock

- Cardiac changes may include a thickened left ventricular wall, decreased elasticity of the myocardium, and more rigid valves. These changes result in a decreased stroke volume and cardiac output, thus decreasing responses to shock in general and increasing the risk of cardiogenic shock.
- Decreased arterial wall elasticity and vasomotor tone reduce the older adult's ability to respond to a decrease in oxygenation.

- Decreased elasticity and turgor of the skin make assessments of skin turgor more difficult.
- Previous medication and blood administration increase the risk of anaphylactic shock.
- Decreased immune system response increases the risk of septic shock.

Altered Tissue Perfusion

As shock progresses, diminished tissue perfusion causes ischemia and hypoxia of major organ systems. As shock worsens, blood flow and oxygenation of the lungs, heart, and brain are also impaired. Hypoxia and ischemia result from decreased tissue perfusion in the kidneys, brain, heart, lungs, gastrointestinal tract, and the periphery.

- Monitor skin color, temperature, turgor, and moisture. *Decreased tissue perfusion is evidenced when the skin becomes pale, cool, and moist; as hemoglobin concentrations decrease, cyanosis occurs.*
- Monitor cardiopulmonary function by assessing/monitoring the following:
  - Blood pressure (by auscultation or by hemodynamic monitoring)
  - Rate and depth of respirations
  - Lung sounds
  - Pulse oximetry and arterial blood gases
  - Peripheral pulses (brachial, radial, dorsalis pedis, and posterior tibial); include presence, equality, rate, rhythm, and quality (If unable to palpate pulses, use a device such as a Doppler ultrasound flowmeter to assess peripheral arterial blood flow.)
  - Jugular vein distention
  - CVP measurements

  Baseline vital signs are necessary to determine trends in subsequent findings. As shock progresses, the blood pressure decreases, and the pulse becomes rapid, weak, and thready. As perfusion of the lungs decreases, crackles, wheezes, and dyspnea are commonly assessed. Capillary refill is prolonged, and peripheral pulses are weak or nonpalpable. Neck veins that cannot be seen when the patient is in the supine position indicate decreased intravascular volume. CVP is an accurate means of determining fluid status in the patient in shock; the findings will be low (5–15 cmH$_2$O or 2–6 mmHG is normal) in hypovolemic shock because of the decreased blood volume. (∞ See Chapter 10 for a discussion of CVP.)
- Monitor body temperature. *An elevated body temperature increases metabolic demands, depleting reserves of bodily energy. It also increases myocardial oxygen demand and may place the patient with previous cardiac problems at even greater risk for hypoperfusion.*
- Monitor urinary output per Foley catheter hourly, using a urimeter. *Urine output is a reliable indicator of renal perfusion.*
- Assess mental status and level of consciousness. *The appropriateness of the patient's behavior and responses reflects the adequacy of cerebral circulation. Restlessness and anxiety are common early in shock; in later stages, the patient may become lethargic and progress to a comatose state. Altered levels of consciousness are the result of both cerebral hypoxia and the effects of acidosis on brain cells.*

Anxiety

Many patients in hypovolemic shock have experienced some form of major trauma and may have multiple life-threatening injuries that result in emergency care and the potential for emergency surgery. Throughout this sequence of crisis events, treatment is invasive, and contact with family is minimal.

Patient and family responses to these situations of uncertainty, instability, and change include anxiety, fear, and powerlessness. These responses are affected by age, developmental level, cultural and ethnic group, experience with illness and the healthcare system, and support systems.

- Assess the cause(s) of the anxiety, and manipulate the environment to provide periods of rest. *Reducing stimuli that cause anxiety is calming and facilitates rest, which is necessary in the patient at risk for bleeding.*
- Administer prescribed pain medications on a regular basis and implement any applicable nonpharmacologic comfort measures. *Pain precipitates and/or aggravates anxiety.*
- Provide interventions to increase comfort and reduce restlessness:
  - Maintain a clean environment.
  - Provide skin and oral care.
  - Monitor the effectiveness of ventilation or oxygen therapy.
  - Eliminate all nonessential activities.
  - Remain with the patient during procedures.
  - Speak slowly and calmly, using short sentences.
  - Use touch to provide support.

  Unfamiliar sounds, sights, and odors can increase anxiety. Damp skin or a dry mouth increases discomfort. Inadequate gas exchange with a decrease in oxygen or an increase in carbon dioxide in the blood may cause the patient to experience a "feeling of doom." Activity increases the body's need for oxygen. Listening and touch provide support in an environment in which the patient often feels alone and abandoned. Severe anxiety interferes with the ability to understand others and to respond appropriately.
- Provide support for the patient and family:
  - Provide time, space, and privacy for family members.
  - Allow family members access to the patient when feasible.
  - Encourage the expression of feelings and concerns. Provide anticipatory guidance to prepare for recovery or death and to support realistic hope.

NANDA, NIC, AND NOC LINKAGES
The Patient in Shock

NANDA	Risk for Ineffective Cerebral Tissue Perfusion

⬇

NIC	Cerebral Perfusion Promotion Central Perfusion Monitoring Fluid/Electrolyte Management Hypovolemia Management Shock Management

⬇

NOC	Tissue Perfusion: Cerebral, Ineffective Circulation Status Vital Signs Neurological Status

Adapted from Bulechek, G., Butcher, H., & Dochterman, J. M. (Eds). (2008). *Nursing interventions classification (NIC)* (5th ed.). St. Louis: Mosby Elsevier; Moorhead, S., Johnson, M., Maas, M., & Swanson, E. (Eds). (2008). *Nursing outcomes classification (NOC)* (4th ed.). St. Louis: Mosby Elsevier; and Nanda International. (2009). *Nursing diagnoses: Definitions and classification 2009–2011*. Oxford, UK: Wiley-Blackwell.

- Acknowledge the beliefs, values, and expectations of the patient and family.

    Allowing the family access to the patient reduces anxiety and gives both the patient and the family some feeling of control. If prognosis is poor, access and involvement allow the family to begin the grieving process. If recovery is expected, contact provides the patient and family with a feeling of hope. Supporting the patient and family facilitates concrete problem solving, promotes acceptance of the illness and its implications, and helps them begin to establish ways of managing the illness experience.

- Provide information about the current setting to both the patient and family; give the family information about available resources (such as pastoral care, social services,

temporary housing, meals). *Knowing what to expect and how to control the environment to meet basic needs reduces anxiety.*

Using NANDA, NIC, and NOC

Linkages between a selected NANDA nursing diagnosis, NIC, and NOC for the patient in shock are shown in the chart on the previous page.

Community-Based Care

Home care for the patient who has experienced shock is highly individualized, depending on the cause and the illness or injury that caused shock. Therefore, topics for consideration are not included in this section.

CHAPTER HIGHLIGHTS

- Trauma is defined as injury to human tissues and organs resulting from the transfer of energy from the environment. Energy sources can be mechanical, gravitational, thermal, electrical, physical, or chemical.
- Trauma types included minor trauma, which causes minimal damage to underlying tissues, or major/multiple trauma, which involves at minimum a serious single system injury or multiple trauma. Trauma can also be categorized as blunt and penetrating trauma. Blunt trauma is caused by forces like deceleration, acceleration, shearing, compression, or crushing. Penetrating trauma is the entrance into the body of a foreign object.
- Maintenance of the airway and cervical spine are the highest priority in the trauma patient, with airway assessment superseding all other interventions.
- The primary assessment conducted by the nurse identifies all life-threatening injuries and performance of appropriate interventions. The secondary assessment is when the nurse identifies all injuries in order to prioritize care.
- Shock is a clinical syndrome characterized by a systemic imbalance between oxygen supply and demand. This imbalance results in a state of inadequate blood flow to body organs and tissues, causing life-threatening cellular dysfunction.
- The symptoms of shock arise from the body's attempts to maintain vital organs (heart and brain) and to preserve life following a drop in oxygen delivery to the cells.
- An important early sign of shock is a change in the level of consciousness with restlessness a common symptom of cerebral hypoxia.

- Shock is defined in 3 stages: compensatory (stage 1), an early and reversible stage; progressive (stage 2), occurring after a fluid loss of 35% to 50% (1800 to 2500 mL of fluid), where the affected cells switch from aerobic to anaerobic metabolism in order to stay alive; and the final stage, refractory/irreversible (stage 3), where tissue anoxia and death becomes widespread.
- Hypovolemic shock is the most common type of shock and is caused by a decrease in circulating blood volume by 15% or greater.
- Cardiogenic shock is caused when the pumping ability of the heart is compromised to the point where adequate cardiac output cannot be maintained.
- Obstructive shock is caused by an obstruction in the heart or great vessels that either impedes venous return or prevents effective cardiac pumping action. Causes can include cardiac tamponade, pneumothorax, pulmonary embolism and aortic stenosis.
- Distributive shock includes several types of shock that result from widespread vasodilatation and decreased peripheral resistance. As the blood volume does not change, relative hypovolemia results, leading to altered cellular metabolism. Examples of distributive shock include septic, neurogenic, and anaphylactic shock.
- Septic shock is part of a progressive syndrome called systemic inflammatory response syndrome (SIRS), a condition most commonly caused by gram-negative infections.
- Anaphylactic shock is caused by a fulminating hypersensitivity reaction to a foreign substance.

TEST YOURSELF NCLEX-RN® REVIEW

1. What is the most common mechanical source of injury in adults of all ages?
    1. firearms
    2. accidental fire
    3. swimming pools
    4. motor vehicles

2. Severe facial injuries, such as those resulting from going through a windshield, increase the risk for all of the following. For which complication would you assess first?
    1. airway obstruction
    2. hemorrhage
    3. shallow respirations
    4. fractures

3. Which hospital intervention would be the priority?
   1. Verify cause of injury.
   2. Assess airway patency.
   3. Evaluate peripheral capillary refill.
   4. Check for hemorrhage.

4. You are monitoring blood administration to a trauma victim in shock. Which of the following assessment findings indicate a dangerous transfusion reaction?
   1. multiple urticaric, pruritic skin lesions
   2. an increase in body temperature by 3°
   3. decreasing dyspnea
   4. increasing blood pressure

5. Which of the following types of shock causes widespread vasodilatation and decreased peripheral resistance?
   1. cardiogenic shock
   2. septic shock
   3. hypovolemic shock
   4. obstructive shock

6. What is the best method to manage uncontrolled bleeding?
   1. Use direct pressure.
   2. Clamp a visible vessel.
   3. Apply a tourniquet.
   4. Elevate the injured part.

7. Trauma is defined as which of the following?
   1. an injury to human tissues from the transfer of energy
   2. the result of random chance vs. intention
   3. an accidental injury
   4. an intentional injury

8. Which of the following is a risk from a blood transfusion?
   1. pregnancy
   2. tuberculosis
   3. transfusion reaction
   4. weight gain

9. Distributive shock is caused from which of the following?
   1. blood loss
   2. widespread vasodilatation
   3. ineffective cardiac pumping action
   4. hypersensitivity reaction

10. Shock is defined as which of the following?
    1. systemic imbalance between oxygen supply and demand
    2. sufficient cardiac output
    3. controlled hemorrhage
    4. abnormal blood pressure

See Test Yourself answers in Appendix C.

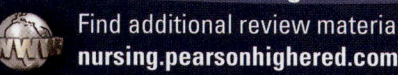

Pearson Nursing Student Resources

Find additional review materials at
nursing.pearsonhighered.com
Prepare for success with additional NCLEX®-style practice questions, interactive assignments and activities, Web links, animations and videos, and more!

BIBLIOGRAPHY

American College of Emergency Physicians. (2009). Domestic Family Violence. Retrieved from http://www.acep.org/practres.aspx?id=29184

American Red Cross. (2003). Cryoprecipitate Transfusion Guidelines. Retrieved from http://www.newenglandblood.org/professional/cryoguide.htm

American Red Cross. (2003). Plasma Transfusion Guidelines. Retrieved from http://www.newenglandblood.org/professional/plasmaguide.htm

American Red Cross. (2003). Platelet Transfusion Guidelines. Retrieved from http://www.newenglandblood.org/professional/plateletguide.htm

American Red Cross. (2003). Red Cell Transfusion Guidelines. Retrieved from http://www.newenglandblood.org/professional/redcellguide.htm

American Red Cross. (2009). Blood types. Retrieved from http://www.givelife2.org/aboutblood/bloodtypes.aspAustralian Red Cross

Bickley, L. S. (2008). *Bates' guide to physical examination and history taking* (7th ed.). Philadelphia: Lippincott Williams & Wilkins.

Carcillo, J., Han, K., Lin, J., & Orr, R. (2007). Goal directed management of pediatric shock in the emergency department. *Clinical Pediatric Emergency Medicine 8*(3), 165–175.

Catenacci, M. H., & King, K. (2008). Severe sepsis and septic shock: Improving outcomes in the emergency department. *Emergency Medicine Clinics of North America, 26*(3), 603–623.

Cocci, M. N., Kimlin, E., Walsh, M., Donnino, M. W. (2007). Identification and resuscitation of the trauma patient in shock. *Emergency Medicine Clinics of North America,* 25(3), 623–642.

Deglin, J. H., & Vallerand, A. H. (2009). *Davis' drug guide* (10th Ed.). Philadelphia: F.A. Davis.

Department of Veterans' Affairs. (2009). Common reactions after trauma. Retrieved from http://ncptsd.va.gov/ncmain/ncdocs/fact_shts/fs_commonreactions.html

Dine, C. J., & Abella, B. S. (2009). Therapeutic hypothermia for neuroprotection. *Emergency Medicine Clinics of North America, 27*(1), 137–149.

Domino, F.J., Baldor, R. A., Golding, J., Grimes, J., & Taylor, J. S. (2010). *The 5-minute clinical consult* (18th ed.). Philadelphia: Lippincott, Williams & Wilkins.

Emergency Nurses Association. (2003). Core curriculum for pediatric emergency nursing. Chicago: Author.

Emergency Nurses Association. (2008). Emergency Nursing Core Curriculum (6th ed.). Philadelphia: Saunders.

Erickson, T. B., Thompson, T. M., Lu, J. J. (2007). The approach to the patient with the unknown overdose. *Emergency Medicine Clinics of North America, 25*(2), 249–281.

Fishman, A. P., Elias, J. A., Fishman, J. A., Grippi, M. A., Senior, S. M., & Pack, A. J. (2008). *Fishman's pulmonary diseases and disorders* (4th ed.). New York: McGraw-Hill Co.

Hildebrand, F., Pape, H. C., van Griensven, M., et al. (2005). Genetic predisposition for a compromised immune system after multiple trauma. *Shock, 24*(6), 518–522.

Huether, S. E., & McCance, K. L. (2008). *Understanding Pathophysiology* (4th ed.). St. Louis: Mosby Elsevier.

McGill, J. (2007). Airway management in trauma: An update. *Emergency Medicine Clinics of North America, 25*(3), 603–622.

Men Stopping Violence. (2009). The art of change. Retrieved from http://www.menstoppingviolence.org/index.php

NANDA International. (2009). *Nursing diagnoses: Definitions and classification 2009–2011* Oxford, UK: Wiley-Blackwell.

National Center of Health Statistics [NCHS]. (2009). *Health, United States,* 2008 with chartbook. Hyattsville, MD: Author.

National Center for Patient Safety. (2004). Falls Toolkit. Retrieved from http://www.patientsafety.gov/SafetyTopics/fallstoolkit/index.html

National Highway Traffic Safety Administration. (2009). Child passenger safety studies and reports. Retrieved from http://www.nhtsa.dot.gov/portal/site/nhtsa/menuitem.9f8c7d6359e0e9bbbf30811060008a0c

National Institute of Mental Health. (2009). Men and depression. Retrieved from http://www.nimh.nih.gov/health/publications/men-and-depression/index.shtml

National Library of Medicine. (2009). Domestic Violence. Retrieved from http://www.nlm.nih.gov/medlineplus/domesticviolence.html

National Library of Medicine. (2009). Suicide. Retrieved from http://www.nlm.nih.gov/medlineplus/suicide.html

Papadakis, M. A., & McPhee, S. J. (2007). *Current consult medicine 2007* New York: McGraw-Hill.

Perrin, K. O. (2009). *Understanding the essentials of critical care nursing.* Upper Saddle River, NJ: Pearson Prentice-Hall.

Sheehy, S. A. B. (1984). Primary trauma survey and immediate intervention with the use of the mnemonic ABC4. *Journal of Emergency Nursing, 10*(4), 220–221.

Transfusion.com (2009). Transfusion update 2009: Cryoprecipitate. Retrieved from http://www.transfusion.com.au/Cryoprecipitate.aspx

Trzeciak, S., Dellinger, P., Abate, N. L., et al. (2007). Translating research to clinical practice: A 1-year experience with implementing early goal-directed therapy for septic shock in the emergency department. *Chest, 129*(2), 225–232.

Van Leeuwen, A. M., Kranpitz, T. R., & Smith, L. S. (2006). *Davis' laboratory and diagnostic tests* (2nd ed.). Philadelphia: F.A. Davis.

LEARNING OUTCOMES

1. Explain the components and functions of the immune system and the immune response.
2. Compare antibody-mediated and cell-mediated immune responses.
3. Describe the pathophysiology of wound healing, inflammation, and infection.

4. Identify factors responsible for nosocomial infections.
5. Discuss the purposes, nursing implications, and health education for medications and treatments used to treat inflammations and infections.
6. Explain the nursing care necessary to prevent and/or monitor the status of infections.

CLINICAL COMPETENCIES

1. Apply standard precautions, particularly hand hygiene, to prevent the spread of infection within the patient, to other patients in the facility, and to members of the interdisciplinary team and visitors.
2. Use the nursing process as a framework to provide safe, effective individualized care for patients with inflammation and infection.
3. Collaborate with the interdisciplinary care team to integrate care of patients with infection.

4. Promote therapeutic levels and complete dosage of anti-inflammatory and anti-infective medication through prompt administration and patient and family teaching.
5. Assess for hypersensitivities to anti-infectives prior to administering and during administration.
6. Participate in quality improvement processes to reduce the rates and risk of infection for a patient group or population.

KEY TERMS

acquired immunity, 281
active immunity, 281
adaptive immune response, 270
anergy, 283
antibodies, 273
antibody-mediated (humoral) immune response, 273
antigens, 273
B lymphocytes (B cells), 272

cell-mediated (cellular) immune response, 273
cytokines, 281
endotoxins, 292
exotoxins, 292
immunity, 281
immunocompetent, 278
immunoglobulin (Ig), 278
infection, 292
innate adaptive immunity, 269

lymphocyte, 272
macrophages, 272
natural killer cells (NK cells, null cells), 272
nosocomial infections, 294
passive immunity, 281
pathogens, 291
phagocytosis, 276
T lymphocytes (T cells), 272
vaccines, 283

The human body is continually threatened by foreign substances, infectious agents, and abnormal cells. The immune system is the body's major defense mechanism against infectious organisms and abnormal or damaged cells. Recent years have seen the emergence of resistant microorganisms such as methicillin-resistant *Staphylococcus aureus* (MRSA) and altered strains of familiar diseases, such as multiple-drug-resistant tuberculosis. Other diseases have also emerged, including Lyme disease, *Clostridium difficile*, and human immunodeficiency virus (HIV).

A thorough knowledge of the immune system increases understanding of the local and systemic inflammatory response, resistance to infectious disease, and the importance of immunization. This foundation can help the nurse teach patients and families to follow recommended treatment regimens, to promote and maintain health, and to prevent disease. In addition, the nurse can prescribe appropriate rehabilitative measures, such as increased rest and attention to optimal nutrition.

Overview of the Immune System

The immune system is a complex and intricate network of specialized cells, tissues, and organs. Cells of the immune system seek out and destroy damaged cells and foreign tissue, yet recognize and preserve host cells (Porth, 2007). The immune system defends and protects the body from infection by bacteria, viruses, fungi, and parasites; removes and destroys damaged or dead cells; and identifies and destroys malignant cells, thereby preventing their further development into tumors.

The immune system is activated by minor injuries, such as small lacerations or bruises, or by major injuries, such as burns, surgeries, and systemic diseases (e.g., pneumonia). The response of the immune system may be innate or adaptive. Innate immunity provides a nonspecific, generic response to harmful events; adaptive immunity provides a specific response to unique organisms and includes memory as well as active and limited responses. **Innate adaptive immunity** responses prevent or limit the entry of invaders into the body, thereby limiting the extent of tissue damage and reducing the workload of the adaptive immune system. Inflammation is an innate, nonspecific response activated by both minor and major injuries. When the inflammatory process is unable to destroy invading organisms or toxins, a more specific response, called the **adaptive immune response**, is activated.

Immune System Components

The immune system consists of molecules, cells, and organs that produce the immune response (Table 12–1). These components may be involved in the innate inflammatory response, the adaptive immune response, or both.

Leukocytes

Leukocytes (white blood cells, WBCs) are the primary cells involved in both innate and adaptive immune system responses. Like all blood cells, leukocytes derive from stem cells, the hemocytoblasts, in the bone marrow (Figure 12–1 ■). Unlike red blood cells (RBCs), which are confined to the circulation, leukocytes use the circulation to transport themselves to the site of an inflammatory or immune response. As the mobile units of the immune system, leukocytes detect, attack, and destroy anything that is recognized as "foreign." They are able to move through tissue spaces, locating damaged tissue and infection by responding to chemicals released by other leukocytes and damaged tissue.

The normal number of circulating leukocytes is 4,500 to 10,000 cells per cubic millimeter (mm^3) of blood. Many more leukocytes are "marginated." Margination refers to adhesion of leukocytes to vascular epithelial cells along the vessel walls, in other tissue spaces, or in the lymph system. Marginated leukocytes migrate into injured areas or areas where pathogens infiltrate as part of the innate immune response. In the presence of an attack such as an infection, additional WBCs are released from the bone marrow, leading to *leukocytosis*, a WBC count of greater than $10,000/mm^3$. As WBCs move out of the bone marrow into the blood, the bone marrow increases its production of additional leukocytes. A decrease in the number of circulating leukocytes, known as *leukopenia*, occurs when bone marrow activity is suppressed or when leukocyte destruction increases.

Leukocytes are divided into three major groups: granulocytes, monocytes, and lymphocytes. The granulocytes and monocytes derive from the myeloid stem cells of the bone marrow and are instrumental in the inflammatory response. Lymphocytes derive from the lymphoid stem cells of the bone marrow and are the primary cells involved in the specific immune response. In laboratory tests, the WBC count indicates the total number of circulating leukocytes. The WBC differential identifies the portion of the total represented by each type of leukocyte.

GRANULOCYTES   Granulocytes constitute 60% to 80% of the total number of normal blood leukocytes. Their cytoplasm has a granular appearance, and their nuclei are distinctively multilobular (see Figure 12–1). Granulocytes have a short life span, measured in hours to days, compared to the life span of monocytes, which is measured in months to years. Granulocytes play a key role in protecting the body from harmful microorganisms

TABLE 12–1 Cells and Tissues of the Immune System

COMPONENT	LOCATION	FUNCTION
Leukocytes		
Granulocytes		
Neutrophils	Circulation	Phagocytosis and chemotaxis
Eosinophils	Circulation, respiratory tract, and gastrointestinal tract	Phagocytosis Protection against parasites Involved in allergic response
Basophils	Circulation	Release of chemotactic substances
Monocytes and macrophages	Circulation (monocytes) and body tissue, such as skin (histiocytes), liver (Kupffer cells), alveoli, spleen, tonsils, lymph nodes, bone, bone marrow, brain	Trapping and phagocytizing of foreign substances and cellular debris Secretion of interleukin-1 to stimulate lymphocyte growth
Lymphocytes	Circulation, lymph system, tissues	Activation of T and B cells
T cells (mature in thymus gland)		Control of viral infections and destruction of cancer cells Involved in hypersensitivity reactions and graft tissue rejection
B cells (mature in bone marrow)	Circulation, spleen	Production of antibodies (immunoglobulins) to specific antigens
NK (natural killer) cells	Circulation	Cytotoxic; killing of tumor cells, fungi, viral-infected cells, and foreign tissue
Lymphoid Tissues		
Primary or central lymphoid structures	Bone marrow and thymus gland	Production of immune cells; sites for cell maturation
Secondary or peripheral lymphoid structures	Lymph nodes, spleen, tonsils, intestinal lymphoid tissue, lymphoid tissue in other organs	Sites for activation of immune cells by antigens

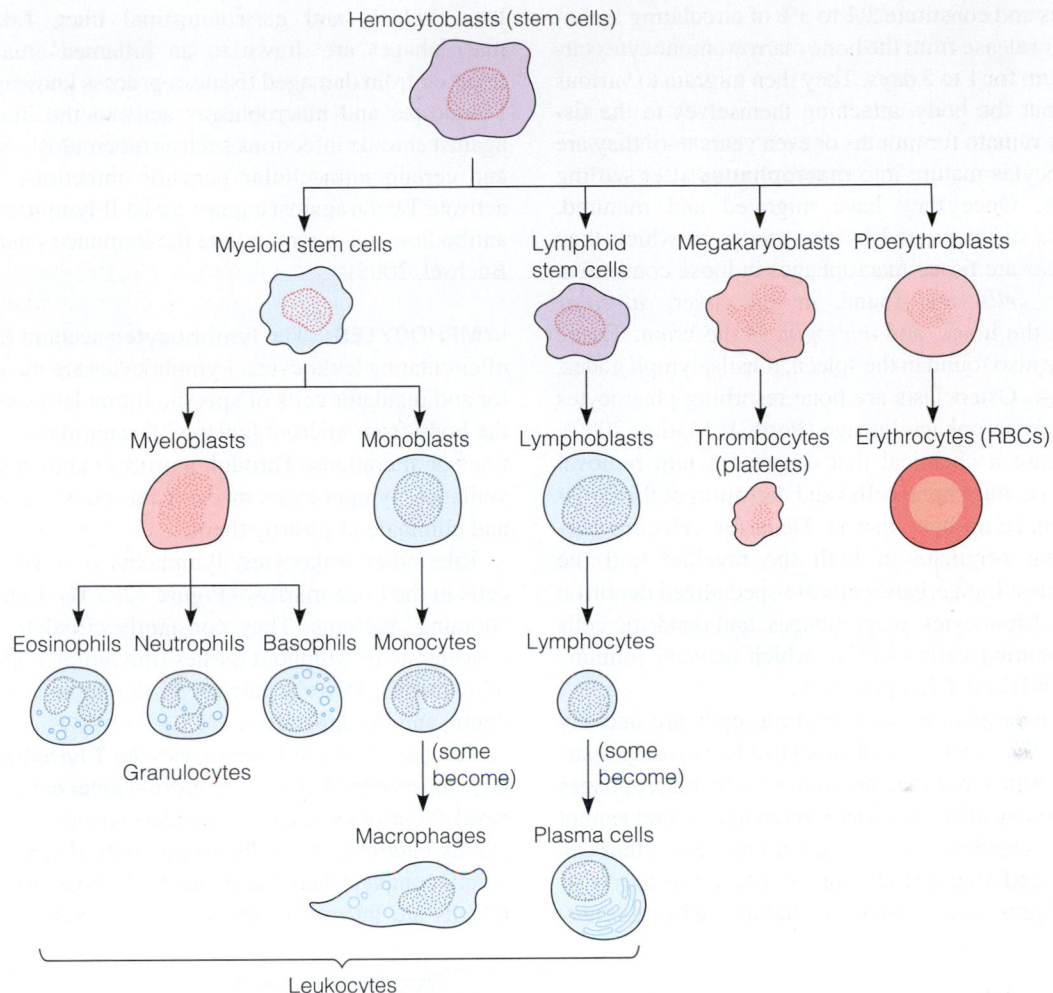

Hemocytoblasts (stem cells)

Myeloid stem cells   Lymphoid stem cells   Megakaryoblasts   Proerythroblasts

Myeloblasts   Monoblasts   Lymphoblasts   Thrombocytes (platelets)   Erythrocytes (RBCs)

Eosinophils   Neutrophils   Basophils   Monocytes   Lymphocytes

Granulocytes

(some become)   (some become)

Macrophages   Plasma cells

Leukocytes

Figure 12–1 ■ The development and differentiation of leukocytes from hemocytoblasts.

during acute inflammation and infection. There are three types of granulocytes: neutrophils, eosinophils, and basophils.

Neutrophils, also called polymorphonuclear leukocytes (PMNs or polys), are the most plentiful of the granulocytes, constituting 55% to 70% of the total number of circulating leukocytes. Neutrophils are *phagocytic* cells, responsible for engulfing and destroying foreign agents, particularly bacteria and small particles. Neutrophils are the first phagocytic cells to arrive at the site of invasion, drawn by chemicals released by damaged tissue and invading organisms.

Neutrophils are produced in the bone marrow and released into the circulation when they mature. Segmented neutrophils (or segs) are mature forms, and usually account for about 55% of total leukocytes. *Bands* are immature neutrophils and usually comprise 5% of leukocytes. As neutrophils mature, their nucleus changes from round to kidney-bean-shaped (banded) and then the nucleus separates into small, attached segments, thus the designations "banded" versus "segmented" neutrophils. It takes about 10 days for a neutrophil to mature and be released into the circulation. Once released, neutrophils have a circulating half-life of 6 to 10 hours. They cannot replicate and must be replaced constantly to maintain adequate numbers in the circulation. They do not return to the bone marrow.

Eosinophils account for 1% to 4% of the total number of circulating leukocytes. They mature in the bone marrow in 3 to

6 days before being released into the circulation. Eosinophils have a circulating half-life of 30 minutes and a tissue half-life of 12 days. They too are phagocytic cells, but are less efficient at this process than neutrophils. Eosinophils are found in large numbers in the respiratory and gastrointestinal tracts, where they are thought to be responsible for protecting the body from parasitic worms, including tapeworms, flukes, pinworms, and hookworms. Eosinophils surround the parasite and release toxic enzymes from their cytoplasmic granules. The parasite, although too large to be phagocytized, is destroyed. Eosinophils are also involved in a hypersensitivity response, inactivating some of the inflammatory chemicals released during the inflammatory response.

Basophils constitute about 0.5% to 1% of the circulating leukocytes. These cells are not phagocytic. Granules within basophils contain proteins and chemicals such as heparin, histamine, bradykinin, serotonin, and a slow-reacting substance of anaphylaxis (leukotrienes). These substances are released into the bloodstream during an acute hypersensitivity reaction or stress response.

MONOCYTES, MACROPHAGES, AND DENDRITIC CELLS

Monocytes, macrophages, and dendritic cells are the mediators of immunity. They recognize foreign matter (from molecules to cells) and initiate immune responses. *Monocytes* are the largest of the leukocytes and constitute 2% to 3% of circulating leuko-cytes. After their release from the bone marrow, monocytes cir-culate in the serum for 1 to 2 days. They then migrate to various tissues throughout the body, attaching themselves to the tis-sues, where they remain for months or even years until they are activated. Monocytes mature into **macrophages** after settling into the tissues. Once they have migrated and matured, macrophages are differentiated by the tissues in which they reside. *Histiocytes* are tissue macrophages in loose connective tissue, *Kupffer cells* are found in the liver, *alveolar macrophages* in the lungs, and *microglia* in the brain. Tissue macrophages are also found in the spleen, tonsils, lymph nodes, and bone marrow. Osteoclasts are bone resorbing phagocytes of the monocyte/macrophage lineage (Porth & Matfin, 2009). These cells release a chemical that causes calcium removal from osteocytes (mature bone cells) and digestion of the colla-gen fibers that make up bone matrix. Dendritic cells are star-shaped cells that originate in both the myeloid and the lymphoid cell lines. Langerhans cells are specialized dendritic cells in the skin. Monocytes, macrophages, and dendritic cells are antigen-presenting cells (APCs), which activate immune responses in both B and T lymphocytes.

Monocytes, macrophages, and dendritic cells are actively phagocytic, with the capacity to phagocytize large foreign par-ticles and cell debris. Once they are in the tissue, macrophages can multiply to encapsulate and trap foreign matter that cannot be phagocytized. Dendritic cells have long processes that can capture antigens and migrate to lymphoid tissue. They serve as sentinels for antigens in most organs including the heart, lungs,

liver, kidney, and gastrointestinal tract. Like neutrophils, macrophages are drawn to an inflamed area by chemicals released from damaged tissue, a process known as chemotaxis. Monocytes and macrophages activate the immune response against chronic infections such as tuberculosis, viral infections, and certain intracellular parasitic infections; dendritic cells activate T cells against cancer, assist B lymphocytes to produce antibodies, and downregulate the immune system (DeMeyer & Buchsel, 2005).

LYMPHOCYTES   The **lymphocytes** account for 20% to 40% of circulating leukocytes. Lymphocytes are the principal effec-tor and regulator cells of specific immune responses to protect the body from microorganisms, foreign tissue, and cell muta-tions or alterations. Through a process known as immune sur-veillance, lymphocytes monitor the body for cancerous cells and eliminate or destroy them.

Like other leukocytes, lymphocytes derive from the stem cells in the bone marrow (Figure 12–2 ■). Lymphocytes have "homing" patterns: They constantly circulate, then return to concentrate in lymphoid tissues (the lymph nodes, spleen, thy-mus, tonsils, Peyer's patches in the submucosa of the distal ileum, and the appendix).

The three types of lymphocytes are **T lymphocytes (T cells)**, **B lymphocytes (B cells)**, and **natural killer cells (NK cells** or **null cells)**. None of these cells acts independently. Their functions are closely interrelated. T cells mature in the thymus gland, whereas B cells complete their maturation in the bone marrow. T cells and B cells are integral to the specific immune response and are

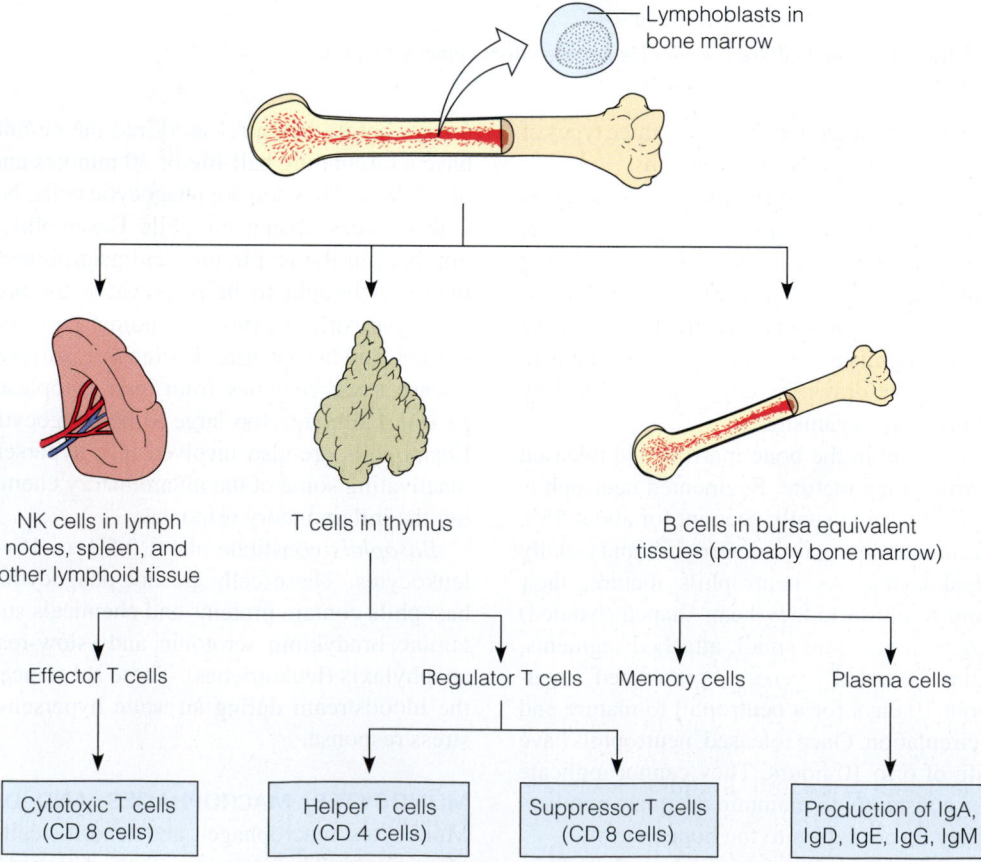

Figure 12–2 ■ The development and differentiation of lymphocytes from the lymphoid stem cell (lymphoblasts).

discussed further in that section of this chapter. On contact with an antigen, B lymphocytes are activated and mature into either plasma cells, which secrete antibodies, or memory cells. On contact with APCs, T lymphocytes mature into active T_{helper} cells, cytotoxic T cells, or memory T cells. Memory cells stay inactive, sometimes for years, but activate immediately with subsequent exposure to the same antigen. They then proliferate rapidly, producing an intense immune response. Memory cells are responsible for providing acquired immunity.

NK cells are large, granular cells found in the spleen, lymph nodes, bone marrow, and blood. They constitute 15% of circulating lymphocytes. NK cells are part of the innate immune system, provide immune surveillance and resistance to infection, and they play an important role in the destruction of early malignant cells. Like B cells and T cells, NK cells are cytotoxic, but unlike T cells do not require connection with an APC to become activated and kill cancer cells, virus-infected cells, and cells infected with microbes (Porth & Matfin, 2009). Fortunately, NK cells are inhibited when contact is made with normal host cells.

ANTIGENS Substances the immune system recognizes as foreign or "nonself" are called **antigens**; they provoke a specific immune response when introduced into the body. Typically, antigens are large protein molecules, although polysaccharides, polypeptides, and nucleic acids may also be antigenic. Many antigens are proteins found on the cell membrane or cell wall of microorganisms or tissues such as transplanted tissue or organs, incompatible blood cells, vaccines, pollen, egg white, and insect or snake venom.

Complete antigens, known as immunogens, have two characteristics: (1) *immunogenicity* is the ability to stimulate a specific immune response and (2) *specific reactivity* is the stimulation of specific immune system components. When an antigen is encountered in the body, generation of an effective immune response involves two major groups of cells: lymphocytes and antigen-presenting cells. Dendritic cells are APCs; two specific types of dendritic cells develop from pluripotent stem cells in the bone marrow. DC1s arise from monocytes, myeloid-type immune cells, and DC2s derive from lymphocyte precursors (DeMeyer & Buchsel, 2005). DC1s activate T cells against cancer cells. DC2s assist B lymphocytes to produce antibodies and to downregulate the immune system (Kimball, 2005). Downregulation of the immune response is very important to avoid autoimmune diseases.

Antigen-presenting cells are recognized by a specific receptor on a lymphocyte, and an immune response is generated by the lymphocytes. Two separate but overlapping immune responses may occur, depending on the antigen itself and the type of immune cell activated by contact with the antigen. The B cell or humoral branch of the immune system mainly eliminates extracellular antigens such as bacteria, bacterial toxins, and free viruses through the production of **antibodies**, molecules that bind with the antigen and inactivate it. There are five classes of antibodies: IgG, IgA, IgM, IgD, and IgE. These proteins make up the **antibody-mediated (humoral) immune response**. Intracellular pathogens, such as viral-infected cells, cancer cells, and foreign tissue, activate T lymphocytes, which are the primary agents of the **cell-mediated (cellular) immune response**.

In this immune response, the lymphocytes themselves, in the form of helper T cells, cytotoxic T cells, and NK cells, inactivate the antigen, either directly or indirectly.

Lymphoid System

The *lymphoid system* consists of the lymph nodes, spleen, thymus, tonsils, lymphoid tissue scattered in connective tissues and mucosa, and the bone marrow. The thymus and bone marrow, in which T cells and B cells mature, are considered central lymphoid organs. The spleen, lymph nodes, tonsils, and other peripheral lymphoid tissue are peripheral lymphoid organs (Figure 12–3 ■). This system exists to recover proteins such as albumin for the vascular system and to protect the bloodstream from invading organisms. Cells of the immune system such as neutrophils, macrophages, and dendritic cells carry antigens from interstitial space to lymph nodes for immune surveillance in the lymphatic circulation. Unlike the vascular tree, which has tight epithelial junctions, lymphatic epithelium is replete with open junctions that promote lymphocyte access and effectively protect the bloodstream from antigen entry.

Lymph nodes, the most numerous elements of the lymphoid system, are small, round or bean-shaped encapsulated bodies that vary in size from 1 mm to 2 cm. Distributed throughout the body, lymph nodes generally occur in groups at the junction of the lymphatic vessels. They can be found in the neck, axillae, abdomen, and groin.

Lymph nodes filter foreign products or antigens from the lymph and house and support proliferation of lymphocytes and macrophages. Lymph, a clear, protein-containing fluid transported within lymph vessels, enters the node through afferent

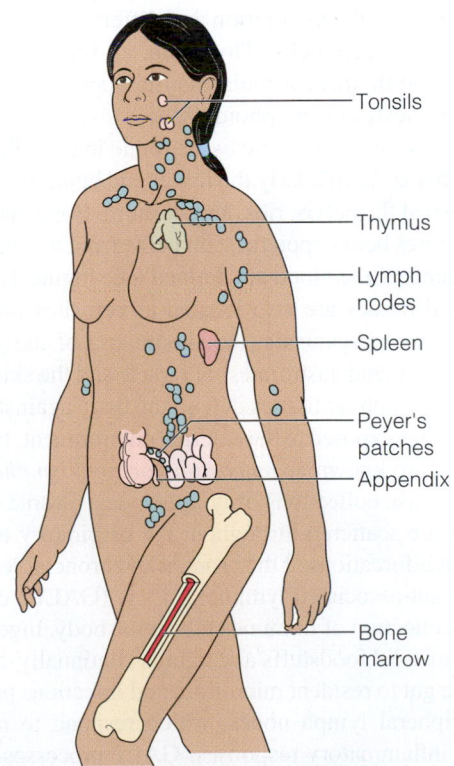

Figure 12–3 ■ The lymphoid system: the central organs of the thymus and bone marrow, and the peripheral organs, including the spleen, tonsils, lymph nodes, and Peyer's patches.

lymphatic vessels. Inside the node, the lymph flows through sinuses in the cortex of the lymph node where T and B lymphocytes and macrophages are abundant, then through sinuses of the medulla of the lymph node, which contains macrophages and plasma cells. The presence of a foreign antigen stimulates lymphocytes and macrophages to proliferate in the lymph nodes. Macrophages destroy the antigen by phagocytosis. Immune cells and lymph then leave the lymph node through efferent vessels. An abundant blood supply to the node also facilitates lymphocyte movement.

The *spleen* is the largest lymphoid organ in the body and the only lymphoid organ that can filter blood. The spleen is located in the upper left quadrant of the abdomen. The spleen has two kinds of tissue, white pulp and red pulp. White pulp is lymphoid tissue that serves as a site for lymphocyte proliferation and immune surveillance. B cells predominate in the white pulp. Blood filtration occurs in the red pulp. In blood-filled venous sinuses, phagocytic cells dispose of damaged or aged RBCs and platelets. Other debris and foreign matter, such as bacteria, viruses, and toxins, are also removed from the blood. The spleen also stores blood and the breakdown products of RBCs for future use. The spleen is not essential for life. If it is removed because of disease or trauma, the liver and the bone marrow assume its functions.

The *thymus gland* is located in the superior anterior mediastinal cavity beneath the sternum. It reaches its maximum size at puberty, then begins to atrophy slowly. By adulthood it is difficult to differentiate from surrounding adipose tissue even though it remains active. In the older adult, the vast majority of thymus tissue has been replaced by adipose and fibrous connective tissue. During fetal life and childhood, the thymus serves as a site for the maturation and differentiation of thymic lymphoid cells, the T cells. Thymosin, an immunoregulatory hormone of the thymus, stimulates lymphopoiesis, the formation of lymphocytes or lymphoid tissue.

Bone marrow is soft organic tissue found in the hollow cavity of the long bones, particularly the femur and humerus, as well as the flat bones of the pelvis, ribs, and sternum. Bone marrow produces and stores hematopoietic stem cells, from which all cellular components of the blood are derived (see Figure 12–1).

Lymphoid tissues are also located at key sites of potential invasion by microorganisms: the submucosa of the genitourinary, respiratory, and gastrointestinal tracts and the skin. Plasma cells in these lymphoid tissues defend the body against bacterial invasion at areas exposed to the external environment. In general, these tissues are known as *mucosa-associated lymphoid tissue* (MALT). Diffuse collections of lymphocytes, plasma cells, and phagocytes are scattered throughout the respiratory tract, concentrating at bifurcations of the bronchi and bronchioles. Peyer's patches, or gut-associated lymphoid tissue (GALT), comprises the largest collection of immune cells in the body. Ingestion and absorption of solid foodstuffs and liquids continually expose the lining of the gut to resident microflora and infectious pathogens. Unlike peripheral lymph nodes, which respond to pathogens with acute inflammatory responses, GALT processes common intestinal antigens without producing acute inflammation. Collections of immune cells make up the GALT. Intraepithelial lymphocytes fill the spaces between mucosal epithelial cells.

Beneath the basement membrane of gut epithelium lie abundant T cells and mature plasma cells, which are sources of IgA. Peyer's patches hold dense collections of lymphocytes in lymphoid nodules. As naïve B and T cells migrate through Peyer's patches, they are sensitized to specific antigens. In mesenteric lymph nodes these sensitized cells proliferate and circulate throughout the vascular tree where they produce secretory IgA. Secretory IgA coats mucosal cells and prevents attachment of intraluminal bacteria in the intestine, upper respiratory tract, the bronchi, mammary ducts, and salivary glands. Thus the GALT collection of immune cells effectively protects mucosa throughout the body that is exposed to resident and foreign pathogens.

Tonsils and adenoids protect the body from inhaled or ingested foreign agents. Skin-associated lymphoid tissue contains lymphocytes and dendritic cells such as Langerhans cells in the epidermis, which transport antigens to regional lymph nodes for destruction and development of specific immunity to the antigen.

Innate Immune Response

Innate immunity is the first line of defense. It is nonspecific and includes skin and mucosal barriers, vascular and cellular responses, and phagocytosis. Cells of the innate system include neutrophils, macrophages, and NK cells. NK cells indiscriminately kill pathogens but recognize self cells and leave them unharmed. Complement proteins and cytokines also function in the innate immune response.

Barrier protection is the body's defense against infection. Intact skin prevents invasion by external organisms. When the skin is damaged or lost (e.g., as a result of injury, surgery, or burns), infection is much more likely. The membranes lining inner surfaces of the body are protected by a barrier of mucus, which traps microorganisms and other foreign substances. These can then be removed by other protective mechanisms, such as ciliary movement or the washing action of tears or urine. In addition, many body fluids contain bactericidal substances that provide barrier protection. These include acid in gastric fluid, zinc in prostatic fluid, and lysozyme in tears, nasal secretions, saliva, and sweat (Porth & Matfin, 2009).

When these defenses are breached, the resulting tissue damage or foreign material entering the body induces inflammation. *Inflammation* is a response to injury that brings fluid, dissolved substances, and blood cells into the interstitial tissues where the invasion or damage has occurred. The response is called nonspecific because the same events occur regardless of cause of the inflammatory process. Through the inflammatory reaction, the invader is neutralized and eliminated, destroyed tissue removed, and the process of healing and repair initiated.

The inflammatory response has two stages: (1) a vascular response characterized by vasodilation and increased permeability of blood vessels, and (2) a cellular response. Phagocytosis sets the stage for healing (tissue repair).

Vascular Response

After tissue cells are damaged, local blood vessels briefly constrict. Vasodilation of the capillary arterioles and venules follows almost immediately as inflammatory mediators such as histamine and kinins are released from damaged tissue (Box 12–1).

Increased blood flow causes vasocongestion at the injury site with resultant redness and heat. The congestion also increases local hydrostatic pressure. This, along with increased vessel permeability that results from chemical mediators, moves fluid out of the capillaries and into the interstitial spaces of the tissue. The escaping fluid, called fluid exudate, contains large amounts of protein. This protein increases osmotic pressure in the interstitial spaces, which draws water and causes local edema. Fluid exudate provides protection to the injured tissue by bringing certain nutrients needed for tissue healing, diluting bacterial toxins, and transporting cells needed for phagocytosis. Mild tissue damage such as a blister produces a *serous* exudate of primarily plasma fluid and a few proteins. With moderate to severe tissue damage, fluid exudate is *sanguineous* or *hemorrhagic*, containing large amounts of RBCs. A mixture of RBCs and serum is referred to as *serosanguineous* exudate. *Fibrinous* exudate forms a thick, sticky meshwork of fibrinogen, in effect "walling off" inflamed tissues and preventing the spread of infection (Porth, 2007). In more severe or acute inflammation, the fluid contains fibrin, RBCs, and dead and live bacteria. This type of exudate, called *purulent* exudate, has an odor and color characteristic of the bacteria present.

Many of the outward manifestations of inflammation result from vasoactive substances such as *histamine*, *serotonin*, and *leukotrienes* (formerly known as slow-reacting substance of anaphylaxis, or SRS-A). Stored in mast cells, basophils, and platelets, histamine is released when an injury occurs or with stimulation by the immune system. An important component of the early inflammatory response, histamine causes vasodilation and vascular permeability in the affected area. Histamine is also

a key factor in many hypersensitivity reactions. Serotonin is released from platelets and produces effects similar to those of histamine. The leukotrienes play a significant vasoactive role in the later stages of the inflammatory response.

Prostaglandins are chemotactic substances that draw leukocytes to the inflamed tissue. In addition, they play a vasoactive role and are pain and fever inducers. Aspirin and other nonsteroidal anti-inflammatory drugs (NSAIDs) as well as the glucocorticoids inhibit prostaglandin synthesis, thereby reducing fever, pain, and inflammation.

Plasma factors such as Hageman factor activate the clotting cascade, plasminogen system (involved in the lysis of clots), and complement system. With activation of the clotting cascade, bacteria and other foreign substances are trapped in the area of tissue damage. Fibrin, which has vasoactive by-products, is also released. (∞ See Chapter 29 for a full description of the clotting process.) The complement system serves a chemotactic role and facilitates the phagocytic process.

Major chemical mediators of inflammation are summarized in Table 12–2.

The vascular response localizes invading bacteria and keeps them from spreading. Increased capillary permeability enhances the release of clotting factors such as fibrinogen, which converts to fibrin threads, entrapping the bacteria and walling them off from contact with the rest of the body.

Cellular Response

The cellular stage of the inflammatory process begins within less than an hour after the injury. This stage is marked by the margination and emigration of leukocytes into the damaged tissue, chemotaxis, and phagocytosis (Porth & Matfin, 2009).

As serous fluid escapes the capillaries, the viscosity of blood in the area increases and its flow becomes more sluggish. Leukocytes marginate, moving to the edges of the blood vessels, and begin to adhere to the capillary endothelium. This process is known as *pavementing*. After margination and pavementing, leukocytes emigrate from the blood vessel into the tissue spaces (Figure 12–4 ■). Within hours, millions of leukocytes emigrate into the area of inflammation.

Once leukocytes have emigrated, they are drawn to the damaged or inflamed tissues by chemotactic signals. Infectious agents, damaged tissues, and activated plasma substances such as complement fractions provide chemotaxic signals that attract an army of neutrophils, monocytes, and macrophages to the injury site.

TABLE 12–2 Major Chemical Mediators of Inflammation

FACTOR	SOURCE	EFFECT
Histamine	Mast cells, basophils, and platelets	Vasodilation and increased capillary permeability, producing tissue redness, warmth, and edema
Kinins (bradykinin and others)	Plasma protein factors	Histamine-like effects; chemotaxis and pain inducers
Prostaglandins	Metabolism of arachidonic acid from cell membranes	Histamine-like effects; chemotaxis, pain, and fever inducers
Leukotrienes	Arachidonic acid metabolism	Smooth muscle constriction (especially bronchoconstriction), increased vascular permeability, chemotaxis

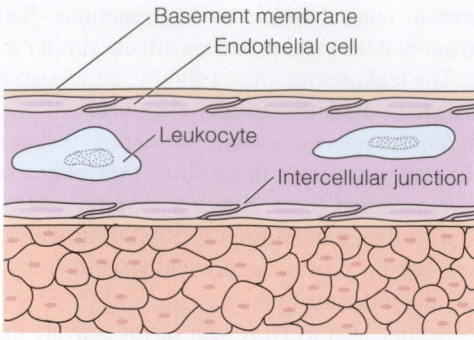

A Leukocytes in circulation

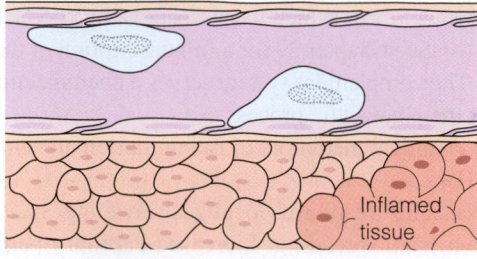

B Margination and pavementing

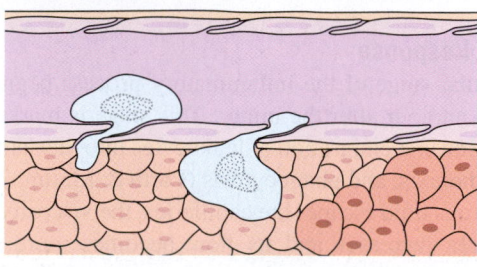

C Emigration

Figure 12–4 ■ The process of leukocyte emigration at the site of inflammation. *A,* Normal blood flow with free movement of formed elements. *B,* As blood flow slows, leukocytes move toward the periphery of stream and begin to cling to capillary endothelium, a process known as margination and pavementing. *C,* Leukocytes emigrate from the vessel into inflamed tissues.

The number of neutrophils around the site increases to about 15,000 to 25,000/mm^3, and they begin their role in phagocytosis within a few hours. Monocytes become transient macrophages to augment the activity of the fixed macrophages and dendritic cells; together they engulf dead cells, damaged tissue, nonfunctioning neutrophils, and invading bacteria.

Phagocytosis

Phagocytosis is a process by which a foreign agent or target cell is engulfed, destroyed, and digested. Neutrophils, macrophages, and dendritic cells, known as *phagocytes,* are the primary cells involved in phagocytosis. Once attracted to the inflammatory site, phagocytes select and engulf foreign material.

The following factors or processes help phagocytes differentiate foreign tissue from normal cells:

■ *Smooth surface.* Normal tissue has a smooth surface that is resistant to phagocytosis, whereas the rough surface of a foreign agent or target cell promotes phagocytosis.

■ *Surface charge.* Healthy body cells present an electronegative surface charge that repels phagocytes. Cellular debris and foreign agents, by contrast, have an electropositive charge that attracts them.

■ *Opsonization.* This immune system process coats the surface of bacteria or target cells with a substance (an opsonin) as in the complement system (Box 12–2). Opsonization enables the phagocyte to bind tightly with the foreign tissue, facilitating phagocytosis (Figure 12–5*A* ■).

Phagocytes engulf the foreign agent or target cell by projecting pseudopodia ("false feet") in all directions around it (Figure 12–5*B*). This produces a chamber called a *phagosome* containing the antigen, which is ingested into the cytoplasm (Figure 12–5*C*). Once the phagosome has been engulfed, lysosomes fuse with the phagosome, killing any live organism and releasing digestive enzymes, which destroy the antigen (Figure 12–5*D*).

Phagocytes—in particular, neutrophils and macrophages—contain bactericidal agents that kill most of the bacteria they ingest before the bacteria can multiply and destroy the phagocyte itself. The phagocyte kills bacteria in a number of ways; for example, it alters the intracellular pH and produces bactericidal agents. Oxidizing agents, such as superoxide, hydrogen peroxide, and hydroxyl ions, are bactericidal. Two lysosomal substances that kill bacteria are lysozyme and phagocytin.

Some antigens, such as the tubercle bacterium, have coats or secrete substances that are resistant to lysosomal and bactericidal agents. To destroy such antigens, lysosomes release digestive enzymes into the phagosome. The lysosomes of neutrophils and macrophages contain an abundance of proteolytic

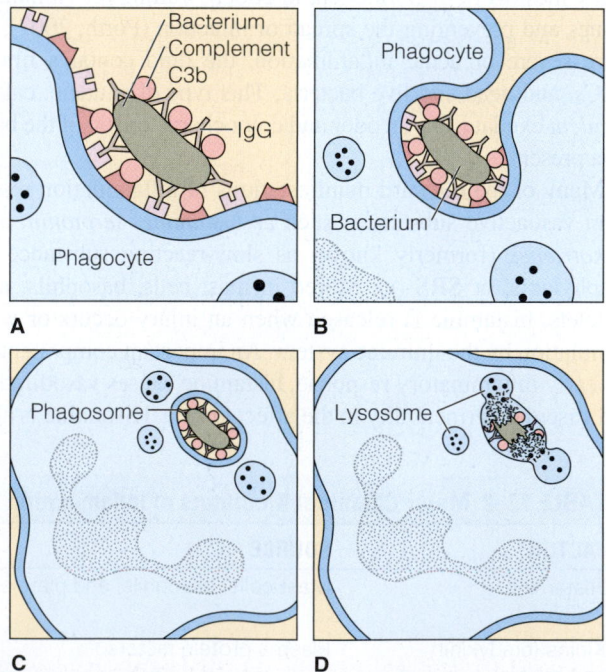

A   **B**

C   **D**

Figure 12–5 ■ The process of phagocytosis. *A,* Opsonization coats the surface of the bacterium with IgG (an antibody) and complement. *B,* The bacterium is bound to and engulfed by the phagocyte. *C,* The phagosome is ingested into the cytoplasm of the phagocyte. *D,* Lysosomes fuse with the phagosome, releasing digestive enzymes and destroying the antigen.

BOX 12–2 The Complement System

The *complement system* consists of approximately 20 complex plasma proteins that are activated by a tissue injury or antigen–antibody reaction. The complement system is involved in both innate and adaptive immune responses. Its activation results in the production of effector molecules that are involved in the processes of inflammation, phagocytosis, and cell lysis or destruction (Porth & Matfin, 2009). Specifically, complement activation leads to the following:

- *Mediation of the inflammatory response.* When the complement system is activated, chemical mediators such as histamine are released from mast cells and basophils, leading to smooth muscle contraction, increased vascular permeability and edema, and the attraction of leukocytes.
- *Opsonization (or coating) of microbes and antigen–antibody complexes to facilitate phagocytosis.*
- *Alteration of the cell membrane or viral capsule.* When the cell surface is altered, a pore or channel is created for complement fluids and ions to enter the phagocytic cell and cause cell lysis and death. Bacteria and viruses are destroyed; certain normal cells, such as RBCs, platelets, and lymphocytes, that are damaged or old may also be destroyed through this process.

The complement system has three "arms," or pathways, of protein and enzyme reactions. The *classic pathway* is activated by antibody-containing immunoglobulins and other substances such as DNA and C-reactive protein. The *alternate* and *lectin pathways* do not use antibodies; are activated by tissue injury, polysaccharides, or enzymes; and are part of the innate immune system (Porth, 2007). When either pathway is activated, the result is mediation of the inflammatory process, attraction of phagocytes, facilitation of phagocytosis, and lysis of microbes.

(protein-destroying) enzymes that digest bacteria and other foreign protein components. The macrophage's lysosomes also contain lipases (fat-splitting enzymes) capable of digesting the thick lipid membranes of such bacteria as *Mycobacterium tuberculosis* and *Mycobacterium leprae.*

Once neutrophils have ingested toxic substances to their capacity, they in turn are killed. Neutrophils have the capacity to phagocytize 5 to 20 bacteria before they become inactive. Macrophages then digest the dead neutrophils. Monocytes or macrophages are capable of phagocytizing up to 100 bacteria. Because of their size, they can ingest larger particles than neutrophils can ingest, such as whole RBCs, necrotic tissue, cell fragments, malarial parasites, and dead neutrophils. Dendritic cells are also phagocytic and secrete Il-12, which is an important cytokine in the maturation of T_{helper} cells (Kimball, 2005). Macrophages have the ability to extrude (release) the toxic substances and lysosomal enzymes within their phagosomes. As a result, they can continue to function for months and even years.

Healing

During the initial inflammatory process, particulate matter, bacteria, damaged cells, and inflammatory exudate are removed by phagocytosis. This process, called *debridement*, prepares the wound for healing. Adequate nutrition is essential for inflammation and healing to proceed. Protein, glucose, and oxygen are needed by leukocytes for chemotaxis, phagocytosis, and intercellular killings. Persons with diabetes are at risk

for poor healing of wounds. Probable causes for this risk may be small vessel disease, which impairs microcirculation, and increased affinity for oxygen common to glycosylated hemoglobin. Oxygen circulation is impaired as well as release of oxygen to the cells.

The second phase of the healing process, known as *reconstruction*, may overlap the inflammatory phase. The ideal result of the healing process is *resolution*, the restoration of the original structure and function of the damaged tissue. Simple resolution occurs when there is no destruction of the normal tissue and the body is able to neutralize and remove the offending agent through the inflammatory process.

Resolution may also occur when the damaged tissue is capable of regeneration. The ability to regenerate, or replace lost *parenchyma* (functional tissue) with new, functional cells varies by tissue and cell type.

- *Labile cells* continue to regenerate throughout life. These cells are found in tissues where there is a daily turnover of cells—namely, bone marrow and the epithelial cells of the skin, mucous membranes, cervix, gastrointestinal tract, and genitourinary tract.
- *Stable cells* normally stop replicating when growth ceases, but are capable of regeneration when stimulated by an injury. Osteocytes (which are found in bone) and parenchymal cells of the kidneys, liver, and pancreas are stable cells.
- *Permanent* or *fixed cells* are unable to regenerate. When these cells are destroyed, they are replaced by fibrous scar tissue. Nerve cells, skeletal muscle cells, and cardiac muscle cells are fixed cells (Porth & Matfin, 2009).

Researchers are searching for signaling molecules that will stimulate repair of permanent cells, allowing regeneration. Paralysis from spinal cord injury is often the stimulus for this research focus. When regeneration and complete resolution are not possible, healing occurs by replacement of the destroyed tissue with collagen scar tissue. This process is known as *repair*. Although tissue that has undergone repair lacks the physiologic function of the destroyed tissue, the scar fills the lesion and provides tensile tissue strength. The healing process is discussed further in ∞ Chapter 4.

Adaptive Immune Response

The introduction of antigens into the body causes a second, more specific reaction than the innate, nonspecific immune response. On the first exposure to an antigen, a change occurs in the host, resulting in a specific and rapid response following subsequent exposures. This specific response is known as the *adaptive immune response.*

The adaptive immune response to an antigen has the following distinctive properties:

- The adaptive immune response typically is directed against materials recognized as foreign (i.e., from outside the body) and is not usually directed against the self (i.e., cells or structures produced by the body). This property is known as *self-recognition.*
- The immune response is *specific*. It is initiated by and directed against particular antigens (such as a specific virus, bacterium, or transplanted tissue).

■ Unlike a localized inflammatory response, the immune response is systemic. Immunity is generalized; it is not restricted to the initial site of infection or entry of foreign tissue.

■ The immune response has memory. Repeated exposures to an antigen produce a more rapid response.

A patient whose immune system is able to identify antigens and effectively destroy or remove them is said to be **immunocompetent**. Health problems may occur when the immune response is altered (∞ see Chapter 13 for further discussion).

Antibody-Mediated Immune Response

The antibody-mediated (humoral) immune response is produced by B lymphocytes (B cells). B cells are constantly replaced through cell division and proliferation in the bone marrow. It is believed that B cells mature in the bone marrow and then migrate to the spleen to await activation. They normally constitute 10% to 15% of circulating lymphocytes.

B cells are activated by contact with an antigen and by T cells (discussed in the next section). Each B cell has receptor

sites for a specific antigen or antigens. When the antigen is encountered, the activated B cell proliferates and differentiates into antibody-producing plasma cells and memory cells (Figure 12–6 ■). Plasma cells are short lived, lasting only about 1 day. While alive, however, they can produce thousands of antibody molecules per second. Memory cells retain antibody-producing information, allowing a rapid response if the antigen is again encountered.

An antibody is an **immunoglobulin (Ig)** molecule with the ability to bind to and inactivate a specific antigen. Immunoglobulins comprise the gamma globulin portion of the blood proteins. The immune system produces numerous antibodies, each active against a specific antigen. As mentioned earlier, antibodies fall into five classes of immunoglobulins: IgG, IgA, IgM, IgD, and IgE. Each has a slightly different structure and function. Their roles are summarized in Table 12–3.

Antibodies are Y-shaped molecules with two light and two heavy polypeptide chains (Figure 12–7 ■). The top portion of the Y, called the *Fab* or *antigen-binding fragment*, is chemically variable and specific to the antigen. The lower portion, the

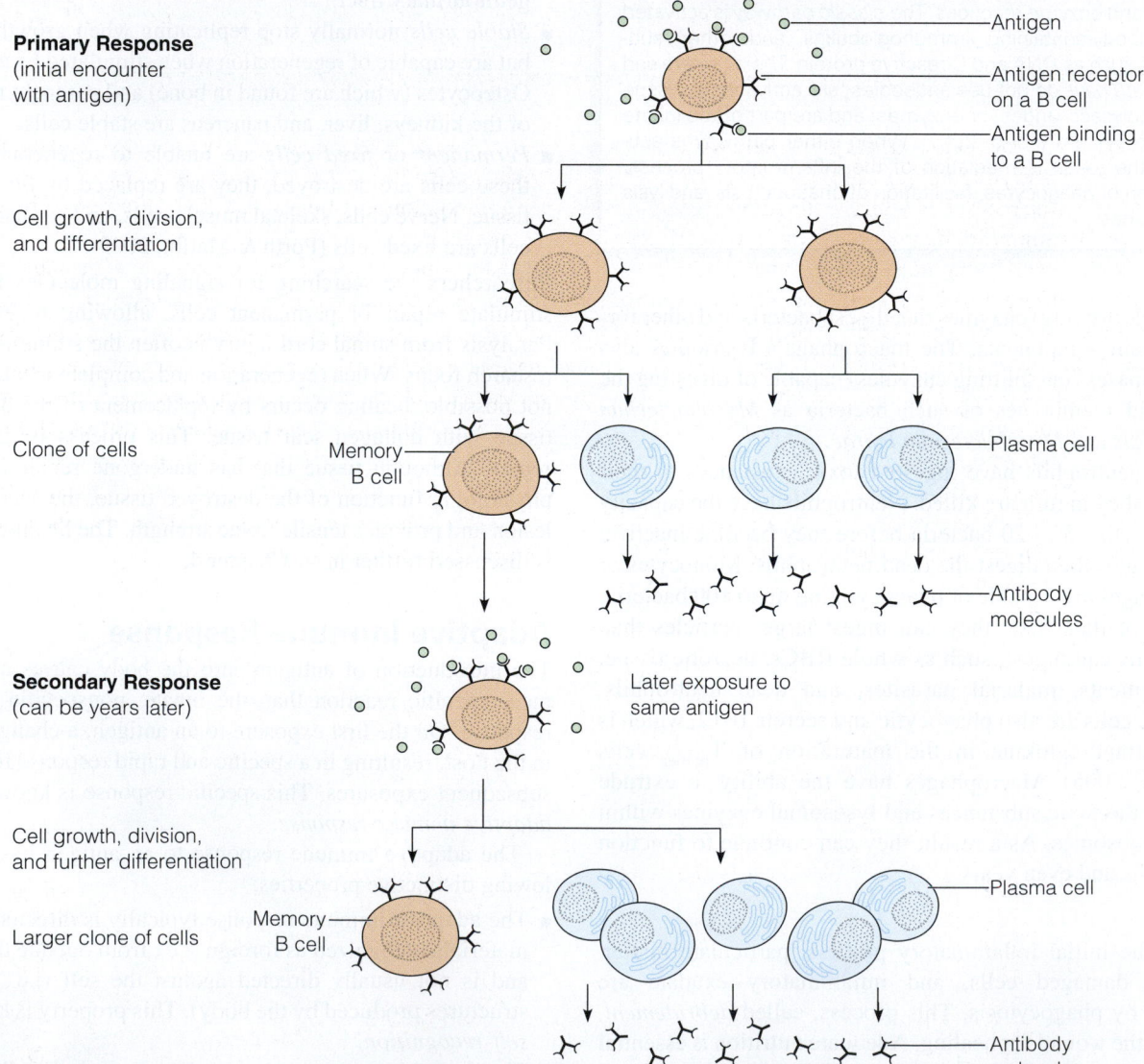

Primary Response
(initial encounter
with antigen)

Antigen

Antigen receptor
on a B cell

Antigen binding
to a B cell

Cell growth, division,
and differentiation

Clone of cells

Memory
B cell

Plasma cell

Antibody
molecules

Secondary Response
(can be years later)

Later exposure to
same antigen

Cell growth, division,
and further differentiation

Larger clone of cells

Memory
B cell

Plasma cell

Antibody
molecules

Figure 12–6 ■ Antibody-mediated (humoral) immunity. On initial exposure to the antigen, B cells with appropriate receptor sites are activated to become plasma cells and produce antibodies or memory cells. This is known as the primary response. With subsequent exposures, memory cells respond rapidly with antibody production. This is known as the secondary response.

TABLE 12–3 Immunoglobulin Characteristics and Functions

CLASS	PERCENTAGE OF TOTAL	CHARACTERISTICS AND FUNCTION
IgG	75%	Most abundant Ig; also known as gamma globulin; found in blood, lymph, and intestines.
		Active against bacteria, bacterial toxins, and viruses.
		Activates complement and binds to macrophages.
		The only Ig to cross the placenta, providing immune protection to neonate.
IgA	10% to 15%	Found in saliva; tears; and bronchial, gastrointestinal, prostatic, and vaginal secretions, as well as blood and lymph.
		Provides local protection on exposed mucous membrane surfaces and potent antiviral activity by preventing binding of the virus to epithelial cells.
		Levels decrease during stress.
IgM	5% to 10%	Found in blood and lymph.
		First antibody produced with primary immune response.
		High concentrations early in infection, decreases within about a week.
		Mediates cytotoxic response and activates complement.
IgD	<1%	Found in blood, lymph, and surfaces of B cells.
		Exact function unknown; may be receptor-binding antigens to B-cell surface.
IgE	<0.1%	Found on mast cells and basophils.
		Involved in release of chemical mediators responsible for immediate hypersensitivity (allergic and anaphylactic) response and parasitic infections.

F_c, or *crystallized fragment*, is constant for its class of immunoglobulin and directs the biologic activity of the immunoglobulin (the manner in which it functions). For example, the lower portion of immunoglobulin molecules produced against hepatitis A and hepatitis B are the same (IgG), but the upper portion is different and specific to the virus.

The antibodies produced by B cells (see Figure 12–6) link with the antigen (Figure 12–8 ■) and inactivate it through one of the following processes:

- Promoting phagocytosis of the antigen by neutrophils
- Precipitation: combining with soluble antigens to form an insoluble complex or precipitate
- Neutralization: combining with a toxin to neutralize its effects; the antigen–antibody complex is then destroyed by the process of phagocytosis

- Lysis of the antigen cell membrane caused by combination with antibodies and complement proteins
- Agglutination (clumping) of antigens to form a noninvasive aggregate
- Opsonization: coating of the antigen with antibodies and complement, making them more susceptible to phagocytosis

The complete antibody-mediated response occurs in two phases. With initial exposure to an antigen, the primary response develops. B cells are activated to proliferate and begin producing antibodies. There is a latency period of 3 to 6 days before antibodies become detectable in the blood. Levels then continue to rise, peaking at 10 to 14 days after the initial exposure. With many illnesses (e.g., chickenpox), this peak correlates with recovery.

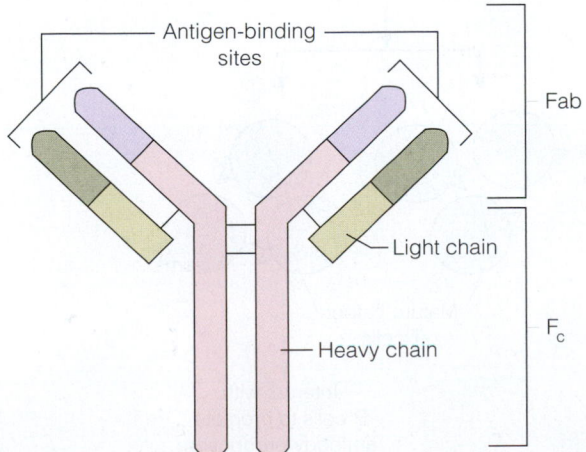

Figure 12–7 ■ An antibody molecule. The Fab section is unique, providing an antigen-specific binding site. The F_c section is common to each class of immunoglobulin (IgG, IgA, IgM, IgD, IgE).

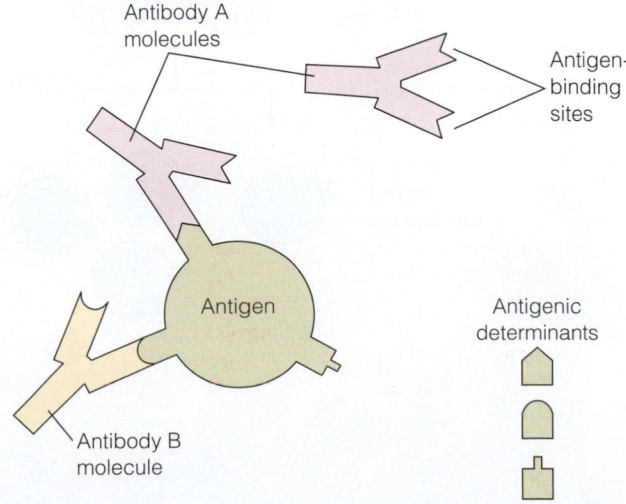

Figure 12–8 ■ Antigen–antibody binding. The unique Fab site on the antibody binds with specific receptor sites on the antigen. As shown, more than one kind of antibody may be produced to an antigen.

Subsequent exposure to the same antigen elicits a secondary response. Memory cells (see Figure 12–6) formed during the primary response stimulate the production of plasma cells, and an almost immediate rise in antibody levels occurs (Figure 12–9 ■). This rapid secondary response is the basis of acquired immunity and is instrumental in preventing disease. It is also the mechanism through which vaccines provide protection from disease.

Cell-Mediated Immune Response

Many antigens cannot stimulate the antibody-mediated response or are "hidden" from it because they live inside the body's cells (viruses and mycobacteria are examples of such antigens). The immune response providing protection against these antigens is the cell-mediated immune response, also called *cellular immunity*. T lymphocytes (T cells) initiate this type of immune response.

Approximately 70% to 80% of circulating lymphocytes are T cells. T cells migrate to the thymus during fetal and early life, establishing the lifetime pool of cells. T cells have a life span measured in years, maintaining their numbers through proliferation, primarily in the lymph nodes. T cells are much more complex than B cells. There are two major classes of T cells, *effector cells* and *regulator cells*. The main effector T cell is the *cytotoxic cell*, also called the *killer T cell*. Regulator T cells are further classified into two groups: *helper T cells* and *suppressor T cells*. T cells are antigen specific; that is, each subset is activated by a particular antigen. The antigens that activate T cells must be presented on another cell surface, such as pieces of virus presented on the surface of an

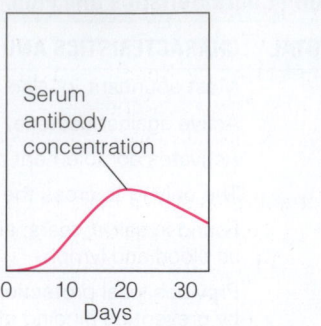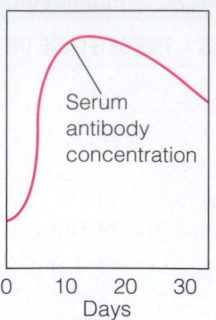

Figure 12–9 ■ Antibody production in the primary and secondary responses of the antibody-mediated immune response. Note the more rapid and effective production following subsequent exposure.

infected cell, or the histocompatibility locus antigen on a cell of transplanted tissue. When activated, T cells divide and proliferate, forming antigen-specific *clones* (Figure 12–10 ■). A clone is an exact copy of another cell.

Cytotoxic T cells bind with cell surface antigens on virus-infected or foreign cells. Killer T cells destroy the identified cell by combining with it and then either destroying its cell membrane or releasing cytotoxic substances into the cell. They are vital in the control of viral and bacterial infections.

Regulator T cells play a key role in controlling the immune response. The majority of regulator T cells are helper T cells. They stimulate the proliferation of other T cells, amplify the cytotoxic activity of killer T cells, and activate B cells to proliferate

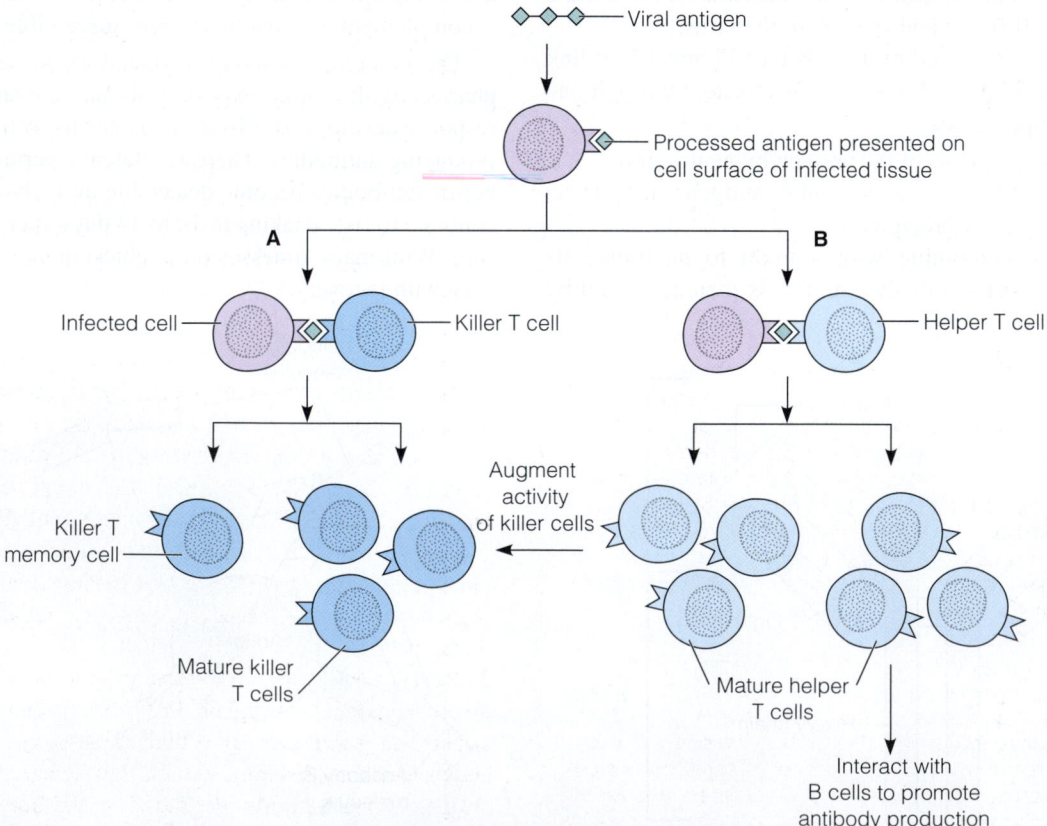

Figure 12–10 ■ Cellular immune response. *A,* An infected cell, abnormal cell, or phagocyte presents antigen on its surface that binds with a receptor site on a killer T cell or a helper T cell. The killer T cell is activated to proliferate into memory cells or mature cytotoxic cells. *B,* The helper T cell is activated to augment the cytotoxic response and stimulate the antibody-mediated immune response.

and differentiate. They interact directly with B cells to promote their multiplication and conversion into plasma cells capable of producing antibodies. The other regulatory T-cell group, suppressor T cells, provides negative feedback, making the immune response a self-limiting process. Suppressor T cells release lymphokines, which inhibit the activity of other T cells and B cells.

On activation, both effector and regulator T cells synthesize and release lymphokines, a type of soluble protein. Lymphokines are a subgroup of nonspecific defense mechanisms known as **cytokines** (Box 12–3). Lymphokines secreted by cytotoxic and helper T cells are important in amplifying the immune response and the inflammatory response. They stimulate the following:

- B cells to become plasma cells and produce antibodies
- Macrophages to become activated macrophages (the most aggressive phagocyte)
- Proliferation of killer T cells

Although T cells can be activated only by specific antigens, much of the resulting effect is nonspecific—in other words, an enhanced inflammatory response. Like the antibody-mediated response, the cell-mediated response has memory. Subsequent exposures to an antigen result in a more rapid and effective inflammatory response and more effective phagocytosis by macrophages. This memory provides the basis for skin testing. A patient previously exposed to tuberculosis, for example, develops a more pronounced inflammatory response when minute amounts are injected under the skin.

BOX 12–3 Cytokines

Cytokines are hormone-like polypeptides produced primarily by cells of the immune system. Cytokines are also produced in small quantities in many different tissues throughout the body. Cytokines act as messengers of the immune system, facilitating communication between the cells to adjust or vary the inflammatory reaction or to initiate immune cell proliferation and differentiation. Cytokines are an essential component of an adequate immune response. The major cytokines and their functions are summarized in Table 12–4.

The inflammatory cytokines contribute to sickness behaviors. Patients respond to increases in these chemicals with increased sleep, seeking warmth, and reduced energy output to obtain and consume food or perform grooming activities. These are considered adaptive responses to illness; interventions to reduce or eliminate the production of certain cytokines are common. Aspirin or NSAIDs to reduce pain and fever are commonly used. Because some cytokines cross the blood–brain barrier, their increase may explain depression and anxiety experienced during illness. Prevention or limitation of these effects by prophylactic antidepressant medication may improve quality of life for patients receiving biologic therapy (cytokines such as Interleukin-2) as part of their treatment for rheumatoid arthritis, Crohn's disease, or cancer (Myers, 2008).

Interferons are a class of cytokine with broad antiviral and anticancer effects. A number of different forms of interferon exist, broadly grouped as alpha, beta, and gamma interferons. Interferon is synthesized by cells infected with a virus and secreted into extracellular fluid. It then binds to specific receptors on uninfected neighboring cells, protecting them from infection. The spread of the virus is thus inhibited, and recovery from infection enhanced. It appears that interferons also moderate the activity of NK cells and may be involved in preventing the spread of abnormal malignant cells.

The Patient with Natural or Acquired Immunity

Immunity refers to the protection of the body from disease. Immunity to disease may be either natural or acquired, active or passive.

Immunity develops from the activation of the body's immune response. Depending on the antigen, antibody-mediated or cell-mediated responses are activated. The immune response typically involves components of both. In the *immunocompetent* (having an immune system capable of responding to pathogens and tissue damage) patient, these responses inactivate and remove the antigen, allowing recovery to occur or preventing the development of disease. Patients with suppressed or impaired immune function are more susceptible to disease and require protection from exposure to environmental elements. Isolation techniques are employed to prevent the spread of disease and to protect immune-suppressed patients.

Pathophysiology

The processes of antibody-mediated and cell-mediated immunity result in the development of **acquired immunity** or **active immunity**. Active immunity occurs when the body produces antibodies or develops immune lymphocytes against specific antigens. Memory cells, which can produce an immediate immune response on re-exposure to the antigen, provide long-term immunity.

Active immunity can be naturally acquired, resulting from contact with the disease-producing antigen and subsequent development of the disease. Naturally acquired immunity is common for diseases such as chickenpox and hepatitis A, making the risk of developing the disease a second time very low.

For many diseases, the potential consequences of a single disease episode on the individual and society make prevention desirable, especially for highly contagious diseases capable of causing epidemics. In these instances, immunization or vaccination is used to provide artificially acquired immunity. The purpose of vaccination is to establish adequate levels of antibody and/or memory cells to provide effective immunity. Vaccination introduces the disease-producing antigen into the body in a manner that will stimulate the immune system to form antibodies and memory cells but will not produce disease. Vaccines may be made of killed organisms or of live organisms that have been *attenuated* or modified to reduce their disease-producing capability. Typhoid is an example of a killed organism vaccine; measles-mumps-rubella (MMR) vaccine, by contrast, is made from attenuated organisms. Many newer vaccines use subunits of the antigen; these are portions of the organism that have antigenic properties but are unable to produce disease.

Passive immunity provides temporary protection against disease-producing antigens. Passive immunity is provided by antibodies produced by other people or animals. These acquired antibodies are used up; they either combine with the antigen or are naturally degraded by the body, and their protection is gradually lost. Naturally acquired passive immunity is provided by the transfer of maternal antibodies via the placenta and breast milk to the infant. Rabies human immune

TABLE 12–4 Major Cytokines and Their Functions

CYTOKINE	WHERE PRODUCED	PRIMARY FUNCTIONS
Interleukin-1 (IL-1)	Monocytes, macrophages, and dendritic cells	Activates T and B cells
		Induces fever and tissue catabolism
		Enhances NK activity
		Attracts neutrophils, macrophages, and lymphocytes
		Stimulates bone marrow and endothelial cell growth, collagen, and collagenases
Interleukin-2 (IL-2)	Helper T cells	Stimulates T and B cell proliferation; aids in discriminating between self and nonself
		Activates killer T and NK cells
Interleukin-3 (IL-3)	T cells	Stimulates growth and differentiation of bone marrow stem cells
Interleukin-4 (IL-4)		Stimulates proliferation of T cells
		Increases IgE secretion by B cells
Interleukin-5 (IL-5)	T cells and activated mast cells	Promotes differentiation of B cells and eosinophils
		Stimulates production of IgA
Interleukin-6	T cells and macrophages	Pro-inflammatory and anti-inflammatory cytokine
		Induces fever
Interleukin-8	Macrophages	Mediator of the innate immune response
		Induces fever
		Angiogenic (stimulates vessel formation)
Gamma interferon	T and NK cells	Stimulates phagocytosis by neutrophils and macrocytes
		Activates NK cells
		Augments B cell proliferation, enhancing both cellular and humoral immune responses
Alpha and beta interferons	Virus-infected cells; macrophages	Activate macrophages and endothelial cells; β interferon induces fever
		Augment NK cell activity
		Act at gene level to protect neighboring cells from invasion by intracellular parasites, such as viruses, rickettsia, malaria
Macrophage inflammatory proteins (MIP-1-4CC)	Macrophages, dendritic cells, and lymphocytes	Chemokines (CC), which are small cytokines
		Promote inflammatory response, chemotaxis, and homeostasis (control migration of cells in maintenance and development)
Tumor necrosis factor (TNF)	Activated macrophages, T cells, and NK cells	Major chemical mediator of inflammatory response
		Stimulates T-cell activation, antibody production, and accumulation of leukocytes at inflammatory site
		Directly cytotoxic to some tumor cells
		Induces fever

globulin and hepatitis B immune globulin (HBIG) are examples of immunizations used to provide artificially acquired passive immunity. The types of active and passive immunity are summarized in Table 12–5.

Interdisciplinary Care

Collaborative care focuses primarily on assessing the patient's immune status and ensuring acquired immunity to prevent disease.

Diagnosis

A number of diagnostic tests can be performed to assess the patient's immune status.

- *Serum protein* measures the total protein in the blood, including albumin and globulins. Normal total protein levels for the adult are 6 to 8 g/dL; albumin is approximately 60% (3.2 to 4.5 g/dL) of the total serum protein, and globulins are normally 2.3 to 3.4 g/dL. Total protein levels, albumin, and globulin are decreased in malnutrition and liver disease. Decreased globulin levels are noted with immunologic deficiencies.

- *Protein electrophoresis* analyzes protein content especially for albumin and gamma globulin and is used to assess immune function. Gamma globulins subjected to further electrophoresis separate into immunoglobulins: IgA, IgD, IgE, IgG, and IgM (see Table 12–2). Analysis of specific levels of each provides clues about the immune status of the patient. IgG levels are increased during acute infection. Decreased levels of IgG, IgA, and IgM are found in malignancies.

- *Antibody testing* is ordered to determine if a patient has developed antibodies in response to an infection or immunization. Antibodies for hepatitis, HIV, rubella, toxoplasmosis, and *Treponema pallidum* (the organism causing syphilis) can be identified. An elevated titer for hepatitis and rubella indicates immunity. For the other disorders and hepatitis, it may also be used to determine if the patient has the disease.

TABLE 12–5 Types of Acquired Immunity

TYPE OF IMMUNITY		HOW DEVELOPED	EXAMPLES
Active Immunity	Natural	Acquired by infection with an antigen, resulting in the production of antibodies	Chickenpox, hepatitis A
	Artificial	Acquired by immunization with an antigen, such as attenuated live virus vaccine	MMR, polio, DPT, hepatitis B vaccines
Passive Immunity	Natural	Acquired by transfer of maternal antibodies to the fetus or neonate via the placenta or breast milk	Neonate initially protected against MMR if mother immune
	Artificial	Acquired by administration of antibodies or antitoxins in immune globulin	Gamma globulin injection following hepatitis A exposure

■ *Skin testing* can assess cell-mediated immunity. A known antigen such as streptokinase, tuberculin purified protein derivative (PPD), or candida is injected intradermally. The site is then observed for induration and erythema, which typically peaks at 24 to 48 hours. An induration of at least 10 mm in diameter is a positive reaction indicating previous exposure and sensitization to the antigen. (∞ See Chapter 13 for further information on skin testing for hypersensitivity reactions.) No reaction, or **anergy**, indicates depressed cell-mediated immunity.

Immunizations

Vaccines are suspensions of whole or fractionated bacteria or viruses that have been treated to make them nonpathogenic. Vaccines are given to induce an immune response and subsequent immunity. Although vaccine development has been a major factor in improving public health, no vaccine is completely effective or entirely safe. Table 12–6 outlines the vaccines recommended for the adult patient to maintain optimal health and immune status (CDC, 2009).

Adults born before 1957 are generally considered to be immune to measles, mumps, and rubella by prior infection. For persons born after 1957 whose immunologic status is unclear or who are at significant risk of exposure to these diseases (e.g., persons entering healthcare careers), reimmunization is recommended by the CDC (Centers for Disease Control and Prevention). Adults who only received one dose of varicella (chickenpox) vaccine should receive a second dose. Adults aged 60 and older should receive zoster vaccine regardless of history of chickenpox or herpes zoster (shingles).

Tetanus and diphtheria (Td) toxoids are combined in a single immunization. The vaccine stimulates active immunity by inducing the production of antibodies and antitoxins. After an initial series of three immunizations, a booster injection is recommended every 10 years to maintain protection. Older patients, particularly those who never entered the workforce (e.g., older female adults), may have never received the initial series of Td vaccine. A resurgence of active cases of pertussis among adults and children has led the CDC to recommend that all adults receive one dose of tetanus/diphtheria/pertussis (Tdap) vaccine.

Hepatitis B (HB) vaccine is given as a series of three immunizations to promote active immunity to hepatitis B. It is mandated by the Occupational Health and Safety Administration (OSHA) for healthcare workers. High-risk populations include intravenous drug users, sexual partners of infected individuals, patients on hemodialysis, prison guards, and athletic coaches.

Influenza vaccine is recommended for persons at high risk for serious sequelae of influenza, including older adults, persons with lung disease or other chronic illness, and immunosuppressed individuals. The antigenic strain included in the influenza vaccine varies each year according to the predicted predominant strains affecting the population. Yearly reimmunization is therefore required. Pneumococcal vaccine is generally recommended for the same populations as influenza vaccine. A single dose of this vaccine confers lifetime immunity, although repeating immunization every 6 years may be considered for high-risk patients (including smokers and those with asthma). Pneumococcal vaccine for all senior citizens is a U.S. public health and Medicare goal. The purpose of immunization is to prevent respiratory infections and hospitalizations.

Human papillomavirus (HPV) vaccine has been shown to significantly reduce the risk for cervical cancer. HPV is recommended for all previously unvaccinated women through age 26 years.

In addition to routine immunizations, people traveling outside the United States and Canada should receive vaccines against diseases that are endemic in certain regions of the world.

Other immunologic substances may be administered as indicated. Immune globulins provide passive immunity as protection against a known or potential exposure to an antigen. Standard immune globulin is given to household contacts of patients with hepatitis A and persons traveling to areas in which it is endemic. HBIG contains higher titers of antibody to hepatitis B virus and is used for persons exposed by blood or sexual contact. Following confirmed or suspected contact with a pathogen, selected vaccines may be administered to stimulate an immediate immune response.

For most vaccines, a sensitivity test should be performed prior to administration to detect sensitivity to substances such as horse serum or eggs. The substance is injected intradermally; if after 20 minutes there is no evidence of a reaction, the selected vaccine can be administered.

Moderate to severe local reactions may occur following administration of an immunization. Common reactions include redness, swelling, tenderness, and muscle ache. Administering the vaccine in the dominant arm of the patient helps minimize local reactions because use and movement of the arm facilitates absorption of the solution. Applying heat to the site is also beneficial. Occasionally local ulcerations occur; when they do, warm, wet pack, or sterile wet-to-dry dressings may be prescribed.

TABLE 12–6 Recommended Immunizations for Adults

VACCINE	TYPE	DOSE	INDICATIONS	PRECAUTIONS AND NURSING IMPLICATIONS
Human papilloma virus (HPV)	Not a live virus	0.5 mL IM	Prior to exposure to HPV through sexual activity.	3 doses for females ≤ 26 years; IM in deltoid.
Measles-mumps-rubella (MMR)	Live virus	0.5 mL SC	All adults born after 1956, particularly those who are at risk for infection, such as college students and military recruits. Measles and mumps vaccination particularly recommended for males without history of previous infection; rubella vaccination recommended for all seronegative females.	As a live virus vaccine, should not be administered to pregnant women or immunocompromised patients. Do not administer to patients with a history of anaphylactic reaction to egg protein or neomycin. Give SC in fatty tissue over triceps.
Tetanus and diphtheria toxoids (Td); pertussis (Tdap)	Inactivated toxins	0.5 mL IM	Initial series of three injections (two doses, 4 to 6 weeks apart; third dose 6 to 12 months after dose 2) if never immunized; booster every 10 years; following a major or contaminated wound if more than 5 years since last booster. Replace one booster with Tdap.	Do not give in first trimester of pregnancy or to patients with a history of anaphylactic reaction to horse serum; administer deep IM in deltoid of dominant arm.
Hepatitis A		1 mL IM	Persons with liver disease or who receive clotting factors; travel to areas with high endemicity; illicit drug use or men who have sex with men.	Give IM in deltoid.
Hepatitis B (HB)	Inactive viral antigen	1.0 mL IM	Series of three doses: initial and at 1 and 6 months. Recommended for anyone at risk for exposure and for postexposure prophylaxis.	Use with caution in pregnant or lactating females, older patients, and patients with active infection; have epinephrine 1:1000 available on unit in case of anaphylaxis and laryngospasm.
Influenza	Inactivated virus or viral components	0.5 mL IM	Yearly for all patients over age 65 and those at risk for complications, including debilitated patients and patients with chronic disease.	Do not administer to acutely ill patients or patients with history of anaphylactic reaction to egg protein.
Pneumococcal	Bacterial polysaccharides	0.5 mL IM or SC	One dose for patients over age 65 and those at risk for pneumococcal pneumonia, including patients with chronic lung disease or other chronic diseases.	Do not administer to pregnant women.
Herpes zoster (shingles)		0.65 mL SC	Adults ≥ 60 years including those who report having had shingles.	Give in fatty tissue over triceps. Do not administer during pregnancy, immunocompromised, or HIV-infected persons.
Meningococcal vaccine (Menactra©)		0.5 mL IM	College students living in dormitories and military recruits.	Give in deltoid muscle; persons previously diagnosed with Guillain-Barré syndrome should not receive this vaccine.

✍ Nursing Care

Maintaining a population that is fully immunized against common, potentially epidemic, and devastating diseases is a major public health task for nursing. Nurses not only recommend and administer vaccines to individual patients and their families, but also plan and implement preventive care for whole communities.

Although this process may appear to be straightforward, multiple issues affect society's ability to immunize the entire population. For some people, for example, religious beliefs may preclude the use of immunizations to prevent disease.

Also, people who are not citizens and the medically indigent population have difficulty accessing immunization services. Lack of immunization not only puts the individual at increased risk for infectious disease, but also increases the cost of medical services and the possibility of exposing immunocompromised people to disease.

Clinically important medical events including fever, injection-site hypersensitivity, unspecified rash, and injection-site edema that occur after vaccination should be reported to the Vaccine Adverse Event Reporting System (VAERS) by calling 1-800-822-7967 or by using the VAERS website. This report needs to be made even if the reporting person is not certain the event was caused by the vaccine. Approximately 14% of all reports describe serious adverse events, including life-threatening illness, hospitalization or prolongation of hospitalization, permanent disability, or death (Stokowski, 2008).

Health Promotion

In the public health setting, the nurse looks at the immunization needs and illness risk for an entire community. Communities include not only cities and localities but also groups of people, such as college populations and employees in a workplace. Public education needs may be met through presentations to groups of people, feature articles in newspapers and other local publications, advertising, radio presentations and public service announcements, and one-to-one discussion and teaching.

Assessment

Collect the following data through the health history and physical examination. Further focused assessments are described with nursing interventions in the next section.

- *Health history:* Age, medication use (corticosteroids and antibiotics) and blood transfusion, nutrition, known allergies, pregnancy status, infection, immunizations, autoimmune disorders, chronic diseases such as asthma, diabetes mellitus, cancer, smoking history.
- *Physical assessment:* Skin lesions or rashes, breath sounds, respiratory rate.

Nursing Diagnoses and Interventions

Nursing care focuses on preventing injury from the immunization and educating the patient. See the accompanying Case Study & Nursing Care Plan.

Health-Seeking Behaviors: Immunization

For individual patients and their families, nurses promote immunocompetence by assessing immune status, recommending appropriate immunizations, and administering vaccines as ordered or indicated. Once a person reaches adulthood, routine immunizations often become a neglected part of health care.

- Determine knowledge level, understanding, attitudes, and religious beliefs about immunization. *This provides a basis for further education and determines if religious beliefs may contraindicate immunization.*
- Discuss the value and reasons for recommended immunizations. *Understanding promotes adherence.*

CASE STUDY & NURSING CARE PLAN A Patient with Acquired Immunity

Terry Adams is a 48-year-old executive who is planning a trip to central Africa. In preparation, he contacts his local healthcare provider to obtain the necessary immunizations. Jane Wong, the registered nurse in the clinic, obtains a nursing history of Mr. Adams.

ASSESSMENT

Mr. Adams's history reveals that he has always been very healthy and active, apart from a mild case of asthma. As an adult, he has had little problem with his asthma "except for those rare occasions on which I am dumb enough to smoke more than one cigarette!" He is divorced and is not currently in a continuing relationship. He has two grown daughters with whom his relationship is good. Since contracting hepatitis A several years ago, he drinks alcohol only rarely, and never more than one or two drinks at any one time. He confesses to little organized exercise but plays golf two or three times a week and states that he is such a hyperactive workaholic that he rarely sits for any length of time. Mr. Adams has not seen a physician since recovering from the hepatitis and is unsure when he last received any immunizations. He does not know if he had all recommended childhood immunizations, but says his mother was "pretty conscientious" about health checkups. His physical examination reveals an alert and healthy individual with no abnormalities noted. His vital signs are as follows: T 97.4°F, P 64, R 14, and BP 142/82.

The physician orders the following immunizations for Mr. Adams:
- Measles-mumps-rubella (MMR)
- Combined tetanus and diphtheria toxoids with pertussis (Tdap)
- Yellow fever vaccine
- Typhoid vaccine
- Meningococcal meningitis vaccine

DIAGNOSES

- *Health-Seeking Behaviors:* Immunization related to impending international travel
- *Ineffective Health Maintenance* related to apparent lapse in immunization status
- *Risk for Injury* related to adverse response to immunization

EXPECTED OUTCOMES

- Obtain necessary immunizations.
- Verbalize a schedule for maintaining up-to-date immunization status.
- Experience no significant adverse effects from immunization.

PLANNING AND IMPLEMENTATION

- Administer MMR, Tdap, and meningococcal meningitis vaccines prior to discharge from clinic.
- Observe closely for 30 minutes following immunization for potential adverse responses.
- Schedule return visit in 1 week for typhoid vaccine.
- Provide referral to a registered vaccination center for yellow fever vaccine and documentation of vaccination.
- Provide instructions for comfort measures to relieve local and systemic adverse effects of vaccines. Provide written instructions on manifestations that should be reported to the physician.
- Document immunizations on a permanent record at the clinic and for the patient.

EVALUATION

Mr. Adams completes his prescribed immunizations without major adverse effects, although he does complain of fever, malaise, and general achiness for several days following the typhoid vaccination. His trip to Africa is successful, and he returns to the United States without contracting any infectious diseases.

CRITICAL THINKING IN THE NURSING PROCESS

1. Explain why it is important for adults to continue receiving immunizations throughout their life span.
2. If a patient says to you, "I don't believe in immunizations. I hear they are dangerous," how would you respond?
3. What manifestations would cause a patient to contact the primary caregiver after receiving an immunization? What is the rationale for the need to do this?

See Evaluating Your Response in Appendix C.

- Reinforce positive health-seeking behaviors. *This will help promote future health maintenance activities.*
- Using recommended immunization schedules, develop a plan to attain optimal immunization status. *Adherence with recommended schedules for immunization is important in preventing disease and disability.*
- Do not administer influenza vaccine if the patient is allergic to eggs, or tetanus antitoxin if sensitive to horse serum. *Vaccines prepared from chicken or duck embryos are contraindicated in patients who are allergic to eggs. Tetanus antitoxin is prepared from horse serum. Both will cause a severe allergic reaction.*
- Withhold administration of active immunologic products in the presence of an upper respiratory infection or other infection. *Active immunizations can cause a greater inflammatory reaction in the presence of infections.*
- Do not administer oral polio vaccine, MMR, or any live virus vaccine to immunosuppressed patients or to patients who are in close household contact with an immunosuppressed person. *Live virus vaccines can cause disease in the immuno-suppressed patient. The virus may be transmitted from close household contacts during the initial postvaccination period.*
- Do not administer vaccines such as MMR, pneumococcal, or varicella to women who are pregnant. *Although the risk to the developing fetus is greatest during the first trimester, these vaccines are avoided throughout pregnancy.*
- Do not administer live attenuated virus vaccines and passive immunizations such as gamma globulin simultaneously. *Passive antibodies interfere with the response of the live attenuated virus.*
- Prior to administering prescribed vaccine, check the expiration date and manufacturer's instructions. *Outdated vaccines cannot provide adequate immunization protection. Certain injection sites have better absorption than others.*
- Keep epinephrine 1:1000 readily available for subcutaneous injection when administering immunizations. *Epinephrine causes vasoconstriction and reduces laryngospasm; in acute anaphylaxis, it can be lifesaving.*

SAFETY ALERT
Observe the patient for 20 to 30 minutes following vaccine administration to monitor for possible adverse reactions.

Helpful resources include state and county health departments, the CDC, and the National Institute of Allergy and Infectious Diseases.

Normal Immune Responses

The Patient with Tissue Inflammation

Inflammation is a nonspecific response to injury that serves to destroy, dilute, or contain the injurious agent or damaged tissue. Inflammation may be either acute or chronic. Acute inflammation is a short-term reaction of the body to all types of tissue damage. It is immediate and aimed at protecting the body and preventing further invasion or injury. Acute inflammation usually lasts less than 1 to 2 weeks. Once the injurious agent is removed, the inflammation subsides. Healing with tissue repair or scar formation occurs, and the body functions in normal or near-normal capacity.

Chronic inflammation is slower in onset and may not have an acute phase. Its clinical manifestations occur over months or years. It involves cell proliferation and is debilitating, with long-term adverse effects. There is increased cellular exudate, necrosis, fibrosis, and sometimes tissue scarring, resulting in severe tissue damage.

Pathophysiology and Manifestations

The tissue damage that evokes an inflammatory response may be caused by specific or nonspecific agents. These agents may be *exogenous*, from outside the body, or *endogenous*, from within the body. Causes of inflammation include the following:

- Mechanical injuries, such as cuts or surgical incisions
- Physical damage, such as burns
- Chemical injury from toxins or poisons
- Microorganisms, such as bacteria, viruses, or fungi
- Extremes of heat or cold
- Immunologic responses, such as hypersensitivity reactions
- Ischemic damage or trauma, such as a stroke or myocardial infarction

Acute Inflammation

Regardless of the cause, location, or extent of the injury, the acute inflammatory response follows the previously outlined sequence of vascular response, cellular and phagocytic response, and healing.

Many of the manifestations of inflammation are produced by inflammatory mediators such as histamine and prostaglandins released when tissue is damaged (see Box 12–1). The primary manifestations of inflammation include the following:

- Erythema (redness)
- Local heat caused by the increased blood flow to the injured area (hyperemia)
- Swelling due to accumulated fluid at the site
- Pain from tissue swelling and chemical irritation of nerve endings
- Loss of function caused by the swelling and pain

The degree of functional loss depends on the location and extent of the injury. With increased tissue damage, more fluid exudate is formed, resulting in increased swelling, pain, and functional impairment. Pain may be immediate or delayed. Prostaglandins intensify and prolong the pain. Kinins cause irritation to the nerve endings and contribute to the pain sensation.

Dead neutrophils, necrotic tissue, and (if the tissue is infected) digested bacteria accumulate as a result of inflammation and phagocytosis, forming *pus*. Pus usually forms and remains until after the infection subsides. Pus may push itself to the surface of the body or become internalized. In the latter case, pus is gradually autolyzed (self-digested) by enzymes over a period of days. The end product is then absorbed by the body. On occasion, pus may remain after the infection is resolved. Pockets of pus, called abscesses, may need to be artificially drained with a procedure called *incision and drainage (I&D)*.

Ectopic calcifications are another possible result of residual collections of pus.

Systemic responses to inflammation include an increase in the size of lymph nodes due to the proliferation of macrophages within the nodes in response to microorganisms in the lymph. Enlarged lymph nodes are usually noted in the groin, axillae, and neck. Fever, often precipitated by inflammatory mediators or bacterial toxins, inhibits the growth of many microorganisms and increases tissue repair functions. Loss of appetite and fatigue may occur in the effort to conserve energy during the inflammatory process. Leukocytosis occurs with increased WBC production to support inflammation and phagocytosis.

Chronic Inflammation

Whereas acute inflammation is a self-limiting process lasting less than 2 weeks, chronic inflammation tends to be self-perpetuating, lasting weeks to months or years. Chronic inflammation may develop when the acute inflammatory process has been ineffective in removing the offending agent. For example, mycobacteria have cell walls with high lipid and wax content, making them resistant to phagocytosis. Chronic inflammation and granuloma formation is common with *Mycobacterium tuberculosis* infection. Persistent irritation by chemicals, particulate matter, or physical irritants such as talc, asbestos, or silica may also result in chronic inflammation.

The chronic inflammatory process is characterized by a dense infiltration of the site by lymphocytes and macrophages. The macrophages mass or coalesce to form a multinucleated giant cell surrounded by lymphocytes, in a lesion called a *granuloma*. The granuloma is effective in walling off the offending agent, isolating it from the rest of the body; however, the infectious agent or offending irritant may not be destroyed and can survive within the granuloma for a long period of time. The granuloma formed in tuberculosis is called a tubercle. *M. tuberculosis* can survive for many years within the tubercle, emerging when the patient's immune system is no longer able to contain it. Rheumatoid arthritis is another condition marked by chronic inflammation. Inflammation in the joint capsule makes movement of the joint painful. The capsule is enlarged by inflammatory exudates, which cause stretching of the capsule.

Complications

Inflammation and wound healing are highly metabolic processes that may be affected by a number of factors. Without adequate nutrition, blood supply, and oxygenation, tissues cannot effectively complete the process. Impaired inflammatory and immune processes can interfere with phagocytosis and preparation of the wound for healing. Infection prolongs the inflammatory process and delays healing.

Chronic diseases may also impair healing. Diabetes mellitus is a prominent example. With high blood glucose levels associated with poorly controlled diabetes, chemotaxic and phagocytic function are decreased. Collagen formation and tensile strength of the wound are also impaired. Small blood vessel disease is common in people with diabetes, a factor that further impairs the healing process.

Drug therapy, particularly corticosteroid medications, may suppress the immune and inflammatory responses, delaying healing (Porth & Matfin, 2009). Other external factors, such as exposure to ionizing radiation and wound cleansing agents, can also affect healing. Table 12–7 summarizes major factors that affect the inflammatory process and wound healing.

Interdisciplinary Care

Management of the patient with inflamed tissue focuses on promoting healing. Care is generally supportive, allowing the patient's own physiologic processes to remove foreign matter and damaged cells. Wound care may be minimal, involving only simple cleaning, or extensive, involving irrigations and debridement. The patient is encouraged to rest, to increase fluid intake, and to eat a well-balanced, nutritious diet. Antibiotics may be prescribed to help eliminate infectious causes of inflammation.

Diagnosis

The following diagnostic tests may be ordered to identify the source and extent of inflammation. An important part of the assessment of the patient with an inflammation is monitoring the results of these tests.

TABLE 12–7 Factors That May Impair Healing

FACTOR	EFFECT
Malnutrition	
Protein deficit	Prolongs inflammation and impairs healing process
Carbohydrate and kilocalorie deficit	Impairs metabolic processes and promotes catabolism; proteins are used for energy rather than for healing
Fat deficit	Impairs cell membrane synthesis in tissue repair
Vitamin deficits	
Vitamin A	Limits epithelialization and capillary formation
B-Complex	Inhibits enzymatic reactions that contribute to wound healing
Vitamin C	Impairs collagen synthesis
Tissue hypoxia	Associated with an increased risk of infection and impaired healing, because oxygen is required to support cell function and collagen synthesis
Impaired blood supply	Inadequate delivery of oxygen and nutrients to healing tissues and removal of waste products
Impaired inflammatory and immune processes	Decreased phagocytosis and wound debridement; increased risk of infection; delayed healing

TABLE 12–8 The White Blood Cell Count and Differential

CELL TYPE AND NORMAL VALUE	INCREASED	DECREASED
Total WBCs: 4,000 to 10,000 per mm³	*Leukocytosis:* Infection or inflammation, leukemia, trauma or stress, tissue necrosis	*Leukopenia:* Bone marrow depression, overwhelming infection, viral infections, immunosuppression, autoimmune disease, dietary deficiency
Neutrophils (segs, PMNs, or polys): 55% to 70%	*Neutrophilia:* Acute infection or stress response, myelocytic leukemia, inflammatory or metabolic disorders	*Neutropenia:* Bone marrow depression, overwhelming bacterial infection, viral infection, Addison's disease
Eosinophils (eos): 1% to 4%	*Eosinophilia:* Parasitic infections, hypersensitivity reactions, autoimmune disorders	*Eosinopenia:* Cushing's syndrome, autoimmune disorders, stress, certain drugs
Basophils (basos): 0.5% to 1%	*Basophilia:* Hypersensitivity responses, chronic myelogenous leukemia, chickenpox or smallpox, splenectomy, hypothyroidism	*Basopenia:* Acute stress or hypersensitivity reactions, hyperthyroidism
Monocytes (monos): 2% to 8%	*Monocytosis:* Chronic inflammatory disorders, tuberculosis, viral infections, leukemia, Hodgkin's lymphoma, multiple myeloma	*Monocytopenia:* Bone marrow depression, corticosteroid therapy
Lymphocytes (lymphs): 20% to 40%	*Lymphocytosis:* Chronic bacterial infection, viral infections, lymphocytic leukemia	*Lymphocytopenia:* Bone marrow depression, immunodeficiency, leukemia, Cushing's syndrome, Hodgkin's lymphoma, renal failure

- *WBC with differential* provides information about the type and extent of inflammatory response. The differential count (the percentage of the total WBC made up by each type of leukocyte) provides further clues about inflammatory processes (Table 12–8).

- *Erythrocyte sedimentation rate* (*ESR* or *sed rate*) is a nonspecific test to detect inflammation. The rate at which RBCs fall to the bottom of a vertical tube is an indicator of inflammation. An increased ESR may indicate acute or chronic inflammation.

- *C-reactive protein (CRP) test* is used to detect CRP. This abnormal glycoprotein is produced by the liver and is excreted into the bloodstream during the acute phase of an inflammatory process. The expected result of this test is negative for CRP. A positive result indicates an acute or chronic inflammatory process. It may also indicate the patient's response to therapy, because it decreases when inflammation subsides.

In addition, cultures of the blood and other body fluids may be ordered to determine if infection is the cause of inflammation.

Medications

Medications may be prescribed for the patient with an inflammatory response to help alleviate distressing manifestations or destroy infectious agents.

Acetaminophen (Tylenol) may be administered to reduce the fever and pain associated with inflammation. Acetaminophen has no anti-inflammatory effect; it will not reduce the inflammatory process but will relieve associated manifestations. Acetaminophen decreases fever by acting directly on the hypothalamus heat-regulating center. It also works on the central nervous system to relieve pain sensations.

Antibiotics may be used either prophylactically to prevent infection from interfering with the healing process of damaged tissue, or therapeutically to treat the infection. If infection is present, the organism and its response or sensitivity to various antibiotics are used to guide therapy. Antibiotic therapy is discussed in the section of this chapter on infectious diseases.

Although inflammation is a beneficial process to prepare acutely injured tissue for healing, it can have damaging effects as well. When these effects are a concern or the manifestations of inflammation are deleterious to the patient, anti-inflammatory medications may be prescribed. Anti-inflammatory medications fall into three broad groups: salicylates, such as aspirin; other nonsteroidal anti-inflammatory drugs (NSAIDs); and corticosteroids.

Aspirin (acetylsalicylic acid, or ASA) is an NSAID that has antipyretic, analgesic, and antiplatelet effects. Its beneficial effects are largely dose related. Low doses (as little as 81 mg/day) inhibit platelet aggregation and normal blood clotting. Higher doses (650 to 1000 mg four to five times per day) are required to accomplish its anti-inflammatory effects. However, 650 mg of aspirin is an effective analgesic and antipyretic dosage. To relieve pain, aspirin acts primarily on peripheral sensory nerves by inhibiting the synthesis of prostaglandins and kinins, which are chemical stimuli of sensory nerves. As an antipyretic, aspirin acts both centrally and peripherally. It inhibits the formation of pyrogenic substances that raise the hypothalamic thermostat. It also dilates peripheral blood vessels and promotes diaphoresis, increasing the dissipation of heat (Wilson et al., 2009).

In therapeutic doses, aspirin mediates the inflammatory process by inhibiting the synthesis of prostaglandins and acting on the mobility and activation of leukocytes. Inflammation is reduced, along with the swelling, redness, and impaired function that accompanies it.

The other NSAIDs have activity similar to that of aspirin. They inhibit prostaglandin synthesis, reducing the inflammatory and pain response. Each NSAID has a slightly different mode of action for prostaglandin inhibition. Patients may have varying degrees of relief with different NSAIDs; sometimes, several different agents must be tried before the most effective is identified. Side effects also differ to a certain extent; however, all have a potential cross-sensitivity with aspirin, all irritate the gastrointestinal tract, and all cause some degree of sodium and water retention. They also are more costly than aspirin, but they have a longer duration of action; therefore, fewer daily doses are required to achieve the desired effect. Indomethacin and phenylbutazone are the most toxic of the NSAIDs. Their use is limited to short-term therapy. (∞ See Chapter 9 for further information on NSAIDs.)

For acute hypersensitivity reactions, such as reactions to poison ivy, or for inflammation that cannot be managed by aspirin or NSAID therapy, corticosteroid therapy may be prescribed. The glucocorticoids are hormones produced by the adrenal cortex that have widespread effects on body metabolism and the immune response. Glucocorticoids inhibit inflammation and may be life-saving in acute fulminating or chronic progressive inflammation. They do not cure disease; they are palliative to manage the inflammatory process. When glucocorticoids are prescribed to manage inflammation, the smallest possible effective dose is used. Whenever possible, a local-acting preparation such as a topical agent or intra-articular injection is prescribed to minimize its systemic effects. The incidence of potentially harmful side effects increases with higher doses and prolonged therapy. Wound healing is impaired, and the metabolism of fats, proteins, and carbohydrates is altered. Blood glucose control is impaired. Fat distribution changes, producing a cushingoid appearance with a moon face, increased truncal fat, and "buffalo hump." Fluid retention and hypertension are potential problems, as are osteoporosis, gastrointestinal bleeding, and emotional disturbances.

Nutrition

Healing depends on cell replication, protein synthesis, and the function of specific organs—the liver, heart, and lungs in particular. Weight loss and protein depletion are risk factors for poor healing and wound complications. Even a few days of severely impaired nutritional intake can noticeably affect healing. The patient with an inflammatory process or healing wound requires a well-balanced diet of sufficient kilocalories to meet the metabolic needs of the body (see Table 12–8). Inflammation often produces catabolism, a state in which body tissues are broken down. Healing, by contrast, is a process of anabolism or building up. Without sufficient kilocalories and nutrients, catabolism may predominate, impairing healing.

Carbohydrates are important to meet energy demands, as well as to support leukocyte function. However, hyperglycemia experienced in diabetes may impair healing. In diabetes, the glucose molecules bind the oxygen more tightly to the hemoglobin molecule and prevent adequate release of oxygen to the tissues for healing. Furthermore, neutrophils have diminished chemotactic and phagocytic functioning in hyperglycemia (Porth & Matfin, 2009). Adequate protein is necessary for tissue healing and the production of antibodies and WBCs. Lack of adequate protein increases the risk of infection. Complete protein sources, those that provide the essential amino acids, are preferred. Dietary fats are used in the synthesis of cell membranes.

Vitamins A, B-complex, C, and K are also important to the healing process. Vitamin A is necessary for capillary formation and epithelialization. B-complex vitamins promote wound healing, and vitamin C is necessary for collagen synthesis. Vitamin K provides a vital component for the synthesis of clotting factors in the liver.

Although it has been established that minerals contribute to the inflammatory and healing processes, less is known about required amounts. Zinc appears to be important for tissue growth, skin integrity, cell-mediated immunity, and other general immune mechanisms (Arnold & Barbul, 2006). However, the use of zinc supplements in smokers is cautioned against and sources in whole foods are recommended over supplements.

Oxygen is an important element in healing. Arterial and venous disorders impair oxygen availability to peripheral tissues and healing. White blood cells and fibroblasts for healing are impaired in ischemic conditions. In trauma, loss of blood flow to tissue causes ischemia and if prolonged, infection and cell death. Hyperbaric chambers increase oxygen above normal atmospheric pressure and promote healing. While 100% oxygen at atmospheric pressure saturates red blood cell hemoglobin, only hyperbaric pressures increase plasma transport of oxygen, making more available to tissues for immune function and healing.

∞ Nursing Care

Acute inflammation may be self-limiting or extensive and require hospitalization. Nursing care includes teaching patients with acute and chronic inflammatory conditions self-management at home.

Health Promotion

Health promotion activities to prevent inflammation focus on reducing the risk for accidents and exposure to harmful agents that can result in subsequent injury. It is important to educate the public about potential hazards in both the work and home environments. In addition, safety education guidelines such as not drinking and driving, wearing a protective helmet when riding a bicycle, and using a safety belt in the car are important areas for discussion. Because most injuries occur at home, it is also important to discuss ways to make the home safer.

Assessment

The following data are collected through the health history and physical examination. Further focused assessments are described with nursing interventions in the next section.

- *Health history:* Risk factors, nutrition, medication use (anti-inflammatory and corticosteroids), location, duration, and type (redness, heat, pain, swelling, and impaired function) of manifestations
- *Physical assessment:* Movement of injured area, pain, circulation, wounds, lymph nodes.

Nursing Diagnoses and Interventions

The nursing care needs of the patient with an inflammation are related to the manifestations and altered tissue integrity. Priority nursing diagnoses include *Acute Pain*, *Impaired Tissue Integrity*, and *Risk for Infection*.

Acute Pain

Along with redness, warmth, swelling, and impaired function, pain is one of the primary manifestations of inflammation. Depending on the cause, affected area, and degree of inflammation, pain may be acute and immobilizing or chronic and demoralizing. It is important to remember that pain is a subjective experience and that patient responses to pain vary. (∞ Refer to Chapter 9 for more information about pain and pain management.)

- Assess pain using a scale of 0 to 10, with 0 being no pain and 10 being the worst pain; note the character, location, and duration of the pain. *Because pain is subjective, the patient provides the most accurate information regarding his or her pain experience.*
- Use physical and nonverbal cues to further assess the level of pain. *This intervention is especially important if the patient is nonverbal or tends to underreport pain.*
- Administer anti-inflammatory medications as prescribed. *These medications help reduce the pain resulting from acute inflammation.*
- Administer analgesic medications as prescribed. *Although most analgesics do little to reduce inflammation, they provide additional pain relief by reducing the perception of pain. Chest infections such as pneumonia may compromise breathing. In addition to administering oxygen at appropriate levels, relieving pain with opioid or NSAID analgesics helps increase the depth and slow the rate of respirations.*

> **PRACTICE ALERT**
> Because opioids can depress respirations, it is important to monitor oxygen saturation and encourage the patient to take deep breaths to keep oxygen saturation adequate.

- Provide comfort measures, such as back rubs, position changes, or relaxation techniques. *These measures reduce muscle tension, relieve areas of pressure, and provide distraction.*
- Encourage activities such as reading, watching television, and taking part in social interactions. *Such activities provide distraction from the pain experience.*
- Encourage rest. *Strenuous activity or exercising an inflamed body part may increase discomfort and tissue damage.*
- Provide cold or heat as pain-relief measures, as ordered. *For an acute injury, cold reduces swelling and relieves pain; after the initial stage, heat increases blood flow to the affected tissue and relieves pain and swelling by promoting absorption of edema. Do not apply either heat or cold for more than 20 minutes at a time and ensure there is a covering between the patient and the application*

> **SAFETY ALERT**
> Use heat or cold application cautiously in older patients who have fragile skin and are at risk for tissue injury.

- Elevate the inflamed area if possible. *Elevation promotes venous return and reduces swelling.*
- Teach about the appropriate use and expected effects of anti-inflammatory medications. *If the patient's pain continues after the initial doses of anti-inflammatory medication, he or she may become discouraged and stop taking the medication before it becomes fully effective.*

Impaired Tissue Integrity

The inflammatory response can either precipitate or result from impairment of the integrity of skin or other tissues. Whatever the cause of the tissue damage, it is vital that the nurse consider this alteration in delivering care.

- Assess general health and nutritional status. *Poor general health or chronic diseases such as diabetes mellitus or renal failure interfere with the healing processes and increase the risk of infection.*
- Assess circulation to the affected area. *Adequate tissue perfusion and oxygenation are necessary for healing.*
- Monitor the skin and surrounding tissue for increased manifestations of inflammation. *Inflammation can spread to adjacent tissues leading to conditions such as cellulitis.*
- Provide protection and support for inflamed tissue. *This reduces discomfort and decreases the risk of further tissue damage.*
- Clean inflamed tissue gently; if possible, use water, normal saline, or nontoxic wound cleansers such as Comfeel (Coloplast Corporation) only. *Soap and harsh cleansers such as povidone-iodine (Betadine) and hydrogen peroxide can cause further drying and tissue damage. Granulation tissue in a healing wound is fragile and easily damaged.* (∞ See Chapters 4 and 16 for further discussion of wound care.)
- Keep the inflamed area dry, and expose it to air as much as possible. *This promotes healing and helps prevent infection.*
- Balance rest with activity. *Rest decreases metabolic demands and allows for cell regeneration, while mobility helps to promote oxygenation and perfusion of the tissues.*
- Provide supplemental oxygen as ordered. *Supplemental oxygen improves tissue oxygenation and reduces hypoxia.*
- Provide a well-balanced diet with adequate kilocalories to meet the body's metabolic and healing needs. If the patient is allowed nothing by mouth (NPO), suggest parenteral or enteral nutrition. For the patient who is unable to consume an adequate diet, consult with a dietitian for between-meal supplements and/or multivitamin supplements. *Careful attention to diet and nutrient intake is important to provide the nutrients necessary for immune function and healing and to prevent catabolism.*

Risk for Infection

The inflammatory response often indicates that body defense mechanisms have been set in motion to protect against invading microorganisms. Wounds, whether traumatic or surgical in nature, are typically contaminated, as attested to by subsequent wound infections. The patient with a healing wound is at particular risk for infection.

- Assess the wound for specific manifestations of infection, including purulent drainage, foul odor, and delayed healing. *The normal inflammatory response can indicate infection and, on occasion, mask its presence.*
- Evaluate complete blood counts for adequate WBC response. *Leukocytosis may indicate infection or healthy response to injury and protection from infection. Immune-impaired patients may not respond with increased WBCs; manifestations of inflammation may be diminished in those individuals.*
- Monitor vital signs and pain level at least every 4 hours. *In response to the inflammatory process the temperature rises,*

usually in the range of 99°F (37.2°C) to 100.9°F (38.2°C). A temperature of 101.0°F (38.3°C) or above indicates infection. Fever is usually accompanied by increased heart and respiratory rates.

- Apply dry or moist heat to the affected area for no longer than 20 minutes several times a day. *Heat increases the circulation of blood to and from the inflamed tissue. Time is limited to prevent burns.*

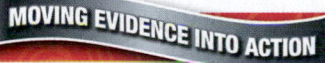

- Provide and encourage fluid intake of 2500 mL/day. Older patients may limit fluid intake when mobility is impaired by illness or injury; high fluid intake increases the need for urination and patients may want to limit bathroom trips. *Teach the purpose and importance of hydration to promote blood flow and nutrient supply to the tissues and also dilution and removal of waste products and heat from the body.*

- Ensure adequate nutrition. *Adequate nutrition enhances the function and production of T cells and B cells, which are important in the immune response.*

- Use good hand hygiene techniques consistently. *Hand hygiene removes transient microorganisms and is the best mechanism to prevent the spread of infection to a susceptible person.*

- Use sterile technique when providing wound care. *Using sterile gloves and aseptic technique helps prevent further contamination of the wound and the spread of infection to other patients.*

Community-Based Care

Patient and family teaching enhances understanding of the inflammatory process, its cause, and its management. Teaching is also important to prevent further compromise that could result in infection.

Instructions, verbal and written, should include the following:

- Increase fluid intake to 2500 mL (approximately 2.5 quarts) per day, including that found in solid foods.
- Eat a well-balanced diet high in vitamins and minerals and with adequate protein and kilocalories for healing.
- Use good hand hygiene, particularly when caring for wounds or inflamed tissue and after using the bathroom.
- Elevate the inflamed area to reduce swelling and pain.
- Apply heat or cold for no longer than 20 minutes at a time to reduce the risk of tissue damage from burns or frostbite.
- Take all medications as prescribed, notifying the physician if adverse effects or hypersensitivity responses are noted. (See Moving Evidence into Action.)
- Rest acutely inflamed tissue; do not engage in strenuous activity until the inflammation has subsided.

The Patient with an Infection

Microorganisms—including bacteria, viruses, fungi, and parasites—often invade the human body and proliferate if undetected and controlled or eliminated by inflammatory and immune responses. In most cases, contact between humans and microorganisms is incidental and may even be beneficial to both organisms. Resident bacteria of the skin, mucous membranes, and gastrointestinal tract are an important part of the body's defense system. However, many microorganisms are virulent; that is, they have the ability to cause disease. **Pathogens** are virulent organisms rarely found in the absence of disease. Some microorganisms, known as opportunistic pathogens, rarely, if ever, cause harm to persons with intact immune systems, but are capable of producing infectious disease in the immunocompromised host (Porth & Matfin, 2009).

Prevention Video

MOVING EVIDENCE INTO ACTION — **Teaching to Take Antibiotics Appropriately**

Nurses discharging patients from outpatient and acute care settings frequently teach patients to take a complete prescribed dose of oral antibiotics to manage acute infectious illness. Ingesting less than complete doses exposes patients to the risk of resistant infections and less than therapeutic outcomes. There are many potential restraining forces to the completion of antibiotic dosing: cost of purchase; difficulty swallowing the pills; multiple, frequent doses; and the potential for adverse, unpleasant side effects.

Because adherence is so important and nurses are patient educators, Aronson (2005) studied the experience of 11 patients who had just completed a short-term antibiotic regimen to treat a variety of acute infectious with various antibiotic regimens. The 11 subjects represent diverse gender and cultural backgrounds. The patients' descriptions, views, and experiences are the unique aspect of this research on adherence to antibiotic self-administration. The central theme that emerged was successful antibiotic self-administration. The patients integrated the dosing into their daily schedules and adapted to any unplanned circumstances. The primary categories involved in self-administration were (1) medication-taking behaviors, (2) factors influencing adherence, and (3) attitudes and beliefs about the medication and the value of completing the prescribed dose.

IMPLICATIONS FOR NURSING

Nurses teach patients about short-term antibiotic self-administration in outpatient and inpatient settings. The findings from this study can be used to guide educational interventions. Based on the findings in this study, encourage patient involvement in the decision to take short-term antibiotic medications to strengthen the relationship with the prescriber. Ask patients to identify the method they will use to remind themselves of each dose; inquire about their knowledge of and plans to manage side effects from the medication.

CRITICAL THINKING IN PATIENT CARE

1. Identify methods that patients can use to remind themselves of dosing schedules.
2. An 86-year-old woman is being discharged to her home following a respiratory infection. Identify the information she will need about short-term antibiotic medication when she is discharged.
3. Make a list of barriers to taking complete doses of antibiotics. What do you think is the single most important (to the patient) reason?
4. Discuss the interrelationship between malnutrition and immune system function (see the previous discussion of immune system function).

Source: Aronson, B. (2005). Medication management behaviors of adherent short-term antibiotic users. *Clinical Excellence for Nurse Practitioners, 9*(1), 23–30.

To a certain extent, modern medicine has contributed to the development of infectious diseases caused by antibiotic-resistant strains of microorganisms. Tuberculosis is on the rise in many countries, partially because organisms have become resistant to standard therapies. Patients receive immunosuppressive therapy following organ or tissue transplant or in the treatment of neoplasms, making them more susceptible to infection. Metal and plastic prosthetic devices are implanted, providing potential sites for colonization by disease-producing organisms. It has also become apparent that many diseases long considered unrelated to microorganisms may actually be infectious; for example, colonization of the gastric mucosa with *Helicobacter pylori* is the predominant cause of peptic ulcer disease, and oncogenic viruses have the ability to transform normal cells into malignant cells.

Pathophysiology

Infection occurs when an organism is able to colonize and multiply within a host. The host can be any organism capable of supporting the nutritional and physical growth requirements of the microorganism—for example, humans. When the host experiences injury, pathologic changes, inflammation, or organ dysfunction in response to an infection or from intoxication by cellular poisons produced by a pathogen, the host is said to have an infectious disease.

For a microorganism to cause infection, it must have disease-causing potential (virulence), be transmitted from its reservoir, and gain entry into a susceptible host. This is known as the chain of infection (Figure 12–11 ■).

PATHOGENS Pathogens capable of infecting and causing disease in a susceptible host include bacteria, viruses, mycoplasma, rickettsia, chlamydia, fungi, and parasites such as protozoa, helminths (worms), and arthropods (Box 12–4). Each organism causes a different specific reaction in the host.

A number of different mechanisms have evolved in pathogens to facilitate their transmission and increase their ability to invade the host and cause disease. Factors influencing the transmission of an organism include its resistance to drying and to variations in environmental temperature. For example, spore-forming organisms are extremely resistant to drying.

Many microorganisms are capable of producing toxins or enzymes to facilitate their invasion of the host, increase their resistance to host defenses, and increase their ability to cause disease. Adhesion factors produced by or incorporated into the cell wall or membrane of the pathogen improve its ability to attach to and colonize the host. Pathogens may also produce enzymes to enhance their spread to local tissues, chemicals to block specific immune processes or deplete neutrophils and macrophages, or extracellular capsules to discourage phagocytosis.

Pathogens are often capable of producing toxins that alter or destroy the normal function of host cells and promote colonization, proliferation, and invasion by the pathogen. Toxins often increase the disease-producing capability of the pathogen and, in some cases, are totally responsible for it; for example, cholera, tetanus, and botulism result from bacterial toxins, not from the direct effects of the infection. **Exotoxins** are soluble proteins secreted into surrounding tissue by the microorganism. Exotoxins are highly poisonous, causing cell death or dysfunction. **Endotoxins** are found in the cell wall of gram-negative bacteria and are released only when the cell is disrupted. Endotoxins have less specific effects than exotoxins, but they act as activators of many human regulatory systems, producing fever; inflammation; and potentially clotting, bleeding, or hypotension when released in large quantities.

RESERVOIR AND TRANSMISSION The reservoir or source, where the pathogen lives and multiplies, may be either endogenous or exogenous. Organisms that reside on skin or mucosal surfaces of the host are endogenous. Exogenous sources can include other humans, animals, soil, water, intravenous fluid, or equipment. Infectious diseases are usually transmitted from human sources, that is, persons who have clinical disease or carriers with subclinical infection. Carriers harbor the pathogen without showing evidence of clinical disease. Pathogens exit human hosts via respiratory secretions, body fluids from the gastrointestinal and genitourinary tracts, skin or mucous membrane lesions, the placenta, and blood.

Organisms may be transmitted from the source to the susceptible host by direct or indirect contact, droplet or airborne transmission, or a vector. Direct contact includes person-to-person spread or contact with infected body fluids, as well as transmission from contaminated food or water. Indirect contact occurs when the infectious agent is contracted by use of inanimate objects, such as dirty eating utensils. Sneezing, talking, and coughing allow transmission by droplet contact when the host is within 2 to 3 feet of the source. Smaller respiratory particles that stay suspended in air and are carried via air currents allow airborne transmission. Vectors are insects and animals such as flies, mosquitoes, or rodents that act as intermediate hosts between the source and host. Microorganisms usually

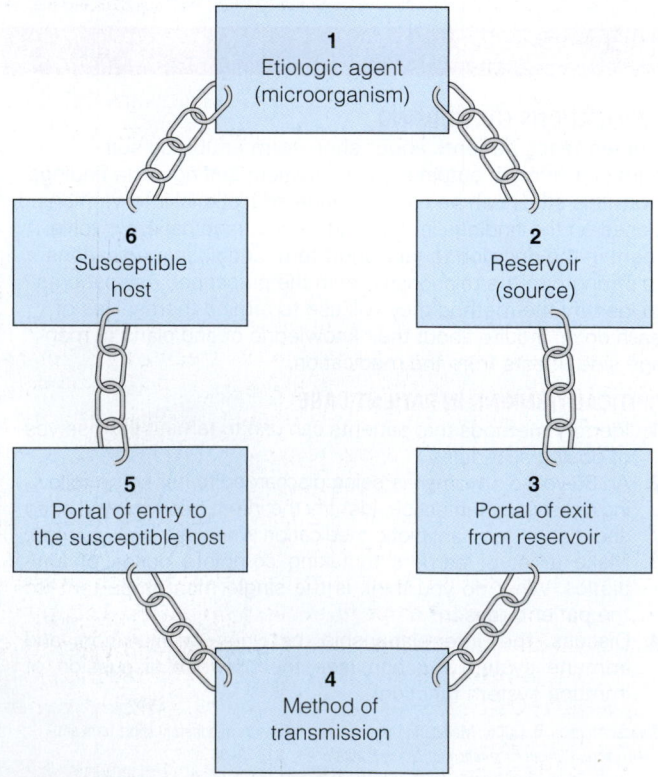

Figure 12–11 ■ The chain of infection.

BOX 12–4 Pathogenic Organisms

Bacteria

Bacteria are single-celled organisms capable of autonomous reproduction. Relatively small and simple organisms, they contain a single chromosome. A flexible cell membrane and rigid cell wall surrounds their cytoplasm, giving them a distinctive shape; some also have an extracellular capsule for additional protection. Bacteria have different characteristics and growth requirements: *aerobes* require oxygen for survival, whereas *anaerobes* cannot survive in the presence of oxygen; *gram-positive* bacteria stain purple when subjected to crystal violet stain, whereas *gram-negative* bacteria do not stain with crystal violet but turn red when subjected to safranin stain; the colonies formed by replicating bacteria differ from one another.

Prions

Prions are not independent organisms but small molecules that can modify host proteins. They primarily affect the neurologic system, causing neurologic degeneration in diseases such as mad cow disease (bovine spongiform encephalopathy) in animals and Creutzfeldt-Jacob in humans. These are slowly progressive, non-inflammatory conditions leading to dementia, lack of coordination, and death. Prion entry into the neurologic cells makes them resistant to the host immune system and anti-bacterial and anti-viral medications. They enter the host by injection, transplantation of contaminated tissue or medical devices, and possibly food (Porth & Matfin, 2009). They are very resistant to disinfection, requiring special procedures for sterilizing instruments, especially those used in CNS surgeries (Prusiner & Miller, 2007).

Viruses

Viruses are obligate intracellular parasites that are incapable of reproducing outside of a living cell. Viruses consist of a protein coat around a core of either DNA or RNA. Some viruses are shed continuously from infected cell surfaces; others, after inserting their genetic material into that of the infected cell, remain latent until they are stimulated to replicate. Viruses may or may not cause lysis and death of the host cell during replication. Oncogenic viruses are able to transform normal cells into malignant cells.

Mycoplasma

Although similar to bacteria, mycoplasma are smaller and have no cell wall, making them resistant to antibiotics that inhibit cell wall synthesis (e.g., penicillins).

Rickettsia and Chlamydia

As obligate intracellular parasites with a rigid cell wall, rickettsia and *Chlamydia* have some features of both bacteria and viruses. Rather than depending on the host cell for reproduction, they use vitamins, nutrients, or products of metabolism (e.g., ATP) from the host. *Chlamydia* are transmitted by direct contact, whereas many rickettsiae infect the cells of arthropods (e.g., fleas, ticks, and lice) and are transmitted from these vectors to humans.

Fungi

Fungi are prevalent throughout the world, but few are capable of causing disease in humans. Most fungal infections are self-limited, affecting the skin and subcutaneous tissue. Some fungi, such as *Pneumocystis jiroveci*, can cause life-threatening opportunistic infections in the immunocompromised host.

Parasites

The term *parasite* is typically applied to members of the animal kingdom that infect and cause disease in other animals. Protozoa, helminths, and arthropods are considered parasites. Protozoa are single-celled organisms transmitted via direct or indirect contact or an arthropod vector. Helminths are wormlike parasites: round-worms, tapeworms, and flukes are examples. They gain entry into humans primarily through ingestion of fertilized eggs or penetration of larvae through the skin or mucous membranes. Arthropod parasites, such as scabies (mites), lice, and fleas, typically infest external body surfaces, causing localized tissue damage and inflammation. Transmission is by direct contact with the arthropod or its eggs.

---

first colonize the portal of entry: nonintact skin; wounds; mucous membranes; and the respiratory, gastrointestinal, or genitourinary tracts.

HOST FACTORS The susceptible host is the final link in the chain of infection. Exposure to pathogens does not automatically cause infection or infectious disease. The outcome of contact with a pathogenic microorganism is determined by the balance of microbial virulence and host resistance. Factors that can enable the host to resist infection include the following:

- Physical barriers, such as intact skin and mucous membranes
- The hostile environment created by acid stomach secretions, urine, and vaginal secretions
- Antimicrobial factors in saliva, tears, and prostatic fluid
- Respiratory defenses, including humidification, filtration, the mucociliary escalator, cough reflex, and alveolar macrophages
- Innate and adaptive immune responses to pathogenic invasion

Stages of the Infectious Process

When infectious disease develops in the host, it typically follows a predictable course with stages based on the progression and intensity of manifestations.

The initial stage is the incubation period, during which the pathogen begins active replication but does not yet cause manifestations. Depending on the organism and host factors, the incubation period may last from hours, as with salmonella, to years, as with HIV infection.

The prodromal stage follows, during which manifestations first begin to appear. At this stage, manifestations are often nonspecific and include general malaise, fever, myalgias, headache, and fatigue.

Maximal impact of the infectious process is felt during the acute phase as the pathogen proliferates and disseminates rapidly. Toxic by-products of microorganism metabolism and cell lysis, along with the immune response, produce tissue damage and inflammation during this stage (Porth & Matfin, 2009). Manifestations are more pronounced and specific to the infecting organism and site during the acute stage. Fever and chills may be significant during this phase. However, alcoholic patients and the very old may respond to severe infection by becoming hypothermic. The patient is often tachycardic and tachypneic because of increased metabolic demands. Localized manifestations include redness, heat, swelling, pain, and impaired function. When the infectious disease affects an internal organ, manifestations are related to inflammatory changes in that organ and surrounding tissue. The patient may experience tenderness to palpation over the site or show manifestations of impaired function, such as the hematuria and proteinuria characteristic of renal infections.

If the infectious process is prolonged, manifestations of the continuing immune response may become apparent. Catabolic and anorexic effects of the infection can lead to loss of body fat and muscle wasting. Immune complexes may be deposited at sites other than the primary infection, resulting in an inflammatory process. Glomerulonephritis (e.g., following strep throat) and vasculitis are possible results. Another possible consequence of prolonged infection and immune response is the triggering of an autoimmune disease process (discussed in ∞ Chapter 13), such as rheumatic cardiomyopathy or celiac disease. Type 1 diabetes mellitus is thought to be the result of such a response (Porth, 2007).

As the infection is contained and the pathogen eliminated, the convalescent stage of the disease occurs. During this stage, affected tissues are repaired and manifestations resolve. Resolution of the infection is total elimination of the pathogen from the body without residual manifestations. If a balance between organism and host factors occurs with neither predominating, chronic disease may develop or the organism may be driven into a protected site, such as an abscess. A carrier state develops when host defenses eliminate the infectious disease but the organism continues to multiply on mucosal sites.

Complications

Multiple and varied complications are associated with infectious diseases. They are typically specific to the infecting organism and the body system affected.

Acute invasion of the blood by certain microorganisms or their toxins can result in septicemia and septic shock. Whereas bacteremia, the presence of bacteria in the blood, may not have serious effects, septicemia refers to systemic disease associated with their presence or toxins. Septic shock indicates a state of hypotension and impaired organ perfusion resulting from sepsis. Unless treated aggressively, septic shock leads to diffuse cell and tissue injury, and potentially to organ failure. ∞ See Chapter 11 for an in-depth discussion of septic shock, other shock syndromes, and their management.

Nosocomial Infections

Nosocomial infections are acquired in a healthcare setting, such as a hospital or nursing home. Also called healthcare-associated infections (HAIs), nosocomial infections account for an estimated 1.7 million infections, 99,000 deaths, and $4.5 billion in excess healthcare costs annually. HAIs add hospital days, reduce admissions by occupying available beds, and add to the cost of health care (CDC, 2010; Klevens et al., 2007; Stone et al., 2005).

> **FAST FACTS**
> - Nosocomial infections typically manifest after 48 hours of hospitalization.
> - Urinary tract infection is the most common type of HAI, followed by surgical site infection and pneumonia (CDC, 2009).
> - *Clostridium difficile*–associated diarrhea is a frequently acquired nosocomial infection. It is an antibiotic-associated diarrhea and the risk of acquiring it increases with length of hospital stay, especially in an intensive care unit (ICU).

Patients entering hospitals are often the least able to mount immune defenses to infection. Immunologic responses may be compromised and normal defenses impaired in patients with, for

example, cancer or chronic diseases, pressure ulcers, or organ transplants (McPhee, Papadakis, & Tierney, 2008). Nosocomial infections also occur when antibiotic therapy has altered natural defenses and impaired resistance to harmful microorganisms. Endogenous organisms outside their normal habitats (such as in *Escherichia coli* in the urinary tract) become a threat to the patient. Other pharmacologic and therapeutic procedures such as chemotherapy, the use of corticosteroids, or radiation therapy also contribute to nosocomial infections. Gram-negative enteric bacteria and gram-positive *Staphylococcus aureus* are the most common bacteria responsible.

Invasive procedures and altered immune defenses are the main factors contributing to infection. Urinary catheterization is the number one cause; cardiac catheterization, peripheral and central intravenous lines, respiratory care procedures, and surgical procedures are also closely linked to nosocomial infection. Consequently, the urinary tract, surgical wounds, respiratory tract, and invasive catheter sites on the skin are most often affected by hospital-acquired infection.

Surgical site infections rank second in frequency of healthcare associated infections (CDC, 2010). Superficial or deep wounds may be contaminated by endogenous or exogenous sources. Infections in body cavities or associated with prosthetics are difficult to diagnose; interventional radiology to obtain specimens of possible infected sites may be necessary (Weinstein, 2007).

Hospital-acquired pneumonia is the third most common nosocomial infection, accounting for 15% to 20% of these serious infections. Usually associated with ICU stays and mechanical ventilation, Sopina and Sobria (2005) found hospital-acquired pneumonia in non-ICU patients with severe underlying disease and a hospital stay greater than 5 days. Organisms causing the infection are often resistant to many drugs, not responding to antibiotics usually effective in treating infections acquired outside the hospital. There are more deaths associated with HA pneumonia than any other site of infection (Weinstein, 2007).

> **SAFETY ALERT**
> Since October 2002, alcohol-based hand rub has been recommended by the CDC as the preferred method for hand hygiene (CDC, 2002a). Antiseptic soaps and detergents are the next most effective agents and nonantiseptic soaps are the least effective. A soap and water wash is recommended for visibly soiled hands. Wearing gloves does not eliminate the need for hand hygiene.

Prevention is the most important control measure for nosocomial infections. The pathogens causing these infections are transmitted primarily by contact with hospital personnel and contaminated inanimate objects (Posani, 2004). *Effective hand hygiene is the single most important measure in infection control (Haas & Larsen, 2008).* Although infections may also be transmitted by the airborne route, contaminated equipment, or from the environment, these are less significant causes. Invasive procedures and equipment should be used only when absolutely necessary; for example, it is not appropriate to insert an indwelling catheter when the only indication is incontinence. Peripheral intravenous equipment and sites must be kept

1. Central venous catheter infections have decreased by using chlorhexidine antiseptic for disinfection and maximal barrier precautions during insertion.
2. Ventilator-associated pneumonia is decreased by weaning patients off ventilators as soon as possible, limiting sedation of the patient, positioning patients to prevent gastric reflux and for maximal ventilation, and proper hand hygiene and sterile technique for all ventilator-associated care.
3. Surgical site infections are reduced by administering a prophylactic antibiotic 1 hour before the incision and discontinuing it within 24 hours after surgery, limiting hair removal (no shaving), controlling perioperative glucose levels (especially in cardiac surgeries), and ensuring normothermia for the patient during the perioperative period (especially in colorectal surgeries) (Weinstein, 2007).

clean and changed regularly: intravenous bags and bottles every 24 hours, tubing every 24 to 96 hours, and sites every 72 to 96 hours according to agency policy.

Antibiotic-Resistant Microorganisms

Antibiotic-resistant microorganisms are increasing at an alarming rate primarily due to prolonged or inappropriate use of antibiotic therapy. Although antibiotic therapy is expected to eradicate all targeted microorganisms, sometimes a few bacteria survive, leading to bacteria that reproduce with antibiotic resistance already encoded into their genetic makeup (Vrtis, 2008). Other bacteria produce enzymes that inactivate drugs, change drug binding sites, or alter their cell membrane to prevent drug absorption. It is important for infectious agents to be identified and treated with effective antibiotics; culture and sensitivity analysis guides prescription of effective antimicrobials. These reports need to be reviewed carefully and appropriate action taken if drug-resistant pathogens are found (Vrtis, 2008).

Standard precautions, most importantly hand hygiene and use of carefully selected antibiotics, are critical actions for stopping the spread of these diseases. Equipment such as stethoscopes, blood pressure cuffs, and thermometers should be restricted to use by each patient identified with one of these diseases. Personal protective gear used and disposed of appropriately are important safeguards.

Interdisciplinary Care

The goals of care for the patient with an infection are to identify the organ system affected by the infection; to identify the causative agent; and to achieve a cure by the least toxic, least expensive, and most effective means. Fortunately, most infectious diseases are self-limiting and will resolve with little or no medical care. However, medical treatment can be lifesaving in an overwhelming infection or immunocompromised host.

The body part or organ system affected by the infection is often obvious from the patient's history and presenting manifestations. Identifying the system allows the range of possible infecting organisms to be narrowed to those known to affect that system. Once the infecting agent has been identified, either positively or by probability, therapy can be specifically tailored to the patient's needs. Viral infections often resolve without treatment other than supportive care, such as providing rest and fluids. Skin infections may respond to a topical agent, avoiding the potential adverse effects of one administered systemically.

Diagnosis

To assess the patient's response to infection, identify the infecting organism, and monitor the progress of therapy, the following diagnostic tests may be ordered:

- *WBC count* provides clues about the infecting organism and the body's immune response to it.
- *WBC differential* is also ordered (see Table 12–8). Neutrophilia, increased numbers of circulating neutrophils (or PMNs), is a common response with infection or inflammation as the bone marrow responds to an increased need for phagocytes. Along with neutrophilia, a shift to the left is common in acute infection. This means that there are more immature neutrophils in circulation than normal, indicating an appropriate bone marrow response.

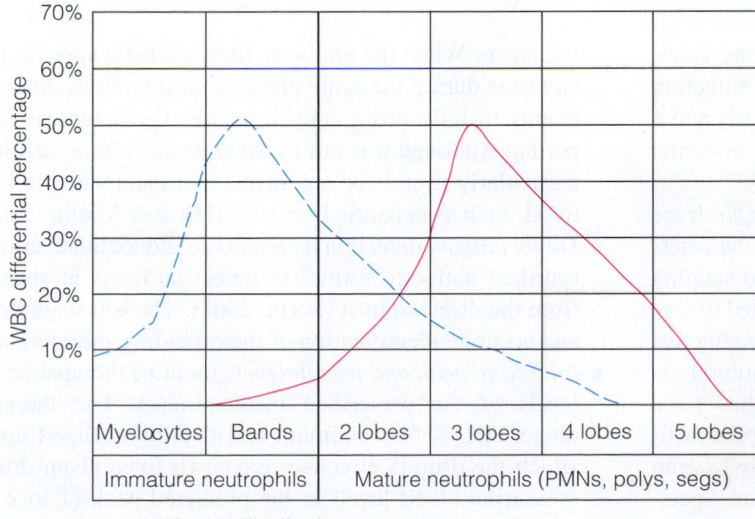

Type of WBC	Normal differential	Shift to left
Myelocytes	0%	Present
Band neutrophils (bands)	3% to 5%	Increased
Segmented neutrophils (segs, polys, PMNs)	50% to 65%	May be stable, increased, or decreased

Figure 12–12 ■ Neutrophils by stage of maturity and normal distribution in the blood.

NURSING CARE OF THE OLDER ADULT   **Infections in Older Adults**

Because immune function declines with aging, older adults are more susceptible to infections. Infections are among the top 10 causes for hospitalization and 1 of the 5 leading causes of death among people over 65 years of age. Additionally, the following changes that occur with aging place the older adult at greater risk of acquiring an infection than younger people.

- *Cardiovascular changes:* decreased cardiac output, loss of capillaries, and decreased tissue perfusion delaying inflammatory response and healing.
- *Respiratory system changes:* decreased mucociliary escalator, decreased elastic recoil, and a diminished cough reflex leading to decreased clearance of respiratory secretions. As a result of physiologic changes, the older adult with pneumonia may not present with cough or sputum production. The leading causes of pneumonia in older adults include *S. pneumoniae*, *Haemophilus influenzae*, *Klebsiella pneumoniae*, *S. aureus*, and pneumococci. Influenza A and B are prevalent in the aged; however, strain A accounts for greater illness severity and death (Eliopoulos, 2009). Older adults are at greater risk for developing pneumonia as a complication of influenza. Both pneumonia and influenza cause high mortality rates in the older person.
- *Genitourinary changes:* loss of muscle tone, reduced bladder contractility, altered bladder reflexes, and prostatic hypertrophy in men leading to reduced bladder capacity and incomplete emptying. Urinary tract infection (UTI) is the most common infection and the leading cause of bacteremia and sepsis in older adults. Factors that contribute to UTI include poor hygiene, incomplete bladder emptying, inadequate fluid intake, and long-term indwelling catheters. In addition, chronic conditions and medications may contribute to retention, which can result in UTI.
- *Gastrointestinal system changes:* impaired swallow reflex, decreased gastric acidity, and delayed gastric emptying, thus increasing the risk of aspiration with subsequent pneumonia.
- *Skin and subcutaneous tissue changes:* thinning of skin, decreased cushioning, and decreased sensation leading to increased risk of injury and ulceration, especially in patients with limited mobility or with urinary or bowel incontinence.
- *Immune changes:* decreased phagocytosis, reduced inflammatory response, and slowed or impaired healing processes. Immunoglobulin levels remain relatively stable,

but primary and secondary antibody responses decline with aging. The thymus gland atrophies and some T-cell populations decrease or decline in function as the person ages. T-cell activation and the ability of T cells to proliferate following activation also decline with advancing age (Porth & Matfin, 2009). With these changes, cell-mediated immune function declines. The patient has reduced resistance to antigens such as *M. tuberculosis*, influenza and varicella-zoster viruses, malignant cells, and tissue grafts.

Other factors, such as a lower activity level, poor nutrition and an increased risk for dehydration, a higher prevalence of chronic diseases such as diabetes, use of multiple medications, and altered mentation contribute to the older adult's risk for infection.

Nosocomial infections are more common in older adults. The nurse must steadfastly adhere to principles of infection control. Nursing interventions should focus on prevention strategies such as (1) avoiding prolonged bed rest unless the medical condition contraindicates mobilization, (2) encouraging patients to take deep breaths, (3) providing adequate fluids, (4) providing regular toileting schedules with good hygiene, and (5) avoiding use of invasive devices such as indwelling catheters unless medically necessary.

The older adult may not exhibit the classic manifestations of inflammation and infection. The manifestations of inflammation—redness, heat, and swelling—tend to be diminished or absent in older adults. The classic manifestations of infection—fever and chills—may be absent altogether because of age-related changes in the immune system, loss of central temperature control mechanisms, decreased muscle mass, and loss of shivering ability. Rather than an elevated temperature to signal an infection, confusion and subtle changes in behavior such as restlessness may be observed. The older adult may have only subtle manifestations of sepsis, including changes in mental status, disorientation, and tachypnea.

In addition to monitoring for changes in the patient's mental status or behavior, the nurse should collect data on the amount of fluids consumed, urinary output, activity levels, complaints of fatigue, and respiratory status. Older adults are at increased risk for dehydration due to such factors as diminished thirst sensation and impaired water conservation by the kidneys. Carefully evaluate intake and output to determine if input is adequate (Spigt et al., 2006). A thorough assessment is necessary to facilitate an early diagnosis and prompt treatment that will improve outcomes for the older adult.

- *Procalcitonin (CTpr)* is a precursor of the hormone calcitonin. Procalcitonin increases dramatically during infection and sepsis and is accepted as both a marker of sepsis and a harmful mediator in lower respiratory tract and systemic infections.
- *Cultures of the wound, blood, or other infected body fluids* are used to identify probable microorganisms by their characteristics, such as shape, growth patterns, and Gram-staining qualities. After the organism is cultured, it is subjected to sensitivity testing using various antibiotics known to be effective against its particular strain to determine which antibiotic is likely to be most effective. Generally 24 to 48 hours are required to grow the organism, potentially delaying the institution of therapy. Because antibiotics (and possibly oxygen therapy) can alter the ability to culture an organism, specimens should be obtained before instituting therapy.
- *Serologic testing* provides an indirect means of identifying infecting agents by detecting antibodies to the suspected

organism. When the antibody titer against a specific organism rises during the acute phase of an infectious disease and begins to fall during convalescence, the diagnosis is supported. Although it is not as accurate as culture, serology is particularly useful for organisms that cannot easily be cultured, such as hepatitis B or HIV (Porth & Matfin, 2009).

- *Direct antigen detection methods* use monoclonal antibodies (purified antibody forms) to detect antigens in specimens from the diseased host (Porth, 2007). These tests offer rapid and accurate identification of the offending microorganism.
- *Antibiotic peak and trough levels* monitor therapeutic blood levels of the prescribed medication(s). The therapeutic range, that is, the minimum and maximum blood levels at which the drug is effective, is known for a given drug. By measuring blood levels at the predicted peak (1 to 2 hours after oral administration, 1 hour after intramuscular administration, and 30 minutes after intravenous administration) and trough (lowest level, usually a few minutes before the next

scheduled dose), healthcare personnel can determine that the patient is maintaining a level within the therapeutic range at all times, ensuring maximal effect from the drug. It is also possible to determine whether the drug is reaching a toxic or harmful level during therapy, increasing the likelihood of adverse effects.

- *Radiologic examination of the chest, abdomen, or urinary system* may be ordered to detect organ abnormalities indicating an inflammatory response or tissue damage.
- *Lumbar puncture* is performed to obtain cerebrospinal fluid (CSF) for examination and culture if a central nervous system (CNS) infection, such as meningitis or encephalitis, is suspected.
- *Ultrasonic examination* is a noninvasive diagnostic test such as an echocardiogram or renal ultrasonography to identify an infectious site or evaluate the effects of infection on organ function.

Medications

After the infecting organism and affected body system have been identified, specific therapy to cure the infectious disease can be instituted. Antimicrobial preparations are broadly classified as bacteriostatic or bactericidal. *Bacteriostatic agents* inhibit the growth of the microorganism, leaving its destruction to the host's immune system. These agents are generally not indicated for the immunocompromised host. Tetracyclines, erythromycin, and chloramphenicol are bacteriostatic preparations. *Bactericidal agents* are capable of killing the organism without immune system intervention. These include the penicillins, cephalosporins, and aminoglycoside antibiotics.

The activity of antimicrobial agents on bacteria, fungi, and viruses falls under five basic mechanisms:

- Impairing cell wall synthesis, leading to lysis and cell destruction
- Inhibiting protein synthesis, causing impaired microbial function
- Altering cell membrane permeability, causing intracellular contents to leak
- Inhibiting the synthesis of nucleic acids
- Inhibiting cell metabolism and growth

Many microorganisms have the ability to develop resistance to an anti-infective agent; that is, the pathogen continues to live and grow in the presence of the anti-infective. Resistance develops as a result of a chance mutation by the pathogen, allowing a subpopulation of cells to survive. The chance of an organism's becoming resistant to an agent is partially related to the dose delivered. Resistance is less likely to occur when a lethal dose is administered; therefore, it is vital that patients understand the need to take all doses of the prescribed drug as ordered.

ANTIBIOTICS Medications used to treat bacterial infections are generally known as antibiotics. Most antibiotics are biologic substances, that is, substances produced by other microorganisms. Antibiotics fall into classes of drugs with related chemical structure and activity. Some are effective against only gram-positive bacteria, and others are effective against only gram-negative organisms. Broad-spectrum antibiotics have activity against a wide variety of bacteria, including both gram-positive

and gram-negative forms. No antibiotic is totally safe. Hypersensitivity responses occur; always check for allergies before administering the first dose. Some drugs are toxic to organ systems, exhibiting hepatotoxicity, nephrotoxicity, ototoxicity, or bone marrow suppression. The antibiotics presented in the following Medication Administration box are organized according to their antibacterial action.

ANTIVIRALS Most antibiotics have little effect on viruses because the virus has no cell wall and no cytoplasm, produces no enzymes, and sequesters itself in a host cell to reproduce. Antiviral agents must be very selective in differentiating normal cellular activity from viral activity. In addition, the immune function of the host is a vital component in fighting viral infections; antiviral therapy may be relatively ineffective in the severely immunocompromised host. Making a timely diagnosis to allow institution of antiviral therapy can be an additional problem because viruses are less easily identified using laboratory techniques. Antiviral agents in common use are summarized in the Medication Administration box on page 298. Antiretroviral agents used in the management of HIV and AIDS are presented in ∞ Chapter 13.

ANTIFUNGALS Antifungal agents are available in both topical and systemic forms. They act by interfering with the cytoplasmic membrane of the fungus. Topical agents include preparations for cutaneous use to treat candidiasis, tineas, and ringworm. Vaginal preparations to treat vulvovaginal candidiasis are also available, as are several nonprescription topical and vaginal antifungal agents.

Amphotericin B (Fungizone) is a systemic antifungal agent for parenteral administration. It is used to treat severe, life-threatening fungal infections including histoplasmosis, blastomycosis, and candidiasis. Another systemic antifungal in current use is flucytosine (Ancobon). Unlike amphotericin B, flucytosine can be administered orally. It is used to treat severe candidiasis infections such as candida septicemia, endocarditis, pulmonary or urinary tract infections, and *Cryptococcus* meningitis.

Fluconazole (Diflucan) has the broadest use as an antifungal agent. It can be administered either orally or parenterally and is used to treat candidiasis infections as well as *Cryptococcus* meningitis. It is generally better tolerated than other systemic antifungal medications.

ANTIPARASITICS Drugs used to treat parasitic infections are as varied as the organisms that cause them. Generally, agents classified as antiparasitic are both expensive and likely to be toxic. Quinine was one of the first antiparasitic drugs developed in the treatment of malaria. Quinine is highly toxic, but newer forms such as chloroquine (Aralen, Chlorcon) and hydroxychloroquine (Plaquenil) are widely used as antimalarial drugs. Metronidazole (e.g., Flagyl) is used to treat infections of protozoan parasites (see the preceding Medication Administration box).

Isolation Techniques

Controlling the spread of infectious diseases in the hospital or long-term care setting is particularly important to preventing nosocomial infection. Hand hygiene remains the single most important factor in preventing the transmission of infections. Not all infectious diseases spread readily, necessitating special techniques or procedures. However, diseases such as chickenpox

MEDICATION ADMINISTRATION — Antibiotic Therapy

I. Cell Wall Synthesis Inhibitors

PENICILLINS

Penicillin G	Dicloxacillin (Dynapen)
Penicillin V	Methicillin (Staphcillin)
Amoxicillin (Amoxil)	Mezlocillin (Mezlin)
Nafcillin (Unipen)	Oxacillin (Prostaphlin)
Ampicillin (Polycillin)	Piperacillin (Pipracil)
Carbenicillin (Geopen, Geocillin)	Ticarcillin (Ticar)

Combination Agents

ampicillin and sulbactam (Unasyn)

ticarcillin and clavulanate (Timentin)

piperacillin and tazobactam (Zosyn)

amoxicillin and clavulanate (Augmentin)

Penicillins are bactericidal and interfere with cell wall synthesis and the enzymes involved in cell division and synthesis. They are more effective on gram-positive than gram-negative organisms. Penicillins are considered to be safe, effective, and of low toxicity. Resistance is now more common among *Streptococci* and *Staphylococci*. Penicillins and related antibiotics such as the cephalosporins (see below) contain a molecular structure known as a beta-lactam ring. Some bacteria produce enzymes (beta-lactamases or penicillinases) that cleave this ring, making the antibiotics ineffective. To combat this resistance, beta-lactamase or penicillinase inhibitors such as sulbactam and clavulanate are combined with some antibiotics to create an antibiotic effective against drug-resistant bacterial strains.

Nursing Responsibilities

■ Monitor for hypersensitivity responses such as local erythema and itching at the site of injection, skin rashes, urticaria (hives), itching, fever, chills, and anaphylaxis.

■ Observe patients receiving parenteral penicillin for at least 30 minutes.

■ Discontinue the drug immediately if any hypersensitivity response occurs. Be prepared to administer antihistamines or corticosteroids for a mild reaction. Anaphylaxis is treated with epinephrine subcutaneously or intravenously and airway support.

■ Do not administer penicillin to anyone with a history of a severe allergic reaction to any form of the drug; a cross-reactivity may occur in patients allergic to cephalosporin or carbapenem antibiotics.

■ Assess for superinfection (vaginitis, stomatitis, or diarrhea) due to elimination of resident bacteria.

Health Education for the Patient and Family

■ Notify the physician if you see white patches on the oral mucosa or if vaginitis develops. An antifungal drug may be prescribed and the antibiotic continued.

■ Consuming yogurt or buttermilk may prevent superinfection. Do not take these products within 1 hour of taking the drug.

CEPHALOSPORINS

1st Generation	2nd Generation
Cephalexin (Keflex)	Cefotetan (Cefotan)
Cefazolin (Ancef)	Cefaclor (Ceclor)
Cefadroxil (Duricef)	Cefoxitin (Mefoxin)
Cefradrine (Velocef)	Cefprozil (Cefzil)
	Cefuroxime (Ceftin)
	Cefixime (Cefixime)
	Cefotaxime (Claforan)

3rd Generation	4th Generation
Cefoperazone (Cefobid)	Cefepime (Maxipime)
Ceftazidime (Fortaz)	
Ceftriaxone (Rocephin)	

Cephalosporins are structurally similar to the penicillins and also inhibit cell wall synthesis. They are divided into four groups, or generations. First-generation cephalosporins act primarily against gram-positive organisms. Second- and third-generation drugs are more effective against gram-negative organisms than against gram-positive ones. Fourth-generation cephalosporins act effectively against both gram-positive and gram-negative organisms.

Nursing Responsibilities

■ Monitor for previous hypersensitivity response to cephalosporins or penicillins.

■ Assess intravenous site for phlebitis; intramuscular injection may cause local pain.

■ Monitor laboratory results for adverse response, such as leukopenia and thrombocytopenia, nephrotoxicity (elevated BUN and serum creatinine), or hepatotoxicity (elevated bilirubin, LDH, ALT, AST, and alkaline phosphatase).

■ Assess for manifestations of superinfections.

Health Education for the Patient and Family

■ Take the medication on an empty stomach, 1 hour before or 2 hours after meals.

■ Avoid alcohol while using cefmetazole, cefoperazone, or cefotetan because alcohol intolerance can develop with these antibiotics. These same drugs intensify bleeding tendencies.

■ Space doses of the medication relatively evenly throughout the day and evening hours.

■ Increase consumption of buttermilk or yogurt to prevent intestinal superinfection.

CARBAPENEMS

Imipenem (Primaxin)

Meropenem (Merrem)

Ertapenem (Invanz)

This newer class of antibiotics includes only three drugs and all must be given parenterally. Imipenem has the broadest antimicrobial spectrum of any drug. This makes it especially useful against mixed organism infections. These antibiotics cross the meninges and achieve therapeutic doses in CSF; they are effective against methicillin-resistant staphylococcus aureus (MRSA). These antibiotics cause bacterial cell wall lysis and subsequent death of the bacteria. Side effects include nausea and vomiting, diarrhea, hypersensitivity reactions, occasional superinfections with bacteria or fungi, and, rarely, seizures.

Nursing Responsibilities

■ Ertapenem should not be mixed with dextrose or other drugs containing dextrose. IV infusions should be given over at least 30 minutes.

■ Check for history of hypersensitivity to cephalosporins and penicillins and monitor for manifestations of reactions.

■ Assess for manifestations of superinfection.

■ Monitor laboratory indicators of renal function.

Health Education for the Patient and Family

■ Report any manifestations of allergy such as skin rash, itching, or hives.

VANCOMYCIN

This antibiotic inhibits cell wall synthesis and is used for serious infections. It is only effective against gram-positive bacteria, especially *S. aureus* and *Staphylococcus epidermidis*, including the strains resistant to methicillin. *C. difficile* is also susceptible to this antibiotic, but infection with *C. difficile* is often treated first with metronidazole to delay emergence of resistance to vancomycin.

Nursing Responsibilities

- Infuse slowly over 60 minutes or more to avoid "red man" syndrome. The syndrome is characterized by erythematous rash, flushing, tachycardia, and hypotension. Patients may become dizzy and agitated. The occurrence is usually associated with a first dose of vancomycin and is seen within 4 to 6 minutes of the start of a dose or after completion.
- Ototoxicity is a serious adverse effect because hearing loss may be irreversible. Notify the physician immediately if the patient reports a sensation of fullness in the ears, as this indicates ototoxicity.

II. Bacterial Protein Synthesis Inhibitors

TETRACYCLINES

Tetracycline HCl (Sumycin)	Minocycline HCl (Minocin)
Doxycycline (Vibramycin)	Oxytetracycline (Terramycin)

Tetracyclines are active against many gram-positive and gram-negative bacteria, such as *Mycoplasma*, *Rickettsia*, and *Chlamydia*. They are bacteriostatic, interfering with microbial protein synthesis. Tetracycline binds readily with metal and solid elements in the bowel, limiting its absorption when administered with food; the other preparations are highly soluble in lipids and can be administered with food.

Nursing Responsibilities

- Schedule doses 1 hour before or 2 hours after meals. Do not give with milk or milk products or antacids.
- Monitor for manifestations of superinfection.
- If the patient is taking an anticoagulant, monitor prothrombin time and for manifestations of bleeding.

Health Education for the Patient and Family

- Avoid excessive sun exposure to reduce the risk of photosensitivity reactions.
- Tetracyclines can stain the enamel of developing teeth when taken during pregnancy; although deciduous (baby) teeth are affected, permanent teeth are not.

MACROLIDES

Erythromycin (E-Mycin, Erythrocin)	Clarithromycin
Azithromycin (Zithromax)	Dirithromycin (Dynabac)
	Troleandomycin (Tao)

Macrolides are bacteriostatic and act effectively against gram-positive and gram-negative organisms. Erythromycin is used to treat *Streptococcal pharyngitis* in patients who are allergic to penicillin, and is the drug of choice for treating pertussis. Clarithromycin and azithromycin produce less nausea than erythromycin, increasing patient adherence.

Nursing Responsibilities

- Administer erythromycin on an empty stomach or immediately before meals.
- Give the drug with a full glass of water. Do not administer with acidic fruit juice.
- Intravenous doses are very irritating to veins; give slowly (20 to 60 minutes per gram).

Health Education for the Patient and Family

- Gastric distress is a common side effect with erythromycin.

AMINOGLYCOSIDES

Amikacin (Amikin)	Gentamicin (Garamycin)
Kanamycin (Kantrex)	Neomycin (Mycifradin)
Streptomycin	Tobramycin (Nebcin)

Aminoglycosides are bactericidal, interfering with protein synthesis in the pathogen. They are especially effective against gram-negative organisms. To provide a broader spectrum of activity, they are often combined with other antibiotics, especially penicillins. Aminoglycosides can be administered in multiple or single daily doses. They are ototoxic and nephrotoxic; the risk is highest for older adults, patients with preexisting renal disease, and persons receiving other ototoxic or nephrotoxic drugs.

Nursing Responsibilities

- Assess renal function before and during aminoglycoside therapy. Monitor intake and output, daily weight, BUN, and serum creatinine.
- Assess for adverse effects on hearing such as loss of perception of high tones, tinnitus, and vertigo.
- Notify the physician if the patient is receiving other nephrotoxic or ototoxic drugs such as furosemide (Lasix) and ethacrynic acid (Edecrin).
- Administer intravenous preparations separately from other drugs; flush tubing before and after administration.

Health Education for the Patient and Family

- Monitor for a sudden weight gain that may indicate adverse effects on the kidney and report it to the physician.

OXAZOLIDINONES

Linezolid (Zyvox) is the first antibiotic in a class of antibiotics called oxazolidinones. This antibiotic inhibits protein synthesis and is effective against organisms that are resistant to both vancomycin and methicillin. Because of its usefulness against those organisms, its use should be reserved for infections caused by vancomycin-resistant enterococci (VRE) and MRSA.

Nursing Responsibilities

- Monitor for side effects including nausea, diarrhea, hypertension, and headache.
- Monitor platelets if patient is at risk for bleeding; this drug may cause thrombocytopenia.

Health Education for the Patient and Family

- It can be taken with or without food.
- Avoid taking ephedrine, pseudoephedrine, methylphenidate, or cocaine with this drug as high blood pressure may develop.

III. Bacterial Nucleic Acid Inhibitors

FLUOROQUINOLONES

Ciprofloxacin (Cipro)	Gatifloxacin (Tequin) (ophthalmic)
Levofloxacin (Levaquin)	

Fluoroquinolones are bactericidal and especially active against gram-negative and some gram-positive organisms. They are used to manage infections of the respiratory, gastrointestinal, and genitourinary tracts. Cipro is approved to treat inhalation anthrax; infected individuals are not contagious (Lane & Fauci, 2008).

Nursing Responsibilities

- Increase fluid intake to 2000 to 3000 mL/day unless contraindicated to prevent crystalluria.
- Monitor laboratory results for hepatotoxicity (elevated ALT, AST).

Health Education for the Patient and Family

- Drink six to eight glasses of water per day.
- Avoid exposure to sunlight while taking these drugs.

SULFONAMIDES AND TRIMETHOPRIM

Sulfamethizole (Thiosulfil Forte)

Sulfamethoxazole (Gantanol; in combination with trimethoprim, TMP-SMZ, Bactrim, Septra)

Sulfisoxazole (Gantrisin)

Sulfadiazine (Coptin)

(continued)

Sulfonamides are bacteriostatic. Trimethoprim is an antibiotic effective against most gram-positive and many gram-negative organisms. It is often combined with sulfamethoxazole to manage urinary tract infections, *P. jiroveci* pneumonia, and otitis media. Skin rashes and pruritus are the most common hypersensitivity reactions. Severe reactions include exfoliative dermatitis and Stevens-Johnson syndrome.

Nursing Responsibilities
- Assess for history of hypersensitivity to sulfonamides and related medications, such as thiazide diuretics and sulfonylurea preparations.
- Monitor intake and output. Maintain a fluid intake of at least 1500 mL/day to prevent crystalluria.
- Assess for evidence of bleeding, easy bruising, or systemic infection, and monitor blood count for possible bone marrow depression.

Health Education for the Patient and Family
- Take medication on an empty stomach with a full glass of water. Maintain a fluid intake of at least 2 quarts per day.
- Protect the skin from excessive sun exposure with clothing and sunscreens to reduce the risk of photosensitivity.

METRONIDAZOLE (FLAGYL)
Metronidazole is effective against anaerobic gram-negative bacteria and protozoan infections caused by amebiasis, giardiasis, and trichomoniasis. It is commonly used to prevent and treat infections following intestinal surgery, and is the drug of first choice with *C. difficile*.

Nursing Responsibilities
- Monitor for CNS effects of dizziness, headache, ataxia, confusion, depression, and peripheral neuropathy.
- Administer with food to minimize gastric distress and metallic taste. Infuse intravenous metronidazole over 60 minutes.
- Discontinue the medication and notify the physician if neurologic reactions occur.
- Increase fluid intake to 2500 mL/day to minimize the risk of nephrotoxicity.

Health Education for the Patient and Family
- This medication may turn urine reddish brown; this is expected and not harmful.
- Stop taking the drug and notify the physician if hypersensitivity reaction or adverse effects occur, such as changes in mentation or coordination, painful or frequent urination, painful or difficult intercourse, impotence.
- Do not drink alcohol while taking this medication; an Antabuse-type reaction (flushing, sweating, headache, vomiting, and abdominal cramps) may occur.
- Maintain a fluid intake of 2.5 to 3 quarts per day.
- When the drug is prescribed for *Trichomonas* infections, treatment of both partners is necessary. Use condoms to prevent cross-contamination during intercourse.

(varicella) are highly contagious and are spread by the airborne route, requiring special precautions to protect other hospitalized patients. Two additional airborne threats are SARS and avian flu. These are addressed in ∞ Chapter 36.

In determining the need for isolation precautions, healthcare personnel consider the usual reservoir or source of the microorganism, the mode of transmission, and susceptibility of hospital staff and other patients. For example, patients with *P. jiroveci* pneumonia do not require isolation, because immunocompetent persons are not susceptible to this infection.

The CDC has published guidelines for isolation precautions to be used in healthcare facilities (CDC, 2007). These guidelines include both *standard precautions* and *category-specific isolation precautions*.

Standard Precautions
Standard Precautions, published by the Hospital Infection Control Practices Advisory Committee of the Centers for Disease Control in 1996, provides guidelines for the handling of blood and other body fluids. These guidelines are used with all patients, regardless of whether they have a known infectious disease. The guidelines were developed in light of the realization that many patients with an infectious disease such as HIV or hepatitis B have no apparent manifestations, but can transmit the disease to others. Standard precautions are used by all healthcare workers who have direct contact with patients or with their body fluids or have indirect contact, such as by emptying trash, changing linens, or cleaning the room.

AMANTADINE (SYMMETREL)
Amantadine is used to prevent and treat influenza A. It has been shown to be 55% to 80% or more effective in preventing the disease. When administered within 24 to 72 hours after the onset of manifestations, it reduces common manifestations of influenza. It is generally well tolerated; minimal CNS side effects, such as dizziness, anxiety, insomnia, and difficulty concentrating, may occur.

ACYCLOVIR (ZOVIRAX) AND GANCICLOVIR (CYTOVENE)
Acyclovir and ganciclovir are related compounds used primarily in the treatment of herpes viruses. Acyclovir is prescribed mainly in the treatment of genital herpes simplex infections. Although it does not kill the virus, acyclovir is effective in reducing the severity, duration, and frequency of recurrence of manifestations. Ganciclovir is indicated primarily in the treatment of cytomegalovirus infection. Although acyclovir is generally well tolerated with little toxicity, ganciclovir may profoundly suppress bone marrow function, and its use is therefore limited.

VIDARABINE (VIRA-A)
Vidarabine inhibits viral DNA synthesis and is effective against many herpesvirus infections. Its primary use is in treatment of herpes simplex encephalitis.

INTERFERONS
Interferons are naturally produced cytokines whose use as antiviral agents is being explored. When administered intranasally, interferons have been shown to be effective in preventing rhinovirus upper respiratory infections. Other uses being explored include treatment of human papillomavirus (genital warts) and preventing or reducing Kaposi's sarcoma in patients with AIDS. They are also used in combination biotherapy regimens for malignant melanoma.

Standard precautions apply to the following:

- Blood
- All body fluids, secretions, and excretions, regardless of whether they contain visible blood
- Nonintact skin
- Mucous membranes

Barrier protection is used to prevent exposing skin and mucous membrane surfaces to blood and body fluids. Barrier protection involves using gloves for touching or handling body fluids, and adding other protection such as gowns, masks, and goggles if splashing or spraying is likely. Needles and other sharp objects are not recapped or bent, but disposed of in puncture-proof containers to prevent inadvertent percutaneous (needle-stick) exposure. Standard precautions are presented in ∞ Appendix A.

Transmission-Based Precautions

In addition to hand hygiene and standard precautions, the nature and spread of some infectious diseases require that special techniques be used to protect uninfected patients and workers. The CDC identifies three types of transmission-based precautions: airborne, droplet, and contact precautions. Transmission-based precautions may be combined for diseases that have multiple routes of transmission. Indications for the use of transmission-based isolation precautions and the specific measures to be taken are outlined in Table 12–9.

∞ Nursing Care

Nursing management related to infectious disease focuses on prevention and health promotion and maintenance. Prevention is facilitated by assessing the patient's risk for infection based on underlying conditions, immune response, and prophylactic measures such as immunizations.

Health Promotion

Preventing infection requires education of not only healthcare personnel but also the general public. Part of an education program includes understanding the importance of immunizations, the guidelines for using antibiotics to prevent drug-resistant microorganisms, and the ways to prevent the spread of infection. Check immunization records for all family members and encourage them to keep immunizations up to date. Increase public awareness regarding appropriate antibiotic use. Guidelines for preventing the spread of infection to others include the following:

- Avoid crowds and contact with susceptible persons, especially those who are immunosuppressed (e.g., persons who have HIV infection, who are undergoing therapy for cancer, or who have had an organ transplant).
- Use disposable tissues to contain respiratory secretions when coughing or sneezing. Cough into the elbow or upper arm instead of the hand if disposable tissues are not available.
- Use appropriate food-handling precautions for diseases spread via the fecal–oral route, such as hepatitis A.
- Avoid contact with or sharing of body fluids. For example, do not share needles or razors; use a condom during sexual activity, or abstain; have each person clean his or her own blood spills or wounds if possible.

Assessment

The following data are collected through the health history and physical examination. Further focused assessments are described with nursing interventions in the next section.

- *Health history:* Current manifestations, age, medication use (antipyretics and anti-infectives), nutrition, exposure to infectious persons, immunizations, invasive procedures and therapies, chronic diseases such as diabetes mellitus, cancer.
- *Physical assessment:* Vital signs, body system(s) where infection is suspected, lymph node enlargement, and tenderness.

TABLE 12–9 Transmission-Based Precautions

CATEGORY	INFECTIOUS DISEASES	PURPOSE	PRECAUTIONS
Airborne precautions	Pulmonary tuberculosis, chickenpox (with contact precautions), measles, respiratory infections (pneumonia)	Reduce risk of airborne transmission of infectious agents. Airborne transmission occurs by dissemination of either airborne droplet nuclei or dust particles containing the infectious agent.	Private room with hand washing and toilet facilities, and special ventilation that does not allow air to circulate to general hospital ventilation; mask or special filter respirator for everyone entering room
Droplet precautions	Meningitis, pertussis	Reduce risk of droplet transmission of infectious agents. Droplet transmission involves contact of conjunctivae of the eyes or mucous membranes of the nose or mouth with large-particle droplets generated during coughing, sneezing, talking, or procedures such as suctioning.	Private room with hand washing and toilet facilities; mask, eye protection, and/or face shields worn by everyone entering room
Contact precautions	Acute diarrhea, chickenpox (with airborne precautions), respiratory syncytial virus (RSV); skin, wound, or urinary tract infection with multidrug-resistant organisms; S. aureus infections	Reduce risk of transmission by direct or indirect contact. Direct contact transmission involves skin-to-skin contact and physical transfer of organisms. It may occur between patients or during direct care activities such as bathing or turning patients. Indirect contact involves contact with a contaminated object.	Private room with hand washing and toilet facilities; gowns and protective apparel to provide barrier protection; disposable supplies or decontamination of all articles leaving room

Nursing Diagnoses and Interventions

Patients with an infection may be managed in the hospital or at home, depending on the severity of the infection. During the acute phase, nursing care includes administering prescribed antibiotics, implementing and maintaining aseptic technique and infection control measures, and encouraging a balance of rest and activity, good nutritional intake, and other general health measures to support immunologic function and healing. The key nursing diagnoses are *Risk for Infection, Anxiety,* and *Hyperthermia.*

Risk for Infection

The spread of infection is a risk in any facility that houses many people. It is a particular risk in hospitals, where many patients have at least some degree of immunosuppression and many drug-resistant strains of pathogens are prevalent. It is vital that nurses use good hand hygiene techniques at all times, employ standard precautions with all patients, and use category-specific isolation techniques as indicated to prevent infectious spread to other patients, themselves, and their families.

- Admit patients with known or suspected infections to a private room. *This is important to minimize the risk to other patients.*
- Perform hand hygiene using hand sanitizer on entering and leaving the patient's room. If visibly soiled, wash hands using a 10- to 15-second vigorous scrub with soap or anti-bacterial scrub solution. *A 10- to 15-second scrub removes transient microorganisms from the skin and helps prevent transmission of infection to or from the patient.*
- Use standard precautions and personal protective devices to reduce the risk of transmission. *Gloves, gowns, and masks are to be worn whenever there is a risk of skin or mucous membrane contamination by direct contact with infectious material, airborne spread of organisms, or droplet nuclei.*
- Explain the reasons for and importance of isolation procedures during hospitalization. *Patients with isolation precautions may feel neglected, dirty, or shunned. Explanation of reasons and procedures can enhance the patient's and family's understanding and acceptance.*
- Place a mask on the patient and/or cover all infectious lesions or wounds completely when transporting the patient to other parts of the facility for diagnostic or treatment procedures. *These measures help minimize air contamination and the risk to visitors and personnel.*
- Collect a culture and sensitivity (C&S) specimen as ordered or indicated by purulent drainage, pyuria, or other manifestations of infection. *C&S is performed to determine the presence and type of infectious organisms as well as antibiotics most likely to be effective in eradicating it.*

> **PRACTICE ALERT**
> Collect the specimen for C&S before the first dose of antibiotics is administered to ensure adequate organisms for culture.

- Administer prescribed anti-infective agents. *Anti-infectives are used to destroy the invading microorganism.*
- Inform all personnel having contact with the patient of the diagnosis. *This is particularly important for a patient with a* disease requiring category-specific isolation so that personnel can take appropriate precautions.
- Ensure that visitors don appropriate protective wear before they enter the patient's room. *Protective wear reduces their risk of infection.*
- Use appropriate measures for disposing of contaminated tissues, dressings, or other material and for removing soiled linens and equipment from the patient's room. *Check hospital policy or published guidelines for category-specific isolation.*
- Teach the importance of complying with prescribed treatment for the entire course of the regimen. *Because anti-infective agents kill only a portion of the pathogen population with each dose, completion of the entire course of therapy is necessary to reduce the risk of relapse and of creating drug-resistant organisms.*

Anxiety

The patient with an infectious disease may experience anxiety related to his or her manifestations, treatment measures, the prognosis, and expected outcome of the disease. The diagnosis of an infection can be traumatic, causing feelings of uneasiness, isolation, guilt (e.g., in regard to sexually transmitted infections), apprehension, or depression.

- Assess level of anxiety. *The level of anxiety influences the patient's response to and interpretation of the situation and degree of threat it poses.*
- Discuss the infection, treatments, prognosis, and outcomes. *Discussions help to allay fears and misconceptions.*
- Support and enhance the patient's coping strategies. *A person uses intrapersonal and interpersonal mechanisms to reduce or relieve anxiety.*
- Include significant others in the plan of care. *Inclusion of the patient and family members provides assurance and confidence, and promotes understanding of the unknown.*
- Explain isolation procedures, and answer any concerns. *Isolation may be necessary to prevent the spread of infection but can cause great anxiety for the patient and family members.*
- Provide referrals as needed for continuing care, for example, to home health agencies or for dressing changes or periodic assessment. *Referrals are often necessary to provide ongoing interventions and maintain continuity of care.*

Hyperthermia

Hyperthermia is an expected consequence of the infectious disease process. Fever may produce mild, short-term effects or, when prolonged, may cause serious life-threatening effects.

- Monitor temperature especially during episodes of chills; note heart rate and rhythm. *Chills indicate a rising temperature. Hyperthermia can cause dysrhythmias.*
- Administer prescribed antipyretic as indicated for elevated temperature. *Although antipyretics lower the temperature and enhance comfort for the patient, this benefit must be weighed against the possible beneficial effect of an elevated temperature in the immune response. Fever increases the motility and activity of WBCs, stimulates the production of interferon, and activates T cells. In addition, temperatures above the normal range inhibit the growth of many microorganisms (Porth & Matfin, 2009).*

- Promote body cooling through lowering the room temperature. *Rapid cooling stimulates the hypothalamus to increase the body's temperature; this increases both shivering and metabolic rate.*

> **PRACTICE ALERT**
> Use ice packs, cool/tepid baths, or a hypothermia blanket with caution to prevent unnecessary shivering.

- Monitor fluid loss; encourage increased fluid and electrolyte intake either orally or intravenously. *Hyperthermia causes fluid loss from evaporation and may result in dehydration and electrolyte imbalance.*
- If diaphoretic, bathe and provide dry clothing and bedding. *These measures increase patient comfort and decrease further water evaporation.*
- Promote rest periods. *Rest increases the energy reserve that is depleted by an increased metabolic, heart, and respiratory rate.*

Using NANDA, NIC, and NOC

Linkages between a selected NANDA nursing diagnosis, NIC, and NOC for the patient with an infection are shown in the chart that follows.

Community-Based Care

Patient and family teaching is directed toward helping the patient recover from the infection or disease, preventing its spread to others, and preventing life-threatening complications. Instructions should include the following points:

- Use good hand hygiene techniques, particularly after touching infected wounds or lesions, coughing, sneezing, blowing the nose, or using the bathroom. Wash hands thoroughly before eating or performing any procedures such as dressing changes. Wash hands with soap and water before and after preparing food or eating and before and after using the toilet or handling diapers. Do not share eating utensils.
- Take all prescribed antibiotics as ordered even after manifestations have subsided. Take the prescription at intervals around the clock as directed.
- Never allow anyone else to use your medications and never use anyone else's prescription even if they appear to be the same.

> **NANDA, NIC, AND NOC LINKAGES**
> The Patient with an Infection
>
> **NANDA** → Delayed Surgical Recovery
>
> **NIC** → Infection Control
> Medication Administration
> Vital Signs Monitoring
> Wound Care
>
> **NOC** → Infection Severity
> Wound Healing: Primary Intention
> Post Procedure Recovery Status
>
> Data from NANDA International. (2009). *Nursing diagnoses: Definitions & classification 2009–2011.* Oxford, UK: Wiley-Blackwell; Bulechek, G. M., Butcher, H. K., & Dochterman, J. M. (Eds.). (2008). *Nursing interventions classification (NIC)* (5th ed.). St. Louis, MO: Mosby; and Moorhead, S., Johnson, M., Maas, M., & Swanson, E. (Eds.). (2008). *Nursing outcomes classification (NOC)* (4th ed.). St. Louis, MO: Elsevier Mosby.

- Notify your healthcare provider if
  - symptoms do not improve within 24 to 48 hours after antibiotic therapy is instituted, or they worsen.
  - manifestations of antibiotic allergy (itching, rash, difficulty breathing or swallowing, swelling of the face or tongue) occur. Discontinue medication and contact prescriber.
  - adverse responses, such as gastrointestinal distress or diarrhea interfere with completion of the prescription.
  - manifestations of infection recur after completing prescribed antibiotic.
- Report redness, swelling, or drainage around wounds or persistent high fever.
- Increase fluid intake to at least 2500 mL (2.5 quarts) per day.
- Report any manifestations of opportunistic infections: loose, watery, and foul-smelling diarrhea; vaginal discharge or itching; fuzzy growth or white plaques in mouth or on tongue; blood in urine; chills; fever; or unusual cough.
- In addition, suggest the following resources: County or public health department, Centers for Disease Control and Prevention.

CHAPTER HIGHLIGHTS

- The human body has a remarkable capacity to survive in an environment of deadly microorganisms and pathogens that can weaken and kill the body. Both natural barriers and the immune system prevent the invasion and replication of pathogens. The lymphatic system provides conduits for pathogens, isolating them from the bloodstream where they would grow rapidly.
- The adaptability and specificity of immune responses is possible because immune cells are genetically encoded to capture pathogens, move them to lymph nodes, and develop specific immune reactions. However, if the immune system's self-recognition fails, highly damaging autoimmune diseases can develop.
- A revolutionary increase in knowledge and understanding of the immune system has enabled progress in clinical medicine. Through scientific research concerning T and B lymphocytes, cytokines, antibodies, and other elements of the immune system, treatments are evolving for cancer, AIDS, organ transplantation, autoimmune diseases, infectious disease, and vaccines.
- Inflammation is a protective mechanism designed to prevent pathogens from entering the bloodstream and populating

functional tissues such as heart, liver, and kidney. Pain acts as a signal that tissue has been damaged and stimulates protective responses such as cleansing wounds and limiting function while healing progresses. Restoration occurs as the inflammatory process isolates the injury and repairs damaged tissue.

■ Localized infections may damage tissue and create pain, but systemic infections are life-threatening if they progress to septic shock. Unfortunately, hospitals are hazardous environments populated with collections of pathogens. Hospital-borne infections are often introduced into the body by medical procedures.

■ Hygiene, protection from harm, and nutrition support the immune defenses. Antimicrobial medications limit the spread of pathogens, but can lose their effectiveness when microbes mutate and develop resistance.

TEST YOURSELF NCLEX-RN® REVIEW

1. When a patient receives gamma globulin following exposure to hepatitis A, the nurse expects the patient to develop which of the following?
   1. natural passive immunity
   2. natural active immunity
   3. acquired passive immunity
   4. acquired active immunity

2. What would be the priority nursing intervention in the treatment of a patient with an infection?
   1. Administer prescribed anti-infective.
   2. Assess for history of hypersensitivities and allergies.
   3. Obtain specimen for culture and sensitivity.
   4. Monitor for reaction to anti-infective.

3. When administering medications, the nurse would know that which one of the following medications inhibits prostaglandin synthesis?
   1. acetaminophen (Tylenol)
   2. prednisone
   3. penicillin
   4. aspirin

4. The patient with an acute infection shows a shift to the left on the WBC differential count. The nurse recognizes a shift to the left because of which laboratory finding?
   1. increased band neutrophils
   2. increased eosinophils
   3. decreased leukocytes
   4. decreased monocytes

5. A patient is admitted with methicillin-resistant *Staphylococcus aureus* in a draining sacral wound. The patient should be placed in which type of isolation precautions?
   1. droplet precautions
   2. contact precautions
   3. airborne precautions
   4. protective precautions

6. The T cells of the immune system adapt to kill which type of organism?
   1. intracellular organisms
   2. interstitial microbes
   3. extracellular viruses
   4. protozoans

7. How would the nurse describe thrombocytosis?
   1. increased platelets
   2. decreased clotting time
   3. decreased platelets
   4. average number of platelets

8. A nurse makes the nursing diagnosis *Risk for Infection*. What group is he or she considering when making this diagnosis?
   1. the infected patient only
   2. healthcare workers in the facility
   3. patients hospitalized at the same time
   4. the infected patient, healthcare workers, and other patients

9. What does the nurse primarily monitor when administering antibiotics?
   1. compliance
   2. therapeutic levels
   3. oxygen desaturation
   4. hypersensitivities and teaching

10. All nurses are expected to follow standard precautions for all hospitalized patients. What do these include?
    1. hand hygiene, use of masks, and recapping needles
    2. use of masks and gowns, and spraying of disinfectant regularly
    3. use of gloves, gowns, and goggles with contaminated body fluids
    4. use of alcohol-based hand rub for visibly dirty or blood-contaminated hands

See Test Yourself answers in Appendix C.

Pearson Nursing Student Resources

Find additional review materials at
nursing.pearsonhighered.com

Prepare for success with additional NCLEX®-style practice questions, interactive assignments and activities, Web links, animations and videos, and more!

BIBLIOGRAPHY

Arnold, M., & Barbul, A. (2006). Nutrition and wound healing. *Plastic and Reconstructive Surgery, 117*(7 Suppl), 42S–58S.

Aronson, B. (2005). Medication management behaviors of adherent short-term antibiotic users. *Clinical Excellence for Nurse Practitioners, 9*(1), 23–30.

Bulechek, G. M., Butcher, H. K., & Dochterman, J. M. (Eds.). (2008). *Nursing interventions classification (NIC)* (5th ed.). St. Louis: Mosby Elsevier.

Centers for Disease Control and Prevention. (2002a). Guidelines for hand hygiene in health-care settings. *MMWR Recommendations and Reports, 51*(RR 16), 1–44.

Centers for Disease Control and Prevention. (2002b). *Guidelines for the prevention of intravascular catheter-related infections.* Retrieved from http://www.cdc.gov/mmwr/preview/mmwrhtml/mm5132a9.htm

Centers for Disease Control and Prevention. (2010). *Estimates of healthcare associated infections.* Retrieved from http://www.cdc.gov/ncidod/dhqp/hai.html

Centers for Disease Control and Prevention. (2007b). *Guideline for isolation precautions: Preventing transmission of infectious agents in healthcare settings.* Retrieved from http://www.cdc.gov/ncidod/dhqp/gl_isolation.html

Centers for Disease Control and Prevention. (2009). Recommended adult immunization schedule—United States, 2009. *MMWR, 57*(53).

Christ-Crain, M., Jaccard-Stolz, D., Bingisser, R., et al. (2004). Effect of procalcitonin-guided treatment on antibiotic use and outcome in lower respiratory tract infections: Cluster-randomised, single-blinded intervention trial. *Lancet, 363*(9409), 600–607.

Eliopoulos, C. (2009). *Gerontological nursing* (7th ed.). Philadelphia: Lippincott Williams & Wilkins.

Fauci, A., Braunwald, E., Kasper, D. L., et al. (Eds.). (2008). *Harrison's principles of internal medicine* (17th ed.). New York: McGraw-Hill.

George, E. L. (2005). Does a high WBC count signal infection? *Nursing2005, 35*(1), 20–21.

Haas, J. P., & Larson, E. L. (2008). Compliance with hand hygiene. *American Journal of Nursing 108*(8), 40–45.

Kee, J. (2009). *Prentice Hall handbook of laboratory and diagnostic tests with nursing implication.* Upper Saddle River, NJ: Pearson Prentice Hall.

Kjonegaard, R., & Myers III, F. E. (2005). Arresting drug-resistant organisms. *Nursing 2005, 35*(6), 48–50.

Lacy, C. F., Armstrong, L. L., Goldman, M. P., & Lance, L. L. (2008). *Drug information handbook: A comprehensive resource for all clinicians and healthcare professionals.* Hudson, Ohio: Lexi-Comp Inc.

Lane, H. C., & Fauci, A. S. (2008). Microbial terrorism. In Fauci, A., Braunwald, E., Kasper, D. L., Hauser, S. L., Longo, D. L., Jameson, J. L., & Loscalzo, J. (Eds.), *Harrison's Principles of Internal Medicine* (17th ed.). New York: McGraw-Hill.

McPhee, S., Papadakis, M., & Tierney, L., (Eds.). (2008). *Current medical diagnosis & treatment* (47th ed.). Stamford, CT: Appleton & Lange.

Moorhead, S., Johnson, M., Maas, M., & Swanson, E. (Eds.). (2008). *Nursing outcomes classification (NOC)* (4th ed.). St. Louis, MO: Mosby Elsevier.

NANDA International. (2009). *Nursing diagnoses: Definitions and classification 2009–2011.* Oxford, UK: Wiley-Blackwell.

Porth, C. (2007). *Essentials of pathophysiology: Concepts of altered health states* (2nd ed.). Philadelphia: Lippincott Williams & Wilkins.

Porth, C., & Matfin, G. (2009). *Pathophysiology: Concepts of altered health states* (8th ed.). Philadelphia: Lippincott Williams & Wilkins.

Posani, T. (2004). *Clostridium difficile*: Causes and interventions. *Critical Care Nursing Clinics of North America, 16*(4), 547–551.

Prusiner, S. B., & Miller, B. (2007). Prion diseases. In Fauci et al., (Eds.), *Harrison's Principles of Internal Medicine* (17th ed.) (2646–2651). New York: McGraw-Hill.

Rakel, R. E., & Bope, E. T. (2008). *Conn's current therapy.* Philadelphia: Sanders Elsevier.

Shorr, A. F. (2005). Preventing pneumonia: The role for pneumococcal and influenza vaccines. *Clinics in Chest Medicine, 26*(1), 123–134.

Skidmore-Roth, L. (2009). *Mosby's nursing drug reference.* St. Louis: Mosby Elsevier.

Spigt, M. G., Knottnerus, J. A., Westerterp, K. R., Rikkert, M., & van Schayck, C. P. (2006). The effects of 6 months of increased water intake on blood sodium, glomerular filtration rate, blood pressure, and quality of life in elderly (Aged 55–75) men. *Journal of the American Geriatric Society 54,* 438–443.

Stokowski, L. A. (2008). Promoting vaccine safety: Answers to common questions. Medscape Nurses; Nursing Perspectives. Retrieved from http://www.medscape.com/viewarticle/568534

Stone, P. W., Hedblom, E. C., Murphy, D. M., & Miller, S. B. (2005). The economic impact of infection control: Making the business case for increased infection control resources. *American Journal of Infection Control, 33*(9), 542–547.

Vrtis, M. C. (2008). Is your patient taking the right antimicrobial? *American Journal of Nursing, 108*(6), 49–55.

Weinstein, R. A. (2007). Healthcare associated infections. In Fauci et al., *Harrison's principles of internal medicine* (17th ed.) (835–841). New York: McGraw-Hill.

White, K. A. (2008). The growing threat of cephalosporin resistance. *American Nurse Today, 3*(4), 9–12.

Wilson, B., Shannon, M., & Shields, K. (2009). *Prentice Hall nurse's drug guide.* Upper Saddle River, NJ: Pearson Prentice Hall.

13 Nursing Care of Patients with Altered Immunity

LEARNING OUTCOMES

1. Review the normal anatomy and physiology of the immune system.
2. Compare and contrast the four types of hypersensitivity reactions.
3. Explain the pathophysiology of autoimmune disorders and tissue transplant rejection.
4. Discuss the characteristics of immunodeficiencies.
5. Identify laboratory and diagnostic tests used to diagnose and monitor immune response.
6. Describe interdisciplinary therapies and medications used to treat patients with altered immunity.
7. Correlate the pathophysiologic alterations with the manifestations of HIV/AIDS infection.

CLINICAL COMPETENCIES

1. Assess functional health status of patients with altered immunity and monitor, document, and report abnormal manifestations.
2. Assess for hypersensitivities and anticipate interdisciplinary interventions if manifestations develop.
3. Provide patient teaching about hypersensitivities, avoidance of sensitizing agents, and prophylactic treatment.
4. Use appropriate interventions to protect patients who are immune suppressed.
5. Recognize the burden and benefit of highly active anti-retroviral drug therapy (HAART) for the patient with HIV infection.
6. Use the nursing process as a framework to provide safe and individualized care to patients with altered immune responses.
7. Revise plan of care as needed to provide safe and knowledgeable interventions to promote or restore functional health status to patients with altered immunity.

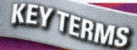

KEY TERMS

acquired immunodeficiency syndrome (AIDS), *324*
allergy, *308*
allograft, *317*
anaphylaxis, *308*

antigenic substances, *306*
autograft, *317*
autoimmune disorder, *315*
histocompatibility, *317*
human immunodeficiency virus (HIV), *324*

hypersensitivity, *308*
immunosuppression, *317*
Kaposi's sarcoma (KS), *328*
seroconversion, *325*

Considering the complexity of the immune system, it is not surprising that abnormal or harmful responses occur. Altered immune system responses include those characterized by hyperresponsiveness of the immune system and those characterized by an impaired immune response. Allergies, autoimmune disorders, and reactions to organ or tissue transplants are all examples of hyperresponsive immune function. AIDS and other immunodeficiency disorders result from impairment of the immune system.

New diseases affecting the immune system have emerged in recent years. These diseases include human immunodeficiency virus (HIV) infection and altered strains of familiar diseases such as multiple-drug-resistant tuberculosis. At the same time, understanding of the components of the immune system and specific immune responses is increasing. Alterations of the immune system affect the functional health status of affected individuals in all areas; knowledge of the prevention and care of patients with disorders of the immune system is increasingly important in today's healthcare system.

Overview of the Immune System

The immune system protects the body from invasion by foreign antigens, identifies and destroys potentially harmful cells, and removes cellular debris. These functions are accomplished by the lymphoid organs and specifically designed lymphocytes through the processes of antibody-mediated immune response and cell-mediated immune response.

The effectiveness of the immune system depends on its ability to differentiate normal host tissue from abnormal or foreign tissue. Body cells, tissues, and fluids have unique antigenic properties recognized by the immune system as "self." **Antigenic substances** stimulate an immune system response, but when identified as "self" the competent immune system does not react. External agents, such as microorganisms, cells and tissues from other humans or animals, and some inorganic substances, have antigenic properties recognized by the immune system as "nonself."

Each body cell displays specific cell surface characteristics, or markers, that are unique to each person. These are known as *human leukocyte antigens (HLAs)*. A person's HLA characteristics are coded within a large cluster of genes known as the major histocompatibility complex (MHC) located on chromosome 6. Chromosomes are paired, with each person inheriting one member of the pair from each parent. A chromosome pair contains multiple genes, each carrying instructions for production of one polypeptide chain. The number of genes in the MHC results in a multitude of HLA combinations. As a result, the possibility of two people having the same HLA type is extremely remote. Identical twins may be the exception, and some siblings have very similar HLA patterns. In tissue grafting and organ transplants, matching the HLA type as closely as possible tends to decrease rejection.

Immunocompetent people have an immune system that identifies antigens and effectively destroys or removes them. When the immune system functions improperly, the result may be an overreaction or a deficiency, resulting in health problems. Overreaction of the immune system leads to hypersensitivity disorders, such as allergies. When the immune system loses the ability to recognize self, autoimmune disorders may ensue (these disorders are discussed in later chapters of this book). Immunodeficiency diseases or malignancies can develop when the immune system is incompetent or unable to respond effectively, as is the case with acquired immunodeficiency disorder. These alterations in immunity are discussed later in this chapter.

As described in Chapter 12, the *antibody-mediated immune response* is accomplished by B lymphocytes (B cells) that are further divided into memory cells and plasma cells. They are activated by contact with an antigen and by T cells. B cells produce antibodies, also known as immunoglobulins (see Table 12–3), and serve to inactivate an invading antigen. One immunoglobulin in particular, IgM, forms natural antibodies, such as those for ABO blood group antigens, and is an important component of the immune system complexes seen in autoimmune disorders. Memory cells "remember" an antigen, and, when exposed to it a second time, immediately initiate the immune response. This action provides the foundation of acquired immunity.

MEMORY CUE
- B lymphocytes produce antibodies and cytokines to cause extracellular immunity and acquired immunity.
- T lymphocytes produce cytokines to cause intracellular immunity and acquired immunity.

The T cell component of the immune system identifies cells containing antigens and signals B cells and other components of the immune system to attack infected cells. T lymphocytes do not secrete antibodies. T lymphocytes are subdivided into effector cells and regulator cells. The cytotoxic cell or killer T cell is the primary effector cell. Regulator T cells are divided into two subsets known as helper T cells and suppressor T cells. In addition to destroying viruses within cells marked as "non self," cytotoxic T lymphocytes also attack malignant cells and are responsible for the rejection of transplanted organs and grafted tissues.

Immune function is also affected with aging, as described in the following Nursing Care of the Older Adult box.

Assessing Altered Immune System Function

Unlike body systems that are composed of closely related organs, the immune system is diverse and scattered. Optimal immune function depends on intact skin and mucous membrane barriers, adequate blood cell production and differentiation, a functional system of lymphatics and the spleen, and the ability to differentiate foreign tissue and pathogens from normal body tissue and flora. Because of this diversity of organs and function, assessment of the immune system is often integrated throughout the history and physical examination.

Health History

Before conducting the health history, review the biographic data, including age, gender, race, and ethnic background. Many autoimmune disorders are more prevalent in women than in men. Family history is also important because there is a genetic component in the etiology of many disorders affecting the immune system.

NURSING CARE OF THE OLDER ADULT   **Changes in Immune Function in the Older Adult**

Immune function declines with aging. External factors, such as nutritional status and the effects of chemical exposure, ultraviolet radiation, and environmental pollution, affect the older adult's immune status. Internal factors affect it as well, including genetics, the function of the neurologic and endocrine systems, chronic and prior illnesses, and individual anatomic and physiologic variations. These influences make it difficult to determine the effect of aging on the immune system. In some older individuals, the immune system is as effective as that of younger persons.

Immunosenescence refers to the decline in immune system effectiveness brought about by aging (Hakim & Gress, 2007). Changes associated with this decline include involution of the thymus with less competent T cell maturation, diminished antibody production and adhesion, and decreased tolerance of self antigens. Increased morbidity and mortality associated with infection and increases in cancer and autoimmune disorders result from these changes. Recent studies show improved immune function when elderly subjects receive a nutritional supplement formulated to stimulate the immune systems (Langkamp-Henken et al., 2006).

Many interview questions related to the immune system and disorders that affect it are of a sensitive nature. Be sure to provide privacy prior to the interview. If family members are present, request that they leave. Ask the least sensitive questions before moving into those that are more sensitive, such as those related to the use of illicit drugs or sexual activity. Cultural sensitivity is necessary for effective communication.

Physical Assessment

The techniques of inspection and palpation are used to assess a patient's immune system.

- Assess the general appearance; evident fatigue or weakness may indicate acute or chronic illness or immunodeficiency. Note whether the stated and apparent age coincide. Assess height, weight, and body type for apparent weight loss or wasting. Observe ease of movement and note any evident stiffness or difficulty moving. Check vital signs. An elevated temperature may indicate an infection or inflammatory response.
- Inspect the mucous membranes of the nose and mouth for color and condition. Pale, boggy (edematous) nasal mucosa is often associated with chronic allergies. Note petechiae, white patches, or lacy white plaques in the oral mucosa; they may indicate hemolysis or immunodeficiency.
- Assess skin color, temperature, and moisture. Pale or jaundiced skin may indicate a hemolytic reaction. Pallor may also indicate bone marrow suppression with accompanying immunodeficiency. Inspect the skin for evidence of rashes or lesions, such as petechiae; numerous bruises; purple or blue patches or lesions indicative of Kaposi's sarcoma; and wounds that are infected, inflamed, or unhealed. Note the location and distribution of any rashes or lesions.
- Inspect and palpate the cervical, axillae, and groin lymph nodes for evidence of lymphadenopathy (swelling) or tenderness.
- Inspect and palpate the joints for redness, swelling, tenderness, or deformity, which may indicate an autoimmune disorder such as rheumatoid arthritis or systemic lupus erythematosus. Assess joint range of motion, including the spine.

The Patient with a Hypersensitivity Reaction

Hypersensitivity is an altered immune response to an antigen that results in harm to the patient. When the antigen is environmental or exogenous, it is called an **allergy**, and the antigen is referred to as an *allergen*. The tissue response to a hypersensitivity reaction may be bothersome, causing a runny nose or itchy eyes, or it may be life threatening, leading to blood cell hemolysis or laryngospasm, an involuntary tightening of the muscles of larynx that causes difficulty inhaling.

Hypersensitivity reactions are primarily classified by the type of immune response that occurs on contact with the allergen. They may also be classified as immediate or delayed hypersensitivity responses. Anaphylaxis and transfusion reactions are examples of immediate hypersensitivity reactions; contact dermatitis is a typical delayed response. Allergies are sometimes referred to by the affected organ system (e.g., allergic rhinitis) or the allergen involved, as in hay fever. More than one type of reaction may occur simultaneously (King et al., 2005).

Pathophysiology

In a hypersensitivity reaction, an antigen–antibody or antigen–lymphocyte interaction causes a response that is damaging to body tissues. Antigen–antibody responses characterize types I, II, and III, also known as immediate hypersensitivity responses. Type IV hypersensitivity is an antigen–lymphocyte reaction, resulting in a delayed hypersensitivity response.

Type I IgE-Mediated Hypersensitivity

Common hypersensitivity reactions, such as allergic asthma, allergic rhinitis (hay fever), allergic conjunctivitis, hives (urticaria), and anaphylactic shock, are typical of type I or IgE-mediated hypersensitivity. This type of hypersensitivity response is triggered when an allergen interacts with IgE bound to mast cells and basophils. The antigen–antibody complex prompts release of histamine and other chemical mediators, complement, acetylcholine, kinins, and chemotactic factors (Figure 13–1 ■).

When a potent allergen such as bee or wasp venom or a drug is injected, resulting in widespread antibody–antigen reaction and response to these chemical mediators, a systemic response such as anaphylaxis, urticaria, or angioedema (localized, rapid swelling beneath the skin) results.

Anaphylaxis is an acute systemic type I response that occurs in highly sensitive persons following injection of a specific antigen. Substances known to trigger anaphylaxis are summarized in Box 13–1. Anaphylaxis rarely follows oral ingestion although this is possible. Food allergies are the cause of approximately 150 deaths per year in the United States (CDC, 2007).

The reaction begins within minutes of exposure to the allergen and may be almost instantaneous. The release of histamine and other mediators causes vasodilation and increased capillary permeability, smooth muscle contraction, and bronchial constriction. These chemical mediators cause the typical manifestations of anaphylaxis. Initially, a sense of foreboding or uneasiness, light-headedness, and itching palms and scalp may be noted. Hives may develop, along with angioedema of the eyelids, lips, tongue, hands, feet, and genitals. Swelling can also affect the uvula and larynx, impairing breathing. This is further complicated by bronchial constriction, manifested by air hunger, stridor and wheezing, and a barking cough. These respiratory effects can be lethal if the reaction is severe and intervention is not provided

BOX 13–1 Substances Known to Trigger Anaphylaxis in Sensitized Persons

- **Hormones:** insulin, vasopressin, parathormone
- **Enzymes:** trypsin, chymotrypsin, penicillinase
- **Pollens:** ragweed, grass, trees
- **Foods:** eggs, seafood, nuts, grains, beans, cottonseed oil, chocolate
- **Vitamins:** thiamine, folic acid
- **Insect Venom:** yellow jacket, hornet, paper wasp, honey bee
- **Occupational Agents:** rubber, latex, industrial chemicals
- **Antibiotics:** penicillins, cephalosporins, amphotericin B, nitrofurantoin
- **Local Anesthetics:** procaine, lidocaine

Hypersensitivity Video

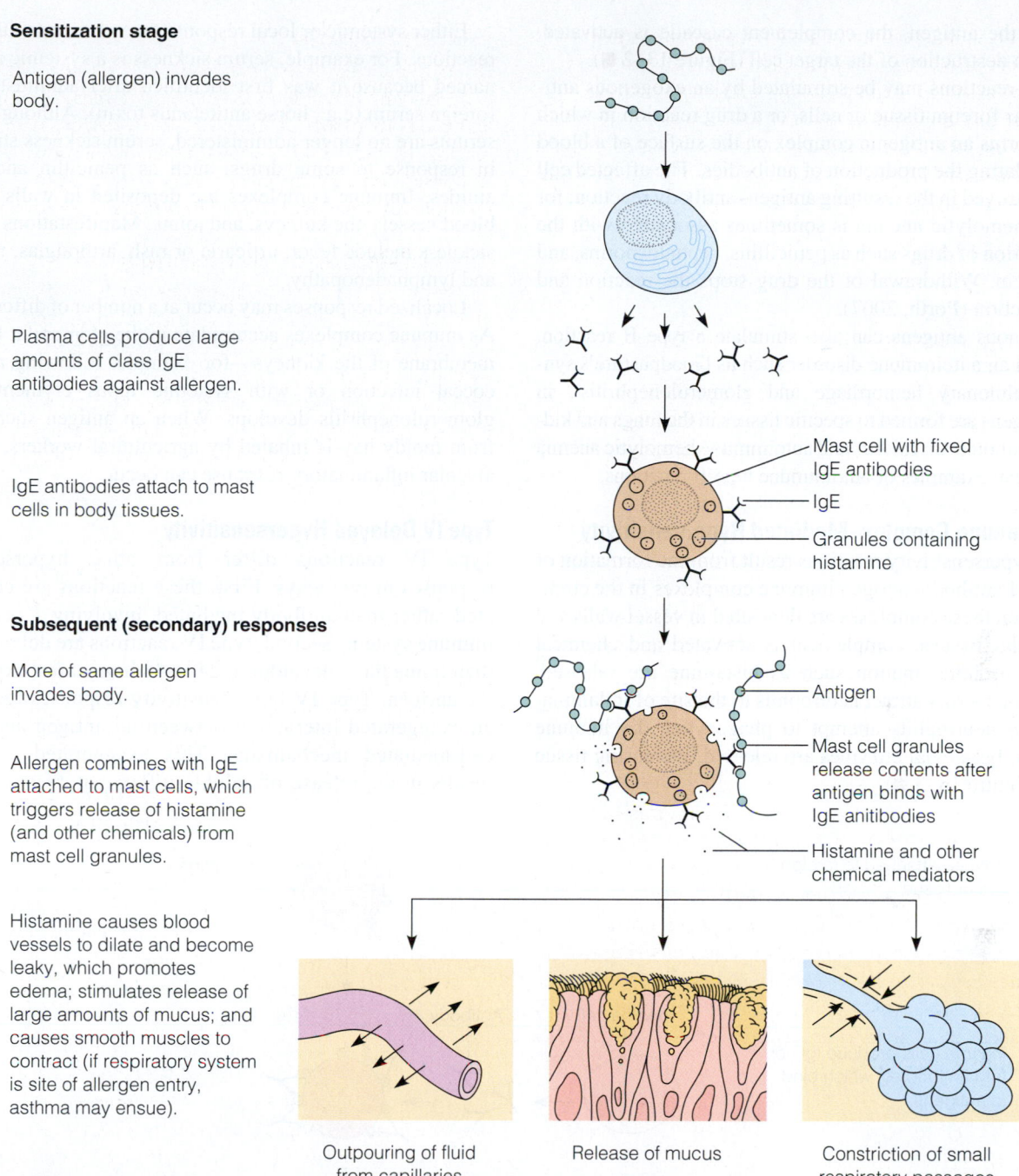

Sensitization stage

Antigen (allergen) invades body.

Plasma cells produce large amounts of class IgE antibodies against allergen.

IgE antibodies attach to mast cells in body tissues.

Subsequent (secondary) responses

More of same allergen invades body.

Allergen combines with IgE attached to mast cells, which triggers release of histamine (and other chemicals) from mast cell granules.

Histamine causes blood vessels to dilate and become leaky, which promotes edema; stimulates release of large amounts of mucus; and causes smooth muscles to contract (if respiratory system is site of allergen entry, asthma may ensue).

Mast cell with fixed IgE antibodies

IgE

Granules containing histamine

Antigen

Mast cell granules release contents after antigen binds with IgE anitbodies

Histamine and other chemical mediators

Outpouring of fluid from capillaries

Release of mucus

Constriction of small respiratory passages (bronchioles)

Figure 13–1 ■ Type I IgE-mediated hypersensitivity response.

immediately. Vasodilation and fluid loss from the vascular system can lead to impaired tissue perfusion and hypotension, a condition known as *anaphylactic shock* (∞ see Chapter 11).

Fortunately, localized responses are more common manifestations of type I hypersensitivity. Atopic reactions, which have a genetic predisposition, are localized, rather than systemic, IgE-mediated responses to an allergen. They are the result of contact of the allergen with cell-bound IgE in the bronchial tree, nasal mucosa, and conjunctival tissues. Chemical mediators are released locally, producing symptoms such as asthma, allergic rhinitis (hay fever), conjunctivitis, or atopic dermatitis. Allergens commonly associated with atopic reactions of this type include pollens, fungal spores, house dust

mites, animal dander, and feathers (Porth & Matfin, 2009). When an allergic response to food occurs in the digestive system, nausea, vomiting, diarrhea, and cramping may develop. If the gastrointestinal mucosa is altered by a local allergic response, then the allergen may be absorbed, leading to a systemic reaction. Urticaria (hives) is the most common systemic response to food allergies.

Type II Cytotoxic Hypersensitivity

A hemolytic transfusion reaction to blood of an incompatible type is characteristic of a type II or cytotoxic hypersensitivity reaction. IgG or IgM type antibodies are formed to a cell-bound antigen such as the ABO or Rh antigen. When these antibodies bind with the antigen, the complement cascade is activated, resulting in destruction of the target cell (Figure 13–2 ■).

Type II reactions may be stimulated by an exogenous antigen, such as foreign tissue or cells, or a drug reaction in which the drug forms an antigenic complex on the surface of a blood cell, stimulating the production of antibodies. The affected cell is then destroyed in the resulting antigen–antibody reaction; for example, hemolytic anemia is sometimes associated with the administration of drugs such as penicillins, cephalosporins, and streptomycin. Withdrawal of the drug stops the reaction and cell destruction (Porth, 2007).

Endogenous antigens can also stimulate a type II reaction, resulting in an autoimmune disorder such as Goodpasture's syndrome (pulmonary hemorrhage and glomerulonephritis), in which antigens are formed to specific tissues in the lungs and kidneys. Hashimoto's thyroiditis and autoimmune hemolytic anemia are additional examples of autoimmune type II reactions.

Type III Immune Complex–Mediated Hypersensitivity

Type III hypersensitivity reactions result from the formation of IgG or IgM antibody–antigen immune complexes in the circulation. When these complexes are deposited in vessel walls and extravascular tissues, complement is activated and chemical mediators of inflammation such as histamine are released. Chemotactic factors attract neutrophils to the site of inflammation. When neutrophils attempt to phagocytize the immune complexes, lysosomal enzymes are released, increasing tissue damage (Figure 13–3 ■).

Either systemic or local responses may be seen with type III reactions. For example, serum sickness is a systemic response, named because it was first identified after administration of foreign serum (e.g., horse antitetanus toxin). Although foreign serums are no longer administered, serum sickness still occurs in response to some drugs, such as penicillin and sulfonamides. Immune complexes are deposited in walls of small blood vessels, the kidneys, and joints. Manifestations of serum sickness include fever, urticaria or rash, arthralgias, myalgias, and lymphadenopathy.

Localized responses may occur at a number of different sites. As immune complexes accumulate in the glomerular basement membrane of the kidneys—for example, following a streptococcal infection or with systemic lupus erythematosus—glomerulonephritis develops. When an antigen such as dust from moldy hay is inhaled by agricultural workers, an acute alveolar inflammatory response can occur.

Type IV Delayed Hypersensitivity

Type IV reactions differ from other hypersensitivity responses in two ways. First, these reactions are cell mediated rather than antibody mediated, involving T cells of the immune system. Second, type IV reactions are delayed rather than immediate, developing 24 to 48 hours after exposure to the antigen. Type IV hypersensitivity responses result from an exaggerated interaction between an antigen and normal cell-mediated mechanisms. This exaggerated interaction results in the release of soluble inflammatory and immune

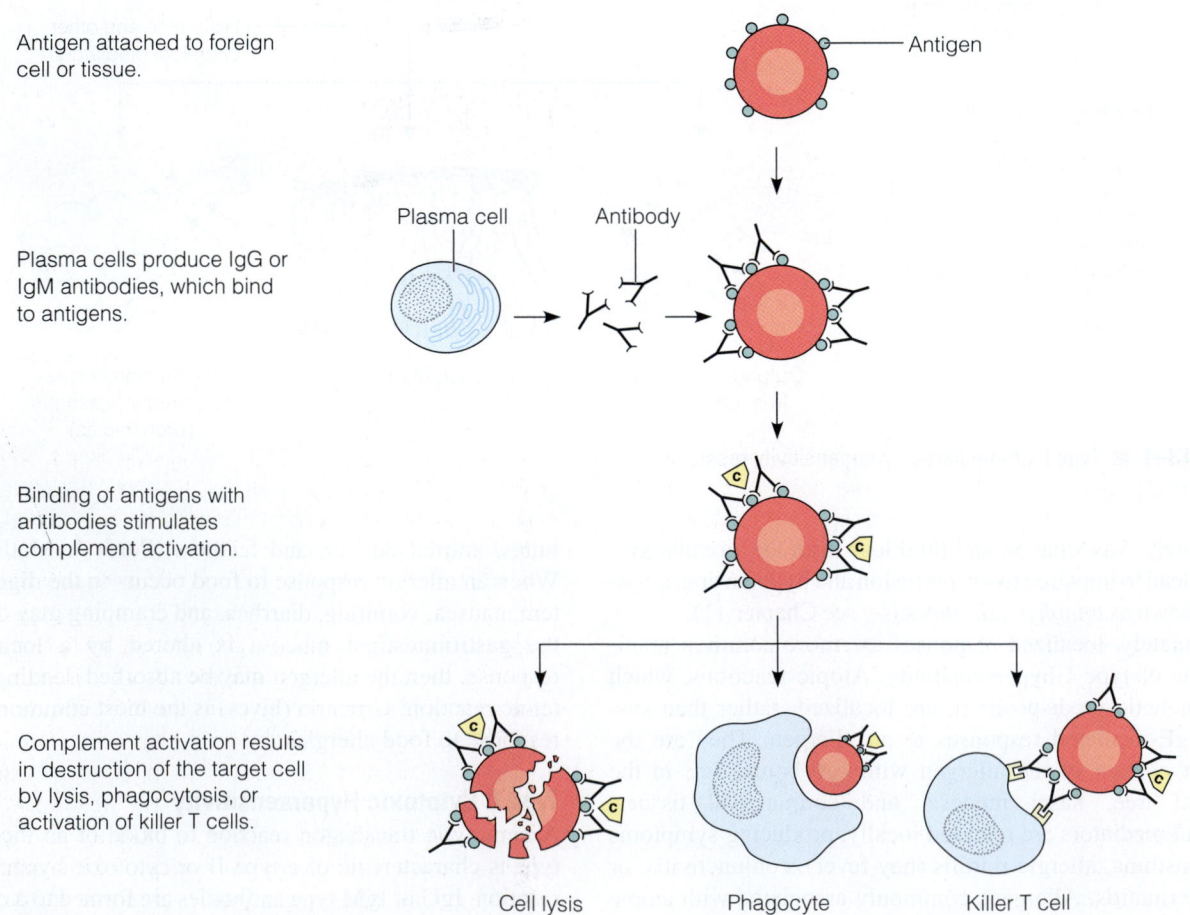

Antigen attached to foreign cell or tissue.

Antigen

Plasma cells produce IgG or IgM antibodies, which bind to antigens.

Plasma cell   Antibody

Binding of antigens with antibodies stimulates complement activation.

Complement activation results in destruction of the target cell by lysis, phagocytosis, or activation of killer T cells.

Cell lysis   Phagocyte   Killer T cell

Figure 13–2 ■ Type II cytotoxic hypersensitivity response.

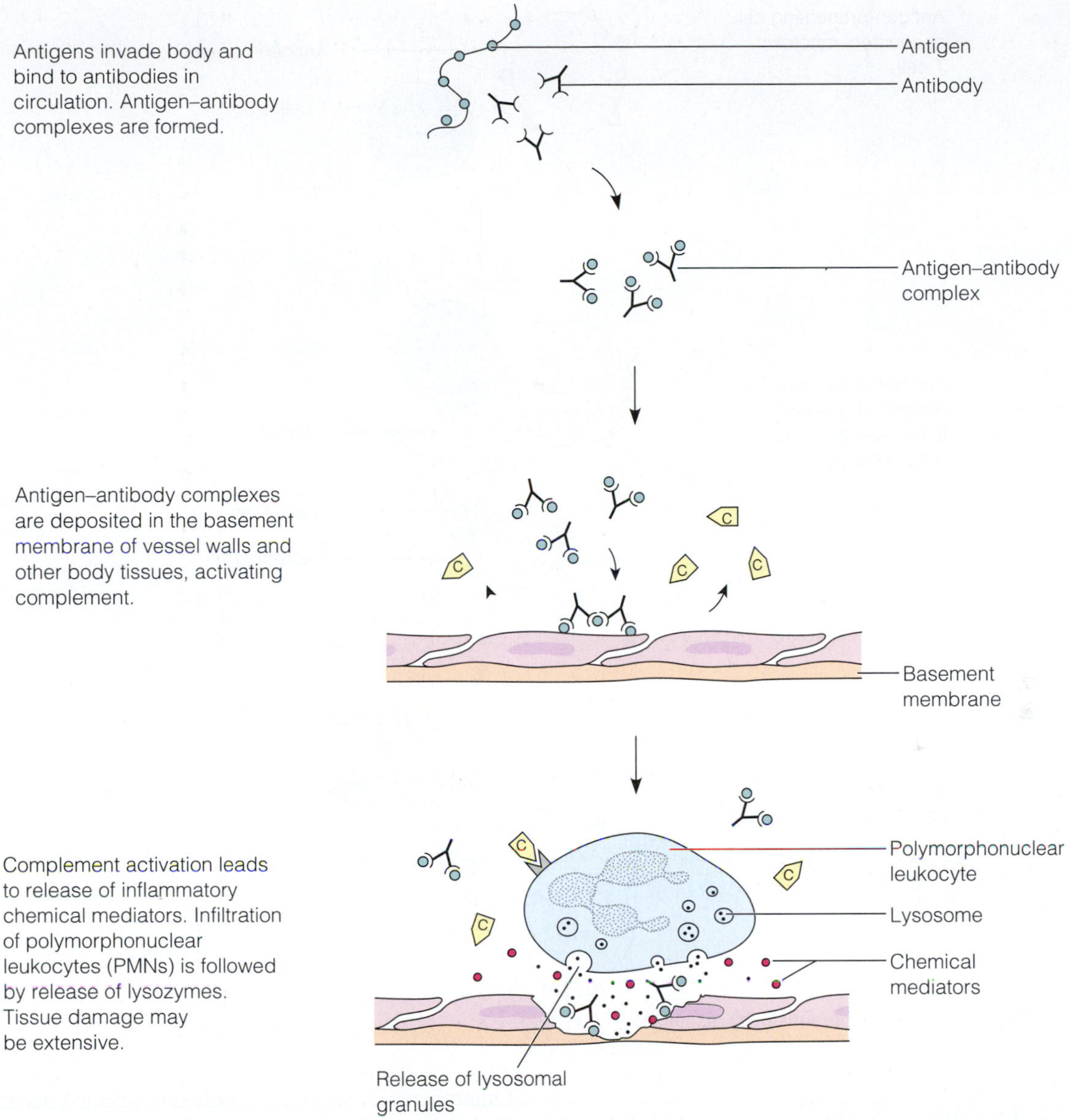

Antigens invade body and bind to antibodies in circulation. Antigen–antibody complexes are formed.

— Antigen

— Antibody

— Antigen–antibody complex

Antigen–antibody complexes are deposited in the basement membrane of vessel walls and other body tissues, activating complement.

— Basement membrane

Complement activation leads to release of inflammatory chemical mediators. Infiltration of polymorphonuclear leukocytes (PMNs) is followed by release of lysozymes. Tissue damage may be extensive.

— Polymorphonuclear leukocyte

— Lysosome

— Chemical mediators

Release of lysosomal granules

Figure 13–3 ■ Type III immune complex–mediated hypersensitivity response.

mediators (from the lysozymes within the macrophages) and recruitment of killer T cells, causing local tissue destruction (Figure 13–4 ■).

Contact dermatitis is a classic example of a type IV reaction. Intense redness, itching, blister formation, and thickening affect the skin in the area exposed to the antigen. Many antigens can provoke this response; poison ivy is a prime perpetrator. In the healthcare setting, an allergic response to latex can also produce contact dermatitis. An estimated 8% to 13% of healthcare workers are allergic to latex and sensitivity remains beyond 5 years, making continued avoidance very important (Smith et al., 2007). Other examples of cell-mediated responses include a positive tuberculin test and graft rejection episodes.

Latex Allergy

Although protective against infection, the repetitive use of latex gloves creates a persistent exposure to latex for healthcare workers. When gloves are powdered with cornstarch to facilitate donning and removing gloves, the cornstarch particles aerosolize when the gloves are removed. The cornstarch includes latex particles. This creates a respiratory exposure as well as dermal exposure to latex. In addition, chemicals used in the manufacture of latex products may be irritating. Products such as balloons, condoms, and rubber bands are commonly made of latex.

Sensitivity to latex develops without the user being aware until a rash appears on the hands. Type IV hypersensitivity (contact dermatitis) can progress to type I systemic allergic reactions without previous symptoms signaling an escalation. It is important to protect the patient and the healthcare worker who is allergic to latex. Prevention is aided by employers who select products free of latex. Nonlatex gloves are recommended for use where there is no contact with infectious materials or blood. Workers should be screened periodically to detect symptoms of allergy and educated about latex sources. Hand hygiene after using latex products limits exposure (NIOSH, 2008).

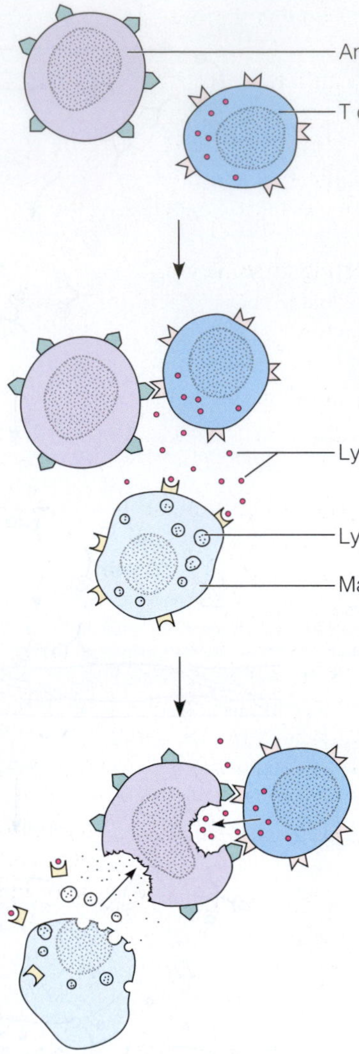

Antigen-presenting cell encounters cytotoxic T cell.

Antigen-presenting cell

T cell

Interaction causes release of lympho-kines, which attract macrophages.

Lymphokines

Lysozymes

Macrophage

Macrophages release lysozymes, resulting in local tissue damage.

Figure 13–4 ■ Type IV delayed hypersensitivity response.

Interdisciplinary Care

The focus of care for patients with allergic responses is to minimize exposure to the allergen, prevent the hypersensitivity response, and provide prompt, effective interventions for allergic responses. Identifying allergens for the individual to reduce the likelihood of exposure is a key aspect of management. A complete history of the patient's allergies is obtained, including medications, foods, animals, plants, and other materials. The type of hypersensitivity response is documented, as is its onset, manifestations, and usual treatment.

When a documented or suspected hypersensitivity reaction occurs, the allergen (e.g., intravenous medication or transfusion) is withdrawn immediately. With a type I hypersensitivity response, managing the patient's airway takes highest priority, followed by maintaining cardiac output. Type II hypersensitivity responses may necessitate aggressive management of bleeding or renal failure. A type III (immune complex) reaction is treated by removing the offending antigen and interrupting the inflammatory response.

With a hypersensitivity response, supportive care is important to relieve discomfort. This often involves the administration of selected antihistamine or anti-inflammatory medications.

Other therapies may be prescribed in selected instances, such as plasmapheresis, a procedure that involves continually withdrawing and reinfusing blood from the patient while removing the allergic components from the plasma portion.

Diagnosis

To identify possible allergens or hypersensitivity reactions, the following laboratory tests may be ordered:

- *White blood cell (WBC) count with differential* can detect high levels of circulating eosinophils. Increased numbers of eosinophils are often present in patients with type I hypersensitivities.
- *Radioallergosorbent test (RAST)* is a blood test that measures the amount of IgE directed toward specific allergens. Test results are compared with control values and used to identify hypersensitivities. RAST may also be used instead of skin testing if a severe allergic response is suspected (American Association of Clinical Chemistry, 2006).
- *Blood type and crossmatch* are ordered prior to any anticipated transfusions. This diagnostic test is described in ∞ Chapter 11. Other blood tests associated with blood transfusions are a *Coombs' Direct* (to detect antibodies on red blood cells [RBCs]) and a *Coombs' Indirect* (to check

recipient's and donor's blood for antibodies before a blood transfusion).

- *Immune complex assays* may be performed to detect the presence of circulating immune complexes in suspected type III hypersensitivity responses. The normal result is a test negative for circulating immune complexes. A negative test does not, however, rule out an immune complex hypersensitivity response.

- *Complement assay* is also useful in detecting immune complex disorders. In these disorders, complement is, in effect, used up by the development of antigen–antibody complexes. Decreased levels are seen on examination. Both total complement level and amounts of individual components of the complement cascade can be determined.

Skin Tests for Allergies

Skin tests are also used to determine causes of hypersensitivity reactions. These tests are used to identify specific allergens to which a person may be sensitive. Allergens for testing are selected according to the patient's history. Test solutions made from extracts of inhaled, ingested, or injected materials, such as pollens, mites, venoms, or some drugs, are used for the prick test and intradermal testing. Epicutaneous testing (prick testing) is generally done first to avoid a systemic reaction; it is followed by intradermal testing of allergens with a negative response to prick testing. Substances that cause a reaction to the prick test should not be tested intradermally.

- *Prick (epicutaneous or puncture) test:* A drop of diluted allergenic extract is placed on the skin, and the skin is then pricked or punctured through the drop. With a positive test, a localized pruritic (itchy) wheal and erythema occur. The response is maximal at 15 to 20 minutes.

- *Intradermal:* A small amount of allergen extract at a 1:500 or 1:1000 dilution is injected intradermally in the forearm or intrascapular area. If several allergens are being tested, injections are spaced 0.25 to 0.5 apart. As control measures, plain diluent (negative control) and histamine (positive control) are injected. If there is no response to a particular allergen at 15 to 20 minutes, the test is negative. The appearance of a wheal and erythema, with a wheal diameter at least 5 mm greater than that produced by the control, indicates a positive response (Figure 13–5 ■).

- *Patch:* A 1-inch patch impregnated with the allergen (e.g., perfume, cosmetics, detergents, or clothing fibers) is applied to the skin for 48 hours. Absence of a response indicates a negative test result. Positive responses are graded from mild (erythema in the exposed area) to severe (erythema, papules, vesicles, or ulceration).

Food Allergy Testing

Food allergy testing is performed when a food allergy is suspected but the source or implicated food item has not been clearly identified. Food allergy symptoms are typically demonstrated within hours of eating. The patient is asked to keep a diary of foods consumed and allergic responses for a week. An elimination diet, excluding most common food allergens and all suspected foods) is then prescribed for one week. If symptoms do not improve, a different variation of the elimination

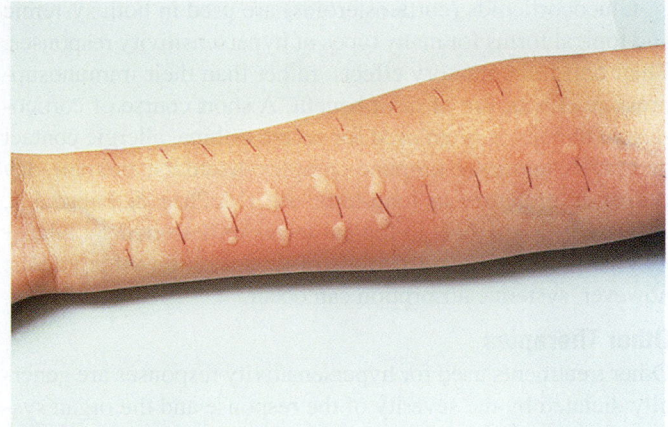

Figure 13–5 ■ Skin testing on the forearm showing induration and erythema typical of a positive response to an antigen.
Source: Southern Illinois University/Photo Researchers, Inc.

diet is prescribed. If symptoms are relieved, foods are reintroduced to the diet one at a time until symptoms recur, indicating allergy to that food.

Medications

When it is impossible to avoid the offending allergen and allergic manifestations are severe or disrupt the patient's activities of daily living (ADLs), medications may be prescribed. *Immunotherapy*, also called hyposensitization or desensitization, consists of injecting an extract of the allergen(s) in gradually increasing doses. Immunotherapy is used primarily for allergic rhinitis or asthma related to inhaled allergens. It has also been shown to be effective in preventing anaphylactic responses to insect venom. With weekly or biweekly subcutaneous injections of the allergen, the patient develops IgG antibodies to the allergen that appear to block effectively the allergic IgE-mediated response. Once a therapy plateau is reached, injections may be discontinued or continued indefinitely either monthly or bimonthly.

Antihistamines are the major class of drugs used in treating the symptoms of hypersensitivity responses, type I in particular. They are also useful to some extent in relieving manifestations (such as urticaria) of some type II and type III reactions. Antihistamines block H_1-histamine receptors, acting as a competitive antagonist to histamine, but they do not affect the production or release of histamine. The prototype antihistamine is diphenhydramine (Benadryl). It and other antihistamines alleviate the systemic effects of histamine such as urticaria and angioedema (localized tissue swelling). They are also useful in relieving allergic rhinitis, drying respiratory secretions through an anticholinergic effect. The preferred route of administration is oral, although diphenhydramine and others can be given parenterally, particularly when immediate action is needed, as in anaphylaxis. Side effects include drowsiness and dry mouth. Antihistamines are not effective in relieving asthmatic responses to allergens and may actually worsen symptoms by their drying effect on respiratory secretions. Antihistamines are often combined with a sympathomimetic agent such as pseudoephedrine to improve their decongestant activity and counteract their sedative effect. Antihistamines and decongestants are discussed further in ∞ Chapter 35.

Hypersensitivity Video

Glucocorticoids (corticosteroids) are used in both systemic and topical forms for many types of hypersensitivity responses. Their anti-inflammatory effects, rather than their immunosuppressive effects, are of most benefit. A short course of corticosteroid therapy is often used for severe asthma, allergic contact dermatitis, and some immune-complex disorders; alternate-day dosing is preferred in long-term use (McPhee & Papadakis, 2009). Corticosteroids in topical forms or delivered by inhaler may be used for longer periods of time with few side effects; however, systemic absorption can occur.

Other Therapies

Other treatments used for hypersensitivity responses are generally dictated by the severity of the response and the organ system affected. Airway management takes highest priority for the patient with an acute anaphylactic reaction. Insertion of an endotracheal tube or emergency tracheostomy may be required to maintain airway patency with severe laryngospasm. Because anaphylaxis places the person at risk for vasomotor collapse and significant hypotension, it is necessary to insert an intravenous line and initiate fluid resuscitation with an isotonic solution such as Ringer's lactate.

Plasmapheresis, removal of harmful components in the plasma (also known as *plasma exchange therapy*), may be used to treat immune complex responses such as glomerulonephritis and Goodpasture's syndrome. Plasma and the glomerular-damaging antibody–antigen complexes are removed by passing the patient's blood through a blood cell separator. The RBCs are then returned to the patient along with an equal amount of albumin or human plasma. This procedure is usually done in a series rather than as a one-time treatment. It is not without risk, and informed consent is required. Potential complications of plasmapheresis include those associated with intravenous catheters, shifts in fluid balance, and alteration of blood clotting.

Treatment of Anaphylaxis

The immediate treatment for anaphylaxis is parenteral epinephrine, an adrenergic agonist (sympathomimetic) drug that has both vasoconstricting and bronchodilating effects. These qualities, combined with its rapid action, make epinephrine ideal for treating an anaphylactic reaction. For mild reactions with wheezing, pruritus, urticaria, and angioedema, a subcutaneous injection of 0.3 to 0.5 mL of 1:1000 epinephrine is generally sufficient. For patients with an injected toxin such as a bee sting, an additional amount equivalent to one-half the above may be injected directly into the site of the sting and a tourniquet applied above it to prevent further systemic absorption. Intravenous epinephrine using a 1:100,000 concentration may be used in the patient with a more severe anaphylactic reaction.

✺ Nursing Care

Nursing care related to hypersensitivity reactions is primarily directed toward prevention, early identification, and providing prompt, effective treatment.

Health Promotion

Health promotion activities include helping patients identify possible allergens that prompt a hypersensitivity response and discussing strategies to avoid these allergens. Anyone with severe food allergies may need referral to a dietitian to discuss necessary dietary changes and ways to continue meeting nutrient needs. It is important that persons with hypersensitivities inform healthcare personnel of all allergens. People who experience anaphylactic reactions should wear a Medic-Alert bracelet or tag at all times to identify the substance(s) that provokes this response. Patients who have experienced an anaphylactic reaction to insect venom or other potentially unavoidable allergens should carry a kit (commonly called a bee sting kit) for immediate treatment of future exposures. This kit typically includes a prefilled syringe of epinephrine and an epinephrine nebulizer, allowing prompt self-treatment.

Assessment

Collect the following data through the health history and physical examination. Further focused assessments are described with nursing interventions in the next section.

- *Health history:* risk factors, hypersensitivities (medications, household dust, bee stings, etc.), reaction (rash, hives, difficulty breathing), type of treatment for hypersensitivity reactions; allergy skin testing; asthma, hay fever, or dermatitis.
- *Physical assessment:* mucous membranes of nose and mouth, skin for lesions or rashes, eyes (tearing and redness), respiratory rate, and adventitious breath sounds.

Nursing Diagnoses and Interventions

Priority nursing diagnoses will vary according to the type of hypersensitivity reaction experienced by the patient. Because nurses are most likely to become involved with a patient experiencing a type I or type II response, this section focuses on diagnoses for these patients. Airway, breathing, and circulation (the ABCs) are of greatest importance for the patient with an anaphylactic reaction.

Ineffective Airway Clearance

In anaphylactic reactions, the airway may be obstructed due to facial angioedema, bronchospasm, or laryngeal edema. Establishing and maintaining a patent airway is of highest priority.

- Administer oxygen per nasal cannula at a rate of 2 to 4 L/min. Apply oxygen emergently and obtain a physician order for oxygen administration. *Providing external oxygen increases the alveolar oxygen and its availability to cells of the body.*
- Assess respiratory rate and pattern, level of consciousness and anxiety, nasal flaring, use of accessory muscles of respiration, chest wall movement, audible stridor; palpate for respiratory excursion; auscultate lung sounds and any adventitious sounds, such as wheezes. *Extreme anxiety or agitation, nasal flaring, stridor, and diminished lung sounds indicate air hunger and possible airway obstruction, necessitating immediate intervention.*
- Position in Fowler's to high Fowler's *to promote optimal lung expansion and ease of breathing.*
- Insert a nasopharyngeal or oropharyngeal airway, and arrange for immediate intubation as indicated. *Ensuring an adequate airway is vital to preserve life.*
- Administer subcutaneous epinephrine 1:1000, 0.3 to 0.5 mL, as prescribed. This may be repeated in 20 to 30 minutes if necessary. Administer parenteral diphenhydramine (deep intramuscular or intravenous) as prescribed. *Epinephrine is a*

potent vasoconstrictor and bronchodilator, counteracting the effects of histamine. Diphenhydramine is an antihistamine that blocks histamine receptors and their effect. These medications can be effective in rapidly reversing manifestations of anaphylaxis.

■ Provide calm reassurance. *Hypoxemia and air hunger are terrifying for the patient. Anxiety can impair the patient's ability to cooperate with treatment and can increase the respiratory rate, making breathing less effective.*

Decreased Cardiac Output

Peripheral vasodilation and increased capillary permeability from the release of histamine can significantly impair cardiac output. When it falls to the degree that tissue perfusion becomes impaired and hypoxia results, a state of anaphylactic shock exists.

■ Monitor vital signs frequently, noting fall in blood pressure, decreasing pulse pressure, tachycardia, and tachypnea. *These vital sign changes may indicate shock.*

■ Assess skin color, temperature, capillary refill, edema, and other indicators of peripheral perfusion. *As cardiac output falls, peripheral vessels constrict and tissue perfusion is impaired.*

■ Monitor level of consciousness. *A change in level of consciousness (lethargy, apprehension, or agitation) is often the first indicator of decreased cardiac output.*

■ Insert one or more large-bore (18-gauge or larger) intravenous catheters as prescribed. *It is important to insert intravenous catheters as soon as possible to provide sites for rapid fluid replacement.*

■ Administer warmed intravenous solutions of lactated Ringer's or normal saline, as prescribed. *These isotonic solutions help maintain intravascular volume. Warmed solutions are used to prevent hypothermia from the rapid administration of large amounts of fluid at room temperature (about 70°F, or 21.1°C).*

■ Insert an indwelling catheter, and monitor urinary output frequently. *As the cardiac output drops, the glomerular filtration rate (GFR) falls. With an output of less than 30 mL/h, the patient is at risk for acute renal failure from ischemia.*

> **PRACTICE ALERT**
> Aggressive fluid therapy may lead to hypervolemia, resulting in pulmonary edema; assess for shortness of breath and crackles in the lungs.

Community-Based Care

Most hypersensitivity responses are appropriately treated by the patient or family members with self-care measures. Teaching is a vital component of care. If the patient is at risk for anaphylaxis, involving the family in teaching is essential because the response may occur with such rapidity that the patient will be unable to provide self-care. Include the following points in teaching the patient and family about managing hypersensitivities:

■ When and how to use an anaphylaxis kit containing epinephrine and antihistamines in injectable, inhaler, and oral forms

■ When to seek medical attention

■ Use and adverse reactions of antihistamines and decongestants

■ Advantages of autologous blood transfusion if future surgery is scheduled

■ Skin care to prevent and care for contact dermatitis, as discussed in ∞ Chapter 16

■ Helpful resources:
  ■ ALERT, Inc., Allergy to Latex Education and Resource Team (Toll free 1-888-97-ALERT)
  ■ Food Allergy and Anaphylaxis Network

The Patient with an Autoimmune Disorder

Maintaining optimal health and preventing disease depend not only on the immune system's ability to recognize and destroy foreign tissues and other antigens, but also on the immune system's ability to recognize self. When self-recognition is impaired and immune defenses are directed against normal host tissue, the result is an **autoimmune disorder**.

Autoimmune disorders can affect any tissue in the body. Some are tissue or organ specific, affecting a particular tissue or a particular organ. Hashimoto's thyroiditis is an example of an organ-specific autoimmune disorder. Circulating antibodies are formed to certain thyroid components, resulting ultimately in destruction of the gland. In other disorders, autoantibodies are formed that are not tissue specific, but tend to accumulate and cause an inflammatory response in certain tissue, for example, the renal glomeruli or the hepatic small bile ductules. Autoimmune disorders may also be systemic, with neither antibodies nor the resulting inflammatory lesions confined to any one organ. Rheumatologic disorders, such as rheumatoid arthritis and systemic lupus erythematosus (SLE), are characteristic of systemic autoimmune disorders.

Pathophysiology

The mechanism that causes the immune system to recognize host tissue as a foreign antigen is not clear. The following factors are under study as possible contributors to the development of autoimmune disorders:

■ The release of previously "hidden" antigens into the circulation, such as DNA or other components of the cell nucleus, which elicits an immune response

■ Chemical, physical, or biologic changes in host tissue that cause self-antigens to stimulate the production of autoantibodies

■ The introduction of an antigen, such as a bacteria or virus, whose antigenic properties closely resemble those of host tissue, resulting in the production of antibodies that target not only the foreign antigen but also normal tissue. This is termed molecular mimicry. Heart damage in rheumatic fever and acute glomerulonephritis following beta-hemolytic streptococcal infections are examples of the development of antibodies against normal tissue (Porth & Matfin, 2009).

■ A defect in normal cellular immune function that allows B cells to produce autoantibodies unchecked

■ Initiation of the autoimmune response by very slow-growing mycobacteria

Although the exact mechanism producing autoimmunity is unclear, several characteristics of autoimmune diseases are known. It is apparent that genetics plays a role because a higher incidence is seen in family members of people with autoimmune disorders. More than one genetic change is likely occurring to cause development of these disorders. Autoimmune disorders are far more prevalent in females than in males. There is evidence that estrogen stimulates the immune response while androgens suppress the immune response (Porth, 2007).

The disorders tend to overlap, so that the patient with one autoimmune disorder may develop another or some manifestations of another. The onset of an autoimmune disorder is frequently associated with a physical or psychologic stressor. Autoimmune disorders are frequently characterized by periods of exacerbation and remission.

Specific autoimmune disorders are discussed in the sections of this textbook related to the affected organ systems or functional disruption.

Interdisciplinary Care

For the most part, the diagnosis of an autoimmune disorder is based on the patient's manifestations. Although the manifestations of these disorders can often be managed, a cure typically is not possible unless the affected target tissue is removed (e.g., colectomy for the patient with ulcerative colitis).

Diagnosis

Serologic assays are used to identify and measure antibodies directed toward host tissue antigens or normal cellular components. Many detectable autoantibodies are not specific to a single autoimmune disorder and are used to establish the autoimmune process rather than the specific disorder. Although healthy people often have low levels of autoantibodies, levels are much higher in patients affected by an autoimmune disorder. The following serologic assays may be ordered:

- *Antinuclear antibody (ANA)* detects antibodies produced to DNA and other nuclear material. These antibodies can cause tissue damage characteristic of autoimmune disorders such as SLE. The patient's serum is combined with nuclear material and tagged antihuman antibody to detect ANA-antihuman antibody complexes. A negative, or normal, result is a titer < 1:20. When complexes are detected at higher titer levels (> 1:20), the test is positive for ANA.
- *Lupus erythematosus (LE) cell test* is used to detect SLE and monitor its treatment. Neutrophils that contain large masses of phagocytized DNA from the nuclei of PMNs are called LE cells. Like the ANA, the LE cell test is nonspecific for SLE. A positive result may also be seen in rheumatoid arthritis (RA) or with medications such as isoniazid, clofibrate, penicillin, phenytoin, procainamide, streptomycin, tetracycline, trazodone, oral contraceptives, or sulfonamide drugs.
- *Rheumatoid factor (RF)* is an immunoglobulin present in the serum of approximately 80% of patients with rheumatoid arthritis. A person with RA may not have detectable RF (Porth & Matfin, 2009). Low titer levels (< 1:20) may normally be present in the older adult. An RF titer 1:80 or higher indicates RA. A titer between 1:20 and 1:80 could indicate SLE, scleroderma, or liver cirrhosis. Results are also reported as IU/ml; above 20 IU/ml is indicative of RA or Sjogren's syndrome, a disease in which autoantibodies attack the moisture-producing glands to cause dry eyes and dry mouth (Delaleu et al., 2009).

- *Complement assay* may also be useful in identifying autoimmune disorders. In these disorders, complement may be consumed in the development of antigen–antibody complexes. Decreased levels are seen on examination. Both total complement level and amounts of individual components of the complement cascade can be determined.
- *Anti CCP antibody test* is a blood test for RA. It measures anti-cyclic citrullinated peptide antibody in blood; the results are specific for RA. These antibodies replace normal protein in the joints of patients with RA.

Medications

Various approaches are used in the treatment of autoimmune disorders.

- Anti-inflammatory medications such as aspirin, nonsteroidal anti-inflammatory drugs (NSAIDs), and corticosteroids may be prescribed to reduce the inflammatory response and minimize tissue damage. When these agents are not effective or well tolerated by the patient, disease-modifying antirheumatic drugs or slow-acting anti-inflammatory medications may be prescribed.
- Cytotoxic drugs (described in the next section) may be used in combination with plasmapheresis in treating many autoimmune disorders.
- Disease-modifying antirheumatic drugs (DMARDs) reduce manifestations, reduce or prevent joint damage, and preserve the structure and function of the joints in patients with RA. The most common DMARDs in current use are methotrexate (Rheumatrex), sulfasalazine (Azulfidine), hydroxychloroquine (Plaquenil), leflunomide (Arava), and cyclosporine (Sandimmune, Neoral).
- Another class of antirheumatic drugs, referred to as *biologicals* or *biological response modifiers*, consists of laboratory-produced proteins that decrease the inflammatory process. These antibodies bind tumor necrosis factor alpha (TNF-α) and interleukin-1, both inflammatory elements. These medications include infliximab (Remicade) or adalimumab (Humira), etanercept (Enbrel), anakinra (Kineret), Rituxan, and abatacept (Orencia).
- Slow-acting anti-inflammatory drugs, including gold salts, hydroxychloroquine (Plaquenil), and penicillamine, may be used when other therapies are ineffective or not tolerated by the patient. These drugs, however, are relatively toxic and less frequently used.

✑ Nursing Care

Nursing interventions for the patient with an autoimmune disorder are individualized and tailored to needs dictated by manifestations of the disorder. Nurses often will be involved with the patient in an outpatient setting, evaluating the patient's response to therapy and self-care management.

Consider the following nursing diagnoses in planning care for the patient with an autoimmune disorder:

- *Activity Intolerance* related to inflammatory effects of autoimmune disorder
- *Ineffective Coping* related to chronic disease process
- *Interrupted Family Processes* related to lack of understanding about autoimmune disorder and its effects
- *Ineffective Protection* related to disordered immune function

Community-Based Care

Because many autoimmune disorders are chronic, teaching the patient and family about the disorder and its management is a key nursing intervention. The patient may be taking drugs with multiple side effects or long-term effects, necessitating effective teaching. Patients with autoimmune disorders often do not appear to be ill, making it difficult for friends and families to understand their care needs. The chronicity of these disorders also puts the patient at high risk for unproven remedies and quackery. Provide psychologic support, listening, and teaching. In addition, suggest resources such as local support groups and the American Autoimmune Related Diseases Association.

The Patient with a Tissue Transplant

Since the first kidney transplant was performed from one identical twin to the other in 1954, organ and tissue transplantation have become increasingly popular and viable treatment options. The transplantation of avascular tissues, such as skin, cornea, bone, and heart valves, is considered routine, with little need for tissue matching and **immunosuppression** (the use of drugs to make the immune response less effective). Transplants of organs (e.g., the kidney, heart, heart and lung, liver, and bone marrow) are increasingly common. Commonly performed organ transplants are outlined in Table 13–1; success rates refer to survival of the transplant recipient.

Transplant success is closely tied to obtaining an organ with tissue antigens as close to those of the recipient as possible. Every body cell has cell surface antigens known as human leukocyte antigens (HLA) that are unique to the individual. Even though identical twins may have the same HLA type, a few of their antigens may be dissimilar enough to cause a transplant between them to be rejected. Matching the HLA type of the donor and recipient as closely as possible decreases the potential for rejection of the transplanted organ or tissue but does not eliminate it. Combining multiple organs for transplant such as liver-kidney, heart-liver, or heart-lung seems to be protective from rejection. The multiplicity of antigens seems to increase tolerance or may produce an "immune paralysis" (Rana et al., 2008).

Pathophysiology

An **autograft**, a transplant of the patient's own tissue, is the most successful type of tissue transplant. Skin grafts are the most common examples of autografts. Increasingly, autologous bone marrow transplants and blood transfusions are being used to reduce immunologic responses. When the donor and recipient are identical twins, the term *isograft* is used. Because of the high likelihood of an HLA match, the success of these grafts is good and rejection episodes are mild.

Few people, however, have an identical twin to provide tissue for donation, and when the need is for an organ such as the heart, liver, or lungs, a living-donor transplantation is not possible. Most often, organ and tissue transplants are **allografts**, which are grafts between members of the same species that have different genotypes and HLA. Allografts may come from living donors; examples are bone marrow, blood, and a kidney. Most often, organs for transplantation are obtained from a cadaver. Donors are typically people who meet the criteria for brain death; are less than 65 years old; and are free of systemic disease, malignancy, or infection, including HIV, hepatitis B, or hepatitis C. The organ is removed immediately before or after cardiac arrest and preserved until it is transplanted into the waiting recipient. Finally, *xenograft* is a transplant from an animal species to a human. These transplants are the least successful but may be used in selected instances, such as the use of pig skin as a temporary covering for a massive burn.

Tissue typing is used to determine **histocompatibility**, the ability of cells and tissues to survive transplantation without immunologic interference by the recipient. Tissue typing is performed in an attempt to match the donor and recipient as closely as possible for HLA type and blood type and to identify preformed antibodies to the donor's HLA.

Both antibody-mediated and cell-mediated immune responses are involved in the complex process of host-versus-graft transplant rejection. Host macrophages process donor antigen, presenting it to T and B lymphocytes. Activated lymphocytes (B and T cells) produce both antibody- and cell-mediated effects. Killer T cells bind with cells of the transplanted organ, resulting in cell lysis. Helper T cells stimulate the multiplication and differentiation of B cells, and

TABLE 13–1 Organ Transplant Indications and Success Rate

ORGAN	GRAFT TYPE	INDICATIONS FOR TRANSPLANT	SUCCESS RATE
Kidney	Allograft; may be isograft	End-stage renal disease	88.1% at 5 years
Heart	Allograft	End-stage cardiac disease refractory to medical management	74.4% at 5 years
Lung	Allograft	Pulmonary hypertension, cystic fibrosis, pulmonary fibrosis, chronic obstructive pulmonary disease	52.6 % at 5 years
Liver	Allograft	Severe liver dysfunction due to chronic active hepatitis, primary biliary cirrhosis, sclerosing cholangitis	73.6 % 5-year survival
Bone marrow	Autograft or allograft	Leukemia, aplastic anemia, congenital immunologic defects	30%–70% cure
Skin	Autograft, allograft, or xenograft	Severe burns, plastic surgery	> 95% at 5 years
Cornea	Allograft	Corneal ulceration and opacification	> 95% at 5 years
Pancreas	Allograft	Pancreatic insufficiency, diabetes	88.1% at 5 years
Islet cells	Allograft (multiple donor)	Type 1 diabetes mellitus	100% > 2 years

Source: US Transplant.org; Scientific registry of transplant recipients, http://www.ustransplant.org/

antibodies are produced to graft endothelium. Complement activation or antibody-dependent cell-mediated cytotoxicity leads to transplant cell destruction. Rejection typically begins after the first 24 hours of the transplant, although it may present immediately. Rejection episodes are characterized as hyperacute, acute, or chronic, as summarized in Table 13–2.

Hyperacute tissue rejection occurs immediately to 2 to 3 days after the transplant of new tissue. Hyperacute rejection is due to preformed antibodies and sensitized T cells to antigens in the donor organ. It is most likely to occur in patients who have had a previous organ or tissue transplant, such as a blood transfusion, and may be evident even before the transplant procedure is completed. The grafted organ initially appears pink and healthy, but soon becomes soft and cyanotic as blood flow is impaired. Organ function deteriorates rapidly, and manifestations of organ failure develop.

Acute tissue rejection is the most common and treatable type of rejection episode. It occurs between 4 days and 3 months after the transplant. Acute rejection is mediated primarily by the cellular immune response, resulting in transplant cell destruction. The patient experiencing acute rejection demonstrates manifestations of the inflammatory process, with fever, redness, swelling, and tenderness over the graft site. Signs of impaired function of the transplanted organ may be noted (e.g., elevated blood urea nitrogen [BUN] and creatinine, liver enzyme and bilirubin elevations, or elevated cardiac enzymes and signs of cardiac failure).

Chronic tissue rejection occurs from 4 months to years after transplant of new tissue. Chronic rejection is most likely the result of antibody-mediated immune responses. Antibodies and complement are deposited in transplant vessel walls, causing narrowing and decreased function of the organ due to ischemia. The gradual deterioration of transplanted organ function is seen with chronic tissue rejection.

Graft-versus-host disease (GVHD) is a frequent and potentially fatal complication of bone marrow transplant, some liver transplants, or transfusions with nonirradiated blood to immunocompromised patients (Porth & Matfin, 2009). When there is no close match between donor and recipient HLA, immunocompetent cells in the grafted tissue recognize host tissue as foreign and mount a cell-mediated immune response. If the host is immunocompromised, as is often the case when a bone marrow transplant is performed, host cells are unable to destroy the graft and instead become the targets of destruction.

Three important strategies for preventing or decreasing the severity of GVHD include (1) deleting donor T cells in the tissue or organ prior to infusion into the patient (however, this may increase the risk of graft failure and infection); (2) using umbilical cord stem cells in adult patients; and (3) closer HLA matching between donor and recipient. Acute GVHD occurs within the first 100 days following a transplant and primarily affects the skin, liver, and gastrointestinal tract. The patient develops a maculopapular pruritic rash beginning on the palms of the hands and soles of the feet. The rash may spread to involve the entire body and lead to desquamation. Gastrointestinal manifestations include abdominal pain, nausea, and bloody diarrhea. GVHD that lasts longer than 100 days is said to be chronic. If it is limited to the skin and liver, the prognosis is good. If multiple organs are involved, the prognosis is poor (Porth & Matfin, 2009).

Interdisciplinary Care

Pretransplant care and post-transplant care are directed toward reducing the risk that transplanted tissue will be rejected or result in GVHD. Diagnostic studies are directed first at identifying the potential recipient's blood type and histocompatibility. Potential donors are identified through diagnostic studies, and the recipient's immune response to the transplant is monitored. Immunosuppressive therapy with medications is a vital part of post-transplant care. The development of effective immunosuppressive drugs as well as improved methods of tissue typing are responsible for the success of organ transplants using allografts.

Diagnosis

Laboratories specializing in transplant are equipped to make the following diagnostic tests prior to organ or tissue transplantation:

- *Blood type* of both the donor and recipient are determined and they must match.
- *DNA sequencing* is made on blood cells to determine histocompatibility. Sequencing can be completed quickly. Quick response is important to minimize cold ischemia in cadaverous organs. Diagnostic testing of recipients can be made less urgently.
- *Crossmatching* of the patient's serum against the donor's lymphocytes is performed to identify any preformed antibodies against antigens on donor tissues. If present, these antibodies would likely result in an immediate or hyperacute graft rejection with probable loss of the transplant.

TABLE 13–2 Transplant Rejection Episodes

TYPE	CAUSE	PRESENTATION	TREATMENT
Hyperacute	Preexisting antibodies to donor ABO or HLA antigens	Occurs within minutes to hours or days of the transplant Rapid deterioration of organ function	The transplant usually cannot be saved; prevent with crossmatch, and use antimetabolites or anti-inflammatory drugs before surgery.
Acute	Primarily a cell-mediated immune response to HLA antigens; antibody-mediated response may also contribute	Occurs within days to months after the transplant Signs of inflammation and impaired organ function	Increase immunosuppression using steroids, cyclosporine, monoclonal antibodies, or anti-lymphocyte globulins.
Chronic	Probably antibody-mediated response; may also involve inflammatory damage to vessel endothelium	Occurs 4 months to years after the transplant Gradual deterioration of organ function	None; loss of graft will occur, requiring retransplant.

■ *HLA histocompatibility testing* identifies donors with an HLA type close to that of the recipient. It is used primarily to identify living donors for bone marrow and kidney transplant. Because of GVHD, histocompatibility tests to identify an identical or very close HLA match are particularly important in bone marrow transplant. HLA tests are performed using lymphocytes from a blood sample. The sample should not be obtained within 72 hours of a blood transfusion, because this will interfere with results.

■ *Mixed lymphocyte culture (MLC) assay tests* also are used to determine histocompatibility between the donor and the allograft recipient. This test identifies whether lymphocytes of the recipient will react against the potential donor's leukocyte antigens (HLA). When a pretransplant test reveals a high potential for reaction, potent immunosuppression may prevent rejection. If the intended recipient is severely immunocompromised, the results may be falsely negative. Patients treated with chemotherapy within 2 weeks of specimen collection are potentially immunocompromised.

■ *Ultrasonography* or *magnetic resonance imaging (MRI)* of the transplanted organ may be performed to evaluate its size, perfusion, and function.

■ *Tissue biopsies* of the transplanted organ are performed routinely to assess for evidence of tissue rejection.

Medications

Prior to transplantation, several antibiotic and antiviral drugs may be prescribed, including the following:

■ Trimethoprim-sulfamethoxazole (Septra, Bactrim) to decrease the incidence of gram-negative bacterial infections

■ Acyclovir (Zovirax) to prevent the development of herpes simplex virus pneumonia in bone marrow transplant recipients

■ Ganciclovir (Cytovene) to prevent the development of cytomegalovirus (CMV) pneumonia with bone marrow transplant recipients

The mainstays of drug therapy for patients following a tissue or organ transplant are immunosuppressive agents. See Figure 13–6 ■. Varying regimens of these drugs are used, depending on the transplanted tissue and the medical center; however, a combination of corticosteroids and cyclosporine is common for maintenance therapy. Antilymphocyte therapy and the use of monoclonal antibodies are increasingly common in the immediate post-transplant period and for treating steroid-resistant rejection episodes.

Corticosteroids, primarily prednisone (Deltasone, others) and methylprednisolone (Solu-Medrol, others) are important agents. The exact anti-inflammatory and immunosuppressive activity of corticosteroids is unknown but they are known to suppress production of interleukin-1 and -2, decrease monocyte migration, and suppress proliferative and cytotoxic T-cell activity. Although they are very effective, large doses of corticosteroids used post-transplant are associated with significant adverse effects. Wound healing is impaired, and the metabolism of fats, proteins, and carbohydrates is altered. Blood glucose increases with steroid use, impairing glucose control. Fat distribution changes, producing a cushingoid appearance with a moon face, increased truncal fat, and "buffalo hump." Fluid retention and hypertension are potential problems, as are osteoporosis, gastrointestinal bleeding, and emotional disturbances.

Cyclosporine inhibits T-cell function and the normal cell-mediated immune response. The incidence of cyclosporine toxicity and side effects is related to blood levels, so blood levels are monitored closely. Cyclosporine is both nephrotoxic and hepatotoxic, especially at high doses. Observable toxic effects include hypertension and central nervous system (CNS) symptoms such as flushing or tingling of the extremities, confusion, visual disturbances, and seizures or coma.

Azathioprine (Imuran) inhibits both cell-mediated and antibody-mediated immunity, although its activity is more specific for T cells than B cells. Because it is rapidly metabolized by the liver, azathioprine can be given to patients with impaired renal function but may not be effective in patients with impaired hepatic function. Bone marrow suppression is the most common adverse effect of this drug, necessitating frequent evaluation of the complete blood count (CBC). Hepatotoxicity, pancreatitis, and increased risk of neoplasm are also associated with azathioprine administration. Nursing responsibilities related to azathioprine are listed in the Medication Administration box on the following pages. Patients who cannot tolerate azathioprine may receive a newer immunosuppressant, mycophenolate mofetil (CellCept). Primarily, it is prescribed following renal and cardiac transplants.

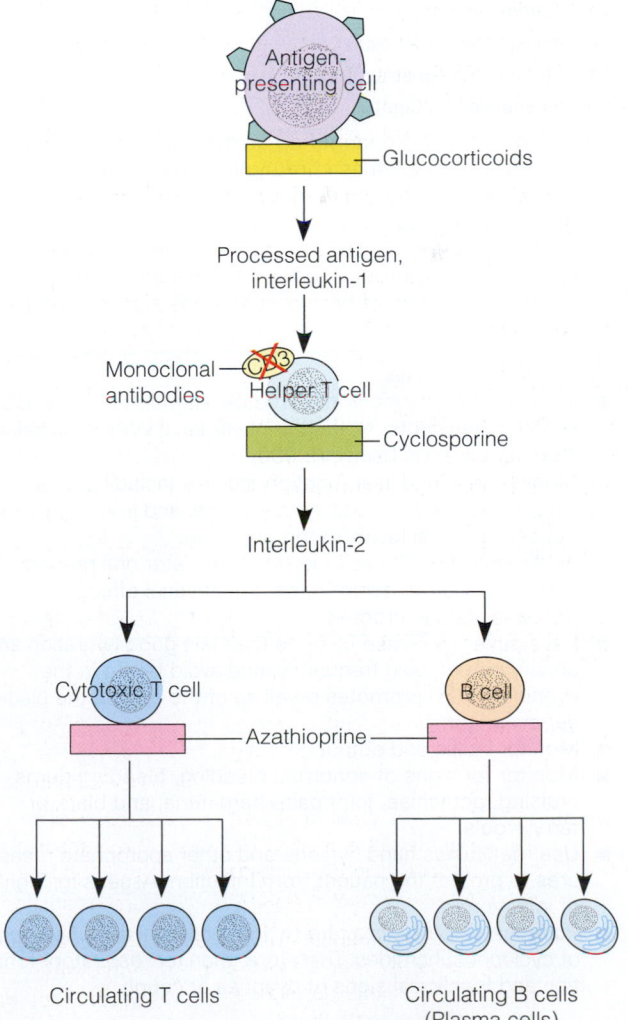

Figure 13–6 ■ Sites of action of immunosuppressive agents.

T-CELL SUPPRESSORS

Cyclosporine (Sandimmune)

Tacrolimus (Prograf)

Sirolimus (Rapamune)

These drugs inhibit T-cell development and activation. They are given concurrently with a glucocorticoid and in combination with other immunosuppressants and inhibit immune system activity and organ rejection.

Nursing Responsibilities

- Monitor BUN and creatinine for evidence of nephrotoxicity.
- Teach the signs and symptoms of infection unique to immune-suppressed individuals. A temperature of 100.6°F is significant evidence of infection. A sore throat may be a manifestation. Other signs and symptoms of inflammation and infection may be absent.
- Teach patients good hygiene to avoid infection with special emphasis on hand hygiene and avoiding infected individuals.
- Monitor blood pressure and availability and use of antihypertensive medications.
- Teach to avoid grapefruit juice, which can raise cyclosporine levels by 50% to 200% and increase the risk of toxicity. Sirolimus should not be taken with grapefruit juice. Sirolimus increases cholesterol and triglycerides. Lipid-lowering drugs may be necessary to prevent hyperlipidemias.

CYTOTOXIC AGENTS

Azathioprine (Imuran)

Cyclophosphamide (Cytoxan)

Methotrexate (Rheumatrex, Trexall)

Mycophenolate (CellCept)

Certain drugs that are identified as cytotoxic or antineoplastic agents are effective as immunosuppressive agents. They act by decreasing the proliferation of cells within the immune system and are widely used to prevent rejection following a tissue or organ transplant. They are usually administered concurrently with corticosteroid therapy, allowing lower doses of both preparations and resulting in fewer side effects.

Nursing Responsibilities

- Monitor blood count, with particular attention to the WBC and platelet counts. Notify the physician if WBCs fall below 4,000 or platelets below 75,000.
- Monitor renal and liver function studies, including creatinine, BUN, eGFR, creatinine clearance, and liver enzymes. Report abnormal levels to the physician.
- Administer the drug as ordered. Administer oral preparations with food to minimize gastrointestinal effects. Antacids may be ordered.
- Have patient increase fluids to maintain good hydration and urinary output, void frequently, and avoid taking in the evening, which promotes dwelling of the drug in the bladder overnight.
- Monitor intake and output.
- Monitor for signs of abnormal bleeding, bleeding gums, bruising, petechiae, joint pain, hematuria, and black or tarry stools.
- Use meticulous hand hygiene and other appropriate measures to protect the patient from infection. Assess for signs of infection.
- Pulmonary fibrosis is a rare (< 1%) potential adverse effect of cyclophosphamides. Therefore, monitor respiratory function and for clinical signs of dyspnea or cough.

Health Education for the Patient and Family

- Avoid large crowds and situations where exposure to infection is probable.
- Report signs of infection, such as chills, fever, sore throat, fatigue, or malaise, to the physician.
- Use contraceptive measures to prevent pregnancy while on immunosuppressive therapy; these drugs are teratogenic.
- Avoid the use of aspirin or ibuprofen while taking these drugs. Report any signs of bleeding to the physician. Check labels: Many over-the-counter products contain aspirin.
- With cyclophosphamide, amenorrhea may occur. The menses may resume after the drug is discontinued.
- If taking cyclophosphamide, report difficulty breathing or cough to the physician.

MONOCLONAL ANTIBODIES

Muromonab-CD3 (Orthoclone OKT3)

Basiliximab (Simulect)

Daclizumab (Zenapax)

Alemtuzumab (Campath)

Monoclonal antibodies are formed by immunizing a mouse with an antigen to produce a specific antibody. Lymphocytes producing the antibody are cloned, and the antibody is harvested. When injected into humans, the antibody binds with a surface antigen on T cells, removing them from circulation and inactivating those bound to allograft cells. Due to the high incidence of adverse effects, the first doses of the monoclonal antibody are administered by a physician and the patient closely observed for 2 hours following each dose. Alemtuzumab is used in bone marrow transplants, renal transplant, and in clinical trials for multiple sclerosis. This drug increases the risk of opportunistic infections such as cytomegalovirus.

Nursing Responsibilities

- Be sure a chest x-ray has been performed within 24 hours preceding initiation of monoclonal antibody therapy and that no pulmonary or cardiovascular congestion is present. The risk of anaphylaxis is greater in the patient with fluid overload.
- Premedicate as ordered with hydrocortisone, acetaminophen, and diphenhydramine to reduce potential adverse effects.
- Position a crash cart or code cart with emergency medications in the patient's room or in close proximity to it.
- After each of the first two doses, monitor vital signs every 15 minutes for 2 hours, then every 30 minutes for 2 hours.
- Observe closely for potential adverse effects, including chills and fever; tachycardia; headache and tremor; hypertension or hypotension; nausea, vomiting, and diarrhea; chest pain, dyspnea, and wheezing.
- OKT3 can also cause anaphylaxis; observe for evidence of urticaria, angioedema, laryngeal edema, wheezing, or other signs of anaphylactic reaction.
- Alemtuzumab infusion is potentially associated with chills, fever, rash, and hypotension. Adverse cardiac events and autoimmune reactions have been reported.
- Monitor CBC for evidence of leukopenia or pancytopenia.
- Assess for infection.

Health Education for the Patient and Family

- Teach about the drug and its purpose.
- Discuss potential adverse and side effects, and emphasize the need to report symptoms promptly.
- Inform the patient that adverse effects are most likely to occur following the first two doses, necessitating close observation at that time. Reassure the patient that this is standard protocol for this medication.

MEDICATION ADMINISTRATION   Immunosuppressive Agents (continued)

ANTILYMPHOCYTE GLOBULINS
Antithymocyte globulin or ATG (ATGAM)

Antilymphocyte globulin or ALG

These globulins containing antilymphocyte antibodies are produced by immunizing horses (the main source), rabbits, or sheep with human lymphocytes to stimulate production of antibodies (see the following figure). Serum from the animal is then recovered, and the active IgG fraction is isolated, purified, and administered parenterally to the patient. It binds with peripheral lymphocytes and mononuclear cells, removing them from circulation.

Lymph nodes   Thymus   Spleen

Human lymphocytes extracted from lymphoid tissues

Injected into horse, rabbit, sheep

Serum recovered

IgG fraction isolated and purified

Purified IgG fraction administered to client

A horse is inoculated with washed human lymphocytes, stimulating the production of immunoglobulin with polyclonal antilymphocyte antibodies. These are then extracted from horse serum, purified, and administered intravenously to the patient.

ATG or ALG is used both to induce immunosuppression immediately following a transplant and to treat steroid-resistant rejection episodes. As with monoclonal antibody, multiple side effects are associated with ATG or ALG.

Nursing Responsibilities
- Perform a skin test for sensitivity to horse serum prior to initial dose. Report any positive reaction to the physician and hold administration until desensitization therapy has been completed.
- Premedicate as ordered with acetaminophen and diphenhydramine prior to each dose. Steroids may also be administered before the initial dose. Have epinephrine and hydrocortisone injections available at the bedside in case of anaphylactic reaction.
- Administer by intravenous infusion into a central line over 4 to 6 hours.
- Monitor vital signs hourly while medication is infusing.
- Assess for adverse effects, including chills and fever, erythema, and pruritus. Notify the physician; these may be treated symptomatically.
- Monitor CBC daily, notify the physician if WBC falls to less than 3000/mm^3 or platelet count to less than 100,000/mm^3. The medication may be stopped or reduced.
- Assess renal function studies to monitor for serum sickness. Report complaints of joint pain.
- Monitor for signs of infection, and report any signs promptly.

CORTICOSTEROIDS
Prednisone

Methylprednisolone (Medrol, Solu-Medrol)

Corticosteroids are immunosuppressants but also have dangerous side effects when high doses are used for a prolonged time. The mechanism of action is not fully identified but cytokine production is reduced, disabling an immune response. Adverse reactions include hypertension, hyperglycemia, and opportunistic infection. Too little corticosteroid can result in graft rejection. A few months after transplantation, patients can be weaned off corticosteroids without increasing the frequency of rejection episodes.

Health Education for the Patient and Family
- Explain the need for special precautions and close monitoring while this drug is being administered.
- Instruct the patient to report any adverse effects, including malaise or joint pain, promptly.
- Ask the patient to report any evidence of easy bruising, bleeding gums, or black stools.
- Teach family members about the importance of not exposing the patient to persons with infectious diseases.

Muromonab-CD3, also known as OKT3 or Orthoclone, is the first monoclonal antibody produced for therapeutic use in humans. As a monoclonal antibody, OKT3 is specific to T cells, blocking their generation and function. It binds with a surface antigen on T cells, inactivating and removing them from circulation. It also blocks killer T cells attached to the graft. Because of significant side effects, the use of OKT3 is limited primarily to treatment of steroid-resistant rejection. Two newer monoclonal antibodies, basiliximab (Simulect)

and daclizumab (Zenapax), are a combination of mouse and human antibodies and cause fewer side effects.

Polyclonal antilymphocyte antibodies are also used as adjunctive immunosuppressant therapy. These are administered as antilymphocyte globulin (ALG) or antithymocyte globulin (ATG). These globulins contain antibodies against both T and B cells, as well as other mononuclear leukocytes. When administered, they deplete circulating lymphocytes, platelets, and granulocytes.

Nursing Care

The patient who has an organ or tissue transplant has both immediate and long-term nursing care needs. Both the patient and the family must be considered in providing nursing care.

Health Promotion

Part of the health promotion activities focus on preventing the need for a tissue transplant. It is important to increase public awareness regarding unhealthy lifestyle behaviors, such as excessive alcohol consumption and illegal drug use, and their relationship to organ failure. Patients with chronic diseases such as diabetes mellitus and hypertension must understand that inadequate management of these disorders could lead to end-stage renal disease. Other risk factors may simply relate to a person's heredity; understanding how heredity could affect future health might influence the patient's lifestyle choices.

Assessment

Assessment data collected following a tissue transplant focus on identifying potential rejection episodes. Further focused assessments are described with nursing interventions in the next section.

Nursing Diagnoses and Interventions

Because of the continuing risk of transplant rejection and the need for immunosuppression, *Ineffective Protection* and *Risk for Impaired Tissue Integrity* are priority nursing diagnoses. The patient's underlying disease process, the transplant, and the continuing need for immunosuppressive drug therapy also have emotional and psychologic consequences. Other nursing diagnoses, such as *Powerlessness* or *Ineffective Coping*, also may be appropriate.

Ineffective Protection

Ineffective protection is a problem for the transplant patient at all stages. Before the transplant occurs, failure of the affected organ may put the patient at risk for infection and other multisystemic problems. Incisions and invasive perioperative procedures impair skin and mucous membrane protection from infectious organisms and other antigens. Immunosuppressive drugs given postoperatively to prevent graft rejection disarm the immune response to a certain extent, increasing the risk of infections and neoplastic growths.

> **SAFETY ALERT**
> Use strict aseptic technique in changing dressings and caring for invasive catheters such as intravenous lines and indwelling urinary catheters to protect against external and resident host microorganisms.

- Wash hands and use hand sanitizer on entering room and before providing direct care. *Hand hygiene removes transient organisms from the skin, reducing the risk of transmission to the patient.*
- Assess frequently for manifestations of infection. Monitor vital signs, including temperature, every 4 hours. Assess for evidence of inflammation, abnormal wound drainage, changes in urine or other body secretions, complaints of pain, or behavior changes that may indicate infection. Culture abnormal wound drainage. *The patient on immunosuppressive therapy is more susceptible to infection, and usual manifestations may not be evident. Both the body temperature and inflammatory response can be suppressed by therapy. Prompt identification and intervention for infection is important in the immunosuppressed patient.*
- Monitor laboratory values, including CBC and tests of organ function; report changes to the physician. *An elevation in the WBC count with increased numbers of immature cells (bands) or a decline in function of the transplanted organ (e.g., a rising BUN and creatinine in the renal transplant patient) may be early indications of infection or transplant failure.*
- Initiate reverse or protective isolation procedures as indicated by the patient's immune status. *These procedures further protect the severely immunocompromised patient from infection.*
- Instruct ill family members and visitors to avoid contact with the patient. *A "minor" upper respiratory infection can be a significant illness in the immunocompromised host.*
- Help ensure adequate nutrient intake, offering supplementary feedings as indicated or maintaining enteral or parenteral nutrition if necessary. *Adequate nutrition is important for healing and immune system function.*
- Change intravenous bags and tubing at least every 24 hours, and change peripheral intravenous sites every 72 to 96 hours, unless contraindicated. Remove invasive catheters and lines as soon as they are no longer necessary. *Changing lines and sites is important to reduce bacterial contamination. Fewer invasive lines provide fewer sites for bacterial invasion of the body.*
- Emphasize the importance of meticulous hand hygiene after using the bathroom and before eating. *This reduces the risk of infection with endogenous organisms.*
- Provide good mouth care. *Good mouth care reduces the population of oral microorganisms and helps maintain an intact mucous membrane lining.*
- Monitor for potential adverse effects of medications:
  - Thrombocytopenia and possible bleeding
  - Fluid retention with edema and possible hypertension
  - Renal or hepatic toxicity
  - Cardiac effects, particularly in the presence of fluid retention and hypervolemia.
  Medications used to maintain immunosuppression and preserve the allograft have many potential adverse effects that can alter normal protective and homeostatic mechanisms.

Risk for Impaired Tissue Integrity: Allograft

The risk for transplant rejection is highest in the initial postoperative period, but it is never completely eliminated for the patient who has had an allograft. The patient who has had a bone marrow transplant has the additional risk of developing GVHD, which can affect the integrity of skin, mucous membranes, and other organs.

- Administer immunosuppressive therapy as prescribed. *Suppression of the immune response is necessary to reduce the risk of graft destruction by normal immune responses and to preserve the graft's function.*
- Assess for evidence of graft rejection, including tenderness, erythema, and swelling over the site; sudden weight gain,

edema, and hypertension; chills and fever; malaise; and an increased WBC count and sedimentation rate. Report any changes immediately. *Early identification of rejection allows adjustment of medication regimens and, possibly, preservation of the graft.*

- Monitor results of laboratory studies for function of the transplanted organ. *With a functional graft, results (e.g., renal or liver function studies) will improve; a functional decline may be an early indicator of rejection.*
- Assess for and report signs of GVHD immediately, including maculopapular rash, erythema of the skin and possible desquamation, hair loss, abdominal cramping and diarrhea, or jaundice with elevated bilirubin and liver enzymes (AST, ALT). *GVHD is a potentially lethal complication in the immunosuppressed patient and necessitates immediate intervention.*
- Stress the importance of maintaining immunosuppressive therapy and reporting signs of graft rejection promptly to the physician. *Continued immunosuppression and prompt treatment of rejection are vital to preserving graft function.*

Anxiety

The patient who undergoes an organ or tissue transplantation often faces the unwelcome choices of death from organ failure or receiving an organ that his or her body will likely attempt to reject. In most cases, the patient understands that to receive this transplant, someone else must die and be willing to give up an organ. When the transplant comes from a living donor (bone marrow or kidney), the patient may worry not only about him- or herself, but also about the condition of the donor. Fear of rejection and guilt may be even greater in this instance.

- Assess level of anxiety by noting such cues as expressions of apprehension, fear, or inadequacy; facial expression, tension, or shakiness; difficulty focusing; helplessness; poor eye contact; and restlessness. *Patients may have difficulty identifying or verbalizing feelings of fear and anxiety. Nonverbal cues are often useful in recognizing states of anxiety.*
- Provide opportunities to express feelings. Use opening statements such as "Facing an organ transplant must be very stressful," or "What concerns you most about this transplant?" Listen attentively. *Encouragement and active listening allow the patient to express feelings of anxiety or fear.*
- Arrange tasks to allow as much time with the patient as possible. When leaving, tell the patient when you will return. *Time spent with the patient facilitates the development of trust.*
- Provide clear, concise directions. *Highly anxious patients have difficulty focusing and retaining information.*
- Encourage involvement in care but do not request unnecessary decisions. *The patient needs to feel a sense of control but

may become irritated if asked to make decisions unrelated to the situation.

- Encourage family members to remain with the patient as much as possible. *This can help reduce the patient's anxiety.*
- Encourage the use of coping behaviors that have been effective for the patient in the past. *Coping mechanisms and behaviors help lower anxiety to a more acceptable level.*
- Reduce or eliminate environmental stressors to the extent possible. *This gives the patient a better sense of control.*
- Assist with stress reduction and relaxation techniques, such as guided imagery, meditation, and muscle relaxation. *These techniques help the patient gain control over physical responses to anxiety.*
- Refer to a counselor, mental health specialist, or spiritual advisor as appropriate. *Counseling can help the patient identify and deal with his or her concerns and fears.*

Community-Based Care

Teaching the patient and family about an organ or tissue transplant begins before the transplant and continues throughout hospitalization and follow-up treatment. Transplant coordinators are nurses specializing in the transplant process and are excellent resources for patients, families, and nursing staff.

Initial teaching focuses on the options, risks, and potential benefits of the transplant itself. Include the procedure by which the organ is selected and obtained, as well as the procedure by which it is transplanted into the patient. If a living related donor is an option, discuss the risks and benefits for both the patient and the donor. Outline the post-transplant treatment regimen, including any lifestyle changes that may be necessary. Waiting for a cadaver organ is a tedious process; the patient must be ready to present for transplant when an organ is available. The transplant process is complex, expensive, and anxiety-provoking.

Following the transplant, provide verbal and written instructions, including the following:

- Manifestations of transplant rejection and the importance of notifying the physician
- Immunosuppressive drug regimen and side effects
- Wound care
- Avoiding exposure to infectious diseases, particularly respiratory infections, and wearing a mask when going outside
- Meticulous personal hygiene, hand hygiene technique, and frequent mouth care
- Wearing a Medic-Alert bracelet or tag
- Follow-up visits to the physician or clinic
- Helpful resources:
  - American Council on Transplantation
  - Local and state support groups related to specific organ transplant, such as the National Kidney Foundation

Impaired Immune Responses

Disorders of impaired immune system responses may be either congenital or acquired. Often the function of either T or B cells is impaired, reducing the body's ability to defend against foreign antigens or abnormal host tissue.

No matter what the cause, patients with immunodeficiency disorders demonstrate an unusual susceptibility to infection.

When the antibody-mediated response is primarily affected, the patient is at particular risk for severe and chronic bacterial infections. These patients do not develop long-lasting immunity to such diseases as chickenpox and are prone to recurrence of the diseases. Patients with a defect of cell-mediated immunity tend to develop disseminated viral infections such as herpes simplex and cytomegalovirus (CMV). Candidiasis (yeast) and other fungal infections are also common. Because T cells are involved with activating antibody-mediated immune responses as well, overwhelming bacterial infections may occur. Immunodeficiency in its most severe form occurs when both antibody-mediated and cell-mediated responses are impaired. Patients with combined immunodeficiency are susceptible to all varieties of infectious organisms, including those not normally considered to be pathogens.

Most immunodeficiency diseases are genetically determined and rare. They affect children more than adults. The noted exception is AIDS, an infectious disease caused by a virus.

The Patient with HIV Infection

In 1981, five cases of *Pneumocystis jiroveci* pneumonia (then known as *P. carinii* pneumonia or PJP) and 26 cases of a rare cancer, Kaposi's sarcoma, were diagnosed in young, previously healthy homosexual males in Los Angeles and New York City. The term **acquired immunodeficiency syndrome (AIDS)** was used to describe the immune system deficits associated with these opportunistic disorders. Prior to this time, both PJP and Kaposi's had been seen only in elderly, debilitated, or severely immunodeficient people. Other groups at risk for AIDS were soon identified: injection drug users, persons with hemophilia, recipients of blood transfusions, and immigrants from Haiti. Research to identify the cause of this apparently new disease progressed feverishly, and in 1983, a common antibody was identified in patients with AIDS. The **human immunodeficiency virus (HIV)** was isolated in 1984. It then became apparent that AIDS was the final, fatal stage of HIV infection. HIV is a retrovirus transmitted by direct contact with infected blood and body fluids. Significant concentrations of the virus are present in blood, semen, vaginal and cervical secretions, and cerebrospinal fluid (CSF) of infected individuals. It is also found in breast milk and saliva.

It began, like so many epidemics, with a few isolated cases, and has become a worldwide plague. (See the accompanying Focus on Cultural Diversity box.) Progression of HIV disease to AIDS has slowed because of the effectiveness of highly active antiretroviral therapy (HAART). Survival with AIDS has improved from 2.03 years with prophylactic treatment for opportunistic infections to more than 13 years with antiretroviral agents (Walensky, 2006).

Although the incidence of HIV has leveled and mortality due to AIDS has declined, the epidemic is far from over. In the United States it continues to disproportionately affect African Americans, men who have sex with men (MSM), people who engage in high-risk heterosexual behavior (sex with individuals known to be infected with HIV or at high risk for having HIV), and injection drug users. Two separate elements are reported in the surveillance data: HIV infection rate and AIDS occurrence. HIV infection is dependent on exposure to the virus; conversion to AIDS is related to access and use of HAART. HIV new cases are highest among MSM and high-risk heterosexuals; AIDS occurrence continues among MSM, high-risk heterosexuals, and African Americans (CDC, 2008).

Incidence and Prevalence

Through 2006, the CDC (2008) estimated that 1,106,400 persons in the United States were living with HIV/AIDS, with 21% undiagnosed and unaware of their HIV infection. There were 56,300 new cases of AIDS in 2006 in the United States. Deaths among people with AIDS had decreased from 50,610 in 1995 to 14,627 in 2006, more than likely the result of improved treatments rather than a decline in spread of the disease. A continued decline in deaths is dependent on access to quality care and treatment and continued development of treatments for those already heavily treated (McPhee & Papadakis, 2009).

The risk factors for HIV infection are behavioral. Among adults in the United States, 60% of reported cases are MSM, including homosexuals, bisexuals, and such groups as prison populations. Unprotected anal intercourse is the major route of transmission in this group. Injection drug use is the second leading risk factor, accounting for approximately 25% of cases, with sharing of needles and other drug paraphernalia the primary route of transmission. Heterosexual intercourse with an infected drug user and exchanging sex for drugs are major risk factors for women. Hemophiliacs who require large amounts of intravenous clotting factors and people infected through blood transfusion account for a small number of cases, approximately 2% (CDC, 2008).

Among risk groups, the most rapid increases are noted in young gay and bisexual men, women, and inner-city injection drug users, especially African Americans and Hispanics. In the United States, the rate of male adult/adolescent HIV/AIDS cases (per 100,000 population) reported was 83.7 among African Americans, 29.3 among Hispanics, 14.6 among Native Americans/Alaska Natives, 19.6 among Caucasians, and 10.3 among Asian and Pacific Islanders. The rapid increase of AIDS cases among women is of special concern: the reported rate of new cases among women in the United States per 100,000 population was 55.7 among African Americans, 14.4 among

(Left margin vertical text: HIV/AIDS Video)

FOCUS ON CULTURAL DIVERSITY
HIV/AIDS

- There are an estimated 33 million people infected with AIDS worldwide, with virtually every country in the world reporting cases (United Nations AIDS/WHO, 2007). The highest incidence is found in sub-Saharan Africa, South and Southeast Asia, the United States, western Europe, South America, and Canada.
- Approximately 67% of all people infected with HIV or who have AIDS live in sub-Saharan Africa, and another 15% live in South and Southeast Asia, largely in Thailand and India.
- The most common mode of transmission is heterosexual intercourse. The cofactors that increase the risk of HIV transmission include the presence of ulcerative or inflammatory sexually transmitted diseases, trauma, menses, and lack of male circumcision (McPhee & Papadakis, 2009; UNAIDS Report, 2007).

Hispanics, and 3.8 among Caucasians. The majority of women are infected through heterosexual contact (75%) with the remaining 25% through injection drug use (CDC, 2008).

In addition, AIDS in adults over age 50 accounts for approximately 29% of persons living with HIV/AIDS in the United States (CDC, 2008). Survival of persons infected earlier in their life accounts for a significant portion of these adults. Declining immune system function in older adults significantly increases their risk for contracting HIV/AIDS, along with the belief that they cannot be affected by it. Just as younger persons with HIV/AIDS contract the diseases primarily through sexual intercourse, so does the aging population. Because older adults are beyond childbearing years, they often fail to use condoms when engaging in sexual activity. Manifestations may be overlooked by healthcare professionals, leading to a delayed diagnosis and increased severity of the disease.

Less than 0.04% of people voluntarily donating blood (a process that generally excludes people with high-risk behavior) are found to be HIV positive. HIV is not transmitted by casual contact, nor is there any evidence of its transmission by vectors such as mosquitoes. Blood donation also poses no risk of contracting HIV to the donor, because only new sterile equipment is used. A small but real occupational risk exists for healthcare workers. Percutaneous exposure to infected blood or body fluids through a needle-stick injury or nonintact skin is the primary route of transmission. Documented evidence indicates that parenteral exposure poses a 1:300 risk of becoming HIV positive (McPhee & Papadakis, 2009). Mucosal exposures, such as splashing in the eyes or mouth, pose a much smaller risk.

Pathophysiology and Manifestations

HIV is a retrovirus, meaning it carries its genetic information in RNA. On entry into the body, the virus infects cells that have the CD4 antigen (T lymphocytes). Once inside the cell, the virus sheds its protein coat and uses an enzyme called *reverse transcriptase* to convert the RNA to DNA (Figure 13–7 ■). This viral DNA is then integrated into host cell DNA and duplicated during normal processes of cell division. Within the cell, the virus may remain latent or become activated to produce new RNA and to form *virions*. The virus then buds from the cell surface, disrupting its cell membrane and leading to destruction of the host cell.

Although the virus may remain inactive in infected cells for years, antibodies are produced to its proteins, a process known as **seroconversion**. These antibodies are usually detectable 6 weeks to 6 months after the initial infection. Helper T or CD4 cells are the primary cells infected by HIV, but it also infects macrophages, dendrites, and certain cells of the CNS. Helper T cells play a vital role in normal immune system function, recognizing foreign antigens and infected cells and activating antibody-producing B cells. They also direct cell-mediated immune activity and influence the phagocytic activity of monocytes and macrophages. The loss

---

PATHOPHYSIOLOGY LINKAGE   HIV Infection/AIDS

MANIFESTATIONS

Acute Retroviral Syndrome (ARS) or Primary HIV infection: fever, sore throat, arthralgias and myalgias, headache, rash, nausea, vomiting, and abdominal cramping. Difficult to diagnose; similar to infectious mononucleosis.

Asymptomatic infection (latency): From 3 years to more than 15 years, depending on availability and adherence to treatment with antiretroviral medications. No vaccine or cure is currently available.

AIDS: HIV-associated neoplasms and opportunistic infections
General malaise, fatigue, low grade fever, night sweats, involuntary weight loss, skin dryness, or rashes.
AIDS Dementia Complex
Opportunistic Infectious Diseases
    Pneumocystis jiroveci pneumonia
    Mycobacterium tuberculosis
    Mycobacterium avium complex
    Candidiasis
    Cryptosporidiosis
    Cryptococcosis
    Toxoplasmosis
    Herpes simplex or herpes zoster
    Cytomegalovirus
Secondary Cancers
    Kaposi's sarcoma
    Hodgkin's & non-Hodgkin's lymphoma
    Cervical dysplasia and cervical cancer
Other Conditions
    Pelvic inflammatory disease
    Human papillomavirus

RELATED PATHOPHYSIOLOGY

This is the first phase in the natural history of HIV/AIDS beginning about 14 days after infection. T_{helper} (CD4) cells are infected with a high load of rapidly replicating HIV RNA during ARS. Persistent generalized lymphadenopathy develops and the lining of the intestine is also damaged very quickly. Antibodies cannot be detected for 6 weeks to 6 months but the infected patient is highly contagious.

A strong cell-mediated and humoral anti-HIV immune defense decreases viral load in the blood. However the virus harbors in lymphoid and neurologic tissues. The level of viral load achieved in this period is predictive of onset of full blown AIDS.

As the T4 cells fall below 200 per mm^3, virus titers rise rapidly and immune activity drops precipitously. It is the loss of immune competence that enables normally benign opportunistic parasites such as viruses, fungi or protozoa to cause infections. Malignancies develop as immune surveillance fails.

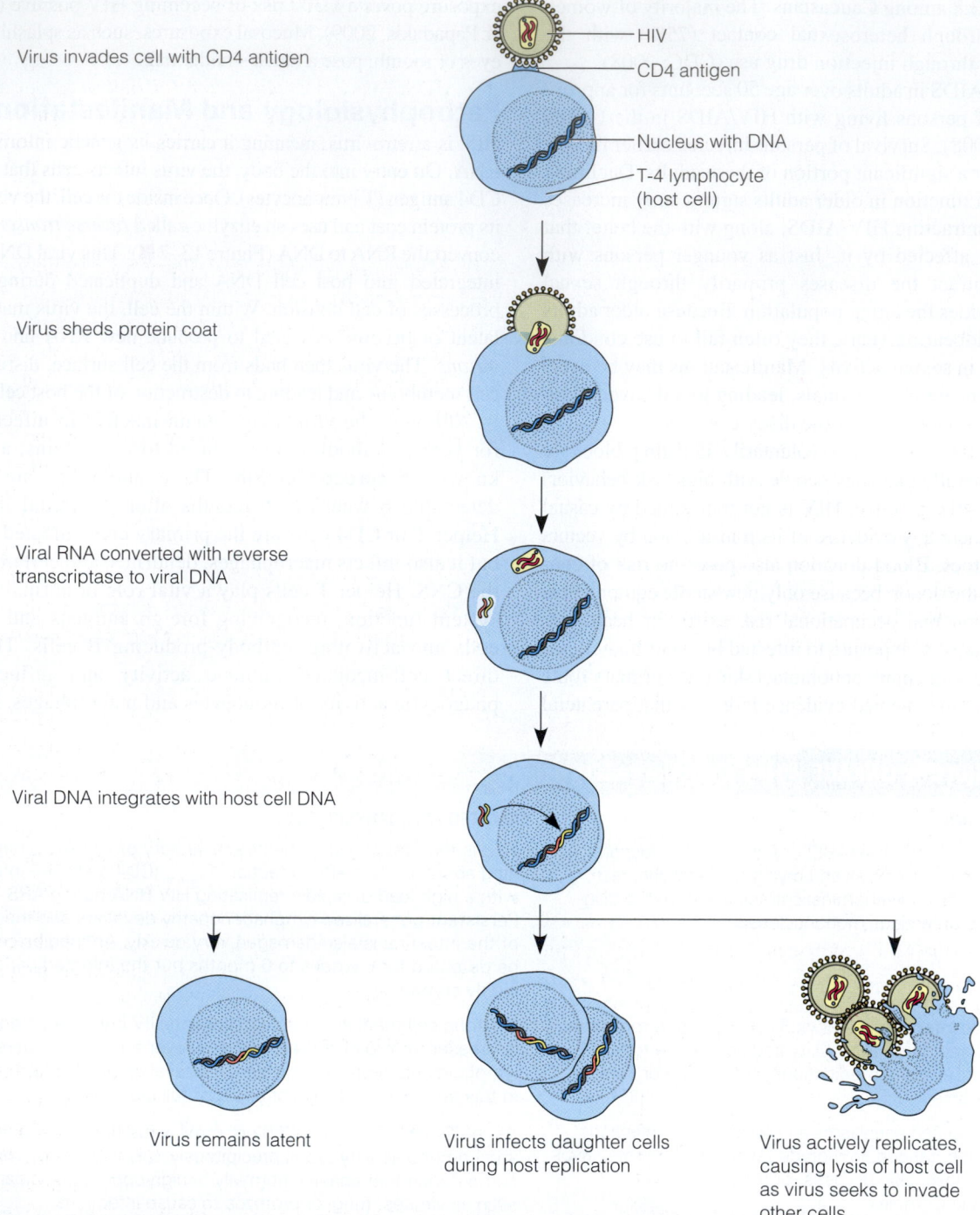

Virus invades cell with CD4 antigen

HIV

CD4 antigen

Nucleus with DNA

T-4 lymphocyte (host cell)

Virus sheds protein coat

Viral RNA converted with reverse transcriptase to viral DNA

Viral DNA integrates with host cell DNA

Virus remains latent

Virus infects daughter cells during host replication

Virus actively replicates, causing lysis of host cell as virus seeks to invade other cells

Figure 13–7 ■ How HIV infects and destroys CD4 cells.

of these helper T cells leads to the immunodeficiencies seen with HIV infection. Figure 13–8 ■ illustrates the typical course of HIV infection.

The manifestations of HIV infection range from no symptoms to severe immunodeficiency with multiple opportunistic infections and cancers (see the Pathophysiology Linkage box on page 325). Most patients develop an acute mononucleosis-type illness within days to weeks after contracting the virus. Typical manifestations include fever, sore throat, arthralgias and myalgias, headache, rash, and lymphadenopathy. Pathologic changes are also noted in the CNS of many infected individuals although the mechanism of neurologic dysfunction is unclear. The patient

may also experience nausea, vomiting, and abdominal cramping. The patient often attributes this initial manifestation of HIV infection to a common viral illness such as influenza, upper respiratory infection, or stomach virus.

Following this acute illness, patients who are treated enter a long-lasting asymptomatic period. Although the virus is present and can be transmitted to others, the infected host has few or no symptoms. Most HIV-infected persons are in this stage of the disease. The length of the asymptomatic period varies widely, but its mean length is estimated to be 8 to 10 years.

Some patients with few other symptoms develop persistent generalized lymphadenopathy. This is defined as enlargement

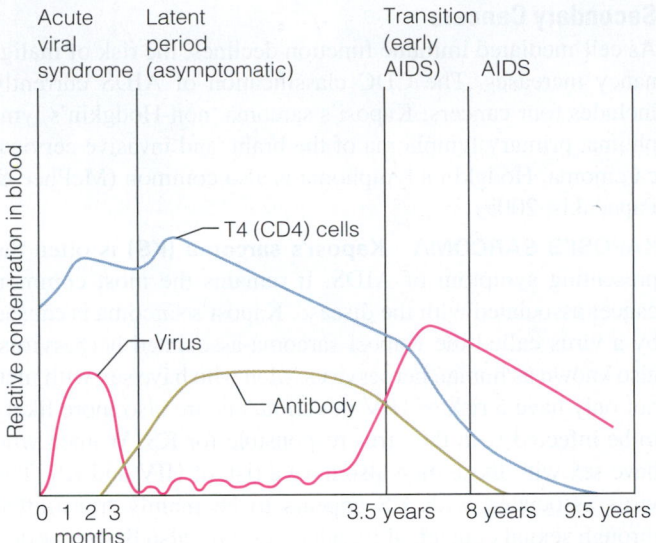

Figure 13–8 ■ The progression of HIV infection. Acute illness develops shortly after the virus is contracted, corresponding with a rapid rise in viral levels. Antibodies are formed and remain present throughout the course of infection. Late in the disease, viral activation results in a marked increase in virus while CD4 (T4) cells diminish as they are destroyed with viral replication. Antibody levels gradually decrease as immune function is impaired.

of two or more lymph nodes outside the inguinal chain with no other illness or condition to account for the lymphadenopathy.

The move from asymptomatic disease or persistent lymphadenopathy to AIDS is often not clearly defined. The patient may complain of general malaise, fever, fatigue, night sweats, and involuntary weight loss (Figure 13–9 ■). Persistent skin dryness and rash may be a problem. Diarrhea is common, as are oral lesions such as hairy leukoplakia, candidiasis, and gingival inflammation and ulceration. The development of advanced HIV varies according to the viral load, rate of disease progression, and the development of resistance to antiretroviral therapy. Estimated survival time for newly-diagnosed patients who are treated with HAART is 20.4 years (Knoll, Lassmann, & Temesgen, 2007). This has increased from about 13 months at the start of the AIDS epidemic. With the development of significant constitutional disease, neurologic manifestations, or opportunistic infections or cancers, the patient has manifestations that are characteristic of

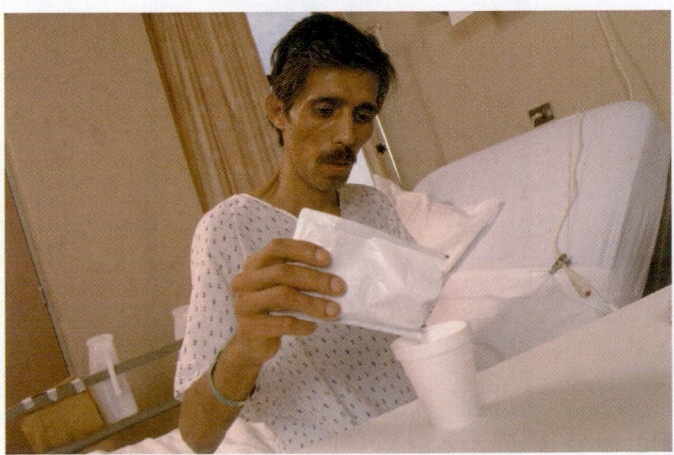

Figure 13–9 ■ Wasting syndrome in a patient with AIDS.

AIDS and a very poor prognosis. When manifestations develop, the outcome varies. With highly active antiretroviral therapy (HAART), many patients are living longer after being diagnosed with AIDS. Today *Pneumocystis carinii* or *jiroveci* pneumonia is most commonly diagnosed in those who are undiagnosed or have a late diagnosis of HIV infection or who fail to take prophylactic antibiotics when their CD4 count is < 200. HAART is credited with decreasing the incidence of opportunistic infections and improving survival (McPhee and Papadakis, 2009).

AIDS Dementia Complex and Neurologic Effects

Neurologic manifestations of HIV include dementia, delirium, and seizures. They result from both the direct effects of the virus on the nervous system and opportunistic infections.

AIDS dementia complex is the most common cause of mental status changes for patients with HIV infection. This dementia results from a direct effect of the virus on the brain and affects cognitive and motor function. Fluctuating memory loss, confusion, difficulty concentrating, lethargy, and diminished motor speed are typical manifestations of AIDS dementia complex. Patients become apathetic, losing interest in work and social and recreational activities. As the complex progresses, the patient develops severe dementia with motor disturbances such as ataxia, tremor, spasticity, incontinence, and paraplegia (Fauci et al., 2008; Porth, 2007).

Infections and lesions common with AIDS may also affect the CNS. Toxoplasmosis and non-Hodgkin's lymphoma are space-occupying lesions that may cause headache, altered mental status, and neurologic deficits. Cryptococcal meningitis and CMV infection also are common in people with AIDS. CNS complications have declined with the use of HAART therapy (McPhee & Papadakis, 2009) Peripheral nervous system manifestations are also common in HIV-infected patients. Sensory neuropathies with manifestations of numbness, tingling, and pain in the lower extremities affect about 30% of patients with AIDS. Weakness and paralysis progress and death occurs within 2 to 4 months (Porth, 2007).

Opportunistic Infections

Opportunistic infections are the most common manifestation of AIDS, often occurring simultaneously. The risk of opportunistic infections is predictable by the T4 or CD4 cell count. The normal CD4 cell count is greater than $1000/mm^3$. When the CD4 count falls to less than $500/mm^3$, manifestations of immunodeficiency are seen. With a count of less than $200/mm^3$, opportunistic infections and cancers are likely.

PNEUMOCYSTIS JIROVECI PNEUMONIA *Pneumocystis jiroveci* (or *Pneumocystis carinii*) pneumonia is the most common opportunistic infection affecting patients with AIDS. When the CD4 count level cannot be maintained above 200 cells/mcl, PJP is likely to develop (McPhee & Papadakis, 2009). It tends to be recurrent, and is a major cause of death in patients with AIDS. PJP is caused by a common environmental fungus that is not pathogenic in patients with intact immune systems. Community-acquired bacterial or viral pneumonia rather than PJP is the most common cause of pulmonary disease in HIV infected persons treated with HAART (McPhee & Papadakis, 2009). Unlike many pneumonias, the manifestations of PJP are nonspecific and may progress insidiously.

Patients often present with fever, cough, dyspnea, tachypnea, and tachycardia. Complaints of mild chest pain and sputum may also be present. Breath sounds may initially be normal. With severe disease, the patient may present with cyanosis and significant respiratory distress.

TUBERCULOSIS (TB) An estimated 4% of patients with AIDS develop TB, contributing significantly to the rise in incidence of this disease in the United States (McPhee & Papadakis, 2009). In some patients, active TB results from reactivation of a prior infection. In other patients, it is a new, primary disease facilitated by impaired immune function. TB is the leading cause of death among HIV infected people (American Lung Association [ALA], 2007). Rapid progression, diffuse pulmonary infiltrates, and disseminated disease occur more commonly in patients with AIDS. Multiple-drug-resistant strains of tuberculosis present a significant problem.

Patients with pulmonary TB present with a cough productive of purulent sputum, fever, fatigue, weight loss, and lymphadenopathy. Disseminated disease affects the bone marrow, bone, joints, liver, spleen, CSF, skin, kidneys, gastrointestinal tract, lymph nodes, brain, and other sites.

OTHER INFECTIONS Herpes virus infections are common in patients with AIDS and may be severe. CMV can affect the retina, the gastrointestinal tract, or lungs. Disseminated herpes simplex or herpes zoster may occur, although severe mucocutaneous manifestations are more common.

Even for patients receiving HAART therapy, sinusitis is common and often frustrating. It manifests as headache, fever, and sinus congestion and discharge. Treatment includes antibiotics and guaifenesin to reduce sinus congestion.

Parasitic infections with *Toxoplasma gondii* and *Cryptococcus neoformans* commonly affect the CNS. Toxoplasmosis occurs as encephalitis or an intracerebral mass lesion. Changes in mental status, focal neurologic signs, and seizures may result. *Cryptococcus* infection may present as either meningitis or disseminated disease, primarily affecting the lungs. *Cryptosporidium*, a protozoon affecting the gastrointestinal tract, is an important cause of prolonged diarrhea in AIDS patients. Bacterial salmonella infections are also a relatively common cause of diarrhea.

Candida albicans infection is a common opportunistic infection in patients with AIDS. It is usually manifested as oral thrush or esophagitis. Oral thrush presents as white, friable plaques on the buccal mucosa or tongue and, in the HIV-infected patient, is often an early indication of progression to AIDS. Patients with esophagitis have difficulty swallowing and substernal pain or burning that increases with swallowing. Vaginal candidiasis is more common and more severe in women with HIV and is treated with topical or systemic medication.

Mycobacterium avium complex (MAC) is a major cause of "wasting syndrome" in persons with AIDS, typically occurring late in the course of the disease when CD4 cell counts are less than 50/mm^3. MAC is caused by organisms commonly found in food, water, and soil. Women with AIDS have a high incidence of pelvic inflammatory disease (PID). Although the pathogens appear to be the same as those in PID affecting non-HIV-infected women, the disease is more severe. Inpatient treatment with intravenous antibiotics is often necessary.

Secondary Cancers

As cell-mediated immune function declines, the risk of malignancy increases. The CDC classification of AIDS currently includes four cancers: Kaposi's sarcoma, non-Hodgkin's lymphoma, primary lymphoma of the brain, and invasive cervical carcinoma. Hodgkin's lymphoma is also common (McPhee & Papadakis, 2009).

KAPOSI'S SARCOMA **Kaposi's sarcoma (KS)** is often the presenting symptom of AIDS. It remains the most common cancer associated with the disease. Kaposi's sarcoma is caused by a virus called the Kaposi sarcoma-associated herpesvirus, also known as human herpesvirus. Men who have sex with men not only have a risk of HIV infection, but are also more likely to be infected with the virus responsible for KS. Women who have sex with these men also have a risk of HIV and KS. The virus associated with KS appears to be mainly transmitted through sexual contact, although cases have also been reported in injection drug users. People whose immune system is suppressed because they have received an organ transplant and are taking immunosuppressive medications are also at risk of developing KS (American Cancer Society, 2005).

A tumor of the endothelial cells lining small blood vessels, KS presents as vascular macules, papules, or violet lesions affecting the skin and viscera (Figure 13–10 ■). In people with dark skin, Kaposi's lesions appear more brown toned. In addition to the palate and toe webs, the face is a common site for skin lesions, especially the tip of the nose and pinnae of the ears. Common sites for visceral disease include the gastrointestinal tract, lungs, and lymphatic system.

The lesions of KS are usually painless initially, but may become painful as the disease progresses. Internally, the tumors may obstruct organ function or cause bleeding. When the lungs are involved, gas exchange may be severely impaired, resulting in pulmonary hemorrhage. This disease may progress slowly or rapidly. Rapidly progressing KS is treated with chemotherapy; milder forms may improve with the initiation of HAART therapy (McPhee & Papadakis, 2009).

LYMPHOMAS Lymphomas are malignancies of the lymphoid tissue, including lymphocytes, lymph nodes, and the lymphoid organs such as the spleen and bone marrow. In AIDS,

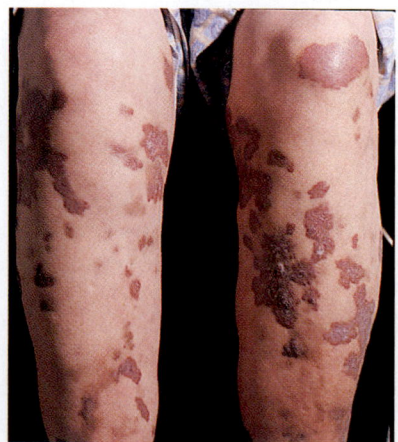

Figure 13–10 ■ Kaposi's sarcoma lesions.
Source: Zeva Oelbaum/Peter Arnold, Inc.

70% of lymphomas are outside the lymphatic system. Hodgkin's disease also occurs five times more frequently in patients with HIV infection than in those without (McPhee & Papadakis, 2009). The CNS is the usual site for these lymphomas, although they may be found in the bone marrow, gastrointestinal tract, liver, skin, and mucous membranes. They are aggressive tumors, growing and spreading rapidly. Headache and changes in mental status are common early symptoms of lymphomas affecting the CNS.

CERVICAL CANCER Cervical cancer develops frequently in women with HIV infection and tends to be aggressive. Women with concurrent HIV infection and cervical cancer usually die of the cervical cancer, not AIDS. Because of this, it is recommended that women with HIV infection have Papanicolaou (Pap) smears every 6 months and aggressive treatment of cervical dysplasia with colposcopic examination and cone biopsy.

CARDIOVASCULAR AND METABOLIC COMPLICATIONS With the advances in HAART, AIDS has become a chronic disease and patients face increased risk for developing cardiovascular disease and metabolic diseases including diabetes. Dyslipidemia (high cholesterol, high triglycerides, low high-density lipoproteins, high levels of low-density lipoproteins) leads to atherosclerosis; these abnormalities develop secondary to some HAART medications, as well as in the absence of HAART. The protease inhibitor drugs make statin (medications used to lower hypercholesterolemia) therapy difficult because they impair metabolism of statins, leading to muscle toxicity.

AIDS NEPHROPATHY Nephropathy is a kidney disorder. HIV-associated nephropathy (HIVAN) manifests as excessive protein in the urine, excessive nitrogen in the blood (azotemia), normal-to-large kidneys on ultrasound images, normal blood pressure, and glomerular lesions revealed by renal biopsy. Before HAART, nephropathy rapidly progressed to renal failure and end-stage renal disease (ESRD), leading to the need for dialysis. HAART taken regularly from the time of diagnosis has decreased the incidence of nephropathy. Nucleoside reverse transcriptase inhibitors (NRTIs) and nonnucleoside reverse transcriptase inhibitors (NNRTIs) may require dose adjustments but are beneficial, even with renal insufficiency. Protease inhibitors may precipitate kidney stones, a painful but nonmetabolic disorder (Salifu, Pani, & Misra, 2007).

Interdisciplinary Care

Although multiple research studies to identify a cure for HIV infection and AIDS are under way, no cure is currently available. This fact, plus the apparent universally fatal nature of the disease, make prevention a vital strategy in HIV care. Search for a vaccine has not been successful to date. HIV infection is different from other viral diseases such as mumps and polio; there is a brief period after entry when viral infected cells are susceptible to the immune system. Following that brief period, latency develops, making an immune response ineffective. The goals of care for the patient with HIV disease are as follows:

- Early identification of the infection
- Promoting health-maintenance activities to prolong the asymptomatic period as long as possible

- Preventing opportunistic infections
- Treating disease complications, such as cancers
- Providing emotional and psychosocial support

Diagnosis

Diagnostic testing is used to screen and identify the infection, as well as to monitor the patient's disease and immune status. False-positive HIV test results are more likely in settings where the prevalence of HIV in the tested population is lower than in settings where the tested population prevalence is higher. When a preliminary, positive rapid test is explained to patients, phrases like "a good chance of being infected" or "very likely infected" can be used to indicate the likelihood of HIV infection, and qualified based on the HIV prevalence in the setting and the patient's individual risk. See Box 13–2 for CDC recommendations for HIV testing.

- *HIV rapid antibody test.* The rapid tests consist of test strips with embedded HIV antigen. If there are antibodies to HIV in the patient's blood, the strip turns a color indicating the test is positive. The results are interpreted visually. Confirmation of positive results is required with the Western blot antibody test. There are six FDA approved rapid tests (see Table 13–3). These tests are widely used because results can be given immediately and three of these can be performed by personnel without formal laboratory training (point-of-care testing). Immediate notification is critical because many patients tested for HIV do not return to learn the results; many cannot be located to receive the test results and be educated about safe behaviors whether they are positive or negative for HIV. Although confirmation of results is dependent on testing with a second source, enzyme-linked immunosorbent assay (ELISA) or Western blot test, learning results immediately gives the patient more information to make wise choices about his or her behaviors and self-care.

BOX 13–2 CDC Recommendations for HIV Testing of Adults and Adolescents

1. All persons aged 13–64, regardless of risk, should receive routine, voluntary screening for HIV in all health-care settings in which the prevalence of undiagnosed HIV infection is at least 0.1%.
2. All patients beginning treatment for TB should be screened for HIV.
3. All patients seeking treatment for sexually transmitted infections should be screened for HIV each time they seek such treatment.
4. Healthcare providers should encourage patients and their prospective sex partners to be tested before initiating a new sexual relationship.
5. Repeat HIV screening should be performed for patients with known risk at least annually. Persons likely to be at high risk include injection-drug users and their sex partners, persons who exchange sex for money or drugs, sex partners of HIV-infected persons, and men who have sex with men (MSM) or heterosexual persons who themselves or whose sex partners have had more than one sex partner since their most recent HIV test.

Source: Centers for Disease Control and Prevention. (2006). *Revised Recommendations for HIV Testing of Adults, Adolescents, and Pregnant Women in Health-care Settings.* Retrieved from http://www.cdc.gov/mmwr/preview/mmwrhtml/rr5514a1.htm

TABLE 13–3 Rapid HIV Tests

TEST	SPECIMEN
OraQuick Advance Rapid HIV 1/2 Antibody Test	Whole blood (venipuncture or fingerstick), oral fluid or plasma
RevealG3 Rapid HIV-1 Antibody Test	Plasma or serum
Uni-Gold Recombigen HIV Test	Whole blood (venipuncture or fingerstick), plasma or serum
Multispot HIV-1/HIV-2 Rapid Test	Serum or plasma
Clearview HIV 1/2 STAT-PAK	Whole blood (venipuncture and fingerstick), serum or plasma
Clearview Complete HIV 1/2	Whole blood (venipuncture and fingerstick), serum or plasma

- *Enzyme-linked immunosorbent assay (ELISA)* is the most widely used screening test for HIV infection. ELISA tests for HIV antibodies; it does not detect the virus. Therefore, a patient may have a negative ELISA test early in the course of infection, before detectable antibodies have developed. The test has a 99.5% or higher sensitivity when performed at least 13 weeks after infection. This means that more than 99.5% of tests performed on blood containing HIV antibodies will show a positive result. False positives can occur; therefore, an initial positive result is always tested repeatedly and confirmed using a different method of antibody detection, usually the Western blot.
- *Western blot antibody testing* is more reliable but more time consuming and more expensive than ELISA. When combined with ELISA, however, a specificity of greater than 99.9% is achieved. Specificity is a measure of the probability that a negative test result indicates that no antibodies are present. In this test, the patient's serum is mixed with HIV proteins to detect reaction. If antibodies to HIV are present, a detectable antigen–antibody response will occur.
- *HIV viral load tests* measure the amount of actively replicating HIV. Levels correlate with disease progression and response to antiretroviral medications. Levels greater than 5,000 to 10,000 copies/mL indicate the need for treatment.
- *CBC* is performed to detect anemia, leukopenia, and thrombocytopenia, which are often present in HIV infection. Lymphopenia (or low levels of lymphocytes) is especially common in this disease.
- Absolute *CD4 lymphocyte count* is the most widely used test to monitor the progress of the disease and guide therapy. The CD4 cell count correlates very closely with the immunodeficiency disorders seen in AIDS. AIDS is now defined not only by the presence of opportunistic infections and other diseases indicative of immunodeficiency, but also by HIV-seropositive status and a CD4 count of less than $200/mm^3$ or a percentage of CD4 lymphocytes of less than 14%. CD4 counts are recommended every 3 to 6 months for all people with HIV disease.

- *Blood culture for HIV* provides the most specific diagnosis but is an expensive and cumbersome test that is not widely available in the United States.

Other diagnostic tests are used primarily to detect secondary cancers and opportunistic infections in the patient with HIV. Tests ordered are both general and specific to the patient's manifestations and may include the following:

- *Tuberculin skin testing* to detect possible tuberculosis infection
- *MRI* of the brain to identify lymphomas
- *Specific cultures and serology examinations for opportunistic infections* such as PJP, toxoplasmosis, and others
- *Pap smears* every 6 months for early detection of cervical cancer in women with cervical dysplasia (McPhee & Papadakis, 2009).

Medications

Pharmacologic management of the patient with HIV disease has four primary goals: (1) to suppress the infection itself, decreasing symptoms and prolonging life, (2) to provide prophylaxis of opportunistic infections, (3) to stimulate hematopoietic response, and (4) to treat opportunistic infections and malignancies. Today the drugs have been combined and dosing schedules simplified, which helps patients adhere to medication administration schedules.

The Panel on Antiretroviral Guidelines for Adults and Adolescents (2008) and the International AIDS Society—US Panel (2008) recommend initiation of treatment when the CD4 count falls to 350 mm^3. Effectiveness of treatment is monitored by viral load and CD4 cell counts; positive results are indicated by a reduction in viral load along with preserving the CD4 count above 350 mm^3. Starting treatment before immune failure, when the CD4 count is above 500 or 1000, may protect the immune system. Patients with a viral load higher than 100,000 copies, a rapidly declining CD4 cell count (> 100/μL per year), hepatitis B or C, cardiovascular disease risk, or HIV-associated nephropathy, and women who are pregnant, are treated regardless of their CD4 level or viral load. Monitoring these individuals may reveal higher levels of CD4 or lower viral load.

Six classes of drugs used in antiretroviral treatment include nucleoside reverse transcriptase inhibitors (NRTIs), nonnucleoside reverse transcriptase inhibitors (NNRTIs), protease inhibitors (PIs), and three types of entry inhibitors. HAART is a combination of three or more antiretroviral drugs. Combination therapies increase the likelihood of decreasing viral load and adherence to administration schedules has been eased by making various combinations available in one pill. Patients beginning the HAART protocol must understand the benefits, risks, costs, and effects on daily life. HAART does not eradicate HIV infection.

HAART medications are expensive; the newer triple combinations such as Trizivir (one pill twice a day) and Atripla (one pill once a day) cost between $1270 and $1600 for a 30-day supply. This cost does not include medications to prevent or treat opportunistic infections or cancer (McPhee & Papadakis, 2009). If medications are scheduled for specific times throughout the day, leading a normal life becomes a challenge. In addition, all HAART medications cause major adverse reactions leading to less than perfect adherence, as with most chronic diseases; in this case, however, the outcome could be fatal.

Each patient must be able to adhere to the treatment regimen. It may be preferable to delay initiating therapy until the patient is able to agree to adhere so irregular dosing does not lead to viral resistance. Some providers gauge patient ability to follow the HAART regimen by the patient's success with prophylaxis for an opportunistic infection. Discontinuation or interruption of HAART is considered dangerous; because of the burden of adverse reactions, patients may desire brief "holidays" from taking the medications. Periods without the drugs may result in acceleration of viral growth, immune failure, and clinical progression of the disease.

Another approach to adherence is the use of electronic monitoring devices (EMD) (Bova et al., 2005). By placing a microprocessor in a medication cap, records are created of the time, date, and frequency of bottle opening. Although this method does not guarantee that the medication will be taken even if the cap is removed, the record created is a source for follow-up and discussion between the provider and the patient. Whether the patient is asked to keep a diary of taking the medication, uses an EMD to keep a record, or relies on pill count, adherence to medication regimen is critically important.

Ingersoll and Heckman (2005) found the most effective provider–patient relationship for fostering adherence is a balance of appropriate challenge and support. Providers who were never confrontational seem to be perceived by patients as giving permission to be less adherent. Although depression, substance use, and financial considerations undoubtedly influence adherence to HAART therapy, and need to be addressed, provider–patient relationships seem to have the most influence on adherence behavior.

NUCLEOSIDE REVERSE TRANSCRIPTASE INHIBITORS The NRTIs (also called nucleoside analogs) inhibit the action of viral reverse transcriptase, a retroviral enzyme that catalyzes the substrates for conversion and copying of viral RNA to DNA sequences. This enzyme is necessary for viral integration into cellular DNA and replication. The nucleoside analogs act as a chemical decoy for building blocks of the formation of the DNA copy, preventing the RNA from being copied into DNA. Each drug substitutes for a particular nucleoside base at different points on the chain. See the accompanying Medication Administration box for this group of drugs.

Zidovudine (Retrovir, AZT), an antiretroviral agent approved for use with HIV infection, is generally reserved for second- or third-line regimens because it causes anemia and neutropenia. Zidovudine is often given in combination with lamivudine (Combivir) and the combination reduces the frequency of dosing. Zidovudine may also be used prophylactically following a documented parenteral exposure to HIV.

Abacavir causes hypersensitivities in genetically predisposed individuals. Before prescribing this medication, HLA B*5701 testing should be done; if the test is positive, the patient will have a hypersensitivity reaction and should not take the medication.

PROTEASE INHIBITORS Protease is a viral enzyme necessary for the formation of specific viral protein needed for viral assembly and maturation. PIs bond chemically with protease to block the function of the enzyme and result in the production of immature, noninfectious viral particles. When combined with other antiviral drugs, these chemicals increase the chance of eliminating the virus by interfering with different stages of its life cycle. However, viral resistance occurs rather quickly. PIs inhibit and induce metabolism of other drugs, so their use with other medications and the dose of those medications must be carefully planned. Some drugs will circulate longer because their metabolism is inhibited; others will be speedily metabolized and eliminated.

Protease inhibitors and nucleoside analogs are associated with serious metabolic derangements. These include elevated cholesterol and triglycerides, insulin resistance and diabetes mellitus, and changes in body fat composition, which are particularly distressing to the patients. These body fat changes are primarily abdominal obesity and skeletal wasting. This set of symptoms is referred to as lipodystrophy (McPhee & Papadakis, 2009). Elevated cholesterol should be treated with pravastatin or atorvastatin. Lovastatin and simvastatin react with PIs, so they need to be avoided. Reduction of dietary sources of cholesterol should be made. Unlike most PIs, atazanavir (Reyataz) has a beneficial effect on lipids, is effective in reducing viral load, and is usually well-tolerated by patients (Kirtin, 2008).

NONNUCLEOSIDE REVERSE TRANSCRIPTASE INHIBITORS Etravirine (Intelence), delavirdine (Rescriptor), efavirenz (Sustiva), and nevirapine (Viramune) are NNRTIs that may be used in combination with nucleoside analogs and protease inhibitors. However, one limitation to NNRTIs is the high incidence of cross-resistance to NRTIs. Some studies have shown that nevirapine and efavirenz may significantly reduce serum levels of the protease inhibitors. Only one NNRTI should be used at the same time. Nevirapine has a reported risk for liver toxicity and severe rash; it should not be used as a first line treatment for women whose CD4 count is > 250 cells/mcl (McPhee & Papadakis, 2009).

ENTRY INHIBITORS These newer antiviral drugs act by binding to the virus or the host cells and preventing viral entry into the host cells. Enfuvirtide (Fuzeon) blocks the HIV virus from entering human cells. This is the first of the entry inhibitors; unfortunately it can only be administered by injection twice a day and it is very expensive. Patients who develop resistance to HAART regimens are candidates for this regimen. Side effects include injection site pain, itching, and hardening of the tissue; allergic reactions; peripheral neuropathy; insomnia; depression; dyspnea; anorexia; and arthralgia (AIDSinfo, 2008).

Maraviroc (Selzentry) is the first antiretroviral drug that targets the host cells rather than targeting the virus directly. CCR5 antagonists block certain HIV viruses from entry to host immune cells. Certain forms of HIV viruses (R5 tropic viruses) require a CCR5 receptor as a "co-receptor" to gain entry to the cell; with this entry inhibitor, the R5 tropic virus cannot interact with the receptor and therefore is blocked from entering human cells. Before prescribing, a blood test is made to identify the type of viruses the patient carries; if the R5 form of the virus is found, the patient may be a candidate for taking this drug. This entry inhibitor is approved for use in treatment-experienced patients only. Preexisting cardiac and liver conditions are associated with adverse reactions (AIDS InfoNet, 2008).

MEDICATION ADMINISTRATION Antiretroviral Drugs

NUCLEOSIDE REVERSE TRANSCRIPTASE INHIBITORS (NRTIs)
Zidovudine (AZT, Retrovir)

emtricitasbine (emtriva)

lamivudine (epivir)

zalcitabine (Hivid)

didanosine (Videx)

tenofovir disoproxil fumarate (Viread)

stavudine (Zerit)

abacavir sulfate (Ziagen)

COMBINATIONS OF NRTIs
lamivudine and zidovudine (combivir)

abacavir and lamivudine (Epzicom)

abacvir, zidovudine, and lamivudine (Trizivir)

Tenofovir disoproxil fumarate and emtricitabine (Truvada)

Nursing Responsibilities
- Assess for possible contraindications to therapy including allergic response, previous episodes of pancreatitis, and impaired renal or liver function.
- Abacavir sulfate causes allergic reactions in some patients. Prior to administering, HLA B*5701 testing should be made and if the test is positive, the patient should not take abacavir. Monitor for an allergic response: sudden fever, skin rash, severe tiredness or achiness, diarrhea, nausea, vomiting, stomach pain, sore throat, shortness of breath, cough, or general ill feeling. Stop the medication and inform the physician immediately.
- Administer with caution to patients taking vincristine (cancer drug), rifampin (Tb), pentamidine (*pneumocystis jiroveci*), ethambutol (Tb), or metronidazole (bacterial and protozoal infections). Concurrent use may increase the risk of acute and fatal pancreatitis.
- Assess for adverse effects. Nausea and headache are common. They may be self-limiting, decreasing with time, or significant and continuing, necessitating a change of therapy. Peripheral neuropathies may develop; these manifest as a sharp burning pain sensation in the hands and/or legs. Anemia and neutropenia are treated with erythropoietin (epoetin alpha) and G-CSF (filgrastim).
- Assess CBC with differential and serum chemistries for evidence of liver or pancreas changes. Lactic acidosis, an indication of liver disease may develop; monitor lactate levels and pH. Notify the physician of significant changes.
- Didanosine interferes with the absorption of ketoconazole and dapsone (given for opportunistic infection prophylaxis or treatment). Doses of these drugs should be scheduled at least 2 hours apart from didanosine doses. Do not use alcohol while taking didanosine; alcohol may increase the risk of pancreatitis.

Health Education for the Patient and Family
- Antiretroviral medications will not cure HIV infection but rather slow its progress and reduce significant symptoms.
- Follow individual drug guidelines for administration with or without food, swallowing whole, and dissolving a powder or chewing a tablet.
- You are still infective and can pass the infection to others. Use safer sex practices and other measures to prevent transmission to partners. Do not donate blood or breastfeed.
- Notify the physician if signs of an infection or adverse response develop: sore throat, swollen lymph glands, fever; unusual fatigue or weakness; easy bruising, bleeding gums, or an injury that will not heal; persistent or intractable nausea; muscle pain or wasting.

- Continue all scheduled follow-up visits and laboratory studies to monitor for drug toxicity.
- Check with the physician before taking any prescription or over-the-counter drug.

PROTEASE INHIBITORS (PIs)
Amprenavir (Agenerase)

Tipranavir (Aptivus)

Indinavir (Crixivan)

Saquinavir mesylate (Invirase)

Fosamprenavir calcium (Lexiva)

Ritonavir (Norvir)

Darunavir (Prezista)

Atazanavir sulfate (Reyataz)

Nelfinavir mesylate (Viracept)

Lopinavir/ritonavir (Kaletra)

Nursing Responsibilities
- Assess for evidence of cardiovascular or liver disease and diabetes mellitus. Most PIs are associated with lipodystrophy (enlarged abdomen, loss of tissue from the face, arms and legs) and diabetes mellitus (elevated blood glucose).
- The protease inhibitors are known to precipitate kidney stones. Monitor creatinine clearance and patient reports of colicky flank pain.
- Ritonavir is combined with other PIs—an approach called "PI boosting." The benefit of taking Ritonavir in combination with other PIs is the added strength and effectiveness of some drugs and decreased food interactions. However, Ritonavir interacts with many drugs, both prescription and over the counter.
- Administer by mouth. Follow individual drug guidelines for administration with or without food, swallowing whole, and dissolving a powder or chewing a tablet.
- Assess for adverse effects. Nausea and intestinal distress are common. Headache and peripheral neuropathies also are common. Skin reactions may be severe in about 1% of patients. Side effects may be self-limiting, decreasing with time, or significant and necessitating a change of therapy.

NONNUCLEOSIDE REVERSE TRANSCRIPTASE INHIBITORS (NNRTIs)
Etravirine (Intelence)

Delavirdine (Rescriptor)

Efavirenz (Sustiva)

Nevirapine (Viramune)

Nursing Responsibilities
- Assess for history of liver disease before administering these drugs.
- Administer by mouth. Follow individual drug guidelines for administering with or without food, swallowing whole, dissolving a powder or chewing a tablet.
- Assess for evidence of severe skin rash accompanied by blisters, fever, joint or muscle pain, redness and swelling of the eyes, sores in the mouth, and swelling; serious kidney problems; anemia; and liver and muscle problems. Individuals should tell a doctor if they have any of these side effects.
- Efavirenz side effects may include abnormal thinking, confusion, depression, hallucinations, memory loss, paranoid thinking, and thoughts of suicide.

MULTICLASS COMBINATION AGENTS
ATRIPLA: Efavirenz (NNRTI), emtricitabine (NRTI), and tenofovir disoproxil fumarate (NRTI)

TRIZIVIR: Abacavir (NRTI), lamivudine (NRTI), and zidovudine (NRTI)

MEDICATION ADMINISTRATION   Antiretroviral Drugs   (continued)

Nursing Responsibilities

- Trizivir contains abacavir sulfate, which causes allergic reactions in some patients. Prior to administering, HLA B*5701 testing should be made and if the test is positive, the patient should not take abacavir. Monitor for an allergic response: sudden fever, skin rash, severe tiredness or achiness, diarrhea, nausea, vomiting, stomach pain, sore throat, shortness of breath, cough, or general ill feeling. Stop the medication and inform the physician immediately.
- NRTIs can cause a sometimes fatal lactic acidosis and liver disease as well as blood problems or muscle weakness. A doctor should be notified if an individual taking this medication experiences digestive system problems, joint or muscle pain and weakness, pain or tingling of hands or feet, headache, dizziness, and unusual tiredness.
- Administer by mouth.
- Assess for evidence of severe skin rash accompanied by blisters, fever, joint or muscle pain, redness and swelling of the eyes, sores in the mouth, and swelling; serious kidney problems; anemia; and liver and muscle problems.

ENTRY INHIBITORS

Enfuvirtide (Fuzeon)

Maraviroc (Selzentry)

Nursing Responsibilities

- Enfuvirtide is injected; Maraviroc is administered orally.
- Both Enfuvirtide and Maraviroc must be given in combination with other antiviral drugs.
- Enfuvirtide is supplied as a powder and must be dissolved in water for injection. Roll but do not shake the mixture because excessive foam may form. Inject when completely dissolved or refrigerate up to 24 hours. Do not inject solution until it warms to room temperature. Rotate sites.
- Side effects may include cough, fever, upper respiratory tract infections, abdominal pain, dizziness, and rash. These may indicate allergy. Musculoskeletal aches, stiffness, or weakness may indicate bone necrosis caused by the drugs. Instruct patient to report these to the doctor immediately.
- Monitor liver function (cirrhosis and hepatitis decrease liver function) tests including bilirubin, amylase, lipase, AST, and ALT.
- Monitor kidney function (serum creatinine and BUN).

INTEGRASE INHIBITORS

Raltegravir (Isentress)

Nursing Responsibilities

- Administer orally with or without food.
- Assess for side effects: headache, dizziness, diarrhea, and nausea.

HIV Integrase Strand Transfer Inhibitor

Raltegravir (Isentress) targets integrase, an HIV enzyme that integrates the viral genetic material into human DNA. Raltegravir is also called a "strand transfer inhibitor," referring to the process of DNA strand transfer from the virus to the host. It is taken orally twice daily and side effects include nausea, diarrhea, and headache. It is approved only for individuals who have developed resistance to HAART combinations. Like other types of HAART, raltegravir is not considered effective if used alone (AIDS InfoNet, 2008).

Other agents may also be administered in combination with antiretroviral therapy. Interferons, which are naturally occurring lymphokines, have been used alone and in combination. Alpha-interferon may be used to treat KS and in combination with zidovudine to slow disease progression. Gamma-interferon is also used. As more drugs become available, the burden to choose the best regimen increases for the healthcare provider. Referral to a physician who specializes in care of patients with HIV/AIDS is recommended. The most important limiting factor when choosing a regimen is patient adherence. Second to that is selecting an effective combination of drugs without overlapping toxicities or toxicities so debilitating that adherence will be further impaired.

Some patients undergoing HAART are developing body composition changes and metabolic abnormalities associated with the therapy, especially the PIs. Increased fat deposition in the midsection, breasts, and neck with atrophy in the face, buttocks, and extremities describes the body composition changes; metabolic abnormalities include increased low-density lipoprotein cholesterol and triglycerides and insulin resistance. The combination of changes is consistent with metabolic syndrome, which increases the risk of cardiovascular disease and diabetes. These conditions are commonly treated with medications. A number of pharmacologic agents are used to prevent and treat opportunistic infections and malignancies in the patient with HIV.

Many patients at some point require an implanted venous access device, such as a Groshong catheter, to facilitate blood sampling, intravenous medication administration, transfusions, and parenteral nutrition. ∞ See Chapter 14 for nursing care of the patient with an intravenous access device implant.

It is recommended that all HIV-infected patients receive pneumococcal, influenza, hepatitis B, and *Haemophilus influenzae b* vaccines. Persons with a positive PPD and negative chest x-ray are given prophylactic isoniazid. When the patient's CD4 cell count falls to less than 200, prophylactic treatment for PJP is begun, usually with trimethoprim-sulfamethoxazole. Patients with a CD4 count of less than 100 are started on prophylactic treatment for MAC.

∞ Nursing Care

The patient with HIV and AIDS has many nursing care needs, including both physical and psychosocial support (see the Moving Evidence into Action box on page 334). Because there is as yet no cure for HIV disease, many of these needs fall within the realm of nursing to promote knowledge and understanding, self-care, comfort, and quality of life. As with many diseases that have an ultimately fatal outcome, the course of HIV infection may well be affected by the patient's social support systems, control, perceived self-efficacy in management, and coping mechanisms.

As the epidemic continues, nurses are providing care for increasing numbers of patients with HIV infection at various stages of disease including the undiagnosed. These patients are not only in special care settings, but also on general units, maternal–child units, hospice, and home settings. As patients with HIV disease live longer, nurses will increasingly encounter patients in whom HIV disease is a secondary diagnosis with another primary diagnosis, for example, seizures, heart disease, diabetes mellitus, or an operative procedure.

Prevention

To stop the spread of HIV it is important to identify those who are infected but undiagnosed (approximately 25% of HIV positive patients) and offer them treatment. In many states, requirements for documented informed consent and formalized counseling seem to discourage patient participation. The CDC has proposed "opt-out" testing for HIV. The test is made after informing the patient that (1) the test will be performed and (2) the patient may elect to decline or defer testing. Consent is inferred unless the patient declines testing. In opt-out testing, consent for screening is part of the general consent for care, without formalized pretest and posttest counseling performed by supplemental staff. Using existing nursing staff to obtain consent, provide pre-and post-test information, and perform point-of-care HIV testing has been tried and found effective in emergency room settings. HIV testing can be offered 24 hours a day, 7 days per week without hiring additional personnel. However, some states require documented informed consent that includes formalized pre- and posttest counseling by staff dedicated to this role (Kirton & Stevens, 2008).

To date, no safe immunization to protect against HIV infection has been developed. Education, counseling, and behavior modification are the primary tools for AIDS prevention. The benefit of education and behavior modification is evident in the homosexual male population. The incidence of new HIV infections in this population has declined dramatically in high-prevalence cities. Nurses play a vital role in providing education about this epidemic and infection prevention for individuals and communities.

All sexually active individuals need to know how HIV is spread. Following are the only *totally* safe sex practices:

- No sex
- Long-term mutually monogamous sexual relations between two uninfected people
- Mutual masturbation without direct contact

Patients who do engage in sexual activity need to know and practice safer sex. (∞ See Chapter 50 for safer sex guidelines.) Reducing the number of sexual partners—for example, by entering into and remaining in a long-term mutually monogamous relationship with an uninfected partner—reduces the risk. Patients should not engage in unprotected sex, especially if the HIV status of the partner is unknown. Latex condoms have been shown to reduce the risk of transmitting HIV. Their effectiveness is improved when nonoxynol-9, a spermicide, is used for lubrication; however, it may cause genital ulcers, which can facilitate HIV transmission. To be effective, condoms must be used with every sexual encounter involving vaginal, oral, or anal intercourse. They also need to be applied and removed properly. A female condom is also available for use.

Healthcare workers exposed to HIV infection or adults who experience a high-risk exposure to HIV may choose postexposure prophylaxis. Risk of exposure for healthcare workers may be through needle sticks or cuts with a sharp object; mucous membrane or nonintact skin contact with semen, vaginal secretions, fluids contaminated with visible blood, and possibly CSF, synovial fluid, and pleural, peritoneal, pericardial, or amniotic fluids. CDC guidelines recommend treatment with HAART, which includes two NRTIs for lower risk exposures

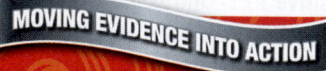

MOVING EVIDENCE INTO ACTION — **Improving Dietary Habits in Disadvantaged Women with HIV/AIDS: The SMART/EST Women's Project**

Women diagnosed with HIV/AIDS in the United States face many stresses. In a study (Segal-Isaacson, Tobin, Weiss et al., 2006), funded by the National Institutes of Mental Health, disadvantaged women with HIV/AIDS living in New York/New Jersey or Miami, Florida, were randomized to four treatment groups for assistance in learning effective coping strategies in phase I and to receive brief nutrition education in phase II. This study was the second SMART/EST (Stress Management and Relaxation Training/Expressive-Supportive Therapy) trial. Researchers learned in the first trial that the strategies they taught decreased depression and anxiety, and improved HIV-related self-care. These results were positively related to increased CD4 levels and decreased viral loads. A SMART/EST II trial was conducted to see if participation in training to improve stress management and expressive therapy would improve the subjects' ability to apply insights and information from health education counseling.

Nutritional practices were evaluated by self reports of intake by food groups (not by calories or nutrients) with a Rapid Eating and Activity Assessment for Patients—Short Version (REAP-S) questionnaire designed for a low literacy level. Significant changes were reported throughout the measurement points.

Improvement in lowering high fat intake and high sugar intake was made; no increase in fruit, vegetable, whole grains, or calcium-source intake was found. Those in groups did not report more change than those trained individually, suggesting that social support did not have a large effect

IMPLICATIONS FOR NURSING

Although wasting is a serious problem for many patients with HIV/AIDS, overweight and obesity are common and may impair quality of life for those living with HIV/AIDS. The researchers in this study observed that when empowered for greater self care, the participants improved their disease conditions. Perhaps the most encouraging aspect of these findings is the effect of brief nutritional information encounters. Nurses can affirm with each interaction that diet and exercise are beneficial and seek to learn the concerns and barriers patients face when attempting to meet their needs. A second and perhaps more urgent implication is the importance of healthy coping and self-care. When patients are discouraged, depressed, and denying the importance of self-care, nurses should help them obtain counseling services to address their needs. Advocating for mental health care is an important nursing intervention.

and the addition of a third drug for higher risk exposure. A 4-week course of treatment is recommended and should be started within 72 hours, preferably within 2 to 3 hours of exposure (Bartlett & Weber, 2005).

The most difficult group of high-risk people to reach and educate has been injection drug users. People in this group should never share needles, syringes, or other drug paraphernalia. Many cities have initiated needle-exchange programs, providing a sterile needle and syringe in exchange for a used one. A fresh solution of household bleach and water in a 1:10 ratio is effective to clean paraphernalia when sterile supplies are not available. It is important to also teach people in this population about safer sex practices, because most heterosexual HIV transmission occurs between injection drug users and their partners.

Screening of voluntary blood donors and donated blood supplies has reduced the risk of transmission by transfusion to 1 in 100,000. Because current blood-screening methods use antibody testing, receiving donated blood continues to carry a small risk. Patients in the *window period* between contraction of the virus and the development of detectable antibodies are able to transmit the virus to others, even though they do not yet test positive for HIV. This window period usually lasts from 6 weeks to 6 months; rarely, it lasts up to 1 year. When possible, encourage patients to use autologous transfusion, donating their own blood prior to an anticipated surgery.

Encourage HIV-positive patients to abstain from donating blood, organs, or sperm. They should understand tactics to avoid exchange of body fluids by not sharing needles or other drug paraphernalia, not sharing razors, and not obtaining a tattoo. Stress the importance of informing all medical personnel providing direct care (especially anyone performing a dental, surgical, or obstetric procedure) about the diagnosis.

Healthcare workers can prevent most exposures to HIV by using standard precautions (∞ refer to Appendix A and see Figure 13–11 ■). Testing to determine HIV status remains voluntary and relies on the use of antibody-screening methods. It is therefore impossible to identify every patient who is HIV positive. With standard precautions, all patients are treated alike, eliminating the need to know the patient's HIV status. All high-risk body fluids are treated as if they are infectious, and barrier precautions are used to prevent skin, mucous membrane, or percutaneous exposure to them. Counseling and testing are provided to healthcare workers with a documented needle-stick exposure. Some clinicians and facilities recommend prophylactic AZT therapy after needle-stick or splash exposure; however, it must be initiated immediately, and its effectiveness has yet to be established.

Assessment

Collect the following data through health history and physical examination. Further focused assessments are described with nursing interventions next.

- *Health history:* Risk factors (transfusion, unprotected sex, needle exposure), infections (sexually transmitted infections, hepatitis, tuberculosis), medications, recreational drug use, foreign travel, pets.
- *Physical assessment:* Height, weight, nutrition, skin and mucous membranes, vision, lymph nodes, breath sounds, abdominal tenderness, motor strength, coordination, cranial nerves, gait, deep tendon reflexes, genitourinary examination, mental status.

Nursing Diagnoses and Interventions

Nursing care needs for the patient with HIV infection change over the course of the disease. Preventive healthcare measures, health maintenance activities, education, and support of coping mechanisms are important in the early stages of the disease. Counseling the patient with a new diagnosis of HIV infection is vital. HIV infection and AIDS continue to carry a social stigma that may interfere with the patient's usual support systems and coping mechanisms. As the disease progresses and the patient experiences more physical symptoms, direct care needs become more important while the need for psychosocial support continues. Acute exacerbation of opportunistic infections may necessitate hospitalization, but typically the patient is managed at home. See the accompanying Nursing Case Study & Care Plan on page 336.

Ineffective Coping

On receiving the test results indicating HIV seropositive status, the person with HIV infection is faced with multiple issues rarely affecting other patients. HIV is a disease for which there is no known cure and which is, at this time, thought to be almost universally fatal. Social support systems, family relationships, and the ability to obtain and retain useful work and

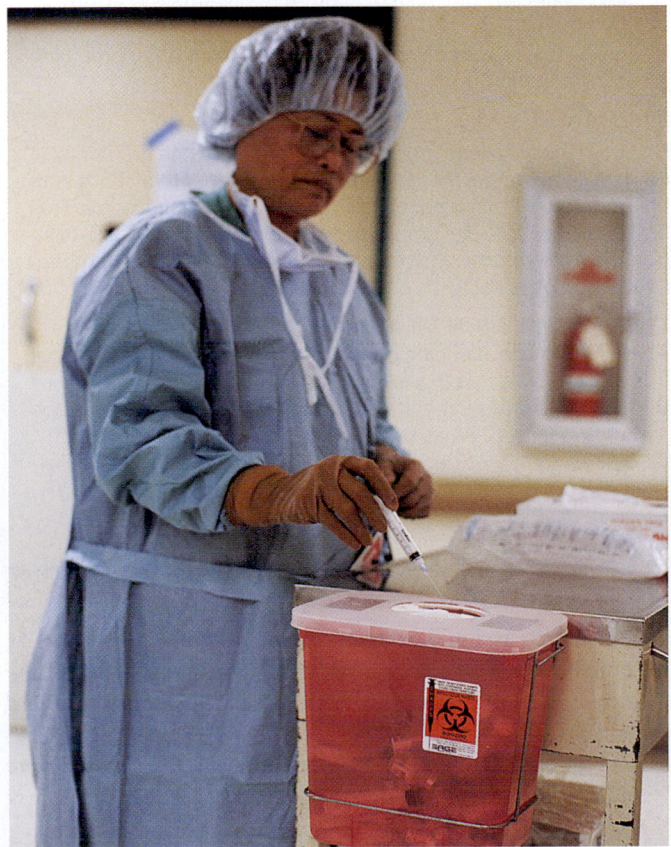

Figure 13–11 ■ This nurse is disposing of a needle and syringe in a special container, a necessary practice to avoid the transmission of HIV through needle sticks with contaminated needles.

CASE STUDY & NURSING CARE PLAN   A Patient with HIV Infection

Sara Lu is a 26-year-old elementary school teacher who lives with her parents and two younger sisters. Ms. Lu is very close to her parents and sisters; they share everything with each other. During the required physical for admission to graduate school, Ms. Lu tells her physician that lately she has felt fatigued. She also states that she has had a persistent sore throat, intermittent bouts of diarrhea, and mild shortness of breath for about a month. She takes no routine medications other than a daily multivitamin and an occasional acetaminophen tablet for a headache. She is active in a drama club in her community, and she jogs 3 miles three to four times a week. She is engaged to be married; her wedding date is 6 months away. Her fiancé is the only person with whom she has had sexual relations. Her sexual activity has been unprotected. Ms. Lu has a history of open heart surgery 7 years ago to correct a congenital valve defect. She has been physically healthy since that time, until about a month or two ago. The physician orders a mononucleosis test, ELISA, Western blot analysis, CD4 T-cell count, a p24 antigen test, and an erythrocyte sedimentation rate (ESR). She has been asked to return in 1 week for follow-up.

ASSESSMENT

On Ms. Lu's follow-up visit, Carole Kee, RN, obtains her nursing history. Ms. Lu continues to have flulike symptoms but has improved somewhat. She states that she just has not been as active as usual and is worried about her health. Her appetite has decreased because of soreness in her mouth, and she has noted some whitish patches on her tongue and cheeks.

A chest x-ray film reveals no abnormality. The results of her laboratory tests are as follows:
- ELISA: positive for antibodies against HIV
- Western blot analysis: positive for antibodies against HIV
- p24 antigen test: positive for circulating HIV antigens
- ESR: increased to 25 mm/h (normal for women is 15 to 20 mm/h; normal for men is 10 to 15 mm/h)
- CD4 T-cell count: 599/mm^3 (normal range is 600 to 1200 mm^3)

Ms. Lu's physical examination reveals that she has enlarged lymph nodes in her neck and white patches on her oral mucosa. Her skin is warm to the touch. Her vital signs are as follows: T 99.9°F (37.7°C), P 84, R 20, and BP 120/78.

Ms. Lu is told of the results of her laboratory tests and the medical diagnosis of HIV infection. Ms. Lu is obviously distressed and wants to know how this happened, its meaning, whether she has infected her loved ones, and whether she will get better.

DIAGNOSES

- *Imbalanced Nutrition: Less than Body Requirements* related to soreness in mouth
- *Risk for Deficient Fluid Volume* related to decreased fluid intake and diarrhea
- *Risk for Infection* related to altered immune protection
- *Anxiety* related to diagnosis and fear

- *Readiness for Enhanced Knowledge* about the HIV disease process and self-care

EXPECTED OUTCOMES

- Maintain adequate nutrition for optimal body and cellular function.
- Consume at least 2500 mL of fluid per day.
- Remain free of infections and their complications.
- Verbalize anxiety and use appropriate coping mechanisms.
- Verbalize and demonstrate knowledge of HIV disease.
- Verbalize measures to prevent HIV transmission to others, including safer sex practices.

PLANNING AND IMPLEMENTATION

- Monitor daily weight and intake and output.
- Monitor dietary habits and serum albumin levels.
- Teach Ms. Lu the importance of consuming a nutritionally balanced diet and maintaining adequate fluid intake.
- Provide dietary consultation referral.
- Encourage oral care before and after meals.
- Assess bowel sounds and monitor elimination pattern.
- Monitor for signs of dehydration, such as poor skin turgor, oliguria, and orthostatic hypotension.
- Increase fluid to 2500 mL daily.
- Use strict aseptic technique for all invasive procedures.
- Teach Ms. Lu to avoid exposure to infection and people with known illnesses.
- Monitor response to prescribed medications.
- Encourage regular physical exercise.
- Provide opportunities for Ms. Lu to verbalize her feelings.
- Avoid false reassurances.
- Provide appropriate and adequate information about HIV/AIDS.
- Teach safer sex practices and other measures to prevent HIV transmission.
- Teach anxiety-controlling techniques, such as deep breathing and meditation.

EVALUATION

Ms. Lu is eager to learn about her illness and wants her family to come with her for further explanation. She states that she is sure her fiancé will be available as well. Ms. Lu is taking home antifungal medication, diet plans, and a schedule for increased exercise. She will return in 1 week for counseling and in 1 month for a follow-up physical.

CRITICAL THINKING IN THE NURSING PROCESS

1. How does age affect the body's response to fighting HIV? What other factors affect the risk of HIV infection and its progression?
2. Are the laboratory results for Ms. Lu a true indication that she is HIV positive? What additional tests might be ordered?
3. Ms. Lu says that her fiancé would like to have a child. How will you counsel her regarding pregnancy and childbearing?

See Evaluating Your Response in Appendix C.

---

health insurance may be disrupted by the disease. The patient may experience guilt about his or her lifestyle and how the disease was contracted. As the disease progresses, social isolation, fatigue, body image changes, medication side effects, and multiple other issues affect the patient's ability to cope.

- Assess social support network and usual methods of coping. *This will help both the nurse and the patient identify people and mechanisms that can help the patient cope more effectively with the disease.*

- If possible, assign a primary nurse, whether the setting is home health, hospice, or acute care. *This helps promote the development of a therapeutic and trusting relationship and provides for continuity of care.*
- Plan for consistent, uninterrupted time with the patient. *Time and a consistent presence encourage the patient to express feelings and work through issues related to HIV infection.*
- Interact at every opportunity outside of providing specific nursing care treatments. *This purposeful interaction communicates caring and acceptance without fear of HIV disease.*

■ Support the patient's social network. *Nontraditional families may offer more support than the traditional family. This in turn may necessitate a liberal interpretation of the term family if unit policy is immediate family only.*

■ Promote interaction between the patient, significant others, and family. *Hospitalization and manifestations of HIV disease may bring about isolation from others and decrease the patient's ability to cope.*

■ Encourage involvement in making care decisions. *This gives the patient a greater sense of self-worth and control over the situation, increasing coping abilities.*

■ Set and maintain limits on manipulative and other destructive behaviors. *The patient who is unable to limit inappropriate behaviors needs the external control established by setting limits.*

■ Assist to accept responsibility for actions without blaming others. *Effective coping cannot occur without accepting responsibility for one's actions.*

■ Support positive coping behaviors, decisions, actions, and achievements. *As self-esteem is enhanced, coping improves* (Côté & Pepler, 2005).

Risk for Situational Low Self-Esteem

■ Assess negative self-evaluation and statements of self-worth. *Statements of self-worth indicate level of self-esteem.*

■ Reinforce personal strengths that are identified. *Focusing on personal strengths enables movement away from negative thoughts.*

■ Assist in setting realistic goals. *Establishing and meeting realistic short-term goals is helpful in increasing self-confidence and decreasing negative self-talk.*

■ Encourage active participation in plan of care. *Active participation reinforces sense of control and independence, increasing self-esteem.*

■ Refer to clergy, social worker, clinical specialist, and/or counselor as appropriate. *Persons with expertise in counseling may be necessary to enable coping with current situation.*

Impaired Skin Integrity

Dryness, malnutrition, immobility from fatigue, and skin lesions on pressure sites contribute to impaired integrity of the skin for the patient with HIV disease. Maintaining skin integrity is important because of the progressive and debilitating nature of the disease. It is also a consideration both as the first line of defense against infection in an immunosuppressed patient and as a site for secondary manifestations such as KS and herpes.

■ Assess the skin frequently for lesions and areas of breakdown. *Early identification of impaired skin integrity allows prompt intervention.*

■ Monitor lesions for signs of infection or impaired healing. *Infection or poor tissue perfusion not only impairs healing but may lead to further skin breakdown.*

■ Turn at least every 2 hours if unable to turn self, more frequently if necessary. *Turning decreases unrelieved pressure on bony prominences and improves circulation to the tissues.*

■ Keep skin clean and dry using mild, nondrying soaps or oils for cleansing. *Night sweats and diarrhea, if present, can cause breakdown and damage to the skin. Frequent cleansing with nondrying products discourages bacterial growth, thus reducing the risk of infection.*

> **PRACTICE ALERT**
> Applying protective creams to reddened areas in the rectal area protects skin from the caustic effects of diarrhea.

■ Massage around but not over affected pressure sites to increase circulation to the surrounding tissue. *Massaging over the affected area can cause skin breakdown.*

■ If blisters are noted, leave intact, and dress with a hydrocolloid (e.g., DuoDERM) dressing. *Blisters provide natural sterile coverings for damaged tissue, improving healing and preventing bacterial invasion.*

■ Caution against scratching. If confused, trim fingernails and use mitts or soft restraints to prevent scratching. Check for circulation of hands and fingers frequently if mitts or restraints are used. *Scratching and skin damage allow bacteria to be introduced into lesions, increasing the risk of infection. Tight or restrictive restraints or mitts may compromise circulation.*

■ Avoid the use of heat or occlusive dressings. *Heat can further dry and damage the skin; occlusive dressings may impair circulation and lead to ulceration.*

■ Prevent skin shearing by using a turnsheet and adequate personnel when repositioning. *Shearing causes tissue trauma that can lead to decubitus ulcers.*

■ Encourage ambulation if possible; if the patient is confined to bed, encourage active or passive range-of-motion exercises. *Activity increases circulation, decreases pressure and skin breakdown, and helps maintain muscle tone.*

■ Monitor nutritional intake and albumin levels. *Maintenance of optimal nutrition decreases the risk of tissue breakdown and improves resistance to infection.*

Imbalanced Nutrition: Less than Body Requirements

Many factors associated with HIV disease, including manifestations of the disease itself, put the patient at risk for altered nutrition and weight loss. Nausea and anorexia may be manifestations of the disease or the result of antiretroviral therapy. Chronic diarrhea is a common manifestation of HIV disease. Wasting syndrome is also common. It is manifested by involuntary weight loss of greater than 10% to 15% of baseline weight, severe diarrhea, fever, and chronic fatigue and weakness. The exact cause of wasting syndrome is unclear, but the diarrhea and fatigue contribute, as does the increased metabolic rate associated with fever. Oral and esophageal candidiasis and KS of the gastrointestinal tract may cause painful swallowing, making eating difficult and thereby contributing to anorexia. Poor nutritional status in the patient with HIV can ultimately result in altered comfort, a change in body image, muscle wasting, increased risk of infection, and higher mortality and morbidity.

■ Assess nutritional status, including weight; body mass; caloric intake; and laboratory studies, such as total protein and albumin levels, hemoglobin, and hematocrit. *These factors provide a baseline to determine the effectiveness of interventions.*

■ Identify possible causes of altered nutrition. *Identification of causes provides direction for planned interventions.*

■ Administer prescribed medications for candidiasis and other manifestations as prescribed. *Eliminating this opportunistic infection improves comfort and facilitates food intake. Topical viscous anesthetic can help reduce pain and improve oral intake.*

■ Administer antidiarrheal medications after stools and antiemetics prior to meals. Provide antipyretics as needed to control fever. *Reducing diarrhea will improve nutrient absorption; preprandial medication with an antiemetic reduces nausea and improves food intake. Reduction of fever lowers the body's metabolic demands.*

> **PRACTICE ALERT**
> High-fiber foods can increase intestinal motility and the incidence of diarrhea.

■ Provide a diet high in protein and kilocalories. *A high-protein, high-kilocalorie diet provides the necessary nutrients to meet metabolic and tissue healing needs.*

■ Offer soft foods and serve small portions. *Soft foods are easily digested. Small portions are more appealing to the anorectic or nauseated patient.*

■ Involve in meal planning and encourage significant others to bring favorite foods from home. *The patient is more likely to consume adequate amounts of preferred foods. Allowing food choices enhances the patient's sense of control.*

■ Assist with eating as needed. *Fatigue and weakness can prevent the patient from eating an adequate amount of food.*

■ Provide supplementary vitamins and enteral feedings, such as Ensure. *This improves nutritional status and caloric intake.*

■ Provide or assist with frequent oral hygiene. *Oral hygiene improves comfort and appetite, and reduces the risk of mucosal lesions.*

■ Administer appetite stimulants, such as megestrol (Megace) and dronabinol (Marinol) as ordered. *Both drugs may increase appetite and promote weight gain.*

Ineffective Sexuality Pattern

The diagnosis of HIV infection can significantly alter the patient's expressions of sexuality. Guilt over the diagnosis may interfere with libido. The patient may be angry with a significant other or partner if that person was the probable source of infection. The patient may fear spreading the disease to others via sexual relations. As the disease progresses, its manifestations can affect body image and self-esteem, impairing sexuality. Other symptoms, such as nausea, fatigue, and weakness, may also interfere with libido and sexual satisfaction. If nurses are not comfortable discussing sexuality, referral to an appropriate counselor is appropriate.

■ Examine own feelings about sexuality, role in dealing with a patient's sexuality, the patient's lifestyle, and sexual preferences. *To deal effectively with the patient's concerns, it is vital that the nurse be comfortable with his or her own feelings of sexuality and be able to accept the patient's lifestyle. Referring the patient to another nurse or counselor may be necessary.*

■ Establish a trusting, therapeutic relationship through the use of time, active listening, caring, and self-disclosure. Maintain a nonthreatening, nonjudgmental attitude toward the patient.

Sexuality is a private issue that will be uncomfortable or impossible for the nurse and patient to discuss without a mutually trusting relationship.

■ Provide factual information about HIV infection and its effects. *This helps the patient separate fears and myths from reality.*

■ Discuss safer sex practices, including hugging, cuddling, nonsexual contact, the use of latex condoms and spermicidal lubricant, and mutual masturbation. *Alternative forms of sexual activity and expressing affection can allow the patient and significant other to remain close throughout the course of the disease.*

■ Encourage discussion of fears and concerns with significant other. *Open communication helps him or her to deal with issues related to sexuality.*

■ For the patient without a significant other, stress the need to continue to meet people and develop social relationships while practicing safer sex. *The risk of isolation is high in the patient with HIV infection, and relationships with others help the patient to cope with the disease.*

■ Refer the patient and significant other to local support groups for people and partners of people with HIV. *Support groups provide a social and support network of people facing the same issues.*

Using NANDA, NIC, and NOC

Linkages between a selected NANDA nursing diagnosis, NIC, and NOC for the patient with an HIV infection are shown in the chart that follows.

Community-Based Care

Teaching needs for both the patient and significant other are extensive. The primary need is information about the disease, its spread, and its expected course. The patient and family need current factual information to plan realistically and to combat myths, misperceptions, and prejudices. At the same time, it is important to include information about current research and progress in treating the disease to maintain a sense of hopefulness.

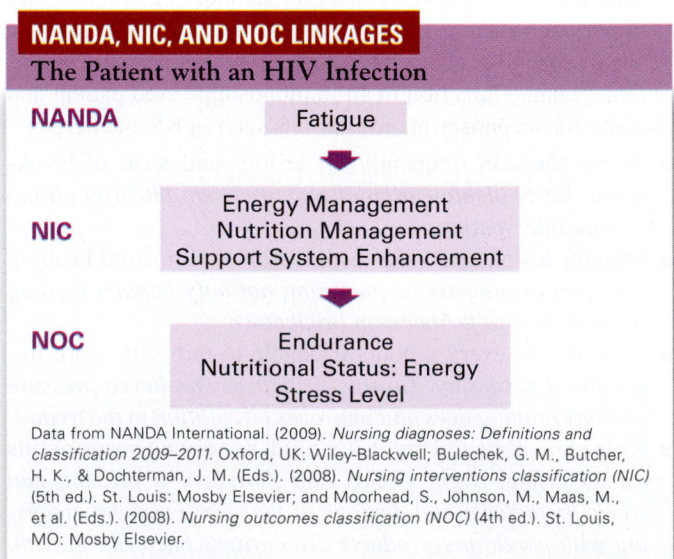

NANDA, NIC, AND NOC LINKAGES
The Patient with an HIV Infection

NANDA	Fatigue
NIC	Energy Management Nutrition Management Support System Enhancement
NOC	Endurance Nutritional Status: Energy Stress Level

Data from NANDA International. (2009). *Nursing diagnoses: Definitions and classification 2009–2011.* Oxford, UK: Wiley-Blackwell; Bulechek, G. M., Butcher, H. K., & Dochterman, J. M. (Eds.). (2008). *Nursing interventions classification (NIC)* (5th ed.). St. Louis: Mosby Elsevier; and Moorhead, S., Johnson, M., Maas, M., et al. (Eds.). (2008). *Nursing outcomes classification (NOC)* (4th ed.). St. Louis, MO: Mosby Elsevier.

The following topics should be discussed with the patient and family to prepare for home care:

- Guidelines for safer sex practices
- Nutrition, rest and exercise, stress reduction, lifestyle changes, and maintaining a positive outlook
- Infection prevention and transmission including hand hygiene and wearing gloves when handling patient's secretions or excretions
- Importance of regular medical follow-up and monitoring of immune status
- Signs and symptoms of opportunistic infections and malignancies, as well as other symptoms that should be reported
- Medications and adverse effects

- Use and care of implanted venous access devices, total parenteral nutrition, intravenous pumps and continuous medication delivery systems, and intravenous or aerosolized medications
- Cessation of smoking, alcohol, and recreational or illicit drug use
- Home health services
- Hospice and respite care services
- Community resources, such as support groups, social agencies, and counselors
- Helpful resources:
  - CDC National AIDS Hotline
  - Gay Men's Health Crisis Network
  - National Association of People with AIDS
  - National Organization on HIV over Fifty

CHAPTER HIGHLIGHTS

- The immune system is a complex combination of cellular and humoral components that protect against disease. Immunity develops when the body recognizes foreign proteins as "nonself" and develops nonspecific inflammatory responses and specific cellular responses to each foreign antigen.
- Patients suffer when the immune system is excessively or inadequately responsive, or when recognition of self fails and reactions escalate against self. The latter occurs in autoimmune diseases.
- With aging, there is a general decline in the sensitivity and regulation of the immune system, which may result in autoimmune disease.
- Hypersensitivities are excessive responses to antigens that result in harm to the patient. These range from benign to severely life threatening. Damage to host tissue is caused by chemicals of the immune response, destruction of cells, or creation of large antigen–antibody complexes that accumulate in the kidney glomerular capillaries.
- Allergic reactions are treated pharmacologically to prevent or moderate allergic responses. Another method of dampening allergic responses is by desensitization, a weekly process of introducing increasing amounts of known allergens subdermally.
- Patients must be taught that the safest practice is to avoid contact with all known allergens.
- Latex allergy is a problem for healthcare professionals. Repeated exposure to latex-containing equipment and gloves results in delayed hypersensitivity.

- Any type of allergic reaction has the potential to escalate to anaphylaxis. Respiratory arrest and cardiac failure are risks with full blown allergic reactions. Nurses must recognize early signs and symptoms and immediately signal for emergency care.
- Intentional immunosuppression is an essential step in preventing transplant rejection. The patient receiving a transplanted organ will be treated with immune-suppressing drugs to prevent initial rejection, to maintain the transplant, and to halt any rejection process that may develop. Patients will take the immune-suppressing, antirejection drugs for their lifetime. The drugs prevent cytokine production that upregulates an immune reaction and targets the transplanted organ. Most immunosuppressing drugs are nephrotoxic; immunosuppression places patients at greater risk for infection and cancers.
- HIV/AIDS continues to spread and many patients are unaware they have the virus. AIDS is a profoundly immune-suppressed condition that results from viral destruction of cellular components of host immunity.
- A major change in the AIDS epidemic is the disease profile, which has benefited from HAART. HAART is a combination of drugs that limits viral replication and host susceptibility to opportunistic infections and cancer. Patients are living much longer with the disease without progression to AIDS. The number of pills needed has decreased significantly by pharmaceutical combinations, but side effects of the combination of drugs that make up HAART are appearing as patients live longer.

TEST YOURSELF NCLEX-RN® REVIEW

1. Which one of the following conditions is caused by a type I IgE-mediated hypersensitivity reaction?
   1. autoimmune hemolytic anemia
   2. systemic lupus erythematosus
   3. graft rejection
   4. anaphylaxis
2. A patient received a liver transplant 1 day ago. If the patient were to develop an acute transplant rejection episode, when should the nurse expect to see the manifestations?
   1. approximately 4 days to 3 months later
   2. approximately 2 days later
   3. within the first 24 hours
   4. within the first 8 hours

3. The nurse notes a cough, shortness of breath, and tachypnea in a patient with AIDS. Which opportunistic infection is probably causing these manifestations?
   1. *Toxoplasma gondii*
   2. cytomegalovirus
   3. *Pneumocystis jiroveci*
   4. *Cryptococcus neoformans*
4. Which of the following explanations should the nurse give to a patient who has tested positive for HIV?
   1. "You have been diagnosed with AIDS."
   2. "At this point, AIDS is not active in your blood."
   3. "This means that you will not develop AIDS in the future."
   4. "Antibodies to the AIDS virus are present in the blood."

5. A patient is taking zidovudine (Retrovir). What would the nurse monitor to identify adverse reactions?
   1. cardiotoxicity
   2. leukopenia
   3. nephrotoxicity
   4. polycythemia

6. The order of administering antigens in allergy testing is based on prevention of anaphylaxis. Which method would a nurse expect to be used first?
   1. inhalation
   2. prick test
   3. intradermal injection
   4. subcutaneous injection

7. A hypersensitivity response is suspected when blood products are infusing. What priority intervention would the nurse perform?
   1. Discard the product immediately.
   2. Replace all tubing and attach a new line with NS.
   3. Backflush the line and run the NS attached at the Y tubing.
   4. Remove the intravenous catheter and establish access distal to the site.

8. Protease inhibitors and nucleoside analogs share correlations to metabolic abnormalities including which of the following?
   1. lactose intolerance
   2. diabetes mellitus
   3. Hashimoto's thyroiditis
   4. systemic lupus erythematosus

9. The priority when initiating or changing HIV drug therapy regimens is which of the following?
   1. cost of therapy
   2. access to dental care
   3. toxicities associated with each drug
   4. patient willingness to adhere to the drug regimen

10. Patients receiving kidney transplants will receive immunosuppressant therapy. What agent is used to induce immunosuppression immediately following a transplant?
    1. azathioprine
    2. corticosteroids
    3. muromonab-CD3
    4. antithymocyte globulin

See Test Yourself answers in Appendix C.

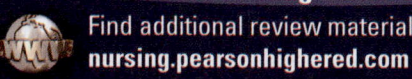

Pearson Nursing Student Resources

Find additional review materials at
nursing.pearsonhighered.com

Prepare for success with additional NCLEX®-style practice questions, interactive assignments and activities, Web links, animations and videos, and more!

BIBLIOGRAPHY

AIDS InfoNet. (2008). *Tropism tests.* Retrieved from http://www.aidsinfonet.org/fact_sheets/view/129

AIDSinfo. (2008). *AIDSinfo Drug Database.* US Department of Health and Human Services. Retrieved from http://www.aidsinfo.nih.gov/DrugsNew/Default.aspx?MenuItem=Drugs&Search=On

American Association for Clinical Chemistry. (2006). Lab Tests Online. Retrieved from http://www.labtestsonline.org/understanding/analytes/allergy/test.html

Bova, C. A., Fennie, K. P., Knafl, G. J., Dieckhaus, K. D., Wtrous, E., & Williams, A. B. (2005). Use of electronic monitoring devices to measure antiretroviral adherence: Practical considerations. *AIDS and Behavior, 9*(1), 103–110.

Branson, B. M. (2008). *Expanded HIV Testing—Implementing the CDC Recommendations: Guidance for Nurses.* Retrieved from http://www.medscape.com/viewarticle/572177

Bulechek, G. M., Butcher, H. K., & Dochterman, J. M. (Eds.). (2008). *Nursing interventions classification (NIC)* (5th ed.). St. Louis: Mosby Elsevier.

Centers for Disease Control and Prevention. (2006). Revised recommendations for HIV testing of adults, adolescents, and pregnant women in health-care settings. Retrieved from http://www.cdc.gov/mmwR/preview/mmwrhtml/rr5514a1.htm

Centers for Disease Control and Prevention. (2007). National Center for Chronic Disease Prevention and Health Promotion: Food Allergies. Retrieved from http://www.cdc.gov/HealthyYouth/foodallergies/

Centers for Disease Control and Prevention. (2008). HIV/AIDS. Retrieved from http://www.cdc.gov/hiv/topics/surveillance/.htm

Côté J. K., & Pepler, C. (2005). Cognitive coping intervention for acutely ill HIV-positive men. *Journal of Clinical Nursing, 14*(3), 321–326.

Department of Health and Human Services. (2008). *Panel on antiretroviral guidelines for adults and adolescents. Guidelines for the use of antiretroviral agents in HIV-1 infected adults and adolescents.* Retrieved from http://www.aidsinfo.nih.gov/ContentFiles/AdultandAdolescentGL.pdf

Fauci, A., Braunwald, E., Kasper, D., Hauser, S., Longo, D., Jameson, J., et al. (2008). *Harrison's principles of internal medicine* (17th ed.). New York, NY: McGraw Hill.

Hakin, F. T., & Gress, R. E. (2007). Immunosenescence: deficits in adaptive immunity in the elderly. *Tissue Antigens, 70*(3), 179–189.

Hammer, S. M., Eron, J. J., Reiss, P., Schooley, R. T., Thompson, M. A., Walmsley, S., Cahn, P., Fischl, M. A., Gatell, J. M., Hirsch, M. S., Jacobsen, D. M., Montaner, J. S., Richman, D. D., Yeni, P. G., & Volberding, P. A. (2008). Antiretroviral treatment of adult HIV infection; 2008 recommendations of the International AIDS Society—USA Panel. *Journal of the American Medical Association, 300*(5), 555–570.

Ingersoll, K. S., & Heckman, C. J. (2005). Patient-clinician relationships and treatment system effects on HIV medication adherence. *AIDS and Behavior, 9*(1), 89–101.

Kee, J. L. (2009). Prentice Hall handbook of laboratory and diagnostic tests with nursing implications. Upper Saddle River, NJ: Pearson Prentice Hall.

King, H. C., Mabry, R. L., Mabry, C. S., Gordon, B. R., & Marple, B. F. (2005). *Allergy in ENT practice: The basic guide* (2nd ed.). New York: Thieme Medical Publisher.

Kirton, C.A. (2008). Managing long-term complications of HIV. *Nursing, 38*(8), 44–50.

Kirton, C. A., & Stevens, L. C. (2008). *Implementing a rapid HIV testing program in the acute care setting: Nurses take the lead.* Retrieved from http://www.medscape.com/viewarticle/572180

Knoll, B., Lassmann, B., & Temesgen, Z. (2007). Current status of HIV infection: A review for non-HIV-treating physicians. *International Journal of Dermatology, 46*(12), 1219–1228.

Langkamp-Henken, B., Wood, S. M., Herlinger-Garcia, K. A., Thomas, D. J., Stechmiller, J. K., Bender, B. S., Gardner, E. M., DeMichele, S. J., Schaller, J. P., & Murasko, D. M. (2006). Nutritional formula improved immune profiles of seniors living in nursing homes. *Journal of the American Geriatric Society, 54*(12), 1861–1870.

McPhee, S. J., & Papadakis, M. (Eds.). (2009). *Current medical diagnosis & treatment* (48th ed.). New York: Lange-McGraw-Hill.

Moorhead, S., Johnson, M., Maas, M., & Swanson, E. (Eds.). (2008). *Nursing outcomes classification (NOC)* (4th ed.). St. Louis, MO: Mosby Elsevier.

NANDA International. (2009). *Nursing diagnoses: Definitions and classification 2009–2011.* Oxford, UK: Wiley-Blackwell.

Porth, C. M. (2007). *Essentials of pathophysiology: Concepts of altered health states* (2nd ed.). Philadelphia: Lippincott Williams & Wilkins.

Porth, C. M., & Matfin, G. (2009). *Pathophysiology: Concepts of altered health states.* (8th ed.). Philadelphia: Lippincott Williams & Wilkins.

Rana, A., Robles, S., Russo, M. J., Halazun, K. J., Woodland, D. C., Witkowski, P., Ratner, L. E., & Hardy, M. A. (2008). The combined organ effect: Protection against rejection? *Annals of Surgery, 248*(5), 871–879.

Robinson, F. P. (2005). Body composition changes in patients with HIV. *American Journal of Nursing, 105*(13), 69–72.

Salifu, M.O., Pani, S., & Misra, N. (2007). *HIV Nephropathy.* Retrieved from http://www.emedicine.com/med/TOPIC3203.HTM

Segal-Issacson, C., Tobin, J., Weiss, S., Brondolo, E., Vaughn, A., Wang, C., Camille, J., Gousse, Y., Ishii, M., Jones, D., LaPerriere, A., Lydston, D., Schneiderman, N., & Ironson, G. (2006). Improving dietary habits in disadvantaged women with HIV/AIDS: The SMART/EST women's project. *AIDS Behavior, 10*(5), 659–670.

Smith, A. M., Amin, H. S., Biagini, R. E., Hamilton, R. G., Arif, S. A., Yeang, H. Y., & Bernstein, D. I. (2007). Percutaneous reactivity to natural rubber latex proteins persists in health-care workers following avoidance of natural rubber latex. *Clinical & Experimental Allergy, 37*(9), 1349–1356.

Walensky, R. P., Paltiel, A. D., Losina, E., Mercincavage, L. M., Schackman, B. R., Sax, P. E., Weinstein, M. C., & Freedberg, K. A. (2006). The survival benefits of AIDS Treatment in the United States. *Journal of Infectious disease, 194*(1), 11–19.

WebMd. (2009). Allergy testing. Retrieved from http://www.webmd.com/allergies/allergy-tests

Wilkinson, J. M. (2008). *Nursing diagnosis handbook.* (9th ed.). Upper Saddle River, NJ: Pearson Prentice Hall.

Wilson, B., Shannon, M., & Shields, K. (2009). *Prentice Hall nurse's drug guide 2009.* Upper Saddle River, NJ: Pearson Prentice Hall.

Nursing Care of Patients with Cancer

LEARNING OUTCOMES

1. Define cancer and differentiate benign from malignant neoplasm.
2. Describe the theories of carcinogenesis.
3. Explain known carcinogens and identify risk factors for cancer.
4. Compare the mechanisms and characteristics of normal cells with those of malignant cells.
5. Describe physical and psychological effects of cancer.
6. Describe and compare laboratory and diagnostic tests for cancer.
7. Discuss the role of chemotherapy in cancer treatment and classify chemotherapeutic agents.
8. Compare and contrast the role of surgery, radiation therapy, and biotherapy in the treatment of cancer.
9. Explain causes and discuss the nursing interventions for common oncologic emergencies.
10. Design an appropriate care plan for patients with cancer and their families regarding cancer diagnosis, treatment, and coping strategies.

CLINICAL COMPETENCIES

1. Assess functional health status of patients with cancer, and monitor, document, and report abnormal manifestations.
2. Incorporate evidence-based research into the plan of nursing care for patients with cancer.
3. Prioritize nursing diagnosis based on assessment data and implement appropriate nursing interventions for patients with cancer during cancer diagnosis, treatment, and rehabilitation.
4. Safely administer medications for pain, nausea and vomiting, mucositis, or anemia.
5. Use the nursing process as a framework for planning and providing individualized care and integrating interdisciplinary care for patients with cancer to meet their healthcare needs.
6. Include cultural variation and diverse values in designing and implementing individualized plans of care for patients with cancer.
7. Design and provide individualized patient and family teaching to restore, promote, and maintain patients' functional status.
8. Revise plan of care as needed to provide effective interventions for patients with cancer and their families.

KEY TERMS

anaplasia, 346
biotherapy, 365
brachytherapy, 365
cachexia, 351
cancer, 341
carcinogenesis, 346
carcinogens, 346
cell cycle, 346

chemotherapy, 360
differentiation, 346
dysplasia, 346
hospice, 380
hyperplasia, 346
metaplasia, 346
metastasis, 348
neoplasm, 348

oncogene, 346
oncologic emergencies, 376
oncology, 342
proto-oncogenes, 346
radiation therapy, 364
tumor marker, 355
xerostomia, 375

Cancer is a group of complex diseases characterized by uncontrolled growth and spread of abnormal cells (American Cancer Society [ACS], 2010a). Cancer can manifest in different ways depending on which body system is affected and the type of tumor cells involved. Cancer can affect people of any age, gender, ethnicity, or geographic region. Although the incidence and mortality rates of cancer have continued to decline since 1990, it remains one of the most feared diseases (ACS, 2010a). The fear engendered by even the suggestion of a cancer diagnosis often evokes feelings of hopelessness and helplessness (Fu, Xu, Liu, & Haber, 2008).

This chapter focuses on the general pathogenesis, pathophysiology, and etiology of cancer; identifies current diagnostic and treatment modalities; and discusses nursing care appropriate for patients with cancer. Discussions of cancers that affect specific body systems can be found in corresponding disorders chapters in the text.

Cancer occurs when normal cells mutate into abnormal cells with uncontrolled growth and spread in the body. Cancer can affect any body tissue. Nursing care of the patient with cancer is holistic and comprehensive, focusing on cancer as not one single disease, but as a constellation of many diseases. The nurse recognizes that cancer is a disruptive and life-threatening process affecting not only the person who is diagnosed with cancer, but also his or her significant others and family members. Nursing interventions are based on the understanding that cancer is a chronic disease with acute episodes, and that the patient is often treated with a combination of treatment modalities and in outpatient settings. Equally important, the nurse recognizes that caring for the patient with cancer involves prevention, early detection, risk reduction, treatment, patient education and counseling, long-term follow-up and rehabilitation, and comprehensive symptom management and palliation (Oncology Nursing Society [ONS], 2009).

Oncology is the study of cancer. The term is derived from the Greek word *oncoma* ("bulk"). Oncologists specialize in caring for patients with cancer; they may be medical doctors, surgeons, radiologists, immunologists, or researchers. The oncology nurse is an important and significant member of the oncology team. Oncology nurses are nurses who have received specialized training in cancer care and treatment. They have special skills in assisting the patient and family with physical and psychosocial issues associated with cancer, treatment, and palliation (ONS, 2009). Collaboration among healthcare professionals (e.g., surgeons, oncologists, nurses, social workers) ensures the most effective care and treatment for the patient with cancer.

Incidence and Mortality

In the United States, cancer is the second most common cause of death and about 1,529,560 new cancer cases are expected to be diagnosed in 2010 (ACS, 2010a). One in every four deaths in the United States is caused by cancer and more than 1500 people die of cancer each day (ACS, 2010a). Mortality rates for different cancers vary. Lung cancer remains the leading cause of all cancer deaths in both men and women, accounting for approximately 28% of all cancer deaths (ACS, 2010a).

Due to advances in cancer prevention, early detection, and treatment, the 5-year survival rate for individuals with cancers continues to improve in the United States. However, minority ethnic groups such as African American and Asian American populations have a disproportionate burden of cancer. African Americans have the highest mortality rate for all cancers and major cancers among all ethnic groups (ACS, 2010). For example, although breast cancer occurs more commonly in Caucasian women than in African American women, the survival rate is 90% for Caucasian women compared to only 77% for African Americans; breast cancer death rates are 32% higher in African American women than in White women (ACS, 2010). Similar disparities are seen in survival rates for colorectal, prostate, and endometrial cancers in these ethnic groups. Research has shown

that lack of health insurance, lower incomes, unequal access to health care, knowledge deficit, and cultural beliefs and attitudes are influential factors contributing to cancer disparity among African Americans (Ward et al., 2008). The Black–White disparity in overall cancer death rates have decreased from the early 1990s through 2004, especially in men. This reduction in disparity may be due to more rapid decreases in mortality from tobacco-related cancers in Black men than White men (DeLancey, Thun, Jemal, & Ward, 2008).

For information about diversity, cancer risk, and incidence see the accompanying Focus on Cultural Diversity box.

FAST FACTS

Cancer in the United States

- Breast cancer is the most frequently diagnosed cancer in women, with an estimated incidence of 207,090 new cases in 2010.
- Prostate cancer is the most frequently occurring cancer in men, with an estimated incidence of 217,730 new cases during 2010. The incidence rates of prostate cancer are significantly higher in African American men than in White men.
- Melanoma occurs mainly among Whites; the incidence rates are more than 10 times higher than African Americans.
- The incidence of bladder cancer is about four times higher in men than in women, and almost two times higher in Whites than in African Americans.

Source: American Cancer Society. (2010a). *Cancer facts and figures—2010*. Atlanta: Author.

Risk Factors

Risk factors are factors that make an individual or a population vulnerable to a specific disease or other unhealthy outcome. Risk factors can be divided into those that are controllable and those that are not controllable. Knowledge and assessment of risk factors are especially important in counseling patients and families about measures to prevent cancer. Figure 14–1 ■ summarizes the interaction of factors that promote cancer.

Heredity

It is estimated that 5% of all cancers have a strong hereditary component (ACS, 2010a). The familial pattern of some breast and colon cancers has been well documented. Lung, ovarian, and prostate cancers have also shown some familial relationships.

FOCUS ON CULTURAL DIVERSITY
Risk and Incidence of Cancer

- Hispanics have higher rates of cancers associated with infection, such as uterine, cervix, liver, and stomach.
- The incidence of liver cancer is almost twice as high in Hispanics compared to non-Hispanic Whites.
- African Americans are more likely to develop cancer than any other ethnic or racial group in the United States.
- African Americans have the highest death rate and shortest survival of any racial and ethnic group in the United States for most cancers.
- African Americans have the highest incidence and mortality for colorectal and lung cancers.
- Breast cancer occurrence is about 10% lower in African American women than in White women, but the mortality rate is approximately 37% higher.
- African American men are at least 59% more likely to develop prostate cancer than men of any other ethnic or racial group.
- Cancer incidence and mortality are lower in Native American men and women than in any other ethnic or racial group.

Sources: American Cancer Society. (2010a). *Cancer facts and figures—2009*. Atlanta: Author. American Cancer Society. (20010b). *Cancer facts and figures for African Americans—2009–2010*. Atlanta: Author. American Cancer Society. (2010c). *Cancer facts and figures for Hispanics/Latinos—2009–2010*. Atlanta: Author.

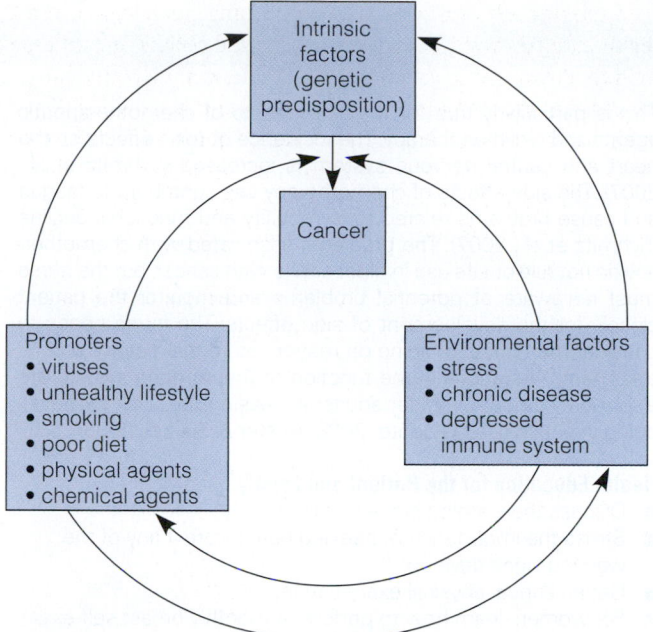

Figure 14–1 ■ Interaction of factors that promote cancer. Most people have immune systems that are competent enough to resist the establishment of cancer from an initiated cell. Cancer takes hold when a number of promotional factors occur together and over enough time to weaken immune resistance. Like factors are grouped together for ease of presentation but may occur in any combination.

The Human Genome Project has identified 50,000 genetic mutations linked to cancer through examination of 4,800 genes and 250,000 tumors (Forbes et al., 2008). For most cancers, research has yet to distinguish true genetic transfer from environmental causes. Although further research is needed to identify cancers that are due to the inheritance of defective genes, familial predisposition to malignancies should be counted among risk factors so that people at risk can reduce behaviors that promote cancer. For example, a patient with a family history of lung cancer should be counseled to avoid smoking, to avoid areas where smoking is allowed, and to avoid working in an occupation that may expose the patient to inhaled carcinogens.

Age

Cancer is a disease associated with aging; about 78% of cancer diagnoses occur after age 55 (ACS, 2010a). A number of factors are associated with this increased risk in older adults. One possible factor is that at least five cycles of genetic mutations seem necessary to cause permanent damage to the afflicted cells. In addition, long-term exposure to high doses of promotional agents is usually necessary to allow the cancer to take hold. In addition, poor overall immune response accompanies aging as a result of a progressive and overall diminution of immune functions that affect all cells and organs of the innate and adaptive immune system (Pfister & Savino, 2008). Another problem is that free radicals (molecules resulting from the body's metabolic and oxidative processes) tend to accumulate in the cells over time. Thus, with aging, the immune cells show an increase in oxidant and inflammatory compounds and a decrease in antioxidant defenses, causing cellular damage and mutation (De la Fuente, 2008).

Hormonal changes that occur with aging can be associated with cancer. Postmenopausal women receiving exogenous estrogen have an increased risk for breast and uterine cancers. Older men are at risk for prostate cancer, possibly due to breakdown of testosterone into carcinogenic forms. See the Nursing Care of the Older Adult box on page 344 for a discussion about older adults and cancer.

Stress resulting from severe and/or cumulative losses also is implicated in promoting cancer (Bauer, 2008). These losses, which are common to older adults, include the death of a spouse or friends, loss of position and status in society, and a decline in physical abilities. These repeated stressors are related to changes in the immune system that may lead to the development of cancer.

Gender

Gender is a risk factor for certain types of cancer. Breast cancer is the most frequently diagnosed cancer in women; prostate cancer in men. The incidence of bladder cancer is about four times higher in men than in women (ACS, 2010a). Thyroid cancer occurs more commonly among females, whereas bladder cancer is seen more often among males (ACS, 2010a). ∞ See Chapters 48 and 49 for more information on gender-specific cancers.

Poverty

The poor are at higher risk for cancer than the population in general. Lack of health insurance and inadequate access to health care, especially preventive screening and counseling, may be major factors (ACS, 2010a). Although other factors that may be involved, such as diet and stress, usually come under the category of controllable risks, these risks are frequently uncontrollable in this population.

Stress

Continuous unmanaged stress that keeps hormones such as epinephrine and cortisol at high levels can result in systematic "fatigue" and impaired immunologic surveillance. When the body attempts to adapt to physiologic and psychologic stressors, it goes through a series of stages called the general adaptation syndrome (Bauer, 2008). First, the "alarm reaction" occurs, in which adrenal hormones increase, allowing the body to cope with the stressor. Eventually, the body reaches the "stage of resistance," in which the stress hormones are significantly reduced, indicating that adaptation has occurred. If the physiologic adaptation is supported by appropriate coping strategies, the stressor is considered managed and body systems return to prealarm functioning. However, if adaptation continues and the stress hormones remain elevated, the "stage of exhaustion" sets in. This stage will maintain life, but at great expense to body systems, resulting in general wear-and-tear and depression of the immune system (Armaiz-Pena, Lutgendorf, Cole, & Sood, 2009).

Diet

Dietary factors appear to be one of the most important factors for cancer risk. A diet that is high in red meat and saturated fat appears to increase risk. Vegetables, fruits, fiber, folate, and calcium may be protective (ACS, 2010a). Some foods are considered genotoxic, such as the nitrosamines and nitrous indoles (a crystalline alkaloid compound) found in preserved meats and pickled, salted foods. Other foods, such as high-fat, low-fiber

NURSING CARE OF THE OLDER ADULT   Older Adults with Cancer

Nurses need to be aware of how cancer and cancer treatments affect older adults. Cancer is the second leading cause of death in people over age 65 (ACS, 2010a). The incidence of cancer increases with advancing age, probably as a result of the accumulated exposure to carcinogens and to age-related declines in the action of the immune system (De la Fuente, 2008; Pfister & Savino, 2008). The most commonly seen cancers in older women are colorectal, breast, lung, pancreatic, and ovarian. In older men, lung, colorectal, prostate, pancreatic, and gastric cancers occur most frequently.

The importance of screening and early detection of cancer does not diminish with age. Unfortunately, older adults may be less likely to undergo cancer screening or seek treatment for cancer due to fear, depression, cognitive impairments, poor access to health care, or financial constraints (Sheinfeld et al., 2008). Some older adults (and healthcare providers) mistake cancer symptoms for normal age-related changes. Believing that little can be done, they do not seek health care for their symptoms. Fear of the cancer diagnosis also keeps older adults from seeking appropriate health care. When they do seek treatment, chronic conditions frequently seen in older adults may make the diagnosis of cancer more difficult by masking or confounding the usual symptoms associated with cancer.

Older adults are at greater risk for side effects associated with cancer treatment because of age-related physiologic changes and chronic conditions associated with aging (Schmitz et al., 2007).

This is particularly true for the side effects of chemotherapeutic agents and radiation therapy. The incidence of toxic effects on the heart and central nervous system is increased (Schmitz et al., 2007). The side effects of chemotherapy can contribute to fatigue and cause problems related to immobility and functional decline (Schmitz et al., 2007). The problems associated with chemotherapy do not rule out its use in older adults with cancer, but the nurse must be aware of potential problems and monitor the patient closely for the development of side effects. The nurse needs to consider the effects of aging on responses to the disease and its treatment. Alterations in the function of the immune system are also more frequent in older adults, increasing their risk for developing infection (De la Fuente, 2008; Pfister & Savino, 2008).

Health Education for the Patient and Family

- Discuss the warning signs of cancer.
- Stress the importance of seeking health care if any of the warning signs develop.
- Get an annual physical examination.
- For women, learn how to perform a monthly breast self-exam (BSE) and emphasize the importance of continuing BSE and regular mammography after menopause.
- Teach men the early signs of prostate cancer, and encourage them to have an annual digital rectal exam.

---

foods—the mainstay of many American diets—promote colon, breast, and sex hormone–dependent tumors. When fish and meat are excessively fried or broiled, potent carcinogenic compounds can form that may cause tumors in the mammary glands, colon, liver, pancreas, and bladder. Also, repeatedly using fat to fry foods at high temperatures produces high levels of polycyclic hydrocarbons, which increase cancer risk considerably. Other food-related substances believed to increase cancer risk include sodium saccharine, red food dyes, and both regular and decaffeinated coffee.

Occupation

Occupational risk might be considered to be either controllable or uncontrollable. For many people, both education and ability limit their choice of occupation; during times of high unemployment, moreover, changing one's occupation because it poses risk factors may not be a viable option. Federal standards are designed to protect workers from hazardous substances, but many believe that these standards are not strict enough and that inspections are not frequent enough to prevent violations.

Specific risks vary according to the occupation. For example, outdoor workers such as farmers and construction workers are exposed to solar radiation, healthcare workers such as x-ray technicians and biomedical researchers are exposed to ionizing radiation and carcinogenic substances, and exposure to asbestos is a problem for people who work in old buildings with asbestos insulation in the walls. Table 14–1 correlates known carcinogens and occupations.

Infection

A number of viruses have been linked to some cancers (Maeda et al., 2008). Avoiding those specific infections will decrease risk. Although some infections may be unavoidable (Epstein-Barr,

for example), others, such as genital herpes and human papillomavirus–induced genital warts, can often be avoided by following safer sex practices (e.g., the use of condoms) or obtaining a human papillomavirus (HPV) vaccine.

Tobacco Use

Smoking-related diseases remain the world's most preventable cause of death (ACS, 2010a). Lung cancer is considered highly preventable because of its relationship to smoking. The genotoxic carcinogenic substances in tobacco are considered weak; therefore, stopping smoking can reverse the damage it causes. However, many other substances in tobacco are highly promotional, so that the larger the dose and longer the use, the higher the risk for developing cancer. Research has shown a significantly lower lung cancer death risk for former smokers compared to current smokers.

Tobacco is also related to other forms of cancer. Smokers face an increased risk for oropharyngeal, esophageal, laryngeal, gastric, pancreatic, and bladder cancers (ACS, 2010a). Pipe and cigar smokers are especially susceptible to oropharyngeal and laryngeal cancers. Oral and esophageal cancers are more common among those who chew tobacco or use snuff. Smokers who have a genetic decrease in alpha-$_1$-antitrypsin (an enzyme that protects lung tissue) that results in emphysema face an even higher cancer risk than smokers without this defect.

Additional research has documented the deleterious effects of secondhand tobacco smoke (Van Hemelrijck et al., 2006). Tobacco-specific nitrosamines were recovered in the urine of children living with smokers. It is now accepted that nonsmokers exposed to tobacco smoke over long periods of time, whether in the workplace or the home, have an increased risk for lung or bladder cancers.

TABLE 14–1 Chemical Carcinogens and Relationship to Occupation

CHEMICAL AGENT	ACTION	OCCUPATION AFFECTED
Polycyclic hydrocarbons (smoke, soot, tobacco, smoked foods)	Genotoxic	Miners, coal/gas workers, chimney sweeps, migrant workers, workers in offices where smoking is allowed in closed areas
Benzopyrene		
Arsenic	Genotoxic	Pesticide manufacturers, mining
Vinyl chloride polymers	Promotional	Plastics workers
		Artists
Methylaminobenzine	Genotoxic	Fabric workers
		Rubber and glue workers
Asbestos	Promotional	Construction workers, workers in old, run-down buildings with asbestos insulation, insulation makers
Wood and leather dust	Promotional	Woodworkers, carpenters, leather toolers
Chemotherapy drugs	Genotoxic	Drug manufacturers, pharmacists, nurses

Alcohol Use

Alcohol promotes cancer by enhancing the contact between carcinogens such as those in tobacco and the stem cells that line the oral cavity, larynx, and esophagus. People who both smoke and drink a considerable amount of alcohol daily have an increased risk for oral, esophageal, and laryngeal cancers.

Recreational Drug Use

Recreational drug use often promotes an unhealthy lifestyle that increases general cancer risk; for example, drug users often do not maintain adequate nutrition. Furthermore, recreational drugs are implicated as promoters because of their suppressive effect on the immune system. Although it has not been directly implicated in cancer development, marijuana has been demonstrated to cause chromosomal damage that may over time also result in cancer-causing DNA damage and genetic mutations. Marijuana smoke is also more injurious to lung tissue than tobacco smoke.

Obesity

Overweight and obesity contribute to 14% to 20% of all cancer-related mortality in the United States (ACS, 2010a). Excessive body fat has been linked to an increased risk of hormone-dependent cancers. Because sex hormones are synthesized from fat, obese people often have excessive amounts of the hormones that feed hormone-dependent malignancies of the breast, bowel, ovary, endometrium, and prostate. Overweight and obesity are clearly associated with increased risk for developing many cancers, including cancers of the breast (in postmenopausal women), colon, endometrium, kidney, and adenocarcinoma of the esophagus (ACS, 2010a).

Sun Exposure

As the protective ozone layer thins, more of the sun's damaging ultraviolet radiation reaches the earth. As a consequence, the rate of skin cancers has increased. Sun-related skin cancers are now considered to be a problem for all people, regardless of skin color, but people of northern European extraction with very fair skin, blue or green eyes, and light-colored hair are most vulnerable. Elderly people with decreased pigment are also more at risk, even those with darker skin.

Pathophysiology

Cancer is a complex disease with hundreds of agents that can contribute to its pathogenesis. Advances in research have greatly increased the understanding of how cancer develops. It is now known that the development of cancer is a process in which normal cells are changed and acquire malignant properties. Before a discussion of the various theories of the causes of cancer, it is useful to review how normal cells divide and adapt to changing conditions.

Normal Cell Growth

Mature normal cells are uniform in size and have nuclei that are characteristic of the tissue to which the cells belong. Within the nucleus of normal cells, chromosomes containing deoxyribonucleic acid (DNA) molecules carry the genetic information that controls the synthesis of polypeptides (proteins). Genes are subunits of chromosomes and consist of portions of DNA that specify the production of particular sets of proteins. Thus, genes control the development of specific traits. The genetic code in the DNA of every gene is translated into protein structures that determine the type, maturity, and function of a cell. Any change or disruption in a gene can result in an inaccurate "blueprint" that can produce an aberrant cell, which may then become cancerous. Box 14–1 lists some of the functions of DNA.

The Cell Cycle

Two coordinated events are responsible for cellular reproduction. Reproduction occurs as the result of replication of cellular DNA and mitosis, when the cell divides into two daughter cells with identical DNA.

BOX 14–1 Functions of DNA

- Orders production of enzymes
- Instructs cells to produce specific chemicals
- Instructs cells to develop specific structures
- Determines individual traits and characteristics
- Controls other DNA by telling a cell to "switch on"

The **cell cycle** consists of four phases. In the gap 1 or G_1 phase, the cell enlarges and synthesizes proteins to prepare for DNA replication. During this phase the cell prepares to replicate and enter into the synthesis phase. During the synthesis (S) phase, DNA is replicated and the chromosomes in the cell are duplicated. During the gap 2 or G_2 phase, the cell prepares itself for mitosis. Finally, with all preparation complete, the cell begins mitosis in the M phase. This phase culminates in the division of the parent cell into two exact copies called daughter cells, each having identical genetic material. The cells then immediately enter G_1 where they begin the cell cycle again, or divert into a resting phase called G_0. The cell cycle is controlled by cyclins, which combine with and activate enzymes called cyclin-dependent kinases. Some cyclins cause a "braking" action and prevent the cycle from proceeding. Checkpoints in the cell cycle ensure that it proceeds in the correct order.

A malfunction of any of these regulators of cell growth and division can result in the rapid proliferation of immature cells. In some cases, these cells are considered cancerous (malignant). Knowledge of cell cycle events is used in the development of chemotherapeutic drugs, which are designed to disrupt the cancer cells during different stages of their cell cycle. These drugs and their use are discussed later in the chapter.

Differentiation

Differentiation is a normal process occurring over many cell cycles that allows cells to specialize in certain tasks. For example, some epithelial cells lining the lungs develop into tall columnar cells with cilia. These columnar cells sweep potentially dangerous debris out of the lungs. When adverse conditions occur in body tissues during differentiation, protective adaptations can produce alterations in cells. Some of these alterations are helpful, but in other cases the cells mutate beyond usefulness and become liabilities. Following are potentially unproductive cellular alterations that occur during cell differentiation:

- **Hyperplasia** is an increase in the number or density of normal cells. Hyperplasia occurs in response to stress, increased metabolic demands, or elevated levels of hormones. Examples include the hyperplasia of myocardial cells in response to a prolonged increase in the body's demand for oxygen, and hyperplasia of uterine cells in response to rising levels of estrogen during pregnancy. Hyperplastic cells are under normal DNA control.
- **Metaplasia** is a change in the normal pattern of differentiation such that dividing cells differentiate into cell types not normally found in that location in the body. The metaplastic cell is normal for its particular type, but it is not in its normal location. Some metaplastic cells are less functional than the cells they replace. Metaplasia is a protective response to adverse conditions. Metaplastic cells are under normal DNA control and are reversible when the stressor or other disruptive condition ceases.
- **Dysplasia** represents a loss of DNA control over differentiation occurring in response to adverse conditions. Dysplastic cells show abnormal variation in size, shape, and appearance and a disturbance in their usual arrangement. Examples of dysplasia include changes in the cervix in response to continued

irritation, such as from HPV, or leukoplakia on oral mucous membranes in response to chronic irritation from smoking.
- **Anaplasia** is the regression of a cell to an immature or undifferentiated cell type. Anaplastic cell division is no longer under DNA control. Anaplasia usually occurs when a damaging or transforming event takes place inside the dividing, still undifferentiated cell, leading to loss of useful function. Anaplasia may occur in response to overwhelmingly destructive conditions inside the cell or in surrounding tissue.

Although hyperplasia, metaplasia, and dysplasia often reverse after the irritating factor is eliminated, they can lead to malignancy under certain conditions. This is especially true of dysplasia, which represents a loss of DNA control. Anaplasia is not reversible, but the degree of anaplasia determines the potential risk for cancer.

Theories of Carcinogenesis

Factors that cause cancer are both external (chemicals, radiation, and viruses) and internal (hormones, immune conditions, and inherited mutations). Causal factors may act together or in sequence to initiate or promote **carcinogenesis**, a process by which normal cells are transformed into cancer cells. Often, more than 10 years pass between exposures or mutations and detectable cancer.

Cellular Mutation

The theory of cellular mutation suggests that certain agents cause mutations in cellular DNA and transform cells into cancer cells. Such agents are called **carcinogens**. It is believed that the carcinogenic process has three stages: initiation, promotion, and progression. The initiation stage involves permanent damage in the cellular DNA as a result of exposure to a carcinogen (e.g., radiation, chemicals) that was not repaired or had a defective repair. Promotion may last for years and includes conditions, such as smoking or alcohol use, that act repeatedly on the already affected cells. In the progression stage further inherited changes acquired during the cell replication develop into a cancer.

Oncogenes

Proto-oncogenes are normal genes that promote cell growth and repair. **Oncogenes** are abnormal genes that promote cell proliferation and are capable of triggering cancerous characteristics. Oncogenes can be classified according to their overall function. Several oncogenes and their relationship to human cancers have been identified. For example, BRCA-1 and BRCA-2 are oncogenes associated with breast cancer (Eccles, 2008).

A decrease in the body's immune surveillance may allow the expression of oncogenes; this can occur during times of stress or in response to certain carcinogens. For example, patients with AIDS, who have a decreased number of T-helper lymphocytes, have a much higher than normal incidence of certain cancers, including non-Hodgkin's lymphoma and Kaposi's sarcoma (Nowicki et al., 2008).

Tumor Suppressor Genes

Tumor suppressor genes normally block cell growth by suppressing oncogenes. They can become inactive by deletion or mutation. Inherited cancers have been associated with tumor suppressor genes. An example is p53, a suppressor gene that has been associated with sarcoma and cancer of the breast and brain.

Central to these theories are two important concepts about the etiology of cancer. First, damaged DNA, whether inherited or from external sources, sets up the necessary initial step for cancer to occur. Second, impairment of the human immune system, from whatever cause, lessens its ability to destroy abnormal cells.

Known Carcinogens

A number of agents are known to cause cancer, or at least are strongly linked to certain kinds of cancers. These known carcinogens include viruses, drugs, hormones, and chemical and physical agents. The National Toxicology Program (NTP) and the International Agency for Research on Cancer (IARC) play an important role in the identification and evaluation of carcinogens. See their respective websites for a list of substances known or reasonably anticipated to be human carcinogens.

Carcinogens can be categorized in two groups: Genotoxic carcinogens directly alter DNA and cause mutations, and promoter substances cause other adverse biologic effects, such as cytotoxicity, hormonal imbalances, altered immunity, or chronic tissue damage. Promoter substances do not cause cancer in the absence of previous cell damage (initiation) and often require high-level and long-term contact with the altered cells (NTP, 2005) (see Table 14–1). Although everyone comes in contact with a vast number of substances considered carcinogenic, not everyone develops cancer. Other factors, such as genetic predisposition, impairment of the immune response, and repeated exposure to the carcinogen, are necessary for a cancer to develop.

Viruses

Several viruses have been associated with the development of cancer. They damage cells and induce hyperplastic cell growth. Viral infection may play a role in cell mutation that can progress to malignant cells. Most people are able to suppress this progression. Box 14–2 identifies these viruses and the cancers with which they are associated. In addition, viruses play a

---

BOX 14–2 Cancers Associated with Different Viruses

Herpes Simplex Virus Types I and II (HSV-1 and HSV-2)
- Carcinoma of the lip
- Cervical carcinoma
- Kaposi's sarcoma

Human Cytomegalovirus (HCMV)
- Kaposi's sarcoma
- Prostate cancer

Epstein-Barr Virus (EBV)
- Burkitt's lymphoma

Human Herpesvirus-6 (HHV-6)
- Lymphoma

Hepatitis B Virus (HBV)
- Primary hepatocellular cancer

Papillomavirus
- Malignant melanoma
- Cervical, penile, and laryngeal cancers

Human T-Lymphotropic Viruses (HTLV)
- Adult T-cell leukemia and lymphoma
- T-cell variant of hairy-cell leukemia
- Kaposi's sarcoma

---

significant role in weakening immunologic defenses against neoplasms. For example, human immunodeficiency virus (HIV), which infects T-helper lymphocytes and monocytes, impairs the person's protection against certain cancers such as lymphoma and Kaposi's sarcoma (Nowicki et al., 2008).

Other viruses have also been associated with human malignancies. Hepatitis B virus integrates its DNA with liver cell DNA and is believed to cause primary hepatocellular carcinoma. Papillomaviruses cause plantar, common, and flat warts, which are benign and usually regress spontaneously; however, they also cause genital warts and laryngeal papillomas, which are associated with malignant melanoma and cervical, penile, and laryngeal cancers. Vaccines to prevent virus-induced cancers are being investigated in various cancers, such as melanoma, lung cancer, and osteosarcoma (Bodles-Brakhop & Draghia-Akli, 2008; di Pietro et al., 2008; Ullenhag et al., 2008). More research is needed to investigate the effectiveness of immunotherapy, such as vaccines.

Drugs and Hormones

Certain drugs can be either genotoxic or promotional. For example, chemotherapeutic drugs used to disrupt the cell cycle of malignant cells can be genotoxic for normal cells. They can also be promotional: By drastically reducing the number of leukocytes, they impair immune function. Examples of these chemotherapeutic drugs include busulfan, chlorambucil, and cyclophosphamide. Some recreational drugs also are implicated as carcinogens. These include the genotoxic betel nut chewed by many Pacific Islanders and the immunosuppressant promoters heroin and cocaine.

Hormones are also potential genotoxic carcinogens or promoters. Gonadotropic hormones often mediate cancers of the reproductive organs. Estrogen, both natural and synthetic, and diethylstilbestrol (DES) have been linked to cervical, endometrial, and breast cancers. Estrogen-containing contraceptive pills have been implicated in breast cancer, but they also have been shown to decrease the risk of ovarian cancer. Investigators have not reached a final conclusion about the cancer risk posed by contraceptives. Newer research suggests that alterations in the molecular structure of testosterone in older men may promote the development of prostate cancer. Also, glucocorticosteroids (cortisone) and anabolic steroids may act as promoters by altering the immune response or endocrine balance.

Chemical Agents

Many chemicals are both genotoxic and promotional. Because many of these substances are encountered in the workplace, they constitute occupational hazards. Examples of industrial and environmental carcinogens include polycyclic hydrocarbons, found in soot; benzopyrene, found in cigarette smoke; and arsenic, found in pesticides. These chemicals have some genotoxic action; some alter DNA replication. Other industrial and environmental chemicals are considered promotional agents, including wood and leather dust, polymer esters (used in plastics and paints), carbon tetrachloride, asbestos, and phenol (NTP, 2005). Polycyclic aromatic hydrocarbons, nitrosamines, phenols, and other chemicals in tobacco act as either carcinogens or promoters of cancer (see Table 14–1).

Natural substances in the body may also be carcinogenic or promotional. For example, end products of metabolism that are produced in excess amounts or are ineffectively eliminated, such as bile acids from a high-fat diet, may promote cancer.

Some foods contain carcinogens added during preparation or preservation. Examples include the sugar substitute sodium saccharine and nitrosamines and nitrous indoles, which are found in pickled, salted foods. In some cases, food contaminants produce carcinogenic chemicals. The *Aspergillus* fungi produce aflatoxin, a highly potent carcinogen. These organisms grow on improperly stored vegetable products, such as grains and peanuts.

Physical Agents

It has been well documented that excessive exposure to radiation causes increased rates of cancer by damaging the DNA in cells, by activating other oncogenetic factors, or by suppressing antitumor activity (protein inhibitors). Both solar radiation from ultraviolet rays and ionizing radiation from industrial or medical sources are carcinogenic. This fact has implications for workers exposed to these agents and for the population in general. Radon, a naturally formed radioactive gas found in the basements of many homes, is also a known carcinogen. People who have lived in areas where nuclear weapons have been tested or whose groundwater has been polluted by nuclear wastes are at risk for developing cancers. The effects of high-dose radiation exposure and subsequent cancer development have been demonstrated in the survivors of the atomic bombs at Nagasaki and Hiroshima and in workers exposed to radiation during the cleanup of nuclear disasters such as Chernobyl.

Types of Neoplasms

A **neoplasm** is a mass of new tissue (a collection of cells) that grows independently of its surrounding structures and has no physiologic purpose. The term *neoplasm* is often used interchangeably with *tumor*, from the Latin word meaning "swelling." Neoplasms are said to be autonomous because they grow at a rate uncoordinated with body needs, they share some of the properties of the parent cells but with altered size and shape, and they do not benefit the host and in some cases are harmful.

Neoplasms are not completely autonomous because they require a blood supply with nutrients and oxygen to sustain their growth. Neoplasms typically are classified as benign or malignant on the basis of their potential to damage the body and on their growth characteristics.

Benign Neoplasms

Benign neoplasms are localized growths. They form a solid mass, have well-defined borders, and frequently are encapsulated. Benign neoplasms tend to respond to the body's homeostatic controls. Thus, they often stop growing when they reach the boundaries of another tissue (a process called *contact inhibition*). They grow slowly and often remain stable in size. Because they are usually encapsulated, benign neoplasms often are easily removed and tend not to recur.

Although typically harmless, benign neoplasms nevertheless can be destructive if they crowd surrounding tissue and obstruct the function of organs. For example, a benign meningioma of the brain or spinal cord can cause increased intracranial pressure (IICP), which progressively impairs the person's cerebral function. Unless the meningioma can be successfully removed, the steadily rising IICP will eventually lead to coma and death.

Malignant Neoplasms

In contrast to benign neoplasms, malignant neoplasms grow aggressively and do not respond to the body's homeostatic controls. Malignant neoplasms are not cohesive, and present with an irregular shape. Instead of slowly crowding other tissues aside, malignant neoplasms cut through surrounding tissues, causing bleeding, inflammation, and necrosis (tissue death) as they grow. This invasive quality of malignant neoplasms is reflected in the word origin of *cancer*, from the Greek *karkinos*, meaning "crab."

Malignant cells from the primary tumor may travel through the blood or lymph to invade other tissues and organs of the body and form a secondary tumor called a **metastasis**. This term also refers to the process by which such spreading of malignant neoplasms—perhaps their most destructive trait—occurs. Malignant neoplasms can recur after surgical removal of the primary and secondary tumors and after other treatments. Table 14–2 compares benign and malignant neoplasms.

Malignant neoplasms vary in their degree of differentiation from the parent tissue. Highly differentiated cancer cells try to mimic the specialized function of the parent tissue, but undifferentiated cancers, consisting of immature cells, have almost no resemblance to the parent tissue and so perform no useful function. Undifferentiated cancers rob the body of its energy and nutrition as they grow. Undifferentiated anaplastic cells have little structural or functional relationship to the parent cells and are the basis of many malignant neoplasms. The degree of differentiation of anaplastic cells is a consideration in the classification and staging of neoplasms, discussed later in this chapter.

Characteristics of Malignant Cells

Malignant neoplasms may be identified by the following predictable cellular characteristics:

- *Loss of regulation of the rate of mitosis.* This leads to rapid cell division and growth of the neoplasm.
- *Loss of specialization and differentiation.* Malignant cells do not perform typical cellular functions. Many produce hormones

TABLE 14–2 Comparison of Benign and Malignant Neoplasms

BENIGN	MALIGNANT
Local	Invasive
Cohesive	Noncohesive
Well-defined borders	Does not stop at tissue border
Pushes other tissues out of the way	Invades and destroys surrounding tissues
Slow growth	Rapid growth
Encapsulated	Metastasizes to distant sites
Easily removed	Not always easy to remove
Does not recur	Can recur

and enzymes similar to those of the parent tissue, but usually in excessive amounts, possibly revealing their presence.

- *Loss of contact inhibition.* Malignant cells do not respect other cellular boundaries. They easily invade and destroy other tissues.
- *Progressive acquisition of a cancerous phenotype.* Cellular mutation seems to be a sequential process involving successive generations of cells, each generation becoming more deviant than the previous one. Additionally, malignant cells seem to be "immortal"; that is, they do not stop growing and die, as do normal cells, which have a genetically determined life span.
- *Irreversibility.* The transformation into a malignant cell is irreversible. Rarely does a malignant neoplasm revert to a benign state.
- *Altered cell structure.* Cytologic examination of malignant cells reveals distinct differences in the cell nucleus and cytoplasm as well as an overall cell shape that differs from that of normal cells of the particular tissue type.
- *Simplified metabolic activities.* The work of malignant cells is simpler than that of normal cells; they show an increased synthesis of substances needed for cell division, and they have no need to create proteins for the specialized functions of the tissues they invade.
- *Transplantability.* Malignant cells often break away from the primary tissue site and travel to other locations in the body, where they establish new growths.
- *Ability to promote their own survival.* Malignant cells may create ectopic sites to produce the hormones they need for their growth. By their very presence and their ability to initiate vascular permeability, malignant cells promote the development of nonneoplastic stroma, a connective tissue framework consisting of collagen and other components, which then supports the neoplasm. They may also create their own blood supply. Through a process called angiogenesis, tumor cells secrete a polypeptide angiogenic growth factor that stimulates blood vessels from surrounding normal tissue to grow into the tumor. Finally, malignant cells divert nutrition from the host to meet their own needs, by diffusion when the tumor is less than 1 mm and thereafter by means of the newly formed blood vessels. If unchecked, malignant cells eventually destroy their host.

The characteristics of malignant cells are summarized in Box 14–3.

BOX 14–3 Characteristics of Malignant Cells

- Loss of regulation of mitotic rate
- Loss of cell specialization
- Loss of contact inhibition
- Progressive acquisition of the cancerous phenotype and immortality
- Irreversibility of cancerous phenotype to greater aggressiveness
- Altered cell structure: differences in cell nucleus and cytoplasm
- Simplified metabolic activity
- Transplantability (metastasis)
- Ability to promote own survival

Tumor Invasion and Metastasis

Metastasis or the ability of cancer cells to invade adjacent tissues and travel to distant organs is considered their most ominous characteristic. This quality makes treatment a considerable challenge.

Invasion

Aggressive tumors possess several qualities that facilitate invasion (Figure 14–2 ■):

- *Ability to cause pressure atrophy.* The pressure of a growing tumor can cause atrophy and necrosis of adjacent tissues. The malignancy then moves into the vacated space.
- *Ability to disrupt the basement membrane of normal cells.* Many cancer cells can bind to elements of the basement membrane and secrete enzymes that degrade that physical barrier, thus facilitating their movement into normal tissues, lymph, and blood circulation.
- *Motility.* Because malignant cells are less tightly bound to each other than normal cells (reduced adhesiveness), they easily separate from the neoplasm and move into surrounding body fluids and tissues.
- *Response to chemical signals from adjacent tissues.* Chemotaxis (the movement of cells in response to a chemical stimulus) calls the tumor cells into the normal tissues, possibly as a result of the degrading of the basement membranes of the normal cells. This breakdown of normal cellular membranes releases the chemical stimulus physiologically designed to draw normal phagocytic cells to clean up the debris. (∞ See Chapter 12 on the inflammatory response for more information on chemotaxis.) Malignant cells are also known to respond chemotactically to the end product of cellular metabolism. Some cancer cells even produce a substance called autocrine motility factor, which calls other malignant cells to a normal tissue. The first invading cells produce this substance, which then actively draws other malignant cells from the primary tumor into the invaded normal tissue.

Metastasis

The factors that favor invasion also contribute to the process of metastasis. Metastasis can occur by means of one or more mechanisms including embolism in the blood or lymph, or spread by way of body cavities.

A blood- or lymph-borne metastasis allows a new tumor to be established in a distant organ. Figure 14–3 ■ shows metastasis through the bloodstream. A tumor's ability to metastasize in this manner requires the following steps:

1. Intravasation of malignant cells through blood or lymphatic vessel walls and into the circulation.
2. Survival of the malignant cells in the blood. (To survive, the cells must escape the notice of the body's immune surveillance; only about 1 in 1000 cells does so.)
3. Extravasation from the circulation and implantation in a new tissue.

The tumor cells tend to clump together, forming an embolus, and continue growing until their size prevents further travel in the vessel or lymph channel. The growing neoplastic mass then uses its invasive abilities (secreting enzymes and motility factor) to move into the nearest organ.

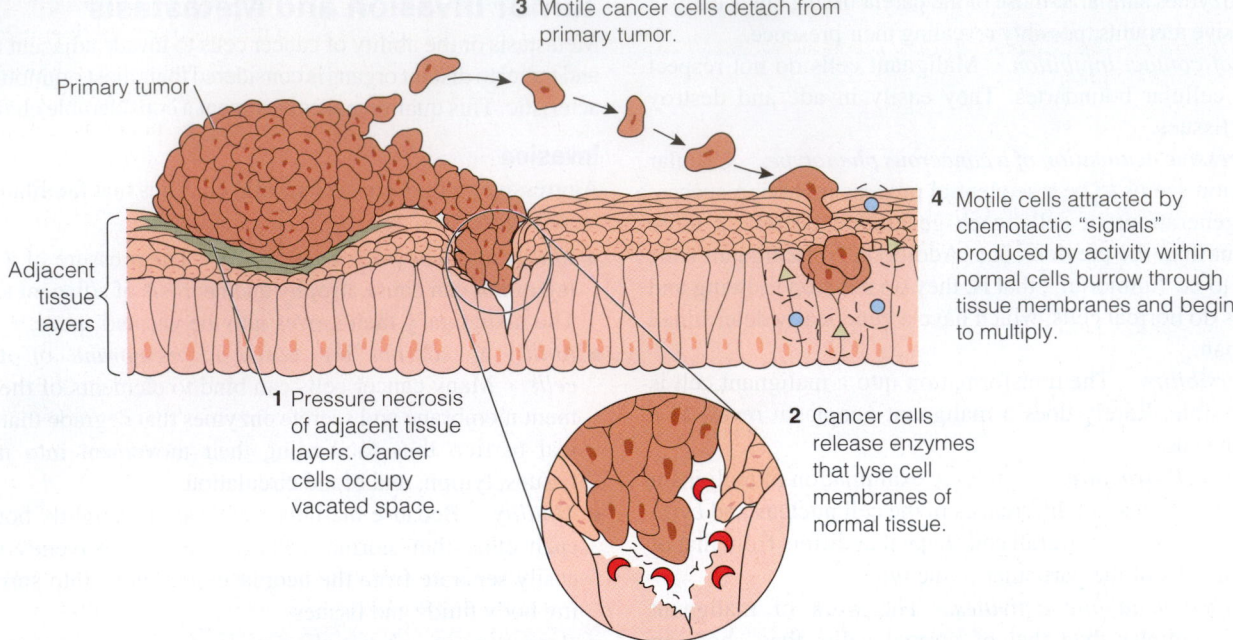

Figure 14–2 ■ How cancer cells invade normal tissue.

3 Motile cancer cells detach from primary tumor.

Primary tumor

Adjacent tissue layers

4 Motile cells attracted by chemotactic "signals" produced by activity within normal cells burrow through tissue membranes and begin to multiply.

1 Pressure necrosis of adjacent tissue layers. Cancer cells occupy vacated space.

2 Cancer cells release enzymes that lyse cell membranes of normal tissue.

About 60% of metastatic lesions tend to occur in a pattern that reflects blood or lymph circulation. However, it has been demonstrated that some malignant cells defy a bloodborne pattern and actually target specific organs to which they prefer to metastasize. For example, lung cancer frequently metastasizes to the adrenal glands, and breast cancer frequently metastasizes to bone. Malignant cells that gain access to

lymph channels may travel to a preferred organ and then move into it the same way they move through blood vessels. Alternatively, the malignant cells may become trapped in the lymph node and continue to grow. Eventually, the malignant cells replace the node's tissues. At this point, emboli from the cancerous node disseminate to other nodes, creating a cascade reaction. The malignant cascade causes widespread transfer of the tumor to uncharacteristic sites.

A malignant tumor may break through the walls of the organ in which it is primarily housed, shedding cells into the nearby body cavity. The cells then are free to establish new tumors in a distant area of that cavity. For example, malignant cells from a colon cancer may be seeded into the peritoneal cavity, establishing a new tumor in the mesenteric epithelium.

Metastatic lesions are differentiated from primary neoplasms by cell morphology: Metastatic cells do not resemble the tissue in which they reside. The most common sites of metastasis are the lymph nodes, liver, lungs, bones, and brain. Table 14–3 lists different cancers and common sites of metastasis.

For metastasis to occur, the cancerous cells must avoid detection by the immune system. Thus, impairment of the immune system is a major factor in the establishment of

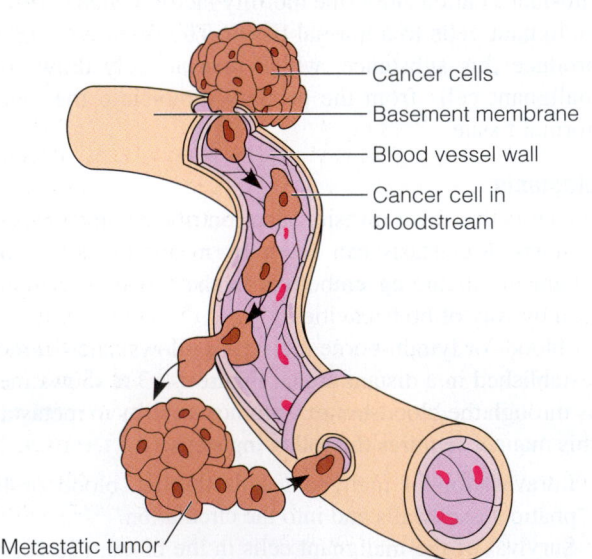

Cancer cells

Basement membrane

Blood vessel wall

Cancer cell in bloodstream

Metastatic tumor

Figure 14–3 ■ Metastasis through the bloodstream. Cancer cells secrete enzymes and a motility factor that disrupt the basement membrane in the blood vessel. In this way, the cancer cells gain access to the circulation. Once in the blood, only about 1 cell in 1000 escapes immune detection, but that can be enough. Undetected cells move out of the blood, again secreting enzymes and cutting through the vessel wall into new tissue. The tissue selected for establishing a new tumor may be downstream from the original tumor, or a chemical attraction may cause the malignant cells to target a specific site. Once in the new site, the malignant cells multiply and establish a metastatic tumor.

TABLE 14–3 Various Cancers and Sites of Metastases

PRIMARY TUMOR	COMMON METASTATIC SITES
Bronchogenic (lung)	Spinal cord, brain, liver, bone
Breast	Regional lymph nodes, vertebrae, brain, liver, lung, bone
Colon	Liver, lung, brain, ovary, bone
Prostate	Bladder, bone (especially vertebrae), liver
Malignant melanoma	Lung, liver, spleen, regional lymph nodes, brain

metastatic lesions. Cells may escape detection in several different ways:

- Aggressive cancer cells may compile a large mass (greater than 1 cm) so rapidly that the immune system is unable to overcome the tumor before it takes hold in a new tissue.
- For tumor cells to be recognized as foreign by the immune system, they must display on their surface a special antigen called tumor-associated antigen (TAA). TAA marks tumor cells for destruction by the lymphocytes. Some oncogenic viruses depress the expression of TAA on infected cells. Also, some tumors in advanced stages of growth no longer display TAA. Thus, such tumor cells escape detection as they travel through the blood or lymph.
- If the person's immune response is weakened or altered, then a metastatic tumor may take hold with little opposition. Factors that may weaken or alter the immune response are listed in Box 14–4.

An estimated 50% to 60% of all cancers have already metastasized by the time the primary tumor is identified. This may account for the current 50% death rate and certainly supports the need for patient education to facilitate early diagnosis. The time it takes for metastasis to occur is extremely variable and often difficult to predict. Some cancers, such as basal cell carcinomas, do not metastasize. The aggressiveness and location of the tumor, and the state of the person's immune system, determine whether and how rapidly metastasis takes place.

Physiologic and Psychologic Effects of Cancer

Much of the nursing care for patients with cancer is related to the effects of cancer disease and the side effects of cancer treatment. Although pathophysiologic effects of the cancer vary with the type and location of the cancer, the following effects usually are observed.

Disruption of Function

Physiologic functioning can be upset by obstruction or pressure. For example, a large tumor in the bowel can stop intestinal motility, resulting in a bowel obstruction. Prostatic tumors can obstruct the bladder neck or urethra, resulting in urine retention. Intracranial pressure can be dangerously increased by a glioma. Obstruction or pressure can cause anoxia and necrosis of surrounding tissues, which in turn cause a loss of function of the involved organ or tissue. For example, a kidney tumor may progress to renal failure. Pressure against the superior vena cava from an adjacent lung tumor or tumor-infiltrated lymph nodes can interrupt the blood flow to the heart.

In the liver, either a primary hepatocellular cancer or metastatic lesion can have several significant effects. In liver parenchymal tissue, it impairs the multiple life-sustaining functions of the liver, such as carbohydrate metabolism, synthesis of plasma proteins, detoxification, and immunologic functions. These functional impairments result in severe nutritional, hormonal, hematologic, and immunologic problems. (∞ See Chapter 25 for a more complete discussion of liver functions and effects of disruption.) Because more than 1 L of blood per minute passes through the liver via the portal vein, obstruction to this flow by a tumor can cause portal hypertension. This results in backup of fluid and increased pressure in the splanchnic circulation. The end result is ascites (third-spaced fluid in the peritoneal cavity) and varices (friable, overdistended blood vessels) of the esophageal, gastric, mesenteric, and hemorrhoidal vessels.

Hematologic Alterations

Hematologic alterations can impair the normal function of blood cells. For example, in leukemia, a malignant proliferative disease of the hematopoietic (blood cell–producing) system, the immature leukocytes cannot perform the normal protective phagocytic functions and immunity is compromised. The excessive numbers of immature leukocytes in the bone marrow diminish erythrocyte and thrombocyte (platelet) production, resulting in secondary anemia, neutropenia, and thrombocytopenia. In addition, gastrointestinal tumors disrupt the absorption of vitamin B_{12} and iron; growing tumors accumulate and store purines, depriving the bone marrow of substances needed for erythropoiesis (red blood cell production); and renal cell carcinoma produces its own erythropoietin hormone, resulting in production of an excessively large number of red blood cells and viscous blood, which impairs circulation, plugs small capillaries, and promotes thrombus formation (polycythemia).

Infection

If the tumor invades and connects two incompatible organs, such as the bowel and bladder, creating a fistula, infection becomes a serious problem. As they destroy viable tissue and thus their source of nutrition, tumors may become necrotic and septicemia may result. Some tumors are less efficient in creating capillaries; as a consequence, the center of the tumor may become necrotic and infected. When a tumor grows near the surface of the body, it may erode through to the surface, breaking down the natural defenses of intact skin and mucous membranes and providing a site for the entry of microorganisms. Any malignant involvement of the organs or tissues of immunity—such as the liver, bone marrow, Peyer's patches in the small intestine, spleen, or lymph nodes—can seriously impair the immune response, allowing infections to develop in vulnerable tissues.

Hemorrhage

Tumor erosion through blood vessels can cause extensive bleeding, giving rise to severe anemia. Hemorrhage can be serious enough to cause life-threatening hypovolemic shock.

Anorexia-Cachexia Syndrome

A characteristic feature of cancer is the wasted appearance of its victims, called **cachexia**. In many cases, unexplained rapid weight loss is the first manifestation that brings the patient to a healthcare provider. This can be due to a variety of problems associated with cancer, such as pain, infection, depression, or the side effects of chemotherapy and radiation. Usually the emaciation, malnutrition, and loss of energy are attributed to the anorexia-cachexia syndrome.

This syndrome is specific to cancer because of the effect of cancer cells on the host's metabolism. The neoplastic cells divert nutrition to their own use while causing changes that reduce the patient's appetite. Early in the disease, altered glucose metabolism leads to an increase in serum glucose levels, which creates negative feedback resulting in *anorexia* (loss of appetite). In addition, the tumor secretes substances that decrease appetite by altering taste and smell and producing early satiety. Pain, infection, and depression also contribute to anorexia. Some types of cancers cause specific food aversions, such as to red meat, coffee, or chocolate.

Avaricious cancer cells support their growth through widespread catabolism of the body's tissue and muscle proteins. This catabolism, coupled with inadequate nutrient intake, results in the typical cachexia. Normally, a starvation state reduces the body's basal metabolic rate. However, in many people with cancer, the metabolic rate is increased, probably because of the hyperactive metabolic and reproductive activities of the malignant cells. One theory suggests that cytokinins the body produces in response to the tumor are responsible for both early satiety and cachexia. One specific cytokine, called tumor necrosis factor alpha or cachectin, is believed to enhance the increased metabolic consumption of nutrients. Cancers of the gastrointestinal system further promote anorexia-cachexia by decreasing absorption and use of nutrients; the side effects of some treatment modalities enhance this effect. Figure 14–4 ■ shows the characteristic appearance of a cachectic person.

Paraneoplastic Syndromes

Paraneoplastic syndromes are indirect effects of cancer. They may be early warning signs of cancer or indicate complications or return of a malignancy. The most frequently occurring paraneoplastic syndromes are endocrine, occurring when cancers set up ectopic sites of hormone production, and neurologic, occurring when cancer damages the nervous system (Toothaker & Rubin, 2009). Table 14–4 lists laboratory indicators of ectopic functioning. These ectopic sites produce excessive amounts of the hormone, which harm the host. Consider the following examples:

■ Breast, ovarian, and renal cancers may set up ectopic parathyroid hormone sites, causing severe hypercalcemia.

■ Oat cell and other lung cancers may produce ectopic secretions of insulin (causing hypoglycemia), parathyroid hormone (PTH), antidiuretic hormone (ADH, which causes excessive fluid retention, hypertension, and peripheral edema), and adrenocorticotropic hormone (ACTH). ∞ See Chapter 19 for the description of the multiple problems caused by excessive secretions of cortisone.

Other paraneoplastic syndromes include hematologic abnormalities such as anemia, thrombocytopenia, and coagulation abnormalities; nephrotic syndrome; cutaneous syndromes; and neurologic syndromes, such as distant tumors that produce IICP (Toothaker & Rubin, 2009).

Pain

Pain is a major healthcare problem for patients with cancer. Despite extensive progress in the scientific understanding of pain, more than 60% patients with cancer experience moderate to severe pain at some time during their illness (Deandrea, Montanari, Moja, Apolone, 2008; Paim et al., 2008). Despite recommendations of the World Health Organization (WHO) and even if effective treatments are available for 70% to 90% of cases, under-treatment is well documented and can involve up to 40% of patients (Deandrea et al., 2008). Under-treatment is usually attributed to an inappropriate use of opioids and barriers related to healthcare provider, patient, family, institution, and society (Eaton & Frieze, 2008). Communication and knowledge deficit are the major barriers to effective pain management. Because pain management for people with cancer has a reputation for being under-treated and ineffective, the anticipation of pain may engender fear in even the most stoic people.

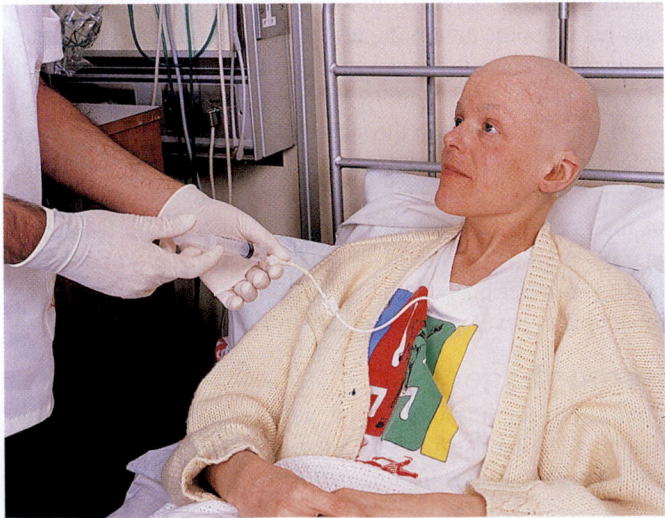

Figure 14–4 ■ Cachectic person. Cancer robs its host of nutrients and increases body catabolism of fat and muscle to meet its metabolic needs.

Source: Simon Fraser/SPL/Photo Researchers, Inc.

TABLE 14–4 Laboratory Indicators of Ectopic Functioning	
HORMONE	**SPECIFIC LABORATORY TEST**
Antidiuretic hormone (ADH)	Serum and urine osmolality
Adrenocorticotropic hormone (ACTH)	Plasma ACTH
	ACTH suppression test
	ACTH stimulation test
	Urine catecholamines
Calcitonin	Serum calcitonin
Insulin	Serum glucose Glucose tolerance test
Parathyroid hormone (PTH)	Serum PTH
	Serum calcium
Thyroxine	Serum thyroid-stimulating hormone (TSH), T_3, T_4

Types of Cancer Pain

Cancer pain can be divided into two main categories, acute and chronic, with subgroupings. These classifications serve to indicate appropriate therapeutic approaches. Acute pain has a well-defined pattern of onset, exhibits common signs and symptoms, and is often identified with hyperactivity of the autonomic system. Chronic pain, which lasts more than 6 months, frequently lacks the objective manifestations of acute pain, primarily because the autonomic nervous system adapts to this chronic stress. Chronic pain often results in personality changes, alterations in functional abilities, and lifestyle disruptions that can seriously affect compliance with treatment and the quality of life.

Most cancer patients who cite acute pain as the primary symptom that led to the diagnosis tend to associate pain with the introduction to their disease. If these patients experience pain during the illness or after treatment, they often perceive the pain as introducing another cancer, a recurrence of the original cancer, or a component of cancer treatments (Rosedale & Fu, 2010).

Chronic pain may be related to treatment or may indicate progression of the disease. Identifying the pain as treatment-related rather than tumor related is extremely important because it has a definite effect on the patient's psychological outlook. For the patient whose pain is due to the advancement of the disease, psychologic factors play an even more important role. Hopelessness and fear of impending death intensify physiologic pain and contribute to overall suffering (which goes well beyond just physical pain).

Three other categories used to classify patients with cancer pain include patients with preexisting pain, those with a history of drug abuse, and dying patients with cancer-related pain. The first two groups may have altered perceptions of pain and may not have the anticipated response to pain medication. For the dying patient, pain is strongly associated with both the patient's and family's confrontation of issues of hopelessness and death. Confronting these issues can intensify the perception of pain.

Causes of Cancer Pain

Direct tumor involvement is the primary cause of the pain experienced by people with cancer. This includes metastatic bone disease, nerve compression, and involvement of visceral organs. The pain from tumor involvement is believed to be mechanical, resulting from stretching of tissues and compression. Chemicals from ischemia or tumor metabolites and toxins that activate and sensitize nociceptors and mechanoreceptors are also responsible for tumor pain. ∞ See Chapter 9 for a more complete discussion of the mechanics of pain.

Side effects or toxic effects of cancer therapies (e.g., surgery, radiation, and chemotherapy) may also cause cancer pain. These are usually the result of traumatized tissue; one example of this is the oropharyngeal ulcerations that occur with some types of chemotherapy. However, these therapies may also be used to manage pain, such as radiation to decrease pain associated with bone metastasis.

Physical Stress

When the immune system discovers a neoplasm, it tries to destroy it using the resources of the body. The body mounts an all-out assault on the foreign invader, calling on many resources, including chemical mediators, hormones and enzymes, blood cells, antibodies, proteins, and inflammatory and immune responses. These protective responses mobilize fluid, electrolytes, and nutritional systems. This massive effort requires tremendous energy. If the neoplasm is small enough (i.e., microscopic), the immune system can destroy it, and a tumor will never manifest. A neoplasm of 1 cm is large enough to overwhelm most immune systems; however, the body will continue to try to fight it until it reaches the stage of exhaustion and is no longer capable (Selye, 1984). Thus, many patients with cancer present with fatigue, weight loss, anemia, dehydration, and altered blood chemistries (e.g., decreases in electrolytes).

Psychologic Stress

People confronted with the diagnosis of cancer exhibit a variety of psychologic and emotional responses. Some people see cancer as a death sentence and experience overwhelming grief, often giving up. Others may feel guilt, considering the cancer a punishment for past behaviors, such as smoking, unhealthy eating habits, or for delaying diagnosis or treatment. They may experience anger, especially if the person believes that he or she had been practicing a healthful lifestyle; beneath that anger may reside feelings of powerlessness. Fear is common: fear of the outcome of the illness, fear of the effects of treatment, fear of pain, fear of death. Some people feel isolated because of the stigma of cancer and old beliefs of contagion. Body image concerns and sexual dysfunction may be present but often are unexpressed, especially if the cancer is of the breast or sexual organs, or causes visible body changes.

Interdisciplinary Care

Interdisciplinary care for the patient with cancer begins with a variety of specialized laboratory and diagnostic tests.

Diagnosis

Several procedures are used to diagnose cancer. X-ray imaging, computed tomography (CT), ultrasonography, and magnetic resonance imaging (MRI) can locate abnormal tissues or tumors. However, only microscopic histologic examination of the tissue reveals the type of cell and its structural difference from the parent tissue. Tissue samples are acquired through biopsy, shedded cells (e.g., Papanicolaou smear), or collections of secretions (e.g., sputum). Lymph nodes are also biopsied to determine whether metastasis has begun. Simple screening procedures can be used to identify substances secreted by the tumor, such as the prostatic-specific antigen (PSA) blood test used to identify early prostatic cancers. Increases in enzymes or hormones released by normal tissues when they are damaged can also contribute to the diagnosis. Increased alkaline phosphatase noted in bone metastases and osteosarcoma is one example of an enzyme increase associated with cancer. Tumor markers are used for early diagnosis, for tracking responses to therapy, and for devising immunologic treatments.

CLASSIFICATION To help standardize diagnosis and treatment protocols, an elaborate identification system has been developed. This consists of naming the tumor (classification) and describing its aggressiveness (grading) and spread within or beyond the tissue of origin (staging).

Tumors are classified and named by the tissue or cell of origin. Tumor nomenclature often incorporates the Latin stem identifying the tissue from which the tumor arises. For example, a carcinoma arises from epithelial tissue; adjectives are added to further specify the location. A glandular malignancy arising from epithelial tissue is classified as an adenocarcinoma. A tumor arising from supportive tissues is called a sarcoma; the specific type of tissue is added as a prefix. For example, a cancer of fibrous connective tissue is called fibrosarcoma, and a smooth muscle cancer is a leiomyosarcoma. A tumor from seminal or germ tissue is called a seminoma. Table 14–5 compares the nomenclature of benign and malignant neoplasms.

Other names for tumors incorporate the name of the discoverer of that particular cancer, such as Burkitt's lymphoma or Hodgkin's disease. Hematopoietic malignancies (also known as "liquid tumors") are usually named by the type of immature blood cell that predominates. An example is myelocytic leukemia, named for the immature form of the granulocyte that is predominant in this malignancy.

GRADING AND STAGING Grading evaluates the amount of differentiation (level of functional maturity) of the cell and estimates the rate of growth based on the mitotic rate. Cells that are the most differentiated—that is, most like the parent tissue and therefore the least malignant—are classified as grade 1 and are associated with a better prognosis. Grade 4 is reserved for the least differentiated

and most aggressively malignant cells. Because of the differences inherent in tumor appearance and biologic behavior, grading criteria may vary with different locations and types of tumors.

Staging is used to classify solid tumors and refers to the relative size of the tumor and extent of the disease. The TNM classification system is an internationally recognized staging system: The T stands for the relative tumor size, depth of invasion, and surface spread; N indicates the presence and extent of lymph node involvement; and M denotes the presence or absence of distant metastases. Table 14–6 shows the basic outline of the TNM system; however, other systems are also used to differentiate types and locations of tumors (e.g., melanomas, cervical cancer, Hodgkin's disease).

CYTOLOGIC EXAMINATION For the malignant tissues to be identified by name, grade, and stage, they must first be subjected to histologic and cytologic examination by light or electron microscope. Specimens are collected by three basic methods:

1. *Exfoliation from an epithelial surface.* Examples include scraping cells from the cervix (Pap smear) or bronchial washings.
2. *Aspiration of fluid from body cavities or blood.* Examples include white blood cells for evaluation of hematopoietic cancers, pleural fluid, and cerebrospinal fluid.
3. *Needle aspiration of solid tumors.* This could include the breast, lung, or prostate.

TABLE 14–5 Nomenclature for Benign and Malignant Neoplasms

	TISSUE OF ORIGIN	BENIGN	MALIGNANT
Ectoderm/Endoderm	Epithelium	Papilloma	Carcinoma
	Gland	Adenoma	Adenocarcinoma
	Liver cells	Hepatocellular adenoma	Hepatocellular carcinoma
	Neuroglia	Glioma	Glioma
	Melanocytes	Melanoma	Malignant melanoma
	Basal cells		Basal cell carcinoma
	Germ cells	Tetroma	Seminoma
Mesoderm	Connective tissue		
	Adipose tissue	Lipoma	Liposarcoma
	Fibrous tissue	Fibroma	Fibrosarcoma
	Bone tissue	Osteoma	Osteosarcoma
	Cartilage	Chondroma	Chondrosarcoma
	Muscle		
	Smooth muscle	Leiomyoma	Leiomyosarcoma
	Striated muscle	Rhabdomyoma	Rhabdomyosarcoma
	Neural tissue		
	Nerve cells	Ganglioneuroma	Neuroblastoma
	Endothelial tissues		
	Blood vessels	Hemangioma	Angiosarcoma
			Kaposi's sarcoma
	Meninges	Meningioma	Malignant meningioma
Hematopoietic Tissues	Granulocytes	Granulocytosis	Leukemia
	Plasma cells		Multiple myeloma
	Lymphocytes		Lymphomas

TABLE 14–6 TNM Staging Classification System

	STAGE	MANIFESTATIONS
Tumor	T_0	No evidence of primary tumor
	T_{IS}	Tumor *in situ*
	T_1, T_2, T_3, T_4	Ascending degrees of tumor size and involvement
Nodes	N_0	No abnormal regional nodes
	N_{1a}, N_{2a}	Regional nodes—no metastasis
	N_{1b}, N_{2b}, N_{3b}	Regional lymph nodes—metastasis suspected
	N_x	Regional nodes cannot be assessed clinically
Metastasis	M_0	No evidence of distant metastasis
	M_1, M_2, M_3	Ascending degrees of metastatic involvement of the host, including distant nodes

Cytologic examination is also carried out on specimens from biopsied tissues or tumors and on collected body secretions, such as sputum or urine.

After collection, specimens are spread on a glass slide, fixed, and stained if necessary. The morphologic features of the cells are examined, with special attention to the nucleus and cytoplasm. Other special pathologic procedures can be carried out on the specimen, but they must be ordered ahead of time if special preparations of the specimen are necessary. Several special diagnostic cytologic procedures, such as cytogenetics, are proving useful in diagnosing and monitoring patient response to treatment.

TUMOR MARKERS   A **tumor marker** is a protein molecule detectable in serum or other body fluids. This marker is used as a biochemical indicator of the presence of a malignancy. Small amounts of tumor marker proteins are found in normal body tissues or benign tumors and are not specific for malignancy.

However, high levels are suspicious and mandate follow-up diagnostic studies. Tumor marker tests are most useful for monitoring the patient's response to therapy and for detecting residual disease. However, one marker, PSA, is a detector of prostate cancer.

Tumor markers fall into two general categories: those derived from the tumor itself and those associated with host (immune) response to the tumor. Examples of tumor markers include the following:

- *Antigens.*   These are present in fetal tissue but normally are suppressed after birth. Thus, their presence in large amounts may reflect an anaplastic process in tumor cells. Alpha-fetoprotein (AFP) and carcinoembryonic antigen (CEA) are oncofetal antigens.
- *Hormones.*   Hormones are present in considerable amounts in human blood and tissues, but very high levels not related to other conditions may signify the presence of a hormone-secreting malignancy. Some common hormones seen as tumor markers include human chorionic gonadotropin (HCG), antidiuretic hormone (ADH), parathyroid hormone (PTH), calcitonin, and catecholamines.
- *Proteins.*   These narrow down the type of tissue that may be malignant, although they can also be increased in hyperplastic disorders. Examples of tissue-specific proteins include serum immunoglobulin and beta-2 microglobulin.
- *Enzymes.*   Rapid, excessive growth of a tissue may cause some of the enzymes and isoenzymes normally present in that particular tissue to spill into the bloodstream. Elevated levels can point to either hyperplasia of the tissue or cancer. Prostatic acid phosphatase (PAP) and neuron-specific enolase (NSE) are examples. Table 14–7 compares selected tumor-derived markers with their presence in neoplasms and other conditions.

ONCOLOGIC IMAGING   Because physical assessment usually cannot detect cancer until the tumor has reached a size that poses a major risk for metastasis, radiologic examination is extremely important in early diagnosis. This diagnostic process

TABLE 14–7 Tumor-Derived Markers Associated with Specific Neoplasms

	TUMOR MARKER	ASSOCIATED NEOPLASM
Oncofetal Antigens	Carcinoembryonic antigen (CEA)	Adenocarcinomas of colon, lung, breast, ovary, stomach, pancreas
	Alpha-fetoprotein (AFP)	Hepatocellular carcinoma, gonadal germ cell tumors (seminoma)
Hormones	Human chorionic gonadotropin (HCG)	Gonadal germ cell tumors
	Calcitonin	Medullary cancer of thyroid
	Catecholamines/metabolites	Pheochromocytoma
Isoenzymes	Prostatic acid phosphatase (PAP)	Adenocarcinoma of prostate
	Neuron-specific enolase (NSE)	Small-cell lung carcinoma, neuroblastoma
Specific Proteins	Prostate-specific antigen (PSA)	Adenocarcinoma of prostate
	Immunoglobin	Multiple myeloma
	CA 125	Epithelial ovarian cancer
	CA 19-9	Adenocarcinoma of pancreas, colon
	CA 15-3	Breast cancer

Source: Adapted from Pfeifer, J. D., & Wick, M. R. (1995). The pathologic evaluation of neoplastic disease. In A. I. Holleb, D. J. Fink, & G. P. Murphy (Eds.), *American Cancer Society textbook of clinical oncology* (pp. 75–95). Atlanta: American Cancer Society.

may involve routine x-ray imaging (usually for screening only), CT, MRI, ultrasonography, nuclear imaging, angiography, and positron emission tomography. These diagnostic tests, including preparation and nursing implications, are discussed in the assessment chapters as well as with specific body system cancers throughout the book.

X-Ray Imaging   Standard x-ray imaging is the method of choice for screening such body areas as the breast (mammography), lung, and bone to identify changes in tissue density that may indicate malignancies. X-ray imaging is still the method of choice for lung cancer, but does not usually reveal tumors until late in their development when they have reached about 1 cm in size.

Computed Tomography (CT)   CT allows the visualization of cross sections of the anatomy. Because CT scans reveal subtle differences in tissue densities, they provide much greater accuracy in tumor diagnosis. This procedure is useful in screening for renal cell and most gastrointestinal tumors. CT scans are especially useful for evaluating possible lymph node involvement.

Magnetic Resonance Imaging (MRI)   During an MRI, the patient is placed within a strong magnetic field, pulsed radio waves are directed at him or her, and transmitted signals based on tissue characteristics are analyzed by a computer. Related diagnostic imaging procedures—positron emission tomography (PET) and single photon emission computed tomography (SPECT)—create visible images by measuring electrical impulses from different body structures. MRI is the diagnostic tool of choice for both screening and follow-up of cranial and head and neck tumors.

Ultrasonography   Ultrasonography measures sound waves as they bounce off various body structures, revealing abnormalities that indicate tumors. For example, transrectal ultrasonography has provided excellent imaging of early prostate cancers and is used to guide needle biopsy. Ultrasound imaging is more useful for detecting masses in the denser breast tissue of young women.

Nuclear Imaging   Nuclear imaging involves the use of a special scanner in conjunction with the ingestion or injection of specific radioactive isotopes. This is an invasive but usually safe diagnostic method for identifying tumors in various body tissues. The procedure is often used to check for possible bone or other organ metastases.

Angiography   Angiography is performed when the precise location of the tumor cannot be identified or there is a need to visualize the tumor's extent prior to surgery. The procedure involves injecting a radiopaque dye into a major blood vessel proximal to the organ or tissue to be examined. The movement of the dye through the vasculature of the organ or tissue is traced by means of fluoroscopy or serial x-ray films. Blockage to the flow of the dye indicates the tumor's location. Dye may be used to identify blood vessels supplying a tumor, allowing the surgeon to know where to safely ligate vessels.

DIRECT VISUALIZATION   Direct visualization procedures are invasive but do not require the use of radiography. Examples include sigmoidoscopy (viewing the sigmoid colon with a fiber-optic flexible sigmoidoscope), cystoscopy (viewing the urethra and bladder), endoscopy (viewing the upper gastrointestinal tract), and bronchoscopy (inspecting the tracheobronchial tree). These methods allow the visual identification of the organs within the limits of the scope and usually permit biopsy of suspicious lesions or masses. Flexible fiber-optic scopes may be more useful because they allow deeper penetration than do traditional scopes. These procedures all require some patient preparation, cause moderate to considerable discomfort, and may require sedation or anesthesia, as in the case of bronchoscopy. Some procedures, such as sigmoidoscopy and cystoscopy, may be performed in the physician's office and therefore cost less, making them more accessible screening procedures.

When the tumor is exposed, a sample of tissue (biopsy) is sent to the pathology laboratory for a "frozen-section" histologic examination. This can be done rapidly while the patient remains on the operating table under anesthesia. If the initial report is negative, the benign mass is usually removed to prevent further symptoms. If the report is positive for cancer, the tumor and often adjacent lymph nodes are dissected, along with any other suspicious tissue. The tumor, nodes, and any other specimens are sent to the pathology laboratory for more in-depth analysis. The patient then receives the usual postoperative care.

LABORATORY TESTS   Most laboratory tests of blood, urine, and other body fluids are used to rule out nutritional disorders and other noncancerous conditions that may be causing the patient's symptoms. In conjunction with other diagnostic studies, some laboratory tests can be quite useful either in screening for other pathologic conditions or for validating the cancer diagnosis. Table 14–8 identifies some useful laboratory tests, their normal values, and their possible indications.

PSYCHOLOGIC SUPPORT DURING DIAGNOSIS   Preparing for and awaiting the results of diagnostic tests can create extreme anxiety. Many patients compare the experience to that of a prisoner awaiting trial and sentencing: After they know what the "sentence" is, then they can prepare for the future. In addition to coping with the possibility of a life-threatening disease, or at least a life-altering one, patients often also face the prospect of uncomfortable, even painful, diagnostic procedures. They have important decisions to make that depend on the outcome of those tests. Many unspoken questions may exist, including the following:

- Do I have cancer?
- If so, what kind, and how serious?
- Has it spread?
- Will I survive?
- What kind of treatment is needed?
- How will this affect my lifestyle?
- How will this affect family members and friends?

Denial or intellectualization can help some patients coping with cancer, but others display signs of anxiety and stress as they attempt to cope. The nurse can provide valuable support during this very difficult stage by helping patients become actively involved in managing their life and disease. Talk with patients as soon as they enter the healthcare system, asking what they know already about what is going to happen and soliciting questions from them. Taking this approach and encouraging patients to share what knowledge and experience

TABLE 14–8 Laboratory Tests Used for Cancer Diagnosis*

TEST	REFERENCE VALUE	ABNORMALITY INDICATED
Acid phosphatase (ACP)	0.0 to 0.8 unit/L	Elevated in prostate, breast, and bone cancer and in multiple myeloma
Adrenocorticotropic hormone (ACTH)	8 to 80 pg/mL	Decreased in adrenal cancer Elevated in pituitary cancer or with tumor that secretes ACTH (bronchiogenic cancer)
Alanine aminotransferase (ALT)	5 to 35 unit/mL (Frankel)	Moderate elevation in liver cancer
Albumin	3.5 to 5.0 g/dL	Decreased in malnutrition, metastatic liver cancer
Alkaline phosphatase (ALP)	20 to 90 unit/L	Elevated in cancer of liver, bone, breast, and prostate; in leukemia; and in multiple myeloma
Alpha-fetoprotein (AFP)	Male and nonpregnant female: < 15 ng/mL	Elevated in germ cell tumors (e.g., seminoma), testicular cancer
Aspartate aminotransferase (AST)	5 to 40 unit/mL (Frankel)	Elevated in liver cancer
Bilirubin	Total: 0.1 to1.2 mg/dL Direct: 0.0 to 0.3 mg/dL	Elevated in liver and gallbladder cancer
Bleeding time	Ivy method: 3 to 7 minutes	Prolonged in leukemia and metastatic liver cancer
Blood urea nitrogen (BUN)	5 to 25 mg/dL	Decreased in malnutrition; increased in renal cancer
Calcitonin	Male: < 40 pg/mL Female: < 20 pg/mL	Elevated to > 500 pg/mL in thyroid medullary cancer, breast cancer, and lung cancer
Calcium (Ca)	4.5 to 5.5 mEq/L 9.0 to 11.0 mg/dL	Elevated in bone cancer and ectopic parathyroid hormone production (paraplastic syndrome)
Carcinoembryonic antigen (CEA)	2.5 ng/mL in nonsmokers 5 ng/mL in smokers; > 12 ng/mL neoplasms	Elevated with GI cancers, lung, breast, bladder, kidney, cervical, leukemias Used to evaluate effectiveness of cancer treatment
Chloride (Cl)	95 to 105 mEq/L	Decreased in vomiting, diarrhea, syndrome of inappropriate antidiuretic hormone (SIADH)
C-reactive protein	> 1:2 titer is positive	Elevated in metastatic cancer and Burkitt's lymphoma
Creatinine	0.5 to 1.5 mg/dL	Decreased in malnutrition; elevated in most cancers
Dexamethasone suppression test	> 50% reduction in plasma cortisol	Nonsuppression in adrenal cancer and ACTH-producing tumors, severe stress
Estradiol-serum	Female: 20 to 300 pg/mL Menopausal female: < 20 pg/mL Male: 15 to 50 pg/mL	Elevated in estrogen-producing tumors and testicular tumors
Fibrinogen	200 to 400 mg/dL	Decreased in leukemia and as a side effect of chemotherapy
Gamma glutamyltransferase (GGT)	Male: 10 to 80 international unit/L Female: 5 to 25 international unit/L	Elevated in cancer of liver, pancreas, prostate, breast, kidney, lung, and brain
Fasting blood sugar	70 to 110 mg/dL	Decreased in malnutrition, cancer of stomach, liver, and lung
Haptoglobin	20 to 240 mg/dL	Elevated in Hodgkin's disease and cancer of lung, large intestine, stomach, breast, and liver
Hematocrit (Hct)	Male: 40% to 54% Female: 36% to 46%	Decreased in anemia, leukemia, Hodgkin's disease, lymphosarcoma, multiple myeloma, and malnutrition and as a side effect of chemotherapy
Hemoglobin (Hgb)	Male: 13.5 to 18 g/dL Female: 12 to 16 g/dL 1:3 ratio of Hgb:Hct	Decreased in anemia, many cancers, Hodgkin's disease, leukemia, and malnutrition and as a side effect of chemotherapy
Human chorionic gonadotropin (HCG)	Nonpregnant female <0.01 international unit/L	Elevated in choriocarcinoma
Insulin	5 to 25 microunit/mL	Elevated in insulinoma (islet cell tumor) and insulin-secreting cancers (e.g., lung cancer)
Lactic dehydrogenase (LDH)	100 to 190 international unit/L	Elevated in liver, brain, kidney, muscle cancers, acute leukemia, anemia
Occult blood	Negative	Positive in gastric and colon cancers

(continued)

TABLE 14–8 Laboratory Tests Used for Cancer Diagnosis* (continued)

TEST	REFERENCE VALUE	ABNORMALITY INDICATED
Serum osmolality	280 to 300 mOsm/kg H_2O	Decreased in SIADH
Urine osmolality	50 to 1200 mOsm/kg H_2O	Increased in SIADH
Parathyroid hormone (PTH)	400 to 900 pg/mL	Increased in PTH-secreting tumors
Platelet (thrombocyte) count	150,000/mm^3 to 400,000/mm^3	Decreased in bone, gastric, and brain cancer, in leukemia, and as a side effect of chemotherapy
Potassium (K)	3.5 to 5.0 mEq/L	Decreased in vomiting and diarrhea and in malnutrition
Prostatic-specific antigen (PSA)	0 to 4 ng/mL	Elevated from 10 to 120+ in prostate cancer
Total protein	6.0 to 8.0 g/dL	Decreased in malnutrition, gastrointestinal cancer, Hodgkin's disease; elevated in vomiting, diarrhea, multiple myeloma
Red blood cells (RBCs)	Male: 4.6 to 6.0 million/mm^3 Female: 4.0 to 5.0 million/mm^3	Decreased in anemia, leukemia, infection, multiple myeloma
Sodium (Na)	135 to 145 mEq/L	Decreased in SIADH, vomiting; elevated in dehydration
Uric acid	Male: 3.5 to 8.0 mg/dL Female: 2.8 to 6.8 mg/dL	Increased in leukemia, metastatic cancer, multiple myeloma, Burkitt's lymphoma, after vigorous chemotherapy
White blood cells (WBC)		
Total leukocytes	4500/mm^3 to 10,000/mm^3	Elevated in acute infection, leukemias, tissue necrosis; decreased as a side effect of chemotherapy
Neutrophils	50% to 70%	Elevated in bacterial infection and Hodgkin's disease; decreased in leukemia and malnutrition and as a side effect of chemotherapy
Eosinophils	1% to 3%	Elevated in cancer of bone, ovary, testes, and brain
Basophils	0.4% to 1.0%	Elevated in leukemia and healing stage of infection
Monocytes	4% to 6%	Elevated in infection, monocytic leukemia and cancer; decreased in lymphocytic leukemia and as a side effect of chemotherapy
Lymphocytes	25% to 35%	Elevated in lymphocytic leukemia, Hodgkin's disease, multiple myeloma, viral infections, and chronic infections; decreased in malnutrition, cancer, and other leukemias and as a side effect of chemotherapy

*All values refer to serum values unless otherwise indicated. Values are approximate; check the reference standards specified by your own agency's laboratory.

they have allows them to maintain control. From there, the nurse can provide the information needed.

As patients begin to feel more comfortable with the nurse, they may express concerns, fears, and other emotions. The nurse should actively listen and be supportive, but avoid giving advice and false reassurance, providing appropriate information when needed. For patients who are not ready to discuss concerns or for those who appear angry, being nonjudgmental and providing nonverbal support may facilitate more open communication. An atmosphere of calmness, warmth, caring, and respect can ease the tension and often unspoken terror of this initial period.

Support of and communication with the patient's significant others is extremely important. Often they try to be strong for the patient but have many fears and emotional concerns that they do not feel comfortable expressing. The nurse needs to be available to the family while the patient is undergoing diagnostic procedures. Allowing them to talk without the need to edit for the patient's benefit can help them manage their own difficulties in coping with their loved one's potential cancer diagnosis.

Cancer Treatment

The goals of cancer treatment are aimed at cure, control, or palliation of symptoms. These goals may overlap. Cancer may be treated through surgery, chemotherapy, radiation therapy, biotherapy, photodynamic therapy, bone marrow and stem cell transplants, hormonal therapy, and complementary therapies. Once cancer is diagnosed, the initial focus is on surgical and medical treatment. The goals of treatment are the following:

- Eliminating the tumor or malignant cells
- Preventing metastasis
- Reducing cellular growth and the tumor burden
- Promoting functional abilities and providing pain relief to those whose disease has not responded to treatment

SURGERY   Surgery remains an important approach in cancer care. Surgical resection is used for diagnosis and staging of more than 90% of all cancers and for primary treatment of more than 60% of cancers. The goals of surgery have also expanded to include prophylaxis, diagnosis, treatment, reconstruction, and palliation.

Prophylactic surgery aims to remove tissues or organs that are likely to develop cancer. Advances in identification of genetic markers make prophylactic surgery an option for individuals with a strong family history and genetic predisposition for the development of cancer. For example, a woman with a strong history of breast cancer, positive findings of BRCA-1 or BRCA-2, and abnormal finding on mammography may consider prophylactic mastectomy as one of the selective options. Other examples of prophylactic operations include colectomy and oophorectomy. With limited research on the long-term physiologic and psychological effects on individuals undergoing prophylactic surgery for cancer, it is vitally important for nurses and other healthcare professionals to discuss thoroughly with the patient and family potential risks and postoperative outcomes of the prophylactic surgery prior to the surgery. Nurses should respect the patient's decision whether or not to pursue the prophylactic surgery. For those patients who choose prophylactic surgery as a preventive measure for cancer, comprehensive preoperative teaching and counseling should be provided and long-term postoperative follow-up should be ensured to monitor the patient's physiologic and psychological adjustment to the surgery.

Diagnostic surgery aims to ensure histological diagnosis and staging of cancer through biopsy, endoscopy, laparoscopy, and open surgical exploration. Table 14–9 provides information about common surgical diagnostic procedures.

As a primary treatment for cancer, the goal of surgery is to remove the entire tumor and involved surrounding tissue and lymph nodes as much as possible and feasible. This sometimes necessitates mutilation of the body and the creation of new structures to assume function of the lost structures. For example, removal of the distal sigmoid colon and rectum requires a new means of bowel elimination, so the remaining healthy segment of the bowel is brought out through a created opening (stoma) in the abdominal wall, resulting in a permanent colostomy (∞ see Chapter 24). In like manner, when the bladder is removed, the ureters are transplanted into a created pouch just under the abdominal wall. This serves as a continent ileostomy, a substitute reservoir for urine (∞ see Chapter 27). Surgery can destroy sensitive nerve plexuses, resulting in alteration or loss of normal functioning; for example, prostate surgery may result in incontinence and impotence. Surgical removal of involved regional lymph nodes can lead to long-term lymphedema (swelling in the affected area) that greatly impacts cancer survivors' quality of life, for instance, lymphedema following surgery for breast cancer and melanoma (Norman et al., 2009).

Not all surgery results in such radical changes in functioning. The following surgeries can eliminate cancer successfully with less distressing results:

- Removing a nonessential portion of the organ or tissue containing the tumor, such as *in situ* small-bowel tumors
- Removing an organ whose function can be replaced chemically, such as the thyroid
- Resecting one of a pair of organs when the unaffected organ can take over the function of the missing one, such as a lung

Although the removal of any major body part has physiologic and psychological consequences, the alternative—terminal disease—is usually less desirable.

If the tumor is in a nonresectable location or deeply invaded with metastases, surgery may be done to achieve palliation to allow the involved organs to function as long as possible, to relieve pain, to provide comfort, or to bypass an obstruction. Surgery may also be done to reduce the bulk of the tumor in advanced disease, both at primary and metastatic sites. Decreasing the tumor size enhances the ability to control the remaining disease through other modalities. Surgery is often used in conjunction with other treatments to effect a cure. In cases when extensive removal of tissue is contraindicated (e.g., in surgical removal of a brain tumor), radiation may be used prior to surgery in an attempt to shrink the tumor before it is removed.

Surgical intervention may be used for reconstruction and rehabilitation to achieve more desirable functional and cosmetic effect after curative or radical surgery. One example is the construction of transabdominal myocutaneous (TRAM) flaps in conjunction with or following modified radical mastectomy (∞ see Chapter 49). For surgical interventions for cancers affecting specific body systems, refer to later chapters.

Surgical oncologists are working with researchers to identify premalignant disease earlier in high-risk populations and to conduct studies on ways to reverse oncogenic cell activity. Surgeons work with molecular biologists using sophisticated techniques to develop monoclonal antibodies. Laser technology is being explored for use in different types of cancer surgery because it minimizes blood loss, reduces deformity, increases the accuracy of tissue resection, and enhances healing. Lasers are currently being used to treat radical prostatectomy in order to preserve urinary continence and sexual functioning.

Another collaborative strategy is intraoperative radiation therapy, in which radiosensitive, nondiseased organs that may be damaged by radiation therapy are moved away from the radiation field and shielded. Radiation is administered while the patient is on the operating table. This technique allows

TABLE 14–9 Surgical Diagnostic Procedures

PROCEDURE	EXPLANATION
Fine-needle biopsy	Use of a very thin needle to aspirate a small amount of tissue from the tumors
Needle core biopsy	Use of a slightly larger needle than that used for a fine-needle biopsy to extract a small amount of tissue from tumors that cannot be aspirated by fine-needle aspiration
Incisional biopsy	Removal of part of a larger tumor by cutting through the skin
Excisional biopsy	Removal of an entire tumor through operation
Endoscopy	Use of a small viewing lens or video camera through natural body openings to view tumors such as cancer of the esophagus, stomach, or colon
Laparoscopy	Use of a small viewing lens or video camera through a small incision in the abdominal wall

more penetrating radiation to be directed to the malignant tumor with less trauma to normal, vulnerable tissues or organs.

Nursing responsibilities focus on preparing the patient physically and psychologically for surgery, as well as teaching routine postoperative care in which the patient is expected to participate (∞ see Chapter 4). Before surgery, the nurse should give the patient the opportunity to ask questions and to discuss concerns and fears. In some cases, the patient may want to discuss alternative treatment options. In the latter case, the nurse should contact the oncologist and the surgeon and set up a conference for the patient before surgery.

CHEMOTHERAPY **Chemotherapy** involves the use of cytotoxic medications to cure liquid and solid cancers, such as leukemias, lymphomas, and breast and prostate cancer; to decrease tumor size, adjunctive to surgery or radiation therapy; or to prevent or treat suspected metastases. Chemotherapy may also be used in conjunction with biotherapy. All chemotherapy has side effects or toxic effects. The type and severity depend on the drugs used.

Chemotherapy disrupts the cell cycle in various phases by interrupting cell metabolism and replication. It also works by interfering with the ability of the malignant cell to synthesize vital enzymes and chemicals. Phase-specific drugs work during only some phases of the cell cycle; non-phase-specific drugs work through the entire cell cycle. Figure 14–5 ■ lists some of the drugs useful in each phase of the cell cycle.

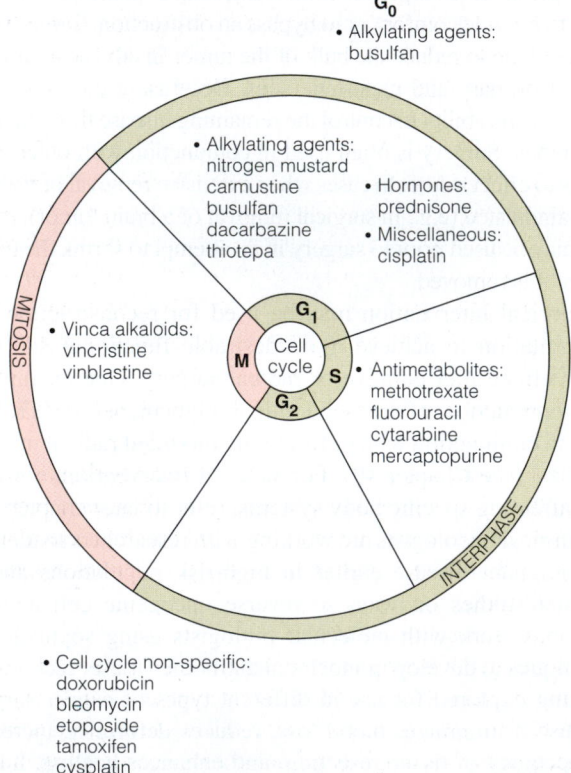

Figure 14–5 ■ Chemotherapeutic drugs useful in each phase of the cell cycle. Based on their chemical makeup and biologic activity, different drugs used for cancer treatment act in specific phases and subphases of the cell cycle. Some drugs, called non-phase-specific drugs, are generalized and act throughout the cycle. Chemotherapy often involves combinations of drugs designed to attack the cancer cells at many different times in the cycle to enhance effectiveness.

Most chemotherapy involves combinations of drugs administered over varying periods of time according to different protocols. One protocol for adult acute lymphocytic leukemia (ALL) uses the acronym DVPA: daunorubicin given on days 1 through 3; vincristine given on days 1, 8, 15, and 22; prednisone given on days 1 through 28, and asparaginase given on days 17 through 28. The treatment regimen is administered in cycles with rest periods, especially if toxic effects such as liver dysfunction or severe neutropenia (abnormally low amounts of neutrophils, a type of white blood cell) occur. The treatment is continued until the remission of the cancer is achieved. If the cancer progresses the particular protocol is abandoned and a new protocol may be tried.

Several courses of chemotherapy are necessary based on the hypothesis of cell-killing. A 1-cm tumor contains about 10^9 (10 billion) total cells, most of which are viable. During each cell cycle, the chemotherapy kills a fixed percentage of cells, always leaving some behind. With each reduction, the tumor burden of cells decreases until the number of viable, clonogenic cells (i.e., those that are able to clone daughter cells) becomes small enough to allow the body's immune system to finish the job. For this reason, oncologists usually give the maximum amount of chemotherapy tolerated by the patient. High-dose chemotherapy remains controversial.

CLASSES OF CHEMOTHERAPY DRUGS Chemotherapeutic agents can be classified either by the effects of the agent on the cell or by the pharmacologic properties of the agent. According to the effects of the agent on the cell, chemotherapeutic agents can be divided into cell cycle–specific and cell cycle–nonspecific agents. Cell cycle–specific agents are effective at a specific phase (for example, S and M phases) in the cell cycle to prevent cell replication by damaging cellular DNA and blocking production of protein necessary for DNA and RNA synthesis. Cell cycle–nonspecific agents are effective throughout all the phases of the cell cycle, including the resting phase. Both cell cycle–specific and cell cycle–nonspecific agents are effective in rapidly dividing cells to prohibit the growth of fast-growing tumors.

The most common way of classifying chemotherapeutic agents is based on pharmacologic properties of the agent. The classifications include alkylating agents, antimetabolites, antitumor antibiotics, mitotic inhibitors, hormones and hormone antagonists, and miscellaneous agents.

Alkylating Agents Alkylating agents are not phase specific and basically act on preformed nucleic acids by creating defects in tumor DNA. They cause crosslinking of DNA strands, which can permanently interfere with replication and transcription.

Alkylating agents work with both proliferating and nonproliferating cells (those in G_0 phase). Their toxicity relates to their ability to kill slowly cycling stem cells and manifests in delayed, prolonged, or permanent bone marrow failure. Toxicity can cause a mutagenic effect on bone marrow stem cells, culminating in a treatment-resistant form of acute myelogenous leukemia. Because of the alkylating agents' effect on stem cells, they also cause irreversible infertility. Other common adverse effects include nephrotoxicity (kidney damage) and hemorrhagic cystitis (bladder damage).

The several subclasses of alkylating agents include nitrogen mustard (mechlorethamine), nitrosoureas (carmustine), alkyl sulfonates (busulfan), triazines (dacarbazine), ethyleneamines (thiotepa), and cisplatin. Cisplatin is an alkylating agent containing platinum and chlorine atoms. It is most active in the G_1 subphase, but it is also not phase specific. Cisplatin binds to DNA and acts much like alkylating agents by forming intrastrand DNA crosslinks (gluing strands of DNA together so that they cannot separate). Its major toxic effect is reversible renal tubular necrosis. Cisplatin may be used alone or in combination with other chemotherapeutic drugs for testicular and ovarian cancers.

Antimetabolites The different types of antimetabolites include folic acid analogues (methotrexate), pyrimidine analogues (5-fluorouracil), cytosine arabinoside (ARA-C), and purine analogues (6-mercaptopurine). Antimetabolites, are phase specific, working best in the S phase and having little effect in G_0. They interfere with nucleic acid synthesis by either displacing normal metabolites at the regulatory site of a key enzyme or by substituting for a metabolite that is incorporated into DNA or RNA molecules. Toxic effects usually do not occur until very high levels of the drug are administered. Toxicity is more likely when the drugs accumulate in third-spaced fluid, such as pleural fluid (a characteristic that also makes them useful in treating malignant pleural effusions). Because the drug diffuses slowly from the third-spaced fluid, exposure of the tissue to the drug is prolonged. Most toxic effects relate to rapidly proliferating cells, such as cells in the gastrointestinal tract, hair, and skin and WBCs. Manifestations include nausea and vomiting, stomatitis, diarrhea, alopecia, and leukopenia. Some of the drugs can also cause liver and lung toxicity.

Antitumor Antibiotics Antitumor antibiotics are derived from natural sources that are generally too toxic to be used as antibacterial agents. They are not phase specific and act in several ways: They disrupt DNA replication and RNA transcription; create free radicals, which generate breaks in DNA and other forms of damage; and interfere with DNA repair. In addition, these drugs bind to cells and kill them, probably by damaging the cell membrane. Their main toxic effect is damage to the cardiac muscle. This limits the amount and duration of treatment. Examples of these antibiotics include actinomycin D, doxorubicin, bleomycin, mitomycin-C, and mithramycin.

Mitotic Inhibitors Mitotic inhibitors are drugs that act to prevent cell division during the M phase. Mitotic inhibitors include the plant alkaloids and taxoids. Plant alkaloids consist of medications extracted from plant sources: Vinca alkaloids (e.g., vincristine and vinblastine) and etoposide (also called VP-16). The Vinca alkaloids are phase specific, acting during mitosis. They bind to a specific protein in tumor cells that promotes chromosome migration during mitosis and serves as a conduit for neurotransmitter transport along axons. The toxicity of these drugs is characterized by depression of deep tendon reflexes, paresthesias (pain and altered sensation), motor weakness, cranial nerve disruptions, and paralytic ileus. Etoposide acts in all phases of the cell cycle, causing breaks in DNA and metaphase arrest. Although etoposide may cause bone marrow suppression and nausea and vomiting, the most common toxic effect is hypotension resulting from too rapid intravenous administration. The taxoids act during the G_2 phase to inhibit cell division. Paclitaxel is used for the treatment of Kaposi's sarcoma and metastatic breast and ovarian

cancer. Taxotere is used for breast cancer. Toxicities associated with these drugs include alopecia, bone marrow depression, and severe hypersensitivity reactions (e.g., hypotension, dyspnea, and urticaria).

Hormones and Hormone Antagonists The main hormones used in cancer therapy are the corticosteroids (e.g., prednisone), which are phase specific (G_1). These act by binding to specific intracellular receptors, repressing transcription of mRNA, and thereby altering cellular function and growth. Corticosteroids have multiple side effects such as impaired healing, hyperglycemia, hypertension, osteoporosis, and hirsutism.

Hormone antagonists work with hormone-binding tumors, usually those of the breast, prostate, and endometrium. They block the hormone's receptor site on the tumor and prevent it from receiving normal hormonal growth stimulation. These drugs do not cure, but cause regression of the tumor in about 40% of breast and endometrial tumors and 80% of prostate tumors. Tamoxifen competes with estradiol receptors in breast tumors. Raloxifene blocks estrogen in the breast. Diethylstilbestrol competes with hormone receptors in endometrial and prostate tumors. Aromatase inhibitors (Arimidex, Femara, and Aromasin) reduce the amount of estrogen produced in post-menopausal women. Antiandrogen (flutamide) and luteinizing hormone–releasing hormone block testosterone synthesis in prostate cancers. The main side effects of these drugs are alterations of the secondary sexual characteristics.

Miscellaneous Agents Several miscellaneous agents act at different phases in the cell cycle. L-Asparaginase and hydroxyurea are examples of miscellaneous agents.

EFFECTS OF CHEMOTHERAPEUTIC DRUGS The side effects and toxic effects of chemotherapy vary with the drug used and the length of treatment. Because most of these drugs act on fast-growing cells, the side effects are manifestations of damage to normal rapidly dividing somatic cells. The side effects of hormones express the action of the hormone used or suppression of the normal hormone, such as the masculinizing effects of male hormones administered for ovarian cancers.

Tissues usually affected by cytotoxic drugs include the following:

- Mucous membranes of the mouth, tongue, esophagus, stomach, intestine, and rectum. This may result in anorexia, loss of taste, aversion to food, erythema and painful ulcerations in any portion of the gastrointestinal tract, nausea, vomiting, and diarrhea.
- Hair cells, resulting in alopecia.
- Bone marrow depression affecting most blood cells (e.g., granulocytes, lymphocytes, thrombocytes, and erythrocytes). This results in an impaired ability to respond to infection, a diminished ability to clot blood, and severe anemia.
- Organs, such as heart, lungs, bladder, kidneys. This kind of damage is related to specific agents, such as cardiac toxicity with doxorubicin or pneumonitis with bleomycin.
- Reproductive organs, resulting in impaired reproductive ability or altered fetal development.

Table 14–10 gives the classifications of chemotherapeutic drugs, common examples, target malignancies, adverse effects

TABLE 14–10 Classifications of Chemotherapeutic Drugs

DRUG CLASSIFICATION	COMMON DRUGS	TARGET MALIGNANCIES	ADVERSE EFFECTS OR SIDE EFFECTS	NURSING IMPLICATIONS
Alkylating agents	Mechlorethamine (Mustargen)	Hodgkin's disease Lymphosarcoma Lung cancer Chronic leukemia	Nausea and vomiting Leukopenia Thrombocytopenia Hyperuricemia	Maintain good hydration. Alkalinize urine. Administer antiemetics prior to chemotherapy. Monitor WBC, uric acid. Assess for infection.
	Busulfan (Myleran)	Chronic myelogenous leukemia	Leukopenia Thrombocytopenia Renal failure Pulmonary fibrosis	Monitor WBCs, BUN. Maintain adequate fluid intake. Assess for infection. Assess lungs for fibrotic (coarse, loud) rales.
	Cyclophosphamide (Cytoxan)	Lymphomas Multiple myeloma Leukemias Adenocarcinoma of lung and breast	Hemorrhagic cystitis Renal failure Alopecia Stomatitis Liver dysfunction	Encourage daily fluid intake of 2 to 3 L during treatment. Monitor WBCs, BUN, liver enzymes. Teach ways to manage hair loss.
Antimetabolites	Methotrexate	Acute lymphoblastic leukemia Osteosarcoma Gestational trophoblastic carcinoma	Oral and gastrointestinal ulcerations Anorexia and nausea Leukopenia Thrombocytopenia Pancytopenia	Monitor CBC, WBC differential, BUN, uric acid, creatinine. Assess oral mucous membranes; treat ulcers prn. Assess for infection, bleeding.
	5-Fluorouracil (5-FU)	Colon carcinoma Rectal carcinoma Breast carcinoma Gastric carcinoma Pancreatic cancer	Stomatitis Alopecia Nausea and vomiting Gastritis Enteritis Diarrhea Anemia Leukopenia Thrombocytopenia	Monitor CBC with differential, BUN, uric acid. Administer antiemetics prn. Assess for bleeding; check stool occult blood. Evaluate hydration and nutrition status. Teach oral care for stomatitis. Assess for infection. Teach care for hair loss.
Antitumor antibiotics	Doxorubicin (Adriamycin)	Acute lymphoblastic leukemia (ALL) Acute myeloblastic leukemia Neuroblastoma Wilms' tumor Breast, ovarian, thyroid, lung cancer	Stomatitis Alopecia Nausea and vomiting Gastritis Enteritis Diarrhea Anemia Leukopenia Thrombocytopenia Cardiac toxicity	Monitor ECG; assess for arrhythmias, gallops, and congestive heart failure (CHF). Monitor CBC with differential, BUN, uric acid. Administer antiemetics prn. Assess for bleeding; check stool for occult blood. Evaluate hydration and nutrition status. Teach oral care for stomatitis. Assess for infection. Teach care for hair loss.
	Bleomycin (Blenoxane)	Squamous cell carcinoma Lymphosarcoma Reticulum cell sarcoma Testicular carcinoma Hodgkin's disease	Mucocutaneous ulcerations Alopecia Nausea and vomiting Chills and fever Pneumonitis and pulmonary fibrosis	Check for fever 3 to 6 hours after administration. Have chest x-ray films taken every 2 to 3 weeks. Assess respiratory status, and check for coarse rales. Evaluate hydration and nutrition status. Teach oral care for stomatitis. Assess for infection. Teach care for hair loss.
Plant alkaloids	Vincristine (Oncovin)	Combination therapy for acute leukemia, Hodgkin's and non-Hodgkin's lymphomas, rhabdomyosarcoma, neuroblastoma, Wilms' tumor	Areflexia Muscle weakness Peripheral neuritis Constipation Paralytic ileus Mild bone marrow Depression	Assess neuromuscular function. Monitor CBC with differential. Evaluate gastrointestinal function. Manage constipation.

TABLE 14–10 Classifications of Chemotherapeutic Drugs (continued)

DRUG CLASSIFICATION	COMMON DRUGS	TARGET MALIGNANCIES	ADVERSE EFFECTS OR SIDE EFFECTS	NURSING IMPLICATIONS
Plant alkaloids (*continued*)	Vinblastine (Velban)	Combination therapy for Hodgkin's disease, lymphocytic and histocytic lymphoma Kaposi's sarcoma, advanced testicular carcinoma, unresponsive breast cancer	Areflexia Alopecia Nausea and vomiting Bone marrow depression	Assess neuromuscular function. Monitor CBC with differential. Administer antiemetics prn. Teach ways to manage hair loss.
	Etoposide, also called VP-16 (VePesid)	Nonresponsive testicular tumors Small-cell lung cancer	Alopecia Hypotension with rapid infusion	Hydrate adequately before administration. Administer for 60 minutes. Monitor vital signs every 15 minutes during administration and every 2 to 4 hours thereafter. Teach ways to manage hair loss.
	Prednisone	Combination therapy for many tumors Leukemia Lymphoma	Fluid retention Hypertension Steroid diabetes Emotional lability Silent bleeding ulcers Increased risk for infection	Monitor vital signs. Administer diuretics prn. Check blood glucose regularly. Evaluate mental status. Administer oral medications with food. Administer hydrogen ion antagonist drugs (antacids) as ordered. Monitor WBC with differential. Check for signs of systemic infection.
	Diethylstilbestrol (DES)	Advanced breast and prostrate cancers	Fluid retention Feminization Uterine bleeding	Monitor vital signs. Administer diuretics prn as ordered. Explain reason for feminization to men, bleeding to women. Monitor for excessive bleeding.
	Tamoxifen (Nolvadex)	Breast cancer	Hot flashes Nausea and vomiting	Teach ways to manage hot flashes. Explain reason for hot flashes. Administer antiemetics as ordered.
Miscellaneous drugs	Cisplatin (CDDP) (Platinol)	Combination and single therapy for metastatic testicular and ovarian cancers, advanced bladder cancer, head and neck tumors, non-small-cell lung carcinoma, osteogenic sarcoma, neuroblastoma	Bone marrow depression: leukopenia and thrombocytopenia Renal tubular damage Deafness	Monitor WBC with differential and platelets, BUN, creatinine, uric acid. Watch for bleeding. Monitor for signs of infection. Evaluate hearing; check for tinnitus. Ensure that patient is well hydrated before drug is administered. Encourage 2 to 3 L of fluid intake daily.

and side effects, and nursing implications. Consult current pharmacology textbooks for additional drugs and for new combination therapies as they are developed.

PREPARATION AND ADMINISTRATION Many states and individual hospitals require that personnel be trained and certified to administer chemotherapy. Pharmacists in large hospitals and independent home care agencies usually prepare chemotherapeutic drugs for parenteral administration under specific safety guidelines established by the federal government or the Oncology Nursing Society. In some agencies, nurses both prepare and administer these drugs. Because of the potential carcinogenic effects, it is usually recommended that the healthcare professional wear gloves, a mask, and gown while preparing and administering the drug and disposing of equipment. The nurse must use care when handling excretory products of patients undergoing chemotherapy and teach patients to dispose of their own body fluids safely. Oral medications pose a lesser risk of exposure, but a risk nonetheless, primarily through excretion in the urine.

Chemotherapeutic drugs can be administered orally, such as cyclophosphamide (Cytoxan) and chlorambucil (Leukeran). Other drugs, such as hormones or hormone-blocking agents, may also be given intramuscularly. However, many drugs require intravenous infusion or direct injection into intraperitoneal or intrapleural body cavities. Intravenous preparations can be given through large peripheral veins, but the risk of extravasation or irritation to the vein may preclude this method for long-term therapy. Many patients now receive vascular access devices (VADs), especially if their treatment requires several cycles over weeks or months. VADs are also useful for adjunctive parenteral nutrition in the patient who needs continuous intravenous infusions to manage pain or frequent blood drawing to monitor blood counts. Different types of VADs are available:

- Catheters that are inserted nonsurgically by threading them through a large peripheral vein into the vena cava. Called peripherally inserted central catheters (PICCs), they have multiple lumens that facilitate blood drawing. Placement is usually monitored by fluoroscopy.
- Catheters tunneled under the skin on the chest into a major vein, such as the subclavian vein. Hickman or Groshong catheters may be used.
- Surgically implanted ports are placed under the skin with a connected catheter inserted into a major vein. These are accessed by means of a special needle with a 90-degree angle inserted through the skin directly into the rubber dome of the port, which has a hard plastic back to prevent tissue damage.

Figure 14–6 ■ shows examples of different catheters and vascular access ports.

Risk of infection, catheter obstruction, and extravasation are the main problems associated with VADs. Nurses must teach patients and family members to observe for redness, swelling, pain, or exudate at the insertion site, which may indicate infection; to observe for swelling of the neck or skin near the VAD for extravasation and infiltration; and to flush catheters and provide site care (cleaning and dressing changes) on a regular basis. During each encounter with the patient, the nurse always inspects the site; observes for infection, infiltration, and catheter occlusion; and provides site care when necessary.

MANAGEMENT OF PATIENTS RECEIVING CHEMOTHERAPY

Nurses also help identify and manage toxic effects or side effects of the drugs and provide psychosocial support. Careful assessment and monitoring of the patient's manifestations, including appropriate laboratory tests, alert the nurse to the onset of toxicity. Nausea and vomiting, diarrhea, inflammation and ulceration of oral mucous membranes, hair loss, skin changes, anorexia, and fatigue require specific medical and nursing actions (discussed later in this chapter under the appropriate nursing diagnoses). Indicators of organ toxicities, such as nephrotoxicity, neurotoxicity, or cardiac toxicity, must be reported immediately to the physician. Another aspect of managing patients undergoing chemotherapy is to teach them how to care for access sites and to dispose of used equipment and excretions safely. Nurses teach patients to increase fluid intake to flush out the drugs; to get extra rest, which can both assist therapy and help the patient avoid other illnesses; to identify major complications of their particular drug protocol; to know when to call the physician or emergency medical services; and, if their WBC count is low, to limit their exposure to other people, especially children or those with infections.

During chemotherapy, a number of psychologic issues that can cause moderate to severe emotional distress may arise. The need to plan activities around chemotherapy treatments and their side effects can impair the patient's ability to work, manage a household or care for family members, function sexually, or participate in social and recreational activities. Weight loss and alopecia may prompt feelings of powerlessness and depression. The nurse can assist by carefully evaluating manifestations, providing specific interventions, and allowing patients opportunities to express their fears, concerns, and feelings. Patients should be encouraged to participate in their care and maintain control over their life as much as possible. Specific interventions will be discussed later in the chapter under the appropriate nursing diagnoses. Table 14–10 includes nursing implications for specific adverse effects of common chemotherapy drugs.

RADIATION THERAPY   Still the treatment of choice for some tumors or by some oncologists, radiation may be used to kill the tumor, to reduce its size, to decrease pain, or to relieve obstruction. Lymph nodes and adjacent tissues are irradiated when beginning metastasis is suspected. **Radiation therapy**

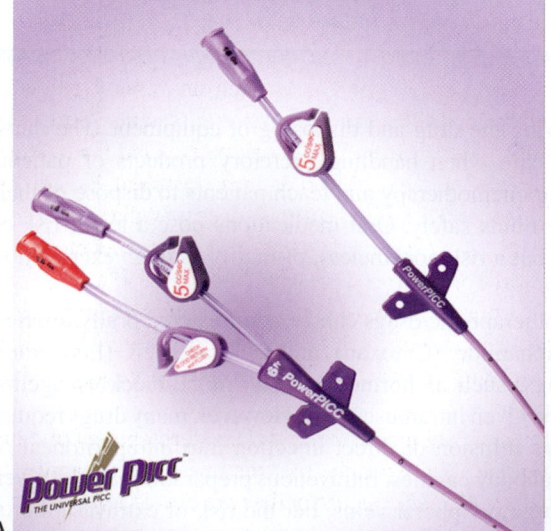
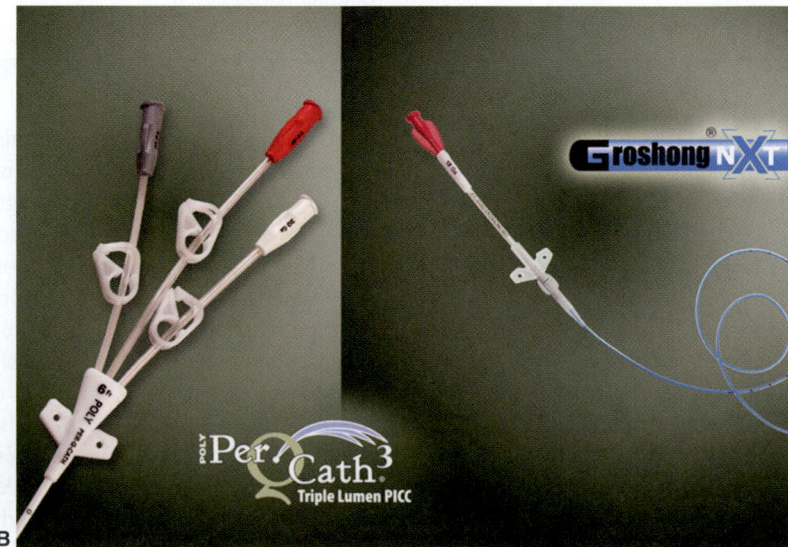

Figure 14–6 ■ Vascular access devices. *A,* Single- and double-lumen catheters. *B,* Triple-lumen and Groshong catheters.

Source: Photos A, B: Courtesy of Bard Access Systems, Salt Lake City, UT.

consists of delivering ionizing radiations of gamma and x-rays in one of two ways:

- *External Radiation.* Also called *teletherapy*, involves delivery of radiation from a source at some distance from the patient. A relatively uniform dosage is delivered to the tumor.
- *Internal Radiation.* Also called **brachytherapy** in which radiation is given inside the body by implanting small amounts of radioactive material directly into a tumor or body cavity while avoiding scattering radiation to the surrounding tissues or organs. This technique allows delivery of high doses of radiation to the tumor while sparing adjacent tissue. Brachytherapy is referred to as internal, interstitial, or intracavitary radiation. The innovation of brachytherapy uses a MammoSite catheter to provide a 5-day accelerated partial breast irradiation and holds promise of reducing the risk of radiation-induced complications.

Lethal injury to DNA is believed to be the primary mechanism by which radiation kills cells, especially cells in faster growing tumors and tissues. As a result, when given over time, radiation can destroy not only rapidly multiplying cancer cells but also rapidly dividing normal cells, such as those of the skin and mucous membranes. A malignant tumor is considered cured when there are no surviving tumor stem cells. The goal of radiation therapy is to achieve maximum tumor control with a minimum of damage to normal tissue.

Implanted or ingested radiation can be dangerous for those living with, taking care of, or treating the patient. Caregivers must use protection by, for example, shielding themselves from the source of radiation, limiting the time of exposure to the patient, increasing the distance from the patient, and using specific safety procedures for handling secretions. Box 14–5 identifies safety principles to be followed by those caring for patients undergoing internal radiation.

BOX 14–5 Safety Principles for Radiation

These recommendations apply to caregivers working with patients receiving internal radiation (brachytherapy).

- Maintain the greatest possible distance from the source of radiation.
- Spend the minimum amount of time close to the radiation source.
- Shield yourself from the radiation with lead gloves and aprons when possible.
- If pregnant, avoid contact with radiation sources.
- If you work routinely near radiation, wear a monitoring device to measure whole-body exposure.
- Avoid direct exposure with radioisotope containers; for example, do not touch the container.
- Keep patients with implanted radioisotopes in a private room with private bath and as far away from other hospitalized persons as possible.
- Dispose of body fluids of patients with unsealed implanted radioisotopes with special care and in specially marked containers.
- Handle bed linen and clothing with care and according to agency protocol.
- Use long-handled forceps to place any dislodged implants into a lead container.
- Consult with the radiation therapy department for any questions or problems in caring for patients with radioactive implants.

Tumors have differing sensitivities to radiation. Tumors that have the greatest number of rapidly proliferating cancer cells usually exhibit the best early response to radiation. The decision to use radiation rather than other modalities is based on balancing the probability of controlling the tumor against the probability of causing complications, such as tissue damage. The decision is usually made by risk–benefit analysis. Planning for radiation therapy includes assessing the disease site, tumor size, and histologic findings. Treatment schedules vary based on these factors. The patient receiving external radiation may experience skin changes such as blanching, erythema, desquamation, sloughing, or hemorrhage. Ulcerations of mucous membranes may cause severe pain; in addition, oral secretions can decrease, making the patient more vulnerable to infection and dental caries. Gastrointestinal effects include nausea and vomiting, diarrhea, or bleeding. Lungs may develop interstitial exudate, a condition called radiation pneumonia. Occasionally, external radiation therapy may cause fistulas or necrosis of adjacent tissues. Implanted radioactive materials can lead to similar problems; moreover, the excretory products of these patients are usually considered dangerous and need special disposal. See the Nursing Care box on page 366 for nursing implications for patients receiving radiation therapy.

BIOTHERAPY **Biotherapy** modifies the biologic processes that result in malignant cells, primarily through enhancing the person's own immune responses. The development of this therapy was based on the immune surveillance hypothesis. Although it has been established that a competent immune system is the body's most important defense against any disease, the role that various immune cells play in combating different types of malignancies continues to be investigated. Currently, biotherapy is used for both hematologic malignancies, such as lymphoma and hairy-cell leukemia, and solid tumors, such as renal cancer, lung cancer, and melanoma (Trinh, 2008; Wu et al., 2008).

Tumor immunology has the following applications: detection screening in high-risk groups, differential diagnosis and classification of tumor cells, monitoring the course of the disease with early detection of recurrence, and active therapies to halt or limit the disease. The theory underlying tumor immunology is that most tumor cells have a structural appearance recognizable by the immune cells. Tumor-associated antigens exist on tumor cells but not on normal cells. TAAs elicit an immune response that, in a person with a competent immune system, destroys or inhibits tumor growth. Thus, TAAs can be isolated from serum and used for both diagnosis and various treatment modalities. The PSA is one such TAA currently in successful diagnostic use.

Tumor cells are often in a stage of arrested development (i.e., in the differentiation stage) for the cell type they represent; thus, they express antigens characteristic of that particular stage of development. The immaturity of the cells provides the physician with information about the relative aggressiveness of the cancer.

Another aspect of immunotherapy is the development of monoclonal antibodies that enhance the immune system's ability to fight the cancer. Monoclonal antibodies are developed by inoculating an animal with tumor antigen and recovering the specific antibodies produced. The antibodies are then given to the person with that cancer to assist in the destruction of the tumor.

Monoclonal antibodies are also re-created, or cloned, in the genetic laboratory by recombining DNA to produce the specific antibody. Techniques involving recombinant DNA have been used to combine these antibodies with toxins and drugs that are then delivered selectively to the tumor sites. For example, approximately one fourth of all women diagnosed with early breast cancer present with tumors that are associated with Her-2/neu receptor overexpression. Overexpression of Her-2/neu results in a high risk of metastasis and poor prognosis, which represents a target for a selective monoclonal antibody therapy with trastuzumab (Herceptin) (Singer, Kostler, & Hudelist, 2008). Trastuzumab (Herceptin) a monoclonal antibody that inhibits Her-2 by binding to extracellular portion of the receptor to inhibit initial signal transduction, thus inhibit growth, proliferation, and angiogenesis. The combination of trastuzumab with chemotherapy has led to a considerable reduction of recurrences and to a significant reduction in breast cancer mortality (Singer et al., 2008).

A number of cytokines (normal growth-regulating molecules) with antitumor activity have been synthesized. Alpha interferon (IFN-α), bacillus Calmette-Guérin (BCG, which has been used for many years as an inoculation against tuberculosis), and interleukin-2 (IL-2) have shown some therapeutic benefit in eliciting increased immune responses. Combination strategies have also helped stimulate the function of macrophages. The use of hematopoietic growth factors (HGF) has been one of the most successful in biotherapy. HGF, such as granulocyte colony-stimulating factor and erythropoietin, offsets the suppression of granulocytes and erythrocytes that results from chemotherapy (Andres et al., 2008).

A promising discovery has been the natural killer (NK) cells. These cells are like large granular lymphocytes, but have a cell surface phenotype different from that of T lymphocytes or macrophages. They have demonstrated a spontaneous cytotoxic effect on some types of cancer cells. They provide a strong resistance to metastasis and secrete cytokines. Combining biotherapy (such as IL-2, IL-12) with chemotherapy show increased tumor destructive activity and treatment responses (Trinh, 2008; Wu, Jiang, Shi, & Xu, 2008).

NURSING CARE OF THE PATIENT   **Receiving Radiation Therapy**

NURSING RESPONSIBILITIES FOR EITHER EXTERNAL OR INTERNAL RADIATION THERAPY

- Assess and manage any complications, usually in collaboration with the radiation oncologist.
- Assist in documenting the results of the therapy; for example, patients receiving radiation for metastases to the spine will show improved neurologic functioning as tumor size diminishes.
- Provide emotional support, relief of physical and psychologic discomfort, and opportunities to talk about fears and concerns. For some patients, radiation therapy is a last chance for cure or even for relief of physical discomfort.

EXTERNAL RADIATION

Prior to the start of treatments, the treatment area will be specifically located by the radiation oncologist and marked with colored semipermanent ink or tattoos. Treatment is usually given 5 days per week for 15 to 30 minutes per day over 2 to 7 weeks.

Nursing Responsibilities

- Monitor for adverse effects: skin changes, such as blanching, erythema, desquamation, sloughing, or hemorrhage; ulcerations of mucous membranes; nausea and vomiting, diarrhea, or gastrointestinal bleeding.
- Assess lungs for rales, which may indicate interstitial exudate. Observe for any dyspnea or changes in respiratory pattern.
- Identify and record any medications that the patient will be taking during the radiation treatment.
- Monitor white blood cell counts and platelet counts for significant decreases.

Health Education for the Patient and Family

- Wash the skin that is marked as the radiation site only with plain water, no soap; do not apply deodorant, lotions, medications, perfume, or talcum powder to the site during the treatment period. Take care not to wash off the treatment marks.
- Do not rub, scratch, or scrub treated skin areas. If necessary, use only an electric razor to shave the treated area.
- Apply neither heat nor cold (e.g., heating pad or ice pack) to the treatment site.
- Inspect the skin for damage or serious changes, and report these to the radiologist or physician.

- Wear loose, soft clothing over the treated area.
- Protect skin from sun exposure during treatment and for at least 1 year after radiation therapy is discontinued. Cover skin with protective clothing during treatment; once radiation is discontinued, use sun-blocking agents with a sun protection factor (SPF) of at least 15.
- External radiation poses no risk to other people for radiation exposure, even with intimate physical contact.
- Be sure to get plenty of rest and eat a balanced diet.

INTERNAL RADIATION

The radiation source, called an implant, is placed into the affected tissue or body cavity and is sealed in tubes, containers, wires, seeds, capsules, or needles. An implant may be temporary or permanent. Internal radiation may also be ingested or injected as a solution into the bloodstream or a body cavity or be introduced into the tumor through a catheter. The radioactive substance may transmit rays outside the body or be excreted in body fluids.

Nursing Responsibilities

- Place the patient in a private room.
- Limit visits to 10 to 30 minutes, and have visitors sit at least 6 feet from the patient.
- Monitor for side effects such as burning sensations, excessive perspiration, chills and fever, nausea and vomiting, or diarrhea.
- Assess for fistulas or necrosis of adjacent tissues.

Health Education for the Patient and Family

- While a temporary implant is in place, stay in bed and rest quietly to avoid dislodging the implant.
- For outpatient treatments, avoid close contact with others until treatment has been discontinued.
- If the radiologist indicates the need for such measures, dispose of excretory materials in special containers or in a toilet not used by others.
- Carry out daily activities as able; get extra rest if feeling fatigued.
- Eat a balanced diet; frequent, small meals often are better tolerated.
- Contact the nurse or physician for any concerns or questions after discharge.

A combination of cytokines, particularly IFN-α and IL-2, with chemotherapy has been used to treat renal cell cancer, metastatic melanoma, and lung patients with promising results. Such a combination is referred to as either biochemotherapy or chemoimmunotherapy (Trinh, 2008; Wu et al., 2008). The rationale for biochemotherapy is based on the independent antitumor activity of both IFN-α and IL-2 against melanoma and their lack of cross-resistance with cytotoxic chemotherapy. Although the precise mechanism of antitumor effect of biochemotherapy regimens is less understood, two hypotheses have been proposed: (1) Chemotherapy enhances the antitumor effect of biologic agents and; (2) the biologic agents enhance the antitumor cytotoxic effect of chemotherapy.

As promising as these biotherapies or biochemotherapies are, they are accompanied by serious side effects and toxicities (Trinh, 2008; Wu et al., 2008). IL-2 can cause acute alterations in renal, cardiac, liver, gastrointestinal, and mental functioning. IFN-α causes mental slowing, confusion, and lethargy and, when used in combination with 5-fluorouracil or IL-2, severe flulike symptoms—chills and fever of 103°F to 106°F (39.4°C to 41.1°C), nausea, vomiting, diarrhea, anorexia, severe fatigue, and stomatitis—may result. The toxic effects are probably exaggerations of the normal systemic effects that these substances cause when fighting infection. For example, IL-2 is known to raise body temperature substantially in an attempt to create a hostile environment for foreign invaders.

The following Nursing Care box discusses nursing implications for patients receiving immunotherapy. For nursing care of specific problems, refer to the appropriate nursing diagnoses later in this chapter.

PHOTODYNAMIC THERAPY (PDT) Photodynamic therapy is a method of treating certain kinds of superficial tumors. It is known by several different names: phototherapy, photoradiation, and photochemotherapy. Patients who have tumors growing on the surface of the bladder, peritoneal cavity, chest wall, pleura, bronchus, or head and neck are candidates for this treatment. The patient is given an intravenous dose of a photosensitizing compound, Photofrin, which is selectively retained in higher concentrations in malignant tissue. This drug is activated by a laser treatment that is started 3 days after the drug injection and administered for 3 days. The drug interacts with oxygen molecules in the tissue to produce a cytotoxic oxygen molecule called singlet oxygen.

At the time of the first intravenous injection, patients are observed for adverse hypersensitivity reactions, such as nausea, chills, and hives. Systemic or long-term toxicities are rare. The main side effects are local skin reactions and temporary photosensitivity, transiently elevated liver enzymes, and inflammatory responses of the tissues being treated, such as peritoneal or pleural tissues.

The major nursing responsibilities associated with photodynamic therapy are to address the patient and family's anxiety and to educate them in managing side effects. The drug remains in the subcutaneous tissues for 4 to 6 weeks after injection. Any direct or indirect exposure to the sun activates the drug, resulting in a chemical sunburn. Patients are taught to protect themselves from sunlight (even on cloudy days) by covering themselves from head to toe in opaque clothing, including a wide-brimmed

---

NURSING CARE OF THE PATIENT
Receiving Immunotherapy

Immunotherapy can consist of various substances used alone, such as IL-2, IL-12, or combination biotherapy, such as IFN-a with 5-fluorouracil. The nurse's role is to enhance the patient's quality of life.

Nursing Responsibilities
- Monitor for side effects: IFN-α may cause mental slowing, confusion, fatigue, and lethargy; combination therapy of 5-fluorouracil or IL-2 and IFN-α may cause severe flulike symptoms, with chills and fever of 103°F to 106°F (39.4°C to 41.1°C), nausea, vomiting, diarrhea, anorexia, severe fatigue, and stomatitis; erythropoietin may cause acute hypertension.
- Monitor enzymes and other appropriate biochemical indicators for acute alterations in renal, cardiac, liver, or gastrointestinal functioning, which can be side effects of IL-2.
- Evaluate response to therapy by conducting a thorough evaluation of patients' symptoms.
- Assess patients' coping behaviors and teach new strategies as needed.
- Manage fatigue and depression.
- Encourage self-care and participation in decision making.
- Provide close supervision for patients with altered mental functioning, either by caretakers or frequent nursing visits to the patient's home.
- If patient is unable to manage alone, teach medication administration and care of equipment to caregivers.

Health Education for the Patient and Family
- Minimize symptoms by managing fever and flulike symptoms: increase fluid intake, take analgesic and antipyretic medications, and maintain bed rest until symptoms abate.
- Seek help for serious problems not managed by usual means, such as dehydration from diarrhea.
- Use correct techniques for providing subcutaneous injections.
- Identify how to work and care for ambulatory pumps when medication is administered through an intercatheter or vascular access device.

---

hat, gloves, shoes and stockings, and sunglasses with 100% ultraviolet block. Long-term care of treated skin includes moisturizing lotions and protection from trauma or irritation.

BONE MARROW AND PERIPHERAL BLOOD STEM CELL TRANSPLANTATIONS Bone marrow transplantation (BMT) is an accepted treatment to stimulate a nonfunctioning marrow or to replace marrow. BMT is given as an intravenous infusion of bone marrow cells from donor to patient. Most commonly used in leukemias, this therapy is being expanded to include treatment of other cancers including melanoma and testicular cancer. ∞ Chapter 33 provides an in-depth discussion of this procedure. Peripheral blood stem cell transplantation (PBSCT) is the process of removing circulating stem cells from the peripheral blood through apheresis and returning these cells to the patient after dose-intensive chemotherapy. PBSCT has fewer side effects, shorter hospitalization, and decreased cost compared to BMT.

COMPLEMENTARY THERAPIES Although advances in cancer treatment have increased 5-year survival rates, the uncertainty of cure of cancer and cancer reoccurrence compels some patients to look for complementary therapies. Complementary therapies refer to therapies that patients choose as a complement to medical treatment. Common complementary therapies for cancer can be categorized into botanical agents, nutritional supplements, dietary regimens, mind–body modalities, energy healing, spiritual approaches, and miscellaneous therapies. Box 14–6 provides information about complementary therapies.

To provide sensitive nursing care, nurses should be knowledgeable about common complementary therapies. It is important for nurses to provide truthful, nonjudgmental responses to the questions or inquiries about complementary therapies from patients with cancer. Nurses should encourage patients to report the use of any complementary therapies to their oncologist to prevent potential interactions of the those therapies with their medical treatment.

Pain Management

Pain management is an important component of oncology care and is considered a crucial part of the collaborative treatment plan. It is estimated that more than 60% of patients with early-stage cancer and up to 95% of patients with advanced cancer experience pain that requires analgesia (Eaton & Frieze, 2008). There are three main categories of pain syndromes in patients with cancer, and the category influences the type of treatment:

- *Pain associated with direct tumor involvement.* The most common causes are metastases to bone, nerve compression or infiltration, and involvement of hollow visceral organs.
- *Pain associated with treatment.* This may include postsurgical incisional or wound pain; peripheral neuropathy, ulceration of mucous membranes, and pain from herpes zoster outbreaks

secondary to chemotherapy; and pain in nerve plexuses, muscles, and peripheral nerves from radiation therapy.

- *Pain from a cause not related to either the cancer or therapy,* such as diabetic neuropathy.

The goal of pain therapy is to provide relief that allows patients to function as they wish and, in the case of terminally ill patients, to die relatively free of pain. With the emphasis on putting evidence into nursing practice, the Oncology Nursing Society (ONS, 2007) conducted a systematic review on cancer pain and concluded combinations of nonopioids, opioids, and coanalgesics are effective management of acute and persistent nociceptive and neuropathic pain that occurs as a result of cancer or cancer treatment. Other therapies include injection of anesthetic drugs into spinal cord or specific nerve plexuses, surgical severing of nerves, radiation to reduce tumor size and pressure, and behavioral approaches. Pharmacologic pain management follows these steps:

1. Conduct careful initial and ongoing assessment of the pain.
2. Evaluate the patient's functional goals.
3. Establish a plan with combinations of nonnarcotic drugs (such as aspirin or ibuprofen) with adjuvants (such as corticosteroids or antidepressants).
4. Evaluate the degree of pain relief.
5. Progress to stronger drugs as needed, from mild narcotics such as oxycodone (Percodan) or propoxyphene (Darvon) to strong narcotics such as morphine or hydromorphone (Dilaudid), and monitor side effects.
6. Continue to try combinations and escalate dosages until maximal pain relief balanced with patient's need to function is achieved.

BOX 14–6 Common Complementary Therapies for Cancer

Type	Description
Botanical agents	Herbs are believed to be the most "natural" and "safe" plants ingested with the hope for a cure of cancer. Commonly used botanical agents include echinacea, Essiac, ginseng, green tea, pau d'arco, and Hoxsey. The safety for many of these botanical agents has not been proven, especially as a complement to medical treatment.
Nutritional supplements	Chemical compounds include vitamins, minerals, enzymes, amino acids, and essential fatty acids, or proteins (such as shark cartilage). They are believed to have the ability to promote health and to help cure cancer. The safety of certain compounds such as vitamins has been established; however, in megadoses, many of the compounds can be toxic and have potential interactions with some therapeutic agents used for cancer such as chemotherapy.
Dietary regimens	The ingestion of only natural substances is believed to have the effect of purifying the body and slowing down the growth of cancer. Popular regimens include the grape diet, the carrot juice diet, and garlic, onions, and liver intake. The effectiveness of these dietary regimens remains to be established.
Mind–body modalities	The harmony of mind and body are believed to facilitate physiologic and psychological healing. Such modalities include relaxation, meditation, or imagery. Recent research has shown that these modalities helped individuals with cancer adjust to the experience of cancer.
Energy healing	The human body is believed to be an energy field and cancer might be the result of a disturbed energy field. Energy therapies, such as therapeutic touch and healing touch, can affect the energy field of the human body and promote physiologic healing. Therapeutic touch uses the hands on or near the body with the intent to promote healing. Healing touch uses energy healing techniques to heal by restoring the harmony and balance of the body. Clinical practice and research on energy healing have shown positive findings of energy healing in a variety of patients.
Spiritual approaches	Faith in God or a higher power of the universe is believed to help cancer healing. Spiritual approaches include faith healing, prayer to God, prayer groups, and chain prayer. Research has shown that faith in God or a higher power helped individuals with cancer to adjust to the experience of cancer.
Miscellaneous therapies	Aromatherapy has been used for patients with cancer to relieve nausea, vomiting, or retching and to decrease anxiety. However, aromatherapy might not be appropriate for patients who are highly sensitive to strong fragrance. Music, art, and humor therapies have been used to help patients with cancer to reduce anxiety, to express feeling of loss, and to promote optimism.

Medication usually is administered by the oral route as long as this route continues to be effective. Medication is given on a regular time schedule (e.g., every 4 hours) with additional medication prescribed to cover breakthrough pain. When the oral route alone becomes inadequate, the primary narcotic can be administered intramuscularly, subcutaneously, or rectally on an intermittent schedule; continuously by transdermal patches; or intravenously by a continuous drip, usually controlled by an infusion pump. Some newer pumps are portable, deliver medication continuously, and allow patients to control their breakthrough pain with a limited number of boluses. When narcotic doses are increased gradually, there is no limit to the amount the patient can receive, as long as adverse reactions can be managed. Patients have received up to 4800 mg daily (200 mg per hour) of morphine sulfate with up to six 200- to 400-mg breakthrough doses daily without major ill effects and with good pain control. The body develops tolerance to the sedative after a short period, and most patients are able to tolerate the level of medication needed to control the pain. Other side effects, such as constipation, nausea and vomiting, and itching, can be managed through the usual means and are discussed under the appropriate nursing diagnoses. If the patient has persistent untoward side effects that do not respond to treatment, or if the patient does not get adequate relief from the narcotic, different narcotics and combinations are tried. Morphine sulfate and transdermal fentanyl are the most commonly used drugs for relief of cancer pain (ONS, 2007). Patients receiving high-dose narcotics should not have the medication abruptly stopped, because withdrawal symptoms will occur. If the drug needs to be stopped, it must be tapered gradually. For more information on pain management, and on alternative therapies in particular, ∞ see Chapter 9.

∞ Nursing Care

Nurses face a major challenge in educating patients about preventive measures and lifestyle changes to reduce the risk of cancer. At the same time, patients with cancer must be reassured that they are not responsible for having acquired cancer.

Once a cancer diagnosis is established, nurses help patients recover and support them during the rehabilitation phase. In cases of terminal cancer, nurses provide comfort and facilitate positive growth for the patient and significant others.

Health Promotion

Early detection and treatment are considered the most important factors influencing the prognosis of those who have cancer. However, many people do not seek early diagnosis and treatment because of denial, fear and anxiety, stigma, or the absence of specific early signs such as pain or weight loss (which usually are late signs). For this reason, screening procedures such as mammograms, PSA, occult blood stool tests, and sigmoidoscopy may be lifesaving.

The ACS promotes early cancer detection through promotion of cancer awareness and guidelines for screening procedures. Although no longer in use by the ACS, the CAUTION model (Box 14–7) is helpful in promoting awareness of common symptoms that may indicate cancer. This model encourages people to seek medical attention when they discover signs and symptoms characteristic of cancer. For people without

---

BOX 14–7 Seven Warning Signs of Cancer

American Cancer Society CAUTION Model
Change in bowel or bladder habits
A sore that does not heal
Unusual bleeding or discharge
Thickening or lump in breast or elsewhere
Indigestion or difficulty swallowing
Obvious change in wart or mole
Nagging cough or hoarseness
If you have a warning signal, see your doctor!

Source: American Cancer Society.

---

symptoms, the ACS recommends incorporating a cancer checkup into periodic health examinations. This general cancer checkup includes health counseling, teaching self-examination techniques when appropriate, and, depending on age and gender, examination for cancers of the thyroid, oral cavity, skin, lymph nodes, testes, and ovaries (ACS, 2009a).

If a person is at special risk due to heredity, environment, occupation, or lifestyle, special tests or more frequent examinations may be necessary. A routine cancer checkup should include counseling to improve health behaviors and physical examination with related tests of the breast, uterus, cervix, colon, rectum, testes, prostate, skin, thyroid, and lymph nodes. Box 14–8 lists the tests recommended for a cancer checkup. Nurses have a special role in public education and should encourage everyone they come in contact with to schedule cancer checkups. Nurses must be familiar with the ACS guidelines so that they can advise patients, their families, and significant others.

Assessment

The assessment chapters in this text contain questions based on functional health patterns that include questions about manifestations and risk factors for cancer. Examples of appropriate questions to elicit information during a health history assessment follow:

Interview Questions

The following are appropriate questions to ask the patient during the initial interview and at subsequent assessments:

- "What brought you in to see the doctor?" Asking this question allows patients to tell their story in their own way, which may elicit more information than asking specific questions. The answer should elicit not only data about the signs and symptoms but also fears or concerns. If the cancer was discovered during a routine physical examination or checkup, the patient may have some difficulty accepting the disease, especially if there were no symptoms. For patients who offer insufficient information in response to this open-ended question, more specific questions may be necessary, such as "Did you have pain or any specific physical problems that caused you to seek health care?"

- "Do you have any other medical conditions or problems that are troubling you at this time?" It may be necessary to ask about specific diseases to help the patient focus. For example, "Do you have high blood pressure?" or "Are you having any problems with your lungs?" Information gained from these questions can help you anticipate problems and formulate potential nursing diagnoses related to other diseases that may interact with the cancer.

BOX 14–8 American Cancer Society Guidelines for Cancer Screening

Breast Cancer

- Yearly mammograms are recommended starting at age 40.
- A clinical breast exam should be part of a periodic health exam, about every 3 years for women in their 20s and 30s, and every year for women 40 and older.
- Women should know how their breasts normally feel and report any breast changes promptly to their healthcare providers. Breast self-exam is an option for women starting in their 20s.
- Screening MRI is recommended for women with an approximately 20% to 25% or greater lifetime risk of breast cancer, including women with a strong family history of breast or ovarian cancer and women who were treated for Hodgkin's disease.

Cervix/Uterus

- Screening should begin approximately three years after a woman begins having vaginal intercourse, but no later than 21 years of age.
- Screening should be done every year with regular Pap tests or every two years using liquid-based tests.
- At or after age 30, women who have had three normal test results in a row may get screened every 2 to 3 years. Doctors may suggest a woman get screened more frequently if she has certain risk factors, such as HIV infection or a weakened immune system.
- Women 70 and older who have had three or more consecutive Pap tests in the last 10 years may choose to stop cervical cancer screening.

- Screening after a total hysterectomy (with removal of the cervix) is not necessary unless the surgery was done as a treatment for cervical cancer.

Colon and Rectum

Beginning at age 50, men and women should follow one of the following examination schedules:

- A guaiac-based fecal occult blood test (FOBT) or a fecal immunochemical test (FIT) every year
- A flexible sigmoidoscopy (FSIG) every 5 years
- A colonoscopy every 10 years
- A double-contrast barium enema every 5 years
- A CT colonography every 5 years
- People who are at moderate or high risk for colorectal cancer should talk with their doctor about a more-frequent testing schedule for a stool DNA test (interval uncertain).

Prostate

- The prostate-specific antigen (PSA) test and the digital rectal examination (DRE) should be offered annually, beginning at age 50, to men who have a life expectancy of at least 10 years.
- Men at high risk (African American men and men with a strong family history of one or more first-degree relatives diagnosed with prostate cancer at an early age) should begin testing at age 45.
- For men at average risk and high risk, information should be provided about what is known and what is uncertain about the benefits and limitations of early detection and treatment of prostate cancer so that they can make an informed decision about testing.

Source: American Cancer Society, 2010a.

- "What kinds of physical problems are you having at this time? Do you have pain? Are you nauseated? Have you lost a great deal of weight? Are you so tired you have difficulty carrying on your daily activities? Are you feeling blue or discouraged because of your illness?" For each positive response, ask follow-up questions to narrow down or define the exact nature of the problem. This data helps identify what nursing diagnoses should be included in the care plan.
- "What options has your physician suggested for treating your cancer?" The answer will indicate patients' knowledge about their treatment and, possibly, their communication with the physician. Often, under the stress of a cancer diagnosis, patients do not hear or understand what the doctor is saying and are afraid to ask questions. Lack of knowledge indicates a need to collaborate with the physician to explain the information to the patient so that the patient can absorb and understand it. If the patient has a good understanding of the treatment plan, discussing how he or she feels about it can be useful in exposing fears, concerns, and emotional responses.
- "What do you expect to happen as a result of this treatment?" The answer may reveal unrealistic expectations or lack of understanding of consequences of the treatment.
- "What effects are the disease and/or treatment having on your ability to carry on with your usual daily activities?" Additional questions may be needed to pinpoint the types of limitations. The response to this question should provide information on the patient's functional status such as those shown in Box 14–9. This information can also be used to identify the need to collaborate with professionals from other disciplines. For example, if the patient is the sole financial

support of the family and is unable to work, a social worker may be able to help with resources; if the patient is extremely weak, referral to a physical therapist may help with energy conservation strategies and strengthening exercises.

- "Who is available to help you at home and run errands for you? Who can provide transportation for you to get to your appointments or treatments? Who can you rely on to be a good listener when you're sad or to be a comfortable companion? Is there someone you would like to make healthcare decisions for you if there is a time when you are unable to make them for yourself?" It often seems that the person with cancer is the one who takes care of everyone else; asking for help may be difficult for this person. This information can identify how much support and help the patient has access to. The last question introduces the concept of advanced directives and durable power of attorney regarding health care (see Chapter 5).
- "How do you manage your stress or your feelings of discomfort? What helps you feel better? Do you think these measures work well for you?" The responses to these questions provide information about the patient's coping strategies and may identify maladaptive strategies such as alcohol or drug use. Lack of appropriate coping methods can interfere with the patient's response to treatment and decrease overall quality of life.

Other assessment questions may be useful at different stages of the patient's illness. For example, if the patient is not expected to survive the cancer, it is important to ask whether the patient has made decisions about last wishes (e.g., for a funeral and burial), whether these have been discussed with significant others, and whether the patient has made out a will.

BOX 14–9 Two Scales of Functional Status for Cancer Patients

I. Karnofsky Scale: Criteria of Performance Status (PS)

100 Normal; no complaints; no evidence of disease.
90 Able to carry on normal activity; minor signs or symptoms of disease.
80 Able to carry on normal activity with effort; some signs or symptoms of disease.
70 Cares for self; unable to carry on normal activity or to do active work.
60 Requires occasional assistance but is able to care for most of own needs.
50 Requires considerable assistance and frequent medical care.
40 Disabled; requires special care and assistance.
30 Severely disabled; hospitalization indicated, although death not imminent.
20 Very sick; hospitalization necessary; active supportive treatment necessary.
10 Moribund; fatal processes progressing rapidly.
0 Dead.

II. Eastern Cooperative Oncology Group Scale (ECOG)

0 Fully active, able to carry on all predisease activities without restriction. (Karnofsky 90 to 100)
1 Restricted in physically strenuous activity, but ambulatory and able to carry out work of a light or sedentary nature, for example, light housework or office work. (Karnofsky 70 to 80)
2 Ambulatory and capable of all self-care, but unable to carry out work activities. Up and about more than 50% of waking hours. (Karnofsky 50 to 60)
3 Capable of only limited self-care, confined to bed or chair 50% or more of waking hours. (Karnofsky 30 to 40)
4 Completely disabled, cannot carry out any self-care, totally confined to bed or chair. (Karnofsky 10 to 20)

"Two Scales of Functional Status for Cancer Patients" from "Nitrogen Mustards in the Palliative Treatment of Carcinoma" by D. A. Kamofsky, L. Craver, & J. Burchenal, 1948. *Cancer,* 1(4), pp. 634-656. © American Cancer Society, reprinted by permission of Wiley-CISS, Inc., a subsidiary of John Wiley & Sons.

Physical Assessment

As soon as the patient is admitted to the healthcare service or agency, conduct a complete physical assessment to establish a baseline for subsequent evaluation of later changes. It is especially important to document the nutritional status of the patient using anthropomorphic measurements (i.e., frame size, height, weight, body fat, muscle mass, body mass index, and body composition), and to evaluate laboratory results and note any specific signs and symptoms. Table 14–11 compares the manifestations of good nutrition with those of malnutrition.

It is also important to assess the patient's hydration status, especially if the patient is not taking oral food and fluids well or is having bouts of vomiting. Box 14–10 lists specific assessments for hydration status. Other recommended assessments are discussed under the specific nursing diagnoses that follow. They can also be found in other chapters that address specific body systems affected by the cancer.

BOX 14–10 Factors to Consider in Assessing Hydration Status

- Intake and output
- Rapid weight changes
- Skin turgor and moisture
- Venous filling
- Vital sign changes
- Tongue furrows and moisture
- Eyeball softness
- Lung sounds
- Laboratory values

Nursing Diagnoses and Interventions

Nursing goals focus on supporting the whole person and providing interventions for specific problems such as pain, poor nutrition, dehydration, fatigue, adverse emotional responses, altered individual and family coping, and the side effects of medical

TABLE 14–11 Signs of Nutritional Status

SYSTEM	GOOD NUTRITION	POOR NUTRITION
General	Alert, energetic, good endurance, psychologically stable Weight within range for height, age, body size	Withdrawn, apathetic, easily fatigued, irritable Over- or underweight
Integumentary	Skin glowing, good turgor, smooth, free of lesions Hair shiny, lustrous, minimal loss	Skin dull, pasty, scaly-dry, bruises, multiple lesions Hair brittle, dull, falls out easily
Head, eyes, ears, nose, and throat	Eyes bright, clear, no fatigue circles Oral mucous membranes pink-red and moist Gums pink, firm Tongue pink, moderately smooth, no swelling	Eyes dull, conjunctiva pale, discoloration under eyes Oral mucous membranes pale Gums red, spongy, and bleed easily Tongue bright to dark red, swollen
Abdomen	Abdomen flat, firm	Abdomen flaccid or distended (ascites)
Musculoskeletal	Firm, well-developed muscles Good posture No skeletal changes	Flaccid muscles, wasted appearance Stooped posture Skeletal malformations
Neurologic	Good attention span, good concentration, astute thought processes Good reflexes	Inattentive, easily distracted, impaired thought processes Paresthesias, reflexes diminished or hyperactive

treatment. Nursing care also focuses on improving quality of life by promoting rehabilitation for survivors of cancer and helping those who succumb to the disease maintain their dignity in the dying process. Because cancer affects the whole family, nursing care includes everyone involved with the patient from the onset of diagnosis through the entire disease and treatment process and the ultimate outcome. Many diagnoses are pertinent to patients with cancer; this section addresses only the most common diagnoses. See the Case Study & Nursing Care Plan on page 378.

Anxiety

Early in the disease process (i.e., during diagnosis and treatment), threats to or changes in health status, physical comfort, role functioning, or even socioeconomic status can cause anxiety. Later, anxiety may result from the anticipation of pain, disfigurement, or the threat of death. In particular, patients whose coping skills have been poor in the past (e.g., in managing anger) may find themselves at a loss to manage this current crisis. The patient may manifest overt signs of anxiety: trembling, restlessness, irritability, hyperactivity, stimulation of the sympathetic nervous system (increased blood pressure, pulse, respiration, excessive perspiration, pallor), withdrawal, worried facial expressions, and poor eye contact. The patient may report insomnia and feelings of tension and apprehension, or express concerns regarding perceived changes brought about by the disease and fear of future events.

- Carefully assess the patient's level of anxiety (moderate anxiety, severe anxiety, or panic) and the reality of the threats represented in the patient's current situation. The level of anxiety and the reality of the perceived threat influence the type of intervention that is appropriate for the patient. *A patient in panic may need medical intervention with appropriate medications, whereas those with moderate or severe anxiety are often managed by the nurse through counseling and teaching new coping skills.*
- Establish a therapeutic relationship by conveying warmth and empathy and listening in a nonjudgmental manner. *A patient who feels safe in the relationship with the nurse more easily expresses feelings and thoughts. The patient will be able to trust the nurse and perhaps be willing to try new behaviors as suggested. The amount of time this relationship may take to develop depends on the patient's current emotional and mental state and the stage of the disease process.*
- Encourage the patient to acknowledge and express feelings, no matter how inappropriate they may seem to the patient. *Just by expressing their feelings, patients often can significantly diminish anxiety. Expressing feelings also allows the patient to direct energy toward healing and thus has a positive therapeutic effect. Moreover, by acknowledging feelings, especially those the patient considers unacceptable, the patient can lay the groundwork for new coping behaviors.*
- Review the coping strategies the patient has used in the past and build on past successful behaviors, introducing new strategies as appropriate. Explain why inappropriate strategies, such as repressing anger or turning to alcohol, are not helpful. *The patient will be more willing to make changes that build on what has already worked in the past. The patient will also be more willing to reject inappropriate strategies if he or she is given a persuasive reason why they have not had the desired effect in managing previous crises.*

- Identify resources in the community (such as crisis hotlines and support groups) that can help the patient manage anxiety-producing situations. *The patient may not have support systems available, or the patient's significant others may be having their own difficulties in dealing with the cancer diagnosis. Programs such as "I Can Cope," sponsored by the ACS in most communities, provide education, counseling, and support in a group setting with other cancer patients.*
- Provide specific information for the patient about the disease, its treatment, and what may be expected, especially for those patients with obvious misinformation. *Knowing what is to come gives the patient a sense of control and enables the patient to make decisions. Also, knowing that every effort will be made to keep the patient as free of pain as possible can do a great deal to relieve anxiety.*
- Provide a safe, calm, and quiet environment for the patient in panic. Remain with the patient and administer anti-anxiety medications as ordered. *Staying with the patient and displaying calmness and confidence can protect the patient from injury and prevent further panic. If the panic does not subside with the nurse's presence and support, referral to the physician for medication management may be necessary.*
- Use crisis intervention theory to promote growth in the patient and significant others, regardless of the outcome of the disease. *During a major crisis, people can, with assistance, transform the experience from one that causes defeat and despair to one that enhances personal and spiritual growth. If you are not skilled in this area, a referral to an appropriate mental health professional may be helpful to the patient and family.*

Disturbed Body Image

Cancer and cancer treatments frequently result in major physiologic and psychological body image changes. Loss of a body part (e.g., amputation, prostatectomy, or mastectomy), skin changes and hair loss from chemotherapy or radiation therapy, disfigurement of body part (e.g., lymphedema in the affected upper and lower extremities), or creation of unnatural openings on the body for elimination (e.g., colostomy or ileostomy) may have a major effect on the person's self-image. The gaunt, wasted appearance of the cachectic patient or draining, malodorous lesions that result when cancer breaks through the skin are other significant etiologies of body image disturbance. This may give rise to fear of rejection, which plays a major role in sexual dysfunction. In addition to all of the other afflictions the cancer brings about, the patient may undergo major changes in appearance and function. The patient may exhibit a visible physical alteration of some portion of the body, verbalize negative feelings about the body and/or fear of rejection by others, refuse to look at the affected site, and depersonalize the body change or lost part (e.g., by calling the colostomy "that thing").

- Discuss the meaning of the loss or change with the patient. *Doing so helps the nurse discover the best approach for this particular patient and involves the patient more actively in interventions. A small, seemingly trivial loss may have a big impact, especially when viewed in light of the other changes that are occurring in the patient's life. Likewise, a major loss may not be as important as the nurse might imagine. To ensure more appropriate and individualized care, evaluate each situation in terms of the reactions of the specific patient.*

■ Observe and evaluate interaction with significant others. *People who are important to the patient may unintentionally reinforce negative feelings about body image; on the other hand, the patient may perceive rejection where none exists.*

■ Allow denial, but do not participate in it; for example, if a patient does not want to look at the wound, the nurse may say, "I am going to change the dressing to your breast incision now." *During the initial stage of shock at the loss of a body part, denial is a protective mechanism and should not be challenged, nor should it be promoted. A matter-of-fact approach and an empathetic attitude will go far to facilitate the eventual acceptance of the change.*

■ Assist the patient and significant others to cope with the changes in appearance:
  a. Provide a supportive environment.
  b. Encourage the patient and significant others to express feelings about the situation.
  c. Give matter-of-fact responses to questions and concerns.
  d. Identify new coping strategies to resolve feelings.
  e. Enlist family and friends in reaffirming the patient's worth. *A supportive, safe environment in which feelings are respected and new coping strategies can be tried promotes acceptance, as does reaffirming that the patient's worth is not diminished by any physical changes.*

■ Teach the patient or significant others to participate in the care of the afflicted body area. Provide support and validation of their efforts. *Active involvement in providing care, such as changing a dressing or emptying a colostomy bag, empowers the patient and/or significant others. This intimate involvement also desensitizes feelings about disfigurement and promotes acceptance. Involving significant others reduces the risk of their rejecting the patient and can promote closeness. Positive reinforcement from the nurse encourages them to continue these behaviors.*

■ Teach strategies for minimizing physical changes, such as providing skin care during radiation therapy and dressing to enhance appearance and minimize change in the body part. *Early intervention can limit the negative side effects of treatment and actually promote recovery. Involving the patient provides an additional way for the patient to be in control of a difficult situation.*

■ Teach ways to reduce the alopecia that results from chemotherapy and to enhance appearance until the hair grows back:
  a. Discuss the pattern and timing of hair loss. *This allows the patient to cope with changes and incorporate them into daily activities.*
  b. Encourage wearing cheerful, brightly colored head coverings; assist in color coordinating them with usual clothing. *Attractive head coverings protect the bald head while allowing the patient to feel stylish and well dressed.*
  c. Refer to a good wig shop before hair loss is experienced. *Hair color and texture can be matched to minimize obvious changes in appearance.*
  d. Refer to support programs such as "Look Good...Feel Better," which is sponsored by the ACS and the Cosmetic, Toilet, and Fragrance Association Foundation. *A support*

group can diminish feelings of isolation and provide practical tips for managing problems. For a list of community resources available to patients with cancer, refer to a local phone book.

  e. Reassure that hair will grow back after chemotherapy is discontinued, but also inform that the color and texture of the new hair may be different. Hair loss has been identified as the most distressing symptom by many patients. *Interventions to reduce that loss can have a significant impact on body image concerns. Moreover, knowing what to expect may decrease anxiety and distress.*

Anticipatory Grieving

Anticipatory grieving is a response to loss that has not yet occurred. Overall, only 50% of people with cancer fully recover, and certain types of cancer have a much higher death rate; thus, the patient with cancer is often confronted with facing death and making preparations for it. This can be a healthy response that allows the patient and family to work through the dying process and achieve growth in the final stage of life. Perceived changes in body image and lifestyle also can prompt anticipatory grieving. The patient or significant others may show sorrow, anger, depression, or withdrawal, expressing distress at the potential loss or verbalizing concern about unfinished life business. (∞ See Chapter 5 for more on nursing care of the patient who is grieving or dying.)

■ Use the therapeutic communication skills of active listening, silence, and nonverbal support to provide an open environment for the patient and significant others to discuss their feelings realistically and to express anger or other negative feelings appropriately. *This helps the patient and family to get in touch with feelings and confront the possibility of the loss or death.*

■ Answer questions about illness and prognosis honestly, but always encourage hope. *This allows for realistic appraisal of the situation and planning, and it also helps combat feelings of hopelessness and depression.*

■ Encourage the dying patient to make funeral and burial plans ahead of time and to be sure the will is in order. Make sure the necessary phone numbers can be easily located. *This gives a sense of control and relieves family members of these concerns at a time when the patient is most in need of their support and when they themselves are extremely stressed.*

■ Encourage the patient to continue taking part in activities he or she enjoys, including maintaining employment as long as possible. *This gives a sense of continuity of life even in the face of severe losses.*

Risk for Infection

Malnutrition, impaired skin and mucous membrane integrity, tumor necrosis, and suppression of the WBCs from chemotherapy or radiation may contribute to the risk for infection. Anorexia, as well as the disease itself, deprives the body of nutrients needed for healing, while impaired integrity of skin and mucous membranes (a result of chemotherapy and/or radiation therapy) compromise the first lines of defense against microbial invasion. Cells in the center of large or not very vascular tumors may die from malnutrition, eventually eroding through tissues to increase the risk of sepsis. Bone marrow depression due to the effects of certain types of cancers and chemotherapy undermine the body's ability to respond to infection. The patient may exhibit the classic signs of infection: lassitude, fever, anorexia, pain in the affected area, and physical evidence of infection, such as a purulent, draining lesion or wound. If the bone marrow is compromised, the usual signs and symptoms of infection may be absent or reduced.

■ Monitor vital signs. *Fever and sympathetic nervous system responses, such as increased pulse and respiration, are usual early signs of infection. However, severely immunosuppressed patients may be unable to mount a fever; therefore, the absence of fever cannot rule out infection.*

■ Monitor WBC counts frequently, especially if the patient is receiving chemotherapy known to cause bone marrow suppression. *This allows the nurse to notify the physician at the first sign of diminishing WBC counts so that corrective action can be taken.*

■ Teach the patient to avoid crowds, small children, and people with infections when WBC count is at nadir (lowest point during chemotherapy) and to practice scrupulous personal hygiene. *During periods of leukopenia, the patient may lose immunity to his or her own natural flora. Careful attention to hygiene reduces the risk of infection. Crowds, which promote contact with a greater variety of infectious agents, and friends with minor infections can be very dangerous for the immunosuppressed. Small children should be avoided because they often have microbes to which most people are usually immune but which the patient may not be able to resist.*

■ Protect skin and mucous membranes from injury. Teach appropriate skin care measures, such as good hygiene, use of a moisturizing lotion to prevent dryness and cracking, frequent changes of position for the bed-bound, and immediate attention to skin breaks or lesions. *Ensuring intact skin strengthens the first line of defense against infection.*

■ Encourage the patient to consume a diet high in protein, minerals, and vitamins, especially vitamin C. *Improving nutrition decreases the risk of infection. Vitamin C has been shown to help prevent certain types of infection, such as colds.*

Risk for Injury

In addition to infection, cancer can pose a risk for injury from, for example, obstruction by a large tumor or one located in a limited body space (e.g., in the brain, bowel, or bronchial airways). If the cancer is one that creates ectopic sites of hormones, elevated levels of hormones that are not under the control of the pituitary gland can injure the patient in a variety of ways. Signs of obstruction depend on the organ involved: Bowel obstruction presents with pain, distention, and cessation of bowel activities; obstruction in the brain gives signs of increased intracranial pressure or personality/behavioral change; bronchial obstruction manifests as respiratory distress, cyanosis, and altered arterial blood gases. Ectopic production of parathyroid hormone manifests as high serum calcium levels as well as signs of hypercalcemia; ectopic production of antidiuretic hormone causes fluid retention and manifests as hypertension and peripheral and pulmonary edema.

■ Assess frequently for signs and symptoms indicating problems with organ obstruction. *Early detection of major problems allows the nurse to seek medical help before the problem evolves into a physiologic crisis.*

■ Teach to differentiate minor problems from those of a serious nature. Encourage the patient to consult with the nurse or physician if in doubt or to call 911 if the patient becomes very ill. Box 14–11 provides guidelines to help patients identify serious problems. *Having guidelines for when to call the doctor provides an anxiety-reducing safety net for the patient and family and promotes early detection of complications.*

■ Monitor laboratory values that may indicate the presence of ectopic functioning and report abnormal findings to physicians immediately. (See Table 14–4 for laboratory indicators of ectopic functions.) *Early detection promotes early medical intervention and prevents serious consequences from the ectopic secretion.*∞ Refer to Chapters 10, 19, and 20 for specific signs and symptoms of electrolyte imbalances and endocrine disorders.

Imbalanced Nutrition: Less than Body Requirements

The anorexia-cachexia syndrome (described earlier in this chapter) is a common cause of malnutrition in cancer patients. Metabolism increases in response to increased cancer cell production while the cancer's parasitic activity reduces the nutrients available to the body. Loss of appetite, food aversion, nausea and vomiting, and painful oral lesions from chemotherapy or radiation may contribute to impaired nutrition. Tumors of the gastrointestinal tract that affect absorption also contribute to the problem. Manifestations include wasted appearance, considerable weight loss over a relatively short period of time, anthropometric measurements below 85% of standard for fat and muscle tissue, decreases in serum proteins, and negative responses to antigen testing.

■ Assess current eating patterns, including usual likes and dislikes, and identify factors that impair food intake. *This allows for a more individualized plan based on needs and preferences.*

■ Evaluate degree of malnutrition:
   a. Check laboratory values for total serum protein, serum albumin and globins, total lymphocyte count, serum

---

BOX 14–11 When to Call for Help

Instruct the patient or family member to call the nurse or physician if any of the following manifestations are experienced:
■ Oral temperature greater than 101.5°F (38.6°C)
■ Severe headache; significant increase in pain at usual site, especially if the pain is not relieved by the medication regimen; or severe pain at a new site
■ Difficulty breathing
■ New bleeding from any site, such as rectal or vaginal bleeding
■ Confusion, irritability, or restlessness
■ Withdrawal, greatly decreased activity level, or frequent crying
■ Verbalizations of deep sadness or a desire to end life
■ Changes in body functioning, such as the inability to void or severe diarrhea or constipation
■ Changes in eating patterns, such as refusal to eat, extreme hunger, or a significant increase in nausea and vomiting
■ Appearance of edema in the extremities or significant increase in edema already present

Instruct the patient or family member to call 911 if the patient
■ is having much difficulty breathing or if the lips or face have a bluish tinge.
■ becomes unconscious or has a convulsion.
■ exhibits unmanageable behavior, such as being physically abusive, hurting self, or engaging in uncontrollable activity.

transferrin, hemoglobin, and hematocrit. *These values represent the laboratory values that are most likely to decrease with malnutrition.*

b. Calculate nitrogen balance and creatinine-height index. Calculate skeletal muscle mass, and compare findings to normal ranges. *Urinary creatinine is an index of lean body mass and decreases in malnutrition. Lean muscle mass is catabolized for energy in patients with cancer.*

c. Take anthropometric measurements and compare them to standards: height, weight, elbow breadth, arm circumference, triceps skinfold thickness, and arm muscle mass. *This estimates the degree of wasting; findings below 85% of standard are considered malnutrition.*

- Teach the principles of maintaining good nutrition by using the Food Guide Pyramid and adapting the diet to medical restrictions and current preferences. *This tailors the food plan to the patient's needs and thereby promotes compliance.*
- Manage problems that interfere with eating:

a. Encourage eating whatever is appealing and consider adding nutritional supplements such as Ensure Plus or Isocal to diet. *It is better to eat something even if it is not nutritionally balanced.*

b. Eat small, frequent meals. *These are more easily digested and absorbed and usually better tolerated by the patient with anorexia.*

c. Encourage to try icy cold foods (such as ice cream) or those that are more highly seasoned if food has no taste. *Chemotherapy and radiation therapy may harm taste buds and prevent distinguishing the taste of foods. Strong seasonings and coldness make food more enjoyable to the patient with diminished taste. However, spicy foods are not recommended for patients with stomatitis.*

d. Encourage cold and bland semisoft and liquid foods with painful oropharyngeal ulcers; use a nonalcohol anesthetic mouthwash prior to eating. *These foods are less irritating to sensitive mucous membranes; deadening the pain can make chewing and swallowing easier.*

e. Manage nausea and vomiting by administering antiemetic drugs (around-the-clock medication may be an effective preventive measure). Encourage patient to eat small, frequent, low-fat meals with dry foods such as crackers and toast, to avoid liquids with meals, and to sit upright for an hour after meals. Remove emesis basins, and encourage oral hygiene before eating. *Dry, low-fat foods are more readily tolerated when nauseated. Removing vomiting cues, such as odor and supplies associated with vomiting, can reduce nausea.*

- Teach to supplement meals with nutritional supplements such as Ensure Plus or Isocal and to take multivitamin and mineral tablets with meals. Suggest increasing calories by adding ice cream or frozen yogurt to the liquid supplement or commercial protein-carbohydrate powders to milk or fruit juice. *Because the food intake is usually less than that needed to maintain or gain weight, these supplements can add calories in a manner often tolerated.*
- Teach to keep a food diary to document daily intake. *If the patient can see how little is being consumed, he or she may eat more. A food diary also helps the nurse keep a calorie count and alert the physician if more drastic nutritional*

measures, such as a feeding tube or parenteral nutrition, need to be instituted.

- Teach to administer parenteral nutrition via a central line or other VAD. Teach safety measures and care of the VAD, and explain how the pump delivering the solution works. Provide an emergency phone number for help with administration problems. (∞ See Chapter 22 for safety guidelines for administering parenteral nutrition.) *The patient with chronic or terminal cancer requiring parenteral nutrition is usually managed at home, so information on how to manage the entire process may be needed.*

Impaired Tissue Integrity

The most common impairment of tissue integrity occurs in the oral-pharyngeal-esophageal mucous membranes. It is secondary to the effects of some chemotherapeutic drugs and radiation treatment to the head and neck. The oral-pharyngeal-esophageal tissues are lined with cells with a high mitotic turnover rate and are therefore vulnerable to many chemotherapeutic drugs. Leukemias, bone marrow transplants, and herpes viral infections are other etiologic factors in the disruption of oral-pharyngeal-esophageal tissue. Manifestations of this problem may include the following:

- Small ulcers occur on the tongue and mucous membranes in the mouth and throat.
- Herpes simplex type 1 lesions or vesicles evolve into ulcerations.
- Fungal infections, such as thrush (due to *Candida* infections), are manifested by a white, yellow, or tan coating with dry, red, fissured tissue underneath.
- Red, swollen, friable gums bleed with minimal or no trauma.
- **Xerostomia** is excessive dryness of the mucous membranes (due to chemotherapy or radiation).

Manage such problems with the following interventions:

- Carefully assess and evaluate the type of tissue impairment present. Identify possible sources, such as chemotherapy or radiation therapy to head and neck. *This allows the nurse to implement corrective measures appropriate to the type of problem.*
- Implement and teach measures for preventing oropharyngeal infection:

a. Observe for systemic signs of infection. Be suspicious of any fever that has no apparent cause. *This facilitates early identification of an infection before it spreads.*

b. Encourage cleaning teeth gently and using a nonalcohol mouthwash several times a day. This can be done after waking up in the morning, after any oral intake, and before bedtime. Soak dentures nightly in hydrogen peroxide and floss gently with waxed floss after meals and bedtime; this measure may be contraindicated for people with leukemia or thrombocytopenia. *Disrupted mucous membranes allow the normal oral bacterial flora into the systemic circulation, which can result in sepsis in the immunocompromised person. Reducing the oral flora by frequent hygiene decreases the risk of infection.*

c. Culture any oral lesions, and report the problem to the physician. Herpes lesions may not follow a typical pattern in immunosuppressed patients. *Identifying the cause of the infection, whether viral, fungal, or bacterial, allows the physician to prescribe the appropriate treatment.*

- Implement and teach measures for reducing trauma to delicate tissues:
  a. Counteract dry mouth (xerostomia) with lubricating and moisturizing agents, such as Gatorade, sugarless gum, and Blistex. *This protects mucous membranes from infection and trauma.*
  b. Avoid putting sharp instruments in the mouth. Use smooth plastic spoons and forks for eating, especially with a bleeding disorder. Dental work should be done by dental oncologists.
  c. Brush teeth with a very soft toothbrush and obtain a new toothbrush monthly. If gums are friable and bleeding, clean teeth with a soft cloth or toothpaste over finger. Chlorhexidine mouthwash (Peridex) may be used. *This protects gums from trauma and decreases risk of hemorrhage.*
- Administer specific medications as ordered to control infection and/or pain:
  a. Acyclovir is often used to treat viral infections.
  b. Systemic antibiotics are used to treat bacterial infections.
  c. Nystatin or clotrimazole solution for "swish and swallow" or lozenges that dissolve slowly in the mouth are used for fungal infections.
  d. Use viscous Xylocaine or various combination mouthwashes before meals and as needed. These agents reduce pain and inflammation. See Box 14–12 for the ingredients of combination mouthwashes. *Knowing the contents of each mouthwash can prevent hypersensitivity reactions (e.g., to lidocaine) and assist in patient teaching.*

Nursing Interventions for Oncologic Emergencies

In caring for patients with cancer, nurses may encounter a number of emergency situations in which their role may be pivotal to the patient's survival. Most of these emergencies require astute observations, accurate judgments, and rapid action once the problem has been identified. A brief description of the more common **oncologic emergencies** with nursing interventions follows. In all cases, immediate notification of the physician or emergency team is the first step.

BOX 14–12 Combination Mouthwashes for Oropharyngeal Pain Control

Kaiser Mouthwash
- Nystatin
- Hydrocortisone
- Tetracycline

Stanford Mouthwash
- Nystatin
- Tetracycline
- Lidocaine
- Hydrocortisone

Xyloxylin Suspension
- Benylin syrup
- Lidocaine
- Maalox suspension

Stomafate Suspension
- Sucralfate
- Sterile water
- Benylin syrup
- Maalox suspension

Pericardial Effusions and Neoplastic Cardiac Tamponade

Malignant pericardial effusion is an accumulation of excess fluid in the pericardial sac that compresses the heart, restricts heart movement, and results in a cardiac tamponade. The signs of cardiac tamponade are caused by compression of the heart, which leads to decreased cardiac output and impaired cardiac function. Signs include hypotension, tachycardia, tachypnea, dyspnea, cyanosis, increased central venous pressure, anxiety, restlessness, and impaired consciousness.

Interventions include the following:

- Start oxygen and alert respiratory therapy for other respiratory support as needed.
- Insert an intravenous catheter if one is not already in place.
- Monitor vital signs and initiate hemodynamic monitoring.
- Prepare vasopressor drugs.
- Bring emergency cart to bedside.
- Set up for and assist physician with a pericardial tap (pericardiocentesis).
- Reassure the patient.

Superior Vena Cava Syndrome

The superior vena cava can be compressed by mediastinal tumors or adjacent thoracic tumors. The most common cause is small-cell or squamous-cell lung cancers. Occasionally the problem is caused by thrombus around a central venous catheter that then plugs up the vena cava, resulting in obstruction and backup of the blood flowing into the superior vena cava.

Obstruction of the venous system causes increased venous pressure, venous stasis, and engorgement of veins that are drained by the superior vena cava. Signs and symptoms may develop slowly; facial, periorbital, and arm edema are early signs. As the problem progresses, respiratory distress, dyspnea, cyanosis, tachypnea, and altered consciousness and neurologic deficits may occur. Figure 14–7 ■ illustrates the superior venal cava syndrome.

Emergency measures include the following:

- Provide respiratory support with oxygen, and prepare for tracheostomy.
- Monitor vital signs.
- Administer corticosteroids (e.g., dexamethasone) to reduce edema.
- If the disorder is due to a clot, administer antifibrinolytic or anticoagulant drugs.
- Provide a safe environment, including seizure precautions.

After the emergency is managed, the patient often receives radiation or chemotherapy to reduce the tumor size.

Sepsis and Septic Shock

Tumor necrosis, immune deficiency, antineoplastic therapy, malnutrition, and comorbid conditions can lead to the development of sepsis. Bacteria gain entrance to the blood, grow rapidly, and produce septicemia. Because malignant tumors are more likely to use anaerobic metabolic pathways, the bacteria of tumor sepsis are usually gram negative and damage the body through a combination of bacterial endotoxins and an uncontrolled immune reaction. Gram-negative sepsis progresses to systemic shock and eventually results in multisystem failure. Signs and symptoms appear in two phases. The first phase is characterized by vasodilation with vascular dehydration, high fever, peripheral edema,

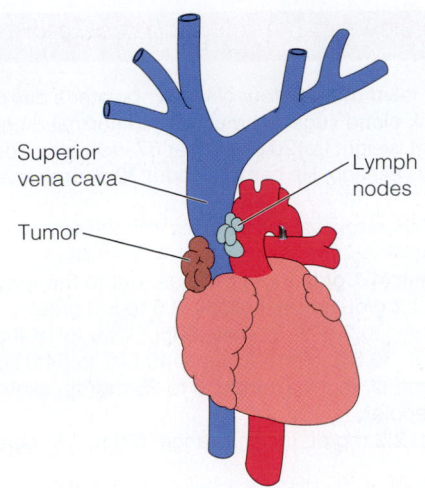

Figure 14–7 ■ The superior vena cava syndrome. The enlargement of a tumor adjacent to the superior vena cava (usually in the lung or mediastinum) compresses that major blood vessel, which leads into the right atrium of the heart. As a result, blood backs up into the venous system behind the obstruction, diminishing blood flow into the heart.

hypotension, tachycardia, tachypnea, hot flushed skin with creeping mottling beginning in the lower extremities, and anxiety or restlessness. Without treatment, the shock progresses to the second phase, which shows the more classic signs of shock: hypotension, rapid thready pulse, respiratory distress, cyanosis, subnormal temperature, cold clammy skin, decreased urinary output, and altered mentation. Identifying the problem while the patient is still in the hyperdynamic state is crucial to the patient's survival. ∞ See Chapter 11 for further discussion of septic shock.

Spinal Cord Compression

Spinal cord compression is most commonly associated with pressure from expanding tumors of the breast, lung, or prostate; lymphoma; or metastatic disease. Spinal cord compression constitutes an emergency because of the potential for irreversible paraplegia. Back pain is the initial symptom in almost all cases of spinal cord compression. This may progress to leg pain, numbness, paresthesias, and coldness. Later, bowel and bladder dysfunction occur and, finally, neurologic dysfunction progressing from weakness to paralysis. Treatment often consists of radiation or surgical decompression, but early detection is essential. ∞ See Chapter 43 for further discussion of spinal cord compression.

Obstructive Uropathy

Patients with intra-abdominal, retroperitoneal, or pelvic malignancies, such as prostate, cervical, or bladder cancers, may experience obstruction of the bladder neck or the ureters. Bladder neck obstruction usually manifests as urinary retention, flank pain, hematuria, or persistent urinary tract infections, but ureteral obstruction is not often evident until the patient is in renal failure. ∞ See Chapter 28 for further discussion of obstructive uropathy.

Hypercalcemia

Hypercalcemia in patients with cancer results from the excessive ectopic production of parathyroid hormone and is most commonly associated with cancers of the breast, lung, esophagus, thyroid, head, and neck and with multiple myeloma. Bone metastases may also cause hypercalcemia. When the rate of calcium mobilization

from the bone exceeds the renal threshold for excretion, serum calcium levels can become dangerously elevated. Patients with hypercalcemia often present with nonspecific symptoms of fatigue, anorexia, nausea, polyuria, and constipation. Neurologic symptoms include muscle weakness, lethargy, apathy, and diminished reflexes. Without treatment, hypercalcemia progresses to alterations in mental status, psychotic behavior, cardiac arrhythmias, seizures, coma, and death (∞ see Chapter 10).

Hyperuricemia

Hyperuricemia usually is a complication of rapid necrosis of tumor cells after vigorous chemotherapy for lymphomas and leukemias. Hyperuricemia may be related to increased uric acid production or to the tumor lysis syndrome associated with Burkitt's lymphoma. Uric acid crystals are deposited in the urinary tract, causing renal failure and uremia. Patients with hyperuricemia manifest with nausea, vomiting, lethargy, and oliguria.

Tumor Lysis Syndrome

Tumor lysis syndrome (TLS) is a life-threatening emergency for patients with cancer. TLS is characterized by a combination of two or more metabolic abnormalities, including hyperuricemia, hyperphosphatemia, hyperkalemia, and/or hypocalcemia (Cairo & Bishop, 2004). The syndrome develops because of massive and rapid destruction or death of cancer cells caused by cytotoxic treatment such as chemotherapy, radiation, biologic therapy, hormonal therapy, and surgery. It can occur spontaneously with sudden death of tumor cells. A high incidence of TLS occurs in patients with bulky, highly proliferating, and chemosensitive tumors such as high-grade lymphomas (Burkitt's lymphoma) and acute leukemia (ALL). Although the incidence of TLS in solid tumors is rare, cases of TLS following chemotherapy have been reported in patients with small-cell lung cancer, breast cancer, neuroblastoma, melanoma, and ovarian cancer.

The major cause of TLS is chemotherapy to tumors with a high proliferative rate, a relatively large tumor burden, and high sensitivity to cytotoxic agents, which leads to massive and rapid cell death. Usually, within a week of initiating chemotherapy, the body no longer can excrete the large amount of metabolic by-products from the cell death, resulting in the release of intracellular contents and metabolic by-products (such as potassium, phosphorus, and nucleic acid) into the bloodstream (Cairo & Bishop, 2004). As a result, a combination of metabolic derangements occurs, including hyperkalemia, hyperuricemia, and hyperphosphatemia with secondary hypocalcemia (Cairo & Bishop, 2004). These metabolic abnormalities put patients at risk for cardiac malfunction and renal failure.

Manifestations of TLS include nausea, vomiting, lethargy, edema, fluid overload, congestive heart failure, cardiac dysrhythmias, seizures, muscle cramps, tetany, syncope, and possible sudden death (Cairo & Bishop, 2004). Diagnosis of TLS mainly depends on laboratory tests and clinical signs and symptoms. Prevention is crucial in management of TLS. Patients at risk for TLS include those with bulky chemosensitive cancer such as high-grade lymphomas and acute leukemia, elevated serum uric acid, potassium, phosphorus, and renal deficiency. Preventive and management measures include identifying patients at risk, administration of allopurinol to inhibit the conversion of nucleic acid to uric acid, hydration and

James Casey, aged 72, is of northern European heritage. He has been receiving medical care for chronic obstructive pulmonary disease, chronic bronchitis, status postmyocardial infarction, and type I diabetes mellitus for over 15 years. He reports that he lost his wife from lung cancer 5 years ago and still "misses her terribly." He describes his bad habits as smoking two packs of cigarettes a day for 52 years (104 packs/year), one to two six-packs of beer a week, one "bourbon and water" a night, and "a lot of sugar-free junk food, like french fries." He assures the nurse that he quit smoking 2 years ago, when he could no longer walk a block without considerable shortness of breath, and just quit drinking alcohol a few weeks ago at his physician's insistence. About a year ago, he had a basal-cell carcinoma removed from his right ear. Six months ago, cancerous tumors were discovered in his bladder, and he underwent two 6-week chemotherapy courses of bladder instillations of BCG. His latest report indicates that the tumors have grown back and no further chemotherapy would be useful. The urologist had considered surgery but believed that Mr. Casey's other medical problems would compromise his chances of survival. Mr. Casey decides to let the disease run its course and to be managed at home through hospice care. Because he lives alone in a modest home, he asks his daughter, Mary, and her family to move in with him to provide care and support during his final months. The daughter accepts, saying she is glad to be able to spend this time with her father; she has been informed of the physical and emotional stress this will entail.

ASSESSMENT

Glynis Jackson, RN, the hospice nurse assigned as case manager for Mr. Casey, completes a health history and physical examination during her first two visits in his home, 1 day apart. She gathers this information over 2 days to conserve his strength and allow more time for Mr. Casey and his daughter to talk about their concerns.

During the physical assessment, Ms. Jackson notes that Mr. Casey is pale with pink mucous membranes, thin with a wasted appearance and a strained, worried facial expression. He complains of severe back pain no longer adequately relieved by Percodan and Vicodin alternating every 2 to 4 hours. His blood pressure is 90/50, right arm in the reclining position with no significant orthostatic change; his apical pulse is 102, regular and strong; respiratory rate 24 and unlabored; breath sounds are clear but diminished in the bases; oral temperature is 96.8°F.

A tunneled Groshong catheter as a VAD is present in the right anterior chest. There is no drainage, redness, or swelling at the site. The catheter was placed last week when the patient was being evaluated at the anesthesiologist's office for pain management, but no medication is running via the VAD. Mary reports that his urinary output is adequate. Approximately 200 mL of yellow, cloudy, nonmalodorous urine is present in the urinal at the bedside from his last voiding.

Mr. Casey states that he spends most of his time either in bed or sitting up in a chair in his room. He reports that he has no energy any more and is unable to walk to the bathroom unassisted, dress himself, or take care of his own personal hygiene. Ms. Jackson rates Mr. Casey's functional level at ECOG level 4: capable of only limited self-care, confined to bed or chair 50% or more of waking hours (Karnofsky 10 to 20). He tells the nurse that his daughter "is working day and night to help me and is looking awfully tired."

Mary reports that Mr. Casey is eating very poorly: He usually eats a small bowl of oatmeal with milk for breakfast and vegetable soup and crackers for lunch, but he tells her that he is too tired for dinner and wants only fruit juice. Mr. Casey tells the nurse that he has no appetite and eats just to please Mary. He does drink at least three to four glasses of water a day plus juice. His fingerstick blood sugars remain within normal range.

His current weight is 120 pounds at 67 inches tall, down from 180 pounds a year ago. He has lost about 30 pounds over the last 2 months.

Available laboratory values from his visit with the doctor show the following:

Total protein: 4.1 g/dL (normal range: 6.0 to 8.0 g/dL)
Albumin: 2.2 g/dL (normal range: 3.5 to 5.0 g/dL)
Hemoglobin: 10.2 g/dL (normal range: 13.5 to 18.0 g/dL)
Hematocrit: 30.5% (normal range: 40.0% to 54.0%)
BUN: 30 mg/dL (normal range: 5 to 25 mg/dL, slightly higher in older people)
Creatinine: 2.2 mg/dL (normal range: 0.5 to 1.5 mg/dL)

DIAGNOSES

- *Imbalanced Nutrition: Less than Body Requirements* related to anorexia and fatigue
- *Risk for Caregiver Role Strain* related to severity of her father's illness and lack of help from other family members
- *Chronic Pain* related to progression of disease process
- *Impaired Physical Mobility* related to pain, fatigue, and beginning neuromuscular impairment
- *Risk for Impaired Skin Integrity* related to impaired physical mobility and malnourished state

EXPECTED OUTCOMES

- Increase oral intake and show improvement in serum protein values.
- Experience minimal pain for the rest of his life.
- Able to continue his current activity level.
- Maintain intact skin.
- Continue receiving support and care from his daughter.

PLANNING AND IMPLEMENTATION

- Ask about favorite foods, and ask Mary to offer a small portion of one of these foods each day.
- Encourage drinking up to four cans of liquid nutritional supplement with fiber a day, sipping them throughout the day.
- Talk with the physician about prescribing a medication to help stimulate the appetite.
- Refer to home health agency to have a home health aide come to the home, give him a shower or bed bath daily, and assist his daughter with some of the household chores.
- Talk with Mary about having her adult son and daughter relieve her of the housework and stay with Mr. Casey so that she can get out of the house occasionally. Offer to talk with them if she is uncomfortable doing so.
- Request a volunteer to spend up to 4 hours a day, twice a week with Mr. Casey so that Mary can attend to outside activities and chores.
- Talk with the anesthesiologist, and work out a pain control program, using the VAD and a CADD-PCA infusion pump with a continuous morphine infusion.
- Call the infusion therapist to set up the equipment and supplies (including the medication) for the morphine infusion.
- Teach how to use the pump and about the side effects of the morphine infusion, including those that require a call to the nurse for assistance. Teach which untoward effects should be reported.
- Request a physical therapy consultation to evaluate current level of functioning and determine how to maintain current level.
- Instruct Mary to allow ample rest periods for Mr. Casey between activities.
- Order a hospital bed with electronic controls to be delivered to the house.

CASE STUDY & NURSING CARE PLAN A Patient with Cancer (continued)

■ Order a special foam pad for bed and chair and a bedside commode from the medical supply house.

■ Instruct Mary and the home health aide to inspect skin daily, give good skin care with emollient lotion after bathing, and report any beginning lesions immediately to the nurse.

EVALUATION

James Casey did increase his oral intake a little, sometimes eating the special treats his daughter prepared and drinking one or two cans of liquid nutritional supplement a day. However, his weight did not increase; it stayed at about 120 pounds until his death 2 weeks later. His daughter was very grateful for the extra help from the home health aide and the volunteer, though she could not bring herself to ask her son and daughter for help and did not want the nurse to do so. She did become more rested and reported that "Dad and I had some wonderful 3:00 AM talks when he couldn't sleep."

Mr. Casey was started on 20 mg of morphine per hour with boluses of 10 mg 4 times a day for breakthrough pain. This medication relieved his pain quite well; after 2 days he was alert enough most of the time to carry on a normal conversation and still walk to the bathroom with help up until 2 days before he died.

The hospital bed simplified Mr. Casey's care and made it much easier for him to rest comfortably and change position. His skin remained intact and in good condition.

Mary reported that Mr. Casey died peacefully in his sleep, about 2 weeks after care was started. She said spending the last weeks of his life together was a healing experience for both of them.

CRITICAL THINKING IN THE NURSING PROCESS

1. What other tests could be done to evaluate Mr. Casey's nutritional status?
2. Mr. Casey had severe back pain. What were the possible pathophysiologic reasons for his pain?
3. One of the specified interventions was to consult the physician regarding medication to increase Mr. Casey's appetite. What medications might fulfill that function? What side effects might they have that would contraindicate these medications for him?
4. If Mr. Casey had developed signs and symptoms of sepsis, what manifestations would you expect to see? As the nurse making the home visits, what would be your nursing actions, and in what order of priority?

See Evaluating Your Response in Appendix C.

---

diuretic therapy to promote urinary excretion of uric acid and phosphate, urine alkalinization to promote the urinary excretion of uric acid, administration of oral phosphate binder such as aluminum hydroxide to promote the excretion of phosphate through the bowel, administration of sodium polystyrene sulfonate (Kayexalate) to promote the excretion of potassium through the bowel, and initiation of hemodialysis to patients unresponsive to standard approaches to hyperkalemia, hyperuricemia, or hyperphosphatemia (Cairo & Bishop, 2004).

Using NANDA, NIC, and NOC

Linkages between a selected NANDA nursing diagnosis, NIC, and NOC for the patient with cancer are shown in the chart that follows.

NANDA, NIC, AND NOC LINKAGES
The Patient with Cancer

NANDA

Chronic Pain

NIC

Pain Management
Medication Management

NOC

Pain Control
Comfort Level
Pain: Disruptive Effects
Pain Occurrence
Pain Severity
Pain Distress
Pain Experience

Adapted from Bulechek, G., Butcher, H., & Dochterman, J. M. (Eds.). (2008). *Nursing interventions classification (NIC)* (5th ed.). St. Louis: Mosby Elsevier; and Moorhead, S., Johnson, M., Maas, M., & Swanson, E. (Eds.). (2008). *Nursing outcomes classification (NOC)* (4th ed.). St. Louis: Mosby Elsevier. A full listing of interventions and outcomes may be found in these books.

Health Education for the Patient
Prevention

The ACS makes specific recommendations for cancer prevention in addition to the screening measures discussed earlier in this chapter (see Box 14–13). Encourage people to report to the public health department any known leaking of chemicals or radioactive materials into the water or air and any noted increase in the incidence of cancer, especially of one specific type, in their communities.

Rehabilitation and Survival

Rehabilitation from cancer not only involves regaining strength, recovering from surgery or chemotherapy, and learning to live with an altered body part or appliance, but also entails recovering from associated psychological and emotional turmoil.

Rehabilitation centers provide physical therapy, occupational therapy, speech therapy, job retraining, and an opportunity to recuperate before resuming full responsibilities. In addition, many patients go home to convalesce and receive in-home support in the form of nursing supervision, direct care, and teaching. Hygiene and home maintenance can be provided

BOX 14–13 American Cancer Society Dietary Guidelines to Prevent Cancer

■ Avoid obesity.
■ Cut down on total fat intake.
■ Include a variety of vegetables and fruits in the daily diet.
■ Eat more high-fiber foods, such as whole-grain cereals, vegetables, and fruits.
■ Limit consumption of alcoholic beverages, if you drink at all.
■ Limit consumption of salt-cured, smoked, and nitrate-cured foods.

Source: From the American Cancer Society, 2010a.

by a certified home health aide. Physical and occupational therapists provide muscle strengthening and mobility training (especially with prostheses), and home safety teaching.

Psychological rehabilitation of cancer survivors addresses quality-of-life issues. Three "seasons of cancer survival" have been described (Mullan, 1985). The first starts with diagnosis but is dominated by treatment. The second stage is one of extended survival, which occurs when treatment ends and the watchful waiting period begins. This period is characterized by fear of recurrence. Permanent survival is said to begin when the survival period has gone on long enough that the risk of recurrence is small. In this period, the patient has to deal with secondary problems related to health and social issues resulting from the cancer experience. Employment may be a problem, health insurance may be canceled, and life insurance may be difficult to get. Relationships may have suffered from the strain of the illness on significant others and the essential self-focusing required for recovery. Both the patient and significant others may have undergone a personal and spiritual growth that ushers in a new and enriching period of their lives.

New self-help groups are emerging in many communities to support others through their "seasons of survival." Many cancer survivors speak to groups about assisting other cancer survivors. Patients and families need to be informed about the resources available through community agencies as well as the survivor support groups.

Community-Based Care

Before the patient is discharged, teach both the patient and significant others or caregivers to manage the patient at home. Discuss problems that may result from the type of cancer and the treatment received, and provide information on how to manage these problems and when to call the physician.

- Teach wound care to the patient with an open wound or draining lesion, and provide a referral to a home health nurse to monitor progress.
- Explain special diets clearly, or refer the patient to a dietitian before discharge.
- Carefully review the physician's instructions with the patient and family, making sure they understand medications to be taken, any other treatments, and when to see the doctor for follow-up care.
- Provide or order equipment and supplies needed for home care, especially any specialized bed or equipment to aid mobility and ensure safety in the home.
- For the patient who will need complex care, such as parenteral nutrition, provide a referral to a home health nurse before discharge.

Because the hospital stay is often short, the patient and family will benefit from follow-up phone calls at home for several days. People do not learn well under the stress of going home; give the patient and family a number to call if they have concerns or questions.

Hospice Care

More and more patients with terminal cancer disease are electing to die at home. This decision has been made easier by the increased availability of **hospice** programs. When a patient and family or significant others elect hospice care, they are usually precluding additional hospitalizations other than those required to manage reversible problems.

Many hospice services are connected with an inpatient respite care unit, where the patient can receive 24-hour care for up to several weeks. This source provides the necessary care to the patient if a family member becomes ill or needs to be relieved temporarily of the tremendous burden of caring for a dying loved one. ∞ Chapter 5 provides more information on hospice care.

CHAPTER HIGHLIGHTS

- One in every four deaths in the United States is caused by cancer and more than 1500 people die of cancer each day. Cancer can affect people of any age, gender, ethnicity, or geographic region.
- Cancer is the second leading cause of death in people over age 65. The incidence of cancer increases with advancing age. The most commonly seen cancers in older women are colorectal, breast, lung, pancreatic, and ovarian. In older men, lung, colorectal, prostate, pancreatic, and gastric cancers occur most frequently.
- Oncogenes are genes that promote cell proliferation and are capable of triggering cancerous characteristics. Several oncogenes, such as BRCA-1 and BRCA-2, are associated with breast cancer.
- Tumor suppressor genes, which normally suppress oncogenes, can become inactive by deletion or mutation. Inherited cancers have been associated with tumor suppressor genes, such as p53, a suppressor gene that has been associated with sarcoma and cancer of the breast and brain.

- The diagnosis and treatment of cancer is a pivotal, life-changing event that prompts individuals to make immediate and ongoing adjustment to this life-threatening illness.
- Effective physical and psychosocial adjustment to cancer diagnosis and treatment has been shown to lead to successful completion of treatment, enhancement of cancer patients' ability to cope with disease, improvement of patients' quality of life, and ultimately, improvement of survival.
- The goals of cancer treatment are aimed at cure and control of cancer as well as management of cancer-related and treatment-related symptoms.
- Chemotherapy uses cytotoxic medications to cure or control cancer by interrupting cell metabolism and replication and by interfering with the ability of the malignant cell to synthesize vital enzymes and chemicals.

- Pain management is an important component of care for cancer patients. It is estimated that 20% to 50% of patients with early-stage cancer and up to 95% of patients with advanced cancer experience pain.
- Complementary therapies are therapies that patients choose as a complement to medical treatment. Common complementary therapies for cancer include botanical agents, nutritional supplements, dietary regimens, mind-body modalities, spiritual approaches, and miscellaneous therapies.

- Tumor lysis syndrome (TLS), a combination of two or more metabolic abnormalities, is a life-threatening emergency for patients with cancer. Patients at risk for TLS include those with bulky chemosensitive cancer such as high-degrade lymphomas and acute leukemia; elevated serum uric acid, potassium, and phosphorus; and renal deficiency.

TEST YOURSELF NCLEX-RN® REVIEW

1. A patient has a history of colon cancer. Cells from the colon tumor have traveled to his liver. What is this process called?
   1. carcinogenesis
   2. dysplasia
   3. metastasis
   4. mutation
2. A patient diagnosed with lung cancer reports he is having difficulty sleeping and often feels tense. What would be the most appropriate initial nursing intervention?
   1. Encourage the patient to express his feelings about the cancer diagnosis.
   2. Document the patient's report of difficulty sleeping and tenseness in the chart.
   3. Obtain an order for medication for sleep from the physician.
   4. Offer an anti-anxiety drug such as Ativan (lorazepam).
3. A patient is receiving external radiation for treatment of lung cancer. What would the nurse teach the patient about care of the skin in the marked area?
   1. Apply antibacterial ointment daily.
   2. Avoid contact with others.
   3. Avoid rubbing or scratching treated skin areas.
   4. Cleanse the skin with plain water.
4. A patient states she is having nausea and vomiting following her daily chemotherapy treatment. What would be the most appropriate nursing intervention?
   1. Keep the patient NPO until her daily chemotherapy is completed.
   2. Provide antiemetic medication 30 to 40 minutes prior to each treatment.
   3. Provide clear liquids until the chemotherapy is completed.
   4. Schedule chemotherapy administration for bedtime.
5. A patient experiences bone marrow depression as a result of chemotherapy. Which of the following assessments would the nurse expect to find?
   1. alopecia
   2. nausea and vomiting
   3. platelet count 50,000
   4. temperature 102°F

6. A 46-year-old businessman with a diagnosis of metastatic lung cancer is going to have chemotherapy tomorrow. To help him better understand the role of chemotherapeutic agents in treating cancer, the nurse has completed teaching him about chemotherapy. The nurse determines that the teaching is effective when the patient states which of the following?
   1. "Chemotherapy uses drugs that promote the normal growth of cells while killing the cancer cells."
   2. "Chemotherapy only uses a single drug to treat cancer because drug resistance is rare."
   3. "Chemotherapy includes drugs that not only attack cancer cells but also normal rapidly dividing cells."
   4. "Chemotherapy is a preferred therapy because it has fewer adverse effects than radiation therapy."
7. During training for new radiation nurses, the nurses learn about the delivery of high-energy radiation (e.g., electrons, x-rays, photons) to kill cancer cells by using a machine to focus a beam of radiation on the body. What is this called?
   1. external radiation therapy
   2. internal-beam radiation therapy
   3. brachytherapy
   4. biochemotherapy
8. A nurse is taking care of a patient who just received the first cycle of chemotherapy for acute leukemia 2 days ago. The patient's laboratory tests of uric acid, potassium, phosphorus, and calcium are closely monitored, based on the knowledge that the patient is at risk for what complication?
   1. spinal cord compression
   2. tumor lysis syndrome
   3. septic shock
   4. superior vena cava syndrome
9. In what phase of the cell cycle does DNA replicate to form two sets of chromosomes?
   1. G_1
   2. G_2
   3. S
   4. M
10. What is a characteristic of oncogenes?
    1. They promote cell growth when activated.
    2. They block cell growth.
    3. They stimulate a complex signaling process.
    4. They are strictly regulated.

See Test Yourself answers in Appendix C.

Pearson Nursing Student Resources

Find additional review materials at
nursing.pearsonhighered.com

Prepare for success with additional NCLEX®-style practice questions, interactive assignments and activities, Web links, animations and videos, and more!

BIBLIOGRAPHY

American Cancer Society. (2010a). *Cancer facts and figures—2009.* Atlanta: Author.

American Cancer Society. (2009). *Cancer facts and figures for African Americans—2009–2010.* Atlanta: Author.

American Cancer Society. (2010b). *Cancer facts and figures for Hispanics/Latinos—2009–2010.* Atlanta: Author.

Andres, E., Federici, L., Weitten, T., Vogel, T., Alt, M. (2008). Recognition and management of drug-induced blood cytopenias: The example of drug-induced acute neutropenia and agranulocytosis. *Expert Opinion on Drug Safety, 7*(4), 481–489.

Armaiz-Pena, G. N., Lutgendorf, S. K., Cole, S. W., Sood, A. K. (2009). Neuroendocrine modulation of cancer progression. *Brain, Behavior, & Immunity, 23*(1), 10–15.

Bauer, M. E. (2008). Chronic stress and immunosenescence: A review. *Neuroimmunomodulation, 15*(4-6), 241–250.

Bodles-Brakhop, A. M., & Draghia-Akli, R. (2008). DNA vaccination and gene therapy: Optimization and delivery for cancer therapy. *Expert Review of Vaccines, 7*(7), 1085–1101.

Cairo, M. S., & Bishop, M. (2004). Tumour lysis syndrome: New therapeutic strategies and classification. *British Journal of Haematology, 127*(1), 3–11.

Deandrea, S., Montanari, M., Moja, L., Apolone, G. (2008). Prevalence of undertreatment in cancer pain. A review of published literature. *Annals of Oncology, 19*(12), 1985–1991.

De la Fuente, M. (2008). Role of neuroimmunomodulation in aging. *Neuroimmunomodulation, 15*(4-6), 213–223.

DeLancey, J. O., Thun, M. J., Jemal, A., & Ward, E. M. (2008). Recent trends in Black-White disparities in cancer mortality. *Cancer Epidemiology, Biomarkers & Prevention. 17*(11), 2908–2912.

di Pietro, A., Tosti, G., Ferrucci, P. F., Testori, A. (2008). Oncophage: Step to the future for vaccine therapy in melanoma. *Expert Opinion on Biological Therapy, 8*(12), 1973–1984.

Dragun, A. E., Harper, J. L., Jenrette, J. M., Sinha, D., & Cole, D. J. (2007). Predictors of cosmetic outcome following MammoSite breast brachytherapy: A single-institution experience of 100 patients with two years of follow-up. *International Journal of Radiation Oncology, Biology, Physics, 68*(2), 354–358.

Eaton, K. D., & Frieze, D. A. (2008). Cancer pain: Perspectives of a medical oncologist. *Current Pain & Headache Reports, 12*(4), 270–276.

Eccles, D. M. (2008). Identification of personal risk of breast cancer: Genetics. *Breast Cancer Research, 10,*(Suppl 4), S12.

Farquhar, C., Marjoribanks, J., Basser, R., Hetrick, S., & Lethaby, A. (2006). High dose chemotherapy and autologous bone marrow or stem cell transplantation versus conventional chemotherapy for women with metastatic breast cancer. *Cochrane Breast Cancer Group Cochrane Database of Systematic Reviews (3).*

Forbes, S. A. Bhamra, G., Bamford, S., Dawson, E., Kok, C., Clements, J., Menzies, A., Teague, J. W., Futreal, P. A., & Stratton, M. R. (2008). The Catalogue of Somatic Mutations in Cancer (COSMIC). *Current Protocols in Human Genetics* (Chapter 10: Unit 10.11).

Fu, M. R., Xu, B., Liu, Y., Haber, J. (2008). "Making the best of it": Chinese women's experiences of adjusting to breast cancer diagnosis and treatment. *Journal of Advanced Nursing, 63*(2), 155–165.

Karnofsky, D., Abelmann, W., Craver, L., & Burchenal, J. (1948). The use of nitrogen mustard in the palliative treatment of carcinoma. *Cancer, 1,* 634–656.

Kwitniewski, M., Juzeniene, A., Glosnicka, R., Moan, J. (2008). Immunotherapy: A way to improve the therapeutic outcome of photodynamic therapy? *Photochemical & Photobiological Sciences, 7*(9), 1011–1017.

Maeda, N., Fan, H., Yoshikai, Y. (2008). Oncogenesis by retroviruses: Old and new paradigms. *Reviews in Medical Virology, 18*(6), 387–405.

Misset, J., & Levi, F. (1995). Chronomodulated chemotherapy combining 5-fluorouracil, folinic acid, and oxaliplatin in advanced colorectal cancer: An overview of seven years of experience (Meeting abstract). *Cancer Investigation, 13*(Suppl 1), 49–50.

Mullan, F. (1985). Seasons of survival: Reflections of a physician with cancer. *New England Journal of Medicine, 313,* 270–273.

National Toxicology Program (NTP). (2005). *11th Report on Carcinogens.* Research Triangle Park. Retrieved from http://ntp.niehs.nih.gov/ntp/roc/toc11.html

Nowicki, M. J., Vigen, C., Mack, W. J., Seaberg, E., Landay, A., Anastos, K., Young, M., Minkoff, H., Greenblatt, R., Levine, A. M. (2008). Association of cells with natural killer (NK) and NKT immunophenotype with incident cancers in HIV-infected women. *AIDS Research & Human Retroviruses, 24*(2), 163–168.

Oncology Nursing Society. (2007).Pain: What are the pharmacologic interventions for nociceptive and neuropathic cancer pain in adults? Putting Evidence Into Practice (PEP Card). Retrieved March 23, 2009, from http://www.ons.org/outcomes/volume3/pain/pdf/ShortCard_pain.pdf

Oncology Nursing Society. (2009). Oncology Nursing Society position paper on quality cancer care. Retrieved March 10, 2009, from http://www.ons.org/publications/positions/QualityCancerCare.shtml

Paim, C. R., de Paula Lima, E. D., Fu, M. R., de Paula Lima, A., Cassali, G. D. (2008). Postlymphadenectomy complications and quality of life among breast cancer patients in Brazil. *Cancer Nursing, 31*(4), 302–309; quiz 310-1.

Pfister, G., & Savino, W. (2008). Can the immune system still be efficient in the elderly? An immunological and immunoendocrine therapeutic perspective. *Neuroimmunomodulation, 15*(4-6), 351–364.

Rosedale, M., & Fu, M. R. (2010). Confronting the unexpected: Temporal, situational, and attributive dimensions of breast cancer survivors' experiences of distressing symptoms. *Oncology Nursing Forum, 37*(1), E28–E33.

Schmitz, K. H., Cappola, A. R., Stricker, C. T., Sweeney, C., & Norman, S. A. (2007). The intersection of cancer and aging: Establishing the need for breast cancer rehabilitation. *Cancer Epidemiology, Biomarkers & Prevention, 16*(5), 866–872.

Selye, H. (1984). *The stress of life* (rev. 2nd ed.). New York: McGraw-Hill.

Sheinfeld, Gorin.S., Gauthier, J., Hay, J., Miles, A., & Wardle, J. (2008). Cancer screening and aging: Research barriers and opportunities. *Cancer, 113*(12 Suppl), 3493–3504.

Singer, C. F., Kostler, W. J., Hudelist, G. (2008). Predicting the efficacy of trastuzumab-based therapy in breast cancer: Current standards and future strategies. *Biochimica et Biophysica Acta, 1786*(2), 105–113.

Toothaker, T. B., & Rubin, M. (2009). Paraneoplastic neurological syndromes: A review *Neurologist, 15*(1), 21–33.

Trinh, V. A. (2008). Current management of metastatic melanoma. *American Journal of Health-System Pharmacy, 65*(24 Suppl 9), S3–8.

Ullenhag, G. J., Spendlove, I., Watson, N. F., Kallmeyer, C., Pritchard-Jones, K., Durrant, L. G. (2008). T-cell responses in osteosarcoma patients vaccinated with an anti-idiotypic antibody, 105AD7, mimicking CD55. *Clinical Immunology, 128*(2), 148–154.

Van Hemelrijck, M. J., Michaud, D. S., Connolly, G. N., Kabir, Z. (2009). Secondhand smoking, 4-aminobiphenyl, and bladder cancer: Two meta-analyses. *Cancer Epidemiology Biomarkers Prevention, 18*(4), 1312–1320.

Van Leeuwen, M. S. (2006). *Davis' comprehensive handbook to laboratory and diagnostic tests with nursing implications* (2nd ed.). St. Louis: C.V. Mosby.

Ward, E., Halpern, M., Schrag, N., Cokkinides, V., DeSantis, C., Bandi, P., Siegel, R., Stewart, A., & Jemal, A. (2008). Association of insurance with cancer care utilization and outcomes. *CA: A Cancer Journal for Clinicians, 58*(1), 9–31.

Wu, C., Jiang, J., Shi, L., Xu, N. (2008). Prospective study of chemotherapy in combination with cytokine-induced killer cells in patients suffering from advanced non-small-cell lung cancer. *Anticancer Research. 28*(6B), 3997–4002.

Functional Health Pattern: Health Perception-Health Management

Think about patients with altered health perception or health management for whom you have cared in your clinical experiences.

- What were their major medical diagnoses? Had they been injured in an accident? Had they or will they be experiencing a loss of body function, loss of an important object, or loss of a family member? Had they had surgery? Did they have a genetic disorder?

- What manifestations did each of these patients have? Were these manifestations similar or different?

- How did the patients' healthcare behaviors interfere with their health status? Did the patient have a genetic disorder? Was there a family history of genetic disorders? Did the patient have genetic studies done? Did the patient complain of pain? If so, what type of pain? In what region of the body was the pain? Did the pain radiate? What was the quality and quantity of pain? What was the severity of the pain? What did the patient do to relieve pain? Did the patient have a significant body fluid loss? If so, what was the loss: vomiting, diarrhea, or hemorrhage? Did the patient have excess body fluid such as edema? Did the patient complain of cardiac dysrhythmias? Did the patient complain of muscle weakness or muscle spasms? Did the patient complain of numbness or tingling around the mouth or of the fingers and toes? Did the patient exhibit changes in respiratory patterns? Did the patient exhibit personality changes or confusion? Did the patient have any seizure activity? Did the patient have any traumatic injuries: multiple trauma injuries, abuse? Did the patient have a blood transfusion? Was the patient treated for shock? Was the patient treated for an infection? Did the patient have a problem with wound healing? Was the patient up-to-date with immunizations? Did the patient have allergies? Did the patient have any autoimmune disorders? Had the patient had an organ or tissue transplant? Had the patient been tested for HIV? Did the patient have HIV or AIDS?

The Health Perception-Health Management Functional Health Pattern includes healthcare behaviors such as health promotion and illness prevention activities, medical treatments, and follow-up care. Early intervention and health-promotion-focused care can result in a longer life and a better quality of life. Health perception and health maintenance are affected by perceived health status in two primary ways:

- Factors that change or disrupt genes are genetic alterations (e.g., Down's syndrome, Turner syndrome, chronic myelogenous leukemia, Alzheimer's disease), autosomal dominant inheritance patterns (e.g., breast and ovarian cancer, neurofibromatosis, Huntington disease), autosomal recessive inheritance patterns (e.g., cystic fibrosis, sickle cell anemia), X-linked recessive inheritance (e.g., hemophilia), and monogenic inheritance (e.g., Prader-Willi syndrome).

- Factors that change or disrupt cells are altered immune response (e.g., hypersensitivity, rheumatoid arthritis, systemic lupus erythematosus, HIV/AIDS), inflammation (e.g., osteoarthritis, *mycobacterium tuberculosis*, infection (e.g., influenza, meningitis), cancer (e.g., leukemia, lymphoma, sarcoma), trauma (e.g., rape, burns, fractures, gunshot wound), shock (e.g., hypovolemic, septic, anaphylactic), fluid volume (e.g., dehydration, edema), electrolyte imbalance (e.g., hyponatremia, hyperkalemia, hypocalcemia), and acid–base imbalance (e.g., respiratory acidosis, metabolic alkalosis).

The human body is continually threatened by foreign substances, infectious agents, and abnormal cells, resulting in alterations that cause abnormalities or disease processes. A patient's perceived pattern of health and well-being affects how health is managed, leading to manifestations such as the following:

- **Rapid weight loss** (*neoplastic cells divert nutrition for own use causes increase in serum glucose and increased metabolic rate resulting in reduced appetite*)

- **Tachycardia** (*shock or trauma causes vasoconstriction and decreased blood volume resulting in rapid, weak, and thready pulse to increase cardiac output*)

- **Tachypnea** (*decreased perfusion of alveoli causes impaired gas exchange resulting in increased carbon dioxide and respiratory acidosis*)

Priority nursing diagnoses within the health perception and health management functional health pattern that may be appropriate for patients include the following:

- *Risk for Infection* as evidenced by traumatized tissue, malnutrition, stasis of body tissue, leucopenia, and decreased hemoglobin

- *Acute pain* as evidenced by guarding, facial grimacing, crying, diaphoresis, restlessness, and pupillary dilation

- *Disturbed Body Image* as evidenced by verbalization of feelings, fear of rejection, preoccupation with loss, feelings of helplessness, and hiding body part

- *Risk for Violence* as evidenced by verbal threats, physical injury to others, refusal to take medications, impulsivity, and clenching fists and jaw

Two nursing diagnoses from other functional health patterns often are of high priority for the patient with deficits in health perception or health maintenance:

- *Impaired Tissue Integrity* (Nutritional-Metabolic Functional Health Pattern)

- *Risk for Post-trauma Syndrome* (Cognitive-Perceptual Functional Health Pattern)

Question

1. Besides administration of medication, what did you do to help your patients manage their health related to pain, fever, inflammation, tachycardia, and tachypnea?

CLINICAL SCENARIO

Directions: *Read the following clinical scenarios and answer the questions that follow. To complete this exercise successfully, you will utilize not only knowledge of the content in this unit but also principles related to priority setting and maintaining patient safety.*

You have been assigned to work with the following four patients for the 0700 shift on a medical-surgical unit. Significant data obtained during report is as follows:

- Allen Barber is a 55-year-old patient with diabetes mellitus who is 4 days postoperative abdominal surgery with an inflammation of the incision site. Temperature is 101°F, pulse 94, respirations 24, blood pressure 138/82. The abdominal incision appears red with warmth and edema around the incision. The patient states his pain level is 8 on a pain scale of 0 to 10. Labs and wound cultures have been ordered.

- Tamra Sanders is a 22-year-old patient with Down syndrome. She is admitted in sickle cell crisis with a temperature of 102°F, pulse 90, respirations 30 and shallow, and blood pressure of 110/84. She is complaining of severe chest pain with shortness of breath. She states her pain scale level is 10 of 10. She has an order to begin morphine PCA.

- Mia Windham is a 26-year-old who was admitted yesterday with a maculopapular rash on her hands and feet that is spreading to her arms and legs. This morning she is complaining of abdominal pain, nausea, and bloody diarrhea. The patient has a history of having a bone marrow transplant 3 months ago as treatment for leukemia.

- Harry Anderson is a 40-year-old in late stages of AIDS. He is confused, incontinent, and is very spastic. He is on seizure precautions. He needs to be turned every 2 hours to prevent pressure sores. He is currently yelling that he needs help.

Questions

Priority Setting

1. In what order would you visit these patients after report?
   A. _____
   B. _____
   C. _____
   D. _____

Health Promotion

1. Harry Anderson, with HIV, has experienced weight loss. The dietician teaches him meal planning in which type of diet?
   A. high protein, high fiber
   B. high protein, high kilocalorie
   C. low fiber, low protein
   D. high carbohydrate, high vitamins

2. Before Allen Barber is discharged, what will the nurse encourage him to do at home to promote healing of his incision?

Nursing Process

1. Besides obtaining vital signs, what diagnosis-specific assessment data should be collected for each patient?
   A. _____
   B. _____
   C. _____
   D. _____

2. Identify one priority nursing diagnosis for each patient presented earlier. What is the rationale for your choices?

	Nursing Diagnosis	Rationale
Allen Barber		
Tamra Sanders		
Mia Windham		
Harry Anderson		

3. In what position should the nurse place Tamra Sanders to ease her breathing?

4. The nurse performs wound cleansing with which procedure?
   A. Cleanse the wound with soap and water.
   B. Use normal saline to cleanse the wound.
   C. Cleanse the wound with povidone-iodine.
   D. Hydrogen peroxide (1/2 strength) is used to cleanse the wound.

5. Due to diarrhea, Mia Windham's arterial blood gas results are pH – 7.30, pCO_2 – 35mmHg, pO_2 – 90mmHg, HCO_3^- 19mEq/L. Which does the nurse interpret these results as being?
   A. metabolic acidosis
   B. metabolic alkalosis
   C. respiratory acidosis
   D. respiratory alkalosis

6. Which laboratory studies would you expect to be drawn on a patient who is 4 days postoperative with an inflammation of the incision site?
   A. white blood cell count/differential, erythrocyte sedimentation rate, C-reactive protein
   B. troponins, metabolic panel for electrolytes, cultures of wound site
   C. blood cultures, hematocrit and hemoglobin, blood glucose level
   D. complete blood cell count, alkaline phosphatase, urine creatinine, and blood urea nitrogen

Communication

1. What information will you report to Mia Windham's doctor regarding her symptoms this morning?

2. The family of the patient with sickle cell anemia asks the nurse how sickle cell anemia is transmitted from one family member to another. Which statement by the nurse is the correct response?
   A. "The mother carries the gene for sickle cell anemia and passes it to the children."
   B. "The father carries the gene for sickle cell anemia and passes it to the children."
   C. "Both parents carry the gene for sickle cell anemia and have a 25% chance of children getting the disease process."
   D. "One parent has the disease and one parent carries the affected gene and they have a 50% chance of passing it to the children."

3. What communication techniques will you use when talking with Tamra Sanders because of her diagnosis of Down syndrome?

Delegation

1. What nursing interventions for each patient can be delegated to a CNA?

   A. _____

   B. _____

   C. _____

   D. _____

Related Questions

1. In which position does the nurse place the patient with hypovolemic shock?

   A. Semi-Fowler's position with legs straight

   B. Trendelenburg position with legs elevated 10 degrees

   C. left lateral position with legs bent toward chest

   D. supine position with legs elevated 20 degrees

2. Prior to administering cytotoxic agents, such as cyclophosphamide (Cytoxan), the nurse needs to notify the physician of which lab results?

   A. hemoglobin of 10.8g/dL, hematocrit of 35%

   B. potassium of 3.4mEq/L, sodium of 130mEq/L

   C. creatinine of 2mg/dL, blood urea nitrogen of 30mg/dL

   D. white blood cell count 3900mm^3, platelets of 74,000mm^3

3. The patient is admitted to the emergency department for a severe anaphylactic reaction to aspirin. Which medication is ordered to be administered?

   A. 0.5 mL of 1:1000 epinephrine subcutaneously

   B. 0.3 mL of 1:10,000 epinephrine subcutaneously

   C. Intravenous infusion of 1:10,000 epinephrine

   D. Intravenous infusion of 1:100,000 epinephrine

4. When administering a blood transfusion, what manifestations indicate a hemolytic reaction to the blood being administered?

5. The nurse teaches patients and families to decrease risk factors of cancer by following which cancer prevention recommendations? **Select all that apply.**

   A. Avoid tobacco and excessive alcohol use.

   B. Eat a diet low in fat and high in carbohydrates.

   C. Increase intake of vitamins A, D, E, and K.

   D. Limit exposure to sun from 11:00 AM to 3:00 PM.

   E. Increase vegetables and fruits in the diet.

   F. Eat meats grilled over charcoal fire instead of fried.

CASE STUDY: Herman Blount

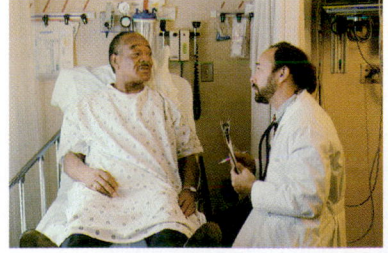

Herman Blount is a 60-year-old African American construction worker who is seen in the physician's office with complaints of dull chest pain, shortness of breath, swelling of his hands and feet, weight loss, fatigue, and weakness. Upon physical assessment, vital signs are temperature 99.8°F, pulse 84, respirations 24, blood pressure 168/92. His height is 5' 11" and weight is 175 pounds. Mr. Blount states this is a loss of 35 pounds over the past 3 months. Wheezing is heard when breath sounds are auscultated. Coughing is noted with deep breathing. Remainder of the physical assessment is unremarkable. He has a medical history of high blood pressure for which he takes diltiazem and ramipril. He has a history of smoking 1 to 2 packs of cigarettes per day since he was 15 years old. He states he has been exposed to asbestos in his employment. Mr. Blount's nutrition assessment indicates that his diet consists of fried meats (especially chicken), green vegetables cooked in fatback, eggs, and bacon for breakfast, and at break time he eats doughnuts or cookies. His fluid intake consists of coffee for breakfast and break time, soda at lunch, and 3 to 4 beers at night.

Blood is drawn for a complete blood count, electrolytes, blood glucose, calcitonin, CEA, haptoglobulin, GGT, and creatinine. A sputum specimen is sent to the laboratory. A chest x-ray and CT scan are done. Based on the results of the chest x-ray, bronchoscopy and needle aspiration biopsies are performed to confirm the diagnosis of lung cancer. The pathophysiology of lung cancer is formation of tumors that begin as mucosal lesions that grow to form masses that obstruct the bronchi and invade adjacent lung tissue. The lung tumor can hemorrhage, causing hemoptysis. The cancer cells can spread via the lymph system to lymph nodes and other organs. Manifestations of lung cancer are chronic cough, hemoptysis, wheezing, shortness of breath, dull and aching chest pain, hoarseness, dysphagia, weight loss, anorexia, fatigue, weakness, bone pain, and clubbing of the fingers and toes. Complications of lung cancer are metastasis to other organs, superior vena cava syndrome, anemia, Cushing's syndrome, syndrome of inappropriate antidiuretic syndrome (SIADH), thrombophlebitis, osteoathropathy, peripheral neuropathy, and cerebellar degeneration.

As Mr. Blount is faced with decisions regarding treatment of his newly diagnosed lung cancer, the nursing diagnosis *Readiness for Enhanced Management of Therapeutic Regimen* is of highest priority at this time.

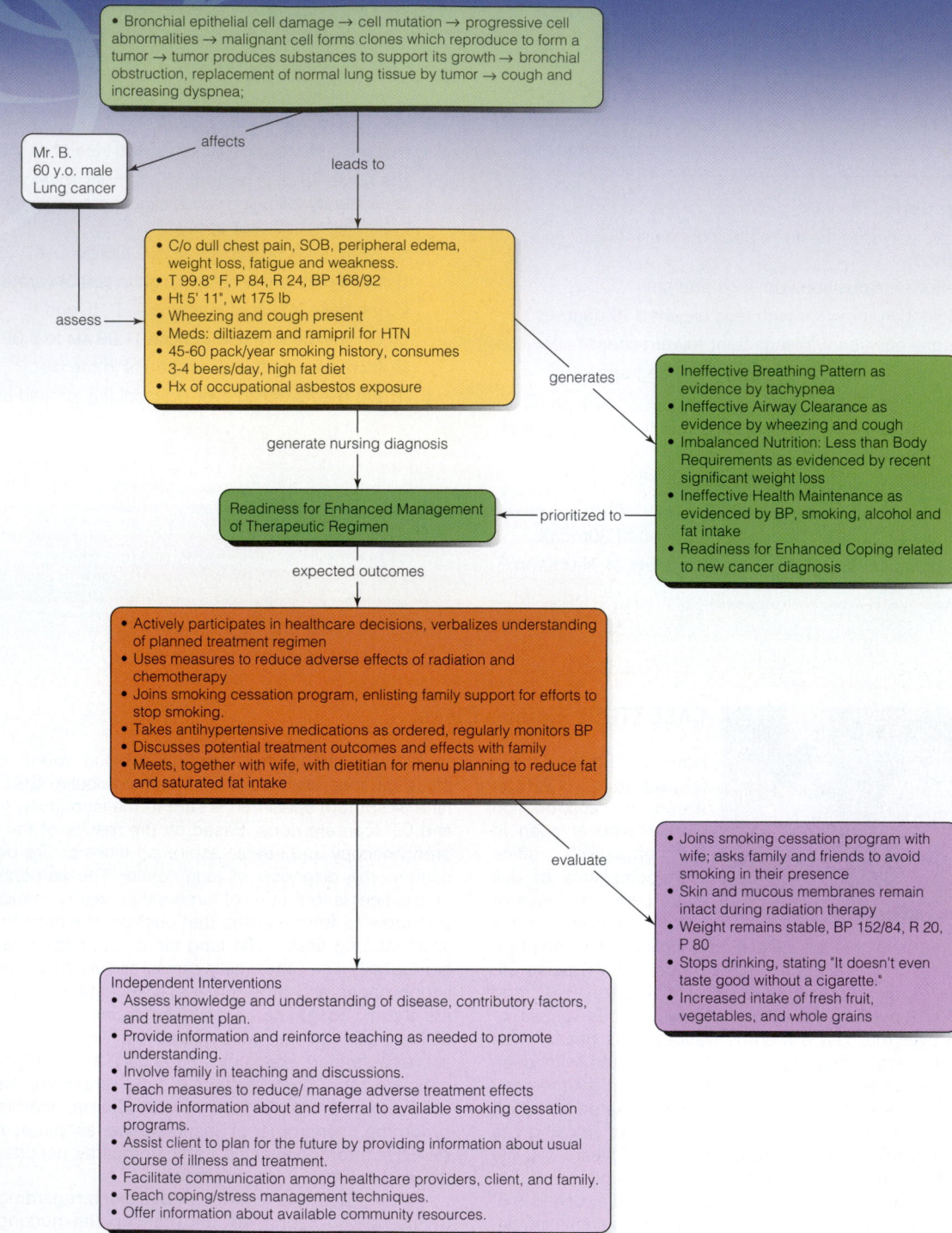

- Bronchial epithelial cell damage → cell mutation → progressive cell abnormalities → malignant cell forms clones which reproduce to form a tumor → tumor produces substances to support its growth → bronchial obstruction, replacement of normal lung tissue by tumor → cough and increasing dyspnea;

Mr. B.
60 y.o. male
Lung cancer

affects

leads to

assess

- C/o dull chest pain, SOB, peripheral edema, weight loss, fatigue and weakness.
- T 99.8° F, P 84, R 24, BP 168/92
- Ht 5' 11", wt 175 lb
- Wheezing and cough present
- Meds: diltiazem and ramipril for HTN
- 45-60 pack/year smoking history, consumes 3-4 beers/day, high fat diet
- Hx of occupational asbestos exposure

generates

- Ineffective Breathing Pattern as evidence by tachypnea
- Ineffective Airway Clearance as evidence by wheezing and cough
- Imbalanced Nutrition: Less than Body Requirements as evidenced by recent significant weight loss
- Ineffective Health Maintenance as evidenced by BP, smoking, alcohol and fat intake
- Readiness for Enhanced Coping related to new cancer diagnosis

generate nursing diagnosis

Readiness for Enhanced Management of Therapeutic Regimen

prioritized to

expected outcomes

- Actively participates in healthcare decisions, verbalizes understanding of planned treatment regimen
- Uses measures to reduce adverse effects of radiation and chemotherapy
- Joins smoking cessation program, enlisting family support for efforts to stop smoking.
- Takes antihypertensive medications as ordered, regularly monitors BP
- Discusses potential treatment outcomes and effects with family
- Meets, together with wife, with dietitian for menu planning to reduce fat and saturated fat intake

evaluate

- Joins smoking cessation program with wife; asks family and friends to avoid smoking in their presence
- Skin and mucous membranes remain intact during radiation therapy
- Weight remains stable, BP 152/84, R 20, P 80
- Stops drinking, stating "It doesn't even taste good without a cigarette."
- Increased intake of fresh fruit, vegetables, and whole grains

Independent Interventions
- Assess knowledge and understanding of disease, contributory factors, and treatment plan.
- Provide information and reinforce teaching as needed to promote understanding.
- Involve family in teaching and discussions.
- Teach measures to reduce/ manage adverse treatment effects
- Provide information about and referral to available smoking cessation programs.
- Assist client to plan for the future by providing information about usual course of illness and treatment.
- Facilitate communication among healthcare providers, client, and family.
- Teach coping/stress management techniques.
- Offer information about available community resources.

Activity:

1. After reviewing the concept map, go to the Pearson Nursing Student Resources for this book at www.nursing.pearson-highered.com to write a concept map based on the nursing diagnosis *Ineffective Breathing Pattern*.

   See answers and hints in Appendix C.

Nutritional and Metabolic Pattern

PART II

Functional Health Patterns with Related Nursing Diagnoses

HEALTH PERCEPTION HEALTH MANAGEMENT

- Perceived health status
- Perceived health management
- Health care behaviors: health promotion and illness prevention activities, medical treatments, follow-up care

VALUE-BELIEF

- Values, goals, or beliefs (including spirituality) that guide choices or decisions
- Perceived conflicts in values, beliefs, or expectations that are health related

COPING-STRESS-TOLERANCE

- Capacity to resist challenges to self-integrity
- Methods of handling stress
- Support systems
- Perceived ability to control and manage situations

NUTRITIONAL-METABOLIC

- Daily consumption of food and fluids
- Favorite foods
- Use of dietary supplements
- Skin lesions and ability to heal
- Condition of the integument
- Weight, height, temperature

PART II

Nutritional–Metabolic, Elimination (bowel) Patterns: Examples of related NANDA Nursing Diagnoses

- Anxiety
- Bowel Incontinence
- Constipation
- Diarrhea
- Disturbed Body Image
- Dysfunctional Gastrointestinal Motility
- Deficient Fluid Volume
- Hypothermia
- Hyperthermia
- Impaired Dentition
- Impaired Oral Mucous Membranes
- Impaired Skin Integrity
- Impaired Swallowing
- Ineffective Thermoregulation
- Impaired Tissue Integrity
- Risk for Electrolyte Imbalance
- Risk for Trauma
- Risk for Unstable Blood Glucose

SEXUALITY-REPRODUCTIVE

- Satisfaction with sexuality or sexual relationships
- Reproductive pattern
- Female menstrual and perimeno-pausal history

ELIMINATION

- Patterns of bowel and urinary excretion
- Perceived regularity or irregularity of elimination
- Use of laxatives or routines
- Changes in time, modes, quality or quantity of excretions
- Use of devices for control

ROLE-RELATIONSHIP

- Perception of major roles, relationships, and responsibilities in current life situation
- Satisfaction with or disturbances in roles and relationships

ACTIVITY-EXERCISE

- Patterns of personally relevant exercise, activity, leisure, and recreation
- ADLs which require energy expenditure
- Factors that interfere with the desired pattern (e.g., illness or injury)

SELF-PERCEPTION– SELF-CONCEPT

- Attitudes about self
- Perceived abilities, worth, self-image, emotions
- Body posture and movement, eye contact, voice and speech patterns

SLEEP-REST

- Patterns of sleep and rest/relaxation in a 24-hr period
- Perceptions of quality and quantity of sleep and rest
- Use of sleep aids and routines

COGNITIVE-PERCEPTUAL

- Adequacy of vision, hearing, taste, touch, smell
- Pain perception and management
- Language, judgment, memory, decisions

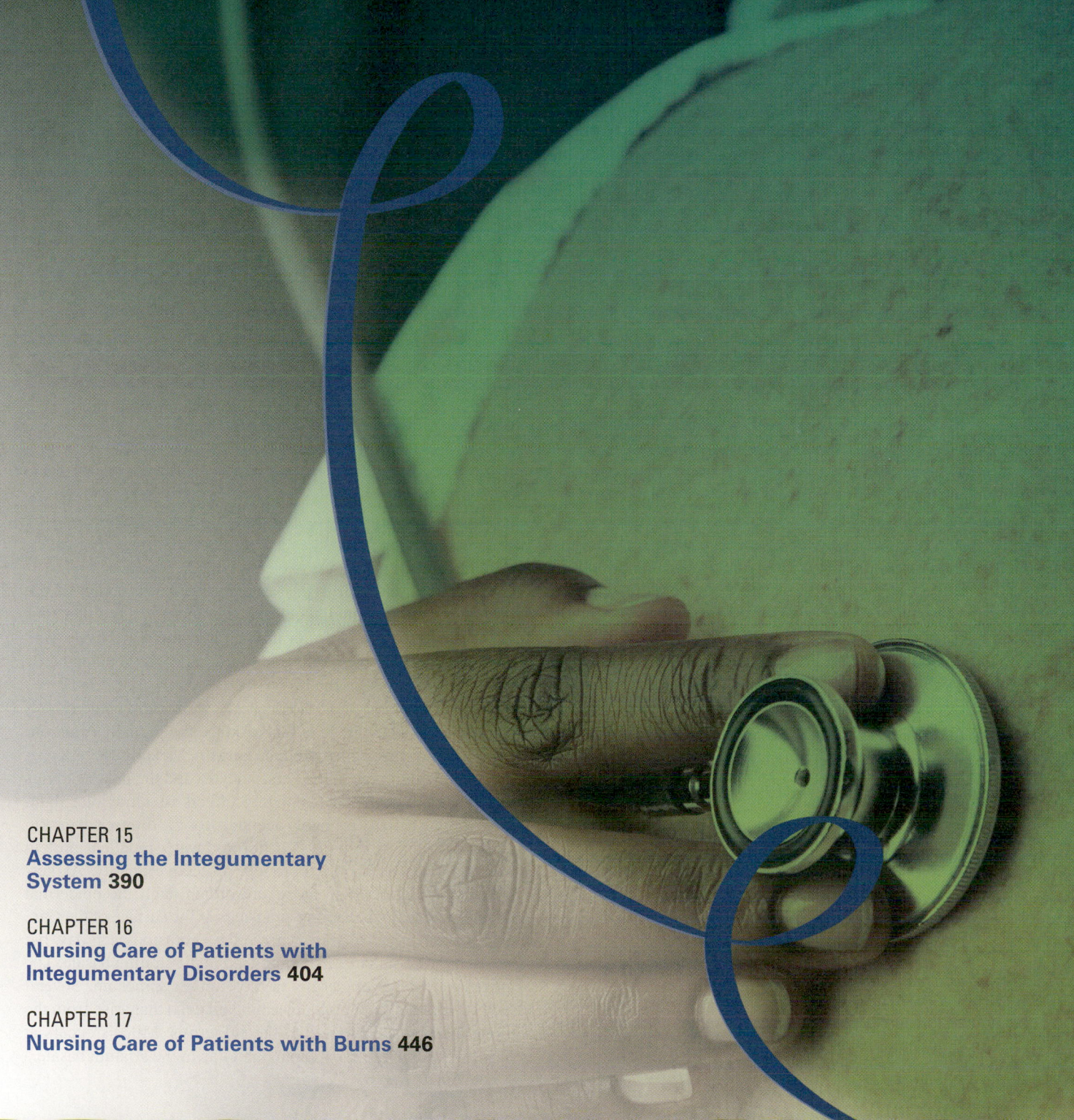

Responses to Altered Integumentary Structure and Function

UNIT 4

LEARNING OUTCOMES

1. Describe the anatomy, physiology, and functions of the skin, hair, and nails.
2. Discuss factors that influence skin color.
3. Identify specific topics for a health history interview of the patient with problems involving the skin, hair, or nails.
4. Explain techniques for assessing the skin, hair, and nails.
5. Give examples of genetic disorders of the integumentary system.
6. Describe normal variations in assessment findings for the older adult.
7. Identify abnormal findings that may indicate impairment of the integumentary system.

CLINICAL COMPETENCIES

1. Conduct and document a health history for patients who have or are at risk for alterations in the skin, hair, or nails.
2. Conduct and document a physical assessment of the integumentary system.
3. Monitor the results of diagnostic tests and report abnormal findings.

EQUIPMENT NEEDED

- Disposable gloves
- Ruler
- Flashlight

KEY TERMS

alopecia, *399*	hirsutism, *399*	sebum, *392*
cyanosis, *392*	jaundice, *392*	urticaria, *398*
ecchymosis, *398*	keratin, *390*	vitiligo, *398*
edema, *398*	melanin, *390*	
erythema, *392*	pallor, *392*	

The skin, the hair, and the nails make up the integumentary system. The skin, the largest organ of the body, provides an external covering for the body, separating and protecting the body's organs and tissues from the external environment. Functions of the skin, hair, and nails are summarized in Table 15–1.

Anatomy, Physiology, and Functions of the Integumentary System

The Skin

The skin has a total surface area of 15 to 20 square feet and weighs about 9 pounds. It has been estimated that each square inch of skin contains 15 feet of blood vessels, 4 yards of nerves, 650 sweat glands, 100 oil glands, 1500 sensory receptors, and more than 3 million cells that are constantly dying and being replaced. The skin is composed of two regions: the epidermis and the dermis (Figure 15–1 ■). Alterations in the skin increase the risk for many physical and psychologic disorders, including fluid and electrolyte balance, temperature regulation, infection, wound healing, and self-concept.

The Epidermis

The epidermis, which is the surface or outermost part of the skin, consists of epithelial cells. The epidermis has either four or five layers, depending on its location; there are five layers over the palms of the hands and the soles of the feet, and four layers over the rest of the body.

The stratum basale is the deepest layer of the epidermis. It contains melanocytes, cells that produce the pigment **melanin**, and keratinocytes, which produce **keratin**. Melanin forms a protective shield to protect the keratinocytes and the nerve endings in the dermis from the damaging effects of ultraviolet light. Melanocyte activity probably accounts for the difference in skin color in humans. Keratin is a fibrous, water-repellent protein that gives the epidermis its tough, protective quality. As keratinocytes mature, they move upward through the epidermal layers, eventually becoming dead cells at the surface of the skin. Millions of these cells are worn off by abrasion each day, but millions are simultaneously produced in the stratum basale. The next layer of the epidermis is the stratum spinosum. Several cells thick, this layer contains abundant cells that arise from the bone marrow and migrate to the epidermis. Mitosis occurs at this layer, although not as abundantly as in the stratum basale.

TABLE 15–1 Functions of the Skin and Its Appendages

STRUCTURE	FUNCTIONS
Epidermis	Protects tissues from physical, chemical, and biologic damage.
	Prevents water loss and serves as a water-repellent layer.
	Stores melanin, which protects tissues from harmful effects of the ultraviolet radiation in sunlight.
	Converts cholesterol molecules to vitamin D when exposed to sunlight.
	Contains phagocytes, which prevent bacteria from penetrating the skin.
Dermis	Regulates body temperature by dilating and constricting capillaries.
	Transmits messages via nerve endings to the central nervous system.
Sebaceous (oil) glands	Secrete sebum, which lubricates skin and hair and plays a role in killing bacteria.
Eccrine sweat glands	Regulate body heat by excretion of perspiration.
Apocrine sweat glands	Remnants of sexual scent gland.
Hair	Cushions the scalp. Eyelashes and cilia protect the body from foreign particles. Provides insulation in cold weather.
Nails	Protect the fingers and toes, aid in grasping, and allow for various other activities, such as scratching the skin, picking up small items, peeling an orange, and so on.

The stratum granulosum is only two to three cells thick. The cells of the stratum granulosum contain a glycolipid that slows water loss across the epidermis. Keratinization, a thickening of the cells' plasma membranes, begins in the stratum granulosum. The stratum lucidum is present only in areas of thick skin. It is made up of flattened, dead keratinocytes. The outermost layer of the epidermis, the stratum corneum, is also the thickest, making up about 75% of the epidermis's total thickness. It consists of about 20 to 30 sheets of dead cells filled with keratin fragments arranged in "shingles" that flake off as dry skin.

The Dermis

The dermis is the second, deeper layer of skin. Made of a flexible connective tissue, this layer is richly supplied with blood cells, nerve fibers, and lymphatic vessels. Most of the

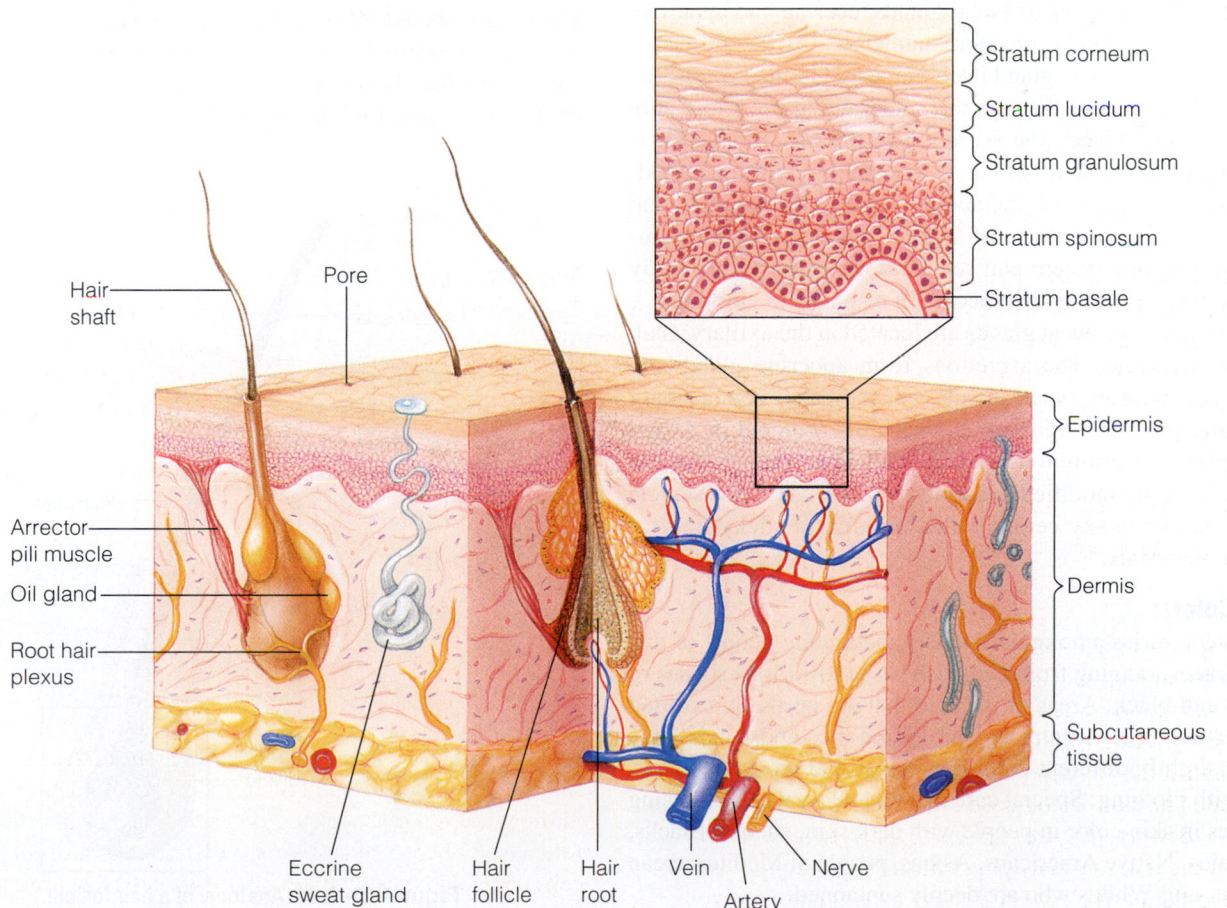

Figure 15–1 ■ Anatomy of the skin.

hair follicles, sebaceous glands, and sweat glands are located in the dermis. The dermis consists of a papillary and a reticular layer. The papillary layer contains capillaries and receptors for pain and touch. The deeper, reticular layer contains blood vessels, sweat and sebaceous glands, deep pressure receptors, and dense bundles of collagen fibers. The regions between these bundles form lines of cleavage in the skin. Surgical incisions parallel to these lines of cleavage heal more easily and with less scarring than incisions or traumatic wounds across cleavage lines.

Superficial Fascia

A layer of subcutaneous tissue called the superficial fascia lies under the dermis. It consists primarily of adipose (fat) tissue and helps the skin adhere to underlying structures.

Glands of the Skin

The skin contains sebaceous (oil) glands, sudoriferous (sweat) glands, and ceruminous glands. Each of these glands has a different function. Sebaceous glands are found all over the body except on the palms and soles. These glands secrete an oily substance called **sebum**, which usually is ducted into a hair follicle. Sebum softens and lubricates the skin and hair and also decreases water loss from the skin in low humidity. Sebum also protects the body from infection by killing bacteria. The secretion of sebum is stimulated by hormones, especially androgens. If a sebaceous gland becomes blocked, a pimple or whitehead appears on the surface of the skin; as the material oxidizes and dries, it forms a blackhead.

There are two types of sweat glands: eccrine and apocrine. Eccrine sweat glands are more numerous on the forehead, palms, and soles. The gland itself is located in the dermis; the duct to the skin rises through the epidermis to open in a pore at the surface. Sweat, the secretion of the eccrine glands, is composed mostly of water but also contains sodium, antibodies, small amounts of metabolic wastes, lactic acid, and vitamin C. The production of sweat is regulated by the sympathetic nervous system and serves to maintain normal body temperature. Sweating also occurs in response to emotions.

Most apocrine sweat glands are located in the axillary, anal, and genital areas. The secretions from apocrine glands are similar to those of sweat glands, but they also contain fatty acids and proteins. Apocrine glands are a remnant of sexual scent glands. Ceruminous glands, located in the skin of the external ear, are modified apocrine sweat glands. They secrete yellow-brown, waxy cerumen that provides a sticky trap for foreign materials.

Skin Color

Skin color varies among individuals and among people of different races, ranging from a pinkish white to various shades of brown and black. Areas of the skin that are normally exposed to the sun and environment, such as the face and hands, may have a slightly different color from areas that are usually covered with clothing. Special care must be taken when assessing changes in skin color in people with dark skin, such as Blacks, Hispanics, Native Americans, Asians, people of Mediterranean descent, and Whites who are deeply suntanned.

The color of the skin is the result of varying levels of pigmentation. Melanin, a yellow-to-brown pigment, is darker and is produced in greater amounts in persons with dark skin color than in those with light skin color. Exposure to the sun causes a buildup of melanin and a darkening or tanning of the skin in people with light skin. Carotene, a yellow-to-orange pigment, is found most in areas of the body where the stratum corneum is thickest, such as the palms of the hands. Carotene is more abundant in the skins of persons of Asian ancestry and, together with melanin, accounts for their golden skin tone. The epidermis in White skin has very little melanin and is almost transparent. Thus, the color of the hemoglobin found in red blood cells (RBCs) circulating through the dermis shows through, lending a pinkish skin tone.

Skin color is influenced by emotions and illnesses. **Erythema**, a reddening of the skin, may occur with embarrassment (blushing), fever, hypertension, or inflammation. It may also result from a drug reaction, sunburn, acne rosacea, or other factors. A bluish discoloration of the skin and mucous membranes, called **cyanosis**, results from poor oxygenation of hemoglobin. **Pallor**, or paleness of skin, may occur with shock, fear, or anger or in anemia and hypoxia. **Jaundice** is a yellow-to-orange color visible in the skin and mucous membranes; it is most often the result of a hepatic disorder. Table 15–2 further defines these terms and compares and contrasts skin color changes in people with light and dark skin.

The Hair

Hair is distributed all over the body, except the lips, nipples, parts of the external genitals, the palms of the hands, and the soles of the feet. Hair is produced by a hair bulb, and its root is enclosed in a hair follicle (Figure 15–2 ■). The exposed part,

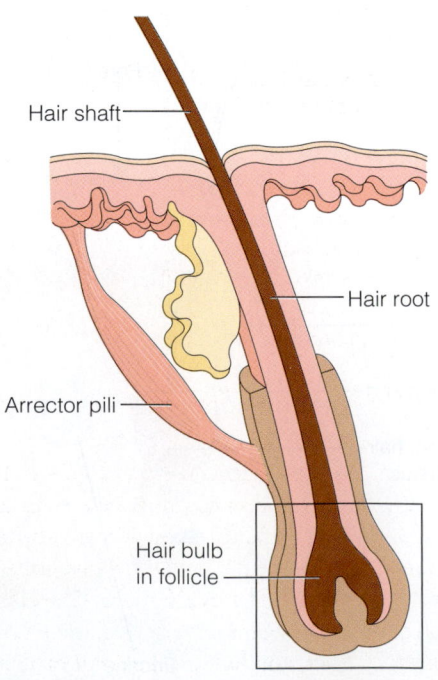

Figure 15–2 ■ Anatomy of a hair follicle.

TABLE 15–2 Skin Color Assessment Variations in People with Light and Dark Skin

PALLOR: *A decrease or absence in skin color as the result of a decrease in tissue perfusion; a decrease in shape, size, or amount of RBCs; or absence of melanin (local or generalized).*

DISORDER AND CAUSE	CHANGE IN LIGHT SKIN	CHANGE IN DARK SKIN
Anemia (decreased or abnormal size and shape of RBCs)	Generalized paleness	Brown skin is dull and has a yellow cast; black skin is dull and has an ashen gray cast.
Hemorrhage (decreased amount of circulating RBCs)	Generalized paleness	Brown skin is dull and has a yellow cast; black skin is dull and has an ashen gray cast
Shock (decreased amount of circulating RBCs or decreased perfusion)	Generalized paleness	Brown skin is dull and has a yellow cast; black skin is dull and has an ashen gray cast
Arterial insufficiency (trauma, acute arterial occlusion, or arteriosclerosis)	Local paleness	Dull, ashen gray
Vitiligo (patchy loss of melanocytes)	Patches of white spots, most often found over skin of the face, hands, or groin	Patches of white spots, most often found over skin of the face, hands, or groin
Albinism (total absence of melanin)	White/pink	Tan, cream, or white

CYANOSIS: *A bluish discoloration of the skin and mucous membranes resulting from a local or generalized excess of deoxygenated hemoglobin or a structural defect in the hemoglobin molecule.*

DISORDER AND CAUSE	CHANGE IN LIGHT SKIN	CHANGE IN DARK SKIN
Acute and chronic disorders of the structure and function of the heart and lungs (arterial insufficiency; exposure to cold, hypothermia)	Dusky blue (may be generalized or local, depending on cause)	Skin may appear darker, but will be dull; cyanosis is more readily assessed in the nail beds, oral mucous membranes, and conjunctivae

ERYTHEMA: *Redness of the skin or mucous membranes that is the result of dilatation and congestion of superficial capillaries.*

DISORDER AND CAUSE	CHANGE IN LIGHT SKIN	CHANGE IN DARK SKIN
Hyperemia (inflammation, increased body temperature, hot environmental temperature, embarrassment, alcohol ingestion)	Red or bright pink	Difficult to assess, skin may have dark red cast
Carbon monoxide poisoning (carbon monoxide displaces oxygen on the hemoglobin molecule, causing hypoxia, carboxyhemoglobinemia)	Cherry red in face and upper torso	Cherry red lips, oral mucous membranes, and nail beds
Venous stasis (inability of veins to return blood to heart; may result from edema, varicose veins, or pressure)	Dusky red	Difficult to assess

JAUNDICE: *Yellowish discoloration of the skin, mucous membranes, and sclerae of the eyes, caused by increased amounts of bilirubin or other pigments in the blood.*

DISORDER AND CAUSE	CHANGE IN LIGHT SKIN	CHANGE IN DARK SKIN
Increased serum bilirubin to >2–3 mg/100 mL (liver disease, pancreatic disease, gallbladder disease, hemolysis, such as following blood transfusion, severe burns or infections)	Yellowing of skin follows yellowing of sclerae and mucous membranes; may also be assessed in the fingernails and palms of the hands	Yellowing is best assessed at the junction of the hard palate and the soft palate or on the palms of the hands. Sclerae may be yellow near the limbus (do not confuse with normal yellow eye pigmentation)
Uremia (retained urochrome pigments in the blood)	Orange-green or gray cast to skin	Difficult to assess; may appear as yellowish green color in the scleral of the eye

called the shaft, consists mainly of dead cells. Hair follicles extend into the dermis and in some places, such as the scalp, below the dermis. Many factors, including nutrition and hormones, influence hair growth. Hair in various parts of the body has protective functions: The eyebrows and eyelashes protect the eyes, hair in the nose helps keep foreign materials out of the upper respiratory tract, and hair on the head protects the scalp from heat loss and sunlight.

The Nails

A nail is a modified scalelike epidermal structure. Like hair, nails consist mainly of dead cells. The body of the nail rests on the nail bed (Figure 15–3 ■). The proximal visible end of the nail has a white crescent, called a lunula. The sides of the nail are overlapped by skin, called nail folds. The proximal nail fold is thickened and is called the eponychium or cuticle. Nails form a protective coating over the dorsum of each digit on the fingers and toes.

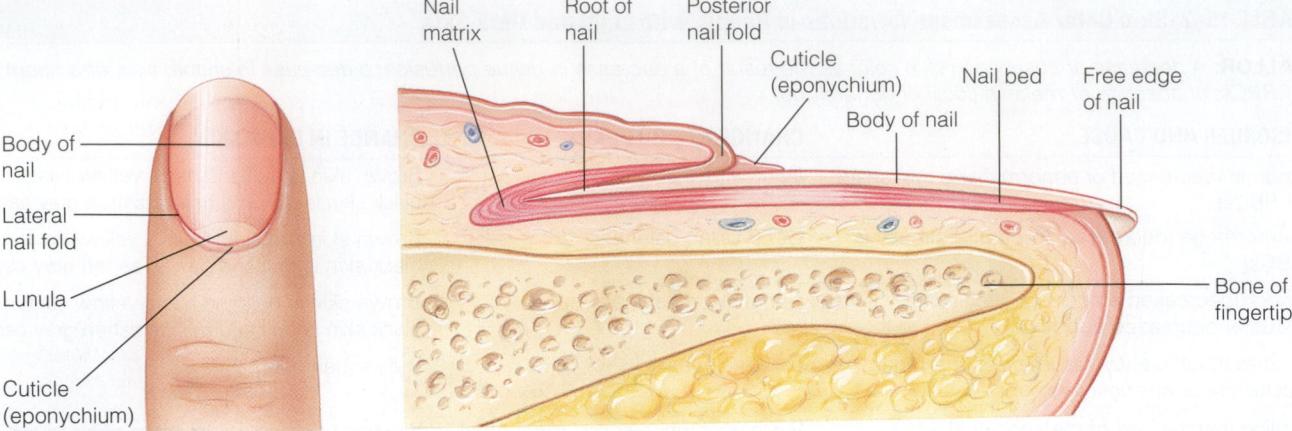

Figure 15–3 ■ Anatomy of a nail.

Assessing the Integumentary System

The structures of the integumentary system are assessed by findings from diagnostic tests, a health assessment interview to collect subjective data, and a physical assessment to collect objective data. See the box that follows the physical assessment information for a sample documentation of an assessment of the integument.

Diagnosis

The results of diagnostic tests of the structure and function of the integumentary system are used to support the diagnosis of a specific injury or disease, to provide information to identify or modify the appropriate medication or treatments used to treat the disease, and to help nurses monitor the patients' responses to nursing care interventions. Some diagnostic tests are conducted to identify bacterial carriers. For example, if patients have repeated bacterial skin infections, or if a healthcare unit or agency experiences numerous bacterial infections of patients, nasal cultures may be performed to determine if the patients or the healthcare workers are carriers of the bacteria.

Regardless of the type of diagnostic test, the nurse is responsible for explaining the procedure and any special preparation needed, for assessing for medication use that may affect the outcome of the tests, for supporting the patient during the examination as necessary, for documenting the procedures as appropriate, and for monitoring the results of the tests.

Diagnostic tests to assess the integumentary system are described in the box on page 395. More information is included in the discussion of specific health problems or injuries in ∞ Chapters 16 and 17.

Genetic Considerations

When conducting a health assessment interview and physical assessment, it is important for the nurse to consider genetic influences on the health of the adult. During the health assessment interview, ask about integumentary disorders or abnormalities in immediate family members and also inquire about their gender. During the physical assessment, assess for any manifestations that indicate a genetic disorder (see the box Genetic Considerations: Examples of Integumentary Disorders). If data are found that indicate genetic risk factors or alterations, ask about genetic testing and refer for appropriate genetic counseling and evaluation. ∞ Chapter 8 provides further information about genetic implications in medical-surgical nursing.

Health Assessment Interview

A health assessment interview to determine problems with the integumentary system may be conducted as part of a health screening or total health assessment, or it may focus on a chief complaint (such as itching or a rash). If the patient has a skin problem, analyze its onset, characteristics and course, severity, precipitating and relieving factors, and note the timing and circumstances of any associated symptoms. For example, ask the patient the following:

- What type of itching have you experienced?
- When did you first notice a change in this mole?
- Did you change to any different kinds of shampoo or other hair products just before you started to lose your hair?

> **GENETIC CONSIDERATIONS**
> ### Examples of Integumentary Disorders
>
> - Oculocutaneous albinism, an autosomal recessive inheritance disorder, causes hypopigmentation (albinism or absence of color) of the skin, hair, and eyes as a result of an inability to synthesize melanin.
> - Keloids, which are elevated scars, have a familial tendency and are more commonly found in Blacks.
> - Vitiligo, the sudden appearance of white patches on the skin, has a familial tendency.
> - Male pattern baldness (the most common cause of baldness in men) is genetically predetermined.
> - Hirsutism (excessive hair in women) may be genetically predetermined.
> - Blacks may have very dry scalps and dry, fragile hair of genetic origin.
> - A family history of skin cancer is a risk factor for skin cancer

DIAGNOSTIC TESTS of the Integumentary System

NAME OF TEST	PURPOSE & DESCRIPTION	RELATED NURSING INTERVENTIONS
Biopsy	A punch biopsy is done to differentiate benign lesions from skin cancers. An instrument is used to remove a small section of dermis and subcutaneous fat. Depending on size, the incision may be sutured with a single suture. An incisional biopsy is done to differentiate benign lesions from skin cancers. An incision is made and the skin lesion or tumor is removed for analysis. The incision is closed with sutures.	Apply dressing and provide information about self-care and when to return for suture removal.
Culture	A culture of scrapings from a lesion, from drainage, or of exudate is done to identify fungal, bacterial, or viral skin infections.	Obtain the culture with a sterile Culturette swab and culture tubes. Maintain strict asepsis while obtaining the culture.
Immunofluorescent Slides	Immunofluorescent studies of samples from skin and/or serum may be done to identify IgG antibodies (present in pemphigus vulgaris) and to identify varicella in skin cells (for herpes zoster). Skin or blood samples are placed on a slide and examined microscopically.	No special preparation is necessary.
Oil Slides	Oil slides are used to determine the type of skin infestation present. Scrapings of the lesion are placed on a slide with mineral oil and examined microscopically.	No special preparation is necessary.
Patch Test, Scratch Tests	These tests are used to determine a specific allergen. In a patch test, a small amount of the suspected material is placed on the skin under an occlusive bandage. In a scratch test, a needle is used to "scratch" small amounts of potentially allergic materials on the skin surface.	Explain to the patient the need to return in 48 hours to have the patched area or scratched areas evaluated.
Potassium Hydroxide (KOH)	A specimen from hair or nails is examined for a fungal infection. The specimen is obtained by placing material from a scraping on a slide, adding a potassium hydroxide solution, and examining it microscopically.	No special preparation is necessary.
Tzanck Test	This test is used to diagnose herpes infections, but it does not differentiate herpes simplex from herpes zoster. Fluid and cells from the vesicles are obtained, put on a slide, stained, and examined microscopically.	
Wood's Lamp	This test uses an ultraviolet light that causes certain organisms to fluoresce (such as *Pseudomonas* organisms and fungi). The skin is examined under a special lamp.	

Ask about any change in health, rashes, itching, color changes, dryness or oiliness, growth of or changes in warts or moles, and the presence of lesions. Precipitating causes, such as medications, the use of new soaps, skin care agents, cosmetics, pets, travel, stress, or dietary changes must also be explored. In assessing hair problems, ask about any thinning or baldness, excessive hair loss, change in distribution of hair, use of hair care products, diet, and dieting. When assessing nail problems, ask about nail splitting or breakage, discoloration, infection, diet, and exposure to chemicals.

The patient's medical history is important. Questions focus on previous problems, allergies, and lesions. Skin problems may be manifestations of other disorders, such as cardiovascular disease, endocrine disorders, hepatic disease, and hematologic disorders. Occupational and social history may provide cues to skin problems; ask the patient about

travel, exposure to toxic substances at work, use of alcohol, and responses to stress.

Assess the presence of risk factors for skin cancer carefully. These include male gender; age over 50; family history of skin cancer; extended exposure to sunlight; tendency to sunburn; history of sunburn or other skin trauma; light-colored hair or eyes; residence in high altitudes or near the equator; and exposure to radiation, x-rays, coal, tar, or petroleum products. (Risks for skin cancer are further discussed in ∞ Chapter 16.) Include specific questions to identify risk factors for malignant melanoma. These include a large number of moles, the presence of atypical moles, a family history of melanoma, prior melanoma, repeated severe sunburns, ease of freckling and sunburning, or inability to tan.

Interview questions categorized by functional health patterns follow. Responses should be documented in the patient's medical record.

FUNCTIONAL HEALTH PATTERN INTERVIEW   Integumentary System

Functional Health Pattern	Interview Questions and Leading Statements
Health Perception-Health Management	■ Describe any health problems, injuries, or surgeries you have had. How were these treated? ■ Describe medications, herbs, and vitamins you currently are taking. ■ Describe your current problem. How long has it lasted? What have you done to treat it? ■ Do you have allergies to foods, plants, pets? Explain how the allergy affects you. ■ Describe what you do each day to care for your skin, hair, and nails.
Nutritional-Metabolic	■ Describe what you eat and how much and type of fluids you drink in a 24-hour period. ■ Do you have a history of food allergies? If so, describe what you are allergic to and how you respond. ■ Have you recently eaten any new foods? ■ Do you take any nutritional supplements, herbs, or vitamins? If so, what are they? ■ How well do your cuts and scratches heal?
Elimination	■ Is your skin and scalp dry or oily? ■ Have you noticed swelling around your eyes or ankles? ■ Do you perspire a lot?
Activity-Exercise	■ Describe your physical activities in a typical day. ■ Do you bruise easily? ■ Do you use a sunscreen when you are outside? If so, what SPF? ■ Do you visit tanning salons?
Sleep-Rest	■ How many hours do you sleep each night? ■ Do you have trouble sleeping because of itching or sweating?
Cognitive-Perceptual	■ Do you have any of the following: pain, discomfort, itching, tingling, burning, tenderness, or numbness? If so, where?
Self-Perception-Self-Concept	■ How does this condition make you feel about yourself?
Role-Relationships	■ How does this condition affect your relationships with others? ■ Is there anything in your work environment that may have caused this condition?
Sexuality-Reproductive	■ Has this condition interfered with your usual sexual activities?
Coping-Stress-Tolerance	■ Have you experienced any type of stress that may have worsened this condition? ■ Has this condition created stress for you? ■ Describe what you do when you feel stressed.
Value-Belief	■ Tell me how specific relationships or activities help you cope with this condition. ■ Describe specific cultural beliefs or practices that affect how you care for and feel about this condition. ■ Is there anything interfering with your spiritual beliefs, needs, or practices as a result of this condition? What can I or another caregiver do to help you with your spiritual needs? ■ Are there any specific treatments that you would not use to treat this condition?

Physical Assessment

Physical assessment of the skin, hair, and nails may be performed either as part of a total assessment or may be a focused assessment of the integument for patients with known or suspected problems. Physical assessment of the skin, hair, and nails is conducted by inspection and palpation. Assess the skin for color, presence of lesions (observable changes from normal skin structure), temperature, texture, moisture, turgor, and presence of edema. Characteristics of lesions to note include location and distribution, color, pattern, edges, size (measure with a ruler in centimeters), elevation, and type of exudate (if present). Common skin lesions of older adults are outlined in Box 15–1; see the box Nursing Care of the Older Adult for age-related integument changes. Examine the hair for color, texture, quality, and scalp lesions. Determine the shape, color, contour, and condition of the nails. Terminology of skin lesions with examples are outlined in Table 15–3.

The examination should be conducted in a warm, private room. The patient removes all clothing and puts on a gown or drape. The areas to be examined should be fully exposed, but protect the patient's modesty by keeping other areas covered. The patient may be standing, sitting, or lying down at various times of the examination. Don disposable gloves when

BOX 15–1 Common Skin Lesions of Older Adults

■ *Skin tags:* soft brown or flesh-colored benign papules
■ *Keratoses:* horny growth of keratinocytes, may be seborrheic (benign) or actinic (premalignant)
■ *Lentigines ("liver spots"):* brown or black benign macule with a defined border
■ *Angiomas (hemangioma):* benign vascular tumors with dilated blood vessels, found in the middle to upper dermis
■ *Telangiectases:* single dilated blood vessels, capillaries, or terminal arteries
■ *Venous lakes:* small, dark blue, slightly raised benign papules
■ *Photoaging:* wrinkling, mottling, pigmented areas, loss of elasticity, benign or malignant lesions

palpating open lesions, skin surfaces suspicious of infections or infestations, or discharge from lesions of the skin and mucous membranes. A ruler is used to measure the size of lesions. A flashlight is used to better visualize lesions.

SAMPLE DOCUMENTATION

Assessment of the Integumentary System

A 50-year-old man with no history of skin lesions, hair loss, or disorders of the nails. Took antibiotic for respiratory infection approximately 10 days ago and reports having a fine, raised, red rash on trunk and arms that itched. Nurse practitioner prescribed antihistamine and rash cleared in 3 days. Skin light brown, warm, dry, and elastic. Patches of vitiligo present over dorsum of hands. No lesions or edema noted. Healed scar on lower left abdomen (appendectomy as a young adult). Hair dark brown with gray at the temples, clean. Nails are smooth, hard, and immobile.

TABLE 15–3 Terminology of Skin Lesions with Associated Disorders

LESION	EXAMPLES OF DISORDERS
Pigmented	Freckle, seborrheic keratosis, nevus, melanoma
Scaly	Psoriasis, dermatitis, xerosis, tinea, actinic keratoses
Pustular	Acne vulgaris, folliculitis, candidiasis
Vesicular	Herpes simplex, herpes zoster, scabies
Nodular	Warts, basal cell carcinoma, acne
Weepy, crusted	Acute contact allergic dermatitis, impetigo
Figurate (shaped) erythema	Urticaria, cellulites
Bullous	Pemphigus, toxic epidermal necrolysis
Pruritic	Xerosis, scabies, pediculosis
Ulcerated	Pressure ulcer, skin cancer, herpes simplex

NURSING CARE OF THE OLDER ADULT — Age-Related Skin Changes

AGE-RELATED CHANGE	SIGNIFICANCE
Epidermis: ↓ thickness and miotic activity	■ Skin is more fragile and at greater risk for tears or injury ■ Delayed wound healing ■ Hyperkeratoses and skin cancers in sun-exposed areas are more evident
Epidermis: ↑ permeability, ↓ Langerhans cells	■ Increased risk of reactions to irritants ■ Decreased inflammatory response
Epidermis: ↓ number of active melanocytes	■ Increased susceptibility to sun exposure
Epidermis: hyperplasia of melanocytes, especially in sun-exposed areas	■ Small areas of hyperpigmentation ("liver spots") and hypopigmentation ("age spots"), especially on the hands
Epidermis: ↓ vitamin D production	■ Increased risk of osteomalacia, osteoporosis
Epidermis: dermal–epidermal junction flattens	■ Increased risk of skin tears, purpura, and pressure ulcers
Dermis: ↓ perfusion	■ More susceptible to dry skin ■ Decreased sensation (pain, touch, temperature, and peripheral vibration) ■ Increased risk of injury
Dermis: ↓ vasomotor response	■ Greater risk of hyperthermia and hypothermia
Dermis: elastic fibers degenerate	■ Decreased tone and elasticity, with wrinkle formation
Dermis: proliferation of capillaries	■ Cherry hemangiomas are common
Subcutaneous skin layer: thins	■ Greater risk of hypothermia ■ Increased risk of pressure ulcers
Subcutaneous skin layer: adipose tissue is redistributed	■ Cellulite forms ■ Bags over and under the eyes ■ Double chin forms ■ Abdominal fat increases ■ Breasts sag ■ Skin returns to normal more slowly when pinched (also called tenting)
Glands: ↓ eccrine and apocrine activity	■ Dry skin is common ■ Absent perspiration

TABLE 15–4 Integumentary Assessments

TECHNIQUE/NORMAL FINDINGS	ABNORMAL FINDINGS
Inspect skin color and note any odors coming from the skin. *Skin color should be even, appropriate to the age and race of the patient, without foul odors.*	■ A strong odor of perspiration may indicate poor hygiene and a need for patient teaching. A foul odor may indicate a disorder of the sweat glands. ■ Pallor and/or cyanosis are seen with exposure to cold and with decreased perfusion and oxygenation. In cyanotic dark-skinned patients, skin loses glow and appears dull. Cyanosis may be more visible in the mucous membranes and nail beds of these patients. ■ In dark-skinned patients, jaundice may be most apparent in the sclerae of the eyes. ■ Redness, swelling, and pain are seen with various rashes, inflammations, infections, and burns. First-degree burns cause areas of painful erythema and swelling. Red, painful blisters appear in second-degree burns, whereas white or blackened areas are common in third-degree burns. ■ **Vitiligo**, an abnormal loss of melanin in patches, typically occurs over the face, hands, or groin. Vitiligo is thought to be an autoimmune disorder.
Inspect the skin for lesions and alterations, including calluses, scars, tattoos, and piercings. Include inspection of skin creases and folds. *Skin should be intact without lesions.*	Primary, secondary, and vascular lesions are described and shown in Tables 15–5 through 15–7. ■ Pearly edged nodules with a central ulcer are seen in basal cell carcinoma. ■ Scaly, red, fast-growing papules are seen in squamous cell carcinoma. ■ Dark, asymmetric, multicolored patches (sometimes moles) with irregular edges appear in malignant melanoma. ■ Circular lesions are usually present in ringworm and in tinea versicolor. ■ Grouped vesicles may be seen in contact dermatitis. ■ Linear lesions appear in poison ivy and herpes zoster. ■ **Urticaria** (hives) appears as patches of pale, itchy wheals in an erythematous area. ■ In psoriasis, scaly red patches appear on the scalp, knees, back, and genitals. ■ In herpes zoster, vesicles appear along sensory nerve paths, turn into pustules, and then crust over. ■ Bruises (**ecchymosis**) are raised bluish or yellowish vascular lesions. Multiple bruises in various stages of healing suggest trauma or abuse.
Palpate skin temperature. *Skin should be warm.*	■ Skin is warm and red in inflammation and is generally warm with elevated body temperature. ■ Decreased blood flow decreases the skin temperature; this may be generalized, as in shock, or localized, as in arteriosclerosis.
Palpate skin texture. *Skin should be smooth.*	■ Changes in the texture of the skin may indicate irritation or trauma. ■ The skin is soft and smooth in hyperthyroidism and coarse in hypothyroidism.
Palpate skin moisture. *Skin should be dry.*	■ Excessively dry skin often is present in the elderly and patients with hypothyroidism. ■ Oily skin is common in adolescents and young adults. Oily skin may be a normal finding, or it may accompany a skin disorder such as acne vulgaris. ■ Excessive perspiration may be associated with shock, fever, increased activity, or anxiety.
Palpate skin turgor. *Skin fold should return rapidly to normal position.*	■ Pinch the patient's skin gently over the back of the hand or collarbone. Tenting, in which the skin remains pinched for a few moments before resuming its normal position, is common in older patients who are thin (Figure 15–4 ■). ■ Skin turgor is decreased in dehydration. It is increased in edema and scleroderma.

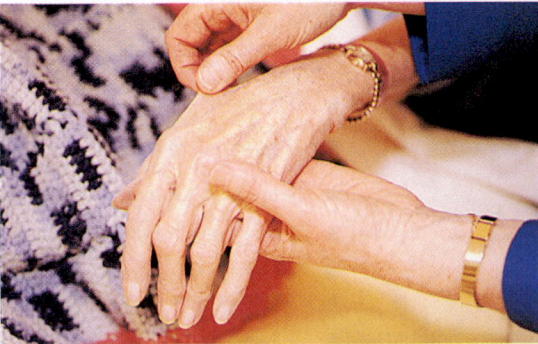

Figure 15–4 ■ Tenting in an older patient.

Assess for edema. *No edema should be present.*	■ Assess **edema** (accumulation of fluid in the body's tissues) by depressing the patient's skin (Figure 15–5 ■). Record findings as follows: 1+ Slight pitting, no obvious distortion 2+ Deeper pit, no obvious distortion 3+ Pit is obvious; extremities are swollen 4+ Pit remains with obvious distortion ■ Edema is common in cardiovascular disorders, renal failure, trauma, and cirrhosis of the liver. It also may be a side effect of certain drugs.

TABLE 15–4 Integumentary Assessments (continued)

TECHNIQUE/NORMAL FINDINGS   ABNORMAL FINDINGS

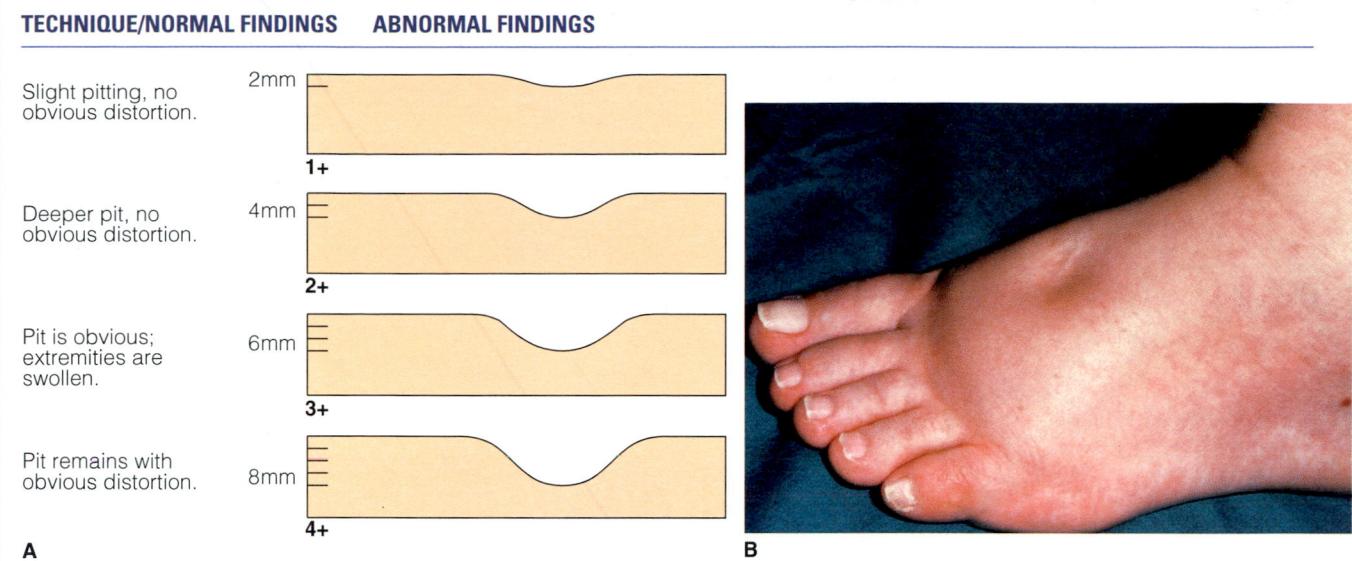

Slight pitting, no obvious distortion.

2mm

1+

Deeper pit, no obvious distortion.

4mm

2+

Pit is obvious; extremities are swollen.

6mm

3+

Pit remains with obvious distortion.

8mm

4+

A

B

Figure 15–5 ■ *A*, Degrees of pitting in edema. *B*, 4+ pitting.

Source: Dr. P. Marazzi/Science Photo Library/Photo Researchers, Inc.

Inspect distribution and quality of hair. *Hair should be evenly distributed for patient's gender.*

- A deviation in the normal hair distribution in the male or female genital area may indicate an endocrine disorder. **Hirsutism** (increased growth of coarse hair, usually on the face and trunk) is seen in Cushing's syndrome, acromegaly, and ovarian dysfunction. **Alopecia** (hair loss) may be related to changes in hormones, chemical or drug treatment, or radiation. In adult males whose hair loss follows the normal male pattern, the cause is usually genetic.

Palpate hair texture. *Hair should be of even texture.*

- Some systemic diseases change the texture of the hair. For instance, hypothyroidism causes the hair to coarsen, whereas hyperthyroidism causes the hair to become fine.

Inspect the scalp for lesions. *There should be no lesions on the scalp.*

- Mild dandruff is normal, but excessive, greasy flakes indicate seborrhea.
- Hair loss, pustules, and scales appear on the scalp in tinea capitis (scalp ringworm).
- Red, swollen pustules appear around infected hair follicles and are called folliculitis.
- Head lice may be seen as oval nits (eggs) adhering to the base of the hair shaft. Head lice are usually accompanied by itching.

Inspect nail curvature. *Nails should not be excessively curved.*

- Clubbing (Figure 15–6 ■), in which the angle of the nail base is greater than 180 degrees, is seen in respiratory disorders, cardiovascular disorders, cirrhosis of the liver, colitis, and thyroid disease. The nail becomes thick, hard, shiny, and curved at the free end.

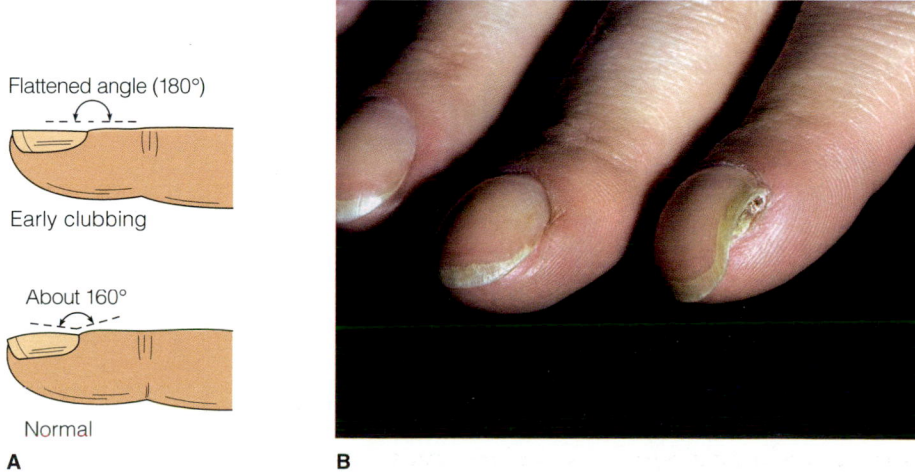

Flattened angle (180°)

Early clubbing

About 160°

Normal

A

B

Figure 15–6 ■ *A*, Assessing clubbing of the nails. *B*, Hand with nail clubbing.

Source: Logical Images, Inc.

Inspect the surface of the nails.

- The nail folds become inflamed and swollen and the nail loosens in paronychia, an infection of the nails.

(continued)

TABLE 15–4 Integumentary Assessments (continued)

TECHNIQUE/NORMAL FINDINGS	ABNORMAL FINDINGS
Nail surfaces should be smooth and nail folds firm, without redness.	■ Inflammation and transverse rippling of the nail are associated with chronic paronychia and/or eczema. ■ The nail plate may separate from the nail bed in trauma, psoriasis, and *Pseudomonas* and *Candida* infections. This separation is called oncholysis. ■ Nail grooves may be caused by inflammation, by planus, or by nail biting. ■ Nail pitting may be seen with psoriasis. ■ A transverse groove (Beau's line) may be seen in trachoma and/or acute diseases. ■ Thin spoon-shaped nails (Figure 15–7 ■) may be seen in anemia.

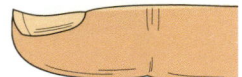

Figure 15–7 ■ Spoon-shaped nails.

Inspect nail color. *Nail color should be even. Pigmented bands are normally found in more than 90% of African Americans.*	■ The sudden appearance of a pigmented band may indicate melanoma in people with light skin. ■ Yellowish nails are seen in psoriasis and fungal infections. ■ Dark nails occur with trauma, *Candida* infections, and hyperbilirubinemia. ■ Blackish-green nails are apparent in injury and in *Pseudomonas* infection.
Inspect nail thickness. *Nails should not be excessively thick.*	■ Trauma to the nails usually causes thickening. Other causes of thick nails include psoriasis, fungal infections, and decreased peripheral vascular blood supply. ■ Thinning of the nails is seen in nutritional deficiencies.

TABLE 15–5 Primary Skin Lesions

Macule, Patch

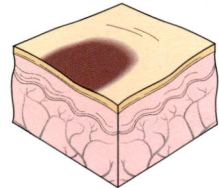

Flat, nonpalpable change in skin color. Macules are smaller than 1 cm, with a circumscribed border, and patches are larger than 1 cm and may have an irregular border.

Examples Macules: freckles, measles, and petechiae. Patches: Mongolian spots, port-wine stains, vitiligo, and chloasma.

Papule, Plaque

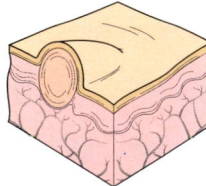

Elevated, solid, palpable mass with circumscribed border. Papules are smaller than 0.5 cm; plaques are groups of papules that form lesions larger than 0.5 cm.

Examples Papules: elevated moles, warts, and lichen planus. Plaques: psoriasis, actinic keratosis, and also lichen planus.

Nodule, Tumor

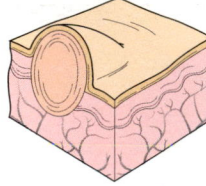

Elevated, solid, hard or soft palpable mass extending deeper into the dermis than a papule. Nodules have circumscribed borders and are 0.5 to 2 cm; tumors may have irregular borders and are larger than 2 cm.

Examples Nodules: small lipoma, squamous cell carcinoma, fibroma, and intradermal nevi. Tumors: large lipoma, carcinoma, and hemangioma.

Vesicle, Bulla

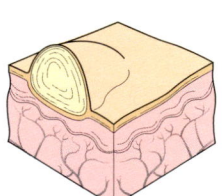

Elevated, fluid-filled, round or oval shaped, palpable mass with thin, translucent walls and circumscribed borders. Vesicles are smaller than 0.5 cm; bullae are larger than 0.5 cm.

Examples Vesicles: herpes simplex/zoster, early chickenpox, poison ivy, and small burn blisters. Bullae: contact dermatitis, friction blisters, and large burn blisters.

Wheal

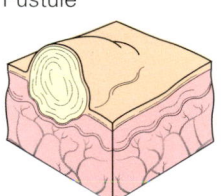

Elevated, often reddish area with irregular border caused by diffuse fluid in tissues rather than free fluid in a cavity, as in vesicles. Size varies.

Examples Insect bites and hives (extensive wheals).

Pustule

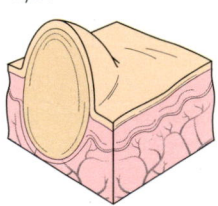

Elevated, pus-filled vesicle or bulla with circumscribed border. Size varies.

Examples Acne, impetigo, and carbuncles (large boils).

Cyst

Elevated, encapsulated, fluid-filled or semisolid mass originating in the subcutaneous tissue or dermis, usually 1 cm or larger.

Examples Varieties include sebaceous cysts and epidermoid cysts.

TABLE 15–6 Secondary Skin Lesions

Atrophy

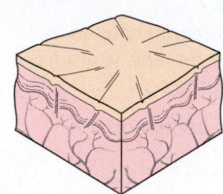

A translucent, dry, paper-like, sometimes wrinkled skin surface resulting from thinning or wasting of the skin due to loss of collagen and elastin.

Examples Striae, aged skin.

Ulcer

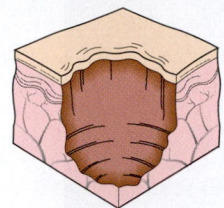

Deep, irregularly shaped area of skin loss extending into the dermis or subcutaneous tissue. May bleed. May leave scar.

Examples Decubitus ulcers (pressure sores), stasis ulcers, chancres.

Erosion

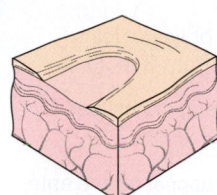

Wearing away of the superficial epidermis causing a moist, shallow depression. Because erosions do not extend into the dermis, they heal without scarring.

Examples Scratch marks, ruptured vesicles.

Fissure

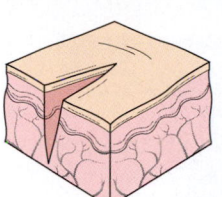

Linear crack with sharp edges, extending into the dermis.

Examples Cracks at the corners of the mouth or in the hands, athlete's foot.

Lichenification

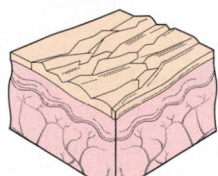

Rough, thickened, hardened area of epidermis resulting from chronic irritation such as scratching or rubbing.

Example Chronic dermatitis.

Scar

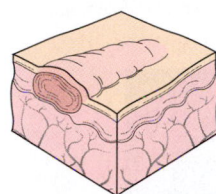

Flat, irregular area of connective tissue left after a lesion or wound has healed. New scars may be red or purple; older scars may be silvery or white.

Examples Healed surgical wound or injury, healed acne.

Scales

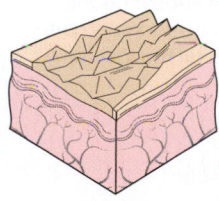

Shedding flakes of greasy, keratinized skin tissue. Color may be white, gray, or silver. Texture may vary from fine to thick.

Examples Dry skin, dandruff, psoriasis, and eczema.

Keloid

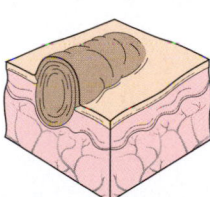

Elevated, irregular, darkened area of excess scar tissue caused by excessive collagen formation during healing. Extends beyond the site of the original injury. Higher incidence in people of African descent.

Examples Keloid from ear piercing or surgery.

Crust

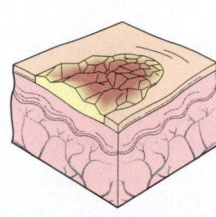

Dry blood, serum, or pus left on the skin surface when vesicles or pustules burst. Can be red-brown, orange, or yellow. Large crusts that adhere to the skin surface are called scabs.

Examples Eczema, impetigo, herpes, or scabs following abrasion.

TABLE 15–7 Vascular Skin Lesions

Spider Angioma

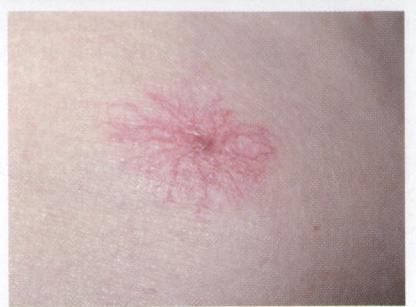

Source: Custom Medical Stock Photo, Inc.

A flat, bright red dot with tiny radiating blood vessels ranging in size from a pinpoint to 2 cm. It blanches with pressure.

Cause A type of telangiectasis (vascular dilatation) caused by elevated estrogen levels, pregnancy, estrogen therapy, vitamin B deficiency, or liver disease, or may not be pathologic.

Localization/Distribution Most commonly appear on the upper half of the body.

Venous Star

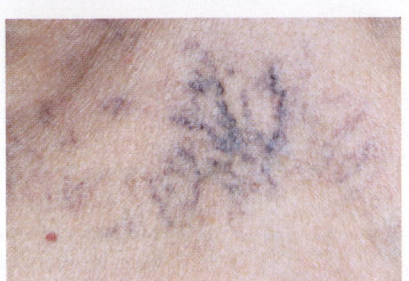

Source: Photo Researchers, Inc.

A flat blue lesion with radiating, cascading, or linear veins extending from the center. It ranges in size from 3 to 25 cm.

Cause A type of telangiectasis (vascular dilatation) caused by increased intravenous pressure in superficial veins.

Localization/Distribution Most commonly appear on the anterior chest and the lower legs near varicose veins.

Petechiae

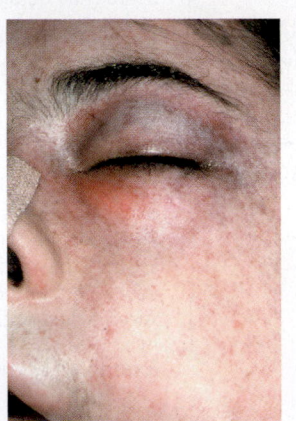

Source: Custom Medical Stock Photo, Inc.

Flat red or purple rounded "freckles" approximately 1 to 3 mm in diameter. Difficult to detect in dark skin. Do not blanch.

Cause Minute hemorrhages resulting from fragile capillaries, petechiae are caused by septicemias, liver disease, or vitamin C or K deficiency. They may also be caused by anticoagulant therapy.

Localization/Distribution Most commonly appear on the dependent surfaces of the body (e.g., back, buttocks). In the patient with dark skin, look for them in the oral mucosa and conjunctivae.

Purpura

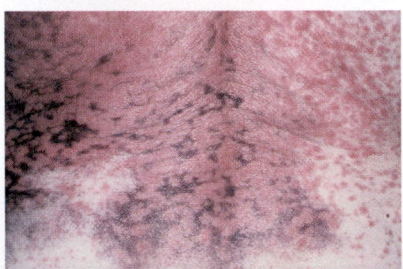

Source: Custom Medical Stock Photo, Inc.

Flat, reddish blue, irregularly shaped extensive patches of varying size.

Cause Bleeding disorders, scurvy, and capillary fragility in the older adult (senile purpura).

Localization/Distribution May appear anywhere on the body, but are most noticeable on the legs, arms, and backs of hands.

Ecchymosis

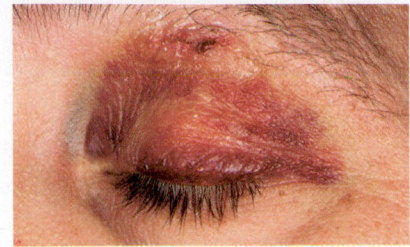

Source: Photo Researchers, Inc.

A flat, irregularly shaped lesion of varying size with no pulsation. Does not blanch with pressure. In light skin, it begins as bluish purple mark that changes to greenish yellow. In brown skin, it varies from blue to deep purple. In black skin, it appears as a darkened area.

Cause Release of blood from superficial vessels into surrounding tissue due to trauma, hemophilia, liver disease, or deficiency of vitamin C or K.

Localization/Distribution Occurs anywhere on the body at the site of trauma or pressure.

TEST YOURSELF NCLEX-RN® REVIEW

1. Following a burn involving several layers of skin, the healed burn area does not grow hair or sweat. Which layer of the skin was a part of the burn?
   1. epidermis
   2. dermis
   3. stratum basale
   4. stratum spinosum

2. What pigment is responsible for skin tanning?
   1. carotene
   2. red blood cells
   3. melanin
   4. sebum

3. Which of the four assessment techniques are used during assessment of the integumentary system? **Select all that apply.**
   1. inspection
   2. palpation
   3. percussion
   4. auscultation

4. A nurse takes a patient's body temperature orally and finds it is elevated by 3 degrees. What other assessment would also be commonly found?
   1. erythema
   2. jaundice
   3. pallor
   4. cyanosis

5. A nurse is assessing a patient who is complaining of severe itching. What would be an appropriate interview question?
   1. "Tell me how this itch feels."
   2. "Why do you keep scratching it?"
   3. "Have you used a new soap?"
   4. "Describe your daily fluid intake."

6. A nurse is assessing the skin of an older adult patient for dehydration. What finding would indicate this condition?
   1. decreased turgor
   2. increased moisture
   3. presence of lesions
   4. pallor or cyanosis

7. A nurse is assessing for edema. What part of the body would he or she palpate?
   1. scalp
   2. fingers
   3. clavicle
   4. ankle/foot

8. A nurse documents that a patient with chronic dermatitis has rough, thickened areas of skin. What term would he or she use?
   1. ulcers
   2. papules
   3. atrophy
   4. lichenification

9. While making a home visit to an older woman, a nurse notices multiple angiomas on her arms and body. What might these indicate?
   1. high intake of vitamin A
   2. poor hygiene
   3. caregiver strain
   4. aging skin

10. While assessing the hair of a family, a nurse notices small white eggs on the hair shaft. What type of infestation is being assessed?
    1. bacterial
    2. viral
    3. head lice
    4. head lichens

See Test Yourself answers in Appendix C.

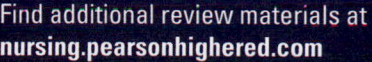

Pearson Nursing Student Resources
Find additional review materials at
nursing.pearsonhighered.com
Prepare for success with additional NCLEX®-style practice questions, interactive assignments and activities, Web links, animations and videos, and more!

BIBLIOGRAPHY

Armstrong, J., & Mitchell, E. (2008). Comprehensive nursing assessment in the care of older people. *Nursing Older People, (20)*1, 36–40.

Bickley, L., & Szilagyi, P. (2007). *Bates' guide to physical examination and history taking* (9th ed.). Philadelphia: Lippincott.

Fletcher, K. (2005). Skin: Geriatric self-learning module. *MEDSURG Nursing, 14*(2), 138–142.

Kee, J. (2009). *Prentice Hall handbook of laboratory & diagnostic tests with nursing implications.* (6th ed.). Upper Saddle River, NJ: Pearson Prentice Hall.

Khachemoune, A., & Ehrsam, E. (2005). Assessing malignant melanoma: A case study. *Dermatology Nursing, 17*(3), 188–190.

Kulkowski, K., & Ratliff, C. (2004). Wounds & skin care: Managing venous and neuropathic ulcers. *Nursing, 34*(8), 68.

Mirmirani, P. (2007). How to approach hair loss in women. *Dermatology Nursing, 19*(6), 531–535.

National Institute of Health. (2008). *Genes and Disease: Skin and Connective Tissue.* Available at http://www.ncbi.nlm.nih.gov/books/bookres.fegi/gnd/pdf.html

Nicol, N. (2005) Anatomy and physiology of the skin. *Dermatology Nursing, 17*(1), 62.

Osman, B., & Kernodle, M. (2007). A new look at pressure ulcers: Ultrasound technology can help detect skin integrity issues that are not apparent in a visual skin assessment. *Provider, 33*(4), 35–37.

Porth, C. (2007). Essentials of *Pathophysiology: Concepts of altered health states* (2nd ed.). Philadelphia: Lippincott.

Pullen, R. (2007). Assessing skin lesions. *Nursing, 37*(8), 44–45.

Rushing, J. (2008). Assessing a patient for lice infestation. *Nursing, 38*(7), 20.

Scanlon, E., & Stubbs, N. (2004). Pressure ulcer risk assessment in patients with darkly pigmented skin. *Professional Nurse, 19*(6), 339–341.

Scott, T. (2008). How do I differentiate normal aging of the skin from pathologic conditions? *Medscape Nurses.* Available at http://www.medscape.com/viewarticle/575293

Smith, M., & Nodorost, S. (2008). Hand dermatitis: Nursing support in the plan of care. *Dermatology Nursing, 20*(2), 121–125.

Snow, M. (2008). Fighting fungal infections: Stopping tinea in its tracks. *Nursing, 38*(7), 62–63.

Weber, J., & Kelley, J. (2006). *Health assessment in nursing* (3rd ed.). Philadelphia: Lippincott Williams &Wilkins.

Yoder, L. (2005). Be sun safe! Understand skin cancer prevention and detection. *MEDSURG Nursing, 14*(4), 254–256.

CHAPTER 16

Nursing Care of Patients with Integumentary Disorders

LEARNING OUTCOMES

1. Describe the manifestations, self-care, and nursing care of common skin problems and lesions.
2. Compare and contrast the etiology, pathophysiology, interdisciplinary care and nursing care of patients with infections and infestations, inflammatory disorders, and malignancies of the skin.
3. Explain the risk factors for, pathophysiology of, and nursing interventions to prevent and care for pressure ulcers.
4. Discuss surgical options for excision of neoplasms, reconstruction of facial or body structures, and cosmetic procedures.
5. Explain the pathophysiology of selected disorders of the hair and nails.
6. Discuss the effects and nursing implications of medications and treatments used to treat disorders of the integument.

CLINICAL COMPETENCIES

1. Assess functional health status of patients with integumentary disorders, and monitor, document, and report abnormal manifestations.
2. Use research to plan and implement evidence-based nursing care for patients with pressure ulcers.
3. Use assessed data, patient values, evidence, and clinical expertise to determine priority nursing diagnoses and select and implement individualized nursing interventions for patients with integumentary disorders.
4. Administer topical, oral, and injectable medications used to treat integumentary disorders knowledgeably and safely.
5. Effectively communicate with and function within the interdisciplinary team to plan and provide care for patients with integumentary disorders.
6. Provide teaching appropriate for prevention and self-care of manifestations and disorders of the integumentary system.
7. Adapt individual and cultural variations, as well as expressed needs and preferences, into the plan of care for patients with integumentary disorders.
8. Revise the plan of care as needed to provide effective interventions to promote, maintain, or restore functional health status to patients with disorders of the integument.

KEY TERMS

acne, 421	frostbite, 439	pemphigus vulgaris, 422
actinic keratosis, 424	furuncle, 411	pressure ulcer, 434
angioma, 407	herpes simplex, 416	pruritus, 405
basal cell cancer, 425	herpes zoster, 416	psoriasis, 407
carbuncle, 411	keloids, 406	scabies, 415
cellulitis, 411	keratosis, 407	skin graft, 440
comedones, 421	lichen planus, 423	squamous cell cancer, 426
cyst, 405	malignant melanoma, 428	toxic epidermal necrolysis (TENS), 423
dermatitis, 419	nevi, 407	warts, 415
dermatophytoses, 413	paronychia, 443	xerosis, 405
folliculitis, 410		

The skin and its accessory structures (the integumentary system) enclose and cover the body, providing protection by serving as a barrier between the internal and external environments. The skin contains receptors for touch and sensation, helps regulate body temperature, and maintains fluid and electrolyte balance. The skin also provides cues to racial and ethnic background, and plays a major role in determining self-concept, roles, and relationships.

Disorders of the integument range from dry skin to life-threatening cancer. Many disorders are treated in an outpatient setting or by self-care. This chapter discusses disorders of the skin, hair, and nails; Chapter 17 discusses the patient with burns. Primary and secondary skin lesions are described and illustrated in Chapter 15, Tables 15–5 and 15–6. These terms are used throughout this and the next chapter.

Common Skin Problems and Lesions

The disorders discussed in this section are those experienced by a large number of people. Although they are considered minor health problems in terms of health care, they may cause major problems for the person experiencing a high level of discomfort and/or chronicity.

The Patient with Pruritus

Pruritus is a subjective itching sensation producing an urge to scratch. Pruritus may occur in a small, circumscribed area, or it may involve a widespread area; it may or may not be associated with a rash. The itch sensation begins in nerve endings in the skin, is carried to the dorsal horn of the spinal cord, and is then transmitted to the somatosensory cortex in the central nervous system (CNS). Itching may also be perceived by the brain but does not exist on the skin. Scratching is a neurologic reflex that can be controlled in varying degrees by the individual (Porth & Matfin, 2009).

Almost anything in the internal or external environment can cause pruritus. Insects, animals, plants, fabrics, metals, medications, allergies, and emotional distress are among the most common causes. Pruritus also may occur as a secondary manifestation of systemic disorders, such as certain types of cancer, diabetes mellitus, liver disease, and renal failure. Although the exact physiology is unknown, it is known that heat and prostaglandins trigger pruritus and that it is increased by histamine and morphine.

The pathophysiologic response of pruritus to stimulation or irritation follows a similar pathway, regardless of cause. The irritating agent stimulates receptors in the junction between the epidermis and dermis, and may also trigger the release of histamine and other chemical mediators that either further stimulate or mediate the itch response. The response of the person experiencing the itch is to scratch or rub the affected area. This may irritate the skin and cause further inflammation, which in turn sets off a cycle of increasingly intense itching and scratching, called the *itch-scratch-itch cycle*.

Secondary effects of scratching include skin excoriation, erythema (redness), wheals, changes in pigmentation, and infections. Persistent pruritus may interrupt sleep patterns because the itching sensation is often more intense at night. Long-term pruritus may be debilitating and increases the risk of infection as excoriation occurs.

Management of pruritus focuses on identifying and eliminating the cause and providing medications to relieve the itch. Antihistamines may relieve pruritus in some patients. Tranquilizers provide sedation, which may in turn relieve the emotional stress associated with pruritus; however, eliminating the stressors produces a more successful result. Topical or systemic antibiotics are used to treat the infection resulting from the scratching and excoriation. Topical medications that contain corticosteroids are often used to relieve the pruritus and inflammation. Topical medications may also be administered through therapeutic baths or soaks with agents that relieve pruritus, such as cornstarch and baking soda or coal tar concentrates. Creams containing a topical anesthetic or antibiotic may also be used. Therapeutic baths are discussed in the Medication Administration on page 406. Table 16–1 lists examples of topical agents used to treat skin disorders.

The Patient with Dry Skin (Xerosis)

Dry skin, also called **xerosis**, is most often a problem in the older adult from a decrease in the activity of sebaceous and sweat glands, reducing the skin's lubrication and moisture retention. However, dry skin may occur at any age from exposure to environmental heat and low humidity, sunlight, excessive bathing, and a decreased intake of liquids.

Two types of severe dry skin are xeroderma and ichthyosis. Xeroderma is a chronic skin condition characterized by dry, rough skin. Ichthyosis is an inherited dermatological condition in which the skin is dry, fissured, and hyperkeratotic; the surface of the skin has the appearance of fish scales.

The primary manifestation of dry skin is pruritus. Other manifestations include visible flaking of surface skin and an observable pattern of fine lines over the area. If the skin has been excessively dry and pruritic for a long period, the patient may have secondary skin lesions and lichenification (thickening).

Nursing care focuses on teaching the patient and family how to reduce the dry skin and relieve the pruritus, as outlined in Box 16–1.

The Patient with Benign Skin Lesions

The skin is subject to many different types and kinds of benign skin lesions, including cysts, keloids, nevi, angiomas, skin tags, and keratoses. Although these benign lesions are often considered more of a nuisance than an illness, they do require monitoring for an increase in size that interferes with the skin's appearance or function. Most benign skin lesions do not require treatment, although excision or laser surgery may be desired or necessary. Cysts may enlarge, skin tags may become irritated and bleed, nevi may change in appearance, or any of the lesions may cause discomfort with appearance.

Cysts

Cysts of the skin are benign closed sacs in or under the skin surface that are lined with epithelium and contain fluid or a semisolid material. Epidermal inclusion cysts and pilar cysts are the most common types.

TABLE 16–1 Medications Used to Treat Skin Disorders

TYPE	USE	EXAMPLES
Creams	Moisturize the skin	Aquacare, Curel, Nutraderm
Ointments	Lubricate the skin and retard water loss	Aquaphor, Vaseline
Lotions	Moisturize and lubricate the skin	Alpha-Keri, Dermassage, Lubriderm
Anesthetics	Relieve itching	Xylocaine
Antibiotics	Treat infection	Bacitracin, Polysporin, Gentamicin, Silvadene
Corticosteroids	Suppress inflammation and relieve itching	Dexamethasone, Clocortolone, Desonide

MEDICATION ADMINISTRATION   Therapeutic Baths

AGENTS USED IN THERAPEUTIC BATHS

Saline or tap water

Antibacterial agents: potassium permanganate, acetic acid, hexachlorophene

Colloid substances: oatmeal (Aveeno), cornstarch, sodium bicarbonate

Coal tar derivatives: Balnetar, Zetar, Polytar

Emollients: Alpha Keri, Lubath, mineral oil

Therapeutic baths have a variety of uses in treating skin disorders. Depending on the agent used, therapeutic baths soothe the skin, lower the skin bacteria count, clean and hydrate the skin, loosen scales, and relieve itching.

Nursing Responsibilities

- Ensure that the bath water is at a comfortable temperature that is neither too hot nor too cool, usually 110°F to 115°F (45°C to 46°C).
- Fill the tub one-third to one-half full.
- Mix the agent well with the water.
- Assist the patient into and out of the tub to prevent falls.
- Dry the patient's skin by blotting with the towel.

Health Education for the Patient and Family

- Use a bath mat in the tub because the medications may cause the tub to become slippery.
- Keep the bathroom warm but adequately ventilated.
- Follow directions carefully for the amount of medication to use in the bath.
- Fill the bath one-third to one-half full of water that is at a comfortable temperature.
- Stay in the bath for 20 to 30 minutes, and immerse the areas to be treated.
- Do not get the bathwater in your eyes.
- Dry by blotting (not rubbing) with the towel.
- If the medications cause staining, use old towels or linens.
- If the itching is not relieved or the skin becomes excessively dry, call your healthcare provider.

Epidermal inclusion cysts may occur anywhere on the body but are most often found on the head and trunk. Although they are painless, they may grow so large that they become irritated by contact with clothing (e.g., if located on the back of the neck) or cause obstruction (e.g., if located on the nose). The cysts contain a semisolid material mainly of keratin. Pilar cysts are found on the scalp and originate from sebaceous glands. They are also painless. Both types of cysts rarely require treatment unless they become large and bothersome.

Keloids

Keloids are elevated, irregularly shaped, progressively enlarging scars. They arise from excessive amounts of collagen in the stratum corneum during scar formation in connective tissue repair. These lesions are more common in young adults and appear within 1 year of the initial trauma.

BOX 16–1 Teaching to Reduce Dry Skin and Relieve Pruritus

- Wash clothing in a mild detergent and rinse twice; do not use fabric softeners.
- Avoid using perfumes and lotions containing alcohol.
- Apply skin lubricants after a bath to help retain moisture.
- Soaps and hot water are drying. Clean the skin with tepid water and either a mild soap or cleansing creams. If soap is used, rinse it off carefully.
- It is not necessary to take a bath every day.
- If bath oils are used, add them to the bath water at the end of the bath (the moist skin is more likely to retain the oil). Use care not to slip in the tub.
- Use a humidifier to humidify the air.
- Apply creams and lotions when the skin is slightly damp after bathing.
- Increase fluid intake.
- Keep nails trimmed short, wear loose clothing, and keep the environment cool.
- A brief application of pressure or cold may relieve pruritus.
- Cotton gloves may be worn at night if scratching during sleep causes skin excoriation.
- Distraction or relaxation techniques may prove helpful.

This abnormal response most often occurs in people of African and Asian descent who sustain burns of the skin, but even seemingly minor trauma can result in keloid formation. There is a familial tendency to develop keloids. Other risk factors for keloid formation include excessive tension on a wound and poor alignment of skin edges following accidental or intentional skin trauma. Certain skin surfaces are also more likely to develop keloids: the chin, ears, shoulders, back, and lower legs.

The excessive scar formation is associated with increased metabolic activity of fibroplasts and increased type III collagen. The swollen appearance of the keloids is the result of an excess of extracellular material. The keloids first appear as red, firm, rubbery plaques that persist for several months after the initial trauma (Figure 16–1 ■). Uncontrolled overgrowth over time causes the keloids to extend beyond the original scar. Eventually, the keloid becomes smooth and hyperpigmented.

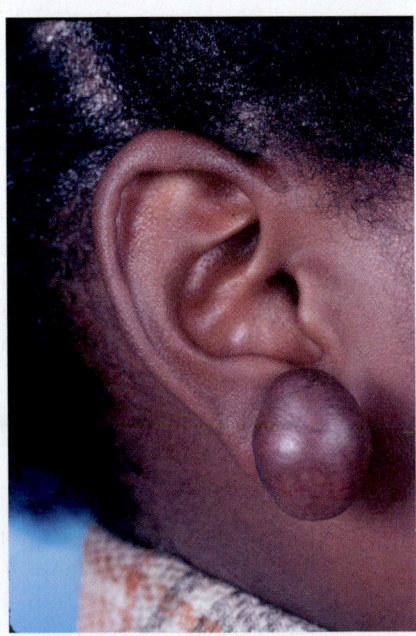

Figure 16–1 ■ Keloids form as a result of deposits of excessive amounts of collagen during scar formation.

Nevi

Nevi, more commonly called *moles*, are flat or raised macules or papules with rounded, well-defined borders (Figure 16–2 ■). Nevi arise from melanocytes during early childhood, with the cells initially accumulating at the junction of the dermis and epidermis. Over time, the cluster of cells moves into the dermis, and the lesion becomes visible. Nevi can occur on any skin surface of the body and may arise as single lesions or in groups. Almost all adults have nevi.

Nevocellular nevi are tan to deep brown, small in size, and grow in groups. Dysplastic nevi are larger than other nevi and may be flat, slightly raised, or appear as lesions with a darker, raised center and irregular border. Dysplastic nevi can transform into malignant lesions (see the later discussion about melanoma). It is important to monitor nevi for changes in size, thickness, color, bleeding, or itching. If any of these changes occur, the person should seek immediate professional assessment.

Angiomas

Angiomas, also called *hemangiomas*, are benign vascular tumors. They appear in the adult in different forms:

- Nevus flammeus (port-wine stain) is a congenital vascular lesion that involves the capillaries. The lesions tend to occur on the upper body or face as macular patches that range from light red to dark purple. These lesions are present at birth and grow proportionately with the child into adulthood.
- Cherry angiomas are small, rounded papules that may occur at any age, but they most commonly arise in the 40s and gradually increase in number. The lesions range in color from bright red to purple. These lesions are often found on the trunk.
- Spider angiomas are dilated superficial arteries. They are common in pregnant women and in patients with hepatic disease. Spider angiomas occur most often on the face, neck, and upper chest. The lesions are usually small, bright red papules with radiating lines.
- Telangiectases are single dilated capillaries or terminal arteries that appear most often on the cheeks and nose. These lesions are more common in older adults and result from photoaged (aging, sun-damaged) skin. The lesions look like broken veins.

- Venous lakes are small, flat, blue blood vessels. They are seen on the exposed skin of the older adult: the ears, lips, and backs of the hands.

Skin Tags

Skin tags are soft papules on a pedicle. They can be as small as a pinhead or as large as a pea and are most often found on the front or side of the neck and in the axillae, as well as in areas where clothing (such as underwear) rubs the skin. These lesions have normal skin color and texture.

Keratoses

A **keratosis** is any skin condition in which there is a benign overgrowth and thickening of the cornified epithelium. These lesions most often appear in adults after age 50. *Seborrheic keratoses* appear as superficial flat, smooth, or warty-surfaced growths, 5 to 20 mm in diameter, most often on the face and trunk. The lesions may be tan, waxy yellow, dark brown, or flesh-colored, and they often appear greasy. They are most often seen in the older adult and do not appear to be related to damage from sun exposure.

The Patient with Psoriasis

Psoriasis is a chronic immune skin disorder characterized by raised, reddened, round circumscribed plaques covered by silvery white scales (Figure 16–3 ■). There are several different forms, but the most common is plaque psoriasis (psoriasis vulgaris), occurring in about 80% of cases (American Academy of Dermatology, 2009). As with any chronic illness, the skin manifestations may occur and disappear throughout life, with no discernible pattern to the recurrence.

As many as 7.5 million people in the United States have psoriasis; about 20% have moderate to severe forms (National Psoriasis Foundation, 2009). The incidence of psoriasis is lower in warm, sunny climates. The average age of onset is in the 30s, but it may occur at any age. Psoriasis occurs more often in Caucasians, and men and women are affected equally. Sunlight, stress, seasonal changes, hormone fluctuations, steroid withdrawal, and certain drugs (such as beta blockers, lithium, and chloroquine [an antimalarial]) appear to act as triggers to

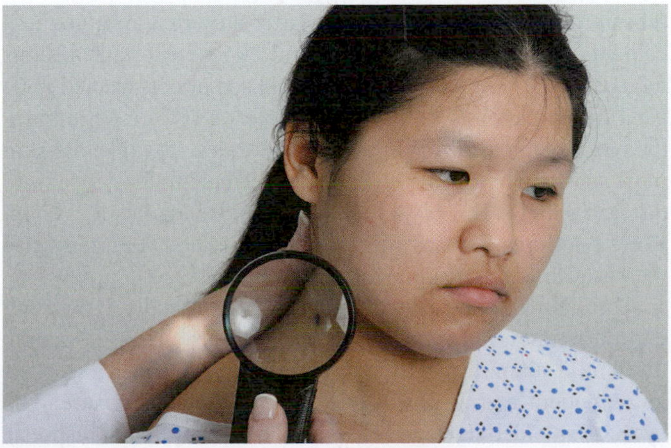

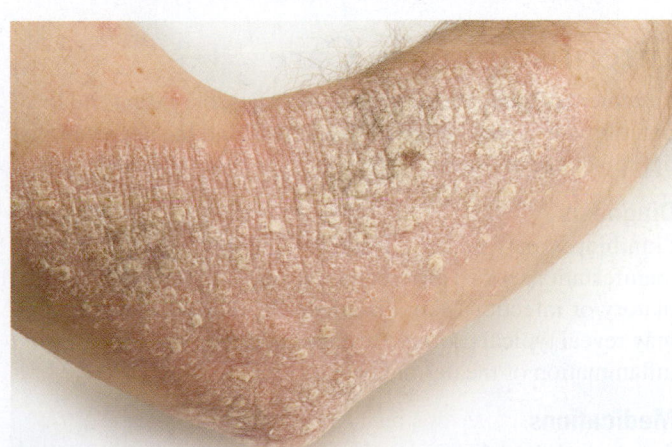

Figure 16–2 ■ Nevi (moles) arise from melanocytes and are common in all adults.

Figure 16–3 ■ The characteristic lesions of psoriasis are raised, red, round plaques covered with thick, silvery scales.

development of the disorder. About one-third of patients have a family history of psoriasis. Trauma to the skin from such events as surgery, sunburn, or excoriation is also a common precipitating factor; lesions that result from trauma are called Koebner's reaction (Porth & Matfin, 2009).

Pathophysiology

Normally, the keratinocyte (an epidermal cell making up 95% of the epidermis) migrates from the basal cell to the stratum corneum (the outer skin layer) in about 14 days and is sloughed off 14 days later. Psoriatic skin cells, by contrast, have a shorter cycle of growth, completing the journey to the stratum corneum in only 4 to 7 days, a condition called hyperkeratosis. These immature cells produce an abnormal keratin that forms thick, flaky scales at the surface of the skin. The increased cell metabolism stimulates increased vascularity, which contributes to the erythema of the lesions.

Although the exact cause is unknown, there is increasing evidence that a T-lymphocyte-mediated reaction results in the production of chemical messengers that stimulate the growth of keratinocytes and dermal blood vessels. The accompanying inflammation further contributes to plaque formation. The lesions can be found anywhere on the skin but most commonly involve the skin over the elbows, knees, and scalp. Lesions involving the hand and foot are especially problematic for the patient. Initially, the lesions are papules that form into well-defined erythematous plaques with thick, silvery scales. The plaques in darker-skinned persons may appear purple.

Manifestations

The characteristic lesions in plaque psoriasis are well-demarcated regions of erythematous plaques that shed thick, silver-gray flakes. Pruritus is common over the psoriatic lesions. If the lesions are located in an intertriginous zone, such as between the toes, under the breasts, or in the perianal region, the psoriatic scales may soften, allowing painful fissures to form. When psoriasis affects the nails, pitting and a yellow or brown discoloration results. The nail may separate from the nail bed, thicken, and crumble. The involved nails, which are more often fingernails than toenails, are at high risk for infection. Psoriatic arthritis is a specific form of arthritis involving not only skin lesions but also inflammation of joints.

Interdisciplinary Care

Treatment is based on the type of psoriasis, the extent and location of the lesions, the age of the patient, and the degree of disfigurement or disability.

Diagnosis

Skin biopsy may be done if the patient presents with atypical manifestations, or to differentiate psoriasis from other inflammatory or infectious skin disorders. In addition, an ultrasound may reveal typical psoriatic changes in the stratus corneum and inflammation of the dermis.

Medications

A variety of medications and treatments may be prescribed, including topical medications and photochemotherapy. Although there is no cure, treatment decreases the severity and pain of the lesions. Corticosteroids, tar preparations, anthralin, calcipotriene (a vitamin D derivative) and tazarotene (a synthetic retinoid) are typically used. Ustekinumab, an injectable monoclonal antibody that decreases the immune response, is in advanced clinical trials for severe psoriasis.

Topical corticosteroids decrease inflammation, suppress mitotic activity of psoriatic cells, and delay the movement of keratinocytes to the surface of the skin (thus giving them time to mature and decreasing hyperkeratinosis). The most effective topical corticosteroids are potent preparations that are well absorbed through the skin and are used under an occlusive dressing. Corticosteroids may also be taken systemically or injected directly into the lesions. However, corticosteroids rarely cause a lasting remission and may cause the psoriasis to become unstable (McPhee, Papadakis, & Tierney, 2008). They are therefore used for repeated short periods of treatment and combined with other measures, such as tar preparations, occlusion, or a topical retinoid.

Tar preparations (such as Estar, Psorigel, and Fototar) suppress mitotic activity and are also anti-inflammatory. Their exact mechanism of action is unknown, but they are effective in removing scales and increasing remission time. Preparations made of coal tar are messy, cause staining, and have an unpleasant odor, but they are an effective form of treatment. Salex shampoo is prescribed for patients with scalp psoriasis to remove plaques and scales. Psorent is a non-prescription cream that is made from coal tar but does not stain or have an odor.

Calcipotriene (Dovonex) has been effective and safe in both the short-term and long-term treatment of psoriasis. It inhibits cell proliferation in the epidermis and facilitates cell differentiation. Although more irritating than calcipotriene, tazarotene gel (Avage, Tarorac) is a topical retinoid that may also be used to treat mild to moderate psoriasis.

Treatments

Psoriasis that is generalized (i.e., involves more than 30% of the body surface) is difficult to treat with topical medications. Treatments for generalized psoriasis include ultraviolet light therapy and photochemotherapy.

PHOTOTHERAPY Ultraviolet-B (UVB) light or narrow band UVB are treatments for generalized psoriasis. UVB light decreases the growth rate of epidermal cells, thereby decreasing hyperkeratosis. Mercury vapor lights or fluorescent UV tubes provide the UVB light; the latter are often arranged in a cabinet so the patient can stand and expose psoriatic lesions more easily. These units may be purchased or constructed to be used in the patient's home. Ultraviolet-A (PUVA) combines the oral or topical administration of psoralen (to make the skin more sensitive to light) with UVA, which penetrates deeper into the skin than UVB. PUVA requires fewer treatments for remission of lesions, but has more side effects and long-term use increases the risk of skin cancers.

The light therapy is administered in gradually increasing exposure times, until the patient experiences a mild erythema, like a mild sunburn. Treatments are given three times a week as an outpatient and are measured in seconds of exposure. The eyes are shielded during the treatment. The erythema response occurs in about 8 hours. Careful assessment is necessary to prevent more severe burning, which could exacerbate the psoriasis. In patients with extensive psoriasis, UVB treatments may be combined with tar preparations, which increase the photosensitivity of the skin.

PHOTOCHEMOTHERAPY In photochemotherapy, a light-activated form of the drug methoxsalen is used. This drug is an antimetabolite that inhibits DNA synthesis and thereby prevents cell mitosis, decreasing hyperkeratosis. Exposure to ultraviolet-A (UVA) rays activates methoxsalen; it is administered orally, and the patient is exposed to UVA 2 hours later. Treatments are administered 2 to 3 times a week, for 10 to 20 total treatments. Treatment causes tanning, and direct sunlight must be avoided for 8 to 12 hours thereafter. Photochemotherapy has had a high success rate in achieving remission of psoriasis, but it can accelerate aging of exposed skin, induce cataract development, alter immune function, and increase the risk of melanoma.

∂♥ Nursing Care

The patient with psoriasis requires nursing care to meet physical and psychologic responses to the illness. The nurse provides teaching for self-care and emotional support through nonjudgmental acceptance.

Nursing Diagnoses and Interventions

The nursing interventions discussed in this section focus on common problems of risk for impaired skin integrity and disturbed body image.

Impaired Skin Integrity

Psoriatic lesions range from several scales to large, open areas. Typical psoriatic skin lesions increase the risk of infection, which can compromise healing. In addition, certain treatments (e.g., the use of UVA or retinoids) may cause erythema or peeling of the skin, further altering skin integrity.

■ Teach methods to reduce injury to the skin when taking therapeutic baths or treatments: Use warm, not hot, water; gently rub lesions with a soft washcloth, using a circular motion; dry the skin with a soft towel, using a blotting or patting motion; and keep the skin lubricated at all times. *Hot water and dry skin increase pruritus, further stimulating the itch-scratch-itch cycle. Dry skin also worsens psoriasis. Washing or drying the skin with rough linens or pressure may excoriate the skin over the psoriatic lesions.*

■ Teach how to apply topical medications (see Box 16–2). *Applying a thin layer of medication more frequently is often more effective than applying a single thick layer of medication. The medications used to treat psoriasis may irritate the eyes and mucous membranes; when applied in skinfolds, they may also cause maceration (skin breakdown due to prolonged exposure to moisture).*

■ Teach manifestations of infection and how to contact the healthcare provider if these occur: elevated temperature, increased swelling, redness, pain, increase in drainage, and any change in the color of the drainage. *The patient with skin lesions is at high risk for infection, as the skin is the body's first line of defense.*

BOX 16–2 General Guidelines for Applying Topical Medications

■ Each time a medication is applied, the skin surface must be clean and dry. Remove the medication from the previous application. Remove creams by washing the skin with tap water; remove ointments by washing the skin first with mineral oil and then with a mild soap and water.
■ To apply gels, creams, and pastes: Squeeze about 1/2 to 1 inch of the gel or cream into the palm of the hand. Rub the hands together until they are covered. Apply gels and creams to the affected areas with long strokes until the skin is thinly covered. Differences from these general guidelines follow:
   a. Corticosteroids are usually applied two to three times a day in small amounts and rubbed directly onto the lesions. Apply the medication after a bath and cover with an occlusive dressing.
   b. Apply medications containing tar in the direction of hair growth. Do not apply these medications to the face, to the genitals, or in skin folds. If the tar is water based or oil based, it will stain clothing.
   c. Wear gloves when applying anthralin stains.
■ To apply lotions: Shake the bottle of lotion well. Pour a small amount into the palm of the hand, and pat the medication onto the skin. If the lotion is thin, apply it with a gauze pad.
■ To apply sprays: Hold the container about 6 inches from the skin and apply the medication in a short spray.
■ To apply medicated shampoo: Rinse out medication from the previous application. Apply the shampoo, massage into the hair and over the scalp carefully, and allow it to remain for the prescribed time. Rinse.
■ To apply pastes: Use enough paste on an applicator (such as a wooden tongue depressor) to cover the lesion thinly.

■ Teach manifestations of the complications of treatment: excoriation, increased erythema, increased peeling, and blister formation. *The topical medications or treatments may damage cells through chemical burns or excessive exposure to ultraviolet light. Times and methods of treatment need to be adjusted if these manifestations occur.*

Disturbed Body Image

The chronic skin lesions of psoriasis may cause patients to isolate themselves from social contacts, withdraw from normal roles and responsibilities, and feel helpless or powerless.

■ Establish a trusting relationship by expressing acceptance of the patient, both verbally and nonverbally. For example, touch the patient during social communications, demonstrating that the lesions are not contagious or offensive. *One's body image is affected not only by self-perception but also by the responses of others. Nonjudgmental acceptance helps the patient adapt to the change in body image. By touching the patient during interactions, the nurse demonstrates acceptance.*

■ Encourage expression of self-perception and the asking of questions about the disease and treatment in view of the chronic nature of psoriasis. *The patient adapts to a changed body image through a process of recognition, acceptance, and resolution. Each person responds individually to disfigurement and loss.*

- Promote social interaction through family involvement in care and referral to support groups of people with psoriasis or other chronic skin conditions. *Acceptance by others is critical to acceptance of self. Psoriasis treatment is lifelong, time consuming, and often unappealing. By becoming involved in care, the family communicates acceptance. Sharing experiences with others who have the same health problem is a source of strength in adjusting to a visible, chronic illness.*

Community-Based Care

Patient and family teaching focuses on treatments and skin care needs. The following topics should be addressed:

- The chronic nature of the disease, factors that may precipitate an exacerbation, and methods to reduce stress.

- Interventions for pruritus and dry skin, and specific care for psoriasis:
  - Expose the skin to sunlight, but avoid sunburn.
  - Avoid trauma to the skin (e.g., do not scrub off scales, and use only an electric razor).
  - Avoid exposure to contagious illnesses such as influenza and colds.
  - Discuss current medications with the healthcare provider. Certain drugs (such as indomethacin [Indocin], lithium, and beta-adrenergic blocking agents) are known to precipitate exacerbations of psoriasis.
- Suggest the National Psoriasis Foundation, the National Institutes of Health, or the American Academy of Dermatology as resources.

Infections and Infestations of the Skin

The skin's resistance to infections and infestations is provided by protective mechanisms, including skin flora, sebum, and the immune response. Although the skin is normally resistant to infections and infestations, these disorders may occur as a result of a break in the skin surface, a virulent agent, and/or decreased resistance due to a compromised immune system. This section discusses skin disorders resulting from bacterial infections, fungal infections, parasitic infestations, and viral infections.

The Patient with a Bacterial Infection of the Skin

A number of bacteria normally inhabit the skin and do not cause an infection. However, when a break in the skin allows invasion by pathogenic bacteria, an infection, called a *pyoderma*, may occur. The most common bacterial infections are caused by gram-positive *Staphylococcus aureus* and beta-hemolytic streptococci. Bacterial infections of the skin may be primary or secondary. Primary infections are caused by a single pathogen and arise from normal skin; secondary infections develop in traumatized or diseased skin.

Most bacterial infections are treated by a primary care provider, and the patient remains at home for care. If the infection becomes more serious, inpatient care may be required. In addition, nosocomial infections of wounds or open lesions in hospitalized patients are often the result of bacterial infections, especially by methicillin-resistant *Staphylococcus aureus (MRSA)*.

Pathophysiology

Bacterial infections of the skin arise from the hair follicle, where bacteria can accumulate and grow and cause a localized infection. However, the bacteria also can enter the body through open wounds, invade deeper tissues, and cause a systemic infection, a potentially life-threatening disorder. Various types of bacterial infections involve the skin, including folliculitis, furuncles and carbuncles, cellulitis, and *staphylococcus aureus*.

Folliculitis

Folliculitis is a bacterial infection of the hair follicle, most commonly caused by *Staphylococcus aureus*. The infection begins at the follicle opening and extends down into the follicle. The bacteria release enzymes and chemical agents that cause an inflammation. The lesions appear as pustules surrounded by an area of erythema on the surface of the skin (Figure 16–4 ■). The lesions are accompanied by discomfort ranging from slight burning to intense itching. A major complication is abscess formation. Folliculitis is found most often on the scalp and extremities. It is also often seen on the face of bearded men (called sycosis barbae), on the legs of women who shave, and on the eyelids (called a stye). Although folliculitis may appear without any apparent cause, contributing factors include poor hygiene, poor nutrition, prolonged skin

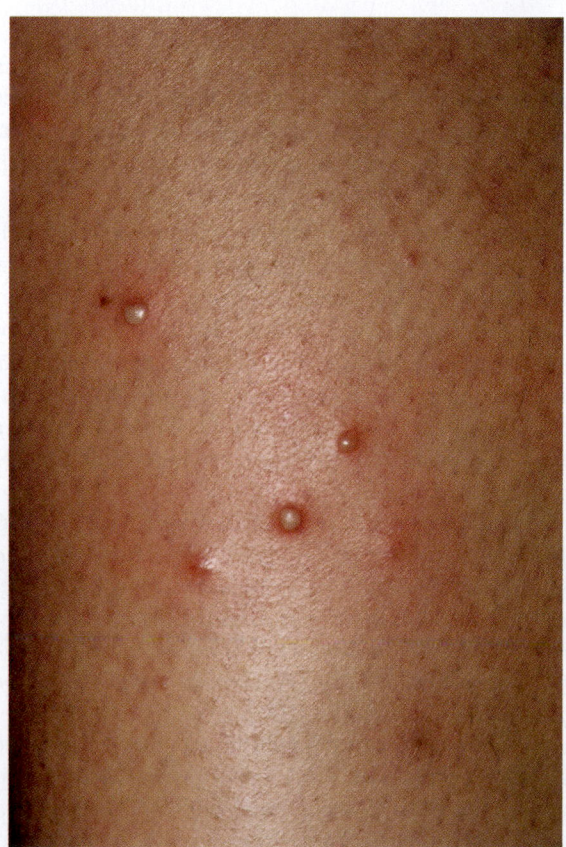

Figure 16–4 ■ The lesions of folliculitis are pustules surrounded by areas of erythema.

moisture, tight heavy fabrics on the upper legs, and trauma to the skin.

Furuncles and Carbuncles

Furuncles, often called boils, are inflammations of the hair follicle. They often begin as folliculitis, but the infection spreads down the hair shaft, through the wall of the follicle, and into the dermis. The causative organism is commonly *Staphylococcus aureus*. A furuncle is initially a deep, firm, red, painful nodule from 1 to 5 cm in diameter (Figure 16–5 ■). After a few days, the nodule changes into a large, painful cystic nodule. The cysts may drain substantial amounts of purulent drainage. One or more furuncles may occur on any part of the body that has hair. Contributing factors include poor hygiene, trauma to the skin, areas of excessive moisture (including perspiration), and systemic diseases such as diabetes mellitus and hematologic malignancies.

A **carbuncle** is a group of infected hair follicles. The lesion begins as a firm mass located in the subcutaneous tissue and the lower dermis. This mass becomes swollen and painful and has multiple openings to the skin surface. Carbuncles are most frequently found on the back of the neck, the upper back, and the lateral thighs. In addition to the local manifestations, the patient may experience chills, fever, and malaise. The contributing factors for carbuncles are the same as for furuncles. Both infections are more common in hot, humid climates.

Cellulitis

Cellulitis is a localized infection of the dermis and subcutaneous tissue. Cellulitis can occur following a wound or skin ulcer or as an extension of furuncles or carbuncles. The infection spreads as a result of a substance produced by the causative organism, called spreading factor (hyaluronidase). This factor breaks down the fibrin network and other barriers that normally localize the infection. The area of cellulitis is red, swollen, and painful (Figure 16–6 ■). In some cases, vesicles may form over the area of cellulitis. The patient may also experience fever, chills, malaise, headache, and swollen lymph glands.

Methicillin-resistant *Staphylococcus aureus* (MRSA) Infection

Methicillin-resistant *Staphylococcus aureus* (MRSA) infection is caused by the *S. aureus* bacteria, an organism resistant to the broad-spectrum antibiotics (such as methicillin, oxacillin, amoxicillin, and penicillin) usually used to treat it. This potentially fatal disease is divided into 2 types: Healthcare-associated infections (acquired in hospitals and other healthcare settings) (HA-MRSA) and community associated infections (acquired in the community in otherwise healthy people) (CA-MRSA). MRSA in hospitalized patients may lead to infections of wounds, skin around invasive tubes or catheters, the blood, the lungs, or the urinary system. MRSA in patients in the community is often manifested as skin infections and a potentially life-threatening pneumonia.

S. aureus are normally found on the skin and in the nose of about one-third of the population. If present, but not causing illness, the person is said to be colonized and capable of spreading the bacteria to other people. The bacteria are spread by direct contact with the bacteria or with contaminated equipment. The Association for Professionals in Infection Control (2007) reported that an estimated 1.2 million hospitalized patients acquired HA-MRSA and more than 425 were colonized (increasing the risk of infecting self or others). The incidence of CA-MRSA is about 5 per 100,000 people, but those numbers are increasing. The rates of both types are highest in healthcare workers, in males, in those over age 65, in Blacks, and in those with HIV and AIDS. The risk for CA-MRSA is increased in those who participate in contact sports, and in people sharing personal items and/or living in crowded or unsanitary conditions.

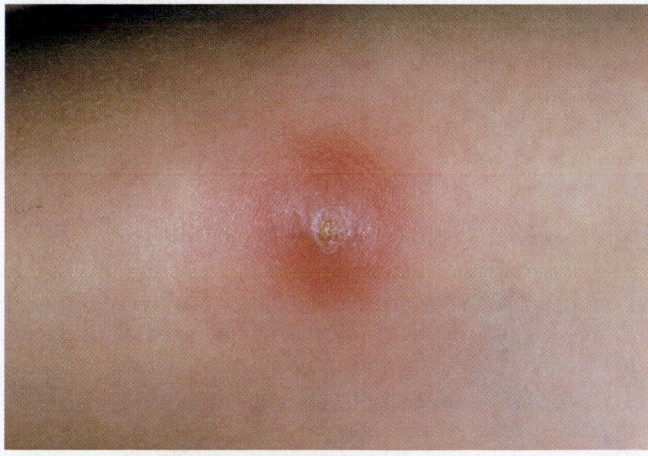

Figure 16–5 ■ A furuncle (boil) is a deep, firm, red, painful nodule.

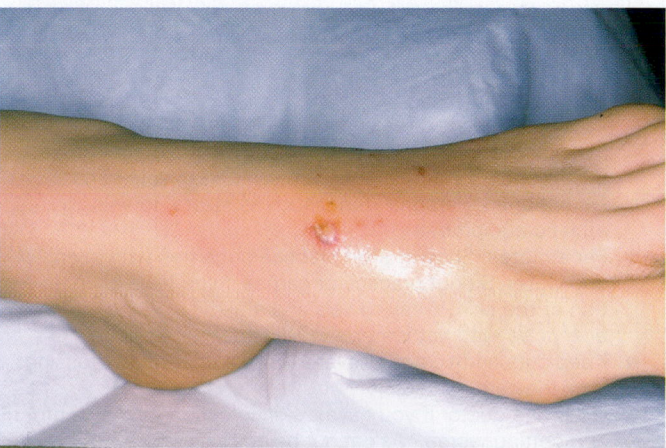

Figure 16–6 ■ Cellulitis is a bacterial infection localized in the dermis and subcutaneous tissue. The involved area is red, swollen, and painful.

The infection usually begins as a small, raised, red nodule on the skin that resembles a pimple or spider bite. The nodule rapidly increases in size, becomes dark red, is painful, contains pus, and may become a deep abscess. Cellulitis involving the area containing the initial infection (such as an extremity) is common. Actions to prevent MRSA are outlined in Box 16–3.

Interdisciplinary Care

The diagnosis of a bacterial infection of the skin is made by assessing the appearance of the lesion and by identifying the causative organism. Antibiotics effective against the organism are used in treatment.

Diagnosis

Drainage from a lesion or a blood culture may be ordered to identify the causative organism and target the most effective antibiotic. People who experience repeated bacterial skin infections, or who provide care for others who exhibit infections, may have a culture taken from the external nares to determine whether they are carriers of bacteria (e.g., MRSA) and are reinfecting themselves or others.

Medications

The primary treatment for bacterial infections of the skin is an antibiotic specific to the organism. The antibiotic is usually taken orally, and may also be applied topically. Multiple furuncles and carbuncles may be treated with cloxacillin (a penicillinase-resistant penicillin); the cephalosporins also are often effective. MRSA infections may be treated with antimicrobial therapy, including trimethoprim-sulfamethoxazole (Bactrim), minocycline (Minocin), doxycycline (Vibramycin), or clindamycin (Cleocin). There are no recommended guidelines for treating colonization. For repeated infections in a household, treatment may include mupirocin ointment (Bactroban Nasal) and an antiseptic body wash (Leung-Chen, 2008).

BOX 16–3 Preventing MRSA in the Hospital and in the Community

In the Hospital:
- Wash your hands frequently.
- Ask all hospital staff to wash their hands or use an alcohol-based hand sanitizer every time before touching you or objects in your environment.
- Ensure all invasive tubes or needles are inserted under sterile conditions.

In the Community:
- Wash your hands often and for as long as it takes to hum the "Happy Birthday" song. Use a hand sanitizer with at least 60% alcohol for times when you can't wash your hands.
- Do not share personal items such as razors, towels, or athletic equipment.
- For athletes: Shower after practice or games with soap and water. Sit out practice or games if you have an infection of the skin. Wash towels and athletic clothing after every use with hot water and bleach.
- Keep cuts and scrapes covered with a dry sterile dressing until they are healed.
- Go to the doctor if you have a skin infection that is painful and getting worse. Ask about being tested for MRSA.
- Use antibiotics appropriately. Take the full prescribed dose. Do not share.

☙ Nursing Care

Nursing care focuses on preventing the spread of infection and restoring normal skin integrity. Many patients provide self-care at home, but need education about preventing CA-MRSA.

Nursing Diagnosis and Interventions

Risk for Infection

- Practice good hand washing (hand hygiene) and teach its importance. *Careful hand hygiene is one of the most effective methods to reduce the spread of infection both in and out of the hospital setting. Healthcare providers must wash their hands with soap and water before and after patient care and between each patient contact. All patients, family members, and visitors (both in the home and hospital setting) should be taught the importance of hand hygiene, but it is even more important for the patient with a bacterial infection.*
- Assess for and teach how to identify an increase in infection, which may be manifested systemically by fever, tachycardia, chills, and malaise. Local manifestations of the spread of the infection include an increase in erythema, the size of the lesion, and drainage. *This assessment is especially important for older, debilitated, or immunosuppressed patients, and for those who have large or dirty wounds.*

> **SAFETY ALERT**
> If a patient with a bacterial skin infection is hospitalized, place him or her on isolation precautions to limit the spread of the organisms to other patients.

- Cover draining lesions with a sterile dressing, and handle soiled dressings or linens according to standard precautions. When changing dressings, always wear disposable rubber gloves and masks. *These actions are necessary to prevent the spread of infection to other areas of the patient's body, to other patients, to visitors, and to the nurse providing care.*

Community-Based Care

The increasing numbers of people with community-associated MRSA have resulted in state laws about reporting of or screening for MRSA. Many state public health departments have guidelines available about the manifestations, prevention, and treatment of CA-MRSA, and the Centers for Disease Control and Prevention (CDC) has treatment guidelines. Teaching for any bacterial infection focuses on facilitating tissue healing and eliminating the infection. Address the following topics:

- The importance of maintaining good nutrition
- The importance of maintaining cleanliness through careful hand hygiene and proper handling and disposal of dressings
- Preventing the spread of infection by not sharing linens and towels and washing clothing and linens in hot water
- The importance of not squeezing or trying to open a pimple or boil
- The importance of taking the full course of prescribed antibiotics

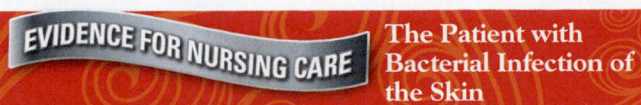

EVIDENCE FOR NURSING CARE | **The Patient with Bacterial Infection of the Skin**

Selected resources that nurses may find helpful when planning evidence-based nursing care follow.

- Casey, M. L., & Chasens, E. R. (2009). Community-associated methicillin-resistant staphylococcus aureus: Implications for emergency department nursing. *Journal of Emergency Nursing, 35*(3), 224–229.
- Haas, J. P., & Larson, E. L. (2008). Compliance with hand hygiene. *The American Journal of Nursing, 108*(8), 40–44.
- Hodgkinson, B., Agnew, J., Godfrey, C., Goldie, B., Kenner, C., González, R. L., Ramirez, B. A., Maria, E. G., McInerney, P., & Robertson-Malt, S. (2007). Topical skin care in aged care facilities. *Best Practice, The Joanna Briggs Institute, 11*(3), 1–4. Retrieved from, http://www.joannabriggs.edu.au/pdf/BPISEng_11_3.pdf
- Johnson, D., Lineweaver, L., & Maze, L. M. (2009). Patients' bath basins as potential sources of infection: A multicenter sampling study. *American Journal of Critical Care, 18*(1), 31–38.

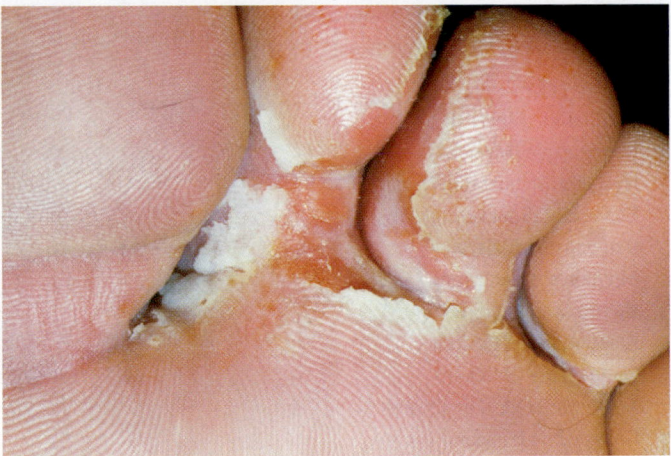

Figure 16–7 ■ Tinea pedis (athlete's foot) is a fungal infection that often occurs between the toes.

The Patient with a Fungal Infection

Fungi are free-living, plantlike organisms that live in the soil, on animals, and on humans. The fungi that cause superficial skin infections are called dermatophytes. In humans, the dermatophytes live on keratin in the stratum corneum, hair, and nails. Fungal disorders are also called *mycoses*.

Pathophysiology

Fungal infections include dermatophytoses (tinea or ringworm) and candidiasis (yeast) infections. The candidiasis infections may affect various parts of the body, but are more commonly seen in women as vaginal infections, discussed and illustrated in ∞ Chapter 50.

Dermatophytoses (Tinea)

Superficial fungal infections of the skin are called **dermatophytoses** or, more commonly, ringworm. Fungal infections occur when a susceptible host comes in contact with the organism. The organism may be transmitted by direct contact with animals or other infected persons or by inanimate objects such as combs, pillowcases, towels, and hats. The most important factor in the development of the infection is moisture; the onset and spread of the fungal infection is greatest in areas where moisture content is high, such as within skinfolds, between the toes, and in the mouth. Other factors that increase the risk of a fungal infection include the use of broad-spectrum antibiotics that kill off normal flora and allow the fungi to grow, diabetes mellitus, immunodeficiencies, nutritional deficiencies, pregnancy, increasing age, and iron deficiency. The dermatophyte infections are named by the body part affected, for example:

- Tinea pedis is a fungal infection of the soles of the feet, the space between the toes, and/or the toenail (Figure 16–7 ■).

More often called athlete's foot, this is the most common tinea infection. The lesions vary from mild scaliness to painful fissures with drainage, and they are usually accompanied by pruritus and a foul odor. The infection is often chronic, absent in winter but reappearing in hot weather when perspiring feet are encased in shoes.

- Tinea corporis is a fungal infection of the body. It can be caused by several different fungi, and the lesions vary according to the causative organism. The most common lesions are large circular patches with raised red borders of vesicles, papules, or pustules. Pruritus and erythema are also present.
- Tinea cruris is a fungal infection of the groin that may extend to the inner thighs and buttocks. Often called "jock itch," it is often associated with tinea pedis and is more common in people who are physically active, are obese, and/or wear tight underclothing.

Interdisciplinary Care

Fungal infections are primarily diagnosed in outpatient settings and treated at home, but may also occur in hospitalized patients. The treatment is the same, regardless of the setting.

Diagnosis

Diagnostic tests are conducted to determine the causative fungi and may include cultures, microscopic examination using KOH and examination of the skin with ultraviolet light (Wood's lamp), described in ∞ Chapter 15.

Medications

Fungal infections of the skin are treated by topical or systemic antifungal medications. The over-the-counter (OTC) medications (such as miconazole, clotrimazole, butenafine, and terbinafine) are often less expensive and are effective (McPhee, Papadakis, & Tierney, 2008). Nursing implications for the antifungal medications are described in the Medication Administration Box on page 414.

MEDICATION ADMINISTRATION — Antifungal Agents

EXAMPLES:
Butenafine (Mentax)
Clotrimazole (Mycelex)
Nystatin (Mycostatin, Nilstat)
Econazole (Spectazole)
Oxiconazole (Oxistat)
Miconazole (Monistat)
Undecylenic acid (Desenex)
Ketoconazole (Nizoral)
Fluconazole (Diflucan)
Amphotericin B (Fungizone)
Griseofulvin (Fulvicin)

Antifungal medications are prepared in a variety of forms, depending on the specific drug: powders, creams, shampoos, suspensions, troches, vaginal suppositories, and oral tablets. Some drugs interfere with the permeability of the fungal cell membrane, others interfere with DNA synthesis. Most of these medications are fungistatic but in large doses they may be fungicidal.

Nursing Responsibilities
- When taking the health history, ask about known hypersensitivity reactions to these agents; document carefully.
- Assess for side effects: skin rash, local irritation, gastrointestinal symptoms (if given PO), and mental status.
- Administer ketoconazole with food to minimize gastrointestinal irritation.
- Shake suspensions well before administration, and ask the patient to swish them around the mouth before swallowing.
- Tell the patient to allow oral tablets to dissolve in the mouth.

Health Education for the Patient and Family
- Therapy usually continues over a long period of time, but regular use of medications for the recommended period is necessary. Do not miss doses, and complete the full treatment.
- For griseofulvin: Take with meals or foods high in fat (such as ice cream) to avoid stomach upset and help with absorption. Avoid alcohol (which may cause rapid pulse and flushing) and exposure to sunlight (this drug causes increased sensitivity).
- For nystatin: Dissolve lozenges completely in the mouth. Hold suspensions in the mouth and swish throughout the mouth as long as possible before swallowing. Insert intravaginal medication high in the vagina. Continue with intravaginal applications throughout the menses.
- For antifungal shampoo: Use two times a week for 4 weeks, allowing at least 3 days between each shampoo. Wet hair, apply shampoo to produce lather, leave in place for 1 minute, and then rinse. Apply shampoo a second time, lather, leave in place for 3 minutes, and then rinse thoroughly.
- For topical application: Rub well into the affected areas, but do not get the medication in your eyes.
- For vaginal candidiasis infections: During therapy, refrain from sexual intercourse or advise partner to use a condom.
- Your sexual partner will need to be treated at the same time so that you do not pass the infection back and forth to each other.

Nursing Care

Many people treat themselves with OTC antifungal medications. It is recommended, however, that the person be professionally diagnosed the first time the infection occurs. If symptoms reappear, self-treatment is usually satisfactory. The interventions discussed for nursing care of the patient with a bacterial infection are also appropriate for the patient with a fungal infection. Teaching topics specific to fungal infections are as follows:

- Fungal diseases are contagious. Do not share linens or personal items with others.
- Use a clean towel and washcloth each day.
- Carefully dry all skinfolds, including those under the breasts, under the arms, and between the toes.
- Wear clean cotton underclothing each day.
- Fungi grow in moist environments, such as on sweaty feet. To prevent further infections, do not wear the same pair of shoes every day, wear socks that permit moisture to wick away from the skin surface, do not wear rubber- or plastic-soled shoes, and use talcum powder or an OTC antifungal powder twice a day.

The Patient with a Parasitic Infestation

Infestations of the skin by parasites are more common in developing countries but may occur in any geographic area of the world. They affect people of all social classes but are associated with crowded or unsanitary living conditions.

Pathophysiology

Two of the more common parasitic infestations of the skin are caused by lice and mites. These parasites do not normally live on the skin, but infest the skin through contact with an infested person or contact with clothing, linens, or objects infested with the parasites.

Pediculosis

Pediculosis is an infestation with lice, parasites that live on the blood of an animal or human host. The louse is a 2- to 4-mm oval organism with a stylet that pierces the skin; an anticoagulant in its saliva prevents host blood from clotting while it eats. The female louse lays its eggs (small pearl-gray or brown eggs, called nits) on hair shafts. The louse within the egg hatches, reaches the adult reproductive stage, and dies in 30 to 50 days (Porth & Matfin, 2009).

Two common types of human pediculosis follow:

- Pediculosis corporis is an infestation with body lice. This infestation is more common in people who do not have access to facilities for bathing or washing clothes, such as the homeless. The lice live in clothing fibers and are transmitted primarily by contact with infested clothing and bed linens. The skin lesions occur at the site of a louse bite; macules appear initially, followed by wheals and papules. Pruritus is common, and scratching often results in linear excoriations. The lesions are most often seen on the shoulders, trunk, and buttocks.
- Pediculosis pubis is an infestation with pubic lice (often called "crabs"). This infestation is spread through sexual activity with someone already infested or by contact with

infested clothing or linens. The lice are found in the pubic region and occasionally spread to the axillae or men's beards. The lice cause skin irritation and intense itching.

Scabies

Scabies is a parasitic infestation caused by a mite (Sarcoptes scabiei). The pregnant female mite burrows into the skin and lays two to three eggs each day for about a month. The eggs hatch in 3 to 5 days, and the larvae migrate to the surface of the skin but burrow into the skin for food or protection. The larvae develop, and the cycle repeats. Scabies infestation affects people of all socioeconomic classes. The infestation is found in webs between the fingers, the inner surfaces of the wrist and elbow, the axillae, the female nipple, the penis, the belt line, and the gluteal crease. The lesions are a small red-brown burrow, about 2 mm in length, sometimes covered with vesicles, which appears as a rash. Pruritus in response to the mite or its feces is common, especially at night, and excoriations may develop. The excoriations predispose the person to secondary bacterial infections. The incidence of scabies in residents of nursing homes and extended care facilities has increased.

Interdisciplinary Care

Parasitic infestations are diagnosed by identifying the organism and are treated with medications that kill the lice or mites.

Diagnosis

When a patient has manifestations of pediculosis, the hair shaft and the clothing are examined to identify the lice or the nits. Microscopic examination of the parasite provides a positive diagnosis. Scabies is diagnosed by skin scrapings and microscopic examination for the mites or their feces.

Medications

Lice are eradicated with agents that kill the parasite. Infestations of the body and pubic area are treated with topical medications that contain gamma benzene hexachloride, malathion (Prioderm lotion), or permethrin (NIX).

Infestations of the hair are treated with shampoos containing lindane, such as Kwell. A fine-toothed comb can be used to comb the dead nits off the hair shaft. Scabies may be eradicated by a single treatment of lindane lotion or Kwell applied to the entire skin surface for 12 hours. The associated itching is treated with systemic or topical medications, including corticosteroids. Secondary bacterial infections are treated with the appropriate antibiotic.

‿ Nursing Care

Nursing care for patients with a parasite infestation most often focuses on teaching to prevent infestation or to eradicate an existing infestation. For a hospitalized patient with pediculosis, isolation procedures are instituted until the patient no longer has the infestation.

Patient and family teaching is necessary to facilitate treatment at home, to prevent the spread of the infestation, and to dispel the myth that lice infest only people in dirty living conditions or with poor hygiene. Specific information includes the following:

- Wash clothing and linens in soap and hot water, or have them dry cleaned.
- Ironing the clothes kills any lice eggs.
- All family members and sexual partners must also be treated.
- Lice and mites may infest anyone.

The Patient with a Viral Infection

Viruses are pathogens that consist of an RNA or DNA core surrounded by a protein coat. They depend on live cells for reproduction and so are classified as intracellular pathogens. The viruses that cause skin lesions invade the keratinocyte, reproduce, and either increase cellular growth or cause cellular death.

An increase in the incidence of viral skin disorders has been attributed to a variety of causes. Some commonly used drugs, such as birth control medications and corticosteroids, are known to have immunosuppressive properties that allow the viruses to multiply. Other drugs, such as antibiotics, kill off normal skin bacteria that would otherwise serve as defense against viral infections.

Pathophysiology

Viral infections cause many different kinds of skin disorders, including warts, herpes simplex infections, and herpes zoster infections.

Warts

Warts, or verrucae, are lesions of the skin caused by the human papillomavirus (HPV). Warts may be nongenital or genital. Nongenital warts are benign lesions; genital warts may be precancerous. Warts are transmitted through skin contact. Wart lesions may be flat, fusiform (tapered at both ends), or round, but most are round and raised and have a rough, gray surface. There are many different types of warts; location and appearance of the warts depend on the causative virus. (Genital warts are discussed in ∞ Chapter 50.) Commonly occuring warts are as follows:

- A common wart (verruca vulgaris) may appear anywhere on the skin and mucous membranes of the body; they most commonly appear on the fingers. Common warts grow above the skin surface and may be dome-shaped with ragged borders (Figure 16–8 ■).
- Plantar warts occur at pressure points on the soles of the feet. The pressure of shoes and walking prevents these warts from growing outward, so they tend to extend deeper beneath the skin surface than do common warts. Plantar warts are often painful.
- A flat wart (verruca plana) is a small, flat lesion, usually seen on the forehead or dorsum of the hand.

Depending on their size, location, and any associated discomfort, warts may be treated with medications, cryotherapy, or electrodesiccation and curettage. A common method of wart removal is acid therapy, using a colloidal solution of 16% salicylic acid and 16% lactic acid. The solution is applied to the wart every 12 to 24 hours; the wart disappears in 2 to 3 weeks.

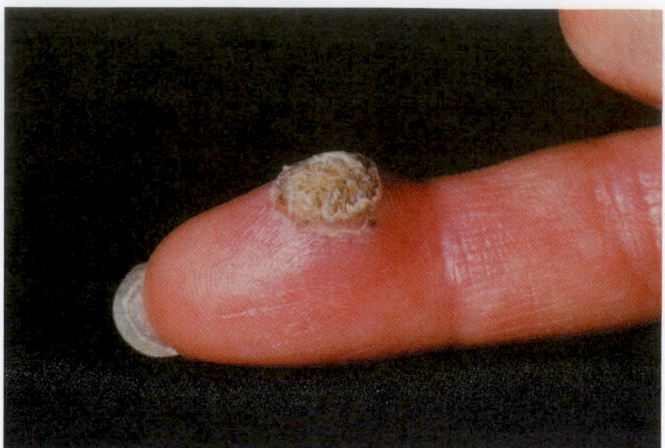

Figure 16–8 ■ The common wart, caused by a virus, appears as a raised, dome-shaped lesion.

Other methods of eradicating warts are cryosurgery, freezing with liquid nitrogen, and electrodesiccation of the wart with an electric current followed by excision of the dead tissue. Warts may also resolve spontaneously when immunity to the virus develops. This response may take up to 5 years.

Herpes Simplex

Herpes simplex (also called a fever blister or cold sore) virus infections of the skin and mucous membranes are caused by two types of herpesvirus: HSV I and HSV II. Most infections above the waist are caused by HSV I, with herpes simplex lesions most often found on the lips, face, and mouth. (Genital herpes infections, caused by HSV II) are discussed in ∞ Chapter 50.) The virus may be transmitted by physical contact, oral sex, or kissing.

The infection begins with a burning or tingling sensation, followed by the development of erythema, vesicle formation, and pain (Figure 16–9 ■). The vesicles progress through pustules, ulcers, and crusting until healing occurs in 10 to 14 days.

The initial infection is often severe and accompanied by systemic manifestations, such as fever and sore throat; recurrences are more localized and less severe. The virus lives in nerve ganglia and may cause recurrent lesions in response to sunlight, menstruation, injury, or stress. Oral acyclovir may be used prophylactically to prevent reoccurrences and to treat recurrent outbreaks.

Herpes Zoster

Herpes zoster, also called *shingles*, is a viral infection of a dermatome section of the skin caused by varicella zoster (the herpesvirus that also causes chickenpox). The infection is believed to result from reactivation of a varicella virus remaining in the sensory dorsal ganglia after a childhood infection of chickenpox. When reactivated, the virus travels from the ganglia to the corresponding skin dermatome area.

Herpes zoster affects more than 1 million people in the United States each year, with more than half of the cases being in adults over the age of 60 (Porth & Matfin, 2009). Patients with Hodgkin's disease, certain types of leukemia, and lymphomas are more susceptible to an outbreak of the disease. Herpes zoster occurs more often in immunocompromised people, such as those with HIV infections, those receiving radiation therapy or chemotherapy, and those who have had major organ transplants. The appearance of the lesions in people with HIV infections may be one of the first manifestations of immune compromise. The herpes eruption lasts for about 2 to 3 weeks and usually does not recur.

Herpes zoster lesions are vesicles with an erythematous base. The vesicles appear on the skin area supplied by the neurons of a single or associated group of dorsal root ganglia (although they may occur beyond this area in immunosuppressed people). The lesions usually appear unilaterally on the face, trunk, and thorax (Figure 16–10 ■). New lesions continue to erupt for 3 to 5 days, then crust and dry. Recovery occurs in 2 to 3 weeks. The patient often experiences severe pain for up to 48 hours before and during eruption of the lesions. The pain may continue for weeks to months after the lesions have disappeared. The older adult is especially sensitive to the pain and often experiences more severe outbreaks of herpes zoster lesions.

Eruption of vesicles over a single dermatome usually only occurs one time. Generalized herpes zoster may indicate an

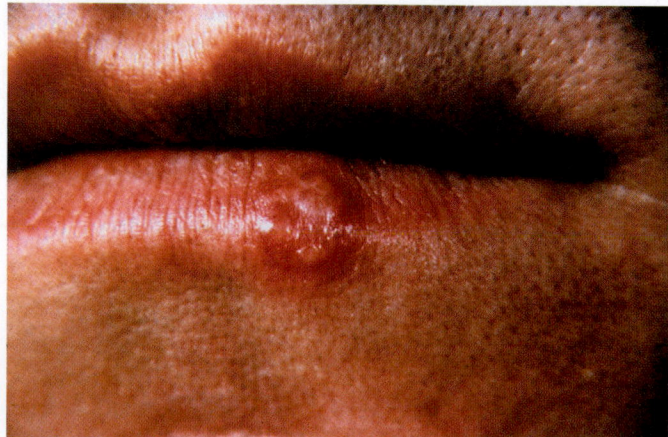

Figure 16–9 ■ Herpes simplex is a viral infection of the skin and mucous membranes.

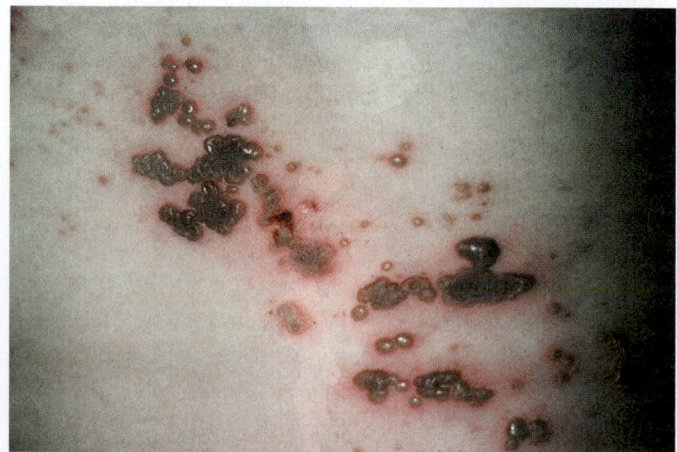

Figure 16–10 ■ Herpes zoster is a viral infection of a dermatome section of the skin. The typical lesions are painful vesicles lying along the path of the nerve.

associated immunocompromised disease, such as Hodgkin's disease or HIV infection. Patients infected with HIV are 20 times more likely to develop herpes zoster (McPhee, Papadakis, & Tierney, 2008).

Complications of herpes zoster include postherpetic neuralgia (a sharp, spasmodic pain along the course of one or more nerves) and visual loss. The neuralgia, described as burning or stabbing, results from inflammation of the root ganglia. Permanent loss of vision may follow occurrence of lesions that arise from the ophthalmic division of the trigeminal nerve. The disease may disseminate in immunocompromised patients, causing lesions beyond the dermatome, visceral lesions, and encephalitis. This serious complication may cause death.

Interdisciplinary Care

The treatment for viral skin infections focuses on stopping viral replication and treating patient responses, such as itching and pain.

Diagnosis

Although diagnosis is usually based on manifestations and appearance of the lesions, laboratory tests may be necessary to differentiate herpes zoster from contact dermatitis and herpes simplex. The laboratory tests include a Tzanck smear, which identifies the herpes virus but does not distinguish herpes zoster from herpes simplex. Cultures of fluid from the vesicles and antibody tests are used to make the differential diagnosis of herpesvirus types. HIV testing should be considered if patients are under age 55 with a history of HIV risk factors. ∞ See Chapter 15 for more information about these tests.

Medications

Antiviral drugs are used to treat herpes zoster infections. Acyclovir (Zovirax) interferes with viral synthesis and replication. Although it does not cure herpes infections, it does decrease the severity of the illness and also decreases pain. It may be administered topically, orally, or parenterally. It is more effective if administration begins within the first 1 to 2 days after the first vesicles appear. Other antiviral medications include famciclovir (Famvir), and valacyclovir (Valtrex). Nerve blocks may be needed to treat initial pain. Narcotic and nonnarcotic analgesics are prescribed for pain management, and antihistamines may be administered for relief of pruritus. Patients with eye involvement are treated with topical steroid ophthalmic ointments and mydriatics.

Zostavax (a weakened form of varicella-zoster virus) is a vaccine used for adults age 60 years or older to prevent herpes zoster. It works by increasing the immune system response; if the patient experiences an outbreak of blisters despite being vaccinated, the nerve pain that follows may be prevented. The vaccine should not be taken by people who are allergic to any of the ingredients, gelatin, or neomycin; have a weaker immune system (such as those with AIDs or leukemia); or take steroids. Side effects include injection site manifestations (such as redness, itching, pain, bruising), headache, fever, hives at the injection site, joint or muscle pain, a rash, and swollen glands.

∞ Nursing Care

Patients with herpes zoster require nursing care for infection, pruritus, and pain. They also require teaching about preventing the spread of the virus to others. See page 418 for a case study and nursing care plan for the patient with herpes zoster.

Nursing Diagnoses and Interventions

This section focuses on the nursing diagnoses of acute pain and risk for infection.

Acute Pain

The patient with herpes zoster often experiences severe pain over the entire dermatome supplied by the affected nerve root. The pain is described as burning, tearing, or stabbing. The patient may avoid movement and does not want clothing or bed linens to touch the affected area.

- Monitor the location, duration, and intensity of the pain. *Each person experiences and expresses pain in his or her own manner. Pain tolerance is also individual. Accurate assessment of the patient's perception and tolerance of pain is essential in facilitating pain management.*
- Explain the rationale for taking prescribed medications on a regular schedule. *Delaying or withholding medications may allow the pain to reach an intensity at which the medication is less effective in promoting relief.*
- Teach measures to relieve pruritus: Take prescribed antipruritic medications, apply calamine lotion or wet compresses if prescribed, keep the room temperature cool, and use a bed cradle to keep sheets off affected areas of the body (see Box 16–10). *Pruritus is a common problem for patients with herpes zoster; scratching may excoriate the skin and increase the risk for secondary infections. Pruritus may intensify the experience of pain.*
- Encourage the use of distraction (such as music) or a specific relaxation technique (such as progressive muscle relaxation or deep breathing). *Noninvasive methods to relieve pain not only help the patient manage the pain experience but also increase the effectiveness of pain medications.*

Risk for Infection

Patients with herpes zoster have impaired skin integrity and pruritus with scratching and possible excoriation. These factors contribute to a high risk for secondary bacterial infection. In addition, the patient is contagious to others who did not have chickenpox as children.

- If hospitalized, monitor white blood cell count and assess for lymph gland enlargement. *Secondary bacterial infections may occur in any patient with impaired skin integrity; if the patient is immunocompromised, the risk is even greater. Fever, changes in lesions or drainage, an increased white blood cell count, and lymph gland enlargement are manifestations of an infection.*
- Teach interventions to decrease the itch-scratch-itch cycle, thereby decreasing the possibility of excoriation (see discussion about nursing care of patients with pruritus and psoriasis earlier in this chapter). *Excoriation from scratching provides an avenue for bacterial invasion.*

CASE STUDY & NURSING CARE PLAN A Patient with Herpes Zoster

Jesus Rivera is a 34-year-old migrant farm worker who currently lives in temporary housing in a rural area of the southwestern United States. His family includes his wife, Marta, who is 3 months pregnant, and two children, ages 3 and 5. He takes his wife to a medical clinic staffed by volunteer nurses, physicians, and students from a nearby university for a prenatal checkup. The clinic is open only on Saturday and provides care on a sliding fee scale or for free if the family is unable to pay. While Mrs. Rivera is being examined, Mr. Rivera asks the nurse to have someone look at some very painful blisters on his chest that developed about a week ago. He is afraid that exposure to pesticides has caused the sores.

ASSESSMENT

Mr. Rivera speaks Spanish and is able to communicate only slightly in English. The initial assessment of Mr. Rivera is performed by Anita Mendez, a student nurse fluent in Spanish. Mr. Rivera's history reveals problems with lower back pain but no significant past medical illnesses. He is not aware of any allergies and cannot remember having had chickenpox as a child. Two years ago, both children were sick and had blisters on their bodies, and a friend told them it was chickenpox. Mrs. Rivera thinks she had chickenpox as a child.

Because Mr. Rivera has not had any medical care for several years, baseline laboratory tests are ordered to screen for any other illnesses. The complete blood count (CBC), blood chemistry, and urinalysis are all within normal limits.

Mr. Rivera says that he did not feel well for several days before the blisters appeared, having experienced chills and general achiness. He had not taken his temperature because the family does not own a thermometer. Current vital signs are as follows: T 99°F (37.2°C), P 74, R 22, and BP 148/88.

Physical examination of the trunk reveals a bandlike pattern of lesions across the left thorax. Some of the lesions are vesicles filled with serous fluid; others are darker in color and are oozing a light yellow drainage. The skin around the lesions is red and inflamed. Mr. Rivera complains of a severe, burning pain with itching across his chest. He is diagnosed with herpes zoster.

DIAGNOSES

- *Risk for Infection* related to open oozing areas on the left thorax
- *Acute Pain* related to the presence of lesions and pruritus
- *Deficient Knowledge* of the cause of the skin disorder and recommended treatment
- *Anxiety* related to need to work in areas of pesticide application
- *Ineffective Health Maintenance* related to limited access to health care due to transitory work conditions and cultural and language barriers

EXPECTED OUTCOMES

- Skin lesions will heal without evidence of a secondary infection.
- Limit exposure (as much as possible) to his wife and children and to persons with debilitating illnesses to prevent the spread of the virus.
- Obtain relief of pain and pruritus with the proper use of medications.

- Verbalize an understanding of the disease process and participate in the treatment plan.
- Obtain follow-up care.
- Make an appointment for a referral for information about occupational hazards.

PLANNING AND IMPLEMENTATION

- Provide verbal and written instructions (in Spanish) for self-care:
  - Wear a clean cotton undershirt each day.
  - Trim the fingernails short, and keep the hands clean.
  - Wash the hands each time the infected area is touched.
  - Wash any soiled clothes or linens in hot water and soap.
  - Do not allow other family members to use your towels.
  - Take medications as prescribed for itching and pain.
  - Take the medicine for your sores every 4 hours, even during nighttime hours, for 7 days.
  - As much as possible, do not touch your wife and children until the sores are covered with scabs. Do not have sex with your wife while you have these sores.
- Teach how to take care of skin lesions:
  - Wear disposable gloves every time you do this treatment.
  - Wash the sores and the skin around them very gently with a soft washcloth and a mild soap.
  - Using your fingers, carefully rub the cream on the sores. Do this once every morning after breakfast and once every evening after supper.
  - Wash your hands carefully before and after each treatment.
- Make a follow-up appointment for the next week.
- Provide Mr. Rivera with the name and phone number of the Occupational Safety and Health Administration (OSHA) and recommend he call for an appointment to discuss his concerns about pesticides.

EVALUATION

Mrs. Rivera explains how she has taken care of her husband, and Mr. Rivera is careful to describe how he has followed the nurse's instructions. The skin lesions are dry and crusty, with no new blister formation. Mr. Rivera says he has not called OSHA and is not sure that he will, but he thanks Miss Mendez for the phone number. The nurses make an appointment in 1 month for a prenatal checkup for Mrs. Rivera and for follow-up of Mr. Rivera's herpes zoster. Mr. Rivera promises to return if they are still living close enough to keep the appointment.

CRITICAL THINKING IN THE NURSING PROCESS

1. Identify barriers to care present in this case study. How may nursing interventions promote healthcare delivery to disadvantaged populations?
2. Although most cases of herpes zoster are self-limiting, what further assessments and interventions might have been indicated had the lesions shown little improvement over time and/or the pain remained severe?
3. If Mr. Rivera is advised not to work until his lesions heal, the family may face economic and sociocultural hardships. Develop a plan of care for Mr. Rivera for the nursing diagnosis *Ineffective Role Performance*.

See Evaluating Your Response in Appendix C.

- Institute infection control procedures for patients who are hospitalized:
  - Maintain strict isolation for immunocompromised patients.
  - Wear gloves and gown if contact with lesions is likely.

  - Instruct pregnant women to avoid exposure until lesions have crusted over.

Isolation procedures are instituted for the immunocompromised patient to prevent patient infection. Wear gloves and gown to prevent spreading the infection to self or others. Pregnant women must avoid exposure to people with herpes zoster because the herpes virus can cross the placental barrier.

Using NANDA, NIC, and NOC

Linkages between a selected NANDA nursing diagnosis, NIC, and NOC for the patient with herpes zoster are shown in the chart that follows.

Community-Based Care

Because most patients with viral infections provide self-care at home, the nurse focuses on teaching the patient and family how to provide the necessary care. With herpes zoster increasing in incidence in patients who are older or have a serious chronic illness, it may also be necessary to make a referral to a community health provider for continued support. Provide the following information and instructions:

- A vaccine is available to help prevent herpes zoster.
- The disease is usually self-limiting and heals completely. Second occurrences of herpes zoster are rare.
- Do not have social contact with children or pregnant women until crusts have formed over the blistered areas with herpes zoster, as the disease is contagious to people who have not had chickenpox.
- Use pain medications regularly.
- Follow suggestions to help reduce itching, scratching, and pain: Use medications as prescribed, wear lightweight cotton

clothing, keep room temperatures cool, wear cotton gloves at night if scratching is a problem, and practice relaxation and distraction activities.
- Report any increase in pain, fever, chills, drainage that smells bad and has pus, or a spread in the blisters to your healthcare provider.

NANDA, NIC, AND NOC LINKAGES
Herpes Zoster

NANDA	Acute Pain
NIC	Pain Management Analgesic Administration Medication Management
NOC	Comfort Status: Physical Pain Control Pain Level

Adapted from data from Bulechek, G., Butcher, H., & Dochterman, J. M. (Eds). (2008). *Nursing interventions classification (NIC)* (5th ed.) (pp. 128–129, 491, 532–533). St. Louis: Mosby Elsevier; Nanda International. (2009). *Nursing diagnoses: Definitions and classification 2009–2010.* Oxford, UK: Wiley-Blackwell; Moorhead, S., Johnson, M., Maas, M., & Swanson, E. (Eds). (2008). *Nursing outcomes classification (NOC).* (4th ed.) (pp. 282, 536, 539–540). St. Louis: Mosby Elsevier.

Inflammatory Disorders of the Skin

The inflammatory skin disorders discussed in this section include dermatitis, acne, pemphigus, lichen planus, and toxic epidermal necrolysis.

The Patient with Dermatitis

Dermatitis is an inflammation of the skin characterized by erythema and pain or pruritus. Dermatitis may be acute or chronic.

Pathophysiology

Various exogenous and endogenous agents can cause an inflammatory response of the skin. Different types of skin eruptions occur, often specific to the causative allergen, infection, or disease. The initial skin responses to these agents or illnesses include erythema, formation of vesicles and scales, and pruritus (Figure 16–11 ■). Subsequently, irritation from scratching promotes edema, a serous discharge, and crusting. Long-term irritation in chronic dermatitis causes the skin to become thickened and leathery and darker in color.

Contact Dermatitis

Contact dermatitis is a type of dermatitis caused by a hypersensitivity response or chemical irritation. The major sources known to cause contact dermatitis are dyes, perfumes, poison plants (ivy, oak, sumac), chemicals, and metals (Box 16–4). A contact dermatitis common in the healthcare field is latex dermatitis.

FAST FACTS
Latex Allergy
- It is estimated that 5% to 10% of healthcare providers are allergic to latex (WebMD, 2009).
- The most common type of allergic response to latex gloves is Type IV, T-cell mediated contact dermatitis.
- Type I, IgE-mediated hypersensitivity, manifested by urticaria, rhinoconjunctivitis, asthma, or anaphylaxis, is far more serious than the T-cell mediated type.

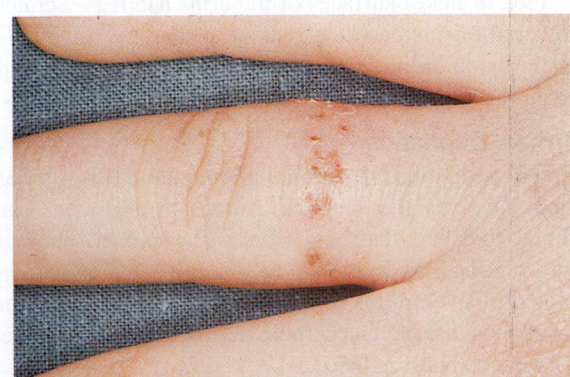

Figure 16–11 ■ Dermatitis, may be a response to allergens, infections, or chemicals. This patient has contact dermatitis resulting from the metal salts in a ring.

Source: Biophoto Associates/Photo Researchers, Inc.

Allergic contact dermatitis is a cell-mediated or delayed hypersensitivity to a wide variety of allergens. Sensitizing antigens include microorganisms, plants, chemicals, drugs, metals, or foreign proteins. On initial contact with the skin, the allergen binds to a carrier protein, forming a sensitizing antigen. The antigen is processed and carried to the T cells, which in turn become sensitized to the antigen. The first exposure is the sensitizing contact and the person does not experience manifestations, which occur with subsequent exposures. The manifestations include erythema, swelling, and pruritic vesicles in the area of allergen contact. For example, a person hypersensitive to metal may have lesions under a ring or watch.

Irritant contact dermatitis is an inflammation of the skin from irritants; it is not a hypersensitivity response. Common sources of irritant contact dermatitis include chemicals (such as acids), soaps, and detergents. The skin lesions are similar to those seen in allergic contact dermatitis.

Atopic Dermatitis

Atopic dermatitis is an inflammatory skin disorder that is also called eczema. The exact cause is unknown, but related factors include depressed cell-mediated immunity, elevated IgE levels, and increased histamine sensitivity. Patients with atopic dermatitis have a family history of hypersensitivity reactions, such as dry skin, eczema, asthma, and allergic rhinitis. Although up to one-third of patients with atopic dermatitis also have food allergies, a positive correlation has not been found.

The dermatitis results from a Type-1 hypersensitive reaction (∞ See Chapter 13). The immune response interacts with the allergen to create a chronic inflammatory condition. In the adult form of atopic dermatitis, characteristic lesions include chronic lichenification, erythema, and scaling, the result of pruritus and scratching. The lesions are usually found on the hands, feet, or flexor surfaces of the arms and legs. Scratching and excoriation increase the risk of secondary infections, as well as invasion of the skin by viruses such as herpes simplex. Serum studies may find elevated eosinophil and IgE levels.

Seborrheic Dermatitis

Seborrheic dermatitis is a chronic inflammatory disorder of the skin that involves the scalp, eyebrows, eyelids, ear canals, nasolabial folds, axillae, and trunk. The cause is unknown. Patients taking methyldopa (Aldomet) for hypertension occasionally develop this disorder, which is also a component of Parkinson's disease. Seborrheic dermatitis is also frequently seen in patients with AIDS.

The lesions are yellow or white plaques with scales and crusts. The scales are often yellow or orange and have a greasy appearance. Mild pruritus is also present. Diffuse dandruff with erythema of the scalp often accompanies the skin lesions.

Exfoliative Dermatitis

Exfoliative dermatitis is an inflammatory skin disorder characterized by excessive peeling or shedding of skin. The cause is unknown in about half of all cases, but a preexisting skin disorder (such as psoriasis, atopic dermatitis, contact dermatitis, or seborrheic dermatitis) is found in up to 63% of the cases (McPhee, Papadakis, & Tierney, 2008). Reactions to medications, such as sulfonamides, account for 20% to 40% of cases. Certain cancers (such as lymphoma) may also cause exfoliative dermatitis.

Both systemic and localized manifestations may appear. Systemic manifestations include weakness, malaise, fever, chills, and weight loss. Scaling, erythema, and pruritus may be localized or involve the entire body. In addition to peeling of skin, the patient may lose his or her hair and nails. Generalized exfoliative dermatitis may cause debility and dehydration. The impairment of skin integrity increases the risk for local and systemic infections.

Interdisciplinary Care

The patient with dermatitis is treated primarily with topical medications and therapeutic baths. If the dermatitis is due to hypersensitivity to an allergen, the patient avoids exposure to environmental irritants and suspected foods. The patient also discontinues as many medications as possible to determine whether the dermatitis is the result of a drug allergy.

Diagnosis

The diagnosis is often based on the manifestations of the disorder and on a history of exposure to a known allergen. Scratch tests and intradermal tests are used to identify a specific allergen.

Medications

The medications used depend on the cause of the dermatitis and the severity of the manifestations. Minor cases are treated with antipruritic medications, whereas more severe cases are treated with oral antihistamines, oral and/or topical corticosteroids, and wet dressings for weeping lesions. Topical immunosuppressive modulators (tacrolimus and pimecrolimus) are effective, but the FDA has published an alert about a possible link with skin cancer and lymphoma. Topical anti-infectives may be prescribed if necessary.

∞ Nursing Care

Nursing care of the patient with dermatitis focuses primarily on providing information for self-care at home. The patient is responsible for managing skin problems and requires education and support. Address the following topics:

■ Medications and treatments do not cure the disease; they only relieve the symptoms.
■ Dry skin increases pruritus, which stimulates scratching. Scratching may in turn cause excoriation, and excoriation increases the risk of infection.
■ It may be necessary to change the diet or environment to avoid contact with allergens.
■ When using steroid preparations, apply only a thin layer to slightly damp skin (e.g., after taking a bath).
■ If occlusive dressings are necessary, a plastic suit may be used.
■ When using oral corticosteroids, never abruptly stop taking the medication. Follow instructions to taper the dosage gradually.

- Advise to discuss use of topical steroids on the face for more than 2 weeks with healthcare provider to avoid adverse reactions, including steroid rosacea and steroid addiction syndrome (Smith, Nedorost, & Tackett, 2007).
- Antihistamines cause drowsiness. When using these medications, avoid alcohol and use caution when driving or working around machinery.

The Patient with Acne

Acne is a disorder of the pilosebaceous (hair and sebaceous gland) structure, which opens to the skin surface through a pore. Sebaceous glands are present over the entire skin surface except the soles of the feet and the palms of the hands, but the largest glands are on the face, scalp, and scrotum. The sebaceous glands, which empty directly into the hair follicle, produce sebum, a lipid substance. Sebum production is a response to direct hormonal stimulation by testicular androgens in men and adrenal and ovarian androgens in women.

Pathophysiology

Acne may be noninflammatory or inflammatory. Noninflammatory acne lesions are primarily **comedones**, more commonly called pimples, whiteheads, and blackheads. Whiteheads are pale, slightly elevated papules categorized as closed comedones. Blackheads are plugs of material that accumulate in the sebaceous glands. They are categorized as open comedones. The color is the result of the movement of melanin into the plug from surrounding epidermal cells. Inflammatory acne lesions include comedones, erythematous pustules, and cysts (Figure 16–12 ■). Inflammation close to the skin surface results in pustules; deeper inflammation results in cysts. The inflammation is believed to result from irritation from fatty acid constituents of the sebum and from substances produced by *Propionibacterium acnes* bacteria, both of which escape into the dermis when the follicular wall of closed comedones ruptures.

Several forms of acne occur at different periods of the life span. The most common are acne vulgaris, acne rosacea, and acne conglobata.

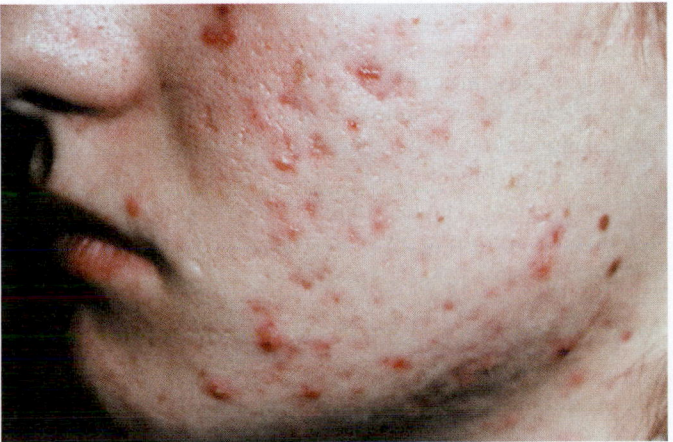

Figure 16–12 ■ Acne vulgaris lesions include comedones, erythematous pustules, and cysts.

Acne Vulgaris

Acne vulgaris is the form of acne common in adolescents and young to middle adults. The actual cause of acne vulgaris is unknown. Possible causes include androgenic influence on the sebaceous glands, increased sebum production, and proliferation of the organism *Propionibacterium acnes*. Many factors once thought to cause acne vulgaris, including high-fat diets, chocolate, infections, and cosmetics, have been disproved.

> ### FAST FACTS
> **Acne Vulgaris**
> - Acne vulgaris is the most common of all skin conditions.
> - Twelve percent of women and 3% of men over the age of 25 have acne vulgaris, and the rate does not begin to decrease until after age 44 (McPhee, Papadakis, & Tierney, 2008).
> - Scarring may be a sequelae of the disease, or may result from picking and manipulating the comedones by the patient.

Mild cases may involve only a few scattered comedones, but severe cases are manifested by multiple lesions of all types. Most acne vulgaris lesions form on the face and neck, but they also occur on the back, chest, and shoulders. Women in their 30s and 40s, often with no prior acne, may develop papular lesions on the chin and around the mouth. The lesions are usually mildly painful and may itch. The complications of acne vulgaris, especially in severe cases, are formation of cysts, pigment changes in persons with dark skin, severe scarring, and lowered self-concept from the skin eruptions.

Acne Rosacea

Acne rosacea is a chronic type of facial acne that occurs more often in middle and older adults. The cause is unknown. The lesions of acne rosacea begin with erythema over the cheeks and nose. Other skin lesions may or may not appear. Over years of time, the skin color changes to dark red, and the pores over the area become enlarged. The soft tissue of the nose may exhibit rhinophyma, an irregular bullous thickening.

Acne Conglobata

Acne conglobata is also a chronic type of acne of unknown cause that begins in middle adulthood. This type causes serious skin lesions: Comedones, papules, pustules, nodules, cysts, and scars occur primarily on the back, buttocks, and chest but may occur on other body surfaces. The comedones have multiple openings and a discharge that ranges from serous to purulent with a foul odor.

Interdisciplinary Care

The management of acne is similar, regardless of type. Because acne vulgaris is most common, the discussions of interdisciplinary and nursing care focus on that type. Treatment is based on the type and severity of the lesions.

Diagnosis

The disease is diagnosed by the typical location and appearance of lesions. If the patient has pustules, a culture of the drainage is performed to differentiate viral or bacterial dermatitis from acne.

TRETINOIN (AVITA, RENOVA, RETIN-A)

- Use the cream in a test area twice at night to test for sensitivity; if no reaction occurs, increase applications gradually to the prescribed frequency.
- A pea-sized amount of the cream is enough to cover the entire face.
- Apply the cream to clean, dry skin.
- Do not apply the cream to the eyes, mouth, angles of the nose, or mucous membranes.
- Wash your face no more than two to three times a day, using a mild soap. Do not use skin preparations (such as

aftershave lotion or perfumes) that contain alcohol, menthol, spice, or lime; they may irritate your skin.
- The medication may cause a temporary stinging or warm sensation but should not cause pain.
- The skin where you apply the cream will be mildly red and may peel; if you experience a more severe reaction, consult your healthcare provider.
- The medication may cause increased sensitivity to sunlight, use sunscreens and wear protective clothing when outdoors.
- Your acne may become worse during the first 2 weeks of treatment; this is an expected response.

Medications

The treatment of acne is tailored to the individual and is based on the severity of the lesions. For acne with comedones, tretinoin (retinoic acid, Retin-A) or benzoyl peroxide preparations are prescribed. Azelaic acid (Azelex) may also be used. The administration of these vitamin A analogues is discussed in the Medication Administration feature shown above. Benzoyl peroxide preparations are found in OTC medications such as Fostex, Acne-Dome, Desquam-X, Benzagel, Clear By Design, and Xerac BP. These products are keratolytic and loosen the comedones. Epiduo (a prescription gel) combines adapalene and benzoyl peroxide to treat acne vulgaris.

Mild forms of papular inflammatory acne are treated with topical clindamycin (Cleocin T), a bacteriostatic agent that decreases the amount of fatty acids on the skin surface. This medication may be combined with tretinoin therapy.

Moderate forms of papular inflammatory acne are treated with oral or topical antibiotics, such as tetracycline, erythromycin, and minocycline. These antibiotics are administered for 3 to 4 months; if the patient's skin is clear, the dose is lowered gradually to a maintenance dose that will maintain clear skin.

Treatments

Acne scars may alter the individual's self-concept. The scars may be removed by dermabrasion and laser treatment. (Dermabrasion is discussed in greater detail later in this chapter.)

✍ Nursing Care

Nursing care is individualized and is conducted primarily through teaching in clinics or healthcare provider offices. Regardless of the patient's age or gender, it is important to remember that almost all patients with acne are embarrassed by and self-conscious of their appearance. Prior to teaching, establish rapport with the patient and clarify beliefs; for example, the patient may believe the lesions result from poor hygiene, masturbation, use of cosmetics, eating the wrong types of foods, or lack of sexual activity. It is critical to teach the patient about the causes of and factors involved in acne prior to teaching self-care.

The teaching plan for the patient with acne includes general guidelines for skin care and health as well as specific guidelines for care of the acne lesions. The following topics should be addressed:

- Wash the skin with a mild soap and water at least twice a day to remove accumulated oils.
- Shampoo the hair often enough to prevent oiliness.
- Eat a regular, well-balanced diet. Foods do not cause or increase acne.
- Expose the skin to sunlight, but avoid sunburn.
- Get regular exercise and sleep.
- Try to avoid putting your hands on your face.
- Do not squeeze a pimple. Squeezing forces the material of the pimple deeper into the skin and may cause the pimple to become larger and infected.
- The treatment for acne lasts months, in some cases for the rest of one's life. It is very important to take the medications each day for the prescribed length of time.

The Patient with Pemphigus Vulgaris

Pemphigus vulgaris is a chronic disorder of the skin and oral mucous membranes characterized by blister formation. The disease is caused by autoantibodies that cause acantholysis (the separation of epidermal cells from one another). The disorder is associated with IgG antibodies and HLA-A10 antigen. Septicemia from an infection of *Staphylococcus aureus* is the most common cause of death. The disease occurs in middle and older adults of all races and ethnic backgrounds. The disorder has been associated with other autoimmune disorders and with the administration of certain drugs, such as penicillamine and captopril.

The blisters that form in pemphigus vulgaris usually appear first in the mouth and on the scalp and then spread in crops or waves to involve large areas of the body, including the face, back, chest, umbilicus, and groin. The blisters form in the epidermis and cause the epidermal cells to separate above the basal layer. These blisters rupture, leaving denuded skin, crusting, and oozing of fluid with a musty odor. The lesions are painful. Pressure on a blister causes it to spread to adjacent skin (Nikolsky's sign). The loss of fluid from the blisters may result in fluid and electrolyte imbalances. Secondary bacterial infections are a serious risk.

Interdisciplinary Care

The goals of treatment are to control the severity of the disease, to prevent infection and loss of fluids, and to promote healing. Patients who experience severe attacks or secondary infections are usually hospitalized. Although the disease cannot be cured, the manifestations can be controlled.

Diagnosis

Pemphigus vulgaris is diagnosed by manifestations and diagnostic tests, including immunofluorescence microscopy, which is done to identify the presence of IgG antibodies in the epidermis and serum, and skin biopsy (∞ see Chapter 15) to determine the presence of acantholysis.

Medications

Early lesions are treated with highly potent topical corticosteroids. As the disease becomes more severe, systemic corticosteroids or immunosuppressive agents (such as azathioprine or methotrexate) are prescribed. Secondary infections are treated with topical and/or systemic antibiotics.

Treatments

Plasmapheresis is occasionally used to treat pemphigus. In this procedure, the plasma is selectively removed from whole blood and reinfused into the patient. This decreases the serum level of antibodies for a period of time. Plasmapheresis with related nursing care is discussed in ∞ Chapter 44.

∞ Nursing Care

The hospitalized patient with pemphigus requires careful assessment of skin lesions and monitoring for manifestations of infection. Provide skin care through bathing and applying dressings to denuded areas, using aseptic technique to prevent infection. The patient may be placed on reverse isolation as a protective measure. Monitor the patient's hydration status to prevent fluid volume deficit and incorporate pain medications and noninvasive pain management techniques in the plan of care. Oral lesions often make eating difficult; the patient requires meticulous oral hygiene and nonirritating foods. The patient often is depressed and fearful; establishing a therapeutic relationship is essential, and referrals for counseling may be necessary.

Teaching the patient and family how to provide care at home also involves skin care, oral care, diet, pain management, prevention of infection and how to take prescribed medications. A referral to a home health agency or local health department may be necessary.

The Patient with Lichen Planus

Lichen planus is an inflammatory disorder of the mucous membranes and skin. It has no known cause but has been associated with exposure to drugs or to film processing chemicals. The disease affects adults of all ages.

The lesions first appear as violet papules, 2 to 10 mm in size, commonly occurring on the wrists, ankles, lower legs, and genitals. The lesions itch intensely. Over time, persistent lesions thicken and become dark red, forming hypertrophic lichen planus. Lesions on the oral mucous membranes appear as white, lacey rings; lesions may also appear on the mucous membranes of the vaginal area and the penis. The nails become thin and may shed.

Lichen planus lesions are self-limiting but last for an average of 12 to 18 months. The disorder is diagnosed by manifestations. Corticosteroids are used to control the inflammation, and antihistamines are used to control the pruritus.

The Patient with Toxic Epidermal Necrolysis

Toxic epidermal necrolysis (TEN) is a rare, life-threatening disease in which the epidermis peels off the dermis in sheets, leaving large areas of denuded skin. Conjunctivitis and mucositis of the mouth, upper airway, esophagus, and sometimes the genitourinary tract are often associated with TEN. The patient usually requires critical care, often in a burn center. The incidence of TEN has not been documented, but it is seen more often in men and in people of African descent. The mortality rate is decreasing because of current methods of care. The cause of death is almost always sepsis.

Although some cases have no known cause, most cases result from a drug reaction, and others are associated with a serious concomitant illness, such as cancer or AIDS. Drugs that have been associated with TEN are the sulfonamides, barbiturates, NSAIDs, phenytoin, allopurinol, and penicillin.

The pathophysiologic process in TEN is not completely understood, but the triggering mechanism is believed to be a hypersensitivity or immune response. TEN begins with a painful, localized erythema of the face and extremities, accompanied by fever, chills, muscle aches, and generalized malaise. A macular rash develops, followed by the formation of large, flaccid blisters over the body surface during the next 24 to 96 hours. The skin begins to slough, leaving the dermal surface exposed. Even in areas without blistering, the skin may peel off in layers. The skin sloughing continues over several days and can expose 95% or more of the dermal surface. Other manifestations include conjunctivitis, pharyngitis, stomatitis, and enlargement of lymph glands. Urethral slough is common, causing such painful voiding that the patient voluntarily retains urine. The patient is often disoriented, may be nearly comatose, and is seriously ill.

The loss of skin leads to fluid and electrolyte imbalances and secondary infections, as well as systemic effects on all other body systems. These complications may cause death. However, if the complications can be prevented, healing by epidermal regeneration occurs in about a month. The long-term complications of TEN include blindness, lacrimal duct occlusion, scarring and contractures, loss of nails, esophageal strictures, and glomerulonephritis.

The patient is hospitalized and requires rapid diagnosis and treatment. Any medication in use by the patient is stopped immediately. Interdisciplinary care involves fluid replacement, correction of electrolyte imbalances, prevention or management of infection, and pain control. The interdisciplinary and nursing care are essentially the same as for the patient with burns, discussed in ∞ Chapter 17.

Malignant Skin Disorders

The skin, despite its ability to protect the internal body from external damage, is a fragile organ and is subject to damage from ultraviolet radiation and chemicals. Over time, this damage results in alterations in cellular structure and function, and malignancies of the skin occur. Many of these lesions are found on skin surfaces that have undergone long-term exposure to the sun or the environment. Malignant skin tumors are the most common of all cancers.

The Patient with Actinic Keratosis

Actinic keratosis, also called senile or solar keratosis, is an epidermal skin lesion directly related to chronic sun exposure and photodamage. The prevalence is highest in people with light-colored skin; these lesions are rare in people with dark skin. About 20% of actinic keratoses convert to squamous cell carcinoma (Porth & Matfin, 2009). However, there is some thought that the lesions are all premalignant.

The lesions are erythematous rough macules a few millimeters in diameter. They are often shiny but may be scaly; if the scales are removed, the underlying skin bleeds. They occur in multiple patches, primarily on the face, dorsa of the hands, the forearms, and sometimes on the upper trunk (Figure 16–13 ■). Enlargement or ulceration of the lesions suggests transformation to malignancy. The lesions are usually treated by cryosurgery (freezing) or with 5-fluorouracil cream, which erodes the lesions.

The Patient with Nonmelanoma Skin Cancer

The nonmelanoma skin cancers are basal cell cancer and squamous cell cancer. Other types of nonmelanoma skin cancers, accounting for less than 1% of cases (ACS, 2008) are Merkel

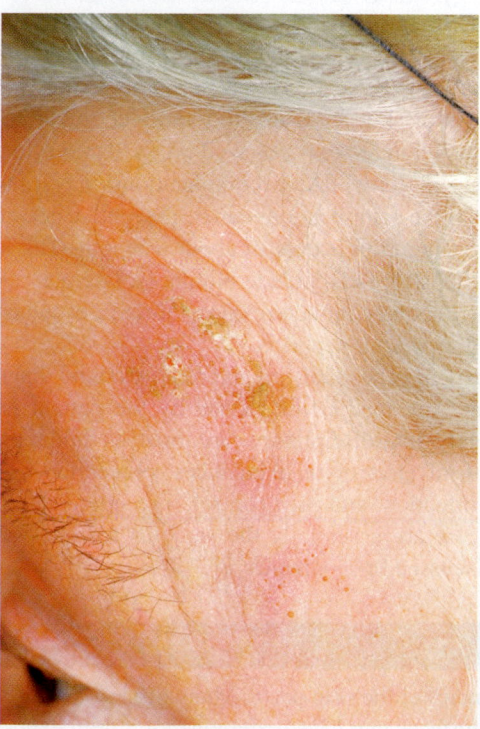

Figure 16–13 ■ The effects of long-term sun exposure are illustrated in this epidermal skin lesion, called actinic keratosis.

cell carcinoma; Kaposi sarcoma; and lymphomas, sarcomas, and adnexal tumors of the skin. These uncommon tumors are not included in this discussion, but information can be found on the American Cancer Society website or the National Cancer Institute website.

Incidence

Nonmelanoma skin cancer is the most common malignant neoplasm found in fair-skinned Americans. The ACS (2008) estimates that more than 1 million new cases of nonmelanoma skin cancer are diagnosed in the United States each year. Of that number, about 80% are basal cell cancers and 20% are squamous cell cancers. Deaths from nonmelanoma skin cancer have dropped by 30% in the past 30 years. Men develop nonmelanoma skin cancer more often than do women, probably because of occupational exposures. Although nonmelanoma skin cancer may occur at any age, the incidence increases with each decade of life. Adults between the ages of 30 and 60 have the majority of these cancers.

Risk Factors

There are multiple etiologic factors involved in the development of nonmelanoma skin cancer, including environmental factors and host factors.

Environmental Factors

Ultraviolet radiation (UVR) from the sun is believed to be the cause of most nonmelanoma skin cancers. Sunlight contains both short-length rays (UVB) and long-length rays (UVA). UVB rays are absorbed by the top layer of skin and cause sunburn. UVA rays penetrate deeper into the skin layers, causing tissue damage. Both types of rays cause DNA alterations and suppress T-cell and B-cell immunity, allowing cancer cells to grow. Researchers have also discovered that many skin cancers contain changes in tumor suppressor genes (these genes normally help keep cells from growing out of control). The damaged gene found in basal cell cancer is p53, a gene that normally causes damaged cells to die. The damaged gene found in squamous cell cancer is the "patched" (PTCH) gene, which normally helps keep cell growth in check (ACS, 2008).

The amount of UVR reaching the earth is increasing, most likely from depletion of the ozone layer surrounding the planet. The U.S. Environmental Protection Agency predicts that for every 1% decrease in the ozone layer, a corresponding 1% to 3% increase in nonmelanoma skin cancer per year will occur.

Geographic, environmental, and lifestyle factors affect the amount of exposure to the sun and the risk for nonmelanoma skin cancer. People who live in latitudes close to the equator and those who live at higher altitudes receive greater UVR exposure. The amount of clothing worn, the time of day, and amount of time in the sun also determine the amount of exposure. Exposure to UVR in tanning booths is also implicated in the development of nonmelanoma skin cancer.

Certain chemicals have long been associated with nonmelanoma skin cancer. Polycyclic aromatic hydrocarbons, found in mixtures of coal, tar, asphalt, soot, and mineral oils, have been linked with skin cancers. Psoralens, used in conjunction with UVA for treatment of psoriasis and cutaneous T-cell lymphoma, increase the risk of squamous cell cancer. Other factors associated with nonmelanoma skin cancer are the use of ionizing radiation, viruses, and physical trauma. X-ray therapy for tinea capitis and the use of radium to treat other malignancies are risk factors. Human papillomavirus is implicated in the development of squamous cell cancer, as is damage to the skin from burns. Organ transplant recipients who undergo immunosuppression to prevent rejection are also at risk for the development of squamous cell cancer.

Host Factors
Skin pigmentation is an important factor in the development of nonmelanoma skin cancer. The amount of melanin pigment produced by the melanocytes determines a person's skin color. The more melanin, the more the skin is protected from the damage produced by ultraviolet rays. Thus, Asian and people of African and Mediterranean descent have a much lower incidence of nonmelanoma skin cancer than do people who have fair complexions and tend to freckle or sunburn easily, such as people of Irish, Scandinavian, or English ancestry.

Although most people have numerous pigmented lesions on their body, almost all of these are normal. However, a major risk factor in the development of nonmelanoma skin cancer is a change in an existing lesion or the presence of a premalignant lesion, such as actinic keratosis.

Pathophysiology
Basal cell cancer and squamous cell cancer arise from epithelial tissue but have different pathophysiology, classifications, and manifestations. These cancers are classified as keratinocyte cancers; when viewed under a microscope they share some features with keratinocytes, the most abundant skin cell type.

Basal Cell Cancer
Basal cell cancer is an epithelial tumor believed to originate either from the basal layer of the epidermis or from cells in the surrounding dermal structures. These tumors are characterized by an impaired ability of the basal cells of the epidermis to mature into keratinocytes, with mitotic division beyond the basal layer. This results in a bulky tumor that grows by direct extension and if untreated, destroys surrounding tissue, including healthy skin, nerves, blood vessels, lymphatic tissue, cartilage, and bone. Basal cell cancer is the most common but least aggressive type of skin cancer, rarely metastasizing. Although once seen only in middle to older adults, it is now being seen in younger people, probably due to increased sun exposure.

Basal cell cancers tend to recur. Tumors greater than 2 cm in diameter have a high recurrence rate. Predisposing factors for metastasis are the size of the tumor and the patient's resistance to treatment with surgery or chemotherapy. Even though they rarely metastasize, untreated basal cell cancers invade surrounding tissue and may destroy body parts, such as the nose or eyelid. Basal cell cancer is classified as nodular, superficial, pigmented, morpheaform, or keratotic.

Nodular basal cell cancer, the most common type of basal cell cancer, most often appears on the face, neck, and head. The tumor is made up of masses of cells that resemble epidermal basal cells and grow in a bulky, nodular form from lack of keratinization. In early stages, the tumor is a papule that looks like a smooth pimple. It is often pruritic and continues to grow at a steady rate, doubling in size every 6 to 12 months. As the tumor grows, the epidermis thins, but it remains intact. The skin over the tumor is shiny, and either pearly white, pink, or flesh colored. Telangiectasis may be visible over the area of the tumor. As the tumor continues to increase in size, the center or periphery may ulcerate, and the tumor develops well-circumscribed borders. It bleeds easily from mild injury.

Superficial basal cell cancer, found most often on the trunk and extremities, is the second most common type of basal cell cancer. This tumor is a proliferating tissue that attaches to the undersurface of the epithelium. The tumor is a flat papule or plaque, often erythematous, with well-defined borders. The tumor may ulcerate and be covered with crusts or shallow erosions (Figure 16–14 ■).

Pigmented basal cell cancer, found on the head, neck, and face, is less common. This tumor concentrates melanin pigment in the center of the basal cancer cells, giving it a dark brown, blue, or black appearance. The border of the tumor is shiny and well defined.

Morpheaform basal cell cancer, the rarest form of basal cell cancer, usually develops on the head and neck. The tumor forms fingerlike projections that extend in any direction along dermal tissue planes. The tumor resembles a flat ivory or flesh-colored scar. This form is more likely to extend into and destroy adjacent tissue, especially muscle, nerve, and bone. It is often more difficult to diagnose because of its appearance.

Keratotic basal cell cancer (basosquamous) is found on the preauricular and postauricular groove. It contains both basal cells and squamoid-appearing cells that keratinize. Its appearance is much like that of nodular basal cell cancer. This type of basal cell cancer tends to recur locally and also is the type most likely to metastasize.

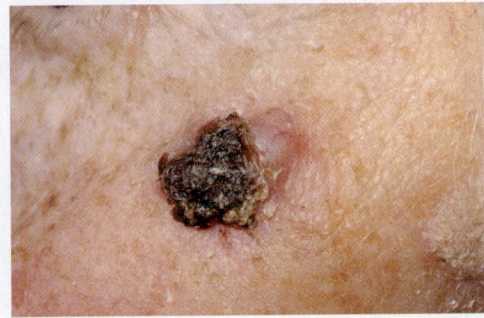

Figure 16–14 ■ A superficial basal cell cancer is characterized by erythema, ulcerations, and well-defined borders.

Squamous Cell Cancer

Squamous cell cancer is a malignant tumor of the squamous epithelium of the skin or mucous membranes. It occurs most often on areas of skin exposed to ultraviolet rays and weather, such as the forehead, helix of the ear, top of the nose, lower lip, and back of the hands. Squamous cell cancer may also arise on skin that has been burned or has chronic inflammation. This is a much more aggressive cancer than basal cell cancer, with a faster growth rate and a much greater potential for metastasis if untreated. The tumors arise when the keratinizing cells of the squamous epithelium proliferate, producing a growth that eventually fills the epidermis and invades the dermal tissue planes. Keratinization of some cells is present, and the formation of keratin "pearls" is common. The keratin formation diminishes as the tumor grows. As the tumor grows, the tumor cells increase in number and rate of mitosis, forming odd shapes. An early form of squamous cell cancer is called Bowen's disease or cancer *in situ*.

Squamous cell cancer begins as a small, firm red nodule. The tumor may be crusted with keratin products. As it grows, it may ulcerate, bleed, and become painful. As the tumor extends into the surrounding tissue and becomes a nodule, the area around the nodule becomes indurated (hardened) (Figure 16–15 ■).

Recurrent squamous cell cancer can be invasive, increasing the risk of metastasis. Invasive squamous cell cancer may arise from preexisting skin lesions, such as scars and actinic keratosis, and extend into the dermis (called intraepidermal squamous cell cancer). This form appears as a slightly raised erythematous plaque with well-defined borders. Metastasis occurs most often via the lymphatics. The degree of risk for metastasis depends on the size and depth of penetration of the tumor.

Interdisciplinary Care

Treatment of nonmelanoma skin cancer focuses on removal of all malignant tissue using such methods as surgery, curettage and electrodesiccation, cryotherapy, or radiotherapy. These modalities offer a greater than 90% cure rate. After the malignant tissue is removed, the patient should have regular examinations for recurrence.

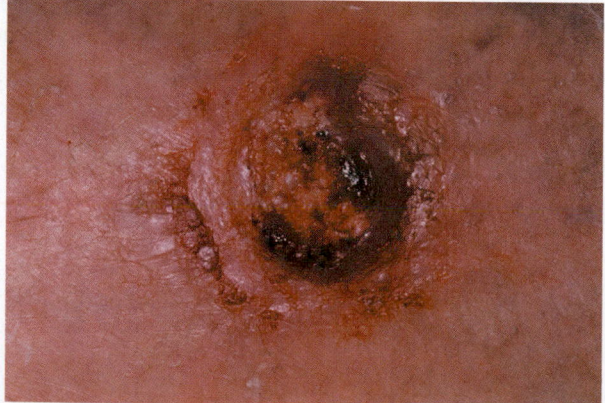

Figure 16–15 ■ As a squamous cell cancer grows, it tends to invade surrounding tissue. It also ulcerates, may bleed, and is painful.

Diagnosis

Nonmelanoma cancer is diagnosed by microscopic examination of tissue biopsied from the tumor. The biopsy is usually done as an office procedure under local anesthesia. The types of biopsy used are shave, punch, incisional, and excisional. Information about skin biopsy is provided in ∞ Chapter 15.

Treatments

Depending on the stage, type, size, and location of a nonmelanoma cancer, it may be treated with surgical excision, Mohs' surgery, curettage and electrodessication, radiation, or other forms of local therapy.

SURGICAL EXCISION Both basal cell and squamous cell cancers are excised surgically. The surgery may be minor or major, depending on the size and location of the tumor. Surgery for small tumors is most often performed in the outpatient surgery department or in the surgeon's office. Surgical excision allows rapid healing and yields good cosmetic results.

The goal of surgical excision is to remove the tumor completely, so some surrounding tissue is excised along with the tumor. If the tumor is on the face, the incision is made along normal wrinkle or anatomic lines so that the scars will be less obvious. The incision is closed in layers to leave the smallest possible scar. A pressure dressing is usually applied over the incision to provide support. If a large tumor is removed, a skin graft or skin flap may be performed to cover the excised area. If grafting is necessary, the patient is hospitalized.

MOHS' SURGERY In Mohs' surgery, thin layers of the tumor are horizontally shaved off. A frozen section of the tissue is stained at each level to determine tumor margins. This method is the most accurate in assessing the extent of nonmelanoma skin cancer and the method that conserves the most normal tissue. It is often used in areas such as the nose, the nasolabial fold, the medial canthus, and the ear.

CURETTAGE AND ELECTRODESICCATION Curettage and electrodesiccation are used to treat basal cell cancers that are less than 2 cm in diameter, are superficial, or recur because of poor margin control. It may also be used for primary squamous cell cancers that are less than 1 cm in diameter and have distinct borders. This type of treatment is most successful for tumors on anatomic sites over a fixed underlying surface, such as the ear, chest, and temple.

Abnormal tissue is scraped away (curettaged) within 1 to 2 mm of the margin and then a low-voltage electrode is used to abrade the tumor base (electrodesiccation). Curettage and electrodesiccation is not used for lesions where the dermis is thin (such as the eyelid) or where the tumor extends into the subcutaneous tissue. Curettage and electrodesiccation provide good cosmetic results and preserve normal tissue. However, healing time is longer, and it is difficult to ensure that all tumor margins have been removed.

Instead of a low-voltage electrode, some physicians use a carbon dioxide laser to vaporize the tumor. When used in conjunction with curettage, this treatment is effective on superficial basal cell cancers. Carbon dioxide vaporization results in minimal thermal injury to adjacent cells, less pain, and quicker healing.

RADIATION THERAPY Radiation is most often used for lesions that are inoperable because of their location (such as tumors on the corner of the nose, the eyelid, the canthus, and the lip) or size (between 1 cm and 8 cm). It is also used for patients who are older and of poor surgical risk. Radiation is painless and can be used to treat areas surrounding the tumor if necessary. However, the treatment is given over 3 to 4 weeks in a clinical facility, does not allow control of tumor margins, and may itself cause skin cancer.

OTHER FORMS OF LOCAL THERAPY Other forms of local therapy include the following:

- Cryosurgery, which involves applying liquid nitrogen to the tumor to freeze and kill abnormal cells.
- Photodynamic therapy (PDT) involves administering a topical or injectable chemical that collects in the tumor cells and makes them more sensitive to light. A light source is then focused on the tumor and the cells die.
- Topical chemotherapy means that an anti-cancer drug (usually 5-fluorouracil [5-FU]) is applied as a cream directly on the skin to kill the tumor cells.
- Immune response modifiers cause an immune response to the cancer, causing it to get smaller and die. The drugs used are imiquimod (Aldara) (a topical cream) and interferon (injected directly into the tumor).
- Laser surgery uses laser light to vaporize cancer cells.

Nursing Care

The increasing number of people with skin cancer means that nurses must be involved in prevention and early detection. Nurses have the opportunity to teach preventive behaviors in all settings, including the hospital, home, community, school, and clinic.

Nursing care for the patient with nonmelanoma skin cancer depends on the treatment used. Surgical excision is the most common form of treatment; nursing care depends on the extent of the procedure. However, regardless of the type of treatment, the patient will have impaired skin integrity, an increased risk for infection, and anxiety about the future following a diagnosis of cancer. Interventions with rationales for the patient with any type of skin cancer are discussed in the following section on melanoma.

Health Promotion

It is well known that cumulative sun exposure positively correlates with nonmelanoma skin cancers. Many skin cancers can be prevented by limiting exposure to risk factors. Primary prevention behaviors recommended by the ACS and the Skin Cancer Foundation are outlined in Box 16–5. In addition to these preventive behaviors, the ACS recommends "Slip! Slop! Slap! Wrap!" method: **slip** on a shirt, **slop** on 15 SPF (or higher) sunscreen, **slap** on a hat, and **wrap** on sunglasses before exposure to the sun. Information about sunscreen is listed in Box 16–6.

Nurses also provide patient and family education for early detection of nonmelanoma skin cancer. Numerous brochures describing the types of skin cancers, photographs of lesions, and prevention behaviors are available from the ACS, health education and support agencies, and pharmaceutical companies that manufacture sunscreen. Most of this literature is free.

BOX 16–5 Health Promotion: Preventing Skin Cancer

- Minimize sun exposure between the hours of 10 AM and 3 PM, when ultraviolet rays are the strongest.
- Cover up with a wide-brimmed hat, sunglasses, long-sleeved shirt, and long pants made of tightly woven materials when in the sun.
- Apply a waterproof or water-resistant sunscreen with an SPF of 15 or more at least 30 minutes before every exposure to the sun. If swimming or sweating heavily, reapply every hour. Apply sunscreen not only on sunny days but also on cloudy days (when ultraviolet rays can penetrate 70% to 80% of the cloud cover.
- Use sunscreen and protective clothing when you are on or near sand, snow, concrete, or water (which can reflect more than 50% of the ultraviolet rays onto your skin).
- Avoid tanning booths; UVR emitted by tanning booths damages the deep skin layers.

The patient or family at risk for or diagnosed with a skin cancer must be taught how to conduct a self-examination of the skin, described in Box 16–7, as well as the importance of conducting the examination on the same day of each month. Family members can help with areas that are hard to examine, such as the ears, scalp, and back.

BOX 16–6 Sunscreen Information

Types of Sunscreen

Chemical
Chemical sunscreens absorb ultraviolet light and act as a radiation filter. Examples follow:
- p-Aminobenzoic acid (PABA)
- Benzophenones
- Anthranilates
- Salicylates

Physical
Physical sunscreens reflect and scatter ultraviolet light. Examples follow:
- Zinc oxide
- Titanium dioxide
- Magnesium silicate
- Ferric chloride
- Kaolin
- Ichthyol

Adverse Reactions Associated with Sunscreens
Adverse reactions associated with sunscreens include contact and photocontact dermatitis. People with previous hypersensitivity reactions to benzocaine, procaine, sulfonamides, or paraphenylenediamine may develop hypersensitivity responses to PABA. People who are also taking systemic thiazide diuretics or sulfonamides may develop eczematous dermatitis.

Sunscreen Ratings
In the United States, the Food and Drug Administration rates commercial sunscreens according to their sun protection factor, or SPF. The SPF value is the ratio of the time required to produce minimal skin redness through a sunscreen product with the time required to produce the same degree of redness without the sunscreen. A person who can tolerate 1/2 hour of sun without a sunscreen should be able to tolerate 3 hours of sun when a sunscreen of SPF 6 is applied to the skin. SPF values of sunscreens range from 2 to 100. An SPF of 15 or greater is recommended.

BOX 16–7 Health Promotion: Skin Self-Examination

1. Choose the same day each month (such as the first day) to do the examination.
2. The best time to do the examination is after you take a bath or shower. Examine yourself in a well-lighted room in front of a full-length mirror. Have a hand mirror, a chair, and a hair dryer available. If you have difficulty seeing your back and scalp (or any other parts of your body), ask someone to help you.
3. Follow the same pattern with each examination:

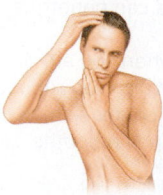

Examine head and face, using one or both mirrors. Use blow dryer to inspect scalp.

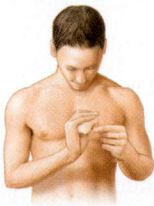

Check hands, including nails. In full-length mirror, examine elbows, arms, underarms.

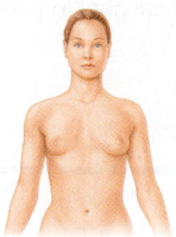

Focus on neck, chest, torso. Women: Check under breasts.

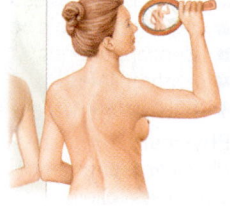

With back to the mirror, use hand mirror to inspect back of neck and back including buttocks.

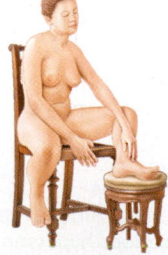

Sitting down, check legs and feet, including soles, heels, and nails. Use hand mirror to examine genitals.

Community-Based Care

Teach the patient and family specific measures for self-care following surgery, including information about

- how and when to change dressings.
- the use of aseptic technique and careful hand hygiene when caring for the wound.
- symptoms to report (such as bleeding, fever, or signs of wound infection), and how to protect the operative site against trauma and irritations.

Malignant Melanoma Video

The Patient with Melanoma

Melanoma (malignant melanoma) arises from melanocytes. This serious skin cancer is increasing in incidence each year. Melanoma accounts for less than 5% of skin cancers, but it causes a large majority of skin cancer deaths (ACS, 2008).

Incidence

This disease is over 10 times more common in fair-skinned people than in dark-skinned people. It is slightly more common in men than in women. Melanoma occurs more often in people who live in sunny climates, burn easily, and patronize tanning parlors. However, it may arise from already present lesions or from skin normally covered with clothing. Melanoma occurs in a wide age range, from adolescents to older adults, with the greatest rates in those over the age of 80.

Risk Factors

Although the exact cause of melanoma is unknown, it is known that certain risk factors are associated with the disease. The risk factors for melanoma are listed in Box 16–8.

Pathophysiology

Melanomas arise from melanocytes, cells located at or near the basal layer (the deepest epidermal layer). These cells produce melanin, the dark skin pigment. Melanin is made in granules and transferred to keratinocytes, where it accumulates on the superficial side of each keratinocyte and forms a shield of pigment over the nucleus as protection against ultraviolet rays. Melanomas can develop wherever there is pigment, but about one-third of them originate in existing nevi (moles).

Almost all melanomas are more than 6 mm in diameter, are asymmetric, and initially develop within the epidermis over a long period. While they are still confined to the epidermis, the lesions (called melanoma *in situ*) are flat and relatively benign. However, when they penetrate the dermis, they mingle with blood and lymph vessels and are capable of metastasizing. At this latter stage, the tumors develop a raised or nodular appearance and often have smaller nodules, called satellite lesions, around the periphery.

The prognosis for survival for people diagnosed with melanoma is determined by several variables, including location, tumor thickness, ulceration, metastasis, site, age, and gender.

BOX 16–8 Risk Factors for Melanoma Skin Cancer

- A high number of moles, or large moles
- Fair skin, freckling, blond hair, or blue eyes
- Close relative with the disease
- Men with gene changes from a family history of breast or ovarian cancer
- Treatment with medications that suppress the immune system
- Too much exposure to UV radiation from sunlight, tanning lamps, or tanning booths
- Over age 50
- Xeroderma pigmentosus, a rare inherited disease in which people are less able to repair damage caused by sunlight
- Past history of melanoma

Younger patients and women have a somewhat better chance of survival. Patients with tumors on the scalp and neck have a lower survival rate.

Precursor Lesions

The three specific precursor lesions for the development of melanoma are congenital nevi, dysplastic nevi, and lentigo maligna. A precursor lesion is also called a premalignant lesion, a name that indicates that the lesion's risk of becoming malignant is greater than normal.

CONGENITAL NEVI Congenital nevi are present at birth. Some lesions are small; others are large enough to cover an entire body area. Their color can range from brown to black. They are often slightly raised, with an irregular surface and a fairly regular border.

DYSPLASTIC NEVI Dysplastic nevi are also called atypical moles. Although dysplastic nevi are not present at birth, they appear as normal nevi during childhood and become dysplastic (having abnormal development) after puberty. A patient with classic dysplastic nevi has more than 100 nevi, at least one of which is larger than 8 mm in diameter, and at least one of which has the characteristics of melanoma (asymmetry, irregular border, color variegation, and a diameter greater than 6 mm). A familial tendency to dysplastic nevi increases the risk for the development of melanoma. Having many moles, whether normal or atypical, is a risk factor for melanoma.

Dysplastic nevi most often appear on the face, trunk, and arms but also are seen on the scalp, female breast, groin, and buttocks. The pigmentation of the nevi is irregular, with mixtures of tan, brown, black, red, and pink. An area of lighter pigmentation is surrounded by a papular area of deeper pigmentation (described as a "fried egg appearance"). The borders of the nevi are irregular.

LENTIGO MALIGNA Lentigo maligna, also called Hutchinson's freckle, is a tan or black patch on the skin that looks like a freckle. It grows slowly, becoming mottled, dark, thick, and nodular. It is usually seen on one side of the face of an older adult who has had a large amount of sun exposure.

Classification

Melanomas are classified into different types. The major types are superficial spreading melanoma, lentigo maligna melanoma, nodular melanoma, and acral lentiginous melanoma. Each of these tumors is characterized by a radial and/or vertical growth phase. During the initial radial phase, which may last from 1 to 25 years (depending on the type), the melanoma grows parallel to the skin surface. During this phase, the tumor rarely metastasizes and is often curable by surgical excision. However, during the vertical growth phase, atypical melanocytes rapidly penetrate into the dermis and subcutaneous tissue, greatly increasing the risk for metastasis and death.

SUPERFICIAL SPREADING MELANOMA Superficial spreading melanoma is the most common type, comprising 70% to 80% of all melanomas (Porth & Matfin, 2009). The lesions are usually flat and scaly or crusty and are about 2 cm in diameter. They often arise from a preexisting nevus. This type of melanoma is found on the trunk and back of men and on the legs

of women. Superficial spreading melanomas occur more often in women than in men. The median age of occurrence is the 50s.

The radial growth phase lasts from 1 to 5 or more years. When the lesion enters the vertical growth phase, it grows rapidly, and its color changes from a mixture of tan, brown, and black to a characteristic red, white, and blue. The lesion also develops irregular borders and often has raised nodules and ulcerations (Figure 16–16 ■).

LENTIGO MALIGNA MELANOMA Lentigo maligna melanoma often arises from the precursor lesion, lentigo maligna. The lesions are large and tan with different shades of brown. This type of melanoma makes up 5% to 10% of malignant melanomas and is the least serious form (Porth & Matfin, 2009). It occurs on skin that has had long-term sun exposure, such as the face, neck, and sometimes the dorsal surface of the hands and lower extremities. Lentigo maligna melanoma affects women more than men. It is typically diagnosed in people in their 60s and 70s.

Lentigo maligna melanoma is characterized by a proliferation of atypical melanocytes parallel to the basal layer of the epidermis. The radial growth phase may last from 10 to 25 years, with the lesion growing to as large as 10 cm. The lesion becomes malignant as soon as the melanocytes invade the dermis. In the vertical growth phase, raised nodules may appear on the surface of the lesion. The lesion tends to acquire a freckled or mottled appearance.

NODULAR MELANOMA Nodular melanoma lesions are raised, dome-shaped, blue-black or red nodules on areas of the head, neck, and trunk that may or may not have been exposed to the sun. The lesions may look like a blood blister, or they may ulcerate and bleed. The lesions arise from unaffected skin rather than from a preexisting lesion. This type makes up 10% to 15% of malignant melanomas and is often diagnosed in people in their 50s (Porth & Matfin, 2009).

Nodular melanoma has only a vertical growth phase, but it grows aggressively during that phase. However, the absence of a radial growth phase makes this type more difficult to diagnose before it metastasizes.

ACRAL LENTIGINOUS MELANOMA Acral lentiginous melanoma, also called mucocutaneous melanoma, is less common in people with fair skin and more common in people with

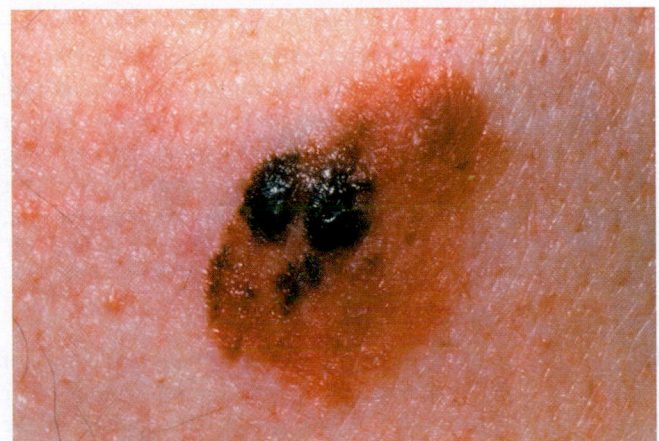

Figure 16–16 ■ Malignant melanoma is a serious skin cancer that arises from melanocytes.

dark skin. The lesions progress from tan, brown, or black flat lesions to elevated nodules and are about 3 cm in diameter. The radial phase lasts from 2 to 5 years, and the lesions are found on the palms of the hands, soles of the feet, the mucous membranes, and the nailbeds. Acral lentiginous melanoma affects both men and women equally and is most often diagnosed in people in their 50s and 60s.

Interdisciplinary Care

The management of the patient with melanoma begins with identification, diagnosis, and tumor staging. If treatable, the tumor is removed through surgical excision. Melanoma is also treated with chemotherapy, immunotherapy, and radiation therapy. Other therapies used with success include biological therapies with interleukin-2 and interferon and therapeutic vaccines containing melanoma antigens.

Identification

Melanoma is most often found on the trunk of men and on the lower extremities of women. Nevertheless, it is important for the patient to have a complete physical examination and total skin assessment. In addition to a visual examination of all skin surfaces, palpation of regional lymph nodes, the liver, and the spleen is essential to assess for metastasis when a melanoma is suspected or found.

A change in the color or size of a nevus is reported in 70% of people diagnosed with a melanoma. The ABCDE rule is used to assess suspicious lesions.

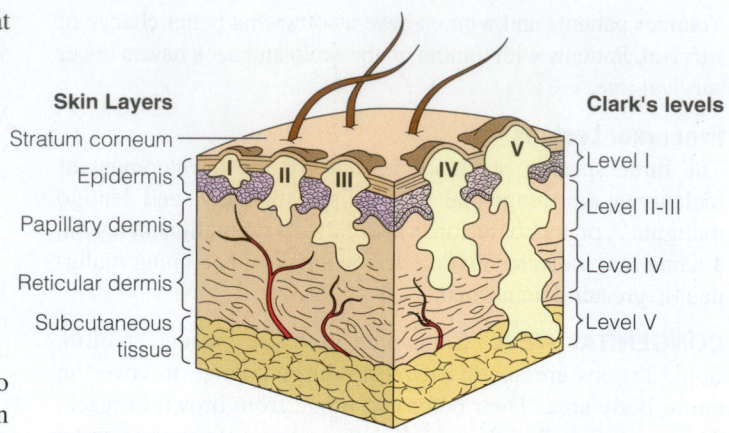

Figure 16–17 ■ Clark's levels for staging measure the invasion of a melanoma from the epidermis to the subcutaneous tissue.

> **FAST FACTS**
>
> **The ABCDE Rule + The Ugly Duckling Sign**
> Using the ABCDE rule to assess for melanoma:
> A = asymmetry (one half of the nevus does not match the other half)
> B = border irregularity (edges are ragged, blurred, or notched)
> C = color variation or dark black color
> D = diameter greater than 6 mm (size of a pencil eraser)
> E = evolving or changing
>
> The Ugly Duckling Sign = a mole that looks or feels different that other moles, or changes differently over time than other moles

Diagnosis

In addition to biopsy of any suspicious lesion, diagnostic tests are conducted to determine whether the tumor has metastasized. Because malignant melanoma may metastasize to any organ or tissue of the body, a variety of tests may be conducted, including microscopic examination, biopsy, and tests for metastasis (liver function tests and CT scan of the liver, a complete blood count, serum blood chemistry profile, chest x-ray, bone scan, and CT scan or MRI of the brain).

Microstaging

The term microstaging describes the assessment of the level of invasion of a malignant melanoma and the maximum tumor thickness. In one method, the Clark system of microstaging, the vertical growth of the lesion is measured from the epidermis to the subcutaneous tissue to determine the level of invasion (Figure 16–17 ■).

Treatments

Surgical excision is the preferred treatment for malignant melanoma. Other methods of treatment include chemotherapy, immunotherapy, and radiation therapy.

SURGERY   If a biopsy identifies the lesion as a melanoma, a wide excision is performed that includes the full thickness of the skin and subcutaneous tissue. Regional lymph nodes are the most common sites for metastasis of melanoma. Standard surgical treatment for clinically suspicious lymph node involvement includes excision of the primary lesions as well as surgical dissection of the involved lymph nodes. Surgery also is indicated for palliative management of isolated metastasis. Removal of metastatic tumors in the brain, liver, lung, gastrointestinal tract, or subcutaneous tissue may relieve symptoms and prolong life. (See the Case Study & Nursing Care Plan that follows.)

IMMUNOTHERAPY   Immunotherapy is a relatively new treatment modality for melanoma. The role of the immunologic response initially was recognized because of the numerous spontaneous remissions seen in patients with melanoma—a higher occurrence than with any other adult tumor. In addition, researchers have recently identified tumor-specific antigen-antibodies in patients with melanoma.

Agents such as interferons, interleukins, monoclonal antibodies, bacille Calmette-Guérin (BCG), levamisole, transfer factors, and tumor vaccines have shown activity in melanoma, with varying response rates. The effectiveness of these agents, used either alone, in combination with chemotherapy, or in combination with each other, is under investigation. The use of immunotherapy in the treatment of melanoma is still new and requires further investigation.

RADIATION THERAPY   Melanoma responds to higher dose radiation, especially if the tumor is small. Response rates to radiation therapy depend on the site of the tumor, the thickness of the tumor, the type of melanoma, and the patient's general health, but may range from 0% to 71%. Radiation frequently is used for palliation of symptoms resulting from metastasis to the brain, bone, lymph nodes, gastrointestinal tract, skin, or subcutaneous tissue. Liver and lung metastases are not treated with radiation therapy because a loss of organ function may result.

BIOLOGICAL THERAPY Biological therapy is used to boost or restore the ability of the immune system to fight the cancer. Agents used include the monoclonal antibodies, growth factors, and vaccines. These agents may also have a direct antitumor effect.

NEW METHODS OF TREATMENT Melanoma skin cancer research is ongoing and directed toward more specific methods of diagnosis and treatment. Examples are as follows:

- *Gene therapy:* Clinical trials are in progress to test the effectiveness of adding certain genes to the malignant cells.
- *Melanoma DNA research*: Genes such as CDKN2A (also known as $_p$16) have been found to be mutated in some families with a high rate of melanoma.
- *Staging*: Very sensitive new tests can better detect the spread of melanoma to lymph nodes and can possibly better identify people who could be helped by a treatment such as immunotherapy after surgery.

Nursing Care

Nurses have the opportunity to assess the skin of patients requiring care for many different health problems and may be the first healthcare provider to identify suspicious lesions. Wide excision and the high risk of metastasis from melanoma usually requires inpatient surgical treatment, with the nurse providing care and teaching. See the Evidence for Nursing Care box for selected resources related to the patient with malignant melanoma.

Health Promotion

The most important aspect of preventing melanoma is a health history and skin assessment. The ACS recommends that people between the ages of 20 and 40 see a skin specialist every 3 years and those over 40 have annual skin checkups. People with actinic keratoses should also have their skin checked regularly for any signs of change. Patients at risk (those with precancerous lesions and with personal risk factors), as well as those over the age of 40, should conduct a monthly skin self-examination (described in Box 16–7). When self-assessing for melanoma, the patient looks for a change in the following:

- Color, especially any lesion that becomes darker or variegated in shades of tan, brown, black, red, white, or blue
- Size, especially any lesion that becomes larger or spreads out

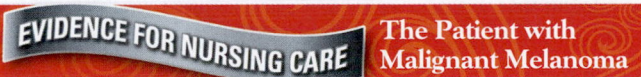

EVIDENCE FOR NURSING CARE The Patient with Malignant Melanoma

Selected resources that nurses may find helpful when planning evidence-based nursing care follow.
- Rubin, K. (2009). Management of metastatic melanoma: Nursing challenges today and tomorrow. *Clinical Journal of Oncology Nursing, 13*(1), 81–89.
- Torrens, R., & Swan, B. A. (2009). Promoting prevention and early recognition of malignant melanoma. *Dermatology Nursing, 21*(3), 115–22. Retrieved from http://www.dermatologynursing.net/ceonline/2011/article21115122.pdf
- Zimmerman, L., & Britton, K. (2009). Prevention through vigilance: Malignant melanoma management. *Nursing Management, 40*(6), 26–29. Retrieved from http://www.nursingcenter.com/prodev/ce_article.asp?tid=865443

- Shape, especially any lesion that protrudes more from the skin or begins to have an irregular outline
- Appearance of a lesion, especially bleeding, drainage, oozing, ulceration, crusting, scaliness, or development of a mushrooming outward growth
- Consistency, especially any lesion that becomes softer or is more easily irritated
- Skin around a lesion, such as redness, swelling, or leaking of color from a lesion into the surrounding skin
- Sensation, such as itching or pain

Assessment

Skin assessment is discussed in ∞ Chapter 15. Specific health history questions and assessments for skin cancer are outlined in Box 16–9.

Nursing Diagnoses and Interventions

Although many different nursing diagnoses may be appropriate for the patient with a melanoma, common responses are impaired skin integrity, hopelessness, and anxiety. These diagnoses are also appropriate for use with patients with nonmelanoma skin cancer.

Impaired Skin Integrity

Melanomas not only destroy skin layers but also invade body structures. Certain types of melanomas may ulcerate prior to diagnosis, and treatment typically involves some type of surgical biopsy and excision. Any open lesion or incision increases the risk for secondary infection.

- Monitor for manifestations of infection: fever, tachycardia, malaise, incisional erythema, swelling, pain, or drainage that increases or becomes purulent. *Intact skin is the first line of defense against infection; impaired skin integrity increases the risk for infection. If infection is present, the patient may have both systemic and local manifestations.*
- Keep the incision line clean and dry by changing dressings as necessary. *Moisture increases the risk of infection.*
- Follow principles of medical and surgical asepsis when caring for patient's incision. Teach family members and visitors the importance of careful hand hygiene. Maintain standard precautions if drainage is present. *Careful hand hygiene is essential in preventing the spread of infection. Aseptic techniques are necessary when caring for any surgical incision to prevent infection.*
- Encourage and maintain adequate caloric and protein intake in the diet. Suggest a consultation with the dietitian if the patient does not want to eat. *Adequate calories and protein are necessary for proper healing. The patient with cancer has increased metabolic needs; if these needs are not met, nutritional problems that impair healing may result.*

Hopelessness

Hopelessness is an emotional state in which a person feels that there is no possibility that life will improve. Patients who experience hopelessness are often withdrawn, passive, and apathetic.

The diagnosis of melanoma threatens the quality and quantity of life as the patient faces the possibility or reality of metastasis; the possibility that the cancer may recur and cause death; and alterations in self-concept, roles, and relationships. Inspiring hope in patients during this health crisis is a legitimate nursing action.

BOX 16–9 Nursing Assessment for Skin Cancer

Interview Questions

- Have any members of your family ever been treated for skin cancer?
- Have you had a skin cancer removed from any part of your body?
- Have you noticed any change in the size, shape, or color of a mole, wart, birthmark, or scar?
- Do you have any moles, warts, birthmarks, or scars that itch, are painful, have crusting, or bleed?
- In what parts of the country or world have you lived?
- Have you ever been badly sunburned?
- Do you visit tanning salons?
- Are you exposed to any hazardous chemicals in your job?
- Have you been taught how to examine your skin? If so, how do you do this examination? How often?

Physical Assessment

1. Ask the patient to remove all clothing and put on an examination gown. Ensure good light; natural, bright light is best for inspection of lesions. The patient may sit, stand, or lie down.
2. Inspect and palpate the skin. Stretching the skin tightly during assessment facilitates assessment of nodular and scaly lesions and lesions in the dermis. Assess for the following:
   a. Obvious lesions
   b. Visible swellings

   c. Alterations in normal contour and borders of nevi
   d. Enlarged lymph glands
   e. Skin or mucosal discolorations
   f. Areas of ulceration, scaling, crusting, or erosion.
3. The order of assessment follows:
   a. Head and neck: entire scalp, eyelids, external ear, auditory canals, external surface of the nose, internal surface of the nose, the oral cavity, facial skin, the facial glands (parotid, submaxillary, sublingual)
   b. Thyroid and neck, including lymph glands
   c. Chest and abdomen, with special attention under pendulous breasts, in skin folds, and in areas covered with hair
   d. Back and buttocks, with special attention to the area between the buttocks
   e. Extremities, with special attention to the axillae, nail beds, webs between the fingers and toes, and soles of the feet
   f. External genitals, with special attention to skin folds, mucous membranes, and areas covered with hair
4. Measure and record a description of all skin lesions on an anatomic chart. Take photographs (if possible) of any suspicious lesion, and include them in the patient's record for future reference.

- Provide an environment that encourages the patient to identify and express feelings, concerns, and goals:
  - Use active listening, ask open-ended questions, and reflect on the patient's statements.
  - Acknowledge and respect feelings of apathy and/or anger as expressions of distress.
  - Convey an empathetic understanding of the fears and concerns.
  - Provide opportunities to express positive emotions: hope, faith, a sense of purpose, and the will to live.
  - Explore the patient's perceptions, and modify or clarify them if necessary by providing information and correcting misconceptions.
  - Encourage the patient to identify support systems and sources of strength and coping in the past.
    Verbalizing feelings, concerns, and goals allows others to validate or correct them, promotes a therapeutic nurse–patient relationship, and fosters feelings of self-worth. Expressing positive emotions and calling on support systems and sources of strength that were effective in coping with past crises help the person resolve the crisis and develop hope.
- Encourage active participation in self-care as well as in mutual decision making and goal setting. *Meeting self-care needs and making decisions about care increase personal confidence in one's capacity for coping.*
- Encourage a focus not only on the present but also on the future: Review past occasions for hope, discuss the patient's personal meaning of hope, establish and evaluate short-term goals with the patient and family, and encourage them to express hope for the future. *The nurse mobilizes the patient's resources to strengthen motivation, hope, and the will to live.*

Anxiety

The intensity of anxiety, aroused by a perceived threat, depends on the severity of the present situation and the patient's ability to handle the threat. Anxiety is one of the most common psychosocial responses in patients with cancer. Anxiety increases at the time of diagnosis and remains a constant emotion throughout the course of treatment, regardless of treatment type or setting. Interventions center on helping the patient recognize the manifestations of anxiety, determining whether the patient wishes to do anything about the anxiety, and facilitating coping strategies.

- Provide reassurance and comfort:
  - Set aside time to sit quietly with the patient.
  - Speak slowly and calmly.
  - Convey empathetic understanding by touch and supporting present coping mechanisms, such as crying and talking.
  - Do not make demands or expect the patient to make decisions.

  Coping behaviors differ from situation to situation and from person to person. Anxiety at moderate to severe levels narrows perceptions and the ability to function.

- Decrease sensory stimuli by using short, simple sentences; focusing on the here and now; and providing concise information. *Higher levels of anxiety result in a focus on the present, inability to concentrate, and difficulty in understanding verbal communications.*
- Provide interventions that decrease anxiety levels and increase coping:
  - Provide accurate information about the illness, treatment, and expected length of recovery.
  - Encourage discussion of expected physical changes and ways to minimize disfigurement through cosmetics and clothing.

Geoff Sanders, aged 69, is retired from the postal service. He has always been an avid participant in outdoor sports: When he was younger he played baseball and tennis, and for the last 10 years he has played golf at least twice a week. He now lives in Connecticut, but as a younger man he lived in Florida for almost 15 years. Mr. Sanders has a variety of warts and moles and rarely pays attention to them. However, after taking a shower one day he noticed that a mole on his left lower leg looked bigger and darker. Mr. Sanders had just seen a public service announcement on television about the dangers of changes in moles, and he immediately called his primary care physician for an appointment at the dermatology clinic.

ASSESSMENT

On arriving at the clinic, Mr. Sanders is interviewed and examined by Tom Hall, a clinical nurse specialist. Following the assessment, Mr. Hall documents the following information.

Mr. Sanders has a family history of skin cancer; his father had several squamous cell cancers removed from his face. He has numerous nevi on his body; the one causing concern is located on the medial anterior left leg, 2 inches below the patella. Mr. Sanders states that the mole has been present for years but that he noticed just yesterday that it has become larger and darker. On further questioning, he states that the mole itches sometimes but has never hurt or bled. Mr. Sanders lived in Florida for 15 years and now experiences a sunburn early each summer before he tans. The sunburn involves the lower legs because Mr. Sanders wears shorts during his twice-weekly golf game.

A complete skin assessment reveals various freckles, warts, and nevi. With the exception of the nevus that prompted Mr. Sanders to come to the clinic, all lesions appear normal. The nevus in question is raised, 3 cm in diameter, with irregular borders and a nodular surface. It is variegated in color, with various shades of brown. The skin surrounding the nevus is slightly erythematous. Inguinal lymph nodes are not enlarged or painful. Mr. Hall takes a photograph of the lesion with Mr. Sanders's permission.

Following the assessment, Mr. Sanders discusses the lesion with a surgeon, who recommends excision. They discuss the possibility of skin cancer and the importance of early detection and treatment. Mr. Sanders is scheduled for a biopsy of the nevus under a local anesthetic the following morning. Following the biopsy, histologic examination reveals lentigo maligna melanoma. Staging of the tumor reveals that it is a melanoma *in situ*, with no metastasis to regional lymph nodes. Mr. Sanders undergoes a wide excision of the lesion the following afternoon.

DIAGNOSES

- *Impaired Skin Integrity* related to excision of melanoma from the left lower leg
- *Risk for Infection* related to surgical wound on left lower leg
- *Acute Pain* related to wide excision of melanoma on left lower leg
- *Anxiety* related to diagnosis of skin cancer

EXPECTED OUTCOMES

- Demonstrate complete healing of the incision without manifestations of infection.
- Verbalize relief of pain by the time the incision is healed.
- Verbalize fears and concerns about the diagnosis.

PLANNING AND IMPLEMENTATION

- Make the first dressing change, but ensure that Mr. Sanders can safely change the dressing himself prior to discharge the day after surgery.
- On discharge, provide adequate dressings and tape for the first home dressing change; include in discharge instructions necessary information about where to buy supplies and how many dressing supplies will be needed.
- Review and provide written instruction for prescribed systemic antibiotic and pain medication.
- Provide written instructions for dressing change, manifestations of infection, and phone number of clinic; stress importance of calling if any abnormal symptoms occur.
- Teach how to protect the incision from bumps and to protect the site from irritants.
- Discuss diagnosis, positive outlook for treatment of melanoma *in situ*, and the patient's concerns.
- Stress importance of lifelong regular healthcare evaluations to identify any recurrence or metastasis.

EVALUATION

Mr. Sanders returned to the dermatology clinic 1 week after his surgical incision. His incision is well approximated and shows no signs of infection. He is taking his antibiotic 4 times a day as prescribed and reports that his need for pain medications is decreasing. During his clinic visit the following week, Mr. Hall removes the sutures and assesses the wound as healed. Mr. Sanders completed his antibiotics and no longer requires pain medications. He says he is still "scared to death" about having cancer, but he has decided to join a local cancer support group. He also says he had gotten a list of skin safety rules from the American Cancer Society and will be sure to cover up and use sunscreens when he plays golf. Mr. Sanders makes an appointment for follow-up care in 3 months.

CRITICAL THINKING IN THE NURSING PROCESS

1. Consider reasons why people who notice a change in a skin lesion put off seeking health care. What can nurses do to effect change?
2. Design a teaching plan for young adults for preventing skin cancers.
3. What would you say to Mr. Sanders if he called the clinic and said that the antibiotics were making him sick and he didn't think he needed them anyway?
4. Design a nursing care plan for Mr. Sanders for the diagnosis *Powerlessness*.

See Evaluating Your Response in Appendix C.

- Include family members in teaching sessions.
- Encourage participation in care.

Although the prognosis and treatment of melanoma depend on various factors, the prognosis of complete cure is decreased with metastasis. Surgical incisions include excision with wide margins, which may cause disfigurement.

Active participation in care give the patient some control over the future and is often an effective means of coping with anxiety.

Using NANDA, NIC, and NOC

Linkages between a selected NANDA nursing diagnosis, NIC, and NOC for the patient with malignant melanoma are shown in the chart that follows.

Community-Based Care

Teaching the patient and family experiencing the diagnosis and treatment of melanoma focuses on self-care and ongoing self-monitoring. Education for the patient and family is specific to the type of treatment. In addition to wound care, patients who have had a lymph node dissection need instructions in how to protect the extremity from bleeding, trauma, and infection. Address the following topics:

- Schedule regular medical checkups every 3 months for the first 2 years, every 6 months for the next 5 years, and yearly thereafter.
- Proper self-care combined with regular medical care can help the patient lead a fairly normal life.
- If assistance for home care is necessary, provide referrals to a community health agency or a home care agency. In addition, refer the patient to a local cancer support group if desired. Other resources are the ACS, the Skin Cancer Foundation, and the National Cancer Institute.

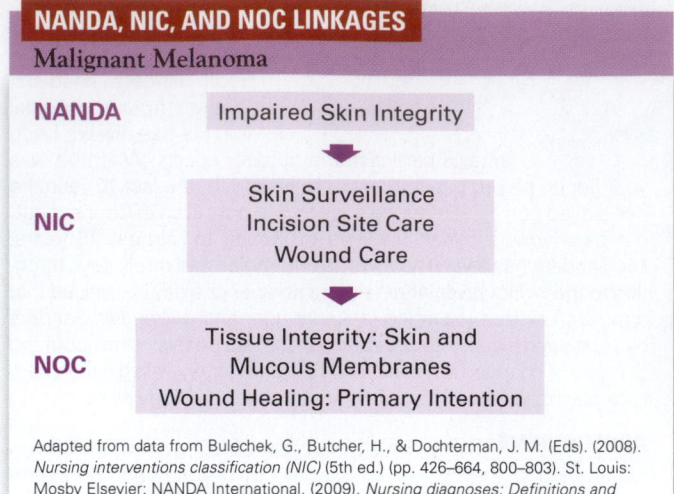

NANDA, NIC, AND NOC LINKAGES
Malignant Melanoma

NANDA → Impaired Skin Integrity

NIC → Skin Surveillance / Incision Site Care / Wound Care

NOC → Tissue Integrity: Skin and Mucous Membranes / Wound Healing: Primary Intention

Adapted from data from Bulechek, G., Butcher, H., & Dochterman, J. M. (Eds). (2008). *Nursing interventions classification (NIC)* (5th ed.) (pp. 426–664, 800–803). St. Louis: Mosby Elsevier; NANDA International. (2009). *Nursing diagnoses: Definitions and classification 2009-2011. Oxford, UK: Wiley-Blackhead;* and Moorhead; S., Johnson, M., Maas, M., & Swanson, E. (Eds). (2008). *Nursing outcomes classification (NOC)* (4th ed.) (pp. 699–700, 730–731). St. Louis: Mosby Elsevier.

Skin Trauma

Trauma to the skin can be unintentional or intentional (as in the case of surgery). Chemicals, radiation, pressure, or thermal changes cause skin trauma. This section discusses pressure ulcers and frostbite, as well as intentional trauma from cutaneous and plastic surgery or treatment. Thermal injury, or burns, is discussed in ∞ Chapter 17.

The Patient with a Pressure Ulcer

Pressure ulcers are ischemic lesions of the skin and underlying tissues caused by unrelieved pressure that impairs the flow of blood and lymph. The ischemia causes tissue necrosis and eventual ulceration. These ulcers, also called bed sores or decubitus ulcers, tend to develop over a bony prominence (such as the heels, greater trochanter, sacrum, and ischia), but they may appear on the skin of any part of the body subjected to external pressure, friction, or shearing forces.

Incidence

The increasing incidence of pressure ulcers in all healthcare settings, but especially in hospitals and long-term care facilities, has resulted in infection, loss of function, and pain for patients. These complications, in turn, have caused increased length of stay and costs. As a result, the Centers for Medicare and Medicaid will no longer make additional reimbursement payments to hospitals to cover the cost of pressure ulcers developed during a hospital stay.

FAST FACTS
Pressure Ulcers
- The incidence of pressure ulcers in hospitals is approximately 8%; the incidence in long-term care ranges from 2.4% to 23%.
- An estimated 60,000 patients die each year from pressure ulcer complications.
- The cost of treating these chronic wounds is about $11 billion a year.

(Ayello & Lyder, 2007; Porth & Matfin, 2009).

The prevention and treatment of pressure ulcers is a public health issue. The national health policy statement *Healthy People 2010* set a target of a 50% decrease in the prevalence of pressure ulcers in long-term care residents. The National Institute for Healthcare Improvement (NHI) has made preventing pressure ulcers one of 12 interventions to save lives. The NHI recommendations are described in the nursing care section that follows. Pressure ulcers are preventable, with nursing care being a major part of prevention.

Pathophysiology

Pressure ulcers develop from external pressure that compresses blood vessels or from friction and shearing forces that tear and injure vessels. Both types of pressure cause traumatic injury and initiate the process of pressure ulcer development.

External pressure that is greater than capillary pressure and arteriolar pressure interrupts blood flow in capillary beds. When pressure is applied to skin over a bony prominence for 2 hours, tissue ischemia and hypoxia from external pressure cause irreversible tissue damage. For example, when the body is in the supine position, the body's weight applies pressure to the sacrum. The same amount of pressure causes more damage when it is applied to a small area than when it is distributed over a large surface.

Shearing forces result when one tissue layer slides over another. The stretching and bending of blood vessels cause injury and thrombosis. Patients in hospital beds are subject to shearing forces when the head of the bed is elevated and the torso slides down toward the foot of the bed. Pulling the patient up in bed also subjects the patient to shearing forces. (For this reason, always lift patients up in bed). In both cases, friction and moisture cause the skin and superficial fascia to remain fixed to the bed sheet, while the deep fascia and bony skeleton slides in the direction of body movement.

When a person lies or sits in one position for an extended length of time without moving, pressure on the tissue between a bony prominence and the external surface of the body distorts capillaries and interferes with normal blood flow. If the pressure is relieved, blood flow to the area increases, and a brief period of reactive hyperemia occurs without permanent damage. However, if the pressure continues, platelets aggregate in the endothelial cells surrounding the capillaries and form microthrombi. These microthrombi impede blood flow, resulting in ischemia and hypoxia of tissues. Eventually, the cells and tissues of the immediate area of pressure and of the surrounding area die and become necrotic.

Alterations in the involved tissue depend on the depth of the injury. Injury to superficial layers of skin results in blister formation, whereas injury to deeper structures causes the pressure ulcer area to appear dark reddish-blue. As the tissues die, the ulcer becomes an open wound that may be deep enough to expose the muscles and bone. The necrotic tissue elicits an inflammatory response, and the patient experiences increases in temperature, pain, and white blood cell count. Secondary bacterial invasion is common. Enzymes from bacteria and macrophages dissolve necrotic tissue, resulting in a foul-smelling drainage.

Pressure ulcers are staged to classify the degree of tissue damage. The updated stages from the National Pressure Ulcer Advisory Panel (2007) are listed in Box 16–10.

BOX 16–10 NPUAP's Updated Pressure Ulcer Staging

STAGE I

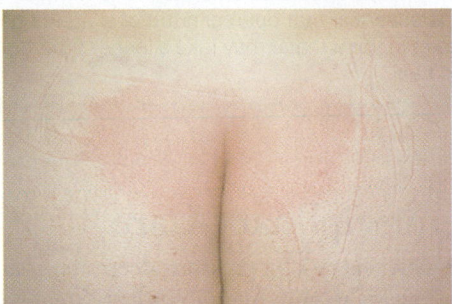

A sign of risk. Intact skin with nonblanchable redness of a localized area, usually over a bony prominence. The area may be painful, firm, soft, warmer or cooler than adjacent tissue. May be difficult to detect in people with dark skin.

STAGE II

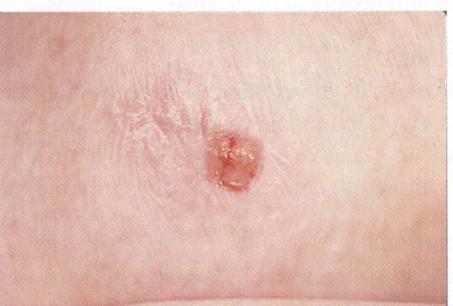

Partial thickness loss of dermis presenting as a shallow open ulcer with a red or pink wound bed. May also present as an intact or open blister. The ulcer may shiny or dry, without bruising or slough (loss of tissue).

STAGE III

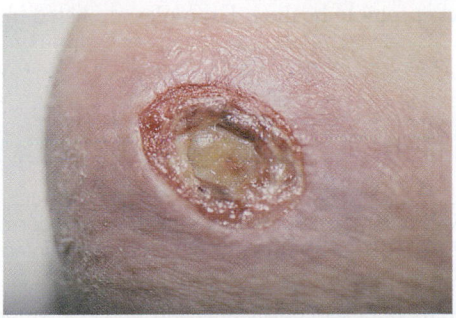

Full-thickness tissue loss. Subcutaneous fat may be visible but bone, tendon, or muscle are *not* exposed. Slough may be present but does not obscure the depth of tissue loss. *May* include undermining and tunneling.

STAGE IV

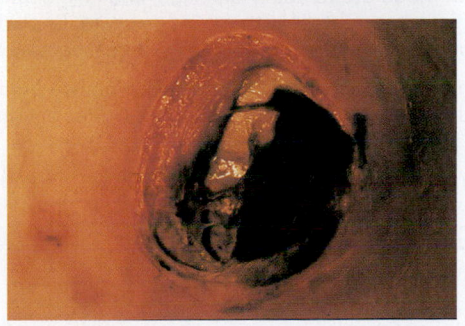

Full-thickness skin loss with exposed bone, tendon or muscle. Slough or eschar (dead tissue such as a scab) may be present on some parts of the wound bed. Often includes undermining and tunneling.

Source: Text is from *Pressure Ulcers in Adults: Prediction and Prevention* by the Agency for Health Care Policy and Research, 1992 Rockville, MD: US Department of Health and Human Services. Photos courtesy of Karen Lou Kennedy, RN, FPN, www.kennedyterminalulcer.com.

Pressure Ulcer Prevention

Older adults are at a greater risk for developing pressure ulcers because of age-related changes in the integumentary system. Cell renewal slows, resulting in skin that has decreased elasticity. The margin between the epidermis and the dermis separates more easily, making the skin more prone to tearing. In addition, thinning subcutaneous tissue provides less cushioning over bony prominences. Water content decreases, and the skin becomes drier. These changes increase the older adult's susceptibility to skin trauma and prolong wound healing.

Chronic conditions associated with immobility and self-care deficit place older adults at risk of developing pressure ulcers. For example, bowel or bladder incontinence can produce regions of wet skin that are prone to infections and breakdown. Furthermore, sensory-perceptual alterations and impaired cognitive functioning may reduce the frequency with which the older adult shifts position when sitting or lying in bed. Finally, undernutrition, which is often seen in older adults, heightens the risk for developing pressure ulcers.

To prevent pressure ulcers, the skin of older adults should be kept clean, dry, and well hydrated. Moisturizers are recommended to keep the skin free of excessive dryness. Older adults should be taught to avoid bumping into furniture and to wear long skirts or pants to help protect the lower extremities from trauma.

When hospitalized, older adults should have a validated risk assessment for pressure ulcers completed on admission and as often as the tool suggests. A daily systematic skin inspection with particular attention to bony prominences should be completed.

Once pressure ulcers develop in older adults, the treatment is the same as for younger patients. However, additional steps may need to be taken. Because local perfusion to tissues is compromised, steps should be taken to prevent under- or overhydration. It is essential that optimal nutritional status be maintained. Also, keep in mind that it may take a longer time for the pressure ulcer to heal.

Risk Factors

Although a pressure ulcer may develop in an adult of any age who has an impairment in mobility, those most at risk are older adults with limited mobility and fractured hips, people with quadriplegia, and patients in the critical care setting (Porth & Matfin, 2009). Other patients prone to develop pressure ulcers are those with fractures of large bones (e.g., hip or femur) or who have undergone orthopedic surgery or sustained spinal cord injury. In addition to deficits in mobility and activity, incontinence and nutritional deficit also increase the risk of pressure ulcer development. Patients with chronic illnesses, such as renal failure and anemia, and those with edema or infection are also at increased risk. See nursing care of the older adult above for information about preventing pressure ulcer development in older adults.

Interdisciplinary Care

For the patient at risk for pressure ulcers, the goal is prevention. Existing ulcers require interdisciplinary treatment to promote healing and restore skin integrity.

Diagnosis

Diagnostic tests are conducted to determine the presence of a secondary infection and to differentiate the cause of the ulcer. If the ulcer is deep or appears infected, drainage or biopsied tissue is cultured to determine the causative organism.

Medications

Topical and systemic antibiotics specific to the infectious organism eradicate any infection present. Additionally, a variety of products promote healing. Examples are listed in Table 16–2.

TABLE 16–2 Products Used to Treat Pressure Ulcers

PRODUCT	PURPOSE
Hydrocolloid Dressings (such as DuoDerm)	May be used for stages I, II, III, and IV with minimal exudate. Forms a gel when coming into contact with wound exudate. Forms an occlusive barrier over the ulcer while maintaining a moist environment and preventing infection. Helps prevent friction and shear.
Alginate Dressings (such as SilvaSorb and Sorbsan)	May be used for stages II, III, and IV with moderate to heavy drainage, and in infected and non-infected wounds. Forms a gel when coming into contact with wound exudate. Should not be applied to dry or minimally draining wounds, as dehydration and delay in healing may result.
Hydrofibers (such as Aquacel)	May be used for stage II, III, and IV with moderate to heavy exudate. Can be used with actual or risk for infection. Combines the absorption of the hydrofiber with 1.2% silver as an antimicrobial agent.
Hydrogel Dressings (such as Intrasite gel)	May be used for stages II, III, IV. Rehydrate the wound bed and decrease pain. Promotes autolytic debridement.
Transparent Adhesive Dressings (such as OpSite and Tegrderm)	May be used in shallow I, II, and III ulcers. Provide a moist wound setting, prevent infection, and promote re-epithelialization. Minimize friction and shear.
Wet-to-Dry Dressings	Provide mechanical debridement.
Vacuum-assisted closure (VAC) sponges	Stimulate wound contracture while removing the exudate and wound edema.

Surgical Treatment

Surgical debridement may be necessary if the pressure ulcer is deep, if subcutaneous tissues are involved, or if an eschar has formed over the ulcer, preventing healing by granulation. Large wounds may require skin grafting for complete closure.

Nursing Care

The patient with one or more pressure ulcers not only has impaired skin integrity but also is at increased risk for infection, pain, and decreased mobility. Pressure ulcers prolong treatment for other health problems, increase healthcare costs, and diminish the patient's quality of life. See the nursing research box below for information on evidence-based interventions.

Nursing Diagnoses and Interventions

The following interventions and rationales are adapted from the clinical guidelines developed by the Agency for Health Care Policy and Research (1992, 1994) in identifying adults at risk and treating those with stage I pressure ulcers.

Risk for Impaired Skin Integrity

- Identify at-risk individuals needing prevention and the specific factors placing them at risk.
- Assess bed- and chair-bound patients, as well as those who are unable to reposition themselves, for additional risk factors: immobility, incontinence, nutritional factors (such as inadequate dietary intake and impaired nutritional status), and altered level of consciousness.
- Assess patients on admission to acute care and rehabilitation hospitals, nursing homes, home care programs, and other healthcare facilities.

- Use a systematic risk assessment by using a validated risk assessment tool (such as the Braden scale). See the information about predicting risk and using the Braden scale at the Nursing Center website (Stotts & Gunning berg, 2007).
- Document all assessments of risk. *Individuals at risk for pressure ulcers must be identified so that risk factors can be reduced through intervention. The primary risk factors for pressure ulcers are immobility and limited activity; therefore, assess patients who cannot reposition themselves or whose activity is limited to bed or chair. Validated tools ensure systematic evaluation of individual risk factors. The patient requires periodic reassessment for pressure ulcers. Accurate and complete documentation of all risk assessments ensures continuity of care and may be used as a foundation for the skin care plan.*
- Conduct a systematic skin inspection at least once a day, paying particular attention to the bony prominences. Systematic, comprehensive, and routine skin care may decrease pressure ulcer incidence Inspect the following to assess a pressure ulcer:
  - Location of any lesion or ulcer
  - Estimation of the stage
  - Dimensions of the ulcer: length, width, depth
  - Presence of any abnormal pathways in the wound:
  - Sinus tract: a cavity or channel underneath the wound
- Tunneling: a passageway or opening that may be visible at skin level, but with most of the tunnel under the surface of the skin
- Undermining: areas of tissue destruction underneath intact skin along wound margins
- Visible necrotic tissue (Slough is necrotic tissue that is in the process of separating from viable tissue.)
- Presence of an exudate

MOVING EVIDENCE INTO ACTION — **Preventing Pressure Ulcers in Acute Care and Home Care Settings**

Despite advances in health care to extend life and improve functional status, older adults with chronic illnesses are at increased risk of developing pressure ulcers. The older adult, with age-related compromised cellular activity is especially vulnerable to impaired healing of injured tissue such as pressure ulcers. This article (Frantz, 2004) describes an evidence-based protocol designed to enhance the healing of pressure ulcers in older patients by using evidence-based interventions. The following interventions are recommended:

- Assess all individuals admitted to a healthcare facility with a pressure ulcer for the risk of developing additional pressure ulcers by using a standardized risk assessment scale.
- Perform a complete history and physical examination, combined with a detailed assessment of the ulcer characteristics (location, stage, type of tissue, presence of tunneling or tracts, exudate, odor, and condition of skin around the ulcer).
- Remove necrotic tissue and debris from the ulcer to decrease the growth of bacteria and remove foreign materials, such as exudates and metabolic wastes.
- Provide a moist wound environment to promote reepithelialization and healing.
- Control bacterial levels in the wound by using cleansing and debridment, as well as systemic and topical antibiotics.
- Supply essential substrates for tissue repair, including protein, calories, vitamins, and minerals. Maintain a positive nitrogen balance.
- Manage tissue loads by positioning to avoid external force on the ulcer.

IMPLICATIONS FOR NURSING

The design and implementation of a pressure ulcer prevention and treatment plan is essential for any person at risk, including older adults, those with debilitating or multiple illnesses, and those with health problems limiting mobility. To effectively implement a plan, it is important to prepare providers to use a standard protocol through educational programs, and to monitor indicators of improvement or deterioration in the ulcer and presence or absence of new ulcers. These outcomes should be assessed and recorded on a weekly basis.

CRITICAL THINKING IN PATIENT CARE

1. Describe the differences and similarities in a pressure ulcer prevention plan of care you would develop for two patients: a 76-year-old man in a nursing home who has had a stroke that paralyzed his left side, and a 36-year-old man with a spinal cord injury from a motorcycle accident who cannot walk and lives at home.
2. Consider the activities to treat pressure ulcers, and answer the following:
   a. What level of healthcare provider would you delegate to care for the patient?
   b. How much time in an 8-hour period would be needed for nursing care?
3. What would you teach family caregivers about providing care at home?

- Presence or absence of granulation tissue
  Skin inspection provides data the nurse uses in designing interventions to reduce risk and in evaluating outcomes of those interventions.
- Clean the skin at the time of soiling and at routine intervals, as frequently as the patient's need or preference dictates. Avoid hot water, use a mild cleansing agent, and clean the skin gently, applying as little force and friction as possible. *Metabolic wastes and environmental contaminants accumulate on the skin; these potentially irritating substances should be removed frequently. Feces and urine cause chemical irritation and should be removed as soon as possible. Hot water may cause skin injury. Mild cleansing agents are less likely to remove the skin's natural barrier.*
- Minimize environmental factors leading to skin drying, such as low humidity and exposure to cold. Treat dry skin with moisturizers. *Well-hydrated skin resists mechanical trauma. Hydration decreases as the ambient air temperature decreases, especially when the air humidity is low. Poorly hydrated skin is less pliable, and severe dryness is associated with fissuring and cracking of the stratum corneum. Moisturizers reduce dry skin.*
- Avoid massage over bony prominences. *Although massage has been practiced for years, evidence now suggests that massage over bony prominences may lead to deep tissue trauma in patients at risk for or with beginning skin manifestations of a pressure ulcer.*
- Minimize skin exposure to moisture due to incontinence, perspiration, or wound drainage. When these sources of moisture cannot be controlled, use underpads or briefs made of materials that absorb moisture and present a quick-drying surface to the skin. Change underpads and briefs frequently. Do not place plastic directly against the skin. *Moisture from incontinence, perspiration, or wound drainage may contain factors that irritate the skin; moisture alone can increase the susceptibility of the skin to injury.*
- To minimize skin injury due to friction and shearing forces, use proper positioning, transferring, and turning techniques. Lubricants (such as cornstarch or creams), protective films (such as transparent dressings and skin sealants), protective dressings (such as hydrocolloids), and protective padding may also reduce friction injuries. *Shear injury occurs when skin remains stationary and the underlying tissue shifts. This shift diminishes the blood supply to the skin and results in ischemia and tissue damage. Proper positioning, however, can eliminate most shear injuries. Friction injuries to the skin occur when it moves across a coarse surface, such as bed linens. Most friction injuries can be avoided by using appropriate techniques to move patients so that their skin is never dragged across the linens. Any agent that eliminates contact or decreases the friction between the skin and the linens reduces the potential for injury.*
- Assess factors involved in inadequate dietary intake of protein or kilocalories. Offer nutritional supplements, and support the patient during mealtimes. If dietary intake remains inadequate, consult with a dietitian about other dietary interventions. *The role nutrition plays in the development of (and to a lesser degree, the healing of) pressure ulcers is not understood, but poor dietary intake of kilocalories, protein, and iron has been associated with the development of pressure ulcers.*
- Maintain the patient's current level of activity, mobility, and range of motion. *Frequent turning, repositioning, and movement are essential in reducing the risk of pressure ulcers.*
- For the patient on bed rest or who is immobile, provide interventions against the adverse effects of external mechanical forces of pressure, friction, and shear:
  - Reposition all at-risk patients at least every 2 hours, using a written schedule for systematic turning and repositioning.
  - For patients on bed rest, use positioning devices, such as pillows or foam wedges, to protect bony prominences.
- For completely immobile patients, use devices to totally relieve pressure on the heels (the most common method is to raise the heels off the bed). Do not use donut-type devices.
- Avoid placing patients in the side-lying position directly on the trochanter.
- Maintain the head of the bed at the lowest degree of elevation consistent with the patient's medical condition and other restrictions. Limit the amount of time the head of the bed is elevated.
- Use assistive devices, such as a trapeze or bed linen, to move patients in bed who cannot assist during transfers and position changes.
- Place any at-risk patient on a pressure-reducing device, such as foam, static air, alternating air, gel, or water mattress. *Data indicate that the more spontaneous movements that bedridden, older adult patients make, the lower the incidence of pressure ulcers and that fewer pressure ulcers develop in at-risk patients who are turned every 2 to 3 hours. Proper positioning can reduce pressure on bony prominences. It is difficult to redistribute pressure under heels; suspending the heels is the best method. Donut cushions are more likely to cause than to prevent pressure ulcers. Shearing forces are exerted on the body when the head of the bed is elevated. Lifting (rather than dragging) is less likely to cause injury from friction. Pressure-reducing devices and beds can decrease the incidence of pressure ulcers.*
- For chair-bound patients, use pressure-reducing devices. Consider postural alignment, distribution of weight, balance and stability, and pressure relief when positioning these patients. Avoid uninterrupted sitting in a chair or wheelchair. Reposition the patient every hour. Teach patients who can do so to shift their weight every 15 minutes. Use a written plan for positioning, movement, and the use of positioning devices. Do not use donut devices. *Prolonged, uninterrupted mechanical pressure results in tissue breakdown. The patient's weight should be shifted at least every hour.*

Community-Based Care

Patient and family teaching for care of a pressure ulcer also focuses on prevention and includes much of the same information presented in the preceding section. Because many patients with pressure ulcers are older or have other serious illnesses, a caregiver may require teaching on such topics as the following:

- Definition and description of pressure ulcers
- Common locations of pressure ulcers
- Risk factors for the development of pressure ulcers

- Skin care
- Ways to avoid injury
- Diet

Depending on the stage of the pressure ulcer, the nurse teaches the patient or caregiver how to care for ulcers that are already present: how to change wet-to-dry dressings, apply skin barriers, and avoid injury and infection. Referrals to a home health agency or community health department can help the family through the lengthy healing process.

The Patient with Frostbite

Frostbite is an injury of the skin from freezing. If the exposure to freezing temperatures is limited, only the skin and subcutaneous tissues become involved. However, as exposure increases, deeper structures freeze. The skin freezes when the temperature drops to 14°F to 24.8°F (210°C to 24°C). Frostbite is most common on exposed or peripheral areas of the body, such as the nose, ears, feet, and hands.

As human tissues freeze, ice crystals form and increase intracellular sodium content. Small blood vessels initially vasoconstrict but then vasodilate and become more permeable, causing cellular and tissue swelling. With continued exposure, vasoconstriction and increased viscosity of the blood cause infarction and necrosis of the affected tissue.

Superficial frostbite causes numbness, itching, and prickling. The skin appears cyanotic, reddened, or white. Deeper frostbite causes stiffness and paresthesias. As the skin and tissues thaw, the skin becomes white or yellow and loses its elasticity. The patient experiences burning pain. Edema, blisters, necrosis, and gangrene may appear.

Rapid thawing may significantly decrease tissue necrosis. General guidelines for rewarming areas of frostbite follow:

- If you are outdoors, treat superficial frostbite by applying firm pressure with a warm hand or by placing frostbitten hands in the axillae. If the feet are frostbitten, remove wet footwear, dry the feet, and put on dry footwear. Do not rub the areas with snow.
- In the hospital, rapidly rewarm affected areas in circulating warm water, 104°F to 105°F (40°C to 40.5°C) for 20 to 30 minutes. Do not rub or massage the areas.

Following rewarming, the patient is kept on bed rest with the affected parts elevated. Pain medications and anti-inflammatory agents are administered. Blisters are debrided. Whirlpool therapy may be used to clean the skin and debride necrotic tissue. Recovery from frostbite is usually complete if the involved area has not become necrotic. Necrotic tissue may require amputation.

The Patient Undergoing Cutaneous and Plastic Surgery

Although many skin disorders are so small and benign that no treatment is necessary, others require some type of surgery of the skin to remove the lesion. Other surgeries and treatments for skin lesions and deformities are used to restore function and change appearance. This section discusses both cutaneous and plastic surgery, as well as other types of treatment modalities used in the care of the patient with a skin disorder.

Cutaneous Surgery and Procedures

The basic types of cutaneous surgery described here are excision, electrosurgery, cryosurgery, curettage, and laser surgery. Two nonsurgical procedures, chemical destruction and sclerotherapy, are also discussed. Most of these procedures are performed in the office or outpatient clinic.

Fusiform Excision

Fusiform excision is the removal of a full thickness of the epidermis and dermis, usually with a thin layer of subcutaneous tissue. It is used to remove tissue for biopsies and for complete removal of benign and malignant lesions of the skin. Excision of small, superficial lesions is performed under a local anesthetic, and care is taken to place the incision in a way that will provide good cosmetic results.

Electrosurgery

Electrosurgery involves the destruction or removal of tissue with high-frequency alternating current. A variety of surgical procedures may be performed, including *electrodesiccation* (which produces superficial skin destruction), *electrocoagulation* (which produces deeper tissue destruction), and *electrosection* (which can cut through skin and tissue). Electrodesiccation is used to remove benign surface lesions, such as skin tags, keratoses, warts, and angiomas. It is also used to produce hemostasis for capillary bleeding. Electrocoagulation is used to remove telangiectases, warts, and superficial nonmelanoma skin cancers. Electrosection is used to make incisions, excise tissue, and perform biopsies.

Cryosurgery

Cryosurgery is the destruction of tissue by cold or freezing with agents such as fluorocarbon sprays, carbon dioxide snow, nitrous oxide, and liquid nitrogen. Cryosurgery is used to treat many skin lesions. The freezing agents are applied topically to the lesion. The effects depend on the degree of freeze. Light freezing causes damage to the epidermis with blistering or crusting that heals without scarring. Deeper freezes, used to treat malignant cells, cause edema, necrosis, and tissue slough. The effects of cryosurgery may not be obvious until 24 hours following the treatment. Postoperatively, infection is prevented by applying a topical antibiotic and keeping the treated areas clean. Healing occurs in 2 to 3 weeks.

Curettage

Curettage is the removal of lesions with a curette (a semisharp cutting instrument). It is used to remove benign and malignant superficial epidermal lesions. Benign lesions removed include keratoses, nevi, and angiomas. Nonmelanoma skin lesions are removed by curettage if they are small, well-defined, primary tumors. Curettage is also used to remove specimens of tissue for biopsy.

Following curettage, the wound may be treated with electrodesiccation to destroy any remaining malignant cells and to provide hemostasis. These wounds are not closed; rather, they are left open to heal by second intention. Topical antibiotic ointments and dressings may be used in the postoperative period.

Laser Surgery

Laser surgery is used to treat a variety of skin disorders. A laser is an intense light that produces a thermal injury on contact with tissue. The injury causes coagulation, vaporization, excision, and ablation (removal of a growth). Argon, pulsed dye, carbon dioxide, and Nd:YAG lasers are used in cutaneous and plastic surgery. A local anesthetic may be used, although pulsed dye laser causes minimal pain and rarely requires anesthesia.

Chemical Destruction

Chemical destruction is the application of a specific chemical to produce destruction of skin lesions. Chemical destruction is used to treat both benign and premalignant lesions. The chemical is applied to the lesion or is used to cause peeling. After application, the treated area forms a thin crust that sloughs off in about a week.

Sclerotherapy

Sclerotherapy is the removal of benign skin lesions with a sclerosing agent that causes inflammation with fibrosis of tissue. Agents that cause therapeutic sclerosis include aethoxysklerol (Sclerodex) and hypertonic sodium chloride. This type of treatment is used for telangiectases and superficial spider veins of the lower extremities. The solution is injected into the affected veins, causing a reaction that closes the lumen of the vein.

Plastic Surgery

Plastic surgery is the alteration, replacement, or restoration of visible portions of the body, performed to correct a structural or cosmetic defect. The word *plastic* comes from the Greek word *plastikos*, which means "able to be molded."

Many skin disorders discussed in this chapter cause changes in appearance. For example, acne may leave deep pitting scars, nevi and keloids are often disfiguring, and skin cancers may require wide excision and skin grafting. These scars, lesions, and wounds often cause embarrassment and alterations in body image. In addition, the removal of lesions may leave unsightly scars or areas of obviously missing tissue.

Cosmetic surgery involves procedures to enhance the attractiveness of normal features. There were almost 12 million surgical and nonsurgical cosmetic procedures performed in 2007 (American Society for Aesthetic Plastic Surgery, 2009). The most frequently performed procedures were Botox injections, liposuction, breast augmentation, and laser hair removal. Reconstructive surgery uses similar techniques; however, its purpose is to improve the function or appearance of parts of the body damaged by trauma, disease, or birth defects.

Many of the plastic surgeries permanently alter body image. To provide the patient with a preview of what surgery will accomplish, some surgeons integrate computer imaging into preoperative teaching. The computer projects a photograph of the targeted area onto a monitor and uses graphics to demonstrate how the size and or shape of the body part or area will change as a result of the surgery.

Skin Grafts and Flaps

Skin grafts and flaps are used to restore function while also maintaining an acceptable appearance. Both of these procedures involve the movement of skin from one part of the body to another part.

A **skin graft** is a surgical method of detaching skin from a donor site and placing it in a recipient site, where it develops a new blood supply from the base of the wound. Skin grafting is an effective way to cover wounds that have a good blood supply, that are not infected, and in which bleeding can be controlled.

Skin grafts may be either split thickness or full thickness. A split-thickness graft contains epidermis and only a portion of dermis of the donor site. A common donor site for a skin graft is the anterior thigh. Skin is removed in sheets from the donor site with a dermatome. A full-thickness graft contains both epidermis and dermis. These layers contain the greatest number of skin elements (sweat glands, sebaceous glands, or hair follicles) and are best able to withstand trauma. Areas of thin skin are the best donor sites for full-thickness skin grafts. The donor site must be surgically closed and will scar.

A skin flap is a piece of tissue whose free end is moved from a donor site to a recipient site while maintaining a continuous blood supply through its connection at the base or pedicle. Flaps carry their own blood supply and are therefore used to cover recipient sites that have a poor blood supply or have sustained a major tissue loss. They are often used for reconstruction or closure of large wounds. Microsurgical techniques, with anastomosis of small blood vessels and nerves, allow reconstruction with free flaps (in which the flap is completely removed from its donor site and moved to the recipient site).

Chemical Peeling

Chemical peeling is the application of a chemical to produce a controlled and predictable injury that alters the anatomy of the epidermis and superficial dermis. The result is skin that appears firmer, smoother, and less wrinkled. This form of cosmetic surgery is more useful in people who have fair, thin skin with fine wrinkling. Chemical agents used for peeling include phenol, trichloroacetic acid (TCA), and alpha-hydroxy acids (AHA).

Liposuction

Liposuction is a method of changing the contours of the body by aspirating fat from the subcutaneous layer of tissue. This treatment is used to remove excess fat from the buttocks, flanks, abdomen, thighs, upper arms, knees, ankles, and chin. It is not a cure for obesity and should not be used as a substitute for weight loss. The procedure is usually done for younger patients because their skin is more elastic. Liposuction may be performed on either an outpatient or inpatient basis.

To aspirate the fat, a small incision is made close to the area, and a suction cannula or curette is inserted and attached to a suction apparatus. The high vacuum pressure caused by the suction machine causes fat cells to emulsify, and they are aspirated out of the body. Following removal of the fat, a pressure dressing is applied to help the skin conform to the new tissue size.

Dermabrasion

Dermabrasion is a method of removing facial scars, severe acne, and pigment from unwanted tattoos. The area is sprayed with a chemical to cause light freezing and is then abraded with sandpaper or a revolving wire brush to remove the epidermis and a portion of the dermis.

Facial Cosmetic Surgery

Many different reconstructive surgeries may be performed to correct deformities or improve cosmetic appearance. Those discussed here are rhinoplasty, blepharoplasty, and rhytidectomy (face-lift).

- A rhinoplasty is conducted to improve the appearance of the external nose. The nasal skeleton is reshaped, and the overlying skin and subcutaneous tissue are allowed to redrape over the new framework. A submucous resection of the nasal septum is often done at the same time; this surgery resects a segment of the septal cartilage to improve the nasal airway and also to alter the appearance of the nose. This surgery is done through incisions within the nose, so no visible scars remain after healing.
- A blepharoplasty is a cosmetic surgery in which loose skin and protruding periorbital fat is removed from the upper and lower eyelids. With aging, the eyelid skin sags, allowing the periorbital fat to bulge; the skin of the upper eyelid can be so lax that it partially obstructs vision. The procedure is performed under local anesthesia, and excess skin and fat are excised. The incision is made in the normal eyelid lines so that scars are not visible after healing.
- A rhytidectomy, or face-lift, is a cosmetic surgery done to improve appearance by removing excess skin (and sometimes fat) from the face and neck. As one ages, the skin of the face and neck tends to become loose and wrinkled. The procedure is usually performed with local anesthesia. To perform the surgery, bilateral incisions are made from the scalp at the temple, in front of the ear in the natural skin line, around the ear lobe, and to the occipital scalp. The skin is then elevated, fat is removed or suctioned, and excess skin is excised. The incision lines are sutured, and a pressure dressing is applied.

∞ Nursing Care

Nursing care for the patient having cutaneous or plastic surgery is highly individualized. It depends on the type of surgery or procedure performed, the type of deficit treated, the reason for the surgery or procedure, the expected results of the treatment, and the response of the patient to the lesion or surgery. Although some surgeries, such as skin grafts and flaps, require in-hospital care, many of the surgeries are carried out in the primary care setting, and the patient provides self-care at home following or between treatments.

Nursing Diagnoses and Interventions

A variety of nursing diagnoses may be appropriate for the patient having cutaneous or plastic surgery or procedures; the most common are Impaired Skin Integrity, Acute Pain, and Disturbed Body Image.

Impaired Skin Integrity

The patient having surgery of the skin has impaired skin integrity. Skin grafts and flaps are performed to repair large wounds, and it is necessary to inflict further wounds to collect the graft or flap from a donor site. Excisions and various cosmetic surgeries cause wounds. Skin is traumatized by freezing, chemicals, abrasion, sclerosing agents, electrical currents, and lasers. Although all of these treatment modalities are conducted to remove lesions, improve function, or improve appearance, they first impair the integrity of the skin. These impairments increase the risk for infection, which would further impair the skin integrity and may negate the benefits of surgery.

Nurses provide preoperative care and teaching, intraoperative assistance, and postoperative care and teaching; in each case, care and teaching are specific to the type of surgical treatment and the individual patient. In all cases, the nurse provides appropriate preoperative interventions to prepare the patient physically and emotionally for surgery and the postoperative period. The following interventions are appropriate for the patient having inpatient skin grafts or flaps.

- Monitor incisions and graft, and flap donor and recipient sites, for manifestations of infection and necrosis:
  - Take and record vital signs every 4 hours.
  - Monitor all wounds for changes in color, consistency, amount, and odor of drainage every 4 to 8 hours.
  - Monitor wounds for increased swelling, redness, and pain every 4 to 8 hours.
  - Monitor and document assessment of graft every 4 hours.
  - Monitor and document temperature, turgor, color, dermal bleeding, and capillary refill of flaps every 4 hours.
  When bacterial infection is present, the inflammatory phase of wound healing is prolonged, retarding healing. Increased body temperature and tachycardia are manifestations of infection. The drainage in wounds that become infected is often increased in amount, purulent, thicker, and has a musty or foul odor. Tissue response to infection includes edema, increased erythema, and pain. Grafts and flaps that do not have adequate blood supply will appear black instead of the normal pink-red color.
- Provide care for the donor site:
  - Position the patient to minimize pressure on the donor site.
  - Use a bed cradle to keep linens off the area.
  - If the donor site is left open and a heat lamp is to be applied to the area, place the lamp no closer than 2 feet from the wound.
  - Avoid moving the body part containing the donor site, if possible.
  - If the donor site is on the posterior portion of the body, place the patient on a special bed (such as a low-pressure or fluidized bed) to decrease pressure and allow air circulation around the donor site.
  Minimizing trauma from pressure and movement facilitates healing of the donor site. Leaving the site open to the air and providing heat increase healing. Special beds minimize ischemia and allow donor sites on the posterior side of the body to dry.
- Encourage a diet high in protein, ascorbic acid, vitamins, and minerals. *An adequate protein intake is necessary to supply amino acids for tissue repair. Vitamin C is necessary for collagen formation and wound strength. Vitamins and minerals contribute to the healing process.*
- Change dressings as prescribed, or if the frequency is not indicated, as necessary. Determine which dressings are not to be removed during the healing process and which are to be changed, and whether the wound is to be kept dry or moist.

Use aseptic technique and follow standard precautions when changing dressings. Remove old dressings carefully and gently.

Donor sites may be covered with an adherent gauze dressing that is allowed to dry and remains adherent through the healing process. Aseptic techniques prevent secondary bacterial infections. Standard precautions protect the nurse from HIV infection. Unless care is taken, the removal of adherent old dressings may damage the wound by traumatizing granulation tissue or wound edges. The use of semipermeable transparent dressings provides an environment that optimizes wound healing by promoting collagen synthesis and the formation of granulation tissue; it also increases cell migration and epithelial resurfacing and prevents the formation of scabs, crusts, and eschar.

Acute Pain

The patient having a graft or flap has two wounds; in fact, the donor site may be more painful than the recipient site. Cutaneous surgeries, dermabrasions, and chemical treatments result in blistering, swelling, and loss of epidermal tissue. The patient having facial reconstructive surgery has edema, with resultant pain.

- Administer pain medications on a regular basis, following guidelines for controlling pain in patients having operative procedures (∞ see Chapter 9). *Established, severe pain is difficult to control and has negative physical and psychological consequences.*
- Use alternative pain relief measures as appropriate and prescribed, such as ice bags or cold compresses. *Cold reduces swelling, acts as a local anesthetic, and decreases pain.*
- Teach noninvasive methods of pain relief, such as deep breathing, relaxation, and guided imagery. *Noninvasive methods of pain relief increase the effectiveness of pain medications and also allow the patient some control and self-management of pain.*

Disturbed Body Image

Cosmetic surgery is performed for a variety of reasons in adult patients of all ages. Changes in appearance, especially in a society that values youth and beauty, affect one's self-perception. Lesions or scars, especially of the face, may decrease self-esteem and cause a person to avoid social interactions and relationships. With aging, the skin becomes looser and wrinkles appear; this can be a source of anxiety and despair, especially to the woman who has always prided herself on her youthful appearance. Most patients cite one reason for having plastic surgery: to "feel better about myself."

- Provide preoperative teaching: Explain that bruising and swelling will be present and that it will be several weeks before these responses to surgery disappear. Explain that it may take a year for healing to complete and the final results to appear. *Expectations differ; many people expect immediate results. Knowledge of postoperative responses is necessary for the patient to adapt to change. The patient may need to make arrangements to take time off from work during the initial healing stage.*
- Provide time for the patient to verbalize feelings and concerns. Be empathetic, and listen nonjudgmentally. *Such nurse–patient interaction facilitates acceptance of changes in body image.*
- Refer to a consultant who can provide information on the use of cosmetics and apparel to enhance personal appearance. *Knowledgeable use of cosmetics and clothing can make scars much less noticeable. If the patient feels better about appearance, body image is improved.*

Community-Based Care

The nurse teaches the patient and family to provide self-care at home after cutaneous and plastic surgery and procedures. The nurse asks about the patient's expectations and stresses that final results will not be seen for several months, providing written instructions about wound care and manifestations of infection.

Hair and Nail Disorders

Disorders of the hair and nails are not serious threats to health, but they may cause embarrassment and a negative body image. Changes in hair growth and pattern as in nail growth and character occur as secondary responses to other illnesses or treatments and are also a part of the aging process.

The Patient with a Disorder of the Hair

Racial characteristics and gender influence the amount and type of hair one has. Caucasians typically have more facial and body hair than do Asians. People of Mongolian or Native American descent usually have straight hair, those of African descent have wavy to curly hair, and whites have straight to curly hair. In addition, male hair growth characteristics (such as facial hair and hair on the lower extremities) are normal in certain women of some races and families.

Pathophysiology

Hair color, growth, and pattern vary from person to person, and they are determined largely by genetic inheritance Changes such as hair loss in men or excess facial hair in women may seem minor, but they may create psychosocial problems for the person experiencing the changes.

Hirsutism

Hirsutism (hypertrichosis), is the appearance of excessive hair in women. Hirsutism most often occurs in a male distribution (that is, on the upper lip, chin, abdomen, and chest) in women. The excess hair is primarily the result of an increase in androgen levels (especially testosterone) that may be due to familial predisposition (considered normal); polycystic ovary syndrome; ovarian, adrenal, or pituitary tumors; Cushing's syndrome (an adrenal disorder); some central system disorders; and medications, such as minoxidil, cyclosporine, phenytoin, certain progestins, and anabolic steroids.

The manifestations of hirsutism include increased male pattern hair growth, acne, and menstrual irregularities. If the androgen excess is great, defeminization (a decrease in breast size and loss of normal adipose tissue) and virilization (frontal balding, increased muscle mass, deepening of the voice, and enlargement of the clitoris) may occur.

Alopecia

Alopecia is loss of hair, or baldness. Alopecia may result from scarring, various systemic diseases, or genetic predisposition. Scarring from trauma, radiation, and severe bacterial, fungal, or viral infections causes permanent and irreversible hair loss over the scarred area. Systemic diseases that may cause alopecia include systemic lupus erythematosus, thyroid disorders, and pituitary insufficiency. The hair loss from these disorders may be reversible. Hair loss from androgenic causes may also occur in the postmenopausal woman. Alopecia may be drug induced and is a side effect of a variety of medications (Box 16–11).

Examples of types of alopecia follow:

- Male pattern baldness is the most common cause of alopecia in men and is genetically predetermined. The hair loss begins at the temples, with recession of the hairline and baldness of the crown.
- Female pattern alopecia begins in women in their 20s and 30s, with progressive thinning and loss of hair over the central part of the scalp. Unlike men, women do not lose hair from the frontal hairline. Many of these women have elevated adrenal androgens.
- Alopecia areata is characterized by round or oval bald patches on the scalp as well as on other hairy parts of the body. The cause is unknown. This type of alopecia is usually self-limiting and reverses without treatment, although it often recurs.

Interdisciplinary Care

The patient with hirsutism is examined for hormone levels and indications of other systemic illnesses. Hirsutism is treated by addressing the underlying systemic disorder and stopping medications that may be causing the problem. Alopecia is diagnosed by assessing the appearance of the hair and hair loss and by assessing the patient for other systemic diseases and the use of medications that may cause hair loss. Various treatments are used to restore hair.

Diagnosis

Diagnostic tests that may be ordered for the woman with hirsutism include serum testosterone levels and an adrenal CT scan. Testosterone levels are measured and levels greater than 200 ng/dL indicate the need for further tests, such as a pelvic examination and tests of ovarian function. Adrenal tumors, a possible cause of hirsutism, are identified with an adrenal CT scan.

Medications

Hirsutism is treated with medications specific to the underlying cause. Oral contraceptives containing estrogen decrease ovarian androgen production and decrease free testosterone levels. Dexamethasone (Decadron) may be prescribed for people with high cortisol levels. Ketoconazole (Nizoral) inhibits androgen production. Antiandrogenic medications cause congenital abnormalities in male infants and are therefore given only to nonpregnant women, who are cautioned to avoid pregnancy while taking the medications.

BOX 16–11 Medications Causing Alopecia

- Thallium
- Retinoids
- Anticoagulants
- Antimitotic agents
- Antithyroid drugs
- Oral contraceptives
- Trimethadone
- Excessive use of vitamin A
- Allopurinol
- Propranolol
- Indomethacin
- Amphetamines
- Salicylates
- Levopdopa
- Gentamicin
- Chemotherapy

Male pattern baldness has been successfully treated with topical minoxidil (Loniten) or Rogaine Extra Strength, a commercial product that contains minoxidil. These drugs, which are vasodilators, stimulate vertex hair growth, probably by stimulating the epithelium of the hair follicle. About 40% of patients treated two times a day for a year will have moderate to dense regrowth of hair at the temples (McPhee, Papadakis & Tierney, 2008).

Surgery

Hair transplant techniques are used to restore hair or reduce the size of areas of alopecia. Transplanting hairs as small hair plugs or single hairs taken from the back or sides of the scalp is an effective means of replacing hair to areas of alopecia. This procedure is done in an outpatient office or clinic. Other types of surgical procedures include scalp reduction and flaps.

Nursing Care

The patient with either hirsutism or alopecia is often self-conscious about appearance and tries a variety of OTC treatments before seeking medical care. Nursing care for the patient with hair disorders focuses on teaching the patient self-care and providing support during long-term care. Women with hirsutism are taught to use various means of removing unwanted hair, such as shaving, applying depilatories, waxing, or undergoing electrolysis. Women with mild hirsutism may bleach facial hair to make it less obvious. Patients with alopecia may wear hair pieces or wigs.

The Patient with a Disorder of the Nails

Nail disorders may be congenital or genetic, or they may be due to systemic diseases, trauma, allergies, or irritants. Nails may be discolored, multicolored, malformed, infected, or separated from underlying tissue.

Pathophysiology

The nail disorders discussed here are separation of the nail, infection, and ingrown toenails.

- Onycholysis is the separation of the distal nail plate from the nail bed. It occurs most often in the fingernails. This disorder may result from many different factors, including excessive or prolonged exposure to water, soaps, detergent, alkalies, and industrial keratolytic agents; Candida infections; nail hardeners; and thyroid disorders. Prolonged application of false fingernails may also cause this disorder.
- A **paronychia** is an infection of the cuticle of the fingernails or toenails. The disorder often follows a minor trauma and secondary infection with staphylococci, streptococci, or Candida. The acute form begins with a painful inflammation that may progress to an abscess. The chronic form is seen most often in people who have frequent exposure to water. In the chronic form, the skin around the nail is painful, edematous, and infected. The nail plate may become ridged and discolored.
- An onychomycosis is a fungal or dermatophyte infection of the nail plate. The nail plate elevates and becomes yellow or white. Psoriasis infections of the nail plate cause the nails to pit.

■ An ingrown toenail (unguis incarnatus) results when the edge of the nail plate grows into the soft tissue of the toe. Pain and infection may occur. The infection, if untreated, may spread to the bone. This disorder is especially dangerous for the person with diabetes mellitus or peripheral vascular disease.

Interdisciplinary Care

The treatment of disorders of the nail vary from pharmacologic treatment to surgical removal. Infections of the nails are treated with antifungal or antibiotic medications. If the causative agent is a fungus or chronic dermatologic disorder, treatment is difficult and may not be effective. Persistently painful and/or infected nails are in some cases surgically removed.

Nursing Care

Nursing care of the patient with a disorder of the nail focuses on teaching self-care. Patients with nail disorders that are caused by frequent exposure to water are taught to protect the hands or feet by wearing rubber gloves or boots and to keep the nails as clean and dry as possible. Patients with ingrown toenails are cautioned not to cut into the lateral nail bed, but rather to soak the nail twice a day and insert a piece of cotton or gauze under the softened nail until the nail has grown out enough to trim.

CHAPTER HIGHLIGHTS

■ Pruritus (itching) accompanies dry skin (xerosis) and many skin disorders and may result in excoriation and infection as a result of scratching.

■ Cysts, keloids, nevi, angiomas, skin tags, and keratoses are benign skin lesions. However, nevi should be monitored for changes indicating transformation into a malignant lesion.

■ Psoriasis is a chronic immune skin disorder arising from keratinocytes. A variety of medications and treatments are used, with ultraviolet light therapy being most effective for generalized lesions.

■ Skin disorders may be caused by a variety of bacteria, fungi, parasites, and viruses. The disorders are treated with organism-specific antibiotics, fungicides, anti-viral agents, or agents that kill the parasites. Herpes zoster, believed to follow a childhood infection with chickenpox, causes acute pain.

■ Inflammatory disorders of the skin range from mild dermatitis to potentially lethal toxic epidermal necrolysis. Acne, a disorder of the hair and sebaceous glands opening to the skin surface, is characterized by comedones, pustules, and cysts.

■ Malignant skin disorders include actinic keratosis, nonmelanoma skin cancer (basal cell cancer and squamous cell cancer), and malignant melanoma skin cancer. Skin cancer is the most common malignancy found in fair-skinned Americans. Prevention by avoiding sunburn, using sunscreen, and maintaining monthly skin self-examination is critical in preventing loss of tissue or metastasis and death.

■ Skin trauma may be intentional (as in the case of cutaneous and plastic surgery) or unintentional (as from trauma, frostbite, and pressure). Older adults with limited mobility, as well as patients who are unable to move or who are in critical care units, are at greater risk for pressure ulcers. Prevention of pressure ulcers is the goal of both interdisciplinary and nursing care.

■ Disorders of the hair include alopecia (loss of hair) and hirsutism (excess hair in women). Nails may be discolored, multicolored, malformed, infected, or separated from underlying tissue.

TEST YOURSELF NCLEX-RN® REVIEW

1. An elderly patient has severe xerosis. What topic should the nurse include in a teaching plan for this patient?
   1. Take a hot bath every day.
   2. Use fabric softeners when laundering clothing.
   3. Apply skin lotions after a bath.
   4. Maintain a warm environment.

2. A nurse assesses the following common skin lesions. Which lesion has the potential of becoming malignant?
   1. nevi
   2. angiomas
   3. skin tags
   4. keloids

3. A nurse has been asked to teach a woman with generalized psoriasis about ultraviolet light therapy (UVB). What should be included in the teaching?
   1. "The exact effect of UVB is unknown, but it decreases severe itching."
   2. "When combined with hot baths, UVB is very effective."
   3. "Treatments with UVB have to be given in the hospital to be safe."
   4. "UVB slows the growth of epidermal cells and decreases keratosis."

4. Which of the following skin lesions, if assessed, is a risk for skin cancer?
   1. lice infestation
   2. actinic keratosis
   3. pressure ulcer
   4. folliculitis

5. What question should the nurse include in a health history of a patient with a linear pattern of painful vesicles over the left thorax?
   1. "Do you remember being sunburned as a child?"
   2. "Are you a regular patron of tanning booths?"
   3. "Have you ever been diagnosed with acne?"
   4. "Did you have chickenpox when you were young?"

6. Which of the following statements would be appropriate for a nurse to make to a patient about a lice infestation?
   1. "Only dirty people have lice."
   2. "Anyone can have lice."
   3. "Lice do not like to live on humans."
   4. "Lice are a form of fungus."

7. Which assessments by the nurse would indicate a greater risk to develop a nonmelanoma skin cancer?
1. blond hair, freckles, fair skin
2. alopecia, thin hair, itching
3. dark hair, dark skin, dry skin
4. tanned skin, dark hair, edema

8. Of the following, which assessment is most significant to the development of a melanoma?
1. a change in the color or size of a nevus
2. sexual contact with a person who has a herpes virus infection
3. inadequate knowledge about infection prevention
4. a dietary intake of high-calorie foods

9. What is the rationale for a nurse lifting, rather than pulling, a patient up in bed?
1. Lifting a patient allows a brief period of increased capillary circulation.
2. Lifting a patient prevents tissue injury from shearing forces.
3. Pulling a patient up in bed decreases tissue ischemia and hypoxia.
4. Pulling a patient up in bed promotes capillary blood flow.

10. A nurse is caring for a young adult with acne scars. The patient asks about treatment to reduce the scarring. Which of the following might the nurse discuss?
1. liposuction
2. skin flap
3. dermabrasion
4. blepharoplasty

See Test Yourself answers in Appendix C.

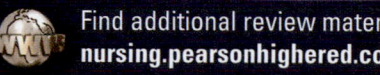

Pearson Nursing Student Resources

Find additional review materials at
nursing.pearsonhighered.com
Prepare for success with additional NCLEX®-style practice questions, interactive assignments and activities, Web links, animations and videos, and more!

BIBLIOGRAPHY

Agency for Health Care Policy and Research. (1992). *Pressure ulcers in adults: Prediction and prevention.* Rockville, MD: USDHHS.

Agency for Health Care Policy and Research. (1994). *Treatment of pressure ulcers.* Rockville, MD: USDHHS.

Allergies: Latex allergy. (2009). *WebMD.* Available at http://www.webmd.com/allergies/guide/latex-allergies

American Cancer Society. (2006). UV radiation & cancer. Retrieved from http://www.cancer.org

American Cancer Society. (2007). Skin cancer. Retrieved from http://www.cancer.org

American Cancer Society. (2008a). Melanoma skin cancer. Retrieved from http://www.cancer.org

American Cancer Society. (2008b). What are the key statistics about melanoma? Retrieved from http://www.cancer.org

American Cancer Society. (2008c). Skin cancer: Basal and squamous cell. Retrieved from http://www.cancer.org

American Society for Aesthetic Plastic Surgery. (2009). Cosmetic procedures in 2007. Retrieved from http://www.surgery.org/public/consumer/trends/cosmetic_procedures_in_2007

Ayello, E. A. (2007). Try this: Best practices in nursing care to older adults. Predicting pressure ulcer risk. *The Hartford Institute for Geriatric Nursing,* Issue 5, College of Nursing, New York University. Retrieved from http://www.hartfordign.org

Barklay, L. (2008). Management of atypical moles reviewed. *Medscape.* Retrieved from http://www.medscape.com/viewarticle/580864

Barclay, L. (2009). Use of topical corticosteroids for dermatologic conditions reviewed. *American Family Physician, 79,* 135–140.

Baron, E., Kirkland, E., & Domingo, D. (2008). Advances in photoprotection. *Dermatology Nursing, 20*(4), 265–273.

Barthel, D., & Crutchfield, C. (2004). Herpes zoster. *Dermatology Nursing, 16*(4), 362.

Black, J., Baharestani, M., Cuddigan, J., Dorner, B., Edsberg, L., Langemo, D., Posthauer, M., Ratliff, C., & Taler, G. (2007). National Pressure Ulcer Advisory Panel's updated pressure ulcer staging system. *Dermatology Nursing, 19*(4), 343–349.

Bolton, L. (2007). Evidence corner: Pressure ulcer risk scales. *Wounds, 19*(6), A15–A23.

Braden, B., & Bergstrom, N. (1988). *Braden scale for predicting pressure sore risk®.* Retrieved from http://www.bradenscale.com

Brown, J., Wimpenny, P., & Maughan, H. (2004). Skin problems in people with obesity. *Nursing Standard, 18*(35), 38–42.

Bulechek, G., Butcher, H., & Dochterman, J. (Eds.). (2008). *Nursing interventions classification (NIC)* (5th ed.). St. Louis: Mosby Elsevier.

Centers for Disease Control and Prevention. (2008a). *Community-associated methicillin resistant Staphylococcus aureus (CA-MRSA).* Retrieved from http://www.cdd.gov/ncidod/dhqp/ar_mrsa_ca.html

Centers for Disease Control and Prevention. (2008b). *Healthcare-associated methicillin resistant Staphylococcus aureus (HA-MRSA).* Retrieved from http://www.cdd.gov/ncidod/dhqp/ar_MRSA.html

Daus, L. (2008). Give them a hand: Patients with hand and foot psoriasis require special attention. *Dermatology Nursing, 20*(4), 291–193.

Gorgos, D. (2004). Top 3 causes of hair disorders identified. *Dermatology Nursing, 16*(4), 367–368.

Gould, D., Gldstone, L., Kelly, D., & Gammon, J. (2004). Examining the validity of pressure ulcer risk scales: A replication study. *International Journal of Nursing Studies, 41*(3), 3331–3339.

Hanson, D., Thompson, P., Langemo, D., Hunter, S., Tinkler, J., & Anderson, J. (2008). What you should know about psoriasis. *Nursing, 20*(6), 58–59.

Hess, C. (2009). Take steps to prevent pressure ulcers. *Nursing, 39*(1), 61.

Khachemoune, A., & Ehrsam, E. (2005). Assessing malignant melanoma: A case study. *Dermatology Nursing, 17*(3), 188–190.

Kucera, K. (2004). Managing common skin problems in the elderly. *Clincial Advisor, 7*(6), 23–24, 27–30.

McPhee, S., Papadakis, M., & Tierney, L. (Eds.). (2008). *Current medical diagnosis & treatment* (47th ed.). Stamford, CT: McGraw Hill Lange.

Moorhead, S., Johnson, M., Maas, M., & Swanson, E. (Eds.) (2008). *Nursing outcomes classification (NOC)* (4th ed.). St. Louis: Mosby Elsevier.

National Pressure Ulcer Advisory Panel. (2007). Pressure ulcer stages updated by NPUAP. Retrieved from http://www.npuap.org/pr2.htm

Nanda International. (2009). *Nursing diagnoses: Definitions & classification 2009–2011.* Oxford, UK: Wiley-Blackwell.

Porth, C. (2007). *Essentials of pathophysiology: Concepts of altered health states* (2nd ed.). Philadelphia: Lippincott Williams & Wilkins.

Porth, C., & Marfin, G. (2009). *Pathophysiology: Concepts of altered health states.* (8th ed.). Philadelphia: Lippincott Williams & Wilkins.

PsoriasisNet. (2008). *What is psoriasis?* Retrieved from http://www.skincarephysicians.com/psoriasisnet/whatis.html

Skin biopsy. (2008). *Harvard Health Publications,* Harvard Medical School. Retrieved from http://www.health.harvard.edu/diagnostic-tests/skin-biopsy.htm

Skin Cancer Foundation. (2008a). *Skin cancer facts.* Retrieved from http://www.skincancer.org/Skin-Cancer-Facts/

Skin Cancer Foundation. (2008b). *Melanoma.* Retrieved from http://www.skincancer.org/Melanoma/

Smith, M. (2008). Healthier aging. Taking a closer look for skin cancer. *Nursing, 37*(10), 58–60.

Smith, M., Nedorost, S., & Tackett, B. (2007). Facing up to withdrawal from topical steroids. *Nursing, 37*(9), 60–61.

Snow, M. (2008). Necrotizing fasciitis: Threatening life and limb. *Nursing, 38*(11), 23.

Stotts, N., & Gunningberg, L. (2007). Predicting pressure ulcer risk. *American Journal of Nursing, 107*(11), 40–48.

Tosanger, M., & Crutchfield, C. (2004a). Tinea corporis. *Dermatology Nursing, 16*(5), 453.

Tonanger, M., & Crutchfield, C. (2004b). Atrophic lichen planus. *Dermatology Nursing, 16*(1), 73–74.

Van Rijswijk, L., & Lyder, C. (2008). Pressure ulcers: Were they there on admission? *American Journal of Nursing, 108*(11), 27–28.

Wilson, B., Shannon, M., & Shields, K. (2010). *Prentice Hall's nurse's drug guide.* Upper Saddle River, NJ: Pearson Prentice Hall.

Wurster, J. (2007). What role can nurse leaders play in reducing the incidence of pressure sores? *Nursing Economics, 25*(5), 267–269.

Yamarmoto, L., & Marten, M. (2007). Listen up, MRSA. The bug stops here. *Nursing, 37*(12), 50–55.

Yarbo, C., Frogge, M., Goodman, M., & Groenwald, S. (Eds.) (2005). *Cancer nursing: Principles and practice.* (6th ed.). Sudbury, MA: Jones & Bartlett.

Zulkowski, K., & Gray-Leach, K. (2009). Staging pressure ulcers: What's the buzz in wound care? *American Journal of Nursing, 109*(1), 27–30.

17 Nursing Care of Patients with **Burns**

LEARNING OUTCOMES

1. Discuss the types and causative agents of burns.
2. Explain burn classification by depth and extent of injury.
3. Compare and contrast the pathophysiology and interdisciplinary care of a minor burn and a major burn.
4. Discuss the systemic pathophysiologic effects of a major burn and the stages of burn wound healing.
5. Explain the interdisciplinary care and nursing implications necessary during the emergent/resuscitative stage, the acute stage, and the rehabilitative stage of a major burn.

CLINICAL COMPETENCIES

1. Assess functional health status of patients with burns, and monitor, document, and report abnormal manifestations.
2. Use evidence-based research to plan and implement nursing care for patients with burns.
3. Determine priority nursing diagnoses, based on assessed data, to select and implement individualized nursing interventions for patient with burns.
4. Administer medications knowledgeably and safely to patients with burns.
5. Integrate interdisciplinary care into care of patients with burns.
6. Provide teaching appropriate for prevention of burns.
7. Revise plan of care as needed to provide effective interventions to promote, maintain, or restore functional health status to patients with burns.

KEY TERMS

allograft, *463*
autografting, *462*
burn, *446*
burn shock, *454*
compartment syndrome, *455*
contractures, *464*
Curling's ulcers, *455*
debridement, *463*

eschar, *454*
escharotomy, *460*
fascial excision, *460*
fasciectomy, *460*
fluid resuscitation, *458*
full-thickness burn, *449*
heterograft, *463*

homograft, *463*
hypertrophic scar, *452*
keloid, *452*
partial-thickness burn, *448*
superficial burn, *448*
surgical debridement, *460*
xenograft, *463*

A **burn** is an injury resulting from exposure to heat, chemicals, radiation, or electric current. A transfer of energy from a source of heat to the human body initiates a sequence of physiologic events that in the most severe cases leads to irreversible tissue destruction. Burns range in severity from a minor loss of small segments of the outermost layer of the skin to a complex injury involving all body systems. Treatments vary from simple application of a topical antiseptic agent in an outpatient clinic to an invasive, multisystem, interdisciplinary team approach in the aseptic environment of a burn center.

It is estimated that 500,000 million burn injuries that require medical intervention occur each year in the United States, and of those, about 40,000 require hospitalization with approximately 4000 of the burn injuries resulting in death (American Burn Association [ABA], 2007). The home is the most common site for fire-related burns (43%). Home fires cause 92.5% of all fire-related deaths. Most residential fires are caused by unattended cooking, resulting from combustible grease, cabinets, wall coverings, curtains, and paper or plastic bags. Smoking materials, including cigarettes, cigars, and pipes, are the leading cause of home fire deaths. Trash, mattresses, and upholstered furniture are frequently ignited materials in the home.

FAST FACTS
Causes of Home Fires
1. Cooking fires
2. Smoking
3. Heating equipment

Factors associated with deaths from burns are age (especially children under 5 and adults 65 and older), careless smoking, alcohol or drug intoxication, and physical and mental disabilities. A common source of burns in young children and older adults is from tap water scalds, while older children receive most burns from flame injuries. Older adults are more susceptible to deep burns from scalds because of their thinner skin. Fire injuries and deaths, occurring among college-age students, usually are due to alcohol use that impairs judgment and hampers escape (NFPA, 2004). Occupations involving work with chemicals, gasoline, or electricity pose another risk factor. Abuse is suspected when scald burns show a clear line of demarcation, indicating deliberate immersion. The presence of small, circular burns may be from cigarette burns inflicted by an abuser.

Older adults are more vulnerable to fire and burn injury because of decreased visual acuity, depth perception, sense of smell, and hearing, in addition to impaired mobility. All of these factors increase the risk for accidentally starting a fire and diminish the ability to survive it.

FAST FACTS

Fire Deaths in Older Adults

- More than 1200 deaths in adults 65 and older occur each year.
- Leading causes of fire-related deaths are smoking, heating, and cooking.
- One-fifth of the deaths occur in bedridden or physically challenged older adults.

Infants and older adults have a greater risk of mortality. Morbidity increases in patients with pre-existing cardiac, pulmonary, or renal disorders, and diabetes mellitus. Patients who are alcoholics have lower survival rates of a major burn injury due to the development of more complications. Men account for 70% of burn patients versus 30% for women (ABA, 2007).

Types of Burn Injury

The four types of burn injury are thermal, chemical, electrical, and radiation. Although all four types can lead to generalized tissue damage and multisystem involvement, the causative agents and priority treatment measures are unique to each (Table 17–1).

Thermal Burns

Thermal burns result from exposure to dry heat (flames) or moist heat (steam and hot liquids). They are the most common burn injuries and occur most often in children and older adults. Direct exposure to the source of heat causes cellular destruction that can result in charring of vascular, bony, muscle, and nervous tissue.

Chemical Burns

Chemical burns are caused by direct skin contact with acids, alkaline agents, or organic compounds. More than 25,000 products found in the home or workplace can cause chemical burns. The chemical destroys tissue protein, leading to necrosis. Burns caused by alkalis (such as lye) are more difficult to neutralize than are burns caused by acids. They also tend to have deeper penetration with a correspondingly more severe burn than from acid. Organic compound burns, such as by petroleum distillates, cause cutaneous damage through fat solvent action and may also cause renal and liver failure if absorbed.

Chemical agents are further classified according to the manner by which they structurally alter proteins. Oxidizing agents, such as household bleach, alter protein configuration through the chemical process of reduction. Corrosives, such as lye, cause extensive protein denaturation. Protoplasmic poisons, such as organic compounds, form salts with proteins, inhibiting calcium and other ions needed for cell viability. The severity of the chemical burn is related to the type of agent, the concentration of the agent, the mechanism of action, the duration of contact, and the amount of body surface area exposed. Box 17–1 lists household cleaning agents that may cause burns.

Electrical Burns

The severity of electrical burns depends on the type and duration of current, and amount of voltage. It is particularly difficult to assess the extent of the electrical burn injury, because the destructive processes initiated by the electrical insult are concealed and may persist for weeks beyond the time of the incident. It is challenging to assess the depth and extent of the burn, as electricity follows the path of least resistance, which in the human body tends to lie along muscles, bone, blood vessels, and nerves. Entry and exit wounds tend to be small, masking widespread tissue damage underneath the wound. Tissue necrosis results from impaired blood flow, secondary to blood coagulation at the site of the electrical injury. Because electrical burn wounds of the extremities often cause severe tissue necrosis, they frequently develop gangrene that necessitates amputation (Bishop, 2004).

Alternating current (AC), as is found in conventional households, produces repeated electrical surges that lead to tetanic muscle contractions. Such sustained muscle contractions inhibit respiratory efforts for the duration of contact and result in respiratory arrest. The contractions also cause the person to clamp down on the power source (such as an electrical cord)

TABLE 17–1 Types, Causative Agents, and Priority Treatment Measures for Burns

TYPE	CAUSATIVE AGENT	PRIORITY TREATMENT
Thermal	Open flame	Extinguish flame (stop, drop, and roll).
	Steam	
	Hot liquids (water, grease, tar, metal)	Flush with cool water.
		Consult fire department.
Chemical	Acids	Neutralize or dilute chemical.
	Strong alkalis	Remove clothing.
	Organic compounds	Consult poison control center.
Electrical	Direct current	Disconnect source of current.
	Alternating current	Initiate CPR if necessary.
	Lightning	Move to area of safety.
		Consult electrical experts.
Radiation	Solar (ultraviolet)	Shield the skin appropriately.
	X-rays	Limit time of exposure.
	Radioactive agents	Move the patient away from the radiation source.
		Consult a radiation expert.

BOX 17–1 Household Cleaning Agents That May Cause Burns

- Drain cleaners
- Lye
- Industrial-strength ammonia
- Household ammonia
- Oven cleaners
- Toilet bowl cleaners
- Dishwasher detergents
- Bleach

and thus may increase the duration of contact with the source. Direct current, as in injury from a lightning bolt, exposes the body to very high voltage for an instantaneous period of time. High voltage (lightning) injury usually results in entry and exit wounds. The flash-over effect, a phenomenon unique to lightning injury, actually saves the patient from death. It is seen in those instances in which the current travels over the moist surface of the skin rather than through deeper structures. Cardiopulmonary arrest is the most common cause of death from lightening.

Radiation Burns

Radiation burns are usually associated with sunburn or radiation treatment for cancer. These kinds of burns tend to be superficial, involving only the outermost layers of the epidermis. All functions of the skin remain intact. Symptoms are limited to mild systemic reactions: headache, chills, local discomfort, nausea, and vomiting. More extensive exposure to radiation or radioactive substances, as in nuclear power accidents, leads to the same degree of tissue damage and multisystem involvement associated with other types of burns.

Factors Affecting Burn Classification

Tissue damage following a burn is determined primarily by two factors: depth of the burn (the layers of underlying tissue affected) and the extent of the burn (the percentage of body surface area involved).

Depth of the Burn

The depth of burn of injury is determined by the elements of the skin that have been damaged or destroyed. Burn depth results from a combination of the temperature of the burning agent and the length of contact. Burns are classified as either superficial, partial thickness, or full thickness. Characteristics of burns are described next, summarized in Table 17–2, and illustrated in Figure 17–1 ■.

Superficial Burns

A **superficial burn** involves only the epidermal layer of the skin. This type of burn most often results from damage from sunburn, ultraviolet light, minor flash injury (from a sudden ignition or explosion), or mild radiation burn associated with cancer treatment. Because the skin remains intact, this degree of burn is not calculated into the estimates of burn injury. The skin color ranges from pink to bright red, and there may be slight edema over the burned area. Superficial burns involving large body surface areas may be manifested by chills, headache, nausea, and vomiting. The injury usually heals in 3 to 6 days, with dryness and peeling of the outer layer of skin. There is no scar formation. Superficial burns are treated with mild analgesics and the application of water-soluble lotions. Extensive superficial burns, especially in older adults, may require intravenous fluid treatment.

Partial-Thickness Burns

Partial-thickness burns may be subdivided into superficial partial-thickness and deep dermal partial-thickness burns. The classification depends on the depth of the burn.

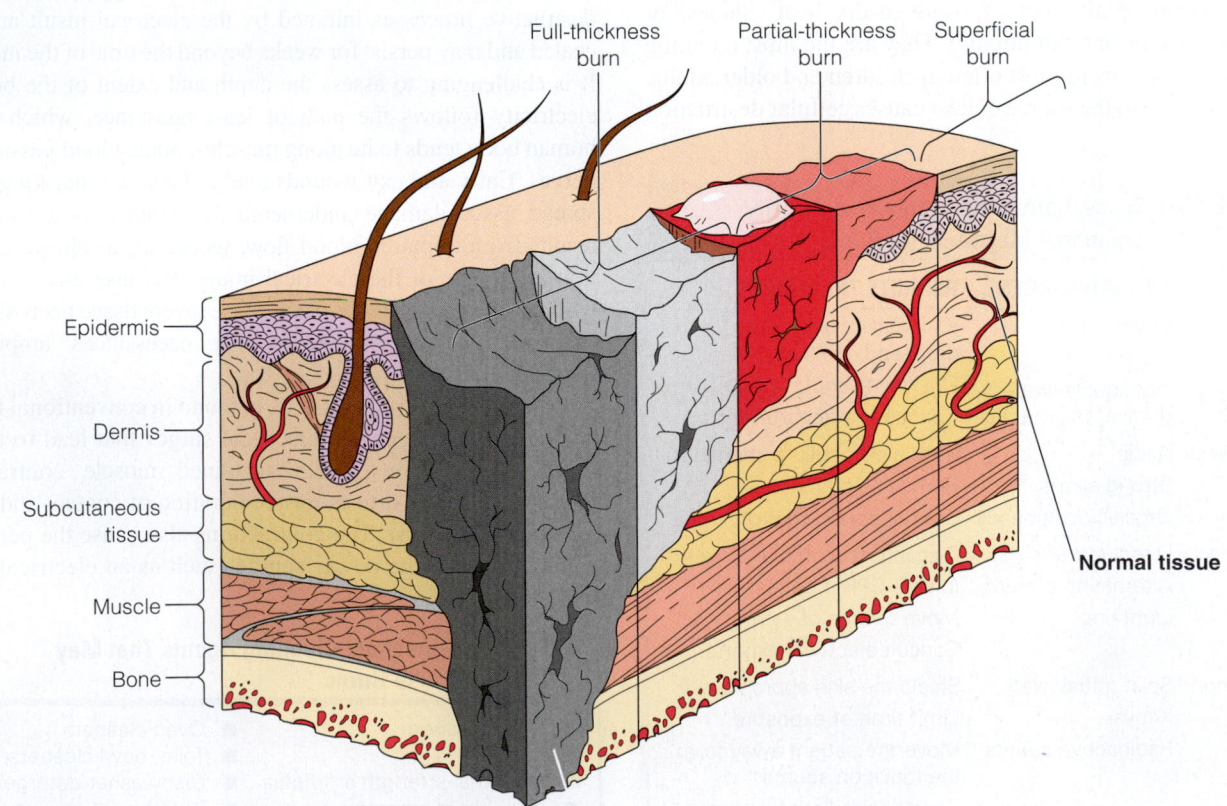

Figure 17–1 ■ Burn injury classification according to the depth of the burn.

TABLE 17–2 Characteristics of Burns by Depth

CHARACTERISTIC	SUPERFICIAL	PARTIAL THICKNESS	FULL THICKNESS
Skin layers lost	Epidermis	Epidermis and dermis	Epidermis, dermis, and underlying tissues
Skin appearance over burn	Pink to red and dry; may have local edema	Fluid-filled blisters; bright pink or red with superficial partial-thickness Pale, mottled, waxy white with deep partial-thickness burns	Waxy white; dry, leathery, charred
Skin function	Present	Absent	Absent
Pain sensation	Present	Present	Absent
Manifestations at the burn site	Pain; local edema	Severe pain; edema; weeping of fluid	Little pain; edema
Treatment	Regular cleaning Topical agent of choice	Regular cleaning Topical agent of choice May require skin grafting with deep partial-thickness burns	Regular cleaning Topical agent of choice Skin substitutes Excision of eschar Skin grafting
Scarring	None	May occur in deep burns	Of grafted area
Time to heal	3 to 6 days	14 to > 21 days	Requires skin grafting to heal

A *superficial partial-thickness burn* involves the entire dermis and the papillae of the dermis. Causes may include such injuries as a brief exposure to flash flame or dilute chemical agents, or contact with a hot surface. This burn is often bright red, but has a moist, glistening appearance with blister formation (Figure 17–2 ■). The burned area will blanch on pressure, and touch and pain sensation remain intact. Pain in response to temperature and air is usually severe. These injuries heal within 21 days with minimal or no scarring, but pigment changes are common. Analgesics are administered, and if large blistered areas are disrupted, skin substitutes may be used.

A *deep partial-thickness burn* also involves the entire dermis, but extends further into the dermis than a superficial partial-thickness burn. Hair follicles, sebaceous glands, and epidermal sweat glands remain intact (Huether & McCance, 2008). Hot liquids or solids, flash flame, direct flame, intense radiant energy, or chemical agents may cause this level of burn wound. The surface of the burn wound appears pale and waxy and may be moist or dry. Large, easily ruptured blisters may be present, or the blisters may look like flat, dry tissue paper. Capillary refill is decreased, and sensation to deep pressure is present. The burn wound is less painful than a superficial partial-thickness burn, but areas of pain and areas of decreased sensation may be present. Deep partial-thickness burn wounds often require more than 21 days for healing and may convert to a full-thickness injury as necrosis extends the depth of the wound. Contractures are possible, as are hypertrophic scarring and functional impairment (Figure 17–3 ■). Excision and grafting may be necessary to decrease scarring and loss of function.

Full-Thickness Burns

A **full-thickness burn** involves all layers of the skin, including the epidermis, the dermis, and the epidermal appendages (Figure 17–4 ■). The burn wound may extend into the subcutaneous fat, connective tissue, muscle, and bone. Full-thickness burns are caused by prolonged contact with flames, steam, chemicals, or high-voltage electric current.

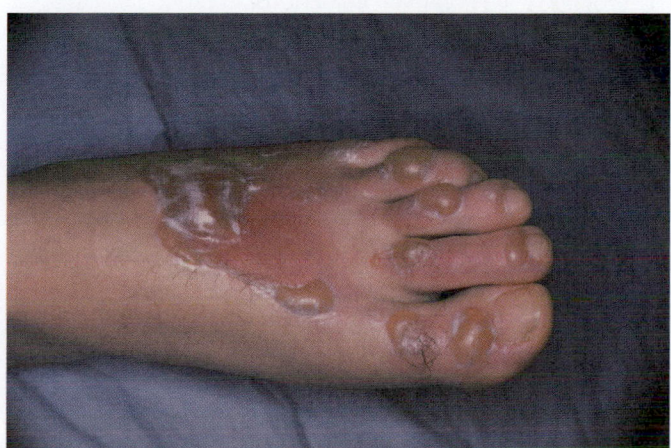

Figure 17–2 ■ Partial-thickness burn injury.

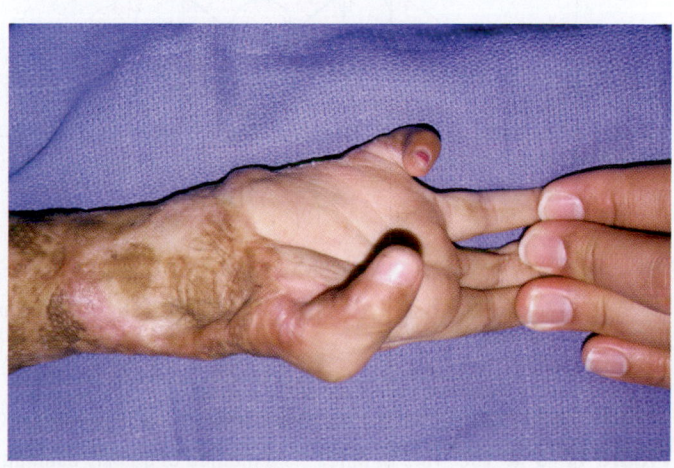

Figure 17–3 ■ Burn contracture.

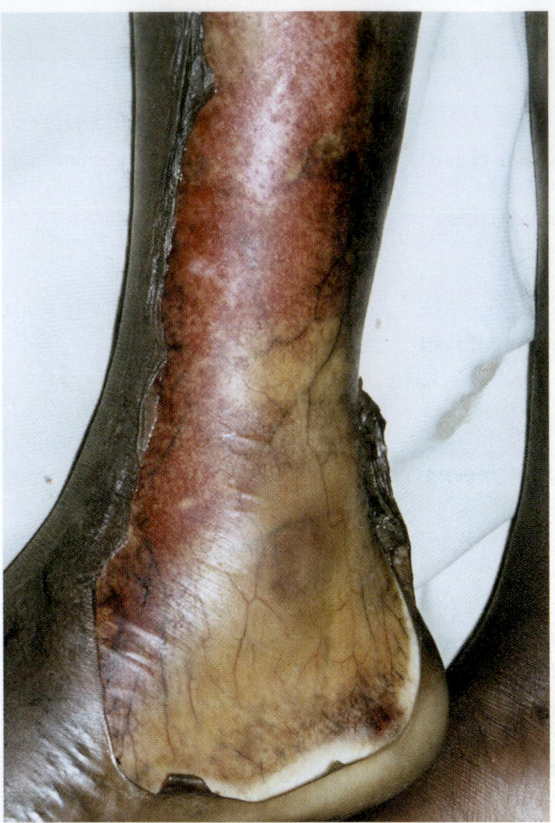

Figure 17–4 ■ Full-thickness burn injury.
Source: Photo Researchers, Inc.

Depending on the cause of injury, the burn wound may appear pale, waxy, yellow, brown, mottled, charred, or non-blanching red. The wound surface is dry, leathery, and firm to the touch. Thrombosed blood vessels may be visible under the surface of the wound. There is no sensation of pain or light touch, as pain and touch receptors have been destroyed. Full-thickness burns require skin grafting to heal.

Extent of the Burn

The extent of the burn injury is expressed as a percentage of the total body surface area (TBSA). There are several methods used for determining the extent of injury. The "rule of nines" is a rapid method of estimation used during the prehospital and emergency care phases. In this method, the body is divided into five surface areas—head, trunk, arms, legs, and perineum—and percentages that equal or total a sum of nines are assigned to each body area (Figure 17–5 ■). For example, a patient with burns of the face, anterior right arm, and anterior trunk has burn injury involving 27% of the total body surface area (in this example, face = 4.5%, arm = 4.5%, and trunk = 18% to total 27%). Only partial- and full-thickness burns are included in the estimation.

On the patient's admission to the hospital, critical care area, or burn center, more accurate methods for estimating the extent of injury are employed. For example, the Lund and Browder method (Figure 17–6 ■) determines surface area measurements for each body part according to the age of the patient.

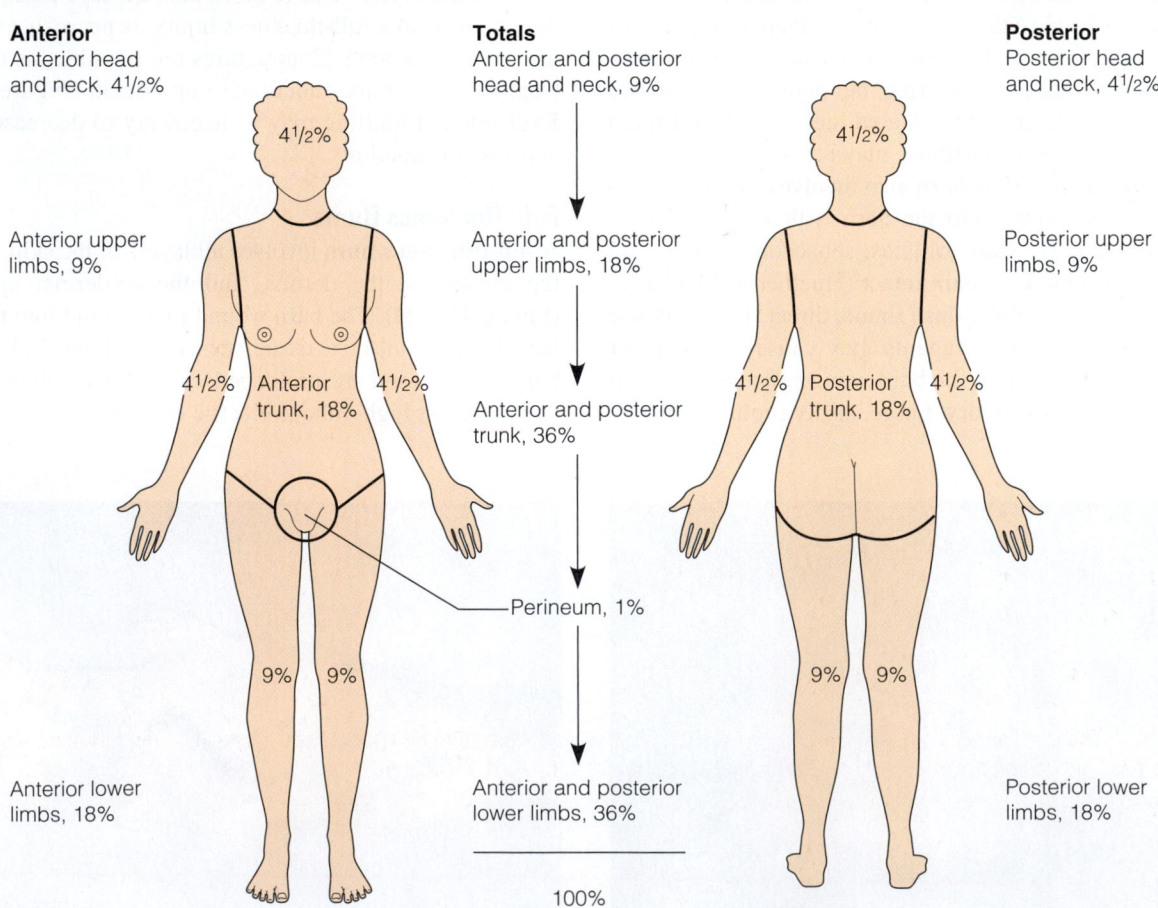

Anterior
Anterior head and neck, 4¹/₂%

Anterior upper limbs, 9%

Anterior trunk, 18%

Anterior lower limbs, 18%

Totals
Anterior and posterior head and neck, 9%

Anterior and posterior upper limbs, 18%

Anterior and posterior trunk, 36%

Perineum, 1%

Anterior and posterior lower limbs, 36%

100%

Posterior
Posterior head and neck, 4¹/₂%

Posterior upper limbs, 9%

Posterior trunk, 18%

Posterior lower limbs, 18%

Figure 17–5 ■ The "rule of nines" is a method of quickly estimating the percentage of TBSA affected by a burn injury. Although useful in emergency care situations, the rule of nines is not accurate for estimating TBSA for adults who are short, obese, or very thin.

Area	Age (years)					% 1°	% 2°	% 3°	% Total
	0–1	1–4	5–9	10–15	Adult				
Head	19	17	13	10	7				
Neck	2	2	2	2	2				
Ant. trunk	13	13	13	13	13				
Post. trunk	13	13	13	13	13				
R. buttock	$2\frac{1}{2}$	$2\frac{1}{2}$	$2\frac{1}{2}$	$2\frac{1}{2}$	$2\frac{1}{2}$				
L. buttock	$2\frac{1}{2}$	$2\frac{1}{2}$	$2\frac{1}{2}$	$2\frac{1}{2}$	$2\frac{1}{2}$				
Genitalia	1	1	1	1	1				
R.U. arm	4	4	4	4	4				
L.U. arm	4	4	4	4	4				
R.L. arm	3	3	3	3	3				
L.L. arm	3	3	3	3	3				
R. hand	$2\frac{1}{2}$	$2\frac{1}{2}$	$2\frac{1}{2}$	$2\frac{1}{2}$	$2\frac{1}{2}$				
L. hand	$2\frac{1}{2}$	$2\frac{1}{2}$	$2\frac{1}{2}$	$2\frac{1}{2}$	$2\frac{1}{2}$				
R. thigh	$5\frac{1}{2}$	$6\frac{1}{2}$	$8\frac{1}{2}$	$8\frac{1}{2}$	$9\frac{1}{2}$				
L. thigh	$5\frac{1}{2}$	$6\frac{1}{2}$	$8\frac{1}{2}$	$8\frac{1}{2}$	$9\frac{1}{2}$				
R. leg	5	5	$5\frac{1}{2}$	6	7				
L. leg	5	5	$5\frac{1}{2}$	6	7				
R. foot	$3\frac{1}{2}$	$3\frac{1}{2}$	$3\frac{1}{2}$	$3\frac{1}{2}$	$3\frac{1}{2}$				
L. foot	$3\frac{1}{2}$	$3\frac{1}{2}$	$3\frac{1}{2}$	$3\frac{1}{2}$	$3\frac{1}{2}$				
					Total				

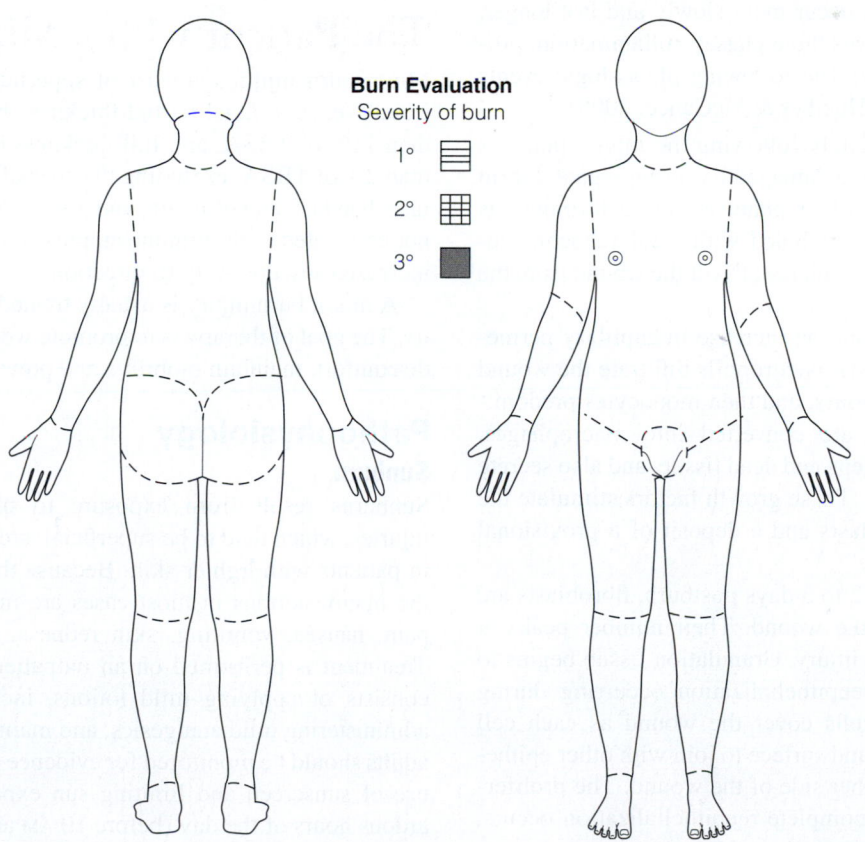

Burn Evaluation
Severity of burn

1°
2°
3°

Figure 17–6 ■ The Lund and Browder burn assessment chart. This method of estimating TBSA affected by a burn injury is more accurate than the "rule of nines" because it accounts for changes in body surface area across the life span.

TABLE 17–3 American Burn Association Classification of Burn Injury

MINOR BURN INJURY	MODERATE BURN INJURY	MAJOR BURN INJURY
Excludes electrical injury, inhalation injury, complicated injuries (such as multiple trauma), and all patients who are considered to be at high risk (such as older adults and those with chronic illnesses)	Excludes electrical injury, inhalation injury, complicated injuries (such as multiple trauma), and all patients who are considered to be at high risk (such as older adults and those with chronic illnesses)	Includes all burns of the hands, face, eyes, ears, feet, and perineum; all electrical injuries, inhalation injuries, multiple trauma injuries, and all patients who are considered to be at high risk
Partial-thickness burns of less than 15% of the total body surface area in adults	**Partial-thickness** burns of 15% to 25% of the total body surface area in adults	**Partial-thickness** burns of greater than 25% of the total body surface area in adults
Full-thickness burns of less than 2% of the total body surface area not involving special care areas (eyes, ears, face, hands, feet, perineum)	**Full-thickness** burns of less than 10% of the total body surface area not involving special care areas (eyes, ears, face, hands, feet, perineum)	All **full-thickness** burns of 10% or greater of the total body surface area

Note: Burn injuries described in this table (except minor burns) should be treated in a specialized burn center. These criteria have been established by the American Burn Association.

A recognized system for describing a burn injury, developed by the ABA, uses both the extent and depth of burn to classify burns as minor, moderate, or major (Table 17–3).

Burn Wound Healing

Burns heal using the same processes as do other wounds, but the wound healing phases occur more slowly and last longer. The healing process involves three phases: inflammation, proliferation, and remodeling. The following physiologic events occur (Carrougher, 2003; Huether & McCance, 2008):

- *Inflammation.* Immediately following the injury, platelets coming in contact with the damaged tissue aggregate. Fibrin is deposited, trapping further platelets, and a thrombus is formed. The thrombus, combined with local vasoconstriction, leads to hemostasis, which walls off the wound from the systemic circulation.

  Local vasodilation and an increase in capillary permeability follow hemostasis. Neutrophils infiltrate the wound and peak in about 24 hours, and then monocytes predominate. The monocytes are converted into macrophages, which consume pathogens and dead tissue, and also secrete various growth factors. These growth factors stimulate the proliferation of fibroblasts and a deposit of a provisional wound matrix.

- *Proliferation.* Within 2 to 3 days postburn, fibroblasts are the major cell within the wound. Their number peaks at about 14 days after the injury. Granulation tissue begins to form, with complete reepithelialization occurring during this stage. Epithelial cells cover the wound as each cell stretches across the wound surface to join with other epithelial cell sheets or the other side of the wound. The proliferation phase lasts until complete reepithelialization occurs, by epithelial cell migration, surgical intervention, or a combination of the two.

- *Remodeling.* This phase may last for years. Collagen fibers, laid down during the proliferative phase, are reorganized into more compact areas. Scars contract and fade in color. In normal healing following a minor burn injury, the newly formed skin closely resembles its neighboring tissue. However, when a burn injury extends into the dermal layer

of skin, two types of excessive scar may develop. A **hypertrophic scar** is an overgrowth of dermal tissue that remains within the boundaries of the wound. A **keloid** is a scar that extends beyond the boundaries of the original wound. People with dark skin are at greater risk for hypertrophic scars and keloids.

The Patient with a Minor Burn

Minor burn injuries consist of superficial burns that are not extensive, superficial partial-thickness burns that involve less than 15% of TBSA, and full-thickness burns that involve less than 2% of TBSA, excluding the special care areas (eyes, ears, face, hands, feet, perineum, and joints). Minor burn injuries are not associated with immunosuppression, hypermetabolism, or increased susceptibility to infection.

A minor burn injury is usually treated in an outpatient facility. The goal of therapy is to promote wound healing, eliminate discomfort, maintain mobility, and prevent infection.

Pathophysiology

Sunburn

Sunburns result from exposure to ultraviolet light. Such injuries, which tend to be superficial, are more commonly seen in patients with lighter skin. Because the skin remains intact, the manifestations in most cases are mild and are limited to pain, nausea, vomiting, skin redness, chills, and headache. Treatment is performed on an outpatient basis and generally consists of applying mild lotions, increasing liquid intake, administering mild analgesics, and maintaining warmth. Older adults should be monitored for evidence of dehydration. Proper use of sunscreen and limiting sun exposure to the less hazardous hours of the day (before 10 AM and after 3 PM) can prevent sunburn.

Scald Burn

Minor scald burns result from exposure to moist heat and involve superficial and superficial partial-thickness burns of less than 15% of TBSA. The goals of therapy are to prevent wound contamination and to promote healing. The nurse teaches the patient to apply antibiotic solutions and light dressings and to maintain adequate nutritional intake. Mild analgesics may be ordered to help the patient carry out activities of daily living. Tetanus toxoid is administered as appropriate.

Interdisciplinary Care

In the outpatient facility, the wound may be washed with mild soap and water. Tetanus toxoid booster is recommended for all patients whose immunization histories are in doubt. Minor burns with blisters may be left intact, or debrided. Follow-up care for the minor burn injury includes twice daily wound cleansing with application of a topical ointment, range-of-motion exercises to affected joints, and weekly clinic appointments until the wound heals completely.

✆ Nursing Care

Although the nurse seldom treats the minor burn in the acute care environment, the burn treatment methods used in the outpatient setting follow the same standard approaches to care. General nursing measures include taking the history, estimating the extent and depth of the injury, cleansing the wound, applying topical agents, dressing the wound, controlling pain, and establishing follow-up care.

Community-Based Care

The nurse should address the following topics to facilitate self-care at home of minor burns.

- How to identify and report manifestations of impaired wound healing:
  - Change in healthy appearance of the wound (altered skin integrity, swelling, blister formation, erythema)
  - Signs of infection (fever, purulent drainage, foul odor)
- Wound care:
  - Daily cleansing with mild soap and water
  - Using sterile technique to change dressings
  - Correct application of ordered topical agents
- Pain management:
  - Use mild analgesics as ordered
  - Use alternative pain management therapies

The Patient with a Major Burn

A major burn involves serious injury to the underlying layers of skin and covers a large body surface area. The ABA defines a major burn as one that involves:

- > 25% TBSA in adults less than 40 years of age
- > 20% TBSA in adults more than 40 years of age
- > 10% TBSA full-thickness burn
- Injuries to the face, eyes, ears, hands, feet, or perineum
- High-voltage electrical injuries
- All burn injuries with inhalation injury or major trauma

Pathophysiology

The pathophysiologic changes that result from major burn injuries involve all body systems. Extensive loss of skin (the body's protective barrier) can result in massive infection, fluid and electrolyte imbalances, and hypothermia. Often the person inhales the products of combustion, thus compromising respiratory function. Cardiac dysrhythmias and circulatory failure are common manifestations of serious burn injuries. A profound catabolic state dramatically increases caloric expenditure and nutritional deficiencies. An alteration in gastrointestinal motility predisposes the patient to developing paralytic ileus, and hyperacidity leads to gastric and duodenal ulcerations. Dehydration slows glomerular filtration rates and renal clearance of toxic wastes and may lead to acute tubular necrosis and renal failure. Overall body metabolism may be profoundly altered. Systemic responses to burns are shown in Figure 17–7 ■ and discussed in the following sections.

Integumentary System

The loss of skin in burn injuries interrupts normal skin functions and its protective mechanisms (∞ see Chapter 15). Key mechanisms lost in burn injuries include the prevention of evaporative water loss and bacteria entry, as well as the maintenance of body warmth.

Heat transfer to skin is a complex phenomenon. If the microcirculation of the skin remains intact during burning, it cools

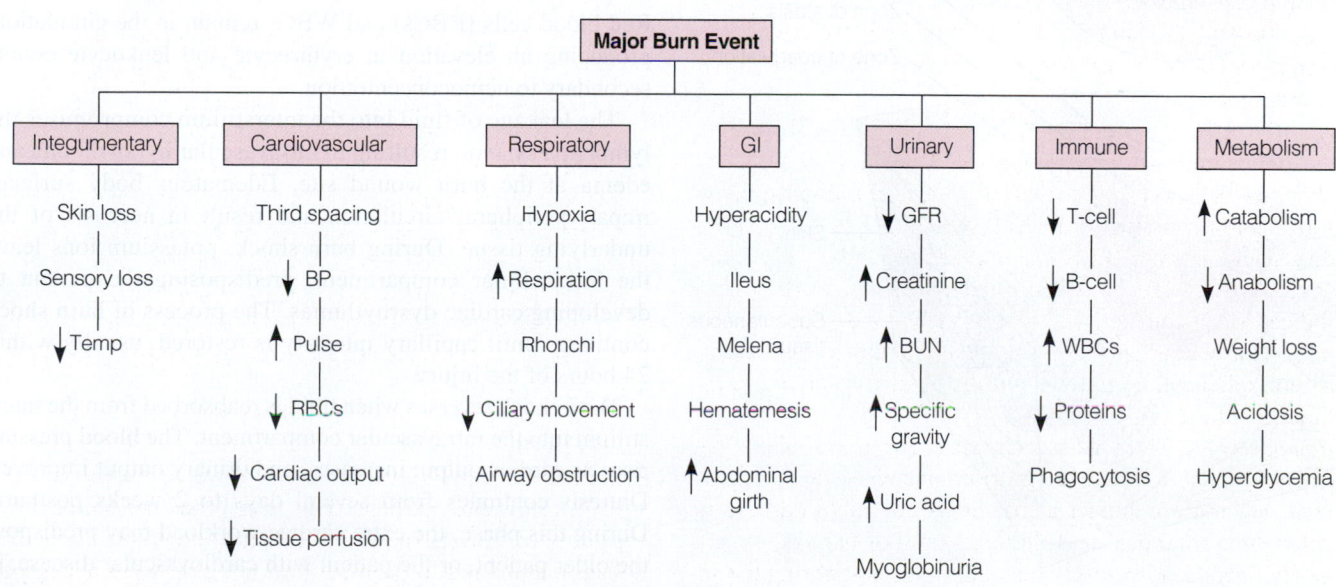

Figure 17–7 ■ Effects of a severe burn on major body systems and metabolism.

and protects the deeper portions of the skin and cools the outer surface once the heat source is removed. With extensive burn injury, the integrity of the microcirculation is lost, and the burning process continues even after the heat source is removed.

Burns have a characteristic skin surface appearance that resembles a bull's-eye, with the most severe burn located centrally and the lesser burns located along the peripheral wound edges. Depending on their intensity, burns consist of one, two, or three concentric three-dimensional zones closely corresponding on the skin surface to the depth of the burn (Figure 17–8 ■).

- The outer zone of hyperemia is unburned tissue, blanches on pressure, and heals in 2 to 7 days postburn.
- The medial zone of stasis is initially moist, red, and blistered and blanches on pressure. It may recover or become pale and necrotic on days 3 to 7 postburn due to decreased perfusion or infection.
- The inner zone of coagulation immediately appears leathery and coagulated. It may merge with the zone of stasis in 3 to 7 days postburn.

The overall thickness of the dermis and epidermis varies considerably from one area of the body to another. Similar temperatures produce different depths of injury to different body parts. For example, in the adult, skin covering the medial aspect of the forearm is thinner and more easily damaged than the skin covering the back of the same person. Skin dissipates heat maximally in areas of greatest vascularization. When heat absorption exceeds the rate of dissipation, cellular temperatures rise, and skin tissue is destroyed.

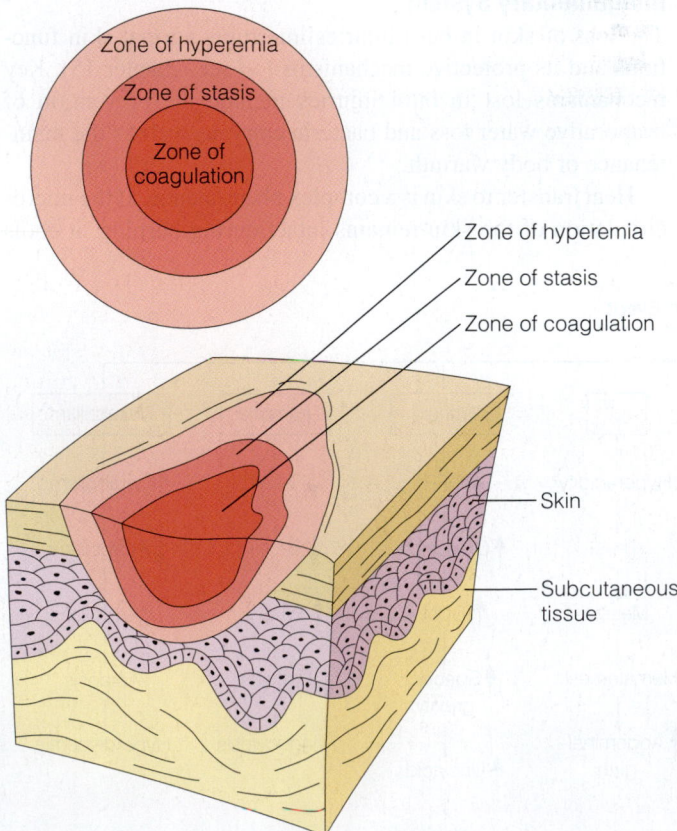

Figure 17–8 ■ The zones of injury.

The burn injury results in the formation of necrotic skin and subcutaneous tissue. During the acute stage of the injury, a hard crust (**eschar**) forms, which covers the wound and harbors necrotic tissue. The eschar is characteristically leathery and rigid. Removal of the eschar facilitates healing.

Cardiovascular System

The effects of a major burn are manifested in all components of the vascular system, and include hypovolemic shock (burn shock), cardiac dysrhythmias (such as ventricular fibrillation), cardiac arrest, and vascular compromise.

HYPOVOLEMIC SHOCK (BURN SHOCK)   Within minutes of the burn injury, a cascade of cellular events is initiated, and a massive amount of fluid shifts from the intracellular and intravascular compartments into the interstitium (third spacing). This shift is a type of hypovolemic shock called **burn shock**, and it continues until capillary integrity is restored, usually within 24 to 36 hours of the injury. Although the pathophysiologic mechanisms of postburn vascular changes and fluid volume shifts are not clearly understood, three processes occur early in the postburn phase in patients with > 40% TBSA:

- Increase in microvascular permeability at the burn wound site
- Generalized impairment of cell wall function, resulting in intracellular edema
- Increase in osmotic pressure of the burned tissue, leading to extensive fluid accumulation

During burn shock, the shifting of fluid is the direct result of a loss of cell wall integrity at the site of injury and in the capillary bed. Fluid leaks from the capillaries into interstitial compartments located at the burn wound site and throughout the body, resulting in a decrease in fluid volume within the intravascular space. Plasma proteins and sodium escape into the interstitium, enhancing edema formation. Blood pressure falls as cardiac output diminishes.

Vasoconstriction results as the vascular system attempts to compensate for fluid loss. Abnormal platelet aggregation and white blood cell (WBC) accumulation result in ischemia in the deeper tissue below the burn, leading to eventual thrombosis. Red blood cells (RBCs) and WBCs remain in the circulation, producing an elevation in erythrocyte and leukocyte counts secondary to hemoconcentration.

The leakage of fluid into the interstitium compromises the lymphatic system, resulting in intravascular hypovolemia and edema at the burn wound site. Edematous body surfaces impair peripheral circulation and result in necrosis of the underlying tissue. During burn shock, potassium ions leave the intracellular compartment, predisposing the patient to developing cardiac dysrhythmias. The process of burn shock continues until capillary integrity is restored, usually within 24 hours of the injury.

Burn shock reverses when fluid is reabsorbed from the interstitium into the intravascular compartment. The blood pressure rises as cardiac output increases, and urinary output improves. Diuresis continues from several days to 2 weeks postburn. During this phase, the extra cardiac workload may predispose the older patient, or the patient with cardiovascular disease, to fluid volume overload.

CARDIAC RHYTHM ALTERATIONS Burns of more than 40% TBSA cause significant myocardial dysfunction, with a decrease in myocardial contractibility and cardiac output. These changes, which occur prior to a decrease in plasma volume, are believed to be due to the release of substances and oxygen-free radicals from the burn wound and from ischemic myocardial cells. Electrical burns often result in cardiac dysrhythmias or cardiopulmonay arrest caused by heat damage to the myocardium or electrical interference with cardiac electrical activity.

PERIPHERAL VASCULAR COMPROMISE Direct heat damage to extremities, especially if circumferential burns are present, results in damage to blood vessels. Circulation to extremities may be further impaired by edema and by peripheral vasoconstriction that occurs during burn shock. In addition, **compartment syndrome** (in which the tissue pressure within a muscle compartment exceeds microvascular pressure, interrupting cellular perfusion) may result from circumferential burns and edema.

Respiratory System

Pulmonary damage may result from either direct inhalation injury or as part of the systemic response to the injury. Inhalation injury is a frequent and often lethal complication of burns. The injury may range from mild respiratory inflammation to massive pulmonary failure such as acute respiratory distress syndrome. Exposure to heat, asphyxiants, and smoke initiates the pathophysiologic process associated with inhalation injury.

Inflammation occurs at localized sites within the airway and is manifested as hyperemia. As a result, cells are destroyed and the bronchial cilia are rendered inactive. Because the mucociliary transport mechanism no longer functions, the patient may develop bronchial congestion and infection.

Interstitial pulmonary edema develops secondary to the escape of fluid from the pulmonary vasculature into the interstitial compartment of the lung tissue. Surfactant is inactivated, resulting in atelectasis and alveolar collapse. Sloughing of the damaged and dead lung tissue occasionally produces debris that may lead to complete airway obstruction.

Upper airway (above the level of the glottis) thermal injury results from the inhalation of heated air or chemicals dissolved in water. Inhalation injury is suspected when the patient has singed facial, scalp, or nasal hair. Physical findings include the presence of soot, charring, edema, blisters, and ulcerations along the mucosal lining of the oropharynx and larynx. The resulting edema in the airway peaks within the first 24 to 48 hours of injury. Ominous signs of hoarseness, labored breathing, or stridor indicate possible airway obstruction due to edema. Lower airway thermal injury is a rare occurrence. Because the lower airway is protected by laryngeal reflexes, thermal injury below the vocal cords is seldom seen. However, when it does occur, it is typically associated with the inhalation of steam or explosive gases or the aspiration of hot liquids. A classic finding is sputum containing soot or carbon particles.

Smoke poisoning results when toxic gases and particulate matter, the products of incomplete combustion, deposit directly onto the pulmonary mucosa. The composition of the products of combustion depends on the combustible material, the rate at which the temperature increases, and the amount of ambient oxygen present. Irritant gases and particulate matter have a direct cytotoxic effect. The degree of injury is determined by their solubility in water, duration of exposure, and the size of the particulate or aerosol droplet.

Carbon monoxide, a common asphyxiant, is a colorless, tasteless, odorless gas that has a 200 times greater affinity for hemoglobin than does oxygen. It displaces oxygen to bind with hemoglobin, forming carboxyhemoglobin. As a result, the decrease in arterial oxyhemoglobin produces tissue hypoxia. Carbon monoxide impairs both oxygen delivery and cellular oxygen use. The clinical manifestations of carbon monoxide poisoning range from mild visual impairment to coma and death (see the following Manifestations box).

Cyanide gas is released when plastics, polyurethane, nylon, or silk are burned. The resultant production of cyanide gas affects cellular respiration. The brain and heart are most vulnerable to cyanide poisoning. Treatment addresses the inability of the body to use oxygen. Hyperbaric oxygen (oxygen delivery in a high pressure chamber) may be used with inhalation of smoke. Hydroxocobalamin (Cyanokit) is a form of vitamin B-12 that converts cyanide to a form that can be excreted from the body.

FAST FACTS
Cyanide Poisoning
- Headache
- Dizziness
- Seizures
- Tachycardia
- Lethal dysrhythmias

Gastrointestinal System

Dysfunction of the gastrointestinal system is directly related to the size of the burn wound. Patients with ≥ 20% TBSA experience decreased peristalsis with resultant gastric distention and increased risk of aspiration. A decrease in or absence of bowel sounds is a manifestation of paralytic ileus (adynamic bowel) secondary to burn trauma. The resulting cessation of intestinal motility leads to gastric distention, nausea, vomiting, and hematemesis.

Stress ulcers (**Curling's ulcers**) are acute ulcerations of the stomach or duodenum that form following the burn injury. Abdominal pain, acidic gastric pH levels, hematemesis, and melana in the stool may indicate a gastric ulcer.

MANIFESTATIONS of Carbon Monoxide Poisoning

LEVEL OF CARBON MONOXIDE	MANIFESTATIONS
10% to 20%	Headache, dizziness, nausea, abdominal pain
21% to 40%	Headache, nausea, drowsiness, dizziness, irritability, confusion, stupor, hypotension, bradycardia, skin color ranging from pale to dark red
41% to 60%	Convulsion, coma, hypotension, tachycardia
> 60%	Death

In addition, ischemia of the intestine from splanchnic vasoconstriction increases the intestinal mucosal permeability. As a result, normal intestinal bacteria move from the lumen of the bowel to extraluminal sites, a process called *bacterial translocation*. This process is believed to be one of the mechanisms causing systemic sepsis and multiple organ dysfunction syndrome.

Urinary System

During the early stages of the burn injury, renal blood flow and glomerular filtration rates are greatly reduced from the decreased intravascular blood volume and the release of antidiuretic hormone (ADH) by the posterior pituitary. Urine output decreases, and serum creatinine and blood urea nitrogen increase.

Dark brown concentrated urine may indicate myoglobinuria or hemoglobinuria, the result of underlying muscle damage or the release of large amounts of dead or damaged erythrocytes after a major burn injury. When large amounts of these pigments are released, the liver cannot keep pace with conjugation and the pigments pass through the glomeruli. The pigments can occlude the renal tubules and cause renal failure, especially when dehydration, acidosis, or shock is also present.

Immune System

The function of the immune system is to protect the human body from invasion by foreign microorganisms. The capillary leak that occurs in the early stages of the burn injury continues throughout the burn shock phase and impairs the active components of both the cell-mediated and humoral immune systems.

The humoral immune system relies on B cells to produce antibodies or immunoglobulins (∞ see Chapter 13). In the burn patient, the serum levels of all immunoglobulins are significantly diminished. Serum protein levels remain persistently low throughout the clinical course until wound closure is effected. A marked decrease in T-cell counts results in a reduction of cytotoxic activity and suppression of the cell-mediated immune system.

The compromise in the humoral and cell-mediated immune systems constitutes a state of acquired immunodeficiency, which places the burn patient at risk for infection. The period of vulnerability is transient and may last from 1 to 4 weeks following the onset of the burn injury. During this time frame, opportunistic infections can be fatal despite aggressive antimicrobial therapy.

Metabolism

Two distinct phases characterize the body's metabolic response to the burn injury. The ebb phase, occurring during the first 3 days of the injury, is manifested by decreased oxygen consumption, fluid imbalance, shock, and inadequate circulating volume. These responses protect the body from the initial impact of the injury.

A second phase, the flow phase, occurs when adequate burn resuscitation has been accomplished. This phase is characterized by increases in cellular activity and protein catabolism, lipolysis, and gluconeogenesis. The basal metabolic rate (BMR) significantly increases, reaching twice the normal rate. Body weight and heat drop dramatically. Total energy expenditure may exceed 100% of normal BMR. Hypermetabolism persists until after wound closure has been accomplished and may reappear if complications occur.

Interdisciplinary Care

The burn team is composed of an interdisciplinary group of healthcare professionals, who together plan the care and treatment of the burn-injured patient during the acute and rehabilitative stages. The burn team consists of the nurse, physician, physical therapist, dietitian, psychiatrist/psychologist, and social worker. The team members meet regularly to discuss patient progress and to determine collaboratively the most effective regimen of care and psychosocial support.

Stages of Interdisciplinary Care

The clinical course of treatment for the burn patient is divided into three stages: the emergent/resuscitative stage, the acute stage, and the rehabilitative stage. Although these stages are useful predictors of the clinical needs of the burn patient, it is important to recognize that the process of burn injury is dynamic and that, in many cases, the clinical stage may not be clearly delineated. Assessment and management of the burn-injured patient are ongoing processes determined by the clinical picture; they last throughout the course of treatment. Figure 17–9 ■ shows the burn patient's progression through the healthcare system during each clinical stage of burn care. During each stage, different groups of nurses, physicians, and other healthcare specialists collaborate to manage the patient's recovery.

THE EMERGENT/RESUSCITATIVE STAGE   The emergent/resuscitative stage lasts from the onset of injury through successful fluid resuscitation. During this stage, healthcare workers estimate the extent of burn injury, institute first-aid measures, and implement fluid resuscitation therapies. The patient is assessed for shock and evidence of respiratory distress. If indicated, intravenous lines are inserted, and the patient may be prophylactically intubated. During this stage, healthcare workers determine whether the patient is to be transported to a burn center for the complex intervention strategies of the professional, interdisciplinary burn team.

Although many burn injuries are treated in local tertiary care facilities, the ABA has developed guidelines for determining whether the patient should be transported to a burn center for interdisciplinary approaches to treatment and rehabilitation. Adult patients who should be treated at burn centers include those with the following:

- Second- or third-degree burns > 10% TBSA in adults older than 50
- Second- or third-degree burns > 20% TBSA in adults younger than 50
- Third-degree burns > 5% TBSA in adults of any age
- Burns involving the hands, feet, face, eyes, ears, or perineum
- Electrical (including lightning), chemical, and inhalation injuries
- Circumferential burns of the extremities and/or chest
- Any burn associated with extenuating problems, preexisting illness, fractures, or other trauma

ACUTE STAGE   The acute stage begins with the start of diuresis and ends with closure of the burn wound (either by natural healing or by using skin grafts). During this stage, wound care management, nutritional therapies, and measures to control infectious processes are initiated. Hydrotherapy and excision

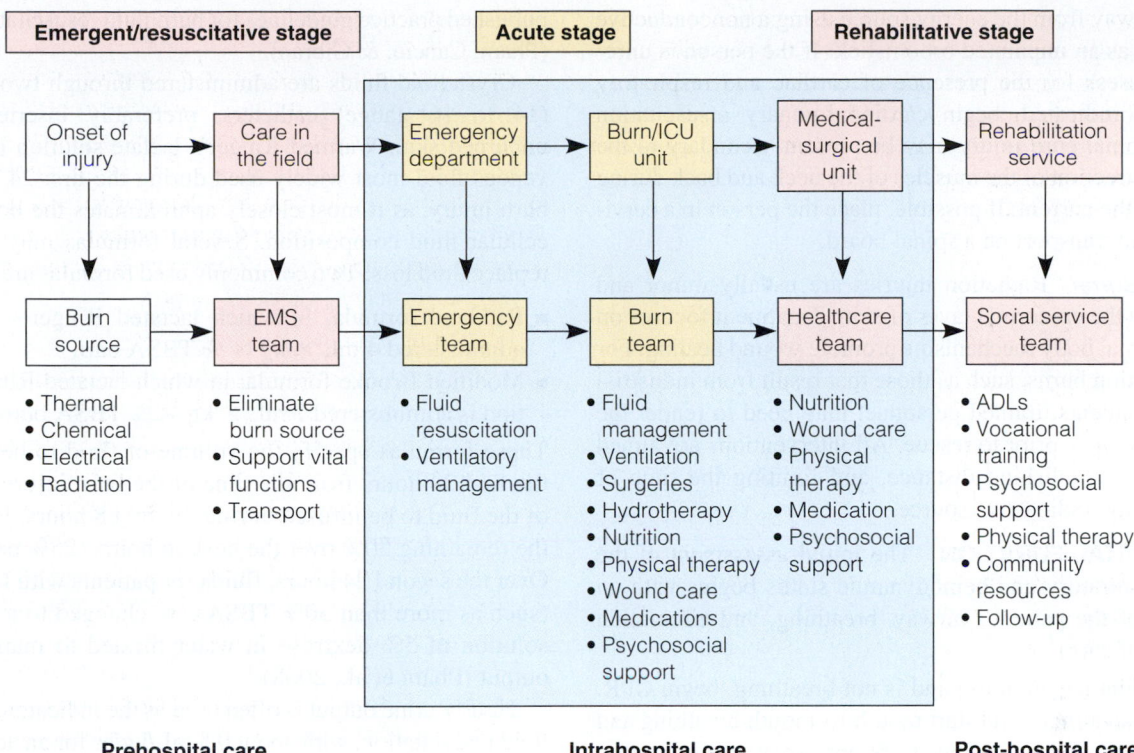

| Emergent/resuscitative stage | | | Acute stage | | | Rehabilitative stage |

Figure 17–9 ■ The patient's progression through the healthcare system during the emergent, acute, and rehabilitative stages of burn injury.

and grafting of full-thickness wounds are performed as soon as possible after injury. Enteral and parenteral nutritional interventions are started early in the treatment plan to address caloric needs resulting from extensive energy expenditure. Measures to combat infection are implemented during this stage, including the administration of topical and systemic antimicrobial agents. Pain management constitutes a significant segment of the nursing care plan throughout the clinical course of the burn-injured patient. The administration of narcotic pharmaceutical agents must precede all invasive procedures to maximize patient comfort and to reduce the anxieties associated with wound debridement and intensive physical therapy.

REHABILITATIVE STAGE The rehabilitative stage begins with wound closure and ends when the patient returns to the highest level of health restoration, which may take years. During this stage, the primary focus is the biopsychosocial adjustment of the patient, specifically the prevention of contractures and scars and the patient's successful resumption of work, family, and social roles through physical, vocational, occupational, and psychosocial rehabilitation. The patient is taught to perform range-of-motion exercises to enhance mobility and to support injured joints.

Prehospital Patient Management

Treatment at the injury scene includes measures to limit the severity of the burn and support vital functions. Before attempting to remove the patient from the source of burn injury, rescuers must ensure their own safety. Depending on the causative agent, rescuers may need to consult with experts to determine the best way to eliminate the source of the injury. Once the safety of the rescuers has been established, all prehospital interventions are aimed at eliminating the heat source, stabilizing

the patient's condition, identifying the type of burn, preventing heat loss, reducing wound contamination, and preparing for emergency transport. Restrictive jewelry and clothing is removed at the scene to prevent circumferential constriction of the torso and extremities.

STOP THE BURNING PROCESS Emergency measures, by type of injury, include the following.

Thermal Burns If the thermal injury has been caused by dry heat, smother inflamed clothing or lavage with water. Help the person "stop, drop, and roll" to extinguish the flame and limit the extent of burn. Once the flame has been extinguished, cover the body to prevent hypothermia. If the thermal injury has been caused by moist heat, lavage the area with cool water. Ice is not used for cooling as it causes vasoconstriction and may result in further injury. Tar and asphalt can be removed with mineral oil, petroleum ointments, Medisol (a citrus and petroleum distillate with hydrocarbon structure), or Crisco.

Chemical Burns For chemical burns, immediately remove the clothing and use a hose or shower to lavage the involved area thoroughly for a minimum of 20 minutes. Many chemicals are in powder form and as much dry chemical needs to be removed as possible before flushing the surface with water. Unusual chemicals may require consultation with the poison control center about appropriate treatment. Protective clothing should be worn during this process to protect the rescuer from chemical exposure. Chemical splashes in or near the eye require immediate eye irrigation with clean, cool water or saline.

Electrical Burns Electrical injuries pose serious potential harm to both rescuer and burn victim. Ensure that the source of electrical current has been disconnected, or move the person to safety and away from the energy source using a nonconductive device such as an unpainted broomstick. If the person is unresponsive, assess for the presence of cardiac and respiratory function. If indicated, begin cardiopulmonary resuscitation (CPR). A spinal cord injury may be present secondary to the forceful contraction of the muscles of the neck and back during exposure to the current. If possible, place the person in a cervical collar and transport on a spinal board.

Radiation Burns Radiation injuries are usually minor and involve only the epidermal layer of skin. Treatment focuses on helping normal body mechanisms promote wound healing. For severe radiation burns, such as those that result from industrial radiation accidents, trained personnel may need to render the area safe for entry prior to rescue. All interventions are aimed at shielding, establishing distance, and limiting the time of exposure to the radioactive source.

SUPPORT VITAL FUNCTION The initial assessment of the patient's respiratory and hemodynamic status begins with an evaluation of the patient's airway, breathing, and circulation (the ABCs of care).

- If the patient has no pulse and is not breathing, begin CPR. Establish an airway, and start mouth-to-mouth breathing and chest compressions. Continue CPR until spontaneous cardiopulmonary function returns or until the emergency management team takes over.
- Position the patient with the head elevated at greater than 30 degrees, and administer 100% humidified oxygen by face mask. Use nasotracheal suction as necessary to maintain a patent airway. Endotracheal intubation may be necessary if the patient has facial edema and inhalation injury. Auscultate the lungs often onsite to monitor respiratory status. Continuous pulse oximetry provides ongoing assessment of the patient's oxygen saturation levels.
- Monitor for cardiac dysrrhythmias or arrest. When available, connect the patient to a cardiac monitor and observe for dysrhythmias. Elevate burned extremities above the level of the heart to facilitate circulation.
- Initiate fluid replacement therapy for burn wounds that involve more than 20% of the total body surface area. Continuously assess heart and lung sounds and observe level of consciousness, cardiac rate and rhythm, blood pressure, and urine output.
- Cover the patient to maintain body temperature and to prevent further wound contamination and tissue damage.

Emergency and Acute Care

Prehospital personnel report to the emergency department staff all findings and medical interventions that occurred at the scene of the injury. The nurse obtains a history of the injury, estimates the depth and extent of the burn, begins fluid resuscitation, and maintains ventilation according to protocol.

FLUID RESUSCITATION **Fluid resuscitation** is the administration of intravenous fluids to restore the circulating blood volume during the acute period of increasing capillary permeability. To counteract the effects of burn shock, fluid resuscitation guidelines are used to replace the extensive fluid and electrolyte losses associated with major burn injuries. Fluid replacement is necessary in all burn wounds that involve ≥ 20% TBSA. The ABA

published practice guidelines for burn fluid resuscitation in 2008 (Pham, Cancio, & Gibran).

Crystalloid fluids are administered through two large-bore (14 to 16 gauge) catheters, preferably inserted through unburned skin. Warmed Ringer's lactate solution is the intravenous fluid most widely used during the first 24 hours after burn injury, as it most closely approximates the body's extracellular fluid composition. Several formulas may be used to replace fluid loss. Two commonly used formulas are as follows:

- Parkland formula, in which lactated Ringer's solution is administered 4 mL × kg × % TBSA burn
- Modified Brooke formula, in which lactated Ringer's solution is administered 2 mL × kg × % TBSA burn

These formulas specify the volume of fluid to be infused in the first 24 hours from the time of the burn injury, with 50% of the fluid to be infused during the first 8 hours, followed by the remaining 50% over the next 16 hours (25% per 8 hours). Over the second 24 hours, fluids for patients with larger burns (such as more than 30% TBSA) are changed to a crystalloid solution of 5% dextrose in water titrated to maintain urine output (Pham et al., 2008).

Hourly urine output is often used as the indicator of effective fluid resuscitation, with about 0.5 mL/kg/hr for an adult considered adequate. Another indicator is heart rate; if fluid resuscitation is adequate, the rate should be fewer than 120 beats per minute or in the upper limits of normal for age. However, fear, anxiety, and pain that accompany burn injuries often increase heart rate. Blood pressure changes are less reliable because significant hypotension does not develop until volume losses exceed 30% due to the body's compensatory mechanisms. Assessment for narrowed pulse pressure, which indicates shock earlier, should be considered along with urine output to monitor adequate fluid resuscitation.

During the fluid resuscitation stage, the patient may require invasive hemodynamic monitoring (∞ see Chapter 29). A pulmonary artery catheter can be used to monitor cardiac output, cardiac index, and pulmonary artery wedge pressures. All measurements must be maintained within normal limits to effect adequate fluid resuscitation.

RESPIRATORY MANAGEMENT Upon the patient's admission to the emergency department, several baseline assessments of respiratory status must be obtained: chest x-ray study, ABGs, vital signs, and carboxyhemoglobin levels. Intubation is indicated for all patients with burns of the chest, face, or neck. The primary treatment plan is oriented toward preventing atelectasis and maintaining alveolar oxygen exchange. The following interventions should be initiated:

- Maintain the head of the bed at 30 degrees or greater to maximize the patient's ventilatory efforts. Turn the patient side to side every 2 hours to prevent hypostatic pneumonia.
- To keep airway passages clear, suction the patient frequently, encourage the patient to use incentive spirometry hourly, and help the patient perform coughing and deep-breathing exercises every 2 hours.
- In the face of impending airway obstruction, the patient will require immediate intubation. Nasotracheal tube placement is the preferred route because it seems to be better tolerated

and can be more effectively secured. If the patient has suffered nasolabial burns, however, the orotracheal route is preferred. Nasotracheal and orotracheal intubation is reserved for short-term ventilatory management. For long-term ventilatory management (i.e., greater than 3 weeks), a tracheostomy is performed.

- Humidification of either room air or oxygen helps prevent the drying of tracheal secretions. Ambient air or oxygen flow is based on ABG results. The patient may be placed on a face mask, steam collar, T-piece, mechanical ventilation with PEEP, pressure support ventilation, or high-frequency jet ventilation. The goal of all therapies is to maintain adequate tissue oxygenation with the least amount of inspired oxygen flow necessary.

- Medications to dilate constricted bronchial passages are administered intravenously and as inhalants to control bronchospasms and wheezing. Mucolytic agents liquefy tenacious sputum and aid in expectoration.

- An arterial line is placed in the patient with major burn injury for continuous assessment of ABGs. Pulmonary artery pressure catheters may be inserted to measure pulmonary vascular resistance (PVR), pulmonary artery pressure (PAP), pulmonary artery wedge pressure (PAWP), and mixed venous oxygen saturation (SVO_2). The PVR and PAP rise in the presence of hypoxia. The SVO_2 is the average percentage of hemoglobin bound with oxygen in the venous blood and reflects overall tissue utilization of oxygen. Pulse oximetry monitors arterial oxygen saturation levels.

- In the presence of carbon monoxide (CO) poisoning, monitor carboxyhemoglobin (COHgb) levels. Pulse oximetry cannot distinguish between oxyhemoglobin and COHgb, thus a false normal or high pulse oximetry reading is seen. High flow 100% oxygen is given immediately by nonrebreather mask. Patients with COHgb greater than 15% may require hyperbaric oxygen therapy to replace the CO.

- Pain medications are administered if the patient is not in shock.

After stabilization in the emergency department, the patient is transferred to the critical care unit or a specialized burn center (a facility that has a burn physician as director of a specialized nursing unit with dedicated burn beds). In both settings, continuous monitoring of diagnostic tests, administration of medications, pain control, wound management, and nutrition support therapies constitute the initial plan of care.

Diagnosis

The following diagnostic tests are used to evaluate the patient's progress and to modify intervention strategies.

- *Urinalysis* indicates the adequacy of renal perfusion and the patient's nutritional status. In catabolic states, nitrogen is excreted in large amounts into the urine. Nitrogen loss is measured through 24-hour urine collections for total nitrogen, urea nitrogen, and amino acid nitrogen. *Myoglobinuria*, which manifests as a dark brown, wine-colored urine, signals the development of acute tubular necrosis. Loss of plasma protein and dehydration lead to proteinuria and elevated urine specific gravity. Glycosuria is a transient development following major burn injury; it indicates a need to adjust the nutritional program.

- The *complete blood count* is monitored regularly. Hematocrit is elevated secondary to hemoconcentration and fluid shifts from the intravascular compartment. Hemoglobin is decreased secondary to hemolysis. White blood cells are elevated if infection is present.

- *Serum electrolytes* are monitored regularly. Sodium levels are decreased secondary to massive fluid shifts into the interstitium. Potassium levels initially are elevated during burn shock, as a result of cell lysis and fluid shifts into the extracellular space. Potassium levels decrease after burn shock resolves, as fluid shifts back to intracellular and intravascular compartments.

- *Renal function* test results are closely monitored. Blood urea nitrogen (BUN) is elevated secondary to dehydration. Creatinine is elevated in the presence of renal insufficiency.

- *Total protein, albumin, transferrin, prealbumin, retinol binding protein, alpha 1-acid glycoprotein, and C-reactive protein* indicate protein synthesis and nutritional status. Because of the fluid shifts that occur during the early stages of the burn injury, they are more useful markers during the rehabilitative phase of care.

- *Creatine phosphokinase (CPK)* is elevated following an electrical burn, secondary to extensive muscle damage. Blood glucose is transiently elevated after major burn injury.

- *Serial ABGs* indicate the presence of hypoxia and acid–base disturbances and indicate patient responses to changes in oxygen therapies. The burn-injured patient may demonstrate elevated or lowered pH, decreased PCO_2, decreased PO_2, and low-normal bicarbonate levels.

- *Pulse oximetry* allows continuous assessment of oxygen saturation levels. The burn-injured patient may have saturation levels below 95%.

- *Serial chest x-ray studies* document changes within the first 24 to 48 hours that may reflect the presence of atelectasis, pulmonary edema, or acute respiratory distress syndrome (ARDS).

- *Serial 12 lead electrocardiograms (EKGs)* are necessary to monitor the development of dysrhythmias, especially those associated with hypokalemic and hyperkalemic states.

Medications

PAIN CONTROL Burns often cause excruciating pain. In the emergent stages of care, intravenously administered narcotics such as morphine, hydromorphone, or fentanyl are the best means of managing pain. Morphine is the drug of choice in a typical dosage of 3 to 5 mg intravenously every 5 to 10 minutes for an adult. Meperidine is avoided because of potential normeperidine accumulation, which can produce tremors and anxiety. Once the patient has been stabilized, it is appropriate to administer narcotics, especially intravenous fentanyl, prior to initiating hydrotherapy or intensive exercising routines. Burn treatments can also produce high levels of anxiety, necessitating the use of anxiolytic agents such as midazolam and lorazepam (Montgomery, 2004). Anxiolytics are especially useful when administered 1 hour before wound care. During the acute stage, opioids are administered around-the-clock to decrease pain that occurs at rest. Patient-controlled analgesia (pca) enhances the patient's ability to cope with pain. The oral, subcutaneous, or intramuscular route of administration should be avoided until hemodynamic stability and unimpaired tissue perfusion returns.

As the patient enters the rehabilitative stage of care, alternative therapies for pain control may be added to the plan of care. Distraction, self-hypnosis, guided imagery, and relaxation techniques are helpful adjuncts in managing pain and coping with loss. ∞ See Chapter 9 for a discussion of strategies for managing pain.

ANTIMICROBIAL AGENTS Systemic infection is a leading cause of death in major burn patients. Gram-positive organisms such as *Staphylococcus* and *Streptococcus* colonize the burn surface during the first week postburn; gram-negative enteric organisms become more common with longer periods of hospitalization. Diagnosing infection is best done through a burn wound biopsy. To eliminate infection on the surface of the burn wound, topical antimicrobial therapy is used, depending on protocol. Generally, topical antimicrobials are not applied until the patient is admitted to a burn unit. Of the many antimicrobial agents available, the three most widely used are mafenide acetate (Sulfamylon) cream, silver sulfadiazine (Silvadene) cream, and silver nitrate 0.5% soaks. All three are broad-spectrum antibiotics. The choice of topical antibiotic is based on the extent of the burn wound, the presence of identified bacterial organisms, whether an open (exposing the wound to the air) or closed (using bulky dressings) method of treatment is used, and patient response. Despite antimicrobial therapy, patients with major burn assault have a greater risk for sepsis and septic shock.

Patients with major burns are usually given prophylactic antibiotics. Systemic antimicrobial therapy is indicated in the immediate preoperative and postoperative period associated with excision and autografting. Postoperatively, the therapy is discontinued as soon as the patient's hemodynamic status returns to normal, usually within the first 24 hours. In the long-term treatment of identified infectious processes, drug administration is limited to the least amount of time required to eradicate the infection. See the following box for nursing implications for topical antimicrobial therapy for the burn patient.

TETANUS PROPHYLAXIS If the patient's immunization status is in doubt, tetanus toxoid is administered intramuscularly early in the acute phase of care to prevent *Clostridium tetani* infection.

PREVENTING GASTRIC HYPERACIDITY Hyperacidity must be controlled to prevent Curling's ulcer. A nasogastric tube is placed during the emergent phase of care, and gastric aspirant is obtained hourly. The gastric pH should be assessed and maintained at levels above 5. To control gastric acid secretion

during the acute phase of care, histamine H_2 blockers (e.g., famotidine [Pepcid]) or proton pump inhibitors (e.g., pantoprazole [Protonix]) can be administered intravenously, either intermittently or as continuous infusions. As soon as bowel sounds become audible, the patient is placed on an antacid regimen.

Treatments

SURGERY Three surgical interventions are commonly employed to manage the burn wound: surgical debridement, escharotomy, and autografting.

Escharotomy When the burn eschar forms circumferentially around the torso or extremities, it acts as a tourniquet, impairing circulation. Left unchecked, the affected body part becomes gangrenous.

To prevent circumferential constriction of the torso or extremity, an **escharotomy** is performed by the physician with a scalpel or by electrocautery (Figure 17–10 ■). A sterile surgical incision is made longitudinally along the extremity or the trunk to release taut skin and allow for expansion caused by edema formation. In the first 24 hours following the procedure, the incision should be gently packed with fine mesh gauze. After 24 hours, the site may be treated with a direct application of a topical antimicrobial agent. See the following box for nursing implications for care of the patient undergoing escharotomy.

Surgical Debridement **Surgical debridement** refers to the process of excising the wound to the level of fascia (fascial excision) or sequentially removing thin slices of the burn wound to the level of viable tissue (tangential excision). Because **fascial excision**, or **fasciectomy**, sacrifices potentially viable fat and lymphatic tissue, its use is reserved for patients with extensive or full-thickness burns. The most common technique is electrocautery with cutting and coagulating current capabilities. Tangential excision is performed with the use of a dermatome. Shallow burns and some of moderate depth bleed briskly after one slice. If bleeding does not occur, the procedure is repeated until a viable bed of dermis or subcutaneous fat is reached. Following surgical debridement, the patient is returned to the burn unit.

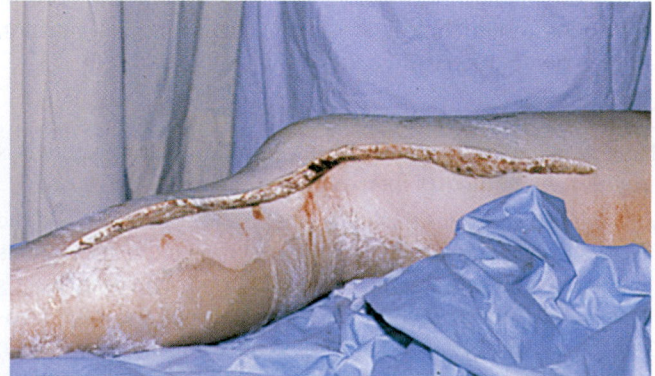

Figure 17–10 ■ Escharotomy. The surgical procedure consists of removing the eschar formed on the skin and underlying tissue following severe burns. The procedure is particularly helpful in restoring circulation to the extremities of patients when scar tissue forms a tight, constrictive band around the circumference of a limb.

TOPICAL ANTIMICROBIAL AGENTS

Mafenide acetate (Sulfamylon)

Silver nitrate

Silver sulfadiazine (Silvadene)

Research shows that the most effective topical agents are those that (1) act against the major pathogens responsible for causing burn wound infection, (2) achieve levels of concentration sufficient to decrease microbial colonization, (3) are rapidly excreted or metabolized, (4) are nontoxic, and (5) are easy to use and inexpensive.

Mafenide Acetate

Mafenide is a synthetic antibiotic closely related chemically, but not pharmacologically, to the sulfonamides. Although the mechanism of action is unclear, the drug appears to interfere with the metabolism of bacterial cells. Mafenide is a bacteriostatic agent effective against many gram-positive and gram-negative organisms.

For topical administration, mafenide is used in an 8.5% cream in a water-miscible base. Following application, the drug is rapidly diffused through the burn eschar and absorbed systemically.

In the general circulation, mafenide metabolizes to a weak carbonic anhydrase inhibitor known as *p*-carboxybenzenesulfonamide, a substance that impairs the renal mechanisms involved in the buffering of blood. Bicarbonate excretion in the urine increases, and ammonia and chloride excretion decreases. To maintain normal acid–base balance, the pulmonary system effects a compensatory hyperventilatory state. If the compensatory hyperventilation is insufficient, the patient develops metabolic acidosis.

Nursing Responsibilities

- Use mafenide with caution in patients with renal or pulmonary disease.
- Approximately 3% to 5% of patients develop a hypersensitivity to mafenide, resulting in a maculopapular rash on the unburned areas. Assess the patient for the following:

Pruritus	Urticaria
Facial edema	Blisters
Swelling	Eosinophilia

  If hypersensitivity reactions occur, discontinue the drug and administer antihistamines.
- Monitor the patient for superinfection within the burn eschar, in the subeschar tissue, or in viable tissue adjacent to the wound.

Health Education for the Patient and Family

- Expect intense pain, stinging, or a burning sensation following drug application. Take appropriate measures to control pain before applying the drug.
- Apply the drug to clean, debrided burn wounds once or twice daily. Continue applications until healing is apparent.
- If any signs of allergy develop, discontinue the drug and notify the physician.
- Report any sudden and prolonged increases in respiratory rate.

Silver Nitrate

Silver nitrate is a bacteriostatic agent that inhibits a wide variety of gram-positive and gram-negative organisms. Its antimicrobial effect is due to the actions of silver ions, which markedly alter the microbial cell wall and membrane. Additionally, the drug denatures bacterial protein, thereby inactivating and precipitating the microbes.

Nursing Responsibilities

- Silver nitrate is used as a 0.5% solution in distilled water. Apply the solution to bulky gauze dressings every 2 hours, and provide complete dressing changes twice daily.
- Silver nitrate has limited penetrating ability and is ineffective if used more than 72 hours following a burn injury.
- At the local tissue level, silver nitrate immediately interacts with chloride ions to form a black silver chloride precipitate that discolors both the burn wound and the adjacent tissues. The discoloration significantly hampers visual inspection of the wound.
- High concentrations of the drug result in cellular toxicity of surrounding healthy tissue.
- Because large amounts of water are systemically absorbed from the dressing site, the patient may demonstrate a hypotonic state. Hyponatremia and hypochloremic alkalosis are common manifestations in burn-injured patients treated with silver nitrate.

Health Education for the Patient and Family

- Watch for and report any signs and symptoms of hypotonicity: swelling, weight gain, difficulty in breathing.
- This drug causes a black discoloration on all skin surfaces and dressings with which it comes into contact.
- Because discoloration can conceal evidence of infection, watch for systemic manifestations of infection fever, malaise, rapid pulse rate, listlessness.
- Saturate the wound dressings every 2 hours with a 0.5% aqueous solution of the drug. Change the dressings completely twice daily.

Silver Sulfadiazine

Silver sulfadiazine, a sulfonamide, is the most commonly used topical agent. The drug acts on the cell membrane and cell wall of susceptible bacteria and binds to cellular DNA. The drug is bactericidal and effective against a wide variety of gram-negative and gram-positive organisms.

Nursing Responsibilities

- Many patients develop a marked leukopenia in response to this drug, which tends to improve spontaneously over the course of therapy. This finding does not contraindicate use of the drug.
- Hypersensitivity to silver sulfadiazine has been reported in a small number of cases. If the patient develops hypersensitivity, administer antihistamine and change the topical agent.
- If sulfa crystals form in the urine, keep the patient well hydrated.
- Treatment with this drug can cause systemic uptake of propylene glycol, which results in an elevated serum osmolality and high urine specific gravity in the patient who is not dehydrated. These findings tend to create confusion during the fluid resuscitative stage of care. Whenever the serum osmolality and urine specific gravity fail to correlate with a clinical picture that reflects fluid volume overload (elevated CVP/PCWP, rhonchi/wheezing, edema), suspect systemic propylene glycol uptake.

Health Education for the Patient and Family

- Apply the drug to clean, debrided wounds once or twice daily, completely covering the burn wound at all times.
- Continue applying the drug until healing is apparent.
- If any signs of allergy develop, discontinue the drug and notify the physician.
- Watch for evidence of concentrated urine, and notify the physician.
- If not contraindicated, drink large amounts of fluids to prevent sulfa crystals from forming in the urine.

BOX 17–2 Nursing Implications for Circumferential Wound Management

Escharotomy

A circumferential burn wound increases the risk for impaired tissue perfusion of the involved area. To prevent arterial occlusion, an escharotomy is performed to release tension and permit unobstructed arterial blood flow. The nurse continuously assesses the involved area and notifies the physician of the need to perform this emergent procedure, which is done at the bedside. Because only the dead burn wound tissue is excised, the patient experiences very little pain.

Nursing Responsibilities

- For circumferential burn wounds of the extremity, assess the extremity for absence of blood flow:
  a. Using a Doppler ultrasound stethoscope, check hourly for the presence of a pulse.
  b. Assess the extremity hourly for warmth, color, sensation, and capillary refill.
  c. Observe for evidence of numbness or tingling.
- For circumferential burn wounds of the torso, assess for evidence of respiratory distress:
  a. Obtain ABGs as needed.
  b. Auscultate lung sounds hourly.

c. Observe for evidence of cyanosis, tachypnea, anxiety, or restlessness.
- For circumferential burn wounds of the neck, assess for evidence of respiratory distress. Prepare the patient for prophylactic intubation.
- Monitor for excessive blood loss, and transfuse the patient if indicated.
- Dress the open wound (escharotomy) with topical antimicrobial agents as ordered.

Patient Teaching

- Teach the patient the importance of reporting any evidence of impaired circulation: numbness, tingling, blue color to the extremity, absence of sensation.
- Assure the patient that the procedure will not be painful and will provide immediate relief.
- Teach the patient the importance of protecting the open wound (escharotomy) from infection.
- Explain the rationale supporting prophylactic intubation for burn wounds involving the head and neck.
- Provide assurance that all blood loss will be replaced and that bleeding at the site will be controlled.

Autografting A procedure performed in the surgical suite, **autografting** is used to effect permanent skin coverage. Early burn wound excision and skin grafting decreases the hospital stay and enhances rehabilitation. Skin is removed from healthy tissue (donor site) of the burn-injured patient and applied to the burn wound (Figures 17–11 ■ and 17–12 ■). (Skin grafts and flaps are discussed in ∞ Chapter 15.) After the autograft is applied, the grafted area is immobilized. The site is assessed daily for evidence of adherence. The patient resumes range-of-motion exercises 5 days postgraft. As the wound heals, the patient may complain of itching, which can be treated with mild lotions.

Cultured epithelial autografting is a technique in which skin cells are removed from unburned sites on the patient's body, then minced and placed in a culture medium for growth. Over a 5- to 7-day period, the cells expand 50 to 70 times the size of the initial biopsies. The cells are again separated out and placed in a new culture medium for continued growth. With this technique, enough skin can be grown over a period of 3 to 4 weeks

to cover an entire human body. The cells are prepared in sheets and attached to petroleum jelly gauze backing, which is applied to the burn wound site. Problems with infection and lack of attachment have occurred.

BIOLOGIC AND BIOSYNTHETIC DRESSINGS The terms *biologic dressing* and *biosynthetic dressing* refer to any temporary material that rapidly adheres to the wound bed, promotes healing, and/or prepares the burn wound for permanent

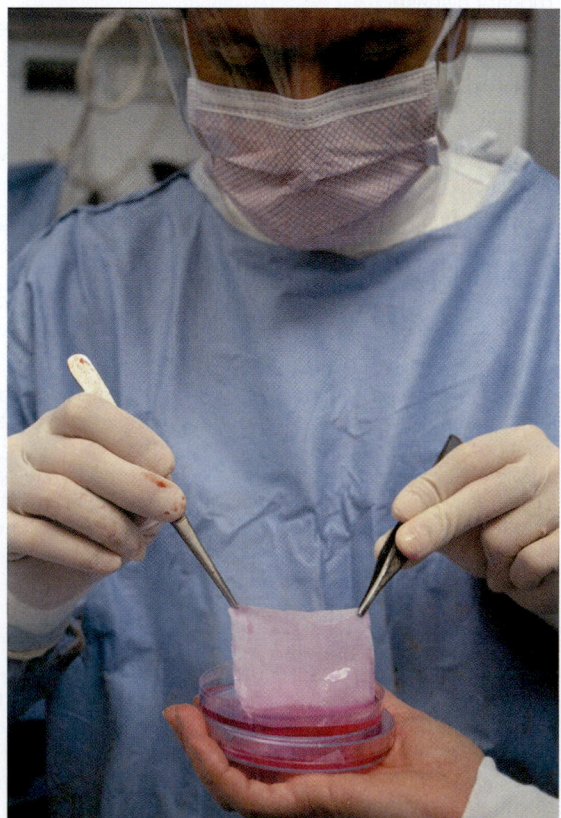

Figure 17–11 ■ Skin graft for burn injury (autograft).

Source: Photo Researchers, Inc.

Figure 17–12 ■ Cultured epithelial autografting of a skin culture.

autograft coverage. Ideally, these kinds of dressings should be easy to apply and remove, inexpensive, nonantigenic, elastic, able to reduce pain, able to serve as a bacterial barrier, and able to enhance the natural healing process. The dressings are applied to the burn wound as soon as possible. Covering the wound eliminates the loss of water through evaporation, reduces infection, and promotes wound healing. Biologic and biosynthetic dressings that are currently in use include homograft (allograft), heterograft (xenograft), amnionic membranes, and synthetic materials.

Homograft, or **allograft**, is human skin that has been harvested from cadavers. It is stored in skin banks located throughout the nation. The development of methods to achieve prolonged storage of frozen, viable skin has increased the use of this dressing; however, its short supply and expense still pose problems. It is manufactured as strips cut to the pattern of the burn and applied using sterile technique. Under normal circumstances, a homograft is rejected within 14 to 21 days following application.

Heterograft, or **xenograft**, is skin obtained from an animal, usually a pig. Although fresh porcine heterograft is available to some centers, frozen heterograft is much more commonly used. Once applied, heterograft appears to undergo early softening and lysis from enzymatic action from the wound. As a result, frequent changes of the heterograft dressing are necessary. Because of the high infection rates associated with this dressing, silver-nitrate-treated porcine heterograft has been developed to retard microbial growth.

The multiple problems associated with the use of biologic dressings have driven the development of synthetic materials. One such material is Biobrane (Smith & Nephew), a composite material consisting of nylon mesh bonded to silicone that has proved successful in the temporary coverage of second- and third-degree burns. Whereas Biobrane adheres well to moderately clean wounds, it cannot adhere to or lower bacterial counts in grossly contaminated wounds. Biobrane dressing is supplied in various sizes, cut to fit the wound site, and secured with tape or Steri-Strips. It spontaneously separates from the wound when the underlying tissue heals. Other biosynthetic wound dressings include Ingrega (Intregra Life Sciences Corp.) and Alloderm (LifeCell Corp.). If dermal thickness is lost in deep partial-thickness or full-thickness burns, several products can serve as a dermal replacement. Integra is a synthetic dermal substitute and Alloderm is human cadaver allograft dermis that is nonimmunogenic. These products are placed in the wound, and split-thickness autografts are then placed over the dermal replacement. These products are used to provide temporary wound coverage, reduce pain, and facilitate healing.

Two recent temporary skin substitutes are TransCyte and Apligraf. TransCyte is a bioengineered substance, derived from human fibroblast cells grown within mesh. As the cells grow, they secrete human dermal collagen, matrix proteins, and growth factors. The product is produced, extensively tested for any infectious agents, and then frozen. It is used for temporary covering for surgically debrided full-thickness and deep partial-thickness burn wounds, and is an alternative to silver sulfadiazine and cadaver skin. TransCyte forms a transparent, protective barrier over the wound surface and is typically applied only once. The best results have been obtained when it was applied within 24 hours of injury. Apligraf is bilayered skin substitute cultured from neonatal foreskin.

Hydrocolloid dressings such as DuoDerm (Convatec) are a type of synthetic material. They are occlusive wafers of gum-like materials that provide a water-resistant outer layer for coverage of the donor site. They protect healing tissue from excessive drying, liquefy necrotic tissue, and absorb wound drainage. Other synthetics are Aquacel (Convatec), a temporary dressing (up to 14 days) that is impregnated with silver, Acticoat (Smith & Nephew), an antimicrobial barrier dressing and Kaltostat (Convatec), a calcium-alginate absorptive dressing. The newest treatment method uses the vacuum-assisted closure (VAC) devise. VAC consists of a sponge placed over the wound and tubing connecting the sponge to a pump. An occlusive, adhesive dressing covers the wound and tubing, sealing the wound to create negative pressure. VAC has shown positive results in reducing wound edema, removing exudate, and improving wound healing in partial-thickness burns and deep hand burns.

WOUND MANAGEMENT The outcomes of care for the patient with a major burn depends on the prevention and treatment of infection through daily topical wound care, wound monitoring, and wound excision and closure. The goals of wound management are as follows:

- Control microbial colonization and prevent wound infection.
- Prevent wound progression.
- Achieve wound coverage as early as possible.
- Promote function of healing skin.

Debriding the Wound Burned tissue releases chemical mediators that stimulate phagocytosis in an attempt to digest debris left by decaying necrotic tissue. Necrotic tissue that remains despite phagocytic action retards healing and prolongs inflammation. **Debridement** is the process of removing all loose tissue, wound debris, and eschar (dead tissue) from the wound. Three methods of debridement are employed: mechanical, enzymatic, and surgical (surgical debridement was previously discussed).

A nurse may perform mechanical debridement by applying and removing gauze dressings (wet-to-dry or wet-to-moist), hydrotherapy, irrigation, or scissors and tweezers. However, removal of gauze dressings can cause pain and possibly damage granulation tissue (Honari, 2004). During hydrotherapy (in an immersion tank, a shower, or on a spray table) the burn injury may be gently washed with a mild, nonperfumed, antimicrobial soap or wound cleaner solution to remove dead skin and separate eschar. The solution is then rinsed off with warm saline or tap water. Body hair (except for eyebrows) should be shaved within the burn and to within 2.5 cm of the wound edges. Blistered skin is grasped with a dry gauze and gently removed. The edges of blisters or eschar are trimmed with blunt scissors. The wound is then covered with a topical antimicrobial agent.

Enzymatic debridement involves the use of a topical agent to dissolve and remove necrotic tissue, as well as lift eschar. An enzyme (such as accuzyme, collagenase [Santyl], or fibrinolysis-deoxyribonuclease [Elase]) is applied in a thin layer only within the wound area and covered with one layer of fine mesh gauze. A topical antimicrobial agent is then applied and covered with a bulky wet dressing; the wound is immobilized with expandable mesh gauze. Enzymatic agents are discontinued once the eschar is removed and granulation tissue appears (Honari, 2004).

DRESSING THE WOUND Once the wound has been cleaned and debrided, it may be dressed using one of two methods. In the open method, the burn wound remains open to air, covered only by a topical antimicrobial agent. This method allows the wound to be easily assessed. Topical agents must be frequently reapplied because they tend to rub off onto the bedding. The open method also increases the risk for hypothermia.

In the closed method, a topical antimicrobial agent is applied to the wound site, which is covered with gauze or a nonadherent dressing and then gently wrapped with a gauze roll bandage (Figure 17–13 ■). With the closed method, burn wounds are usually dressed twice daily and as needed. Dressings are applied circumferentially in a distal-to-proximal manner. All fingers and toes are wrapped separately. Dressings are held in place with stockinettes rather than tape to prevent further skin injury. The closed method decreases heat loss but may impair range of motion (ROM).

Positioning, Splints, and Exercise **Contractures** are a common problem for patients with burn injuries. During therapy, the patient must be maintained in positions that prevent contractures from forming. Because flexion is the natural resting position of joints and extremities, early physical therapy includes maintaining antideformity positions. Splints immobilize body parts and prevent contractures of the joints. They are applied as soon as possible after the injury and removed according to schedules established by the physical therapist.

Early in the acute phase of care, the physical therapist prescribes active and passive ROM exercises, which are performed every 2 hours at the bedside, most often by physical therapy.

Ideally an exercise program is initiated on admission and continued until wounds are healed. Early ambulation is also part of the plan of care once the patient's condition becomes stable.

Support Garments Applying uniform pressure can prevent or reduce hypertrophic scarring. Tubular support bandages are applied 5 to 7 days postgraft to maintain a tension ranging from 10 to 20 mmHg to control scarring. The patient wears custom-made elastic pressure garments such as a Jobst garment for 6 months to a year postgraft (Figure 17–14 ■).

NUTRITIONAL SUPPORT The patient with a major burn is in a hypermetabolic and catabolic state. The resting energy expenditure after severe burn injury can increase by as much as 100% above normal levels, depending on the extent of catabolism and the patient's physical activity, size, age, and gender. This increase is believed due to heat loss from the burn wound, an increase in beta-adrenergic activity, pain, and infection. As a result, total caloric needs may be as great as 4000 to 6000 kcal per day.

Traditional dietary management based on oral intake seldom meets the kcal requirements necessary to reverse negative nitrogen balance and begin the healing process. Enteral feedings with a nasointestinal feeding tube are therefore instituted within 24 to 48 hours of the burn injury to offset hypermetabolism, improve nitrogen balance, decrease sepsis, and decrease length of hospital stay. A nasointestinal feeding tube is placed under fluoroscopy, with the tip extending past the pylorus to prevent reflux and aspiration.

Although enteral feeding is the preferred nutritional therapy, it is contraindicated in Curling's ulcer, bowel obstruction, feeding intolerance, pancreatitis, or septic ileus. When the enteral route cannot be used, a central venous catheter is inserted via the subclavian or jugular vein for the administration of total parenteral nutrition (TPN).

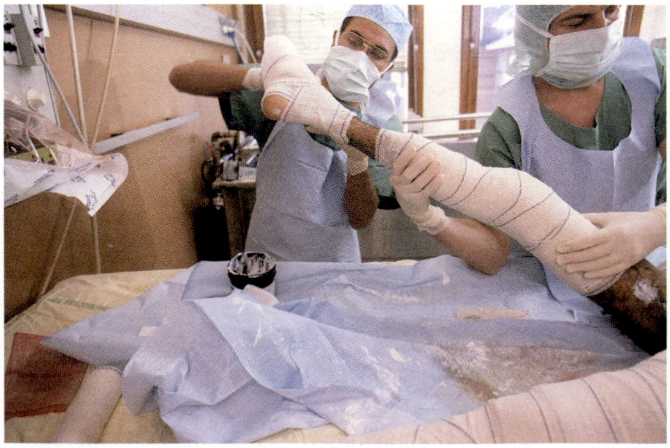

Figure 17–13 ■ Closed method of dressing a burn.
Source: Photo Researchers, Inc.

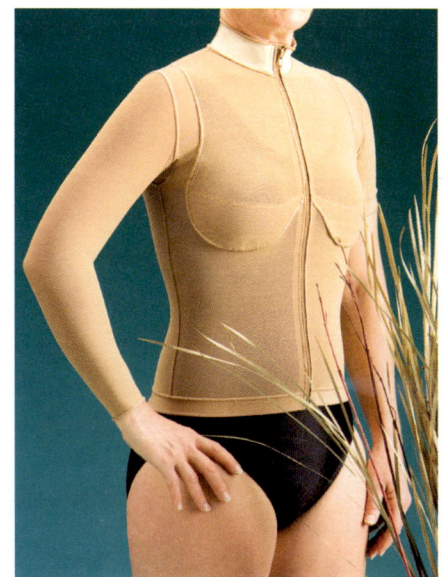

Figure 17–14 ■ The patient wears custom-made elastic pressure garments such as a Jobst garment for 6 months to a year postgraft.
Source: © Gottfried Medical, Inc., used with permission.

∽ Nursing Care

The patient with a major burn has complex, multisystem needs. Table 17–4 lists overall nursing interventions for the emergent, acute, and rehabilitative stages of burn injury. See the Nursing Care Plan on page 470.

Health Promotion

Although treatments have improved significantly over the last several decades, there is no cure for burns. Prevention remains the primary goal. With the public's increasing attention to health promotion and disease prevention, the nursing profession currently is well positioned to collaborate with other disciplines to develop initiatives to reduce the number of burn injuries. For example, as patient advocates, nurses can alert political leaders to the need to pass legislation aimed at reducing the incidence of burns. Appropriate legislative themes might center on safety in the workplace (e.g., requirements for smoke alarms and sprinkler systems), on the highways (e.g., regulations regarding the transportation of flammable liquids), and in the home (e.g., requirements for safety devices for water heaters and wood-burning stoves, and for self-extinguishing cigarettes). As educators, nurses can develop teaching plans for families and communities to heighten awareness of the problem. As researchers, nurses can investigate conditions leading to burn injury and suggest methods to reduce its prevalence. Working together with health care policy makers and community leaders, nurses can join the effort to lower the number of annual burn cases.

Nursing Assessment

Nursing assessment is continuous from the initial contact with the patient with a burn injury. This section describes the survey conducted when the patient arrives at the emergency department. Once there, the staff must act quickly to obtain the patient's history of the burn injury, including the time of injury, causative agents, early treatment, medical history, and patient's age and body weight. In most cases, the patient is awake and oriented and able to relate the information during the emergent phase of care. Because changes in sensorium will become evident within the first few hours following a major burn injury, the nurse obtains as much information as is possible immediately on the patient's arrival.

- *Time of injury.* In many cases, the patient is admitted to the ED an hour or more after the injury occurred. The time of the burn injury must be documented as precisely as possible at the scene, because all fluid resuscitation calculations are based on the time of the burn injury, not on the patient's time of arrival at the ED.
- *Cause of the injury.* Because the type of burn injury determines which nursing measures take priority, identify the specific causative agent to establish the appropriate plan of care.
- *First-aid treatment.* Prior to the arrival of medical personnel, the patient or family may have applied home remedies to treat the burn wound. It is important for the nurse to ascertain and document the nature of all home treatment interventions, including the application of neutralizing agents, liquids, and immobilizing devices used to splint associated injuries.

TABLE 17–4 Interventions in Various Stages of Burn Injury

STAGE OF BURN INJURY	ONSET	END POINT	INTERVENTIONS
Emergent/Resuscitative	Occurrence of burn injury	Successful fluid resuscitation	Remove patient from heat source. Initiate first aid. Assess extent of burn injury. Prevent hypothermia. Assess for shock. Determine need for intubation. Determine need for intravenous therapy. Follow protocol for fluid resuscitation. Obtain history. Transport to tertiary care facility.
Acute	Diuresis	Wound closure	Begin hydrotherapy. Determine need for excision of burn wound. Control spread of infection. Institute wound care. Start nutrition support. Graft burn wound. Initiate physical therapy. Manage pain.
Rehabilitative	Wound closure	Return to highest level of health restoration	Prevent scar formation. Continue physical therapy. Address psychosocial, cultural, and spiritual needs. Consider occupational therapy. Consider vocational training. Assess home maintenance management.

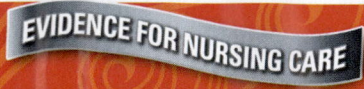

MEETING INDIVIDUALIZED NEEDS Burns in the Older Adult

Older adults are at greater risk for burns of all degrees of severity, with burns and fires being a major cause of death. Most burns are accidental, the result of slower reaction times, decreased mobility, visual deficits, a decreased sense of smell, forgetfulness, and impaired sensation. Many older adults are burned by stoves, hot water, hot food, irons, cookware, and heating pads. Older adults with cognitive impairments or dementias may start fires by leaving foods cooking unattended. The most common burns in this age group are the result of catching clothing on fire and scalding from tap water that is too hot.

The care of the older adult with burns presents unique challenges. They may delay seeking treatment, thus increasing the risk of infection. Their care is often complicated by the presence of other chronic illnesses. They may live alone, and have no one to care for them during rehabilitation. Even small burns have the potential to become lethal in older adults.

Burn prevention topics for older adults are as follows:
- Have a relative or neighbor routinely check for the odor of gas.
- Check the smoke detector battery once a month.
- Wear close-fitting clothing when cooking.
- Use a cooking timer with a loud alarm.
- Never lay anything over a heating device.
- Set the temperature of the hot water heater no higher than 120°F.
- Install antiscald devices in bathroom plumbing.
- Encourage no smoking in the house.

- *Past medical history.* Patients with histories of respiratory, cardiac, renal, metabolic, neurologic, gastrointestinal, or skin diseases; alcohol abuse; or altered immune states require more intense observation. Known allergies are obtained.
- *Age.* Older adults tend to require more supportive care (see the following box).
- *Medications.* Drugs, either prescribed or recreational, taken by the patient prior to the burn injury may further complicate the treatment regimen. Drugs that affect any of the major body systems or cause mood alterations will need to be factored into the treatment plan. As part of the early assessment, obtain and document blood levels of therapeutic pharmaceutical agents and mood-altering substances.
- *Body weight.* During the acute and rehabilitative phases of the burn injury, the patient will lose as much as 20% of preburn weight. This fact will have significant implications for all patients, especially for those who are underweight or cachectic at the time of the injury.

EVIDENCE FOR NURSING CARE The Patient with Compartment Syndrome

Selected resources that nurses may find helpful when planning evidence-based nursing care follow.

- An, G., & West, M. A. (2008). Abdominal compartment syndrome: A concise clinical review. *Critical Care Medicine, 36*(4), 1304–1310.
- Brush, K. A. (2007). Abdominal compartment syndrome: The pressure is on. *Nursing2007, 37*(7), 36–40.
- Forrant, J. A. (2009). Understanding abdominal compartment syndrome. *Nursing2009, 39*(12), 58–59.
- Kumar, V., Saeed, K., Panagopoulos, A., & Parker, P. J. (2007). Gluteal compartment syndrome following joint arthroplasty under epidural anaesthesia: A report of 4 cases. *Journal of Orthopaedic Surgery, 15*(1), 113–117. Retrieved from http://www.josonline.org/pdf/v15i1p113.pdf
- Pirrung, J. M., & Woods, P. (2009). An upward trend in motorcycle crashes. *Nursing2009, 39*(2), 28–33.
- Wolfe, T. R. (2008). Preventing the high-pressure complications of abdominal compartment syndrome. *American Nurse Today, 3*(9), 8–11.

Nursing Diagnoses and Interventions

A major burn affects virtually every body system, as well as social, cultural, economic, psychological, and spiritual well-being. Immediate treatment in an intensive care setting is followed by years of rehabilitation and a lifetime of change in what was possible for an individual before the injury. Many nursing diagnoses are appropriate for the patient with a major burn injury; those described here are *Impaired Skin Integrity, Deficient Fluid Volume, Acute Pain, Risk for Infection, Impaired Physical Mobility, Imbalanced Nutrition: Less than Body Requirements,* and *Powerlessness.*

Impaired Skin Integrity

The burn injury significantly impairs skin integrity. The severity of wounds varies according to the depth and extent of the burn. General treatment measures are designed to restore normal skin function as quickly as possible. Nursing care focuses on assessing and cleansing the wound and controlling infection.

- Estimate the extent and depth of the burn wound and recalculate extent of unhealed burns weekly. *The severity of the burn injury is the basis for determining which types of interventions are appropriate. Reassessment on a regular basis is necessary to monitor the healing process.*
- Provide daily wound care (including debridement method, dressing method, and medication administration) as prescribed *to remove dead tissue, control infection, and promote reepithelialization as soon as possible.*

PRACTICE ALERT
When cleansing wounds, avoid cross-contamination of the patient's wounds.

- Elevate burned or newly skin grafted extremities at or above heart level *to increase venous return and to prevent edema formation.*
- Immobilize skin graft sites for 3 to 5 days or as ordered *to promote graft adherence and to prevent loss of newly grafted skin.*

PRACTICE ALERT
Move patients slowly and carefully across bed sheets to prevent shearing or dislodgement of the new skin grafts.

EVIDENCE FOR NURSING CARE — The Patient with Curling's Ulcers

Selected resources that nurses may find helpful when planning evidence-based nursing care follow.

- Guillamondegui, O. D., Gunter, O. L., Bonadies, J. A., Coates, J. E., Kurek, S. J., DeMoya, M. A., Sing, R. F., & Sori, A. J. (2008). Practice management guidelines for stress ulcer prophylaxis. *National Guideline Clearinghouse.* Retrieved from http://www.guideline.gov
- Judd, W. R., Davis, G. A., Winstead, P. S., Steinke, D. T., Clifford, T. M., & Macaulay, T. E. (2009). Evaluation of continuation of stress ulcer prophylaxis at hospital discharge. *Hospital Pharmacy, 44*(10), 888–893. Retrieved from http://www.factsandcomparisons.com/assets/hpdatenamed/20091001_Oct2009_peer4.pdf
- Liberman, J. D., & Whelan, C. T. (2006). Reducing inappropriate usage of stress ulcer prophylaxis among internal medicine residents: A practice-based educational intervention. *Journal of General Internal Medicine, 21*(5), 498–500. Retrieved from http://www.ncbi.nlm.nih.gov/pmc/articles/PMC1484795/
- Spirt, M. J., & Stanley, S. (2006). Update on stress ulcer prophylaxis in critically ill patients. *Critical Care Nurse, 26*(1), 18–28. Retrieved from http://ccn.aacnjournals.org/cgi/reprint/26/1/18.pdf
- Zeigler, A. J., McAllen, K. J., Slot, M. G., & Barletta, J. F. (2008). Medication reconciliation effect on prolonged inpatient stress ulcer prophylaxis. *The Annals of Pharmacotherapy, 42*(7), 940–946.

- Provide special skin care to sensitive body areas:
  - Clean burns involving the eyes with normal saline or sterile water *to prevent corneal and conjunctival drying and adherence.* If contracture of the eyelid develops, apply drops or ointment to the eye *to prevent corneal abrasion.*
  - Gently wipe burns of the lips with saline-soaked pads. Apply an antibiotic ointment as prescribed. Assess the mouth frequently, and perform mouth care routinely. If an oral endotracheal tube is in place, reposition it often *to prevent pressure ulcer formation.*
  - Gently debride burns of the nose, and apply mafenide acetate (Sulfamylon) cream. Position nasogastric and nasotracheal tubes *to prevent excessive pressure.*

EVIDENCE FOR NURSING CARE — The Patient with Full Thickness Burns

Selected resources that nurses may find helpful when planning evidence-based nursing care follow.

- Cutting, K. F. (2007). Honey and contemporary wound care: An overview. *Ostomy Wound Management, 53*(11), 49–54. Retrieved from http://www.o-wm.com/article/8058
- Hyett, J. M. (2009). How to respond when lightning strikes. *Nursing2009, 39*(7), 32–35.
- Samies, J., & Gehling, M. (2008). Acoustic pressure wound therapy for management of mixed partial- and full-thickness burns in a rural wound center. *Ostomy Wound Management, 54*(3), 56–59. Retrieved from www.o-wm.com/article/8487

EVIDENCE FOR NURSING CARE — The Patient with Partial Thickness Burns

Selected resources that nurses may find helpful when planning evidence-based nursing care follow.

- Jull, A. B., Rodgers, A., & Walker, N. (2008). Honey as a topical treatment for wounds. *Cochrane Database of Systematic Reviews 2008,* (4). Art. No.: CD005083. DOI: 10.1002/14651858.CD005083.pub2.
- Mphande, A. N., Killowe, C., Phalira, S., Jones, H. W., & Harrison, W. J. (2007). Effects of honey and sugar dressings on wound healing. *Journal of Wound Care, 16*(7), 317–319.

- Apply mafenide acetate (Sulfamylon) cream to burns of the ear. Gently debride and thoroughly clean the wound with a water spray. Do not cover ears with dressings. Do not use pillows; to reduce pressure to the area, use a foam doughnut instead. *Burns of the ears are prone to infection; special positioning devices are necessary to decrease pressure ulcer formation.*

Deficient Fluid Volume

Fluid resuscitation rates are adjusted periodically throughout the emergent stage of care. The nurse should be particularly aware of several situations that may warrant the administration of fluids at rates in excess of the calculations needed to maintain adequate urine output: initial underestimation of the burn size, sequestration of fluid into the lung tissue in inhalation injury, electrical injury (which tends to cause more extensive damage than is immediately visible), full-thickness burns, and inordinately delayed starts of fluid resuscitation.

- Assess blood pressure and heart rate frequently. *Vital signs rapidly deteriorate when fluid resuscitation is inadequate.*

PRACTICE ALERT
Tachycardia in the burn patient is not considered until the heart rate is greater than 120 beats per minute.

- Monitor hemodynamic status, including CVP and PCWP. *Inadequate fluid resuscitation is manifested by a drop in the central venous pressure and pulmonary capillary wedge pressure.*
- Follow prescribed protocols for intravenous fluid resuscitation. *Therapy for burn shock is aimed at supporting the patient through the period of hypovolemic instability.*
- Monitor intake and output hourly. *Report urine outputs of less than 50 mL/h. Intake and output measurements indicate the adequacy of fluid resuscitation, and should range from 30 to 50 mL per hour in an adult.*
- Weigh daily. *Body weight is used to calculate fluid requirements.*
- Test all stools and emesis for the presence of blood. *Occult blood in emesis or stool indicates gastrointestinal bleeding.*
- Maintain a warm environment. *Hypothermia leads to shivering and further loss of body fluid through increased energy expenditure and catabolism.*
- Monitor for fluid volume overload. *Older patients and those with underlying cardiac disease may demonstrate symptoms of heart failure during the fluid resuscitation stage.*

Acute Pain

The patient experiences excruciating pain with extensive superficial and all partial-thickness burns. Intense pain is also experienced during wound care and physical therapy. In addition, increased levels of anxiety about treatments and outcomes may further increase the perception of pain.

- Measure the patient's level of pain, using a consistent measurement tool. *Pain tolerance is the duration and intensity of pain that the patient is able to endure. Pain tolerance differs from one patient to the next and may vary in the same patient in different situations.*
- Medicate before painful procedures and determine when PCA is appropriate. *The inability to manage pain results in feelings of despair and frustration.*
- Administer intravenous narcotic analgesics as prescribed. *Nurses' fear of precipitating addiction often makes them reluctant to administer narcotics. During the acute stage of burn injury, however, invasive procedures and exposed neurosensory nerve endings dictate the need for narcotic pharmaceutical agents.*
- Explain all procedures and expected levels of discomfort. *Patients who are prepared for painful procedures and know beforehand the actual sensations they will feel experience less stress.*
- Use methods of nonnarcotic pain control in combination with medications for pain. *Noninvasive pain relief measures (e.g., relaxation, massage, distraction) can enhance the therapeutic effects of pain relief medications.* See the Moving Evidence into Action box on page 469.
- Allow the patient to verbalize the pain experience. *Each person experiences and expresses pain in his or her own manner, using various sociocultural adaptation techniques.*

Risk for Infection

From the onset of the burn injury, loss of the body's natural barrier to the external environment increases the risk of infection. Nursing interventions focus on controlling infectious processes. Monitor the results of diagnostic tests, maintain nutritional therapies, and apply antimicrobial agents to monitor and prevent the spread of infection, a major complication of the burn injury.

- Monitor daily for manifestations of wound infection. Remove topical medications and wound exudate and examine the entire wound. *Early manifestations of wound infection include swelling and inflammation in intact skin surrounding the wound; a change in the color, odor, or amount of exudate; increased pain; and loss of previously healed skin grafts.*
- Monitor for positive blood cultures, *which indicate bacteremia.*
- Monitor for hyperermia, cough, chest pain, wheezing, rhonchi, decreased oxygen saturation, and purulent sputum, *which are manifestations of pneumonia.*
- Monitor for the presence of bacteria in the urine, fever, urgency, frequency, dysuria and superpubic pain, *which are manifestations of urinary tract infections.*
- Obtain daily WBC counts. *Leukocyte counts are indicators of immune system function, and increase in the presence of infection.*
- Determine tetanus immunization status. *Burn patients are at risk for anaerobic infection caused by* Clostridium tetani.
- Maintain high kcal intake. *Nutritional support provides the nutrients needed to maintain the body's defense mechanisms.*
- Maintain an aseptic environment, using standard precautions (including gloving, gowning, and sterile procedures). *Strict isolation technique deters the development of nosocomial infection.*
- Culture all wounds and body secretions per protocol. *Culture and sensitivity reports identify the presence of infectious microbes and indicate appropriate antimicrobial therapies.*
- Administer prescribed antimicrobial medications *to decrease invasive wound infections.*

Impaired Physical Mobility

As the burn wound heals and new skin tissue forms, the involved area tends to shrink. Contractures form at the site and significantly limit mobility, especially when a joint is involved. Physical therapy is important, beginning in the early stages of treatment. The nurse institutes ambulation and planned exercise regimens as soon as the patient's condition stabilizes.

- Perform active or passive ROM exercises to all joints every 2 hours. Ambulate when stable. *Regular exercise prevents further loss of motion, restores movement, and improves functional status.*
- Apply splints as prescribed. Maintain antideformity positions, and reposition the patient hourly. *Splinting and positioning retard the formation of contractures.*
- Maintain limbs in functional alignment *to preserve joint mobility.*
- Anticipate the need for analgesia. *Administering analgesics promotes the patient's comfort during exercising sessions.*

MOVING EVIDENCE INTO ACTION   The Patient with a Major Burn

Patients with major burn injuries experience significant pain related to the injury and treatment. While pain medications significantly reduce pain, other interventions should be considered for use.

De Jong and colleagues (2007) conducted a systematic review of nonpharmacological and nursing interventions for pain relief during burn procedures. Twenty-six articles were included. The interventions fell under two domains of the Nursing Intervention Classification system: behavioral (17 studies) and physical interventions (9 studies). Interventions most commonly used were hypnosis and rapid induction analgesia. Other interventions included combinations of relaxation, guided imagery, attention, information, distraction and/or music. Of the 26 studies, 17 found that the interventions had a positive effect on perceived pain. The authors also report that one underlying concept that explains the intervention effectiveness is the sense of "control" provided to the patient during painful procedures.

IMPLICATIONS FOR NURSING
The use of nonpharmacological interventions gains attention and acceptance as adjuncts to pain medication. Nurses are in the unique position to use such interventions within their scope

of practice. Nonpharmacological interventions are *feasible* (ease of use, minimal time and effort expenditure both while learning and using the intervention), and *acceptable* (related to patient preference). Use of such interventions must be individualized to the patient. Re-evaluation of these interventions should continue over time with continued burn procedures so they can be modified to meet the patient's current needs. The interventions discussed in the review are low risk for adverse events and can be used with appropriate training of the nurses delivering them.

CRITICAL THINKING IN PATIENT CARE
1. When planning pain relief interventions for the burn patient, what salient points should be considered?
2. How should the nurse determine with the patient what nonpharmacological interventions may be effective?
3. Develop a teaching plan for instructing nurses on two commonly used nonpharmacological interventions that can be used in conjunction with pain medications during burn care procedures.

PRACTICE ALERT
Assess all patients, but especially the older adult, for indications of pressure ulcer formation under a splint.

Imbalanced Nutrition: Less than Body Requirements
The burn injury initiates a complex series of events that have a profound effect on the body's use of nutrients and expenditure of energy. Daily kcal requirements are determined by the dietitian, and as soon as possible, enteral feedings are initiated. Nasointestinal tubes are placed to enhance intestinal absorption and retard gastric reflux. Parenteral nutrition is reserved for instances in which enteral feedings are contraindicated. Nursing measures focus on assessing feeding tolerance and use of nutrients.

- Maintain nasogastric/nasointestinal tube placement. *Correct tube placement ensures appropriate absorption of nutrients and prevents aspiration.*
- Maintain enteral/parenteral nutritional support as prescribed. Observe and report any evidence of feeding intolerance: diarrhea, vomiting, excessive gastric residual, abdominal distention, absent bowel sounds, and constipation. *The dietitian, in collaboration with the physician, selects and individualizes the feeding formula according to the patient's daily energy expenditure requirements and feeding tolerance. Failure to maintain rates of infusion predisposes the patient to continued catabolism and negative nitrogen balance.*
- Weigh the patient daily. *Weight indicates the adequacy of nutritional support therapies.*
- Obtain daily laboratory values for protein, iron, CBC, glucose, and albumin. *Decreased serum values indicate inadequate nutritional intake.*

Powerlessness
Usually, the patient with a major burn injury endures a lengthy hospital stay involving many treatments and care protocols that are beyond his or her control. During the early stages, much of

the care regimen involves excruciating pain. Further, the foreign environment of the burn unit makes it difficult for the patient to relate to the immediate surroundings. For example, the need to control infection in the burn unit requires hospital personnel and family members to don sterile clothing prior to coming to the patient's bedside. Family members and nursing personnel appear radically different when they are masked and gowned, and their odd appearance can add to the burn-injured patient's sense of alienation. The patient's body-image is often altered, depending on the extent and location of the burn injury.

- Allow the patient as much control over the surroundings and daily routine as possible. For example, allow the patient to choose times of dressing changes. *Powerlessness derives from the belief that one is unable to influence the outcome of a situation.*
- Keep needed items within reach, such as call bell, urinal, water pitcher, and tissues, *to reinforce the patient's feelings of control.*
- Encourage the patient to express feelings. *The nurse can help the patient cope by therapeutically listening, displaying a caring presence, clarifying misconceptions, and providing positive feedback.*
- Set short-term, realistic goals (e.g., set a goal for the patient to ambulate from bedside to chair twice daily). *Small incremental gains are easier to achieve and allow for frequent positive reinforcement.*

Using NANDA, NIC, and NOC
Linkages between a selected NANDA nursing diagnosis, NIC, and NOC for the patient with a major burn are shown in the chart that follows.

Community-Based Care
Patient and family teaching is an important component of all phases of burn care. As treatment progresses, the nurse encourages family members to assume more responsibility in providing

CASE STUDY & NURSING CARE PLAN   A Patient with a Major Burn

Craig Howard, a 39-year-old truck driver, is admitted to the hospital following an accident in which the cab of his truck caught on fire. He was freed from the truck by a passing motorist, who stayed with him until the rescue team arrived and transported him to a local emergency department (ED). Mr. Howard's wife, Mary, and twin daughters, Jessica and Jane, aged 10, have been notified.

ASSESSMENT

On his admission to the ED, Mr. Howard is diagnosed with deep partial-thickness and full-thickness burns of the anterior chest, arms, and hands. A quick assessment based on the rule of nines estimates the extent of his burn injury at 36% of TBSA. His vital signs are as follows: T 96.2°F (35.6°C), P 140, R 40, and BP 98/60. In the field, the paramedics had inserted a large-bore central line into Mr. Howard's right subclavian vein and started the rapid infusion of lactated Ringer's solution. Mr. Howard is receiving 40% humidified oxygen via face mask. Initial ABGs are pH 7.49, PO_2 60 mmHg, PCO_2 32 mmHg, and bicarbonate 22 mEq/L. Lung sounds indicate inspiratory and expiratory wheezing, and a persistent cough reveals sooty sputum production. A Foley catheter is inserted and initially drains a moderate amount of dark, concentrated urine. A nasogastric tube is connected to low-intermittent suction. Mr. Howard is alert and oriented and complains of severe pain associated with the burn injuries. The burn unit is notified, and Mr. Howard is transferred there.

DIAGNOSIS

- *Risk for Ineffective Airway Clearance*, related to increasing lung congestion secondary to smoke inhalation
- *Deficient Fluid Volume*, related to abnormal fluid loss secondary to burn injury
- *Risk for Ineffective Tissue Perfusion (Peripheral)*, related to peripheral constriction secondary to circumferential burn wounds of the arms

EXPECTED OUTCOMES

- Demonstrate a patent airway, as evidenced by clear breath sounds; absence of cyanosis; and vital signs, chest x-ray findings, and ABGs within normal limits.

- Demonstrate adequate fluid volume and electrolyte balance, as evidenced by urine output, vital signs, mental status, and laboratory findings within normal limits.
- Demonstrate adequate tissue perfusion, as evidenced by palpable pulses, warm extremities, normal capillary refill, and absence of paresthesia.

PLANNING AND IMPLEMENTATION

- Prepare for prophylactic nasotracheal intubation to maintain airway patency.
- Initiate fluid resuscitation therapy using the Parkland formula to calculate intravenous fluid rate for the first 24 hours postburn.
- Assist the physician to perform escharotomies of both upper extremities.

EVALUATION

The nurse anesthetist inserted a nasotracheal tube and connected Mr. Howard to a T-piece delivering 40% oxygen. Vigorous respiratory toileting has significantly improved his ABGs. Bronchodilators have been parenterally administered and mucolytic agents added to his respiratory treatments. His tracheal secretions have begun to show evidence of clearing. Hourly urine outputs indicate adequate fluid resuscitation. Urine output has been maintained at 50 mL/h, and color and concentration have improved. CVP readings have been maintained at 6 cm H_2O, and blood pressure has increased to 100/64. The pulse rate has decreased to 100.

To improve tissue perfusion of both arms, the physician has performed bilateral escharotomies and the wounds are dressed, using sterile procedure. The extremities have demonstrated improved circulation.

CRITICAL THINKING IN THE NURSING PROCESS

1. Explain the rationale for the immediate insertion of a Foley catheter and nasogastric tube.
2. An escharotomy was performed on both arms. Why was this procedure necessary in Mr. Howard's case?
3. What is the rationale supporting the intravenous administration of narcotics to control Mr. Howard's pain?
4. Explain the sequence of events that led to a fluid and electrolyte shift during the first 24 to 48 hours after Mr. Howard sustained his injury.

See Evaluating Your Response in Appendix C.

NANDA, NIC, AND NOC LINKAGES
The Patient with a Major Burn

NANDA   Impaired Skin Integrity

⬇

NIC   Skin Surveillance
Wound Care: Burns
Infection Protection

⬇

NOC   Tissue Integrity: Skin & Mucous Membranes
Wound Healing; Primary Intention

Adapted from Bulechek, G., Butcher, H., & Dochterman, J. M. (Eds.). (2008). *Nursing interventions classification (NIC)* (5th ed.). St. Louis: Mosby Elsevier; Moorhead, S., Johnson, M., Maas, M., & Swanson, E. (Eds.). (2008). *Nursing outcomes classification (NOC)* (4th ed.). St. Louis: Mosby Elsevier; and Nanda International. (2009). *Nursing diagnoses: Definitions and classification 2009–2011.* Oxford, UK: Wiley-Blackwell.

care. From admission to discharge, the nurse teaches the patient and family to assess all findings, implement therapies, and evaluate progress. The following topics should be addressed in preparing the patient and family for home care.

- The long-term goals of rehabilitation care: to prevent soft tissue deformity, protect skin grafts, maintain physiologic function, manage scars, and return the patient to an optimal level of independence
- Avoiding exposure to people with colds or infections and following aseptic technique meticulously when caring for the wound
- The need for progressive physical activity
- How to apply splints, pressure support garments, and other assistive devices
- Dietary requirements with required kcal
- Alternative pain control therapies, such as guided imagery, relaxation techniques, and diversional activities

- Care of the graft and donor sites
- Referral for occupational therapy, social service, clergy, and/or psychiatric services as appropriate

- Helpful resources:
  - American Burn Association
  - International Society for Burn Injuries
  - American Academy of Facial Plastic and Reconstructive Surgery

CHAPTER HIGHLIGHTS

- Four types of burn injuries are thermal, chemical, electrical, or radiation. The depth of the burn injury determines whether it is classified as a superficial, partial-thickness, or full-thickness burn.
- The "rule of nines" is used to estimate the extent of a burn by assigning percentages to different parts of the body.
- Major burns involve multiorgan pathophysiological alterations. Most critical is the fluid shift from the intracellular and intravascular compartments into the interstitium, resulting in a type of hypovolemic shock called burn shock. Other pathologic processes include an impaired immune system, disturbed functions of the skin, inhalation injury, gastrointestinal ulcerations and ileus, renal failure, and hypermetabolism.
- Interdisciplinary care focuses on manginag the patient during the emergent/resuscitative, acute, and rehabilitative stages. To counter the effects of burn shock, fluid resuscitation using

guidelines such as the Parkland formula are initiated to replace fluid and electrolyte losses.

- Additional management for the patient with major burns includes preventing atelectasis, maintaining respiratory function, controlling pain, preventing infection and Curling's ulcer, promoting nutrition, and providing wound care.
- Extensive echar of an extremity or the torso, called circumferential wounds, can potentially occlude arterial flow or decrease respiratory function. An excharotomy is used to release tension, preventing additional complications.
- Surgical management of burn wounds include debridement and skin grafting. Biologic and biosynthetic dressings provide temporary covering and prepare the wound for permanent autografts.
- Continual psychological support of the patient and family is essential throughout convalescence and rehabilitation.

TEST YOURSELF NCLEX-RN® REVIEW

1. During the emergent phase of burn management, what diagnostic test result should the nurse expect to find?
   1. increased hematocrit
   2. serum albumin
   3. decreased serum potassium
   4. decreased blood urea nitrogen (BUN)

2. A patient is admitted with severe burns to the face and chest. The injured skin is dry and leathery, with no pain sensations present. The nurse recognizes that this burn is classified as which of the following?
   1. superficial
   2. superficial partial thickness
   3. deep partial thickness
   4. full thickness

3. Which of the following patients is at greatest risk for developing burn shock?
   1. 21-year-old with 90% superficial burn from a tanning bed
   2. 30-year-old with 10% TBSA from a gasoline explosion
   3. 39-year-old with radiation burns following treatment for cancer
   4. 48-year-old with > 50% TBSA from a high-voltage electrical accident

4. A patient with a major burn is receiving silver sulfadiazine (Silvadene) to the burns. What nursing action should be implemented when using this medication?
   1. premedicate for pain prior to application
   2. monitor WBC count daily
   3. observe for signs of dehydration
   4. monitor serum electrolyte levels daily

5. A patient with full-thickness burns over 50% of the body arrives in the ED. The patient weighs 70 kg. Using the Parkland formula, calculate the amount of fluid replacement that the nurse should deliver in the first 8 hours.
   1. 3500 mL
   2. 7000 mL
   3. 10,500 mL
   4. 14,000 mL

6. For a patient with a major burn, which of the following evaluation criteria indicate that fluid resuscitation is effective during the first 24 hours of care?
   1. urine output of 30 to 50 ml per hour
   2. central venous pressure of 18
   3. heart rate of 130 BPM
   4. blood pressure 96/70

7. A patient has deep partial-thickness burns to the entire left arm and left side of the back. What finding should be reported to the physician immediately?
   1. fluid-filled vesicles on the left arm
   2. pain in the left arm
   3. blanching when pressure applied to the left hand
   4. decreased left radial pulse

8. A patient received deep partial thickness burns to the anterior trunk, perineum, and left arm anterior and posterior. Using the "rule of nines," what is the percent of TBSA that was burned?
   1. 18%
   2. 28%
   3. 36%
   4. 40%

9. Which of the following topics should be included in a presentation on burn prevention at a senior citizen center? **Select all that apply.**
   1. Wear close-fitting clothing when cooking.
   2. Use a solar-powered nightlight.
   3. Set the water heater no higher than 120°F.
   4. Check smoke detectors annually.
   5. Install antiscald devices in bathroom plumbing.
   6. Have a neighbor routinely check for the odor of gas.

10. A patient has possible carbon monoxide poisoning secondary to smoke inhalation. What manifestation should the nurse expect to find in a patient with a 15% carbon monoxide level?
    1. dark red skin color
    2. drowsiness
    3. dizziness
    4. hypotension

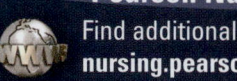

Pearson Nursing Student Resources

Find additional review materials at
nursing.pearsonhighered.com

Prepare for success with additional NCLEX®-style practice questions, interactive assignments and activities, Web links, animations and videos, and more!

BIBLIOGRAPHY

American Burn Association. (2003). Senior safety. Retrieved from http://ameriburn.org

American Burn Association. (2007). Burn incidence and treatment in the US: 2007 fact sheet. Retrieved January 2, 2009, from, http://www.americanburn.org/resources_factsheet.php?

Bishop, J. F. (2004). Burn wound assessment and surgical management. *Critical Care Nursing Clinics of North America, 16,* 145–177.

Bulechek, G., Butcher, H., & Dochterman, J. M. (Eds.). (2008). *Nursing interventions classification (NIC)* (5th ed.). St. Louis: Mosby Elsevier.

Carrougher, G. J., Ptacek, J. T., Sharer, S. R., et al. (2003). Comparison of patient satisfaction and self-reports of pain in adult burn-injured patients. *Journal of Burn Care and Rehabilitation, 24*(1), 1–8.

Deglin, J. H., & Vallerand, A. H. (2009). *Davis' drug guide* (10th ed.). Philadelphia: F.A. Davis.

DeJong, A. E. E., Middlekoop, E., Faber, A. W., & Von Loey, N. E. E. (2007). Non-pharmacological nursing interventions for procedural pain relief in adults with burns: a systematic literature review. *Burns, 33,* 811–827.

Domino, F. J., Baldor, R. A., Golding, J., Grimes, J., & Taylor, J. S. (2010). *The 5-minute clinical consult* (18th ed.). Philadelphia: Lippincott, Williams & Wilkins.

Honari, S. (2004). Topical therapies and antimicrobials in the management of burn wounds. *Critical Care Nursing Clinics of North America, 16,* 1–11.

Huether, S. E., & McCance, K. L. (2008). *Understanding Pathophysiology* (4th ed.). St. Louis: Mosby Elsevier.

Joint Commission. (2009). *2006 patient safety goals.* Retrieved from http://www.jointcommission.org/patientsafety/nationalpatientsafetygoals/

Montgomery, R. K. (2004). Pain management in burn injury. *Critical Care Nursing Clinics of North America, 16,* 39–49.

Moorhead, S., Johnson, M., Maas, M., & Swanson, E. (Eds.). (2008). *Nursing outcomes classification (NOC)* (4th ed.). St. Louis: Mosby Elsevier.

NANDA International. (2009). *Nursing diagnoses: Definitions and classification 2009–2011.* Oxford, UK: Wiley-Blackwell.

National Fire Protection Association. (2004). *Leaving home: College fire safety and burn prevention campaign.* Quincy, MA: NFPA.

National Fire Protection Association. (2005). *Smoking material-related fires.* Retrieved from http://www.nfpa.org/itemDetail.asp?categoryID=294&itemID19303&URL=Research%20&%20Reports/Fact%20sheets/Home%20safety/Smoking%20material-related%20fires

Osborn, K. (2003). Nursing burn injuries. *Nursing Management, 34*(5), 49–56.

Papadakis, M. A., & McPhee, S. J. (2007). *Current consult medicine 2007.* New York: McGraw-Hill.

Perrin, K. O. (2009). *Understanding the essentials of critical care nursing.* Upper Saddle River, NJ: Pearson Prentice-Hall.

Pham, T. N., Cancio, L. C., & Giban, N. S. (2008). American Burn Association practice guidelines burn shock resuscitation. *Journal of Burn Care and Research 29*(1), 257–266.

Supple, K. G. (2004). Physiologic response to burn injury. *Critical Care Nursing Clinics of North America, 16,* 119–126.

Van Leeuwen, A. M., & Poelhuis-Leth, D. J. (2009). *Davis' laboratory and diagnostic tests* (3rd ed.). Philadelphia: F.A. Davis.

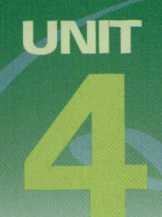

Functional Health Pattern: Nutritional-Metabolic

Think about patients with altered nutrition for whom you have cared in your clinical experiences.

- What were their major medical diagnoses (e.g., psoriasis, cysts, folliculitis, cellulitis, candidiasis, pediculosis, herpes zoster, seborrheic dermatitis, acne vulgaris, nonmelanoma skin cancer, malignant melanoma, basal cell carcinoma, pressure ulcers, hirsutism, alopecia, paronychia, or burn trauma)?

- What kinds of manifestations did each of these patients have? Were these manifestations similar or different?

- How did the patients' healthcare behaviors interfere with their integumentary system? What was their daily intake of foods and fluids? Were they gaining or losing weight? What medications or dietary supplements were they taking? What was the condition of their skin, hair, and nails? Did they complain of dry skin, itching, rashes, bruising easily, or hair loss? Had they noted any changes in moles or warts? Did they have any pressure areas on the sacrum, hips, or ankles? Did they have any previous skin disorders, and how were they treated? Did they use preventative measures to protect against temperature extremes?

The Nutritional-Metabolic Functional Health Pattern includes food and fluid consumption as needed to maintain the nutrition and metabolic needs that supply nutrients to the integumentary system. Breakdown of skin and its accessory structures leads to decreased protection between internal and external environments. Integumentary disorders are affected by nutritional and metabolic status in two primary ways:

- Lack of proper nutrients lowers the body's resistance to disorders and can result in integumentary disorders such as infection (e.g., viral, bacterial) or skin breakdown (e.g., pressure ulcers).

- Exposure to extremes of cold or heat can result in trauma to the skin and accessory structures (e.g., frostbite, burn trauma).

- Use of certain medications to treat disorders can result in hair distribution changes (e.g., hirsutism, alopecia).

Nutrients are used by the body to promote maintenance and repair. Improper intake of nutrients affects the integumentary system's ability to maintain protection, regulate body temperature, and maintain fluid and electrolyte balance. Exposure to environmental extremes breaks down the protective mechanism of the skin and interferes with sensory function. Due to these factors, the patient can develop skin, hair, and nail disorders, leading to manifestations such as the following:

- **Skin ulcerations** (*external pressure impairs the flow of blood and lymph or friction and shearing from sliding tears and injures vessels, causing tissue ischemia and hypoxia to occur, and resulting in tissue death and necrosis*)

- **Infection** (*microorganisms invade tissue and replicate, causing toxic by-products of microorganism metabolism, cell lysis, and immune response to occur, and resulting in inflammation and tissue damage*)

- **Alopecia** (*scarring from trauma, infection, radiation, medications affects rapidly growing cells in hair follicles; affected hair follicle cells slow down hair production, resulting in loss of hair*)

Priority nursing diagnoses within the Nutritional-Metabolic Health Pattern that may be appropriate for patients with integumentary disorders include the following:

- *Impaired Skin Integrity* as evidenced by disruption of skin surface, edema, delayed wound healing, itching, rashes

- *Risk for Infection* as evidenced by breakdown of skin, erythema of skin, warmth, edema, pain, red streaks from injury, fever, chills

- *Deficient Fluid Volume* as evidenced by draining wounds, limited intake of fluids, dry skin, increased skin turgor

- *Disturbed Body Image* as evidenced by altered body appearance, feelings of hopelessness, powerlessness

Two nursing diagnoses from other functional health patterns often are of high priority for the patient with integumentary disorders:

- *Acute Pain* (Cognitive-Perceptual Functional Health Pattern)

- *Ineffective Protection* (Activity-Exercise Functional Health Pattern)

Question

1. When the patient does not have adequate intake of food and fluids, what specifically can the nurse do to encourage nutrition?

CLINICAL SCENARIO

Directions: *Read the following clinical scenarios and answer the questions that follow. To complete this exercise successfully, you will utilize not only knowledge of the content in this unit, but also principles related to priority setting and maintaining patient safety.*

You have been assigned to work with the following four patients for the 0700 shift on a medical-surgical unit. Significant data obtained during report is as follows:

- Mr. Johnson is a 46-year-old who is hospitalized for surgery to release contractures at his elbows that resulted from a flash burn from a grill fire 3 years ago. He is scheduled for surgery at 0800 and needs vital signs, preoperative medication and the preoperative checklist completed.
- Mrs. Carter is a 35-year-old who was hospitalized 2 days ago with cellulitis in the right calf. Vital signs are temperature 100.4°F, pulse 80, respirations 20, and blood pressure 116/76. She is complaining of a headache and pain in the right calf. She was last medicated for pain at 0300.
- Mr. Jenkins is an 86-year-old with herpes zoster. He was admitted 4 days ago with lesions on his left neck and trunk areas. Vital signs are temperature 99°F, pulse 88, respirations 26, and blood pressure 158/90. He is complaining of burning pain across his back and is concerned more lesions are forming.
- Rami Ugandi is a 34-year-old African male who has a history of AIDS. He was transferred from the burn ICU to the medical-surgical unit at 0600 after being treated for toxic epidermal necrolysis for the past month. He will be discharged to his home with limited activity.

Questions

Priority Setting

1. In what order would you visit these patients after report? What is the rationale for your choice?

    A. _____

    B. _____

    C. _____

    D. _____

Health Promotion

1. A diet high in protein and iron may help to prevent pressure ulcers on the patient who is on prolonged bed rest. Which foods should you encourage Mr. Ugandi to eat to help prevent pressure ulcers?

    A. eggs and chicken

    B. broccoli and oranges

    C. oatmeal and bananas

    D. whole-grain bread and kidney beans

2. Mr. Jenkins is being discharged to home. About which of the following related to herpes zoster does the nurse need to teach Mr. Jenkins upon discharge?

    A. "Continue taking the antiviral medication to cure the herpes zoster."

    B. "You can attend church functions as herpes zoster is not contagious."

    C. "Use narcotic pain medications only for severe pain so you do not become addicted to the medication."

    D. "Wear cotton clothing and keep room temperatures cool to decrease the pain and itching from the herpes zoster lesions."

Nursing Process

1. What top priority nursing diagnoses would you choose for each of the patients presented earlier? What is the rationale for your choices?

	Nursing Diagnosis	Rationale
Mr. Johnson		
Mrs. Carter		
Mr. Jenkins		
Mr. Ugandi		

2. Mr. Johnson received partial-thickness and full-thickness flash burns on both anterior and posterior arms and his anterior trunk from a grill fire. Using the "rule of nines," what is the percentage of total body surface (TBSA) burned? _____ %

3. Mrs. Carter was admitted with cellulitis in the right calf. Which clinical manifestations did the nurse assess for on admission?

    A. redness, edema, and pain in the right calf

    B. purulent drainage, pale skin, and pain in right calf

    C. rash, redness, and swelling in right calf

    D. itching, rash, and pain in right calf

4. The nurse applies mafenide acetate (Sulfamylon) to Mr. Ugandi's open skin wounds caused by toxic epidermal necrolysis. Which hypersensitivity reactions would require the nurse to discontinue the drug?

    A. tachycardia and tachypnea

    B. nausea and vomiting

    C. facial edema and pruritis

    D. diarrhea and *candidiasis*

Communication

1. Mr. Jenkins states, "I am tired of having these sores all over. Once they heal they won't ever come back will they? I think I would rather die than go through this again." How will you answer this question?

Delegation

1. What data collection and interventions can be delegated to a CNA for each patient?

    A. _____

    B. _____

    C. _____

    D. _____

Content-Specific Questions

1. Which serum laboratory values are decreased with inadequate nutritional intake, such as in a patient with severe burns? **Select all that apply.**

    A. protein

    B. potassium

    C. iron

    D. complete blood cell count

    E. glucose

    F. calcium

2. When a patient is admitted to the burn unit for treatment of severe burns, it is most important for the nurse to monitor the patient for which of the following?
   A. acute pain
   B. nausea and vomiting
   C. hypothermia
   D. fluid and electrolyte imbalance

3. Which of these patients is most at risk for skin breakdown leading to pressure ulcers?
   A. a 70-year-old who had a stroke with left-sided paralysis
   B. a quadriplegic admitted to the hospital with pneumonia
   C. a 56-year-old patient on dialysis three times a week
   D. an 84-year-old patient in traction for a hip fracture

4. Health promotion teaching for a patient at risk for skin cancer includes which interventions? **Select all that apply.**
   A. Wear long-sleeved shirts and a wide-brimmed hat in the sun.
   B. Apply sunscreen once a day.
   C. Avoid tanning booths or prolonged exposure to the sun.
   D. Minimize exposure to the sun between 1:00 PM and 4:00 PM.
   E. Apply sunscreen before and after swimming.

5. Morphine sulfate is a drug of choice for pain. Which clinical manifestation requires immediate nursing intervention?
   A. vomiting once after medication administered
   B. respiratory rate below 8 breaths per minute
   C. blood pressure of 110/70 after a baseline blood pressure of 120/80
   D. peripheral pulse of 68 after a baseline pulse of 78

CASE STUDY: Stephanie Chelen

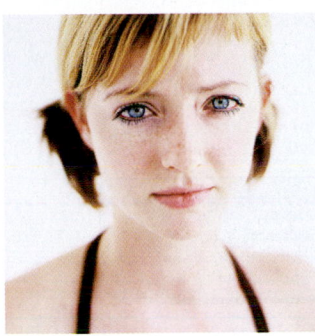

Stephanie Chelen is a 23-year-old who is admitted to the medical-surgical unit after being exposed to the sun for a prolonged period of time. Due to the extent of the burns, she is admitted for observation and treatment. Upon admission, Ms. Chelen stated she fell asleep lying on her stomach while sunbathing at the beach. Her vital signs are temperature 100.6°F, pulse 94, respirations, 26, and blood pressure 116/76. Her height is 5'2" and weight is 125 lbs. Assessment shows that her back is red and slightly edematous with an area ~ 6 by 3 cm between the scapula that is beginning to develop blisters. The backs of her arms and legs and the soles of her feet are red and slightly edematous. She is complaining of pain on her back, arms, legs, and feet. She stated that she feels chilled, is nauseated, and has a headache. Labs are drawn for a complete blood count and electrolytes for baseline assessment. IV therapy is instituted to maintain hydration. The burn areas are washed with soap and water and an antibiotic ointment is applied. A mild analgesic is administered as ordered. The patient is covered to prevent further chilling and to prevent burned areas from exposure to air.

She is diagnosed with first degree and second degree burns. Using the "rule of nines," the partial thickness burned area on her back is classified as approximately 5% total body surface area. The superficial burns over the rest of the reddened areas are not classified. Superficial burns involve the epidermis layer of the skin. Superficial partial thickness burns involve the entire dermis and the papillae of the dermis. The pathophysiology of superficial and superficial partial thickness is the result of exposure to the sun for a prolonged time. An inflammatory response occurs caused by tissue injury. Platelets aggregate at the burn injury site, fibrin is deposited, and thrombus is formed. The thrombus along with vasoconstriction walls off the burn injury site. Then vasodilation occurs and with increased capillary permeability leads to redness and edema. Injury to the dermis from the superficial partial thickness burned area develops a moist, glistening appearance as blisters form. The burned area will blanch on pressure. There is pain in response to touch and temperature changes. The burned area should heal within 14 to 21 days with minimal or no scarring, but may have pigment changes. Manifestations of superficial and superficial partial thickness burns are skin redness, blister formation, local pain, headache, chills, nausea, and vomiting. Complications of superficial and superficial partial thickness burns are infection, hypothermia, dehydration, and fluid and electrolyte imbalances.

Due to the severity of tissue injury from the burns, the nursing diagnosis of *Impaired Skin Integrity* is appropriate for guiding nursing care.

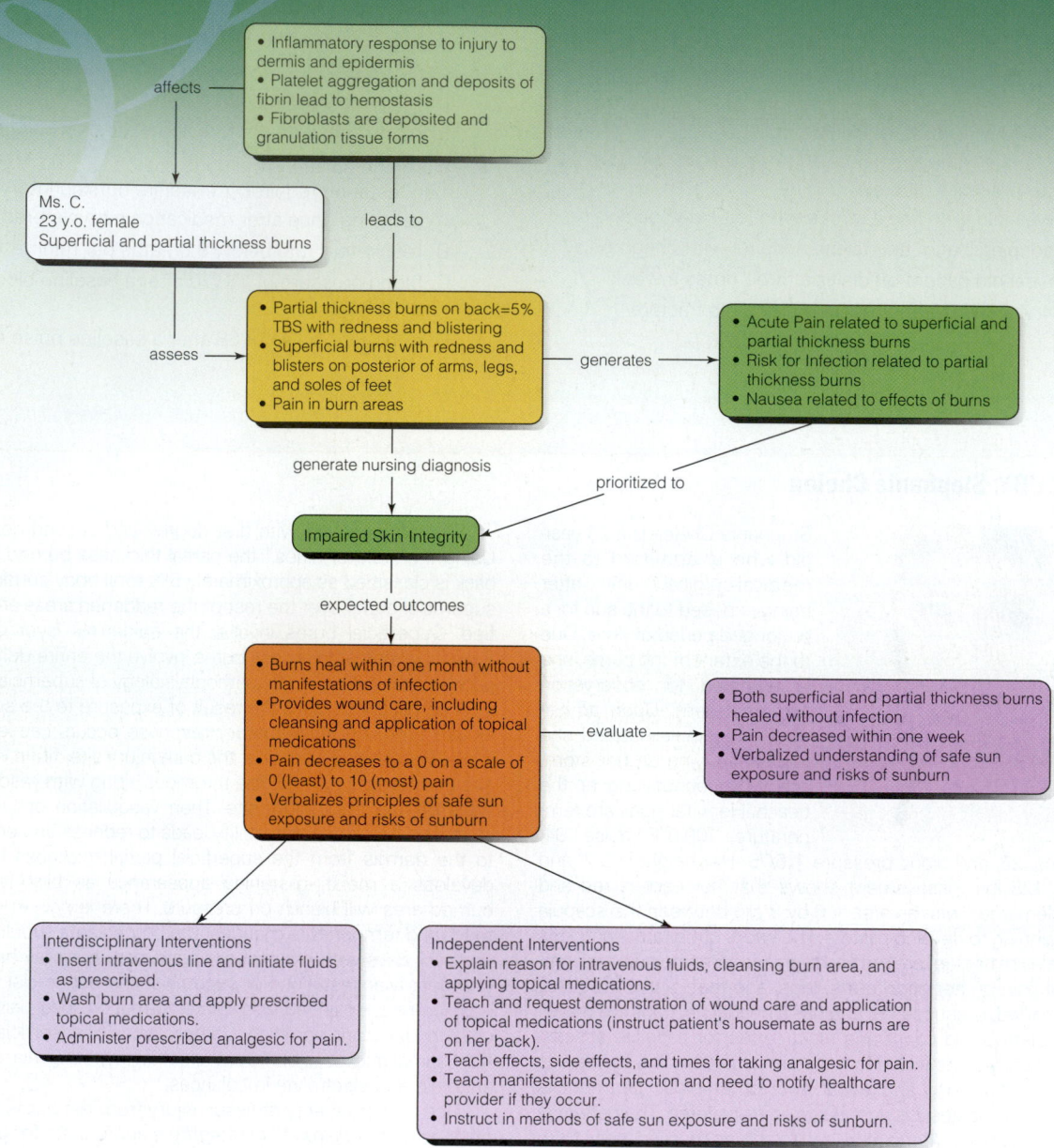

- Inflammatory response to injury to dermis and epidermis
- Platelet aggregation and deposits of fibrin lead to hemostasis
- Fibroblasts are deposited and granulation tissue forms

affects

leads to

Ms. C.
23 y.o. female
Superficial and partial thickness burns

assess

- Partial thickness burns on back=5% TBS with redness and blistering
- Superficial burns with redness and blisters on posterior of arms, legs, and soles of feet
- Pain in burn areas

generates

- Acute Pain related to superficial and partial thickness burns
- Risk for Infection related to partial thickness burns
- Nausea related to effects of burns

generate nursing diagnosis

prioritized to

Impaired Skin Integrity

expected outcomes

- Burns heal within one month without manifestations of infection
- Provides wound care, including cleansing and application of topical medications
- Pain decreases to a 0 on a scale of 0 (least) to 10 (most) pain
- Verbalizes principles of safe sun exposure and risks of sunburn

evaluate

- Both superficial and partial thickness burns healed without infection
- Pain decreased within one week
- Verbalized understanding of safe sun exposure and risks of sunburn

Interdisciplinary Interventions
- Insert intravenous line and initiate fluids as prescribed.
- Wash burn area and apply prescribed topical medications.
- Administer prescribed analgesic for pain.

Independent Interventions
- Explain reason for intravenous fluids, cleansing burn area, and applying topical medications.
- Teach and request demonstration of wound care and application of topical medications (instruct patient's housemate as burns are on her back).
- Teach effects, side effects, and times for taking analgesic for pain.
- Teach manifestations of infection and need to notify healthcare provider if they occur.
- Instruct in methods of safe sun exposure and risks of sunburn.

Activity:

1. After reviewing the concept map above, is there anything you would change to make it more understandable? Would the care be different if patient was male, weighed 270 pounds, and was burned by an electric wire touching his back?

2. Go to the Pearson Nursing Student Resources for this book at www.nursing.pearsonhighered.com to write a concept map for this male patient.

See answers and hints in Appendix C.

Responses to Altered Endocrine Function

18 Assessing the **Endocrine System**

LEARNING OUTCOMES

1. Describe the anatomy and physiology of the endocrine glands.
2. Summarize the functions of the hormones secreted by the endocrine glands.
3. Describe specific topics to consider during a health history interview of the patient with health problems involving endocrine function.
4. Explain techniques for assessing the thyroid gland and the effects of altered function of thyroid hormones.

5. Describe normal variations in endocrine assessment findings for the older adult.
6. Give examples of genetic disorders of the endocrine glands.
7. Identify abnormal findings that may indicate malfunction of the glands of the endocrine system.

CLINICAL COMPETENCIES

1. Conduct and document a health history for patients who have or are at risk for alterations in the structure or function of the endocrine glands.
2. Monitor the results of diagnostic tests and report abnormal findings.

3. Conduct and document a physical assessment of the structure of the thyroid gland and the effects of altered endocrine function on other body structures and functions.

EQUIPMENT NEEDED

- Reflex hammer
- Safety pin, cotton ball, containers with hot and cold water, tuning fork

- Blood pressure cuff
- Stethoscope

KEY TERMS

acromegaly, *490*	dwarfism, *491*	tetany, *491*
carpal spasm, *491*	exophthalmos, *490*	Trousseau's sign, *491*
Chvostek's sign, *491*	goiter, *490*	

The endocrine system is essential to the regulation of the body's internal environment. Through hormones secreted by its glands, the endocrine system regulates such varied functions as growth, reproduction, metabolism, fluid and electrolyte balance, and gender differentiation. It also has a role in adapting to constant alterations in the internal and external environment.

Disorders of the endocrine system primarily result from either too much or too little hormone production. These alterations in hormone levels affect a wide variety of human functions, including activity and exercise, nutrition and metabolism, elimination, self-perception and self-concept, sexuality and reproduction, coping with stress, and role-relationships.

Anatomy, Physiology, and Functions of the Endocrine System

The endocrine system is comprised of the pituitary gland, thyroid gland, parathyroid glands, adrenal glands, pancreas, and gonads (reproductive glands). The locations of these glands are illustrated in Figure 18–1 ■. Table 18–1 summarizes the functions of the endocrine glands and their hormones. Specific information about the ovaries and testes is found in ∞ Chapters 47 through 49.

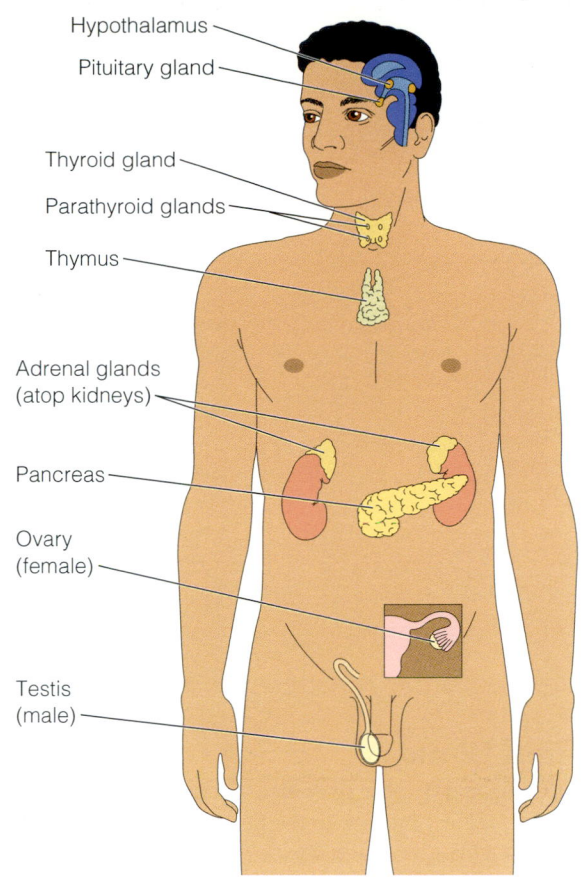

Hypothalamus
Pituitary gland

Thyroid gland
Parathyroid glands

Thymus

Adrenal glands
(atop kidneys)

Pancreas

Ovary
(female)

Testis
(male)

Figure 18–1 ■ Location of the major endocrine glands.

Pituitary Gland

The pituitary gland (hypophysis) is located in the skull beneath the hypothalamus of the brain (Figure 18–2 ■). It often is called the "master gland" because its hormones regulate many body functions. The pituitary gland has two parts: the anterior pituitary (or adenohypophysis) and the

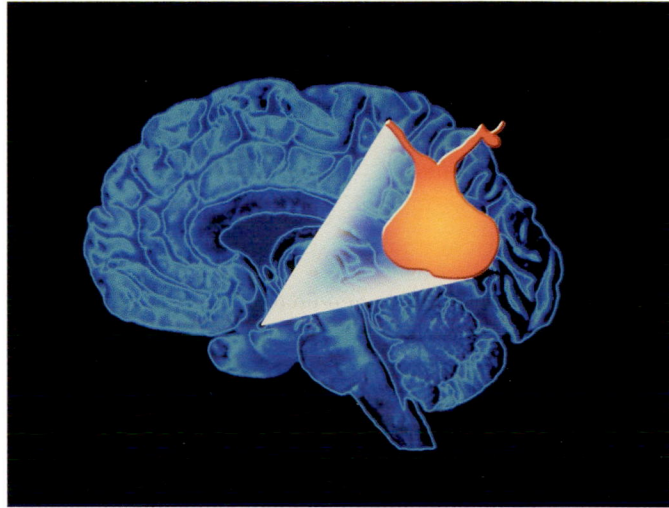

Figure 18–2 ■ Location of the pituitary gland.
Source: Photo Researchers, Inc.

TABLE 18–1 Organs, Hormones, Functions, and Feedback Mechanisms of the Endocrine System

ENDOCRINE GLAND	HORMONE SECRETED	TARGET ORGAN AND FEEDBACK MECHANISM
Thyroid gland	Thyroid hormone (TH): thyroxine (T_4) is the major hormone secreted by the thyroid gland. It is converted to triiodothyronine (T_3) at the target tissues.	Maintains metabolic rate and growth and development of all tissues. T_3 and T_4 are secreted in response to TSH.
	Calcitonin	Maintains serum calcium levels by decreasing bone resorption and decreasing resorption of calcium in the kidneys whenever levels of plasma calcium are elevated.
Parathyroid gland	Parathyroid hormone (PTH)	Maintains serum calcium levels by stimulating bone resorption and formation and by stimulating kidney resorption of calcium in response to falling levels of plasma calcium.
Adrenal cortex	Mineralocorticoids (e.g., aldosterone)	Promotes kidney tubule reabsorption of sodium and water and excretion of potassium in response to elevated levels of potassium and low levels of sodium, thereby increasing blood pressure and blood volume.
	Glucocorticoids (e.g., cortisol)	Helps regulate metabolism of carbohydrates, fats, and proteins. Activates anti-inflammatory responses to stressors. Low cortisol levels stimulate hypothalamic secretion of corticotropin-releasing hormone (CRH), which stimulates the anterior pituitary gland to release ACTH, which in turn stimulates the adrenal cortex to secrete cortisol.
	Gonadocorticoids (androgens and small amounts of estrogen and progesterone)	The quantity of sex hormones produced here is small, and the mechanism is not well understood.
Adrenal medulla	Catecholamines (epinephrine and norepinephrine)	Stimulates the heart, constricts blood vessels, inhibits visceral muscles, dilates bronchioles, increases respiration and metabolism, promotes hyperglycemia. Secreted in response to physical or psychologic stress.
Anterior pituitary (adenohypophysis)	Growth hormone (GH)	Promotes growth of body tissues by enhancing protein synthesis and promoting use of fat for energy and thus conserving glucose. Release is stimulated by growth hormone releasing hormone (GHRH) in response to low GH levels, hypoglycemia, increased amino acids, low fatty acids, and stress.

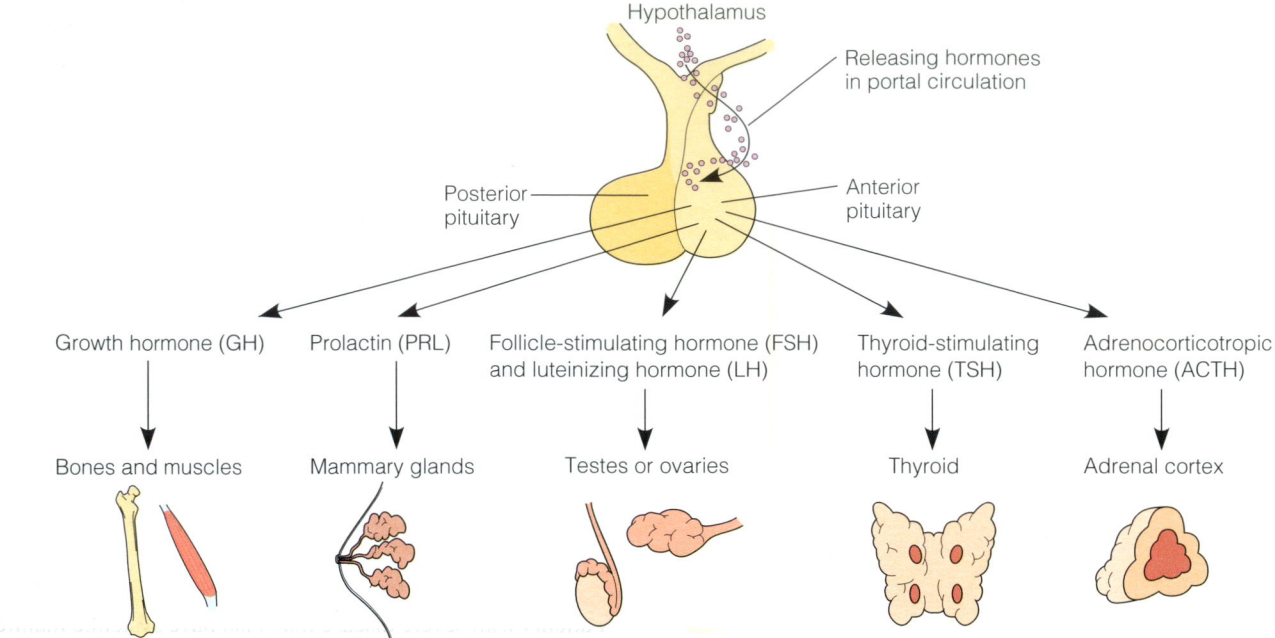

Figure 18–3 ■ Actions of the major hormones of the anterior pituitary.

posterior pituitary (or neurohypophysis). The anterior pituitary is glandular tissue; the posterior pituitary is an extension of the hypothalamus.

Anterior Pituitary

The anterior pituitary has several types of endocrine cells and secretes at least six major hormones (Figure 18–3 ■).

- Somatotropic cells secrete growth hormone (GH) (also called somatotropin). GH stimulates growth of the body by signaling cells to increase protein production and by stimulating the epiphyseal plates of the long bones.
- Lactotropic cells secrete prolactin (PRL). Prolactin stimulates the production of breast milk.
- Thyrotropic cells secrete thyroid-stimulating hormone (TSH). TSH stimulates the synthesis and release of thyroid hormones from the thyroid gland.
- Corticotropic cells secrete adrenocorticotropic hormone (ACTH). ACTH stimulates release of hormones, especially glucocorticoids, from the adrenal cortex.
- Gonadotropic cells secrete the gonadotropin hormones, follicle-stimulating hormone (FSH), and luteinizing hormone (LH). These hormones stimulate the ovaries and testes (the gonads).

Posterior Pituitary

The posterior pituitary is made of nervous tissue. Its primary function is to store and release antidiuretic hormone (ADH) and oxytocin, produced in the hypothalamus:

- ADH, also called vasopressin, decreases urine production by causing the renal tubules to reabsorb water from the urine and return it to the circulating blood.
- Oxytocin induces contraction of the smooth muscles in the reproductive organs. In women, oxytocin stimulates the myometrium of the uterus to contract during labor. It also induces milk ejection from the breasts.

Thyroid Gland

The thyroid gland (Figure 18–4 ■) is anterior to the upper part of the trachea and just inferior to the larynx. This butterfly-shaped gland has two lobes connected by a structure called the isthmus.

The glandular tissue consists of follicles filled with a jelly-like colloid substance named thyroglobulin, a glycoprotein-iodine complex. Cells within the follicles secrete thyroid hormone (TH), a general name for two similar hormones: thyroxine (T_4) and triiodothyronine (T_3). The primary role of thyroid hormones in adults is to increase metabolism. TH secretion is initiated by

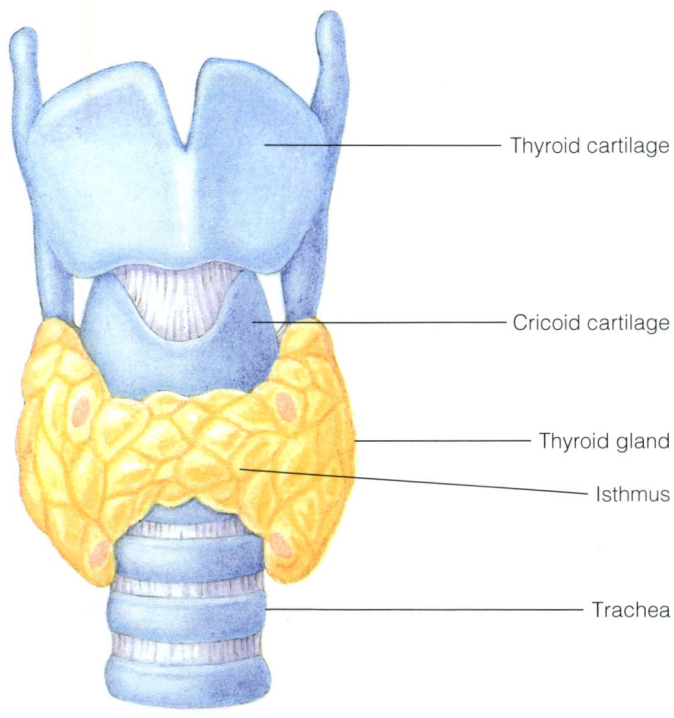

Figure 18–4 ■ The thyroid gland.

Source: Dorling Kindersley Media Library.

the release of TSH by the pituitary gland and is dependent on an adequate supply of iodine.

The thyroid gland also secretes calcitonin, a hormone that decreases excessive levels of calcium in the blood by slowing the calcium-releasing activity of bone cells, serves as a marker for sepsis, and is believed to be a mediator of inflammatory responses.

Parathyroid Glands

The parathyroid glands (usually four to six in number) are embedded on the posterior surface of the lobes of the thyroid gland. They secrete parathyroid hormone (PTH), or parathormone. When calcium levels in the plasma fall, PTH secretion increases. PTH also controls phosphate metabolism. It acts by increasing renal excretion of phosphate in the urine, by decreasing the excretion of calcium, and by increasing bone reabsorption to cause the release of calcium from bones. Normal levels of vitamin D are necessary for PTH to exert these effects on bone and kidneys.

Adrenal Glands

The two adrenal glands are pyramid-shaped organs that sit on top of the kidneys (Figure 18–5 ■). Each gland consists of two parts, an inner medulla and an outer cortex.

The adrenal medulla produces two hormones (also called catecholamines): epinephrine (adrenalin) and norepinephrine (noradrenalin). These hormones are similar to substances also released by the sympathetic nervous system and thus are not essential to life. Epinephrine increases blood glucose levels and stimulates the release of ACTH from the pituitary; ACTH in turn stimulates the adrenal cortex to release glucocorticoids. Epinephrine also increases the rate and force of cardiac contractions; constricts blood vessels in the skin, mucous membranes, and kidneys; and dilates blood vessels in the skeletal muscles, coronary arteries, and pulmonary arteries. Norepinephrine increases heart rate, increases the force of cardiac contractions, and vasoconstricts blood vessels throughout the body.

The adrenal cortex secretes several hormones, all corticosteroids. They are classified into two groups: mineralocorticoids and glucocorticoids. These hormones are essential to life.

The release of the mineralocorticoids is controlled primarily by renin (an enzyme). When a decrease in blood pressure or sodium is detected, specialized kidney cells release renin to act on angiotensinogen, manufactured by the liver. Angiotensinogen is modified by renin and other enzymes to become angiotensin, which stimulates the release of aldosterone from the adrenal cortex. Aldosterone prompts the distal tubules of the kidneys to release increased amounts of water and sodium back into the circulating blood to increase circulating blood volume and pressure. This system (the renin–angiotensin–aldosterone system) is illustrated in ∞ Chapter 10 with the discussion of body fluid regulation.

The glucocorticoids include cortisol and cortisone. These hormones affect carbohydrate metabolism by regulating glucose use in body tissues, mobilizing fatty acids from fatty tissue, and shifting the source of energy for muscle cells from glucose to fatty acids. Glucocorticoids are released in times of stress. An excess of glucocorticoids in the body depresses the inflammatory response and inhibits the effectiveness of the immune system.

Pancreas

The pancreas, located behind the stomach between the spleen and the duodenum, is both an endocrine gland (producing hormones) and an exocrine gland (producing digestive enzymes). The digestive enzymes produced by the pancreas are discussed in ∞ Chapter 21. The content in this chapter discusses the endocrine pancreatic hormones.

The endocrine cells of the pancreas produce hormones that regulate carbohydrate metabolism. They are clustered in structures called pancreatic islets (or islets of Langerhans) scattered throughout the pancreas. Pancreatic islets have at least four different cell types:

- Alpha cells produce glucagon, which decreases glucose oxidation and promotes an increase in the blood glucose level by signaling the liver to release glucose from glycogen stores.
- Beta cells produce insulin, which facilitates the uptake and use of glucose by muscle, liver, and fat cells and prevents an excessive breakdown of glycogen in the liver and muscle. In this way, insulin decreases blood glucose levels. Insulin also facilitates lipid formation, inhibits the breakdown and mobilization of stored fat, and helps amino acids move into cells to promote protein synthesis. In general, the actions of glucagon and insulin oppose one another, helping to maintain a stable blood glucose level.
- Delta cells secrete somatostatin, which inhibits the secretion of glucagon and insulin by the alpha and beta cells.
- F cells secrete pancreatic polypeptide, which is believed to inhibit the exocrine activity of the pancreas.

Gonads

The gonads are the testes in men and the ovaries in women. These organs are the primary source of steroid sex hormones in the body. The hormones of the gonads are important in regulating body growth and promoting the onset of puberty. The structure and functions of the gonads are discussed in ∞ Chapter 47.

An Overview of Hormones

Hormones are chemical messengers secreted by the endocrine organs and transported throughout the body, where they exert their action on specific cells called target cells. Hormones do not cause reactions directly but rather regulate tissue responses. They may produce either generalized effects or local effects.

Hormones are transported from endocrine gland cells to target cells in the body in one of four ways:

- Endocrine glands release most hormones, including TH and insulin, into the bloodstream. Some hormones require a protein carrier.

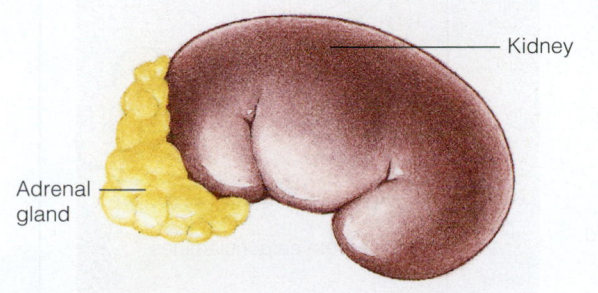

Adrenal gland

Kidney

Figure 18–5 ■ Location of the adrenal glands.

Source: Dorling Kindersley Media Library.

- Neurons release some hormones, such as epinephrine, into the bloodstream. This is called the neuroendocrine route.
- The hypothalamus releases its hormones directly to target cells in the posterior pituitary by nerve cell extension.
- With the paracrine method, released messengers diffuse through the interstitial fluid. This method of transport involves a number of hormonal peptides that are released throughout various organs and cells and act locally. An example is endorphins, which act to relieve pain.

Hormones that are released into the bloodstream circulate as either free, unbound molecules or as hormones attached to transport carriers. Peptide and protein hormones (such as insulin) circulate unbound, while steroid and thyroid hormones are carried by specific transport carriers synthesized by the liver. Hormone receptors are complex molecular structures, located on or inside target cells. They act by binding to specific receptor sites located on the surfaces of the target cells. These receptors recognize a specific hormone and translate the message into a cellular response. The receptor sites are structured so that they respond only to a specific hormone; for example, receptors in the thyroid gland are responsive to TSH but not to LH. Drugs that compete with a hormone for binding with transport carrier molecules increase hormone action by increasing the availability of the free, unbound hormone.

Hormone levels are controlled by the pituitary gland and by feedback mechanisms. Although most feedback mechanisms are negative, a few are positive. Negative feedback is controlled much as the thermostat in a house regulates temperature. Sensors in the endocrine system detect changes in hormone levels and adjust hormone secretion to maintain normal levels. When the sensors detect a decrease in hormone levels, they begin actions to cause an increase in hormone levels; when hormone levels rise above normal, the sensors cause a decrease in hormone production and release. For example, when the hypothalamus or

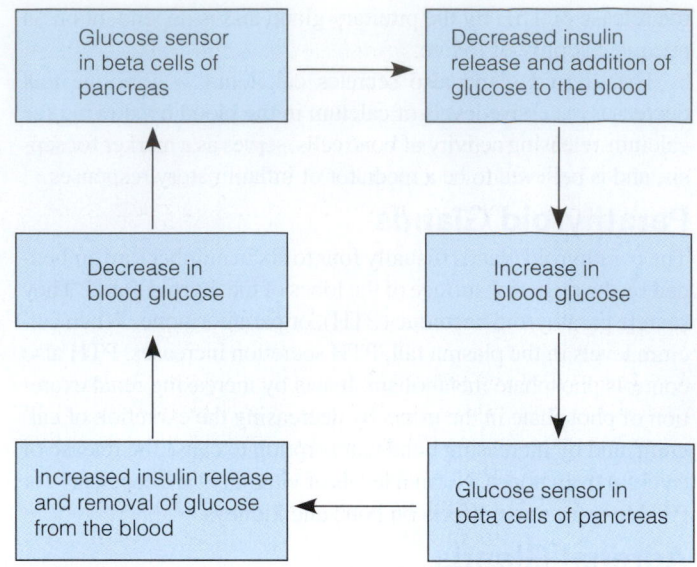

Figure 18–6 ■ Negative feedback.

anterior pituitary gland senses increased blood levels of TH, it releases hormones, causing a reduction in the secretion of TSH, which in turn prompts a decrease in the output of TH by the thyroid gland. See Figure 18–6 ■.

In positive feedback mechanisms, increasing levels of one hormone cause another gland to release a hormone. For example, the increased production of estradiol (a female ovarian hormone) during the follicular stage of the menstrual cycle in turn stimulates increased FSH production by the anterior pituitary gland. Estradiol levels continue to increase until the ovarian follicle disappears, eliminating the source of the stimulation for FSH, which then decreases.

Stimuli for hormone release may also be classified as hormonal, humoral, or neural (Figure 18–7 ■). In hormonal release,

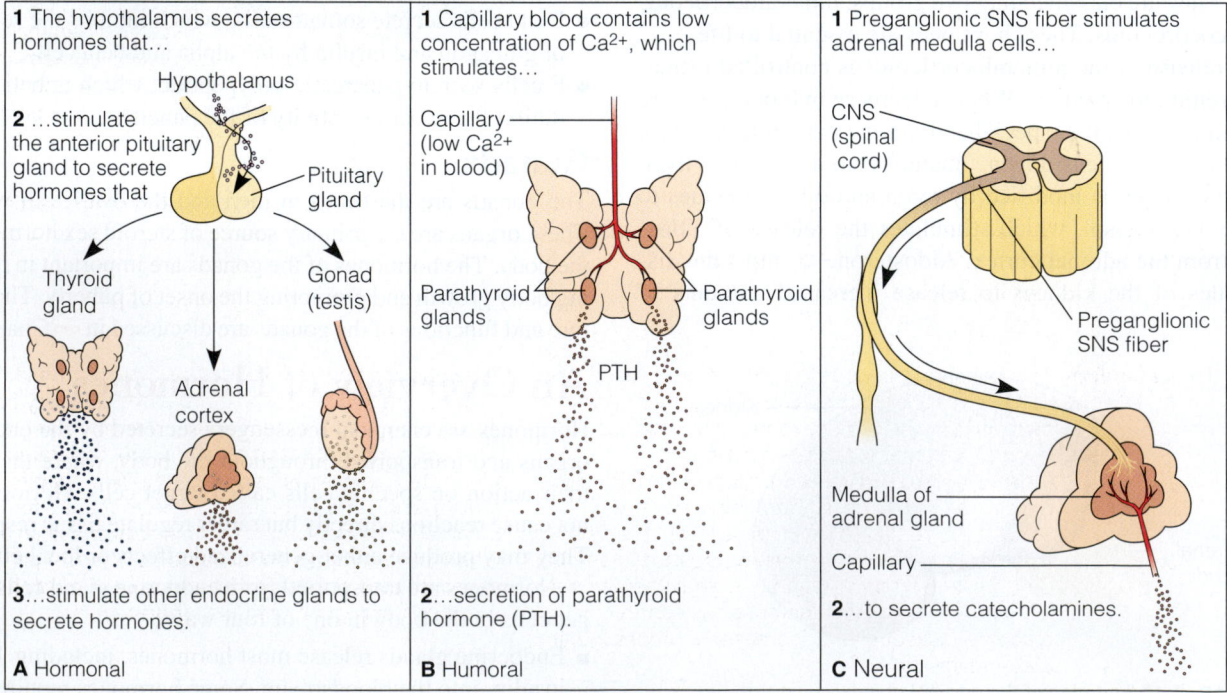

1 The hypothalamus secretes hormones that...

Hypothalamus

2 ...stimulate the anterior pituitary gland to secrete hormones that

Pituitary gland

Thyroid gland

Adrenal cortex

Gonad (testis)

3 ...stimulate other endocrine glands to secrete hormones.

A Hormonal

1 Capillary blood contains low concentration of Ca2+, which stimulates...

Capillary (low Ca2+ in blood)

Parathyroid glands

Parathyroid glands

PTH

2 ...secretion of parathyroid hormone (PTH).

B Humoral

1 Preganglionic SNS fiber stimulates adrenal medulla cells...

CNS (spinal cord)

Preganglionic SNS fiber

Medulla of adrenal gland

Capillary

2 ...to secrete catecholamines.

C Neural

Figure 18–7 ■ Examples of three mechanisms of hormone release: *A,* hormonal; *B,* humoral; or *C,* neural.

hypothalamic hormones stimulate the anterior pituitary to release hormones. Fluctuations in the serum level of these hormones in turn prompt other endocrine glands to release hormones. In humoral release, fluctuations in the serum levels of certain ions and nutrients stimulate specific endocrine glands to release hormones to bring these levels back to normal. In neural release, nerve fibers stimulate the release of hormones.

Assessing Endocrine Function

The function of the endocrine glands is assessed by findings from diagnostic tests, a health assessment interview to collect subjective data, and a physical assessment to collect objective data. Hormones affect all body tissues and organs, and manifestations of dysfunction are often nonspecific, making assessment of endocrine function sometimes more difficult than assessment of other body systems.

Diagnostic Tests

The results of diagnostic tests of the endocrine system are used to support the diagnosis of a specific disease, to provide information to identify or modify the appropriate medication or therapy used to treat the disease, and to help nurses monitor the patient's responses to treatment and nursing care interventions. Diagnostic tests to assess the structure and function of the glands of the endocrine system are described in the following table. More information is included in the discussion of specific disorders in ∞ Chapters 19 and 20.

Regardless of the type of diagnostic test, the nurse is responsible for explaining the procedure and any special preparation needed, for assessing for medication use that may affect the outcome of the tests, for ensuring the consent form is signed (if necessary), for supporting the patient during the examination as necessary, for documenting the procedures as appropriate, and for monitoring the results of the tests. The nurse is also responsible for post-procedure care and patient teaching for self-care at home.

DIAGNOSTIC TESTS of the Endocrine System

PITUITARY TESTS

NAME OF TEST	PURPOSE & DESCRIPTION	RELATED NURSING INTERVENTIONS
Growth Hormone (GH), Human Growth Hormone (hGH)	In this blood serum test, GH levels (affected by food, stress, and activity) are measured to identify GH deficiency (dwarfism) or GH excess (gigantism, acromegaly). Normal value: Men: < 5 ng/mL Women: < 10 ng/mL	Tell patient not to eat or drink 8 to 10 hours prior to having blood drawn. Have patient rest for 30 to 60 minutes before blood is drawn.
Magnetic Resonance Imaging (MRI)	This radiographic study is done to identify tumors of the hypothalamus or pituitary gland.	Tell patient of need to lie still during the examination. Assess for any metallic implants (such as pacemakers, clips on brain aneurysms, body piercings, tattoos, shrapnel). If present, notify imaging physician. Remove transdermal medication patches (both OTC and prescribed) unless otherwise ordered (FDA, 2009). Replace the patch following the procedure. Ask the patient to tell the staff about the patch when making the appointment and when completing the admission information. Ask if patient is pregnant; if so the test is not performed. Ask about claustrophobia; if a problem, request patient to ask for a relaxing medication to take prior to the MRI.
Somatomedin C (Insulin-Like Growth Factor or IGF-1)	The results of this serum test are used to evaluate secretion of growth factor and to identify GH deficiency or excess (as discussed earlier). Normal value: 125–250 ng/mL	None; overnight fasting is preferred but not necessary.
Water Deprivation Test	This combination of blood and urine tests is used to identify causes of polyuria (increased urine output), including central diabetes insipidus, neurogenic diabetes insipidus, syndrome of inappropriate antidiuretic hormone (SIADH), and psychogenic polydipsia (drinking excessive amounts of fluids). ADH or vasopressin is given IM or subcutaneously. In patients without pathology, there is no change in urine and plasma osmolality. Urine osmolality increases in central diabetes insipidus and decreases in nephrogenic diabetes insipidus.	Tell patient not to smoke, eat, or drink after midnight, and that the test will take up to 8 hours. Every hour for ordered length of test assess weight, take postural BP (lying and standing measures separated by 2 minutes), assess urine for volume and specific gravity, and send samples of urine to the lab for osmolality. Blood samples for osmolality are taken when urine samples are collected and when patient demonstrates orthostatic hypotension. Coordinate specimen collection with the laboratory.

(continued)

DIAGNOSTIC TESTS of the Endocrine System (continued)

THYROID TESTS

NAME OF TEST	PURPOSE & DESCRIPTION	RELATED NURSING INTERVENTIONS
Magnetic Resonance Imaging (MRI)—thyroid	This radiographic study is done to identify tumors of the thyroid gland.	See information for MRI of the pituitary.
Radioactive Iodine Uptake (RIA)	This test provides a direct measure of thyroid activity and is useful in evaluating the activity of solitary thyroid nodules. Based on the rationale that the thyroid gland takes up iodine in any form, radioactive iodine is given orally or IV, and the thyroid gland uptake is measured with a scanner at several hourly intervals and at 24 hours. Normal value for uptake: 2–4 hours: 3%–19% 24 hours: 11%–30%	The patient should not eat or drink for 6 to 8 hours before the test, but can have food 1 hour after the oral dose is given. Tell patients not to take supplemental iodine several weeks before the test and thyroid medications should be discontinued.
Thyroid Antibodies (TA)	A blood test used to identify thyroid immune disease (Graves' disease, chronic thyroiditis, Hashimoto's thyroiditis). Normal values: Antithyroglobulin: negative to titer < 1:20 Antimicrosomal: negative to titer < 1:100	Assess for family history of thyroid disease and ask about recent viral infection (which could trigger autoimmune disease).
Thyroid Scan	This radiologic study evaluates thyroid nodules. Radioactive isotopes are given orally and a scanner is passed over the thyroid to make a graphic record of the radiation emitted. A normal thyroid scan has a homogeneous pattern of radiation with symmetric lobes. Benign lesions appear as warm spots (take up more radiation); malignant tumors appear as cold spots (less radiation taken up).	No special preparation is needed.
Thyroid-Stimulating Hormone (TSH)	In this blood test, levels of T_4 are measured to identify the circulating TSH, with levels above or below normal indicating thyroid disease. It is also used to compare TSH results with T_4 results to differentiate between pituitary and thyroid dysfunction. A decreased T_4 level and a normal or increased TSH level can indicate a thyroid disorder. A decreased T_4 level and a decreased TSH level can indicate a pituitary disorder. Normal value: < 3ng/ml	Tell patients to avoid shellfish for several days prior to the test. Assess medications: TSH value may be increased by aspirin, steroids, dopamine, and heparin; and decreased by lithium and potassium iodide.
Thyroid Suppression Test	Triiodothyronine (T_3) is taken for 7 to 10 days, and a reduction of its uptake to less than half of the initial uptake after that time is considered normal. The test is used to diagnose hyperthyroidism and hypothyroidism.	Explain the importance of taking the triiodothyronine for the length of time prescribed.
Thyrotropin-Releasing Hormone (TRH) Stimulation Test	A baseline TSH is measured; followed by an injection of TRH to stimulate the pituitary to release TSH. A second blood sample is drawn 20 to 30 minutes later and the TSH level is again measured. Levels higher or lower than normal are indicative of thyroid disease.	No special preparation is needed.
Thyroxine (T_4)	The results of this serum test are used to determine thyroid function and aid in the diagnosis of hyperthyroidism and hypothyroidism. Normal value: free T_4 1.0–2.3 ng/dL	Assess medications: Value may be decreased by cortisone, chlorpromazine (Thorazine), phenytoin (Dilantin), heparin, lithium, sulfonamides, reserpine (Serpasil), testosterone, propranolol (Inderal), tolbutamide (Orinase), and salicylates in high doses. Values may be increased by oral contraceptives, estrogen, clofibrate, and perphenazine (Trilafon).
Triiodothyronine (T_3)	The results of this blood serum test are used to diagnose hyperthyroidism and to compare T_3 with T_4 for diagnosis of thyroid disorder. Normal value: 80–200 ng/dL	Assess medications: Value can be decreased by propylthiouracil, methimazole (Tapazole), lithium, phenytoin (Dilantin), propranolol (Inderal), reserpine (Serpasil), large doses of aspirin, steroids, and sulfonamides. Value can be increased by estrogen, progestins, oral contraceptives, T_3, and methadone.

DIAGNOSTIC TESTS of the Endocrine System (continued)

NAME OF TEST	PURPOSE & DESCRIPTION	RELATED NURSING INTERVENTIONS
Triiodothyronine Resin Uptake (T$_3$RU)	This test is an indirect measure of free thyroxine (T$_4$). The patient's blood is mixed with radioactive T$_3$ and synthetic resin, and the radioactive T$_3$ will bind with available thyroid-binding globulin sites. The unbound radioactive T$_3$ is added to resin for T$_3$ uptake. In hyperthyroidism there are few binding sites left, more T$_3$ is taken up by the resin, and a high T$_3$ resin uptake results. The opposite occurs in hypothyroidism. Normal value: 25%–35% uptake	No special preparation is needed.

PARATHYROID TESTS

NAME OF TEST	PURPOSE & DESCRIPTION	RELATED NURSING INTERVENTIONS
Calcium (Ca)	This blood serum test is used to check for serum calcium excess or deficit in parathyroid and bone disorders, and to monitor calcium levels. Normal value: 9.0–11.0 mg/dL, 4.5–5.5 mEq/L, or 2.3–2.8 mmol/L (SI units)	Assess for manifestations of tetany, including positive Chvostek's and Trousseau's signs, if hypocalcemia is present (∞ see Chapter 10).
Magnetic Resonance Imaging (MRI)—parathyroid glands	This radiographic study is done to identify tumors of the parathyroid glands. See information for MRI of the pituitary for related nursing interventions.	
Parathyroid Hormone (PTH)	This blood test is used to identify hypoparathyroidism or hyperparathyroidism, and is also used to monitor response to PTH therapy. Normal value: Intact PTH: 11–54 pg/mL C-terminal PTH: 50–330 pg/mL N-terminal PTH: 8–24 pg/mL	Tell patients not to eat or drink for 8 hours before the test.

ADRENAL TESTS

NAME OF TEST	PURPOSE & DESCRIPTION	RELATED NURSING INTERVENTIONS
ACTH Stimulation	This test is conducted to check for pituitary hypofunction. The drug metyrapone (Metopirone) is given to block the production of cortisol, thus causing an increased ACTH secretion. If the ACTH level does not increase, the problem is pituitary insufficiency.	Assess medications as for ACTH test.
ACTH Suppression	This test is used to check for the origin of an endocrine disorder. The drug dexamethasone (Decadron) is given to suppress ACTH production. If an extremely high dose is needed, the cause is of pituitary origin; if the plasma cortisol continues to be high with ACTH suppression, the cause could be adrenal cortex hyperfunction (Cushing's syndrome). Normally, the plasma cortisol level should double in 1 hour.	Tell patients to avoid tea, caffeinated coffee, and chocolates; no other food or fluid restriction is needed. Assess medications: False positives may be caused by phenytoin, barbiturates, meprobamate, and carbamazepine. If dexamethasone causes gastric irritation, milk or antacids may be required.
Aldosterone	This blood test is done to identify a deficit or an excess of aldosterone, and to compare blood and urine levels with other lab data to evaluate overhydration with increased sodium and adrenal malfunction. Normal value: < 16 mcg/dL (fasting) A 24-hour urine test is considered a more reliable measure of aldosterone than a random aldosterone test. Normal value: 6–25 mcg/24 hours	Assess diet and lab results: Levels are increased by hyponatremia, hyperkalemia, and a low-salt diet. Assess medications: Values are increased by diuretics, hydralazine (Apresoline), diazoxide (Hyperstat), nitroprusside, and oral contraceptives. If a urine test is ordered, assess diet and lab results as for blood test. Assess medications: Urine aldosterone levels are increased by diuretics, lithium, and oral contraceptives. Refrigerate specimen during collection.

(continued)

DIAGNOSTIC TESTS of the Endocrine System (continued)

NAME OF TEST	PURPOSE & DESCRIPTION	RELATED NURSING INTERVENTIONS
Adrenocorticotropic Hormone (ACTH)	This blood serum test is used to determine if a decreased plasma level of cortisol is due to adrenal cortex hypofunction or pituitary hypofunction. Normal value: 7–10 AM: 8–80 pg/mL 4 PM: 5–30 pg/mL 10–12 PM: < 10 pg/mL	Tell the patient that food and fluids may be restricted, and to eat a low-carbohydrate diet for 24 hours prior to the test. Assess medications: ACTH values may be increased by metyrapone, vasopressin, and insulin, and decreased by steroids, estrogen amphetamines, and alcohol.
Computerized Tomography (CT) of the abdomen	This radiologic study is used to assess the adrenal gland for tumors (including size and metastasis).	Determine if contrast medium will be used; if so, assess patient for allergy to iodine (shellfish).
Cortisol	This blood serum test is used to measure the amount of total cortisol in the serum and to evaluate adrenal cortex function. Values are decreased in Addison's disease and hypothyroidism, and increased in Cushing's syndrome and hyperthyroidism. Normal value: 8–10 AM: 138–635 nmol 4–6 PM: 83–359 nmol A 24-hour urine test may be conducted to measure free (unbound) cortisol Normal value: < 100 mcg/24 hours	Tell patient not to eat or drink and to rest for 2 hours before the test. Evaluate medications: Cortisol is decreased by androgens, phenytoin (Dilantin), and increased by oral contraceptives, estrogen, spironolactone (Aldactone), and triparanol. Teach patient how to save urine for 24-hour period, to eat a low-sodium diet before the test, and to avoid stressful situations and physical activity for at least 24 hours prior to the test. Assess medications; values may be increased by reserpine (Serpasil), diuretics, phenothiazines, and amphetamines.
Late Night Cortisol Test	This test is used to differentiate the cause of adrenal disorders. A saliva specimen is collected at 11 PM and then dexamethasone 1 mg is administered orally. A serum cortisol is collected at 8 AM the next morning. The dexamethasone suppresses ACTH. If an extremely high dose of dexamethasone is required to suppress ACTH, the primary disorder is adrenal cortex hyperplasia (Cushing's disease). If ACTH is not suppressed with the synthetic cortisol, an adrenal tumor is suspected.	
17-Ketosteroids	This 24-hour urine test is done to measure metabolites in urine and evaluate adrenal cortex function. Normal value: Men: 5–25 mg in 24 hours Women: 5–15 mg in 24 hours	Instruct patient how to save urine (urine must contain a preservative and be refrigerated). Assess medications: Levels are affected by a variety of drugs (check information in agency protocol for test); if possible, these should be discontinued for 48 hours before the test. Women cannot have the test while menstruating because blood can cause a false-positive finding.
Magnetic Resonance Imaging (MRI)—adrenal glands	This radiographic study is done to identify tumors of the adrenal glands.	See information for MRI of the pituitary.
MIBG Scan	This nuclear medicine scan is used to detect the presence and location of adrenal pheochromocytomas. A special radioactive dye is given and concentrates on the tumor in the adrenal gland; the tumor can then be seen on x-ray.	Explain that the test takes about an hour a day for 3 or 4 days.

PANCREATIC ENDOCRINE TESTS

NAME OF TEST	PURPOSE & DESCRIPTION	RELATED NURSING INTERVENTIONS
Computed Tomography (CT) of the abdomen	This radiographic test is done to identify pancreatic tumors or cysts.	If contrast medium is used, assess for allergy to iodine (shellfish).

DIAGNOSTIC TESTS of the Endocrine System (continued)

NAME OF TEST	PURPOSE & DESCRIPTION	RELATED NURSING INTERVENTIONS
Fasting Blood Sugar (FBS)	This test of serum or plasma is used to identify or confirm a diagnosis of diabetes mellitus. It is also used to monitor treatment of diabetes mellitus. A finding of greater than 125 mg/dL, if confirmed with a repeated test on a different day, indicates diabetes mellitus. **Normal value:** Serum/plasma: 70–110 mg/dL (value varies in individual laboratories)	Tell the patient not to eat or drink for 12 hours before the test. Do not administer insulin until blood specimen is taken. Assess medications: FBS may be increased by cortisone, diuretics, ACTH, levodopa, epinephrine, anesthetics, and phenytoin (Dilantin).
Oral Glucose Tolerance Test (OGTT)	This blood and urine test is used to diagnose diabetes mellitus if prior fasting blood sugar (FBS) findings are increased or inconsistent.	**Nursing Implications for Oral Glucose Tolerance Test** The tests will not be done if patient's FBS is consistently high (> 200 mg/dL). The patient drinks a solution of 75 to 100 grams of glucose and samples of blood and urine are taken immediately and at 30, 60, and 120 minutes (or it may extend from 3 to 6 hours). Values for 2-hour plasma at 139 or below are considered normal; values at 200 or greater, if confirmed with a second test on a different day, are diagnostic of diabetes mellitus. Tell the patient not to eat or drink (except water) for 12 hours before the test. Assess medications: Drugs that may increase OGTT levels are steroids, oral contraceptives, estrogens, thiazide diuretics, and salicylates. Explain to the patient that he or she may feel weak and may perspire during the test and that these symptoms should be reported to the nurse. Although they usually are transitory, they may be manifestations of hyperinsulinism.
Glycosylated Hemoglobin (Hb A_1C)	This serum test is used to measure the effectiveness of treatment of diabetes mellitus. The results represent an average blood glucose level during a 1- to 4-month period; an elevated level indicates uncontrolled diabetes mellitus and increased risk for complications. **Normal value:** In most labs, the normal range is 4% to 5.9%. In poorly controlled diabetes, its 8.0% or above, and in well controlled patients it is less than 7.0%.	Monitor findings: Decreased levels can be caused by anemia, long-term blood loss, and chronic renal failure. Increased levels may result from hyperglycemia, alcohol ingestion, pregnancy, hemodialysis, and prolonged cortisone intake.
Magnetic Resonance Imaging (MRI)— pancreas	This radiographic study is done to identify tumors of the pancreas.	See information for MRI of the pituitary.

Genetic Considerations

When conducting a health assessment interview and physical assessment, it is important for the nurse to consider genetic influences on the health of the adult. During the health assessment interview, ask about endocrine disorders in immediate family members, including the family members' age of onset and gender. Ask the patient about a family history of such diseases as diabetes mellitus, diabetes insipidus, thyroid disorders, growth problems, hypertension, and obesity. Ask women about problems with pregnancy, menstruation, and/or menopause.

During the physical assessment, assess for any manifestations that might indicate a genetic disorder (see the following box). If data are found to indicate genetic risk factors or alterations, ask about genetic testing and refer for appropriate genetic counseling and evaluation. ∞ Chapter 8 provides further information about genetics in medical-surgical nursing.

Health Assessment Interview

A health assessment interview to determine problems with the endocrine system may be part of a health screening or total health assessment, or it may focus on a chief complaint (such as increased urination or changes in energy levels). If the patient has a problem with endocrine function, the nurse analyzes its onset, characteristics and course, severity, precipitating and relieving factors, and any associated symptoms, noting the timing and circumstances. For example, the nurse may ask the patient the following:

- "Describe the swelling you noticed in the front of your neck. When did it begin? Have you noticed any changes in your energy level? If so, describe them."
- "When did you first notice that your hands and feet were getting larger?"
- "Have you noticed that your appetite has increased even though you have lost weight?"

Thyroid Disorders Video

GENETIC CONSIDERATIONS
Examples of Endocrine System Disorders

- Type 1 and type 2 diabetes mellitus are classified as multifactorial inheritance disorders because both genetic and environmental factors are necessary for onset of the disorder.
- Pendred syndrome is an inherited disorder in which people have deafness and a thyroid goiter.
- Hashimoto's disease (chronic thyroiditis) is believed to have a genetic component.
- Multiple endocrine neoplasia is a group of rare diseases caused by genetic defects leading to hyperplasia and hyperfunction of two or more components of the endocrine system (especially the parathyroid, pancreas, and pituitary glands).
- Fragile X syndrome is a genetic condition that causes developmental problems including learning disabilities and mental retardation. Males are usually more severely affected than females.

The health history includes information about the patient's medical history, family history, and social and personal history. Ask the patient about any changes in normal growth and development as well as in height and weight. Changes in the size of extremities can often be detected by asking whether the patient has had to have rings enlarged or to buy increasingly larger gloves and shoes. Enlargement of the neck may be identified by asking whether the patient has difficulty finding shirts or blouses with a collar that fits. Also explore changes such as difficulty swallowing; increased or decreased thirst, appetite, and/or urination; visual changes; sleep disturbances; altered patterns of hair distribution (such as increased facial hair in women); changes in menstruation; changes in memory or ability to concentrate; and changes in hair and skin texture. Ask the patient about any injury or surgery of the head, as well as previous hospitalizations,

chemotherapy, radiation (especially to the neck), and the use of medications (especially hormones or steroids).

The nurse also asks about the patient's occupational and social history. Include questions about the patient's satisfaction with occupation, personal relationships, and lifestyle. Other areas of assessment include the patient's usual means of coping; use of alcohol, smoking, or drugs; diet (including weight gain or loss); exercise patterns; and sleep patterns. Although the patient may not recognize changes in behavior, family members may be able to provide important information.

Interview questions categorized by functional health patterns are listed on page 489.

Physical Assessment

Physical assessment of the endocrine system may be performed as part of a total health assessment or it may be a focused assessment of patients with known or suspected problems with endocrine function. Sample documentation of an assessment of the thyroid gland is included in the following box.

The only endocrine organ that can be palpated is the thyroid gland; however, other assessments that provide information about endocrine pathophysiology include inspection of the skin, hair, nails, facial appearance, reflexes, and musculoskeletal system. Measuring and monitoring trends in height and weight and vital signs also provide clues to altered endocrine system function.

The patient may sit during the examination. A reflex hammer is used to test deep tendon reflexes. Prior to the examination, the nurse collects the necessary equipment and explains the techniques to the patient to decrease anxiety. Additional techniques for assessing hypocalcemic tetany, a complication of endocrine disorders or surgery, are included here in the examination sequence. Normal age-related changes in assessment findings are described in Table 18–2.

NURSING CARE OF THE OLDER ADULT — Age-Related Endocrine Changes

AGE-RELATED CHANGE	SIGNIFICANCE
Pituitary: ⬇ production of ACTH, TSH, FSH	■ Decreased secretion of glucocorticoids, 17-ketosteroids, progesterone, androgen, and estrogen (and thus lower levels on diagnostic tests)
Thyroid: ⬆ in fibrosis and nodularity, ⬇ in gland activity	■ Lower basal metabolic rate ■ Increased incidence of hypothyroidism ■ Palpable nodules on palpation
Adrenal medulla: ⬆ secretion and level of norepinephrine, ⬇ beta-adrenergic response to norepinephrine	■ Decreased response to beta-adrenergic and receptor blockers (medications) ■ May contribute to increased incidence of hypertension
Pancreas: calcification of blood vessels and distention and dilation of pancreatic ducts	■ Decreased production of lipase with reduced fat absorption and digestion, leading to intolerance of fatty foods and indigestion ■ Decreased absorption of fat-soluble vitamins
Pancreas: delayed and decreased insulin release; believed accompanied by decreased sensitivity to circulating insulin	■ Decreased ability to metabolize glucose with higher and more prolonged blood glucose levels may contribute to increased incidence of type 2 diabetes mellitus with aging (however, higher than normal blood glucose levels are not unusual in nondiabetic older adults)

FUNCTIONAL HEALTH PATTERN INTERVIEW   Endocrine System

Functional Health Pattern	Interview Questions and Leading Statements
Health Perception-Health Management	■ Describe your overall state of health, rating it on a scale of 1 to 10 with 10 being the best health you have had. ■ Describe any problems you have had with an endocrine gland (pituitary, thyroid, parathyroid, adrenal, pancreas, ovaries, testes). ■ If you had a problem with any of these glands, how was it treated (medications, surgery, diet, hormone replacement)? ■ Do you smoke, drink alcohol, and/or use recreational drugs? If so, how much and what kind? ■ Have you ever been tested for high or low blood sugar?
Nutritional-Metabolic	■ Describe what you eat and how much (and type of) fluid you drink in a 24-hour period. ■ Do you take any nutritional supplements, herbs, or vitamins? ■ Have you noticed any change in your hunger or thirst? ■ Has your weight changed? If so, how many pounds and over what time period? ■ Have you noticed any change in your energy level? If so, explain. ■ Have you noticed any change in your ability to tolerate heat or cold? If so, describe the change. ■ Have you noticed any difficulty swallowing? Explain. ■ Have you noticed any changes in the texture of your skin? If so, what were they?
Elimination	■ Have you noticed any change in the color, odor, amount, or frequency of urination? If so, describe it. ■ Have you ever had kidney stones? If so, how were they treated? ■ Has there been a change in your bowel elimination (such as diarrhea or constipation)? If so, explain the change.
Activity-Exercise	■ Describe your physical activities in a usual day. ■ Has your energy level increased or decreased? Explain. ■ Do some activities make you very tired? Explain how you feel.
Sleep-Rest	■ How many hours of sleep do you get each night? ■ Do you feel nervous and unable to rest? Explain. ■ Have you ever sweated at night? Describe if so.
Cognitive-Perceptual	■ Have you noticed any problem with your memory? What was it? ■ Do you feel restless, anxious, or confused? Explain. ■ Have you noticed any change in your voice? Explain. ■ Have you noticed any change in the color or condition of your skin and hair (color, dryness, oiliness, bruises)? Describe if so. ■ Have you had any headaches, memory loss, changes in sensation, depression? Describe if so. ■ Have you noticed any change in your vision? Describe if so. ■ Have you had any heart palpitations? When did they occur? ■ Have you had any abdominal pain? What is it like and where is it located? ■ Have you had any pain or stiffness in your muscles and joints?
Self-Perception-Self-Concept	■ How does this condition make you feel about yourself? ■ How do you feel about taking medications?
Role-Relationships	■ How does this condition make you feel about yourself? How does this condition affect your relationships with others? ■ Does anyone in your family have an endocrine disorder? If so, when did it begin and how does it affect them? What family member is affected and at what age did it begin?
Coping-Stress-Tolerance	■ Does stress seem to make your condition worse? Explain. ■ Has this condition created stress for you? ■ Describe what you do when you feel stressed.
Value-Belief	■ Tell me how specific relationships or activities help you cope with this condition. ■ Describe specific cultural beliefs or practices that affect how you care for and feel about this condition. ■ Is there anything interfering with your spiritual beliefs, needs, or practices during your illness? What can I or another caregiver do to help you with your spiritual needs? ■ Are there any specific treatments that you would not use to treat this condition?

Endocrine Assessments

TABLE 18–2 Endocrine Assessments

TECHNIQUE/NORMAL FINDINGS	ABNORMAL FINDINGS
Skin Assessments	
Inspect skin color. *Skin color should be even and appropriate to age and race of the patient.*	■ Hyperpigmentation may be seen in patients with Addison's disease or Cushing's syndrome. ■ Hypopigmentation may be seen in diabetes mellitus, hyperthyroidism, or hypothyroidism. ■ A yellowish cast to the skin might indicate hypothyroidism. ■ Purple striae over the abdomen and bruising may be present in the patient with Cushing's syndrome.
Palpate the skin, assessing texture, moisture, and the presence of lesions. *Skin color should be appropriate to the patient's race, smooth, warm, dry, and intact without lesions.*	■ Rough, dry skin is often seen in patients with hypothyroidism, whereas smooth and flushed skin can be a sign of hyperthyroidism. ■ Lesions (such as ulcerations) on the lower extremities might indicate diabetes mellitus.
Nails and Hair Assessment	
Assess texture, distribution, and condition of nails and hair. *Hair should be of normal texture, appropriately distributed for gender; nail surfaces should have even color with smooth surfaces.*	■ Increased pigmentation of the nails is often seen in patients with Addison's disease. ■ Dry, thick, brittle nails and hair may be apparent in hypothyroidism; thin, brittle nails and thin, soft hair may be apparent in hyperthyroidism. ■ Hirsutism (excessive facial, chest, or abdominal hair) may be seen in Cushing's syndrome.
Facial Assessments	
Inspect the symmetry and form of the face. *Face should be bilaterally symmetrical.*	■ Variations of form and structure may indicate growth abnormalities such as **acromegaly** (continued growth of bone from growth hormone hypersecretion).
Inspect position of eyes. *Eyes should be equal in position on both sides of the face. Eyelids should close over eyes.*	■ **Exophthalmos** (protruding eyes) may be seen in hyperthyroidism.
Thyroid Gland Assessment	
Palpate the thyroid gland for size and consistency.	■ The thyroid may be enlarged in patients with Graves' disease or a **goiter** (enlarged thyroid gland).
Stand behind the patient and place your fingers on either side of the trachea below the thyroid cartilage (Figure 18–8 ■). Ask the patient to tilt his or her head to the right. Now ask the patient to swallow. As the patient swallows, displace the left lobe while palpating the right lobe. Repeat to palpate the left lobe. *Thyroid gland is not usually palpable. If it is, lobes should feel smooth, rubbery, and free of nodules.*	■ Multiple nodules may be seen in metabolic disorders, whereas the presence of only one nodule may indicate a cyst or a benign or malignant tumor. ■ A single enlarged nodule suggests malignancy. 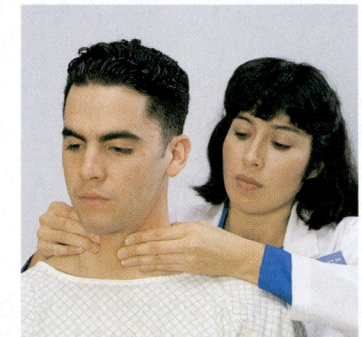 **Figure 18–8 ■** Palpating the thyroid gland from behind the patient.
Motor Function Assessment	
Assess the deep tendon reflexes. Deep tendon reflexes are assessed with the reflex hammer, and include the biceps reflex, brachioradialis reflex, triceps reflex, patellar reflex, and Achilles reflex. *Normal values range from 1+ (present, but decreased) to 2+ (normal) to 3+ (increased).* ∞ *See Chapter 43 for guidelines and illustrations of deep tendon reflex assessment.*	■ Increased reflexes may be seen in hyperthyroidism; decreased reflexes may be seen in hypothyroidism.

TABLE 18–2 Endocrine Assessments (continued)

TECHNIQUE/NORMAL FINDINGS	ABNORMAL FINDINGS
Sensory Function Assessment Test the patient's sensitivity to pain, temperature, vibration, light touch, and stereognosis (the ability to identify an object by touch). Compare symmetric areas on both sides of the body, and compare the distal to the proximal regions of the extremities. Ask the patient to close his or her eyes. *Sensory function should be bilaterally intact.* ■ To test pain, use the blunt and sharp ends of a new safety pin. Discard the pin after use. ■ To test temperature, use cups or other containers of cold and hot water. ■ To test vibration, use a tuning fork over one of the patient's finger or toe joints. ■ To test light touch, use a cotton wisp. ■ To test stereognosis, place in the patient's hand a simple, familiar object, such as a rubber band, cotton ball, or button. Ask the patient to identify the object.	■ Peripheral neuropathy and paresthesias (altered sensations) may occur in diabetes, hypothyroidism, or acromegaly.
Musculoskeletal Assessment Inspect the size and proportions of the patient's body structure. *Size and proportion of body structures should be bilaterally equal.*	■ Extremely short stature may indicate **dwarfism** (a condition characterized by short stature); insufficient pituitary growth hormone is one cause. ■ Extremely large bones may indicate acromegaly, caused by excessive growth hormone.
Assessing for Hypocalcemic Tetany Assess for **Trousseau's sign** (a test for hypocalcemia) with resulting **tetany** (tonic muscle spasms) by inflating a blood pressure cuff above the antecubital space to a point greater than systolic blood pressure for 2 to 5 minutes. Trousseau's sign is discussed in relation to hypocalcemia in ∞ Chapter 10. *A normal finding is no carpal spasm in response to compression of the arm by the blood pressure cuff.*	■ Decreased calcium levels cause the patient's hand and fingers to contract (**carpal spasm**).
Assess for **Chvostek's sign** (a test for hypocalcemia) by tapping your finger in front of the patient's ear at the angle of the jaw. A positive Chvostek's sign causes facial grimacing due to repeated contractions of the facial muscle. Chvostek's sign is discussed and illustrated in relation to hypocalcemia in ∞ Chapter 10. *A normal finding is no facial grimacing in response to tapping the patient's face in front of the ear.*	■ Decreased calcium levels cause the patient's lateral facial muscles to contract.

SAMPLE DOCUMENTATION

Assessment of the Thyroid Gland

A 37-year-old female presents at a community clinic for complaints of "always feeling so hot," "always hungry but losing weight," and "can't sleep at night—too jittery." Weight 110 lb (loss of 12 pounds in last 3 months). BP 90/78 (averages 84/72), P 96. Skin very warm and moist. Anterior neck has diffuse enlargement. Thyroid gland enlarged bilaterally on palpation. Referral made to endocrine clinic for further evaluation.

TEST YOURSELF NCLEX-RN® REVIEW

1. What assessment would the nurse expect if the pituitary produces an increased amount of ADH?
   1. increased output of urine
   2. decreased output of urine
   3. increased facial hair growth in women
   4. decreased production of testosterone

2. What assessment might a nurse make to identify low calcium levels?
   1. Save urine to measure 7-ketosteroids.
   2. Palpate turgor of skin.
   3. Conduct a Trousseau's sign test.
   4. Observe color of skin.

3. Excessive amounts of glucocorticoids, produced by the adrenal cortex, result in what pathophysiologic health problem?
   1. inhibited immune response
   2. increased response to glucagon
   3. delayed onset of puberty
   4. decreased metabolic rate

4. A nurse is conducting a health history focused on the endocrine system. Which of the following questions should be included?
   1. "When did you first notice the pain in your abdomen?"
   2. "Do your children have problems with urination?"
   3. "Have you noticed a change in your thirst?"
   4. "How did you get this scar on your leg?"

5. What assessments are made when the nurse palpates the thyroid gland?
   1. edema and movement
   2. size and consistency
   3. character and texture
   4. pain and pulse rate

6. Decreased calcium levels can be assessed with Chvostek's sign. What does the nurse do to conduct this assessment?
   1. inflates a blood pressure cuff above the antecubital space
   2. taps the finger in front of the patient's ear
   3. depresses the skin over the shin
   4. pinches a fold of skin over the sternum

7. Which of the following tests is the most accurate indicator of thyroid function?
   1. GH
   2. FBS
   3. aldosterone
   4. TSH

8. A nurse is conducting an assessment of the endocrine system in an older adult woman. What assessment is the result of aging?
   1. pituitary enlarged and firm
   2. normal heart tones
   3. thyroid nodules present
   4. decreased facial hair

9. A nurse is caring for a patient with newly diagnosed hypothyroidism. What skin assessment might be expected?
   1. increased hair growth
   2. rough, dry skin
   3. smooth, flushed skin
   4. cold and clammy skin

10. What endocrine disorder might the nurse assess by testing deep tendon reflexes?
    1. Cushing's syndrome
    2. acromegaly
    3. tetany
    4. hyperthyroidism

See Test Yourself answers in Appendix C.

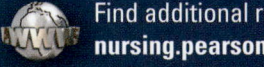

Pearson Nursing Student Resources

Find additional review materials at
nursing.pearsonhighered.com

Prepare for success with additional NCLEX®-style practice questions, interactive assignments and activities, Web links, animations and videos, and more!

BIBLIOGRAPHY

Armstrong, J., & Mitchell, E. (2008). Comprehensive nursing assessment in the care of older people. *Nursing Older People, (20)*1, 36–40.

Bald, H. (2006). The process of conducting a physical assessment: A nursing perspective. *British Journal of Nursing, 15*(13), 710–714.

Bickley, L., & Szilagyi, P. (2007). *Bates' guide to physical examination and history taking* (9th ed.). Philadelphia: Lippincott.

Costello, T., & Coyne, I. (2008). Nurses' knowledge of mouth care practices. *British Journal of Nursing, 17*(4), 264–268.

Daddario, D. (2007). A review of the use of the health belief model for weight management. *MEDSURG Nursing, 16*(6), 363–366.

D'Amico, D., & Barbarito, C. (2007). *Health & physical assessment in nursing.* Upper Saddle River, NJ: Pearson Prentice Hall.

Dufour, D. (2007). Laboratory tests of thyroid function: Uses and limitations. *Endocrinology and Metabolism Clinics of North America, 36*(3), 579–594.

Eliopoulos, C. (2005). *Gerontological nursing* (6th ed.). Philadelphia: Lippincott.

Fletcher, J. (2006). Full nursing assessment of patients at risk of diabetic foot ulcers. *British Journal of Nursing, 15*(15). Tissue Viability Supplement: S18, S20–S21.

Galland, L. (2008). Mystery illness: When fatigue just won't go away. *Bottom Line/Health, 22*(4), 15.

Harrison, S., Cochrane, L., Abboud, R., & Leese, G. (2007). Do patients with diabetes wear shoes of the correct size? *International Journal of Clinical Practice, 61*(11), 1900–1904.

Karnath, B. M., & Hussain, N. (2006). Signs and symptoms of thyroid dysfunction. *Hospital Physician, 42*(10), 43–48.

Kee, J. (2009). *Prentice Hall handbook of laboratory & diagnostic tests with nursing implications* (6th ed.). Upper Saddle River, NJ: Pearson Prentice Hall.

Levin, N., & Greer, K. (2004). Cutaneous manifestations of endocrine disorders. *Dermatology Nursing, 13*(3), 185–186, 189–196, 201–202.

Lie, D. (2008). MRI may be more accurate than fine-needle biopsy in detection of thyroid cancer. Retrieved from http//www.medscape.com/viewarticle/566491

Lloyd, H., & Craig, S. (2007). A guide to taking a patient's history. *Nursing Standard, 22*(13), 42–48.

McClane, K. (2006). Screening instruments for use in a complete geriatric assessment. *Clinical Nurse Specialist, 20*(4), 201–207.

National Institute of Health. (2008). *Genes and disease: Nutritional and metabolic diseases; glands and hormones.* Retrieved from http://www.ncbi.nlm.nih.gov/books/bookres.fegi/gnd/pdf.html

Porth, C. M. (2007). *Essentials of pathophysiology: Concepts of altered health states* (2nd ed.). Philadelphia: Lippincott.

Porth, C. M., & Matfin, G. (2009). *Concepts of altered health states* (8th ed.). Philadelphia: Lippincott Williams & Wilkins.

Pullen, R. L. (2008). Preparing a patient for magnetic resonance imaging. *Nursing, 38*,10, 22.

U. S. Food and Drug Administration [FDA]. (2009). *FDA warns about risk of wearing medicated patches during MRIs.* Retrieved from http://www.fda.gov/bbs/topics/news/2009/new01967.html

Weber, J., & Kelley, J. (2009). *Health assessment in nursing* (4th ed.). Philadelphia: Lippincott Williams & Wilkins.

Nursing Care of Patients with Endocrine Disorders

LEARNING OUTCOMES

1. Apply knowledge of normal anatomy, physiology, and assessments of the thyroid, parathyroid, adrenal, and pituitary glands when providing nursing care for patients with endocrine disorders.
2. Compare and contrast the manifestations of disorders that result from hyperfunction and hypofunction of the thyroid, parathyroid, adrenal, and pituitary glands.
3. Explain the nursing implications for medications prescribed to treat disorders of the thyroid and adrenal glands.
4. Provide appropriate nursing care for the patient before and after a subtotal thyroidectomy and an adrenalectomy.
5. Use the nursing process as a framework for providing individualized care to patients with disorders of the thyroid, parathyroid, adrenal, and pituitary glands.

CLINICAL COMPETENCIES

1. Assess functional health status of patients with endocrine disorders and monitor, document, and report abnormal manifestations.
2. Use assessed data, patient values, clinical expertise, and evidence to determine priority nursing diagnoses and select and implement nursing interventions.
3. Effectively communicate with and function within the interdisciplinary team to plan and provide patient care.
4. Administer medications knowledgeably and safely.
5. Plan and provide patient and family teaching to promote, restore, and maintain functional health status.
6. Monitor for respiratory problems and tetany in patients having a thyroidectomy.
7. Adapt individual and cultural values and variations as well as expressed needs and preferences into the plan of care.
8. Evaluate responses to care and use data to revise plan as needed.

KEY TERMS

acromegaly, 516
Addisonian crisis, 512
diabetes insipidus, 517
euthyroid, 496
exophthalmos, 494
gigantism, 516
goiter, 494

hyperparathyroidism, 505
hypoparathyroidism, 506
myxedema, 500
myxedema coma, 502
proptosis, 494
syndrome of inappropriate ADH
    secretion (SIADH), 516

tetany, 506
thyroid storm or crisis, 496
thyroidectomy, 497
thyroiditis, 496
thyrotoxicosis, 494

The thyroid, parathyroid, adrenal, and pituitary glands are part of the endocrine system. Disorders of the structure and function of these glands alter normal hormone levels and the way body tissues use those hormones. When hormone production increases or decreases, people experience alterations in health.

Patients with disorders of the glands discussed in this chapter require nursing care for multiple functional problems. They often face exhausting diagnostic tests, changes in physical appearance and emotional responses, and permanent alterations in lifestyle. Nursing care is directed toward meeting physiologic needs, providing education, and ensuring psychologic support for the patient and family. A holistic approach to the complex needs of patients with these endocrine disorders is an essential component of nursing care.

Disorders of the Thyroid Gland

Altered thyroid hormone (TH) production or use affects all major organ systems. In the adult, TH changes primarily affect metabolism, cardiovascular function, gastrointestinal function, and neuromuscular function. Thyroid disorders—both hyperthyroidism and hypothyroidism—are among the most common endocrine disorders.

The Patient with Hyperthyroidism

Hyperthyroidism (also called **thyrotoxicosis**) is a disorder caused by excessive delivery of TH to the tissues. Because the primary effect of TH is to increase metabolism and protein synthesis, hyperthyroidism affects all major organ systems of the body. The increase in metabolic rate and the alterations in cardiac output, peripheral blood flow, oxygen consumption, and body temperature are similar to those found in increased sympathetic nervous system activity (Porth & Matfin, 2009).

Pathophysiology and Manifestations

The effects of hyperthyroidism are the result of increased circulating levels of TH. This hormonal excess increases the metabolic rate and heightens the sympathetic nervous system's physiologic response to stimulation. The sensitizing effect of abnormally elevated TH levels increases the cardiac rate and stroke volume. As a result, cardiac output and peripheral blood flow increase. Elevated TH levels also increase carbohydrate, protein, and lipid metabolism. Lipids are depleted, and glucose tolerance decreases. Protein degradation increases, resulting in a negative nitrogen balance. Over time, the hypermetabolic effects of excess TH result in caloric and nutritional deficiencies.

Hyperthyroidism results from many different factors, including autoimmune stimulation (as in Graves' disease), excess secretion of thyroid-stimulating hormone (TSH) by the pituitary gland, thyroiditis, neoplasms (such as toxic multinodular goiter), side effect of certain drugs, and an excessive intake of thyroid medications. The most common etiologies of hyperthyroidism are Graves' disease and toxic multinodular goiter.

The patient with hyperthyroidism typically has an increased appetite and may gain weight, although weight loss is more typical, and may have hypermotile bowels and diarrhea. Additional manifestations related to hypermetabolism include emotional liability, heat intolerance, insomnia, palpitations, and increased sweating. The skin is smooth and warm, hair may become fine, and hair loss in the scalp, eyebrow, axilla, or pubic region is common.

Graves' Disease

Graves' disease, the most common cause of hyperthyroidism, is an autoimmune disorder, sometimes associated with the presence of other autoimmune disorders such as myasthenia gravis, diabetes mellitus, celiac, and pernicious anemia (McPhee & Papadakis, 2009). The serum of patients with Graves' disease has an antibody that binds to TSH receptors in the thyroid follicles and causes the thyroid cells to hyperfunction. When this antibody binds to the TSH receptors, it stimulates hormone synthesis and secretion, enlarging the gland. The cause is unknown, but there is a hereditary link. Graves' disease is seen eight times more often in women than in men and occurs most frequently between the ages of 20 and 40 (McPhee & Papadakis, 2009).

Patients with Graves' disease have an enlarged thyroid gland (**goiter**) and manifestations of hyperthyroidism. The goiter can result from excess TSH stimulation (when the amount of circulating TH is deficient), abnormal growth-stimulating immunoglobulins, or substances that inhibit TH synthesis. A goiter may be present in hyperthyroidism or hypothyroidism.

The eye pathophysiology of Graves' disease is manifested as proptosis and visual dysfunction. **Proptosis** (forward displacement) of the eye occurs in about one-third of cases (Porth, 2007). The forward protrusion of the eyeballs (**exophthalmos**) results from an accumulation of inflammation by-products in the retro-orbital tissues. The sclera may be visible above the iris, the upper lids may be retracted, and the person has a characteristic unblinking stare (Figure 19–1 ■). Exophthalmos is usually bilateral, but it may involve only one eye. The patient may experience blurred vision, diplopia, eye pain, lacrimation, and photophobia. The inability to close the eyelids completely over the protruding eyeballs increases the risk of corneal dryness, irritation, infection, and ulceration. Infiltration of the muscles that move the eye and of the optic nerve lead to paralysis and vision loss. The treatment of Graves' disease may stabilize the manifestations but generally does not reverse these changes in the eyes.

Other manifestations include fatigue, difficulty sleeping, hand tremors, and changes in menstruation ranging from decreased flow to amenorrhea. Older patients may present with atrial fibrillation, angina, or congestive heart failure.

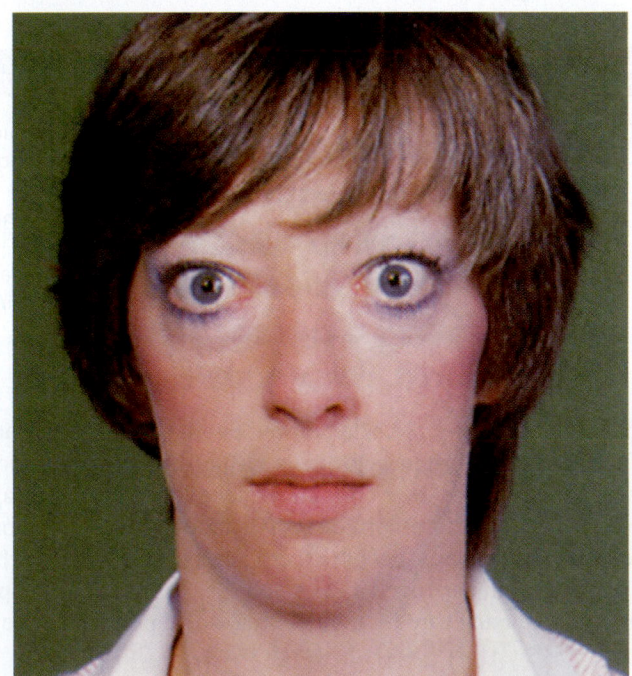

Figure 19–1 ■ Exophthalmos in a patient with Graves' disease. The disease causes edema of fat deposits behind the eyes and inflammation of the extraocular muscles. The accumulating pressure forces the eyes outward from their orbits.

Source: University of Illinois, Custom Medical Stock Photo, Inc.

MULTISYSTEM EFFECTS OF
Hyperthyroidism

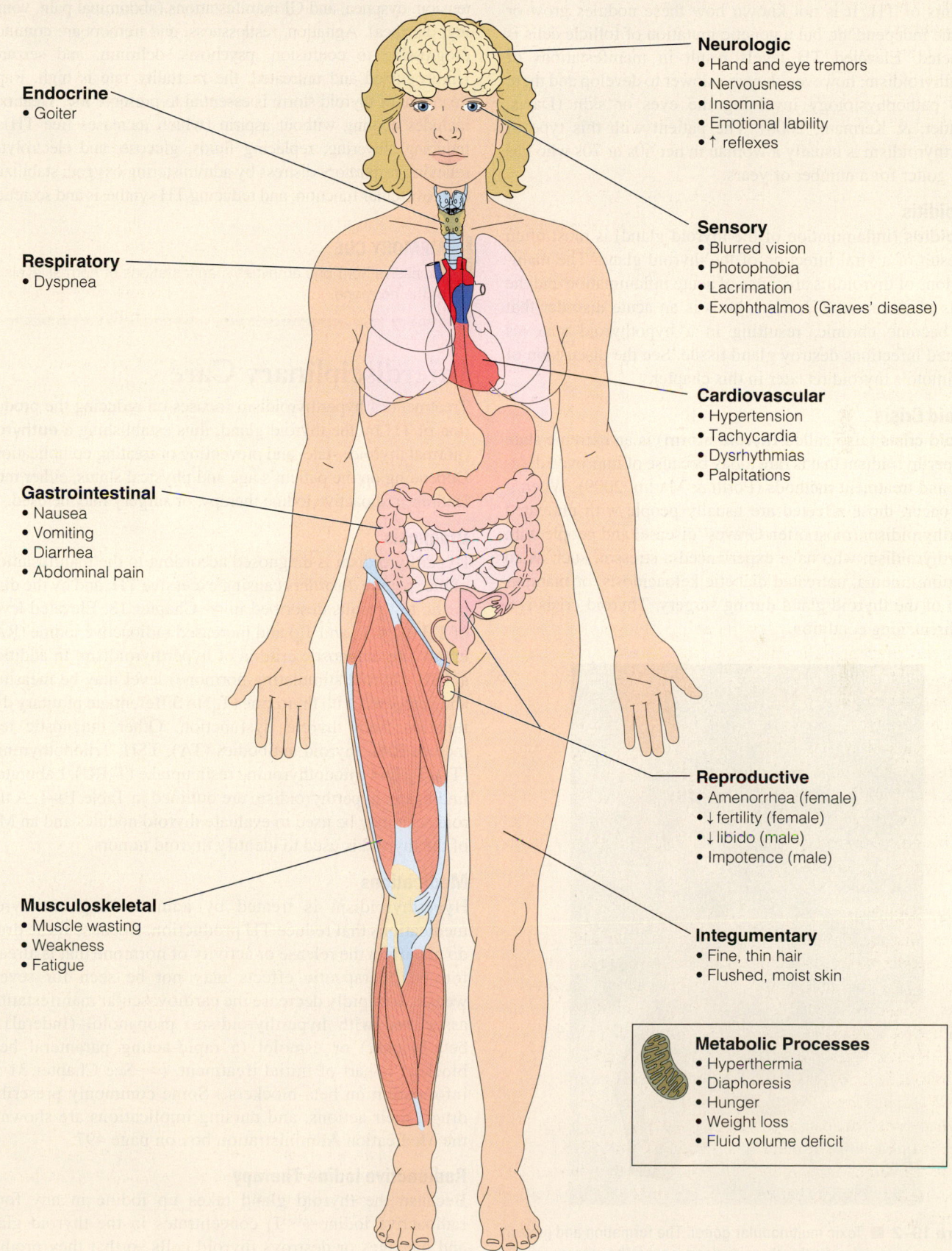

Endocrine
• Goiter

Respiratory
• Dyspnea

Gastrointestinal
• Nausea
• Vomiting
• Diarrhea
• Abdominal pain

Musculoskeletal
• Muscle wasting
• Weakness
• Fatigue

Neurologic
• Hand and eye tremors
• Nervousness
• Insomnia
• Emotional lability
• ↑ reflexes

Sensory
• Blurred vision
• Photophobia
• Lacrimation
• Exophthalmos (Graves' disease)

Cardiovascular
• Hypertension
• Tachycardia
• Dysrhythmias
• Palpitations

Reproductive
• Amenorrhea (female)
• ↓ fertility (female)
• ↓ libido (male)
• Impotence (male)

Integumentary
• Fine, thin hair
• Flushed, moist skin

Metabolic Processes
• Hyperthermia
• Diaphoresis
• Hunger
• Weight loss
• Fluid volume deficit

Toxic Multinodular Goiter

Toxic multinodular goiter (Figure 19–2 ■) is a thyroid tumor characterized by small, discrete, independently functioning nodules in the thyroid gland tissue that secrete excessive amounts of TH. It is not known how these nodules grow or become independent, but a genetic mutation of follicle cells is suspected. Elevated TH levels result in manifestations of hyperthyroidism; however, they are slower to develop and there is no pathophysiology involving the eyes or skin (Davis, Orlander, & Kermani, 2008). The patient with this type of hyperthyroidism is usually a woman in her 60s or 70s who has had a goiter for a number of years.

Thyroiditis

Thyroiditis (inflammation of the thyroid gland) is most often the result of a viral infection of the thyroid gland. The manifestations of thyroiditis are those of acute inflammation and the effects of increased TH. Thyroiditis is an acute disorder that may become chronic, resulting in a hypothyroid state as repeated infections destroy gland tissue. See the discussion of Hashimoto's thyroiditis later in this chapter.

Thyroid Crisis

Thyroid crisis (also called **thyroid storm**) is an extreme state of hyperthyroidism that is rare today because of improved diagnosis and treatment methods (Porth & Matfin, 2009). When it does occur, those affected are usually people with untreated hyperthyroidism (most often Graves' disease) and people with hyperthyroidism who have experienced a stressor, such as an infection, trauma, untreated diabetic ketoacidosis, or manipulation of the thyroid gland during surgery. Thyroid crisis is a life-threatening condition.

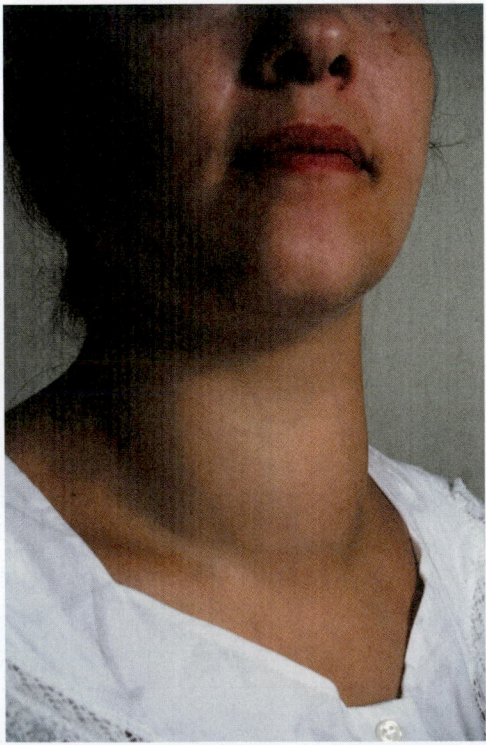

Figure 19–2 ■ Toxic multinodular goiter. The formation and growth of numerous nodules in the thyroid gland cause the characteristic massive enlargement of the neck.

The rapid increase in metabolic rate that results from the excessive TH causes the manifestations of thyroid crisis. The manifestations include hyperthermia, with body temperatures ranging from 102°F to 106°F (39°C to 41°C), tachycardia, systolic hypertension, dyspnea, and GI manifestations (abdominal pain, vomiting, diarrhea). Agitation, restlessness, and tremors are common, progressing to confusion, psychosis, delirium, and seizures. Unrecognized and untreated, the mortality rate is high. Rapid treatment of thyroid storm is essential to preserve life. Treatment includes cooling without aspirin (which increases free TH) or inducing shivering; replacing fluids, glucose, and electrolytes; relieving respiratory distress by administering oxygen; stabilizing cardiovascular function; and reducing TH synthesis and secretion.

> **MEMORY CUE**
> Excessive hormone amplifies manifestations of normal levels of the hormone.

Interdisciplinary Care

Treatment of hyperthyroidism focuses on reducing the production of TH by the thyroid gland, thus establishing a **euthyroid** (normal thyroid) state, and preventing or treating complications. Depending on the patient's age and physical status, either medications, radioactive iodine therapy, or surgery may be used.

Diagnosis

Hyperthyroidism is diagnosed according to the manifestations of the specific disorders causing excessive TH, and by the diagnostic test results described in ∞ Chapter 18. Elevated levels of TH (both T_3 and T_4) and increased radioactive iodine (RAI) uptake are diagnostic criteria of hyperthyroidism. In addition, a TSH (thyroid stimulating hormone) level may be measured and compared with thyroxine (T_4) to differentiate pituitary dysfunction from thyroid dysfunction. Other diagnostic tests include RAI, thyroid antibodies (TA), TSH, Triiodothyronine (T_3), T_4, and triiodothyronine resin uptake (T_3RU). Laboratory findings in hyperthyroidism are outlined in Table 19–1. A thyroid scan may be used to evaluate thyroid nodules and an MRI of the thyroid is used to identify thyroid tumors.

Medications

Hyperthyroidism is treated by administering antithyroid medications that reduce TH production. Because these drugs do not affect the release or activity of hormone that is already formed, therapeutic effects may not be seen for several weeks. To rapidly decrease the cardiovascular manifestations associated with hyperthyroidism, propanolol (Inderal) (a beta-blocker) or esmolol (a rapid-acting parenteral beta-blocker) is part of initial treatment. (∞ See Chapter 31 for information on beta-blockers.) Some commonly prescribed drugs, their actions, and nursing implications are shown in the Medication Administration box on page 497.

Radioactive Iodine Therapy

Because the thyroid gland takes up iodine in any form, radioactive iodine (^{131}I) concentrates in the thyroid gland and damages or destroys thyroid cells so that they produce less TH. Radioactive iodine is given orally. Results typically

TABLE 19–1 Laboratory Findings in Thyroid Disorders

TEST	NORMAL VALUES	HYPERTHYROIDISM	HYPOTHYROIDISM
Serum TA	Negative to 1:20	Increased	Normal
Serum TSH (sensitive assay)	2 to 10 mU/ml	Decreased in primary hyperthyroidism	Increased in primary hypothyroidism
Serum T_4	5 to 12 mcg/dL	Increased	Decreased
Serum T_3	80 to 200 ng/dL	Increased	Decreased
T_3 uptake (T_3RU)	25 to 35 relative percentage	Increased	Decreased
Thyroid suppression		Increased RAI uptake and T_4 levels	No change

occur in 6 to 8 weeks. In most instances, the patient is not hospitalized during treatment and does not require radiation precautions. This type of therapy is contraindicated in pregnant women because radioactive iodine crosses the placenta and can have negative effects on the developing fetal thyroid gland. Because the amount of gland destroyed is not readily controllable, the patient may develop hypothyroidism and require lifelong TH replacement. Adverse reactions include thyroiditis and cardiac instability due to liberation of stored thyroid hormone in the gland (Holcomb, 2006).

Surgery

Some hyperthyroid patients have such enlarged thyroid glands that pressure on the esophagus or trachea causes breathing or swallowing problems. In these cases, removal of all or part of the gland (**thyroidectomy**) is indicated. A subtotal thyroidectomy is usually performed. This procedure leaves enough of the gland in place to produce an adequate amount of TH. A total thyroidectomy is performed to treat cancer of the thyroid; the patient then requires lifelong hormone replacement (McPhee & Papadakis, 2009).

Before surgery, the patient should be in as nearly a euthyroid state as possible. The patient may be given antithyroid drugs to reduce hormone levels and iodine preparations to decrease the vascularity and size of the gland (which also reduces the risk of hemorrhage during and after surgery). Nursing care of the patient having a subtotal thyroidectomy is discussed in the box on page 499.

Nursing Care

Health Promotion

Although hyperthyroidism is not preventable, it is important to teach patients the importance of regular healthcare provider visits and medication intake.

MEDICATION ADMINISTRATION   Hyperthyroidism

IODINE SOURCES

Strong Iodine Solution (Lugol's Solution)

Potassium iodide (SSKI, Thyro-Block, Pima)

Large doses of iodine for a short term inhibit TH synthesis and release. Iodine also makes the hyperplastic thyroid less vascular prior to surgery and hastens the ability of other antithyroid drugs to reduce natural hormone output. It is also used in thyroid storm.

Nursing Responsibilities
- Assess for hypersensitivity to iodine before giving medication; for example, ask patient about allergies to shellfish.
- Dilute liquid iodine sources in water or orange juice to disguise bitter taste.
- Monitor for increased bleeding tendencies if the patient is also taking anticoagulants; iodine increases their effect.

Health Education for the Patient and Family
- The maximum effect of iodine in large doses usually occurs in 10 to 15 days.
- Long-term iodine therapy is not effective in controlling hyperthyroidism.

ANTITHYROID DRUGS

Methimazole (Tapazole)

Carbimazole (converted to methimazole when absorbed)

Propylthiouracil (PTU, Propyl-Thyracil)

Antithyroid drugs inhibit TH production. They do not affect already formed hormones; thus, several weeks may elapse before the patient experiences therapeutic effects. Methimazole crosses the placenta and cannot be taken during pregnancy (Cooper, 2005).

Nursing Responsibilities
- Monitor for side effects: agranulocytosis (reduction in neutrophils, eosinophils, or basophils), hypothyroidism, pruritus rash, elevated temperature, (for iodides) periorbital edema, anorexia, loss of taste, hair loss, changes in menstruation.
- Administer drugs at the same time each day with meals to maintain stable blood levels.
- Monitor for manifestations of hypothyroidism: fatigue, weight gain.

Health Education for the Patient and Family
- Watch for unusual bleeding, redness, swelling, nausea, loss of taste, or epigastric pain. Report any such manifestations to the physician.
- Propylthiouracil is associated with weight changes; check weight daily when starting this medication to determine effect. Report significant changes to physician.
- If you are also taking warfarin, report any signs of bleeding.
- If you are taking lithium, be aware of manifestations of hypothyroidism.
- It may take up to 12 weeks before you experience the full effects of the drugs. Take the medication regularly and exactly as prescribed. Do not discontinue abruptly.

Assessment

The following data are collected through the health history and physical examination. Further focused assessments are described with nursing interventions.

- *Health history:* Other diseases, family history of thyroid disease, when manifestations began, severity of manifestations, intake of thyroid medications, menstrual history, changes in weight, bowel elimination.
- *Physical assessment:* Muscle strength, tremors, vital signs, cardiovascular and peripheral vascular systems, integument, size of thyroid, presence of bruit over thyroid, eyes and vision.

Nursing Diagnoses and Interventions

In planning and implementing nursing care for the patient with hyperthyroidism, the nurse considers the patient's responses to the systemic effects of the disorder. Although each patient may have different needs, nursing diagnoses discussed in this section focus on the most common health problems: cardiovascular problems, visual deficits, altered nutrition, and disturbed body image. See the accompanying Case Study & Nursing Care Plan on page 500.

Risk for Decreased Cardiac Output

The patient with hyperthyroidism is at risk for alterations in cardiac output. Excess TH directly affects the heart, resulting in increased rate and stroke volume. Increases in the metabolic demands and oxygen requirements of peripheral tissues increase the demands on the heart, and systolic hypertension, angina, dysrhythmias, or cardiac failure may occur. The patient often has palpitations and shortness of breath and is easily fatigued. The risk of complications is greater in patients with preexisting cardiovascular disorders.

- Monitor blood pressure, pulse rate and rhythm, respiratory rate, and breath sounds. Assess for peripheral edema, jugular vein distention, and increased activity intolerance. *Increased TH increases cardiac rate, stroke volume, and tissue demand for oxygen, causing stress on the heart. This may result in hypertension, arrhythmias, tachycardia, and congestive heart failure.*
- Suggest keeping the environment as cool and free of distraction as possible. Decrease stress by explaining interventions

EVIDENCE FOR NURSING CARE — The Patient with Thyroid Disorders (Hypo, Hyper, or Both)

Selected resources that nurses may find helpful when planning evidence-based nursing care follow.

- Kulie, T., Groff, A., Redmer, J. Hounshell, J., & Schrager, S. (2009). Vitamin D: An evidence-based review. *The Journal of the American Board of Family Medicine, 22*(6), 698–706.
- Surks, M. I., Ortiz, E., Daniels, G. H., Sawin, C. T., Col, N. F., Cobin, R. H., et al. (2004). Subclinical thyroid disease: Scientific review and guidelines for diagnosis and management. *National Clearinghouse Guideline.* Retrieved from http://www.guideline.gov/summary/summary.aspx?doc_id=5916&nbr=003902&string=hyperthyroid

and teaching relaxation procedures. *A physically comfortable and psychologically calm environment can reduce stimuli and stressors. Stress increases circulating catecholamines, which further increase cardiac workload.*

- Encourage a balance of activity with rest periods. *Rest periods decrease energy expenditure and tissue requirements for oxygen, decreasing demands cardiac workload.*

Disturbed Sensory Perception: Visual

Visual changes that occur in patients with hyperthyroidism include difficulty focusing, diplopia (double vision), or visual loss. If the patient is unable to close the eyelids because of exophthalmos, the risk of corneal dryness with resultant infection or injury increases. Visual deficits may also result from pressure on the optic nerve from retro-orbital edema. Although treatment of hyperthyroidism may stop the progression of eye changes, not all manifestations are reversible.

- Monitor visual acuity, photophobia (excessive sensitivity to light), integrity of the cornea, and lid closure. *The cornea is at risk for dryness, injury, conjunctivitis, and corneal infections. Injury and infection of the cornea can result in further loss of visual acuity.*
- Teach measures for protecting the eye from injury and maintaining visual acuity:
  - Use tinted glasses or shields as protection.
  - Use artificial tears to moisten the eyes.
  - Use cool, moist compresses to relieve irritation.
  - Promptly report any pain or changes in vision.

PRACTICE ALERT

Teach the patient to cover the eyes at night if they do not close, and to sleep with the head of the bed elevated 45 degrees (to decrease periorbital fluid accumulation).

The measures outlined decrease the risk of injury, provide comfort, decrease periorbital edema that can further compromise vision, and ensure immediate care for problems, thereby minimizing the risk of further visual loss.

Imbalanced Nutrition: Less than Body Requirements

The hypermetabolic state that occurs in hyperthyroidism causes gastrointestinal hypermotility, with nausea, vomiting, diarrhea, and abdominal pain. Although the patient may have an increased appetite and eat more than usual, weight loss continues.

- Ask the patient to weigh daily (at the same time each day), and keep a record of results. *The inability to meet metabolic demands results in loss of body weight.*
- In collaboration with a dietitian, teach the patient the need for a diet high in carbohydrates and protein and including between-meal snacks. Six small meals a day may be more desirable than three large meals. Caloric intake may need to be increased to 4000 kcal/day if weight loss exceeds 10% to 17% for height and frame. *Increased nutrients as part of a well-balanced diet are necessary to meet metabolic demands. Patients are often better able to increase food*

NURSING CARE OF THE PATIENT
Having a Subtotal Thyroidectomy

PREOPERATIVE CARE

■ Administer ordered antithyroid medications and iodine preparations, and monitor their effects. *Antithyroid drugs are given before surgery to promote a euthyroid state. Iodine preparations are given to the patient before surgery to decrease vascularity of the gland, thereby decreasing the risk of hemorrhage.*

■ Teach the patient to support the neck by placing both hands behind the neck when sitting up in bed, while moving about, and while coughing. *Placing the hands behind the neck eases tension on the suture line in the front of the neck.*

■ Answer questions, and allow time for the patient to verbalize concerns. *Because the incision is made at the base of the throat, patients (especially women) are often concerned about their appearance after surgery. Explain that the scar will eventually be only a thin line and that jewelry or scarves may be used to cover the scar.*

■ Teach the patient to expect hoarseness due to generalized swelling at the suture line. *This is expected to diminish with healing and is not caused by laryngeal nerve damage.*

POSTOPERATIVE CARE

■ Provide comfort measures: Administer analgesic pain medications as ordered, and monitor their effectiveness; place the patient in a semi-Fowler's position after recovery from anesthesia; support head and neck with pillows. *Analgesic medications reduce the perception of pain and reduce physical stress during the postoperative period. Positioning the patient in a semi-Fowler's position and supporting the head and neck decrease strain on the suture line.*

■ Perform focused assessments to monitor for complications:
  a. **Hemorrhage.** Assess dressing (if present) and the area behind and under the patient's neck and shoulders for drainage. Monitor blood pressure and pulse for manifestations of hypovolemic shock. Assess tightness of dressing (if present). *The vascularity of the gland increases the risk of hemorrhage. The location of the incision and the*

position of the patient may cause the drainage to run back and under the patient. The danger of hemorrhage is greatest in the first 12 to 24 hours after surgery.

  b. **Respiratory distress.** Assess respiratory rate, rhythm, depth, and effort. Maintain humidification as ordered. Assist the patient with coughing and deep breathing. Have suction equipment, oxygen, and a tracheostomy set available for immediate use. *Respiratory distress may result from hemorrhage and edema, which may compress the trachea; from tetany and laryngeal spasms resulting from decreased hormones due to removal or damage to the parathyroid glands; and from damage to the laryngeal nerve, causing spasms of the vocal cords. Stridor is heard in acute obstructions. This is a high-pitched, squeaky sound and is a sign of airway obstruction. Equipment must be immediately available if the patient experiences respiratory distress that requires interventions and treatment.*

  c. **Laryngeal nerve damage.** Assess for the ability to speak aloud, noting quality and tone of voice. *The location of the laryngeal nerve increases the risk of damage during thyroid surgery. Although hoarseness may be due to edema or the endotracheal tube used during surgery and will subside, permanent hoarseness or loss of vocal volume is a potential danger.*

  d. **Tetany.** Assess for manifestations of latent tetany due to calcium deficiency, including tingling of toes, fingers, and lips; muscular twitches; positive Chvostek's and Trousseau's signs; and decreased serum calcium levels. Serum calcium levels will be monitored in the postoperative period. Keep calcium gluconate or calcium chloride available for immediate IV use, if necessary. *The parathyroid glands are located in and near the thyroid gland; surgery of the thyroid gland may injure or remove parathyroid glands, resulting in hypocalcemia and tetany. Tetany may occur in 1 to 7 days after thyroidectomy.*

---

intake by eating frequent, small meals. A 1 lb weight gain requires approximately 3500 extra kilocalories.

■ Monitor nutritional status through results of laboratory data. Serum albumin, transferrin, and total lymphocyte counts are commonly lower than normal in nutritional deficits. *A negative nitrogen balance signifies a catabolic state in which protein is lost and metabolic demands are not being met.*

Disturbed Body Image and Anxiety

Physical changes common in hyperthyroidism include exophthalmos, goiter, tremors, hair loss, increased perspiration, loss of strength, fatigue, weight loss, and changes in reproductive and sexual function (amenorrhea in women and impotence in men). In addition, the patient often has mood changes and insomnia and is constantly nervous and anxious. There may even be periods of psychosis. These changes are frightening not only for the patient but also for family members.

■ Establish a trusting relationship; encourage the patient to verbalize feelings about self and to ask questions about the

illness and treatment. Provide reliable information and clarify misconceptions. *Establishing trust facilitates open sharing of feelings and perceptions.*

Community-Based Care

Patients with hyperthyroidism primarily provide self-care at home. Teaching is individualized to meet the patient's needs. Address the following topics:

■ The patient taking oral medications must understand the need for lifelong treatment.

■ The patient who has a thyroidectomy requires information about postoperative wound care.

■ The patient having radioactive iodine therapy needs to know the manifestations of hypothyroidism.

■ Depending on the age of the patient and the support systems available, referral to community healthcare agencies may be necessary.

■ In addition, suggest the following resources, which are accessible via the Internet: the American Thyroid Association, the Thyroid Foundation of Canada, and the Endocrine Society.

CASE STUDY & NURSING CARE PLAN   A Patient with Graves' Disease

Mrs. Juanita Manuel is a 33-year-old mother of four small children. She is a second-year student at the local community college, within one semester of completing the requirements for an associate's degree in child care. For the past 3 months, Mrs. Manuel has been constantly hungry and has eaten more than usual, but she has still lost 15 lb (6.8 kg). She has repeated bouts of diarrhea and often feels nauseated. Her hands shake, she can feel her heart beating rapidly, and she finds herself laughing or crying for no apparent reason.

Mrs. Manuel makes an appointment with her family physician. The nurse at the office completes a health history and physical assessment. When asked how she has been feeling, Mrs. Manuel replies, "Well, I don't know what's wrong with me—but I keep losing weight and I cry at the drop of a hat. I am also just so hot all the time, and I've never had that problem before. I hope I find out what's wrong and it's nothing serious."

ASSESSMENT

The health history indicates that although her appetite has increased, Mrs. Manuel has lost 15 lb (6.8 kg). She states that she has had diarrhea, nausea, palpitations, heat intolerance, and mood changes. Physical assessment findings include the following: T 101°F (38.3°C), P 110, R 24, and BP 162/86. Her skin is moist and warm, her hair thin and fine. She has visible tremors in her hands. Her eyeballs protrude, and she is unable to close her eyelids completely. Her thyroid is enlarged and palpable. Diagnostic tests reveal the following abnormal results: T_3, 350 g/dL (normal range: 80 to 200 ng/dL), T_4, 15.1 mg/dL (normal range: 5 to 12 mg/dL). A thyroid scan demonstrates an enlarged thyroid with increased iodine uptake. After the medical diagnosis of Graves' disease is made, Mrs. Manuel is started on the antithyroid medication propylthiouracil, 150 mg orally every 8 hours.

DIAGNOSES

- *Risk for Imbalanced Nutrition: Less than Body Requirements* related to weight loss of 15 lb (6.8 kg), with present weight 10% less than normal for height
- *Diarrhea* related to increased peristalsis as evidenced by 8 to 10 liquid stools per day
- *Risk for Disturbed Sensory Perception: Visual* related to an inability to close the eyelids completely
- *Anxiety* related to a lack of knowledge about disease process

EXPECTED OUTCOMES

- Gain at least 1 lb (0.45 kg) every 2 weeks.
- Regain normal bowel elimination patterns.
- Maintain normal vision (with no evidence of corneal damage) and verbalize measures to protect her eyes.
- Verbalize medical treatment and self-care needs.
- Verbalize a decrease in anxiety.

PLANNING AND IMPLEMENTATION

- Request that she keep a record of daily weight.
- Discuss adopting a high-kilocalorie diet. Identify food likes and dislikes, as well as foods that increase diarrhea, before instituting a plan to increase food intake.
- Request that she keep a stool chart, noting the time, type, and precipitating factors for diarrhea stools. Teach comfort measures for irritated anal area (clean washcloth and soap, nonirritating ointment).
- Teach how to apply eyedrops (artificial tears).
- Explain the need to elevate the head of the bed to 45 degrees at night, and tape eye shields over eyes before sleep.
- Teach about Graves' disease, the medication's effects and side effects, and the need for continued medical care.

EVALUATION

By her next office visit, Mrs. Manuel has gained 1 lb (0.45 kg) and has discussed her dietary needs with the nurse and her husband. She is having diarrhea less often. She has safely applied the eyedrops and states that she uses the eye shields and elevates the head of her bed at night. The office nurse reviewed the written and verbal information about Graves' disease and the medication prescribed. Mrs. Manuel verbalizes her understanding, stating, "I'll always take my medicine—I never want to feel like that again!" She says that she feels much less anxious now that she understands what has happened.

CRITICAL THINKING IN THE NURSING PROCESS

1. What is the pathophysiologic basis for Mrs. Manuel's abnormal vital signs?
2. What is the rationale for having the patient with exophthalmos elevate the head of the bed at night?
3. Outline a teaching plan that could be given to patients for home care following a subtotal thyroidectomy.

See Evaluating Your Response in Appendix C.

The Patient with Hypothyroidism

Hypothyroidism is a disorder that results when the thyroid gland produces an insufficient amount of TH. Because a decrease in TH levels decreases metabolic rate and heat production, hypothyroidism affects all body systems. Hypothyroidism is common in women between ages 30 and 60, with the incidence increasing after age 50. However, the disorder can occur at any stage of life. Careful evaluation of manifestations is important in the older adult because manifestations of hypothyroidism are often thought to be the result of aging instead of a pathologic process. The chronic, untreated hypothyroid state in adults is termed **myxedema**. The term reflects the characteristic accumulation of nonpitting edema in the connective tissues throughout the body. The edema is the result of water retention in mucoprotein (hydrophilic proteoglycans) deposits in the interstitial spaces. The face of a patient with myxedema appears puffy, the tongue is enlarged, and the voice is hoarse and husky (Porth & Matfin, 2009).

Pathophysiology and Manifestations

Hypothyroidism may be either primary or secondary. Primary hypothyroidism (which is more common) may be caused by congenital defects in the gland, loss of thyroid tissue following treatment for hyperthyroidism with surgery or radiation, antithyroid medications, thyroiditis, or endemic iodine deficiency. The cardiac drug amiodarone (Cordarone), which contains iodine, is increasingly being implicated in causing thyroid problems, especially hypothyroidism (Porth, 2007). Anabolic steroids, androgens, lithium, phenytoin, propanolol, interferon alpha, and interleukin-2 decrease T_4. The antithyroid drugs propylthiouracil and methimazole decrease T_4 measurement. Secondary hypothyroidism may result from pituitary TSH deficiency or peripheral resistance to thyroid hormones. (McPhee & Papadakis, 2009). Hypothyroidism has a slow onset, with manifestations occurring over months or even years. With treatment, the mental and physical manifestations rapidly reverse in patients of all ages.

MULTISYSTEM EFFECTS OF
Hypothyroidism

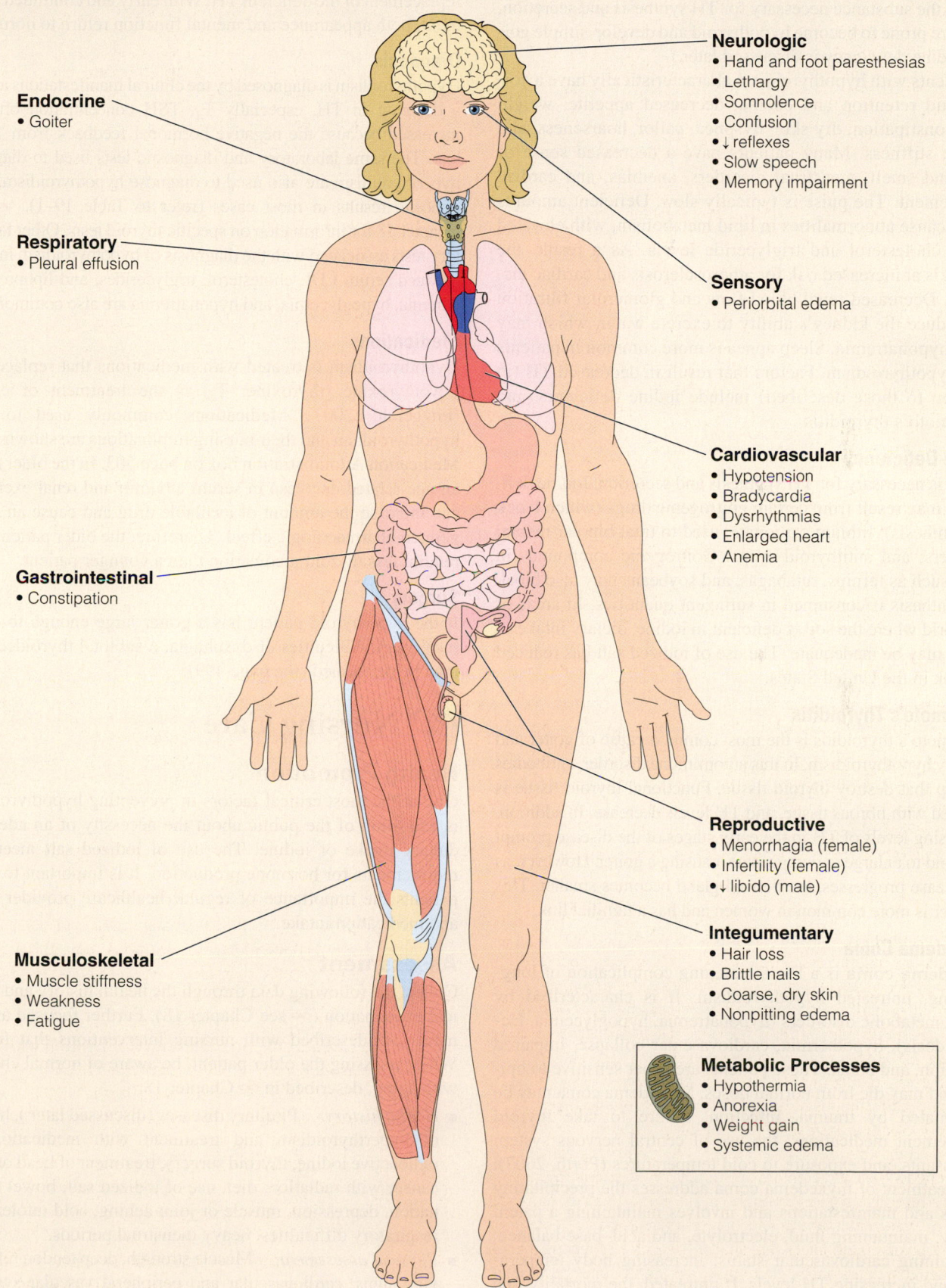

Endocrine
• Goiter

Respiratory
• Pleural effusion

Gastrointestinal
• Constipation

Musculoskeletal
• Muscle stiffness
• Weakness
• Fatigue

Neurologic
• Hand and foot paresthesias
• Lethargy
• Somnolence
• Confusion
• ↓ reflexes
• Slow speech
• Memory impairment

Sensory
• Periorbital edema

Cardiovascular
• Hypotension
• Bradycardia
• Dysrhythmias
• Enlarged heart
• Anemia

Reproductive
• Menorrhagia (female)
• Infertility (female)
• ↓ libido (male)

Integumentary
• Hair loss
• Brittle nails
• Coarse, dry skin
• Nonpitting edema

Metabolic Processes
• Hypothermia
• Anorexia
• Weight gain
• Systemic edema

When TH production decreases, the thyroid gland enlarges in a compensatory attempt to produce more hormone. The goiter that results is usually a simple or nontoxic form. People living in certain areas of the world where the soil is deficient in iodine, the substance necessary for TH synthesis and secretion, are more prone to become hypothyroid and develop simple goiter. (Iodine deficiency is discussed later.)

Patients with hypothyroidism characteristically have a goiter, fluid retention and edema, decreased appetite, weight gain, constipation, dry skin, dyspnea, pallor, hoarseness, and muscle stiffness. Many patients have a decreased sense of taste and smell, menstrual disorders, anemias, and cardiac enlargement. The pulse is typically slow. Deficient amounts of TH cause abnormalities in lipid metabolism, with elevated serum cholesterol and triglyceride levels. As a result, the patient is at increased risk for atherosclerosis and cardiac disorders. Decreased renal blood flow and glomerular filtration rate reduce the kidney's ability to excrete water, which may cause hyponatremia. Sleep apnea is more common in patients with hypothyroidism. Factors that result in decreased TH (in addition to those described) include iodine deficiency and Hashimoto's thyroiditis.

Iodine Deficiency

Iodine is necessary for TH synthesis and secretion. Iodine deficiency may result from certain goitrogenic drugs (which block TH synthesis); lithium carbonate, used to treat bipolar mental disorders; and antithyroid drugs. Goitrogenic compounds in foods such as turnips, rutabagas, and soybeans may also block TH synthesis if consumed in sufficient quantities. In areas of the world where the soil is deficient in iodine, dietary intake of iodine may be inadequate. The use of iodized salt has reduced this risk in the United States.

Hashimoto's Thyroiditis

Hashimoto's thyroiditis is the most common cause of goiter and primary hypothyroidism. In this autoimmune disorder, antibodies develop that destroy thyroid tissue. Functional thyroid tissue is replaced with fibrous tissue, and TH levels decrease. In addition, decreasing levels of TH in the early stages of the disease prompt the gland to enlarge to compensate, causing a goiter. However, as the disease progresses, the thyroid gland becomes smaller. This disorder is more common in women and has a familial link.

Myxedema Coma

Myxedema coma is a life-threatening complication of long-standing, untreated hypothyroidism. It is characterized by severe metabolic disorders (hyponatremia, hypoglycemia, lactic acidosis), hypothermia, cardiovascular collapse, impaired cognition, and coma. These patients are super sensitive to opioids and may die from normal doses. Myxedema coma may be precipitated by trauma, infection, failure to take thyroid replacement medications, the use of central nervous system depressants, and exposure to cold temperatures (Porth, 2007). The treatment of myxedema coma addresses the precipitating factors and manifestations and involves maintaining a patent airway; maintaining fluid, electrolyte, and acid–base balance; maintaining cardiovascular status; increasing body temperature; and increasing TH levels. If untreated, the mortality rate is high (Shah & Lettieri, 2007).

Interdisciplinary Care

The treatment of the patient with hypothyroidism focuses on diagnosis, prevention or treatment of complications, and replacement of the deficient TH. With early and continued treatment, both appearance and mental function return to normal.

Diagnosis

Hypothyroidism is diagnosed by the clinical manifestations and by a decrease in TH, especially T_4. TSH concentration often is increased because the negative hormonal feedback from TH is lost. The same laboratory and diagnostic tests used to diagnose hyperthyroidism are also used to diagnose hypothyroidism, with opposite results in most cases (refer to Table 19–1). ∞ See Chapter 18 for information on specific thyroid tests. Other laboratory tests associated with the diagnosis of hypothyroidism include elevated serum LDL cholesterol, triglycerides, and lipoproteins. Anemia, hypoglycemia, and hyponatremia are also common.

Medications

Hypothyroidism is treated with medications that replace TH. Levothyroxine (thyroxine, T_4) is the treatment of choice (Fitzgerald, 2007). Medications commonly used to treat hypothyroidism and their nursing implications are shown in the Medication Administration box on page 503. In the older adult, an age-related decrease in serum albumin and renal excretion can increase the amount of available drug and cause an exaggerated pharmacologic effect. Therefore, the older patient may require less thyroid medication than a younger patient.

Surgery

If the hypothyroid patient has a goiter large enough to cause respiratory difficulties or dysphagia, a subtotal thyroidectomy may be performed (see page 499).

∞ Nursing Care

Health Promotion

One of the most critical factors in preventing hypothyroidism is education of the public about the necessity of an adequate dietary intake of iodine. The use of iodized salt meets the requirements for hormone production. It is important to teach patients the importance of regular healthcare provider visits and medication intake.

Assessment

Collect the following data through the health history and physical examination (∞ see Chapter 18). Further focused assessments are described with nursing interventions that follow. When assessing the older patient, be aware of normal changes with aging, described in ∞ Chapter 18.

- *Health history:* Pituitary diseases (discussed later), history of hyperthyroidism and treatment with medications or radioactive iodine, thyroid surgery, treatment of head or neck cancer with radiation, diet, use of iodized salt, bowel elimination, depression, muscle or joint aching, cold intolerance, respiratory difficulties, heavy menstrual periods.
- *Physical assessment:* Muscle strength, deep tendon reflexes, vital signs, cardiovascular and peripheral vascular systems, integument, thyroid gland, weight.

MEDICATION ADMINISTRATION Hypothyroidism

THYROID PREPARATIONS
Levothyroxine sodium (T_4) (Levoxyl, Levothroid, Synthroid)
Liothyronine sodium (T_3) (Cytomel)
Liotrix (T_3–T_4) (Euthyroid, Thyrolar)

Thyroid preparations increase blood levels of TH, thus raising the patient's metabolic rate. As a result, cardiac output, oxygen consumption, and body temperature increase. Levothyroxine speeds the elimination of vitamin K–dependent clotting factors enhancing the effects of warfarin (Coumadin). Patients are at increased risk of bleeding if warfarin dosages are not appropriately reduced. The dosage depends on the drug chosen and the patient's degree of thyroid dysfunction, sensitivity to TH, age, body size, and health. The older adult may require lower doses.

Nursing Responsibilities
- Give 1 hour before meals or 2 hours after meals for best absorption.
- Thyroid preparations potentiate the effect of anticoagulant drugs. If the patient is also receiving an anticoagulant, monitor for bruising, bleeding gums, and blood in the urine.
- Thyroid medications potentiate the effect of digitalis. If the patient is also receiving a digitalis preparation, monitor for signs of digitalis toxicity.
- Monitor for manifestations of coronary insufficiency: chest pain, dyspnea, tachycardia.

- If the patient has insulin-dependent diabetes, monitor the effects of insulin. The effect of the insulin may change as thyroid function increases.
- During dose adjustment, take pulse before administering drug. Report pulse > 100.

Health Education for the Patient and Family
- Do not substitute brands of drugs or use generic equivalents without the physician's approval.
- The medications must be taken for the rest of one's life.
- Report manifestations of excess thyroid hormone to the physician: excess weight loss, palpitations, leg cramps, nervousness, or insomnia.
- If you have diabetes and use insulin, monitor blood glucose levels closely; the thyroid medications may alter the amount of insulin required.
- Thyroid preparations increase the risk of iodine toxicity. Do not use iodized salt or over-the-counter drugs containing iodine.
- If you are also taking an anticoagulant, report any signs of bleeding.
- Report any changes in menstrual periods.
- Take the thyroid preparation in the morning 30 minutes before eating to decrease the possibility of insomnia; take other medications such as calcium carbonate, iron, or antacids at least 4 hours before or after taking thyroid drugs; these medications may prevent absorption.
- Closely monitor blood pressure and pulse (older patients).
- Avoid excessive intake of foods that are known to inhibit TH utilization such as walnuts and high-fiber foods.

Nursing Diagnoses and Interventions

In planning and implementing care for patients with hypothyroidism, the nurse takes into account that the disorder affects all organ systems. Although many nursing diagnoses might be valid, this section focuses on patient problems with cardiovascular function, elimination, and skin integrity. See the accompanying Case Study & Nursing Care Plan on page 504.

Decreased Cardiac Output

A TH deficit causes a reduction in heart rate and stroke volume, resulting in decreased cardiac output. There may also be an accumulation of fluid in the pericardial sac (from the edema characteristic of hypothyroidism), and coronary artery disease may be present, further compromising cardiac function.

- Monitor blood pressure, rate and rhythm of apical and peripheral pulses, respiratory rate, and breath sounds. *Hypotension indicates decreasing peripheral blood flow. Fluid in the pericardial sac restricts cardiac function. Monopolysaccharide deposits in the respiratory system decrease vital capacity and hypoventilation.*
- Suggest the patient avoid chilling; increase room temperature, use additional bed covers, and avoid drafts. *Chilling increases metabolic rate and puts increased stress on the heart.*
- Explain the need to alternate activity with rest periods. Ask the patient to report any breathing difficulties, chest pain, heart palpitations, or dizziness. *Activity increases demands on the heart and should be balanced with rest. Manifestations of cardiac stress include dyspnea, chest pain, palpitations, and dizziness.*

Constipation

The hypothyroid patient is likely to have a reduced appetite and decreased food intake, a diminished activity level because of muscle aches and weakness, and reduced peristalsis to the point that fecal impactions may occur.

- Encourage a fluid intake of up to 2000 mL per day. Discuss preferred liquids and the best times of day to drink fluids. If kilocalorie intake is restricted, ensure that liquids have no or low kilocalories. *Sufficient fluid intake is necessary to promote proper stool consistency.*
- Discuss ways to maintain a high-fiber diet. *Diets high in fiber and fluid produce soft stools. Fiber that is not digested absorbs water, which adds bulk to the stool and assists in the movement of fecal material through the intestines. High fiber foods include beans, fruits, breads, cereals, popcorn, and rice. Consult nutritional labels for fiber content. Instruct not to eat high fiber foods within 4 hours of taking a thyroid hormone medication. These foods decrease absorption of thyroid hormone medications.*
- Encourage activity as tolerated. *Activity influences bowel elimination by improving muscle tone and stimulating peristalsis.*

Risk for Impaired Skin Integrity

The patient with hypothyroidism is at risk for impaired skin integrity related to the accumulation of fluid in the interstitial spaces and to dry, rough skin. Decreased peripheral circulation, decreased activity levels, and slow wound healing further increase the risk. These interventions are outlined here for the older patient who is hospitalized for surgery or severe hypothyroidism.

- Monitor skin surfaces for redness or lesions, especially if the patient's activity is greatly reduced. Use a pressure ulcer risk assessment scale to identify patients at risk. *Hypothyroidism causes dry, rough, edematous skin conditions that increase the risk of skin breakdown.*
- Provide or teach the immobile patient measures to promote optimal circulation:
  - Use a turning schedule if the patient is on bed rest, or teach the patient to change position every 2 hours.
  - Limit the time for sitting in one position; shift weight or lift the body using arm rests every 20 to 30 minutes.
  - Use pillows, pads, or sheepskin or foam cushions for bed and/or chair.
  - Teach and implement a schedule of range-of-motion exercises.
    Prolonged pressure, especially in patients with edema and circulatory impairment, can occlude capillaries and cause hypoxic tissue damage.
- Provide or teach the patient measures to maintain skin integrity:
  - Take baths only as necessary; use warm (not hot) water.
  - Use gentle motions when washing and drying skin.
  - Use alcohol-free skin oils and lotions.

Dry skin and edema increase the risk of skin breakdown. Hot water, rough massage, and alcohol-based preparations may increase skin dryness, further impairing the body's ability to maintain skin integrity.

Community-Based Care

Patients with hypothyroidism require lifelong care, primarily at home. Address the following topics:

- The need to take medications for the rest of one's life
- The need for periodic dosage reassessments
- If the patient is older or does not have a support system, helpful community resources
- Additional resources are the same as for the patient with hyperthyroidism.

The Patient with Cancer of the Thyroid

Thyroid cancer has an estimated incidence of slightly more than 37,200 new cases and accounted for more than 1,600 cancer deaths in 2009 (National Cancer Institute, 2009). The most consistent risk factor is exposure to ionizing radiation to the head and neck during childhood. For example, many adults in

---

CASE STUDY & NURSING CARE PLAN   A Patient with Hypothyroidism

Jane Lee is a 60-year-old retired nurse living with her husband and daughter on a farm that has been in the family for four generations. Mrs. Lee has gained 10 lb (4.5 kg) in the past few months, even though she is rarely hungry and eats much less than normal. She is always tired and weak—so tired that she has not even been able to help with the chores on the farm or do housework. She is concerned about her appearance and the way she sounds when she talks. Her face is puffy, and her tongue always feels thick. Mr. Lee convinces his wife to make an appointment at a health center in a nearby town.

ASSESSMENT
Brian Henning, RN, completes the health assessment for Mrs. Lee at the health center. He finds that she now weighs 150 lb (68 kg), an increase of 10 lb (4.5 kg) over her weight at her last visit 6 months earlier. Mrs. Lee states that she always feels cold, tired, and weak. She also states that she is constipated, has difficulty remembering things, and looks different. Physical assessment findings include a palpable and bilaterally enlarged thyroid; dry, yellowish skin; nonpitting edema of the face and lower legs; and slow, slurred speech. Diagnostic tests revealed the following abnormal findings: T_3, 56 ng/dL (normal range: 80 to 200 ng/dL); T_4, 3.1 (normal range: 5 to 12 mg/dL); TSH increased. The medical diagnosis of hypothyroidism is made, and Mrs. Lee is started on levothyroxine 0.05 mg daily.

DIAGNOSES
- *Constipation* related to decreased peristalsis, as evidenced by hard, formed stools every 4 days
- *Impaired Verbal Communication* related to changes in speech patterns and enlarged tongue
- *Situational Low Self-Esteem* related to changes in physical appearance and activity intolerance

EXPECTED OUTCOMES
- Regain normal bowel elimination patterns, having a soft, formed stool at least every other day.
- Experience improvement in verbal communication.
- Regain positive self-esteem as medication reduces physical changes and fatigue.

PLANNING AND IMPLEMENTATION
- Teach to increase fluids, bulk, and fiber in the diet to help regain a normal bowel elimination pattern of a soft, formed stool every other day.
- Take medication as prescribed and do not expect immediate reversal of manifestations affecting speech.
- Plan activities around rest periods. Encourage husband and daughter to help with housecleaning and cooking.

EVALUATION
On return to the health center 2 months later, Mrs. Lee reports that she is no longer constipated but that she is continuing to drink six glasses of water and eating oatmeal every day. She no longer feels cold, is regaining her normal energy, and even feels well enough to plant her garden. Her speech is clear and easy to understand. As she leaves the examining room, Mrs. Lee says, "It's hard to believe that I have changed so much—now I look and feel like the 'old' me!"

CRITICAL THINKING IN THE NURSING PROCESS
1. What physical changes that normally occur with aging are similar to the manifestations of hypothyroidism?
2. Describe the factors that put Mrs. Lee's safety at risk. What alterations in her home environment would you suggest to promote safety until the prescribed medication takes effect?
3. The patient taking oral thyroid medications may develop hyperthyroidism. List the manifestations you would include in a teaching plan to signal this condition.

See Evaluating Your Response in Appendix C.

their 60s, 70s, and 80s received x-ray treatments for colds, tonsillitis, acne, and sinus infections during childhood.

Of the several types of thyroid cancer, the most common types are listed here:

- Papillary thyroid carcinoma is the most common thyroid malignancy. It is usually detected as a single nodule, but may arise from a multinodular goiter. It is most often diagnosed in women between ages 30 and 50 (National Cancer Institute, 2009). Risks for the development of this form are exposure to external x-ray treatments to the head or neck as a child, childhood exposure to radioactive isotopes of iodine in nuclear fallout, and a family history. Papillary thyroid carcinoma is the least aggressive type, but does metastasize to local and regional lymph nodes and lungs.

- Follicular thyroid cancer is the second most common thyroid malignancy. It is diagnosed at a slightly older age (40 to 60) than papillary and more commonly in women. This form is more aggressive than papillary, with potential for vascular invasion and spread to lung and bone. Exposure to radiation is not considered a risk factor for this type of thyroid cancer.

- Medullary thyroid cancer arises from the cells of the thyroid that produce the hormone calcitonin; these cells do not uptake iodine and, therefore, are not susceptible to treatment with radioactive iodine. Persons with a family history of thyroid cancer have a change in a gene named RET and this can be passed from parent to child.

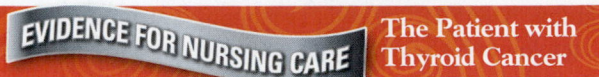

EVIDENCE FOR NURSING CARE — **The Patient with Thyroid Cancer**

Selected resources that nurses may find helpful when planning evidence-based nursing care follow.

- Cooper, D. S., Doherty, G. M., Haugen, B. R., Kloos, R. T., Lee, S. L., Mandel, S J., et al. (2009). Revised American Thyroid Association management guidelines for patients with thyroid nodules and differentiated thyroid cancer. *Thyroid, 19*(11). DOI: 10.1089/thy.2009.0110. Retrieved from http://www.thyroid.org/professionals/publications/documents/ATA_Guidelines_DTC_2009.pdf

Thyroid cancer is manifested by a palpable, firm nontender nodule in the thyroid. If undetected, the tumor may grow and impinge on the esophagus or trachea, causing difficulty in swallowing or breathing. Most people with thyroid cancer do not have elevated thyroid hormone levels. The diagnosis is made by measuring thyroid hormones, performing thyroid scans, and by fine-needle biopsy of the nodule. The usual treatment is subtotal or total thyroidectomy. TSH suppression therapy with levothyroxine may be conducted prior to surgery. Radioactive iodine therapy (^{131}I) and chemotherapy are additional therapeutic options. While standard chemotherapy is not used often, new biologic chemotherapies offer promise of remission or cure for the more aggressive or refractory types of thyroid cancer (Pfister & Fagin, 2008). Nursing care for the patient with cancer is discussed in ∞ Chapter 14.

Disorders of the Parathyroid Glands

Disorders of the parathyroid glands, hyperparathyroidism and hypoparathyroidism, are not as common as those of the thyroid gland. Hypercalcemia and hypocalcemia (the primary results of alterations in parathyroid function) are discussed in ∞ Chapter 10.

The Patient with Hyperparathyroidism

Hyperparathyroidism results from an increase in the secretion of parathyroid hormone (PTH), which regulates normal serum levels of calcium. The increase in PTH affects the kidneys and bones, resulting in increased resorption of calcium and excretion of phosphate by the kidneys (increasing the risk of hypercalcemia and hypophosphatemia), increased bicarbonate excretion and decreased acid excretion by the kidneys (increasing the risk of metabolic acidosis and hypokalemia), increased release of calcium and phosphorus by bones with resultant bone decalcification, and deposits of calcium in soft tissues and the formation of renal calculi.

Pathophysiology and Manifestations

Hyperparathyroidism occurs more often in older adults and is three times more common in women. The disorder itself is not common. Primary hyperparathyroidism occurs when there is hyperplasia or an adenoma in one of the parathyroid glands. Secondary hyperparathyroidism is a compensatory response to chronic hypocalcemia. The tertiary form is most often seen in patients with chronic renal failure.

Many patients with hyperparathyroidism are asymptomatic. When manifestations occur, they are related to hypercalcemia and various musculoskeletal, renal, and gastrointestinal manifestations. Bone reabsorption results in pathologic fractures, while elevated calcium levels alter neural and muscular activity, leading to muscle weakness and atrophy. Proximal renal tubule function is altered, and metabolic acidosis, renal calculi formation, and polyuria occur.

Manifestations of the effect of hypercalcemia on the gastrointestinal tract include abdominal pain, constipation, anorexia, and peptic ulcer formation. Hypercalcemia also affects the cardiovascular system, causing dysrhythmias, hypertension, and increased sensitivity to cardiotonic glycosides (e.g., digitalis preparations).

Interdisciplinary Care

Hyperparathyroidism is diagnosed by excluding all other possible causes of hypercalcemia, by at least a 6-month history of manifestations, and by laboratory analysis of levels of serum calcium and PTH levels (McPhee & Papadakis, 2009).

Treatment of hyperparathyroidism focuses on decreasing the elevated serum calcium levels. Patients with mild hypercalcemia are urged to drink fluids and keep active. They should avoid immobilization, thiazide diuretics, large doses of vitamins A and D, antacids containing calcium, and calcium supplements. Severe hypercalcemia requires hospitalization and intensive treatment with intravenous saline. Medications to inhibit bone resorption and reduce hypercalcemia, such as pamidronate (Aredia), alendronate (Fosamax), and zoledronate (Zometa), are used for short-term treatment, improve bone density, and may relieve bone pain (Fitzgerald, 2007). Calcitonin, a hormone produced by the thyroid gland, decreases plasma levels of calcium by inhibiting bone resorption and increasing calcium excretion by the kidney (Lehne, 2004). A form of calcitonin from salmon is available as a nasal spray or IM/SQ injection. A medication for patients with hyperparathyroidism secondary to renal failure or parathyroid cancer is a calcimimetic. This drug increases the sensitivity of the calcium-sensing receptors of the parathyroid gland to serum calcium. The effect is decreased secretion of PTH and reduced serum calcium and phosphorus.

Surgical removal of the parathyroid glands affected by hyperplasia or adenoma treats primary hyperparathyroidism. The preoperative and postoperative nursing care of the patient having surgery of the parathyroids is essentially the same as that for the patient having a thyroidectomy (see page 499). Manipulation of the thyroid while removing the parathyroids may result in TH release, causing increased cardiac rate and stroke volume.

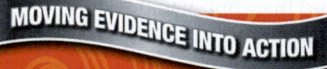 Nursing Care

Nursing care of the patient with hypercalcemia is discussed in ∞ Chapter 10.

The Patient with Hypoparathyroidism

Hypoparathyroidism results from abnormally low PTH levels. The most common cause is damage to or inadvertent removal of all of the parathyroid glands during thyroidectomy. The lack of circulating PTH causes hypocalcemia and an elevated blood phosphate level.

Pathophysiology and Manifestations

Reduced levels of PTH result in impaired renal tubular regulation of calcium and phosphate. In addition, decreased activation of vitamin D results in decreased absorption of calcium by the intestines. The low calcium levels cause changes in neuromuscular activity, affecting peripheral motor and sensory nerves. Hypocalcemia lowers the threshold for nerve and muscle excitability; a slight stimulus anywhere along a nerve or muscle fiber initiates an impulse.

The neuromuscular manifestations that result include numbness and tingling around the mouth and in the fingertips, muscle spasms of the hands and feet, convulsions, and laryngeal spasms. **Tetany**, a continuous spasm of muscles, is the primary symptom of hypocalcemia. In severe cases of tetany, death may occur. Assessments for tetany include Chvostek's sign and Trousseau's sign (∞ see Chapter 18). The manifestations of hypoparathyroidism are summarized in the box on page 507.

Interdisciplinary Care

Hypoparathyroidism is diagnosed by low serum calcium levels and high phosphorous levels in the absence of renal failure, an absorption disorder, or a nutritional disorder.

Treatment of hypoparathyroidism focuses on increasing calcium levels. Intravenous calcium gluconate is given immediately to reduce tetany. Long-term therapy includes supplemental calcium, increased dietary calcium, and vitamin D therapy.

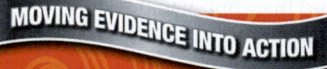 Nursing Care

Nursing care for the patient with hypocalcemia is discussed in ∞ Chapter 10.

Disorders of the Adrenal Glands

Disorders of the adrenal cortex or adrenal medulla result in changes in the production of adrenocorticotropic hormone (ACTH). Hormones of the adrenal cortex are essential to life. They maintain homeostasis in response to stressors. Disorders of the adrenal cortex result in complex physical, psychologic, and

---

MOVING EVIDENCE INTO ACTION | **Serum Parathyroid Hormone Levels Predict Falls in Older Adults with Diabetes Mellitus**

In a retrospective analysis of data, Houston et al. (2008) found a positive correlation between higher levels of PTH and fall incidents in 492 independent-living older persons with an average age of 73.6 years who had diabetes mellitus (DM). The purpose of the study was to determine associations between body composition, weight-related health conditions, and reports of initial incidents causing functional limitations in older adults. Baseline assessments of physical performance and parathyroid hormone were among the data collected. Houston et al. found a positive correlation between increased parathyroid hormone level and the number of falls the subjects reported during the study period. They found no correlation between the physical performance scores of the subjects and the number of falls they reported. Neither gender nor race significantly affected the number of falls reported. However, participants with the highest PTH levels were more likely to be Black, to be sedentary, and have a higher body mass index (BMI).

IMPLICATIONS FOR NURSING

Falls are disconcerting to older adults even when no serious injury occurs. Nurses seek to prevent falls and would benefit from more precisely identifying those at risk for falling as well as decreasing fall potential. If correcting PTH to normal levels could prevent falls, treatment would be reasonable. The precise connection between serum PTH and falls is unknown; more studies are needed to reveal this important detail.

CRITICAL THINKING IN PATIENT CARE

1. What normal changes with aging combined with an increased parathyroid hormone level would increase the risk for falls?
2. What correlation might be considered between obesity, increased PTH levels, and falls?
3. What type of teaching is necessary to prevent falls in the home? How would this differ in the hospital or long-term care facility?

MANIFESTATIONS of Hypoparathyroidism

MUSCULOSKELETAL SYSTEM
- Muscle spasms
- Facial grimacing
- Carpopedal spasms
- Tetany or convulsions

INTEGUMENTARY SYSTEM
- Brittle nails
- Hair loss
- Dry, scaly skin

GASTROINTESTINAL SYSTEM
- Abdominal cramps
- Malabsorption

CARDIOVASCULAR SYSTEM
- Dysrhythmias

CENTRAL NERVOUS SYSTEM
- Paresthesias (lips, hands, feet)
- Mood disorders (irritability, depression, anxiety)
- Hyperactive reflexes
- Psychosis
- Increased intracranial pressure

metabolic alterations that are potentially life threatening. Hormones of the adrenal medulla are not essential to life, because the sympathetic nervous system produces similar body responses. The disorders that occur are hyperfunction and hypofunction of the adrenal cortex and hyperfunction of the adrenal medulla.

The Patient with Hypercortisolism (Cushing's Syndrome)

Cushing's syndrome is a chronic disorder in which hyperfunction of the adrenal cortex produces excessive amounts of circulating cortisol or ACTH. Cushing's syndrome is more common

in women, with the average age of onset between 30 and 50 years (Figure 19–3 ■). However, the disorder may occur at any age, especially as the result of pharmacologic therapy. People who take steroids for long periods of time (e.g., for the treatment of arthritis, after an organ transplant, or as an adjunct to chemotherapy) are at increased risk for developing the disorder.

Pathophysiology

Cushing's syndrome may be the result of various causes. By far the most common cause is iatrogenic; only 2.6 new cases of Cushing's disease per million population are diagnosed yearly (McPhee & Papadakis, 2009). The most common etiologies of the disorder are as follows:

- Iatrogenic Cushing's syndrome, resulting from long-term therapy with potent pharmacologic glucocorticoid preparations.
- The pituitary form, with ACTH hypersecretion by a benign tumor of the pituitary (called *Cushing's disease*). This is most commonly caused by a small pituitary adenoma, with persistent but disorderly and random overproduction of ACTH. Forty-three percent of Cushing's disease is due to hypersecretion of ACTH by the pituitary.
- The ectopic form, caused by ACTH-secreting tumors (such as small-cell lung cancer). In this form, the ACTH is also random and episodic, but greater than in Cushing's disease.
- The adrenal form, resulting from excessive cortisol secretion by a benign or malignant adrenal tumor. The excess secretion suppresses pituitary ACTH production, resulting in atrophy of the uninvolved adrenal cortex.

Manifestations

The manifestations of Cushing's syndrome result from the ACTH or cortisol excess, and manifest as exaggerated cortisol actions. Obesity and a redistribution of body fat result in fat deposits in the

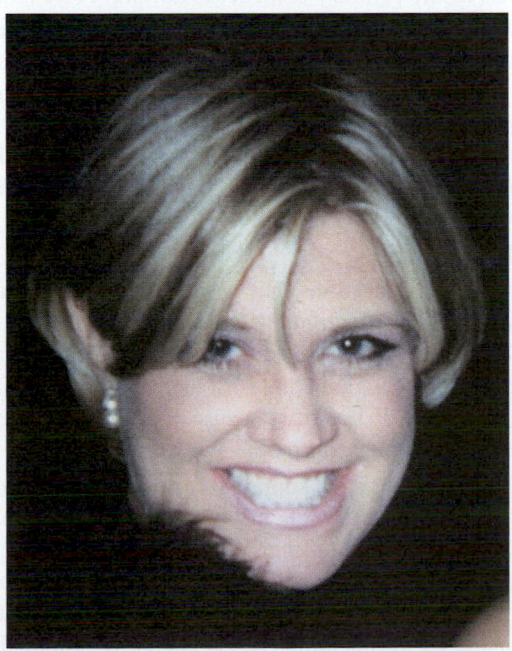
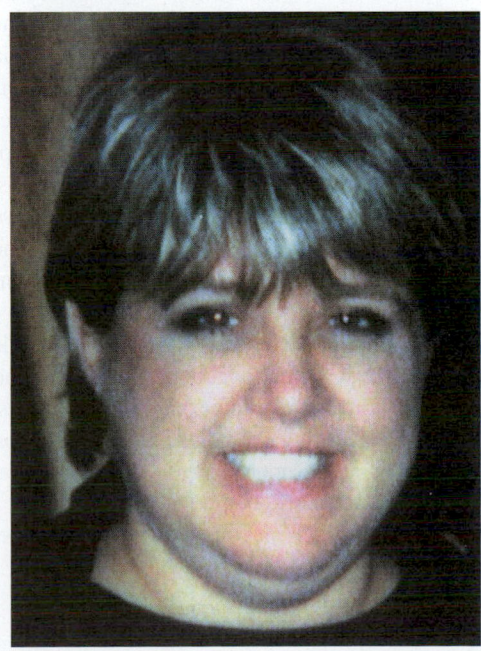

A   B

Figure 19–3 ■ A woman before and after developing Cushing's syndrome. In the photo at the right, notice the swollen facial features.
Courtesy of Dr. Charles Wilson, University of California, San Francisco.

PATHOPHYSIOLOGY LINKAGE   Cushing's Syndrome

MANIFESTATIONS	PATHOPHYSIOLOGY
Fat deposits in the abdominal region (central obesity), fat pads under the clavicles, a "buffalo hump" over the upper back, and a round "moon" face	Excess glucocorticoids affect normal carbohydrate metabolism, resulting in a redistribution of body fat and a breakdown of fats to fatty acids.
Muscle weakness and wasting, especially in the extremities	Excess cortisol results in changes in protein metabolism and protein catabolism from mobilization of amino acids for gluconeogenesis.
Thinning of skin, abdominal striae (purple "stretch marks"), easy bruising, poor wound healing, and frequent skin infections	Inhibition of fibroplasts by excess glucocorticoids with loss of collagen and connective tissue. Excess glucocorticoids depress the inflammatory response and inhibit immune system effectiveness.
Osteoporosis, compression fractures of the vertebrae, rib fractures	Excessive mineralocorticoids result in changes in absorption of calcium.
Hypokalemia	Loss of potassium.
Hypertension and hypernatremia	Excess aldosterone alters the absorption of sodium by the distal tubules of the kidneys (via the renin–angiotensin–aldosterone system) and sodium is retained. As potassium is lost, sodium is retained.
Hyperglycemia, polyuria, polydipsia	Altered glucose metabolism.
Increased risk of gastric ulcers	Increased gastric acid secretion.
Hirsutism (excessive hair growth; especially on the face in women), acne, menstrual irregularities	Increased androgen levels.
Emotional instability	Decreased response to stress.

abdominal region (central obesity), fat pads under the clavicle, a "buffalo hump" over the upper back, and a round "moon" face. Changes in protein metabolism cause muscle weakness and wasting, especially in the extremities. Glucocorticoid excess inhibits fibroblasts, resulting in loss of collagen and connective tissue. Thinning of skin, abdominal striae (reddish purple "stretch marks"), easy bruising, poor wound healing, and frequent skin infections result. Glucose metabolism is altered in the majority of patients, and diabetes mellitus may occur. Electrolyte imbalances also occur with the increased hormone levels. Changes in calcium absorption result in osteoporosis, compression fractures of the vertebrae, fractures of the ribs, and renal calculi. Hypokalemia and hypertension occur as potassium is lost and sodium is retained. Inhibited immune responses increase the risk of infection, and increased gastric acid secretion increases the risk of peptic ulcers. Emotional changes range from depression to psychosis. In women, increasing androgen levels cause hirsutism (excessive facial hair in particular), acne, and menstrual irregularities. The manifestations with related pathophysiology of Cushing's syndrome are outlined in the accompanying box.

The complications of untreated Cushing's syndrome include electrolyte imbalances (hyperglycemia, hypernatremia, and hypokalemia), hypertension, and emotional disturbances. Increased susceptibility to infections is also a factor. Compression fractures from osteoporosis and aseptic necrosis of the femoral head may result in serious disability. If the patient undergoes a bilateral adrenalectomy as a treatment for Cushing's syndrome, an acute deficit of cortisol (Addisonian crisis) may result.

Interdisciplinary Care

The treatment of Cushing's syndrome includes medications, radiation therapy, or surgery, depending on the etiologic origin of the disorder.

Diagnostic Tests

Cushing's syndrome is diagnosed through a variety of diagnostic tests. In addition to the laboratory tests described in ∞ Chapter 18 and in Table 19–2, a late night salivary cortisol test may be performed. A saliva specimen is collected at 11 PM; following the collection, dexamethasone 1 mg is given orally. A serum cortisol is collected at 8 AM the following morning. The dexamethasone *suppresses ACTH*. If an extremely high dose of cortisol is necessary to suppress ACTH, the primary disorder is adrenal cortex hyperplasia. If ACTH is not suppressed with the synthetic cortisol, an adrenal tumor is suspected. If the dexamethasone test is positive, a test for urinary free cortisol is made. This measures the amount of cortisol in the urine over 24 hours. Other diagnostic studies, including a CT scan or MRI of the abdomen, may be conducted to assess the adrenal gland for tumors.

Medications

Cushing's syndrome that results from a pituitary tumor is treated by medications as an adjunct to surgery or radiation. Medications are also used for patients with inoperable pituitary or adrenal malignancies. Although the drugs control manifestations, they do not effect a cure. Examples of some commonly prescribed drugs follow:

- Mitotane directly suppresses activity of the adrenal cortex and decreases peripheral metabolism of corticosteroids. It is used to treat metastatic adrenal cancer.
- Aminoglutethimide or ketoconazole (or both) inhibit cortisol synthesis by the adrenal cortex and may be administered to patients with ectopic ACTH-secreting tumors that cannot be surgically removed.
- Somatostatin analog (octreotide) suppresses ACTH secretion in some patients.

TABLE 19–2 Laboratory Findings in Adrenal Disorders

	TEST	NORMAL VALUES	HYPERFUNCTION (CUSHING'S SYNDROME)	HYPOFUNCTION (ADDISON'S DISEASE)
Serum	Cortisol	8 AM to 10 AM: 138 to 635 mmol	Increased	Decreased
		4 PM to 6 PM: 83 to 359 mmol		
	Blood urea nitrogen (BUN)	5 to 25 mg/dL	Normal	Increased
	Sodium	135 to 145 mEq/L	Increased	Decreased
	Potassium	3.5 to 5.0 mEq/L	Decreased	Increased
	Glucose (serum)	70 to 100 mg/dL	Increased	Decreased
Urine	Urinary free cortisol (UFS)	10 to 50 mcg/24 h	Increased	Low/absent
	17-KS	Male: 5 to 25 mg/24 h	Increased	Decreased
		Female: 5 to 15 mg/24 hr		
		Age > 65: 4 to 8 mg/24 hr		

Surgery

When Cushing's syndrome is caused by an adrenal cortex tumor, an adrenalectomy may be performed to remove the tumor. Only one adrenal gland is usually involved; however, if an ACTH-producing ectopic tumor is involved, a bilateral adrenalectomy is performed. Lifelong hormone replacement is necessary if both adrenal glands are removed. Nursing care of the patient having an adrenalectomy is discussed later.

Surgical removal of the pituitary gland (hypophysectomy) is indicated when Cushing's syndrome is the result of a pituitary disorder. The gland is removed either by a transsphenoidal route or by a craniotomy. Nursing care for the patient having cranial surgery is discussed in ∞ Chapter 42.

∞ Nursing Care

Health Promotion

Stress the risk of developing Cushing's syndrome for patients taking long-term steroids. The risk of abruptly discontinuing the medications is an essential component of teaching. For a review of glucocorticoid administration ∞ see Chapter 13.

Assessment

Collect the following data through the health history and physical examination (∞ see Chapter 18). Further focused assessments are described with nursing interventions later.

- *Health history:* History of pituitary, adrenal, pancreatic, or pulmonary tumor; frequent infections; gastrointestinal bleeding; stress fractures; pain; changes in weight distribution; change in height; fatigue; weakness; change in appearance; bruising; skin infections; menstrual history; sexual function.
- *Physical assessment:* Vital signs, behavior, appearance, fat distribution, face, skin, hair quantity and distribution, muscle size and strength, gait.

Nursing Diagnoses and Interventions

The nurse caring for the patient with Cushing's syndrome must take a holistic approach to plan and implement interventions for a wide variety of responses, including problems related to fluid and electrolyte balance, injury, infection, and body image. For additional information about patients with alterations in fluid and electrolyte balance, ∞ see Chapter 10. Also, see the Case Study & Nursing Care Plan on page 511.

NURSING CARE OF THE PATIENT
Having an Adrenalectomy

PREOPERATIVE CARE
- Request a dietary consultation with the patient to discuss a diet high in vitamins and proteins. If hypokalemia exists, include foods high in potassium. *Glucocorticoid excess increases catabolism. Vitamins and proteins are necessary for tissue repair and wound healing following surgery.*
- Use medical and surgical asepsis when providing care and treatments. *Cortisol excess increases the risk of infection.*
- Monitor the results of laboratory tests of electrolytes and glucose levels. *Electrolyte and glucose imbalances are corrected before the patient has surgery.*
- Teach the patient to turn, cough, and perform deep-breathing exercises. *Although they are important for all surgical patients, these activities are even more important for the patient who is at risk for infection. Having the patient practice and demonstrate the activities increases postoperative compliance.*

POSTOPERATIVE CARE
- Take and record vital signs, measure intake and output, and monitor electrolytes on a frequent schedule, especially during the first 48 hours after surgery. *Removal of an adrenal gland, especially a bilateral adrenalectomy, results in adrenal insufficiency. Addisonian crisis and hypovolemic shock may occur. Cortisol is often given on the day of surgery and in the postoperative period to replace inadequate hormone levels. Intravenous fluids are also administered.*
- Assess body temperature, white blood cell (WBC) levels, and wound drainage. Change dressings using sterile technique. *Impaired wound healing increases the risk of infection in patients with adrenal disorders. Use aseptic technique to decrease this risk.*

Fluid Volume Excess

The excess cortisol secretion associated with Cushing's syndrome results in sodium and water reabsorption, causing fluid volume excess (Porth & Matfin, 2009). The patient will have weight gain, edema, and hypertension.

- Ask the patient to weigh at the same time each day, and maintain a record of results. *Body weight is an accurate indicator of fluid status. One liter of fluid retention corresponds to about 2 lb (0.9 kg) of body weight.*
- Monitor blood pressure, rate and rhythm of pulse, respiratory rate, and breath sounds. Assess for peripheral edema and jugular vein distention. *Extracellular fluid volume excess resulting from sodium and water retention is manifested by hypertension and a bounding, rapid pulse. There may also be crackles and wheezes, dependent edema, and venous distention.*
- Teach the patient and family the reasons for restricting fluid and the importance of limiting fluids if ordered. *Restricting fluid can help decrease the risk of fluid volume excess. Involving the patient and family in the plan of care and teaching the rationale for interventions helps achieve goals.*

Risk for Injury

The patient with Cushing's syndrome is at risk for injury from several causes. Excess cortisol causes increased absorption of calcium and demineralization of bones, resulting in risk of pathologic fractures. Muscle weakness and fatigue are common, increasing the potential for accidental falls. Teach the patient the following:

- Keep unnecessary clutter and equipment out of the way and off the floor.
- Ensure adequate lighting, especially at night.
- Use assistive devices for ambulation or to ask for help if needed.
- Be sure corrective lenses are available and clean.
- Use nonskid slippers or shoes.
- Watch for signs of fatigue (increased pulse and respirations); plan rest periods.
  A well-lighted environment free of clutter decreases the risk of falls and injury. Sensory and motor deficits increase the risk of falls; corrective lenses, assistive devices, and nonslip footwear can decrease this risk. Rest relieves fatigue. To reduce energy expenditure, include alternating periods of rest and activity in daily schedules.

Risk for Infection

Elevated cortisol levels impair the immune response and put the patient with Cushing's syndrome at increased risk for infection. Increased cortisol also affects protein synthesis, causing delayed wound healing, and inhibits collagen formation, which results in epidermal atrophy, further inhibiting resistance to infection. In addition, impaired blood flow to edematous tissue results in altered cellular nutrition, which increases the potential for infection. The following interventions are outlined for the patient with Cushing's syndrome who is hospitalized:

- Place in a private room, and limit visitors. *The patient must avoid exposure to environmental infection.*
- Monitor vital signs and verbalizations of subjective manifestations (e.g., the patient's response to "How do you feel?") every 4 hours. *Increased body temperature and pulse are systemic indicators of infection; however, because Cushing's syndrome impairs the normal inflammatory response, the usual indicators of inflammation may not be present.*
- Use principles of medical and sterile asepsis when caring for the patient, conducting procedures, or providing wound care. *Impaired skin and tissues make aseptic techniques even more necessary to decrease the risk of infection. Intact skin is the first line of defense against infection; if invasive procedures are performed or a wound is present, this defense is lost.*
- If wounds are present, assess the color, odor, and consistency of wound drainage, and look for increased pain in and around the wound. *Cortisol excess delays wound healing and closure.*
- Teach the importance of increasing intake of protein and vitamins C and A. *Protein, vitamin C, and vitamin A are necessary to collagen formation; collagen helps support and repair body tissues.*

> **PRACTICE ALERT**
> A generalized feeling of malaise may be the primary manifestation of infection, especially in the older adult.

Disturbed Body Image

The patient with Cushing's syndrome has obvious physical changes in appearance. The abnormal fat distribution, moon face, buffalo hump, striae, acne, and facial hair (in women) all contribute to disruptions in the way patients with this disorder perceive themselves.

- Encourage patients to express feelings and to ask questions about the disorder and its treatment. *The loss of one's normal body image may prompt feelings of hopelessness, powerlessness, anger, and depression. Understanding the disease and adapting to changes from that disease are the first steps in regaining control of one's own body.*
- Discuss strengths and previous coping strategies. Enlist the support of family or significant others in reaffirming the patient's worth. *Disturbances in body image are often accompanied by low self-esteem. Self-esteem derives from one's perception of competence and from appraisals of others.*
- Discuss signs of progress in controlling manifestations; for example, decreased facial edema or increased activity tolerance. *Many physical changes from cortisol excess disappear with treatment. Clearly communicate this fact, because the patient may believe changes are permanent.*

Using NANDA, NIC, and NOC

Linkages between a selected NANDA nursing diagnosis, NIC, and NOC for the patient with Cushing's syndrome are shown in the chart that follows.

Community-Based Care

The patient with Cushing's syndrome requires education about self-care at home specific to the type of treatment given. Address the following topics:

- Safety measures to prevent falls if fatigue, weakness, and osteoporosis are present.
- Taking medications as prescribed, with information about side effects. Patients often require medications for the rest of their lives, and dosage changes are highly likely.

NANDA, NIC, AND NOC LINKAGES
The Patient with Cushing's Syndrome

NANDA

Risk for Injury

NIC

Risk Identification
Health Education
Infection Protection

NOC

Risk Control
Infection Status
Safe Home Environment

Data from NANDA International. (2009). *NANDA-1 nursing diagnoses: Definitions and classifications 2007–2008.* Oxford, UK: Wiley-Blackwell; Bulechek, G. M., Butcher, H. K., & Dochterman, J. M. (Eds.). (2008). *Nursing interventions classification (NIC)* (5th ed., pp. 389–390, 432–433, 621–624). St. Louis: Mosby Elsevier; and Moorhead, S., Johnson, M., Maas, M., et al. (Eds.). (2008). *Nursing outcomes classification (NOC)* (4th ed., pp. 600–601, 614–615). St. Louis, MO: Mosby Elsevier.

- Having regular health assessments.
- Wearing a medical ID indicating the patient has Cushing's syndrome.
- Helping the older patient with referrals to social services or community health services because of the complexity of the treatment and care required.
- Providing helpful resources: The American Association of Clinical Endocrinologists, the Endocrine Society.

The Patient with Chronic Adrenocortical Insufficiency (Addison's Disease)

Addison's disease is a disorder resulting from destruction or dysfunction of the adrenal cortex. The result is chronic deficiency of cortisol, aldosterone, and adrenal androgens, accompanied by skin pigmentation. It can occur at any age, although it is more common in adults under the age of 60. Like

---

CASE STUDY & NURSING CARE PLAN   A Patient with Cushing's Syndrome

Sara Domico is a 30-year-old lawyer living in a major metropolitan area. She has never been married, and she shares her life with her cat, Beau, and her parents, who live nearby. Her physician recently diagnosed Ms. Domico as having Cushing's syndrome and admits her to the hospital for surgery for an adrenal cortex tumor (adrenalectomy). She has been having increased muscle weakness, so much so that she has difficulty climbing the one flight of stairs to her apartment. She has also had difficulty sleeping, irregular menstrual periods, and hypertension. Ms. Domico is especially concerned about her protruding abdomen, round face, development of facial hair, and the numerous bruises that have appeared on her skin.

ASSESSMENT
When Ms. Domico arrives at the hospital the morning of surgery, she is admitted by her case manager, Ann Sprengel, RN, CNS. Ms. Sprengel completes a physical assessment that includes abnormal findings of thin lower extremities, an enlarged abdomen, purple striae over the abdomen and buttocks, a round face, and obvious facial hair. Her blood pressure is 160/96. Ms. Domico tells Ms. Sprengel that she is always tired and that sometimes it "just wears me out to walk from the bedroom to the kitchen." Diagnostic tests conducted prior to admission reveal the following abnormal findings (all except cortisol levels are corrected before surgery):

Glucose: 186 mg/dL (normal range: 70 to 110 mg/dL)
Sodium: 152 mEq/L (normal range: 135 to 145 mEq/L)
Potassium: 3.2 mEq/L (normal range: 3.5 to 5.0 mEq/L)
Calcium: 4.3 mEq/L (normal range: 4.5 to 5.5 mEq/L)
UFS > 100ug/24 hours (normal range 0–50 ug/24 hours)

DIAGNOSES
- *Fluid Volume Excess* related to sodium retention causing edema and hypertension
- *Risk for Injury* related to generalized fatigue and weakness
- *Risk for Infection* related to impaired immune response and edema
- *Disturbed Body Image* related to physical changes secondary to Cushing's syndrome

EXPECTED OUTCOMES
- Regain a normal body fluid balance.

- Remain free of injury.
- Remain free of infection.
- Verbalize understanding of the physical effects of the disease process and realistic expectations of desired changes in appearance.

PLANNING AND IMPLEMENTATION
- Weigh each morning, using the same scale.
- Maintain an accurate record of intake and output.
- Ensure adequate lighting in the room, and wear glasses and shoes when getting out of bed.
- Develop a written schedule of rest and activity periods.
- If agreeable, provide a private room, and restrict visitors to parents at this time.
- Use strict medical and surgical asepsis when providing care.
- Provide time for discussion of the disease and treatment; encourage verbalization of feelings and identify successful coping mechanisms used in the past.
- Encourage turning, coughing, and deep breathing and/or incentive spirometry every 2 to 4 hours.

EVALUATION
Ms. Domico states that she is "ready to have surgery and start feeling better." She has not fallen or injured herself, and she has remained free of infection. Although edema is still present, she has lost 8 lb (3.6 kg), and her blood pressure is decreased. Ms. Domico has openly discussed her concerns about the way she looks and feels; she understands that manifestations will improve following surgery. She has strong religious beliefs and family support, both of which provide strength and help her cope with the effects of the disorder and the need for any further treatment.

CRITICAL THINKING IN THE NURSING PROCESS
1. When Ms. Domico was admitted to the hospital, several of her test results were abnormal. Describe the pathophysiologic reason for those results.
2. List the assessments that nurses can make to determine body fluid balance.
3. Develop a plan of care for this patient for the nursing diagnosis *Fatigue*.

See Evaluating Your Response in Appendix C.

many endocrine disorders, Addison's disease is more common in women.

Pathophysiology

There are many possible causes of Addison's disease. The etiologies include the following:

- Autoimmune destruction of the adrenals. This is the most common cause. It may occur alone, or as part of a polyglandular autoimmune syndrome (PGA). Type 2 PGA is seen in adults, often associated with autoimmune thyroid disease (usually hypothyroidism), type 1 diabetes, primary ovarian or testicular failure, and pernicious anemia.
- Patients who are taking anticoagulants, have major trauma, sepsis, or are having open heart surgery may have bilateral adrenal hemorrhage.
- Adrenoleukodystrophy, an X-linked disorder characterized by an accumulation of very long chain fatty acids in the adrenal cortex, testes, brain, and spinal cord.
- ACTH deficit, resulting from pituitary tumors, pituitary surgery or irradiation, and the use of exogenous steroids.
- Abrupt withdrawal from long-term, high-dose steroid therapy, and tuberculosis or acquired immune deficiency syndrome (AIDS); the pathogens responsible for either disease can infiltrate and destroy adrenal tissue.

Adrenocortical destruction initially causes a decrease in adrenal glucocorticoid reserve. Basal glucocorticoid secretion is normal, but does not increase in response to stress and surgery. Trauma or infection can precipitate an adrenal crisis. As the destruction of the adrenal cortex continues, even basal secretion of glucocorticoids and mineralocorticoids is deficient. Decreasing plasma cortisol reduces the feedback inhibition of pituitary ACTH and plasma ACTH rises.

Secondary adrenocortical insufficiency occurs when either large doses or prolonged therapy with glucocorticoids are given for their anti-inflammatory and immunosuppressive effects to treat diseases such as arthritis and asthma. If the steroid medications are suddenly discontinued, the hypothalamus and pituitary cannot respond normally to the reduced level of circulating glucocorticoids.

Manifestations

The onset of Addison's disease is slow in most cases; the patient experiences manifestations after about 90% of the function of the gland is lost. The primary manifestations are the result of elevated ACTH levels and decreased aldosterone and cortisol (see the accompanying box). Aldosterone deficiency affects the ability of the distal tubules of the nephron to conserve sodium. Sodium is lost, potassium is retained, extracellular fluid is depleted, and the blood volume is decreased. Postural hypotension and syncope are common, and hypovolemic shock may occur. Hyponatremia causes dizziness, confusion, and neuromuscular irritability. Hyperkalemia causes cardiac dysrhthmias.

Cortisol insufficiency also causes decreased hepatic glyconeogenesis with hypoglycemia. The patient tolerates stress poorly and experiences lethargy, weakness, anorexia, nausea, vomiting, and diarrhea. The increased ACTH levels stimulate hyperpigmentation in more than 90% of patients with

---

MANIFESTATIONS of Addison's Disease

INTEGUMENTARY SYSTEM
- Delayed wound healing
- Hyperpigmentation

CARDIOVASCULAR SYSTEM
- Postural hypotension
- Arrhythmias
- Tachycardia

CENTRAL NERVOUS SYSTEM
- Lethargy
- Tremors
- Emotional lability
- Confusion

MUSCULOSKELETAL SYSTEM
- Weakness
- Muscle wasting
- Joint pain
- Muscle pain

GASTROINTESTINAL SYSTEM
- Anorexia
- Nausea and vomiting
- Diarrhea

REPRODUCTIVE SYSTEM
- Menstrual changes

METABOLIC EFFECTS
- Hyperkalemia
- Hyponatremia
- Hypoglycemia

Addison's disease (Porth & Matfin, 2009). In Caucasian patients, the skin looks deeply suntanned or bronzed in both exposed and unexposed areas.

Addisonian Crisis

Addisonian crisis is a life-threatening response to acute adrenal insufficiency. Triggers include surgery, acute systemic illness, trauma, or abrupt withdrawal of long-term corticosteroid therapy. The disorder is chronic after the acute episode resolves.

This response can occur in any person with Addison's disease; however, it is most commonly precipitated by major stressors, especially if the disease is poorly controlled. Addisonian crisis may also occur in patients who are abruptly withdrawn from glucocorticoid medications or who have hemorrhage into the adrenal glands from either septicemia or anticoagulant therapy.

The patient with Addisonian crisis may have any of the manifestations of Addison's disease, but the primary manifestations develop rapidly and are a high fever; weakness; severe, penetrating pain in the abdomen, lower back, and legs; severe vomiting; diarrhea; hypotension; and circulatory collapse, shock, and coma.

Treatment of the crisis is rapid intravenous replacement of fluids and glucocorticoids. Fluid balance is usually restored in 4 to 6 hours.

Interdisciplinary Care

The patient with Addison's disease requires early diagnosis and treatment. Medical treatment includes cortisol replacement therapy.

Diagnostic Tests

Addison's disease is diagnosed through findings of decreased levels of cortisol, aldosterone, and urinary 17-KS. Dehydration may result in increased hematocrit and blood urea nitrogen (BUN). Blood glucose levels are decreased, and potassium is increased. A list of laboratory findings in Addison's disease is shown in Table 19–2. The following diagnostic tests are used:

- *Serum cortisol levels,* which are decreased in adrenal insufficiency

- *Blood glucose levels*, which are decreased in adrenal insufficiency
- *Serum sodium levels*, which are decreased in adrenal insufficiency
- *Serum potassium levels*, which are increased in adrenal insufficiency
- *BUN levels*, which are increased in adrenal insufficiency
- *Urinary 17-hydroxycorticoids* and *17-KS levels*, which are decreased in adrenal insufficiency
- *Plasma ACTH levels*, which are increased in primary adrenal insufficiency (adrenal gland does not produce cortisol) but decreased in secondary adrenal insufficiency (ACTH is not adequately produced by the pituitary.)
- *ACTH stimulation test* is the most specific diagnostic test for Addison's disease. (Cortisol levels rise with pituitary deficiency but do not rise in primary adrenal insufficiency.)
- *CT scans* of the head, which identify any intracranial lesion impinging on the pituitary gland

Medications

The primary medical treatment of Addison's disease is replacement of corticosteroids and mineralocorticoids, accompanied by increased sodium in the diet. Hydrocortisone (Cortef) is given orally to replace cortisol; fludrocortisone (Florinef) is given orally to replace mineralocorticoids. Nursing implications in cortisol replacement are given in the following box.

Nursing Care

Health Promotion

Health promotion interventions for the patient with or at risk for Addison's disease focus on careful assessments during anticoagulant therapy, open heart surgery, and trauma treatment. If the disease is present, teaching to prevent or treat an Addisonian crisis is essential.

Assessment

Collect the following data through the health history and physical examination (∞ see Chapter 18). Further focused assessments are described with nursing interventions in the following text.

- *Health history:* Weight loss, changes in skin color, nausea and vomiting, anorexia, diarrhea, abdominal pain, weakness, amenorrhea, changes in sexual desire, confusion, intolerance of stress.
- *Physical assessment:* Height and weight, vital signs, skin, hair quality and distribution, muscle size and strength.

MEDICATION ADMINISTRATION Addison's Disease

CORTISOL REPLACEMENTS

Cortisone (Cortone, Cortogen)

Hydrocortisone (Cortisol, Hydrocortone, Cortef)

Fludrocortisone acetate (Florinef, F-Cortef)

Dexamethasone (Decadron, Hexadrol, Dexasone)

Prednisone (Meticorten, Deltasone, Orasone)

Prednisolone (Meticortelone)

Methylprednisolone (Medrol, Solu-Medrol)

Adrenocorticosteroids are used for replacement therapy in acute and chronic adrenal insufficiency. These drugs have anti-inflammatory and immunosuppressant effects. They also facilitate coping with stress.

Because corticosteroids are immunosuppressants, their use is contraindicated when an infection is suspected because they mask the signs of infection. Immunizations with live vaccines should not be attempted. Corticosteroids are contraindicated in many other disorders, including peptic ulcer, Cushing's syndrome, cardiac disease, hyperthyroidism, hypothyroidism, and tuberculosis. Concurrent use with NSAIDs is contraindicated because of the effect on the gastrointestinal tract.

When these drugs are administered in small doses for replacement therapy, side effects are uncommon. Large doses or prolonged therapy may cause a Cushing's-like syndrome, with atrophy of the adrenal cortex. Older patients, especially postmenopausal women, are more prone to develop hypertension and osteoporosis when undergoing glucocorticoid therapy. These drugs are used with caution in children and the older adult and are not usually administered to pregnant women.

Nursing Responsibilities
- Establish baseline data, including mental status, neurologic function, vital signs, and weight.

- Identify medications that might interact with corticosteroids: antidiabetic agents, cardiac glycosides, oral contraceptives, anticoagulants, NSAIDs.
- Document and report increased blood pressure, edema or weight gain, bleeding or bruising, weakness, or manifestations of Cushing's syndrome.
- Administer oral forms of the drug with food to minimize its ulcerogenic effect.
- Monitor electrolyte levels for increased sodium and decreased potassium.
- Monitor capillary blood glucose for hyperglycemia in the diabetic patient.

Health Education for the Patient and Family
- Take medications with food or milk, and report any gastric distress or dark stools.
- Most people need to take the medications for the rest of their lives.
- Consume a diet that is low in potassium, and higher in sodium and protein.
- Weigh yourself each day at the same time, and report any consistent weight gain, which indicates fluid retention.
- Use safety measures in the home to prevent falls and injuries.
- Corticosteroids may impair the effectiveness of oral contraceptives.
- Take the medication regularly and continuously. *Abruptly discontinuing the medication is dangerous.*
- Obtain a Medic-Alert bracelet.
- Monitor for increased stressors (infection, dental work, personal crisis) and increase the dose as indicated by the physician.
- Anticoagulant drugs or insulin may decrease the effectiveness of corticosteroids.
- Report the following to the physician: dizziness on sitting or standing, nausea and vomiting, pain, thirst, feelings of anxiety, malaise, infections.

Nursing Diagnoses and Interventions

The patient with Addison's disease requires nursing care for a wide variety of responses to the decrease in cortisol levels. Nursing diagnoses discussed in this section are directed toward problems with fluid and electrolyte balance and compliance with lifelong self-care. See the accompanying Case Study & Nursing Care Plan on page 515.

Deficient Fluid Volume

Fluid volume deficit in the patient with Addison's disease results from loss of water and sodium, as well as from vomiting and diarrhea. Extracellular fluid volume deficit, decreased cardiac output, hypotension, and hypovolemic shock may occur, especially in crisis situations. Interventions for this diagnosis are outlined for the patient who is hospitalized.

- Monitor intake and output, and assess for signs of dehydration: dry mucous membranes; thirst; poor skin turgor; sunken eyeballs; scanty, dark urine; increased urine specific gravity; weight loss; and increased hemoconcentration (increased hematocrit and BUN). *Glucocorticoid and mineralocorticoid depletion causes fluid volume deficit. Fluid volume deficit may reach crisis levels if undetected, causing altered tissue perfusion and hypovolemic shock.*

- Monitor cardiovascular status: Take and record vital signs, assess character of pulses, monitor potassium levels and ECGs. *Fluid volume deficit may lead to hypotension and a rapid, weak, or thready pulse. As aldosterone levels fall, renal excretion of potassium decreases, increasing blood levels of potassium.*

- Weigh the patient daily at the same time and in the same clothing. *Dehydration is manifested by weight loss.*

- Encourage an oral fluid intake of 3000 mL per day and an increased salt intake. *Cortisol deficiency increases fluid loss, leading to extracellular fluid volume depletion. Oral fluid replacement is necessary to balance this loss. An increase in dietary sodium can decrease the hyponatremia characteristic of adrenal insufficiency.*

- Teach to sit and stand slowly, and provide assistance as necessary. *Extracellular fluid volume deficit causes orthostatic hypotension, dizziness, and possible loss of consciousness. These manifestations increase the risk of injury from falls.*

> **PRACTICE ALERT**
> Hyperkalemia causes changes in cardiac muscle function, which are reflected in ECG changes. (ECGs are discussed in ∞ Chapter 30.)

Risk for Ineffective Therapeutic Regimen Management

Patients with Addison's disease must learn to provide lifelong self-care that involves varied components: medications, diet, and recognizing and responding to responses to stress. Changes in lifestyle are difficult to maintain permanently.

- Teach the effects of illness and treatment. Discuss patient and family concerns. *Lack of knowledge about the illness, as well as the possibility of complications from disregarding or altering the treatment, can negatively affect compliance.*

- Include the following in the teaching plan:
  - Self-administration of steroids
  - The importance of carrying at all times an emergency kit containing parenteral cortisone and a syringe/needle
  - Wearing a Medic-Alert bracelet that says "Adrenal insufficiency—takes hydrocortisone"
  - Increasing oral fluid intake and maintaining a diet high in sodium and low in potassium
  - The necessity of altering the medication dose when experiencing emotional or physical stressors
  - The importance of continuing health care
  One of the most important components of caring for the patient with Addison's disease is teaching both the patient and family to provide care. The length of treatment and the side effects of medications can discourage adherence to the regimen.

Community-Based Care

The patient with Addison's disease provides self-care at home. One of the most important components of caring for the patient with Addison's disease is teaching both the patient and family to provide care. Family stability, an awareness of the serious nature of the disease, and the effectiveness of treatment all promote adherence. The length of treatment and the side effects of medications, however, can discourage adherence. In addition to the information in the teaching topics included with nursing diagnoses and interventions, include the following topics:

- Referral to social worker, if appropriate
- Referral to community agencies for continued education and support
- Helpful resources: National Institute of Diabetes and Digestive and Kidney Diseases (Addison's disease), Endocrine Society, American Association of Clinical Endocrinologists

The Patient with Pheochromocytoma

Pheochromocytomas are tumors of chromaffin tissues in the adrenal medulla. These tumors, which are usually benign, produce catecholamines (epinephrine or norepinephrine) that stimulate the sympathetic nervous system. Although many organs are affected, the most dangerous effects are peripheral vasoconstriction and increased cardiac rate and contractility with resultant paroxysmal hypertension. Systolic blood pressure may rise to 200 to 300 mmHg, the diastolic to 150 to 175 mmHg. Attacks are often precipitated by physical, emotional, or environmental stimuli. This condition is life threatening.

A pheochromocytoma is diagnosed by increased catecholamine levels in the blood or urine, by x-ray studies, and by surgical exploration. Vanillylmandelic acid is the end product of metabolism of all catecholamine substances and is collected in a 24-hour urine sample. Removal of the tumor(s) by adrenalectomy is the treatment of choice.

CASE STUDY & NURSING CARE PLAN   Addison's Disease

A 51-year-old unemployed salesman, Don Sardoff, is brought to the emergency room by his wife, Ellen, at 8 AM. Mrs. Sardoff tells the emergency room nurse that her husband has not been feeling well for the last week, but that when he got up this morning, he was so weak he couldn't dress himself and didn't know where he was. Mrs. Sardoff tells the nurse that her husband has been taking a cortisone drug for treatment of his rheumatoid arthritis for the past 2 years, but notes, "We didn't have the money to buy it this month."

ASSESSMENT

On admission to the emergency room, Mr. Sardoff is dehydrated, with dry oral mucous membranes and tongue, poor skin turgor, and sunken eyeballs. His blood pressure is 94/44, and his pulse is rapid and thready. He is weak, dizzy, and disoriented about time and place. Diagnostic tests reveal the following abnormal findings at 8:30 AM:

- EKG: widening QRS complex and increased PR interval
- Sodium: 129 mEq/L (normal range: 135 to 145 mEq/L)
- Glucose: 54 mg/dL (normal range: 70 to 110 mg/dL)
- Potassium: 5.3 mEq/L (normal range: 3.5 to 5 mEq/L)
- Cortisol: 2 mg/dL (normal for AM: 5 to 23 mg/dL)

The medical orders for Mr. Sardoff include intravenous administration of 5% dextrose in normal saline (D_5NS) at 250 mL/h and hydrocortisone (Solu-Cortef) 200 mg. After the fluids and medication are initiated, Mr. Sardoff is moved to an in-hospital medical bed.

DIAGNOSES

- *Deficient Fluid Volume* related to hypovolemia secondary to adrenal insufficiency
- *Ineffective Tissue Perfusion: Peripheral* related to fluid volume deficit
- *Anxiety* related to lack of knowledge about the effects and treatment of adrenal insufficiency

EXPECTED OUTCOMES

- Regain normal fluid balance.

- Regain normal peripheral perfusion with blood pressure within normal range.
- Verbalize knowledge of the causes and effects of adrenal insufficiency.

PLANNING AND IMPLEMENTATION

- Monitor intake and output closely.
- Take and record weight at the same time daily.
- Monitor blood pressure, pulses, and skin turgor every 2 hours until stable, then four times a day.
- Monitor electrolytes, and report abnormal results.
- Discuss a diet that is high in sodium, low in potassium, and has an increased fluid intake (3000 mL per day). Discuss the types of fluids desired and the best times for intake of increased fluids.
- Assist during activity to prevent falls.
- Provide verbal and written instructions, and encourage verbal feedback about the causes and effects of the disease, the effects of medications, the effects of not taking long-term cortisone drugs, the diet, and self-care at home.

EVALUATION

Following treatment for acute adrenal insufficiency, Mr. Sardoff is no longer dehydrated, and his blood pressure has returned to his normal reading of 132/88. He is alert and oriented, and anxious to learn to care for himself at home. After dietary instructions and teaching for self-care that included his wife, Mr. Sardoff verbalizes an understanding of his illness and the need to take his medication carefully and accurately. A referral is made to a social worker for assistance with costs of medications.

CRITICAL THINKING IN THE NURSING PROCESS

1. Adrenal insufficiency is often diagnosed only when the patient becomes seriously ill in response to a stressor. Explain why this statement is or is not true.
2. Describe the physical assessments that are found in the severely dehydrated patient.
3. Outline a teaching plan for Mr. Sardoff with foods for a high-sodium, low-potassium diet.

See Evaluating Your Response in Appendix C.

Disorders of the Pituitary Gland

The pituitary gland produces hormones that affect multiple body systems through regulation of endocrine function. Target tissues include the thyroid, adrenal cortex, ovary, uterus, mammary glands, testes, and kidneys. Disorders result from an excess or deficiency of one or more of the pituitary hormones due to a pathologic condition within the gland itself or to hypothalamic dysfunction.

Although disorders of the pituitary cause diverse and serious problems, they are not as common as disorders of other endocrine glands. Hyperpituitarism and hypopituitarism are discussed in this section.

The Patient with Disorders of the Anterior Pituitary Gland

Hyperfunction of the anterior pituitary gland, characterized by excess production and secretion of one or more trophic hormones, is usually the result of a pituitary tumor or pituitary

hyperplasia. The most common cause of hyperpituitarism is a benign adenoma. The manifestations result from pressure on the optic nerve causing visual changes or an excess of growth hormone (GH), prolactin (PRL), ACTH, or TSH.

Hypofunction of the anterior pituitary gland results in a deficiency of one or more of the gland's hormones. Conditions causing hypopituitarism include pituitary tumors; surgical removal of the pituitary gland; radiation; and pituitary infarction, infection, or trauma.

Pathophysiology and Manifestations

Growth hormone (somatotropin) is produced by cells in the anterior pituitary throughout life. GH stimulates the production of IGF-1 (an insulin-like growth factor) by the liver. GH is necessary for growth and also contributes to metabolic regulation. GH stimulates all aspects of cartilage growth, and one of its major effects is to stimulate the growth of the epiphyseal cartilage plates of long bones. In addition, other body tissues respond to the metabolic effect of GH and IGF-1 with increases in bone width and the growth of visceral and endocrine organs, skeletal and cardiac muscle, skin, and connective tissue. Gigantism and acromegaly (discussed next) result from overstimulation. Growth retardation and short stature result from deficient production of GH.

Hypersecretion of PRL affects reproductive and sexual function. Women may have irregular or absent menses, difficulty becoming pregnant, and decreased libido. Men may be impotent and have decreased libido. PRL deficiency in postpartal women causes a failure to lactate.

An excess secretion of ACTH overstimulates the adrenal cortex, which in turn increases secretion of adrenal hormones. The result is Cushing's syndrome. Deficiencies of TSH are uncommon, but cause hypothyroidism.

Gigantism

Gigantism occurs when GH hypersecretion begins before puberty and the closure of the epiphyseal plates. The person becomes abnormally tall, often exceeding 7 ft (213 cm) in height, but body proportions are relatively normal. Most often the result of a tumor, the condition is rare today as a result of improved diagnosis and treatment.

Acromegaly

Acromegaly, which literally means "enlarged extremities," occurs when sustained GH and IGF-1hypersecretion begins during adulthood, most commonly because of pituitary tumors. IGF-1 causes most of the clinical manifestations of acromegaly (Porth, 2007). As a result of constant stimulation, the small bones of the hands and feet, the membranous bones of the skull, connective tissue, and soft tissues continue to grow. The forehead enlarges, the maxilla lengthens, the tongue enlarges, and the voice deepens. Overgrowth of bone and soft tissue in the hands and feet causes patients to buy increasingly larger rings, gloves, and shoes. This condition is different from Marfan's syndrome, a genetic disorder that results in elongated bones, optic changes, and severe cardiovascular effects. (∞ See Chapter 31 for nursing care of patients with cardiovascular disorders.)

Other manifestations include peripheral nerve damage from entrapment of nerves, headache, hypertension, congestive heart failure, skin thickening and copious sweating, seizures, and visual disturbances. Changes in appearance are subtle and diagnosis is usually made 10 years or more after onset of GH hypersecretion. Impaired glucose tolerance and diabetes may also develop. Arthralgias in the large joints develop secondary to the bone and connective tissue growth; manifestations may be relieved by treatment that halts excessive GH and IGF-1 production.

Interdisciplinary Care

Acromegaly is treated by surgical removal or irradiation of the pituitary tumor. A transsphenoidal or transfrontal surgical procedure is most commonly used. Somatostatin receptor

binding drugs (SRBDs) suppress the anterior pituitary gland and decrease GH levels. These are administered by injection, and gastrointestinal side effects are common for the first couple of weeks. Gallstones may occur within a year of beginning treatment. Growth hormone receptor antagonists lower IGF-1 production and are used if manifestations persist with SRBDs. Radiation therapy is used when GH-producing tumors persist despite surgery or become resistant to medical therapies (Ben-Shlomo & Melmed, 2008).

Nursing Care

Patients with anterior pituitary disorders require interventions to help in coping with physical and emotional changes, as well as to prevent complications involving other organs and functions of the endocrine system. Nursing care for the patient having cranial surgery is discussed in ∞ Chapter 42.

The Patient with Disorders of the Posterior Pituitary Gland

Disorders of the posterior pituitary are related primarily to excessive or deficient antidiuretic hormone (ADH) secretion. The disorders discussed here are the syndrome of inappropriate ADH secretion and diabetes insipidus.

Pathophysiology and Manifestations

Antidiuretic hormone is secreted in response to low circulatory volume, which is monitored by osmoreceptors in the hypothalamus. When a condition of hyperosmolality occurs, ADH secretion increases, and renal water is reabsorbed. Hypoosmolality causes the suppression of ADH, and renal water excretion increases. ADH, also known as vasopressin, causes the kidney to reabsorb water from the collecting ducts to increase circulatory volume.

Syndrome of Inappropriate ADH Secretion

The **syndrome of inappropriate ADH secretion (SIADH)** is characterized by high levels of ADH in the absence of serum hypo-osmolality. This disorder is most often caused by the ectopic production of ADH by malignant tumors (e.g., oat cell carcinoma of the lung, pancreatic carcinoma, leukemia, and Hodgkin's disease). A transient form may follow a head injury, pituitary surgery, or the use of medications such as barbiturates, anesthetics, or diuretics.

Manifestations of SIADH occur as a result of water retention, hyponatremia, and serum hypo-osmolality. Blood volume expands, but the plasma is diluted. Aldosterone is suppressed; as a result, renal excretion of sodium increases. Water moves from the hypotonic plasma and the interstitial spaces into the cells. Urinary output decreases and the urine becomes very concentrated.

Manifestations of SIADH (∞ see Chapter 10) are usually nonspecific but are related to hyponatremia and water intoxication. Despite fluid retention, the patient may experience thirst. Brain cells may swell, causing neurologic manifestations including headache, changes in mental status or personality, lethargy, and irritability. Weight gain results from the retention of fluid. Usually no edema is present, because water is distributed between the intracellular and extracellular spaces.

Treatment addresses the low serum sodium and intracellular swelling. Besides keeping the patient safe, nursing care involves teaching the patient about restricting fluids to 1 L/day. Fluid restriction continues until the source of ADH is successfully identified and if malignancy is the cause, destroyed. Furosemide and an intravenous infusion of half normal saline decrease circulatory volume and prevent sodium excretion (McAdams-Jones, 2008).

Demeclocycline (Declomycin) is a tetracycline antibiotic with the unique property of creating excessive urine flow. It is used as a treatment for SIADH when patients cannot adequately restrict water intake. Vasopressin antagonists may be given for SIADH. These drugs are especially beneficial for SIADH in persons with heart failure (McPhee & Papadakis, 2009). Sodium levels should be monitored and corrections of hyponatremia must be done cautiously to prevent cerebral osmotic demyelination.

Diabetes Insipidus

Diabetes insipidus is the result of ADH insufficiency. The two types are as follows:

- *Neurogenic diabetes insipidus* can either result from a disruption of the hypothalamus and pituitary gland (as from trauma, irradiation, or cranial surgery) or be idiopathic.
- *Nephrogenic diabetes insipidus* is a disorder in which the renal tubules are not sensitive to ADH. This may be familial in origin or the result of renal failure.

Diabetes insipidus may result from brain tumors or infections, pituitary surgery, cerebral vascular accidents, and renal and organ failure. It is also a complication of closed-head trauma with increased intracranial pressure.

A deficit of ADH causes excretion of large amounts of dilute urine (*polyuria*), in some instances as much as 12 L/day. The patient has extreme thirst and drinks large volumes of water (*polydipsia*). If unable to replace the water loss, the patient becomes dehydrated and hypernatremic. Even though

TABLE 19–3 Comparison of Posterior Pituitary Gland Disorders	
SIADH	**DIABETES INSIPIDUS**
Excessive ADH	Deficient ADH
Fluid volume excess	Fluid volume deficit
Restrict fluid intake	Encourage fluid intake
Demeclocycline (Declomycin) (oral agent) causes excessive urination	Desmopressin (DDAVP) (nasal spray) causes increased water reabsorption

hyperosmolality is present, the urine is dilute and has a low specific gravity.

If this disorder is caused by cerebral injury, manifestations commonly appear 3 to 6 days after the initial injury and last for 7 to 10 days. If the increased intracranial pressure is relieved, manifestations of diabetes insipidus usually disappear. However, diabetes insipidus may also be a chronic illness requiring lifelong treatment and care. See Table 19–3 for a comparison of posterior pituitary gland disorders.

Interdisciplinary Care

SIADH is treated by correcting underlying causes, treating the hyponatremia with intravenous hypertonic saline, and restricting oral fluids to less than 800 mL/day.

Diabetes insipidus is treated by correcting underlying causes, if possible. Other medical interventions include administering intravenous hypotonic fluids, increasing oral fluids, and replacing ADH hormone. Desmopressin acetate, administered intranasally, orally, or parenterally, is the treatment of choice.

∽ Nursing Care

Nursing care for the patient with SIADH and diabetes insipidus focuses on patient problems with fluid and electrolyte balance, as discussed in ∞ Chapter 10.

CHAPTER HIGHLIGHTS

- Hormones regulate growth, development, and metabolism. Homeostasis is dependent on a balanced level of each type of hormone. Not only do hormones affect organ function, but they also interact, and when excesses or deficits occur, manifestations of other endocrine disorders may occur.
- The pituitary gland, in conjunction with the hypothalamus, is the master gland of the body. Fifteen hormones and regulatory factors are synthesized in the anterior pituitary and hypothalamus; many are trophic hormones that stimulate the release of other hormones.

- Thyroid disorders are the most common endocrine disorders. Occurring mainly among women, these diseases change body image and impose upsets to energy levels, creating fatigue and exhaustion.
- Diagnostic tests and therapies are available to identify and treat thyroid disorders. Surgery, radiation therapy, and medications support good quality of life, but the medications must be used throughout the lifetime.
- The parathyroid glands synthesize parathormone, which maintains serum calcium. Thyroid tissues surrounding the parathyroids

synthesize a hormone, calcitonin, which decreases serum calcium to normal levels. These glands provide the proper level of serum calcium, which is vital for cardiac function, bone stability, nerve conduction, and muscle contraction.

■ The adrenal glands regulate energy and fluid balance through corticosteroids and mineralocorticoids. Cushing's and Addison's disease are polar opposites. Treatment eliminates the manifestations of one and creates the manifestations of the other. Patients with these diseases require patient education until they fully grasp the significance of the condition and the importance of adhering to the treatment plan.

TEST YOURSELF NCLEX-RN® REVIEW

1. Graves' disease, the most common cause of hyperthyroidism, is categorized as what type of disorder?
   1. autoimmune
   2. infectious
   3. allergic
   4. genetic

2. What principle supports the treatment of hyperthyroidism with radioactive iodine?
   1. Radioactive iodine reduces the vascularity of the thyroid gland.
   2. Doses of radioactive iodine are too small to be hazardous to other body parts.
   3. The thyroid gland takes up iodine in any form.
   4. Irradiation of the thyroid gland decreases the risk of hypothyroidism.

3. You assess a patient with newly diagnosed hypothyroidism as having an enlarged thyroid gland (goiter). What physiologic process causes this enlargement?
   1. an excess of TH stimulates thyroid follicles
   2. an increased dietary iodine intake
   3. a compensatory effort to produce more TH
   4. tissue hypertrophy in response to increased TH

4. Mrs. Jonah has taken cortisone for her rheumatoid arthritis for several years. What endocrine disorder is she most at risk for developing?
   1. hyperthyroidism
   2. hypothyroidism
   3. acromegaly
   4. Cushing's syndrome

5. Which statement illustrates that the patient with Addison's disease understands your teaching?
   1. "I will be sure to stop taking my medications when I have an infection."
   2. "I have purchased an emergency kit and keep it with me all the time."
   3. "I know I should never alter my dose of medications."
   4. "I wonder why I look suntanned all the time."

6. Manifestations of hyponatremia found in SIADH include which of the following?
   1. weight loss
   2. irritability
   3. hyperkalemia
   4. constipation

7. A home health nurse is caring for a patient with hyperparathyroidism and osteoporosis. Which nursing diagnosis has priority with this patient?
   1. *Risk for Fear*
   2. *Risk for Injury*
   3. *Risk for Isolation*
   4. *Risk for Chronic Low Self-Esteem*

8. A nurse is monitoring a patient for signs of hypercalcemia. Which of the following is a sign of hypercalcemia?
   1. oliguria
   2. positive Chvostek's sign
   3. diminished bowel sounds
   4. hyperactive deep tendon reflexes

9. A patient with increased ACTH levels and Addison's disease is likely to manifest which of the following?
   1. tremor
   2. hair loss
   3. gingival hyperplasia
   4. dermal hyperpigmentation

10. Patients treated with glucocorticoids may be at risk for Addisonian crisis due to which of the following?
    1. rapid withdrawal of glucocorticoids
    2. excessive ACTH
    3. sodium retention
    4. hypokalemia

See Test Yourself answers in Appendix C.

Pearson Nursing Student Resources

Find additional review materials at **nursing.pearsonhighered.com**

Prepare for success with additional NCLEX®-style practice questions, interactive assignments and activities, Web links, animations and videos, and more!

BIBLIOGRAPHY

American Cancer Society. (2007). Making treatment decisions: DHEA. Retrieved from http://www.cancer.org/docroot/ETO/content/ETO_5_3X_Dhea.asp?sitearea=ETO

American Thyroid Association. (2008). Thyroid function tests. Retrieved from http://www.thyroid.org/patients/patient_brochures/function_tests.html

Ben-Shlomo, A., & Melmed, S. (2008). Acromegaly. *Endocrinology and Metabolism Clinics, 37*(1), 101–122.

Bulechek, G. M., Butcher, H. K., & Dochterman, J. M. (Eds.). (2008). *Nursing interventions classification (NIC)* (5th ed.). St. Louis: Mosby Elsevier.

Davis, A. B., Orlander, P. R., & Kermani, A. (2008). Goiter, toxic nodular. eMedicine, WebMD. Retrieved from http://www.emedicine.com/MED/topic920.htm

Elamin, M. B., Murad, M. H., Mullan, R., Erickson, D., Harris, K., et al. (2008). Accuracy of diagnostic tests for Cushing's syndrome: A systematic review and meta-analyses. *The Journal of Clinical Endocrinology and Metabolism, 93*(5), 1553–1562.

Fatourechi, V. (2005). Pretibial myxedema: Pathophysiology and treatment options. *American Journal of Clinical Dermatology, 6*(5), 295–309.

Holcomb, S. S. (2006). Hospital nursing: Do the clues add up to Addison's disease? *Nursing, 36*(3), 64hn1–64hn4.

Houston, D. K., Schwartz, A. V., Cauley, J. A., Tylavsky, F. A., Simonsick, et al. (2008). Serum parathyroid hormone levels predict falls in older adults with diabetes mellitus. *Journal of the American Geriatric Society, 56*(11), 2027–2032.

Kee, J. L. (2010). *Handbook of laboratory and diagnostic tests with nursing implications.* Upper Saddle River, NJ: Pearson Prentice Hall.

McAdams-Jones, D. (2008). Rapid response: Reversing SIADH. *American Nurse Today, 3*(9), 40.

McPhee, S. J. Papadakis, M. A. (Eds.). (2009). *Current medical diagnosis & treatment* (48th ed.). New York: Lange Medical Books/McGraw-Hill.

Moorhead, S., Johnson, M., Maas, M., & Swanson, E. (Eds.). (2008). *Nursing outcomes classification (NOC)* (4th ed.). St. Louis, MO: Mosby Elsevier.

NANDA International. (2009). *Nursing diagnoses: Definitions and classification 2009–2011.* Oxford, UK: Wiley-Blackwell.

National Cancer Institute. (2009). Thyroid cancer. Retrieved from http://www.cancer.gov/cancertopics/types/thyroid

Nieman L. K., Biller, B. M., Findling, J. W., Newell-Price, J., Savage, M. O. et al. (2008). The diagnosis of Cushing's syndrome: An endocrine society clinical practice guideline. *The Journal of Clinical Endocrinology & Metabolism, 93*(5), 1526–1540.

Pfister, D. G., & Fagin, J. A. (2008). Refractory thyroid cancer: a paradigm shift in treatment is not far off. *Journal of Clinical Oncology, 26*(29), 4701–4704.

Porth, C. (2007). *Essentials of pathophysiology: Concepts of altered health states* (2nd ed.). Philadelphia: Lippincott, Williams and Wilkins.

Porth, C., & Matfin, G. (2009). *Pathophysiology: Concepts of altered health states* (8th ed.). Philadelphia: Lippincott Williams and Wilkins.

Shah, A. A., & Lettieri, C. J. (2007). Endocrine emergencies. Medscape Nurses. Retrieved from http://www.medscape.com/viewarticle/567307

Torres, P. U. (2006). Cinacalcet HCl: A novel treatment for secondary hyperparathyroidism caused by chronic kidney disease. *Journal of Renal Nutrition, 16*(3), 253–258.

Wilson, B., Shannon, M., & Shields, K. (2010). *Pearson's nurse's drug guide 2010.* Upper Saddle River, NJ: Pearson Prentice Hall.

20 Nursing Care of Patients with Diabetes Mellitus

LEARNING OUTCOMES

1. Describe the prevalence and incidence of diabetes mellitus (DM).
2. Explain the pathophysiology, risk factors, manifestations, and complications of type 1 and type 2 DM.
3. Provide rationale for diagnostic tests used for screening, diagnosis, and monitoring of DM.
4. Discuss the nursing implications for insulin and oral hypoglycemic agents used to treat patients with DM.
5. Discuss best practices of self-care management of DM related to diet planning, sick day management, and exercise.
6. Compare and contrast the manifestations of hypoglycemia, diabetic ketoacidosis (DKA), and hyperosmolar hyperglycemic state (HHS).

CLINICAL COMPETENCIES

1. Assess blood glucose levels and patterns of hyper- and hypoglycemia in patients with DM.
2. Use assessed data, patient values, clinical expertise, and evidence to determine priority nursing diagnoses and select and implement individualized nursing interventions.
3. Administer oral and injectable medications used to treat DM knowledgeably and safely.
4. Assess patients' ability to read markings on syringes and to identify correct insulin doses.
5. Provide individualized care to patients with hypoglycemia, diabetic ketoacidosis, and hyperosmolar hyperglycemic state.
6. Effectively communicate with and function within the interdisciplinary team to plan and provide patient care.
7. Provide appropriate teaching to facilitate self blood glucose monitoring, administration of oral and injectable hypoglycemic medications, diabetic diet, appropriate exercise, and effective foot care.
8. Adapt individual and cultural values and variations as well as expressed needs and preferences into the plan of care for patients with DM.
9. Revise plan of care as needed to provide effective interventions to promote, maintain, or restore normal glucose levels.

KEY TERMS

diabetes mellitus (DM), *520*
diabetic ketoacidosis (DKA), *541*
gastroparesis, *545*
gluconeogenesis, *521*
glucosuria, *523*
glycogenolysis, *521*
hyperglycemia, *522*
hyperosmolar hyperglycemic state (HHS), *542*
hypoglycemia, *543*
ketosis, *522*
polydipsia, *524*
polyphagia, *524*
polyuria, *523*

Diabetes Mellitus

Diabetes mellitus (DM) is a common chronic disease of adults requiring continuing medical supervision and patient self-care education. However, depending on the type of DM and the age of the patient, both patient needs and nursing care may vary greatly. Consider the following examples:

- Cheryl Draheim is a 45-year-old schoolteacher. She developed DM at age 34 after an automobile crash caused severe pancreatic injuries. Cheryl has always been very careful about taking her insulin, following her diet, and exercising regularly. However, she is beginning to notice that her vision is getting worse and that she is having increasing pain in her legs, especially after standing for long periods of time. Cheryl says that sometimes she believes the disease controls her more than she controls it.
- Tom Chang is 53 years old. Early in his 40s, Tom was diagnosed with type 2 DM. Although Tom was taught about the disease and the importance of taking his oral medications, following his diet plan, and getting exercise, he rarely did more than take the medication. Five years ago, he was hospitalized for hyperglycemia and started taking insulin. Last year Tom had a stroke, leaving him unable to walk. Now, he has been admitted to the hospital for treatment of gangrene of the large toe on his left foot.
- Grace Staples is an independent 82-year-old woman who lives alone and happily takes care of her two cats. She is slightly overweight. Last year, during Grace's annual eye examination, eye changes typical for DM were found. She was referred to her family doctor, who diagnosed type 2 DM and started her on oral medications. Grace sticks to her diet, walks a mile every day, and plans to live to be 100.

As illustrated in these examples, DM is not a single disorder but a group of chronic disorders of the endocrine pancreas, all categorized under a broad diagnostic label. The condition is characterized by inappropriate hyperglycemia caused by a relative or absolute deficiency of insulin or by cellular resistance to the action of insulin. Of the several classifications of DM, this chapter will focus on type 1 and type 2. Type 1 DM is the result of pancreatic islet cell destruction and a total deficit of circulating insulin; type 2 DM results from insulin resistance with a defect in compensatory insulin secretion.

DM has been recognized as a disease for centuries, but it was not until 1921 that techniques were developed for extracting insulin from pancreatic tissue and for measuring blood glucose. At the same time, researchers discovered that insulin, when injected, produces a dramatic drop in blood glucose. This meant that DM was no longer a terminal illness, because hyperglycemia could now be controlled. Since that time, oral hypoglycemic drugs, human insulin products, insulin pumps, home blood glucose monitoring, and transplantation of the pancreas or of pancreatic islet or beta cells have advanced the treatment and care of people with DM.

Patients with DM face lifelong changes in lifestyle and health status. Nursing care is provided in many settings for the diagnosis and care of the disease and treatment of complications. A major role of the nurse is that of educator in both hospital and community settings.

Incidence and Prevalence

Approximately 1.6 million new cases of DM are diagnosed each year in the United States. This chronic illness affects an estimated 23.6 million people, of that number, 17.9 million have been diagnosed and an estimated 5.7 million are undiagnosed (National Institutes of Health [NIH], 2008). There is an increased prevalence of DM (especially type 2 DM) among older adults and in minority populations. See the following Focus on Cultural Diversity box.

DM is the sixth leading cause of death by disease in the United States, primarily because of the widespread cardiovascular effects that result in atherosclerosis, coronary artery disease, and stroke (CDC, 2009). People with DM are two to four times more likely to have heart disease, and two to four times more likely to have a stroke than people who do not have the disease. DM is the leading cause of end-stage renal disease (kidney failure), and the major cause of newly diagnosed blindness in people ages 20 to 74. DM also is the most frequent cause of nontraumatic amputations, with an estimated 71,000 amputations each year in people with DM (NIH, 2008).

Americans with DM use a disproportionate share of the nation's healthcare services. They visit outpatient services and physicians' offices more often than people who do not have the disease, and they require more frequent hospitalizations with longer days of in-hospital treatment. The cost of illness and resulting loss of productivity for people with DM exceeds $174 billion per year, according to an estimate by the American Diabetes Association (NIH, 2008).

Overview of Endocrine Pancreatic Hormones and Glucose Homeostasis

The hormones produced by several different cells of the endocrine pancreas, along with hormones produced by the small intestine, are responsible for glucose homeostasis in the body.

HORMONES The endocrine pancreas produces hormones necessary for the metabolism and cellular utilization of carbohydrates, proteins, and fats. The cells that produce these hormones are clustered in groups of cells called the islets of Langerhans. These islets have three different types of cells:

- Alpha cells produce the hormone *glucagon*, which stimulates the breakdown of glycogen in the liver, the formation of carbohydrates in the liver, and the breakdown of lipids in both the liver and adipose tissue. The primary function of glucagon is to decrease glucose oxidation and to increase blood glucose levels. Through **glycogenolysis** (the breakdown of liver glycogen) and **gluconeogenesis** (the formation of glucose from fats and proteins), glucagon prevents blood glucose from decreasing below a certain level when the body is fasting or in between meals. The action of glucagon is initiated in most people when blood glucose falls below about 70 mg/dL.

- Beta cells secrete the hormone *insulin*, which facilitates the movement of glucose across cell membranes into cells, decreasing blood glucose levels. Insulin prevents the excessive breakdown of glycogen in the liver and in muscle, facilitates lipid formation while inhibiting the breakdown of stored fats, and helps move amino acids into cells for protein synthesis. After secretion by the beta cells, insulin enters the portal circulation, travels directly to the liver, and is then released into the general circulation. Circulating insulin is rapidly bound to receptor sites on peripheral tissues (especially muscle and fat cells) or is destroyed by the liver or kidneys. Insulin release is regulated by blood glucose; it increases when blood glucose levels increase, and it decreases when blood glucose levels decrease. When a person eats food, insulin levels begin to rise in minutes, peak in 3 to 5 minutes, and return to baseline in 2 to 3 hours (Porth & Matfin, 2009). Amylin is a glucose-regulating hormone

FOCUS ON CULTURAL DIVERSITY
Estimates of Prevalence of Diabetes Mellitus

- 14.9 million (9.8%) of all non-Hispanic Whites aged 20 years or older have DM.
- 3.7 million (14.7%) of non-Hispanic African Americans aged 20 years or older have DM and are 1.6 times more likely than non-Hispanic Whites to have DM. Higher rates of kidney disease and amputations occur in this population. There is a 50% lower rate of blindness compared to rates among non-Hispanic Whites.
- 2.5 million (9.5%) of Hispanic/Latino Americans aged 20 years or older have DM and are 1.7 times more likely than non-Hispanic Whites to have DM.
- 7.5% of Asian Americans aged 20 years or older have DM and are two times more likely than non-Hispanic Whites to have DM.
- 105,000 (16.5%) American Indians and Alaska Natives have DM and are 2.6 times more likely than non-Hispanic Whites to have DM. The rate varies; only 6% of Alaska natives have DM while 29.3% of Native Americans in southern Arizona have DM (CDC, 2007).

also secreted by the beta cells with insulin that affects post-prandial (postmeal) glucose levels. It impairs glucagon secretion and slows the rate at which glucose travels to the small intestine for absorption.

- Delta cells produce *somatostatin*, which acts within the islets of Langerhan to inhibit the production of both glucagon and insulin. It also slows gastrointestinal motility, allowing more time for food to be absorbed.

In addition, the small intestine produces hormones that lower blood glucose following the intake of a meal. Glucagon-like peptide-1 (GLP-1) and glucose-dependent insulinotropic polypeptide (GIP) are secreted from the small intestine to increase insulin release after a meal has been ingested. This hormone-stimulated insulin increase following ingestion of food is called an incretin effect. An injectable form of these hormones, exenatide (Byetta), is an incretin mimetic used in the treatment of type II DM.

BLOOD GLUCOSE HOMEOSTASIS All body tissues and organs require a constant supply of glucose; however, not all tissues require insulin for glucose uptake. The brain, liver, intestines, and renal tubules do not require insulin to transfer glucose into their cells. Skeletal muscle, cardiac muscle, and adipose tissue do require insulin for glucose movement into the cells.

Normal blood glucose is maintained in healthy people primarily through the actions of insulin and glucagon. Increased blood glucose levels, amino acids, and fatty acids stimulate pancreatic beta cells to produce insulin. As cells of cardiac muscle, skeletal muscle, and adipose tissue take up glucose, plasma levels of nutrients decrease, suppressing the stimulus to produce insulin. If blood glucose falls, glucagon is released to raise hepatic glucose output, raising glucose levels. Epinephrine,

growth hormone, thyroxine, and glucocorticoids (often referred to as glucose counterregulatory hormones) also stimulate an increase in glucose in times of hypoglycemia, stress, growth, or increased metabolic demand. The regulation of blood glucose levels by insulin and glucagon is illustrated in Figure 20–1 ■.

Pathophysiology of DM

DM is a group of metabolic diseases characterized by hyperglycemia resulting from defects in the secretion of insulin, the action of insulin, or both. There are four major types of DM. Type 1 DM (5% to 10% of diagnosed cases), type 2 DM (90% to 95% of diagnosed cases), gestational DM (2% to 5% of all pregnancies), and other specific types of DM (1% to 2% of diagnosed cases). The classification and characteristics of the four types are described in Table 20–1.

Type 1 Diabetes

Type 1 DM most often occurs in childhood and adolescence, but it may occur at any age, even in the 80s and 90s. This disorder is characterized by **hyperglycemia** (elevated blood glucose levels), a breakdown of body fats and proteins, and the development of **ketosis** (an accumulation of ketone bodies produced during the oxidation of fatty acids). Type 1 DM is the result of the destruction of the beta cells of the islets of Langerhans in the pancreas. When beta cells are destroyed, insulin is no longer produced. Although type 1 DM may be classified as either an autoimmune or idiopathic disorder, 90% of the cases are immune mediated. The disorder begins with insulitis, a chronic inflammatory process that occurs in response to the autoimmune destruction of islet cells. This process slowly destroys production of insulin, with the onset of hyperglycemia occurring when 80% to 90% of beta cell

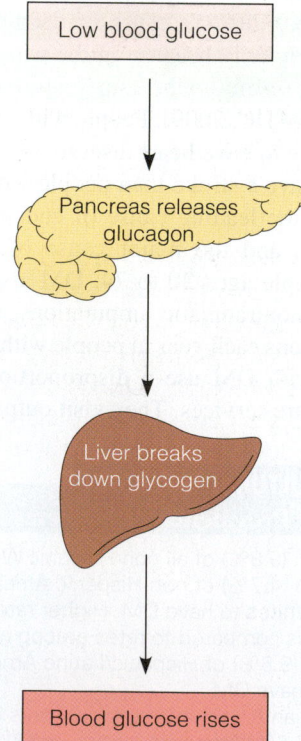

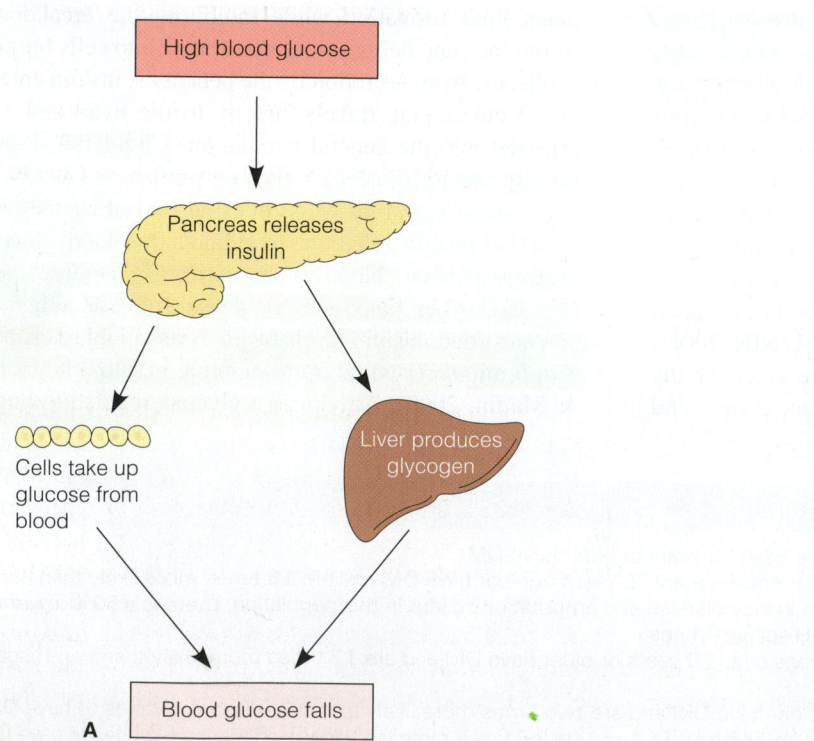

Figure 20–1 ■ Regulation (homeostasis) of blood glucose levels by insulin and glucagon. *A,* High blood glucose is lowered by insulin release. *B,* Low blood glucose is raised by glucagon release.

TABLE 20–1 Classification and Characteristics of Diabetes Mellitus

	CLASSIFICATION	CHARACTERISTICS
I. Type 1 DM	A. Immune-mediated	Beta cells are destroyed, usually leading to absolute insulin deficiency. Markers to the immune destruction of the beta cells include islet cell autoantibodies (ICAs) and insulin autoantibodies (IAAs). The rate of beta cell destruction is variable, usually more rapid in infants and children and slower in adults. Destruction of the beta cells has genetic predispositions and is also related to environmental factors as yet undefined.
	B. Idiopathic	Has no known etiologic causes. Most patients are of African or Asian descent. Is strongly inherited. Need for insulin may be intermittent.
II. Type 2 DM		May range from predominantly insulin resistance with relative insulin deficiency to a predominantly secretory defect with insulin resistance. There is no immune destruction of beta cells. Initially, and in some cases for the entire life, insulin is not necessary. Most people with this form are obese, or have an increased amount of abdominal fat. Risks for development include increasing age, obesity, and a sedentary lifestyle. Occurs more frequently in women who have had gestational DM, and in people with lipid disorders or hypertension. There is a strong genetic predisposition.
III. Other specific types	A. Genetic defects of beta cell	Hyperglycemia occurs at an early age (usually before age 25). This type is referred to as maturity-onset DM of the young (MODY).
	B. Genetic defects in insulin action	Are genetically determined. Dysfunctions may range from hyperinsulinemia to severe DM.
	C. Diseases of the exocrine pancreas	Acquired processes causing DM include pancreatitis, trauma, infection, pancreatectomy, and pancreatic cancer. Severe forms of cystic fibrosis and hemochromatosis may also damage beta cells and impair insulin secretion.
	D. Endocrine disorders	Excess amount of hormones (e.g., growth hormone, cortisol, glucagon, and epinephrine) impair insulin secretion, resulting in DM in people with Cushing's syndrome, acromegaly, and pheochromocytoma.
	E. Drug or chemical induced	Many drugs impair insulin secretion, precipitating DM in people with predisposing insulin resistance. Examples are nicotinic acid, glucocorticoids, thyroid hormone, thiazides, and phenytoin.
	F. Infections	Certain viruses may cause beta cell destruction, including congenital measles, cytomegalovirus, adenovirus, and mumps.
IV. Gestational diabetes mellitus (GDM)		Any degree of glucose intolerance with onset or first recognition during pregnancy.

function is lost. This process usually occurs over a long pre-clinical period. It is believed that both alpha-cell and beta-cell functions are abnormal, with a lack of insulin and a relative excess of glucagon resulting in hyperglycemia.

RISK FACTORS Genetic predisposition plays a role in the development of type 1 DM. Although the risk in the general population ranges from 1 in 400 to 1 in 1000, the child of a person with DM has a 1 in 20 to 1 in 50 risk. Genetic markers that determine immune responses have been found in most people diagnosed with type 1 DM. Although the presence of these markers does not guarantee that the person will develop type 1 DM, they do indicate increased susceptibility (Porth & Matfin, 2009).

Environmental factors are believed to trigger the development of type 1A DM. The trigger can be a viral infection (mumps, rubella, or coxsackievirus B4) or a chemical toxin, such as those found in smoked and cured meats. As a result of exposure to the virus or chemical, an abnormal autoimmune response occurs in which antibodies respond to normal islet beta cells as though they were foreign substances, destroying them. The manifestations of type 1 DM appear when approximately 90% of the beta cells are destroyed. However, manifestations may appear at any time during the loss of beta cells if an acute illness or stress increases the demand for insulin beyond the reserves of the damaged cells. The actual cause and exact sequence are not completely understood, but research continues to identify the genetic markers of this disorder and to investigate ways of altering the immune response to prevent or cure type 1 DM.

Type IB DM, a rare form, is strongly inherited and affects people of African and Asian descent. It is not an autoimmune disorder; beta cell destruction varies and periods of ketoacidosis develop.

MANIFESTATIONS The manifestations of type 1 DM are the result of a lack of insulin to transport glucose across the cell membrane into the cells (Figure 20–2 ■). Glucose molecules accumulate in the circulating blood, resulting in hyperglycemia. Hyperglycemia causes serum hyperosmolality, drawing water from the intracellular spaces into the general circulation. The increased blood volume increases renal blood flow, and the hyperglycemia acts as an osmotic diuretic. The resulting osmotic diuresis increases urine output. This condition is called polyuria. When the blood glucose level exceeds the renal threshold for glucose—usually about 180 mg/dL—glucose is excreted in the urine, a condition called glucosuria. The decrease in intracellular volume and the increased urinary

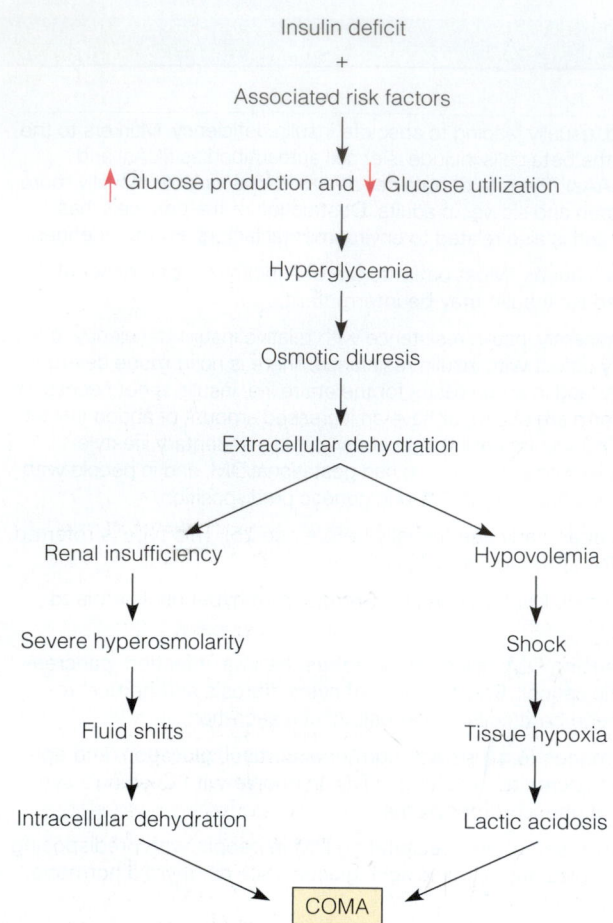

Insulin deficit

+

Associated risk factors

↓

↑ Glucose production and ↓ Glucose utilization

↓

Hyperglycemia

↓

Osmotic diuresis

↓

Extracellular dehydration

Renal insufficiency   Hypovolemia

↓   ↓

Severe hyperosmolarity   Shock

↓   ↓

Fluid shifts   Tissue hypoxia

↓   ↓

Intracellular dehydration   Lactic acidosis

COMA

Figure 20–2 ■ Pathophysiologic results of type 1 DM.

output cause dehydration. The mouth becomes dry and thirst sensors are activated, causing the person to drink increased amounts of fluid (**polydipsia**).

Because glucose cannot enter the cell without insulin, energy production decreases. This decrease in energy stimulates hunger, and the person eats more food (**polyphagia**). Despite increased food intake, the person loses weight as the body loses water and breaks down proteins and fats in an attempt to restore energy sources. Malaise and fatigue accompany the decrease in energy. Blurred vision is also common, resulting from osmotic affects that cause swelling of the lenses of the eyes.

Thus, the classic manifestations are polyuria, polydipsia, and polyphagia, accompanied by weight loss, malaise, and fatigue. Depending on the degree of insulin lack, the manifestations vary from slight to severe. People with type 1 DM require an exogenous (external) source of insulin to maintain life.

Type 2 DM

Type 2 DM is a condition of fasting hyperglycemia that occurs despite the availability of endogenous insulin. Type 2 DM can occur at any age but it is usually seen in middle age and older people. It is the most common form of DM. Heredity plays a role in its transmission. The level of insulin produced varies in type 2 DM, and despite its availability, its function is impaired by insulin resistance in peripheral tissues.

The liver produces more glucose than normal, dietary carbohydrates are not metabolized well, and eventually the pancreas secretes less than adequate amounts of insulin (Porth, 2007). Whatever the cause, there is sufficient insulin production to prevent the breakdown of fats with resultant ketosis; thus, type 2 DM is characterized as a nonketotic form of DM. However, the amount of insulin available is not sufficient to lower blood glucose levels through the uptake of glucose by muscle and fat cells.

A major factor in the development of type 2 DM is cellular resistance to the effect of insulin. This resistance is increased by obesity, inactivity, illnesses, medications, and increasing age. In obesity, insulin has a decreased ability to influence glucose absorption and metabolism by the liver, skeletal muscles, and adipose tissue. Hyperglycemia increases gradually and may exist over a long time before DM is diagnosed, thus approximately half the newly diagnosed type 2 diabetics already have complications (Capriotti, 2005). Treatment usually begins with prescriptions for weight loss and increased activity. If these changes can be sustained, no further treatment will be necessary for many individuals. Hypoglycemic medications are begun when lifestyle changes are insufficient. Often, a combination of insulin and hypoglycemic medication is used to achieve the best glycemic control in the patient with type 2 DM.

RISK FACTORS   The major risk factors for type 2 DM are the following:

- History of DM in parents or siblings. Although there is no identified HLA linkage, the children of a person with type 2 DM have a two to fourfold increased risk of developing type 2 DM and a 30% risk of developing a glucose intolerance (the inability to metabolize carbohydrate normally).
- Obesity, defined as being at least 20% over desired body weight or having a body mass index (BMI) of at least 27 kg/m². Obesity, especially visceral obesity (abdominal fat), is associated with increased insulin resistance.
- Physical inactivity.
- Race/ethnicity (see the box on page 521).
- In women, a history of gestational DM, polycystic ovary syndrome, or delivering a baby weighing more than 9 lb.
- Hypertension (≥ 130/85 in adults), HDL cholesterol of ≥ 35 mg/dL, and/or a triglyceride level of ≥ 250 mg/dL.
- Metabolic syndrome, a cluster of manifestations associated with type 2 DM. Hypertension, visceral obesity, low levels of high-density lipoproteins, high levels of triglycerides, elevated C-reactive protein, and a fasting blood glucose greater than 110 mg/dL increases the risk of DM, coronary heart disease, and stroke (Porth & Matfin, 2009).

MANIFESTATIONS   The person with type 2 DM experiences a slow onset of manifestations and is often unaware of the disease until seeking health care for some other problem. The hyperglycemia in type 2 DM is usually not as severe as in type 1 DM, but similar manifestations occur, especially polyuria and polydipsia. Polyphagia is not often seen, and weight loss is uncommon. Other manifestations are also the result of hyperglycemia: blurred vision, fatigue, paresthesias, and skin infections.

MULTISYSTEM EFFECTS OF
Diabetes Mellitus

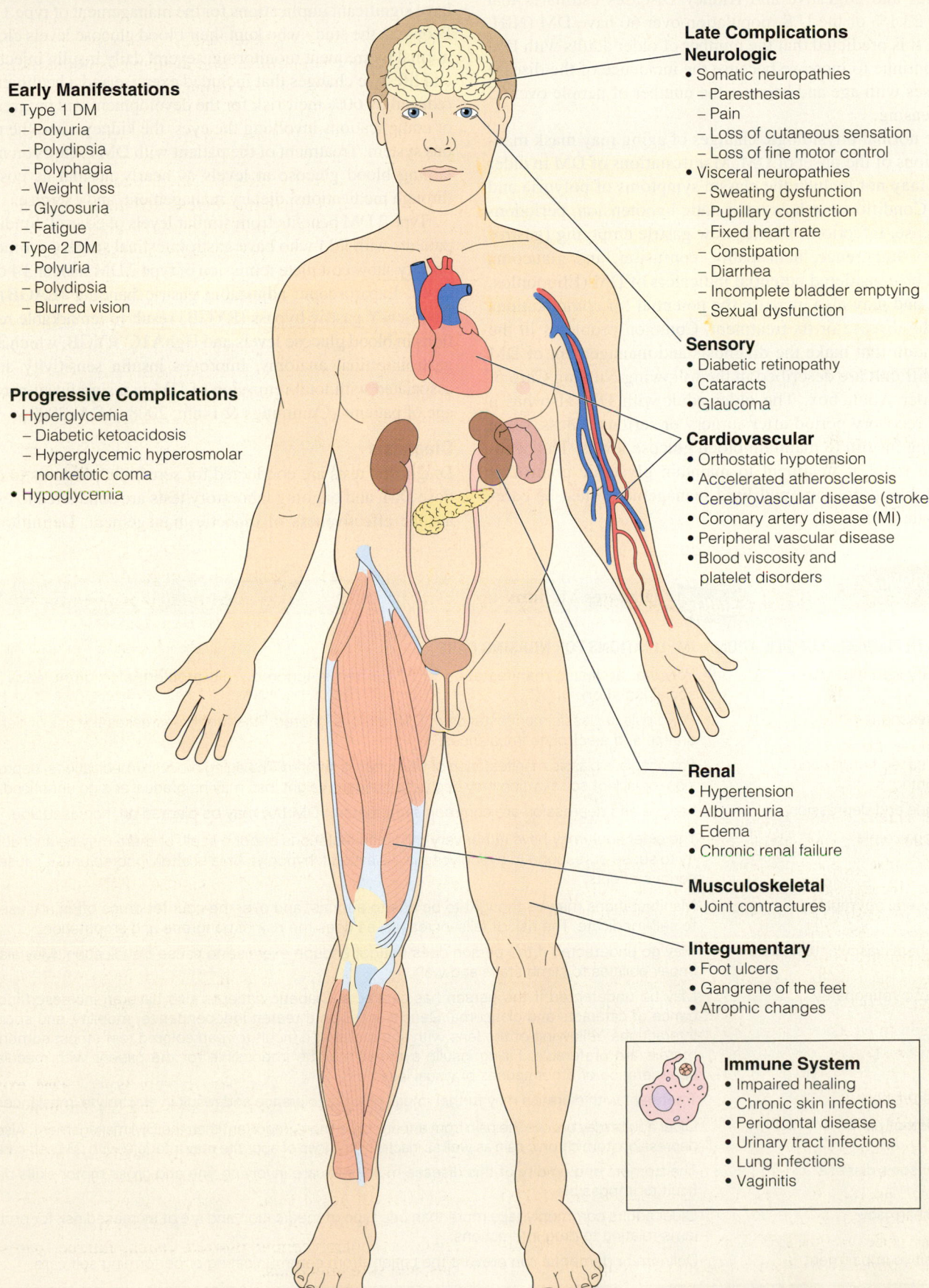

Early Manifestations
- Type 1 DM
  - Polyuria
  - Polydipsia
  - Polyphagia
  - Weight loss
  - Glycosuria
  - Fatigue
- Type 2 DM
  - Polyuria
  - Polydipsia
  - Blurred vision

Progressive Complications
- Hyperglycemia
  - Diabetic ketoacidosis
  - Hyperglycemic hyperosmolar nonketotic coma
- Hypoglycemia

Late Complications
Neurologic
- Somatic neuropathies
  - Paresthesias
  - Pain
  - Loss of cutaneous sensation
  - Loss of fine motor control
- Visceral neuropathies
  - Sweating dysfunction
  - Pupillary constriction
  - Fixed heart rate
  - Constipation
  - Diarrhea
  - Incomplete bladder emptying
  - Sexual dysfunction

Sensory
- Diabetic retinopathy
- Cataracts
- Glaucoma

Cardiovascular
- Orthostatic hypotension
- Accelerated atherosclerosis
- Cerebrovascular disease (stroke)
- Coronary artery disease (MI)
- Peripheral vascular disease
- Blood viscosity and platelet disorders

Renal
- Hypertension
- Albuminuria
- Edema
- Chronic renal failure

Musculoskeletal
- Joint contractures

Integumentary
- Foot ulcers
- Gangrene of the feet
- Atrophic changes

Immune System
- Impaired healing
- Chronic skin infections
- Periodontal disease
- Urinary tract infections
- Lung infections
- Vaginitis

DM in the Older Adult

Although the older adult may have either type 1 or type 2 DM, most often he or she has type 2. The National Institute of Diabetes and Digestive and Kidney Diseases estimates that nearly 23.1% of the U.S. population over 60 have DM (NIH, 2008). It is predicted that the number of older adults with DM will continue to increase because the incidence of the disease increases with age and because the number of people over 65 is increasing.

The normal physiologic changes of aging may mask manifestations of the onset of DM. Manifestations of DM in older adults may not include the classic symptoms of polyuria and thirst. Conditions such as orthostatic hypotension, periodontal disease, infections, stroke, slow gastric emptying (gastroparesis), impotence, neuropathy, confusion, and glaucoma should be considered potential indicators of DM (Eliopoulos, 2005), and may also increase the potential for complications from the disease or its treatment. Common problems in the older adult that make the diagnosis and management of DM more difficult are described in the following Nursing Care of the Older Adult box. The older adult with DM also has a longer recovery period after surgery or serious illness, often requiring insulin to maintain blood glucose levels. The benefits and risks of treatment to maintain glycemic control as well as blood pressure and lipid management must be carefully balanced.

Interdisciplinary Care

The results of a 10-year DM Control and Complications Trial (DCCT), sponsored by the National Institutes of Health (NIH), have significant implications for the management of type 1 DM. People in the study who kept their blood glucose levels close to normal by frequent monitoring, several daily insulin injections, and lifestyle changes that included exercise and a healthier diet reduced by 60% their risk for the development and progression of complications involving the eyes, the kidneys, and the nervous system. Treatment of the patient with DM focuses on maintaining blood glucose at levels as nearly normal as possible through medications, dietary management, and exercise.

Type 2 DM benefits from similar levels of control. Studies of patients with DM who have gastrointestinal surgery for morbid obesity show complete remission of type 2 DM in over 3⁄4 of the cases. Laparoscopic adjustable gastric banding (LAGB) and Roux-en-Y gastric bypass (RYGB) result in remarkable reductions in blood glucose levels and HgbA1C. RYGB, which alters gastrointestinal anatomy, improves insulin sensitivity and is associated with total remission of DM in a significant percentage of patients (Cummings & Flum, 2008; ADA, 2009).

Diagnosis

Diagnostic tests are conducted for screening purposes to diagnose DM, and ongoing laboratory tests are conducted to evaluate the effectiveness of diabetic management. Definitions of

---

NURSING CARE OF THE OLDER ADULT   Diabetes Mellitus

HEALTH PROBLEM/COMPLICATION	IMPLICATIONS FOR NURSING CARE
Urinary incontinence	Polyuria, a classic manifestation of DM, often is ignored. This problem also often leads to social isolation.
Decreased thirst	Polydipsia, a classic manifestation of DM, often is ignored. This further increases the risk of dehydration and electrolyte imbalances.
Decreased hunger and weight loss	Polyphagia, a classic manifestation of DM, often is ignored. The aging process, medications, depression, or lack of socialization may decrease hunger. Weight loss may be gradual and go unnoticed.
Fatigue and depression	Fatigue and depression are common symptoms of DM but may be blamed on increased age.
Hypoglycemia	The older adult may have either very mild manifestations or none at all, or there may be an inability to sense or respond to hypoglycemia. As a result, hypoglycemia is often ignored until it causes serious effects.
Peripheral neuropathy	Manifestations may be thought to be due to arthritis, and over-the-counter drugs often are used to self-medicate. The risk of falls increases, as does the risk of gangrene and amputation.
Peripheral vascular disease	May go undetected if the person does not get enough exercise to cause claudication. May also impair abilities to climb stairs and walk.
Diabetic retinopathy	May be undetected if the person has cataracts. Diabetic patients also have an increased incidence of cataracts and glaucoma. Deficits in vision threaten independence, mobility, and social interactions. Yellowing of the lens with age makes it difficult to read colored test strips; numeric meters are preferable. Filling insulin syringes may be impossible for the patient with macular degeneration or other causes of visual loss.
Hypertension	Treatment with diuretics may further impair glucose tolerance and result in electrolyte imbalances.
Persistent pain	Older adults may believe the pain from arthritis to be more important than the DM management. Also, depression from chronic pain as well as inactivity and loss of appetite may interfere with DM self-care.
Parkinson's disease	The tremors and rigidity of this disease make self-care involving fine and gross motor skills difficult or impossible.
Polypharmacy	Older adults commonly take more than one type of medication and are at increased risk for problems relating to drug interactions.
Cognitive impairment	Delirium or dementia can prevent the patient from communicating or performing self care.

normal blood glucose levels vary in clinical practice, depending on the laboratory that performs the assay.

DIAGNOSTIC SCREENING   Three diagnostic tests may be used to diagnose DM, and each must be confirmed, on a subsequent day, with one of the three tests. The diagnostic criteria recommended by the American Diabetes Association (ADA) (2009) are the following:

1. Manifestations of hyperglycemia (polyuria, polydipsia, and unexplained weight loss) and a casual plasma glucose (PG) concentration > 200 mg/dL (11.1 mmol/L). Causal is defined as any time of day without regard to time since last meal.
2. Fasting plasma glucose (FPG) > 126 mg/dL (7.0 mmol/L). Fasting is defined as no caloric intake for 8 hours.
3. Two-hour PG > 200 mg/dL (11.1 mmol/L) during an oral glucose tolerance test (OGTT). The test should be performed with a glucose load containing the equivalent of 75 anhydrous glucose dissolved in water. See Procedure 20–1 on the following page.

When using these criteria, the following levels are used for the FPG:

- Normal fasting glucose = 100 mg/dL (6.1 mmol/L)
- Impaired fasting glucose (IFG) = > 100 (6.1 mmol/L) and < 126 mg/dL (7.0 mmol/L)
- Diagnosis of DM = > 126 mg/dL (7.0 mmol/L)

When using these criteria, the following levels are used for the OGTT:

- Normal glucose tolerance = 2-hr PG: < 140 mg/dL (7.8 mmol/L)
- Impaired glucose tolerance (IGT) = 2-hr PG: ≥ 140 (7.8 mmol/L) and < 200 mg/dL (11.1 mmol/L)
- Diagnosis of DM = 2-hr PG: ≥ 200 mg/dL (11.1 mmol/L)

In addition, the ADA (2010) recommends measuring levels of glycosylated hemoglobin (A1C), with a level of 6.5% enough to make a diagnosis of diabetes. Levels of 5.7% to 6.49% indicate a high risk for developing both diabetes and cardiovascular disease, and are a marker for prediabetes.

Prediabetes   Prediabetes is a term used to describe people who are at increased risk of developing DM. Prediabetes is characterized by increased levels of A1C, increased fasting blood glucose (IFG), and impaired (IGT) plasma glucose. The results of these tests may not be high enough to be classified as DM. These test results indicate there is a risk for progression to DM, but it is not inevitable. Studies suggest that weight loss and increased physical activity may prevent or delay DM and may return blood glucose levels to normal. People with prediabetes are already at increased risk for other adverse health outcomes such as heart disease and stroke (ADA, 2009).

DIAGNOSTIC TESTS TO MONITOR DM MANAGEMENT   Diagnostic tests used to diagnose and monitor DM include a fasting blood glucose (FBG), an oral glucose tolerance test, and a glycosylated hemoglobin (A1C). Normal values for these tests as well as nursing implications are described in ∞ Chapter 18.

Other tests that may be used are urine tests for glucose, ketones, and albumin. Although not as accurate as blood tests, urine analysis for increased glucose and ketones indicate hyperglycemia. Urine tests for albumin are used to detect the early inset of kidney damage. Serum cholesterol and tyiglyceride levels, if elevated, indicate an increased risk of cardiovascular impairments.

Monitoring Blood Glucose

People with DM must monitor their condition daily by testing glucose levels. Two types of tests are available. The first type, long used prior to the development of devices to directly measure blood glucose, is urine testing for glucose and ketones. Urine testing is less commonly used today. The second type, direct measurement of blood glucose, is widely used in all types of healthcare settings and in the home.

URINE TESTING FOR KETONES AND GLUCOSE   Urine testing for glucose and ketones was at one time the only available method for evaluating the management of DM. An inexpensive, noninvasive, and painless test, it has unpredictable results and cannot be used to detect or measure hypoglycemia. In the healthy state, glucose is not present in the urine because insulin maintains serum glucose below the renal threshold of 180mg/dl. The accuracy of this measurement is not reliable in DM because the renal threshold may rise with aging or secondary to DM. Urine testing is recommended to monitor hyperglycemia and ketoacidosis in people with type 1 DM who have unexplained hyperglycemia during illness or pregnancy. Ketones may be detected through urine testing and reflect the presence of DKA. People who choose not to self-monitor blood glucose by other methods may use urine testing. (See Procedure 20–1.)

SELF-MONITORING OF BLOOD GLUCOSE   Self-monitoring of blood glucose (SMBG) allows the person with DM to monitor and achieve metabolic control and decrease the danger of hypoglycemia. The ADA recommends that all patients with DM be taught some method of monitoring glycemic control. The timing of SMBG is highly individualized, depending on the person's diagnosis, general disease control, and physical state. SMBG is recommended three or more times a day for patients with type 1 DM using multiple insulin injections or insulin pump therapy. Monitoring by patients with type 2 DM who are not using insulin should be sufficient to help them reach glucose goals. Postprandial blood glucose is often the most useful information for evaluating level of glycemic control in the type 2 DM patient (ADA, 2009). If patients only check their fasting glucose, they would be unaware of the postprandial results.

When adding or modifying therapy, patients with both types of DM should test more often than usual. SMBG is also useful when the person is ill or pregnant, or has manifestations of hypoglycemia or hyperglycemia. Both hypoglycemia and hyperglycemia may contribute to complications and decrease quality of life. With the information assessed with SMBG, patients can alter their diet, their physical activity, and even their medication to reduce the postprandial increases, reduce their risk for complications, and feel better because they are no longer experiencing wide swings in glucose levels (Pearson, 2009).

The ADA annually publishes a comprehensive list of currently available blood glucose monitoring machines and strips with approximate prices in *Diabetes Forecast*. Most medical insurance policies cover the cost of these machines and the test strips. Many companies provide a machine free of cost. Testing

PROCEDURE 20–1 Testing Urine for Ketones and Glucose

TO TEST THE URINE FOR KETONES

1. Ask the patient to void, discard the urine, and drink a full glass of water.
2. Thirty minutes later, collect a urine sample.
3. For acid test tablets: Place the tablet on a white paper towel, place one drop of urine on the tablet, and wait

30 seconds. If the tablet turns any shade from lavender to deep purple, the test is positive for ketones.

4. For Ketostix: Dip the reagent stick into the urine sample. Wait 15 seconds, and compare the color of the pad at the end of the stick to an accompanying color chart. Purple is indicative of ketones.

TO TEST THE URINE FOR GLUCOSE

1. Follow the same procedure to collect a urine sample.
2. Dip the reagent stick into the urine sample, and wait the time indicated. Compare the color of the pad on the end of

the reagent stick with an accompanying color chart. The glucose is expressed as a percentage (for example, 0.5%, 1%, 2%). Remember that normally no glucose is found in the urine, so the presence of glucose is an abnormal manifestation indicating hyperglycemia.

---

supplies are specific to each machine and this obligates the recipient to purchase supplies for that machine.

A new technology for continuous blood glucose monitoring (CGM) is available. The CGM has a sensor that is inserted under the skin. This sensor continuously sends data useful as a warning for high or low glucose levels. Finger-stick measurements are required before making therapy adjustments (McPhee & Papadakis, 2009). The CGM may be used for diagnostic evaluation; patients wear the pump for 3 days under the supervision of physicians and nurses. The data reveal patterns of glycemic control useful for treatment.

Following is the equipment needed for SMBG:

- Some type of lancet device to perform a finger-stick for obtaining a drop of blood (such as an Autolet, Penlet, or Soft Touch).
- Chemically impregnated test strips that change color when they come into contact with glucose or that can be read by machine (e.g., Glucostix and Chemstrip bG). The strip may also be read by comparing its color with a color chart on the side of the container or on an insert packed with the strips (Figure 20–3 ■).
- A blood glucose monitor (e.g., the Glucometer, the AccuChek, or the One Touch) if the most accurate measurement is desired

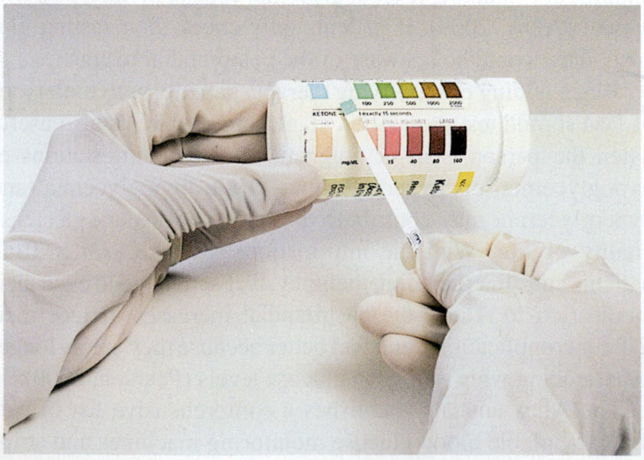

Figure 20–3 ■ Determination of blood glucose levels by visual reading. The color of the strip is compared with the color chart on the side of the container.

or recommended. The manufacturer's instructions must be followed carefully. If the timing of the blood on the strip is not exact, the test will not be accurate. In addition, the machine must be cleaned according to the manufacturer's directions to ensure accuracy. Monitors that use no-wipe technology improve the accuracy of glucose measurement. Other monitors are computerized and/or include a memory of previous glucose readings to show a pattern of control.

FACTORS THAT AFFECT GLUCOSE METER PERFORMANCE

According to the U.S. Food and Drug Administration (FDA), several factors affect the accuracy of blood glucose test results. The quality of the meter and test strips, and training to use the meter contribute to the degree of accuracy. Other factors can create falsely positive or negative readings.

Hematocrit Patients with higher hematocrit values will usually test falsely low in blood glucose and patients with lower hematocrit will test falsely higher. Anemia and sickle cell anemia are two conditions that can affect hematocrit values.

Other Substances Overdoses of many medications will cause inaccurate results. Meters and supplies vary in sensitivity to medications. Uric acid (a natural substance in the body that can be more concentrated in some people with DM), glutathione (an anti-oxidant also called GSH), and ascorbic acid (vitamin C) are known to interfere.

Using Correct Supplies and Sample Volume The test strips must be compatible with the glucose meter, are not outdated, or have been exposed to air and humidity, which can alter strip sensitivity. Insufficient amounts of blood on the testing strip causes inaccurate results. Although a meter may indicate a sufficient amount of blood on the test strip, it is best to observe that the recepticle is full of capillary blood. Yared, Aljaberi, Renouf, and Yale (2005) found that meters read significantly smaller than reference volumes and gave results varying 40% to 68% from the reference volume results. The erroneous results underestimated the true glucose value.

Medications

The pharmacologic treatment for DM depends on the type of DM. People with type 1 must have insulin; those with type 2 are usually able to control glucose levels with an oral hypoglycemic medication, but they may require insulin if control is inadequate or if they are subjected to a stressor, such as surgery.

INSULIN The person with type 1 DM requires a lifelong exogenous source of the insulin hormone to maintain life. Insulin is not a cure for DM; rather, it is a means of controlling hyperglycemia. Insulin is also necessary in other situations, such as the following:

- People who are unable to control glucose levels with oral antidiabetic drugs and/or diet
- People who are experiencing physical stress (such as an infection or surgery) or who are taking corticosteroids
- Women with gestational DM who are unable to control glucose with diet
- People with DKA or HHS
- People who are receiving high-calorie tube feedings or parenteral nutrition

Sources of Insulin Preparations of insulin are derived from animal (pork pancreas) or synthesized in the laboratory from either an alteration of pork insulin or recombinant DNA technology, using strains of *E. coli* to form biosynthetic human insulin. Insulin analogs have been developed by modifying the amino acid sequence of the insulin molecule. Although different types are prescribed on an individualized basis, it is standard practice to prescribe human insulin.

Insulin Preparations Insulins are available in rapid-acting, short-acting, intermediate-acting, and long-acting preparations. The trade names and times of onset, peak, and duration of action are listed in Table 20–2.

Insulin lispro (Humalog) is a human insulin analog that is derived from genetically altered *E. coli* that includes the gene for insulin lispro. It is classified as rapid-acting or ultra-short-acting insulin. Compared to regular insulin, lispro has a more rapid onset (< 15 minutes), an earlier peak of glucose lowering (30 to 60 minutes), and a shorter duration of activity (3 to 4 hours). This means that lispro should be administered within 15 minutes before a meal (rather than 30 to 60 minutes before as recommended for regular insulin). Patients with type 1 DM usually also require concurrent use of a longer-acting insulin product. Lispro is much less likely than regular insulin to cause tissue changes

and may lower the risk of nocturnal hypoglycemia in patients with type 1 DM.

Regular insulin is unmodified crystalline insulin, classified as a short-acting insulin. Regular insulin is clear in appearance and is the only insulin preparation that can be given by the IV route; the other types are suspensions and could be harmful if given by this route. Regular insulin is also used to treat DKA, to initiate treatment for newly diagnosed type 1 DM, and in combination with intermediate-acting insulins to provide better glucose control.

The onset, peak and duration of action of insulin can be changed by adding acetate buffers and protamine. Zinc and protamine are added to NPH insulin to prolong their action, and they are classified as intermediate- or long-acting insulins. These preparations appear cloudy when properly mixed prior to injection. Protamine and zinc are foreign substances and may cause hypersensitivity reactions. Insulin detemir, the newest long acting insulin (17–24 hours), is a clear insulin and must not be mixed with other insulins and cannot be used in insulin pumps. Doses may be administered once or twice daily. Insulin glargine (Lantus) is a 24-hour long-acting DNA human insulin analog that is given subcutaneously once or twice a day, usually at bedtime, to treat patients with both type 1 and type 2 DM. It has a relatively constant effect (meaning it does not have a peak time of effect). It is not recommended for use in pregnancy. Glargine should not be mixed with other insulins; the pH is incompatible (McPhee & Papadakis, 2009). Glargine cannot be used in insulin pumps.

SAFETY ALERT
Insulin glargine and insulin detemir are clear, unlike other intermediate or long-acting insulins. Do not mistake these for regular insulin. Do not mix with *any* other insulins. Do not inject IV, only subcutaneously.

Concentrations of Insulin Insulin is dispensed as 100 U/mL (U-100) and 500 U/mL (U-500) in the United States. U-100 is the standard insulin concentration used; there are 100 units of insulin in 1 mL. U-500 insulin is only used in rare cases of insulin resistance when patients require very large doses.

TABLE 20–2 Insulin Preparations

PREPARATION	NAME	ONSET (h)	PEAK (h)	DURATION (h)
Rapid acting	Lispro	0.25	1–1.5	3–4
	Aspart (NovoLog)	0.25	40–50 minutes	3–5
	Glulisine (Apidra)	0.25	1–1.5	3–5
Short acting	Regular (Novolin-R, Humulin-R)	0.5–1.0	2–3	4–6
Intermediate acting	NPH (Humulin (N) NPH	2	6–8	12–16
	detemir (Levemir)	(onset and peak not defined)		17–24
Long acting	glargine (Lantus)	(onset and peak not defined)		24
Combinations	Humulin 50/50	0.5	3	22–24
	Humulin 70/30	0.5	4–8	24
	Novolin 70/30	0.5	4–8	24

U-500 and the insulin analog lispro are the only insulins that require a prescription.

Insulin Administration   Nursing implications for administering insulin are outlined in the following Medication Administration box and further discussion follows in the chapter. The considerations for administering insulin include routes of administration, syringe and needle selection, preparing the injection, sites of injection, mixing insulins, and insulin regimens.

Routes of Administration   All insulins are given parenterally, although current research is investigating the development of a nasal spray and an oral preparation of insulin. Only regular insulin is given by both subcutaneous and IV routes; all others are given only subcutaneously. If the IV route is not available, regular insulin may also be administered IM in an emergency situation.

CONTINUOUS SUBCUTANEOUS INSULIN INFUSION Regular or rapid-acting insulins are used in continuous subcutaneous insulin infusion (CSII) devices, often called insulin pumps (e.g., MiniMed and Disetronic pumps). CSII devices have a small pump that holds a syringe of insulin, connected to a subcutaneous needle by tubing. The pump is about the size of a pager and can be worn on a belt or tucked into a pocket. The needle is placed in the skin, usually in the abdomen, and is changed every 3 days. This device delivers a constant amount of programmed insulin throughout each 24-hour period. It also can be used to deliver a bolus of insulin manually (e.g., before meals).

MEDICATION ADMINISTRATION   Insulin

Nursing Responsibilities
- Discard vials of insulin that have been open for several weeks or whose expiration date has passed.
- Refrigerate extra insulin vials not currently in use, but do not freeze them.
- Store insulin in a cool place, and avoid exposure to temperature extremes or sunlight.
- Store compatible mixtures of insulin for no longer than 1 month at room temperature or 3 months at 36°F to 46°F (2°C to 8°C).
- Discard any vials with discoloration, clumping, granules, or solid deposits on the sides.
- If breakfast is delayed, also delay the administration of rapid-acting insulin.
- Monitor and maintain a record of blood glucose readings 30 minutes before each meal and bedtime (or as prescribed).
- Monitor food intake, and notify the physician if food is not being consumed.
- Monitor electrolytes (especially potassium) and creatinine.
- Observe injection sites for manifestations of hypersensitivity, lipodystrophy, and lipoatrophy.
- If manifestations of hypoglycemia occur, confirm by testing blood glucose level, and administer an oral source of a fast-acting carbohydrate, such as juice, milk, or crackers. Hypoglycemic manifestations are described later under complications, but commonly include feelings of shakiness, hunger, and/or nervousness accompanied by sweating, tachycardia, or palpitations.
- If manifestations of hyperglycemia occur, confirm by testing blood glucose level, and notify the physician.

Health Education for the Patient and Family
- The manifestations of DM.
- Self-administration of insulin, with a return demonstration.
  a. Wash hands carefully.
  b. Have a vial of insulin, the insulin syringe with needle, and alcohol pads ready to use.
  c. Remove the cover from the needle.
  d. Fill the syringe with an amount of air equal to the number of units of insulin, and insert the needle into the vial.
  e. Push air into the vial, invert the vial, and withdraw the prescribed units of insulin.
  f. Replace the cover over the needle.
  g. Wipe the selected site with alcohol. The injection is less likely to be painful if the alcohol is allowed to dry.
  h. Pinch up a fold of skin, and insert the needle into the tissue at the recommended angle.
  i. Insert the insulin.
  j. Withdraw the needle; if desired, apply firm pressure to the site for a few seconds.
  k. Recap the needle. Many people with DM reuse disposable syringes with attached needles without adverse effects. The primary reason for discarding after several uses is that the needle becomes dull and makes the injection painful.
  l. Insulin pens may be more convenient to us. The dose is selected with a dial on the pen. Needles should be changed with each use and insulins, except commercially-mixed such as 70/30, cannot be mixed in a pen.
- Follow instructions for mixing insulins (refer to the box on page 542).
- Always keep an extra vial or cartridge of insulin available; refrigerate insulins not in use. Discard insulin pens kept at room temperature for current use at 28 days. Discard vials of insulin kept at room temperature for 30 days. Stored, refrigerated vials and cartridges should be discarded if their expiration date is exceeded.
- Always have a vial of regular insulin available for emergencies.
- Be aware of the signs of hypersensitivity responses, hypoglycemia, and hyperglycemia.
- Keep candy or a sugar source available at all times to treat hypoglycemia, if it occurs. Eat within 15 minutes of injecting rapid-acting insulins.
- Vision may be blurred during the first 6 to 8 weeks of insulin therapy; this is the result of fluid changes in the eye and should clear up in 8 weeks.
- Avoid alcoholic beverages, which may cause hypoglycemia.
- Follow these guidelines for sick days:
  a. Never omit insulin.
  b. Always monitor blood glucose and/or urine ketones at least every 2 to 4 hours.
  c. Always drink plenty of fluids, try to drink at least one glass of water or other calorie-free, caffeine-free liquid each hour.
  d. Get as much rest as possible.
  e. Contact the physician if there is persistent fever, vomiting, shortness of breath, severe pain in the abdomen, dehydration, loss of vision, chest pain, persistent diarrhea, blood glucose levels above 250, or ketones in the urine.
- Establish a plan for rotating injection sites, and observe closely for changes in tissues such as hardness, dimpling, or sunken areas.

CORRECTIONAL DOSES OF INSULIN Maintaining normal blood glucose prior to and during hospitalization decreases the risk of postoperative infections and shortens hospital stays. Healing is impaired when hemoglobin is glycosylated as glycosylated Hgb has an increased affinity for oxygen, putting tissues at risk for ischemia and decreases the effectiveness of white blood cells (increasing the risk of infection).

Treatment of hospitalized type 1 and type 2 patients requires a medication regimen that is responsive to glycemic changes secondary to the admitting condition and its treatment, including surgery (Braithwaite et al., 2007). People with type 2 DM may not be able to manage with oral medications during hospitalization because of the risk of hypoglycemia from not eating and the slow response of these medications to correct hyperglycemia. Researchers found significantly less mortality and significantly reduced acquired kidney injury when normal blood glucoses (80–110 mg/dl) were maintained by intensive insulin therapy (intravenous regular insulin) in surgical ICU patients; in critically ill surgical patients, blood glucoses should be kept close to 110 mg/dl and not exceed 140 mg/dl (ADA, 2009). It is recommended that critically ill patients maintain blood glucose levels equal to or < 140 mg/dl (ADA, 2009).

When hospitalized patients who are eating or have some source of oral intake experience periods of hyperglycemia outside the ICU, it is preferable to provide subcutaneous basal-prandial-correction therapy (Umpierrez et al., 2007).

The basal dose is a once or twice daily subcutaneous insulin such as insulin glargine (once daily) or NPH (twice daily). The prandial or mealtime dose is a portion of 1/2 the total daily dose of insulin. Correctional doses are combined with prandial doses, based on carbohydrate intake and are given postprandially. This method is employed to keep serum glucose below 180 mg/dl (ADA, 2009; Braithwaite et al., 2007). If the patient is requiring correction doses, the prandial dose needs to be increased until correction doses are eliminated. See Box 20–1 for methods to calculate basal, prandial, and correction doses for hospitalized patients on scheduled subcutaneous insulin doses and patients with insulin pumps.

Programming the amount of insulin to be delivered with a pump is determined by frequent blood glucose monitoring. Several different pumps are available, and each has rechargeable batteries, a syringe, a programmable computer, and a motor and drive mechanism. The rapid-acting insulin analog lispro is an appropriate insulin for insulin pumps, and short-acting regular insulin may also be used. Lispro is not approved for use in pregnancy.

Many people with DM believe the pump allows more normal regulation of blood glucose and provides greater lifestyle flexibility. Pumps are as safe as multiple-injection therapy when recommended procedures are followed. A potential complication is an undetected interruption in insulin delivery, which may result in a rapid onset of DKA. The needle site

BOX 20–1 Insulin Total Daily Dose (ITDD)

1. The total amount of insulin that the patient administered daily by injection (rapid- or short-acting with intermediate- or long-acting); for example, 48 units (30 units NPH and 18 units regular insulin).
   OR
2. 0.5–1 units/kg (normal kidney/liver function already on insulin) 48 units for 96-kg patient
   OR
3. 0.3–0.5 units/kg (reduced kidney/liver function or initial insulin therapy)
   Test blood glucose with test strip AC and HS.

Basal Dose: 40%–50% of the ITDD
1. Insulin pump. Multiply the ITDD by 50% ($48.0 \times 0.5 = 24$ units). The basal insulin pump dose for this patient is 24 units. Divide the basal insulin pump dose by 24 to get the hourly basal pump dose and rate ($24/24 = 1.0$ unit/hour). Use rapid-acting or regular insulin.
2. Subcutaneous Insulin. Multiply the ITDD by 50% ($48.0 \times 0.5 = 24$ units). This will be administered as one insulin glargine SQ injection daily or NPH injections of 12 units each twice daily. These basal doses are made with long-acting or intermediate-acting insulins.

Mealtime Bolus Dose
1. Insulin pump: To calculate bolus doses, take the remaining 50% of insulin and divide it by four doses according to the patient's meal plan for the day. For example, the remaining 50% could be divided thus: 20% at breakfast = 10 units; 10% at lunch = 5 units; 15% at dinner = 8 units, and 5% with a bedtime snack = 2 units.
   To calculate the units for each of these four daily bolus doses, multiply the percent of each meal bolus times the

total daily insulin pump dose. For example, for 48 units for a total daily dose:
Breakfast dose is 20% (or 0.2) $\times$ 48 units = 10 units
Lunch dose is 10% (or 0.1) $\times$ 48 units = 5 units
Dinner dose is 15% (or 0.15) $\times$ 48 units = 8 units
Bedtime snack dose is 5% (or 0.05) $\times$ 48 = 2 units (Nursing, 2005)
Correction doses may be needed if the patient is hyperglycemic.
2. Subcutaneous insulin mealtime dose: Divide half of the ITDD into three mealtime doses.
Breakfast = 8 units; Lunch = 8 units; Supper = 8 units. No bedtime dose is given.
Rapid-acting insulin (regular or aspart) is given in conjunction with the meal.

Mealtime Correction Dose
This is different from sliding scale dosing because it is given before hyperglycemia develops and with a scheduled insulin dose. It is given with rapid-acting insulin combined with the mealtime dose.
1. Test blood glucose prior to each meal.
   If blood glucose mg/dl is < 80 or symptomatic for hypoglycemia follow hypoglycemia protocol.

81–100	no correction dose needed
101–150	add 1 unit or 2 units if mealtime dose is > 20 units
151–200	add 2 units or 3 units if mealtime dose is > 20 units
201–250	add 3 units or 4 units if mealtime dose is > 20 units
251–300	add 4 units or 5 units if mealtime dose is > 20 units
> 300	add 5 units or 10 units if mealtime dose is > 20 units

Note: When correction doses are needed, the scheduled doses of rapid-acting insulin need to be re-ordered at higher doses.

must be kept clean and changed on a regular basis (usually every 2 to 3 days) to prevent inflammation and infection. Although the patient who chooses an insulin pump has more to learn, many are very satisfied with having more normal glucose control.

SYRINGE AND NEEDLE SELECTION   Insulin is administered by sterile, single-use needles and either disposable insulin syringes or a multiple dose insulin pen (Figure 20–4 ■), calibrated in units per milliliter. This means that in U-100 insulin, there are 100 U of insulin in 1 mL. Syringes for administering U-100 insulin can be purchased in either 0.3 mL (30 U), 0.5 mL (50 U), or 1.0 mL (100 U) size. The advantage of the 0.3 mL and 0.5 mL sizes is that the distance between unit markings is greater, making it easier to measure the dose accurately.

Most insulin syringes are manufactured with the needle permanently attached in a 25- to 27-gauge, 0.5-inch size. If this type of syringe is not available, an insulin syringe and a 25-gauge, 0.5-inch, or 0.75-inch needle should be used. Some hospitals and many patients are using insulin pens instead of insulin syringes to administer insulin. The pens, either reusable or disposable, contain prefilled cartridges of insulin; the desired dose is adjusted on the pen's dial prior to injection. A disposal needle is replaced for each injection and handling the needles creates a risk of needle sticks. Insulin types cannot be mixed in a pen; separate injections must be made if more than one type of insulin is needed (BDdiabetes.com).

Insulin pens are convenient to use, eliminating the need to carry an insulin vial and fill a syringe. The insulin in the cartridges is more stable than insulin packaged in vials. Cartridges in use should be stored at room temperature and must be discarded at 28 days. Cartridges not in current use may be stored in the refrigerator.

Other special injection products are available for people with physical handicaps. These products include automatic injectors and jet spray injectors. Prefilled syringes or pens are useful for people who are visually impaired or traveling. Prefilled syringes are stable for up to 30 days if stored in the refrigerator.

PREPARING THE INJECTION   The vial of insulin in use may be kept at room temperature for up to 4 weeks. Stored vials should be kept in the refrigerator and brought to room temperature prior to administration.

Regular insulin does not require mixing. If the solution is cloudy or discolored, the vial should be discarded. The other types of insulin must be mixed to disperse the particles evenly throughout the solution. Mix the vial by gently rolling it between the hands; vigorous shaking causes bubble formation, which makes the dose inaccurate. It is critical that no air bubbles remain in the prepared dose, because even a small bubble can displace several units of insulin.

SITES OF INJECTION   Although in theory any area of the body with subcutaneous tissue may be used for injections of insulin, certain sites are recommended (Figure 20–5 ■). The rate of absorption and peak of action of insulin differs according to the site. The site that allows the most rapid absorption is the abdomen, followed by the deltoid muscle, then the thigh, and then the hip. Because of the rapid absorption, the abdomen is the recommended site. See Box 20–2 for techniques to minimize painful injections.

When administering insulin, gently pinch a fold of skin and inject the needle at a 90-degree angle. If the person is very thin, a 45-degree angle may be required to avoid injecting into muscle. Aspiration to check for blood is not necessary. Do not massage the site after administering the injection, because this may interfere with absorption; rotation within sites is recommended. The distance between injections should be about 1 inch (avoiding the area within a 2-inch radius around the umbilicus). Insulin should not be injected into an area to be exercised (such as the thigh before a vigorous walk) or to which heat will be applied; exercise or heat may increase the rate of absorption and cause a more rapid onset and peak of action.

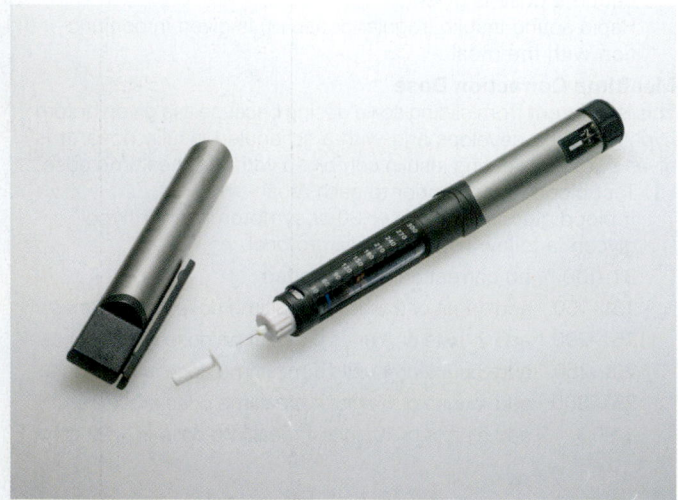

Figure 20–4 ■ Insulin pen with adjustable dose.

Source: Courtesy of Novo Nordisk Inc.

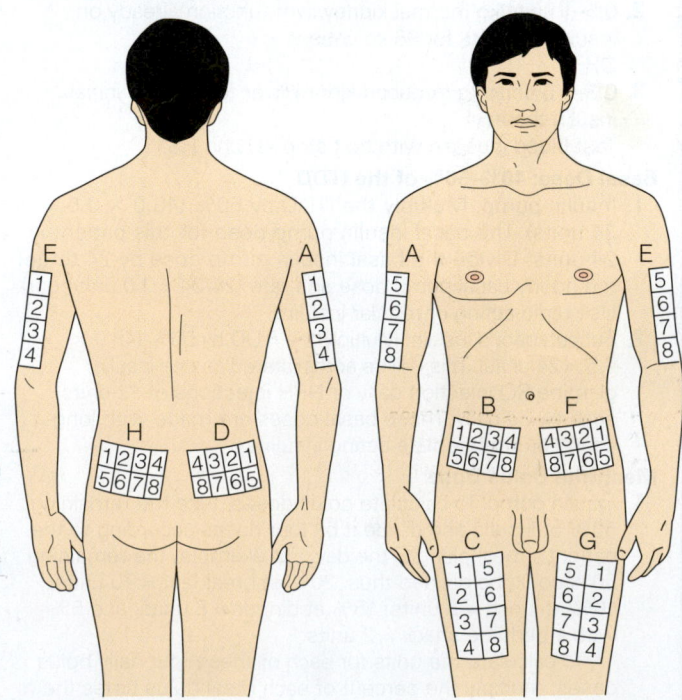

Figure 20–5 ■ Sites of insulin injection. The abdomen is the preferred site.

BOX 20–2 Techniques to Minimize Painful Injections

- Inject insulin that is at room temperature.
- Make sure no air bubbles remain in the syringe before the injection.
- Wait until alcohol on the skin completely dries before the injection.
- Relax muscles in the injection area.
- Penetrate the skin with the needle quickly.
- Don't change the direction of the needle during insertion or withdrawal.
- Don't reuse dull needles.

Note: Adapted from American Diabetes Association. (2004). Insulin administration. *DM Care, 27*(Supplement 1), S108.

Lipodystrophy   Lipodystrophy (hypertrophy of subcutaneous tissue) or lipoatrophy (atrophy of subcutaneous tissue) may result if the same injection sites are used repeatedly. The tissues become hardened and have an orange-peel appearance. The use of refrigerated insulin may trigger the development of tissue atrophy or hypertrophy. These problems rarely occur with the use of human insulins. Lipodystrophy and lipoatrophy alter insulin absorption, delaying its onset or retaining the insulin in the tissue for a period of time instead of allowing it to be absorbed into the body. Lipodystrophy usually resolves if the area is unused for a minimum of 6 months.

MIXING INSULINS   When a person with DM requires more than one type of insulin, mixing is recommended to avoid administering two injections per dose. Two different concentrations are administered, because a single dose of intermediate-acting or long-acting insulin rarely provides adequate control of blood glucose levels. The procedure for mixing insulins is described in Box 20–3. Following are some general guidelines:

- Commercially mixed insulins are recommended if the insulin ratio is appropriate for the requirements of the patient.
- Regular insulin may be mixed with all types of insulin except glargine and detemir; it may be injected immediately after mixing or stored for future use.
- NPH insulin and PZI insulin may be mixed only with regular insulin.
- Always withdraw regular insulin first to avoid contaminating the regular insulin with intermediate-acting insulin.

INSULIN REGIMENS   Individualizing the appropriate insulin dosage is achieved through a balance among insulin, diet, and exercise. For most people with DM, the timing of insulin action requires two or more injections each day, often a mixture of rapid-acting and intermediate-acting insulins. Timing of the injections depends on blood glucose levels, food consumption, exercise, and types of insulin used. The objective is to avoid daytime and nighttime hypoglycemia while achieving adequate blood glucose control. Typical insulin regimens are outlined in Table 20–3.

HYPERSENSITIVITY RESPONSES   When injected, insulin may cause local and systemic hypersensitivity responses. Manifestations of local reactions are a hardening and reddening of the area that develops over several hours. Local reactions result from a contaminant in the insulin and are more likely to occur when less purified insulin products are used.

Systemic reactions occur rapidly and are characterized by widespread red, intensely pruritic welts. Respiratory difficulty may occur. Systemic responses are due to an allergy to the insulin

BOX 20–3 Mixing Insulins: 10 Units of Regular and 20 Units of NPH

1. Wash hands.
2. Inspect regular insulin for clarity.
3. Gently rotate NPH insulin to mix well.
4. Wipe off the top of both vials with an alcohol pad.
5. Draw 20 U of air into the syringe, and inject air into the NPH vial (Figure *A*). Withdraw needle.
6. Draw 10 U of air into the syringe, and inject air into the regular vial (Figure *B*).
7. Invert the vial, and withdraw 10 U of regular insulin (Figure *C*). Withdraw the needle.
8. Insert the needle into the NPH vial, and carefully withdraw 20 U of NPH insulin (Figure *D*).
9. Don disposable gloves.
10. Administer the insulin.
11. Discard gloves, wash hands, and properly dispose of the syringe.
12. Document insulin administration.

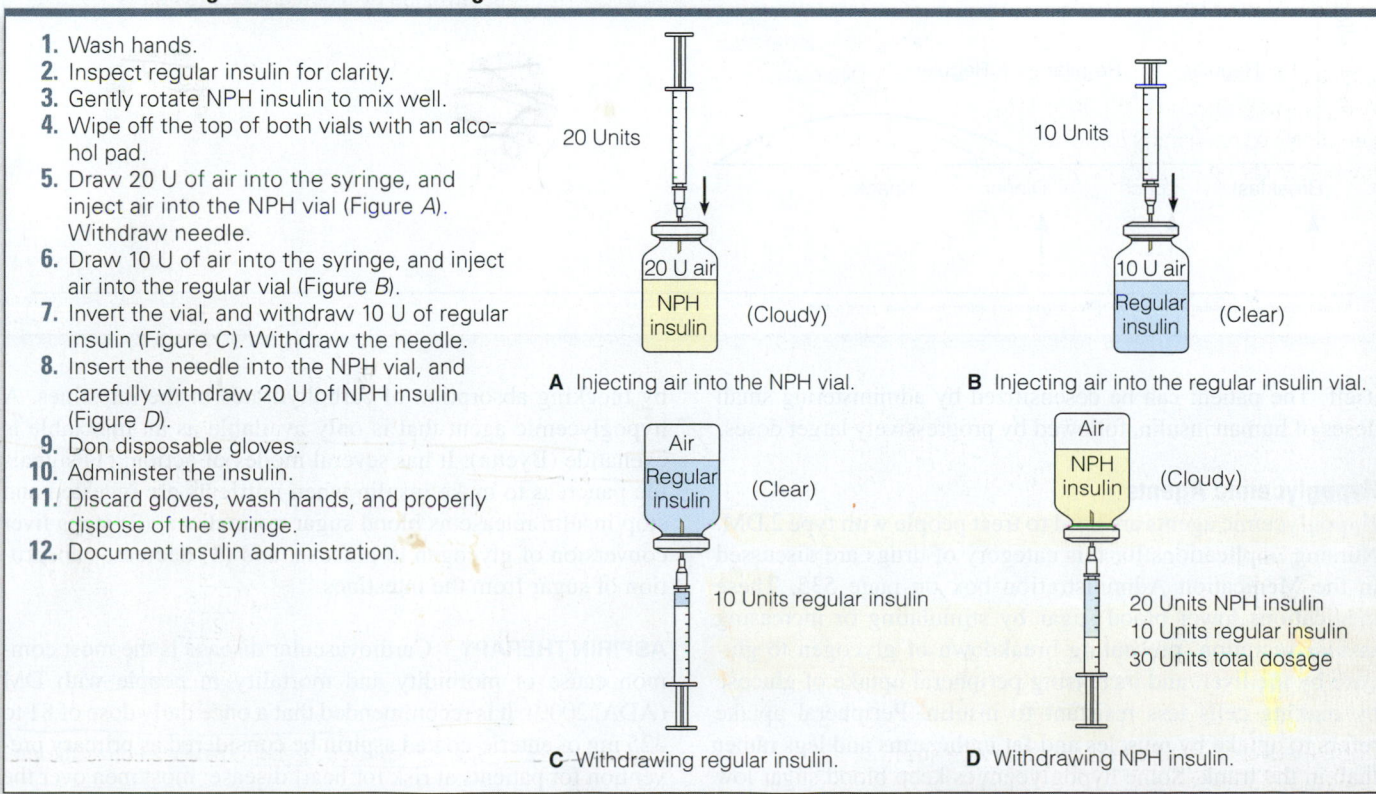

A   Injecting air into the NPH vial.

B   Injecting air into the regular insulin vial.

C   Withdrawing regular insulin.

D   Withdrawing NPH insulin.

TABLE 20–3 Insulin Regimens

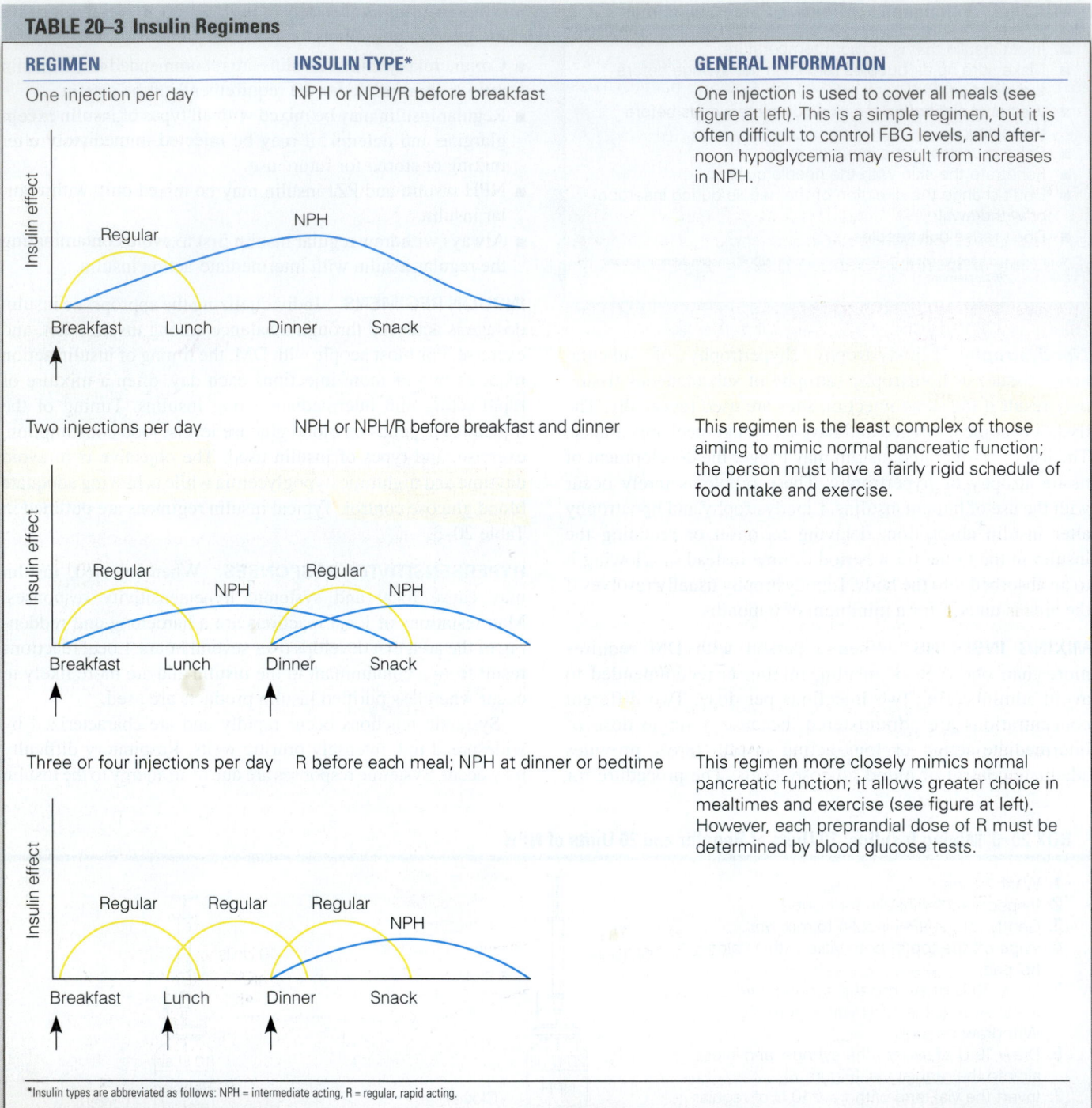

REGIMEN	INSULIN TYPE*	GENERAL INFORMATION
One injection per day	NPH or NPH/R before breakfast	One injection is used to cover all meals (see figure at left). This is a simple regimen, but it is often difficult to control FBG levels, and afternoon hypoglycemia may result from increases in NPH.
Two injections per day	NPH or NPH/R before breakfast and dinner	This regimen is the least complex of those aiming to mimic normal pancreatic function; the person must have a fairly rigid schedule of food intake and exercise.
Three or four injections per day	R before each meal; NPH at dinner or bedtime	This regimen more closely mimics normal pancreatic function; it allows greater choice in mealtimes and exercise (see figure at left). However, each preprandial dose of R must be determined by blood glucose tests.

*Insulin types are abbreviated as follows: NPH = intermediate acting, R = regular, rapid acting.

itself. The patient can be desensitized by administering small doses of human insulin, followed by progressively larger doses.

Hypoglycemic Agents

Hypoglycemic agents are used to treat people with type 2 DM. Nursing implications for this category of drugs are discussed in the Medication Administration box on page 535. These medications lower blood sugar by stimulating or increasing insulin secretion, preventing breakdown of glycogen to glucose by the liver, and increasing peripheral uptake of glucose by making cells less resistant to insulin. Peripheral uptake refers to uptake by muscles and fat in the arms and legs rather than in the trunk. Some hypoglycemics keep blood sugar low by blocking absorption of carbohydrates in the intestines. A hypoglycemic agent that is only available as an injectable is exenatide (Byetta). It has several modes of action: (1) signals the pancreas to make insulin when nutrients are ingested and stop insulin release as blood sugar normalizes, (2) stops liver conversion of glycogen to glucose, and (3) decreases absorption of sugar from the intestines.

ASPIRIN THERAPY Cardiovascular disease is the most common cause of morbidity and mortality in people with DM (ADA, 2009). It is recommended that a once daily dose of 81 to 325 mg of enteric-coated aspirin be considered as primary prevention for patients at risk for heart disease: most men over the age of 50 and most women over the age of 60 with at least one additional risk factor (family history of cardiovascular disease, smoking, hypertension, dyslipidemia, or albuminuria) (ADA, 2010). Aspirin therapy is contraindicated for patients with aspirin allergy, bleeding tendency, anticoagulant therapy, recent gastrointestinal bleeding, or active liver disease.

Nutrition

The management of DM requires a careful balance between the intake of nutrients, the expenditure of energy, and the dose and timing of insulin or oral antidiabetic agents. Although everyone has the same need for basic nutrition, the person with DM must eat a more structured diet to prevent hyperglycemia. The goals for dietary management for adults with DM, based on guidelines established by the ADA, are as follows:

- Achieve and maintain as near normal blood glucose levels as safely possible by balancing food intake with insulin or oral glucose.
- Achieve and maintain optimal serum lipid levels to reduce the risk of vascular disease.
- Achieve and maintain blood pressure levels in the normal range.

MEDICATION ADMINISTRATION Non-Insulin Hypoglycemic Agents

SULFONYLUREAS

Glimepiride (Amaryl)
Glipizide (Glucotrol, Glucotrol XL)
Glyburide (Diabeta, Micronase)
Tolazamide (Tolinase)
Tolbutamide (Orinase)

These drugs are used primarily to treat mild, nonketotic type 2 DM in people who are not obese. Glyburide, glipizide, and glimepiride are 100 to 200 times more potent than tolbutamide. These patients cannot control the manifestations by diet alone, but they do not require insulin. The drugs act by stimulating the pancreatic cells to secrete more insulin and by increasing the sensitivity of peripheral tissues to insulin. Dose adjustments must be made gradually and therefore these drugs are not useful for meeting acute changes that occur in illness or surgery. The most common side effect is hypoglycemia and this is exacerbated by NPO status. They are also associated with weight gain. These drugs are usually suspended during hospitalization (ADA, 2009).

MEGLITINIDES

Repaglinide (Prandin)

This drug lowers blood glucose levels by stimulating release of insulin from the pancreatic islet cells.

BIGUANIDES

Metformin (Glucophage)

Metformin reduces both the FBG and the degree of postprandial hyperglycemia in patients with type 2 DM. It primarily decreases the overproduction of glucose by the liver, and may also make insulin more effective in peripheral tissues. If renal insufficiency develops, metformin must be discontinued. It is used as an adjunct to diet, especially in patients who are obese or not responding to the sulfonylureas. Because of an increased risk of metformin-induced lactic acidosis, metformin is usually suspended during hospitalization. It should be discontinued temporarily before and for 48 hours after using intra-arterial iodinated contrast media for diagnostic imaging and anesthesia due to a small but significant risk of renal failure. In the Diabetes Prevention Program, some people treated with metformin reduced their risk of developing DM. An ADA panel recommends Metformin for prevention only for very-high-risk individuals (those with combined IGT and IFG, BMI > 35, and under 60 years of age with at least one other risk factor for DM). Lifestyle changes including diet and regular moderate exercise are part of preventing or delaying the onset of DM (ADA, 2009).

ALPHA-GLUCOSIDE INHIBITORS

Acarbose (Precose)
Miglitol (Glyset)

These drugs work locally in the small intestine to slow carbohydrate digestion and delay glucose absorption. As a result, postprandial glucose and glycosylated hemoglobin are better controlled, reducing the risk of long-term complications. They do not cause hypoglycemia but diminishing gastrointestinal side effects such as flatulence, diarrhea, and abdominal discomfort may occur.

D-PHENYLALANINE (AMINO ACID) DERIVATIVE

Nateglinide (Starlix)
Repaglinide (Prandin)

This is a new class of oral medications for treatment of type 2 DM. They stimulate rapid and short insulin secretion from the pancreatic beta cells to decrease spikes in glucose following meals and also reduce the overall blood glucose level. They should be taken shortly before meals; without a meal, hypoglycemia is a risk. Side effects may occur and diminish with nateglinide; these include nausea, vomiting, diarrhea, joint pain, and flu-like symptoms. Repaglinide is associated with temporary weight gain, diarrhea, and joint pain.

INCRETIN MIMETICS

Exenatide (Byetta) Injectable only

This medication signals the pancreas to make the right amount of insulin after meals to help lower blood sugar closer to normal levels. It limits liver conversion of glycogen to glucose, and slows the rate at which sugar enters the bloodstream, avoiding high blood sugar spikes.

DPP-4 INHIBITORS

Sitagliptin (Januvia)
Saxagliptin (Onglyza)

The enzyme DPP-4 degrades incretin hormones. Incretin is described in the discussion of exenatide and promotes insulin secretion. These drugs inhibit the DPP-IV enzyme, causing more stable glucose levels by decreasing liver release of glucose and increasing insulin secretion. Side effects may include headache, nasopharyngitis, and urinary tract infections; there may also be allergic-like reactions such as rash and hives. They are taken once daily in combination with diet and exercise.

SYNTHETIC AMYLIN HORMONE

Pramlintide (Symlin)

This medication is a synthetic form of Amylin, a hormone co-secreted with insulin from the B cells in the pancreas. It complements the role of insulin in limiting glucose levels by delaying gastric emptying and suppressing glucagon secretion after food intake. Patients with type 1 DM almost totally lack this hormone. It is used with insulin as a subcutaneous injection at mealtime for type 1 and type 2 DM and increases the risk of severe hypoglycemia.

Nursing Responsibilities

- Assess patients taking oral hypoglycemic agents closely for the first 7 days to determine therapeutic response.

(continued)

MEDICATION ADMINISTRATION   Non-Insulin Hypoglycemic Agents (continued)

- Administer the drug with food.
- Teach the patient the importance of maintaining a prescribed diet and exercise program.
- Monitor for hypoglycemia if the patient is also taking nonsteroidal anti-inflammatory agents (NSAIDs), sulfonamide antibiotics, ranitidine, cimetidine, or beta blockers; these drugs intensify the action of sulfonylureas.
- Monitor for hyperglycemia if the patient is also taking calcium channel blockers, oral contraceptives, glucocorticoids, phenothiazines, or thiazide diuretics; these drugs decrease the hypoglycemic responses to sulfonylureas.
- Do not administer these drugs to pregnant or lactating women.
- Assess for side effects: nausea, heartburn, diarrhea, dizziness, fever, headache, jaundice, skin rash, urticaria, photophobia, thrombocytopenia, leukopenia, or anemia.
- If the patient is to have a thyroid test, determine whether the drug has been taken; sulfonylureas interfere with the uptake of radioactive iodine.
- Monitor for hypoglycemia with concurrent administration of an oral antidiabetic agent and insulin.

- Temporarily hold metformin for 2 days prior to injection of any radiocontrast agent to avoid potential lactic acidosis if renal failure occurs.

Health Education for the Patient and Family
- Maintain prescribed diet and exercise regimen.
- You may need insulin if you have surgery, trauma, fever, or infection.
- Follow instructions to monitor blood glucose.
- Report illness or side effects to the healthcare provider.
- Undergo periodic laboratory evaluations as prescribed by your healthcare provider.
- Avoid alcohol intake, which may cause a reaction involving flushing, palpitations, and nausea.
- The medication interferes with the effectiveness of oral contraceptives; other birth control measures may be required.
- Mild manifestations of hyperglycemia may appear if a different agent is begun.
- Take medications as prescribed; for example, once a day at the same time each day. If you are taking acarbose, take the pill with the first bite of food at breakfast, lunch, and dinner.

- Prevent or at least slow the rate of development of chronic complications of DM by modifying nutrient intake and lifestyle.
- Prevent and treat the acute complications of insulin-treated DM, short-term illnesses, and exercise-related problems.
- Address individual nutrition needs, taking into account personal and cultural preferences and willingness to change.
- Maintain the pleasure of eating by only limiting food choices when indicated by scientific evidence (ADA, 2008).

CARBOHYDRATES The ADA recommends that carbohydrates should be individualized to the patient's needs, with recommended allowances of 45% to 65% of the daily diet. Carbohydrates contain 4 kcal per gram and intake should not be restricted to less than 130 g/day (ADA, 2008). This group of nutrients consists of plant foods (grains, fruits, vegetables), milk, and some dairy products. Carbohydrates can be divided into simple sugars and complex carbohydrates. Glycemic index is the rate a food raises blood glucose, and thus insulin. Proponents of low carbohydrate diets use the glycemic index as the scientific foundation for decreasing intake of foods with a high glycemic index. However, many factors effect the digestion of carbohydrates; to date research does not support using glycemic index as a basis for therapy.

The use of sucrose as part of the total carbohydrate content in the diet does not impair blood glucose control in people with DM. Sucrose and sucrose-containing foods must be substituted for other carbohydrates gram for gram. Dietary fructose (from fruits and vegetables or from fructose-sweetened foods) produces a smaller rise in plasma glucose than sucrose and most starches, so it may offer an advantage as a sweetening agent. However, large amounts of fructose have potentially adverse effects on serum cholesterol and LDL cholesterol, so amounts used should be controlled.

PROTEIN The recommended daily protein intake is 15% to 20% of total daily kcal intake. Protein has 4 kcal per gram. Sources of protein should be low in fat, low in saturated fat, and low in cholesterol. Although this amount of protein is much less than that which most people normally consume, it is recommended to help prevent or delay renal complications. To help the patient accept the decrease in the amount of protein, the nurse may suggest a less severe restriction at diagnosis with a gradual decrease to take place over a period of years.

FATS Dietary fats should be low in saturated fat, trans fatty acids, and cholesterol. Saturated and trans fatty acids are the principal dietary determinants of plasma LDL cholesterol. Saturated fats should be no higher than 10% of the total kcal allowed per day, intake of trans fatty acids should be minimal, and dietary cholesterol intake less than 300 mg per day. Fat has 9 kcal per gram. Sources of the different types of fat include the following:

- *Saturated fat.* Animal meats (butter fats, lard, bacon), cocoa butter, coconut oil, palm oil, and hydrogenated oils.
- *Polyunsaturated fat.* Oils of corn, safflower, sunflower, soybean, sesame seed, and cottonseed.
- *Trans fatty acids.* Partially hydrogenated vegetable oils such as shortenings and in animal fats. Trans fats lower HDL cholesterol and increase LDL cholesterol leading to coronary heart disease.
- *Monosaturated fat.* Peanut oil, olive oil, and canola oil.

Limiting fat and cholesterol intake may help prevent or delay the onset of atherosclerosis, a common complication of DM.

FIBER Dietary fiber may be helpful in treating or preventing constipation and other gastrointestinal disorders, including colon cancer. It also helps provide a feeling of fullness, and large amounts of soluble fiber may be beneficial to serum lipids. Soluble fiber is found in dried beans, oats, barley, and in some vegetables and fruits (e.g., peas, corn, zucchini, cauliflower, broccoli, prunes, pears, apples, bananas, oranges). Insoluble fiber, which is found in wheat, corn, and in some vegetables and fruits (e.g., carrots, brussels sprouts, eggplant, green beans, pears, apples, strawberries), does facilitate intestinal motility and give a feeling of fullness.

The ideal level of fiber has not been determined, but an intake of 14 g/1000 kcal per day is recommended (ADA, 2008). An increase in fiber may cause nausea, diarrhea or constipation, and increased flatulence, especially if the person does not also increase fluid intake. Fiber should be increased gradually.

SODIUM Although the body requires sodium, most people consume much more than is needed each day, especially in processed foods. The recommended daily intake is 1000 mg of sodium per 1000 kcal, not to exceed 3000 mg per day, with lower levels (1500 mg) for people with hypertension. The primary concern with sodium is its association with hypertension, a common health problem in people with DM. It is suggested that table salt (which is 40% sodium) and processed foods high in sodium be avoided in the DM meal plan.

SWEETENERS The diet plan for people with DM restricts the amount of refined sugars. As a result, many people use noncaloric sweeteners and foods or drinks made with noncaloric sweeteners. The Food and Drug Administration (FDA) has approved commercially produced nonnutritive sweeteners. Although questions have been raised about the safety of these substances in laboratory animal studies, they are considered safe for use by humans. Included in this category of sweeteners are saccharin (Sweet & Low), aspartame or neotame (NutraSweet, Equal), sucralose (Splenda), and acesulfame potassium (Sunnette). The nonnutritive sweeteners have negligible amounts of or no kilocalories, do not produce dental caries, and produce very little or no changes in blood glucose levels.

People with DM also use nutritive sweeteners, including fructose, sorbitol, and xylitol. The kcal content of these substances is similar to that of table sugar (sucrose), but they cause less elevation in blood glucose. They are often included in foods labeled as "sugar free." Sorbitol may cause flatulence and diarrhea.

Researchers are continuing to study the safety and effectiveness of the sweeteners. In addition, the FDA recommends that the food industry label products with the amount of each ingredient in milligrams per serving and the number of servings per container. When teaching patients about diet, the nurse should include information about the kilocalorie content of sweeteners and the meaning of such words as sugar free and dietetic on labels.

ALCOHOL Although drinking alcoholic beverages is not encouraged, neither is it totally prohibited for the patient with DM. Alcohol consumption may potentiate the hypoglycemic effects of insulin and oral agents. The ADA recommends that men with DM consume no more than two drinks and women with DM no more than one drink per day.

In the following list are guidelines for people who include alcohol in their diet plan.

- The signs of intoxication and hypoglycemia are similar; thus, the person with type 1 DM is at increased risk for an insulin reaction.
- Two oral hypoglycemic agents (chlorpropamide and tolbutamide) may interact with the alcohol, causing headache, flushing, and nausea.
- Liqueurs, sweet wines, wine coolers, and sweet mixes contain large amounts of carbohydrate.
- Light beer is the recommended alcoholic drink.
- Alcohol should be consumed with meals and added to the daily food intake. In most instances, the alcohol is substituted for fat in calculating the diet; a drink with 1.5 oz of alcohol is the equivalent of two fat exchanges (90 kcal). (Food exchanges are discussed next.)

MEAL PLANNING Several different systems for meal planning are available to the person with DM. These systems include a consistent-carbohydrate DM meal plan, exchange lists, point systems, food groups, carbohydrate counting, and calorie counting. No matter what system is used, however, it must take into account the person's individualized eating habits, diet history, food values, and special needs. Altering foods and meal patterns are often one of the most difficult parts of DM management; careful consideration of individualized preferences enhances compliance with the diet. Although the ADA recommends that a registered dietitian provide the nutrition prescription, nurses must know what is prescribed and be able to reinforce teaching and answer questions.

The Consistent-Carbohydrate DM Meal Plan The consistent-carbohydrate DM meal plan, which is replacing the traditional exchange list plan, focuses on carbohydrate content. The patient eats a similar amount of carbohydrates at each meal or snack each day, based on an individual diet prescription and the food guide pyramid. Carbohydrates in a meal have the most effect on postprandial (after meals) blood glucose levels. They also determine, to a greater extent than do proteins and fats, insulin requirements before meals. Patients should be taught to count carbohydrates so they can administer 1 unit of regular insulin or insulin lispro for each 10 or 15 g of carbohydrate eaten at a meal. This method provides a better connection between food, medications, and exercise.

The Exchange Lists The exchange list diet is based on the person's ideal (or reasonable) weight, activity level, age, and occupation. These factors determine the total kilocalories that the person may consume each day. After the calories have been determined, the proportions of carbohydrates, proteins, and fats are calculated, using guidelines established by the American Diabetes Association and the American Dietetic Association.

The distribution of foods throughout the day is based on exchange lists. The name and quantity of food that make up one exchange (or serving) are listed; standard household measurements are used. One food portion on the list can be substituted (exchanged) for another with very little difference in calories or amount of carbohydrates, proteins, and fats. The meal plan prescribes how many exchanges are allowed for each food group per meal and snacks.

Diet Plan for Type 1 DM   Diet and insulin prescription must be integrated for optimal energy metabolism and the prevention of hyperglycemia or hypoglycemia. The goals of the diet plan are to achieve optimal glucose and lipid levels, improve overall health, and maintain reasonable body weight. To meet these goals, the following strategies must be implemented:

■ Glucose regulation requires correlating eating patterns with insulin onset and peak of action.
■ Meals, snacks, and insulin regimens should be based on the person's lifestyle.
■ Meal planning depends on the specific insulin regimen prescribed.
■ Snacks are an important consideration in relation to the amount and timing of exercise.
■ The diet plan must consider the availability of foods, based on occupational, financial, religious, and ethnic constraints.
■ SMBG levels help the patient make adjustments for planned and unplanned changes in routines.

Diet Plan for Type 2 DM   The goals of the diet plan are to improve blood glucose levels, improve overall health, prevent or delay complications, and attain or maintain reasonable body weight. Because the majority of these patients are overweight, weight loss is important and facilitates achieving the other goals.

There are no specific guidelines for the type 2 diet, but in addition to decreasing kilocalories, it is recommended that the patient consume three meals of equal size, evenly spaced approximately 4 to 5 hours apart, with one or two snacks. The person with type 2 DM should also decrease fat intake. If the exchange list is difficult to use, calorie counting or designing the diet by grams of fat may be more useful.

SICK-DAY MANAGEMENT   When the person with DM is sick or has surgery, blood glucose levels increase, even though food intake decreases. The person often mistakenly alters or omits the insulin dose, causing further problems. The guidelines for dietary management during illness focus on preventing dehydration and providing nutrition for promoting recovery. In general, sick-day management includes the following:

■ Monitoring blood glucose at least four times a day throughout an illness
■ Testing urine for ketones if blood glucose is greater than 240 mg/dL
■ Continuing to take the usual insulin dose or oral hypoglycemic agent
■ Sipping 8 to 12 oz of fluid each hour
■ Substituting easily digested liquids or soft foods if solid foods are not tolerated (The substituted liquids and foods should be carbohydrate equivalents, for example, 1/2 cup sweetened gelatin, 1/2 cup fruit juice, one Popsicle, 1/4 cup sherbet, and 1/2 cup regular soft drink.)
■ Calling the healthcare provider if the patient is unable to eat for more than 24 hours or if vomiting and diarrhea last for more than 6 hours

DIET PLAN FOR THE OLDER ADULT   The majority of older adults with diabetes have type 2 DM and should follow the general guidelines for that diet plan. However, special considerations for the older adult are important if the diet plan is to be followed, including dietary likes and dislikes, changes in taste perception, dental health, available income, and who prepares the food. Other factors to consider in planning the diet for the older adult include the age-related decline in kcal requirements, decline in physical activity due to age and/or chronic illnesses, and the onset or progression of other chronic illnesses. The older adult who is overweight should reduce kcal intake to ensure weight loss, but at the same time, careful monitoring for malnutrition is necessary. It is possible for the older adult to revert to normal glucose tolerance if ideal body weight is regained.

Exercise

The third component of DM management is a regular exercise program consisting of at least 150 minutes per week (ADA, 2009). The benefits of exercise are the same for everyone, with or without DM: improved physical fitness, improved emotional state, weight control, and improved work capacity. In people with DM, exercise increases the uptake of glucose by muscle cells, potentially reducing the need for insulin. Exercise also decreases cholesterol and triglycerides, reducing the risk of cardiovascular disorders. People with DM should consult their primary healthcare provider before beginning or changing an exercise program. The ability to maintain an exercise program is affected by many different factors, including fatigue and glucose levels. It is as important to assess the person's usual lifestyle before establishing an exercise program as it is before planning a diet. Factors to consider include the patient's usual exercise habits, living environment, and community programs. The exercise that the person enjoys most is probably the one that he or she will continue throughout life. Use proper footwear, inspect the feet daily and after exercise, avoid exercise in extreme heat or cold, and avoid exercise during periods of poor glucose control.

TYPE 1 DM   In the person with type 1 DM, glycemic responses to exercise vary according to the type, intensity, and duration of the exercise. Other factors that influence responses include the timing of exercise in relation to meals and insulin injections, and the time of day of the activity. Unless these factors are integrated into the exercise program, the person with type 1 DM has an increased risk of hypoglycemia and hyperglycemia. Following are general guidelines for an exercise program.

■ People who have frequent hyperglycemia or hypoglycemia should avoid prolonged exercise until glucose control improves.
■ The risk of exercise-induced hypoglycemia is lowest before breakfast, when free-insulin levels tend to be lower than they are before meals later in the day or at bedtime.
■ Exercise should be moderate and regular; brief, intense exercise tends to cause mild hyperglycemia, and prolonged exercise can lead to hypoglycemia.
■ Exercising at a peak insulin action time may lead to hypoglycemia.
■ SMBG is essential both before and after exercise.
■ Food intake may need to be increased to compensate for the activity.
■ Fluid intake, especially water, is essential.

Young adults may continue participating in sports with some modifications in diet and insulin dosage. Athletes should begin training slowly, extend activity over a prolonged period, take a carbohydrate source (such as a drink consisting of 5% to 10% carbohydrate) after about 1 hour of exercise, and monitor blood glucose levels for possible adjustments. In addition, a snack should be available after the activity is completed. It may be necessary to omit the usual regular insulin dose prior to an athletic event; even if the athlete is hyperglycemic at the beginning of the event, blood glucose levels will fall to normal after the first 60 to 90 minutes of exercise.

TYPE 2 DM An exercise program for the person with type 2 DM is especially important. The benefits of regular exercise include weight loss in those who are overweight, improved glycemic control, increased well-being, socialization with others, and a reduction of cardiovascular risk factors. A combination of diet, exercise, and weight loss often decreases the need for oral hypoglycemic agents. This decrease is due to an increased sensitivity to insulin, increased kcal expenditure, and increased self-esteem. Regular exercise may prevent type 2 DM in high-risk individuals (ADA, 2009).

Following are general guidelines for an exercise program:

- Before beginning the program, have a medical screening for previously undiagnosed hypertension, neuropathy, retinopathy, and nephropathy.
- Begin the program with mild exercises, and gradually increase intensity and duration.
- Exercise at least 150 minutes a week in regular, shorter time sessions.
- Include resistance exercise (muscle-strengthening) and low-impact aerobic exercises in the program.

Treatments

SURGERY Surgical management of DM includes surgically revising the GI tract as well as replacing or transplanting the pancreas, pancreatic cells, or beta cells. Although it is still in the investigative stage, many researchers believe that transplantation of the tail of the pancreas is the most promising technique for achieving long-term disease control. Islet cell transplantation has had moderate success, and research is continuing. A diabetic patient can receive a portion of a pancreas from a living relative, often as part of a kidney transplant. The transplanted pancreas may protect the new kidney from damage. Transplants of more than one organ survive better than solo transplants (ADA, 2008). Other research is being conducted in the use of an internally implanted artificial pancreas, or closed-loop artificial beta cell.

Surgery is a stressor that often alters self-management and glycemic control in people with DM. In response to stress, levels of catecholamines, cortisol, glucagon, and growth hormones increase, as does insulin resistance. Hyperglycemia occurs, and protein stores are decreased. In addition, diet and activity patterns change, and medication types and dosages vary. As a result, surgical patients who have DM are at increased risk for postoperative infection, delayed wound healing, fluid and electrolyte imbalances, hyper- and hypoglycemia, and DKA (Loh-Trivedi & Rothenberg, 2008). Preoperatively, all patients should be in the best possible metabolic state. Screening for complications and regular blood glucose monitoring are part of preoperative preparation. Oral hypoglycemic agents may be withheld for 1 or 2 days before

surgery, and regular insulin is often administered to the patient with type 2 DM, and those with hyperglycemia but not diagnosed with DM, during the perioperative period. All patients with hyperglycemia whether diagnosed with DM or not follow a carefully prescribed insulin regimen individualized to specific needs.

The insulin regimen in the perioperative period is individualized. When the patient is NPO, short-acting insulin should not be given without intravenous glucose. Patients with type 1 DM and type 2 DM, and patients with hyperglycemia who are critically ill in the perioperative period should receive IV glucose and insulin infusion in an intensive care unit. The target blood glucose level during surgery is between 110 and 140 mg/dL. This avoids hypoglycemia, which is difficult to detect under anesthesia, and prevents glycosuria, dehydration, and impaired wound healing. IV infusion of glucose, insulin, and added potassium is appropriate for all hyperglycemic patients undergoing surgery (ADA, 2009).

The surgical procedure should be scheduled for as early as possible in the morning to minimize the length of fasting. If there is no food intake after surgery, intravenous dextrose should be administered, accompanied by subcutaneous regular insulin every 6 hours for the noncritically ill surgical patient. The dose can be adjusted to blood glucose levels. Although kcal intake is decreased postoperatively, stress can increase insulin requirements. Glucose control is also affected postoperatively by nausea and vomiting, anorexia, and gastrointestinal suction.

During the postoperative period, the patient with type 2 DM may continue to require insulin or may resume oral medications, depending on glucose control. The patient with type 1 DM may require reduced insulin as healing progresses and stress diminishes. Regular blood glucose monitoring is essential, as are assessments for hypoglycemia.

Complications of Diabetes Mellitus

The person with DM, regardless of type, is at increased risk for complications involving many different body systems. Alterations in blood glucose levels, alterations in the cardiovascular system, neuropathies, an increased susceptibility to infection, and periodontal disease are common. In addition, the interaction of several complications can cause problems of the feet. The Multisystem Effects of Diabetes Mellitus illustration on page 525 shows the progression from cardinal signs to acute and late complications for the patient with DM. A discussion of each of these complications follows; related interdisciplinary care and nursing care are discussed later in the chapter.

Acute Complications: Alterations in Blood Glucose Levels

The following discussion provides additional information about hyperglycemia and hypoglycemia. Table 20–4 compares DKA, HHS, and hypoglycemia.

HYPERGLYCEMIA The major problems resulting from hyperglycemia in the person with DM are DKA and HHS. Two other problems are the dawn phenomenon and the Somogyi phenomenon.

TABLE 20–4 DKA, HHS, and Hypoglycemia Compared

		DKA	HHS	HYPOGLYCEMIA
DM Type		Primary Type 1	Type 2	Both
Onset		Slow	Slow	Rapid
Cause		↓ Insulin	↓ Insulin	↑ Insulin
		Infection	Older age	Omitted meal/snack
				Error in insulin dose
Risk Factors		Surgery	Surgery	Surgery
		Trauma	Trauma	Trauma
		Illness	Illness	Illness
		Omitted insulin	Dehydration	Exercise
		Stress	Medications	Medications
			Dialysis	Lipodystrophy
			Hyperalimentation	Renal failure
				Alcohol intake
Assessments	Skin	Flushed; dry; warm	Flushed; dry; warm	Pallor; moist; cool
	Perspiration	None	None	Profuse
	Thirst	Increased	Increased	Normal
	Breath	Fruity	Normal	Normal
	Vital signs	BP ↓	BP ↓	BP ↓
		P ↑	P ↑	P ↑
		R Kussmaul's	R normal	R normal
	Mental status	Confused	Lethargic	Anxious; restless
	Thirst	Increased	Increased	Normal
	Fluid intake	Increased	Increased	Normal
	Gastrointestinal effects	Nausea/vomiting; abdominal pain	Nausea/vomiting; abdominal pain	Hunger
	Fluid loss	Moderate	Profound:	Normal
	Level of consciousness	Decreasing	Decreasing	Decreasing
	Energy level	Weak	Weak	Fatigue
	Other	Weight loss	Weight loss	Headache
		Blurred vision	Malaise	Altered vision
			Extreme thirst	Mood changes
			Seizures	Seizures
Laboratory Findings	Blood glucose	> 300 mg/dL	> 600 mg/dL	< 50 mg/dL
	Plasma ketones	Increased	Normal	Normal
	Urine glucose	Increased	Increased	Normal
	Urine ketones	Increased	Normal	Normal
	Serum potassium	Abnormal	Abnormal	Normal
	Serum sodium	Abnormal	Abnormal	Normal
	Serum chloride	Abnormal	Abnormal	Normal
	Plasma pH	< 7.3	Normal	Normal
	Osmolality	> 340 mOsm/L	> 340 mOsm/L	Normal
Treatment		Insulin	Insulin	Glucagon
		Intravenous fluids	Intravenous fluids	Rapid-acting carbohydrate
		Electrolytes	Electrolytes	Intravenous solution of 50% glucose

The dawn phenomenon is a rise in blood glucose between 4 AM and 8 AM that is not a response to hypoglycemia. This condition occurs in people with both type 1 and type 2 DM. The exact cause is unknown but is believed to be related to nocturnal increases in growth hormone, which decreases peripheral uptake of glucose. The Somogyi phenomenon is a combination of hypoglycemia during the night with a rebound morning rise in blood glucose to hyperglycemic levels. The hyperglycemia stimulates the counterregulatory hormones, which stimulate gluconeogenesis and glycogenolysis and also inhibit peripheral glucose use. This may cause insulin resistance for 12 to 48 hours.

Diabetic Ketoacidosis   As the pathophysiology of untreated type 1 DM continues, the insulin deficit causes fat stores to break down to provide energy, resulting in continued hyperglycemia and mobilization of fatty acids with a subsequent ketosis (see Figure 20–2). **Diabetic ketoacidosis (DKA)** develops when there is an absolute deficiency of insulin and an increase in the insulin counterregulatory hormones (cortisol). Glucose production by the liver increases, peripheral glucose use decreases, fat mobilization increases, and ketogenesis (ketone formation) is stimulated. Increased glucagon levels activate the gluconeogenic and ketogenic pathways in the liver.

In the presence of insulin deficiency, hepatic overproduction of beta-hydroxybutyrate and acetoacetic acids (ketone bodies) causes increased ketone concentrations and an increased release of free fatty acids. As a result of a loss of bicarbonate (which occurs when the ketone is formed), bicarbonate buffering does not occur, and a metabolic acidosis occurs, called DKA. Depression of the central nervous system (CNS) from the accumulation of ketones and the resulting acidosis may cause coma and death if left untreated (Porth & Matfin, 2009). The impact of DKA is illustrated in Figure 20–6 ■.

DKA also may occur in a person with diagnosed DM when energy requirements increase during physical or emotional stress. Stress states initiate the release of gluconeogenic hormones, resulting in the formation of carbohydrates from protein or fat. The person who is sick, has an infection (the most frequent cause of DKA), or who decreases or omits insulin doses is at a greatly increased risk for developing DKA.

DKA involves four metabolic problems:

- Hyperosmolarity from hyperglycemia and dehydration
- Metabolic acidosis from an accumulation of ketoacids
- Extracellular volume depletion from osmotic diuresis
- Electrolyte imbalances (such as loss of potassium and sodium) from osmotic diuresis

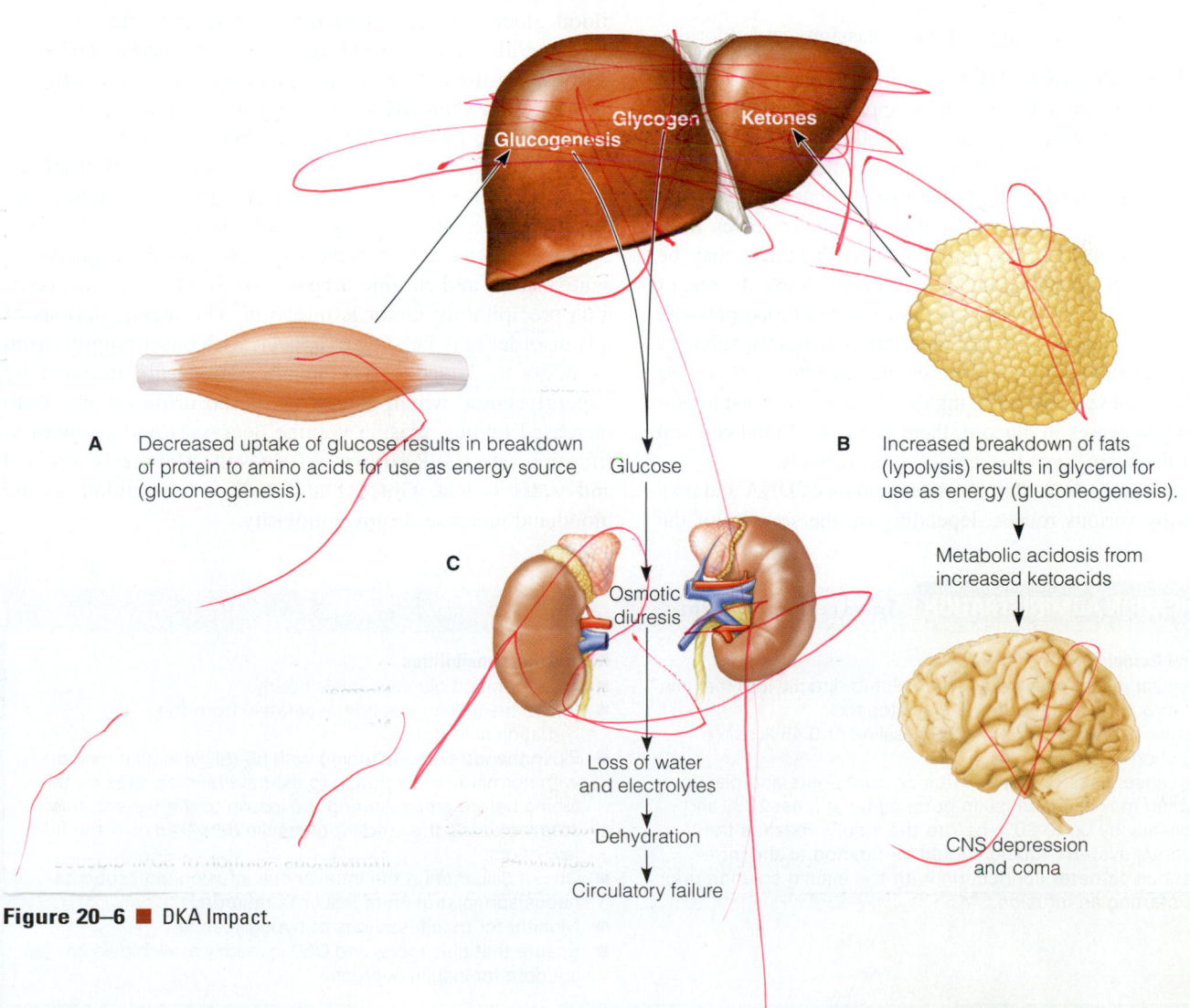

A Decreased uptake of glucose results in breakdown of protein to amino acids for use as energy source (gluconeogenesis).

Glucogenesis   Glycogen   Ketones

Glucose

B Increased breakdown of fats (lypolysis) results in glycerol for use as energy (gluconeogenesis).

C

Osmotic diuresis

Metabolic acidosis from increased ketoacids

Loss of water and electrolytes

Dehydration

Circulatory failure

CNS depression and coma

Figure 20–6 ■ DKA Impact.

MANIFESTATIONS of Diabetic Ketoacidosis (DKA)

DEHYDRATION (FROM HYPERGLYCEMIA)
- Thirst
- Warm, dry skin with poor turgor
- Soft eyeballs
- Dry mucous membranes
- Weakness
- Malaise
- Rapid, weak pulse
- Hypotension

METABOLIC ACIDOSIS (FROM KETOSIS)
- Nausea and vomiting
- Ketone (fruity, alcohol-like) breath odor
- Lethargy
- Coma

OTHER MANIFESTATIONS
- Abdominal pain (cause unknown)
- Kussmaul's respirations (increased rate and depth of respirations, with a longer expiration; a compensatory response to prevent a further decrease in pH)

Manifestations of DKA result from severe dehydration and acidosis. These manifestations are summarized in the box above. Laboratory findings include the following:

- Blood glucose levels higher than 250 mg/dL
- Plasma pH less than 7.3
- Plasma bicarbonate less than 15 mEq/L
- Presence of serum ketones
- Presence of urine ketones and glucose
- Abnormal levels of serum sodium, potassium, and chloride

TREATMENT OF DKA DKA requires immediate medical attention. Admission to the hospital is appropriate when the person has a blood glucose of greater than 250 mg/dL, a decreasing pH, and ketones in the urine. If the patient is alert and conscious, fluids may be replaced orally. In the first 12 hours of treatment, adults usually require 8–10 L of fluid to replace losses from polyuria and vomiting. The initial fluid replacement may be accomplished by administering 0.9% saline solution at a rate of 500 to 1000 mL/h. After 2 to 3 hours (or when blood pressure is returning to normal), the administration of 0.45% saline at 200 to 500 mL/h may continue for several more hours. When the blood glucose levels reach 250 mg/dL, dextrose is added to prevent rapid decreases in glucose; there is a risk of fatal cerebral edema if fluids are given too rapidly or excessively.

Regular insulin is used in the management of DKA and may be given by various routes, depending on the severity of the

condition. Mild ketosis may be treated with subcutaneous insulin, whereas severe ketosis requires intravenous insulin infusion. Nursing responsibilities for the patient receiving intravenous insulin are described in the following Medication Administration box.

When renal function and blood pressure are restored, potassium and sodium can be corrected. The electrolyte imbalance of primary concern is depletion of body stores of potassium. Initially, serum potassium levels may be normal, but they decrease during treatment. Insulin causes potassium to be shifted into the cells, increasing hypokalemia. In DKA (and from rehydration), the body loses potassium from increased urinary output, acidosis, catabolic state, and vomiting or diarrhea. Potassium replacement is begun early in the course of treatment, usually by adding potassium to the rehydration fluids. Replacement is essential for preventing cardiac dysrhythmias secondary to hypokalemia. Cardiac rhythms and potassium levels must be monitored every 2 to 4 hours.

Hyperosmolar Hyperglycemic State (HHS) The metabolic problem called **hyperosmolar hyperglycemic state (HHS)** occurs in people who have type 2 DM. HHS is characterized by a plasma osmolarity of 340 mOsm/L or greater (the normal range is 280 to 300 mOsm/L), greatly elevated blood glucose levels (over 600 mg/dL and often 1000 to 2000 mg/dL), and altered levels of consciousness. HHS is a serious, life-threatening medical emergency and has a higher mortality rate than DKA. Mortality is high not only because the metabolic changes are serious but also because people with DM are usually older and have other medical problems that either cause or are caused by HHS. The precipitating factors associated with HHS include infection, therapeutic agents that cause hyperglycemia, therapeutic procedures, acute illness, and chronic illness (Box 20–4). The most common precipitating factor is infection. The manifestations of this disorder may be slow to appear, with onset ranging from 24 hours to 2 weeks. The manifestations are initiated by hyperglycemia, which causes increased urine output. With increased output, plasma volume decreases and glomerular filtration rate (GFR) drops. As a result, glucose is retained and water is lost. Glucose and sodium accumulate in the blood and increase serum osmolarity.

MEDICATION ADMINISTRATION Intravenous Insulin

General Guidelines
- Regular insulin may be given undiluted directly into the vein or through a Y-tube or three-way stopcock.
- Insulin is usually diluted in 0.9% saline or 0.45% saline solution for infusion.
- Because glass or plastic infusion containers and plastic tubing may reduce insulin potency by at least 20% and possibly by up to 80% before the insulin reaches the venous system, tubing should be flushed to the intravenous catheter connection with the insulin solution prior to starting an infusion.

Nursing Responsibilities
- Monitor blood glucose levels hourly.
- Infuse the insulin solution separately from the hydration solution.
- Flush the intravenous tubing with 50 mL of insulin mixed with normal saline solution to saturate binding sites on the tubing before administering the insulin to the patient; this step increases the amount of insulin delivered over the first few hours.
- Do not discontinue the intravenous infusion until subcutaneous administration of insulin is resumed.
- Monitor for manifestations of hypoglycemia.
- Ensure that glucagons and D50 is readily available as an antidote for insulin overdose.

BOX 20–4 Factors Associated with Hyperosmolar Hyperglycemic State (HHS)

Therapeutic Agents
- Glucocorticoids
- Diuretics
- Beta-adrenergic blocking agents
- Immunosuppressants
- Chlorpromazine
- Diazoxide

Therapeutic Procedures
- Peritoneal dialysis
- Hemodialysis
- Hyperosmolar alimentation (oral or parenteral)
- Surgery

Acute Illness
- Infection
- Gangrene
- Urinary infection
- Burns
- Gastrointestinal bleeding
- Myocardial infarction
- Pancreatitis
- Stroke

Chronic Illness
- Renal disease
- Cardiac disease
- Hypertension
- Previous stroke
- Alcoholism

Serum hyperosmolarity results in severe dehydration, reducing intracellular water in all tissues, including the brain. The person has dry skin and mucous membranes, extreme thirst, and altered levels of consciousness (progressing from lethargy to coma). Neurologic deficits may include hyperthermia, motor and sensory impairment, positive Babinski's sign, and seizures. Metabolic acidosis is not part of the pathology; despite elevated blood glucose, sufficient insulin is present to prevent metabolism of fats with the resulting fatty acids and ketones of DKA. Treatment is directed toward correcting fluid and electrolyte imbalances, lowering blood glucose levels with insulin, and treating underlying conditions.

TREATMENT OF HHS HHS is a serious, life-threatening metabolic condition. The patient admitted to the intensive care unit for treatment typically manifests blood glucose levels over 700 mg/dL, increased serum osmolarity, and altered levels of consciousness or seizures. Treatment is similar to that of DKA: correcting fluid and electrolyte imbalances and providing insulin to lower hyperglycemia. In general, treatment modalities include the following:

- Establishing and maintaining adequate ventilation
- Correcting shock with adequate intravenous fluids
- Instituting nasogastric suction if comatose to prevent aspiration
- Maintaining fluid volume with intravenous isotonic or colloid solutions
- Administering potassium intravenously to replace losses
- Administering insulin to reduce blood glucose, usually discontinuing administration when blood glucose levels reach 250 mg/dL (Because ketosis is not present, there is no need to continue insulin, as with DKA.)

Hypoglycemia

Hypoglycemia (low blood glucose levels) is common in people with type 1 DM and occasionally occurs in people with type 2 DM who are treated with certain oral hypoglycemic agents. This condition is often called insulin shock, insulin reaction, or "the lows" in patients with type 1 DM. Hypoglycemia results primarily from a mismatch between insulin intake (e.g., an error in insulin dose), physical activity, and lack of carbohydrate availability (e.g., omitting a meal). The intake of alcohol and drugs such as chloramphenicol (Chloromycetin), Coumadin, monoamine oxidase (MAO) inhibitors, probenecid (Benemid), salicylates, and sulfonamides can also cause hypoglycemia.

The manifestations of hypoglycemia (see the following box) result from a compensatory autonomic nervous system (ANS) response and from impaired cerebral function due to a decrease in glucose available for use by the brain. The manifestations vary, particularly in older adults. The onset is sudden, and blood glucose is usually less than 45 to 60 mg/dL. Severe hypoglycemia may cause death.

People who have type 1 DM for 4 or 5 years fail to secrete glucagon in response to a decrease in blood glucose. They then depend on epinephrine to serve as a counterregulatory response to hypoglycemia. However, this compensatory response can become absent or blunted. The person then develops a syndrome called hypoglycemia unawareness. The person does not experience manifestations of hypoglycemia, even though it is present. Because treatment is not initiated in the absence of manifestations, the person is likely to have episodes of severe hypoglycemia.

TREATMENT OF HYPOGLYCEMIA

Mild Hypoglycemia When mild hypoglycemia occurs, immediate treatment is necessary. People experiencing hypoglycemia should take about 15 g of a rapid-acting sugar. This amount of sugar is found, for example, in three glucose tablets, 1/2 cup (4 ounces) of fruit juice or regular soda, 8 oz of skim milk, five Life Savers candies, three large marshmallows, or 3 tsp of sugar or honey. Sugar should not be added to fruit juice. Adding sugar to the fruit sugar already in the juice could cause a rapid rise in blood glucose, with persistent hyperglycemia.

MANIFESTATIONS of Hypoglycemia

MANIFESTATIONS CAUSED BY RESPONSES OF THE AUTONOMIC NERVOUS SYSTEM
- Hunger
- Nausea
- Anxiety
- Pale, cool skin
- Sweating
- Shakiness
- Irritability
- Rapid pulse
- Hypotension

MANIFESTATIONS CAUSED BY IMPAIRED CEREBRAL FUNCTION
- Strange or unusual feelings
- Headache
- Difficulty in thinking
- Inability to concentrate
- Change in emotional behavior
- Slurred speech
- Blurred vision
- Decreasing levels of consciousness
- Seizures
- Coma

If the manifestations continue, the 15/15 rule should be followed: Wait 15 minutes, monitor blood glucose, and, if it is low, eat another 15 g of carbohydrate. This procedure can be repeated until blood glucose levels return to normal (McPhee & Papadakis, 2009). BG should be tested 1 hour after the BG has reached ≥ 70 mg/dl because BG levels will start to fall again after 1 hour (Anthony, 2007). People with DM should have some source of carbohydrate readily available at all times so that hypoglycemic manifestations can be quickly reversed. If hypoglycemia occurs more than two or three times a week, the DM management plan should be adjusted.

Severe Hypoglycemia People with DM who have severe hypoglycemia are often hospitalized. The criteria for hospitalization are one or more of the following:

- Blood glucose is less than 50 mg/dL, and the prompt treatment of hypoglycemia has not resulted in recovery of sensorium.
- The patient has coma, seizures, or altered behavior.
- The hypoglycemia has been treated, but a responsible adult cannot be with the patient for the following 12 hours.
- The hypoglycemia was caused by a sulfonylurea drug.

If the patient is conscious and alert, 10 to 15 g of an oral carbohydrate may be given. If the patient has altered levels of consciousness, parenteral glucose or glucagon is administered. Glucose is administered intravenously as a 50 ml of 50% (D50) solution, usually at a rate of 10 mL over 1 minute by intravenous push (McPhee & Papadakis, 2009). This is the most rapid method of increasing blood glucose levels.

Glucagon is an antihypoglycemic agent that raises blood glucose by promoting the conversion of hepatic glycogen to glucose. It is used in severe insulin-induced hypoglycemia and may be given in the recommended dose of 1 mg by the subcutaneous, intramuscular, or intravenous route. Glucagon has a short period of action; an oral (if the patient is conscious) or intravenous carbohydrate should be administered following the glucagon to prevent a recurrence of hypoglycemia. If the patient has been unconscious, glucagon may cause vomiting when consciousness returns.

Chronic Complications

Alterations in the Cardiovascular System

The macrocirculation (large blood vessels) in people with DM undergoes changes due to atherosclerosis; abnormalities in platelets, red blood cells and clotting factors; and changes in arterial walls. It has been established that atherosclerosis has an increased incidence and earlier age of onset in people with DM (although the reason is unknown). Other risk factors that contribute to the development of macrovascular disease of DM are hypertension, hyperlipidemia, cigarette smoking, and obesity. Alterations in the vascular system increase the risk of the long-term complications of coronary artery disease, cerebral vascular disease, and peripheral vascular disease.

Alterations in the microcirculation in the person with DM involve structural defects in the basement membrane of smaller blood vessels and capillaries. (The basement membrane is the structure that supports and serves as the boundary around the space occupied by epithelial cells.) These defects cause the capillary basement membrane to thicken, eventually resulting in decreased tissue perfusion. The effects of alterations in the microcirculation affect all body tissues but are seen primarily in the eyes and the kidneys.

CORONARY ARTERY DISEASE Coronary artery disease is a major risk factor in the development of myocardial infarction in people with DM, especially in the middle to older adult with type 2 DM. Coronary artery disease is the most common cause of death in people with type 2 DM (McPhee & Papadakis, 2009). People with DM who have myocardial infarction are more prone to develop congestive heart failure as a complication of the infarction and are also less likely to survive in the period immediately following the infarction. (Myocardial infarction is discussed in ∞ Chapter 30.)

HYPERTENSION Hypertension is a common complication of DM. It affects 75% of all people with DM, and is a major risk factor for cardiovascular disease and microvascular complications such as retinopathy and nephropathy. Hypertension may be reduced by weight loss, exercise, and decreasing sodium intake and alcohol consumption. If these methods are not effective, treatment with antihypertensive medications is necessary.

STROKE (CEREBROVASCULAR ACCIDENT) People with DM, especially older adults with type 2 DM, are two to four times more likely to have a stroke (CDC, 2007). Although the exact relationship between DM and cerebral vascular disease is unknown, hypertension (a risk factor for stroke) is a common health problem in those who have DM. In addition, atherosclerosis of the cerebral vessels develops at an earlier age and is more extensive in people with DM (Porth & Matfin, 2009).

The manifestations of impaired cerebral circulation (∞ see Chapter 42) are often similar to those of hypoglycemia or HHS: blurred vision, slurred speech, weakness, and dizziness. People with these manifestations have potentially life-threatening health problems and require medical attention.

Peripheral Vascular Disease

Peripheral vascular disease of the lower extremities accompanies both types of DM, but the incidence is greater in people with type 2 DM. Atherosclerosis of vessels in the legs of people with DM begins at an earlier age, advances more rapidly, and is equally common in both men and women. Impaired peripheral vascular circulation leads to peripheral vascular insufficiency with intermittent claudication (pain) in the lower legs and ulcerations of the feet. Occlusion and thrombosis of large vessels and small arteries and arterioles, as well as alterations in neurologic function and infection, result in gangrene (necrosis, or the death of tissue). Gangrene from DM is the most common cause of nontraumatic amputations of the lower leg. In people with DM, dry gangrene is most common, manifested by cold, dry, shriveled, and black tissues of the toes and feet. The gangrene usually begins in the toes and moves proximally into the foot.

DIABETIC RETINOPATHY Diabetic retinopathy is the name for the changes in the retina that occur in the person with DM. The retinal capillary structure undergoes alterations in blood flow, leading to retinal ischemia and a breakdown in the blood-retinal barrier. Diabetic retinopathy is the leading cause of blindness in people between ages 20 and 74 (CDC, 2007).

After 20 years of DM, almost all patients with type 1 DM and more than 60% of patients with type 2 DM will have some degree of retinopathy, in most cases without vision loss (Porth& Matfin, 2009). If exudate, edema, hemorrhage, or ischemia occurs near the fovea, the person experiences visual impairment at any stage. In addition, the person with DM is at increased risk for developing cataracts (opacity of the lens) as a result of increased glucose levels within the lens itself. Screening for retinopathy is important, as laser photo-coagulation surgery has proven beneficial in preventing loss of vision.

DIABETIC NEPHROPATHY   Diabetic nephropathy is a disease of the kidneys characterized by the presence of albumin in the urine, hypertension, edema, and progressive renal insufficiency. This disorder accounts for 44% of new cases of end stage renal disease; 40% of patients requiring dialysis or transplantation in the United States have DM (Porth & Matfin, 2009). Nephropathy occurs in 30%–40% of people with type 1 DM and 15%–20% of those with type 2 (McPhee & Papadakis, 2009).

Despite research, the exact pathologic origin of diabetic nephropathy is unknown, but it is known that thickening of the basement membrane of the glomeruli eventually impairs renal function. It is suggested that an increased intracellular concentration of glucose supports the formation of abnormal gly-coproteins in the basement membrane and mesangium. The accumulation of these large proteins stimulates glomerulosclerosis (fibrosis of the glomerular tissue). Glomerulosclerosis thickens the basement membrane and simultaneously makes it functionally leaky, allowing large molecules such as protein to be lost in the urine. Kimmelstiel-Wilson syndrome is a type of glomerulosclerosis found only in people with DM. In advanced nephropathy, tubular atrophy occurs, and end-stage renal disease results. (Renal failure is discussed in ∞ Chapter 28.)

The first indication of nephropathy is microalbuminuria, an abnormal level of albumin in the urine. Without specific interventions, people with type 1 DM with sustained micro-albuminuria will develop nephropathy, accompanied by hypertension, over a period of 10 to 15 years. People with type 2 DM often have microalbuminuria and nephropathy shortly after diagnosis, because the DM has often been present but undiagnosed for many years. Because the hypertension accelerates the progress of diabetic nephropathy, aggressive antihypertensive management should be instituted. Management includes control of hypertension with ACE inhibitors such as captopril (Capoten), weight loss, reduced salt intake, and exercise.

Alterations in the Peripheral and Autonomic Nervous Systems

Peripheral and visceral neuropathies are disorders of the peripheral nerves and the autonomic nervous system. In people with DM, these disorders are often called diabetic neuropathies The etiology of diabetic neuropathies involves (1) a thickening of the walls of the blood vessels that supply nerves, causing a decrease in nutrients; (2) demyelination of the Schwann cells that surround and insulate nerves, slowing nerve conduction; and (3) the formation and accumulation of sorbitol within the Schwann cells, impairing nerve conduction. The manifestations depend on the locations of the lesions.

The peripheral neuropathies (also called *somatic neuropathies*) include polyneuropathies and mononeuropathies. *Polyneuropathies*, the most common type of neuropathy associated with DM, are bilateral sensory disorders. The manifestations appear first in the toes and feet and progress upward. The fingers and hands may also be involved, but usually only in later stages of DM. The manifestations of polyneuropathy depend on the nerve fibers involved. The lack of sensation prevents awareness of injury and for this reason, people with diabetes must be taught to visually inspect their feet and legs daily, looking for evidence of injury.

The person with polyneuropathy commonly has distal paresthesias (a change in sensation, such as numbness or tingling); pain described as aching, burning, or shooting; and feelings of cold feet. Other manifestations may include impaired sensations of pain, light touch, two-point discrimination, and vibration. There is no specific treatment for polyneuropathy.

Mononeuropathies are isolated peripheral neuropathies that affect a single nerve. Depending on the nerve involved, manifestations may include the following:

- Palsy of the third cranial (oculomotor) nerve, with headache, eye pain, and an inability to move the eye up, down, or medially
- Radiculopathy, with pain over a dermatome and loss of cutaneous sensation, most often located in the chest
- Diabetic femoral neuropathy, with motor and sensory deficits (pain, weakness, areflexia) in the anterior thigh and medial calf
- Entrapment or compression of the medial nerve at the wrist, resulting in carpal tunnel syndrome with pain and weakness of the hand; the ulnar nerve at the elbow, with weakness and loss of sensation over the palmar surface of the fourth and fifth fingers; and the peroneal nerve at the head of the fibula, with foot drop.

VISCERAL NEUROPATHIES   The visceral neuropathies (also called autonomic neuropathies) cause various manifestations, depending on the area of the ANS involved. These neuropathies may include the following:

- Sweating dysfunction, with an absence of sweating (anhidrosis) on the hands and feet and increased sweating on the face or trunk
- Abnormal pupillary function, most commonly seen as constricted pupils that dilate slowly in the dark
- Cardiovascular dysfunction, resulting in such abnormalities as a fixed cardiac rate that does not change with exercise, postural hypotension, and a failure to increase cardiac output or vascular tone with exercise
- Gastrointestinal dysfunction, with changes in upper GI motility (**gastroparesis**) resulting in dysphagia, anorexia, heartburn, nausea, and vomiting and altered blood glucose control. Constipation is one of the most common GI manifestations associated with DM, possibly a result of hypomotility of the bowel. Diabetic diarrhea is not as common, but it does occur and is often associated with fecal incontinence during sleep due to a defect in internal sphincter function.

- Genitourinary dysfunction, resulting in changes in bladder function and sexual function. Bladder function changes include an inability to empty the bladder completely, loss of sensation of bladder fullness, and an increased risk of urinary tract infections. Sexual dysfunctions in men include ejaculatory changes and impotence. Sexual dysfunctions in women include changes in arousal patterns, vaginal lubrication, and orgasm. Alterations in sexual function in people with DM are the result of both neurologic and vascular changes.

MOOD ALTERATIONS Persons with DM, both type 1 and type 2, endure the chronic strains of living with complex self-care and are at increased risk for depression and DM-specific emotional distress. Major depression and depressive symptoms affect 20% of people with DM making it twice as prevalent among people with DM as among the general population (Weinger, 2007). Depression affects the ability to self manage DM; depressed patients tend to forget to take their medications or run out of medications because they forget to refill their prescriptions in a timely manner. Treating depression has been associated with better control of serum glucose so screening for depression is an important part of assessing the individual's ability to manage the disease. Tests to identify the scope of depression are available (ADA, 2009; Weinger, 2007).

Interventions to help patients with depression include antidepressant medications and psychotherapy focused on restoring logical thinking and problem solving skills. But treating the depression alone does not improve self-management. Stress management programs and self-management of DM education are positively correlated with improved self care (Weinger, 2007). Nurses can assist depressed patients by correcting misconceptions about depression, identifying individual strengths in managing DM, acknowledging negative feelings that may be expressed, suggesting problem-solving behaviors to better manage the disease, and referring to appropriate resources.

INCREASED SUSCEPTIBILITY TO INFECTION The person with DM has an increased risk of developing infections. The exact relationship between infection and DM is not clear, but many dysfunctions that result from diabetic complications predispose the person to develop an infection. Vascular and neurologic impairments, hyperglycemia, and altered neutrophil function are believed to be responsible (Porth & Matfin, 2009).

The person with DM may have sensory deficits resulting in inattention to trauma, and vascular deficits that decrease circulation to the injured area; as a result, the normal inflammatory response is diminished and healing is slowed. Nephrosclerosis and inadequate bladder emptying with retention of urine predispose the person with DM to pyelonephritis and urinary tract infections. Bacterial and fungal infections of the skin, nails, and mucous membranes are common. Tuberculosis is more prevalent in people with DM than in the general population. Surgical patients with a blood glucose value greater than 220 mg/dL have higher infection rates (ADA, 2009).

PERIODONTAL DISEASE Although periodontal disease does not occur more often in people with DM, it does progress more rapidly, especially if the DM is poorly controlled. It is believed to be caused by microangiopathy, with changes in vascularization of the gums. As a result, gingivitis (inflammation of the gums) and periodontitis (inflammation of the bone underlying the gums) occur.

Complications Involving the Feet

The high incidence of both amputations and problems with the feet in people with DM is the result of angiopathy, neuropathy, and infection. People with DM are at high risk for amputation of a lower extremity, with increased risk in those who have had DM for more than 10 years, are male, have poor glucose control, or have cardiovascular, retinal, or renal complications.

Vascular changes in the lower extremities of the person with DM result in arteriosclerosis. DM-induced arteriosclerosis tends to occur at an earlier age, occurs equally in men and women, is usually bilateral, and progresses more rapidly. The blood vessels most often affected are located below the knee. Blockages form in the large, medium, and small arteries of the lower legs and feet. Multiple occlusions with decreased blood flow result in the manifestations of peripheral vascular disease (see the box on page 547). Peripheral vascular disease is discussed in ∞ Chapter 32.

Diabetic neuropathy of the foot produces multiple problems. Because the sense of touch and perception of pain is absent, the person with DM may have some type of foot trauma without being aware of it. The person thus is at increased risk for trauma to tissues of the feet, leading to ulcer development. Infections commonly occur in traumatized or ulcerated tissue (see Figure 20–7 ■).

Despite the many potential sources of foot trauma in the person with DM, the most common are cracks and fissures caused by dry skin or infections such as athlete's foot, blisters caused by improperly fitting shoes, pressure from stockings or shoes, ingrown toenails, and direct trauma (cuts, bruises, or burns). It is important to remember that the person with diabetic neuropathy who has lost the perception of pain may not be aware that these injuries have occurred. In addition, when a part of the

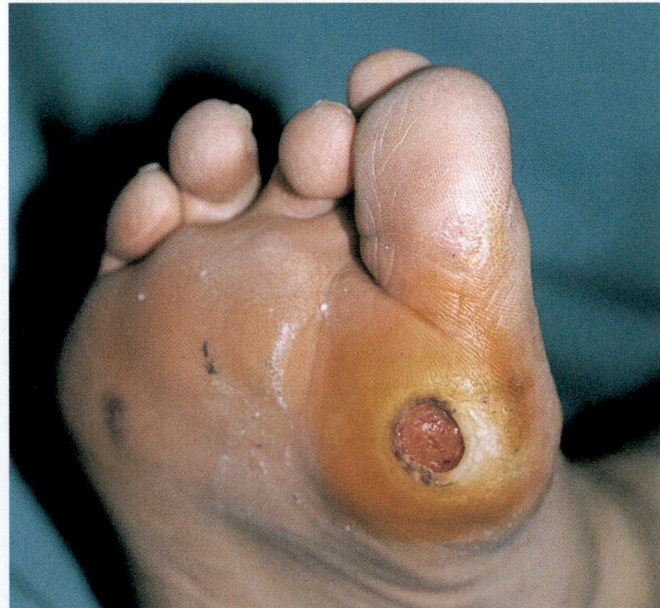

Figure 20–7 ■ Ulceration following trauma in the foot of the person with diabetes.

Source: Harry Przekop, Medichrome/The Stock Shop, Inc.

MANIFESTATIONS of Peripheral Vascular Disease

- Loss of hair on lower leg, feet, and toes
- Atrophic skin changes: shininess and thinning
- Cold feet
- Feet and ankles darker than leg
- Dependent rubor, blanching on elevation
- Thick toenails
- Diminished or absent pulses
- Nocturnal pain
- Pain at rest, relieved by standing or walking
- Intermittent claudication
- Patchy areas of gangrene on feet and toes

body loses sensation, the person tends to dissociate from or ignore the part, so that an injury may go unattended for days or weeks. The injury may even be forgotten entirely.

Foot lesions usually begin as a superficial skin ulcer. In time, the ulcer extends deeper into muscles and bone, leading to abscess or osteomyelitis. Gangrene can develop on one or more toes; if untreated, the whole foot eventually becomes gangrenous. (Care of the feet, an essential part of patient and family education, is discussed later in the chapter.)

✍ Nursing Care

DM is a chronic condition and the plan of care is dedicated to preventing complications and maintaining or improving quality of life. The responses of the person with DM to the illness are often complex and individual, involving multiple body systems. Assessments, planning, and implementation differ for the person with newly diagnosed DM, the person with long-term DM, and the person with acute complications of DM. The plan of care and content of teaching also differ according to the type of DM, the person's age and culture, and the person's intellectual, psychological, and social resources. Nurses who are DM specialists and generalists are relied upon to teach patients to successfully manage living with DM. In order to teach and support patients in their efforts to manage DM, all nurses need to understand DM, learn effective behavioral change strategies, and know appropriate interventions (Seley & Weinger, 2007). The following box describes a nursing study of hypoglycemia in hospitalized adults.

MOVING EVIDENCE INTO ACTION   Hypoglycemia in Hospitalized Adults

Until recently most hospitalized patients with type 2 DM or hyperglycemia were treated with supplemental insulin prescribed by a sliding-scale protocol when they experienced hyperglycemia. These patients are at risk for hypoglycemic events, usually because of inadequate carbohydrate (CHO) intake relative to insulin administration or oral hypoglycemic medications. Newer strategies for tighter control of blood glucose in hospitalized patients increase the incidence of hypoglycemic events. Nurses are the professionals who usually detect the onset of hypoglycemia, either by its manifestations or through routine blood glucose monitoring.

In a study at two midwestern hospitals, Anthony (2007) discovered that nurses failed to provide fully appropriate responses to all of the 410 incidents of hypoglycemia that occurred in 105 patients at each hospital. The acceptable, accurate response to a hypoglycemic event (blood glucose ≤ 70mg/dl) defined at both institutions by their hospital-approved practice guidelines involves five elements: (1) administration of 15 g of CHO, (2) blood glucose (BG) retest performed in 15 minutes, (3) BG performed 1 hour after hypoglycemia resolved, (4) physician notified, and (5) hypoglycemic event documented in the patient record. Step 1 is repeated until the BG is ≥ 70 mg/dl.

There were failures to adhere to each of these five guidelines. First, the correct dose of CHO was only given to 17% of the patients in hospital A and 3% in hospital B. Follow-up BG tests confirming that hypoglycemia had been successfully treated was only recorded in 9% of cases at hospital A and 6% at hospital B. In both institutions, some patients were discharged following a hypoglycemic event without a follow-up BG test. The recommended BG test 1 hour after evidence of normal BG was documented in 25% of events at hospital A and in 16% of events at hospital B. None of the recorded tests was drawn within the 50- to 70-minute window defined for the 1 hour post test. At hospital A, 54% of the events were documented in the patients' medical records; at hospital B, documentation was made in 71% of the events. Physician notification was only documented in 15% of events at hospital A and 28% of events at hospital B.

IMPLICATIONS FOR NURSING

Multiple and complex issues characterize the clinical care of patients with hypoglycemia. Because of the nearly epidemic rise in type 2 DM, and the prevalence of tighter blood glucose control among hospitalized patients, caring correctly for patients with hypoglycemia is very important. This includes preventing hypoglycemia as well as responding to it. Giving the incorrect dose of CHO is attributable to lack of knowledge. Verification that BG has returned to a normal level may be based on the patient's self report that he or she is "fine now." In the hurried practice of staff nursing, accepting a self report as evidence of normal BG is understandable but not acceptable. Someone may feel fine with a blood glucose that is climbing to 200 mg/dl or dropping below 70. Monitoring BG is a professional nursing responsibility, although performing the test can be delegated to trained assistants. Today's DM climate is crowded with new and improved ideas and thousands of newly diagnosed patients who need to adapt to increased levels of self-care and who require expert healthcare guidance. Each nurse must be knowledgeable and willing to teach, mentor, support and refer patients to appropriate professionals in the DM team.

CRITICAL THINKING IN PATIENT CARE

1. You are caring for two patients with DM who are receiving home care for complications of long-term DM. One patient follows the medical regimen faithfully, the other adapts it to his own schedule and needs. What differences can you identify in your own reaction to these two different patients? How would these reactions affect your relationship with the patients?

2. Imagine you have just been diagnosed with type 1 DM. Make a list of the questions you would have and the areas that would cause you the most difficulty in complying with your medical care.

3. How would you respond if your patient tells you, "Sometimes I eat whatever I want to for several days." What do you think this behavior indicates?

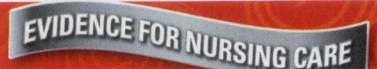

EVIDENCE FOR NURSING CARE   The Patient with Type 1 DM

Selected resources that nurses may find helpful when planning evidence-based nursing care follow.

■ Holzinger, U., Feldbacher, M., Bachlechner, A., Kitzberger, R., Fuhrmann, V., & Madl, C. (2008). Improvement of glucose control in the intensive care unit: An interdisciplinary collaboration study. *American Journal of Critical Care, 17*(2), 150–156. Retrieved from http://ajcc.aacnjournals.org/misc/journalclub.shtml

Health Promotion

Health promotion activities primarily focus on preventing the onset and complications of DM. The prevention of type 2 disease has been shown in randomized controlled trials to be achievable in a significant number of persons at risk. A combination of lifestyle changes (weight loss and increased physical activity) and medications (especially metformin) prevents or delays the onset of type 2 DM (ADA, 2009). Prevention of progression to DM is dependent on at-risk persons accepting responsibility to learn and sustain life style changes through self management education, counseling and coaching. Blood glucose screening at 3-year intervals beginning at age 45 is recommended for those not in the high-risk group.

Assessment

The following data are collected through the health history and physical examination (∞ see Chapter 18). Further focused assessments are described next with nursing interventions. When assessing the older patient, be aware of normal aging changes in all body systems that may alter interpretation of findings.

■ *Health history:* Family history of DM; history of hypertension or other cardiovascular problems; history of any change in vision (e.g. blurring) or speech, dizziness, numbness or tingling in hands or feet; pain when walking; frequent voiding; change in weight, appetite, infections, and healing; problems with gastrointestinal function or urination; or altered sexual function.

■ *Physical assessment:* Height/weight ratio, vital signs, visual acuity, cranial nerves, sensory ability (touch, hot/cold, vibration) of extremities, peripheral pulses, skin and mucous membranes (hair loss, appearance, lesions, rash, itching, vaginal discharge).

Nursing Diagnoses and Interventions

Although many different nursing diagnoses are appropriate for the person with DM, those discussed in this section address problems with skin integrity, infection, injury, sexuality, coping, and health maintenance. The goals of care are to maintain function, prevent complications, and teach self-management. See the accompanying Case Study & Nursing Care Plan for more information.

Risk for Impaired Skin Integrity

The person with DM is at increased risk for altered skin integrity as a result of decreased or absent sensation from neuropathies, decreased tissue perfusion from cardiovascular complications, and infection. In addition, poor vision increases the risk of trauma, and an open lesion is more prone to infection

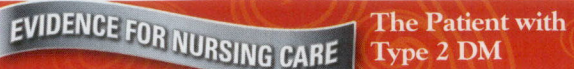

EVIDENCE FOR NURSING CARE   The Patient with Type 2 DM

Selected resources that nurses may find helpful when planning evidence-based nursing care follow.

■ Gazmararian, J., Zimmer, D., & Barnes, C. (2009). Perception of barriers to self-care management among diabetic patients. *The Diabetes Educator, 35*(5), 778–788.

and delayed healing. Impaired skin and tissue integrity, with resultant gangrene, is especially common in the feet and lower extremities. Conduct baseline and ongoing assessments of the feet, including the following:

■ Musculoskeletal assessment that includes foot and ankle joint range of motion, bone abnormalities (bunions, hammertoes, overlapping digits), gait patterns, use of assistive devices for walking, and abnormal wear patterns on shoes.

■ Neurologic assessment that includes sensations of touch and position, pain, and temperature.

■ Vascular examination that includes assessment of lower-extremity pulses, capillary refill, color and temperature of skin, lesions, and edema.

■ Hydration status, including dryness or excessive perspiration.

■ Lesions, fissures between toes, corns, calluses, plantar warts, ingrown or overgrown toenails, redness over pressure points, blisters, cellulitis, or gangrene.
People with DM are at significant risk for lower-extremity gangrene. Peripheral neuropathies may result in alterations in the perception of pain, loss of deep tendon reflexes, loss of cutaneous pressure and position sensation, foot drop, changes in the shape of the foot, and changes in bones and joints. Peripheral vascular disease may cause intermittent claudication, absent pulses, delayed venous filling on elevation, dependent rubor, and gangrene. Injuries, lesions, and changes in skin hydration potentiate infections, delayed healing, and tissue loss in the person with DM.

■ Teach foot hygiene. Wash the feet daily with lukewarm water and mild hand soap; pat dry, and dry well between the toes. Always test the water temperature in the shower or bath before stepping in. Apply a very thin coat of lubricating cream if dryness is present (but not between the toes). *Proper hygiene decreases the chance of infection. Temperature receptors may be impaired, so the water should always be tested before use.*

■ Discuss the importance of not smoking if patient smokes. *Nicotine in tobacco causes vasoconstriction, further decreasing the blood supply to the feet.*

■ Discuss the importance of maintaining blood glucose levels through prescribed diet, medication, and exercise. *Hyperglycemia promotes the growth of microorganisms.*

■ Conduct foot care teaching sessions as often as necessary (see the previous box). If the person has visual deficits, is obese, or cannot reach the feet, teach the caregiver how to inspect and care for the feet. Feet should be inspected daily. *Foot care is a priority in DM management to prevent serious problems. Many people with DM are unaware of lesions or injury until infection and compromised circulation are far advanced. The hows and whys of each component must*

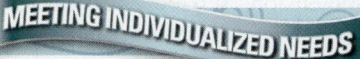
MEETING INDIVIDUALIZED NEEDS   Foot Care Teaching Session

BUYING AND WEARING SHOES AND STOCKINGS

- Shoes that allow 1/2 to 3/4 inch of toe room are best; there should be room for toes to spread out and wiggle. The lining and inside stitching should be smooth, and the insole soft. The sole should be flexible and cushion the foot. The heel should fit snugly, and the arch support should give good support.
- Do not wear open-toed shoes, sandals, high heels, or thongs; they increase the risk of trauma.
- Buy shoes late in the afternoon, when feet are at their largest; always buy shoes that feel comfortable and do not need to be "broken in."
- Shoes made of natural fibers (leather, canvas) allow perspiration to escape.
- Check the shoes before each wearing for foreign objects, wrinkled insoles, and cracks that might cause lesions.
- Stockings made of wool or cotton allow perspiration to dry.
- Do not wear garters, knee stockings, or panty hose; they may interfere with circulation.
- Wear insulated boots in the winter.

INSPECTING THE FEET

- Check the feet daily for red areas, cuts, blisters, corns, calluses, or cracks in the skin. Check between the toes for cracks or reddened areas.
- Check the skin of the feet for dry or damp areas.
- Use a mirror to check each sole and the back of each heel.
- If you are unable to inspect the feet daily, be sure that someone else does so.

CARE OF TOENAILS

- Cut the toenails after washing, when they are softer and easier to trim.
- Cut the nails straight across with a clipper, and smooth edges and corners with an emery board.
- Do not use razor blades to trim the toenails.
- If you are unable to see well or to reach the feet easily, have someone else trim the nails. If the nails are very thick or ingrown, if the toes overlap, or if circulation is poor, get professional care from a podiatrist.

GENERAL INFORMATION

- Never go barefoot. Wear slippers when leaving the bed during the night.
- Do not use commercial corn medicines or pads, chemicals (such as boric acid, iodine, or hydrogen peroxide), or over-the-counter cortisone medications on the feet.
- Do not put heating pads, hot water bottles, or ice packs on the feet. If the feet become cold at night, wear socks or use extra blankets.
- Do not allow the feet to become sunburned.
- Do not put tape on the feet.
- Do not sit with the legs crossed at the knees or ankles.

---

be included in teaching. *A variety of methods may be used, including demonstration, return demonstration, audiovisual aids, and written lists. If the person is wearing shoes and socks, ask him or her to remove them to practice foot care effectively.*

> **PRACTICE ALERT**
> Suggest the use of a hand mirror to check the bottom of the feet and the back of the heels.

Risk for Infection

The person with DM is at increased risk for infection. The risk of infection is believed to be due to vascular insufficiency that limits the inflammatory response, neurologic abnormalities that limit the awareness of trauma, and a predisposition to bacterial and fungal infections.

- Use and teach meticulous hand hygiene. *Hand hygiene is the single most effective method for preventing the spread of infection.*
- Monitor for manifestations of infection: increased temperature, pain, malaise, swelling, redness, discharge, cough. *Early diagnosis and treatment of infections can control their severity and decrease complications.*
- Discuss the importance of skin care. Keep the skin clean and dry, using lukewarm water and mild soap. *People with DM are more prone to develop furuncles and carbuncles; the infection often increases the need for insulin. Clean, intact skin and mucous membranes are the first line of defense against infection.*

- Teach dental health measures:
  - Obtain a dental examination every 4 to 6 months.
  - Maintain careful oral hygiene, which includes brushing the teeth with a soft toothbrush and fluoridated toothpaste at least twice a day and flossing as recommended.
  - Be aware of the manifestations requiring dental care: bad breath; unpleasant taste in the mouth; bleeding, red, or sore gums; and tooth pain.
  - If dental surgery is necessary, monitor for need to make adjustments in insulin. *All people with DM need to be taught proper oral hygiene, the risk of periodontal disease, and the importance of obtaining dental care for manifestations of oral or dental problems.*
- Teach women with DM about the manifestations and preventive measures for vaginitis caused by *Candida albicans*. The manifestations are an odorless, white or yellow cheeselike discharge and itching. *DM is a predisposing factor for* Candida albicans *vaginitis, the most common form of vaginitis. Poor personal hygiene and wearing clothing that keeps the vaginal area warm and moist increase the risk of vaginitis. The infection may spread to the urinary tract, resulting in urinary tract infections; preventing and treating vaginitis decrease this risk.*

> **PRACTICE ALERT**
> Teach women with DM to take preventive measures by maintaining good personal hygiene, wiping front to back after voiding, wearing cotton underwear, avoiding tight jeans and nylon pantyhose, and avoiding douching.

Risk for Injury

The person with DM is at risk for injury from multiple factors. Neuropathies may alter sensation, gait, and muscle control. Cataracts or retinopathy may cause visual deficits. Hyperglycemia often causes osmotic changes in the lenses of the eye, resulting in blurred vision. In addition, changes in blood glucose alter levels of consciousness and may cause seizures. The impaired mobility, sensory deficits, and neurologic effects of complications of DM increase the risk of accidents, burns, falls, and trauma.

- Assess for the presence of contributing or causative factors that increase the risk of injury: blurred vision, cataracts, decreased adaptation to dark, decreased tactile sensitivity, hypoglycemia, hyperglycemia, hypovolemia, joint immobility, unstable gait. *A knowledge base is necessary to develop an individualized plan of care. The risk of injury increases with the number of factors identified.*
- Reduce environmental hazards in the healthcare facility, and teach the patient about safety in the home and in the community.

IN THE HEALTHCARE FACILITY

- Orient the patient to new surroundings on admission.
- Keep the bed at the lowest level.
- Keep the floors free of objects.
- Use a night light.
- Check the temperature of the bath or shower water before the patient uses it.
- Instruct the patient to wear shoes or slippers when out of bed.
- Monitor blood glucose levels regularly.
- Monitor for side effects of prescribed medications, such as dizziness or drowsiness.

IN THE HOME AND COMMUNITY

- Use a night light, preferably one with a soft, nonglare bulb.
- Turn the head away when switching on a bright light.
- Avoid directly looking into headlights when driving at night.
- Test the temperature of the bath or shower water before use.
- Conduct a daily foot inspection.
- Wear shoes and slippers with nonskid soles.
- Do not use throw rugs.
- Install hand grips in the tub and shower and next to the toilet.
- Wear a seat belt when driving or riding in a car.
  Strange environments and the presence of hazardous environmental factors increase the risk of falls or other accidents. Glare is often responsible for falls in people with visual deficits. The nurse can reduce factors that increase the risk of injury by implementing care and teaching safe practices during the activities of daily life.
- Monitor for and teach the patient and family to recognize and seek care for the manifestations of DKA in the patient with type 1 DM: hyperglycemia, thirst, headaches, nausea and vomiting, increased urine output, ketonuria, dehydration, and decreasing level of consciousness. *Blood glucose levels increase if the insulin need is unmet or insufficiently met; the cellular use of fats for fuel results in ketosis. Osmotic diuresis increases urinary output, resulting in thirst and dehydration.*
- Monitor for and teach the patient and family to recognize and seek care for the manifestations of HHS in the patient with type 2 DM: extreme hyperglycemia, increased urinary output, thirst, dehydration, hypotension, seizures, and decreasing level of consciousness. *HHS is a life-threatening condition requiring recognition and treatment.*
- Monitor for and teach the patient and family to recognize and treat the manifestations of hypoglycemia: low blood glucose, anxiety, headache, uncoordinated movements, sweating, rapid pulse, drowsiness, and visual changes. Teach patient and family to carry some form of rapid-acting sugar source at all times. *Severe hypoglycemia causes a decrease in the level of consciousness. The decrease in blood glucose most often results from too much insulin, too little food, or too much exercise.*
- Recommend that the patient wear a MedicAlert bracelet or necklace identifying self as a person with DM. *In case of sudden, severe illness or accident, a MedicAlert bracelet can allow immediate medical attention for DM to be instituted.*

Sexual Dysfunction

Sexuality is a complex and inseparable part of every person. It involves not only physical sexual activities but also a person's self-perception as male or female, roles and relationships, and attractiveness and desirability. Changes in sexual function and in sexuality have been identified in both men and women with DM.

Alterations in erectile ability occur in approximately 50% of all men with DM. The incidence of impotence increases with the duration of the DM and is often associated with peripheral neuropathy. Libido is usually unaffected, even when impotence is present. Women with DM also have alterations in sexual function, although the reason is less clear. The problems reported by women involve decreased desire and decreased vaginal lubrication. Women with DM are also at increased risk for vaginitis and may avoid sexual intercourse in order to avoid pain.

- Include a sexual history as a part of the initial and ongoing assessment of the patient with DM. A specific history form may be used that addresses sexual development, personal and family values, current sexual practices and concerns, and changes desired. Ask a nonthreatening, open-ended question to elicit information, such as, "Tell me about your experience with sexual function since you have been diagnosed with DM." *Obtaining accurate information to assess the sexual health of a patient is necessary before counseling can begin or referrals can be made. Patients may not discuss problems with sexual function unless the nurse initiates the conversation.*
- Provide information about the actual and potential physical effects of DM on sexual function. Include the effect of poor control of blood glucose on sexual function as part of any teaching plan. *Patients benefit from basic information about male and female anatomy and the sexual response cycle, and how DM can affect this part of the body. Changes in blood glucose levels not only may cause changes in desire and physical response but also may alter sexual responses as a result of depression, anxiety, and fatigue.*
- Provide counseling or make referrals as appropriate. The nurse is responsible for knowing about sexuality and sexual health throughout the life span and provides information based on knowledge of the effects of illness and treatment on sexual function. For example, men who are impotent may regain the ability to have sexual intercourse through penile implants, suction apparatus, the use of drugs that facilitate gaining and maintaining an erection, such as sildenafil citrate

(Viagra), or injections of medications (such as yohimbine, an alpha-2 adrenergic blocker) that increase vascular blood flow into the corpus of the penis. Women with decreased vaginal lubrication can decrease painful intercourse by using vaginal lubricants (such as K-Y Jelly) or estrogen creams.

The nurse may make specific suggestions to facilitate positive sexual functioning, referring the patient to the appropriate healthcare provider as necessary for intensive therapy.

Ineffective Coping

Coping is the process of responding to internal or environmental stressors or potential stressors. When coping responses are ineffective, the stressors exceed the individual's available resources for responding. The person diagnosed with DM is faced with lifelong changes in many parts of his or her life. Diet, exercise habits, and medications must be integrated into the person's lifestyle and be carefully controlled. Daily injections may be a reality. Fear of potential complications and of negative effects on the future is common.

If the person is unable to cope successfully with these changes, emotional stress can interfere with glycemic control. In addition, unsuccessful coping often results in noncompliance with prescribed treatment modalities, further impairing glycemic control and increasing the potential for acute and chronic complications.

- Assess the patient's psychosocial resources, including emotional resources, support resources, lifestyle, and communication skills. *Chronic illness affects all dimensions of a person's life, as well as the lives of family members and significant others. A comprehensive assessment of strengths and weaknesses is the first step in developing an individualized plan of care to facilitate coping.*
- Explore with the patient and family the effects (actual and perceived) of the diagnosis and treatment of DM on finances, occupation, energy levels, and relationships. *Common frustrations associated with DM are the disease itself, the treatment modalities, and the healthcare system. Effective coping involves maintaining a healthy self-concept and satisfying relationships, emotional balance, and handling emotional stress.*
- Teach constructive problem-solving techniques. *Problem-focused behaviors include setting attainable and realistic goals, learning about all aspects of the problem, learning new procedures or skills that increase self-esteem, and reaching out to others for support.*
- Provide information about support groups and resources, such as suppliers of products, journals, books, and cookbooks for people with DM. *Sharing with others who have similar problems provides opportunities for mutual support and problem solving. Using available resources improves the ability to cope.*

Using NANDA, NIC, and NOC

Linkages between a selected NANDA nursing diagnosis, NIC, and NOC for the patient with DM are shown in the chart that follows.

Community-Based Care

Teaching the patient and family to self-manage DM is a healthcare team responsibility. Nurses are very important resources and must be knowledgeable and up-to-date on their understanding of

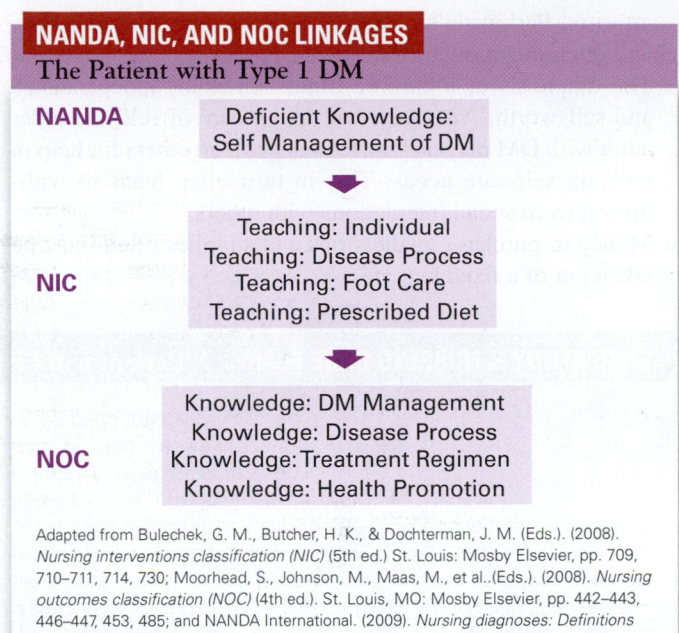

NANDA, NIC, AND NOC LINKAGES
The Patient with Type 1 DM

NANDA — Deficient Knowledge: Self Management of DM

NIC — Teaching: Individual / Teaching: Disease Process / Teaching: Foot Care / Teaching: Prescribed Diet

NOC — Knowledge: DM Management / Knowledge: Disease Process / Knowledge: Treatment Regimen / Knowledge: Health Promotion

Adapted from Bulechek, G. M., Butcher, H. K., & Dochterman, J. M. (Eds.). (2008). *Nursing interventions classification (NIC)* (5th ed.) St. Louis: Mosby Elsevier, pp. 709, 710–711, 714, 730; Moorhead, S., Johnson, M., Maas, M., et al.(Eds.). (2008). *Nursing outcomes classification (NOC)* (4th ed.). St. Louis, MO: Mosby Elsevier, pp. 442–443, 446–447, 453, 485; and NANDA International. (2009). *Nursing diagnoses: Definitions and classification 2009–2011.* Oxford: Wiley-Blackwell.

DM care. Even if a formal teaching plan is developed and implemented by diabetes nurse educators, all nurses must be able to reinforce knowledge and answer questions. Teaching is necessary for both the person who is newly diagnosed and for the person who has had DM for years. In fact, the latter may need almost as much teaching as the newly diagnosed person. Products for DM care, especially insulins, have changed dramatically and knowledge about risk reduction to prevent complications has increased.

The American Diabetes Association recommends that teaching be carried out on three levels. The first level focuses on survival skills, with the person learning basic knowledge and skills to be able to provide DM management for the first week or two while adjusting to the idea of having the disease. The second level focuses on home management, emphasizing self-reliance and independence in the daily management of DM. The third level aims at improving lifestyle and educating patients to individualize self-management of the illness.

Teaching may have to be adapted to the special needs of the older adult. Because 40% of all people with DM are over the age of 65, considering the special needs of this population is essential. Uncontrolled DM in the older adult increases the potential for functional loss, social disengagement, and increased morbidity and mortality. Education for self-care allows the older adult to be more actively involved in his or her DM management and decreases the potential for acute and long-term complications from the disease. Considerations for teaching the older adult with DM include the following:

- Changes in diet may be difficult to implement for many reasons. Balanced meals at regular intervals may not have been part of the patient's lifestyle. Purchasing, storing, and preparing foods may be a problem. Dentures may not fit well. Changes in taste sensation often cause the patient to increase the use of salt and sugar.
- Exercise of any type may not have been part of the activities of daily living. Exercise must be individualized for any physical limitations imposed by other chronic illnesses, such as

arthritis, Parkinson's disease, chronic respiratory diseases, and/or cardiovascular diseases.

■ The diagnosis of a chronic illness threatens independence and self-worth. After years of taking care of self, the older adult with DM may now have to depend on others for help in meeting self-care needs. This in turn often leads to withdrawal from social interactions with others.

■ Money to purchase medications and supplies often must be taken out of a fixed income.

■ Visual deficits make insulin administration difficult or impossible. Visual deficits also interfere with blood glucose monitoring, food preparation, exercises, and foot care.

It is important that the nurse and patient mutually establish goals based on the assessment data. Inquiries about patient and family priorities can be made effectively with the simple question, "What concerns you most about having diabetes?" The topics of concern range from medications to economics. Addressing topics of greatest concern first increases

---

CASE STUDY & NURSING CARE PLAN   A Patient with Type 1 DM

Jim Meligrito, aged 24, is a third-year nursing student at a large midwestern university. Mr. Meligrito also works 20 hours a week as a campus student security guard. His working hours are 8 PM to midnight, five nights a week. He lives with his father, who is also a student. Neither of the two men likes to cook, and they usually eat "whatever is handy." Mr. Meligrito has smoked 8 to 10 cigarettes a day for 5 years. He was diagnosed with type 1 DM at age 12. Although his insulin dosage has varied, he currently takes a total of 32 units of insulin each day, 10 U of NPH and 6 U of regular insulin each morning and evening. He monitors his blood glucose about three times a week. He feels that he is too busy for a regular exercise program and that he gets enough exercise in clinicals and in weekend sports activities. He has not seen a healthcare provider for over a year.

One day during a 6-hour clinical laboratory in pediatrics, Mr. Meligrito notices that he is urinating frequently, is thirsty, and has blurred vision. He also is very tired but blames all his manifestations on drinking a couple of beers and having had only 4 hours of sleep the night before while studying for an examination, and the stress he has been under lately from school and work. When he remembers that he had forgotten to take his insulin that morning, he realizes he must have hyperglycemia but decides that he will be all right until he gets home in the afternoon. Around noon, he begins having abdominal pain, feels weak, has a rapid pulse, and vomits. When he reports his physical manifestations to his clinical instructor, she sends him immediately to the hospital emergency department, accompanied by another student.

ASSESSMENT

As soon as Mr. Meligrito arrives at the emergency department, his blood glucose level is measured at 300 mg/dL. Urine samples and additional blood samples are sent to the laboratory for analysis. Blood glucose is 330 mg/dL, HgbA1c is 9.5%, urine shows the presence of ketones, electrolytes are normal, and pH is 7.1. His vital signs are as follows: T 99°F (37.2°C), P 140, R 28, and BP 102/52. An intravenous infusion of 1000 mL normal (0.9%) saline with 40 mEq of KCl is started at a rate of 400 mL/h. Intravenous regular insulin at 5 U/h (diluted in 0.9% saline) is begun. Hourly blood glucose monitoring is initiated. Mr. Meligrito is nauseated and lethargic but remains oriented. Three hours later, he has a blood glucose level of 160, and his pulse and blood pressure are normal. He is dismissed from the emergency department after making an appointment for the next morning with the hospital's DM nurse educator. When he meets with the DM educator, he says that he no longer feels in control of the DM or his future goal to become a nurse anesthetist.

DIAGNOSIS

■ *Powerlessness* related to a perceived lack of control of DM due to present demands on time
■ *Deficient Knowledge*: Self-management of DM
■ *Risk for Ineffective Role Performance* related to uncertainty about capacity to achieve desired role as registered nurse

EXPECTED OUTCOMES

■ Identify those aspects of DM that can be controlled and participate in making decisions about self-managing care.
■ Demonstrate an understanding of DM self-management through planned medication, diet, exercise, and blood glucose self-monitoring activities.
■ Explore and clarify Mr. Meligrito's perceptions of his role as a student nurse, verbalizing his ability to meet his expectations.

PLANNING AND IMPLEMENTATION

■ Mutually establish specific and individualized short-term and long-term goals for self-management of blood glucose.
■ Provide opportunities to express feelings about himself and his illness.
■ Explore perceptions of his own ability to control his illness and his future, and clarify these perceptions by providing information about resources and support groups.
■ Facilitate decision-making abilities in self-managing his prescribed treatment regimen.
■ Provide positive reinforcement for increasing involvement in self-care activities.
■ Provide relevant learning activities about insulin administration, dietary management, exercise, self-monitoring of blood glucose, and healthy lifestyle.

EVALUATION

After taking an active part in the weekly educational meetings for 2 months, Mr. Meligrito has greatly enhanced his understanding of and compliance with self-management of his DM. He states that he finally understands how insulin, food, and exercise affect his body, having previously thought they were "just things I should do when I wanted to." He decides to perform self-management activities one week at a time, rather than think too far into (and thereby feel overwhelmed by) the future. Both son and father have developed a workable meal schedule and weekly grocery list, and they have begun eating breakfast and dinner together. Mr. Meligrito and a friend have arranged to walk 2 to 3 miles three times a week on a community hiking trail. To gain a sense of control over his illness, he has also worked out a schedule that allows time for school, health care, and himself.

CRITICAL THINKING IN THE NURSING PROCESS

1. What is the pathophysiologic basis for the changes in temperature, pulse, respirations, and blood pressure that occurred on Mr. Meligrito's admission to the hospital emergency department?
2. How can smoking and poor self-management of DM increase the risk of long-term complications?
3. Is powerlessness a common response to a chronic illness? Why or why not?
4. Consider that you are teaching Mr. Meligrito and another patient, Mr. McDaniel (aged 75, newly diagnosed with type 2 DM). What components of your teaching plan would be the same and what components would be different?

See Evaluating Your Response in Appendix C.

the patient's and family's confidence that the information provided will be useful. It is equally important that family members understand that the responsibility for daily management lies with the patient and that the primary role of the family is supportive. The patient is the person with the disease, and it is the patient who each day must take medications or inject insulin, test blood or urine, calculate and balance foods, exercise, adjust medications, inspect the body for injury, and determine whether and when medical assistance is needed. However, family members require the same knowledge so that they can provide emotional support as well as physical care if necessary.

The following should be included in teaching the patient and family about care at home:

- Information about normal metabolism, DM, and how DM changes metabolism
- Diet plan: how diet helps keep blood glucose in normal range; number of kcal required and why; amount of carbohydrates, meats, and fats allowed and why; and how to calculate the diet, integrating personal food preferences

- Exercise: how it helps lower blood glucose, the importance of a regular program, types of exercise, integrating personal exercise preferences, how to handle increased activity
- Self-monitoring of blood glucose: how to perform the tests accurately, how to care for equipment, what to do for high or low blood glucose
- Medications:
  - Insulin: type, dosage, mixing instructions (if necessary), times of onset and peak actions, how to get and care for equipment, how to give injections, where to give injections
  - Oral agents: type, dosage, side effects, interaction with other drugs
- Manifestations of acute complications of hypoglycemia and hyperglycemia; what to do when they occur
- Hygiene: skin care, dental care, foot care
- Sick days: what to do about food, fluids, and medications
- Helpful resources: The American Diabetes Association, the American Dietetic Association, National Diabetes Information Clearinghouse, Indian Health Service, and the National Council of La Raza.

CHAPTER HIGHLIGHTS

- Approximately 1.3 million new cases of DM are diagnosed each year in the United States. DM is the sixth leading cause of death by disease in the United States, primarily due to widespread cardiovascular effects.
- The incidence of type 2 diabetes mellitus (DM) is increasing in epidemic proportions in all racial and ethnic groups in the United States.
- Type 2 DM has a hereditary link and is characterized by obesity and sedentary lifestyles. Unlike Type 1 DM, in which the onset is often sudden, the development of type 2 manifestations that bring patients to their healthcare providers for evaluation is slow; it is estimated that 50% of newly diagnosed

type 2 DM have already developed complications secondary to hyperglycemia.
- Tighter, more intensive glycemic control is increasingly the focus of care for hospitalized patients with hyperglycemia.
- New products for patients with DM include insulins, noninsulin hypoglycemics, and blood glucose monitoring devices. Nurses must be familiar with these products and help patients become proficient in their use.
- Motivation for self-care by the patient with DM continues to be a challenge because treatment commonly includes life style changes. Through education and support, patients can achieve control of DM and avoid complications.

TEST YOURSELF NCLEX-RN® REVIEW

1. Increased susceptibility to the development of type 1 DM is indicated by which of the following?
   1. genetic markers that determine immune response
   2. persistent obesity throughout the adolescent years
   3. delivery of a baby that weighs less than 6 lb
   4. excessive amounts of plasma glucagon
2. Diabetic ketoacidosis is the result of which pathologic process?
   1. An excess amount of insulin drives all glucose into the cells.
   2. A decreased amount of glucagon causes low protein levels.
   3. A deficit of insulin causes fat stores to be used as an energy source.
   4. An increase occurs in the breakdown of glucose molecules with hypoglycemia.

3. Which of the following patients would be most at risk for the development of type 2 DM?
   1. young adult who is a professional basketball player
   2. middle-aged man who maintains normal weight
   3. middle-aged woman who is the sole caretaker of her parents
   4. woman over age 70 who is overweight and sedentary
4. A nurse notes that a patient has a nursing diagnosis of *Peripheral Neurovascular Dysfunction* involving both feet. Which of the following assessments would support this diagnosis?
   1. normal sensation to touch
   2. loss of normal reflexes
   3. states "I can't feel my feet anymore."
   4. states "I have been having chest pain."

5. Which of the following statements would indicate that a patient understands teaching about foot care at home?
   1. "I will walk barefooted as long as I am in the house."
   2. "I always buy my shoes as soon as the stores open."
   3. "I will check my feet for cuts and bruises every night."
   4. "If I get a blister, I just put alcohol on it and bandage it."

6. Lantus and detemir insulin, long-acting insulins, have a unique insulin characteristic that increases the risk for administration error. The nurse understands that which of the following applies to this long-acting insulin?
   1. It is combined with glucose to raise energy levels.
   2. It is subject to being inactivated by light and must be kept cold.
   3. It is a clear solution like regular insulin, unlike other intermediate and long-acting insulins.
   4. It is activated by vigorous agitation.

7. The nurse is preparing an insulin infusion for a patient in diabetic ketoacidosis (DKA). She is careful to select which type of insulin that can be administered intravenously?
   1. glargine
   2. NPH
   3. regular
   4. Humalog

8. Glycosylated hemoglobin (A1C) is useful for evaluating the degree of blood glucose control the patient with DM has been maintaining for the previous 2 to 3 months. The ADA recommends a diagnosis of DM at what A1C level?
   1. > 15%
   2. > 9%
   3. > 6.5%
   4. > 2.25%

9. When the insulin-dependent patient is NPO on the day of surgery, which of the following should be done with short-acting regular insulin?
   1. It should be given intravenously.
   2. It should be chilled to slow absorption.
   3. It should be given with intravenous glucose.
   4. It should be combined with long-acting insulin.

10. Subcutaneous injections of insulin can be made in several locations in the body. The nurse teaches the patient that the most rapid absorption occurs in which of the following?
    1. hip
    2. thigh
    3. deltoid
    4. abdomen

See Test Yourself answers in Appendix C.

Pearson Nursing Student Resources

Find additional review materials at
nursing.pearsonhighered.com

Prepare for success with additional NCLEX®-style practice questions, interactive assignments and activities, Web links, animations and videos, and more!

BIBLIOGRAPHY

American Diabetes Association (ADA). (2008a). Pancreas transplantation. Retrieved from http://www.diabetes.org/

American Diabetes Association (ADA). (2008b). Nutrition recommendations for DM. *Diabetes Care, 31*(Supplement 1), S61–S78.

American Diabetes Association (ADA). (2009). Standards of medical care in diabetes—2009. *Diabetes Care, 32*(Supplement 1), S13–S41.

American Diabetes Association (ADA). (2010). Standards of medical care in diabetes—2010. *Diabetes Care, 33*(Supplement 1), S11–S61.

Anthony, M. (2007). Treatment of hypoglycemia in hospitalized adults. *The Diabetes Educator, 33*(4), 709–715.

BD Diabetes. (2009). *Insulin pens.* Retrieved from http://www.bddiabetes.com/US/main.aspx?cat=1&id=254

Boulton, A. J., & Malik, R. A. (2010). Neuropathy of impaired glucose tolerance and its measurement. *Diabetes Care, 33*(1), 207–209.

Braithwaite, S. S., Robertson, B., Mehrotra, H. P., McElveen, L. M., &Thompson, C. L. (2007). Managing hyperglycemia in hospitalized patients. *Clinical Cornerstone 8*(2), 55–57.

Bulechek, G. M., Butcher, H. K., & Dochterman, J. M. (Eds.). (2008). *Nursing interventions classification (NIC)* (5th ed.). St. Louis: Mosby Elsevier.

Centers for Disease Control and Prevention (CDC). (2007). *National diabetes fact sheet 2007.* Retrieved from http://www.cdc.gov/diabetes/pubs/pdf/ndfs_2007.pdf

Centers for Disease Control and Prevention (CDC). (2008). State-specific incidence of diabetes among adults— participating states, 1995–1997 and 2005–2007. *Morbidity and Mortality Weekly Reports,* October 31, 2008/57(43), 1169–1173.

Cummings, D. E., & Flum, D. R. (2008). Gastrointestinal surgery as a treatment for diabetes. *Journal of the American Medical Association (JAMA), 299*(3), 341–343.

Dixon, J. B., O'Brien, P. E., Playfair, L. J., Chapman, L., Schachter, L. M., et al. (2008). Adjustable gastric banding and conventional therapy for type 2 diabetes: A randomized controlled trial. *Journal of the American Medical Association, 299*(3), 316–323.

Green, D. E. (2007). New therapies for diabetes. *Clinical Cornerstone, 8*(2), 58–63.

Haas, L. (2007). Functional decline in older adults with diabetes. *American Journal of Nursing, 107*(6S), 50–54.

Jain, V., Sharma, D., Prabhakar, H., & Dash, H. H. (2008). Metformin-associated lactic acidosis following contrast media-induced nephrotoxicity. *European Journal of Anaesthesiology, 25*(2), 166–167.

Kitabchi, A. E., Umpierrez, G. E., Murphy, M. B., Barrett, E. J., Kreisberg, R. A., et al (2004). American Diabetes Association Position Statement: Hyperglycemic crises in diabetes. *Diabetes Care, 27*(S1), S94–S102.

Loh-Trivedi, M., & Rothenberg, D. M. (2008). Perioperative management of the diabetic patient. Retrieved from http://emedicine.medscape.com/article/284451-overview

McPhee, S., & Papadakis, M. (Eds.). (2009). *Current medical diagnosis & treatment* (48th ed.). New York: McGraw Hill Medical.

Medtronic MiniMed, Inc. (2006). *MiniMed Paradigm® REAL-Time Insulin Pump and Continuous Glucose Monitoring System.* Retrieved from http://www.minimed.com/ products/insulinpumps/realtime/index.html

Miller, D. K. (2009). Are you ready to care for a patient with an insulin pump? *Nursing, 10*(39), 57–60.

Moorhead, S., Johnson, M., Maas, M., & Swanson, E. (Eds.). (2008). *Nursing outcomes classification (NOC)* (4th ed.). St. Louis: Mosby Elsevier.

NANDA International. (2009). *Nursing diagnoses: Definitions and classification 2009–2011.* Oxford: Wiley-Blackwell.

National Eye Institute. (2006). Diabetic retinopathy. Retrieved from http://www.neil.nih.gov

National Institutes of Health (NIH). (2008). *Diabetes statistics in the United States.* Retrieved from http://diabetes.niddk .nih.gov/dm/pubs/statistics/

Pearson, T. L. (2009). Motivating patients to monitor their blood glucose. Retrieved from http://www.medscape.com/ viewarticle/588565?src=mp&spon=24&uac=116901HG

Peeples, M, & Seley, J. J. (2007). Diabetes care: The need for change. *American Journal of Nursing, 107*(6S), S13–S15, S17–S19.

Porth, C. (2007). *Essentials of Pathophysiology: Concepts of altered health states* (2nd ed.). Philadelphia: Lippincott Williams & Wilkins.

Porth, C., & Matfin, G. (2009). *Pathophysiology: Concepts of altered health states* (8th ed). Philadelphia: Lippincott Williams & Wilkins.

Seley, J. J., & Weinger, K. (2007). Executive summary: The state of the science on nursing best practices for diabetes self-management. *American Journal of Nursing, 107*(6S), 6–11.

Umpierrez, G. E., Smiley, D., Zisman, A., Prieto, L. M., et al. (2007). Randomized study of basal-bolus insulin therapy in the inpatient management of patients with type 2 diabetes. *Diabetes Care, 30,* 2181–2186.

Van Praet, J. T. & De Vriese, A. S. (2007). Prevention of contrast-induced nephropathy: A critical review. *Current Opinion in Nephrology & Hypertension, 16*(4), 336–347.

WebMD, Diabetes Health Center. (2009). *New type 2 diabetes drug Onglyza approved.* Retrieved from http://diabetes.webmd.com/news/20090731/new-type-2-diabetes-drug-onglyza-approved

Weinger, K. (2007). Psychosocial issues and self-care. *American Journal of Nursing, 107*(6S), 34–38.

Wiener, R. S., Wiener, D. C., & Larson, R. J. (2008). Benefits and risks of tight glucose control in critically ill adults: A meta-analysis. *JAMA, 300*(8), 933–944.

Yared, Z., Aljaberi, K., Renouf, N., & Yale, J. (2005). The effect of blood sample volume on 11 glucose monitoring systems. *Diabetes Care, 28,* 1836–1837.

Building Clinical Competence
Responses to Altered Endocrine Function

Functional Health Pattern: Nutritional-Metabolic

Think about patients with altered endocrine function for whom you have cared in your clinical experiences.

- What were their major medical diagnoses (e.g., Graves' disease, myxedema coma, cancer of the thyroid, hyperparathyroidism, hypoparathyroidism, Cushing's syndrome, Addison's disease, pheochromocytoma, gigantism, syndrome of inappropriate antidiuretic hormone secretion, diabetes insipidus, and diabetes mellitus)?

- What kinds of manifestations did each of these patients have? Were these manifestations similar or different?

- How did the patients' healthcare behaviors interfere with their nutritional and metabolic status? Were they on a prescribed diet? What was their daily intake of foods and fluids? Did they have an increased appetite with loss of weight? Did they notice their hands and feet getting larger? Did they have difficulty swallowing or notice swelling in the front of their neck? Did they note an increase or decrease in urination? Did they note a change in energy levels? Had they noticed any visual changes? Did they complain of sleep disturbances? Had they had any changes in hair distribution, such as facial hair or changes in skin texture? Had there been a change in memory or the ability to concentrate? Did the patients use hormones or steroids? Was there a family history of diabetes mellitus, diabetes insipidus, thyroid problems, hypertension, or obesity?

The Nutritional-Metabolic Functional Health Pattern includes metabolism, which is the biochemical processes that take place in the body due to hormones produced and released by the endocrine glands. These processes relate to the distribution of nutrients after digestion of carbohydrates, proteins, and fats. The endocrine system regulates growth, reproduction, metabolism, fluid and electrolyte balance, and gender differentiation. Endocrine disorders affect the metabolic status in two primary ways:

- Lack of hormones can result in endocrine disorders of the thyroid gland (e.g., hypothyroidism), disorders of the parathyroid gland (e.g., hypoparathyroidism), disorders of the adrenal gland (e.g., chronic adrenocortical insufficiency), disorders of the pituitary gland (e.g., hypopituitarism, diabetes insipidus), or disorders of the pancreas (e.g., hypoglycemia).

- Excess hormones can result in endocrine disorders of the thyroid gland (e.g., hyperthyroidism), disorders of the parathyroid gland (e.g., hyperparathyroidism), disorders of the adrenal

gland (e.g., hypercortisolism), disorders of the pituitary gland (e.g., hyperpituitarism, SIADH) or disorders of the pancreas (e.g., hyperglycemia).

Hormones are chemical substances, secreted by the endocrine glands, that initiate or regulate functioning of a target organ by binding to a receptor site located on the surface of the target organ. They are regulated by a negative or positive feedback system in which decreased or increased hormone levels signal the release of hormones to maintain homeostasis of the body's internal environment. Imbalance of hormones can result in endocrine disorders, leading to manifestations such as the following:

- **Weight loss** (*increased thyroid hormones cause an increase in metabolism of carbohydrates, proteins, and lipids resulting in caloric and nutritional deficiencies*)

- **Blurred vision** (*lack of insulin production by the pancreas causes osmotic effects to the eye tissue resulting in swelling of the lenses of the eyes*)

- **Increased urination** (*deficit of antidiuretic hormones causes excretion of large amounts of urine resulting in dehydration and hypernatremia*)

Priority nursing diagnoses within the Nutritional-Metabolic Functional Health Pattern that may be appropriate for patients with endocrine disorders include the following:

- *Imbalanced Nutrition: Less than Body Requirements* as evidenced by increased food intake with weight loss or loss of appetite

- *Deficient Fluid Volume* as evidenced by dry mucous membranes, increased skin turgor, thirst, and decreased urine output

- *Hyperthermia* as evidenced by body temperatures ranging from 102°F (39°C) to 106°F (41°C)

- *Impaired Skin Integrity* as evidenced by dry, rough, reddened, and edematous skin

Two nursing diagnoses from other functional health patterns often are of high priority for the patient with endocrine disorders:

- *Disturbed Body Image* (Self-Perception-Self-Concept Functional Health Pattern)

- *Ineffective Therapeutic Regimen Management* (Health Perception, Health Management, Functional Health Pattern)

Question

1. What did you do to help your patient manage his or her nutritional needs?

CLINICAL SCENARIO

Directions: *Read the following clinical scenarios and answer the questions that follow. To complete this exercise successfully, you will utilize not only knowledge of the content in this unit, but also principles related to priority setting and maintaining patient safety.*

You have been assigned to work with the following four patients for the 0700 shift on a medical-surgical unit. Significant data obtained during report is as follows:

- Mr. Blew is a 54-year-old who is admitted with complaints of polydipsia, polyuria, and polyphagia. There is a fruity odor to his breath and he seems confused at times. Vital signs on admission are temperature 99°F, pulse 90, respirations 30 and deep, and blood pressure 110/68. His blood glucose is 650 on admission at 0630.
- Mrs. Rant is a 65-year-old who is admitted with severe back pain in the flank area on the right side, nausea, and vomiting. She is being evaluated for treatment due to renal calculi. She has a history of hyperparathyroidism. Vital signs are temperature 97.6°F with clammy skin, pulse 100, respirations 24, and blood pressure of 168/94. She is requesting pain medication for the back pain.
- Mrs. Fox is an 86-year-old who was transferred from the medical ICU yesterday. She was admitted after being found in a comatose state by her daughter. On admission her blood sugar was 45, serum sodium was 128, temperature was 96.6°F, and she had a heart rate of 50. Vital signs this AM are temperature 98.4°F, pulse 78, respirations 18, and blood pressure 140/86. She is due for electrolytes to be drawn at 0730.
- Mr. Rite is a 56-year-old who was admitted 4 days ago after falling from a ladder and hitting his head. He is complaining of a headache and thirst even after drinking 2000 ml of fluids during the night. Vital signs are temperature 100°F, pulse 98, respirations 14, and blood pressure 114/84.

Questions

Priority Setting

1. In what order would you visit these patients after report?
   A. _____
   B. _____
   C. _____
   D. _____

Health Promotion

1. Mr. Blew is diagnosed with diabetes mellitus. Besides diet and medication administration, what other teaching is necessary in order for him to maintain a high level of health?

2. The nurse explains to Mrs. Rant the dietary treatment for hyperparathyroidism. Which is the appropriate dietary teaching for this patient?
   A. Increase fluids in the diet and avoid taking vitamin D supplements.
   B. Increase potassium in the diet and avoid taking vitamin C supplements.
   C. Decrease sodium in the diet and take vitamin B6 supplements.
   D. Decrease phosphorus in the diet and take vitamin A supplements.

Nursing Process

1. What top priority nursing diagnoses would you choose for each of the patients presented earlier? Explain the rationale for your choices.

	Nursing Diagnosis	Rationale
Mr. Blew		
Mrs. Rant		
Mrs. Fox		
Mr. Rite		

2. If Mr. Blew's blood glucose drops to 50, which manifestations might he exhibit?
   A. Bradycardia, nausea, and vomiting
   B. Tachycardia, hypotension, and shakiness
   C. Thirst, diarrhea, and fatigue
   D. Hypertension, edema, and dyspnea

3. Due to the manifestations of headache and excessive thirst that Mr. Rite is exhibiting 4 days after his fall, the nurse should monitor for symptoms of which complication?
   A. Migraine headache
   B. Hypertensive crisis
   C. Increased intracranial pressure
   D. Infection

4. A prescription for levothyroxine sodium (Synthroid) is given to Mrs. Fox after being diagnosed with hypothyroidism. The patient voices understanding of how to take the medication when she states which of the following?
   A. "I must take the medication with meals."
   B. "I must take my pulse before taking the medication and report to the doctor a pulse > 100."
   C. "I will only need to take this medication until my thyroid blood levels are back to normal."
   D. "I can eat any food I choose as foods do not interfere with the medications."

5. Which laboratory studies would be conducted for Mr. Blew to monitor his diabetes management? **Select all that apply.**
   A. Fasting blood glucose
   B. Glycosylated hemoglobin (c)
   C. Urinalysis
   D. Complete blood cell count
   E. Serum electrolytes
   F. Serum cholesterol and triglyceride levels

Communication

1. Mr. Blew understands diabetic teaching implemented by the nurse when he states which of the following?
   - A. "I will check my blood glucose before every meal."
   - B. "If I follow my prescribed diet, I will not have to check my blood sugar."
   - C. "If my blood glucose drops below 60, I can drink juice or milk to raise it."
   - D. "If my blood sugar is over 200, I can eat graham crackers to lower it."

2. Mrs. Fox's daughter asks if her mother will be able to go home alone or if she will need to be sent to a nursing home to live. How will you answer?

Delegation

1. For each patient, what assessment data and nursing interventions can be delegated to a certified nursing assistant (CNA)?

Related Questions

1. The nurse assessing a patient with hyperthyroidism may find which manifestations?
   - A. diaphoresis, diarrhea, alopecia, weight loss
   - B. dry skin, constipation, hirsutism, obesity
   - C. hypertension, abdominal pain, constipation, anorexia
   - D. dry skin, numbness around mouth and fingertips, tetany

2. In postoperative thyroidectomy nursing care, it is most important for the nurse to monitor the patient for which of these complications?
   - A. bleeding
   - B. laryngeal nerve damage
   - C. tetany
   - D. respiratory distress

3. Metabolic syndrome is a cluster of manifestations associated with type 2 diabetes mellitus. Which manifestations are indicative of metabolic syndrome?
   - A. hypertension, abdominal obesity, blood glucose > 110 mg/dL
   - B. tachycardia, weight gain, blood glucose < 110 mg/dL
   - C. hypotension, weight loss, blood glucose >150 mg/dL
   - D. bradycardia, stomach obesity, blood glucose < 100 mg/dL

4. Which of the following laboratory value results may be seen in a patient with untreated Cushing's syndrome?
   - A. serum sodium level of 150 mEq/L, serum potassium level of 2.8 mEq/L
   - B. blood glucose of 68mg/dL, blood urea nitrogen level of 28 mg/dL
   - C. serum calcium level of 9.0 mg/dL, serum sodium level of 130 mEq/L
   - D. blood glucose of 350mg/dL, serum potassium level of 5.2 mEq/L

CASE STUDY: Louis Gregg

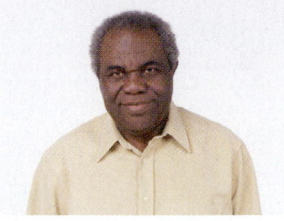

Louis Gregg is a 65-year-old African American male who was admitted with complaints of increased urination, increased thirst, fatigue, blurred vision, and numbness in his feet. He states that he retired 9 months ago after 45 years as a construction worker. He now leads a sedentary lifestyle and doesn't have as much energy as he used to have. He has gained 50 pounds since retirement. Upon assessment, Mr. Gregg weighs 255 pounds and is 5'11" tall. Vital signs are T 98.8°F, P 88, R 20, and BP 150/90. Decreased pulses are noted in dorsal pedis and posterior tibial pulses. Both feet are pale pink in color and cool to touch. Assessment findings are documented in the patient's record and reported to the physician. The following laboratory studies are ordered to determine the diagnosis of type 2 diabetes mellitus: plasma glucose concentration, fasting blood glucose, and oral glucose tolerance test.

Type 2 DM is a disease of fasting hyperglycemia, with some but not enough insulin production by the endocrine pancreas. With increased age, obesity, and a sedentary lifestyle, cells become resistant to insulin. Glucose uptake by muscle and fat cells is not sufficient to lower blood glucose, while insulin has a decreased ability to influence glucose metabolism by the liver, skeletal muscles, and adipose tissue. The manifestations of type 2 DM include polyuria, polydipsia, blurred vision, fatigue, paresthesias, and skin infections. In times of physical stress, the patient may develop HHS. Complications include myocardial infarction, hypertension, stroke, peripheral vascular disease, renal disease, and blindness.

Based on Mr. Gregg's manifestations and weight gain, a nursing diagnosis of *Imbalanced Nutrition: More than Body Requirements* is appropriate for guiding nursing care for this patient.

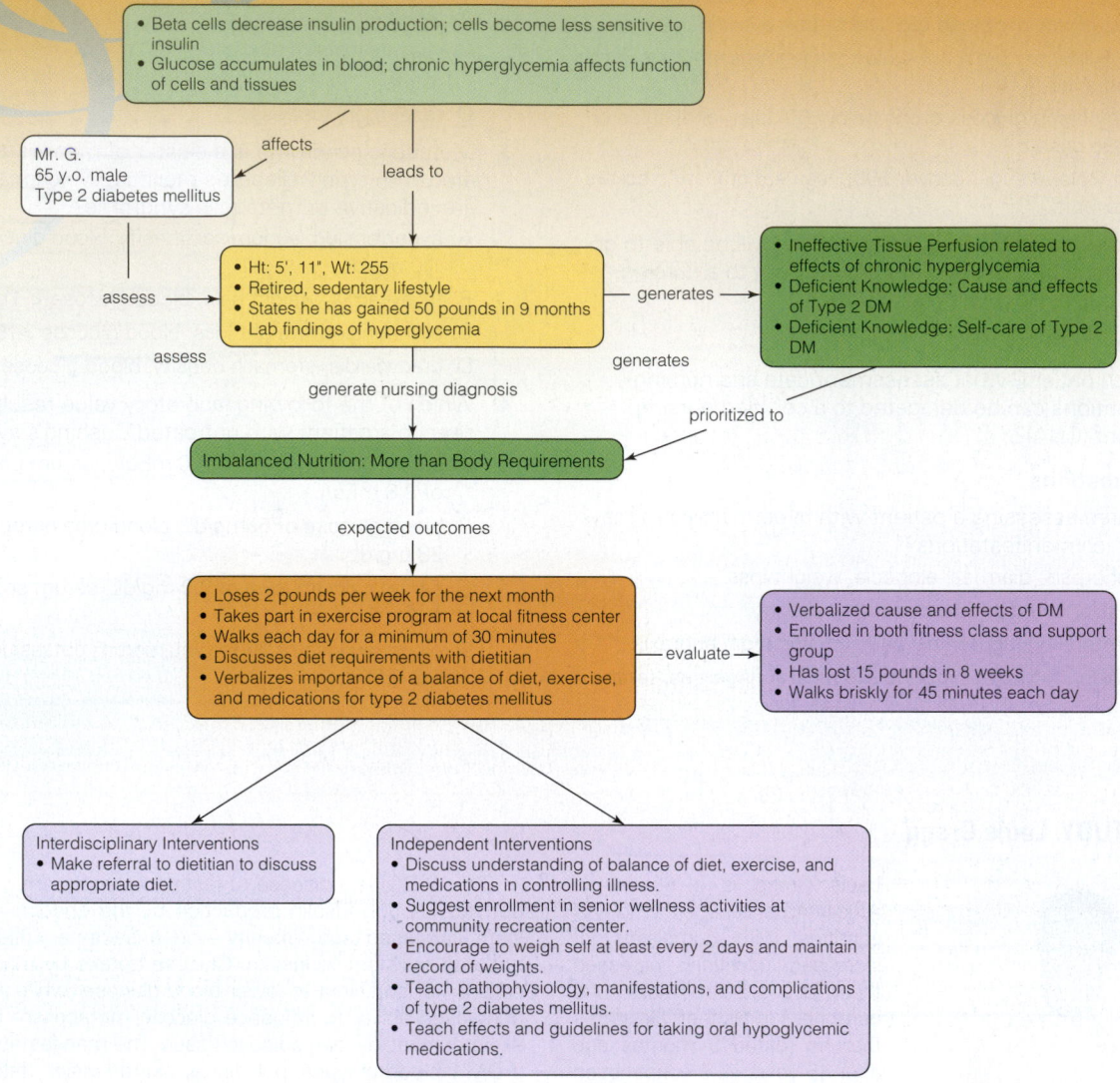

- Beta cells decrease insulin production; cells become less sensitive to insulin
- Glucose accumulates in blood; chronic hyperglycemia affects function of cells and tissues

Mr. G.
65 y.o. male
Type 2 diabetes mellitus

affects

leads to

assess

- Ht: 5', 11", Wt: 255
- Retired, sedentary lifestyle
- States he has gained 50 pounds in 9 months
- Lab findings of hyperglycemia

generates

- Ineffective Tissue Perfusion related to effects of chronic hyperglycemia
- Deficient Knowledge: Cause and effects of Type 2 DM
- Deficient Knowledge: Self-care of Type 2 DM

assess

generate nursing diagnosis

generates

prioritized to

Imbalanced Nutrition: More than Body Requirements

expected outcomes

- Loses 2 pounds per week for the next month
- Takes part in exercise program at local fitness center
- Walks each day for a minimum of 30 minutes
- Discusses diet requirements with dietitian
- Verbalizes importance of a balance of diet, exercise, and medications for type 2 diabetes mellitus

evaluate

- Verbalized cause and effects of DM
- Enrolled in both fitness class and support group
- Has lost 15 pounds in 8 weeks
- Walks briskly for 45 minutes each day

Interdisciplinary Interventions
- Make referral to dietitian to discuss appropriate diet.

Independent Interventions
- Discuss understanding of balance of diet, exercise, and medications in controlling illness.
- Suggest enrollment in senior wellness activities at community recreation center.
- Encourage to weigh self at least every 2 days and maintain record of weights.
- Teach pathophysiology, manifestations, and complications of type 2 diabetes mellitus.
- Teach effects and guidelines for taking oral hypoglycemic medications.

Activity:
1. After reviewing the concept map, is there anything you would change to make it more understandable?
2. Go to the Pearson Nursing Student Resources for this book at www.nursing.pearsonhighered.com to write a concept map using the nursing diagnosis *Risk for Peripheral Neurovascular Dysfunction*.

See answers and hints in Appendix C.

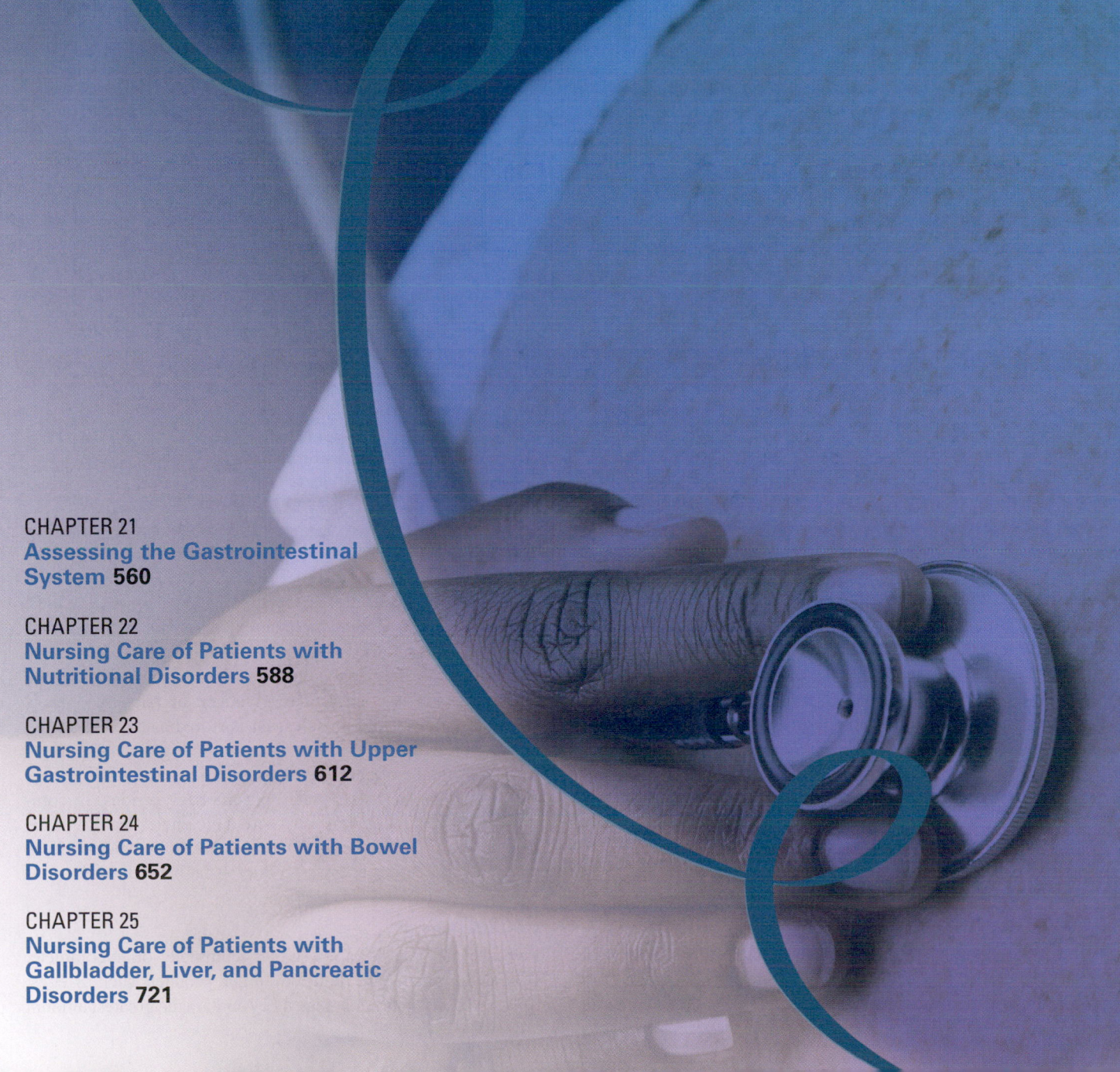

Responses to Altered Gastrointestinal Function

UNIT 6

CHAPTER 21

Assessing the **Gastrointestinal System**

LEARNING OUTCOMES

1. Describe the anatomy, physiology, and functions of the gastrointestinal (GI) system and the accessory digestive organs.
2. Identify specific topics to consider during a health history interview of the patient with GI disorders.
3. Explain techniques used for assessing nutritional status and GI function.
4. Give examples of genetic disorders of the GI system.
5. Describe normal variations in GI assessment findings for the older adult.
6. Identify abnormal findings that may indicate alterations in GI function.

CLINICAL COMPETENCIES

1. Conduct and document a health history for patients who have or are at risk for alterations in GI function.
2. Conduct and document a physical assessment of nutritional status and the GI system.
3. Monitor the results of diagnostic tests and report abnormal findings.

EQUIPMENT NEEDED

- Stethoscope
- Balance scale with height measuring attachment
- Tape measure
- Skin fold calipers
- Water-soluble lubricant
- Occult blood test, such as Occultest or Hemocult II
- Disposable gloves

KEY TERMS

bile, 567	gingivitis, 579	nutrition, 560
borborygmus, 581	glossitis, 579	ostomy, 569
bruit, 581	hernia, 584	steatorrhea, 585
cheilosis, 579	leukoplakia, 579	striae, 580
flatus, 569	melena, 585	Valsalva's maneuver, 567

The GI system consists of the mouth, pharynx, esophagus, stomach, small intestine, and large intestine. The accessory digestive organs include the liver, gallbladder, and pancreas (Figure 21–1 ■). **Nutrition** is the process by which the body, via the GI system and the accessory digestive organs, ingests, absorbs, transports, uses, and eliminates nutrients in food.

Nutrients

Nutrients are substances found in food and are used by the body to promote growth, maintenance, and repair. The categories of nutrients are carbohydrates, proteins, fats, vitamins, minerals, and water.

Carbohydrates

The primary sources of carbohydrates (sugars and starches) are plant foods. Monosaccharides and disaccharides come from milk, sugar cane, sugar beets, honey, and fruits. Polysaccharide starch is found in grains, legumes, and root vegetables. Following ingestion, digestion, and metabolism, carbohydrates are converted primarily to glucose, the molecule body cells use to make adenosine triphosphate (ATP). Excess glucose in the healthy person is converted to glycogen or fat. Glycogen is stored in the liver and muscles; fat is stored as adipose tissue. Carbohydrate use by the body is shown in Figure 21–2A ■.

Excess intake of carbohydrates over time can result in obesity, dental caries, and elevated plasma triglycerides. In comparison, long standing carbohydrate deficiencies lead to tissue wasting from protein breakdown and metabolic acidosis from an excess of ketones as a by-product of fat breakdown.

Proteins

Proteins are classified as either complete or incomplete. Complete proteins are found in animal products such as eggs, milk, milk products, and meat. They contain the greatest amount

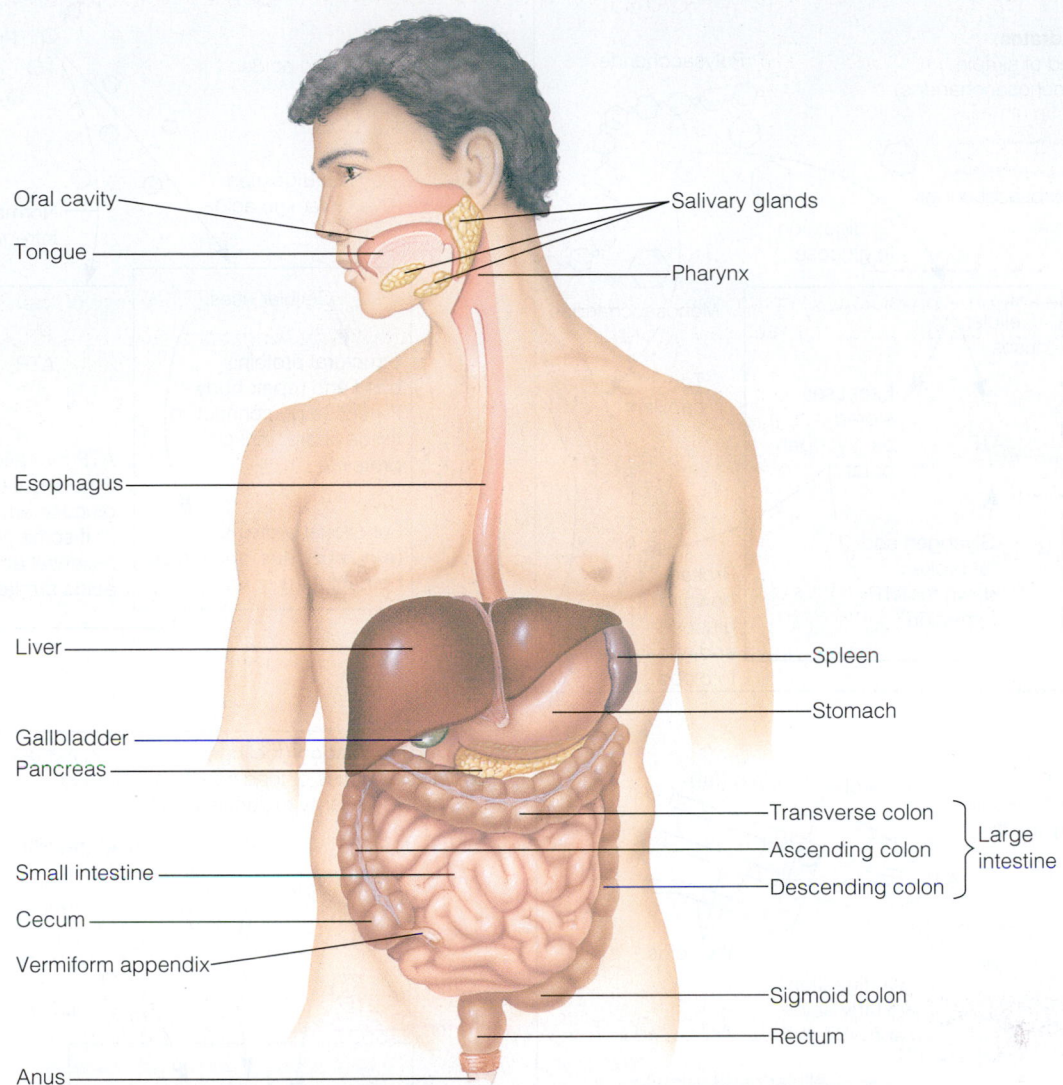

Oral cavity
Tongue
Salivary glands
Pharynx
Esophagus
Liver
Spleen
Stomach
Gallbladder
Pancreas
Transverse colon
Ascending colon
Descending colon
Large intestine
Small intestine
Cecum
Vermiform appendix
Sigmoid colon
Rectum
Anus

Figure 21–1 ■ Organs of the gastrointestinal system and accessory digestive organs.

of amino acids and meet the body's requirements for tissue growth and maintenance. Incomplete proteins are found in legumes, nuts, grains, cereals, and vegetables. These sources are low in or lack one or more of the amino acids essential for building complete proteins.

The body uses proteins to build many different structures, including skin keratin, the collagen and elastin in connective tissues, and muscles. They also are used to make enzymes, hemoglobin, plasma proteins, and some hormones. Protein use by the body is shown in Figure 21–2B.

Healthy people with adequate caloric intake have an equal rate of protein synthesis and protein breakdown and loss, reflected as nitrogen balance. If the breakdown and loss of proteins exceed intake, a negative nitrogen balance results. This may be due to starvation, altered physical states (e.g., from injury or illness), and altered emotional states (such as depression or anxiety). A positive nitrogen balance, which results when protein intake exceeds breakdown, is normal during growth, tissue repair, and pregnancy. Anabolic steroids affect the rate of protein use; for example, the adrenal corticosteroids are released in times of stress to increase protein breakdown and conversion of amino acids to glucose. Excessive intake of

proteins may lead to obesity, whereas deficits cause weight loss and tissue wasting, edema, and anemia.

Fats (Lipids)

Fats (lipids) include phospholipids, steroids (such as cholesterol), and neutral fats, more commonly known as triglycerides. Neutral fats are the most abundant fats in the diet. They may be either saturated or unsaturated. Saturated fats are found in animal products (milk and meats) and in some plant products (such as coconut). Unsaturated fats are found in seeds, nuts, and most vegetable oils. Sources of cholesterol include meats, milk products, and egg yolks. Fat use by the body is shown in Figure 21–2C.

When a person consumes more fats than the body requires, the excess is stored as adipose tissue, increasing the risk of obesity and other chronic illnesses, including cardiovascular disease. A deficit of fats may cause excessive weight loss and skin lesions.

Fats are a necessary part of the structure and function of the body. For example,

■ Phospholipids are a part of all cell membranes.
■ Triglycerides are the major energy source for hepatocytes and skeletal muscle cells.

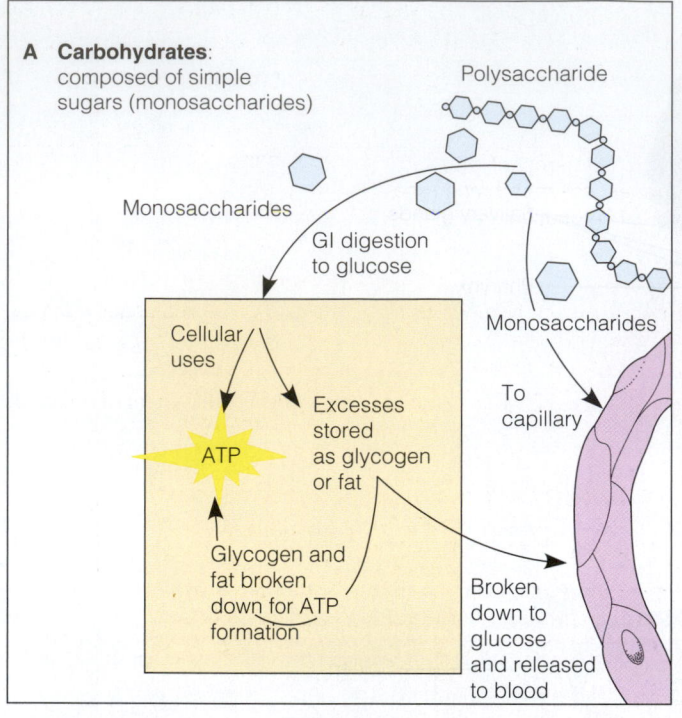

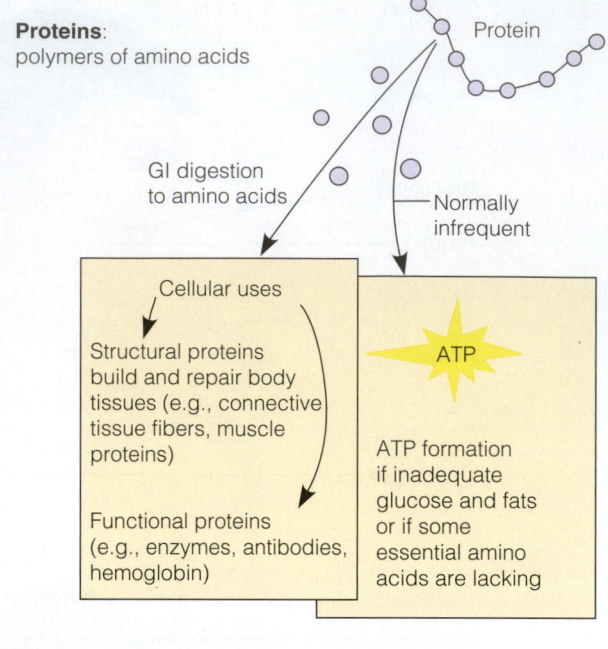

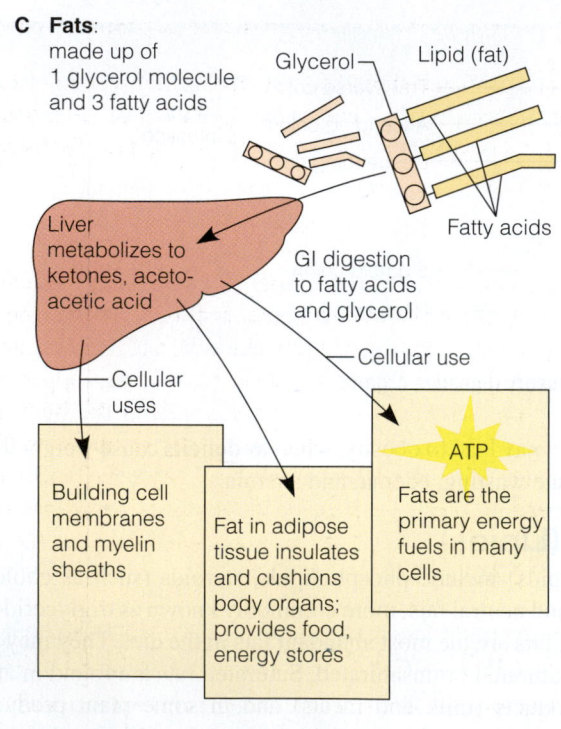

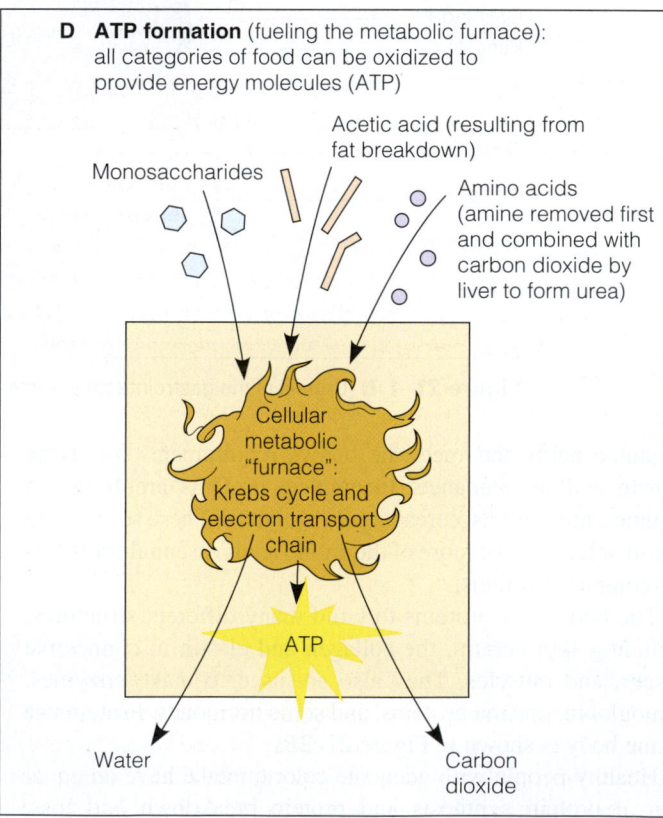

Figure 21–2 ■ A schematic overview of nutrient use by body cells, including *A,* carbohydrates; *B,* proteins; *C,* fats; and *D,* ATP formation.

- Dietary fats facilitate absorption of fat-soluble vitamins.
- Linoleic acid, an essential fatty acid, helps form prostaglandins, regulatory molecules that assist in smooth muscle contraction, maintenance of blood pressure, and control of inflammatory responses.
- Cholesterol is the essential component of bile salts, steroid hormones, and vitamin D.

- Adipose tissue serves as a protection around body organs, as a layer of insulation under the skin, and as a concentrated source of fuel for cellular energy.

Vitamins

Vitamins are organic compounds that facilitate the body's use of carbohydrates, proteins, and fats. All of the vitamins except vitamins D and K must be ingested in foods or taken as supplements.

TABLE 21–1 Recommended Daily Intake of Fat-Soluble Vitamins

NAME	SOURCE	FUNCTION	MINIMUM RECOMMENDED DAILY INTAKE (M = MEN, W = WOMEN)
Vitamin A (retinol)	■ Fish liver oils ■ Egg yolk ■ Liver ■ Fortified milk ■ Margarine	Necessary for vision, integrity of skin and mucous membranes, cell membrane function, and reproductive function	M = 900 mcg W = 700 mcg
Vitamin D	■ The action of sunshine on cholesterol in the skin	Necessary for blood calcium homeostasis (in turn necessary for blood clotting), bone formation, and neuromuscular function	M and W, 50 and under = 5 mcg M and W, 51 to 70 years of age = 10 mcg M and W, 70+ years of age = 15 mcg
Vitamin E	■ Vegetable oils ■ Margarine ■ Whole grains ■ Dark green leafy vegetables	As an antioxidant, helps prevent the oxidation of vitamins A and C in the intestines and decreases the oxidation of unsaturated fatty acids to facilitate cell membrane integrity	M and W = 15 mg
Vitamin K	■ Synthesized by coliform bacteria in the large intestine ■ Green, leafy vegetables ■ Cabbage ■ Cauliflower ■ Pork	Essential for the formation of clotting proteins in the liver	M = 120 mcg W = 90 mcg

Vitamin D is made by ultraviolet irradiation of cholesterol molecules in the skin, and vitamin K is synthesized by bacteria in the intestine.

Vitamins are categorized as either fat soluble or water soluble. The fat-soluble vitamins (A, D, E, and K) bind to ingested fats and are absorbed as the fats are absorbed. Water-soluble vitamins (the B complex and C) are absorbed with water in the GI system (however, vitamin B_{12} must become attached to intrinsic factor to be absorbed). Fat-soluble vitamins are stored in the body, and excesses may cause toxicity; water-soluble vitamins in excess of body requirements are excreted in the urine.

The recommended amounts of vitamins are labeled by the National Academy of Sciences as dietary reference intakes (DRIs) per day. The source, function, and minimum daily recommended intake levels are provided for each vitamin in Table 21–1 and Table 21–2. The recommended DRIs serve as a reference point and should be individualized to each person's lifestyle, medical status, and current knowledge of research about vitamins. It should also be noted that DRIs differ by recommending source.

Minerals

Minerals work with other nutrients to maintain the structure and function of the body. An adequate supply of calcium, phosphorus, potassium, sulfur, sodium, chloride, and magnesium—as well as other trace elements such as iron, iodine, copper, and zinc—is necessary to health. Most minerals in the body are found in body fluids or are bound to organic compounds. The best sources of minerals are vegetables, legumes, milk, and some meats. Dietary sources for the major minerals are discussed in ∞ Chapter 10. The recommended daily intake for minerals is outlined in Table 21–3.

Anatomy, Physiology, and Functions of the GI System

The GI system is a continuous hollow tube, extending from the mouth to the anus. Once foods are placed in the mouth, they are subjected to a variety of processes that move them and break them down into end products that can be absorbed from the lumen of the small intestine into the blood or lymph. These digestive processes are ingestion of food; movement of food and wastes; secretion of mucus, water, and enzymes; mechanical and chemical digestion of food; and absorption of digested food.

The Mouth

The mouth, also called the oral or buccal cavity, is lined with mucous membranes and is enclosed by the lips, cheeks, palate, and tongue (Figure 21–3 ■).

The lips and cheeks are skeletal muscle covered externally by skin. Their function is to keep food in the mouth during chewing. The palate consists of the hard palate and the soft palate. The hard palate covers bone in the roof of the mouth and provides a hard surface against which the tongue forces food. The soft palate, extending from the hard palate and ending at the back of the mouth as a fold called the uvula, is primarily muscle. When food is swallowed, the soft palate rises as a reflex to close off the oropharynx.

The tongue, composed of skeletal muscle and connective tissue, contains mucous and serous glands, taste buds, and papillae. The tongue mixes food with saliva during chewing, forms the food into a bolus (a mass) and initiates swallowing. Some papillae provide surface roughness to facilitate licking and moving food; other papillae house the taste buds.

TABLE 21–2 Recommended Daily Intake of Water-Soluble Vitamins

NAME	SOURCE	FUNCTION	MINIMUM RECOMMENDED DAILY INTAKE (M = MEN, W = WOMEN)
Vitamin B_1 (thiamin)	■ Lean meats ■ Liver ■ Eggs ■ Green leafy vegetables ■ Legumes ■ Whole grains	An essential coenzyme for carbohydrate metabolism and use; also for healthy function of nerves, muscles, and the heart	M = 1.5 mg W = 1.1 mg
Vitamin B_2 (riboflavin)	■ Liver ■ Egg white ■ Whole grains ■ Meat ■ Poultry ■ Fish ■ Milk	Involved in the catabolism and use of carbohydrates, fats, and proteins; the use of other B vitamins; and is important for the production of adrenal hormones	M = 1.8 mg W = 1.4 mg
Vitamin B_6 (pyridoxine)	■ Meat ■ Poultry ■ Fish ■ Potatoes ■ Tomatoes ■ Sweet potatoes ■ Spinach	Necessary for amino acid metabolism, formation of antibodies, and formation of hemoglobin	M = 2.0 mg W = 1.5 mg
Vitamin B_{12} (cyanocobalamin)	■ Liver ■ Meat ■ Poultry ■ Dairy foods (except butter) ■ Eggs	Essential for the production of nucleic acids and red blood cells in the bone marrow; also plays an important role in the use of folic acid and carbohydrates, and in healthy function of the nervous system	M and W = .2.0 mcg
Vitamin C (ascorbic acid)	■ Citrus fruits ■ Potatoes ■ Tomatoes ■ Green leafy vegetables	Acts as an antioxidant and vasoconstrictor; also serves in the formation of connective tissue, conversion for cholesterol to bile salts, iron absorption and use, and conversion of folic acid to an active form	M and W = 60 mg
Vitamin B_3 niacin (nicotinamide)	■ Meat ■ Poultry ■ Fish ■ Liver ■ Peanuts ■ Green leafy vegetables	Plays an important role in the metabolism of carbohydrates and fats; inhibits cholesterol synthesis; important for integumentary, nervous, and digestive system health; assists in the manufacture of reproductive hormones	M = 20 mg W = 14 mg
Biotin	■ Liver ■ Eggs ■ Nuts ■ Legumes	Essential for the catabolism of fatty acids and carbohydrates, and helps dispose of the waste products of protein catabolism	M and W = 30 mcg
Pantothenic acid	■ Meats ■ Whole grains ■ Egg yolk ■ Liver ■ Yeast ■ Legumes	Assists in the synthesis of steroids and of the heme in hemoglobin; is essential for the metabolism of carbohydrates and fats, and for the manufacture of reproductive hormones	M and W = 5 mg
Folic acid (folate)	■ Liver ■ Dark green vegetables ■ Lean beef ■ Eggs ■ Veal ■ Whole grains ■ Synthesized by bacteria in the intestine	The basis of a coenzyme necessary to the manufacture of nucleic acids and so is essential for the formation of red blood cells, growth and development, and nervous system health	M = 200 mcg W = 180 mcg

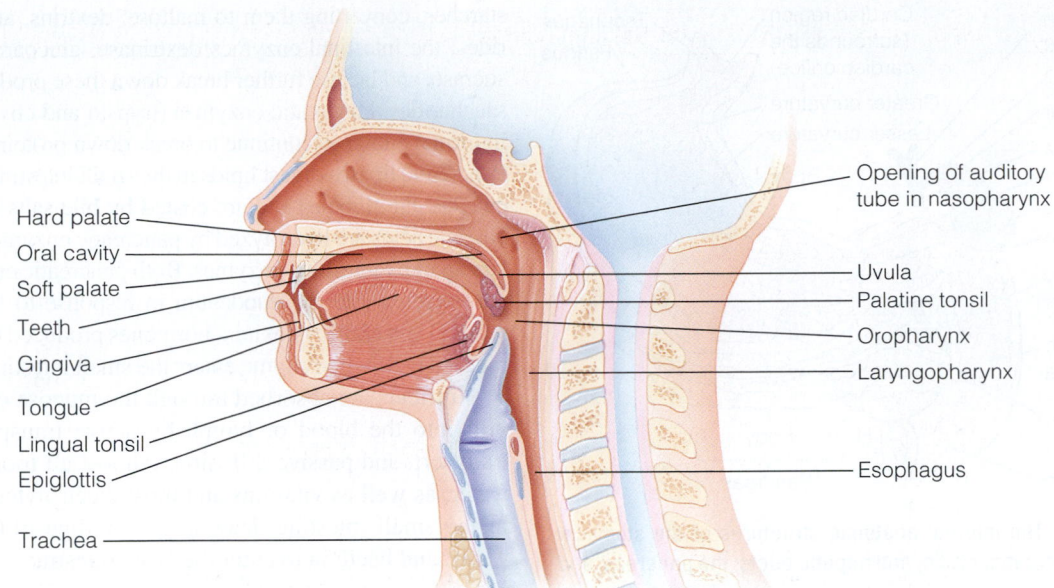

Figure 21–3 ■ Structures of the mouth, the pharynx, and the esophagus.

Saliva moistens food so it can be made into a bolus, dissolves food chemicals so they can be tasted, and provides enzymes (such as amylase) that begin the chemical breakdown of starches. Saliva is produced by salivary glands (parotid, submaxillarly, and sublingual), most of which lie superior or inferior to the mouth and drain into it. Adults have 32 permanent teeth. The teeth chew (masticate) and grind food to break it down into smaller parts, mixed with saliva.

The Pharynx

The pharynx consists of the oropharynx and the laryngopharynx (see Figure 21–3). Both structures provide passageways for food, fluids, and air. The pharynx is made of skeletal muscles and is lined with mucous membranes. The skeletal muscles move food to the esophagus via the pharynx through peristalsis (alternating waves of contraction and relaxation of involuntary muscle). The mucosa of the pharynx contains mucous-producing glands that provide fluid to facilitate the passage of the bolus of food as it is swallowed.

The Esophagus

The esophagus, a muscular tube about 10 inches (25 cm) long, serves as a passageway for food from the pharynx to the stomach (see Figures 21–1 and 21–3). The epiglottis, a flap of cartilage over the top of the larynx, keeps food out of the larynx during swallowing. The esophagus descends through the thorax and diaphragm, entering the stomach at the cardiac orifice. The gastroesophageal sphincter surrounds this opening. This sphincter, along with the diaphragm, keeps the orifice closed when food is not being swallowed.

The Stomach

The stomach, located high on the left side of the abdominal cavity, is connected to the esophagus at the upper end and to the small intestine at the lower end (Figure 21–4 ■). Normally about 10 inches (25 cm) long, the stomach is a distensible organ that can expand to hold up to 4 L of food and fluid. The stomach may be divided into the cardiac region, fundus, body, and pylorus (see Figure 21–4). The pyloric sphincter controls emptying of the stomach into the duodenal portion of the small intestine. The stomach is a storage reservoir for food, continues the mechanical breakdown of food, begins the process of protein digestion, and mixes the food with gastric juices into a thick fluid called chyme.

The stomach is lined with columnar epithelial, mucous-producing cells. Millions of openings in the lining lead to gastric glands that can produce 4 to 5 L of gastric juice each day. The gastric glands contain a variety of secretory cells that produce substances to protect the stomach from being digested

TABLE 21–3 Recommended Daily Intake of Minerals	
NAME	**MINIMUM RECOMMENDED DAILY INTAKE (M = MEN, W = WOMEN)**
Calcium	M and W = 1000 mg, W > menopause = 1200 mg
Phosphorus	M and W = 1000 mg
Iron	M = 8 mg/d, W = 18 mg
Zinc	M = 11 mg/d, W = 8 mg
Manganese	M = 2.3 mg/d, W = 1.8 mg
Molybdenum	M and W = 45 mcg
Chromium	M = 35 mcg/d, W = 25 mcg
Iodine	M and W = 150 mcg
Selenium	M and W = 70 mcg
Magnesium	M and W = 400 mg
Copper	M and W = 900 mcg
Chloride	M and W = 3400 mg
Sodium	M and W = 1100 to 3000 mg, depending on health status and recommending body

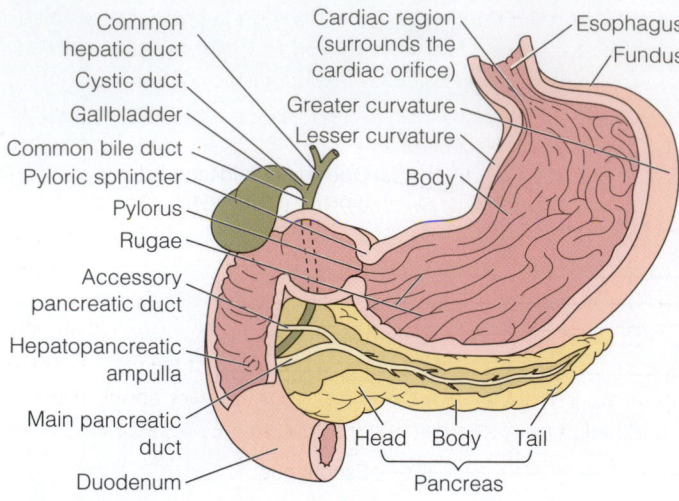

Figure 21–4 ■ The internal anatomic structures of the stomach, including the pancreatic, cystic, and hepatic ducts; the pancreas; and the gallbladder.

by gastric juice, secrete hydrochloric acid and intrinsic factor, and help regulate gastric motility.

The secretion of gastric juice is under both neural and endocrine control. Stimulation of the parasympathetic vagus nerve increases secretory activity; in contrast, stimulation of sympathetic nerves decreases secretions. Mechanical digestion is accomplished by peristaltic movements that churn and mix the food with the gastric juices to form chyme. After a person eats a well-balanced meal, the stomach empties completely in approximately 4 to 6 hours. Gastric emptying depends on the volume, chemical composition, and osmotic pressure of the gastric contents. The stomach empties large volumes of liquid content more rapidly, while gastric emptying is slowed by solids and fats.

The Small Intestine

The small intestine begins at the pyloric sphincter and ends at the ileocecal junction at the entrance of the large intestine (see Figure 21–1). The small intestine is about 20 ft (6 m) long but only about 1 inch (2.5 cm) in diameter. This long tube hangs in coils in the abdominal cavity, suspended by the mesentery and surrounded by the large intestine. The small intestine has three regions: the duodenum, the jejunum, and the ileum. The duodenum begins at the pyloric sphincter and extends around the head of the pancreas for about 10 inches (25 cm). Both pancreatic enzymes and bile from the liver enter the small intestine at the duodenum. The jejunum, the middle region of the small intestine, extends for about 8 ft (2.4 m). The ileum, the terminal end of the small intestine, is approximately 12 ft (3.6 m) long and meets the large intestine at the ileocecal valve.

Food is chemically digested and most of it absorbed as it moves through the small intestine. Circular folds containing villi (finger-like projections of the mucosa cells), and microvilli (tiny projections of the mucosa cells) increase the surface area of the small intestine to enhance absorption of food. Although up to 10 L of food, liquids, and secretions enter the GI system each day, less than 1 L reaches the large intestine.

Enzymes in the small intestine break down carbohydrates, proteins, lipids, and nucleic acids. Pancreatic amylase acts on starches, converting them to maltose, dextrins, and oligosaccharides; the intestinal enzymes dextrinase, glucoamylase, maltase, sucrase, and lactase further break down these products into monosaccharides. Pancreatic enzymes (trypsin and chymotrypsin) and intestinal enzymes continue to break down proteins into peptides. Pancreatic lipases digest lipids in the small intestine. Triglycerides enter as fat globules and are coated by bile salts and emulsified. Nucleic acids are hydrolyzed by pancreatic enzymes and then broken apart by intestinal enzymes. Both pancreatic enzymes and bile are excreted into the duodenum in response to the secretion of secretin and cholecystokinin, hormones produced by the intestinal mucosa cells when chyme enters the small intestine.

Nutrients are absorbed through the mucosa of the intestinal villi into the blood or lymph by active transport, facilitated transport, and passive diffusion. Almost all food products and water, as well as vitamins and most electrolytes, are absorbed in the small intestine, leaving only indigestible fibers, some water, and bacteria to enter the large intestine.

The Large Intestine

The large intestine (colon) begins at the ileocecal valve and terminates at the anus (Figure 21–5 ■). It is about 5 feet (1.5 m) long. The large intestine includes the cecum, the appendix, the colon, the rectum, and the anal canal. The colon is divided into ascending, transverse, and descending segments. The rectum is a mucosa-lined tube approximately 12 cm in length (Figure 21–6 ■). The rectum ends at the anal canal, which terminates at the anus, a hairless, dark-skinned area. The anorectal junction separates the rectum from the anal canal and may be the site of internal hemorrhoids (clusters of dilated veins in swollen anal tissue).

The major function of the large intestine is to eliminate indigestible food residue from the body. The large intestine absorbs water, salts, and vitamins formed by the food residue and bacteria. The semiliquid chyme that passes through the ileocecal valve is formed into feces as it moves through the large intestine by peristalsis. Goblet cells lining the large intestine secrete mucous to facilitate the lubrication and passage of feces.

The defecation reflex is initiated when feces enter the rectum and stretch the rectal wall. This spinal cord reflex causes the walls of the sigmoid colon to contract and the anal sphincters to relax. This reflex can be suppressed by voluntary control of the external sphincter. Closing the glottis and contracting the diaphragm and abdominal muscles to increase intra-abdominal

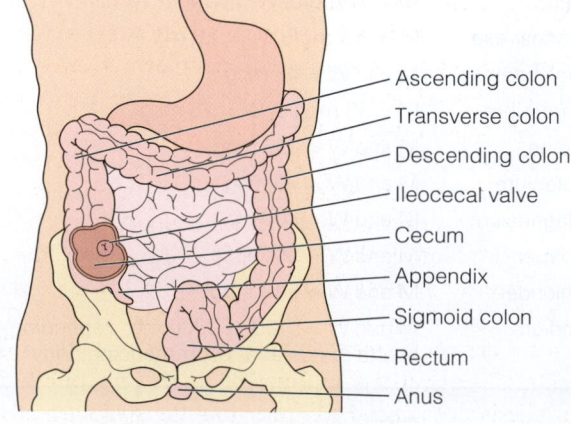

- Ascending colon
- Transverse colon
- Descending colon
- Ileocecal valve
- Cecum
- Appendix
- Sigmoid colon
- Rectum
- Anus

Figure 21–5 ■ Anatomy of the large intestine.

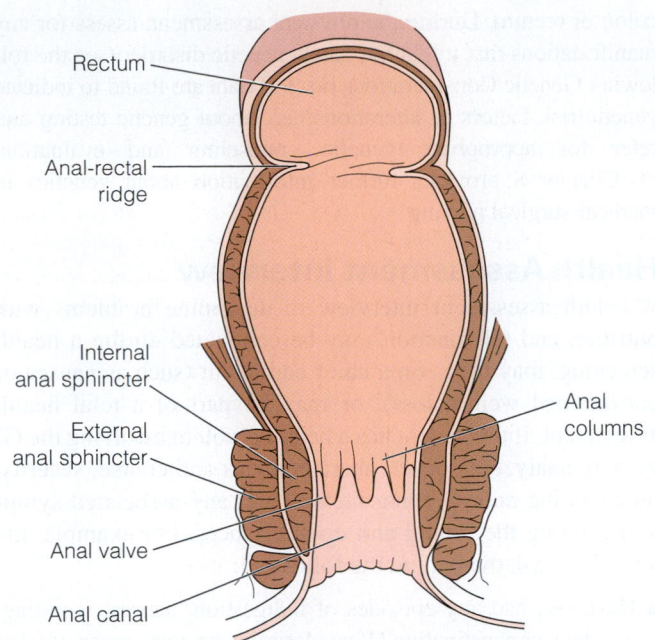

Rectum

Anal-rectal
ridge

Internal
anal sphincter

External
anal sphincter

Anal
columns

Anal valve

Anal canal

Figure 21–6 ■ Structure of the rectum and anus.

pressure (**Valsalva's maneuver**) facilitates expulsion of feces. Prolonged suppression of defecation can result in a weakened reflex that may in turn lead to constipation (infrequent and often uncomfortable passage of hard, dry stool). Frequent bouts of constipation may lead to external hemorrhoids.

The Accessory Digestive Organs

The liver, gallbladder, and exocrine pancreas are accessory digestive organs. The liver produces bile, necessary for fat digestion and absorption, and stores it in the gallbladder. The liver also receives nutrients absorbed by the small intestine and metabolizes or synthesizes these nutrients so they are in a form that can be used by the cells of the body. The exocrine pancreas produces enzymes necessary for digestion of fats, proteins, and carbohydrates.

The Liver and Gallbladder

The liver weighs about 3 lb (1.4 kg) in the average-sized adult. It is located in the right side of the abdomen, inferior to the diaphragm and anterior to the stomach (see Figure 21–1). A mesenteric ligament separates the right and left lobes and suspends the liver from the diaphragm and anterior abdominal wall. The liver is encased in a fibroelastic capsule, called the Glisson capsule. This capsule contains blood vessels, lymphatics, and nerves.

Liver tissue consists of units called lobules, which are composed of plates of hepatocytes (liver cells). A branch of the hepatic artery, a branch of the hepatic portal vein, and a bile duct communicate with each lobule. Sinusoids, blood-filled spaces within the lobules, are lined with Kupffer cells. These phagocytic cells remove debris from the blood.

Bile production is the liver's primary digestive function. **Bile** is a greenish, watery solution containing bile salts, cholesterol, bilirubin, electrolytes, water, and phospholipids. These substances are necessary to emulsify and promote the absorption of fats. Liver cells make from 700 to 1200 mL of bile daily. When bile is not needed for digestion, the sphincter of Oddi (located at the point at which bile enters the duodenum) is

closed, and the bile backs up the cystic duct into the gallbladder for storage. Bile is concentrated and stored in the gallbladder, a small sac cupped in the inferior surface of the liver. When food containing fats enters the duodenum, hormones stimulate the gallbladder to secrete bile into the cystic duct. The cystic duct joins the hepatic duct to form the common bile duct, from which bile enters into the duodenum (see Figure 21–4).

The major digestive and metabolic functions of the liver are outlined in Box 21–1. These functions require a large amount of blood, with the liver receiving blood from both venous and arterial blood vessels. The hepatic artery, branching from the abdominal aorta, provides oxygenated blood at the rate of 400 to 500 mL/min. The hepatic portal vein delivers about 1000 to 1200 mL/min of deoxygenated blood to the liver from the inferior and superior mesenteric veins and the splenic vein.

The Exocrine Pancreas

The pancreas, a gland located between the stomach and small intestine, is the primary enzyme-producing organ of the digestive system. It is a triangular gland extending across the abdomen, with its tail next to the spleen and its head next to the duodenum (see Figure 21–4). The body and tail of the pancreas are retroperitoneal, lying behind the greater curvature of the stomach. The pancreas is actually two organs in one, having both exocrine and endocrine structures and functions. The exocrine portion of the pancreas, through secretory units called acini, secretes alkaline pancreatic juice containing many different enzymes. The acini, clusters of secretory cells surrounding ducts, drain into the pancreatic duct. The pancreatic duct joins with the common bile duct just before it enters the duodenum (so that pancreatic juice and bile from the liver enter the small intestine together). The endocrine functions of the pancreas are discussed in ∞ Chapter 18.

The pancreas produces from 1 to 1.5 L of pancreatic juice daily. Pancreatic juice is clear and has high bicarbonate content. This alkaline fluid neutralizes the acidic chyme as it enters the duodenum, optimizing the pH for intestinal and pancreatic

BOX 21–1   Major Metabolic and Digestive Functions of the Liver

- Secretes bile
- Stores fat-soluble vitamins (A, D, E, and K)
- Metabolizes bilirubin
- Stores blood and releases blood into the general circulation during hemorrhage
- Synthesizes plasma proteins to maintain plasma oncotic pressure
- Synthesizes prothrombin, fibrinogen, and factors I, II, VII, IX, and X, which are necessary for blood clotting
- Synthesizes fats from carbohydrates and proteins to be either used for energy or stored as adipose tissue
- Synthesizes phospholipids and cholesterol necessary for the production of bile salts, steroid hormones, and plasma membranes
- Converts amino acids to carbohydrates through deamination
- Releases glucose during times of hypoglycemia
- Takes up glucose during times of hyperglycemia and stores it as glycogen or converts it to fat
- Alters chemicals, foreign molecules, and hormones to make them less toxic
- Stores iron as ferritin, which is released as needed for the production of red blood cells

enzyme activity. The secretion of pancreatic juice is controlled by the vagus nerve and the intestinal hormones secretin and cholecystokinin. Pancreatic juice contains enzymes that aid in the digestion of all categories of foods: lipase promotes fat breakdown and absorption; amylase completes starch digestion; and trypsin, chymotrypsin, and carboxypeptidase are responsible for half of all protein digestion. Nucleases break down nucleic acids.

Metabolism

After carbohydrates, fats, and proteins are ingested, digested, absorbed, and transported across cell membranes, they must be metabolized to produce and provide energy to maintain life. Metabolism is the process of biochemical reactions occurring in the body's cells. Metabolic processes are either catabolic or anabolic. Catabolism involves the breakdown of complex structures into simpler forms, for example, the breakdown of carbohydrates to produce ATP, an energy molecule that fuels cellular activity. In the process of anabolism, simpler molecules combine to build more complex structures; for example, amino acids bond to form proteins.

The biochemical reactions of metabolism produce water, carbon dioxide, and ATP (see Figure 21–2D on page 562). The energy value of foods is measured in kilocalories (kcal). A kilocalorie is defined as the amount of heat energy needed to raise the temperature of 1 kilogram (kg) of water 1 degree centigrade.

Assessing Gastrointestinal Function

The GI system is assessed by findings from diagnostic tests, a health assessment interview to collect subjective data, and a physical assessment to collect objective data.

Diagnostic Tests

The results of diagnostic tests of nutritional status and GI function are used to support the diagnosis of a specific disease, to provide information to identify or modify the appropriate medication or therapy used to treat the disease, and to help nurses monitor the patient's responses to treatment and nursing care interventions. Diagnostic tests to assess nutritional status and function of the GI system and the accessory organs are described on pages 571–574. More information, including specific laboratory tests, is included in the discussion of disorders in ∞ Chapters 22, 23, 24, and 25.

Regardless of the type of diagnostic test, the nurse is responsible for explaining the procedure and any special preparation needed, ensuring the consent form is signed (if necessary), supporting the patient during the examination as necessary, documenting the procedure as appropriate, and monitoring the results of the test. The nurse is also responsible for postprocedure care and patient teaching for self-care at home.

Genetic Considerations

When conducting a health assessment interview and physical assessment, it is important for the nurse to consider genetic influences on the health of the adult. During the health assessment interview, ask about family members with known abnormalities of copper accumulation in the body, hypercholesteremia, abnormal cholesterol or fat metabolism, obesity, or cancer of the pancreas,

colon or rectum. During the physical assessment, assess for any manifestations that might indicate a genetic disorder (see the following Genetic Considerations box). If data are found to indicate genetic risk factors or alterations, ask about genetic testing and refer for appropriate genetic counseling and evaluation. ∞ Chapter 8 provides further information about genetics in medical-surgical nursing.

Health Assessment Interview

A health assessment interview to determine problems with nutrition and GI function may be conducted during a health screening, may focus on a chief complaint (such as nausea or unexplained weight loss), or may be part of a total health assessment. If the patient has a health problem involving the GI system, analyze its onset, characteristics and course, severity, precipitating and relieving factors, and any associated symptoms, noting the timing and circumstances. For example, the nurse may ask the patient the following:

- Have you had any episodes of indigestion, nausea, vomiting, diarrhea, or constipation? If so, describe the appearance of what was vomited or the stools and anything that makes these problems better or worse. How long have you had these problems?
- What is your usual dietary intake pattern during a 24-hour period?
- Have you ever had bleeding from your rectum? If so, describe the amount and color of the blood (for example, was it bright red or dark red?).

When collecting information about the patient's current health status, ask about any changes in weight, appetite, and the ability to taste, chew, or swallow. What is the patient's perception of the role of nutrition in maintaining health? Who buys and prepares the food? What medications (prescribed, over-the-counter, or vitamins) is the patient currently taking? Does the patient take any vitamins, herbal supplements, or other "health food" items? Does the patient consume alcohol (how much and type)? If the patient has experienced nausea or vomiting, ask whether the vomitus contains bright red blood, dark (old) blood, bile, or fecal material. If the patient is very thin or verbalizes concerns about body size incongruent with the ratio of height to weight, ask whether the patient induces vomiting or uses laxatives to control weight. Ask whether the patient has braces, bridges, or dentures, and what self-care measures are used for such appliances, as well as oral hygiene practices and frequency of dental visits. Ask about any medical conditions that may influence the patient's bowel elimination pattern, such as a stroke or spinal cord impairment, inflammatory GI diseases, endocrine disorders, and allergies. Note any recent travel to other countries. Assess the patient's lifestyle for any patterns of psychologic stress and/or depression, which may alter bowel elimination. Depression may be associated with constipation, whereas diarrhea (frequent passage of loose, watery stools) may occur in situations of high stress and anxiety. Explore the patient's activities of daily living (ADLs), including exercise, sleep–rest patterns, and dietary and fluid intake. Ask the patient to describe the frequency and character of the stools. Ask about any history of diarrhea, constipation, or bleeding from the rectum, and collect information about the use of medications, laxatives, suppositories, or enemas. Anticholinergic drugs, antihistamines, tranquilizers, or narcotics may cause constipation.

Determine whether the patient has had any lower abdominal pain or rectal pain. Crampy, colicky pains occur with diarrhea and/or constipation. A sudden onset of lower abdominal cramping occurs in obstruction of the colon. Left lower abdominal pain is associated with diverticulitis. Rectal pain may occur with stool retention and/or hemorrhoids. ∞ See Chapter 9 for further information about pain assessment.

If the patient has an **ostomy** (surgical opening into the bowel), ask about skin care problems, consistency of stool, foods that cause problems with diarrhea or **flatus** (intestinal gas), the number of times that the patient empties the appliance bag each day, and irrigation habits. It is also important to explore the patient's feelings about the appliance.

Explore any family history of colon cancer, colitis, gallbladder disease, or malabsorption syndromes, such as lactose intolerance and celiac sprue. Assess the patient's risk factors for cancer, including age greater than 50; family member with colon cancer; history of endometrial, ovarian, or breast cancer; and previous diagnoses of colon inflammation, polyps, or cancer.

Ask the patient to describe any heartburn, indigestion, abdominal discomfort, or pain. Explore the location of the pain, the type of pain, the time it occurs, foods that aggravate or relieve it, and how it is relieved. Abdominal pain is often referred to other sites (∞ see Chapter 9). For example, a patient with a liver disorder may experience pain over the right shoulder (Kehr's sign). Epigastric (middle upper abdominal) pain is experienced in cases of acute gastritis, obstruction of the small intestine, and acute pancreatitis. Pain in the right upper quadrant is associated with cholecystitis. Pain in the left upper quadrant may be related to a gastric ulcer.

The health history should include questions about any prior surgeries or trauma of the GI system. Explore the past history of any medical condition that may affect the patient's ingestion, digestion, and/or metabolism (for example, Crohn's disease, diabetes mellitus, irritable bowel syndrome, peptic ulcers, or pancreatitis). Other areas significant to assessment are food allergies (especially to milk, which is evidenced as lactose intolerance with abdominal cramping, excessive flatus, and loose stools) and a family history that may provide clues to increased risk for health problems.

In addition to other factors assessed in the health history, culture and ethnicity are important components of nutritional status and GI health. Nutritional diversity is common among cultural and ethnic groups and questions should be included to identify specific customs, food likes and dislikes, and how foods are prepared and served. For example, in some ethnic groups, dietary substances are used to protect health, such as eating raw garlic or onions (Spector, 2009). In other cultures, dietary balance is believed to be necessary to keep the body in balance or harmony. It is necessary that nurses know about specific culturally related nutritional values and practices, and ask questions to identify health-related concerns specific to individualized dietary intake.

Interview questions categorized by functional health patterns are listed in the box on page 575.

Physical Assessment

Physical assessment of the GI system may be performed as part of a total health assessment, as a focused assessment of patients with known or suspected health problems, in combination with assessment of the urinary and reproductive systems (problems that may cause manifestations similar to those of the GI system), or alone for patients with known or suspected health problems. The techniques of inspection, auscultation, percussion, and palpation are used. Palpation is the last method used in assessing the abdomen. Figure 21–11 ■ illustrates the four quadrants of the abdomen with the organs contained in each quadrant.

GENETIC CONSIDERATIONS
Examples of Gastrointestinal Disorders

- An autosomal recessive disorder, Wilson's disease is an abnormality of copper transport, resulting in copper accumulation and toxicity to the liver and grain. Neurologic disease results in adults.
- Lynch syndrome (hereditary nonpolyposis colorectal cancer) is a type of inherited cancer of the GI system, especially the colon and rectum. Colon polyps occur at an earlier age and are more likely to become malignant.
- Tangier disease is a disease of cholesterol transport, leading to characteristic orange tonsils, very low levels of high-density lipoprotein, and an enlarged liver and spleen.
- Hypercholesterolemia has a familial tendency.
- About 90% of human pancreatic cancers show a chromosome defect.
- Obesity is believed to result from a variety of factors, including genetics.
- Familial adenomatous polyposis (FAP) and hereditary non-polyposis colorectal cancer (HNPCC) are inherited disorders in which there is progressive development of colorectal adenomas. Unless treated, colorectal cancer inevitably occurs by the fourth or fifth decade of life.
- In about 20% of cases, Crohn's disease (an inflammatory bowel disease) appears to be familial in origin.
- Colon cancer is one of the most common inherited cancer syndromes.
- Celiac disease (CD) is a genetic, inheritable disease responsible for the malabsorption of nutrients resulting in malnutrition. If people with CD eat certain types of proteins (glutens, found in wheat, barley, rye, and oats) an autoimmune response causes damage to the small intestine, so that nutrients are not absorbed.
- Gaucher disease, more common in descendants of Jewish people from eastern Europe, results in lack of an enzyme to break down fats. Fats accumulate in the liver, spleen, and bone marrow, causing pain, fatigue, jaundice, bone damage, anemia, and even death.

PRACTICE ALERT
When assessing the abdomen, use palpation last, because pressure on the abdominal wall and contents may interfere with bowel sounds and cause pain, ending the examination.

Collect objective data by obtaining anthropometric measurements (height, weight, triceps skin folds, and midarm circumference) and by examining the mouth and abdomen. Prior to the examination, collect all necessary equipment and explain techniques to the patient to decrease anxiety. Ask the patient to void.

The patient may be seated during assessment of the mouth, but is supine during the abdominal assessment. Have the patient turn to the left lateral (Sims') position for the rectal examination. The older patient or the patient with limited mobility may need assistance in assuming this position. The patient should be standing to assess for an inguinal hernia.

FUNCTIONAL HEALTH PATTERN INTERVIEW   Nutritional Status and Gastrointestinal System

Functional Health Pattern	Interview Questions and Leading Statements
Health Perception-Health Management	■ Have you had any illness or surgery that affects your nutrition, digestion, or bowel elimination? If so, how were these treated? ■ Describe your current problem; how long has it lasted; what have you done to treat it? ■ (Depending on age): Have you had your colon screened for cancer (such as a colonoscopy)? When was it last done? ■ What medications do you take? Do you take antacids? Do you take laxatives or use enemas? If so, what do you use them for and how often do you take them? ■ Do you have allergies to foods? What are they and how do you react? ■ Do you have tooth or gum pain that interferes with your ability to eat? When was your last dental examination? Describe what you do each day to take care of your teeth. ■ Do you use any treatment for hemorrhoids? Describe.
Nutritional-Metabolic	■ Describe what you eat and how much (and type) of fluids you drink in a 24-hour period. ■ Describe herbs, vitamins, and dietary supplements you currently are taking. ■ Have you noticed any change in your appetite? Explain. ■ What is your current weight? What do you feel your ideal weight would be? Have you had a recent gain or loss? Explain. ■ If patient has an ostomy: Do certain foods cause gas or diarrhea? Descibe. Describe your skin around the stoma. ■ Do you have any of the following: indigestion, belching, nausea, vomiting, difficulty swallowing? If so, what causes this and how do you treat it? ■ Do you drink alcohol? If so, what type? Describe your average number of drinks each day. ■ Questions specific to the patient's culture and ethnic group would be included in this functional health pattern area, such as what types of food are preferred or not eaten, what types of foods are never eaten together, and what types of foods are eaten to remain healthy.
Elimination	■ How often do you have a bowel movement? Are your bowel movements affected by what you eat? Explain. ■ Have you noticed any change in the color of your bowel movements? Explain. Have you noticed bright red blood in your bowel movement? ■ Have you ever used laxatives or made yourself vomit to control your weight? Explain.
Activity-Exercise	■ Describe your activities on a typical day. ■ What type of exercise do you get and how often? ■ Do you smoke? If so, what and how many cigarettes per day?
Sleep-Rest	■ Do you wake up hungry during the night? ■ Does abdominal pain, cramping, nausea, or diarrhea ever interfere with your sleep? Explain.
Cognitive-Perceptual	■ Describe the amount and type of foods you should eat each day. ■ Rate your ability to taste and smell foods on a scale of 1 to 10 (with 10 being excellent). ■ Describe any pain you have had in your mouth, stomach, abdomen, or rectum. What type of pain was it (dull, crampy, achy, burning)? What seems to cause it? What do you do to relieve it?
Self-Perception-Self-Concept	■ Are you satisfied with your appearance in terms of weight? If no, why? ■ Have you been successful in the past in gaining or losing weight? ■ How does this condition make you feel about yourself?
Role-Relationships	■ How does this condition affect your relationships with others? ■ Do you eat with others regularly? If so, who?
Sexuality-Reproductive	■ Has this condition interfered with your usual sexual activities?
Coping-Stress-Tolerance	■ Have you experienced any type of stress that may have worsened this condition? ■ Has having this condition created stress for you? ■ Describe what you do when you feel stressed.
Value-Belief	■ Tell me how specific relationships or activities help you cope with this problem. ■ Describe specific cultural beliefs or practices that affect how you care for and feel about this condition. ■ Is there anything interfering with your spiritual beliefs, needs, or practices during your illness? What can I or another caregiver do to help you with your spiritual needs? ■ Are there any specific treatments that you would not use to treat this condition?

DIAGNOSTIC TESTS of the Gastrointestinal System

THE ESOPHAGUS AND STOMACH

NAME OF TEST	PURPOSE & DESCRIPTION	RELATED NURSING INTERVENTION
Barium Swallow or Upper GI Series	These tests are conducted to diagnose esophageal varices, inflammation, ulcerations, hiatal hernia, foreign bodies, polyps, diverticula, and tumors of the esophagus, stomach, and duodenal bulb. The patient drinks 16 to 20 ounces of a chalky liquid (barium sulfate or meglumine diatrizoate [Gastrografin]) before the exam. These radiologic studies are done by observing the movement of a contrast medium with a fluoroscope (Figure 21–7 ■).	Instruct the patient not to eat or drink fluids or smoke for 8 to 12 hours before the test. Tell the patient not to take narcotics or anticholinergic medications for 24 hours pretest and not to take any medications for 8 hours pretest. Following the test, ensure the patient eliminates the barium by taking laxatives and forcing fluids as appropriate.

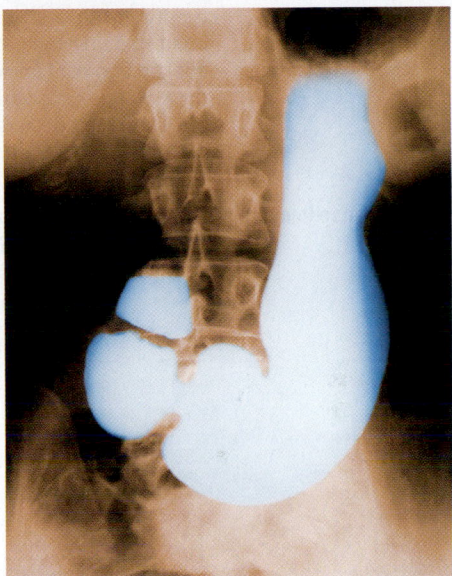

Figure 21–7 ■ A barium x-ray of a healthy stomach.

Source: Biophoto Associates/Photo Researchers, Inc.

Esophageal Acidity, Esophageal Manometry, Acid Perfusion (Bernstein Test)	Esophageal acidity is measured to diagnose problems of the lower esophageal sphincter and chronic reflux esophagitis. A catheter with a pH electrode is inserted into the esophagus through the mouth. The measurement may be one time, or over a 24-hour period. Esophageal manometry is done to measure esophageal sphincter pressure and peristaltic contractions for diagnosis of esophageal motility problems, such as achalasia. A manometric catheter with a pressure transducer is inserted into the esophagus through the mouth and esophageal pressure is measured before and after swallowing. Acid perfusion (Bernstein test) tests are done to distinguish between gastric acid reflux and cardiac involvement. A catheter is inserted through the nose into the esophagus. A saline solution, followed by an HCL solution, is dripped into the catheter and the patient is asked to indicate when pain occurs. Normal esophageal pH is 5 to 6.	Advise the patient to be NPO and to avoid alcohol intake for 8 to 12 hours prior to the exam. Assess medications: Results of the tests may be affected by antacids, anticholinergics, and cimetidine-like drugs, which increase the pH, reducing acidity and causing false test results.

(continued)

DIAGNOSTIC TESTS of the Gastrointestinal System (continued)

NAME OF TEST	PURPOSE & DESCRIPTION	RELATED NURSING INTERVENTION
Gastric Analysis Normal values: Fasting: 1.0–5.0 mEq/L/per hour Stimulation: 10–25 mEq/L/per hour	This test is used to evaluate gastric secretions for an increase or decrease of free hydrochloric acid by inserting a nasogastric tube into the stomach and aspirating stomach fluids. A stimulation gastric analysis may follow, with a gastric stimulant (such as Histalog or pentagastrin) administered and several gastric samples aspirated.	Instruct the patient to not smoke, eat, or drink fluids for 8 to 12 hours prior to the test. Assess medications and fluid intake: Anticholinergics, cholinergics, adrenergic blockers, antacids, steroids, alcohol, and coffee can alter results. Remove loose dentures. Insert nasogastric tube. Aspirate gastric contents at 15- to 20-minute intervals as ordered.
Gastric Emptying Studies	To evaluate the ability of the stomach to empty liquids or solids. In this nuclear imaging study, the patient is asked to eat a cooked egg containing Tc-^{99m} (solids) or to drink orange juice with Tc^{99m} (liquids). Sequential images are recorded with a gamma camera every 2 minutes for up to an hour.	Explain to the patient that the substances contain only very small amounts of radioactivity and are not hazardous.
Magnetic Resonance Imaging (MRI)—Stomach	An MRI of the stomach may be conducted to identify the source of gastric bleeding.	Inform the patient of the need to lie still during the examination. Assess for any metallic implants (such as pacemakers, clips on brain aneurysms, body piercing, tattoos, shrapnel). If present, notify imaging physician. Remove transdermal medication patches (both OTC and prescribed) unless otherwise ordered (FDA, 2009). Replace the patch following the procedure. Tell the patient to inform the staff about the patch when making the appointment and when completing the admission information. Ask if the patient is pregnant; if so the test is not performed. Ask about claustrophobia; if a problem, request that the patient ask for a relaxing medication to take prior to the MRI.
Upper GI Endoscopy (Esophagogastroduodenoscopy [EGD]), Gastroscopy	These tests directly visualize the mucous membrane lining of the esophagus, stomach, and duodenum. A flexible fiber-optic endoscope is used to visualize inflammations, ulcerations, tumors, or varices, and video imaging may illustrate gastric motility. They may also be combined with an ultrasound examination by attaching an ultrasound transducer to the endoscope.	Schedule this test at least 2 days after a barium swallow or upper GI series. Remove dentures and eyeglasses. Inform the patient not to eat food or drink fluids for 6 to 8 hours before the procedure. Tell the patient that the procedure takes about 20 to 30 minutes and that a local anesthetic will be administered to the throat to help prevent discomfort. After the procedure the patient is allowed to eat and drink as soon as he or she can swallow safely. Mild bloating, belching, or flatulence may occur after the procedure. Tell the patient to contact the physician postexamination for difficulty swallowing; epigastric, substernal, or shoulder pain; fever; vomiting blood; or having black tarry stools.

THE INTESTINES

NAME OF TEST	PURPOSE & DESCRIPTION	RELATED NURSING INTERVENTION
Abdominal Ultrasound	This test is used to identify abdominal masses, ascites, and disorders of the appendix. A lubricant gel is applied to the skin and a transducer is placed over the area of interest. High-frequency sound waves pass through the body structures and are recorded as they are reflected.	Tell the patient not to eat, drink, smoke, or chew gum for 6 hours prior to the examination and to eat a fat-free meal the evening before the test. Ensure that the patient has not had any other tests that might interfere with results, such as an upper GI series.
Barium Enema (Ba Enema)	A barium enema is conducted to identify structural abnormalities of the rectum and colon. This fluoroscopic radiologic examination of the colon is done by administering a contrast medium rectally. Double-contrast or air-contrast studies are the examination of choice, with air being infused after the barium is evacuated.	Inform the patient to follow a clear liquid diet for 24 hours and then to not eat or drink fluid for 8 hours before the procedure. Instruct in the administration of the prescribed laxatives, enemas, or suppositories the evening before the procedure. Following the procedure, the patient should increase fluid intake and take a laxative, if prescribed. Stools may be white until all the barium is expelled.

DIAGNOSTIC TESTS of the Gastrointestinal System (continued)

NAME OF TEST	PURPOSE & DESCRIPTION	RELATED NURSING INTERVENTION
Colonoscopy	A visual examination of the entire colon to the ileocecal valve is conducted to identify tumors, polyps, and inflammatory bowel disease and to dilate strictures. A flexible endoscope is inserted anally and advanced through the colon. Polyps are removed during the procedure to prevent future malignancies.	Tell the patient to follow the examining physician's order for preparation (this varies by physician or clinic), which may include a liquid diet the day prior to the examination, remaining NPO for 8 hours before the procedure, and a bowel preparation by, for example, citrate of magnesia, laxatives, or polyethylene glycol. (Be aware that the FDA has issued a "black box" warning for oral phosphate solutions sometimes used as bowel preparation; these drugs may damage kidney function, especially in older adults, or those who are dehydrated, have kidney disease or colitis, or are taking medications that affect kidney function [Khurana et al., 2008]). Explain that sedation is usually given during the procedure and that polyps (if present) will be removed. Instruct the patient to refrain from eating prepared foods that contain olestra (a synthetic fat additive used in products such as potato chips); the chemical may cover tissue lesions and also cause adhesive plaques to form on the colonoscopy instruments. Inform the patient that after the procedure increased flatus is common, and to report to the healthcare provider any abdominal pain, chills, fever, rectal bleeding, or mucopurulent discharge. If polyps were removed, the patient should avoid high-fiber foods for 1 to 2 days and do no heavy lifting for 7 days.
Guaiac Fecal Occult Blood Test (G-FOBT)	In this test, feces are tested for occult (hidden) blood. This is often done as a screening test for colon cancer. A stool specimen may be sent to the laboratory, or the test may be done with a commercial kit such as Hemoccult II or Occultest.	When testing for occult blood with a commercial kit, place a smear of stool on the designated area and drop the reagent on the area. A blue color that develops in response to the reagent indicates the presence of blood. If the test is done at home, tell the patient to avoid (if recommended by the healthcare provider) taking aspirin, NSAIDs, anticoagulants, red meats, fish, broccoli and other high fiber vegetables, mushrooms, vitamin C supplements, and iron supplements for 3 days prior to the stool collection.
Immunochemical Fecal Occult Blood Test (I-FOBT)	An I-FOBT is a test used to test for blood in the stool, and is considered to be more effective in detecting colon cancer than is the guaiac fecal occult blood test. A brush is used to collect water drops around the surface of a stool while it is still in the toilet bowl. The sample is then sent to the laboratory for analysis.	No special preparation is necessary. The specimen is collected and sent to the laboratory.
Magnetic Resonance Imaging (MRI)—Abdominal	An abdominal MRI may be done to identify sources of GI bleeding and to stage colon cancer.	See previous information about MRI of the stomach.
Sigmoidoscopy	A sigmoidoscopy is a visual examination of the anus, rectum, and sigmoid colon to identify tumors, polyps, infections, inflammations, hemorrhoids, and fissures. The test is done by using a flexible sigmoidoscope. Specimens are obtained and polyps removed during the procedure.	Instruct the patient to eat a clear liquid or light diet the evening before the procedure and to take prescribed laxatives. An enema or rectal suppository may be required the morning of the procedure. Explain to the patient that after the procedure large amounts of flatus may be expelled if air was instilled into the bowel, and to report any abdominal pain, fever, or rectal bleeding to the healthcare provider. If a polyp is removed, the patient should avoid heavy lifting for 7 days, and avoid high-fiber foods for 1 to 2 days.
Small-Bowel Series	This radiologic examination is done to diagnose abnormalities of the small intestine. The patient drinks a contrast medium and films are taken every 20 minutes until the medium reaches the terminal ileum. It may also be done in conjunction with an upper GI series or barium swallow.	Inform the patient that a low-residue diet should be eaten as prescribed (usually up to 48 hours pre-procedure), and not to eat for 8 hours or drink fluids for 4 hours before the test. Tell the patient about the procedure: it takes several hours to complete, and barium may be given orally, into the bowel via an endoscope, or through a weighted tube. Following the procedure the patient should increase oral fluid intake and take a prescribed laxative to facilitate evacuation of the barium. The stools will be white for up to 72 hours after the examination; normal color will return when all the barium is evacuated.

(continued)

DIAGNOSTIC TESTS of the Gastrointestinal System (continued)

NAME OF TEST	PURPOSE & DESCRIPTION	RELATED NURSING INTERVENTION
Stool Specimen, Stool Culture	A sample of stool is collected for gross and microscopic examination, as well as for form, consistency, and color. Gross examination includes volume and water content, and the presence of any blood, pus, mucus, or excess fat. Microscopic examination identifies the presence of WBCs, unabsorbed fat, and parasites. When an enteric pathogen is suspected, a stool culture is done.	Ask the patient to provide a fresh stool sample. A sterile container should be used to collect a stool sample for a culture. Ask women of childbearing age if they are having their menstrual period; if so, note this on the laboratory request.
Stool DNA test (sDNA)	This test involves examining a stool specimen for DNA changes. Premalignant polyps and malignant lesions of the bowel shed cells that have been identified as DNA markers for bowel and rectal cancer. The patient uses a kit containing an ice pack (that must be frozen for several hours before use), collects one bowel movement in a special container, then mails or brings the container with the ice pack in a provided box to the laboratory.	No special preparation is needed. Explain the procedure to the patient.
Virtual Colonoscopy (VC)	A VC is used to diagnose polyps, diverticulosis, and cancer. X-rays and computers are used to produce two- and three-dimensional images of the colon on a screen. If abnormalities are found, a conventional colonoscopy may be needed (such as to remove polyps or do a biopsy).	Explain to the patient that laxatives or other oral agents are taken the day before the procedure and a rectal suppository used the morning of the procedure. Inform the patient that a tube is inserted into the rectum, air is instilled to inflate the colon, and scans are taken.

THE GALLBLADDER AND PANCREAS

NAME OF TEST	PURPOSE & DESCRIPTION	RELATED NURSING INTERVENTION
Abdominal Ultrasound, Hepatobiliary Ultrasound, Gallbladder Ultrasound	Abdominal ultrasound is used to detect abdominal tumors, cysts, and ascites. Hepatobiliary ultrasound is used to visualize the biliary ducts, and to detect subphrenic abscesses, cysts, tumors, and cirrhosis of the liver. Gallbladder ultrasound is used to detect gallstones. These noninvasive procedures record ultrasound waves as they are reflected off body structures. A conductive gel is applied to the skin and a transducer placed on the area of interest.	Instruct the patient to remain NPO for 8 to 12 hours prior to the test.
Cholangiography ■ Percutaneous Transhepatic Cholangiogram (PTC) ■ Surgical Cholangiogram	A PTC is done to evaluate filling of the hepatic and biliary ducts. Using local anesthesia, the liver and bile duct is entered with a long needle (using fluoroscopy), bile is withdrawn, and a contrast medium is injected into the bile duct. During a surgical cholangiogram with general anesthesia, contrast medium is injected into the common bile duct to evaluate filling of the duct.	Assess for allergy to iodine, seafood, or x-ray dye (many contain iodine). Assess medications: Oral hypoglycemic agents are contraindicated for use with iodinated contrast. Monitor for bile leakage or hemorrhage following the tests.
Cholecystography (Oral) (GB Series)	The test is used to detect gallbladder stones, inflammation or tumors, and obstruction of the cystic duct. Radiopaque tablets (for example, iopanoic acid [Telepaque], sodium ipodate [Oragrafin], iodoalphionic acid [Priodax], or iodipamide meglumine [Cholografin]) are given the evening before the test; x-rays are taken the following morning. A high-fat meal may be given after the fasting x-rays are completed and further x-rays taken to determine how rapidly the GB expels the dye.	*If the patient is also having GI x-rays with barium, the GB tests should be done first, because barium would interfere with the test.* Instruct the patient to eat a fat-free diet 24 hours prior to test. No food or fluids except sips of water should be taken 12 hours before the test. Radiopaque tablets are to be taken 2 hours after the evening meal. Assess for allergy to iodine, seafood, or x-ray dye (many contain iodine). Assess medications: Oral hypoglycemic agents are contraindicated for use with iodinated contrast.

DIAGNOSTIC TESTS of the Gastrointestinal System (continued)

NAME OF TEST	PURPOSE & DESCRIPTION	RELATED NURSING INTERVENTION
Computed Tomography (CT)	This is a noninvasive procedure using radio-frequency waves and a magnetic field is used to evaluate disorders of the GB, pancreas, and liver.	No special preparation is needed.
Endoscopic Retrograde Cholangiopancreatography (ERCP)	An ERCP is done to directly visualize GI structures, and to retrieve gallstones from the distal common bile duct, dilate structures, and biopsy tumors. A fiber-optic endoscope is inserted through the mouth, the esophagus, stomach, and descending duodenum, and the common bile ducts and pancreatic ducts. Contrast medium is injected into the ducts and structures are visualized.	Tell the patient not to drink fluids or eat for 8 hours before the test. Assess patient for allergy to iodine, seafood, or x-ray dye (many contain iodine). Assess medications: Oral hypoglycemic agents are contraindicated for use with iodinated contrast. Assess gag reflex prior to giving food or fluids. If atropine was given, assess for manifestations of urinary retention. Tell the patient that a sore throat may be present for a few days after the test; suggest warm saline gargles to ease discomfort.
Magnetic Resonance Cholangiopancreatography (MRCP)	This noninvasive MRI study is done to evaluate the biliary and pancreatic ducts.	See previous information for MRI of the stomach.
Serum Amylase Normal value: 0–130 Unit/L	This blood test is used to measure the secretion of amylase by the pancreas. It is used to diagnose acute pancreatitis, when amylase level peaks in 24 hours and then drops to normal in 48 to 72 hours.	No special preparation is needed.
Serum Lipase Normal value: 0–160 Unit/L	This blood test is used to measure the secretion of lipase by the pancreas.	No special preparation is needed.

THE LIVER

NAME OF TEST	PURPOSE & DESCRIPTION	RELATED NURSING INTERVENTION
Liver Biopsy	A liver biopsy is performed to rule out metastatic cancer or to detect a cyst or cirrhosis of the liver. The procedure is considered minor surgery, and is done at a hospital. Using ultrasound, a biopsy needle is inserted into the liver and guided to the pathologic site. See Figure 21–8 ■.	Inform the patient to tell the doctor about any anticoagulants taken, and to withhold aspirin and ibuprofen for a week before the procedure. Food and fluids are withheld for 4 to 6 hours before the procedure, assess and record baseline vital signs, and review prothrombin time and platelet count. Administer vitamin K as prescribed. Ask the patient to void immediately before the procedure. After the needle is removed, pressure is applied; place the patient on the right side for 1 to 2 hours to maintain pressure on the insertion site. Explain to the patient that pain may be experienced in the right shoulder as the local anesthetic loses effect, that the dressing will be assessed frequently, that food and fluids are withheld for 2 hours after the biopsy, and that coughing, lifting, or straining should be avoided for 1 to 2 weeks. The patient will not be allowed to drive home, and must go directly to bed for 8 to 10 hours (or as prescribed by the physician).

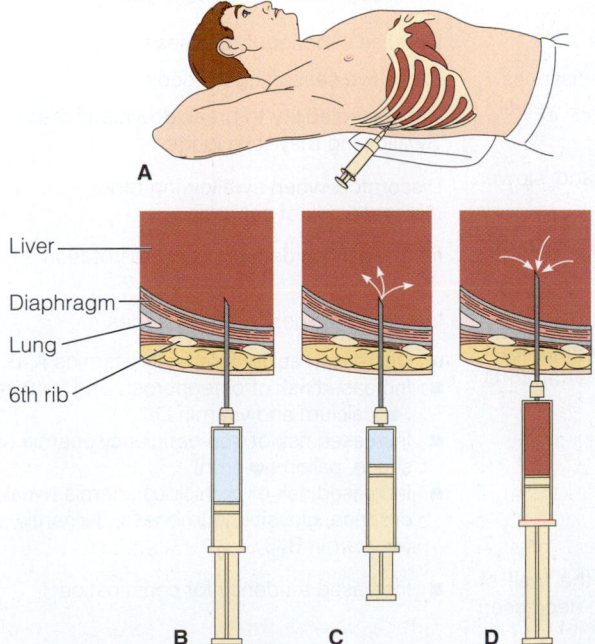

Liver

Diaphragm

Lung

6th rib

A

B   C   D

Figure 21–8 ■ Liver biopsy. *A*, The patient exhales completely, and then holds his or her breath. This brings the liver and diaphragm to their highest position. *B*, The biopsy needle is inserted into the liver. *C*, Approximately 1 mL of saline is injected to clear the needle of blood and tissue. *D*, The needle is advanced, and a tissue sample is aspirated. Pressure is applied to the site immediately after the needle is withdrawn. The specimen is sent to the laboratory for analysis.

Note: A wide variety of blood tests are used to diagnose and monitor liver disease. These are discussed in appropriate interdisciplinary care sections in ∞ Chapter 25.

Explain what will happen during the examination, and encourage the patient to take deep, regular breaths to increase relaxation. Explain that during the rectal examination, it may feel as though the patient is about to have a bowel movement and sometimes flatus (gas) is passed. Assure the patient that this is normal. Ensure that the examination area is private and the patient is draped properly to prevent unnecessary exposure.

Physical assessment of the integumentary system, nervous system, musculoskeletal system, cardiovascular system, and respiratory system may reflect the patient's nutritional status. Table 21–4 summarizes abnormal nutritional assessment findings related to these body systems. Normal age-related findings for the older adult are summarized in the Nursing Care of the Older Adult box.

TABLE 21–4 Assessment Findings Due to Malnutrition

BODY SYSTEM	ASSESSMENT FINDINGS
Nails	Soft and spoon shaped in iron deficiency. Splinter hemorrhages in vitamin C deficiency.
Hair	Dry, dull, and scarce in zinc, protein, and linoleic acid deficiencies.
Skin	Flaky and dry in vitamin A, vitamin B, and/or linoleic acid deficiency. Cracks and/or hyperpigmentation in niacin deficiency. Bruising in vitamin C or vitamin K deficiency.
Eyes	Eyes become dry and soft with decrease in vitamin A. Conjunctiva is pale with a decrease in iron, and red with a decrease in riboflavin.
Nervous system	Reflexes are decreased and patient may have peripheral neuropathies with thiamine deficiency. Patient may be irritable and/or disoriented with thiamine deficiency.
Musculoskeletal system	Muscle wasting is seen with deficits in protein, carbohydrate, and fat metabolism. Calf pain occurs with thiamine deficiency; joint pain may occur with vitamin C deficiency.
Cardiovascular system	Heart size and rate may increase with thiamine deficiency. Diastolic blood pressure may be increased with a high intake of fat. Lowered cardiac output and decreased blood pressure may occur with caloric deficiencies over a long time period.
GI system	Cheilosis (sores at corner of mouth) seen in vitamin B-complex deficiencies, especially riboflavin. Stomatitis and spongy, bleeding gums may also be seen in malnutrition.

NURSING CARE OF THE OLDER ADULT   Age-Related Gastrointestinal Changes

AGE-RELATED CHANGE	SIGNIFICANCE
Teeth: ▲ number of root cavities and cavities around existing dental work; tooth enamel harder and more brittle; dentin is more fibrous; tooth cusps flatten; root pulp shrinks; ▲ loss of bone supporting teeth	Increase in periodontal disease and tooth loss Increase in fractures of teeth Increased incidence of dentures
Gums: Gingiva retracts	Increase in periodontal disease
Taste: Less acute as tongue atrophies, especially for sweet sensations	Excessive seasoning of foods
Saliva: ▼ amount is produced (1/3 of that produced in younger years)	Decreased ability to break down starches Swallowing may take longer
Esophageal motility: ▼ intensity of propulsive waves and slower emptying time, weaker gag reflex	Discomfort when swallowing food Increased risk of aspiration
Stomach: Mucosa atrophies, ▼ production of hydrochloric acid and pepsin leading to higher pH in stomach	Increase in incidence of gastric irritation
Liver: Less efficient handling of cholesterol	Increased incidence of gallstones
Small intestine: ▼ number of absorbing cells on intestinal wall, slowed fat absorption, faulty absorption of vitamin B_{12}, vitamin D, calcium, and iron	▪ Decreased ability to absorb vitamins A, D, E, and K ▪ Increased risk of osteoporosis and fractures (▼ calcium and vitamin D) ▪ Increased risk of iron-deficiency anemia (weakness, lassitude, pallor) (▼ iron) ▪ Increased risk of pernicious anemia (weakness, dyspnea, glossitis, numbness, dementia, depression) (▼ vitamin B_{12})
Large intestine: ▼ mucous secretion and elasticity of the wall of the rectum, loss of tone in internal sphincter with decreased awareness of need to defecate	▪ Increased tendency for constipation

Gastrointestinal Assessments

Technique/Normal Findings	Abnormal Findings

Anthropometric Assessment

Weigh the patient and measure the patient's height. Compare the patient's actual weight to ideal body weight (IBW) (Table 21–5). *Weight should be appropriate to height as indicated on a standardized table.*

- A weight 10% to 20% less than ideal body weight indicates malnutrition.
- A weight 10% above ideal body weight is considered overweight.
- A weight 20% above ideal body weight is considered obese.

TABLE 21–5 Example of a Height and Weight Table

	HEIGHT		WEIGHT		
	FEET	INCHES	SMALL FRAME	MEDIUM FRAME	LARGE FRAME
Men (ages 25–29)	5	2	128–134	131–134	138–150
	5	3	130–136	133–143	140–153
	5	4	132–138	135–145	142–156
	5	5	134–140	137–148	144–160
	5	6	136–142	139–151	146–164
	5	7	138–145	142–154	149–168
	5	8	140–148	145–157	152–172
	5	9	142–151	148–160	155–176
	5	10	144–154	151–163	158–180
	5	11	146–157	154–166	161–184
	6	0	149–160	157–170	164–188
	6	1	152–164	160–174	168–192
	6	2	155–168	164–178	172–197
	6	3	158–172	167–182	176–202
	6	4	162–176	171–187	181–207
Women (ages 25–29)	4	10	102–111	109–121	118–131
	4	11	103–113	111–123	120–134
	5	0	104–115	113–126	122–137
	5	1	106–118	115–129	125–140
	5	2	108–121	118–132	128–143
	5	3	111–124	121–135	131–147
	5	4	114–127	124–138	134–151
	5	5	117–130	127–141	137–155
	5	6	120–133	130–144	140–159
	5	7	123–136	133–147	143–163
	5	8	126–139	136–150	146–167
	5	9	129–142	139–153	149–170
	5	10	132–145	142–156	152–173
	5	11	135–148	145–159	155–176
	6	0	138–151	148–162	158–179

Technique/Normal Findings	Abnormal Findings

Calculate the patient's percentage of ideal body weight (%IBW). To calculate IBW, (1) determine the height and weight of the patient, (2) multiply the height times 2, (3) divide the body weight by the answer obtained in step 2, and (4) multiply the answer from step 3 by 703. The result is the patient's IBW.
Ideal body weight should be within normal range (19–25).

A healthy IBW is from 19 to 25. Underweight is considered anything below 18, 25 to 29 is considered overweight, and anything over 30 is considered obese.
Note: This is one of several ways used to calculate IBW.

Measure body mass index (BMI). Determine BMI by using one of the following formulas. *BMI should be between 20 and 25.*

- A BMI of 25 to 29.9 kg/m^2 indicates overweight.
- A BMI of 30 kg/m^2 indicates obesity.

$$\frac{\text{Weight in kilograms}}{\text{Height in meters}^2} = \text{BMI}$$

$$\frac{\text{Weight in pounds} \times 705}{\text{Height in inches}^2} = \text{BMI}$$

Measure triceps skinfold thickness (TSF). Find the midpoint between the patient's olecranon and acromion processes. Grasp the skin and fat, and pull it away from the muscle. Apply skinfold calipers for 3 seconds, and record the reading (Figure 21–9 ■). Repeat three times, and average the three readings. Compare the patient's reading to the standard values shown in Table 21–6. *TSF should be within normal range as compared to standard values.*

- Triceps readings are 10% or more below standards in malnutrition and 10% or more above standards in obesity or overnutrition.

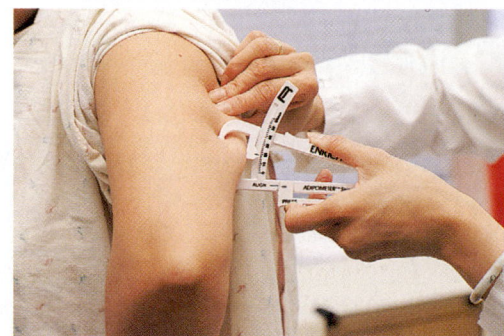

Figure 21–9 ■ Measuring the triceps skinfold thickness with calipers.

TABLE 21–6 Values for Anthropometric Measurements

| MEASUREMENT | STANDARD VALUE | |
	MALE	FEMALE
Triceps skinfold thickness	12.5 mm	16.5 mm
Midarm circumference	29.3 cm	28.5 cm
Midarm muscle circumference	25.3 cm	23.2 cm

Measure midarm circumference (MAC). Find the midpoint between the patient's olecranon and acromion processes. Wind tape measure around arm (Figure 21–10 ■). Compare the patient's reading to the standard values shown in Table 21–6. *MAC should be within normal range as compared to standard values.*

- MAC decreases with malnutrition and increases with obesity.

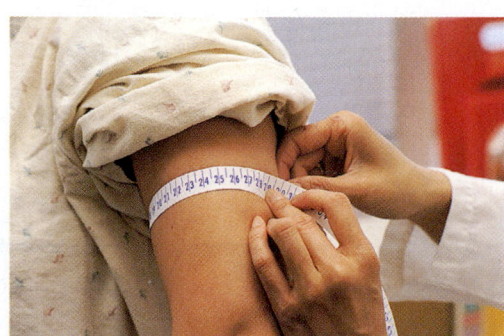

Figure 21–10 ■ Measuring MAC with a tape measure.

Technique/Normal Findings	Abnormal Findings

Calculate midarm muscle circumference (MAMC). Use the patient's triceps skinfold measurement and midarm circumference readings to calculate the patient's MAMC.

Compare the result to the standard values shown in Table 21–6. *MAMC should be within normal range as compared to standard values.*

- In mild malnutrition, the MAMC is 90% of the standard; in moderate malnutrition, 60% to 90%. In severe malnutrition (muscle wasting), the MAMC is less than 60% of the standard.

$$MAMC = MAC - (0.314 \times TSF)$$

Determine waist-to-hip ratio. With the patient standing, measure the waist, and then measure the hips midway between the iliac crest and the greater trochanter. Use the following formula to calculate the waist-to-hip ratio. *Normal findings: females, waist ratio less than or equal to 0.80; males, waist ratio less than or equal to 1.0.*

- Females with a ratio greater than 0.80 and males with a ratio greater than 1.0 have a three to five times greater risk for having a heart attack or stroke (Weber & Kelley, 2009).

$$\frac{\text{Waist circumference}}{\text{Hip circumference}} = \text{waist-to-hip ratio}$$

SAMPLE DOCUMENTATION

Assessment of Nutritional Status

Twenty-two-year-old female visiting health clinic for regular check-up. Height 5 feet, 5 inches (165 cm); Weight 128 pounds (58 kg). BMI: 24. MAC: 28 cm. Waist-to-hip ratio: 0.6. Skin is warm, moist, and smooth without lesions other than well-healed scar on RLQ of abdomen from appendectomy, age 15. Oral mucosa and tongue pink and moist. No breath odor. All teeth present with evidence of dental care. Abdomen slightly concave when lying on back, bowel sounds present in all four quadrants, liver nonpalpable, tympany over lower abdomen on percussion.

Oral Assessment

Inspect and palpate the lips. *Lips should be of normal color for race without lesions.*

- **Cheilosis** (painful lesions at corners of mouth) is seen with riboflavin and/or niacin deficiency.
- Cold sores or clear vesicles with a red base are seen in herpes simplex 1.

Inspect and palpate the tongue. *Tongue should be pink, smooth, and have good turgor.*

- Atrophic smooth **glossitis** is characterized by a bright red tongue. It is seen in B_{12}, folic acid, and iron deficiencies.
- Vertical fissures are seen in dehydration.
- A black, hairy tongue may be seen following antibiotic therapy.

Inspect and palpate the buccal mucosa. *Mucosa should be moist, without lesions and of appropriate color.*

- **Leukoplakia** (small white patches) may be a sign of a premalignant condition.
- A reddened, dry, swollen mucosa may be seen in stomatitis.
- Candidiases (white cheesy patches that bleed when scraped) may be seen in immune-suppressed patients receiving antibiotics or chemotherapy and in terminally ill patients.

Inspect and palpate the teeth. *Teeth should be in a state of good hygiene without caries.*

- Cavities and excessive plaque are seen with poor nutrition and/or poor oral hygiene.

Inspect and palpate the gums. *Gums should be of even color without swelling.*

- Swollen, red gums that bleed easily (**gingivitis**) are seen in periodontal disease, vitamin C deficiencies, or with hormonal changes.

Inspect the throat and tonsils. *Tonsils (if present) should be of appropriate color and size.*

- In acute infections, tonsils are red and swollen and may have white spots.

Note the patient's breath. *Breath should not have unusual or foul odors.*

- Sweet, fruity breath is noted in diabetic ketoacidosis.
- Acetone breath may be a sign of uremia.
- Foul breath may result from liver disease, respiratory infections, and poor oral hygiene.

Abdominal Assessment

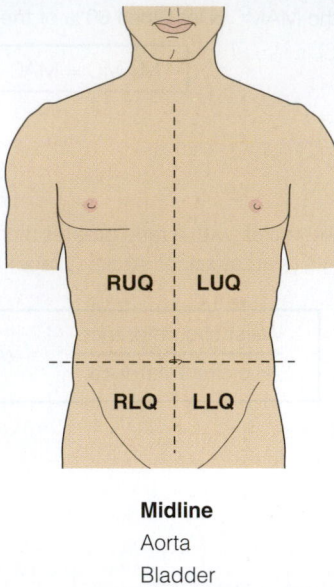

Right Upper Quadrant
Liver and gallbladder
Pylorus
Duodenum
Head of pancreas
Right adrenal gland
Portion of right kidney
Hepatic flexure of colon
Portions of ascending and
    transverse colon

Left Upper Quadrant
Left lobe of liver
Spleen
Stomach
Body of pancreas
Left adrenal gland
Portion of left kidney
Splenic flexure of colon
Portions of transverse and
    descending colon

Right Lower Quadrant
Lower pole of right kidney
Cecum and appendix
Portion of ascending colon
Bladder (if distended)
Right ovary and salpinx
Right spermatic cord
Right ureter

Left Lower Quadrant
Lower pole of left kidney
Sigmoid colon
Portion of descending colon
Bladder (if distended)
Left ovary and salpinx
Uterus (if enlarged)
Left spermatic cord
Left ureter

Midline
Aorta
Bladder
Uterus

◯ = Umbilicus

Figure 21–11 ■ The four quadrants of the abdomen.

BOX 21–2 Guidelines for Assessing the Abdomen

Ask the patient to empty the bladder before beginning the examination. Assist the patient to the dorsal recumbent (supine) position, with a small pillow under the head, a pillow under the knees (if desired), and the arms at the sides of the body. Warm the stethoscope before applying it to the patient's skin. Ask the patient to point to areas that are painful, and explain that those areas will be examined last. Expose the abdomen from below the breasts to the pubic symphysis, and drape the patient's thoracic and genital areas. When you document your findings, specify the location by abdominal quadrant.

General guidelines for abdominal assessment are as follows:
1. Inspect the abdomen under a good light source that is shining across the abdomen. Sit at the right side of the patient, and note symmetry, distention, masses, visible peristalsis, and respiratory movements. If masses are detected, ask the patient to take a deep breath, which decreases the size of the abdominal cavity and makes any abnormality more visible.
2. Auscultate each quadrant of the abdomen, using the diaphragm of the stethoscope. Listen for bowel sounds, arterial bruits, venous hums, and friction rubs.

3. Percuss several areas within each quadrant of the abdomen, using a systematic path. (For example, always begin in the lower left quadrant, then proceed to the lower right quadrant, upper right quadrant, and upper left quadrant, respectively). The predominant percussion tones for the entire abdomen are tympany and dullness. Tympany is present over gas-filled intestines. Dullness is present over the liver, the spleen, an enlarged kidney, or a full stomach. Percuss for fluid, gaseous distention, and masses.
4. Palpate each quadrant of the abdomen for shape, position, mobility, size, consistency, and tenderness of the major abdominal organs. Begin this part of the assessment with light palpation, and increase the depth of palpation to elicit tenderness or better identify organ size and shape. Deep palpation should be conducted only by nurses with considerable experience. Remember to palpate areas of indicated tenderness last and to use gentle pressure. Palpation may be difficult or impossible if the patient exhibits muscle guarding from pain or is ticklish. The gallbladder and the spleen are normally not palpable.

Technique/Normal Findings	Abnormal Findings
Inspect abdominal contour, skin integrity, venous pattern, and aortic pulsation. *Abdomen should be slightly concave or rounded with intact skin. There should not be distended veins or obvious aortic pulsations.*	■ Generalized abdominal distention may be seen in gas retention or obesity. ■ Lower abdominal distention is seen in bladder distention, pregnancy, or ovarian mass. ■ General distention and an everted umbilicus are seen with ascites and/or tumors. ■ A scaphoid (sunken) abdomen is seen in malnutrition or when fat is replaced with muscle. ■ **Striae** (whitish-silver stretch marks) are seen in obesity and during or after pregnancy. ■ Spider angiomas may be seen in liver disease. ■ Dilated veins are prominent in cirrhosis of the liver, ascites, portal hypertension, or venocaval obstruction. ■ Pulsation is increased in aortic aneurysm.

Technique/Normal Findings	Abnormal Findings

Auscultate all four quadrants of the abdomen with the diaphragm of the stethoscope (Figure 21–12 ■). Begin in the lower right quadrant, where bowel sounds are almost always present. If bowel sounds are not heard, ask a colleage to check your findings. *Normal bowel sounds (gurgling or clicking) occur every 5 to 15 seconds. Listen for at least 5 minutes in each of the four quadrants to confirm the absence of bowel sounds.*

- **Borborygmus** (hyperactive high-pitched, tinkling, rushing, or growling bowel sounds) is heard in diarrhea or at the onset of bowel obstruction.
- Bowel sounds may be absent later in bowel obstruction, with an inflamed peritoneum, and/or following surgery of the abdomen

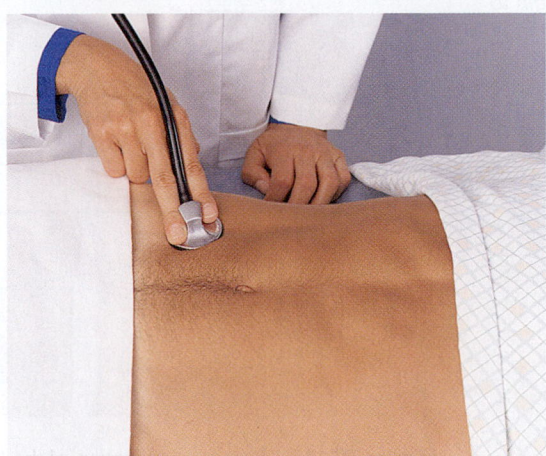

Figure 21–12 ■ Auscultating the abdomen with the diaphragm of the stethoscope.

Auscultate the abdomen for vascular sounds with the bell of the stethoscope (Figure 21–13 ■). *No sounds (bruits, venous hum, or friction rub) other than bowel sounds should be auscultated.*

- **Bruits** (blowing sound due to restriction of blood flow through vessels) may be heard over constricted arteries. A bruit over the liver may be heard in hepatic carcinoma.
- A venous hum (continuous medium-pitched sound) may be heard over a cirrhotic liver.
- Friction rubs (rough grating sounds) may be heard over an inflamed liver or spleen.

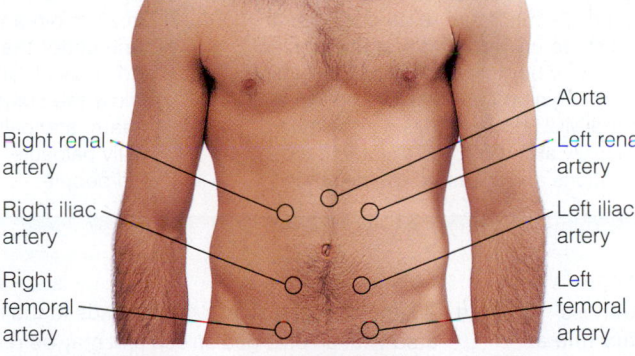

Figure 21–13 ■ Location of placement of the stethoscope for auscultation of arteries of the abdomen.

Percuss the abdomen in all four quadrants (Figure 21–14 ■). *Normally, tympany is heard over the stomach and gas-filled bowels.*

- Dullness is heard when the bowel is displaced with fluid or tumors or filled with a fecal mass.

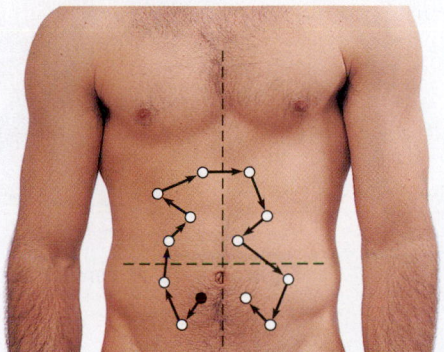

Figure 21–14 ■ Location of sites for systematic percussion of all four quadrants.

Technique/Normal Findings	Abnormal Findings

Percuss the liver (see Box 21–3 for guidelines for liver percussion and palpation; see Figure 21–15 ■ for landmarks). *The lower border of liver dullness is located at the costal margin to 1 to 2 cm below.*

■ In cirrhosis and/or hepatitis, the liver is greater than 6 to 10 cm in the MCL and greater than 4 to 8 cm in the midsternal line (MSL).

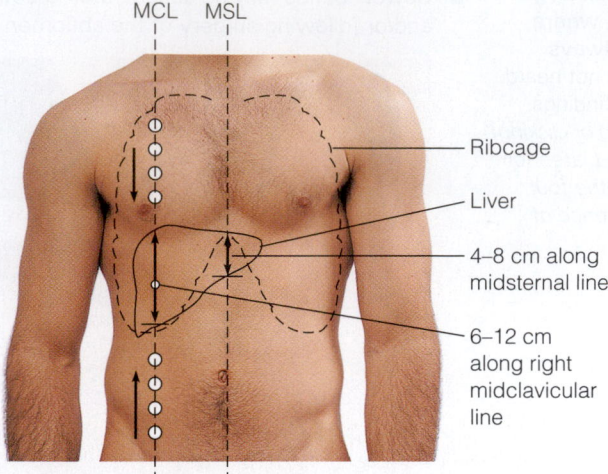

MCL   MSL

Ribcage

Liver

4–8 cm along midsternal line

6–12 cm along right midclavicular line

Figure 21–15 ■ Anatomic location of the liver, with the midclavicular line (MCL) and midsternal line (MSL) superimposed. The normal liver span is 6 to 12 cm.

BOX 21–3 Guidelines for Percussing and Palpating the Liver

The size of the liver may be determined by percussion and palpation, as follows:

1. Percuss, in the midclavicular line (MCL), beginning below the umbilicus (see Figure 21–15). Begin to percuss over a region of tympany, and move upward. The first dull percussion tone occurs at the lower border of the liver. Determine the upper liver border by beginning percussion over an area of lung resonance (in the MCL) and percussing downward to the first dull tone, usually at the 5th to 7th interspace. Mark each of these locations and measure the distance

from one mark to the other to determine liver size. The normal liver size is 6 to 12 cm in the MCL; however, men have larger livers than women.

2. Conduct bimanual palpation of the liver by placing your left hand under the patient at the level of the 11th to 12th ribs and applying upward pressure. Place your right hand below the costal margin, ask the patient to take a deep breath, and palpate for the liver border. The liver is not normally palpable in a healthy adult, although it may be in very thin people.

Percuss the spleen for dullness posterior to the midaxillary line at the level of the 6th to 11th rib (Figure 21–16 ■). *The spleen is percussed as an oval area of dullness approximately 7 cm wide near the left 10th rib and slightly posterior to the midaxillary line.*

■ A large area of dullness that extends to the left anterior axillary line on inspiration is associated with an enlarged spleen and may be related to trauma, infection, or mononucleosis.

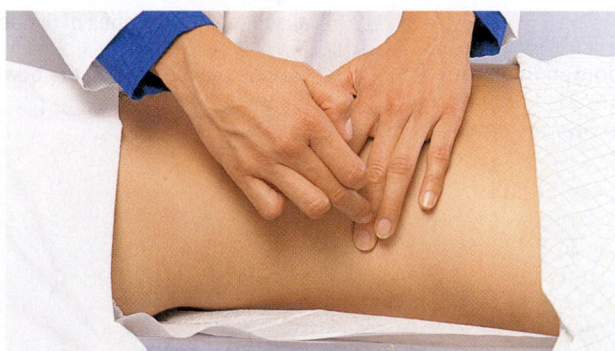

Figure 21–16 ■ Percussing the spleen.

Technique/Normal Findings	Abnormal Findings

Percuss for shifting dullness (Figure 21–17 ■). *If ascites is not present, the borders between tympany and dullness remain relatively constant despite position changes.*

- In a patient with ascites, the level of dullness increases when the patient turns to the side.

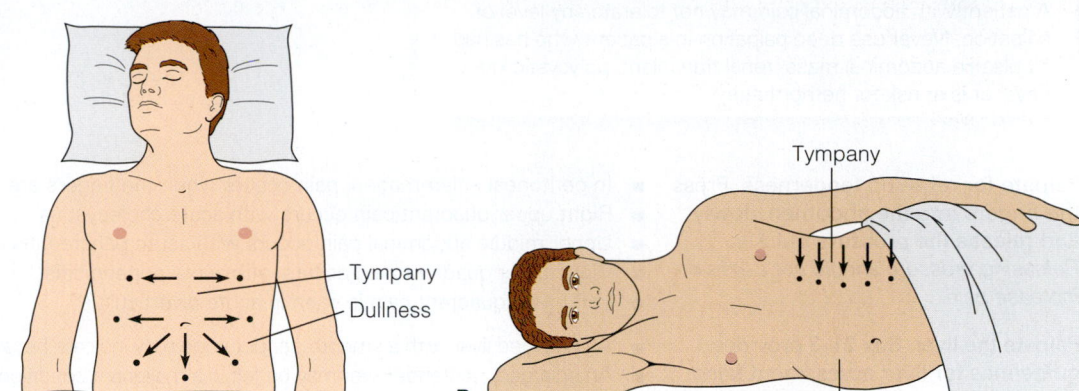

A

B

Figure 21–17 ■ Percussing for shifting dullness in ascites. *A,* Common percussion tones when the patient is lying supine; *B,* changes in percussion tones (shifting dullness) when the patient turns to the side.

Palpate the abdomen in all four quadrants (Figure 21–18 ■). If the patient tightens the abdominal muscles (called "guarding") flexing the knees may relax the muscles. *There should be no abdominal masses or pain on palpation.*

- In cases of peritoneal inflammation, palpation causes abdominal pain and involuntary muscle spasms.
- Abnormal masses include aortic aneurysms, neoplastic tumors of the colon or uterus, and a distended bladder or distended bowel due to obstruction.
- A rigid, boardlike abdomen may be palpated when the patient has a perforated duodenal ulcer.

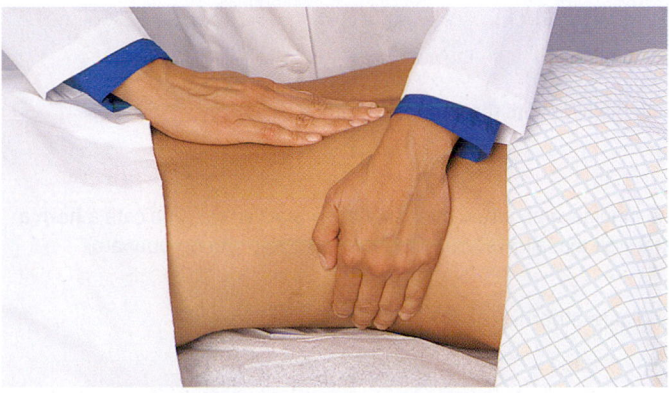

A

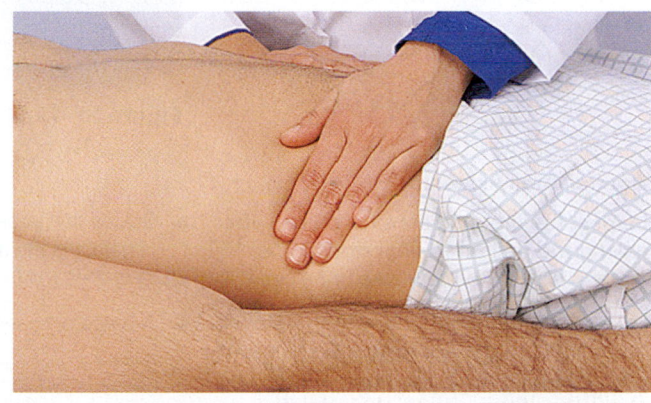

B

Figure 21–18 ■ Light to moderate palpation of the abdomen. *A,* In light palpation, the examiner, keeping the fingers approximated, gently depresses the abdominal wall about 1 cm to assess for large masses, slight tenderness, and muscle guarding. *B,* The examiner performs moderate palpation by using the palm or the side of the hand to depress the abdominal wall to a slightly greater depth than in light palpation. This technique is useful for assessing abdominal organs that move with respiration (such as the liver and the spleen).

Use a circular motion to move the abdominal wall over underlying structures, Feel for masses and note any tenderness or pain the patient may have during this part of the exam. Palpate lightly at first (0.5 to 5 inch), then deeply (1.5 to 2 inches) with caution. If a mass is palpated, ask the patient to raise head and shoulders. A mass in the abdomen may become more prominent with this maneuver, as will a ventral abdominal wall hernia. If the mass is no longer palpable, it is deeper in the abdomen. *There should be no palpable masses or pain.*

Technique/Normal Findings	Abnormal Findings

Palpate for rebound tenderness. Press the fingers into the abdomen slowly and release the pressure quickly. *Releasing pressure should not cause or increase pain.*

- In peritoneal inflammation, pain occurs when the fingers are withdrawn.
- Right upper quadrant pain occurs with acute cholecystitis.
- Upper middle abdominal pain occurs with acute pancreatitis.
- Right lower quadrant pain occurs with acute appendicitis.
- Left lower quadrant pain is seen in acute diverticulitis.

Palpate the liver. Box 21–3 provides guidelines for liver assessment (also see Figure 21–19 ■). Note whether the patient guards the abdomen or reports any sharp pain, especially on inspiration. *The abdomen should be nontender, and the liver is usually nonpalpable.*

- An enlarged liver with a smooth, tender edge may indicate hepatitis or venous congestion.
- An enlarged, nontender liver may be felt in a malignant condition.
- The patient with inflammation of the gallbladder feels sharp pain on inspiration and stops inspiring. This is called Murphy's sign.

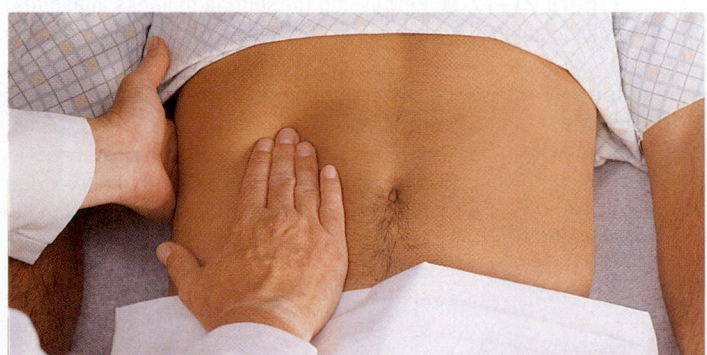

Figure 21–19 ■ Palpating the liver with the bimanual method.

Inguinal Area Assessment

Inspect the inguinal area for bulges after asking the patient to bear down. *The inguinal area is normally free of bulges.*

- Bulges that appear in the inguinal area when the patient bears down may indicate a **hernia** (a defect in the abdominal wall that allows abdominal contents to protrude outward).

Palpate the inguinal area with the gloved hand. Ask the patient to shift weight to the left to palpate the right inguinal area and vice versa. Place your right index finger upward into the inguinal area and ask the patient to bear down or cough. *Bulging or masses are normally not palpable.*

- A bulge or mass may indicate a hernia.

Perianal Assessment

Inspect the perianal area. Wearing gloves, spread the patient's buttocks apart. Observe the area, and ask patient to bear down as if trying to have a bowel movement. *The perianal area should be intact, without obvious lesions.*

Palpate the anus and rectum.

- Swollen, painful, longitudinal breaks in the anal area may appear in patients with anal fissures. (These are caused by the passing of large, hard stools or by diarrhea.)
- Dilated anal veins appear with hemorrhoids.
- A red mass may appear with prolapsed internal hemorrhoids.
- Doughnut-shaped red tissue at the anal area may appear with a prolapsed rectum.

Technique/Normal Findings	Abnormal Findings

Lubricate the gloved index finger and ask the patient to bear down. Touch the tip of your finger to the patient's anal opening. Flex the index finger, and slowly insert it into the anus, pointing the finger toward the umbilicus (Figure 21–20 ■). Rotate the finger in both directions to palpate any lesions or masses. *There should be no masses in the anus or rectum.*

- Movable, soft masses may be polyps.
- Hard, firm, irregular embedded masses may indicate carcinoma.

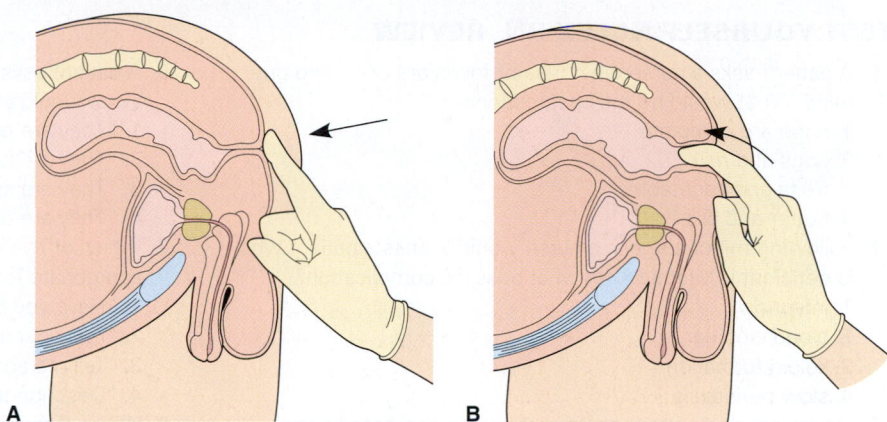

Figure 21–20 ■ Digital examination of the *A,* anus, and *B,* rectum.

Fecal Assessment

Inspect the patient's feces. After palpating the rectum, withdraw your finger gently. Inspect any feces on the glove. Note color and/or presence of blood. Also use gloved fingers to note consistency. *Stool should be soft with no blood present.*

- See Box 21–4 for information about stool characteristics.

Test the feces for occult blood. Use a testing kit such as Occultest or Hemoccult II. *There should be no occult blood in the feces.*

- A positive occult blood test requires further testing for colon cancer or GI bleeding due to peptic ulcers, ulcerative colitis, or diverticulosis.

Note the odor of the feces. *No distinctly foul odors should be present.*

- Distinctly foul odors may be noted with stools containing blood or extra fat or in cases of colon cancer.

SAMPLE DOCUMENTATION

Abdominal Assessment

Seventy-two-year-old female, currently a resident in an extended care facility, states she has not had a bowel movement for a week, and normally has one every other day. She also says she has lost her appetite and "just feels terrible." Abdominal assessment reveals a firm, slightly distended abdomen. Bowel sounds are active with gurgles in all four quadrants. Slight dullness to percussion in LLQ (sigmoid colon). States she has some generalized abdominal discomfort with moderate palpation. Hard stool present in rectum. Stool negative for occult blood.

BOX 21–4 Assessing Stool Characteristics

Inspect feces for color, odor, and consistency after the rectal exam or after defecation. Both hands are gloved.

Color

- Blood *on* the stool results from bleeding from the sigmoid colon, anus, or rectum. Blood *within* the stool indicates bleeding from the colon due to ulcerative colitis, diverticulosis, or tumors. Black, tarry stools, called **melena**, occur with upper GI bleeding. Oral iron may turn stools black and mask melena.
- Grayish or whitish stools can result from biliary obstruction due to lack of bile in stool.
- Greasy, frothy, yellow stools, called **steatorrhea**, may appear with fat malabsorption.

Odor

- Distinct, foul odors may be noted with stools containing blood or extra fat or in cases of colon cancer.

Consistency

- Hard stools or long, flat stools may result from a spastic colon or bowel obstruction due to a tumor or hemorrhoids. Hard stools may also result from ingestion of oral iron.
- Mucousy, slimy feces may indicate inflammation and occur in irritable bowel syndrome.
- Watery, diarrhea stools appear with malabsorption problems, irritable bowel syndrome, emotional or psychologic stress, ingestion of spoiled foods, or lactose intolerance.

TEST YOURSELF NCLEX-RN® REVIEW

1. A patient asks a nurse what type of foods are complete proteins. What would be the best response?
   1. none are complete
   2. eggs and milk
   3. fruits and vegetables
   4. butter and oils

2. Following minor surgery, a nurse would assess a patient who is deficient in vitamin K for what possible complication?
   1. infection
   2. blood clotting
   3. keloid formation
   4. slow peristalsis

3. On monitoring a patient's lab results, a nurse noted a very high serum amylase level. What disease does this indicate?
   1. cheilosis
   2. gastric reflux
   3. gallstones
   4. acute pancreatitis

4. While assessing an older woman, the nurse noticed her teeth have obvious caries and she has difficulty swallowing. She says, "My mouth is so dry." What health problem might result from these findings?
   1. nutritional deficit
   2. acute pain
   3. altered elimination
   4. risk for infection

5. What percussion sound would the nurse expect to hear when assessing the abdomen of a patient with ascites?
   1. flatness
   2. resonance
   3. alternating amplitude
   4. shifting dullness

6. A patient asks you to tell her what internal hemorrhoids are. What would you say?
   1. "They are part of the arteries of the body."
   2. "They are just bits of tissue that occur for no reason."
   3. "They are swollen veins in the anal canal."
   4. "They are part of the lymphatic system."

7. Which of the following questions or statements would be appropriate for the patient with an ostomy?
   1. "Have you had any bleeding from your hemorrhoids?"
   2. "Has your appetite changed lately?"
   3. "Tell me about your family."
   4. "Describe the consistency of your stools."

8. Which diagnostic test would be most appropriate to detect intestinal parasites?
   1. colonoscopy
   2. CT of the abdomen
   3. barium enema
   4. stool specimen

9. Why is removal of polyps during a colonoscopy important?
   1. to identify genetic disorders
   2. to prevent the development of cancer
   3. to facilitate further examination of the bowel
   4. to decrease future problems with constipation

10. A nurse is conducting a health history and states, "Tell me about any colon cancer in your family." Is this an appropriate question?
    1. No, colon cancer is rarely found in family members.
    2. No, this question should only be asked by physicians.
    3. Yes, but it should wait for further diagnostic testing.
    4. Yes, colon cancer is a common inherited disorder.

See Test Yourself answers in Appendix C.

Pearson Nursing Student Resources
Find additional review materials at
nursing.pearsonhighered.com
Prepare for success with additional NCLEX®-style practice questions, interactive assignments and activities, Web links, animations and videos, and more!

BIBLIOGRAPHY

Amella, E. (2007). Assessing nutrition in older adults. *Best Practices in Nursing Care to Older Adults*. The Hartford Institute for Geriatric Nursing. Retrieved from www .hartfordign.org

American Cancer Society. (2009). *American Cancer Society guidelines for the early detection of cancer (colon and rectal cancer)*. Retrieved from http://cancer.org/docroot/ ped/content/ped_2_3x_acs_cancer_detection_ guidelines_3

American Society for Gastrointestinal Endoscopy. (2008). *Colonoscopy*. Manchester, MA: American Society for Gastrointestinal Endoscopy.

Armstrong, J., & Mitchell, E. (2008). Comprehensive nursing assessment in the care of older people. *Nursing Older People, (20)*1, 36–40.

Ayden, N., & Karaoz, S. (2008). Nutritional assessment of patients before gastrointestinal surgery and nurses' approach to this issue. *Journal of Clinical Nursing, 17*(5), 608–617.

Bazensky, I., Shoobridge-Moran, C., & Yoder, L. (2007). Colorectal cancer: An overview of the epidemiology, risk factors, symptoms, and screening guidelines. *MEDSURG Nursing, 16*(1), 46–52.

Berman, H., Brooks, L., & Silver, S. (2007). A rational approach to constipation. *Geriatrics & Aging, 10*(10), 654–660.

Camillo, P. (2007). Should a rectal exam be a routine part of a pelvic examination? *Medscape Nurses*. Retrieved from http://www.medscape.com/viewarticle?562990

Costello, T., & Coyne, I. (2008). Nurses' knowledge of mouth care practices. *British Journal of Nursing, 17*(4), 264–268.

Daly, J., Merchant, M., & Barcey, T. L. (2009). Colorectal cancer screening. *American Journal of Nursing, 10*(109), 60–62.

D'Amico, D., & Barbarito, C. (2007). *Health & physical assessment in nursing*. Upper Saddle River, NJ: Pearson Prentice Hall.

Eliopoulos, C. (2005). *Gerontological nursing* (6th ed). Philadelphia: Lippincott Williams & Wilkins.

Foster, D., Parr, J., & Wright, L. (2005). Tackling malnutrition. *Nursing Management, 12*(5), 28–30.

Grams, L., & Spremulli, M. (2008). Assessing a patient for dysphagia. *Nursing, 38*(8), 15.

Greenwald, B. (2006). A pilot study evaluating two alternate methods of stool collection for the fecal occult blood test. *MEDSURG Nursing, 15*(2), 89–94.

Holcomb, S. S. (2008). Acute abdomen: What a pain! *Nursing, 38*(9), 34–40.

Kee, J. (2009). *Prentice Hall handbook of laboratory & diagnostic tests with nursing implications* (6th ed.). Upper Saddle River, NJ: Pearson Prentice Hall.

Khurana, A., McLean, L., Atkinson, S., & Foulks, C. (2008). The effects of oral sodium phosphate drug products on renal function in adults undergoing bowel endoscopy. *Archives of Internal Medicine, 168*(6), 593–597.

Lee, D. (2008). Colon cancer: The genetic factor. *MedicineNet.com.* Retrieved from http://www.medicinenet.com/script/main/art.asp?article key=46105&pf=3&page=1

Lou, M., Dai, Y., Huang, G., & Yu, P. (2007). Nutritional status and health outcomes for older people with dementia living in institutions. *Journal of Advanced Nursing, 60*(5), 470–477.

McCarron, K. (2007). Jaundice: More than meets the eye. *Nursing Made Incredibly Easy! 5*(3), 25–27.

MedicineNet.com. (2008). Colon cancer: The genetic factor. Retrieved from http://www.medicinenet.com

Molle, E. (2005). Healthier aging: Caring for older adults. Getting down to the lower GI tract. *Nursing, 35*(11), 20–21.

National Digestive Diseases Information Clearinghouse. (2004). Liver biopsy. NIH Publication No. 05-4731.

National Institute of Health. (2008). *Genes and disease: Nutritional and metabolic diseases; The digestive system.* Retrieved from http://www.ncbi.nlm.nih.gov/books/bookres.fegi/gnd/pdf.html

Nelson, R., & Vega, C. (2007). Virtual colonoscopy may be used first in screening for colorectal cancer. *Medscape Medical News.* Retrieved from http://www.medscape.com/viewarticle/564041

Porth, C. M., & Matfin, (2009). *Concepts of altered health states* (8th ed.). Philadelphia: Lippincott Williams & Wilkins.

Pullen, R. L. (2008). Preparing a patient for magnetic resonance imaging. *Nursing, 38*(10), 22.

Schoch, L., & Whiteman, K. (2007). Monitoring liver function. *Nursing, 37*(11), 22–23.

Spector, R. E. (2009). *Cultural diversity in health and illness* (7th ed.). Upper Saddle River, NJ: Pearson Prentice Hall.

U.S. Department of Health. (2005). *Dietary guidelines for Americans 2005. Key recommendations for the general population.* Retrieved from http://www.health.gov/dietaryguidelines/dga2005/recommendations.htm

U. S. Food and Drug Administration [FDA]. (2009). *FDA warns about risk of wearing medicated patches during MRIs.* Retrieved from http://www.fda.gov/bbs/topics/news/2009/new01967.htm

Weber, J., & Kelley, J. (2009). *Health assessment in nursing* (4th ed.). Philadelphia: Lippincott Williams & Wilkins.

22 Nursing Care of Patients with Nutritional Disorders

LEARNING OUTCOMES

1. Compare and contrast the pathophysiology and manifestations of nutritional disorders.
2. Identify causes and predict effects of nutritional disorders on patient health status.
3. Explain interdisciplinary care for patients with nutritional disorders.
4. Develop strategies to promote nutrition for patient populations.

CLINICAL COMPETENCIES

1. Assess the functional health status of patients with nutritional disorders.
2. Monitor nutritional status and responses to care; document and report abnormal or unexpected responses.
3. Use assessed data to determine priority nursing diagnoses and implement evidence-based nursing interventions.
4. Administer medications and enteral and parenteral nutrition knowledgeably and safely.
5. Integrate interdisciplinary care in the plan of care.
6. Adapt cultural values and variations into the plan of care for patients with nutritional disorders.
7. Plan and provide patient-centered teaching to restore, promote, and maintain functional health status.
8. Evaluate responses to care and use data to revise plan of care as needed.

KEY TERMS

anorexia nervosa, *607*
bariatrics, *588*
basal metabolic rate (BMR), *590*
binge-eating disorder, *607*
body mass index (BMI), *588*
bulimia nervosa, *607*

catabolism, *599*
enteral nutrition, *600*
lower body obesity, *590*
malnutrition, *598*
nutrients, *589*
obesity, *588*

parenteral nutrition (PN), *604*
protein-calorie malnutrition (PCM), *599*
starvation, *599*
triglycerides, *590*
upper body obesity, *590*
very low calorie diet (VLCD), *593*

Obesity and malnutrition, the major nutritional disorders in the world today, affect many systems and organs. They often cause serious health problems, such as hypertension, heart disease, fluid and electrolyte imbalances, disability, and death.

Patients with nutritional disorders require complex, skilled nursing care. Developmental, sociocultural, psychologic, and physiologic factors may play a role in these disorders: A holistic approach to nursing care is vital. Before proceeding with the discussion of obesity and malnutrition, review the sections on metabolism and nutrients in ∞ Chapter 21.

The Patient with Obesity

Obesity, an excess of adipose tissue, is one of the most prevalent, preventable health problems in the United States. Obesity has serious physiologic and psychologic consequences, and is associated with increased morbidity and mortality. It contributes to poor health-related quality of life to a greater extent than smoking, excess alcohol use, or poverty. The obesity epidemic has prompted rapid growth in **bariatrics**, the healthcare science that focuses on patients who are extremely obese.

Health-related problems associated with obesity are listed in Table 22–1.

While obesity is often defined by weight, it is more accurately defined by the **body mass index (BMI)**, an indirect measure of the amount of body fat, or adipose tissue. Adipose tissue is created when energy consumption exceeds energy expenditure. A BMI of 25 to 29.9 kg/m^2 is classified as *overweight*; obesity is a BMI of 30 kg/m^2 or greater (Centers for Disease Control and Prevention [CDC], 2009). The terms *overweight* and *obese* are not mutually exclusive; a patient who is obese also is overweight.

FAST FACTS

Prevalence of overweight and obesity in the United States:

- Women
  - Black: 78.2%
  - Hispanic: 76.1%
  - White: 61.2%
- Men
  - Black: 68.5%
  - Hispanic: 79.3%
  - White: 72.6%

TABLE 22–1 Health-Related Problems Associated with Obesity

BODY SYSTEM	OBESITY-RELATED PROBLEMS
Cardiovascular	Atherosclerosis, hypercholesterolemia
	Coronary heart disease
	Heart failure
	Hypertension
	Stroke
	Varicosities
	Venous thrombosis
Respiratory	Asthma
	Sleep apnea
Gastrointestinal	Gallbladder disease
	Hiatal hernia
	Colon cancer
Genitourinary	Prostate cancer
	Stress incontinence
Musculoskeletal	Low back pain
	Muscle strains and sprains
	Osteoarthritis
Endocrine and Reproductive	Diabetes mellitus, type 2
	Breast and endometrial cancers
	Polycystic ovarian syndrome
	Complications of pregnancy
Other	Depression
	Postoperative complications

Incidence and Prevalence

More than 30% of the adult population in the United States is obese; nearly two-thirds of all adults in the United States are overweight. The prevalence of obesity is higher in women and in economically disadvantaged people of all races. While the prevalence of overweight has been increasing since 1960, the prevalence of obesity is increasing to a greater extent, particularly during the past 10 to 15 years (Weight-control Information Network [WIN], 2010). Of particular concern is the increasing incidence of obesity in children and young adults. The prevalence of overweight and obesity varies among ethnic and cultural groups. Adults of Asian heritage generally have a lower incidence of overweight and obesity. See the Focus on Cultural Diversity box that follows.

Risk Factors

Many factors contribute to obesity, including genetic, physiologic, psychologic, environmental, and sociocultural factors. Heredity may contribute up to 40% of the risk for obesity (NHLBI, 1998). The inheritance of obesity does not usually follow a clear Mendelian pattern. There is, however, a strong correlation between the weight of adopted children and their biologic parents, and identical twins tend to have similar BMIs, whether raised together or apart. While several genes that contribute to appetite and fat deposition have been identified, obesity as a purely genetic condition is rare (Fauci et al., 2008).

Physical inactivity is probably the most important factor contributing to obesity. Inactive people may consume fewer calories than active people and continue to gain weight due to lack of energy expenditure. Cultural and environmental factors such as reliance on the automobile for transportation and increased time spent using the computer contribute to decreased energy expenditure among adults in the United States. Increased time spent watching television is seen as a major contributing factor to the increased incidence of obesity among children and adolescents (Fauci et al., 2008).

Environmental influences, such as an abundant and readily accessible food supply, fast-food restaurants, advertising, and vending machines, contribute to increased food intake. Sociocultural influences that contribute to obesity include increased consumption of restaurant meals, overeating at family meals, rewarding behavior with food, religious and family gatherings that promote food intake, and sedentary lifestyles. Socioeconomic status also tends to correlate with the risk for overweight and obesity: In the United States, women with low incomes are more likely to be obese than those of higher socioeconomic status (NHLBI, 2010). The association between socioeconomic status and obesity is less clear in men.

Psychologic factors, such as low self-esteem, also play a role in obesity. Low self-esteem may precipitate unhealthy eating behaviors, and the resulting weight gain in turn may diminish self-image even further. A person may overeat as a result of anxiety, depression, guilt, or boredom, or as a means of getting attention. Some experts characterize overeating as a food addiction and as a coping mechanism for stressful life events.

Overview of Normal Physiology

All body activities require energy, including activities of daily living, as well as those necessary to maintain cell and tissue function. **Nutrients** in food (or enteral or parenteral feedings) provide this energy and are the building blocks for growth and tissue repair. The body stores excess nutrients and energy (measured as kilocalories) to meet the body's needs when required nutrients are unavailable. This ability to store and release energy is important to maintaining body function. A significant portion of daily energy expenditure is fixed: More than 70% of the energy expended each day goes to maintaining the **basal metabolic rate (BMR)**, essentially the "cost" (in kilocalories) of being alive. Physical activity accounts for only 5% to 10% of the energy spent daily (Fauci et al., 2008).

Energy is primarily stored as fat in adipose tissue. Although mature fat cells (adipocytes) do not multiply, the immature cells in adipose tissue can multiply, particularly when exposed to estrogen during puberty, in late adolescence, during breastfeeding, and in middle-aged adults who are overweight. Fat cells store excess energy as **triglycerides**, formed from dietary fats and carbohydrates. The body breaks down the triglycerides in fat cells when needed to provide energy (Porth & Matfin, 2009).

Pathophysiology

Obesity occurs when excess calories are stored as fat. It can result from excess energy intake, decreased energy expenditure, or a combination of both. The etiology of obesity is not as simple as excess kilocalorie intake in relation to energy expenditure.

Energy intake and energy expenditure are regulated by a complex interaction of endocrine and neural signals. In the absence of external influences, these regulatory mechanisms increase appetite and reduce energy expenditure when weight loss occurs, and suppress appetite and increase energy expenditure after overfeeding. In a society where food is abundant and physical activity is limited, the latter is less effective.

Appetite, which affects food intake, is regulated by the central nervous system and by emotional factors. The hunger center in the hypothalamus stimulates appetite in response to stimuli such as hypoglycemia and peptides produced in the gut. As nutrient levels rise, the satiety center (also in the hypothalamus) sends the message to stop eating. Gastrointestinal filling and hormonal factors also signal *satiety* (a sensation of fullness). Appetite may have little relationship to hunger or physical signals, however, people may eat to relieve depression or anxiety.

Several hormones are involved in regulating obesity, including thyroid hormone, insulin, and leptin (a peptide produced by fatty tissue that suppresses appetite and increases energy expenditure). Some studies suggest that leptin resistance is a cause of obesity. Insulin is associated with body fat distribution. The two major types of body fat distribution are upper body and lower body obesity.

Upper body obesity (also called *central obesity*) is identified by a waist-to-hip ratio of greater than 1 in men or 0.8 in women. (∞ See Chapter 21 for a method to calculate the waist-to-hip ratio.) People with upper body obesity tend to have more intra-abdominal fat and higher levels of circulating free fatty acids (Porth & Matfin, 2009). As a result, upper body obesity is associated with a greater risk of complications such as hypertension, abnormal blood lipid levels, heart disease, stroke, and elevated insulin levels. Men tend to have more intra-abdominal fat than women, although women develop a central fat distribution pattern after menopause.

Lower body obesity (also known as *peripheral obesity*), in which the waist-to-hip ratio is less than 0.8, is more commonly seen in women. The risk for hyperinsulinemia, abnormal lipids, and heart disease is lower in people with lower body obesity than in those with upper body obesity. Lower body obesity may be more difficult to treat, however.

Complications of Obesity

Obesity is a major health risk factor, increasing the risk of mortality from all causes over that of normal-weight people. As obesity increases, so does the risk of dying.

CARDIOVASCULAR DISEASE   Obesity is a significant risk factor for cardiovascular disease, including hypertension, coronary heart disease (CHD), and heart failure. The prevalence of hypertension in obese men and women is approximately twice that in people with a BMI of less than 25 (NHLBI, 1998). Several factors contribute to hypertension in obese individuals, including sodium retention with associated increased vascular resistance, blood volume, and cardiac output. The increases in blood pressure seen with obesity increase the risk for CHD and stroke.

Patients who are obese, particularly those who have abdominal obesity, often have a lipid profile that promotes atherosclerosis. Levels of low-density lipoprotein (LDL) and very low density lipoprotein (VLDL) cholesterol and triglycerides are increased, and levels of high density lipoprotein (HDL or desirable) cholesterol are reduced. Furthermore, adipose tissue secretes cytokines that stimulate the liver to produce C-reactive protein (CRP), now recognized as a risk factor for CHD.

These factors account for the fact that many obese individuals have *metabolic syndrome*, a constellation of cardiovascular risk factors, including increased waist circumference, hypertension, elevated blood triglycerides and fasting blood glucose, and low HDL cholesterol. The metabolic syndrome is an identified risk factor for atherosclerosis and CHD.

Obesity increases the risk for heart failure. Left ventricular muscle mass increases, and the ventricle dilates in obese individuals, possibly related to increased blood volume and cardiac output.

RESPIRATORY DISORDERS   Overweight and obesity increase the risk for developing asthma in both adults and children. The relationship between obesity and asthma is not clear, but may be related to genetic factors and the connection between obesity and inflammation. Obesity is the major risk factor for obstructive sleep apnea, intermittent airflow obstruction due to upper airway collapse during sleep. Not only is obesity a risk factor for sleep apnea, the reverse also may be true: sleep apnea may predispose patients for weight gain (NHLBI, 2004).

DIABETES MELLITUS   Obesity increases the risk of insulin resistance and type 2 diabetes. While not all obese people develop diabetes, up to 80% of people with type 2 diabetes are obese. Both weight gain in adulthood and abdominal (central) obesity are positively correlated with the risk for developing type 2 diabetes (Fauci et al., 2008).

OTHER DISORDERS   Obesity affects reproductive function in both men and women. Androgen (male sex hormone) levels are reduced in obese men; menstrual irregularities and polycystic ovarian syndrome (PCOS) are more common in obese women. PCOS is an additional risk factor for hyperinsulinemia and insulin resistance. Increased weight increases the risk for developing gallstones in both men and women. The risk for developing several types of cancer, including colon, breast, and endometrial, increases in obesity. Increased weight places abnormal stress on joints, increasing the prevalence of joint pain and osteoarthritis, particularly in weight-bearing joints (especially the knee joints). Other health-related problems associated with obesity are listed in Table 22–1.

Interdisciplinary Care

Obesity treatment is far more complex than just reducing food consumption. Most experts recommend an individualized program of exercise, diet, and behavior modification designed to meet the patient's specific needs.

Diagnosis

Although body weight may be used to identify obesity, measures of body fat are more accurate. Males at ideal body weight have 10% to 20% body fat, whereas females at ideal body weight have 20% to 30% body fat.

- *Body mass index* is used to identify excess adipose tissue. BMI is calculated by dividing the weight (in kilograms) by the height in meters squared (m^2). See Box 22–1. BMI calculations may not as accurately reflect the extent of adipose tissue in people who are highly muscular (e.g., body builders) or in those who have lost muscle mass (e.g., older adults).
- *Anthropometry* includes measurements of height, weight, bone size, and skinfold to estimate subcutaneous fat. ∞ See Chapter 21 for more information about anthropometric measurements.
- *Underwater weighing (hydrodensitometry)* is considered the most accurate way to determine body fat. This technique involves submerging the whole body and then measuring the amount of displaced water.
- *Bioelectrical impedance* uses a low-energy electrical impulse to determine the percentage of body fat by measuring the electrical resistance of the body.
- *Waist circumference* is measured to determine body fat distribution. Men with a waist measurement of 40 inches (102 cm) or greater and women with a waist measurement of 35 inches (88 cm) or greater have a higher risk for complications of obesity.

Other diagnostic tests may be done to help identify a physiologic cause of obesity, as well as complications of obesity.

- A *thyroid profile* is done to rule out thyroid disease (∞ see Chapter 18).
- *Serum glucose* is measured to identify coexisting diabetes mellitus.

- *Serum cholesterol* is measured to assess for elevated levels.
- A *lipid profile* is ordered; high-density lipoprotein (HDL) levels may be reduced in obese patients, whereas low-density lipoprotein (LDL) levels are elevated.
- An *electrocardiogram (ECG)* is performed to detect effects of obesity on the heart, such as rate or rhythm disruptions, myocardial infarction, or heart enlargement.

Medications

Drug therapy may be used when the patient is at increased medical risk as a result of obesity; it is not recommended for "cosmetic" weight loss. When used in combination with diet and exercise, drugs can help promote weight loss. Prescription weight loss drugs are approved for use only in patients with a BMI of 30 and above, and those with a BMI of 27 or higher and an obesity-related condition such as hypertension, type 2 diabetes, or an abnormal lipid profile. Weight-loss drugs generally fall into one of two classes: appetite suppressants and lipase inhibitors.

Sibutramine (Meridia) is an appetite suppressant that acts on the CNS. Sibutramine may increase the metabolic rate, promoting weight loss, and it has an antidepressant effect. Sibutramine increases the pulse rate and blood pressure, potentially limiting its use in patients with hypertension, CHD, or heart failure. Other drugs used as appetite suppressants include amphetamines and nonamphetamines, and antidepressants such a bupropion (Wellbutrin, Zyban) and fluoxetine (Prozac). None of these drugs are approved for long-term use as appetite suppressants. Amphetamines carry a high abuse potential and are not approved for treating obesity. Nonamphetamines such as diethylpropion (Tenuate) and phentermine (Adipex-P) may be used, but also increase pulse rate and blood pressure.

Orlistat (Xenical) is a lipase inhibitor, reducing fat absorption from the GI tract, leading to weight loss. It reduces blood glucose and total and LDL cholesterol levels, and lowers blood pressure. The adverse effects of orlistat relate to its inhibition of fat absorption: oily stools, flatulence, and fecal urgency. These effects tend to diminish when dietary fat intake is limited. See the Medication Administration box on page 593 for the nursing implications of these drugs.

Rimonabant (Acomplia) is a new drug currently under review by the FDA for use in weight loss, smoking cessation, and to lower cholesterol. The drug works in the brain to suppress appetite and the craving for nicotine, and in the periphery to decrease insulin resistance and improve the lipid profile (Lehne, 2007).

Treatments

Successful treatment of obesity (sustained achievement of normal body weight without adverse consequences) is rarely achieved. Treatment focuses on reducing the health risks associated with obesity by changing both eating and exercise habits. A pound of body fat is equivalent to 3500 kcal. To lose 1 pound a person must reduce daily caloric intake by 500 kcal for 7 days or increase activity enough to burn the equivalent kilocalories. A weight loss goal of 1 to 2 pounds per week and a 10% reduction in body weight in 6 months of therapy is recommended (NHLBI, 2000). A combination of physical activity, dietary therapy, behavior modification, pharmacology, and, in some cases, surgery is required to achieve and maintain weight loss (Table 22–2).

BOX 22–1 Calculating Body Mass Index (BMI)

BMI = weight (kg)/height^2 (m^2)
Normal = BMI 18.5–24.9 kg/m^2
Overweight = BMI 25–29.9 kg/m^2
Obese = BMI > 30 kg/m^2
Extreme obesity = BMI > 40 kg/m^2

MEDICATION ADMINISTRATION Drugs to Treat Obesity

APPETITE SUPPRESSANTS

Phentermine (Adipex-P, Fastin, Ionamin, Obestin-30, Oby-Trim, others)

Sibutramine (Meridia)

Phentermine acts directly on the appetite-control center in the CNS to suppress the appetite and reduce hunger. Sibutramine reduces hunger and increases sensations of satiety by inhibiting the uptake of serotonin, norepinephrine, and dopamine. These drugs may be used to treat obesity in patients with a BMI of > 30 kg/m^2 and obese patients who have risk factors such as diabetes or hypertension.

Nursing Responsibilities

- Assess for contraindications, such as pregnancy or lactation, use of other appetite suppressants, impaired liver or kidney function, history of CHD, or alcohol abuse.
- Regularly monitor blood pressure and heart rate during treatment. Increases may indicate need to reduce dose or discontinue treatment.

Health Education for the Patient and Family

- Take as directed; do not exceed recommended dose. Do not take if you may be pregnant or are nursing.
- Take your last dose no later than 4 PM to avoid insomnia.
- You may experience difficulty sleeping, nervousness, or palpitations while taking this drug.

- Increase your fluid intake to reduce possible side effects of dry mouth and constipation.
- This drug does not replace diet and exercise for weight loss; continue to follow your prescribed regimen.

LIPASE INHIBITOR

Orlistat (Alli, Xenical)

Orlistat inhibits lipases necessary for the breakdown and absorption of fat, thus decreasing the absorption of dietary fat. Its action is primarily local, within the GI tract, with few systemic effects.

Nursing Responsibilities

- Administer with meals or up to 1 hour following a meal.
- Provide a fat-soluble vitamin supplement (A, D, E, and K) daily. Separate administration time from orlistat by at least 2 hours.

Health Education for the Patient and Family

- Take as directed; do not increase dose. You may skip a dose if you do not consume a meal.
- Use in conjunction with a low-calorie, low-fat diet.
- Common gastrointestinal side effects include oily or fatty stools, flatulence, oily discharge, or frequent stools with difficulty controlling defecation. These side effects may diminish with time or increase if a meal high in fat is consumed.
- Notify your healthcare provider if you become pregnant while taking this medication.

EXERCISE Exercise is a critical element in weight loss and maintenance. Physical activity increases energy consumption and promotes weight loss while preserving lean body mass. Physical activity improves physical fitness, decreases appetite, promotes self-esteem, and increases the basal metabolic rate. The Centers for Disease Control and Prevention (CDC) recommend that all adults engage in both aerobic and muscle-strengthening activities each week. Table 22–3 outlines CDC activity recommendations and gives example activities to achieve goals. Activities should be spread throughout the week, and may be spread over the course of the day; however, it is important to expend moderate or vigorous effort for at least 10 minutes at a time when exercising (CDC, 2008).

Because fitness levels differ, patients may be taught to use their target heart rate or perceived exertion to "measure" the vigor of activities. The *target heart rate* is calculated based on maximum heart rate; in turn, maximum heart rate is estimated

using the formula 220 minus age in years. For example, while the maximum heart rate for a 35-year-old is 185 beats per minute (bpm), it would be 155 bpm for someone who is 65 years old. While the target heart rate for the 35-year-old engaging in vigorous intensity activity would be 130 to 157 bpm, it would be 108 to 132 bpm for the older adult. Perceived exertion is a subjective rating of activity intensity, using self evaluation of factors such as heart and respiratory rate, sweating, and muscle fatigue (CDC, 2008).

NUTRITION The diet is planned to create a daily 500- to 1000-kcal deficit. Ideally, the diet should be low in kilocalories and fat and contain adequate nutrients, minerals, and fiber. The patient should eat regular meals with small servings. A gradual, slow weight loss of no more than 1 to 2 pounds per week is recommended. This means a diet of 1000 to 1200 kcal/day for most women, and 1200 to 1600 kcal/day for most men. Fewer

TABLE 22–2 Treatment Recommendations for Overweight and Obesity

TREATMENT	BMI				
	25–26.9	27–29.9	30–34.9	35–39.9	≥40
Diet, exercise, and behavior modification	With two or more comorbidities[1]	With two or more comorbidities[1]	Yes	Yes	Yes
Pharmacotherapy[2]		With two or more comorbidities[1]	Yes	Yes	Yes
Surgery				With two or more comorbidities[1]	

[1] For example, hypertension, hyperlipidemia, diabetes, and other obesity-related complications.

[2] Considered when 6 months of combined therapy has not produced a loss of 1 pound per week.

Source: Adapted from National Institutes of Health; National Heart, Lung, and Blood Institute; North American Association for the Study of Obesity. (2000). *The practical guide: Identification, evaluation, and treatment of overweight and obesity in adults*. Bethesda, MD: NIH.

TABLE 22–3 CDC Physical Activity Recommendations for Adults

ACTIVITY	RECOMMENDATION	EXAMPLES
Aerobic activity:	Engage in moderate- or vigorous-intensity activity for at least the recommended amount of time weekly, or in an equivalent combination of moderate- and vigorous-intensity activity.	
■ Moderate-intensity aerobic activity (target heart rate of 50% to 70% of maximum heart rate)	2 hours and 30 minutes (150 minutes) every week	■ Walking fast ■ Water aerobics ■ Bicycle riding on level ground ■ Doubles tennis ■ Ballroom dancing ■ Pushing a lawn mower ■ General gardening
■ Vigorous-intensity aerobic activity (target heart rate of 70% to 85% of maximum heart rate)	1 hour and 15 minutes (75 minutes) every week	■ Race walking, jogging, running ■ Swimming laps ■ Singles tennis ■ Aerobic dancing ■ Bicycling 10 mph or faster ■ Heavy gardening (continuous hoeing or digging) ■ Hiking uphill
Muscle-strengthening activities	2 or more days per week: at least one set of 8 to 12 repetitions for all major muscle groups	■ Lifting weights ■ Using resistance bands ■ Exercises that use body weight for resistance (push-ups, sit-ups) ■ Heavy gardening ■ Yoga

Source: Centers for Disease Control and Prevention (CDC). (2008). *Physical activity for everyone.* Atlanta, GA: Author.

than 1200 kcal each day may lead to loss of lean tissue and nutritional deficiencies. The recommended diet generally is low in fat and high in dietary fiber (Table 22–4). Recent research shows equivalent weight loss among different diets (e.g., low-fat, low-carbohydrate, or high-protein diets); adherence to the diet and participation in group sessions were shown to be the significant factors (Sacks et al., 2009). Excessive calorie restrictions can lead to failure to follow the prescribed diet, feelings of guilt, and

TABLE 22–4 Recommended Nutrient Intake for Weight Loss

NUTRIENT	RECOMMENDED INTAKE
Calories	1000 to 1600 per day or approximately 500 to 1000 less than usual daily intake
Total fat	30% or less of total calories
Saturated fats	10% or less of total calories
Cholesterol	< 300 mg/day
Protein (from plant and lean animal sources)	Approximately 15% of total calories
Carbohydrate (complex carbohydrates from vegetables, fruits, and whole grains)	55% or more of total calories
Fiber (e.g., oat bran, legumes, barley, most fruits and vegetables)	20 to 30 g/day
Sodium chloride	< 2.4 g sodium or 6 g sodium chloride/day
Calcium	1000 to 1500 mg/day

Source: Adapted from National Institutes of Health; National Heart, Lung, and Blood Institute; North American Association for the Study of Obesity. (2000). *The practical guide: Identification, evaluation, and treatment of overweight and obesity in adults.* Bethesda, MD: NIH.

overeating. "Yo-yo" dieting (repeated cycles of weight loss and gain) may lead to a metabolic deficiency that makes subsequent weight loss efforts increasingly difficult.

Very low calorie diets (VLCDs) are generally reserved for patients who have a BMI greater than 30 (WIN, 2008). This type of program offers a protein-sparing modified fast (800 kcal/day or less) under close medical supervision. VLCDs typically use commercially prepared formulas (liquid shakes or bars) to replace all food intake for several weeks or months, resulting in rapid weight loss while maintaining lean body mass. Exercise, nutrition, and behavior modification counseling should accompany the diet. Benefits include decreased blood pressure, blood glucose, and cholesterol and triglyceride levels, along with improved exercise tolerance. VLCDs may not be appropriate for use in people over age 50 due to normal loss of lean body mass and adverse effects such as fatigue, constipation, nausea, diarrhea, and gallstone formation. In the long term, weight gain is common, and VLCDs may be no more effective for weight loss than a diet that includes 800 to 1000 daily kcal (WIN, 2008).

BEHAVIOR MODIFICATION Behavior modification is a critical component of successful weight management. See the research box on p. 592. Strategies such as keeping food records, eliminating cues that precipitate eating, and changing the act of eating are often helpful.

Recording food intake, amount, location of eating, and situations that induce eating often help the patient gain self-control. Researchers have found that most overweight people are stimulated to eat by external cues, such as the proximity to food and the time of day. In contrast, hunger and satiety are the cues that regulate eating in adults of normal weight. Strategies to control food cues include keeping food out of view, eliminating snack

MOVING EVIDENCE INTO ACTION   The Overweight Patient

What are the most effective strategies to promote weight loss? The type and number of strategies are as diverse as the population, with avid proponents of each. Recent research by Sacks et al. (2008) of the Harvard School of Public Health showed virtually no difference in the amount of weight loss, satiety, hunger, or satisfaction with the diet for groups following diets that emphasized specific nutrients (fat, protein, or carbohydrate). All participants lost weight and their cardiovascular risk factors improved. The strongest predictor of weight loss was attendance at group sessions. A study by Turner, Thomas, Wagner, & Moseley (2008) produced further evidence to support the importance of behavior change to effective weight loss. In their study, patients were allowed to choose their preferred diet from among a low-calorie, low-fat, or low-carbohydrate plan. All patients participated in weekly groups presenting behavior change strategies; fitness activities and a group session with an aerobics instructor were available as part of the program. No significant difference in weight loss was found among the different diet plans. Participating in exercise, on the other hand, made a significant difference. Average weight loss ranged from 2.1 lbs for participants who did not attend the exercise program at all to 9.4 lbs for those who attended three sessions.

IMPLICATIONS FOR NURSING

Achieving and maintaining significant weight loss is a struggle for most overweight and obese patients. Patients frequently seek advice from nurses and other healthcare practitioners about the "best" diet and the "best" way to meet their weight-loss goals. Current evidence points to the importance of using a multidisciplinary approach to behavior change and weight loss: reduced calorie intake, regular exercise, and support groups or programs to help identify and maintain changes in eating behaviors.

CRITICAL THINKING IN PATIENT CARE

1. Although research shows that reducing total calorie intake is more important than emphasizing or limiting intake of fats, carbohydrate, or protein, many people "swear by" a specific diet plan. What factors do you think contribute to the belief that one specific diet is more effective than another?
2. Exercise is consistently shown to be a significant factor in achieving and maintaining weight loss. How does exercise contribute to weight loss?
3. Develop a teaching plan to help a 72-year-old woman with osteoarthritis of her knees achieve CDC recommendations for aerobic and muscle-strengthening activities (see Table 22–4).

foods, and eating only in designated areas. See Box 22–2 for a list of behavior modification strategies.

Other strategies focus on helping patients examine factors such as lifestyle, personality, and environment that affect eating behaviors. The goal is to empower the overweight individual to choose activities that are not related to food.

Social support and group programs such as Weight Watchers, Overeaters Anonymous, and Take Off Pounds Sensibly (TOPS) promote weight loss success through peer support. Most organized programs require participants to pay a fee, which may improve compliance.

SURGERY Surgical treatment of obesity (*bariatric surgery*) generally is limited to extremely obese patients (BMI of over 40 kg/m^2) or those who have serious obesity-related problems such as type 2 diabetes, coronary heart disease, or severe sleep apnea (WIN, 2008). In addition, patients must be able to tolerate surgery and be free of addiction to alcohol or other drugs. The benefits of surgery include major weight loss and improved blood pressure, plus a reduced risk of diabetes, sleep apnea, angina, heart failure, blood lipid levels, and venous disease. Bariatric surgery, however, is not without risk, and the decision to undergo surgery is a significant one.

The most common bariatric surgical procedures are adjustable gastric banding, gastric bypass, gastric sleeve, and biliopancreatic bypass with duodenal switch. These procedures restrict stomach capacity, limiting food intake, and, in most cases, bypass a portion of the small intestine to restrict absorption of calories and nutrients. In many cases, they can be performed laparoscopically.

In the Roux-en-Y gastric bypass (RGB, Figure 22–1A ■), a small stomach pouch is created to restrict food intake. A Y-shaped section of the jejunum is then attached to the pouch to allow food to bypass the lower stomach and duodenum. As

BOX 22–2 Behavioral Change Strategies for the Obese Patient

Controlling the Environment
- Purchase low-calorie foods.
- Shop from a prepared list and on a full stomach.
- Keep all foods in the kitchen.
- Store all foods in the refrigerator or in the cabinets in opaque containers.
- Prepare exact portions of food to eliminate leftovers.
- Eat all foods in the same place, avoid eating in the kitchen.
- Avoid eating when watching television or reading.
- Reduce frequency of eating out at restaurants, parties, and picnics.

Controlling Physiologic Responses to Food
- Eat slowly by taking small bites, allowing 20 minutes for a meal.
- Eat a salad or drink a hot beverage before a meal.
- Chew each bite thoroughly and slowly.
- Put eating utensils or food down between bites.
- Concentrate on the eating process, savor the food.
- Stop eating with the first feelings of fullness.

Controlling Psychologic Responses to Food
- Appreciate the aesthetic experience of eating.
- Use attractive dinnerware, and prepare a formal setting for eating.
- Use small plates and cups to make servings of food look larger.
- Concentrate on conversations and socialization during the meal.
- Use nonfood rewards for meeting a goal.
- Acknowledge small successes and improvements in all behavior.
- Substitute other activities for eating (e.g., reading, exercise, hobbies).

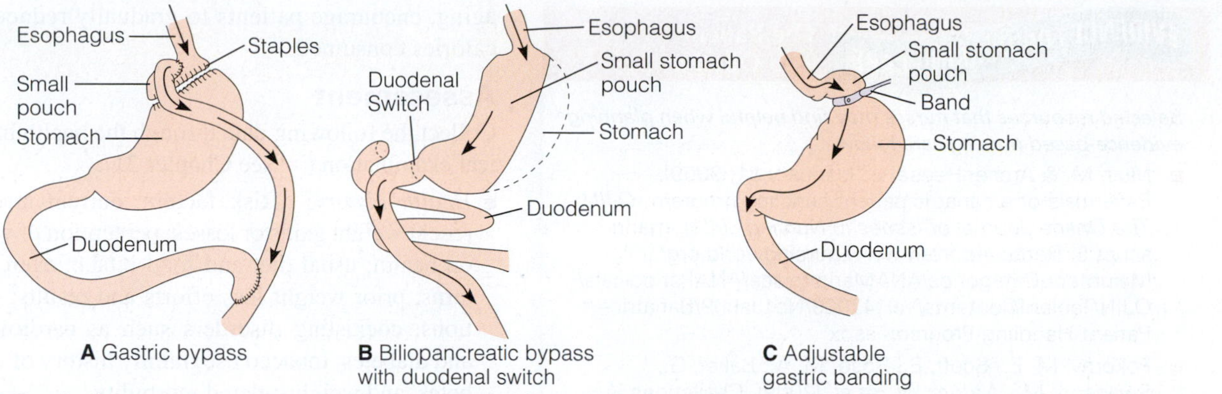

Figure 22–1 ■ Surgical procedures to treat obesity. *A,* Roux-en-Y gastric bypass surgery; *B,* Biliopancreatic diversion; *C,* Adjustable gastric banding.

a result, calorie and nutrient absorption is limited. The biliopancreatic diversion (BPD, Figure 22–1*B*) is a more complex procedure and carries a higher risk of nutritional deficiencies. This surgery may be performed in two stages, with the majority of the stomach removed and a gastric sleeve created during the first stage. In BPD, the duodenum and jejunum are bypassed by connecting the ileum directly to the stomach pouch or just distal to the pyloric valve.

These surgeries that restrict nutrient intake and absorption produce rapid weight loss that is maintained over time. Many patients maintain a significant weight loss for 10 years or more, with improvement in obesity-associated health problems such as type 2 diabetes, hypertension, and sleep apnea. Because these procedures allow food to bypass the duodenum and jejunum, nutrient deficiencies are common, particularly of iron, calcium, vitamin B_{12}, and, possibly, the fat-soluble vitamins.

Restrictive procedures, such as adjustable gastric banding (AGB, Figure 22–1*C*), are safer but generally less effective in the long term. In AGB, a hollow band of silicone rubber is placed around the upper (proximal) portion of the stomach. The band is inflated with saline solution to create a small stomach pouch with a narrow passage through to the rest of the stomach. The amount of band inflation can be adjusted using a port implanted under the skin. Few nutritional deficiencies are associated with restrictive bariatric procedures. Vomiting is a common postoperative risk with restrictive procedures. The band may slip or break, necessitating a return to surgery. While patients typically lose about 50% of their excess body weight within the first year after these procedures, fewer maintain that weight loss over a 10-year period than those undergoing gastric bypass.

Although the risk for postoperative complications is high, the mortality rate for bariatric procedures is low (less than 1% for restrictive surgeries and up to 5% for combination procedures). Possible postoperative complications include anastomosis leak with peritonitis, abdominal wall hernia, gallstones, wound infections, deep venous thrombosis, nutritional deficiencies, and gastrointestinal symptoms. Dumping syndrome, which can be precipitated by a meal high in simple carbohydrates, may develop following gastric bypass surgeries. In dumping syndrome, stomach contents move rapidly through

the small intestine, drawing fluid into the intestine by osmosis. The patient experiences nausea, bloating, abdominal pain, weakness, sweating, and possibly syncope. ∞ See Chapter 23 for more information about dumping syndrome.

Nursing care for the patient who has undergone bariatric surgery is substantially the same as for a patient who has undergone a gastric resection. ∞ See Chapter 23 for more information about gastric resection and associated nursing care. Bariatric patients have additional nursing care needs related to their obesity. See the box on page 596.

Maintaining Weight Loss

Losing weight and maintaining that loss are two separate but related issues. Most experts agree that the majority of dieters regain lost weight within a 2-year period. The potential risks associated with regaining weight make maintenance a critical issue. Patients are encouraged to continue exercise, self-monitoring, and treatment support. Long-term weight loss and maintenance mean a lifelong commitment to significant lifestyle changes, including food and eating habits, activity and exercise routines, and behavior modification. Failure to maintain weight loss can lead to feelings of inadequacy, powerlessness, and hopelessness.

✆ Nursing Care

Health Promotion

Maintaining a healthy weight throughout the life span begins in childhood. Obese children and teenagers become obese adults. Promote healthy eating, including a diet rich in whole grains, fruits, and vegetables and low in fat. The USDA Food Guide Pyramid (∞ Chapter 2) and the Healthy Eating Pyramid provide visual guidance for appropriate food choices to maintain a healthy, well-balanced diet. Encourage all children and adults to maintain an active lifestyle, engaging in at least 30 minutes of aerobic activity daily. Encourage parents to limit time children spend watching television, using the computer, and playing video games. Discuss the effects of smoking and excess alcohol use on nutrition and activity. To reduce weight gain commonly associated with

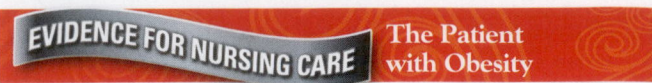

Selected resources that nurses may find helpful when planning evidence-based nursing care follow.

■ Muir, M. & Archer-Heese, G. (January 31, 2009). Essentials of a bariatric patient handling program. *OJIN: The Online Journal of Issues in Nursing, 14*(1), manuscript 5. Retrieved from www.nursingworld.org/MainMenuCategories/ANAMarketplace/ANAPeriodicals/OJIN/TableofContents/Vol142009/No1Jan09/Bariatric-Patient-Handling-Program-.aspx

■ Pokorny, M. E., Scott, E., Rose, M. A., Baker, G., Swanson, M., Waters, W., et al. (2009). Challenges in caring for morbidly obese patients. *Home Healthcare Nurse: The Journal for the Home Care and Hospice Professional, 27*(1), 43–52.

aging, encourage patients to gradually reduce the amount of calories consumed.

Assessment

Collect the following data through the health history and physical examination (∞ see Chapter 21):

■ *Health history:* Risk factors; current and usual weight; recent weight gains or losses; perception of weight and effect on health; usual diet and food intake; exercise/activity patterns; prior weight loss efforts and results; current medications; coexisting disorders such as cardiovascular disease and diabetes; tobacco use; family history of overweight, diabetes, and weight-related morbidity.

■ *Physical examination:* Vital signs; weight (use a scale of adequate capacity) and height; skinfold measurements; waist-to-hip ratio; BMI; inspect skin under the breasts and abdominal folds.

NURSING CARE
The Bariatric Patient Undergoing Surgery

Severely obese patients undergoing bariatric or general surgery have unique nursing care needs to ensure personal and caregiver safety.

■ Obtain a thorough preoperative health history and physical assessment (including skin assessment). Note any limitations of mobility or assistive devices used. *Bariatric patients often have multiple chronic health problems that may affect postoperative assessment and recovery. Skin folds are at high risk for fungal infections that may compromise immune protection. Knowing about and providing assistive devices to accommodate mobility limitations will help promote early postoperative mobilization and reduce the risk for complications.*

■ Obtain equipment of appropriate size and weight capacity, including bed, mechanical lifts, expanded-capacity wheelchair, walker, commode, bedside chair (without arms), sphygmomanometer, and scale. Clearly label any equipment provided by the patient. *Appropriately sized equipment is vital to promote the patient's comfort and safety. Equipment made to meet the needs of patients who are within normal weight and BMI measurements may fail or the patient may not be able to sit or recline without the risk of falling.*

■ Provide friction-reducing devises such as sliders, foam, or pressure-reducing mattresses. *Following surgery, mobility may be limited. Special equipment facilitates skin care while helping maintain patient and caregiver safety.*

■ Ensure training and availability of nursing staff in adequate numbers to ensure patient and caregiver safety during position changes, transfers, and caregiving activities such as hygiene. *Even with use of appropriate lifts, sliders, and other devices, as many as six to eight caregivers may be necessary to safely move and transfer the bariatric patient.*

■ Elevate the head of the bed. Apply continuous positive airway pressure (CPAP) device as ordered. *Thoracic and abdominal fat may restrict lung capacity, particularly when the patient is supine. Elevating the head of the bed*

reduces the pressure of abdominal fat on the diaphragm. Patients who are obese are at risk for obstructive sleep apnea due to upper airway collapse; CPAP helps maintain upper airway patency.

■ Frequently monitor level of consciousness and respiratory status (rate, breath sounds, oxygen saturation). *The postsurgical bariatric patient may sequester anesthetic agents in fatty tissue, increasing the risk for respiratory depression after surgery.*

■ Initiate cardiac monitoring and compare heart rhythm to preoperative ECG. Promptly report changes in rate or rhythm, such as frequent PVCs (∞ see Chapter 30). *The obese patient is at significant risk for coronary heart disease; surgery and anesthesia place an additional risk for cardiovascular complications. Development of dysrhythmias not seen preoperatively may indicate myocardial ischemia, hypoxia, or electrolyte imbalance.*

■ Assess peripheral pulses, skin color, and temperature of extremities. Apply elastic compression stockings or sequential compression device of appropriate size for the patient. Teach and remind to perform foot and leg exercises. *The obese patient is at significant risk for developing deep venous thrombosis due to alterations in clotting and immobility. Furthermore, multiple risk factors for atherosclerosis increase the likelihood of peripheral vascular disease and impaired circulation.*

■ Assess pain level and analgesic effectiveness frequently. *Maintaining adequate pain relief is important to promote lung expansion and prevent respiratory complications in the bariatric patient.*

■ Regularly monitor blood glucose levels, administering insulin as ordered. *Surgery is a physiologic stressor that causes increased cortisol levels that, in turn, can increase blood glucose levels.*

■ Provide meticulous wound care, using strict aseptic technique and frequently assessing for signs of infection. *Excess adipose tissue impairs healing and immune function. Wound infection further delays healing and can be difficult to eradicate.*

Nursing Diagnoses and Interventions

Nursing care for overweight and obese patients is community based and holistic, focusing on both physiologic and psychologic responses to weight and appearance. See the following Case Study & Nursing Care Plan for the patient with obesity.

Imbalanced Nutrition: More than Body Requirements

Although many factors contribute to obesity, it always involves an imbalance of kcal consumption to energy expenditure.

- Encourage the patient to identify the factors that contribute to excess food intake. *Identification of cues to eating helps the patient eliminate or reduce these cues.*
- Establish realistic weight loss goals and exercise/activity objectives. *Small, reasonable goals, such as loss of 1 to 2 pounds per week, increase the likelihood of success.*
- Assess the patient's knowledge and discuss diet plan options. Provide necessary teaching about diet. *Current research (Sacks et al., 2009) shows no significant difference in the efficacy of selected diet plans. Offering a selection of appropriate diet plans empowers the patient to choose a plan that best matches food preferences and lifestyle.*
- Discuss behavior modification strategies, such as self-monitoring and environmental management. *Behavior modification, diet, and exercise are critical to promoting successful, long-term weight loss.*
- Monitor weight loss, blood pressure, and laboratory data, including blood glucose and lipid levels. *Continuing assessment not only is important to evaluate the safety of weight loss strategies, but also to reinforce positive benefits of weight loss.*

Activity Intolerance

Obese patients may experience excess fatigue, tachycardia, and shortness of breath with activity due to the physiologic effects of excess weight as well as a sedentary lifestyle. A medical evaluation may be needed before beginning an exercise program.

- Assess current activity level and tolerance of that activity. Assess vital signs. *This provides baseline information to plan an activity program and assess response to that activity.*
- After medical clearance, plan with the patient a program of regular, gradually increasing exercise. If desired, plan several 10 to 15 minute exercise periods over the course of the day. Develop plans for gradually increasing the duration and intensity of exercise. Consider a consultation with an exercise physiologist. *An individualized exercise program promotes activities within the patient's physical capabilities.*

Ineffective Therapeutic Regimen Management

Most overweight or obese patients experience some difficulty integrating all the components of a weight loss program into a daily routine. To be successful, the overweight patient must modify dietary intake in a world of daily temptations. There may be many obstacles to exercise, including a busy schedule, activity intolerance, impaired physical mobility, lack of equipment, and the embarrassment of being fat.

- Discuss ability and willingness to incorporate changes into daily patterns of diet, exercise, and lifestyle. *This provides data from which to set realistic goals with the patient.*
- Help the patient identify behavior modification strategies and support systems for weight loss and maintenance. *Weight loss and maintenance are most successful if the patient establishes lifestyle patterns that promote interest and motivation and thus exercise and diet management. Family and social support is critical to successful adherence to the therapeutic regime (Turner, Thomas, Wagner, & Moseley, 2008).*
- Have the patient establish strategies for dealing with "stress" eating or interruptions in the therapeutic regime. *A sense of failure associated with overeating or lack of exercise can lead to further overeating. Identifying positive strategies to deal with these situations promotes self-acceptance and limits self-punishment through overeating.*

Chronic Low Self-Esteem

Most overweight and obese individuals verbalize the experience of "fat prejudice," ridicule, embarrassment, and health problems attributed to being "fat." These experiences, coupled with problems such as finding attractive clothing or a chair large enough to sit on can affect self-esteem. Many patients report that "fat" jokes or comments contribute to a sense of negative self-worth.

- Encourage the patient to verbalize the experience of being overweight, and validate the patient's experience. *This provides baseline data to use in developing individualized interventions to address self-esteem issues.*
- Set small goals with the patient and offer positive feedback and encouragement. *Small goals provide more opportunities for success. Positive feedback and encouragement provide a comfortable environment in which to develop self-esteem.*
- Refer for counseling as appropriate. *Many patients benefit from counseling for issues related to self-esteem.*

Using NANDA, NIC, and NOC

Linkages between a selected NANDA nursing diagnosis, NIC, and NOC for the patient for obese patients are shown in the chart that follows.

Community-Based Care

Weight reduction usually occurs in community-based settings. Weight loss and maintenance require a long-term commitment by the patient, family, and support systems. Address the following topics with the patient and family:

- Lifestyle changes are more effective than diets. Fad diets promote rapid weight loss but often are not nutritionally sound or may be difficult to maintain for a lifetime.

NANDA, NIC, AND NOC LINKAGES
The Patient with Obesity

NANDA — Imbalanced Nutrition: More than Body Requirements

NIC — Nutrition Management
Weight Reduction Assistance
Behavior Modification
Body Image Enhancement
Self-Esteem Enhancement

NOC — Nutrition Status
Nutritional Status: Nutrient Intake
Weight Loss Behavior
Body Image
Self-Esteem

Data from NANDA International. (2009). *Nursing diagnoses: Definitions & classification 2009–2011.* Oxford, UK: Wiley-Blackwell; Bulechek, G., Butcher, H., & Dochterman, J. (Eds.). (2008). *Nursing interventions classification (NIC)* (5th ed.). St. Louis, MO: Mosby; and Moorhead, S., Johnson, M., Maas, M., & Swanson, E. (Eds.). (2008). *Nursing outcomes classification (NOC)* (4th ed.). St. Louis, MO: Mosby.

- All household members should consume a diet that is nutritionally sound, low in fat, and high in fiber.
- Establish realistic weight loss goals and a system of nonfood rewards for achieving each goal.
- Identify an "exercise buddy" or support system to promote continued physical activity.
- Expect occasional failures. Resume prescribed diet and exercise routine as soon as possible; the goal is long-term weight management.
- Community resources such as Weight Watchers, TOPS, or health-care-based programs provide information, strategies, and support for successful weight management.

The Patient with Malnutrition

Malnutrition results from inadequate intake of nutrients. There may be a lack of major nutrients (calories, carbohydrates, proteins, and fats) or micronutrients such as vitamins and minerals. Malnutrition may be caused by inadequate nutrient intake; impaired absorption and use of nutrients; loss of nutrients due to diarrhea, hemorrhage, or renal failure; or increased metabolic needs (e.g., infection or physiologic stressors).

CASE STUDY & NURSING CARE PLAN   A Patient with Obesity

Sam Elliott, aged 57, has gained 30 pounds since his retirement 2 years ago. The most active thing he does each day is "puttering around" and "walking to the end of the driveway to get the mail." His diet includes juice, oatmeal, muffin, and coffee with cream for breakfast; donuts and coffee with friends mid-morning; a bologna-and-cheese sandwich with chips and a root beer for lunch; and cheese, crackers, and wine before a dinner of meat, potatoes, vegetables, and dessert. He tells the nurse, "I have never had to diet. I just don't know how to get this weight off."

ASSESSMENT
Mr. Elliott is 5' 8" (173 cm) tall and weighs 201 lb (91.2 kg). His BMI is 30.1 kg/m². His cholesterol is 240 mg/dL (normal 150 to 200 mg/dL) with an HDL of 37 mg/dL (normal male value > 45 mg/dL) and an LDL of 180 mg/dL (normal < 130 mg/dL). His BP is 138/90. His fasting blood glucose is normal at 103 mg/dL. His ECG shows normal sinus rhythm. He reports fatigue and shortness of breath with activity. His healthcare provider has advised a weight loss of 30 pounds and a regular exercise program.

DIAGNOSES
- *Imbalanced Nutrition: More than Body Requirements* related to food intake in excess of energy expenditure
- *Risk for Ineffective Therapeutic Regimen Management* related to knowledge deficit
- *Activity Intolerance* related to sedentary lifestyle

EXPECTED OUTCOMES
- Lose 1 pound each week.
- Walk 30 minutes 5 days each week.
- Verbalize an understanding of the relationship between weight loss, weight control, and exercise.
- Identify behavior modification strategies to avoid overeating.
- Identify support systems for behavior modification.

PLANNING AND IMPLEMENTATION
- Assess weight and blood pressure once or twice each week.
- Discuss current eating habits and strategies to reduce fat and calorie intake.
- Discuss cues that promote eating. Identify strategies to eliminate or reduce eating cues.
- Teach to keep a food diary to examine and change eating habits.
- Discuss the role of regular exercise in weight loss and weight control. Instruct to maintain an exercise record to track the intensity and duration of activity.
- Discuss lifestyle and behavior modification strategies to promote successful weight loss and control.

EVALUATION
Two weeks after changing his diet and beginning to exercise, Mr. Elliott has lost 2 pounds. He has maintained a food diary. He has identified boredom as a cue to eating. In light of that fact, he has started volunteering at the local hospital, where he is working with children. He is walking for 30 minutes 5 days a week. He plans to increase his activity periods to 45 minutes. He verbalizes commitment to a lifelong plan of exercising and eating a low-fat diet. His BP has ranged from 132/76 to 136/84. He plans to have the employee health nurse at the hospital check his weight and BP each week and to join Weight Watchers for ongoing support.

CRITICAL THINKING IN THE NURSING PROCESS
1. What are some possible pathophysiologic bases for Mr. Elliott's abnormal cholesterol, HDL, and LDL levels?
2. Develop a teaching plan for a group of overweight men and women.
3. Identify potential barriers to losing weight and strategies to reduce or eliminate these barriers.

See Evaluating Your Response in Appendix C.

Incidence and Prevalence

Malnutrition is a widespread cause of disease and mortality throughout the world. It is endemic in regions affected by famine. Groups at risk for malnutrition in the United States include the young, poor, elderly, homeless, low-income women, and ethnic minorities. Even when food is plentiful, patients may be undernourished because of poor food choices.

It is estimated that one-third to one-half of all hospitalized patients are malnourished (Fauci et al., 2008). Malnutrition may be present on admission or develop as a result of surgery or serious illness. Malnutrition increases both mortality and the incidence of complications in both medical and surgical patients. The incidence of malnutrition is even higher in long-term care residents, where up to 85% of residents may be malnourished (DiMaria-Ghalili & Amella, 2005).

Risk Factors

Risk factors for malnutrition include the following:

- Age—older adults are at greater risk for malnutrition due to a variety of factors (See the accompanying Meeting Individualized Needs box.)
- Poverty, homelessness, inadequate food storage and preparation facilities
- Functional health problems that limit mobility or vision
- History of weight loss of more than 20% of usual weight
- Oral or gastrointestinal problems that affect food intake, digestion, and absorption
- Inability to eat for 5 or more days
- Chronic pain or chronic diseases such as pulmonary, cardiovascular, renal, or endocrine disorders, or cancer
- Dementia, mental health disorders, eating disorders
- Medications or treatments that affect appetite
- Alcohol or drug addition
- Acute problems such as infection, surgery, or trauma

Pathophysiology

Carbohydrates and fats in the diet are the body's primary energy source. Approximately 15% to 25% of the body is fat, the body's energy reservoir. The remainder (muscles, bones, other body tissues and organs) is lean body mass, metabolically active tissue. Proteins in the diet primarily are used to maintain this tissue. Glycogen and proteins in this lean body mass also act as energy stores.

When dietary intake of nutrients does not meet the body's energy needs, the body uses glycogen, body proteins, and lipids (fats) to support metabolism. In **starvation** (inadequate dietary intake), glycogen initially is used to provide energy. After the first 24 hours of starvation, gluconeogenesis (formation of glucose from proteins) is the major source of energy. As starvation continues, the body breaks down fats into free fatty acids and ketones, which provide energy for the brain. The size of all body compartments is reduced as body fats and muscle proteins are used to meet energy needs. As lean body mass is reduced, metabolically active tissue is lost, and energy expenditure decreases.

The stress of acute illness, surgery, or trauma produces a different response. The acute stress response produces a state of hypermetabolism and **catabolism** (cell and tissue breakdown). This hypermetabolic state increases energy expenditure and nutrient needs, resulting in **protein-calorie malnutrition (PCM)**. In PCM, both protein and calories are deficient. Lean body mass is broken down to meet these needs. If untreated, up to half of the body's protein stores can be used within 3 weeks. Visceral protein stores also are converted to energy, with loss of protein from organs such as the liver, gastrointestinal tract, kidneys, and heart. Loss of protein from the liver affects its ability to produce plasma proteins. Immune cells decrease, and wound healing is impaired. Atrophy of gastrointestinal mucosa leads to malabsorption, further compounding the protein deficit. Myocardial contractility and cardiac output decline, and respiratory function is compromised (Porth & Matfin, 2009).

Chronic protein deficiency with adequate calories to meet energy needs is called *kwashiorkor*. When both proteins and calories are insufficient to meet the body's needs, PCM is known as *marasmus*.

Manifestations

The manifestations of malnutrition may vary among patients. Weight loss is the most apparent manifestation: The malnourished patient may have a body weight of less than 90% of ideal. Body mass also is reduced (see Box 22–1), as is skinfold thickness. Other manifestations include a wasted appearance, dry

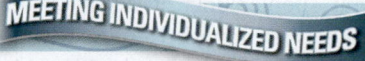

Nutrition for the Older Adult

Older adults are at greater risk for malnutrition. Age-related changes that contribute to this problem include changes in taste and smell, poor oral health, loss of teeth or ill-fitting dentures, medication-related anorexia, and functional limitations that impair the ability to shop and cook. Older adults living on fixed incomes may not be able to afford well-balanced meals. Depression, social isolation, and loneliness often contribute to loss of appetite. Eating is a social event, and older adults who eat alone may not eat as well as those who share meals with companions.

Conduct a thorough assessment to determine nutritional status. Assess psychologic factors that influence eating habits, such as loneliness, isolation, and depression. Note the patient's general appearance and obtain a diet history, including information about foods and nutrients the patient consumes, and recent weight loss or gain. Review laboratory values, including complete blood count, total protein, prealbumin, and albumin levels.

TEACHING FOR HOME CARE
To maintain nutritional status, advise the older patient to do the following:

- Eat a well-balanced diet with fresh fruits and vegetables.
- Shop wisely to get the most value for the money.
- Avoid processed foods and foods high in fat.
- Drink adequate fluids.
- Exercise regularly.
- Contact local agencies for the availability of congregate meals (e.g., at local senior centers) or home-delivered meals (e.g., Meals on Wheels).

and brittle hair, and pale mucous membranes. Peripheral or abdominal edema may be present. Older adults may show general symptoms of frailty, including weakness, slow walking speed, low physical activity level, unintentional weight loss, and exhaustion. Manifestations of specific nutrient deficiencies may be present (see the accompanying box). See page 601 for the Multisystem Effects of Malnutrition.

Subcutaneous fat and muscle proteins are broken down in PCM, impairing mobility and increasing the risk for skin and tissue breakdown (pressure ulcers). Protein synthesis is inhibited and wound healing delayed. Serum albumin levels fall, leading to abdominal edema, diarrhea, and impaired nutrient absorption. Immune function is impaired, increasing the risk of infection. Cardiac output falls, and the risk for postural hypotension increases.

Interdisciplinary Care

The goal of treatment for the malnourished patient is to restore ideal body weight while replacing and restoring depleted nutrients and minerals. The patient's age, severity of malnutrition, and coexisting health problems help determine interventions. Treatment may include oral supplementation, tube feedings, or parenteral nutrition.

Diagnosis

A nutrition screening tool such as the one in Box 22–3 can help identify patients at risk for malnutrition. As with obesity, the standard measurements to assess for malnutrition include height, weight, calculation of BMI, and skinfold measurements. A BMI of less than 18 to 20 kg/m^2 may indicate malnutrition. The following laboratory studies also may be ordered:

- *Serum albumin* is reduced in PCM, and may be below 3.0 g/dL.
- *Prealbumin* (also known as *transthyretin*) is a transport protein and precursor to albumin. It has a short (2-day) half-life, and is sensitive to acute changes in nutritional status. A prealbumin level of less than 10 mg/dl indicates severe nutritional deficiency; a level lower than 5 mg/dl is seen in severe protein depletion (Kee, 2009).
- The *total lymphocyte count* is reduced in PCM.
- *Serum electrolytes* are measured. Potassium levels are low in severe malnutrition.

The following specialized procedures to evaluate the extent of malnutrition may be ordered:

- *Bioelectric impedance analysis* measures body fat and total body water.
- *Total daily energy expenditure* (which includes resting energy expenditure, energy needed for digestion, plus physical activity needs) may be measured to help determine the patient's calorie intake needs.

Medications

Malnourished patients generally require supplemental vitamins and minerals to restore these essential micronutrients. A multivitamin and mineral supplement may be given, or therapy may be tailored to correct specific deficiencies. See the Medication Administration box on page 602 for nursing implications of vitamin and mineral supplements.

MANIFESTATIONS of Specific Nutrient Deficiencies

DEFICIENCY	ASSESSMENT DATA
Calorie	Weight loss
	Weakness, listlessness
	Loss of subcutaneous fat
	Muscle wasting
Protein	Thin or sparse hair
	Flaking skin
	Hepatomegaly
Vitamin A	Night blindness
	Altered taste and smell
	Dry, scaling, rough skin
Thiamine	Confusion, apathy
	Cardiomegaly, dyspnea
	Muscle cramping and wasting
	Paresthesias, neuropathy
	Ataxia
Riboflavin	Cheilosis, stomatitis
	Neuropathy, glossitis
Vitamin C	Swollen, bleeding gums
	Delayed wound healing
	Weakness, depression
	Easy bruising
Iron	Smooth tongue
	Listlessness, fatigue
	Dyspnea

Nutrition

Fluids and nutrients are carefully reintroduced in severely malnourished patients. Refeeding can precipitate fluid and electrolyte imbalances, heart failure, malabsorption, and diarrhea.

First, fluid and electrolyte imbalances are corrected, with particular attention paid to restoring normal potassium, magnesium, and calcium levels, as well as acid–base balance. Once fluid and electrolyte imbalances are corrected, protein and calories are gradually reintroduced into the diet. Initial feedings are limited amounts (100 mL) of liquid formula to prevent diarrhea. Vitamin and mineral supplements at about twice the Dietary Reference Intake (DRI) are provided along with refeeding. Fat and lactose are reintroduced into the diet last. Lactose intolerance may develop in severely malnourished patients; yogurt may be tolerated better than a milk-based formula.

Food intake is gradually increased until the patient is able to consume about 5000 kcal per day, and is gaining 3 to 5 pounds (1.5 to 2.0 kg) weekly. Commercially available nutritional supplements (such as Ensure or Sustacal) may supplement protein and calorie intake.

ENTERAL NUTRITION **Enteral nutrition**, or tube feeding, may be used to meet calorie and protein requirements in patients unable to consume adequate food. Indications for tube feedings include difficulty swallowing, unresponsiveness, oral or neck surgery or trauma, anorexia, or serious illness. Tube feedings

MULTISYSTEM EFFECTS OF
Malnutrition

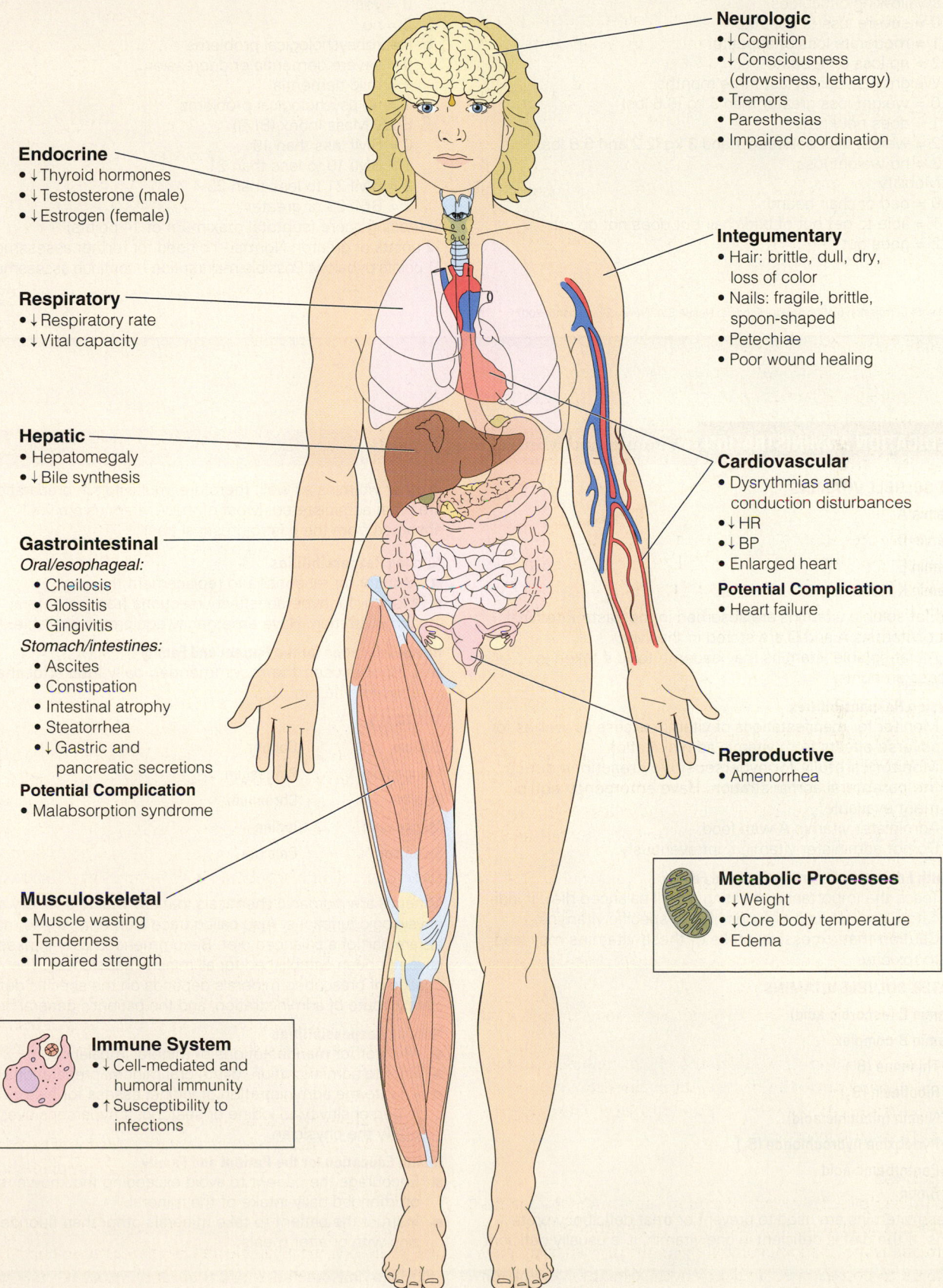

Neurologic
- ↓ Cognition
- ↓ Consciousness (drowsiness, lethargy)
- Tremors
- Paresthesias
- Impaired coordination

Integumentary
- Hair: brittle, dull, dry, loss of color
- Nails: fragile, brittle, spoon-shaped
- Petechiae
- Poor wound healing

Cardiovascular
- Dysrythmias and conduction disturbances
- ↓ HR
- ↓ BP
- Enlarged heart

Potential Complication
- Heart failure

Reproductive
- Amenorrhea

Metabolic Processes
- ↓ Weight
- ↓ Core body temperature
- Edema

Endocrine
- ↓ Thyroid hormones
- ↓ Testosterone (male)
- ↓ Estrogen (female)

Respiratory
- ↓ Respiratory rate
- ↓ Vital capacity

Hepatic
- Hepatomegaly
- ↓ Bile synthesis

Gastrointestinal
Oral/esophageal:
- Cheilosis
- Glossitis
- Gingivitis
Stomach/intestines:
- Ascites
- Constipation
- Intestinal atrophy
- Steatorrhea
- ↓ Gastric and pancreatic secretions

Potential Complication
- Malabsorption syndrome

Musculoskeletal
- Muscle wasting
- Tenderness
- Impaired strength

Immune System
- ↓ Cell-mediated and humoral immunity
- ↑ Susceptibility to infections

BOX 22–3 Mini-Nutritional Assessment MNA®

A. Has food intake declined over the past three months due to loss of appetite, digestive problems, chewing or swallowing difficulties?
0 = severe loss of appetite
1 = moderate loss of appetite
2 = no loss of appetite

B. Weight loss during last three months
0 = weight loss greater than 3 kg (6.6 lbs)
1 = does not know
2 = weight loss between 1 and 3 kg (2.2 and 6.6 lbs)
3 = no weight loss

C. Mobility
0 = bed or chair bound
1 = able to get out of bed/chair but does not go out
2 = goes out

D. Has suffered psychological stress or acute disease in the past three months
0 = yes
2 = no

E. Neuropsychological problems
0 = severe dementia or depression
1 = mild dementia
2 = no psychological problems

F. Body Mass Index (BMI)
0 = BMI less than 19
1 = BMI 19 to less than 21
2 = BMI 21 to less than 23
3 = BMI 23 or greater

Screening score (subtotal maximum of 14 points)
12 points or greater: Normal—no need for further assessment
11 points or below: Possible malnutrition – continue assessment

Used with permission by Société des Produits Nestlé S.A., Vevey Switzerland, 2007.

MEDICATION ADMINISTRATION   **Vitamin and Mineral Supplements**

FAT-SOLUBLE VITAMINS

Vitamin A

Vitamin D

Vitamin E

Vitamin K

The fat-soluble vitamins are absorbed in the gastrointestinal tract. Vitamins A and D are stored in the liver.

All fat-soluble vitamins may become toxic if taken in excess amounts.

Nursing Responsibilities
- Monitor for manifestations of vitamin excess as well as for adverse effects from vitamin administration.
- Monitor carefully for hypersensitivity reactions during the parenteral administration. Have emergency equipment available.
- Administer vitamin A with food.
- Do not administer vitamin K intravenously.

Health Education for the Patient and Family
- Teach the importance of eating a well-balanced diet. If indicated, provide lists of foods high in specific vitamins.
- Caution that excessive intake of these vitamins may lead to toxicity.

WATER-SOLUBLE VITAMINS

Vitamin C (ascorbic acid)

Vitamin B complex:

Thiamine (B_1)

Riboflavin (B_2)

Niacin (nicotinic acid)

Pyridoxine hydrochloride (B_6)

Pantothenic acid

Biotin

These vitamins are used to prevent or treat deficiency problems. If the diet is deficient in one vitamin, it is usually deficient in other vitamins as well; therefore, multivitamin preparations are often administered. Most of these vitamins are well absorbed from the gastrointestinal tract.

Nursing Responsibilities
- Monitor for responses to replacement therapy.
- Monitor for hypersensitivity reactions from parenteral administration. Have emergency equipment available.

Health Education for the Patient and Family
- Do not exceed the recommended daily intake for the specific vitamin.

MINERALS

Sodium	Copper
Manganese	Potassium
Fluoride	Chromium
Magnesium	Iodine
Selenium	Calcium
Zinc	

Minerals are inorganic chemicals that are vital to a variety of physiologic functions. Also called trace elements, these minerals are part of a balanced diet. Recommended daily intakes have not been established for all mineral substances. The dosage of prescribed minerals depends on the specific deficiency, route of administration, and the patient's general health.

Nursing Responsibilities
- Monitor for manifestations of mineral imbalance.
- Prior to administration, dilute oral mineral preparations.
- Prior to the administration of iodine, assess for history of hypersensitivity to iodine or seafood; if hypersensitive, notify the physician.

Health Education for the Patient and Family
- Encourage the patient to avoid exceeding the known recommended daily intake of the mineral.
- Instruct the patient to take minerals other than fluoride and zinc with or after meals.

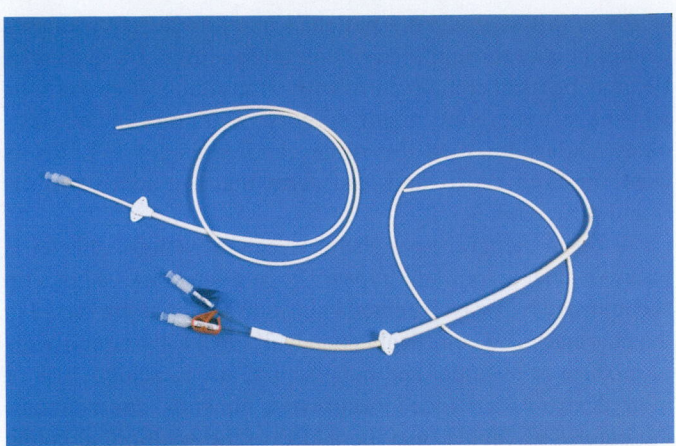

Figure 22–2 ■ A nasoduodenal tube and a jejunostomy tube.
Courtesy of Michal Heron/Pearson Education/PH College

may provide part or all of a patient's nutritional needs. Enteral feedings provide nutrients directly to the gut and other digestive organs, support immune function, promote blood flow to the gut, and support other functions of the GI tract such as the release of hormones and epidermal growth factor (Fauci et al., 2008).

Tube feedings are usually administered through a soft, small-caliber nasogastric or nasoduodenal tube with a weighted tip (Figure 22–2 ■). They also can be administered through a gastrostomy or jejunostomy tube. Small-bore feeding tubes are easily displaced; appropriate tube placement should be periodically checked by aspirating the tube and checking the pH of aspirated contents. A pH of < 4 indicates placement in the stomach; pH > 6 indicates the tube is in the jejunum. See Box 22–4.

Most tube feeding formulas provide 1 kcal/mL with approximately 14% of the calories from protein, 60% from carbohydrates, and 25% to 30% from fat. Administering 1500 mL per day provides the recommended daily intake of all vitamins and minerals. Formulas that provide more calories per milliliter, more grams of protein, added fiber, or

lower fat also are available (Table 22–5). Commercial products provide instructions for initiating therapy. Enteral feedings may initially be started with smaller volumes to prevent diarrhea, with the volume gradually increased to provide the required calories for maintenance and healing. Formulas may be administered as a bolus feeding or as a continuous-drip feeding regulated by a feeding pump (Figure 22–3 ■).

Aspiration and diarrhea are the most common complications of enteral feedings. Continuous infusion of the formula reduces the risk of aspiration. The risk also is reduced by placing the feeding tube in the jejunum rather than the stomach. To avoid aspiration, the nurse elevates the head of the bed at least 30 degrees during feeding and for at least 1 hour after feeding. Dual-lumen tubes that allow gastric suction with simultaneous instillation of an enteral feeding into the jejunum also reduce the risk for aspiration. Formulas that contain fiber can reduce the incidence of diarrhea. Fluid and

TABLE 22–5 Selected Enteral Feeding Formulas

FORMULA TYPE	CONTAINS	EXAMPLES
Complete—suitable for most patients requiring enteral feedings	■ 1 kcal/mL ■ Protein: ~ 14% total kcal ■ Fat: ~ 30% total kcal ■ Carbohydrate: ~ 60% total kcal ■ Recommended daily intake of all minerals and vitamins in 1500 mL/day	Compleat, Ensure, Isocal, Nutren, Isolan, Sustacal, Resource
High-calorie complete—appropriate for patients on fluid restriction	As above; provides 1.5 to 2 kcal/mL	Ensure Plus, Sustacal HC, Comply, Nutren 1.5, Resource Plus, Isocal HCN, Magnacal, TwoCal HN
Complete lactose-free, high-residue—used to prevent/treat diarrhea, constipation	As above; provides fiber	Jevity, Profiber, Nutren 1.0 with fiber, Fiberlan, Sustacal with fiber, Ultracal, Ensure with fiber, Fibersource, Accupep HPF, Reabfin, others
Disease-specific formulas:		
Renal failure	Contain essential amino acids	Amin-Aid, Travasorb Renal, Aminess
Respiratory failure	Fat: > 50% total kcal	Pulmocare, NutriVent
Liver failure with hepatic encephalopathy	High amounts of branched-chain amino acids	Hepatic-Acid II, Travasorb Hepatic

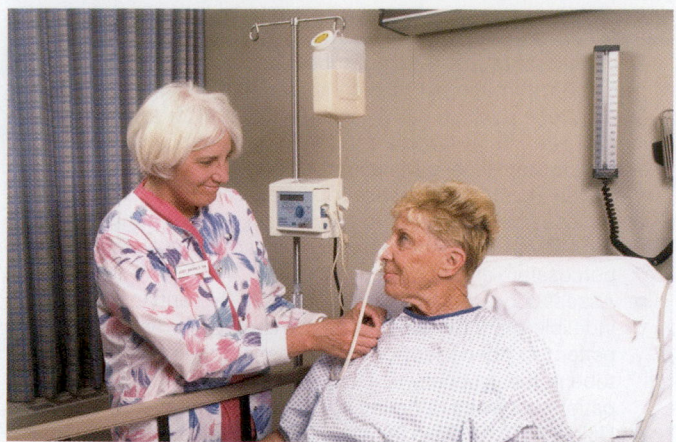

Figure 22–3 ■ The nurse secures the feeding tube of a patient receiving a continuous enteral feeding.

Courtesy of Michal Heron/Pearson Education/PH College

electrolyte status is monitored carefully, and additional water is administered as needed.

PARENTERAL NUTRITION Parenteral nutrition (PN) is the intravenous administration of amino acids, often with added carbohydrates, fats, electrolytes, vitamins, and minerals. These hypertonic solutions usually are administered through a central vein, such as the subclavian vein (Figure 22–4 ■), particularly when therapy may be prolonged. A peripherally inserted central catheter (PICC) line may be used for short-term PN.

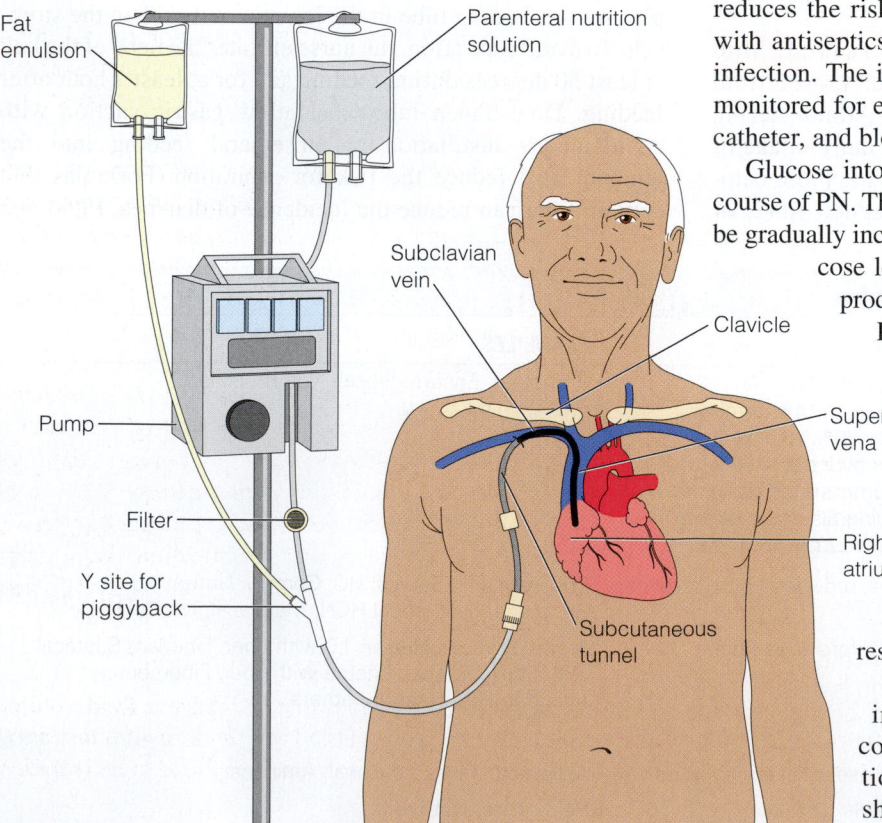

Figure 22–4 ■ Parenteral nutrition infusing through a catheter in the right subclavian vein.

PN is initiated when a patient's nutritional requirements cannot be met through diet or enteral feedings. Increasingly, PN may be used concurrently with enteral nutrition. Patients who have undergone major surgery or trauma or are seriously undernourished are often candidates for PN. PN is used for both short- and long-term management of nutritional deficiencies.

To begin therapy, a peripheral or central venous catheter is inserted under aseptic conditions. The location of the catheter tip is confirmed by x-ray. Parenteral nutrition solutions are mixed in the pharmacy and commonly contain 3% to 11.4% amino acids (a mixture of essential and nonessential amino acids), 10% or more dextrose, and added electrolytes, minerals, and vitamins. Fat emulsions (lipids) may be added to the solution, although they often are administered separately. The sterility of the solution is maintained, and no medication is added to the solution after it is mixed or to the lumen through which the PN is being administered. When given separately, fat emulsions may be administered either through a peripheral vein or via the same intravenous catheter as PN. PN solutions are always administered with an infusion pump to ensure the correct rate of infusion.

Complications The patient receiving parenteral nutrition is at risk for infectious, metabolic, and mechanical complications. Disruption of the skin barrier and administration of a solution high in glucose presents a risk for infection in patients receiving PN. Infection may be local, limited to the insertion site or the catheter itself, or may be systemic. Meticulous sterile technique when inserting the catheter, preparing and administering PN solutions, and during site and catheter care reduces the risk for infection. Using a catheter impregnated with antiseptics and an in-line filter also reduce the risk for infection. The insertion site and the patient's temperature are monitored for evidence of infection. Cultures of the solution, catheter, and blood may be obtained if infection is suspected.

Glucose intolerance may develop, particularly early in the course of PN. The concentration of glucose in PN solutions may be gradually increased to reduce this risk. Blood and urine glucose levels are measured every 6 hours until insulin production adjusts to the increased glucose load. Patients with impaired kidney function or liver disease may develop excessively high blood urea nitrogen (BUN) levels or metabolic acidosis. Hyperlipidemia is a common complication of fat infusions; these solutions are given intermittently to allow fats to clear from the blood between infusions. Fluid overload or dehydration may develop, particularly in older adults. PN formulas can cause electrolyte shifts, with resulting imbalances.

Pneumothorax, brachial plexus injury, and improper position are possible mechanical complications of central venous catheter insertion. Once in place, a thrombus (clot) or fibrin sheath may form within or around the catheter. The catheter also can be mechanically occluded, or may dislodge, leak, or break and become an embolus.

∞ Nursing Care

Health Promotion

Aggressive nursing assessment and interventions can help prevent malnutrition associated with hospitalization or long-term care. In hospitalized patients, carefully monitor food intake. When the patient is placed on NPO status for surgery or tests, ask the care provider to restore diet orders as soon as possible. If allowed, encourage family members to provide favorite foods to promote intake. In long-term care settings, promote socialization during meals. Assess food likes and dislikes for patients, and provide foods they are likely to eat.

Assessment

Collect nutritional assessment data on admission and periodically (once or twice a week) during long-term institutionalization.

- *Health history:* Usual daily dietary pattern (type and amount of foods consumed); usual weight and recent changes; appetite and food tolerance; specific food likes and dislikes; difficulty swallowing; problems such as anorexia, nausea, diarrhea, or constipation; history of surgery and/or chronic diseases (e.g., chronic lung disease) and medications.
- *Physical examination:* Height, weight, skinfold thickness, BMI; vital signs; general appearance, muscle wasting, mobility; skin and mucous membranes; bowel sounds; laboratory studies.

Use of a nutritional assessment tool can help identify patients (older adults in particular) at risk for malnutrition (see Box 22–3).

Nursing Diagnoses and Interventions

The complex effects of malnutrition on multiple body systems place the patient at high risk for a number of other problems. This section addresses problems with nutrition, infections, fluid

---

EVIDENCE FOR NURSING CARE | **The Patient with Malnutrition**

Selected resources that nurses may find helpful when planning evidence-based nursing care follow.

- Capra, S., Collins, C., Lamb, M., Vanderkroft, D., & Chan, S. W-C. (2007). Effectiveness of interventions for undernourished older inpatients in the hospital setting. *Best Practice, The Joanna Briggs Institute, 11*(2), 1–4. Retrieved from http://www.joannabriggs.edu.au/pdf/ BPISEng_11_2.pdf
- Johnson, A. D. (2009). Assessing gastric residual volumes. *Critical Care Nurse, 29*(5), 72–73.
- DiMaria-Ghalili, R. (2008). *Nutrition in the elderly: Nutrition standard of practice protocol: Nutrition in aging.* New York, NY: Hartford Institute for Geriatric Nursing, New York University College of Nursing. Retrieved from www.consultgerirn.org/topics/nutrition_in_the_elderly/ want_to_know_more
- Winkelman, C., & Best, K. (2009). Formula for success: Deliver enterable nutrition using best practices. *American Nurse Today, 4*(3), 18–23.

---

volume, and skin integrity. See page 607 for a Case Study & Nursing Care Plan for the patient with malnutrition.

Imbalanced Nutrition: Less than Body Requirements

The nurse plays a critical role in the ongoing assessment of the malnourished patient, while collaborating with the multidisciplinary team to provide nutritional therapies.

- If the patient is able to eat, provide an environment and nursing measures that encourage eating, for example, adequate staff to assist with meals, sitting at the bedside or in a common area, and providing favorite foods. *Measures to promote a more "normal" and social dining experience support the patient's intake (DiMaria-Ghalili, 2008).*
- Eliminate foul odors, provide oral hygiene before and after meals, make meals appetizing, and offer frequent, small meals including preferred foods. Consult with the nutrition support team to provide adequate protein, calories, minerals, and vitamins. *Oral hygiene and a pleasant environment make food more appetizing. Small, frequent meals are generally more appealing and less overwhelming to a patient with anorexia. Many patients require complicated nutritional therapy such as enteral or parenteral therapy to meet nutritional needs.*
- Provide a rest period before and after meals. *Eating requires energy, and the malnourished patient may have decreased physical strength and energy.*
- Assess knowledge and provide appropriate teaching. *Lack of knowledge often contributes to undernutrition. Education empowers the patient to make healthy choices.*

Risk for Infection

Malnourished patients have a much higher risk for infection than well-nourished people. Malnutrition affects many components of the immune system, including the skin, mucous membranes, and lymph tissue and cells.

- Monitor temperature and assess for manifestations of infection every 4 hours. *Although the baseline temperature may be subnormal in malnourished patients, any elevation from baseline may indicate infection. Manifestations of infection may include chills, malaise, erythema, and leukocytosis. Early detection of infection may prevent complications.*
- Maintain medical asepsis when providing care and surgical asepsis when carrying out procedures. *Hand hygiene is the best strategy to prevent the spread of pathogens. Sterile technique is required for procedures such as inserting central lines and changing dressings.*
- Teach the signs and symptoms of infection, hand hygiene, and factors that increase the risk for infection. *Knowledge empowers the patient to participate in self-care, thus reducing exposure to infectious pathogens.*

Risk for Deficient Fluid Volume

The patient with malnutrition may also have a fluid volume deficit. Difficulty swallowing food and fluids or administration of hyperosmolar nutritional solutions may lead to dehydration or electrolyte disturbances.

- Monitor oral mucous membranes, urine specific gravity, level of consciousness, and laboratory findings every 4 to 8 hours. *Dry mucous membranes, increased urine specific gravity, decreased level of consciousness, and electrolyte imbalances may indicate dehydration.*

■ Weigh daily and monitor intake and output. *Daily weights and intake and output measurements help monitor fluid balance.*

■ If allowed, offer fluids frequently in small amounts, considering the patient's preferences. *Frequent, small amounts of fluids are better tolerated and promote adequate intake.*

Risk for Impaired Skin Integrity

Skin integrity depends on adequate nutrition. Loss of subcutaneous tissue and muscle increase the risk of pressure ulcers. In addition, healing is impaired in malnourished patients.

■ Assess skin every 4 hours. *Baseline and ongoing assessments allow prompt identification of early manifestations of skin breakdown.*

■ Turn and reposition at least every 2 hours. Encourage passive and active range-of-motion exercises. *These measures reduce pressure and promote oxygenation of cells.*

■ Keep skin dry and clean, and minimize shearing forces. Keep linens smooth, clean, and dry. Provide therapeutic beds, mattresses, or pads. *These nursing measures promote comfort and reduce the risk of skin breakdown.*

Using NANDA, NIC, and NOC

Linkages between a selected NANDA nursing diagnosis, NIC, and NOC for the patient with malnutrition are shown in the chart that follows.

Community-Based Care

Community-dwelling older adults, homeless people, and other disadvantaged populations are at particular risk for being malnourished. See the accompanying nursing research box.

Patients with malnutrition may be cared for at home or in the hospital with diet, enteral, or parenteral therapy. Each year, it is

---

NANDA, NIC, AND NOC LINKAGES
The Patient with Malnutrition

NANDA Imbalanced Nutrition: Less than Body Requirements

NIC Weight Gain Assistance
Fluid/Electrolyte Management
Nutrition Therapy
Infection Protection

NOC Nutritional Status
Nutritional Status: Nutrient Intake
Electrolyte & Acid/Base Balance
Immune Status

Data from NANDA International. (2009). *Nursing diagnoses: Definitions & classification 2009–2011.* Oxford, UK: Wiley-Blackwell; Bulechek, G., Butcher, H., & Dochterman J. (Eds.). (2008). *Nursing interventions classification (NIC)* (5th ed.). St. Louis, MO: Mosby; and Moorhead, S., Johnson, M., Maas, M., & Swanson, E. (Eds.). (2008). *Nursing outcomes classification (NOC)* (4th ed.). St. Louis, MO: Mosby.

---

more common to see patients managing tube feeding or PN at home. Teaching for the patient and family includes the following topics:

■ Diet recommendations and use of nutritional supplements

■ Where to obtain recommended foods and nutritional supplements

■ If continuing enteral or parenteral nutrition, (1) how to prepare and/or handle solutions, (2) how to add them to either the feeding tube or central line, (3) how to manage infusion pumps, (4) how to care for the feeding tube or central catheter, (5) how to recognize and manage problems and complications, and (6) how and when to notify the healthcare provider of problems

---

MOVING EVIDENCE INTO ACTION   Patients with Malnutrition

The percentage of older adults who have risk factors for malnutrition is higher than in young and middle adults. These risk factors include functional limitations, chronic disease, and psychosocial factors. A study of community-dwelling low- and underweight older adults by Martin, Kayser-Jones, Stotts, Porter, & Froelicher (2007) found three variables in particular to have a clear association with being severely underweight: an illness or condition that affected food intake, a 10-lb or greater unintentional weight loss within the past 6 months, and an inability to travel outside the home without assistance.

IMPLICATIONS FOR NURSING

This study provides information that can be especially useful for nurses in community-based care settings. Using a brief nutritional screening tool (see Box 22–3) and weighing the patient on a regular basis can alert the nurse to the need for referral or additional support to prevent malnutrition. A patient whose food intake has been affected by chronic disease

should be referred to a dietician for assistance with meal planning. Measures such as encouraging use of nutritional supplements (e.g., Ensure) can help stop or even reverse unintentional weight loss.

CRITICAL THINKING IN PATIENT CARE

1. What essential information should you collect from patients in an ambulatory care setting (e.g., physician's office or clinic) to screen for those who are at risk for becoming malnourished?

2. This study found that participants who needed assistance traveling outside the home were at significant risk for being underweight. Identify nursing interventions and community resources to reduce this risk for an older adult in your community.

3. Develop a teaching plan to prepare caregivers in a residential care facility to use the Mini Nutritional Assessment Screening tool outlined in Box 22–3 for screening residents.

CASE STUDY & NURSING CARE PLAN   A Patient with Malnutrition

Rose Morris is an 88-year-old widow who lives alone. She typically rises early and has a cup of tea before spending her morning puttering in her garden. She consumes her main meal of the day at lunch, which usually includes rice and some vegetables. For dinner, she generally eats a bowl of rice with "whatever seems to be in the refrigerator." She admits to little interest in cooking or eating since her husband died 10 years ago and her group of friends has been "dying off too."

ASSESSMENT

Mrs. Morris weighs 95 lb (43.1 kg) and is 5'3" (160 cm) tall, for a BMI of 16.8. She reports weighing 118 lb (53.5 kg) 5 years ago. Her triceps skinfold thickness measurement is 11 mm (normal values for a female: > 13 mm). Her skin is pale, and she appears thin and wasted. Her temperature is 97°F (36.°C). Diagnostic test results include serum albumin 2.9 g/dL (normal 3.4 to 4.8 g/dL) and serum cholesterol 130 mg/dL (normal 150 to 200 mg/dL). A diagnosis of protein-calorie malnutrition is made, and a 1500-calorie per day diet is recommended.

DIAGNOSES

- *Imbalanced Nutrition: Less than Body Requirements* related to lack of knowledge and inadequate food intake
- *Risk for Infection* related to protein-calorie malnutrition
- *Impaired Social Interaction* related to widowhood and reduced social support group

EXPECTED OUTCOMES

- Gain at least 1 pound per week.
- Verbalize understanding of nutritional requirements and identify strategies to incorporate requirements into daily diet after discharge.

- Remain infection free, evidenced by normal vital signs.
- Identify strategies to increase social interaction, such as participating in senior citizens' lunches at local senior center.

PLANNING AND IMPLEMENTATION

- Weigh weekly at a consistent time of day.
- Refer to dietitian for evaluation of nutritional needs.
- Teach about nutritional requirements, and plan an eating program that includes high-calorie, high-protein foods and supplements and reflects her food preferences. Encourage small, frequent meals.
- Encourage to keep a food intake diary.
- Teach strategies to reduce risks for infection.
- Provide information about communal meals available to seniors in the community, and help Mrs. Morris develop a plan to participate.

EVALUATION

One month later, Mrs. Morris has gained 3 pounds and reports feeling "more energetic." A friend is helping her shop to ensure that she purchases foods to maintain her protein, calorie, and nutrient intake. She has begun attending senior lunches twice a week, and is enjoying "being around people again." Although she still doesn't enjoy cooking like she used to, she is using prepared foods and supplements to maintain her nutrient intake.

CRITICAL THINKING IN THE NURSING PROCESS

1. What is the physiologic basis for Mrs. Morris's low albumin and cholesterol levels?
2. Mrs. Morris asks, "Can I get better by just taking more vitamins?" How will you respond?
3. Design a teaching plan for a Hispanic patient with protein-calorie malnutrition.

See Evaluating Your Response in Appendix C.

The Patient with an Eating Disorder

Eating disorders are characterized by severely disturbed eating behavior and weight management. Eating disorders are more common in affluent societies where food is plentiful. Women are much more commonly affected than men. **Anorexia nervosa** is characterized by a refusal to maintain a minimally normal body weight, a distorted body image, and an intense fear of gaining weight or of loss of control over food intake. Anorexia nervosa affects about 1% of women in the United States at some time in their lives (Fauci et al., 2008). **Bulimia nervosa**, which affects 1% to 3% of women in the United States, is characterized by recurring episodes of binge eating followed by purge behaviors such as self-induced vomiting, use of laxatives or diuretics, fasting, or excessive exercise. A third eating disorder, **binge-eating disorder**, is believed to affect many more people than either anorexia or bulimia. Binge-eating disorder is characterized by recurrent episodes of binge eating—eating an excessive amount of food during a defined period of time and a sense of loss of control over eating during binge episodes (National Institute of Mental Health [NIMH], 2007).

Anorexia Nervosa

Anorexia nervosa typically begins during mid to late adolescence. Patients with anorexia nervosa have a distorted body image and irrational fear of gaining weight. Refusal to maintain body weight at or above a minimally normal level for height and body type is a common manifestation of anorexia nervosa. Patients maintain weight loss by restricted calorie intake, often accompanied by excessive exercise. Some may exhibit binge–purge behavior.

Although its cause is unknown, psychologic, biologic, genetic, and cultural risk factors have been identified for anorexia nervosa. A history of sexual or physical abuse and family history of mood disorders are nonspecific risk factors. Abnormal levels of neurotransmitters and other hormones may play a role. Genetic factors are suggested by a higher incidence within families and in the monozygotic twin of an affected individual. Women who develop anorexia nervosa tend to be obsessive and perfectionistic, and often feel inadequate or unable to maintain control in their lives. Family, social, or occupational (e.g., a career in modeling or ballet) pressures to maintain low body weight also contribute.

The manifestations and complications of anorexia nervosa are listed in the box on page 608. Patients who engage in binge–purge behavior have a higher risk for complications.

Eating Disorder Video

MANIFESTATIONS AND COMPLICATIONS of Eating Disorders

DISORDER	MANIFESTATIONS	COMPLICATIONS
Anorexia Nervosa	■ Weight < 85% of normal, muscle wasting ■ Fear of weight gain, refusal to eat ■ Disturbed body image, excessive exercise ■ Amenorrhea ■ Skin and hair changes ■ Hypotension, bradycardia ■ Hypothermia, cold intolerance ■ Constipation ■ Insomnia	■ Electrolyte and acid–base disturbances ■ Reduced cardiac output, dysrhythmias ■ Elevated BUN, serum creatinine levels ■ Anemia ■ Hypoglycemia, elevated serum uric acid levels ■ Osteoporosis ■ Enlarged salivary glands ■ Delayed gastric emptying ■ Abnormal liver function
Bulimia Nervosa	■ Weight often normal; may be slightly overweight ■ Binge–purge behavior ■ Oligomenorrhea or amenorrhea ■ Lacerations of palate; callous on fingers or dorsum of hand	■ Enlarged salivary glands ■ Stomatitis, loss of dental enamel ■ Fluid, electrolyte, and acid–base imbalances ■ Dysrhythmias ■ Esophageal tears, stomach rupture

Binge-Eating Disorder	■ Usually overweight or obese
	■ Recurrent episodes of binge eating (2 or more days a week for 6 months)
	■ Episodes characterized by the following:
	  ■ Eating more rapidly than usual
	  ■ Eating until uncomfortably full
	  ■ Eating large amounts of food when not physically hungry
	  ■ Eating alone due to embarrassment over quantity
	  ■ Disgust, depression, or guilt following a binge episode
	  ■ Marked distress about binging behavior
		■ Type 2 diabetes
		■ Hypertension, hyperlipidemia
		■ Coronary heart disease, heart failure
		■ Gallbladder disease
		■ Depression, social isolation

Bulimia Nervosa

Bulimia nervosa develops in late adolescence or early adulthood. Unlike patients with anorexia nervosa, the weight of patients with bulimia is within or above the normal range. Like anorexia nervosa, however, the cause likely is multifactorial, including cultural, psychosocial, and biologic factors. The patient with bulimia often restricts caloric intake, leading to increased hunger and overeating. Foods consumed during a binge often are high calorie, high fat, and sweet. After binge eating, the patient induces vomiting (usually by stimulating the gag reflex), or may take excessive quantities of laxatives or diuretics. Fluid and electrolyte balance may be severely disrupted by loss of fluid and gastrointestinal secretions. The complications of bulimia nervosa (see the preceding box) primarily result from the purging behavior.

Binge-Eating Disorder

Binge-eating disorder (BED) shares many of the characteristics of bulimia; however, patients with BED do not purge. BED commonly affects obese middle-aged adults. It affects Blacks and Whites equally. The cause of BED is unknown, although genetics may play a role in its development. Psychosocial factors contribute; people with BED often are depressed, anxious, or have a personality disorder. People with BED consume an excessive amount of food during binging episodes, eating even when not hungry and continuing to eat until uncomfortably full. Binging often occurs when the person is alone. After overeating, the patient may feel disgusted or guilty about the amount of food consumed, and depressed about the inability to control eating.

Interdisciplinary Care

Eating disorders, anorexia nervosa in particular, are difficult to effectively treat. Because of the intense fear of weight gain and the distorted body image of patients with anorexia, they strongly resist increasing food intake. While community-based care is appropriate for most patients with an eating disorder, complications of the disorder or resistance to treatment may necessitate hospitalization for some patients. In all cases, a comprehensive treatment plan for eating disorders includes medical care and monitoring, psychosocial interventions, and nutrition counseling.

Diagnosis

There is no specific diagnostic test for anorexia, bulimia, or binge-eating disorder. Laboratory studies in patients with anorexia or bulimia may show anemia and leukopenia on CBC, abnormal serum electrolyte levels, and elevated BUN and serum creatinine. In patients with BED, the blood glucose and lipid levels may be elevated. The BMI usually is above the normal range, and may identify the patient as obese.

A mental health evaluation is indicated for patients with eating disorders to identify contributing factors and help direct treatment.

Treatment

Patients with anorexia nervosa may require hospitalization, particularly if their weight is less than 75% of normal. Refeeding is gradually introduced to avoid complications such as heart failure. Multivitamins are given along with calcium and vitamin D supplements to minimize bone loss. Meals must be supervised and a firm but empathetic attitude conveyed about the importance of adequate food intake. Intravenous feeding may be required in some cases. Psychologic treatment focuses on providing emotional support during weight gain and helping patients base their self-esteem on factors other than weight (e.g., personal relationships, satisfaction with achieving occupational goals) (Fauci et al., 2008). Cognitive-behavioral therapy or psychotherapy may be used; families often are included in the treatment program. A tricyclic antidepressant, selective serotonin reuptake inhibitor (SSRI) such as fluoxetine (Prozac) or sertraline (Zoloft), or lithium carbonate may be prescribed to facilitate weight maintenance and reduce anxiety.

The goal of bulimia treatment is to reduce or eliminate binge eating and purging behavior. A combination of nutritional counseling and therapy, psychosocial interventions, and medications may be used. Nutritional counseling is directed at establishing a regular meal pattern and encouraging an appropriate amount of regular exercise. An antidepressant drug such as fluoxetine (Prozac) may benefit the patient with bulimia nervosa and help prevent relapse. Cognitive-behavioral therapy also is used to treat bulimia, focusing on excessive concerns about weight, persistent dieting, and binge–purge behaviors.

Treatment for patients with binge-eating disorder focuses on establishing healthy eating patterns, psychosocial therapy (including cognitive-behavioral therapy and group counseling) to address underlying issues, and management of obesity and its complications. Patients with BED also may benefit from an SSRI or other antidepressant drug.

✍ Nursing Care

Nurses can be instrumental in identifying patients with eating disorders and referring them for treatment. It is particularly important to identify these disorders early to prevent adverse effects on growth and increase the success of treatment.

The nurse is an integral part of the eating disorders treatment team. *Imbalanced Nutrition: Less than Body Requirements* is a primary nursing diagnosis for patients with anorexia or bulimia, and *Imbalanced Nutrition: More than Body Requirements* is a priority nursing diagnosis for patients with binge-eating disorder. The following nursing diagnoses also should be considered:

- *Ineffective Therapeutic Regimen Management*
- *Chronic Low Self-Esteem*
- *Disturbed Body Image*
- *Dysfunctional Family Processes*
- *Powerlessness*

When planning and implementing care, consider the following nursing activities.

- Regularly monitor weight, using standard conditions. *Weight gain or loss provides information about the effectiveness of care, as well as the patient's risk for complications.*
- Monitor food intake during meals, recording percentage of meal and snack consumed. Maintain close observation for at least 1 hour following meals; do not allow patient alone in bathroom. *Observing the patient during and after meals helps prevent disposal of food and purging behavior after eating. Recording actual food intake allows accurate calculation of calorie intake.*
- Serve balanced meals, including all nutrient groups. Increase serving size gradually. *The patient may find "normal" food servings overwhelming, reducing the desire to eat. Calorie intake is initially limited to prevent complications associated with refeeding, then gradually increased.*
- Serve frequent, small feedings of cold or room temperature foods. *Cool foods reduce sensations of early satiety, promoting greater food intake at a meal or snack.*
- Administer a multivitamin and mineral supplement to replace losses.

Patients with eating disorders require extended treatment of the disorder. Involvement of the family and social support persons is vital to success. Encourage family members to participate in teaching and nutritional counseling sessions. Discuss the value of family therapy to address issues that have contributed to the disorder. Emphasize the need to provide consistent messages of support for healthy eating habits. Discuss using rewards for food and calorie intake rather than weight gain. Provide referrals to a dietitian, nutritional support team, counseling, and support groups for people with eating disorders.

CHAPTER HIGHLIGHTS

- Nutritional disorders are common, affecting people worldwide, and contributing significantly to mortality and morbidity. While malnutrition is a serious problem in underdeveloped nations, obesity and its consequences are more prevalent in the United States and other industrialized societies.
- Obesity, defined as excess adipose tissue and a BMI greater than 30 kg/m^2, is linked with many disorders, including type 2 diabetes, coronary heart disease, gallbladder disease, and osteoarthritis.
- Exercise and reduced kilocalorie intake are the mainstays of obesity treatment. Drugs that suppress the appetite or interfere with fat absorption in the gut may be used to facilitate weight loss in patients with multiple risk factors for obesity complications or people who have had difficulty achieving weight loss through diet and exercise.

- Bariatric surgery is a treatment option for morbidly obese patients. The primary types of bariatric surgery used in the United States are restrictive procedures that limit stomach capacity and food consumption, and combination restrictive/malabsorptive procedures that limit both capacity and nutrient absorption.
- Nursing care for obese patients focuses on health promotion, education, and support of the prescribed treatment plan.
- In the United States, protein-calorie malnutrition is a common problem among hospitalized patients. Malnutrition increases the risk for complications and impairs healing. Early identification and prevention are the primary focuses of treatment; nurses can be instrumental in identifying at-risk patients (e.g., the elderly, patients living alone, people on extended NPO status).

- Refeeding of malnourished patients is a gradual process. Enteral feedings (oral or by feeding tube) are preferred whenever possible. Parenteral nutrition may be required when enteral feeding is not possible or not tolerated by the patient.
- Eating disorders, including anorexia nervosa, bulimia nervosa, and binge-eating disorder, can be difficult to effectively treat and maintain in remission. While patients with anorexia typically are underweight and malnourished, resisting efforts to achieve a

normal weight, patients with bulimia are more likely to be of normal weight and those with binge-eating disorder are more likely to be overweight or obese.
- Treatment for eating disorders is multifaceted, including physical care to restore electrolyte balance and treat complications, nutritional counseling and therapy, psychosocial therapy, family support, and possibly medications.

TEST YOURSELF NCLEX-RN® REVIEW

1. Of the following noted in a patient's history, which does the nurse identify as the greatest risk factor for obesity?
   1. adopted at 2 months of age
   2. usual diet includes "fast-food" lunches twice a week
   3. does not engage in regular activity
   4. allergic to chocolate and strawberries

2. A patient on a reduced-calorie diet asks the nurse what she can do to lose weight faster, because most weeks she loses no more than 0.5 lb. "At this rate, it will take me years to get to my goal!" The most appropriate response by the nurse would be which of the following?
   1. "Let's reevaluate your long-term goal. Perhaps it was set too low for you."
   2. "A pound of body fat equals 3500 calories. Let's reevaluate your diet and exercise plan for calorie intake and expenditure."
   3. "Perhaps we should look into a diet supplement since you are unable to stick with your prescribed diet plan."
   4. "You sound frustrated. Would you like to take some time off from your diet and exercise plan?"

3. An expected finding in a patient admitted with a diagnosis of protein-calorie malnutrition would be which of the following?
   1. recent 5-lb weight loss
   2. increased skinfold thickness measurements
   3. hyperactive bowel sounds
   4. anxiety and agitation

4. Before administering an intermittent enteral feeding, the nurse confirms placement of the small-bore feeding tube in the stomach by doing which of the following?
   1. instilling water and listening for the gastric gurgle
   2. withdrawing the tube slightly, then reinserting it
   3. aspirating gastric contents and checking for a pH of < 4
   4. obtaining a flat-plate x-ray of the stomach

5. The nurse identifies which of the following as a realistic goal for a patient with anorexia nervosa?
   1. Will consume 100% of a 2500-calorie diet.
   2. Will gain 2 pounds per week.
   3. Will rest alone in room following meals.
   4. Will participate in family counseling.

6. The nurse identifies which nursing diagnosis as high priority for a patient with a BMI of 30.4 kg/m² and a waist–hip ratio of 1.1?
   1. *Health-Seeking Behaviors: Weight Loss*
   2. *Risk for Impaired Tissue Perfusion: Cardiovascular*
   3. *Ineffective Coping*
   4. *Deficient Knowledge: Diet*

7. The nurse teaching a patient about sibutramine (Meridia) includes which of the following instructions? **Select all that apply.**
   1. You may skip a dose of the drug if you skip a meal.
   2. Do not consume alcohol while taking this drug.
   3. Do not drive while taking this drug because the drug may increase sleepiness.
   4. Increase your intake of water and other fluids while taking this drug.
   5. Continue to follow your prescribed diet while taking this drug.

8. The nurse caring for a home-bound older adult who is losing an unplanned 1 to 2 pounds monthly plans for which of the following? **Select all that apply.**
   1. Meals on Wheels deliveries
   2. Ensure nutritional supplements
   3. placement in a residential care facility
   4. transportation to congregate senior meals
   5. follow-up by primary care physician
   6. referral for diagnostic studies

9. Which of the following is a high-priority nursing intervention to prevent malnutrition in the surgical patient?
   1. aggressive pain management
   2. daily weights
   3. maintaining intravenous flow
   4. requesting early restoration of oral intake

10. Three days after gastric bypass surgery, the patient complains of increasing abdominal pain. Bowel sounds are absent; the abdomen is firm and very tender. The nurse should do which of the following?
    1. Report findings to the surgeon.
    2. Ambulate the patient to promote peristalsis.
    3. Chart assessment data and continue to monitor.
    4. Evaluate the effectiveness of analgesia.

See Test Yourself answers in Appendix C.

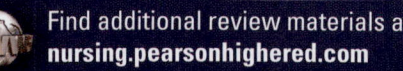

Pearson Nursing Student Resources

Find additional review materials at
nursing.pearsonhighered.com

Prepare for success with additional NCLEX®-style practice questions, interactive assignments and activities, Web links, animations and videos, and more!

BIBLIOGRAPHY

Amella, E. (2007). Assessing nutrition in older adults. *Try this: Best practices in nursing care to older adults, 9*(2007). The Hartford Institute for Geriatric Nursing, New York University, College of Nursing. Retrieved from www.ConsultGeriRN.org

American Psychiatric Association. (2006). Practice guideline for the treatment of patients with eating disorders. (3rd ed.) Washington, DC: American Psychiatric Association (APA);

Arzouman, J., Lacovara, J., Blackett, A., McDonald, P., Traver, G., & Bartholomeaux, F. (2006). Developing a comprehensive bariatric protocol: A template for improving patient care. *MEDSURG Nursing, 15*(1), 21–26.

Baugh, N., Zuelzer, H., Meador, J., & Blankenship, J. (2007). Wounds in surgical patients who are obese. *American Journal of Nursing, 107*(6), 40–50.

Brown, A., & Siahpush, M. (2007). Risk factors for overweight and obesity: Results from the 2001 National Health Survey. *Public Health, 121*, 603–613.

Budd, G. (2007). Disordered eating: Young women's search for control and connection. *Journal of Child and Adolescent Psychiatric Nursing, 20*(2), 96–106.

Centers for Disease Control and Prevention [CDC]. (2008). *2008 Physical activity guidelines for Americans.* Atlanta, GA: Author. Retrieved from www.cdc.gov./physicalactivity

CDC. (2009a). Obesity. Halting the epidemic by making health easier. National Center for Chronic Disease Prevention and Health Promotion. Retrieved from www.cdc.gov/nccdphp

CDC. (2009b). Obesity. Introduction. Retrieved from www.cdc.gov

CDC. (2009c). Preventing obesity and chronic diseases through good nutrition and physical activity. Retrieved from www.cdc.gov

Clinical update. Effectiveness of interventions for undernourished older inpatients in the hospital setting. (2007). *Australian Nursing Journal, 15*(5), 28–31.

Differences in prevalence of obesity among Black, White, and Hispanic adults – United States, 2006–2008. (2009, July 17). *MMWR: Mortality and Morbidity Weekly Report, 58*(27). Retrieved from www.cdc.gov/mmwr

DiMaria-Ghalili, R. (2008). Nutrition in the elderly. Nursing standard of practice protocol: Nutrition in aging. Hartford Institute for Geriatric Nursing, New York University College of Nursing. Retrieved from consultgerirn.org/topics/nutrition_in_the_elderly

DiMaria-Ghalili, R., & Guenter, P. (2008). The mini nutritional assessment. *American Journal of Nursing, 108*(2), 50–59.

Dorner, B. (2007). The obesity challenge. Retrieved from www.nursinghomesmagazine.com

Fauci, A. S., Braunwald, E., Kasper, D. L., Hauser, S. L., Longo, D. L., Jameson, J. L., et al. (Eds.). (2008). *Harrison's principles of internal medicine* (17th ed.). New York: McGraw-Hill.

Flegal, K., Carroll, M., Ogden, C., & Curtin, L. (2010, January 20). Prevalence and trends in obesity among US adults, 1999–2008. *JAMA, 303*(3), 235–241.

Flood, M., & Newman, A. (2007). Obesity in older adults: Synthesis of findings and recommendations for clinical practice. *Journal of Gerontological Nursing, December 2007,* 19–35.

Grindel, M., & Grindel, C. (2006). Nursing care of the person having bariatric surgery. *MEDSURG Nursing, 15*(3), 129–145.

Harrington, L. (2006). Postoperative care of patients undergoing bariatric surgery. *MEDSURG Nursing, 15*(6), 357–363.

Jarosz, P., & Bellar, A. (2008). Age-appropriate obesity treatment. *The Nurse Practitioner, 33*(5), 24–31.

Kumanyika, S., Obarzanek, E., Stettler, N., Bell, R., Field, A., Fortmann, S., et al. (2008). Population-based prevention of obesity: The need for comprehensive promotion of healthful eating, physical activity, and energy balance: A scientific statement from American Heart Association Council on Epidemiology and Prevneion, Interdisciplinary Committee for Prevention. *Circulation, 118,* 428–464. Retrieved from www.circ.ahajournals.org

Lehne, R. (2007). *Pharmacology for nursing care* (6th ed.). St. Louis, MO: Saunders.

Martin, C., Kayser-Jones, J., Stotts, N., Porter, C., & Froelicher, E. (2007). Risk for low weight in community-dwelling, older adults. *Clinical Nurse Specialist, 21*(4), 203–211.

McPhee, S. J., Papadakis, M. A., & Tierney, L. M. (2008). *Current medical diagnosis & treatment* (47th ed.). New York: Lange Medical Books/McGraw-Hill.

McWilliams, B. (2008). Assessing the benefits of a malnutrition screening tool. *Nursing Times: NT, 104*(24), 30–32.

Menifield, C., Doty, N., & Fletcher, A. (2008). Obesity in America. *The ABNF Journal, Summer 2008,* 83–88.

Metheny, N. A., Dahms, T. E., Stewart, B. J., Stone, K. S., Frank, P. A., & Clouse, R. E. (2005). Verification of inefficacy of the glucose method in detecting aspiration associated with tube feedings. *MEDSURG Nursing, 14*(2), 112–121.

Muir, M., Heese, G., McLean, D., Bodnar, S., & Rock, B. (2007). Handling of the bariatric patient in critical care: A case study of lessons learned. *Critical Care Nursing Clinics of North America, 19*(2), 223–240.

National Center for Health Statistics [NCHS]. (2008). NCHS Data on eating behaviors. Retrieved from www.cdc.gov/nchs

National Heart, Lung, and Blood Institute [NHLBI]. (1998). *Clinical guidelines on the identification, evaluation, and treatment of overweight and obesity in adults: The evidence report* (National Institutes of Health: Publication No. 98-4083). Retrieved from http://www.nhlbi.nih.gov

NHLBI. (2009). *Overweight and obesity.* Retrieved from www.nhlbi.nih.gov/health/dci/Diseases/obe/obe_all.html

NHLBI. (2000). *The practical guide. Identification, evaluation, and treatment of overweight and obesity in adults* (NIH Publication No. 00-4084). Retrieved from www.nhlbi.nih.gov

NHLBI. (2004). *Think tank on enhancing obesity research at the National Heart, Lung, and Blood Institute.* (NIH Publication No. 04-5249). Retrieved from www.nhlbi.nih.gov

National Institute of Diabetes and Digestive and Kidney Diseases [NIDDK]. (2008). Longitudinal assessment of bariatric surgery (LABS). (NIH Publication No. 04-5573). Retrieved from www.win.niddk.nih.gov

National Institute of Mental Health [NIMH]. (2007). Eating disorders. (NIH Publication No. 07-4901). Retrieved from www.nimh.nih.gov

Noble, K. (2008). The obesity epidemic: The impact of obesity on the perianesthesia patient. *Journal of PeriAnesthesia Nursing, 23*(6), 418–425.

North American Nursing Diagnosis Association. (2009). *Nursing diagnoses: Definitions & classification 2009–2011.* Oxford, UK: Wiley-Blackwell.

The Obesity Society. (2009a). Obesity, bias, and stigmatization. Retrieved from www.obesity.org

The Obesity Society. (2009b). Obesity statistics. Retrieved from www.obesity.org

Obden, C., Carroll, M., McDowell, M., & Flegal, K. (2007). Obesity among adults in the United States—No statistically significant changes since 2003–2004. NCHS Data Brief No 1. Hayattsville, MD: National Center for Health Statistics.

Pettit, E. (2009). Treating morbid obesity. *RN, 72*(2), 30–34.

Porth, C. M., & Matfin, G. (2009). *Pathophysiology: Concepts of altered health states* (7th ed.). Philadelphia: Lippincott.

Price, D. (2008). Protein-energy malnutrition among the elderly: Implications for nursing practice. *Holistic Nursing Practice, 22*(6), 355–360.

Sacks, F., Bray, G., Carey, V., Smith, S., Ryan, D., Anton, S., et al. (2009). Comparison of weight-loss diets with different compositions of fat, protein, and carbohydrates. *New England Journal of Medicine, 360*(9), 859–873.

Thomas, A., Moseley, G., Stallings, R., Nichols-English, G., & Wagner, P. (2008). Perceptions of obesity: Black and White differences. *Journal of Cultural Diversity, 15*(4), 174–180.

Tozzo, M. (2007). Battling obesity: Small steps, big rewards. *Nursing2007, 37*(3), 68–69.

Turner, S., Thomas, A., Wagner, P., & Moseley, G. (2008). A collaborative approach to wellness: Diet, exercise, and education to impact behavior change. *Journal of the American Academy of Nurse Practitioners, 20*(2008), 339–344.

Weight-control Information Network [WIN]. (2007a). *Medical care for obese patients.* (NIH Publication No. 03-4159). Bethesda, MD: National Institutes of Health.

WIN. (2007b). *Prescription medications for the treatment of obesity.* (NIH Publication No. 07-4191). Bethesda, MD: National Institutes of Health.

WIN. (2010). Overweight and obesity statistics. Bethesda, MD: National Institutes of Health. Retrieved from www.win.niddk.nih.gov

WIN. (2008a). *Bariatric surgery for severe obesity.* (NIH Publication No. 08-4006). Bethesda, MD: National Institutes of Health.

WIN. (2008b). *Very low-calorie diets.* (NIH Publication No. 03-3894). Bethesda, MD: National Institutes of Health.

Wilkinson, J., & Ahern, N. (2009). *Nursing diagnosis handbook* (9th ed.). Upper Saddle River, NJ: Pearson Prentice Hall.

23 Nursing Care of Patients with Upper Gastrointestinal Disorders

LEARNING OUTCOMES

1. Describe the pathophysiology of common disorders of the mouth, esophagus, and stomach.
2. Relate manifestations and diagnostic test results to the pathophysiologic processes involved in upper gastrointestinal disorders.
3. Explain interdisciplinary care for patients with upper gastrointestinal disorders.
4. Describe the role of the nurse in interdisciplinary care of patients with upper gastrointestinal disorders.

CLINICAL COMPETENCIES

1. Assess the functional health status of patients with upper gastrointestinal disorders.
2. Monitor, document, and, as needed, report manifestations of upper gastrointestinal disorders and their complications.
3. Plan patient-centered nursing care using an evidence base, research, and, as appropriate, decision-support technology.
4. Determine priority nursing diagnoses and interventions based on assessed data.
5. Administer medications and prescribed care knowledgeably and safely.
6. Coordinate and integrate interdisciplinary care into plan of care.
7. Construct and revise individualized plans of care considering the culture and values of the patient.
8. Plan and provide patient and family teaching to promote, maintain, and restore functional health.

KEY TERMS

achalasia, *627*
anorexia, *642*
Curling's ulcers, *642*
Cushing's ulcers, *642*
dumping syndrome, *645*
dysphagia, *627*
erosive (stress-induced) gastritis, *642*
gastric mucosal barrier, *630*

gastritis, *641*
gastroesophageal reflux, *622*
hematemesis, *630*
hematochezia, *630*
melena, *630*
nausea, *612*
occult bleeding, *630*
partial gastrectomy, *645*

peptic ulcer disease (PUD), *633*
peptic ulcers, *633*
steatorrhea, *635*
stomatitis, *616*
total gastrectomy, *645*
ulcer, *634*
vomiting, *612*
Zollinger-Ellison syndrome, *635*

The upper gastrointestinal tract includes the mouth, esophagus, stomach, and proximal small intestine. Food and fluids, ingested through the mouth, move through the esophagus to the stomach. The stomach and upper intestinal tract (duodenum and jejunum) are responsible for the majority of food digestion. When an acute or chronic condition or disease process interferes with the function of this portion of the gastrointestinal (GI) tract, nutritional status can be affected and the patient may experience symptoms that interfere with functional status and lifestyle.

Nurses provide acute care for the hospitalized patient, coordinate care in ambulatory and long-term care settings, and teach the skills and knowledge needed to manage these conditions at home.

The Patient with Nausea and Vomiting

Nausea and vomiting are common gastrointestinal symptoms. **Nausea** is a vague but unpleasant sensation of sickness or queasiness. It may or may not be accompanied by (and possibly relieved by) vomiting. **Vomiting** is the forceful expulsion of the contents of the upper GI tract resulting from contraction of muscles in the gut and abdominal wall. Nausea and vomiting without abdominal pain are commonly associated with food poisoning, infectious gastroenteritis (discussed in Chapter 24), gallbladder disease, or ingestion of toxins (such as drugs or alcohol). When associated with severe abdominal pain, they may indicate a serious disorder such as peritonitis, acute gastrointestinal obstruction, or pancreatitis.

Pathophysiology

Nausea, an unpleasant subjective sensation, occurs when the vomiting center in the medulla of the brain is stimulated. Distention of the duodenum is a common stimulus for nausea. The vomiting center can be stimulated by input from several different sources:

- The GI tract, produced by distention, irritation, or infection
- The vestibular system of the ear
- Higher central nervous system centers in response to certain sights, smells, or emotional experiences

- Chemoreceptors outside the blood–brain barrier that are stimulated by drugs, chemotherapeutic agents, toxins, systemic disorders, and pregnancy
- Disorders such as acute myocardial infarction and heart failure commonly produce nausea and vomiting, possibly due to direct stimulation of the vomiting center by hypoxia
- Increased intracranial pressure (e.g., due to intracranial bleeding or a tumor) produces vomiting that may or may not be accompanied by nausea

Anorexia, loss of appetite, commonly precedes nausea, just as nausea frequently precedes vomiting. Vomiting, a response that requires coordinated movements of the thorax and abdominal wall, the gut, the pharynx, and muscles of the mouth and face, is coordinated by the brainstem. *Emesis* (or *vomitus*) is produced when inspiratory muscles of the thorax (including the diaphragm) and abdomen contract, increasing intrathoracic and intra-abdominal pressures. The gastroesophageal sphincter relaxes, and the larynx moves upward to facilitate oral expulsion of gastric contents.

In addition to the subjective sensation of queasiness, nausea frequently is accompanied by autonomic nervous system manifestations such as pallor, sweating, tachycardia, and increased salivation. Vomiting, which stimulates the vagus nerve and parasympathetic nervous system, may be accompanied by dizziness, light-headedness, hypotension, and bradycardia.

Potential complications of vomiting include dehydration, hypokalemia, metabolic alkalosis (from loss of hydrochloric acid from the stomach), aspiration with resulting pneumonia, and rupture or tears of the esophagus.

Interdisciplinary Care

In most cases, nausea and vomiting are self-limited and require no treatment. If vomiting is severe or accompanied by other symptoms, acute care may be required to determine the underlying problem and prevent or treat complications.

Diagnostic tests may include serum electrolytes; pregnancy testing if indicated; liver, pancreatic, and renal function studies; and imaging studies (flat plate of the abdomen, abdominal CT scan) to detect gastrointestinal obstruction. An upper endoscopy may be performed (∞ see Chapter 21 for nursing care of the patient undergoing upper endoscopy). CT scan or MRI of the head may be ordered if an intracranial problem is suspected as the cause. Specialized testing such as gastrointestinal motility studies may be indicated when other diagnostic studies are negative for an anatomic cause of nausea and vomiting.

Food is initially withheld, although clear liquids in small quantities are encouraged to prevent dehydration. Dry foods such as soda crackers may reduce nausea and promote comfort.

Medications

Unless vomiting is associated with pregnancy, antiemetic medications may be prescribed to prevent or control nausea and vomiting. These drugs fall into a number of different classes, and often are more effective when given in combination.

- Serotonin receptor antagonists are the most effective drugs available for patients experiencing nausea and vomiting due to chemotherapy. They are effective when given only once or

twice a day, an additional advantage. Ondansetron (Zofran) is a prototype drug in this class.
- Dopamine antagonists include the phenothiazines (e.g., prochlorperazine [Compazine] and thiethylperazine [Torcan]), butyrophenones (haloperidol [Haldol] and droperidol [Inapsine]), and other drugs such as metoclopramide (Reglan). These drugs, while effective, can produce extrapyramidal symptoms, sedation, and hypotension.
- Antihistamines such as meclizine (Antivert), hydroxyzine (Vistaril, Atarax), and dimenhydrinate (Dramamine) are primarily used to treat nausea and vomiting arising from vestibular center stimuli (e.g., motion sickness).
- Two drugs classed as cannabinoids, related to marijuana, are approved to treat nausea and vomiting associated with chemotherapy. These drugs, dronabinol (Marinol) and nabilone (Cesamet), may produce unpleasant psychiatric effects such as dissociation and dysphoria, and are contraindicated for patients with psychiatric disorders. Tachycardia and hypotension are additional possible side effects.
- While corticosteroids are not approved as a class for treating nausea and vomiting, methylprednisolone (Solu-Medrol) and dexamethasone (Decadron) may be used in combination to treat vomiting associated with cancer treatment.
- Lorazepam (Ativan) is a benzodiazepine drug approved for use as an antiemetic. It produces a degree of sedation, but can suppress anticipatory vomiting (e.g., before chemotherapy). It also helps control extrapyramidal symptoms associated with the phenothiazine antiemetics.
- A new class of antiemetics, neurokinin receptor antagonists, primarily are used to prevent nausea and vomiting associated with chemotherapy. Aprepitant (Emend) is a prototype of this class.

Nursing responsibilities and patient education for antiemetic drugs are outlined in the accompanying Medication Administration box.

Complementary and Alternative Medicine

Mind–body interventions such as biofeedback, guided imagery, music therapy, and hypnosis may be effective for some patients with nausea. Biofeedback uses machinery to translate physiologic processes into audible or visible signals to teach the patient to exert conscious control over those processes. In guided imagery, the patient uses imagination to invoke specific images to modify physiologic responses. Music therapy employs creating or listening to music to affect physiologic and psychologic responses. In hypnosis, an altered mind state is induced to make the patient receptive to suggestions. A study by Suzanne Dibble and colleagues (2007) suggests that acupressure may help relieve chemotherapy-induced nausea and vomiting when combined with standard therapies. See the accompanying box.

Ginger, an aromatic root frequently used in cooking, may also be helpful in relieving nausea and vomiting, particularly when due to motion sickness (Fontaine, 2005; Spencer & Jacobs, 2003). In limited clinical trials, it has been shown to be safe for reducing nausea associated with pregnancy. It may help relieve nausea associated with cancer chemotherapy. Ginger can inhibit platelet aggregation, and may increase the risk of bleeding in patients taking antiplatelet or anticoagulant drugs (Lehne, 2007).

MOVING EVIDENCE INTO ACTION | Chemotherapy-Induced Nausea and Vomiting

Patients undergoing chemotherapy regimens for cancer treatment often experience treatment-related nausea and vomiting. While newer antiemetic drugs are increasingly effective in preventing and treating chemotherapy-induced nausea and vomiting (CINV), many patients still experience both acute and delayed CINV. A study by Suzanne Dibble and colleagues (2007) looked at the effectiveness of acupressure in relieving CINV in women undergoing treatment for breast cancer.

Acupressure is a noninvasive Chinese medicine technique used to restore energy (*Qi*) balance in the body. It is believed that acupressure on P6, a specific point on the wrist, restores energy balance, relieving nausea. Acupressure may be applied using the thumbs, fingers, hands, or passive devices such as wrist bands.

All women in the study received standard CINV therapy. The study group was taught to apply acupressure to P6; a placebo group applied acupressure to a point on the side of the hand (S13), and the control group received standard therapy without acupressure. Although no significant differences were found in the acute nausea experiences among the groups, acupressure on the P6 point was found to be useful in

reducing delayed nausea and vomiting and hastening recovery after chemotherapy.

IMPLICATIONS FOR NURSING

Several studies have found acupressure to be an effective adjunct for relieving CINV. Nurses working in oncology units or with patients undergoing chemotherapy can teach patients how to use this noninvasive technique to promote comfort. Furthermore, patients may be less reluctant to start and continue chemotherapy if they perceive the ability to help control at least some of its unpleasant adverse effects.

CRITICAL THINKING IN PATIENT CARE

1. What are the mechanisms by which chemotherapy produces nausea and vomiting? Why are some regimens associated with more CINV than others?
2. Why is *preventing* CINV from the onset of chemotherapy so important?
3. Do you think acupressure is likely to be effective in a patient who doesn't "believe in all that alternative medicine stuff?" Why or why not?
4. Develop a teaching plan for a patient who will be starting chemotherapy using a drug known to produce nausea and vomiting in most patients who receive it.

Nursing Care

Assessment of the patient is vital to help determine the cause of nausea and vomiting, and to rule out underlying systemic disease or acute conditions that require immediate care (e.g., bowel obstruction). When the cause is known or no other acute symptoms are present, nursing interventions can promote comfort and prevent complications.

Nausea

The nursing diagnosis of nausea is defined as a subjective, unpleasant, wavelike sensation in the throat, epigastric region, or abdomen that may lead to vomiting (Wilkinson & Ahern, 2009).

- Monitor subjective complaints of nausea. *Nausea is a subjective sensation best described by the patient.*
- Monitor vital signs, skin turgor and condition, and weight. Maintain accurate intake and output records. Monitor amount, color, and specific gravity of urine. *Nausea can cause aversion to food and fluids, leading to dehydration even when it is not accompanied by vomiting.*
- Administer antiemetic medication as ordered, prior to meals and before treatments or procedures known to stimulate nausea. *Preventing nausea is particularly important for patients receiving chemotherapy, to avoid the association between the treatment and nausea.*
- Instruct to deep breathe to voluntarily suppress the vomiting reflex. *Controlling vomiting helps prevent dehydration and other complications associated with prolonged or severe vomiting.*
- Instruct to consume small quantities of clear fluids and dry foods at separate times. *Separating the intake of dry foods and fluids helps reduce the nausea stimulus.*

Community-Based Care

Instruct the patient to restrict intake to small quantities of clear liquids (tea, apple juice, broth, Jell-O) and dry foods such as soda crackers to help reduce nausea and prevent vomiting. Teach to avoid food-preparation odors if they produce nausea. Advise to restrict fluid intake for 1 hour before and after meals. Stress the need to maintain fluid intake to prevent dehydration and the importance of seeking additional medical help if unable to take in fluids or keep food down. Provide information about electrolyte replacement solutions such as sports drinks and commercially available electrolyte replacement solutions.

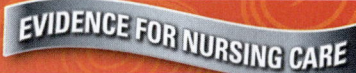

EVIDENCE FOR NURSING CARE | The Patient with Nausea and Vomiting

Selected resources that nurses may find helpful when planning evidence-based nursing care follow.

- Association of Comprehensive Cancer Centres (ACCC). (2006, Jan 12). *Editorial Board Palliative Care: Practice Guidelines. Nausea and vomiting.* Utrecht, The Netherlands. Retrieved from http://www.guideline.gov/summary/summary.aspx?doc_id=11793&nbr=006067&string=
- Abraham, J. (2008 December). Acupressure and acupuncture in preventing and managing postoperative nausea and vomiting in adults. *Journal of Perioperative Practice, 18*(12), 543–551.
- Dibble, S., Lucy, J., Cooper, B., Israel, J., Cohen, M., Nussey, B., et al. (2007). Acupressure for chemotherapy-induced nausea and vomiting: A randomized clinical trial. *Oncology Nursing Forum, 34*(4), 813–820.

SEROTONIN RECEPTOR ANTAGONISTS
Dolasetron (Anzemet)
Granisetron (Kytril)
Ondansetron (Zofran)
Palonosetron (Aloxi)

The serotonin receptor antagonists suppress nausea and vomiting by blocking the effect of serotonin on vagal afferent nerves that stimulate the vomiting center. Their primary uses are to prevent vomiting associated with chemotherapy, radiation therapy, and surgery.

Nursing Responsibilities
■ Administer 30 to 60 minutes prior to chemotherapy or surgery as directed.
■ May be given orally or intravenously (push or infusion; follow directions specific to the drug used).
■ Monitor liver function and clotting studies; report abnormal levels to the physician.

Health Education for the Patient and Family
■ Take this drug exactly as directed.
■ This drug may be taken without regard to food intake.
■ Headache is a common side effect of these drugs, use acetaminophen or another mild analgesic as directed by your physician.

DOPAMINE ANTAGONISTS
Chlorpromazine (Thorazine)
Perphenazine (Trilafon)
Prochlorperazine (Compazine)
Promethazine (Phenergan)
Thiethylperazine (Torcan)
Haloperidol (Haldol)
Droperidol (Inapsine)
Metoclopramide (Reglan)

These drugs act by blocking dopamine receptors in the chemoreceptor trigger zone (CTZ). Their primary uses are to suppress nausea and vomiting associated with surgery, cancer chemotherapy, and toxins. The major adverse effects associated with these drugs are sedation, hypotension, and extrapyramidal reactions. Older adults are more sensitive to the effects of these drugs; a lower dose often is indicated.

Nursing Responsibilities
■ Administer orally or parenterally as ordered before surgery or before meals and procedures known to produce nausea and vomiting.
■ These drugs may interact with a number of other medications, often increasing their sedative and hypotensive effects.
■ Administer with caution to older adults, closely monitoring for adverse effects such as confusion, agitation, changes in vital signs.
■ Monitor for evidence of extrapyramidal symptoms, including tremor, restlessness, hyperactivity, anxiety, impaired coordination; notify physician if symptoms develop.

Health Education for the Patient and Family
■ Use the drug as ordered; do not increase your dose without consulting your primary care provider.
■ These drugs may cause drowsiness. Avoid using other central nervous system (CNS) depressants such as alcohol while taking these drugs.
■ Change positions from lying to sitting and sitting to standing slowly because these drugs can cause lightheadedness or dizziness.

■ Promptly report changes in coordination, tremors, difficulty speaking or swallowing, or weakness to your physician.

SUBSTANCE P/NEUROKININ RECEPTOR ANTAGONIST
Aprepitant (Emend)

Aprepitant is a new drug that can prevent both acute and delayed chemotherapy-induced nausea and vomiting when given in combination with other antiemetic drugs. It is well-absorbed when given orally, and has a prolonged duration of action.

Nursing Responsibilities
■ Administer daily for 3 days, giving the first dose 1 hour before chemotherapy.
■ Can be given with food or on an empty stomach.
■ Monitor for toxic and desired effects of other drugs, including chemotherapy drugs, corticosteroids, and warfarin (Coumadin), as aprepitant can affect their metabolism and blood levels.

Health Education for the Patient and Family
■ Use barrier contraception while taking this drug as oral contraceptives will be less effective.
■ Promptly contact your physician if you develop skin rash, difficulty breathing, changes in heart beat or blood pressure, dizziness or confusion, leg or abdominal pain, or rectal bleeding.
■ Contact your physician before taking any new prescription, over-the-counter, or herbal preparations.

ANTIHISTAMINES
Buclizine (Bucladin-S)
Cyclizine (Marezine)
Dimenhydrinate (Dramamine)
Diphenhydramine (Benadryl)
Hydroxyzine (Vistaril, Atarax)
Meclizine (Antivert)

Antihistamines are primarily used to treat nausea and vomiting associated with motion sickness. They act by blocking histamine and acetylcholine (muscarinic) receptors in the neural pathway from the inner ear to the vomiting center in the brainstem.

Nursing Responsibilities
■ Do not administer these drugs to patients for whom anticholinergic drugs are contraindicated: people with narrow-angle glaucoma, urinary retention, bowel obstruction.
■ May be administered orally, parenterally, or rectally, depending on the preparation and the patient's ability to tolerate oral preparations.
■ Use with caution in patients who are taking other CNS depressants or antihistamine preparations, tricyclic antidepressants, or monoamine oxidase inhibitors.

Health Education for the Patient and Family
■ These drugs frequently cause drowsiness. Use caution when operating machinery or performing tasks requiring mental alertness.
■ Avoid using alcohol or other substances that cause drowsiness or sedation while taking these drugs.
■ The medication may cause dry mouth. Sips of water, ice chips, hard candies, and sugarless gum can be used for comfort.
■ Use sunscreen and protective clothing to protect from sunburn while using these drugs.

(continued)

CANNABINOIDS

Dronabinol (Marinol)

Nabilone (Cesamet)

Drugs in this class, which contain the same active ingredient as marijuana, are reserved for use to relieve nausea and vomiting associated with cancer chemotherapy in patients who have not responded to treatment with other antiemetics. Their action is thought to result from inhibition of the vomiting center in the medulla.

Nursing Responsibilities
- Use with caution in older adults and people with a history of cardiovascular disease or substance abuse. These drugs are contraindicated for patients with a history of psychiatric disorders.

- Monitor for adverse effects such as dizziness, tachycardia, hypotension, impaired thinking and judgment, incoordination, irritability, depersonalization, distorted vision, and hallucinations.

Health Education for the Patient and Family
- Take the drug 1 to 3 hours before chemotherapy.
- Change positions slowly after taking this drug to prevent dizziness.
- You may experience distorted thinking, visual disturbances, confusion, and other mental symptoms while taking this drug.
- Keep this and all drugs out of the reach of children. Do not share this drug with anyone else.

Disorders of the Mouth

Inflammations, infections, and neoplastic lesions of the mouth affect food ingestion and nutrition. Oral lesions may have a variety of causes, including infection, trauma, irritants such as alcohol, and hypersensitivity. Appropriate treatment of the disorder, any underlying factors, and associated symptoms is essential.

The Patient with Stomatitis

Stomatitis, inflammation and ulcers of the oral mucosa, is a common disorder of the mouth. Viral infection is the most common cause. Other causes include bacterial or fungal infections, mechanical trauma (e.g., cheek biting), irritants (e.g., tobacco or ill-fitting dentures), nutritional deficiencies, and chemotherapeutic agents. Stomatitis often affects people who are immunocompromised (e.g., patients with HIV disease or who have cancer, and frail older adults). Box 23–1 lists common risk factors for stomatitis.

FAST FACTS
- Herpes simplex ("cold sore") is the most frequent viral cause of stomatitis; others include primary varicella zoster (chickenpox), Epstein-Barr virus, influenza, cytomegalovirus, and HIV.
- Overgrowth of *Candida albicans* is the most frequent fungal cause of stomatitis, usually following antibiotic or corticosteroid therapy.
- About 40% of people undergoing chemotherapy to treat cancer experience *oral mucositis*, a type of stomatitis; 75% of those undergoing chemotherapy in preparation for bone marrow or stem cell transplant develop oral mucositis.
- Most patients undergoing radiation therapy of the head and neck develop oral mucositis.

Pathophysiology and Manifestations

The oral mucosa, which lines the oral cavity, is a relatively thin, fragile layer of stratified squamous epithelial cells that constantly is being replaced. The blood supply to the oral mucosa is rich. As epithelial cells slough, stem cells in the submucosa develop into epithelial cells to replace those that are lost.

Frequent exposure to the environment, a rich blood supply, and the oral mucosa's delicate nature increase the risk of infection or inflammation, reaction to toxins, and trauma. Stomatitis results from persistent damage to oral mucosal cells. Damage is initially superficial, progressing to ulceration and involvement of the entire epithelium. Finally, healing begins within 2 to 4 weeks.

Oral mucositis progresses through identifiable stages. Radiotherapy and chemotherapy damage the DNA of epithelial cells, resulting in necrosis and death of some cells. This stimulates the release of inflammatory mediators that further damage tissues, causing additional epithelial cells to die. As a result, the oral mucosa thins. Tumor necrosis factor alpha (TNF-α) is released, which activates additional inflammatory cytokines. Tissues below the mucosa are damaged as well. In the ulcerative stage of oral mucositis, irregular ulcers that extend from the epithelium into the submucosa develop. As nerve endings are exposed, this stage is accompanied by significant pain. During the final healing stage, cells in the epithelium proliferate, and the normal thickness of the oral mucosa is restored.

The clinical manifestations of stomatitis vary according to its cause. Table 23–1 outlines common causes of stomatitis with their manifestations and treatment. Chemotherapy or chemical irritation may result in initial generalized redness and swelling, followed by development of deep, irregular ulcerations. Ulcers may be covered with pseudomembranes. Oral pain associated with stomatitis can interfere with the ability to eat, drink, and swallow normally.

Potential complications of stomatitis include malnutrition, fluid and electrolyte imbalance, sepsis, and bacterial endocarditis.

BOX 23–1 Risk Factors for Stomatitis
- Age > 65 years
- Impaired immune status (HIV disease, cancer, diabetes)
- Chronic renal failure or heart failure
- Chemotherapy, radiation therapy, stem cell transplant
- Oxygen therapy, mouth breathing
- Medications (antibiotics, phenytoin, anticholinergics, corticosteroids)
- Poor oral hygiene, ill-fitting dentures
- Tobacco or alcohol use

TABLE 23–1 Manifestations and Treatment of Common Stomatitis Conditions

TYPE	CAUSE	MANIFESTATIONS	TREATMENT
Cold sore, fever blister	Herpes simplex virus	■ Initial burning at site ■ Clustered vesicular lesions on lip or oral mucosa	■ Self-limiting ■ Acyclovir, famciclovir, valacyclovir to shorten course
Aphthous ulcer (canker sore, ulcerative stomatitis)	Unknown; may be type of herpes virus	■ Well-circumscribed, shallow erosions with white or yellow center encircled by red ring ■ Less than 1 cm in diameter ■ Painful	■ Topical steroid ointment ■ Amlexanox oral paste (Aphthasol) ■ Oral prednisone
Candidiasis (thrush)	*Candida albicans*	■ Creamy white, curdlike patches ■ Red, erythematous mucosa	■ Fluconazole (Diflucan) ■ Ketoconazole (Nizoral) ■ Clotrimazole troches ■ Nystatin vaginal troches (dissolved orally) or mouth rinse
Necrotizing ulcerative gingivitis (trench mouth, Vincent's infection)	Infection with spirochetes and bacilli or systemic infection	■ Acute gingival inflammation and necrosis ■ Bleeding, halitosis ■ Fever ■ Cervical lymphadenopathy	■ Correct any underlying disorders ■ Warm, half-strength peroxide mouthwashes ■ Oral penicillin
Oral mucositis	Damage to epithelial cells and stem cells in the submucosa caused by chemotherapy or radiation therapy	■ Erythema and inflammation of oral mucosa ■ Painful, irregularly shaped ulcerations, initially superficial, progressing to deep ulcers that may be confluent (overlapping with one another) ■ Pseudomembranes covering ulcers ■ Tissue necrosis with spontaneous bleeding, potential sepsis	■ Regular oral hygiene with brushing and flossing ■ Saline or sodium bicarbonate solution mouth rinses after and between meals ■ Gelclair mouth rinse before meals for analgesia ■ Palifermin, an epithelial cell growth factor ■ Low-level laser therapy

Interdisciplinary Care

Stomatitis is diagnosed by direct physical examination and, if indicated, cultures, smears, and evaluation for systemic illness. Treatment addresses both the underlying cause and any coexisting illnesses. An undiagnosed oral lesion present for more than 1 week and that does not respond to therapy must be evaluated for malignancy.

Direct smears and cultures of lesions may be obtained to identify causative organisms. If systemic illness is suspected, a variety of diagnostic tests may be ordered to identify the underlying cause.

General treatment measures include providing meticulous oral hygiene, with brushing using a soft brush and flossing (as tolerated). A solution of saline, sodium bicarbonate, or a combination of saline/bicarbonate promotes comfort and healing when used after and between meals.

Medications

Using a topical anesthetic, such as a mouthwash of 2% viscous lidocaine diluted with water, diphenhydramine (Benadryl) solution, or benzocaine spray or gel can promote comfort and the ability to consume oral food and fluids.

> **SAFETY ALERT**
> Instruct patients to expectorate lidocaine solution, not swallow it, to avoid impairment of swallowing.

Amlexanox (Aphthasol, OraDisc A) or Orabase, a protective paste, may be applied to oral ulcers to promote comfort.

Amlexanox speeds healing of aphthous ulcers as well. Triamcinolone acetonide may be mixed in Orabase to reduce inflammation and promote healing. Other coating agents include Amphojel or Kaopectate. Sodium bicarbonate mouthwashes may provide relief and promote cleansing, whereas alcohol-based mouthwashes may cause pain and burning and should be avoided. Agents that form a film over exposed nerve endings and deep ulcerations (e.g., Zilactin, Gelclair) may be used in patients with oral mucositis.

Fungal infections often are treated with a nystatin oral suspension; patients are instructed to "swish and swallow" the solution. Clotrimazole lozenges also treat oral fungal infections. If the infection does not resolve, oral antifungal medications such as fluconazole or ketoconazole may be used. Antifungals are usually continued for at least 3 days after symptoms disappear.

Herpetic lesions may be treated with topical or oral acyclovir (Zovirax), famciclovir (Famvir), or valacyclovir (Valtrex). Acyclovir ointment provides comfort and lubrication while limiting the spread of the virus. Oral preparations reduce the severity of symptoms and the duration of the lesions.

Bacterial infections are treated with antibiotics based on cultures and smears. Oral penicillin is the treatment of choice if the patient is not allergic and the cultured bacteria are sensitive. Nursing implications for selected drugs used to treat stomatitis are outlined on page 618.

An epithelial cell growth-stimulating factor, palifermin (Kepivance), reduces the incidence and duration of oral mucositis in patients undergoing high-dose chemotherapy in preparation for bone marrow or stem cell transplant.

Nursing Care

Health Promotion

Nurses can help prevent stomatitis by identifying patients at risk and suggesting measures to reduce the likelihood that stomatitis will develop. Teach and encourage all patients to regularly perform mouth care, including teeth brushing and flossing. Provide frequent mouth care with nondrying agents for patients who are unable to provide self-care. Encourage patients with ill-fitting dentures or other dental prostheses (such as partial plates) to see a qualified dentist or denturist. Suggest patients taking an extended course of antibiotic therapy or who have impaired immune function consume 8 oz of yogurt containing live bacterial cultures or 8 oz of buttermilk daily unless contraindicated. Discuss dietary modifications, such as limiting consumption of highly spiced or acidic foods and avoiding very hot beverages. Patients undergoing chemotherapy or radiation therapy should avoid use of alcohol and tobacco because these substances further damage oral mucosa, increasing the risk for oral mucositis.

Assessment

Oral assessment is important not only for patients who have been diagnosed with stomatitis, but also for those with risk factors, manifestations, or evidence of possible complications (e.g., recent weight loss).

- *Health history:* Complaints of mouth pain, altered taste, lack of appetite, malaise; presence of dentures, regularity of dental care; current health status including chronic diseases; current medications; use of alcohol or tobacco.
- *Physical examination:* Inspect lips, gums, teeth, interior cheeks, tongue and base of tongue, soft and hard palate; tonsils, and oral pharynx. Observe and assess general health status including temperature, weight.
- *Diagnostic tests:* WBC, sedimentation rate, serum albumin.

Nursing Diagnoses and Interventions

Nursing care for the patient with stomatitis or oral mucositis focuses not only on the oral inflammation, but also on any underlying systemic diseases and the effects of the condition on the patient's comfort and nutrition.

Impaired Oral Mucous Membrane

Stomatitis and oral mucositis disrupt the integrity of the oral mucous membrane. Regardless of cause, the pain and symptoms must be relieved to promote comfort as well as food and fluid intake.

- Assess and document oral mucous membranes and the character of any lesions every 4 to 8 hours. *Baseline and ongoing assessment data provide the basis for evaluation.*
- Assist with thorough mouth care after meals, at bedtime, and every 2 to 4 hours while awake. If unable to tolerate a toothbrush, offer sponge or gauze toothettes. Avoid using alcohol-based mouthwashes or lemon-glycerin swabs. Provide saline or sodium bicarbonate rinse or a combined saline/sodium bicarbonate rinse after every meal and between meals. *Mouth care promotes hygiene, comfort, and healing. Alcohol-based mouthwashes and lemon-glycerin swabs may dry and irritate mucous membranes, causing pain and further tissue*

MEDICATION ADMINISTRATION   **Drugs Used to Treat Stomatitis**

TOPICAL ORAL ANESTHETICS
Orajel

Viscous lidocaine

Anbesol

Triamcinolone acetonide

These drugs reduce the pain associated with mucous membrane lesions or stomatitis. They provide temporary relief of pain. Any oral lesion that persists longer than 1 week should be evaluated by an oral surgeon.

Nursing Responsibilities
- Instruct the patient to seek medical attention for any oral lesion that does not heal within 1 week.
- Monitor for local hypersensitivity reactions, and discontinue use if they occur.

Health Education for the Patient and Family
- Apply every 1 to 2 hours as needed.
- Perform oral hygiene after meals and at bedtime.

TOPICAL ANTIFUNGAL AGENTS
Clotrimazole

Nystatin

These products help in the topical treatment of candidiasis. Their effects are primarily local rather than systemic.

Nursing Responsibilities
- Instruct the patient to dissolve lozenges in the mouth.

- Instruct the patient to rinse mouth with oral suspension for at least 2 minutes and expectorate or swallow as directed.
- These drugs are contraindicated in pregnancy.

Health Education for the Patient and Family
- Take medication as prescribed.
- Do not eat or drink 30 minutes after medication.
- Contact physician if symptoms worsen.
- Perform good oral hygiene after meals and at bedtime; remove dentures at bedtime.

ANTIVIRAL AGENTS
Acyclovir (Zovirax)

Famciclovir (Famvir)

Valacyclovir (Valtrex)

Acyclovir, famciclovir, and valacyclovir are useful in the treatment of oral herpes simplex virus. They help reduce the severity and frequency of infections. These antiviral agents interfere with the DNA synthesis of herpes simplex virus.

Nursing Responsibilities
- Start therapy as soon as herpetic lesions are noted.
- Administer with food or on an empty stomach.

Health Education for the Patient and Family
- The virus remains latent and can recur during stressful events, fever, trauma, sunlight exposure, and treatment with immunosuppressive drugs.
- Take the medication as ordered, and contact the physician if symptoms worsen.

damage, whereas saline or bicarbonate rinses promote comfort and healing *(Cawley & Benson, 2005).*

- Assess knowledge and teach about condition, mouth care, and treatments. Instruct to avoid alcohol, tobacco, and spicy or irritating foods. *Knowledge promotes patient participation in the plan of care and compliance. Alcohol, tobacco, and hot, spicy, or rough foods may injure the inflamed mucous membranes.*

Imbalanced Nutrition: Less than Body Requirements

Oral lesions and pain may limit oral intake, which may in turn lead to nutritional deficits. Anorexia and general malaise may also contribute to decreased intake.

- Assess food intake as well as the patient's ability to chew and swallow. Weigh daily. Provide appropriate assistive devices such as straws or feeding syringes. *Adequate nutrition is essential for healing. Daily weights allow monitoring of the adequacy of food intake. Assistive devices may allow food intake while avoiding irritation of ulcerations or lesions.*
- Encourage a high-calorie, high-protein diet considerate of food preferences. Offer soft, lukewarm, or cool foods or liquids such as eggnogs, milk shakes, nutritional supplements, popsicles, and puddings frequently in small amounts. Obtain nutritional consultation. *Oral intake may be limited, and enriched foods and liquids enhance nutrition. A nutritional consultation can help ensure an adequate diet and assist in meeting nutritional needs.*
- Provide analgesics for pain relief as needed. *Significant pain associated with stomatitis or oral mucositis can interfere with effective mouth care and food and fluid intake. Pain management is a vital part of nursing care.*

Using NANDA, NIC, and NOC

Linkages between a selected NANDA nursing diagnosis, NIC, and NOC for the patient with stomatitis are shown in the chart that follows.

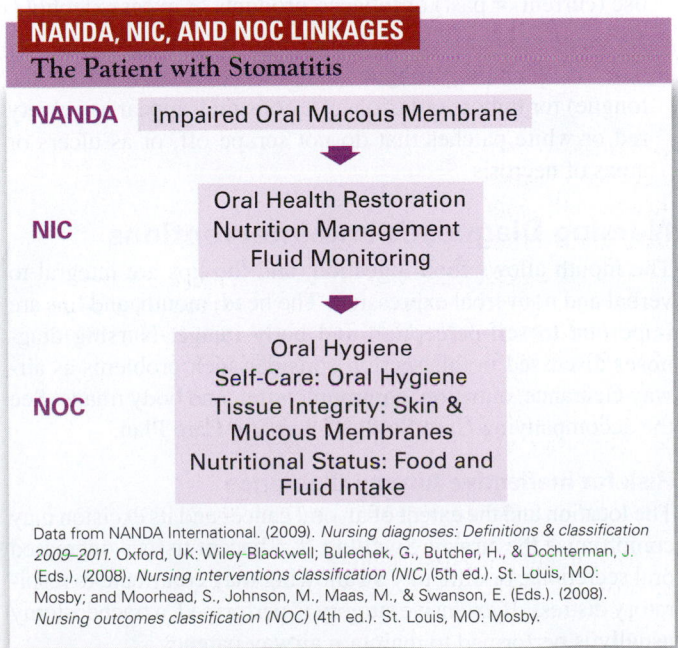

NANDA, NIC, AND NOC LINKAGES
The Patient with Stomatitis

NANDA Impaired Oral Mucous Membrane

NIC
Oral Health Restoration
Nutrition Management
Fluid Monitoring

NOC
Oral Hygiene
Self-Care: Oral Hygiene
Tissue Integrity: Skin & Mucous Membranes
Nutritional Status: Food and Fluid Intake

Data from NANDA International. (2009). *Nursing diagnoses: Definitions & classification 2009–2011.* Oxford, UK: Wiley-Blackwell; Bulechek, G., Butcher, H., & Dochterman, J. (Eds.). (2008). *Nursing interventions classification (NIC)* (5th ed.). St. Louis, MO: Mosby; and Moorhead, S., Johnson, M., Maas, M., & Swanson, E. (Eds.). (2008). *Nursing outcomes classification (NOC)* (4th ed.). St. Louis, MO: Mosby.

Community-Based Care

Patients with mild stomatitis generally provide self-care. While patients with cancer-treatment-related oral mucositis may require more aggressive therapy, the patient and caregivers often are able to manage the regimen in home- or community-based settings. Include the following topics in teaching for home care:

- Managing any underlying health conditions and ongoing treatments such as chemotherapy
- The recommended diet and oral hygiene regime, including foods and substances (e.g., alcohol, tobacco products) to avoid
- Nutritional supplements to help meet nutritional requirements
- Prescribed medication, its route, side effects, frequency of administration, and signs and symptoms to report
- The importance of completing the full course of antibiotic, antiviral, or antifungal treatment
- Manifestations to report and the importance of follow-up care

The Patient with Oral Cancer

Oral cancer, malignancy of the oral mucosa, may develop on the lips, tongue, floor of the mouth, or other oral tissues. It is uncommon, accounting for only 3% of all new cancers diagnosed in men and 2% in women during 2008. It has, however, a high rate of morbidity and mortality. It is seen more often in people over age 40. Although a lesion can develop in any area of the mouth, the most common sites are the lower lip, tongue, and floor of the mouth. The stage of an oral cancer determines the prognosis, treatment, and degree of disability. The primary risk factors for oral cancer are smoking, drinking alcohol, and chewing tobacco. Marijuana use, occupational exposures to chemicals, and viruses such as human papilloma virus (HPV) also may contribute to the risk for oral cancer.

Pathophysiology and Manifestations

More than 90% of oral and oropharyngeal tumors are a squamous cell carcinoma. Most early cancers present as inflamed areas with irregular, ill-defined borders. These lesions typically are not painful. More advanced cancers appear as deep ulcers that are fixed to deeper tissues. Early lesions involve the mucosa or submucosa, whereas more advanced tumors may invade and destroy underlying tissues, including muscles and bones of the face. Tumors frequently metastasize to regional lymph nodes. Other cancerous lesions, including lymphoma, malignant melanoma, and Kaposi's sarcoma, may

MANIFESTATIONS of Oral Cancer

- White patches (leukoplakia)
- Red patches (erythroplakia)
- Ulcers
- Masses
- Pigmented areas (brownish or black)
- Fissures
- Asymmetry of the head, face, jaws, or neck

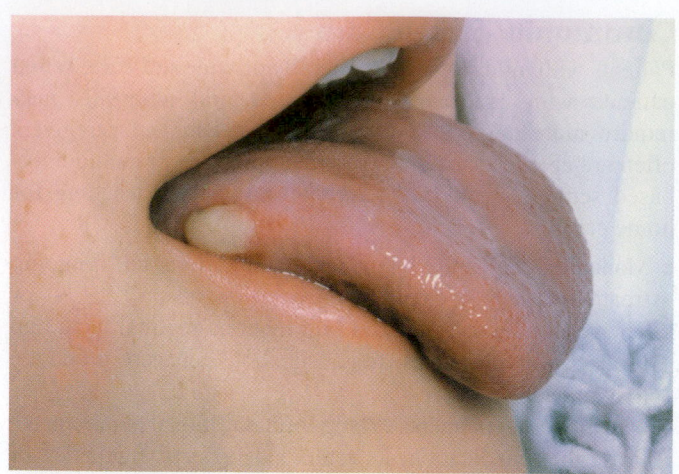

Figure 23–1 ■ Oral cancer.
Source: Biophoto Associates/Photo Researchers, Inc.

BOX 23–2 Oral Cancer Staging

Stage 0	Carcinoma *in situ*
Stage I	Tumor ≤ 2 cm; no regional node involvement
Stage II	Tumor > 2 cm to ≤ 4 cm; no regional node involvement
Stage III	Tumor ≤ 2 cm to > 4 cm; one involved lymph node
Stage IVA & B	Tumor may invade adjacent structures; one or more nodes involved
Stage IVC	Distant metastasis present

develop in the mouth, although less frequently than squamous cell carcinoma.

The earliest symptom of oral cancer is a painless oral ulceration or lesion (Figure 23–1 ■). Later symptoms vary and may include difficulty speaking, swallowing, or chewing; swollen lymph nodes; and blood-tinged sputum. See the accompanying box for other manifestations of oral cancer. Any oral lesion that does not heal or respond to treatment within 1 to 2 weeks should be evaluated for malignancy.

Interdisciplinary Care

The first component of treatment is eliminating any causative factors such as chewing tobacco, smoking, or drinking alcohol. Tumor staging then determines therapy. The TNM (tumor, nodes, metastasis) classification is used to stage oral cancer. See Box 23–2. A biopsy of the oral lesion allows direct visualization of cells to determine the presence or absence of cancerous cells. Staging may require additional diagnostic studies such as computed tomography (CT) scans or magnetic resonance imaging (MRI).

Early cancers (stages I and II) are highly curable using surgery or radiation therapy. The treatment choice is based on the expected functional and cosmetic results of treatment. More advanced tumors (stages III and IV) generally require a treatment combination of surgery, radiation, and possibly chemotherapy. ∞ See Chapter 14 for more information about radiation and chemotherapy to treat cancer.

Following biopsy and staging of the tumor, surgery is often indicated, although an advanced or extensive tumor may be considered unresectable. If the tumor involves surrounding tissues, the cosmetic effects of surgery are important considerations. The goal of surgery is removal of the lesion and potentially cancerous surrounding tissue or lymph nodes. Advanced carcinomas may require extensive excision or a *radical neck dissection*, a potentially disfiguring procedure in which the lymph nodes and muscles of the neck are removed. A tracheostomy is performed at the time of surgery. The tracheostomy may be temporary, but often is permanent. ∞ See Chapter 35 for more information about caring for a patient following radical neck dissection and a tracheostomy.

Nursing Care

Health Promotion

Reducing or eliminating tobacco use (smoking and smokeless tobacco) and excess alcohol consumption can significantly reduce the incidence of oral cancer. Teach children and adolescents about the dangers of using tobacco and alcohol. Emphasize the relationship between smokeless tobacco and oral cancer. Discuss strategies to deal with peer pressure to use tobacco and alcohol.

To promote early identification of and intervention for oral cancer, teach patients about the risk factors for and manifestations of the disease. This is a particularly important nursing strategy in older men who have the highest incidence, and in populations in whom the disease often is advanced when detected (people of lower socioeconomic status, people who rarely see a dentist, and African American men).

Assessment

Early precancerous oral lesions are very treatable. Unfortunately, these lesions usually are painless, so diagnosis and treatment often is delayed. Assess the oral cavity of all patients, particularly those with risk factors for oral cancer.

- *Health history:* Complaints of oral lesions that fail to heal; use (current or past) of tobacco products or excess alcohol.
- *Physical examination:* Inspect and palpate lips and oral mucosa (including tongue and floor of mouth under the tongue) for tumors or lesions. Lesions may appear as velvety red or white patches that do not scrape off, or as ulcers or areas of necrosis.

Nursing Diagnoses and Interventions

The mouth allows food ingestion, and the lips are integral to verbal and nonverbal expression. The head, mouth, and lips are important to self-perception and body image. Nursing diagnoses discussed in this section consider such problems as airway clearance, nutrition, communication, and body image. See the accompanying Case Study & Nursing Care Plan.

Risk for Ineffective Airway Clearance

The location and the extent of an oral cancer and its excision may compromise the airway. Swelling of adjacent tissues, increased oral secretions, or difficulty swallowing may contribute to respiratory distress. If extensive surgery is performed, a tracheostomy usually is performed to maintain airway patency.

CASE STUDY & NURSING CARE PLAN   A Patient with Oral Cancer

Juan Chavez, a married 44-year-old farmer, has two adult children. He and his wife raise and sell fruits and vegetables. Two months ago, Mr. Chavez developed a sore on his tongue that would not heal. Mr. Chavez tells his admission nurse, Sara Bucklin, "The doctor says he will have to remove part of my tongue," and anxiously asks, "Will I ever look the same? How will I be able to talk?"

ASSESSMENT

Mr. Chavez's admission history reveals that he has been healthy, but has smoked two packs of cigarettes a day for more than 20 years, and usually drinks two to four beers per day. He admits to being anxious and fearful of surgery and its outcomes. He says he quit smoking and drinking 2 weeks ago. The biopsy report is positive for squamous cell carcinoma of the tongue. Mr. Chavez has no enlarged cervical nodes and says he has no bloody sputum or saliva, difficulty swallowing, chewing, or talking. His weight is in the normal range for his height. A wide excision of the oral lesion is planned.

DIAGNOSES

- *Risk for Ineffective Airway Clearance* related to oral surgery
- *Risk for Imbalanced Nutrition: Less than Body Requirements* related to oral surgery
- *Impaired Verbal Communication* related to excision of a portion of the tongue
- *Disturbed Body Image* related to surgical excision of the tongue

EXPECTED OUTCOMES

- Maintain a patent airway and remain free of respiratory distress.
- Maintain a stable weight and level of hydration.
- Effectively communicate with staff and family using a magic slate and flash cards.
- Communicate an increased ability to accept changes in body image.

PLANNING AND IMPLEMENTATION

- Assess airway patency and respiratory status every hour until stable.

- Maintain semi-Fowler's position, supporting arms. Encourage to turn, cough, and deep breathe every 2 to 4 hours.
- Teach the importance of activity, turning, coughing, and deep breathing.
- Monitor daily weights.
- Consult with dietitian to assess calorie needs and plan appropriate enteral feeding. Assess response to enteral feedings.
- Demonstrate and allow to practice using magic slate and flash cards prior to surgery.
- Allow adequate time for communication efforts.
- Keep emergency call system in reach at all times and answer light promptly. Alert all staff of inability to respond verbally.
- Encourage expression of feelings regarding perceived and actual changes.
- Provide emotional support and encourage self-care and participation in decision making.

EVALUATION

At the time of discharge, Mr. Chavez has maintained his weight and has started on oral liquids, including supplements and enriched liquids. His airway has remained clear, and he is effectively coughing and deep breathing. He has used the magic slate to communicate throughout his hospital stay. He is regaining use of his tongue, and can speak a few words. Although initially distressed, he is communicating an increased ability to cope with loss of part of his tongue. He and his wife say they understand his discharge instructions, including diet, activity, follow-up care, and signs and symptoms to report.

CRITICAL THINKING IN THE NURSING PROCESS

1. What measures can you, as a nurse, implement to reduce the incidence of oral cancer?
2. Plan a health education program for young athletes who chew tobacco.
3. Mr. Chavez's wife calls you 2 weeks after discharge. She tells you that he refuses to try to talk and is relying on his magic slate to communicate. How will you respond?

See Evaluating Your Response in Appendix C.

PRACTICE ALERT

In the initial postoperative period, assess airway patency and respiratory status at least hourly. A patent airway is vital to maintain respirations and oxygenation of tissues. Frequent assessment allows early identification of possible airway compromise.

- Unless contraindicated, place in Fowler's position, supporting arms. Assist the patient to turn, cough, and deep breathe at least every 2 to 4 hours. *Fowler's position promotes lung expansion. Turning, coughing, and deep breathing help maintain a patent airway by preventing pooling of secretions.*
- Maintain adequate hydration (2000 to 3000 mL per day unless contraindicated) and humidity of inspired air. *Adequate hydration helps thin and loosen secretions.*

Imbalanced Nutrition: Less than Body Requirements

Surgery affects oral food and fluid intake. Enteral feedings or parenteral nutrition may be required. A gastrostomy tube usually is inserted during surgery to maintain nutrition. If an oral diet is permitted, anorexia or pain may affect intake.

- Weigh daily. Assess oral intake for adequacy of protein, calories, and nutrients. *Daily weights and nutritional assessments provide information about the adequacy of diet.*
- Offer soft, bland foods with supplements as indicated. Provide small, frequent feedings, making mealtimes pleasant. *Soft, bland foods may be better tolerated following oral surgery. Large meals may be overwhelming; small, frequent meals promote food and nutrient intake.*
- Provide enteral feedings per gastrostomy tube as ordered. Elevate the head of the bed 30 to 40 degrees. *Enteral feedings maintain nutritional status in the patient who is unable to consume foods orally. Elevating the head of the bed reduces the risk of regurgitation and aspiration of gastric contents.*
- Assess for gastric residual volume per facility protocol for the type of feeding (intermittent or continuous). Notify the physician of volumes greater than 200 mL or 50% of previous feeding if feeding is intermittent. *Excess residual volume may increase the risk for aspiration.*
- Consider a nutritional consultation to assess diet and plan appropriate supplements. *A registered dietitian can calculate energy requirements and develop an individualized diet plan to meet nutritional requirements.*

Impaired Verbal Communication

Oral surgery can interfere with communication. Effective communication is vital to postoperative recovery and prevention of complications.

- Before surgery, establish and practice a communication plan such as using a magic slate or flash cards. *Practicing communication techniques reduces fear and anxiety while promoting communication.*
- Provide ample time for communication efforts and do not answer for the patient. Be alert for nonverbal communications. Use yes/no questions and simple phrases. *Providing adequate time allows the patient opportunity to express ideas and thoughts. Nonverbal communication provides cues regarding comfort or other needs. Simple yes/no questions are easily answered nonverbally.*
- If indicated, refer to or consult with a speech therapist. *A speech therapist can help promote or restore effective communication.*

> **PRACTICE ALERT**
> Provide an emergency call system and respond promptly. Make all staff aware that the patient cannot respond over an intercom system by posting an alert on the intercom. Nonverbal patients rely on an emergency call system to summon help. Answering promptly reduces fear and anxiety and maintains safety.

Disturbed Body Image

Radical surgery of the head or neck seriously affects body image. An altered speech pattern and any disfigurement affect the ability to feel attractive or effective in work or social roles.

Patients may defer lifesaving surgery to postpone disfiguring interventions or therapies.

- Assess coping style, self-perception, and responses to altered appearance or function. *This information can be used to identify appropriate interventions and care.*
- Encourage verbalization of feelings regarding perceived and actual changes. *Nonjudgmental acceptance of feelings and fears helps establish trust.*
- Provide emotional support, encourage self-care, and provide decision-making opportunities. *Self-care promotes self-acceptance and independence. Giving choices empowers the patient to participate in care.*

Community-Based Care

Discharge planning for the patient with oral cancer depends on the type of treatment planned and surgery performed. Depending on the patient's age, condition, and availability of support systems, referral to a rehabilitation center and community healthcare agencies may be an essential component of care. Visits from home care nurses can assist in meeting healthcare needs.

Discuss the following topics with the patient and family members or care providers:

- Diagnosis and prescribed care
- Monitoring for new lesions or recurrences
- Diet, nutrition, and activity
- Pain management
- Airway management, care of incision, and signs and symptoms to report

Disorders of the Esophagus

The esophagus plays an essential role in the ingestion of food and liquids. Disorders of the esophagus can be inflammatory, mechanical, or cancerous. Because of its location and neighboring organs, the symptoms of esophageal disorders may mimic those of a variety of other illnesses.

The Patient with Gastroesophageal Reflux Disease

Gastroesophageal reflux is the backward flowing of gastric contents into the esophagus. When this occurs, the patient experiences heartburn. Many people with gastroesophageal reflux have few symptoms, while others develop inflammatory esophagitis as a result of exposure to gastric juices. *Gastroesophageal reflux disease (GERD)* is a common gastrointestinal disorder.

> **FAST FACTS**
> - GERD affects 15% to 20% of adults.
> - Up to 7% of people experience daily symptoms such as heartburn, regurgitation, and indigestion, and as many as 15% to 20% have symptoms weekly (Fauci et al., 2008; McPhee et al., 2008).

(side margin) Gastrointestinal Reflux Disease Video

Pathophysiology

Normally, the lower esophageal sphincter remains closed except during swallowing. Reflux (backflow) of gastric contents into the esophagus is prevented by pressure differences between the stomach and the lower esophagus. The diaphragm, the lower esophageal sphincter, and the location of the gastroesophageal junction below the diaphragm help maintain this pressure difference (Figure 23–2 ■).

Gastroesophageal reflux may result from transient relaxation of the lower esophageal sphincter, an incompetent lower esophageal sphincter, and/or increased pressure within the stomach. Factors contributing to gastroesophageal reflux include increased gastric volume (e.g., after meals), positioning that allows gastric contents to remain close to the gastroesophageal junction (e.g., bending over, lying down), and increased gastric pressure (e.g., obesity or wearing tight clothing). A hiatal hernia may contribute to GERD.

Gastric juices contain acid, pepsin, and bile, which are corrosive substances. Esophageal peristalsis and bicarbonate in salivary secretions normally clear and neutralize gastric juices in the esophagus. During sleep and in patients with impaired esophageal peristalsis or decreased salivation, the esophageal mucosa is damaged by gastric juices, causing an inflammatory response (Figure 23–3 ■). With prolonged exposure, reflux esophagitis develops. In nonerosive reflux disease, the mucosa remains normal or mildly inflamed. Erosive esophagitis, however,

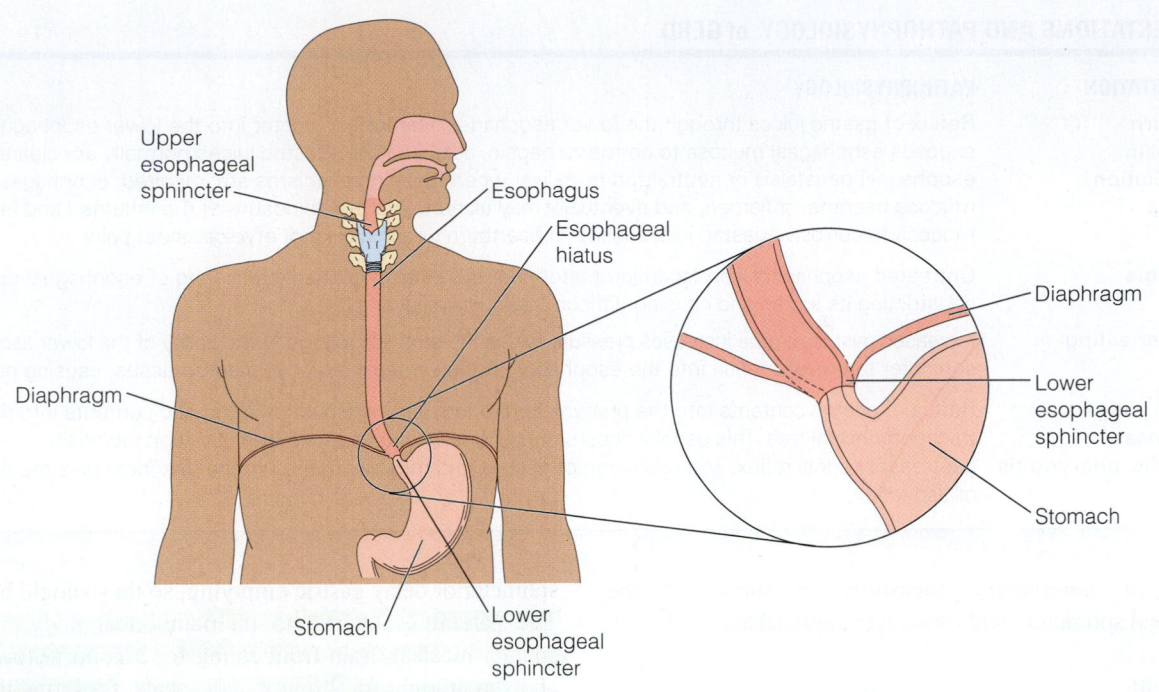

Figure 23–2 ■ The esophagus. The inset shows a closer view of the lower esophageal sphincter.

is characterized by red, friable (easily torn) mucosa and superficial ulcers. If untreated, scarring occurs, and esophageal stricture may develop.

Manifestations

GERD causes heartburn, usually after meals, with bending over, or when reclining. Regurgitation of sour material into the mouth, or difficulty and pain with swallowing may develop. Other manifestations may include atypical chest pain, sore throat, and hoarseness. See the following table illustrating links between the pathophysiology of GERD and its symptoms. Aspiration of gastric contents can cause hoarseness or respiratory symptoms.

Complications include esophageal strictures and Barrett's esophagus. Strictures, caused by scar tissue, edema, and spasm, can lead to dysphagia. Barrett's esophagus is characterized by changes in the cells lining the esophagus and an increased risk of developing esophageal cancer (Porth & Matfin, 2009).

Interdisciplinary Care

Often the diagnosis of GERD is made by the history of symptoms and predisposing factors. Interdisciplinary care focuses on lifestyle changes, diet modification, and for more severe cases, drug therapy. Surgery is reserved for patients who develop serious complications.

Diagnosis

Diagnostic tests that may be ordered for patients with manifestations of GERD include the following:

- *Barium swallow* to evaluate the esophagus, stomach, and upper small intestine.
- *Upper endoscopy* to permit direct visualization of the esophagus. Tissue may be obtained for biopsy to establish the diagnosis and rule out malignancy. ∞ See Chapter 21 for nursing care of the patient undergoing an upper endoscopy.

- In the *Bernstein test*, saline and dilute acid solutions are instilled into the esophagus. In patients with GERD, the acid solution produces symptoms of heartburn, whereas the saline solution does not; neither solution produces symptoms in patients who do not have GERD.
- *24-hour ambulatory pH monitoring* may be performed to establish the diagnosis of GERD. For this test, a small tube with a pH electrode is inserted through the nose into the esophagus. The electrode is attached to a small box worn on the belt that records the data. The data are later analyzed by computer.

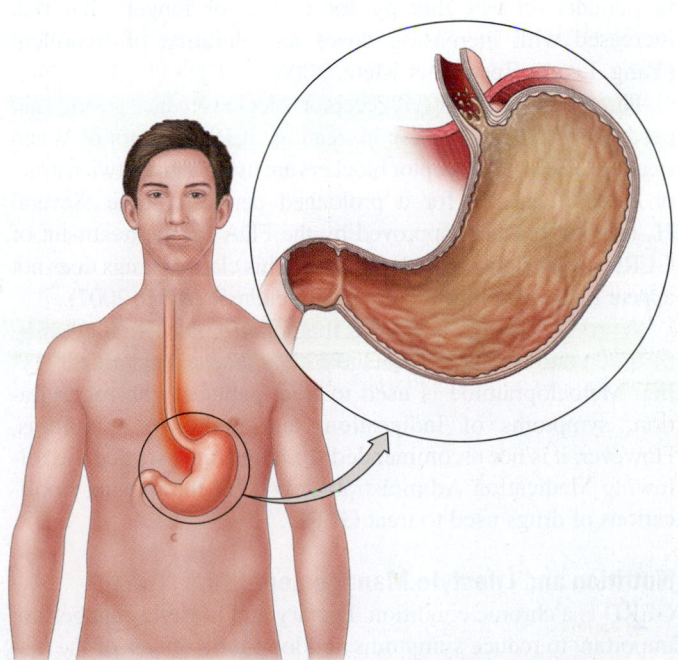

Figure 23–3 ■ In gastroesophageal reflux disease, reflux of corrosive gastric secretions into the lower esophagus causes inflammation of esophageal mucosa.

MANIFESTATIONS AND PATHOPHYSIOLOGY of GERD

MANIFESTATION	PATHOPHYSIOLOGY
Heartburn Chest pain Regurgitation Belching	Reflux of gastric juices through the lower esophageal (cardiac) sphincter into the lower esophagus exposes esophageal mucosa to corrosive pepsin, acid, and bile. Gastric juices normally are cleared by esophageal peristalsis or neutralized by saliva; when these mechanisms are impaired, esophageal mucosa becomes inflamed, and eventually may ulcerate. Further exposure of the inflamed and ulcerated mucosa to corrosive gastric juices leads to heartburn or angina-like or atypical chest pain.
Dysphagia	Untreated esophagitis leads to inflammatory cell infiltrates, fibrosis, and scaring of esophageal tissue, constricting its lumen and causing difficult, painful swallowing.
Pain after eating	Increased gastric volume increases pressure within the stomach relative to the ability of the lower esophageal sphincter to prevent reflux into the esophagus. Reflux irritates already inflamed tissue, causing pain.
Chronic cough Hoarseness Laryngitis, pharyngitis	Reflux of gastric contents into the pharynx and mouth allows aspiration of gastric contents into the tracheobronchial tree. This usually occurs during sleep, when a recumbent position increases gastroesophageal reflux, and relaxation of tissues and muscles in the oropharynx increases the risk of aspiration.

- *Esophageal manometry* measures pressures of the esophageal sphincters and esophageal peristalsis.

Medications

Antacids, such as Mylanta or Maalox, relieve mild or moderate symptoms by neutralizing stomach acid. Gaviscon, which forms a floating barrier between the gastric contents and the esophageal mucosa when the patient is upright, may be used.

Proton-pump inhibitors (PPIs) such as omeprazole (Prilosec) and lansoprazole (Prevacid) reduce gastric secretions. PPIs promote healing of erosive esophagitis and relieve symptoms. An 8-week course of treatment is initially prescribed, although some patients may require 3 to 6 months of therapy. Relapse is common after PPI therapy is discontinued. Although these drugs have minimal side effects, they may interfere with absorption of calcium and vitamin B_{12}. A study by Yang and associates showed an increased risk of hip fracture in patients on PPI therapy for a year or longer. The risk increased with increasing doses and duration of treatment (Yang, Lewis, Epstein, & Metz, 2006).

Histamine$_2$-receptor (H_2-receptor) blockers reduce gastric acid production and are effective in treating GERD symptoms. When treating GERD, H_2-receptor blockers are usually given twice a day or more frequently for a prolonged period of time. Several H_2-receptor blockers approved by the FDA for the treatment of GERD are available over the counter. This class of drugs does not appear to increase hip-fracture risk (Gendreau-Webb, 2007).

A promotility agent, such as metoclopramide (Reglan), may be ordered to enhance esophageal clearance and gastric emptying. Metoclopramide is used to treat patients with regurgitation, symptoms of indigestion, and nighttime symptoms. However, it is not recommended for long-time use. See the following Medication Administration box for the nursing implications of drugs used to treat GERD.

Nutrition and Lifestyle Management

GERD is a chronic condition. Dietary and lifestyle changes are important to reduce symptoms and long-term effects of the disorder. Acidic foods such as tomato products, citrus fruits, spicy foods, and coffee are eliminated from the diet. Fatty foods, chocolate, peppermint, and alcohol relax the lower esophageal sphincter or delay gastric emptying, so they should be avoided. The patient is advised to maintain ideal body weight, eat smaller meals, refrain from eating for 3 hours before bedtime, and stay upright for 2 hours after meals. Elevating the head of the bed on 6- to 8-inch blocks often is beneficial. Stopping smoking is a necessary lifestyle change. Avoiding tight clothing and avoiding bending may help to relieve symptoms.

Surgery

Surgery may be used for patients who do not respond to pharmacologic and lifestyle management. Antireflux surgeries increase pressure in the lower esophagus, inhibiting gastric content reflux. Laparoscopic fundoplication, a procedure in which the gastric fundus is wrapped around the distal esophagus, is the treatment of choice for GERD. An open surgical procedure known as Nissen fundoplication also may be done (Figure 23–4 ■). Other laparoscopic procedures to tighten the lower esophageal sphincter may include use of an endoscopic suturing system or burning spots on the muscle surrounding the sphincter to create scar tissue. Surgery or ablation therapy also is recommended to reduce the risk of esophageal cancer in patients with persistent cell changes in the distal esophagus.

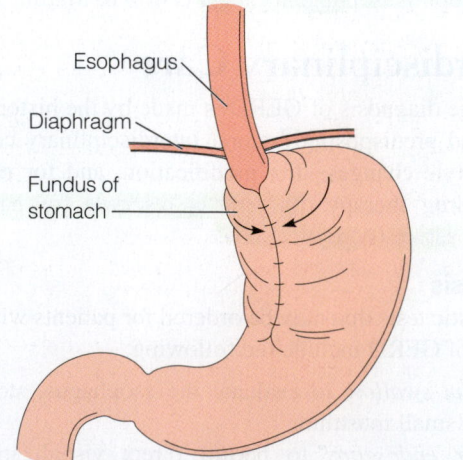

Esophagus

Diaphragm

Fundus of stomach

Figure 23–4 ■ Nissen fundoplication. The fundus of the stomach is wrapped around the lower esophagus and the edges are sutured together.

MEDICATION ADMINISTRATION | Drugs Used to Treat GERD, Gastritis, and Peptic Ulcer Disease

PROTON-PUMP INHIBITORS

Esomeprazole (Nexium)

Lansoprazole (Prevacid)

Omeprazole (Prilosec)

Pantoprazole (Protonix)

Rabeprazole (AcipHex)

Proton-pump inhibitors are the drugs of choice for severe GERD. PPIs inhibit the hydrogen-potassium-ATP pump, reducing gastric acid secretion. If the patient's symptoms do not improve with treatment, the dose may be increased.

Nursing Responsibilities

- Administer 30 minutes before breakfast (and at bedtime if ordered twice a day).
- Do not crush tablets.
- Monitor liver function tests for possible abnormal values, including increased AST, ALT, alkaline phosphatase, and bilirubin levels.

Health Education for the Patient and Family

- Take the drug as ordered for the full course of therapy, even if symptoms are relieved.
- Do not crush, break, or chew tablets.
- Increase your calcium intake or take a calcium supplement while using this drug as it can interfere with calcium absorption.
- Avoid cigarette smoking, alcohol, aspirin, and NSAIDs while taking this drug because these substances may interfere with healing.
- Report black tarry stools, diarrhea, or abdominal pain to your primary care provider.

H₂-RECEPTOR BLOCKERS

Cimetidine (Tagamet)   Ranitidine (Zantac)

Famotidine (Pepcid)   Nizatidine (Axid)

H$_2$-receptor blockers reduce acidity of gastric juices by blocking the ability of histamine to stimulate acid secretion by the gastric parietal cells. As a result, both the volume and concentration of hydrochloric acid in gastric juice are reduced. H$_2$-receptor blockers are given orally or intravenously. Both prescription and over-the-counter preparations are available.

Nursing Responsibilities

- To ensure absorption, do not give an antacid within 1 hour before or after giving an H$_2$-receptor blocker.
- When administered intravenously, do not mix with other drugs. Administer in 20 to 100 mL of solution over 15 to 30 minutes. Rapid intravenous injection as a bolus may cause dysrhythmias and hypotension.
- Monitor for interaction with such drugs as oral anticoagulants, beta-blockers, benzodiazepines, tricyclic antidepressants, and others. H$_2$-receptor blockers may inhibit the metabolism of other drugs, increasing the risk of toxicity.

Health Education for the Patient and Family

- Take the drug as directed, even if pain and gastric discomfort are relieved early in the course of therapy.
- Take at bedtime if once-a-day dosing is ordered. If spaced through the day, take before meals. Avoid taking antacids for 1 hour before and 1 hour after taking this drug.
- To promote healing, avoid cigarette smoking (which increases gastric acid secretion) and gastric mucosal irritants such as alcohol, aspirin, and NSAIDs.

- Long-term use of these drugs can lead to gynecomastia (breast enlargement) and impotence in men and breast tenderness in women. Discontinuing the drug will reverse these effects.
- Report possible adverse effects such as diarrhea, confusion, rash, fatigue, malaise, or bruising to your care provider.

ANTIULCER AGENT

Sucralfate (Carafate)

Sucralfate reacts with gastric acid to form a thick paste that adheres to damaged gastric mucosal tissue. It protects gastric mucosa and promotes healing through this local action.

Nursing Responsibilities

- Administer on an empty stomach, 1 hour before meals and at bedtime.
- Do not crush tablets.
- Separate administration time from antacids by at least 30 minutes.

Health Education for the Patient and Family

- Take as directed, even after symptoms have been relieved.
- Do not crush or chew tablets; shake suspension well.
- Increase your intake of fluids and dietary fiber to prevent constipation.

ANTACIDS

Maalox   Gaviscon   Gelusil   Tums

Mylanta   Aludrox   Riopan   Amphojel

Antacids buffer or neutralize gastric acid, usually acting locally. Antacids are used in GERD, gastritis, and peptic ulcer disease to relieve pain and prevent further damage to esophageal and gastric mucosa.

Nursing Responsibilities

- Antacids interfere with the absorption of many drugs given orally; separate administration times by at least 2 hours.
- Monitor for constipation or diarrhea resulting from antacid therapy. Notify the physician should either develop; a different antacid may be ordered.
- Although most antacids have little systemic effect, electrolyte imbalances can develop. Monitor serum electrolytes, particularly sodium, calcium, and magnesium levels.

Health Education for the Patient and Family

- Take your antacid frequently as prescribed, 1 to 3 hours after meals and at bedtime. To be effective, the antacid must be in your stomach.
- Avoid taking an antacid for approximately 2 hours before and 1 hour after taking another medication.
- Shake suspensions well prior to administration.
- Chew tablets thoroughly, and follow with 4 to 6 ounces of water.
- Report worsening symptoms, diarrhea, or constipation to your primary care provider.
- Continue taking the antacid for the duration prescribed. Although pain and discomfort often are relieved soon after treatment begins, healing takes 6 to 8 weeks.

PROMOTILITY AGENT

Metoclopramide (Reglan)

By acting on the central nervous system, metoclopramide stimulates upper gastrointestinal motility and gastric emptying. As a result, nausea, vomiting, and symptoms of GERD are reduced.

(continued)

MEDICATION ADMINISTRATION   Drugs Used to Treat GERD, Gastritis, and Peptic Ulcer Disease (continued)

Nursing Implications

- Do not administer this drug to patients with possible gastrointestinal obstruction or bleeding, or a history of seizure disorders, pheochromocytoma, or Parkinson's disease.
- Monitor for extrapyramidal side effects (e.g., difficulty speaking or swallowing, loss of balance, gait disruptions, twitching or twisting movements, weakness of arms or legs) or manifestations of tardive dyskinesia (uncontrolled rhythmic facial movement, lip-smacking, tongue rolling). Report immediately.
- Give oral doses 30 minutes before meals and at bedtime.
- May be given by direct intravenous push over 1 to 2 minutes, or diluted by slow infusion over 15 to 30 minutes.

Health Education for the Patient and Family

- Take this drug as directed. If you miss a dose, take as soon as you remember unless it is close to the time for the next dose.
- Do not drive or engage in other activities that require alertness if this drug makes you drowsy.
- Avoid using alcohol or other CNS depressants while you are taking this drug.
- Immediately contact your healthcare provider if you develop involuntary movements of your eyes, face, or limbs.

✍ Nursing Care

Assessment

Assessment data related to GERD include the following:

- *Health history:* Manifestations such as frequent heartburn or atypical chest pain; intolerance of foods that are acidic, spicy, or fatty; regurgitation of acidic gastric juice; increased symptoms when bending over, lying down, or wearing tight clothing; difficulty swallowing; possible hoarseness.
- *Physical assessment:* Epigastric tenderness.

Nursing Diagnoses and Interventions

Relieving the discomfort associated with GERD is the priority of nursing care. Teaching focuses on preventing symptoms and long-term consequences of the disorder.

Acute Pain

The epigastric pain associated with GERD can be severe, interfering with rest and causing anxiety.

- Provide small, frequent meals. Restrict intake of fat, acidic foods, coffee, and alcohol. *Limiting the size of meals reduces pressure in the stomach, reducing esophageal reflux. Fatty, acidic foods, coffee, and alcohol increase gastric acidity and interfere with gastric emptying, increasing the incidence of gastroesophageal reflux.*

- Instruct to stop smoking. Refer to a smoking cessation clinic or program as needed. *Cigarette smoking increases gastric acidity and interferes with healing of damaged mucosa.*
- Administer antacids, H_2-receptor blockers, and PPIs as ordered. Instruct patient to continue therapy as prescribed, even after symptoms have been relieved. *These drugs neutralize or reduce gastric acid secretion, relieving symptoms and promoting healing.*
- Discuss the long-term nature of GERD and its management. *Lifestyle changes need to be continued after healing and symptom relief to manage the long-term effects of GERD.*

Using NANDA, NIC, and NOC

Linkages between a selected NANDA nursing diagnosis, NIC, and NOC for the patient with GERD are shown in the chart that follows.

Community-Based Care

GERD is a lifelong condition best managed by the patient. Teach the patient and family about continuing management strategies, including dietary changes, remaining upright after meals, and avoiding eating for at least 3 hours before bedtime. Suggest elevating the head of the bed on 6- to 8-inch wooden blocks placed under the legs. Discuss the need for continued gastric acid reduction using antacids, H_2-receptor blockers, or

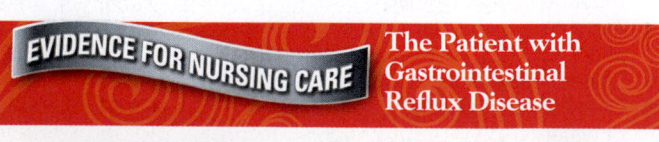

EVIDENCE FOR NURSING CARE   **The Patient with Gastrointestinal Reflux Disease**

Selected resources that nurses may find helpful when planning evidence-based nursing care follow.

- Kahrilas, P., Shaheen, N., Vaezi, M., Hiltz, S., Black, E., Modlin, I., et al. (2008, October). American Gastroenterological Association Medical Position Statement on the management of gastroesophageal reflux disease. *Gastroenterology*, 135(4), 1383–1391. Retrieved from www.guideline.gov/summary/summary .aspx?doc_id=13315&nbr=006759&string=heartburn
- Scottish Intercollegiate Guidelines Network (SIGN). (2003; reaffirmed 2007). *Dyspepsia. A national clinical guideline*. Edinburgh, Scotland: Scottish Intercollegiate Guidelines Network. Retrieved from www.guideline.gov/summary/ summary.aspx?doc_id=3723&nbr=002949&string= dyspepsia

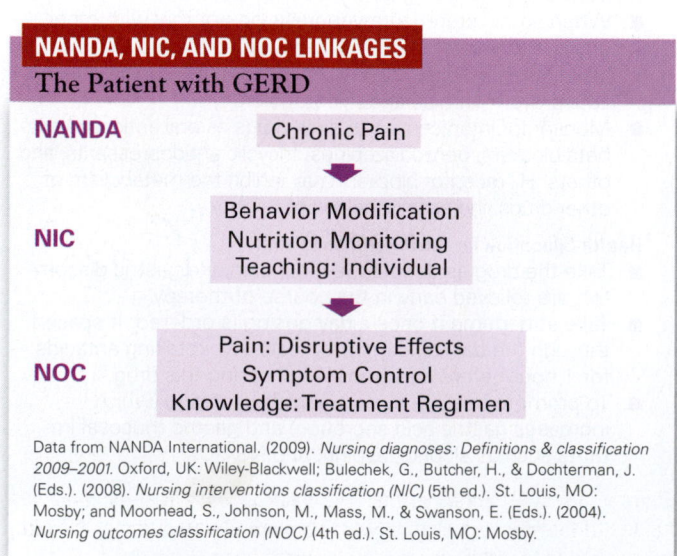

NANDA, NIC, AND NOC LINKAGES
The Patient with GERD

NANDA	Chronic Pain
NIC	Behavior Modification Nutrition Monitoring Teaching: Individual
NOC	Pain: Disruptive Effects Symptom Control Knowledge: Treatment Regimen

Data from NANDA International. (2009). *Nursing diagnoses: Definitions & classification 2009–2001*. Oxford, UK: Wiley-Blackwell; Bulechek, G., Butcher, H., & Dochterman, J. (Eds.). (2008). *Nursing interventions classification (NIC)* (5th ed.). St. Louis, MO: Mosby; and Moorhead, S., Johnson, M., Mass, M., & Swanson, E. (Eds.). (2004). *Nursing outcomes classification (NOC)* (4th ed.). St. Louis, MO: Mosby.

PPIs. All are effective to reduce the acidity of gastric juices. Antacids, the most cost-effective measure, require frequent doses to neutralize gastric acid. H₂-receptor blockers, also available over the counter, are a cost-effective management strategy that require only twice-a-day dosing.

The Patient with Hiatal Hernia

A *hiatal hernia* occurs when part of the stomach protrudes through the esophageal hiatus of the diaphragm into the thoracic cavity. Although hiatal hernia is thought to be a common problem, most affected individuals are asymptomatic. The incidence of hiatal hernia increases with age.

In a *sliding hiatal hernia*, the gastroesophageal junction and the fundus of the stomach slide upward through the esophageal hiatus (Figure 23–5 ■). Several factors may contribute to a sliding hiatal hernia, including weakened anchors of the gastroesophageal junction to the diaphragm, shortening of the esophagus, or increased intra-abdominal pressure. Small sliding hiatal hernias produce few symptoms.

In a *paraesophageal hiatal hernia*, the junction between the esophagus and stomach remains in its normal position below the diaphragm while a part of the stomach herniates through the esophageal hiatus. A paraesophageal hernia can become incarcerated (constricted) and strangulate, impairing blood flow to the herniated tissue. Patients with paraesophageal hernia may develop gastritis, or chronic or acute gastrointestinal bleeding. The manifestations of hiatal hernias are listed in the following box.

A barium swallow or an upper endoscopy may be done to diagnose hiatal hernia. Many patients with hiatal hernia require no treatment. If symptoms are present, treatment

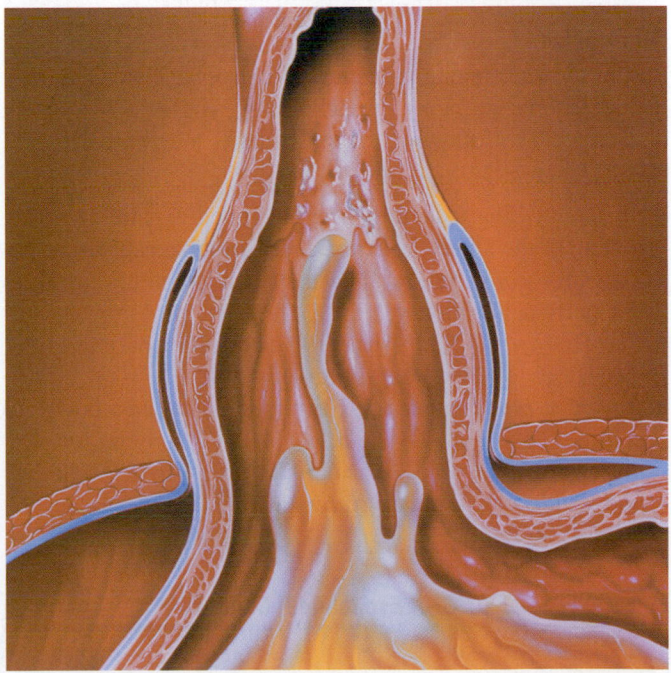

Figure 23–5 ■ Hiatal hernia. The gastroesophageal junction and fundus of the stomach slide upward through the diaphragm, allowing gastric juices to reflux into the lower esophagus.

MANIFESTATIONS of Hiatal Hernia

- Reflux, heartburn
- Feeling of fullness
- Substernal chest pain
- Dysphagia
- Occult bleeding
- Belching, indigestion

measures such as those for patients with GERD may be ordered. If medical management is ineffective or the hernia becomes incarcerated, surgery may be required. The most common surgical procedure is the Nissen fundoplication (see Figure 23–4). This surgery, which may be done laparoscopically, prevents the gastroesophageal junction from slipping into the thoracic cavity.

Nursing care for the patient with a hiatal hernia is similar to that for the patient with GERD. If surgery is performed, nursing care is similar to that for patients undergoing gastric or thoracic surgery (∞ see Chapter 4).

The Patient with Impaired Esophageal Motility

Disorders of esophageal motility can cause **dysphagia** (difficult or painful swallowing) or chest pain. It is estimated that nearly 75% of patients hospitalized with stroke experience dysphagia. Other neurologic disorders such as Parkinson's disease, amyotrophic lateral sclerosis, and Alzheimer's disease also can cause dysphagia.

Primary disorders of swallowing are less common. **Achalasia**, a disorder of unknown etiology, is characterized by impaired peristalsis of the smooth muscle of the esophagus and impaired relaxation of the lower esophageal sphincter (LES). The patient experiences gradually increasing dysphagia with both solid foods and liquids. Fullness in the chest during meals, chest pain, and nighttime cough are additional manifestations. Other patients may experience *diffuse esophageal spasm* that causes nonperistaltic contraction of esophageal smooth muscle. This disorder causes chest pain and/or dysphagia. The chest pain can be severe, and usually occurs at rest.

Treatment of achalasia may include endoscopically guided injection of botulinum toxin into the lower esophageal sphincter or balloon dilation of the LES. Botulinum toxin injection lowers LES pressure, but may need to be repeated every 6 to 9 months. Balloon dilation tears muscle fibers in the LES, reducing its pressure (Figure 23–6 ■). A laparoscopic myotomy (incision into the circular muscle layer of the LES) also reduces pressure and relieves symptoms.

The Patient with Esophageal Cancer

Cancer of the esophagus is a relatively uncommon malignancy in the United States. It does, however, have a high mortality rate, primarily because symptoms often are not recognized until late in the course of the disease.

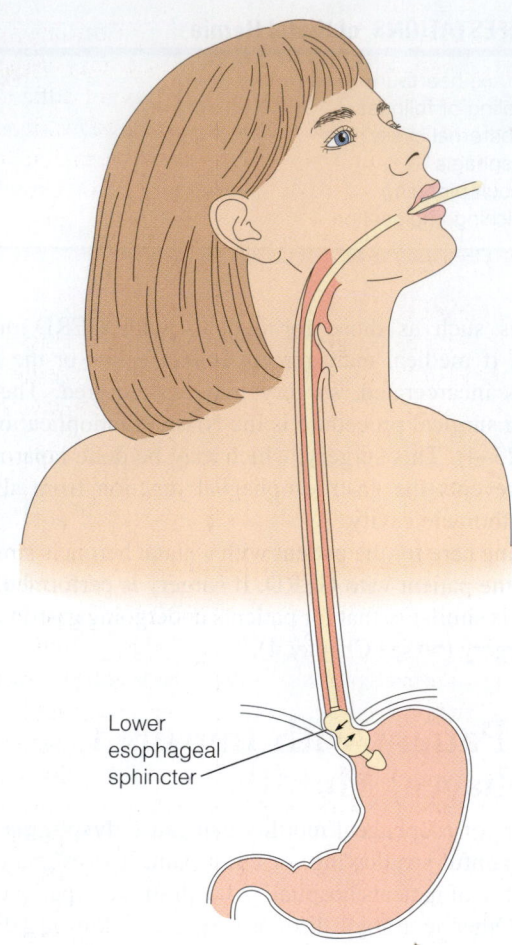

Lower
esophageal
sphincter

Figure 23–6 ■ Balloon dilation of the lower esophageal sphincter.

FAST FACTS

- Esophageal cancer is the seventh leading cause of death in men.
- It accounted for an estimated 11,490 deaths in 2009 (American Cancer Society, 2008).
- Esophageal cancer usually occurs after age 50; it is more common in men than in women and in Blacks than in Whites.
- Most esophageal tumors develop in the lower third of the esophagus.

Pathophysiology

There are two types of esophageal tumors, adenocarcinoma and squamous cell carcinoma. Over the past two decades, the incidence of squamous cell tumors of the esophagus has been decreasing, whereas the incidence of adenocarcinoma has increased dramatically, particularly among white males (Fauci et al., 2008). Cigarette smoking and chronic alcohol use are strong risk factors for squamous cell esophageal tumors, and also appear to contribute to the risk of developing adenocarcinoma. Box 23–3 lists major identified risk factors for esophageal cancer.

Only about 10% of esophageal tumors develop in the upper portion of the esophagus; about 35% develop in the midportion. The lower third of the esophagus is the most common site, accounting for about 55% of tumors. Adenocarcinomas tend to develop in dysplastic (abnormal) columnar epithelium in the

BOX 23–3 Risk Factors for Esophageal Cancer

- Excess alcohol consumption
- Cigarette smoking
- Ingested carcinogens such as nitrates and industrial chemicals
- Smoked opiates
- Physical mucosal damage (e.g., hot tea, lye ingestion, radiation damage, chronic achalasia)
- Congenital disorders
- Chronic gastric reflux

distal esophagus. It is commonly associated with Barrett's esophagus, a possible complication of chronic GERD and achalasia.

The disease usually spreads to adjacent and supraclavicular lymph nodes, the liver, lungs, and the pleura.

Manifestations

The most common symptoms of esophageal carcinoma are progressive dysphagia and recent weight loss. Other manifestations are listed in the box that follows. The cancer often is advanced and incurable by the time the disease is diagnosed because symptoms such as difficulty swallowing don't develop until more than 60% of the circumference of the esophagus is affected by tumor (Fauci et al., 2008).

Tracheoesophageal fistulas may develop as the disease progresses, leading to aspiration and pneumonia. Paraneoplastic symptoms such as hypercalcemia may accompany advanced esophageal cancer.

Interdisciplinary Care

Controlling dysphagia and maintaining nutritional status are essential goals of therapy for patients with esophageal cancer, regardless of the stage of the disease. Treatment may involve surgery, radiation therapy, and/or chemotherapy.

Diagnosis

Diagnostic and staging procedures for esophageal cancer may include esophagography, bronchoscopy, and scans to detect metastasis. The following diagnostic tests may be performed (∞ see Chapter 21):

- *Barium swallow* to identify irregular mucosal patterns or narrowing of the lumen, which suggests esophageal cancer.
- *Esophagoscopy* to allow direct visualization of the tumor and obtain tissue for biopsy.
- *Chest x-ray*, *CT scans*, or *MRI* to identify possible tumor metastases to other organs or tissues.
- *Complete blood count (CBC)* may indicate anemia due to chronic blood loss. *Serum albumin levels* may be low due to malnutrition, and *liver function tests (ALT, alkaline phosphatase, AST, and bilirubin)* are elevated if liver metastases are present.

MANIFESTATIONS of Esophageal Cancer

■ Dysphagia	■ Regurgitation
■ Anemia	■ Anorexia
■ Weight loss	■ Chest pain
■ GERD-like symptoms	■ Persistent cough

Treatments

The treatment of esophageal cancer is challenging; fewer than 5% of patients survive 5 years after it is diagnosed (Fauci et al., 2008). A combination of chemotherapy and radiation, followed by surgery to resect the tumor appears to be more effective than any single form of therapy.

Surgery involves resection of the affected portion of the esophagus (*esophagectomy*) and possible anastomosis of the stomach to the remaining esophagus. Mediastinal lymph nodes may be resected at the time of surgery. Esophagectomy is not without risk; potential surgical complications include anastomosis leak, respiratory complications such as pneumonia or acute respiratory distress syndrome, gastric necrosis or bleeding, cardiac dysrhythmias, and infection and sepsis. Intensive nursing care is required postoperatively to prevent and rapidly identify and treat complications that do develop.

The effectiveness of primary radiation therapy is similar to that with radical surgery. Complications associated with radiation therapy to the esophagus include perforation, hemorrhage, and strictures. When used, combination chemotherapy regimens are more effective in reducing tumor mass than single-drug regimens. When the tumor has spread locally or to distant sites, palliative therapy relieves dysphagia and pain (McPhee et al., 2008). Palliative therapy may include local treatments such as endoscopic dilation, wire stents or laser therapy to keep the esophagus patent, and placement of a gastrostomy or jejunostomy for enteral feeding and fluids.

∾ Nursing Care

Health Promotion

Health promotion measures to reduce the risk for and incidence of esophageal cancer include educating people (especially young people) about the dangers of cigarette smoking and excess alcohol use. Refer to smoking cessation and alcohol treatment programs as indicated. Educate patients with GERD about the relationship between chronic damage to the esophagus due to reflux and esophageal cancer, and stress the importance of effective disease management.

Assessment

Early diagnosis and treatment of esophageal cancer can make a difference in the patient's prognosis. Collect the following assessment data related to esophageal cancer:

- *Health history:* Current symptoms such as chest pain, dysphagia, odynophagia (pain with swallowing), coughing or hoarseness; duration of symptoms; recent weight loss; smoking history; current and past patterns of alcohol consumption.
- *Physical examination:* Weight; general health status; skin color; supraclavicular and cervical lymph nodes for lymphadenopathy.

Nursing Diagnoses and Interventions

Disruption of the integrity and function of the esophagus and the discomfort associated with swallowing in patients with esophageal cancer affect the patient's ability to maintain adequate nutritional status, and, potentially, a patent airway.

Imbalanced Nutrition: Less than Body Requirements

The patient diagnosed with esophageal cancer may already suffer from some degree of malnutrition because of difficulty and pain with swallowing. Enteral nutrition via nasogastric feeding tube or gastrostomy tube or parenteral nutrition maintain nutritional status after surgery or if the tumor is inoperable and obstruction occurs. ∾ See Chapter 22 for nursing interventions related to enteral and parenteral feedings.

Risk for Ineffective Airway Clearance

After surgery for esophageal cancer, the patient is at high risk for aspiration and difficulty maintaining a patent airway due to disruption of the esophagus and incision into the thoracic cavity.

- Assess mental and respiratory status (including rate, depth, breath sounds, and oxygen saturation levels) at least every hour during the initial postoperative period. *Altered mental status increases the risk for aspiration. An increased respiratory rate, dyspnea, diminished breath sounds, or decreased oxygen saturation levels may indicate impaired airway clearance or possible aspiration pneumonia.*
- Provide aggressive pulmonary hygiene measures, including endotracheal suctioning and chest physiotherapy as indicated or ordered. Following extubation, encourage frequent coughing, deep breathing, and use of the incentive spirometer. *Respiratory complications are a frequent complication of esophagectomy. Aggressive nursing care helps mobilize secretions and prevent atelectasis and possible pneumonia.*
- If present, monitor chest tube function and drainage. Promptly report drainage that is bright red and excessive in amount (> 70 mL/h) or purulent. Maintain patency of chest tubes per unit protocol or physician's order. *If a thoracic incision has been used, chest tubes are placed to promote lung reinflation. Proper chest tube function is necessary to prevent pneumothorax and impaired lung inflation.*
- Monitor cardiopulmonary status and hemodynamic pressures. Administer intravenous fluids and fluid boluses as ordered. *Fluid volume imbalances that compromise cardiopulmonary status may develop following esophagectomy. Maintaining adequate fluid intake and preventing fluid overload are important postoperatively. The patient also is at risk for acute respiratory distress syndrome, a critical complication that can further compromise ventilation, gas exchange, and circulation.*
- Do not move or manipulate the nasogastric tube. Maintain low gastric suction as ordered. *Manipulating or moving the nasogastric tube may disrupt suture lines, resulting in a leak into the mediastinum.*
- Verify enteral tube feeding placement by checking the pH of gastric aspirate (∾ see Chapter 22). Stop enteral feedings if feelings of fullness or nausea occur. Suction gastrointestinal contents as needed, positioning the patient on the side. *Overdistention of the stomach or delayed gastric emptying may result in regurgitation of stomach contents. Nausea or a feeling of fullness may indicate stomach overdistention. Suctioning and positioning limit the risk of aspiration.*

Anticipatory Grieving

Upon a diagnosis of cancer, the patient and family may experience a grief reaction. The pessimistic prognosis associated with esophageal cancer and the disruptions in relationships may result in an intense sense of loss. ∞Chapter 5 discusses care of patient experiencing grief and loss.

Community-Based Care

Most care for patients with esophageal cancer is provided in community-based and home settings. Include the following topics in patient and family teaching for home care:

■ Planned treatment options including the risks, benefits, and potential adverse effects of each

■ Wound and follow-up care following surgery
■ Prevention and manifestations of complications such as wound or chest infection, anastomosis leak, deep venous thrombosis
■ How to prepare, implement, and care for tube feedings or home parenteral nutrition

Based on the patient's needs and prognosis, referral to a home health agency and/or hospice may be appropriate.

Disorders of the Stomach and Duodenum

The stomach and upper small intestine (duodenum and jejunum) are responsible for the majority of food digestion. The major disorders that affect digestion are nausea and vomiting, gastritis, peptic ulcer disease, and cancer of the stomach. Nursing roles in managing these disorders include both acute care for the hospitalized patient and teaching to give the patient the skills and knowledge to manage these conditions at home.

Overview of Normal Physiology

Normally, the stomach is protected from the digestive substances it secretes—namely, hydrochloric acid and pepsin—by the **gastric mucosal barrier**. The gastric mucosal barrier includes the following:

■ An impermeable hydrophobic lipid layer that covers gastric epithelial cells. This lipid layer prevents diffusion of water-soluble molecules, but substances such as aspirin and alcohol can diffuse through it.
■ Bicarbonate ions secreted in response to hydrochloric acid secretion by the parietal cells of the stomach. When bicarbonate (HCO_3^-) secretion is equal to hydrogen ion (H^+) secretion, the gastric mucosa remains intact. Prostaglandins, chemical messengers involved in the inflammatory response, support bicarbonate production and blood flow to the gastric mucosa.
■ Mucous gel that protects the surface of the stomach lining from the damaging effects of pepsin and traps bicarbonate to neutralize hydrochloric acid. This gel also acts as a lubricant, preventing mechanical damage to the stomach lining from its contents.

When an acute or chronic irritant disrupts the mucosal barrier, or when disease alters the processes that maintain the barrier, the gastric mucosa becomes irritated and inflamed. Lipid-soluble substances such as aspirin and alcohol penetrate the gastric mucosal barrier, leading to irritation and possible inflammation. Bile acids also break down the lipids in the mucosal barrier, increasing the potential for irritation (Porth & Matfin, 2009). In addition, aspirin and other nonsteroidal anti-inflammatory drugs (NSAIDs) inhibit prostaglandins. Aspirin and NSAIDs alter the nature of gastric mucus, affecting its protective function.

The Patient with Gastrointestinal Bleeding

Because of its constant exposure to the environment, the gastrointestinal tract can be subjected to trauma, exposure to toxins, infection with pathogens such as *Helicobacter pylori*,

inflammatory processes, and insults such as ischemia due to systemic diseases. While the mucosal lining of the GI tract is remarkably able to withstand these insults and heal rapidly, its rich supply of blood can result in significant bleeding when a vessel is eroded or abnormally distended (*varices*). Gastrointestinal hemorrhage is a relatively common admitting diagnosis and complication of critical illnesses. It is a medical emergency requiring aggressive medical and nursing care.

Although bleeding and hemorrhage can occur anywhere in the GI tract, the upper portion of the tract is more commonly affected. The three primary disorders leading to upper (UGI) hemorrhage are erosive gastritis, peptic ulcer disease, and esophageal varices. Erosive gastritis and peptic ulcer disease are discussed in the following sections of this chapter; esophageal varices, usually seen as a complication of cirrhosis of the liver, are discussed in ∞Chapter 25.

> **FAST FACTS**
> ■ About 50% of UGI bleeds are due to peptic ulcer disease.
> ■ Erosive gastritis is the second leading cause of UGI hemorrhage, responsible for about 20% of bleeds.
> ■ The third leading cause, esophageal varices, has the highest mortality rate, between 40% and 70%.

Pathophysiology

Blood in the GI tract has several effects. It is irritating to the stomach, and typically leads to nausea and vomiting (**hematemesis**, vomiting blood). If the blood has been present in the stomach for a period of time and is partially digested, it may have a "coffee-grounds" appearance, rather than presenting as bright red blood. The accumulation of blood in the GI tract stimulates peristasis, leading to hyperactive bowel sounds and diarrhea. Stools may be black and tarry (**melena**) or frankly bloody (**hematochezia**); stool containing partially digested blood has a characteristic odor. With significant upper GI bleeding, digestion of blood proteins increases blood urea nitrogen (BUN) levels.

Physiologic responses to an upper GI bleed depend on the rapidity and magnitude of the blood loss. GI bleeding resulting from erosion of a small vessel typically is slow, and may not be identified until the patient presents with manifestations of blood loss anemia due to depletion of iron stores. (∞ See Chapter 33 for further discussion of blood loss anemia.) Although no visible blood may be present in the stool, **occult** (or hidden) **bleeding** may be detected by chemical means.

GI hemorrhage, with loss of a significant amount of blood within a few hours, rapidly depletes blood volume, producing manifestations of decreased cardiac output: tachycardia, hypotension, pallor, and decreased urine output. Peripheral blood vessels constrict to maintain perfusion of vital organs. Unless the blood volume is restored, hypovolemic shock progresses, leading to acidosis, renal failure, bowel infarction, acute coronary syndrome, coma, and death. ∞ See Chapter 11 for more information about shock and its management.

Interdisciplinary Care

The acuity of the bleed and the patient's condition dictate the timing and extent of diagnostic testing and interventions. A patient with a massive GI hemorrhage is admitted to the critical care unit and aggressively treated to stem bleeding, restore blood volume, and stabilize the cardiovascular system. Identifying the cause of the bleeding is postponed in many cases until the patient's condition has been stabilized.

When the bleeding is slow or chronic, diagnostic testing and treatment may be managed in a community-based setting.

Diagnosis

Diagnostic testing focuses on determining the extent and effects of the bleed, as well as its cause.

- A *complete blood count with hemoglobin and hematocrit* are obtained. In an acute bleed, the CBC, hemoglobin, and hematocrit may not initially indicate the extent of blood loss because plasma is lost along with blood cells.
- *Blood type and crossmatch* are performed to prepare for transfusion as necessary.
- *Serum electrolytes*, *osmolality*, and *BUN* are obtained to determine the effects of the blood loss and protein digestion on blood chemistries.
- *Liver function studies* and a *coagulation profile* may be obtained to help determine the cause of the bleeding.
- An *upper endoscopy* is performed as soon as possible to identify and, if possible, treat the source of bleeding. ∞ See Chapter 21 for nursing care of the patient undergoing upper endoscopy.

Treatments

In acute GI hemorrhage, initial treatment focuses on stemming the bleeding and restoring cardiovascular stability. Intravenous fluids such as normal saline or a balanced electrolyte solution are administered through a large-bore intravenous catheter. Fresh whole blood, which contains clotting factors, is administered to restore blood volume and components in an acute hemorrhage. In less acute situations, packed red cells may be administered to restore the oxygen-carrying capacity of the blood.

Hemostasis is achieved using upper endoscopy whenever possible. A sclerosing agent may be injected into the bleeding vessel, or the vessel may be sealed using a heated probe, electrocautery, or laser. Rarely, emergency surgery is required to stop hemorrhage.

GASTRIC LAVAGE Gastric lavage, washing out of stomach contents, may be done in patients with upper GI hemorrhage to remove blood from the GI tract, prevent vomiting, and prepare for upper endoscopy. See Procedure 23–1 for nursing responsibilities related to gastric lavage.

℘ Nursing Care

Health Promotion

Preventing gastrointestinal bleeding is the most important step in reducing the mortality and morbidity associated with an acute GI hemorrhage. Identifying patients at risk and instituting regular gastric pH monitoring and maintenance of drug therapy to reduce gastric acidity are important preventive measures. All critically ill patients should be considered to be at risk for stress-related erosive gastritis.

Assessment

Assessment of the patient experiencing an acute GI hemorrhage is very focused on the immediate crisis. The ability to obtain subjective information may be limited; however, it is important to identify possible contributing factors such as use of aspirin, other platelet inhibitors, or anticoagulant medications and the presence of any acute or chronic conditions that may contribute to bleeding (e.g., hypertension, a clotting disorder, peptic ulcer disease, chronic hepatitis, or cirrhosis of the liver). If possible, identify all current medications and their purpose, as well as any allergies to medications or other substances.

Physical examination focuses on the effect of the bleeding on cardiovascular status. Obtain vital signs and orthostatic vital signs (an early sign of hypovolemia). Place the acutely ill patient on a cardiac monitor and obtain a rhythm strip. Obtain oxygen saturation level. Assess peripheral pulse strength, as well as color, temperature, and capillary refill of extremities. Evaluate mental status, including level of consciousness and orientation. An indwelling catheter may be inserted to evaluate urine output.

Nursing Diagnoses and Interventions

Nursing care priorities for the patient with an acute GI bleed focus on restoring and maintaining an effective cardiac output and tissue perfusion, and on stopping the hemorrhage and preventing further bleeding.

Risk for Shock

Significant amounts of blood may be lost in a very short time with an acute GI hemorrhage. Because some of the blood enters the bowel, it may be difficult to accurately estimate the amount of blood lost by measuring emesis, gastric suction return, and blood expelled as feces. As blood volume drops, venous return decreases. The heart rate increases to maintain the cardiac output, and peripheral blood vessels constrict to improve venous return and cardiac output.

- Frequently assess and document vital signs, including blood pressure, pulse rate and cardiac rhythm, respiratory rate, and oxygen saturation levels. Obtain hemodynamic pressure measurements as ordered, reporting trends and changes. *The vital signs, oxygen saturation levels, and hemodynamic pressure values provide indicators of the effectiveness of peripheral tissue perfusion, oxygenation, and fluid replacement.*
- Monitor for and report changes in skin color, temperature, and moisture, or slow capillary refill. *Peripheral vasoconstriction and activation of the sympathetic nervous system typically cause pale, cool, and moist or diaphoretic skin. Development of cyanosis or mottling indicates a further decrease in tissue perfusion and oxygenation.*

When it is important to remove or dilute gastric contents rapidly, gastric lavage (irrigation or washing out of the stomach) may be indicated. In acute poisoning or ingestion of a caustic substance, a large-bore 30- to 36-Fr. nasogastric tube is inserted, and lavage performed. An 18-Fr. nasogastric tube may be used when the procedure is performed to remove blood from the upper GI tract. Because the GI tract is not sterile, clean technique is appropriate for use, although the solution used will generally be sterile.

- Obtain baseline assessment, including vital signs, abdominal inspection, girth, and bowel sounds. *It is important to have assessment data documented prior to instituting the procedure for comparison.*
- Explain the procedure, answering questions and clarifying perceptions. Instruct to report any pain, difficulty breathing, or other problems during the procedure. *A patient who is able to understand and cooperate with the procedure will tolerate lavage better. The patient may be aware of symptoms of complications such as perforation or tube displacement before they are evident to the nurse.*
- Place in semi-Fowler's or Fowler's position. If unable to tolerate elevation of the head of the bed because of hypotension, place in left side-lying position. *Elevating of the head of the bed or sidelying position will minimize the risk of aspiration.*
- Insert a nasogastric tube if one is not already in place. Verify tube placement by aspirating gastric contents and test pH of aspirate. *Proper placement is vital to prevent aspiration or overdistention of the small bowel with irrigating solution.*
- Irrigate the stomach, using either a closed or an open system technique.

CLOSED-SYSTEM IRRIGATION

- Wearing clean gloves, connect bag or bottle of normal saline irrigating solution to nasogastric tube using a Y connector. Attach drainage or suction tube to other arm of connector (Figure 23–7 ■). Empty the stomach, clamp drain tube or turn off suction, and allow 50 to 200 mL of solution to run into stomach by gravity. Stop solution and allow to drain or

suction out. Repeat until ordered amount has been used or desired results are obtained, for example, no further clots and solution returns clear or light pink. Measure the amount of drainage, subtracting the amount of irrigant instilled, to obtain gastric output. *The closed system minimizes the risk of contact with body fluids for the nurse. Measuring gastric output is important in monitoring fluid balance.*

INTERMITTENT OPEN SYSTEM

- Wearing clean gloves and other personal protective equipment as necessary (gown and face protection), empty the stomach using suction or a 50-mL catheter-tip syringe. Measure and discard the aspirate. Using the syringe, draw up approximately 50 mL of irrigation solution, and instill it using gentle pressure. Aspirate the nasogastric tube, and discard the solution into a measuring container. Continue this procedure until the desired amount of irrigant has been instilled or desired results have been obtained. *Manual irrigation with a catheter-tip syringe may be more effective than gravity flow in removing clots from the stomach and nasogastric tube.*
- Continue to monitor vital signs (including temperature), tolerance of the procedure, and other assessment data. *The patient may be unstable and require continuous reevaluation. Gastric lavage may cause hypothermia; therefore, monitor temperature and indications of hypothermia, such as lethargy and changes in cardiac rate and rhythm.*
- If the aspirate has not cleared to light pink or pink tinged after 20 to 30 minutes of lavage or if the patient is unable to tolerate the procedure, notify the physician. *Medical or surgical intervention may be necessary to stop hemorrhage in some instances.*
- On completion of lavage, provide mouth and nares care. Continue to monitor vital signs, abdominal status, and other assessment data.
- Document the procedure, including the amount and type of irrigant used, gastric output character and amount, and the patient's condition and tolerance of the procedure.

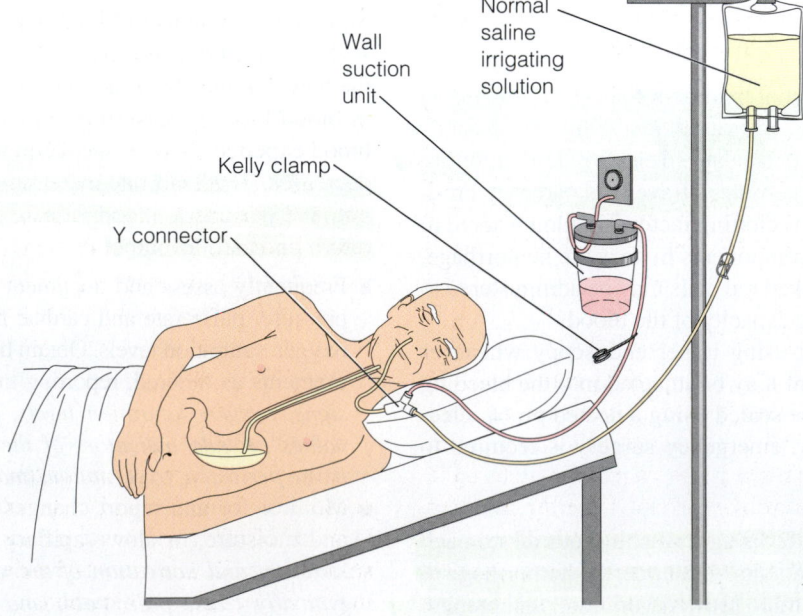

Normal saline irrigating solution

Wall suction unit

Kelly clamp

Y connector

Figure 23–7 ■ The patient with a closed-system gastric lavage.

- Insert an indwelling urinary catheter and measure urine output hourly. Report an output of less than 30 mL for two consecutive hours. *A fall in urine output may indicate further reduction in cardiac output. As cardiac output falls, the kidneys become ischemic and acute renal failure may develop.*
- Unless contraindicated, insert a nasogastric tube and connect to low suction. Measure gastric output hourly unless otherwise directed. *Measuring gastric output provides information about the amount of blood and fluid lost. This information helps determine fluid and blood replacement needs.*
- Maintain two peripheral intravenous lines with large-bore catheters or a central venous catheter for fluid and blood administration as ordered. Frequently monitor vital signs, respiratory status, and hemodynamic pressure measurements, reporting changes in status. *Rapid administration of isotonic intravenous fluids, blood, and blood products can lead to fluid overload and potential heart failure.*
- Replace gastric drainage with balanced electrolyte intravenous solutions as ordered. *GI losses are replaced in addition to fluids given to meet daily requirements to prevent fluid volume deficiency.*

Risk for Bleeding

- Maintain gastric suction and drainage and patency of nasogastric tube. *Blood is irritating to the GI tract, precipitating vomiting and stimulating peristalsis, leading to diarrhea. In addition, digested blood can increase BUN levels, potentially leading to confusion and altered mental status.*
- Irrigate the nasogastric tube with room temperature saline or tap water as ordered. Calculate intake and output, subtracting the amount of irrigant from gastric output. *Irrigation of the nasogastric tube helps remove irritating blood from the gut and produces a degree of vasoconstriction in stomach mucosa, slowing bleeding.*
- Prepare for upper endoscopy or surgery as planned. *Endoscopy or emergency surgery may be performed to repair the bleeding site or sclerose bleeding vessels.*
- Following an acute bleed and in patients at risk for GI bleeding, monitor gastric pH as ordered and check vomitus and feces for the presence of occult blood. Maintain infusions of drugs to reduce gastric acidity as ordered. *The patient remains at risk for GI bleeding. Monitoring for occult blood helps identify slow bleeding or recurrent hemorrhage. Reducing the acidity of gastric secretions reduces irritation of the gastric mucosa, reducing the risk of bleeding.*

Community-Based Care

Following an acute GI hemorrhage, continuing care focuses on resolving the underlying disease process if possible and preventing future episodes of GI bleeding. If a bleeding gastric ulcer was identified, testing for *H. pylori* infection will be done, and a treatment regimen prescribed to eradicate the infection (see the section on peptic ulcer disease later that follows). The patient who experienced an episode of erosive stress gastritis will often be discharged with instructions to continue taking a gastric acid–reducing medication and avoid known gastric irritants such as aspirin and alcohol. The patient with esophageal varices due to cirrhosis or chronic hepatitis needs additional instructions (∞ see Chapter 25).

Patients with minor or slow GI bleeding often are managed in the community. Provide teaching about the cause of the bleeding and measures to prevent future episodes. Provide verbal and written instructions for prescribed medications such as acid reducers and oral iron supplements. Discuss appropriate nutrition; while a special diet to "soothe the stomach" rarely is indicated, foods rich in iron may be recommended to treat the resulting anemia.

Discuss indicators of GI bleeding to be reported to the physician. If the source of bleeding has not been identified, provide instructions about prescribed follow-up diagnostic testing.

The Patient with Peptic Ulcer Disease

Peptic ulcer disease (PUD), a break in the mucous lining of the gastrointestinal tract where it comes in contact with gastric juice, is a chronic health problem. PUD affects approximately 10% of the population or 4 million people in the United States every year, primarily those between ages 25 and 64 years. Furthermore, its complications account for an estimated 15,000 deaths annually (Fauci et al., 2008; Ramakrishnan & Salinas, 2007).

Peptic ulcers occur in any area of the gastrointestinal tract exposed to acid-pepsin secretions, including the esophagus, stomach, or duodenum. *Duodenal ulcers* are the most common. They usually develop between the ages of 30 and 55, and are more common in men than women. *Gastric ulcers* more often affect older patients, between the ages of 55 and 70. Ulcers are more common in people who smoke and who are chronic users of NSAIDs. Alcohol and dietary intake do not seem to cause PUD, and the role of stress is uncertain. Although the incidence of PUD has dramatically decreased, the incidence of gastric ulcers is increasing, believed due to the widespread use of NSAIDs (McPhee et al., 2008).

Risk Factors

Chronic *H. pylori* infection and use of aspirin and NSAIDs are the major risk factors for PUD. Contributing risk factors are listed in Box 23–4. Overall, an estimated 10% to 15% of patients infected with *H. pylori* develop PUD. Of the NSAIDs, aspirin is the most ulcerogenic. A strong familial pattern suggests a genetic factor in the development of PUD. Cigarette smoking is a significant risk factor, doubling the risk of PUD. Cigarette smoking inhibits the secretion of bicarbonate by the pancreas and possibly causes more rapid transit of gastric acid into the duodenum.

Pathophysiology

The innermost layer of the stomach wall, the gastric mucosa, consists of columnar epithelial cells, supported by a middle layer of blood vessels and glands, and a thin outer layer of smooth muscle. The mucosal barrier of the stomach, a thin coating of mucous gel and bicarbonate, protects the gastric mucosa. The mucosal barrier is maintained by bicarbonate secreted by the epithelial cells, by mucous gel production stimulated by

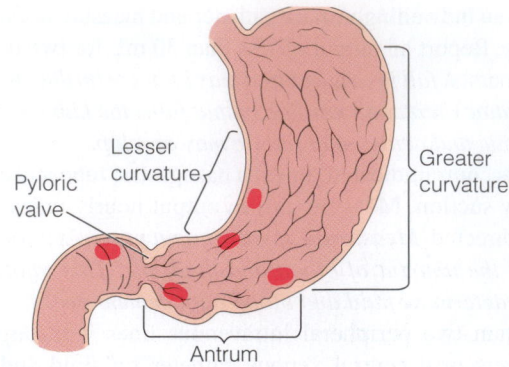

Figure 23–8 ■ Common sites affected by peptic ulcer disease.

prostaglandins, and by an adequate blood supply to the mucosa (see the overview of normal physiology on page 630).

An **ulcer**, or break in the gastrointestinal mucosa, develops when the mucosal barrier is unable to protect the mucosa from damage by hydrochloric acid and pepsin, the gastric digestive juices. See the accompanying Pathophysiology Illustrated: Peptic Ulcer Disease feature on pages 636–637.

H. pylori infection, found in about 50% of people who have PUD, is unique in colonizing the stomach. It is spread person to person (oral–oral or fecal–oral), and contributes to ulcer formation in several ways. The bacteria produce enzymes that reduce the efficacy of mucous gel in protecting the gastric mucosa. In addition, the host's inflammatory response to *H. pylori* contributes to gastric epithelial cell damage without producing immunity to the infection. Although the gastric mucosa is the usual site for *H. pylori* infection, this infection also contributes to duodenal ulcers. This is possibly related to increased gastric acid production associated with *H. pylori* infection.

NSAIDs contribute to PUD through both systemic and topical mechanisms. Prostaglandins are necessary for maintaining the gastric mucosal barrier. NSAIDs interrupt prostaglandin synthesis by disrupting the action of the enzyme cyclooxygenase (COX). The two forms of this enzyme are COX-1 and COX-2. The COX-1 enzyme is necessary to maintain the integrity of the gastric mucosa, but the anti-inflammatory effects of NSAIDs are due to their ability to inhibit the COX-2 enzyme. The COX-2–selective NSAIDs may be less damaging to the gastric mucosa because they have less effect on the COX-1 enzyme. In addition to their systemic effect, aspirin and many NSAIDs cross the lipid membranes of gastric epithelial cells, damaging the cells themselves.

The ulcers of PUD may affect the esophagus, stomach, or duodenum. They may be superficial or deep, affecting all layers of the mucosa (see Pathophysiology Illustrated: Peptic Ulcer Disease). Duodenal ulcers, the most common, usually develop in the proximal portion of the duodenum, close to the pylorus (Figure 23–8 ■). They are sharply demarcated and usually less than 1 cm in diameter (Figure 23–9 ■). Gastric ulcers often are found on the lesser curvature and the area immediately proximal to the pylorus. Gastric ulcers are associated with an increased incidence of gastric cancer.

Peptic ulcer disease may be chronic, with spontaneous remissions and exacerbations. Exacerbations of the disease may be associated with trauma, infection, or other physical or psychologic stressors.

Manifestations

Pain is the classic symptom of peptic ulcer disease. The pain is typically described as gnawing, burning, aching, or hunger-like and is experienced in the epigastric region, sometimes radiating to the back. The pain occurs when the stomach is empty (2 to 3 hours after meals and in the middle of the night) and is relieved by eating with a classic "pain–food–relief" pattern. The patient may complain of heartburn or regurgitation and may vomit.

The presentation of peptic ulcer disease in the older adult is often less clear, with vague and poorly localized discomfort, perhaps chest pain or dysphagia, weight loss, or anemia. In the older adult, a complication of PUD such as upper GI hemorrhage or perforation of the stomach or duodenum may be the presenting symptom.

Complications

The complications associated with peptic ulcers include hemorrhage, obstruction, and perforation. See the following box for the manifestations of these complications.

Among people with PUD, 10% to 20% experience hemorrhage as a result of ulceration and erosion into the blood vessels of the gastric mucosa. Bleeding is the most frequent complication in older adults. It is the presenting symptom in up to 20% of people with PUD (Fauci et al., 2008). When small blood vessels erode, blood loss may be slow and insidious, with occult blood in the stool the only initial sign. If

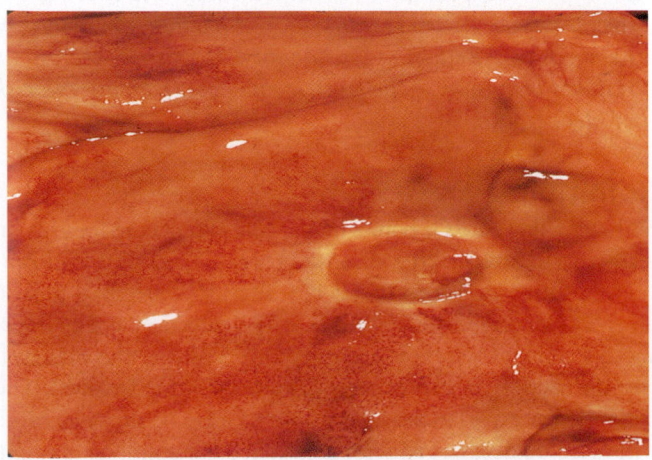

Figure 23–9 ■ A superficial peptic ulcer.
Source: SPL/Photo Researchers, Inc.

bleeding continues, the patient becomes anemic and experiences symptoms of weakness, fatigue, dizziness, and orthostatic hypotension. Erosion into a larger vessel can lead to sudden and severe bleeding with hematemesis, melena, or hematochezia (blood in the stool), and signs of hypovolemic shock.

Gastric outlet obstruction may result from edema surrounding the ulcer, smooth muscle spasm, or scar tissue. Generally, obstruction is a gradual rather than an acute process. Symptoms include a feeling of epigastric fullness, accentuated ulcer symptoms, and nausea. If the obstruction becomes complete, vomiting occurs. Hydrochloric acid, sodium, and potassium are lost in vomitus, potentially leading to fluid and electrolyte imbalance and metabolic alkalosis.

The most lethal complication of PUD is perforation of the ulcer through the mucosal wall. When perforation occurs, gastric or duodenal contents enter the peritoneum, causing an inflammatory process and peritonitis. Chemical peritonitis from the hydrochloric acid, pepsin, bile, and pancreatic fluid is immediate; bacterial peritonitis follows within 6 to 12 hours from gastric contaminants entering the normally sterile peritoneal cavity. When an ulcer perforates, the patient has immediate, severe upper abdominal pain, radiating throughout the abdomen and possibly to the shoulder. The abdomen becomes rigid and boardlike, with absent bowel sounds. Signs of shock may be present, including diaphoresis, tachycardia, and rapid, shallow respirations. Classic symptoms of perforation may not be present in an older adult. The older adult may instead present with mental confusion and other nonspecific symptoms. This atypical presentation can lead to delays in diagnosis and treatment, increasing the associated mortality rate.

Zollinger-Ellison Syndrome

Zollinger-Ellison syndrome is peptic ulcer disease caused by a gastrinoma, or gastrin-secreting tumor of the pancreas, stomach, or intestines. More than 60% of gastrinomas are malignant tumors. Gastrin is a hormone that stimulates the secretion of pepsin and hydrochloric acid. The increased gastrin levels associated with these tumors result in hypersecretion of gastric acid, which in turn causes mucosal ulceration.

The peptic ulcers of Zollinger-Ellison syndrome may affect any portion of the stomach or duodenum, as well as the esophagus or jejunum. Characteristic ulcer-like pain is common. The high levels of hydrochloric acid entering the duodenum may cause diarrhea and **steatorrhea** (excess fat in the feces) from impaired fat digestion and absorption. Complications of bleeding and perforation are often seen with Zollinger-Ellison syndrome. Fluid and electrolyte imbalances may result from persistent diarrhea with resultant losses of potassium and sodium in particular.

Interdisciplinary Care

Treatment for PUD focuses on eradicating *H. pylori* infection and treating or preventing ulcers related to use of NSAIDs.

Diagnosis

- *Upper GI series* using barium as a contrast medium can detect 80% to 90% of peptic ulcers. It commonly is the diagnostic procedure chosen first; it is less costly and less invasive than endoscopy. Small or very superficial ulcers may be missed, however.
- *Endoscopy* allows visualization of the esophageal, gastric, and duodenal mucosa and direct inspection of ulcers. Tissue also can be obtained for biopsy. Nursing care of the patient undergoing endoscopy is outlined in ∞ Chapter 21.
- Biopsy specimens obtained during an endoscopy can be tested for the presence of *H. pylori* using a *biopsy urease test*, which is more than 90% accurate in diagnosing the infection. It is, however, invasive and costly.
- Noninvasive methods of detecting *H. pylori* infection include fecal *H. pylori* antigen tests (to detect antigens to *H. pylori* in the feces), and the *urea breath test*. In this test, radiolabeled urea is given orally. The urease produced by *H. pylori* bacteria converts the urea to ammonia and radiolabeled carbon dioxide, which can then be measured as the patient exhales. These tests also can be used to evaluate the effectiveness of treatment to eradicate *H. pylori*. Treatment with PPIs interferes with urea breath test and fecal antigen test results, so these drugs should be discontinued for 7 or more days prior to testing (McPhee et al., 2008).
- If Zollinger-Ellison syndrome is suspected, *gastric analysis* may be performed to evaluate gastric acid secretion. Stomach contents are aspirated through a nasogastric tube and analyzed. In Zollinger-Ellison syndrome, gastric acid levels are very high.

Medications

The medications used to treat PUD include agents to eradicate *H. pylori*, drugs to decrease gastric acid content, and agents that protect the mucosa. Nursing responsibilities related to selected drugs to treat GERD, gastritis, and PUD are found in the Medication Administration box on pages 625–626.

Eradication of *H. pylori* generally requires 14 days of therapy using a combination of two antibiotics with a proton-pump inhibitor or a bismuth compound (e.g., a PPI, clarithromycin, and amoxicillin, or a PPI, bismuth subsalicylate, tetracycline, and metronidazole). With complete eradication of *H. pylori*, reinfection rates are less than 0.5% per year.

MANIFESTATIONS of PUD Complications

HEMORRHAGE
- Occult or obvious blood in the stool
- Hematemesis
- Fatigue
- Weakness, dizziness
- Orthostatic hypotension
- Hypovolemic shock

OBSTRUCTION
- Sensations of epigastric fullness
- Nausea and vomiting
- Electrolyte imbalances
- Metabolic alkalosis

PERFORATION
- Severe upper abdominal pain, radiating to the shoulder
- Rigid, boardlike abdomen
- Absence of bowel sounds
- Diaphoresis
- Tachycardia
- Rapid, shallow respirations
- Fever

PATHOPHYSIOLOGY ILLUSTRATED
Peptic Ulcer Disease

Normal gastric mucosa

In the stomach and duodenum, the mucosal barrier protects the gastric mucosa (including the epithelial, vascular, and smooth muscle layers) from damage. Specialized mucous cells throughout the gastric mucosa produce a mucus (a mixture of water, lipids, and glycoproteins) that serves as a barrier to the diffusion of ions (such as hydrogen ion) and molecules (such as pepsin). A thin layer of bicarbonate, secreted by surface epithelial cells, forms between the mucus and cell membranes. Blood flow to the gastric mucosa is vital to maintain this barrier. Prostaglandins and nitric oxide stimulate mucus and bicarbonate production, helping maintain it as well. The mucosal barrier constantly bathes surfaces of the gastric epithelial lining.

pH 2

Mucosal barrier

pH 7

Gastric mucosa

Mucus gel layer

Bicarbonate layer

Epithelial layer

• Growth factors (e.g. nitric oxide)

• Prostaglandins

Subepithelial layer

Muscularis mucosae

Submucosa (vascular) layer

Oblique muscle layer

Circular muscle layer

Longitudinal muscle layer

Serosa (visceral peritoneum)

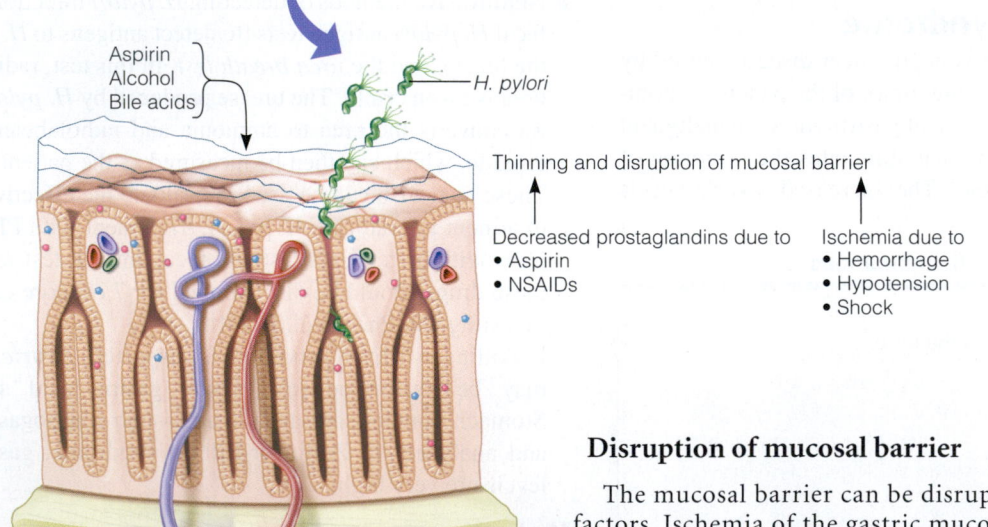

Aspirin
Alcohol
Bile acids

H. pylori

Thinning and disruption of mucosal barrier

Decreased prostaglandins due to
• Aspirin
• NSAIDs

Ischemia due to
• Hemorrhage
• Hypotension
• Shock

Vasoconstriction

Disruption of mucosal barrier

The mucosal barrier can be disrupted by a number of factors. Ischemia of the gastric mucosa (e.g., due to hemorrhage, hypotension, or shock) impairs mucous production, increasing the risk of damage to the mucosa. Aspirin disrupts the mucosal barrier, and, along with other nonsteroidal anti-inflammatory drugs, inhibits prostaglandins which are necessary to maintain mucous production. Alcohol and bile acids also damage the mucous barrier. *Helicobacter pylori*, a common pathogen to infect the gastric mucosa, disrupts the mucosal barrier.

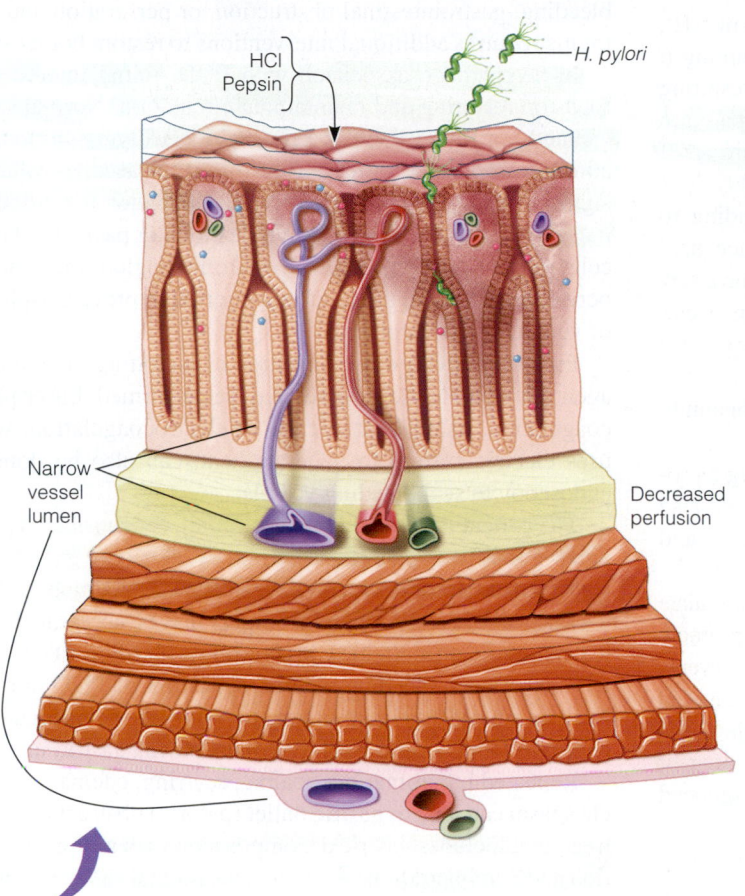

Inflammatory process

When the mucosal barrier is damaged, gastric acid and digestive juices disrupt the epithelial cell membranes, allowing acid to diffuse into cell walls. An acute inflammatory process results. Gastric epithelial cells migrate to the damaged area, a process known as restitution. Adequate blood flow and an alkaline environment are necessary for this repair process. Prostaglandins play an important role in epithelial repair. In the presence of *H. pylori* infection, excess acid production, inadequate blood flow, inhibition of prostaglandins, and other factors that are less clear, the inflammatory process further damages gastric and duodenal epithelial cells, leading to ulceration of the mucosa.

Erosion and ulcer formation

Superficial ulcers (erosions) erode the mucosa, but do not penetrate the muscularis mucosae. True ulcers extend through the muscularis mucosae and into deeper layers of the gastrointestinal wall, damaging blood vessels and potentially penetrating the entire wall. Hemorrhage and peritonitis are potential acute complications of peptic ulcers.

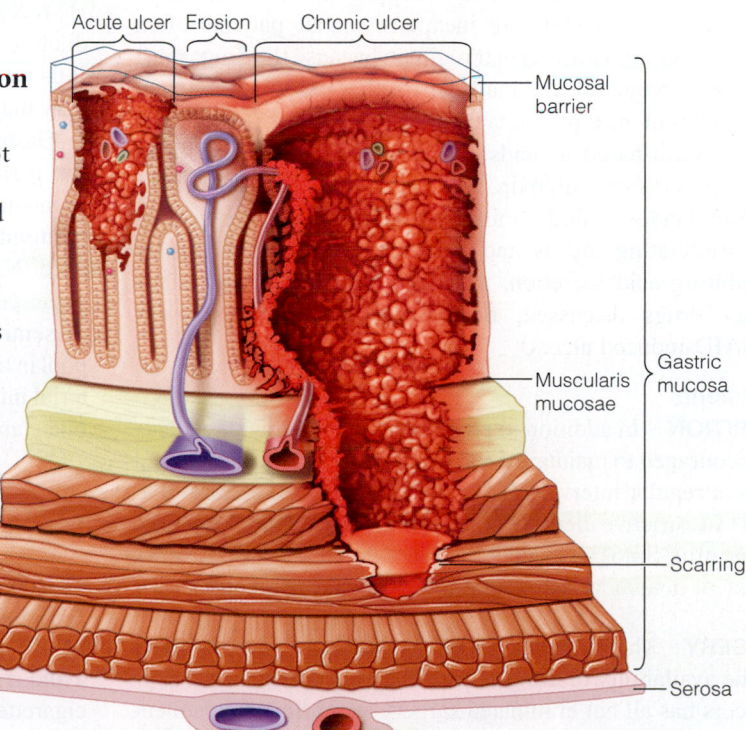

In patients who have NSAID-induced ulcers, the NSAID in use should be discontinued if at all possible. If this is not possible, twice-daily PPIs enable ulcer healing.

Medications that decrease gastric acid content include PPIs and the H_2-receptor antagonists.

- Proton-pump inhibitors bind the acid-secreting enzyme (H^+, K^+ ATPase) that functions as the proton pump, disabling it for up to 24 hours. These drugs are very effective, resulting in more than 90% ulcer healing after 4 weeks. Compared to the H_2-receptor blockers, the PPIs provide faster pain relief and more rapid ulcer healing.
- Histamine$_2$-receptor blockers inhibit histamine binding to the receptors on the gastric parietal cells to reduce acid secretion. These drugs are very well tolerated and have few serious side effects; however, drug interactions can occur. These drugs must be continued for 8 weeks or longer for ulcer healing.

Agents that protect the mucosa include sucralfate, bismuth, antacids, and prostaglandin analogs.

- Sucralfate binds to proteins in the ulcer base, forming a protective barrier against acid, bile, and pepsin. Sucralfate also stimulates the secretion of mucus, bicarbonate, and prostaglandin.
- Bismuth compounds (e.g., Pepto-Bismol, CBS, BBS) stimulate mucosal bicarbonate and prostaglandin production to promote ulcer healing, and likely provide a coating action that prevents further damage by HCl and pepsin. In addition, bismuth has an antibacterial action against *H. pylori*. There are very few side effects, other than constipation and a harmless darkening of stools and the tongue. When used in high doses for a prolonged period, bismuth compounds may be neurotoxic.
- Antacids stimulate gastric mucosal defenses, thereby aiding in ulcer healing. They provide rapid relief of ulcer symptoms, and are often used as needed to supplement other antiulcer medications. Antacids are inexpensive, but patients often have difficulty with a regular regimen because the drugs must be taken frequently and may cause either constipation (from the aluminum-type antacids) or diarrhea (from the magnesium-based antacids). Antacids also interfere with the absorption of iron, digoxin, some antibiotics, and other drugs.
- Prostaglandin analogs (misoprostol) promote ulcer healing by stimulating mucus and bicarbonate secretions and by inhibiting acid secretion. Although not as effective as the other drugs discussed, misoprostol is used to prevent NSAID-induced ulcers.

Treatments

NUTRITION In addition to pharmacologic treatment, patients are encouraged to maintain good nutrition, consuming balanced meals at regular intervals. It is important to teach patients that bland or restrictive diets are unnecessary. Mild alcohol intake is not harmful. Smoking should be discouraged, because it slows the rate of healing and increases the frequency of relapses.

SURGERY The identification of *H. pylori* as a cause of PUD and the availability of drugs to treat the infection and heal peptic ulcers has all but eliminated surgery as a primary treatment option for peptic ulcer disease. Surgery may be required to treat a complication of PUD, such as hemorrhage, perforation, or gastric outlet obstruction. See the section on gastric cancer for more information about gastric surgery and related nursing care.

Treatment of Complications

The patient hospitalized with a complication of PUD such as bleeding, gastrointestinal obstruction, or perforation and peritonitis requires additional interventions to restore homeostasis.

In hemorrhage associated with PUD, initial interventions focus on restoring and maintaining circulation. Normal saline, lactated Ringer's, or other balanced electrolyte solutions are administered intravenously to restore intravascular volume if signs of shock (tachycardia, hypotension, pallor, low urine output, and anxiety) are present. Whole blood or packed red blood cells may be administered to restore hemoglobin and hematocrit levels. A nasogastric tube is inserted to prevent aspiration of vomited gastric contents.

Endoscopy with direct injection of a clotting or sclerosing agent into the bleeding vessel may be performed. Laser photocoagulation, using light energy, or electrocoagulation, which uses electric current to generate heat, can also be done via endoscopy to seal bleeding vessels.

The patient is kept NPO until bleeding is controlled. Proton-pump inhibitors are administered intravenously (e.g., 40 mg of pantoprazole [Protonix] per intravenous push or admixture daily) to reduce the risk of rebleeding. Surgery may be necessary if medical measures are ineffective in controlling bleeding. Older adults who experience bleeding as a complication of PUD are more likely to rebleed or require surgery to control the hemorrhage. See page 646 for nursing care of the patient having gastric surgery.

Repeated inflammation, healing, scarring, edema, and muscle spasm can lead to gastric outlet (pyloric) obstruction. Initial treatment includes gastric decompression with nasogastric suction and administration of intravenous normal saline and potassium chloride to correct fluid and electrolyte imbalance. H_2-receptor blockers are given intravenously as well. Balloon dilation of the gastric outlet may be done via upper endoscopy. If these measures are unsuccessful in relieving obstruction, surgery may be required.

Gastric or duodenal perforation resulting in contamination of the peritoneum with gastrointestinal contents often requires immediate intervention to restore homeostasis and minimize peritonitis. Intravenous fluids maintain fluid and electrolyte balance. Nasogastric suction removes gastric contents and minimizes peritoneal contamination. Placing the patient in Fowler's or semi-Fowler's position allows peritoneal contaminants to pool in the pelvis. Intravenous antibiotics aggressively treat bacterial infection from intestinal flora. Laparoscopic surgery or an open laparotomy may be performed to close the perforation.

✍ Nursing Care

Health Promotion

Although it is difficult to predict which patients will develop peptic ulcer disease, promote health by advising patients to avoid risk factors such as excessive aspirin or NSAID use and cigarette smoking. In addition, encourage patients to seek treatment for manifestations of GERD or chronic gastritis, both of which are associated with *H. pylori* infection.

Assessment

Collect the following subjective and objective data when assessing the patient with peptic ulcer disease:

- *Health history:* Complaints of epigastric or left upper quadrant pain, heartburn, or discomfort; its character, severity, timing and relationship to eating; measures used for relief; nausea or vomiting, presence of bright blood or "coffee-grounds" material in vomitus; current medications including use of aspirin or other NSAIDs; cigarette smoking and use of alcohol or other drugs.
- *Physical examination:* General appearance including height and weight relationship; vital signs including orthostatic measurements; abdominal examination including shape and contour, bowel sounds, and tenderness to palpation; presence of obvious or occult blood in vomitus and stool.

Nursing Diagnoses and Interventions

The priorities of nursing care for the patient with peptic ulcer disease are reducing discomfort, maintaining nutritional status, and preventing or rapidly identifying and intervening for potential complications. See the accompanying Case Study & Nursing Care Plan.

Acute Pain

The pain of peptic ulcer disease is often predictable and preventable. Pain is typically experienced 2 to 4 hours after eating, as high levels of gastric acid and pepsin irritate the exposed mucosa. Measures to neutralize the acid, minimize its production, or protect the mucosa often relieve this pain, minimizing the need for analgesics.

- Assess pain, including location, type, severity, frequency, and duration, and its relationship to food intake or other contributing factors.

> **PRACTICE ALERT**
> Avoid making assumptions about pain. Acute pain may indicate a complication, such as perforation (often heralded by sudden, severe epigastric pain and a rigid, boardlike abdomen) or it may be totally unrelated to PUD (e.g., angina, gallbladder disease, or pancreatitis).

- Administer PPIs, H_2-receptor antagonists, antacids, or mucosal protective agents as ordered. Monitor for effectiveness and side effects or adverse reactions. *The pain associated with PUD is generally caused by the effect of gastric juices on exposed mucosal tissue. These medications reduce pain and promote healing by reducing acid production, neutralizing acid, or providing a barrier for the damaged mucosa.*
- Teach relaxation, stress reduction, and lifestyle management techniques. Refer for stress management counseling or classes as indicated. *Although there is no clear relationship between stress and PUD, measures to relieve stress and promote physical and emotional rest help reduce the perception of pain and may reduce ulcer genesis.*

Disturbed Sleep Pattern

Nighttime ulcer pain, which typically occurs between 1:00 and 3:00 AM, may disrupt the sleep cycle and result in inadequate rest. Anticipation of pain may lead to insomnia or other sleep disruptions.

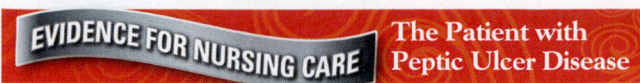

EVIDENCE FOR NURSING CARE — The Patient with Peptic Ulcer Disease

Selected resources that nurses may find helpful when planning evidence-based nursing care follow.

- University of Michigan Health System. (2005). *Peptic ulcer disease.* Ann Arbor, MI: University of Michigan Health System. Retrieved from http://www.guideline.gov/summary/summary.aspx?doc_id=7406&nbr=004376&string=peptic+AND+ulcer+AND+disease
- Stanley, A. J., Ashley, D., Dalton, H. R., Mowat, C., Gaya, D. R., Thompson, E., et al. (2009). Outpatient management of patients with low-risk upper-gastrointestinal haemorrhage: Multicentre validation and prospective evaluation. *Lancet, 373*(9657), 42–7. doi:10.1016/S0140-6736(08)61769-9
- Yang, Y., Lewis, J., Epstein, S., & Metz, D. (2006, December 27). Long-term proton pump inhibitor therapy and risk of hip fracture. *JAMA: Journal of the American Medical Association, 296*(24), 2947–2953.

- Stress the importance of taking medications as prescribed. *The bedtime dose of PPI or H_2-receptor blocker minimizes hydrochloric acid production during the night, reducing nighttime pain.*
- Instruct to limit food intake after the evening meal, eliminating any bedtime snack. *Eating before bed can stimulate the production of gastric acid and pepsin, increasing the likelihood of nighttime pain.*
- Encourage use of relaxation techniques and comfort measures such as soft music as needed to promote sleep. *Once the pain associated with PUD has been controlled, these measures help reduce anxiety and reestablish a normal sleep pattern.*

Imbalanced Nutrition: Less than Body Requirements

In an attempt to avoid discomfort, the patient with peptic ulcer disease may gradually reduce food intake, sometimes jeopardizing nutritional status. Anorexia and early satiety are additional problems associated with PUD.

- Assess current diet, including pattern of food intake, eating schedule, and foods that precipitate pain or are being avoided in anticipation of pain. *The patient may not realize the extent of self-imposed dietary limitations, especially if symptoms have persisted for an extended time. Assessment increases awareness and also helps identify the adequacy of nutrient intake.*
- Refer to a dietitian for meal planning to minimize PUD symptoms and meet nutritional needs. Consider normal eating patterns and preferences in meal planning. *Although no specific diet is recommended for PUD, patients should avoid foods that increase pain. Six small meals per day often help increase food tolerance and decrease postprandial discomfort.*
- Monitor for complaints of anorexia, fullness, nausea, and vomiting. Adjust dietary intake or medication schedule as indicated. *PUD and resultant scarring can lead to impaired gastric emptying, necessitating a treatment change.*

■ Monitor laboratory values for indications of anemia or other nutritional deficits. Monitor for therapeutic and side effects of treatment measures such as oral iron replacement. Instruct the patient taking oral iron replacement to avoid using an antacid within 1 to 2 hours of taking the iron preparation. *Anemia can result from poor nutrient absorption or chronic blood loss in patients with PUD. Oral iron supplements may cause GI distress, nausea, and vomiting; if these side effects are intolerable, notify the physician for a possible change of therapy. Antacids bind with oral iron preparations, blocking absorption.*

Risk for Bleeding

Erosion of a blood vessel with resultant hemorrhage is a significant risk for the patient with peptic ulcer disease. Acute bleeding can lead to hypovolemia and fluid volume deficit, which can lead to a decrease in cardiac output and impaired tissue perfusion.

■ Monitor stools and gastric drainage for overt and occult blood. Assess gastric drainage (vomitus or from a nasogastric tube) to estimate the amount and rapidity of hemorrhage. *Drainage is bright red with possible clots in acute hemorrhage; dark red or the color of coffee grounds when blood has been in the stomach for a period of time.* Hematochezia *(stool containing red blood and clots) is present in acute hemorrhage;* melena *(black, tarry stool) is an indicator of less acute bleeding. When small vessels are disrupted, bleeding may be slow and not overtly evident. With chronic or slow gastrointestinal bleeding, the risk of a fluid volume deficit is minimal; anemia and activity intolerance are more likely.*

■ Maintain intravenous therapy with fluid volume and electrolyte replacement solutions; administer whole blood or packed cells as ordered. *Both fluids and electrolytes are lost through vomiting, nasogastric drainage, and diarrhea in an episode of acute bleeding. To prevent shock, it is essential to maintain a blood volume and cardiac output sufficient to perfuse body tissues. Whole blood and packed cells replace both blood volume and red blood cells, providing additional oxygen-carrying capacity to meet cell needs.*

■ Insert a nasogastric tube and maintain its position and patency. Initially, measure and record gastric output every hour, then every 4 to 8 hours. *Nasogastric suction removes blood from the gastrointestinal tract, preventing vomiting and possible aspiration. Gastric output is replaced milliliter for milliliter with a balanced electrolyte solution to maintain homeostasis.*

■ Monitor hemoglobin and hematocrit, serum electrolytes, BUN, and creatinine values. Report abnormal findings. *Hemoglobin and hematocrit are lower than normal with acute or chronic GI bleeding. In acute hemorrhage, initial results may be within normal range because both cells and plasma are lost. Loss of fluids and electrolytes with gastric drainage and diarrhea will alter normal levels. Digestion and absorption of blood in the GI tract may result in elevated BUN and creatinine levels.*

■ Assess abdomen, including bowel sounds, distention, girth, and tenderness every 4 hours and record findings. *Borborygmi or hyperactive bowel sounds with abdominal tenderness are common with acute GI bleeding. Increased distention, increasing abdominal girth, absent bowel sounds, or extreme tenderness with a rigid, boardlike abdomen may indicate perforation.*

■ Maintain bed rest with the head of the bed elevated. Ensure safety. *Loss of blood volume may cause orthostatic hypotension with resultant syncope or dizziness upon standing.*

Using NANDA, NIC, and NOC

Linkages between a selected NANDA nursing diagnosis, NIC, and NOC for the patient with peptic ulcer disease are shown in the chart that follows.

Community-Based Care

Peptic ulcer disease is managed in home and community-based settings; only its complications typically require treatment in an acute care setting. Provide the following information when preparing the patient for home care:

■ Prescribed medication regimen, including desired and potential adverse effects
■ Importance of continuing therapy even when symptoms are relieved
■ Relationship between peptic ulcers and factors such as NSAID use and smoking. If indicated, refer to a smoking cessation clinic or program.

NANDA, NIC, AND NOC LINKAGES
The Patient with Peptic Ulcer Disease

NANDA | Ineffective Health Maintenance

↓

NIC | Bleeding Reduction: Gastrointestinal
Medication Management
Fluid/Electrolyte Management
Teaching: Disease Process

↓

NOC | Nutritional Status: Food and Fluid Intake
Hydration
Knowledge: Treatment Regimen
Treatment Behavior: Illness or Injury

Data from NANDA International. (2009). *Nursing diagnoses: Definitions & classification 2009–2011.* Oxford, UK: Wiley-Blackwell; Bulechek, G. M., Butcher, H., & Dochterman, J. (Eds.). (2008). *Nursing interventions classification (NIC)* (5th ed.). St. Louis, MO: Mosby; and Moorhead, S., Johnson, M., Mass, M., & Swanson, E. (Eds.). (2008). *Nursing outcomes classification (NOC)* (4th ed.). St. Louis, MO: Mosby.

CASE STUDY & NURSING CARE PLAN   A Patient with Peptic Ulcer Disease

Sean O'Donnell is a 47-year-old police officer who lives and works in a metropolitan area. Mr. O'Donnell has had "heartburn" and abdominal discomfort for years, but thought it went along with his job. Last year, after becoming weak, light-headed, and short of breath, he was found to be anemic and was diagnosed as having a duodenal ulcer. He took omeprazole (Prilosec) and ferrous sulfate for 3 months before stopping both, saying he had "never felt better in his life." Mr. O'Donnell has now been admitted to the hospital with active upper GI bleeding.

ASSESSMENT

Rachel Clark is Mr. O'Donnell's admitting nurse and case manager. On initial assessment, Mr. O'Donnell is alert and oriented, though very apprehensive about his condition. Skin pale and cool; BP 136/78, P 98; abdomen distended and tender with hyperactive bowel sounds; 200 mL bright red blood obtained on nasogastric tube insertion. Hemoglobin 8.2 g/dL and hematocrit 23% on admission. Mr. O'Donnell is taken to the endoscopy lab where his bleeding is controlled using laser photocoagulation. On his return to the nursing unit, he receives two units of packed RBCs and intravenous fluids to restore blood volume. A 5-day course of high-dose oral omeprazole (40 mg bid) is ordered to prevent rebleeding, and Mr. O'Donnell is allowed to begin a clear liquid diet 24 hours after his endoscopy. Tissue biopsy obtained during endoscopy confirms the presence of *H. pylori* infection.

DIAGNOSES

- *Deficient Fluid Volume* related to acutely bleeding duodenal ulcer
- *Risk for Injury* related to acute blood loss
- *Fear* related to threat to well-being
- *Ineffective Self Health Management* related to lack of knowledge regarding PUD and its treatment

EXPECTED OUTCOMES

- Maintains normal blood pressure, pulse, and urine output (> 30 mL/h)
- Remains free of injury
- Seeks information to reduce fear
- Identifies and uses coping strategies to manage fear
- Describes prescribed therapeutic regimen
- Verbalizes ability to manage prescribed regimen

PLANNING AND IMPLEMENTATION

- Place call light within reach and encourage to ask for help when getting up or ambulating. Remind to rise slowly from lying to sitting and sitting to standing.
- Discuss situation and provide information about all procedures and treatments.
- Reassure about the effectiveness of treatment in reducing the risk for further bleeding.
- Discuss current and planned treatment measures; stress the importance of completing the prescribed treatment to reduce the risk of further ulcer development.
- Encourage to avoid using aspirin or NSAIDs in the future; suggest alternative medications such as acetaminophen.
- Discuss stress reduction techniques and refer for stress reduction counseling or workshops as indicated.

EVALUATION

Mr. O'Donnell is discharged 48 hours after admission. He has had no further evidence of bleeding, and has resumed a regular diet. His hemoglobin and hematocrit remain low, and he has a prescription for ferrous sulfate. He will complete the prescribed high-dose omeprazole regimen at home, then begin treatment with omeprazole, amoxicillin, and clarithromycin (Biaxin) to eradicate the *H. pylori* infection detected during endoscopy. After 2 weeks of this regimen, he will continue taking omeprazole at bedtime for 4 to 8 weeks. He verbalizes a good understanding of his treatment and the importance of completing the entire regimen. Mr. O'Donnell expresses concern about his ability to "keep his cool on the inside" when under stress. Ms. Clark, his case manager, gives him the names of several resources to help with stress management in case he wants help.

CRITICAL THINKING IN THE NURSING PROCESS

1. How does *H. pylori* infection contribute to the development of peptic ulcers?
2. Describe the physiologic responses to fear and anxiety. Why is it important to alleviate fear and its physical consequences in patients with PUD?
3. What suggestions can you make to help Mr. O'Donnell manage his complex treatment regimen during the next 3 months?
4. Develop a teaching plan that includes stress reduction techniques Mr. O'Donnell can use while performing his duties as a police officer.

See Evaluating Your Response in Appendix C.

- Importance of avoiding aspirin and other NSAIDs; stress the necessity of reading the labels of over-the-counter medications for possible aspirin content
- Manifestations of complications that should be reported to the care provider, including increased abdominal pain or distention, vomiting, black or tarry stools, light-headedness, or fainting
- Stress and lifestyle management techniques that may help prevent exacerbation. Refer to resources for stress management, such as classes, counseling, and formal or informal groups.

The Patient with Gastritis

Gastritis, inflammation of the stomach lining, results from irritation of the gastric mucosa. Gastritis is common, and may be caused by a variety of factors. The most common form of gastritis, *acute gastritis*, is generally a benign, self-limiting disorder associated with the ingestion of gastric irritants such as aspirin, alcohol, caffeine, or foods contaminated with certain bacteria. Manifestations of acute gastritis may range from asymptomatic to mild heartburn to severe gastric distress, vomiting, and bleeding with hematemesis (vomiting blood).

Chronic gastritis is a separate group of disorders characterized by progressive and irreversible changes in the gastric mucosa (Porth & Matfin, 2009). Chronic gastritis is more common in the elderly, chronic alcoholics, and cigarette smokers. When symptoms of chronic gastritis occur, they are often vague, ranging from a feeling of heaviness in the epigastric region after meals to gnawing, burning, ulcer-like epigastric pain unrelieved by antacids.

Pathophysiology

Acute Gastritis

Acute gastritis is characterized by disruption of the mucosal barrier by a local irritant. This disruption allows hydrochloric acid and pepsin to come into contact with the gastric tissue, resulting in irritation, inflammation, and superficial erosions. The gastric mucosa rapidly regenerates, generally making acute gastritis a self-limiting disorder, with resolution and healing occurring within several days.

The ingestion of aspirin or other NSAIDs, corticosteroids, alcohol, and caffeine is commonly associated with the development of acute gastritis. Accidental or purposeful ingestion of a corrosive alkali (such as ammonia, lye, Lysol, and other cleaning agents) or acid leads to severe inflammation and possible necrosis of the stomach. Gastric perforation, hemorrhage, and peritonitis are possible results. Iatrogenic causes of acute gastritis include radiation therapy and administration of certain chemotherapeutic agents.

Erosive Gastritis

A severe form of acute gastritis, **erosive (stress-induced) gastritis**, occurs as a complication of other life-threatening conditions such as shock, severe trauma, major surgery, sepsis, burns, or head injury. When these erosions follow a major burn, they are called **Curling's ulcers**, after Thomas Curling, a British physician, who first described them in 1842. When stress ulcers occur following head injury or CNS surgery, they are referred to as **Cushing's ulcers**, after Harvey Cushing, a U.S. surgeon.

The primary mechanisms leading to erosive gastritis appear to be ischemia of the gastric mucosa resulting from sympathetic vasoconstriction, and tissue injury due to gastric acid. As a result, multiple superficial erosions of the gastric mucosa develop. Maintaining the gastric pH at greater than 3.5 and inhibiting gastric acid secretion with medications help prevent erosive gastritis.

MANIFESTATIONS   The patient with acute gastritis may have mild symptoms such as **anorexia** (loss of appetite), or mild epigastric discomfort relieved by belching or defecating. More severe manifestations include abdominal pain, nausea, and vomiting. Gastric bleeding may occur, with hematemesis or melena (black, tarry stool that contains blood). Erosive gastritis is not typically associated with pain. The initial symptom often is painless gastric bleeding occurring 2 or more days after the initial stressor. Bleeding typically is minimal, but can be massive. Corrosive gastritis can cause severe bleeding, signs of shock, and an *acute abdomen* (severely painful, rigid, boardlike abdomen) if perforation occurs. See the following Manifestations box.

MANIFESTATIONS of Acute and Chronic Gastritis

ACUTE GASTRITIS

Gastrointestinal	Systemic
■ Anorexia	■ Possible shock
■ Nausea and vomiting	
■ Hematemesis	
■ Melena	
■ Abdominal pain	

CHRONIC GASTRITIS

Gastrointestinal	Systemic
■ Vague discomfort after eating; may be asymptomatic	■ Anemia
	■ Fatigue

Chronic Gastritis

Unrelated to acute gastritis, chronic gastritis is a progressive disorder that begins with superficial inflammation and gradually leads to atrophy of gastric tissues. The initial stage is characterized by superficial changes in the gastric mucosa and a decrease in mucus. As the disease evolves, glands of the gastric mucosa are disrupted and destroyed. The inflammatory process involves deep portions of the mucosa, which thins and atrophies. There are several types of chronic gastritis; *H. pylori* gastritis and autoimmune gastritis are the most commonly seen.

H. pylori gastritis is the most common form of chronic gastritis. Its incidence increases with age, and is significantly higher in developing countries than in industrialized countries (Porth & Matfin, 2009). It is caused by chronic infection of the gastric mucosa by *H. pylori*, a gram-negative spiral bacterium. *H. pylori* infection causes inflammation of the gastric mucosa, with infiltration by neutrophils and lymphocytes. The outermost layer of gastric mucosa thins and atrophies, providing a less effective barrier against the autodigestive properties of hydrochloric acid and pepsin.

Infection with *H. pylori* also is associated with peptic ulcer disease and an increased risk of developing gastric cancer.

Autoimmune gastritis is a less common form of chronic gastritis, accounting for about 10% of patients with chronic gastritis (Porth & Matfin, 2009). In autoimmune gastritis, the body produces antibodies to parietal cells and intrinsic factor. These antibodies destroy gastric mucosal cells, resulting in tissue atrophy and the loss of hydrochloric acid and pepsin secretion. Production of intrinsic factor also is affected in most cases. Because intrinsic factor is required for the absorption of vitamin B_{12}, this immune response results in pernicious anemia. For further discussion of pernicious anemia, ∞ see Chapter 33.

MANIFESTATIONS   Chronic gastritis is often asymptomatic until atrophy is sufficiently advanced to interfere with digestion and gastric emptying. The patient may complain of vague gastric distress, epigastric heaviness after meals, or ulcer-like symptoms. These symptoms typically are not relieved by antacids. In addition, the patient may experience fatigue and other symptoms of anemia. If intrinsic factor is lacking, paresthesias and other neurologic manifestations of vitamin B_{12} deficiency may be present. See the previous Manifestations box.

Interdisciplinary Care

Acute gastritis is usually diagnosed by the history and clinical presentation. In contrast, the vague symptoms of chronic gastritis may require more extensive diagnostic testing.

Patients with acute and chronic gastritis are generally managed in community settings. The patient requires acute care only when nausea and vomiting are severe enough to interfere with normal fluid and electrolyte balance and nutritional status. If hemorrhage results, surgical intervention may be required.

Diagnosis

Diagnostic tests that may be ordered for the patient with gastritis include the following:

■ *Testing* for *H. pylori* infection, including urea breath tests, serologic testing, and fecal antigen testing.

- *Gastric analysis* to assess hydrochloric acid secretion. Secretion may be decreased in patients with chronic gastritis.
- *Hemoglobin, hematocrit*, and *red blood cell (RBC) indices* are evaluated for evidence of anemia. The patient with gastritis may develop pernicious anemia because of parietal cell destruction, or iron-deficiency anemia because of chronic blood loss.
- *Serum vitamin B$_{12}$ levels* are measured to evaluate for possible pernicious anemia. Normal values for vitamin B$_{12}$ are 200 to 1000 pg/mL, with lower levels seen in older adults.
- *Upper endoscopy* may be done to inspect the gastric mucosa for changes, identify areas of bleeding, and obtain tissue for biopsy. Bleeding sites may be treated with electro- or laser coagulation or injected with a sclerosing agent during the procedure.

∞ See Chapter 21 for patient preparation and teaching related to diagnostic tests for upper GI disorders.

Medications

Drugs such as a PPI, H$_2$-receptor blocker, or sucralfate may be ordered to prevent or treat acute stress gastritis. PPIs and H$_2$ receptor blockers reduce the amount or effects of hydrochloric acid on the gastric mucosa. Lansoprazole (Prevacid), esomeprazole (Nexium), and omeprazole (Prilosec) are examples of PPIs. H$_2$-receptor blockers include cimetidine (Tagamet), ranitidine (Zantac), famotidine (Pepcid), and nizatidine (Axid). These drugs also are available in nonprescription strength. Sucralfate (Carafate) works locally to prevent the damaging effects of acid and pepsin on gastric tissue. It does not neutralize or reduce acid secretion. Nursing implications for drugs commonly used in managing gastritis are included in the Medication Administration box on pages 625–626.

Chronic *H. pylori* infection may be treated using combination therapy that includes two antibiotics (such as metronidazole, amoxicillin, clarithromycin, or tetracycline), a bismuth compound, and possibly a PPI. In some cases, eradication of the infection is not warranted, and the patient is treated symptomatically.

Treatments

In acute gastritis, gastrointestinal tract rest is provided by 6 to 12 hours of NPO status, then slow reintroduction of clear liquids (broth, tea, gelatin, carbonated beverages), followed by ingestion of heavier liquids (cream soups, puddings, milk), and finally a gradual reintroduction of solid food.

If nausea and vomiting threaten fluid and electrolyte balance, intravenous fluids and electrolytes are ordered.

GASTRIC LAVAGE Acute gastritis resulting from ingestion of a poisonous or corrosive substance (acid or strong alkali) is treated with immediate dilution and removal of the substance. Vomiting is not induced because it might further damage the esophagus and possibly the trachea; instead, gastric lavage, washing out of the stomach contents, is performed. See Procedure 23–1.

COMPLEMENTARY THERAPIES Complementary therapies such as herbal remedies or aromatherapy may be appropriate to recommend for patients with gastritis. Refer the patient to a healthcare provider trained in natural and herbal remedies or to an aromatherapist for an individualized treatment plan. Recommendations may include the following:

- Chamomile tea or the essential oil used in aromatherapy
- Garlic; one clove chopped fine and taken daily at bedtime
- Ginger, powdered or in capsules or made into a tea taken before or after meals
- Mint oil aromatherapy via a diffuser, in a bath, or diluted with a carrier oil and used for a soothing massage

∞ Nursing Care

Health Promotion

Teach all patients and community members about measures to prevent acute gastritis. Food contaminated with bacteria is a significant cause of acute gastritis. Discuss food safety measures such as fully cooking meats and egg products, and promptly refrigerating foods after cooking to avoid bacterial growth. Stress that food contaminated with potential pathogens often looks, smells, and tastes good, making it difficult to identify. Teach patients to abstain from eating or drinking anything during an acute episode of vomiting, then reintroduce clear liquids gradually once vomiting has stopped (2 to 4 hours after the last episode of vomiting). Suggest using liquids such as Pedialyte or a sport drink to replace lost electrolytes and fluid. Instruct patients to avoid milk and milk products until they easily tolerate clear liquids and solid foods such as dry toast or saltine crackers.

Assessment

Assessment data to collect for patients with acute or chronic gastritis include the following:

- *Health history:* Current symptoms and their duration; relieving and aggravating factors; history of ingestion of toxins, contaminated food, alcohol, aspirin, or NSAIDs; other medications.
- *Physical examination:* Vital signs including orthostatic vitals if indicated; peripheral pulses; general appearance; abdominal assessment including appearance, bowel sounds, and tenderness.

Nursing Diagnoses and Interventions

In planning and implementing nursing care for the patient with acute or chronic gastritis, consider both the direct effects of the disorder on the gastrointestinal system and nutritional status as well as its effects on lifestyle and psychosocial integrity. This section focuses on problems related to nausea and anorexia associated with gastritis.

Nausea

Nausea, vomiting, and abdominal distress are the primary manifestations of acute gastritis. Patients with chronic gastritis often experience anorexia and nausea that can interfere with food intake and nutritional status.

- Monitor subjective complaints of nausea. *Nausea is a subjective sensation best described by the patient.*
- For the patient with acute gastritis, monitor vital signs, skin turgor and condition, and weight. Maintain accurate intake and output records. Monitor amount, color, and specific

gravity of urine. *Nausea and vomiting associated with acute gastritis can significantly affect food and fluid intake, leading to dehydration.*

■ Administer antiemetic medication as ordered, prior to meals and before treatments or procedures known to stimulate nausea. *Preventing nausea is particularly important for patients receiving chemotherapy to avoid the association between the treatment and nausea.*

■ Instruct to consume small quantities of clear fluids and dry foods at separate times. *Separating the intake of dry foods and fluids helps reduce the nausea stimulus.*

Imbalanced Nutrition: Less than Body Requirements

Manifestations of chronic gastritis may lead to reduced food intake and malnutrition. The patient often associates these unpleasant sensations with eating, and may gradually reduce food intake. Associated anorexia also contributes to poor food intake.

■ Monitor and record food and fluid intake and any abnormal losses (such as vomiting). *Careful monitoring can help in developing a dietary plan to meet the caloric needs of the patient.*

■ Monitor weight and laboratory studies such as serum albumin, hemoglobin, and RBC indices. *Weights and laboratory values provide data regarding nutritional status and the effectiveness of interventions.*

■ Arrange for dietary consultation to determine caloric and nutrient needs and develop a dietary plan. Consider food preferences and tolerances in menu planning. *A diet high in protein, vitamins, and minerals may be prescribed to meet nutritional needs of the patient with chronic gastritis. In addition, specific food intolerances may need to be considered. Planning to include preferred foods in the diet helps ensure consumption of the prescribed diet.*

■ Provide nutritional supplements between meals or frequent small feedings as needed. *Many patients with chronic gastritis tolerate small, frequent feedings better than three large meals per day.*

■ Maintain tube feedings or parenteral nutrition as ordered. ∞ Refer to Chapter 22 for further information on enteral and parenteral feedings.

Community-Based Care

Because acute or chronic gastritis is usually managed in community-based settings, teaching is vital. For the patient with acute gastritis, teaching focuses on managing acute symptoms, reintroducing fluids and solid foods, identifying indicators of possible complications (e.g., continued vomiting, signs of fluid and electrolyte imbalance), and preventing future episodes.

Provide the following information for patients with chronic gastritis:

■ Maintaining optimal nutrition
■ Helpful dietary modifications
■ Using prescribed medications
■ Avoiding known gastric irritants, such as aspirin, alcohol, and cigarette smoking

Referral to smoking cessation classes or programs to treat alcohol abuse may be necessary.

The Patient with Cancer of the Stomach

Worldwide, cancer of the stomach is the most common cancer (after skin cancer), but it is less common in the United States.

> **FAST FACTS**
> ■ An estimated 21,130 new cases of stomach cancer are diagnosed annually in the United States (ACS, 2009).
> ■ Its incidence is highest in Hispanics, African Americans, and Asian Americans.
> ■ Men are affected nearly twice as often as women.

Older adults are more likely to develop gastric cancer: The mean age at time of diagnosis is 63. People in lower socioeconomic groups are more often affected by gastric cancer.

Risk Factors

H. pylori infection is a major risk factor for cancer of the distal portion of the stomach; 35% to 89% of cases can be attributed to this infection. Other risk factors are a genetic predisposition, chronic gastritis, pernicious anemia, gastric polyps, and carcinogenic factors in the diet (such as smoked foods and nitrates). Achlorhydria, a lack of hydrochloric acid in the stomach, is a known risk factor. The risk for gastric cancer also is increased in people who have had a partial gastric resection.

Pathophysiology

Adenocarcinoma, which involves the mucus-producing cells of the stomach, is the most common form of gastric cancer. These carcinomas may arise anywhere on the mucosal surface of the stomach but are most frequently found in the distal portion. More than half of all gastric cancers occur in the antrum or pyloric region (Porth & Matfin, 2009). Gastric cancer begins as a localized lesion (*in situ*), then progresses to involve the

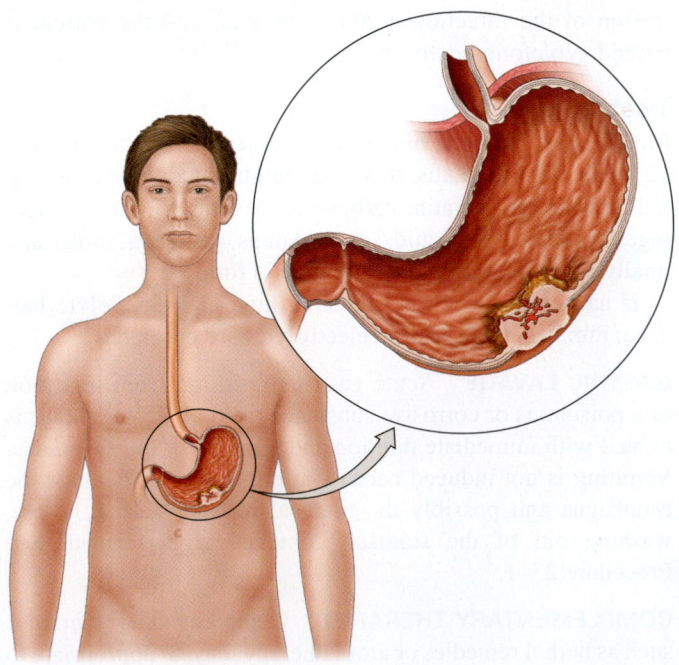

Figure 23–10 ■ Gastric cancer affecting the antrum of the stomach.
Source: Robert Margulies/Phototake NYC.

mucosa or submucosa (early gastric carcinoma). Lesions may spread by direct extension to tissues surrounding the stomach, the liver in particular. The lesion may ulcerate or appear as a polypoid (polyp-like) mass (Figure 23–10 ■). Lymph node involvement and metastasis occur early due to the rich blood and lymphatic supply to the stomach. Metastatic lesions are often found in the liver, lungs, ovaries, and peritoneum.

Manifestations

Gastric cancer has few manifestations. Unfortunately, the disease is often quite advanced and metastases are usually present at the time of diagnosis. Early symptoms are vague, including feelings of early satiety, anorexia, indigestion, and possibly vomiting. The patient may experience ulcer-like pain unrelieved by antacids, typically occurring after meals. As the disease progresses, weight loss occurs, and the patient may be *cachectic* (in very poor health and malnourished) at the time of diagnosis. An abdominal mass may be palpable, and occult blood may be present in the stool, indicating gastrointestinal bleeding.

Interdisciplinary Care

Diagnosis

Anemia detected by a CBC often is the first indication of gastric cancer. An upper GI x-ray with barium swallow is useful to identify lesions, and ultrasound or other radiologic techniques may identify a mass. Upper endoscopy with visualization and biopsy of the lesion provides the definitive diagnosis.

Surgery

When gastric cancer is identified prior to the development of metastasis, surgical removal of part or all of the stomach and regional lymph nodes is the treatment of choice. **Partial gastrectomy** involves removal of a portion of the stomach, usually the distal half to two-thirds. In partial gastrectomy, the surgeon constructs an anastomosis from the remainder of the stomach directly to the duodenum or to the proximal jejunum. The *gastroduodenostomy* (Billroth I) and the *gastrojejunostomy* (Billroth II) are commonly used partial gastrectomy procedures (Figures 23–11A and B ■).

A **total gastrectomy**, removal of the entire stomach, may be done for diffuse cancer that is spread throughout the

gastric mucosa but limited to the stomach. In a total gastrectomy, the surgeon constructs an anastomosis from the esophagus to the duodenum or jejunum. Total gastrectomy with *esophagojejunostomy* is illustrated in Figure 23–11C.

Nursing care of the patient who has undergone gastric surgery is outlined in the following box.

COMPLICATIONS Several long-term complications may develop following gastrectomy procedures. **Dumping syndrome** is the most common problem. It may follow a partial gastrectomy with duodenal or jejunal anastomosis. When the pylorus has been resected or bypassed, a hypertonic, undigested food bolus may rapidly enter the duodenum or jejunum. Water is pulled into the lumen of the intestine by the hyperosmolar character of the chyme, resulting in decreased blood volume and intestinal dilation. Peristalsis is stimulated, and intestinal motility is increased.

Early symptoms of dumping syndrome occur within 5 to 30 minutes after eating. These symptoms result from intestinal dilation, peristaltic stimulation, and hypovolemia caused by undigested food in the proximal small intestine. Manifestations include nausea with possible vomiting, epigastric pain with cramping and *borborygmi* (loud, hyperactive bowel sounds), and diarrhea. Systemic symptoms from the hypovolemia and reflex sympathetic stimulation include tachycardia, orthostatic hypotension, dizziness, flushing, and diaphoresis.

The entry of hyperosmolar chyme into the jejunum also causes a rapid rise in the blood glucose. This stimulates the release of an excessive amount of insulin, leading to hypoglycemic symptoms 2 to 3 hours after the meal. The pathogenesis and clinical manifestations of dumping syndrome are represented in Figure 23–12 ■. Dumping syndrome is typically self-limiting, lasting 6 to 12 months after surgery; however, a small percentage of people continue to experience long-term symptoms.

Dumping syndrome is managed primarily by a dietary pattern that delays gastric emptying and allows smaller boluses of undigested food to enter the intestine. Meals should be small and more frequent. Liquids and solids are taken at separate times instead of together during a meal. The amount of proteins and fats in the diet is increased, because they exit the stomach more slowly than carbohydrates. Carbohydrates, especially simple sugars, are reduced. The patient is instructed to rest in a recumbent or semirecumbent

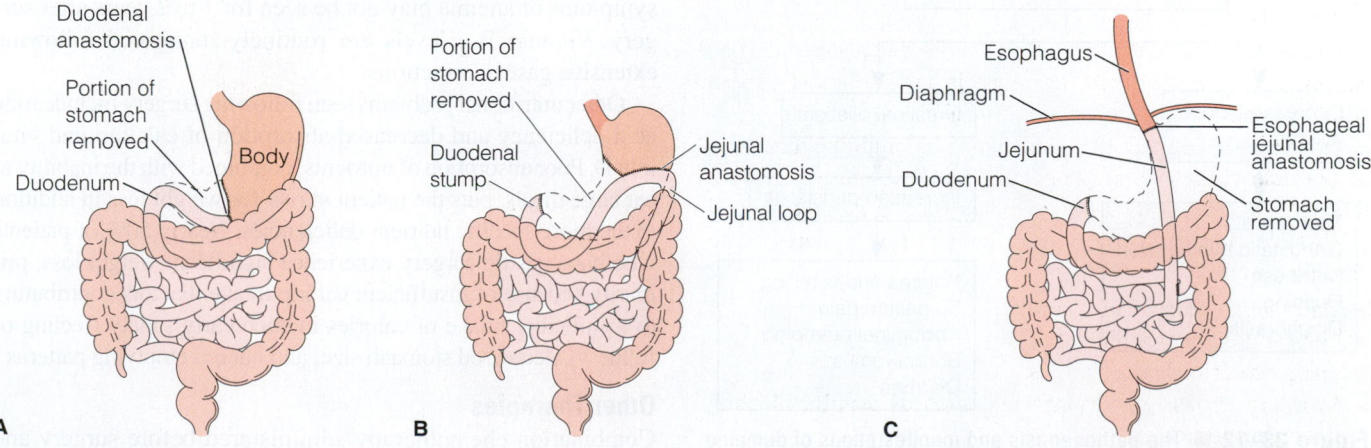

Figure 23–11 ■ Partial and total gastrectomy procedures. *A*, Partial gastrectomy with anastomosis to the duodenum. *B*, Partial gastrectomy with anastomosis to the jejunum. *C*, Total gastrectomy with anastomosis of the esophagus to the jejunum.

NURSING CARE OF THE PATIENT   Having Gastric Surgery

PREOPERATIVE NURSING CARE

- ∞ See Chapter 4 for routine preoperative care and teaching.
- Insert a nasogastric tube if ordered preoperatively. *Although it is often inserted in the surgical suite just prior to surgery, the nasogastric tube may be placed preoperatively to remove secretions and empty stomach contents.*

POSTOPERATIVE NURSING CARE

- Provide routine care for the surgical patient as outlined in ∞ Chapter 4.
- Assess position and patency of nasogastric tube, connecting it to low suction. Gently irrigate with sterile normal saline if tube becomes clogged. *The nasogastric tube will be placed in surgery to avoid disruption of the gastric suture lines and should be well secured. If repositioning or tube replacement is needed, notify the surgeon. Patency must be maintained to keep the stomach decompressed, reducing pressure on sutures.*
- Assess color, amount, and odor of gastric drainage, noting any changes in these parameters or the presence of clots or bright bleeding. *Initial drainage is bright red. It becomes dark, then clear or greenish-yellow over the first 2 to 3 days. A change in the color, amount, or odor may indicate a complication such as hemorrhage, intestinal obstruction, or infection.*
- Maintain intravenous fluids while nasogastric suction is in place. *The patient on nasogastric suction is not only unable to take oral food and fluids but also is losing electrolyte-rich fluid through the nasogastric tube. If replacement fluid and electrolytes are not maintained, the patient is at risk for dehydration; imbalances of sodium, potassium, and chloride; and metabolic alkalosis.*

- Provide antiulcer and antibiotic therapy as ordered. *These medications may be ordered for the postoperative patient, depending on the procedure performed. Antibiotic therapy is a common preventive measure for infection that may result from contamination of the abdominal cavity with gastric contents.*
- Monitor bowel sounds and abdominal distention. *Bowel sounds indicate resumption of peristalsis. Increasing distention may indicate third spacing, obstruction, or infection.*
- Resume oral food and fluids as ordered. Initial feedings are clear liquids, progressing to full liquids and then frequent small feedings of regular foods. Monitor bowel sounds and for abdominal distention frequently during this period. *Oral feedings are reintroduced slowly to minimize trauma to the suture lines by possible gastric distension.*
- Encourage ambulation. *Ambulation stimulates peristalsis.*
- Begin discharge planning and teaching. Consult with a dietitian for diet instructions and menu planning; reinforce teaching. Teach the patient about potential postoperative complications, such as abdominal abscess, dumping syndrome, postprandial hypoglycemia, or pernicious anemia. Also, teach the patient to recognize signs and symptoms and preventive measures. *The patient's gastric capacity is reduced after partial gastrectomy, necessitating a corresponding reduction in meal size. Changes in gastric emptying and reduction in gastric secretions may change the patient's tolerance for many foods, requiring slow reintroduction of these foods. Dumping syndrome, postprandial hypoglycemia, and pernicious anemia are possible long-term complications of partial gastrectomy. For most patients, dietary modifications can control both dumping syndrome and postprandial hypoglycemia.*

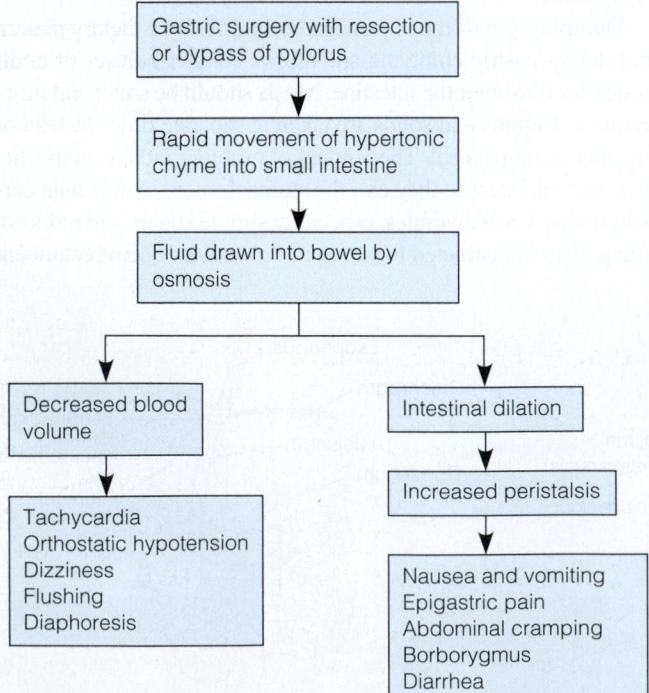

Figure 23–12 ■ The pathogenesis and manifestations of dumping syndrome.

position for 30 to 60 minutes after meals. Anticholinergics, sedatives, and antispasmodics may be prescribed.

Anemia may be a chronic problem after a major gastric resection. Iron is absorbed primarily in the duodenum and proximal jejunum; rapid gastric emptying or a gastrojejunostomy may interfere with adequate absorption.

The cells of the stomach produce intrinsic factor, required for the absorption of vitamin B_{12}. Vitamin B_{12} deficiency leads to pernicious anemia. Because of hepatic stores of vitamin B_{12}, symptoms of anemia may not be seen for 1 to 2 years after surgery. Vitamin B_{12} levels are routinely monitored following extensive gastric resections.

Other nutritional problems seen following surgery include folic acid deficiency and decreased absorption of calcium and vitamin D. Poor absorption of nutrients, combined with the inability to eat large meals, puts the patient at risk for weight loss in addition to the more specific nutrient deficiencies. Nearly 50% of patients who have gastric surgery experience significant weight loss, primarily because of insufficient calorie intake. Factors contributing to insufficient intake of calories include early satiety (feeling of fullness), decreased stomach size, and altered emptying patterns.

Other Therapies

Combination chemotherapy administered before surgery and in combination with radiation therapy after surgery has been found to reduce tumor recurrence and prolong survival (Fauci

NURSING CARE OF THE PATIENT With a Gastrostomy or Jejunostomy Tube

Patients who have had extensive gastric surgery or who require long-term enteral feedings to maintain nutrition may have a gastrostomy or jejunostomy tube inserted.

PROCEDURE
Gastrostomy tubes are surgically placed in the stomach, with the stoma in the epigastric region of the abdomen (see Figure 23–13 ■). Jejunostomy tubes are placed in the proximal jejunum. Immediately following the procedure, the tube may be connected to low suction or plugged. If the patient has been receiving tube feedings, these may be reinitiated shortly after tube placement.

NURSING CARE
- Assess tube placement by aspirating stomach contents and checking the pH of aspirate to determine gastric or intestinal placement. A pH of 5 or less indicates gastric placement; the pH is generally 7 or higher with intestinal placement. *Recent studies show auscultation to be ineffective in determining feeding tube placement. Measuring the pH of aspirate from the tube is more reliable as a means of determining tube placement.*
- Inspect the skin surrounding the insertion site for healing, redness, swelling, and the presence of any drainage. If drainage is present, note the color, amount, consistency, and odor. *Changes in the insertion site, drainage, or lack of healing may indicate an infection.*
- Assess the abdomen for distention, bowel sounds, and tenderness *to evaluate functioning of the gastrointestinal tract.*
- Until the stoma is well healed, use sterile technique for dressing changes and site care. Clean technique is appropriate for use once healing is complete. *Sterile technique reduces the risk of wound contamination by pathogens that can lead to infection. Once healing has occurred, clean technique is acceptable because the gastrointestinal tract is not a sterile body cavity.*
- Wearing clean gloves, remove old dressing. Cleanse the site with saline or soap and water, and rinse as appropriate. A well-healed stoma may be cleansed in the shower with the tube clamped or plugged. Pat dry with 4 × 4 gauze pads, and allow to air dry. Apply Stomahesive, karaya, or other protective agents around tube as needed to protect the skin. *Gastric acid and other wound drainage is irritating to the skin. Meticulous care is important to maintain the integrity of the skin surrounding the stoma.*
- Redress the wound using a stoma dressing or folded 4 × 4 gauze pads. *Do not cut gauze pads, because threads may enter the wound, causing irritation and increasing the risk of inflammation.*
- Irrigate the tube with 30 to 50 mL of water, and clean the tube inside and out as indicated or ordered. Soft gastric tubes may require cleaning of the inner lumen with a special brush to maintain patency. *Tube feeding formulas may coat the inside of the gastrostomy tube and eventually cause it to become occluded. Regular irrigation with water and brushing as indicated maintain tube patency.*
- Provide mouth care or remind the patient to do so. *When feedings are not being taken orally, the usual stimulus to do mouth care is lost. In addition, salivary fluids may not be as abundant, and oral mucous membranes may become dry and cracked.*
- If indicated, teach the patient and family how to care for the tube and feedings. Refer to a home health agency or visiting nurse for support and reinforcement of learning. *Gastrostomy tubes are often in place long term. When the patient and family are able to assume care, independence and self-image are enhanced.*

et al., 2008). For the patient with more advanced disease, treatment is palliative and may include surgery, radiation therapy, and chemotherapy. These patients may require a gastrostomy or jejunostomy feeding tube (Figure 23–13). See the box on for nursing care of the patient with a gastrostomy or jejunostomy tube.

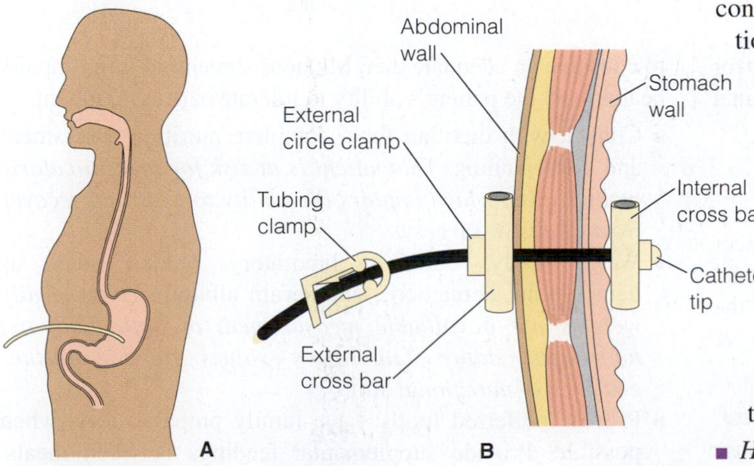

Figure 23–13 ■ Gastrostomy. *A,* Gastrostomy tube placement. *B,* The tube is fixed against both the abdomen and stomach walls by cross bars.

Because gastric cancer is generally advanced by the time of diagnosis, the prognosis is poor. The 5-year survival rate of all patients treated for gastric carcinoma is 10%.

Nursing Care

Health Promotion
Although the exact causes of gastric cancer are unknown, contributing factors such as *H. pylori* infection and consumption of foods preserved with nitrates have been identified. To reduce their risk of developing gastric cancer, encourage patients with known *H. pylori* infection to complete the prescribed course of treatment and verify that it has eradicated the infection. With all patients, discuss the relationship between gastric cancer and consumption of foods preserved with nitrates (such as bacon and other processed meats), and encourage limited consumption of these products.

Assessment
Assessment data related to gastric cancer include the following:
- *Health history:* Manifestations such as anorexia, early satiety, indigestion, or vomiting; epigastric pain after meals; recent unintentional weight loss.

CASE STUDY & NURSING CARE PLAN   A Patient with Gastric Cancer

George Harvey is a 61-year-old estate attorney who lives with his wife, Harriet. For the last 3 months, Mr. Harvey has had increasing anorexia and difficulty eating. He has lost 10 pounds. His physician has diagnosed gastric cancer, and Mr. Harvey is admitted for a partial gastrectomy and gastrojejunostomy. The oncologist has recommended postoperative chemotherapy and radiation. Mr. Harvey reports that the doctor told him "that will give me the best chance for cure."

ASSESSMENT

On admission before surgery, Mr. Harvey tells his nurse, Lauren Walsh, that he has eaten very little in the past few weeks. He asks, "What will happen to my wife if something happens to me? I'm afraid this cancer will get me." Mr. Harvey weighs 147 lb (67 kg) and is 72 inches (183 cm) tall. He is pale and thin; his vital signs are BP 148/86, P 92, R 18, and T 97.8°F PO. A firm mass is palpable in the left epigastric region. The rest of his physical assessment data are within normal limits. Mr. Harvey's hemoglobin is 12.8 g/dL, hematocrit is 39%, and serum albumin level is 3.2 g/dL, indicating that he is mildly malnourished. All other preoperative laboratory and diagnostic studies are within normal limits.

DIAGNOSES

- *Imbalanced Nutrition: Less than Body Requirements* related to anorexia and difficulty eating
- *Acute Pain* related to surgical incision and manipulation of abdominal organs
- *Risk for Ineffective Airway Clearance* related to upper abdominal surgery
- *Grieving* related to recent diagnosis of cancer

EXPECTED OUTCOMES

- Maintain present weight during hospitalization.
- Resume a high-calorie, high-protein diet by time of discharge.
- Verbalize effective pain management, maintaining a reported pain level of 3 or less on a scale of 1 to 10.
- Maintain a patent airway and clear breath sounds.
- Verbalize feelings regarding diagnosis and participate in decision making.

PLANNING AND IMPLEMENTATION

- Weigh daily.
- Maintain nasogastric tube placement, patency, and suction as ordered.

- Maintain intravenous fluids and parenteral nutrition as ordered until oral food intake is resumed.
- Arrange for diet teaching, including strategies to prevent dumping syndrome, before discharge.
- Maintain patient-controlled analgesia until able to take oral analgesics.
- Assess respiratory status including rate, depth, and breath sounds every hour initially, then every 4 hours.
- Assist to cough, deep breathe, and use inspirometer every 2 to 4 hours and as needed. Splint abdomen during coughing.
- Encourage verbalization of feelings about diagnosis and perceived losses.
- Encourage participation in decision making.

EVALUATION

Mr. Harvey's weight remained stable through his hospitalization. On discharge he is taking a high-protein, high-calorie diet in six small feedings per day. He and his wife have reviewed his diet with the dietitian and are planning on using some dietary supplements at home to meet protein needs. He verbalizes an understanding of measures to prevent dumping syndrome, including separating his intake of solid foods and liquids. Mr. Harvey is using oral analgesics in the morning and at bedtime to control his pain. He and his wife have begun to discuss the meaning of his diagnosis. Mrs. Harvey tells the discharge nurse, "We are going to go to a support group called 'Coping with Cancer' when George is stronger."

CRITICAL THINKING IN THE NURSING PROCESS

1. What is the rationale for maintaining nasogastric suction after gastrojejunostomy?
2. Develop a preoperative teaching plan for a patient undergoing a partial gastrectomy.
3. Mr. Harvey calls you just before the initial dose of chemotherapy and says, "Everyone tells me that chemotherapy will cause vomiting, and I don't think I can take being sick again." How would you respond?
4. Design interventions to ensure adequate nutrition for people with advanced gastric cancer.

See Evaluating Your Response in Appendix C.

- *Physical assessment:* General appearance, weight for height; abdominal distention or a palpable upper abdominal mass; occult blood in stool or vomitus.

Nursing Diagnoses and Interventions

Priorities of nursing care for the patient with gastric cancer focus on effects of the disease and its treatment on nutritional status, and on the effects of a potentially fatal disease on the patient and family. See the accompanying Case Study & Nursing Care Plan above.

Imbalanced Nutrition: Less than Body Requirements

The patient with gastric cancer may be malnourished because of anorexia, early satiety, and increased metabolic needs related to the tumor. Extensive gastric resection also makes it difficult

to consume an adequate diet. Malnourishment, in turn, impairs healing and the patient's ability to tolerate cancer treatment.

- Consult with dietitian for a complete nutrition assessment and diet planning. *The patient is at risk for protein-calorie malnutrition, which impairs the ability to heal and recover from extensive surgery.*
- Weigh daily. Monitor laboratory values such as hemoglobin, hematocrit, and serum albumin levels. *Daily weights are a valuable measurement of both fluid and nutritional status. Laboratory values provide further evidence of nutritional status.*
- Provide preferred foods; have family prepare meals when possible. Provide supplemental feedings between meals. *Small, frequent feedings and preferred foods encourage intake of nutrients.*

- Arrange for visitors to be present during meals. *Eating is a social function as well as a physiologic one. Companionship often improves food intake.*
- Administer pain and antiemetic medications as needed before meals. *Pain and nausea suppress the appetite; relief promotes food intake.*

Grieving

- Encourage family members to spend as much time as possible with the patient. *The family may feel helpless and ineffectual. Supporting family members' presence can encourage this vital interaction.*
- Do not negate denial if present. *Denial is a coping mechanism that protects the patient from hopelessness.*
- Allow patients to talk openly if desired about their condition and the prognosis. *Acceptance of the patients' fears helps reduce anxiety and promote coping behaviors.*

- Actively listen to the patient's and family's expressions of grieving. Avoid interrupting or offering meaningless words of consolation. *Being present and listening actively are often the most effective interventions for the grieving patient.*

Community-Based Care

Although the patient with gastric cancer may be hospitalized for surgery, most care is provided in the home and community-based settings such as hospice care. When preparing the patient and family for home care, discuss the following topics:

- Care of incision and feeding tube (if present) or central venous line
- Maintaining nutrition and preventing complications of surgery such as dumping syndrome
- Pain management
- Provide referrals to home care agencies, hospice, and cancer support groups as appropriate
- Provide information about services available through the local chapter of the American Cancer Society

CHAPTER HIGHLIGHTS

- Nausea and vomiting, common GI symptoms, may be indicative of disorders affecting many organ systems, including the GI tract, inner ear, CNS, or heart. Nausea and vomiting also are frequently related to medical interventions, such as drugs and cancer therapies. Complications such as dehydration, electrolyte imbalance, and aspiration of gastric contents are primary concerns in treating nausea and vomiting.
- Stomatitis and oral mucositis are common disorders of the mouth, potentially having a significant effect on comfort and nutrition. In most cases, management is symptomatic and supportive, directed toward promoting comfort and maintaining nutritional status.
- Tobacco and alcohol use contribute to a number of upper GI disorders, including GERD, oral and esophageal cancers, and peptic ulcer disease. Encourage all patients to stop smoking or using smokeless tobacco and to consume alcohol in moderate amounts if at all to reduce their risk or these disorders.
- Gastroesophageal reflux disease (GERD) is common. While it often is considered to be a benign condition, prolonged exposure of the lower esophagus to gastric juices can lead to esophagitis, hemorrhage, and scarring.
- Both esophageal and gastric cancer often are diagnosed late in the disease because their symptoms may be vague. Encourage patients with complaints of dysphagia, a sensation of gastric fullness, or heartburn to seek medical evaluation. Surgical resection

of the cancerous portion of the esophagus or stomach is the treatment of choice when the tumor is diagnosed early.
- Upper gastrointestinal bleeding can lead to significant blood loss and shock. Peptic ulcer disease accounts for the majority of UGI hemorrhage, although erosive gastritis and esophageal varices also are common causes. Nursing care focuses on monitoring and promoting cardiovascular stability and preventing further hemorrhage.
- Acute gastritis, often associated with aspirin or NSAID use, is generally benign and self-limited. Erosive gastritis, a complication of critical conditions such as shock, trauma, a major burn, or head injury, can lead to unexpected gastric hemorrhage. Prophylactic therapy with proton pump inhibitors or H_2-receptor blockers is important to prevent erosive gastritis in at risk patients. Chronic gastritis is an unrelated disorder usually associated with *H. pylori* infection.
- *H. pylori* infection also is a major risk factor for peptic ulcer disease and gastric cancer. Effectively treating the infection can reduce or eliminate the risk of future exacerbations of PUD.
- An acute change in the nature of abdominal pain in a patient with PUD, especially when accompanied by vomiting, guarding of the abdomen, or a change in bowel sounds, could indicate an obstruction or perforation and release of gastric contents into the peritoneal cavity.

TEST YOURSELF NCLEX-RN® REVIEW

1. The nurse assessing for oral cancer risk factors in a patient with a persistent sore on his tongue asks about which of the following?
   1. consumption of highly spiced foods
   2. thumb sucking or pacifier use as a child
   3. regular use of dental floss
   4. tobacco use in any form

2. The nurse teaching a patient with gastroesophageal reflux disease includes which of the following instructions? **Select all that apply.**
   1. This is a benign disease requiring no treatment.
   2. Elevate the head of the bed on 6- to 8-inch blocks.
   3. Stop taking the prescribed proton-pump inhibitor once symptoms are relieved.
   4. Peppermint and chocolate candies can help relieve symptoms.
   5. Avoid lying down for several hours after eating.

3. The nurse evaluates his teaching of a patient with acute stress gastritis as effective when the patient states that she will do which of the following?
   1. Avoid using aspirin or NSAIDs for routine pain relief.
   2. Consume only bland foods.
   3. Return for yearly upper endoscopy exams.
   4. Fully cook all meat, poultry, and egg products.

4. The nurse identifies which of the following nursing diagnoses as highest priority for the patient admitted with peptic ulcer disease and possible perforation?
   1. *Acute Pain*
   2. *Ineffective Health Maintenance*
   3. *Nausea*
   4. *Impaired Tissue Integrity: Gastrointestinal*

5. Following a partial gastrectomy for gastric cancer, a patient complains of nausea, abdominal pain and cramping, and diarrhea after eating. Recognizing manifestations of dumping syndrome, the nurse recommends which of the following?
   1. fasting for a period of 6 to 12 hours before meals
   2. decreasing the protein content of meals
   3. frequent small meals that contain solid foods or liquids, but not both
   4. a diet rich in carbohydrates to maintain blood glucose levels

6. The nurse caring for a patient with esophageal cancer affecting the middle portion of the esophagus would immediately report which of the following?
   1. crackles in the base of the right lung
   2. bright bleeding from the mouth
   3. weight loss
   4. difficulty swallowing solid foods

7. The physician has ordered omeprazole 20 mg twice daily, clarithromycin 500 mg twice daily, and amoxicillin 1 g daily for a patient with peptic ulcer disease. It is most important for the nurse to instruct the patient to do which of the following?
   1. Stop the drugs immediately and notify the physician if a rash, hives, or itching develop.
   2. Consume 8 oz of yogurt or buttermilk daily while taking these drugs.
   3. Take the drugs on an empty stomach, 1 hour before breakfast and at least 2 hours after dinner.
   4. Take the drugs with a full glass of water.

8. When planning care for a patient with stomatitis, the nurse identifies which of the following as a priority intervention?
   1. Assist to cleanse mouth with mouthwash following meals.
   2. Allow patient to select appealing foods from a menu.
   3. Provide viscous lidocaine to relieve mouth pain before meals.
   4. Refer the patient to a smoking cessation program.

9. The evening following a gastric resection, the nurse notes that there has been no drainage from the nasogastric tube for the past 3 hours. The nurse should do which of the following?
   1. Chart the finding.
   2. Reposition the nasogastric tube.
   3. Gently irrigate the tube with normal saline.
   4. Notify the surgeon.

10. A patient with a history of peptic ulcer disease suddenly begins to complain of severe abdominal pain. The nurse should do which of the following? **Select all that apply.**
    1. Administer the prescribed proton-pump inhibitor.
    2. Obtain an order for a narcotic analgesic.
    3. Withhold oral food and fluids.
    4. Place the patient in Fowler's position.
    5. Notify the physician.

See Test Yourself answers in Appendix C.

BIBLIOGRAPHY

Abraham, J. (2008 December). Acupressure and acupuncture in preventing and managing postoperative nausea and vomiting in adults. *Journal of Perioperative Practice, 18*(12), 543–551.

Adams, M. P., Holland, L. N., Jr., & Bostwick, P. M. (2008). *Pharmacology for nurses: A pathophysiologic approach* (2nd ed.). Upper Saddle River, NJ: Pearson Prentice Hall.

Agarwal, K., & Agarwal, S. (2008 February). *Helicobacter pylori* vaccine: From past to future. *Mayo Clinic Proceedings, 83*(2), 168–175.

American Cancer Society. (2009). *Cancer facts and figures 2009.* Atlanta: Author.

American College of Physicians (ACP). (2008 August). In the clinic. Gastroesophageal reflux disease. *Annals of Internal Medicine, 5 August 2008,* ITC2-1– ITC2-14.

American Medical Directors Association (AMDA) (2006). *Gastrointestinal disorders.* Columbia, MD: AMDA.

Barba, A., Fitzgerald, P., & Wood, S. (2007 July). Managing peptic ulcer disease. *Nursing2007.* Retrieved from www.nursing2007.com

Barclay, L., & Vega, C. (2007 April). Peppermint oil may relieve digestive symptoms, headaches. *Medscape Medical News, 2007.* Retrieved from www.medscape.com

Boparai, V., Rajagopalan, J., & Triadafilopoulos, G. (2008). Guide to the use of proton pump inhibitors in adult patients. *Drugs 2008, 68*(7), 925–947.

Bulechek, G. M., Butcher, H. K., & Dochterman, J. M. (Eds.). (2008). *Nursing interventions classification (NIC)* (5th ed.). St. Louis, MO: Mosby.

Cawley, M. M., & Benson, L. M. (2005). Current trends in managing oral mucositis. *Clinical Journal of Oncology Nursing, 9*(5), 584–594.

Copstead, L. C., & Banasik, J. L. (2010). *Pathophysiology* (4th ed.). St. Louis, MO: Elsevier/Saunders.

Dibble, S., Lucy, J., Cooper, B., Israel, J., Cohen, M., Nussey, B., et al. (2007). Acupressure for chemotherapy-induced nausea and vomiting: A randomized clinical trial. *Oncology Nursing Forum, 34*(4), 813–820.

Dodd, V., Watson, J., Choi, Y., Tomar, S., & Logan, H. (2008). Oral cancer in African Americans: Addressing health disparities. *American Journal of Health Behavior, 32*(6), 684–692.

Edmondson, D., & Schiech, L. (2008 April). Esophageal cancer: A tough pill to swallow. *Nursing2008, 38*(4), 44–48.

Edwards, S. J., & Metheny, N. A. (2000). Measurement of gastric residual volume: State of the science. *MEDSURG Nursing, 9*(3), 125–128.

Fauci, A. S., Braunwald, E., Kasper, D. L., Hauser, S. L., Longo, D. L., Jameson, J. L., et al. (2008). *Harrison's principles of internal medicine* (17th ed.). New York: McGraw-Hill.

Fontaine, K. L. (2005). *Healing practices: Alternative therapies for nursing* (2nd ed.). Upper Saddle River, NJ: Prentice Hall Health.

Gendreau-Webb, R. (2007 October). Bone up on proton pump inhibitors and fracture risk. *Nursing2007, 37*(10), 60–61.

Harris, D., Eilers, J., Harriman, A., Cashavelly, B., & Maxwell, C. (2008 February). Putting evidence into practice®: Evidence-based interventions for the management of oral mucositis. *Clinical Journal of Oncology Nursing, 12*(1), 141–152.

Kahrilas, P. (2008 October). Gastroesophageal reflux disease. *New England Journal of Medicine, 359*(16), 1700–1707.

Kee, J. L. (2009). *Handbook of Laboratory and diagnostic tests with nursing implications* (6th ed.). Upper Saddle River, NJ: Pearson Prentice Hall.

Khvorova, Y., & Neill, J. (2008 July). A review of the effect of peppermint oil in various gastrointestinal conditions. *J. GENCA, 18*(3), 6–15.

Knudtson, M., & Davis, Jr., R. H. (2005). Frequent heartburn: An evidence-based approach to cost-effective management. *American Journal for Nurse Practitioners, 9*(1), 137–144.

Lehne, R. A. (2007). *Pharmacology for nursing care* (6th ed.). St. Louis, MO: Elsevier.

Mackenzie, D. J., Popplewell, P. K., & Billingsley, K. G. (2004). Care of patients after esophagectomy. *Critical Care Nurse, 24*(1), 16, 18–31.

McCance, K. L., & Huether, S. E. (2006). *Pathophysiology* (5th ed.). St. Louis, MO: Mosby.

McGinley, S. R. (2003). The other tobacco threat. Smokeless does not mean harmless. *Advance for Nurse Practitioners, 11*(4), 29–30, 34, 90.

McPhee, S. J., Papadakis, M. A., & Tierney, L. M. (2008). *Current medical diagnosis & treatment* (47th ed.). New York: Lange Medical Books/McGraw-Hill.

Moorhead, S., Johnson, M., Maas, M., & Swanson, E. (Eds.). (2008). *Nursing outcomes classification (NOC)* (4th ed.). St. Louis, MO: Mosby.

National Cancer Institute. (2008). Lip and oral cavity cancer treatment (PDQ®). Health professional version. Retrieved from www.cancer.gov

National Cancer Institute. (2008). Oral cancer prevention (PDQ®). Health Professional version. Retrieved from www.cancer.gov

NANDA International. (2009). *Nursing diagnoses: Definitions & classification 2005–2006.* Philadelphia: Author.

Palmer, J. L., & Metheny, N. A. (2008 February). Preventing aspiration in older adults with dysphagia. *American Journal of Nursing, 108*(2), 40–48.

Porth, C. M., & Matfin, G. (2009). *Pathophysiology: Concepts of altered health states* (8th ed.). Philadelphia: Lippincott.

Ramakrishnan, K. (2007 October). Peptic ulcer disease. *American Family Physician, 76*(7), 1005–1012.

Rothrock, J. C. (2007). *Alexander's care of the patient in surgery* (13th ed.). St. Louis, MO: Mosby.

Schlansky, B., & Hwang, J. H. (2009). Prevention of nonsteroidal anti-inflammatory drug-induced gastropathy. *Journal of Gastroenterology, 44*(Suppl XIX), 44–52.

Spencer, J. W., & Jacobs, J. J. (2003). *Complementary and alternative medicine: An evidence-based approach* (2nd ed.). St. Louis, MO: Mosby.

Stovall, M. (2008 April). Diagnosing gastric carcinoma. *Clinical Journal of Oncology Nursing, 12*(2), 209–212.

Sugano, K. (2008 July). Gastric cancer: Pathogenesis, screening, and treatment. *Gastrointestinal Endoscopy Clinics of North America, 18*(3), 513–522.

Treister, N. S., & Woo, S. B. (2008). Chemotherapy-induced oral mucositis. Medscape. Retrieved from www.emdicine.medscape.com

University of Michigan Health System. (2005). Peptic ulcer disease. Ann Arbor, MI: Author. Retrieved from www.guidline.gov

Urden, L. D., Stacy, K. M., & Lough, M. E. (2006). *Thelan's critical care nursing* (5th ed). St. Louis, MO: Mosby.

Use evidence-based clinical guidelines to prevent and treat oral mucositis. *ONS News, 20*(2), 7.

Way, L. W., & Doherty, G. M. (2003). *Current surgical diagnosis & treatment* (11th ed.). New York: McGraw-Hill.

White, G., O-Rourke, F., Ong, B., Cordato, D., & Chan, D. (2008 May). Dysphagia: Causes, assessment, treatment, and management. *Geriatrics, 63*(5), 15–20.

Wilkinson, J. M., & Ahern, N. R. (2009). *Nursing diagnosis handbook* (9th ed.). Upper Saddle River, NJ: Prentice Hall Health.

Yang, Y., Lewis, J., Epstein, S., & Metz, D. (2006 December 27). Long-term proton pump inhibitor therapy and risk of hip fracture. *JAMA: Journal of the American Medical Association, 296*(24), 2947–2953.

Nursing Care of Patients with Bowel Disorders

LEARNING OUTCOMES

1. Compare and contrast the causes, pathophysiology, manifestations, interdisciplinary and nursing care of patients with disorders of bowel motility.
2. Explain the pathophysiology, manifestations, complications, interdisciplinary care, and nursing care of patients with acute or chronic inflammatory bowel disorders, neoplastic disorders, and structural and obstructive bowel disorders.
3. Discuss the purposes, nursing implications, and health education for the patient and family related to medications used to treat bowel disorders.
4. Explain the rationale for using selected diets, including those for diarrhea and constipation and low-residue, gluten-free, and high-fiber diets.
5. Describe selected surgical procedures of the bowel, including colectomy, colostomy, ileostomy, and perianal surgery.

CLINICAL COMPETENCIES

1. Assess the functional status of patients with bowel disorders, and recognize, document, and report unexpected or abnormal findings.
2. Use assessed data to determine priority nursing diagnoses, identify and implement patient-centered evidence-based nursing interventions, and revise the plan of care for patients with bowel disorders.
3. Integrate interdisciplinary care and administer medications knowledgeably and safely for patients with bowel disorders.
4. Provide skilled care to patients having bowel surgery, an ostomy, or perianal surgery.
5. Provide culturally appropriate teaching to promote nutrition, prevent acute and chronic bowel disorders, encourage screening, and facilitate community-based care related to bowel disorders.

KEY TERMS

borborygmi, *656*
colectomy, *684*
colostomy, *704*
constipation, *657*
diarrhea, *652*

hematochezia, *690*
ileostomy, *686*
inflammatory bowel disease (IBD), *679*
malabsorption, *695*

paralytic ileus, *669*
peritonitis, *667*
steatorrhea, *655*
stoma, *686*

Disorders of intestinal absorption and bowel elimination can affect functional elimination status and other health patterns such as health perception-health management, nutritional-metabolic, activity-exercise, self-perception-self-concept, and sexuality-reproductive. Bowel function can be affected by inflammations, infections, tumors, obstructions, or changes in structure.

Patients with intestinal disorders often face extensive diagnostic testing, surgery, and permanent changes in physical appearance and lifestyle. Nursing care is directed toward meeting the patient's physiologic needs, providing emotional support, and educating the patient to adapt to changes in lifestyle.

Disorders of Intestinal Motility

Few body functions respond as readily to internal and external influences as the process of defecation. Factors affecting the gastrointestinal (GI) tract directly, such as food intake and bacterial population, affect the number and consistency of stools. Indirect factors, such as psychologic stress or voluntary postponement of defecation, also affect elimination.

In modern society, normal bowel elimination patterns vary widely. For some patients, two to three stools per day is the usual pattern. Others may normally have as few as three stools per week. It is important to evaluate each patient's bowel elimination against his or her own normal pattern.

The Patient with Diarrhea

Diarrhea is an increase in the frequency, volume, and fluid content of the stool. In diarrhea, the water content of feces is increased, usually due to either malabsorption or water secretion in the bowel. It is a manifestation rather than a primary disorder.

Diarrhea may be acute or chronic. Acute diarrhea, which lasts less than a week, is usually due to an infectious agent. Chronic diarrhea (diarrhea that persists longer than 3 to 4 weeks) may be caused by inflammatory bowel disorders, malabsorption, or endocrine disorders.

Pathophysiology

About 1500 mL of digested material enters the large intestine daily. Normally, most of the water and some of the solutes are reabsorbed in the bowel, leaving only about 200 mL of feces to be eliminated.

Large-volume diarrhea, characterized by both increased numbers and volume of stools, is caused by increased water content of the stool. This increased water content may result from either osmotic or secretory processes. Water may be pulled into the bowel lumen by osmosis when the feces contain osmotically active molecules. Some stool softeners and laxatives work on this principle. When the lactose in milk is not broken down and absorbed, the lactose molecules exert an osmotic pull, causing diarrhea. The diarrhea associated with cholera and *Escherichia coli* infection is caused by increased water secretion in the small and large intestines. Unabsorbed dietary fat, some cathartics and other drugs, and other factors can cause secretory diarrhea.

Small-volume diarrhea, characterized by frequent small stools, is usually caused by inflammation or disease of the colon. Diseases that affect the intestinal mucosa, such as inflammatory bowel disease, cause an exudative diarrhea. The mucosal inflammation causes plasma, serum proteins, blood, and mucus to accumulate in the bowel, increasing fecal bulk and fluidity. An increased rate of propulsion within the bowel can also decrease the amount of water normally absorbed from the chyme, leading to diarrhea. For this reason, laxatives that increase bowel motility and bowel resection or bypass can lead to diarrhea.

Antibiotic-associated diarrhea may occur as a result of disruption of normal intestinal flora by antibiotic therapy. Loss of normal flora can affect food digestion, leading to diarrhea, or can allow overgrowth of pathogens such as *Clostridium difficile* (see the section on gastroenteritis for more information about *C. difficile*). The accompanying nursing research box presents information about other possible causes of diarrhea in hospitalized patients.

Manifestations

The manifestations of diarrhea depend on its cause, duration, and severity, as well as the area of bowel affected and the patient's general health. Diarrhea can present as several large, watery stools daily, or very frequent small stools that contain blood, mucus, or exudate.

Complications

Diarrhea can have devastating effects. Water and electrolytes are lost in diarrheal stool. This can lead to dehydration, particularly in the very young, the older adult, or the debilitated patient unable to respond to thirst. With severe diarrhea, vascular collapse and hypovolemic shock may occur. Potassium and magnesium are lost, potentially leading to hypokalemia and hypomagnesemia. The loss of bicarbonate in the stool can lead to metabolic acidosis. ∞ See Chapter 10 for further discussion of the effects of these imbalances.

SAFETY ALERT
Monitor orthostatic vital signs, skin turgor, serum electrolytes and osmolality, and urinalysis to identify and respond to possible adverse effects of diarrhea.

Interdisciplinary Care

Management of diarrhea focuses on identifying and treating the underlying cause. In addition, the diarrhea itself may need to be treated to promote comfort and to prevent complications. The history (including the onset and associated circumstances of

---

MOVING EVIDENCE INTO ACTION — Diarrhea

Hospitalized patients often have a number of risk factors for diarrhea. *Clostridium difficile* is now recognized as the cause of a significant portion of treatment-related diarrhea; it does not, however, account for all cases. Previous studies have demonstrated a relationship between diarrhea and enteral tube feedings, medications containing sorbitol, lactose intolerance, and other factors. A prospective study by Thorson, Bliss, and Savik (2008) looked at the risk for developing diarrhea among patients receiving enteral tube feeding and a control group without enteral tube feeding. Findings of the study illustrate the contributory effects of severe illness and the combination of sorbitol-containing medications and enteral tube feeding.

IMPLICATIONS FOR NURSING
Severely ill patients often require enteral tube feedings for nutritional support. Healing and immune function require adequate nutrition; other studies point to the beneficial effects of enteral nutrition for the majority of patients. Discontinuing enteral feedings due to diarrhea is not a desirable option. In some cases, changing the enteral feeding formula or adding probiotic (cultures of beneficial yeasts or bacteria) supplements may help

normalize bowel function. Other options include antidiarrheal medications or soluble fiber supplements.

CRITICAL THINKING IN PATIENT CARE
1. Administering medications containing sorbitol, a sugar that is not absorbed by the gut, are associated with an increased risk of developing diarrhea among hospitalized patients. How does sorbitol increase the risk for diarrhea? What would you do if you realized that your seriously ill patient is receiving enteral tube feeding and medications containing sorbitol?
2. The position of the feeding tube tip in the gut also is identified as a risk factor for diarrhea associated with enteral tube feedings. Thinking about the functions of the stomach, pyloric valve, duodenum, and jejunum, which type of tube (gastric, duodenal, or jejunal) might carry the highest risk for diarrhea? The lowest? What other enteral tube feeding risk factors are considered in tube placement?
3. Your patient is being discharged home with a gastrostomy tube and directions for enteral feedings. What teaching will you provide to the patient and family regarding tube care, feeding administration, and bowel management?

the diarrhea) and physical examination often provide enough information to identify its cause.

Diagnosis

Diagnostic tests that may be ordered to help identify the cause of diarrhea include a stool specimen analysis and culture. A sigmoidoscopy may be conducted to directly visualize the bowel mucosa. (∞ See Chapter 21 for further information on diagnostic tests.) Tissue biopsy may be performed to identify chronic inflammatory processes, infection, and other causes of diarrhea. In addition, laboratory tests of serum electrolytes, serum osmolality, and arterial blood gases (ABGs) may be ordered to assess for adverse effects of diarrhea. Increased serum osmolality indicates water loss and dehydration.

Medications

Antidiarrheal medications are used sparingly or not at all until the cause of diarrhea has been identified. In diarrhea associated with botulism or bacillary dysentery, giving an antidiarrheal agent can worsen or prolong the disease by slowing elimination of the toxin from the bowel. Once the underlying cause for diarrhea has been established, specific medications may be ordered to treat the underlying cause. Antibiotics are used with caution because they alter the normal bacterial population of the bowel and may actually worsen diarrhea. A balanced electrolyte solution may be required to replace fluid losses. Intravenous or oral potassium preparations may be prescribed.

Opium and some of its derivatives, anticholinergics, absorbents, and demulcents are commonly used as antidiarrheal preparations. Specific preparations, their method of action, and the nursing implications for these medications are outlined in the Medication Administration box on page 655.

Nutrition

Fluid replacement is of primary importance in managing the patient with diarrhea. If the patient is able to tolerate oral fluids (i.e., if the patient is not experiencing nausea and vomiting), an oral glucose/balanced electrolyte solution provides the best fluid replacement. Commercial preparations such as Gatorade and other sports drinks are available, as are pediatric solutions (e.g., Pedialyte), which can be used for adults as well as children. A solution of 5 mL (1 teaspoon) each of table salt and baking soda and 4 teaspoons (20 mL) of granulated sugar added with desired flavoring (such as lemon extract or juice) to 1 quart (1 L) of water can be made at home to replace water and electrolytes.

Solid food is withheld in the first 24 hours of acute diarrhea to rest the bowel. After that time, frequent, small, soft feedings can be added. Milk and milk products are added last, because the lactose they contain frequently aggravates the diarrhea. Raw fruits and vegetables, fried foods, bran, whole-grain cereals, condiments, spices, coffee, and alcoholic beverages are avoided during the recovery period.

Patients with chronic diarrhea may benefit by eliminating specific foods from the diet. Foods and nonfood substances that may aggravate diarrhea are outlined in Table 24–1. The diet should be high in calories and nutritional value. Vitamin supplements may be necessary, particularly the fat-soluble vitamins (A, D, E, and K). Patients with severe chronic diarrhea may require parenteral nutrition (∞ see Chapter 21).

Complementary and Alternative Therapies

Herbal or homeopathic therapies may be used to help relieve diarrhea. Patients who are lactose intolerant (discussed later in the chapter) may use lactase enzyme tablets or drops when consuming milk products. Herbal treatments may include a strong tea of black pepper, chamomile, coriander, rosemary, sandalwood, or thyme. Ginger in the form of tea or capsules can be helpful in reducing intestinal inflammation and lessens the effects of food poisoning. Homeopathic practitioners may use podophyllum tablets to treat diarrhea. Probiotics, live microorganisms similar to those normally found in the gut, may be used to prevent or treat antibiotic-associated diarrhea (National Center for Complementary and Alternative Medicine [NCCAM], 2008; Rowland et al., 2008). Probiotics are available as dietary supplements and foods (e.g., yogurt, yogurt drinks). Refer the patient to a qualified practitioner for more information about using complementary and alternative therapies to treat diarrhea.

∞ Nursing Care

Diarrhea is a common problem that may complicate patient care.

Health Promotion

Teach all patients about the importance of hand hygiene as a measure to prevent the spread of infectious diseases, including those that cause diarrhea. Teach safe food handling techniques

TABLE 24–1 Foods That May Aggravate Chronic Diarrhea

FOODS	REASON
Milk, ice cream, yogurt, soft cheeses, cottage cheese	Contain lactose; not tolerated by patients with lactase deficiency who cannot digest lactose.
Apple juice, pear juice, grapes, honey, dates, nuts, figs, fruit-flavored soft drinks	Contain fructose; when consumed in large quantities, fructose may not be totally absorbed, causing an osmotic pull of fluid into the bowel.
Table sugar	Contains sucrose; not tolerated by patients with sucrase deficiency.
Apple juice, pear juice, sugarless gums, and mints	May contain sorbitol or mannitol, sugars that are not absorbed and can cause osmotic draw.
Antacids	Magnesium-containing antacids decrease bowel transit time and contain poorly absorbed salts that can exert an osmotic draw.
Coffee, tea, cola drinks, over-the-counter analgesics	Contain caffeine, which can decrease bowel transit time.

to prevent bacterial contamination, and discuss measures to ensure safe drinking water. For patients planning to travel outside the United States or to wilderness areas, teach measures to purify water for drinking and cooking.

Assessment

The nursing assessment can help identify the cause of the patient's diarrhea, as well as early signs of complications. Collect the following assessment data:

- *Health history:* Duration and extent of diarrhea; associated manifestations; dietary intake; recent travel out of the country or to wilderness areas; previous history of diarrhea; chronic diseases; prescription and nonprescription medications.
- *Physical examination:* Vital signs (including orthostatic blood pressure); peripheral pulses; skin temperature, moisture, turgor; color and moisture of mucous membranes; abdominal contour and girth; bowel sounds; stool for obvious or occult blood, pus, mucus, or **steatorrhea** (bulky, foul-smelling stool).

Nursing Diagnoses and Interventions

Nursing care of the patient with diarrhea focuses on identifying the cause, relieving the manifestations, preventing complications, and preventing the potential spread of infection to others.

Diarrhea

Nursing interventions for diarrhea are provided to help the patient recover a normal elimination pattern without adverse consequences.

- Monitor and record the frequency and characteristics of bowel movements *to provide a measure of the effectiveness of treatment.*

MEDICATION ADMINISTRATION   **Antidiarrheal Preparations**

ABSORBENTS AND PROTECTANTS
Kaolin and pectin (Kaopectate, Donnagel-MB)

Polycarbophil (FigerNorm, Equalactin)

Absorbent preparations act locally in the intestines to bind substances that can cause diarrhea. Absorbents are safe and are generally available over the counter, although their efficacy has not been proved.

Nursing Responsibilities
- Assess for contraindications to antidiarrheal therapy, such as some infections or chronic inflammatory bowel disease, including ulcerative colitis.
- If fever is present, check with physician before giving the medication.
- Administer these medications at least 1 hour before or 2 hours after other oral medications; they may interfere with the absorption of other drugs.
- Observe the patient's response to the medication. Constipation is a potential problem.

Health Education for the Patient and Family
- Take the recommended dosage at the onset of diarrhea and after each loose stool.
- Do not take any of these preparations for more than 48 hours. If diarrhea persists, notify the physician.
- Do not give antidiarrheal medications to debilitated older patients without physician supervision.

ANTISECRETORY
Bismuth subsalicylate (Pepto-Bismol)

Bismuth subsalicylate, available without a prescription, has antisecretory, anti-inflammatory, and antibacterial effects. It is widely used to control traveler's diarrhea. Although it is generally safe at recommended doses, bismuth subsalicylate has potential toxic effects and interacts with drugs such as aspirin and oral anticoagulants.

Nursing Responsibilities
- Administer as ordered.
- Do not administer within 1 hour of other drugs, as it may interfere with their absorption.
- Monitor for increased anticoagulant effect when given with Coumadin or aspirin.

Health Education for the Patient and Family
- Chew bismuth subsalicylate tablets, rather than swallowing them whole, for maximal effectiveness.

- This drug may cause harmless darkening of your tongue and stools.
- If you are allergic to aspirin, use bismuth subsalicylate with caution. Do not use aspirin while you are taking this drug unless directed to do so by your physician. Contact your physician if diarrhea persists for more than 2 days.

OPIUM AND OPIUM DERIVATIVES
Camphorated tincture of opium (Paregoric)

Tincture of opium (laudanum, opium tincture)

Difenoxin (Motofen)

Diphenoxylate (Lomotil, Lotrol, others)

Loperamide hydrochloride (Imodium)

Opium and its derivatives act on the central nervous system (CNS) to decrease the motility of the ileum and colon, slowing transit time and promoting more water absorption. They also decrease the sensation of a full rectum and increase anal sphincter tone. Paregoric and tincture of opium have a greater potential for abuse and are prescription drugs subject to controls under the federal Controlled Substance Act of 1970. Difenoxin, diphenoxylate, and loperamide are derivatives of opium with few analgesic, euphoric, or abuse-promoting effects and are in more common use today.

Nursing Responsibilities
- Assess for contraindications to antidiarrheal or narcotic medications prior to giving these drugs.
- Administer paregoric undiluted with water.
- Do not administer difenoxin and diphenoxylate to patients receiving monoamine oxidase inhibitors (MAOIs); hypertensive crises may occur.
- Observe closely for increased effects of other CNS depressants, such as alcohol, narcotic analgesics, or barbiturate sedatives.
- Observe for abdominal distention; toxic megacolon may occur if these drugs are given to the patient with ulcerative colitis.

Health Education for the Patient and Family
- Take the medication as recommended at the onset of diarrhea and after each loose stool.
- These drugs may be habit forming; use for no more than 48 hours.
- Avoid using alcohol and over-the-counter cold preparations while taking these drugs.
- These preparations may cause drowsiness; avoid driving or operating machinery while taking them.

- Measure abdominal girth and auscultate bowel sounds every 8 hours as indicated. Loud, rushing bowel sounds (**borborygmi**) indicate increased peristalsis, and may be heard in patients with acute diarrhea. *Diminished or absent bowel sounds may indicate a complication of treatment, such as constipation or toxic megacolon.*
- Use standard precautions, including gloves and hand hygiene. *Standard precautions help prevent the spread of infection to others.*
- Provide ready access to bathroom, commode, or bedpan. *The patient may have little warning of the need to defecate. Easily accessed toileting facilities reduce the risk for soiling or injury.*
- Administer antidiarrheal medications as prescribed *to promote comfort and prevent excess fluid loss.*
- Limit food intake if the diarrhea is acute, reintroducing solid foods slowly, in small amounts, *to allow the bowel to rest and mucosa to heal in acute diarrhea states.*

Risk for Deficient Fluid Volume

The increased water content of diarrheal stool places the patient at risk for fluid deficit.

- Record intake and output; weigh daily; assess skin turgor, mucous membranes, and urine specific gravity every 8 hours. *These assessments are used to monitor fluid volume.*

> **PRACTICE ALERT**
> Assess skin turgor over the sternum in the older adult. Loss of subcutaneous fat associated with aging makes skin turgor assessment on the arms or hands less reliable.

- Monitor vital signs, including orthostatic blood pressures. *Orthostatic hypotension is identified by a drop in BP of more than 10 mmHg and pulse increase of 10 beats per minute (bpm) when changing from a lying to a sitting position or from a sitting to a standing position. It is an indicator of fluid volume deficit.*

> **SAFETY ALERT**
> Institute safety precautions such as providing assistance when ambulating the patient with orthostatic hypotension. The fall in blood pressure with position changes can cause light-headedness and syncope.

- Provide fluid and electrolyte replacement solutions as indicated. Ensure ready access to fluids; assist the debilitated patient with fluid intake. Notify the care provider if the patient is unable to tolerate oral fluids. *Oral fluids are encouraged as tolerated to prevent dehydration. Intravenous fluids are necessary if oral fluids are not tolerated. An intake of 3000 mL/day or more is often needed to replace fluid losses.*

Risk for Impaired Skin Integrity

Decreased extracellular fluid volume and the irritating effects of diarrheal stool increase the risk for skin breakdown.

- Assist with cleaning the perianal area as needed. Use warm water, a gentle cleanser, and soft cloths. *Cleansing removes*

irritating substances in the stool. Gentle cleansing helps maintain integrity of dehydrated skin.
- Apply protective ointment to the perianal area. *Moisture-barrier ointments or creams protect the skin from excoriation and help prevent tissue breakdown.*

Using NANDA, NIC, and NOC

Linkages between a selected NANDA nursing diagnosis, NIC, and NOC for the patient with diarrhea are shown in the chart that follows.

Community-Based Care

Acute and chronic diarrhea generally are managed by the patient in the home. Teach the patient and family members about the following subjects:

- Causes of diarrhea (as directed by the diagnosis)
- Importance of hand washing and other hygiene measures
- Importance of maintaining adequate fluid intake to replace lost water and electrolytes
- Use of a balanced electrolyte solution such as Gatorade or a similar product (purchased or home prepared) for fluid replacement
- Recommendations to limit food intake during acute diarrhea, and resume gradually with small feedings of foods that have a constipating effect: applesauce, bananas, crackers, rice, potatoes
- To avoid foods high in fiber, milk products, and caffeine
- Ways to maintain nutrition if chronic diarrhea is a problem: frequent small meals, nutritional supplements, vitamin supplements
- Precautions and limitations of antidiarrheal preparations
- Importance of seeking medical intervention if diarrhea continues or recurs

---

NANDA, NIC, AND NOC LINKAGES
The Patient with Altered Bowel Motility

NANDA
Diarrhea

NIC
Diarrhea Management
Electrolyte Monitoring
Fluid/Electrolyte Management
Medication Management
Perineal Care

NOC
Bowel Continence
Electrolyte & Acid–Base Balance
Fluid Balance
Medication Response
Symptom Severity

Data from NANDA International. (2009). *Nursing diagnoses: Definitions & classification 2009–2011.* Oxford, UK: Wiley-Blackwell; Bulechek, G., Butcher, H., & Dochterman, J. (Eds.). (2008). *Nursing interventions classification (NIC)* (5th ed.). St. Louis, MO: Mosby; and Moorhead, S., Johnson, M., Maas, M., & Swanson, E. (Eds.). (2008). *Nursing outcomes classification (NOC)* (4th ed.). St. Louis, MO: Mosby.

The Patient with Constipation

Constipation is defined as the infrequent (two or fewer bowel movements weekly) or difficult passage of stools. Constipation affects older adults more frequently than younger people. Recent studies indicate that approximately 20% to 35% of people over age 65 report recurrent constipation and laxative use. Although fecal transit in the large intestine slows with aging, the increased incidence of constipation is thought to relate more to impaired general health status, increased medication use, and decreased physical activity in the older adult.

Pathophysiology

Constipation may be a primary problem or a manifestation of another disease or condition. Acute constipation, a definite change in the bowel elimination pattern, often is caused by an organic process. A change in bowel patterns that persists or becomes more frequent or severe may be due to a tumor or other partial bowel obstruction. With chronic constipation, functional causes that impair storage, transport, and evacuation mechanisms impede the normal passage of stools. Common causes of constipation are listed in Table 24–2.

Psychogenic factors are the most frequent causes of chronic constipation. These factors include postponing defecation when the urge is felt, and the perception of satisfaction with defecation. Patients often use laxatives and enemas to stimulate a bowel movement when constipation is perceived. Overuse of these measures can lead to real intestinal problems that worsen the condition. For example, *cathartic colon* (impaired colonic motility and changes in bowel structure) mimics ulcerative colitis in that the normal pouchlike or saccular appearance of the colon is lost. *Melanosis coli* is a brownish-black discoloration of the colon mucosa. Both conditions may be caused by long-term laxative use.

TABLE 24–2 Selected Causes of Constipation

FACTOR	RELATED CAUSE
Activity	Lack of exercise: bed rest
Dietary	Highly refined, low-fiber foods; inadequate fluid intake
Drugs	Antacids containing aluminum or calcium salts; narcotic analgesics; anticholinergics; many antidepressants, tranquilizers, and sedatives; antihypertensives, such as ganglionic blockers, calcium-channel blockers, beta-adrenergic blockers, and diuretics; iron salts
Large bowel	Diverticular disease, inflammatory disease, tumor, obstruction; changes in rectal or anal structure or function
Psychogenic	Voluntary suppression of urge; perceived need to defecate on schedule; depression
Systemic	Advanced age; pregnancy; neurologic conditions (trauma, multiple sclerosis, tumors, cerebrovascular accident, parkinsonism); endocrine and metabolic disorders (hypothyroidism, hypercalcemia, uremia, porphyria)
Other	Chronic laxative or enema use

Manifestations and Complications

The manifestations of constipation include having bowel movements less often than the usual pattern, frequent flatus, abdominal discomfort, anorexia, straining to have a bowel movement, and the passage of hard, dry stools.

With significant constipation or long-term dependence on laxatives or enemas, fecal impaction may develop. Impaction may also occur following barium administration for radiologic exam. The impaction is felt as a rock-hard or putty-like mass of feces in the rectum. Abdominal cramping and a full sensation in the rectal area may be manifestations of impaction. Watery mucus or foul-smelling liquid stool may be passed around the impaction, causing the patient to complain of diarrhea.

Interdisciplinary Care

Initial evaluation of constipation is based on the history and physical examination. The abdomen may appear somewhat distended, and bowel sounds may be reduced. If an impaction is present, digital examination of the rectum reveals a palpable, hard or putty-like fecal mass.

Simple or chronic constipation is treated with education (a daily bowel movement is not necessary for health), and modification of diet and exercise routines. If the problem is acute or does not resolve, further diagnostic examination may be ordered.

Diagnosis

A barium enema may be ordered to identify bowel structure, tumors, or diverticula. If the problem is acute, a sigmoidoscopy or colonoscopy may be used for evaluation and biopsy. (∞ See Chapter 21 for nursing implications of these tests.)

Medications

Laxative and cathartic preparations are used to promote stool evacuation. Milder preparations are generally known as laxatives; cathartics have a stronger effect. Most laxatives are appropriate only for short-term use. Cathartics and enemas interfere with normal bowel reflexes and should not be used for simple constipation. Laxatives should not be given if a patient has an undiagnosed intestinal obstruction, abdominal pain, fecal impaction, rectal fissures, ulcerated hemorrhoids, Crohn's disease, ulcerative colitis, or chronic inflammatory bowel disease. When the bowel is obstructed, laxatives or cathartics may cause serious mechanical damage and perforate the bowel.

The only laxatives that are appropriate and safe for long-term use are bulking agents, such as psyllium seed, calcium polycarbophil, and methylcellulose. These agents act by increasing the bulk of the feces and drawing water into the bowel to soften it. Commonly prescribed laxatives and cathartics are discussed in the following Medication Administration box.

Nutrition

Foods that have a high fiber content are recommended. Vegetable fiber is largely indigestible and unabsorbable, so it increases stool bulk. Fiber also helps draw water into the fecal mass, softening the stool and making defecation easier. Raw fruits and vegetables are good sources of dietary fiber, as is cereal bran. Use 2 to 3 teaspoons of unprocessed bran with meals (sprinkled on fruit or cereal) or up to 1/4 cup daily to supply adequate fiber.

MEDICATION ADMINISTRATION   Laxatives and Cathartics

BULK-FORMING AGENTS

Calcium polycarbophil (Fibercon, others)

Methylcellulose (Citrucel)

Psyllium (Metamucil, others)

Bulk-forming agents contain vegetable fiber, which is not digested or absorbed in the gut. This natural fiber creates bulk and draws water into the intestine, softening the stool mass.

Nursing Responsibilities

- Mix the agent with a full glass of cool liquid just prior to administering.
- Do not administer to patients with possible stool impaction or bowel obstruction.

Health Education for the Patient and Family

- Drink at least 6 to 8 full glasses of nonalcoholic fluid per day. Adequate hydration is necessary to produce the drug's laxative effect.
- These agents may be mixed with water, milk, or fruit juice.
- Take the drug in the morning or with meals. To reduce the risk of impaction, do not take at bedtime.
- Because of the increased risk of impaction, check with the physician before increasing dietary fiber while you are taking these agents.

WETTING AGENTS

Docusate (Colace, Surfak, Doxidan, others)

Wetting agents reduce stool surface tension and form an emulsion of fat and water, softening the stool. They are used primarily to prevent straining and reduce the discomfort of expelling hard stools.

Nursing Responsibilities

- Administer with ample fluids to promote softening effect.
- Wetting agents may alter the absorption of other drugs. Do not administer within 1 hour of other oral medications.
- Do not attempt to crush or open caplets; a liquid form is available for patients who cannot swallow pills or capsules.

Health Education for the Patient and Family

- Do not use for more than 1 week unless specifically recommended by the physician.
- Take the medication in the morning or evening, but avoid taking it with other medications.
- Adequate fluid is necessary to obtain the beneficial effect of the drug. Drink 6 to 8 glasses of nonalcoholic fluid per day.

OSMOTIC AND SALINE LAXATIVES/CATHARTICS

Lactulose (Rhodialose)

Sorbitol

Magnesium hydroxide (Milk of Magnesia)

Polyethylene glycol (Klean-Prep)

Laxatives in this group contain poorly absorbed salts or carbohydrates that remain in the bowel, increasing osmotic pressure and drawing water into the intestine. Stool volume increases, consistency decreases, and peristalsis is stimulated. Many of these agents also have an irritant effect on the bowel, further stimulating peristalsis. They are used to stimulate rapid or complete bowel evacuation to relieve constipation and to prepare the bowel for diagnostic and surgical procedures. They should be limited to acute, short-term use; chronic use may suppress normal bowel reflexes.

Nursing Responsibilities

- Assess for possible contraindications to osmotic or saline laxatives, including bowel ulceration or obstruction, dehydration, electrolyte imbalances, heart failure (which may be aggravated by the sodium content), or renal failure.
- Administer with a full glass of liquid, preferably in the morning to avoid sleep disturbance.
- Monitor fluid and electrolyte status: skin turgor, mucous membranes, intake and output; daily weight; and laboratory studies, such as hemoglobin and hematocrit levels, serum osmolality and electrolytes, and urine specific gravity.

Health Education for the Patient and Family

- Do not use these agents on a routine basis to treat or prevent constipation.
- Chill the solution to increase its palatability.
- Expect some abdominal cramping.
- Use only as directed. Increase fluid intake to at least 6 to 8 glasses of nonalcoholic fluid.
- Notify the physician if adverse effects occur, including abdominal pain, bloody stool, excessive skin or mucous membrane dryness, rapid weight loss, dizziness, or other unusual symptoms.
- These agents work in 3 to 6 hours; take them in the morning or early evening to avoid sleep disturbance.

IRRITANT OR STIMULANT LAXATIVES

Bisacodyl (Dulcolax, Bisco-Lax, Carter's Liver Pills, Codylax, others)

Phenolphthalein (Evac-U-Gen, Evac-U-Lax, Feen-A-Mint, Phenolax, others)

Senna (Senna laxative, Fletcher's Castoria)

Castor oil

Stimulant laxatives work by stimulating the motility and secretion of intestinal mucosa. Their use results in watery stool, often accompanied by abdominal cramping and pain. They are used to relieve constipation, although they should not be used as the initial treatment. Stimulant laxatives are also used for preparing the bowel for diagnostic testing.

Nursing Responsibilities

- Assess for potential contraindications to these laxatives, including abdominal pain and cramping, nausea and vomiting, and anal or rectal fissures.
- Administer on an empty stomach to minimize the effects of food on its dissolution and absorption.
- Do not crush enteric-coated bisacodyl tablets or administer with alkaline products. This may hasten their dissolution in the stomach, leading to gastric distress.

Health Education for the Patient and Family

- Discourage the use of this type of laxative, even in over-the-counter preparations, for the initial or continuing relief of constipation.
- Do not use the laxative for more than 1 week; chronic use can be habit forming and may suppress normal bowel reflexes.
- These laxatives are excreted in breast milk and should not be used by lactating women.
- Phenolphthalein-containing products may discolor the urine pink or red. Report possible hypersensitivity manifestations, such as difficulty breathing, dizziness or light-headedness, or skin rashes, to the primary care provider, and stop taking the medication.

LUBRICANTS

Mineral oil

Mineral oil acts by forming an oily coat on the fecal mass, preventing the reabsorption of water, and resulting in softer stool. Problems associated with the use of mineral oil as a laxative include reduced absorption of the fat-soluble vitamins A, D, E, and K; possible damage to the liver and spleen due to systemic absorption; and potential pneumonitis from aspiration of oil droplets into the lungs.

MEDICATION ADMINISTRATION Laxatives and Cathartics (continued)

Nursing Responsibilities
■ Assess for possible contraindications to use of mineral oil, including advanced age, preexisting lung disease, and hemorrhoids or other rectal lesions.
■ Do not give mineral oil concurrently with wetting agents or stool softeners, because these increase the potential for systemic absorption and increase the effects of the mineral oil.
■ Administer mineral oil in the evening before bedtime to reduce the effect on the absorption of fat-soluble vitamins and minimize the risk of aspiration.

■ Assess for manifestations of vitamin deficiency. Monitor the patient taking oral anticoagulants for evidence of increased bleeding, such as bleeding gums, easy bruising, or melena.

Health Education for the Patient and Family
■ Long-term use of mineral oil is not recommended because of its risks and adverse effects.
■ Do not use mineral oil if hemorrhoids or rectal lesions are present; leakage of the oil through the anal sphincter may cause itching and interfere with healing.
■ Suck on a lemon or orange slice after taking oral mineral oil to reduce the oily aftertaste.

Fluids are also important to maintain bowel motility and soft stools. The patient should drink 6 to 8 glasses of fluid per day. It is important to advise the patient to increase fluid intake when dietary fiber is initially increased to decrease flatus and help maintain softer stools.

In older adults, constipation may be due to inadequate food intake. Carefully evaluate diet history and usual daily intake.

Enemas

Significant or chronic constipation or a fecal impaction may require the administration of an enema. As a general rule, enemas are used only in acute situations and only on a short-term basis. They may also be ordered to prepare the bowel for diagnostic testing or examination. The following types of enemas may be prescribed:

■ A *saline enema* using 500 to 2000 mL of warmed physiologic saline solution is the least irritating to the bowel.
■ *Tap-water enemas* use 500 to 1000 mL of water to soften feces and irritate the bowel mucosa, stimulating peristalsis and evacuation.
■ *Soap-suds enemas* consist of a tap-water solution to which soap is added as a further irritant.
■ *Phosphate enemas* (e.g., Fleet) use a hypertonic saline solution to draw fluid into the bowel and irritate the mucosa, leading to evacuation.
■ *Oil retention enemas* instill mineral or vegetable oil into the bowel to soften the fecal mass. The instilled oil is retained overnight or for several hours before evacuation.

The repeated use of enemas can lead not only to impaired bowel function, but also to fluid and electrolyte imbalances. Tap-water and phosphate enemas are particularly likely to cause these problems. In acute conditions with risk of bowel obstruction, perforation, ulceration, or other problem, enemas should not be administered until their safe use can be established.

Complementary and Alternative Therapies

Herbal or homeopathic therapies may be used to help relieve constipation. Flaxseed oil lubricates the colon for easier passage of stool. Patients are instructed to take 1 to 2 tablespoons daily. Flax seeds are a lesser known but a highly concentrated source of fiber, and 1 to 2 tablespoons of ground flaxseeds can be sprinkled on cereals or salads daily, followed by 10 ounces of water.

Acupressure, massage, reflexology, aromatherapy, and stress management therapies can also be very beneficial in relieving constipation (Balch & Stengler, 2004). Other recommendations include exercise to stimulate intestinal contractions.

∞ Nursing Care

Health Promotion

Education can prevent constipation. Teach patients the importance of maintaining a diet high in natural fiber. Foods such as fresh fruits, vegetables, whole-grain products, and bran provide natural fiber. Encourage reducing consumption of meats and refined foods, which are low in fiber and can be constipating. Emphasize the need to maintain a high fluid intake every day, particularly during hot weather and exercise. Discuss the relationship between exercise and bowel regularity. Encourage patients to engage in some form of exercise, such as walking daily.

Discuss normal bowel habits, and explain that a daily bowel movement is not the norm for all people. Encourage patients to respond to the urge to defecate when it occurs. Suggest setting aside a time, usually following a meal, for elimination.

Assessment

To assess the patient with real or perceived constipation, collect the following data:

■ *Health history:* Usual and current pattern of defecation, including time of day, amount, and stool consistency; usual diet, fluid intake, and activity pattern; possible contributing factors such as opioid analgesics, activity limitations, painful hemorrhoids, perianal surgery; chronic diseases such as endocrine or neurologic disorders; prescribed and nonprescription medications.
■ *Physical examination:* Abdominal girth and shape, bowel sounds, tenderness, and percussion tone; digital exam of the rectum if impaction is suspected.

For discussion of constipation in the older adult see Meeting Individualized Needs on page 660.

Nursing Diagnoses and Interventions

Nursing interventions for the patient with constipation focus chiefly on education.

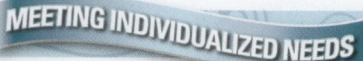

Constipation and perceived constipation are common problems in older adults. Although constipation is not a normal consequence of aging, factors such as slowed peristalsis, lowered activity levels, reduced food and fluid intake, and decreased sensory perception contribute to the higher incidence of constipation seen in the elderly. Chronic diseases such as diabetes, mobility problems, and medications also increase the risk of constipation in older adults.

Cultural influences and advertising lead many older adults to believe that a daily bowel movement is important for health. This belief contributes to an increased incidence of perceived constipation in the elderly. Because of this perception, the older adult may come to rely on laxatives, suppositories, or enemas to facilitate regular bowel movements. These external aids to defecation can further impair the ability to maintain "normal" bowel habits: a movement of soft stool every 2 to 3 days.

(margin, rotated) Irritable Bowel Syndrome Animation

Constipation

Whether real or perceived, constipation is disruptive to the patient's activities of daily living (ADLs) and life satisfaction.

- Monitor pattern of defecation and stool consistency. *This information helps establish the patient's usual pattern of defecation and differentiate between actual and perceived constipation.*
- Provide additional fluids to maintain an intake of at least 2500 mL per day. *A generous fluid intake helps maintain soft stool consistency and promote intestinal motility.*
- Encourage drinking a glass of warm water before breakfast. Provide time and privacy following breakfast for bowel elimination. *This helps develop a pattern of natural elimination; the warm water provides mild stimulation of bowel peristalsis.*
- Consult with the dietitian to provide a diet high in natural fiber unless contraindicated. Provide foods such as natural bran, prunes, or prune juice. *Natural fiber adds bulk to the stool and has a mild stimulant effect.*
- Encourage activities such as ambulation or chair exercises (e.g., range of motion, stretching, wheelchair lifts) as tolerated. *Activity stimulates peristalsis and strengthens abdominal muscles, facilitating elimination.*
- If indicated, consult with primary care provider about the use of bulk laxatives, stool softeners, or other laxatives as needed. *Laxatives may be necessary to relieve acute constipation. Patients with long-term activity or diet restrictions or impaired abdominal muscle strength may need a bulk-forming laxative to maintain normal elimination patterns and prevent constipation.*

Community-Based Care

Include the following topics when teaching self-care measures to prevent and treat constipation:

- Increasing dietary fiber intake by including fresh fruits and vegetables, whole grains, high-fiber breakfast cereals, and unprocessed bran in the diet (Bran can be sprinkled on cereals, mixed into bread or muffin recipes, or mixed with fruit juice to increase its palatability.)
- Maintaining fluid intake of 6 to 8 glasses of water per day (unless contraindicated)
- Suggestions for remaining physically active to promote bowel function and maintain muscle tone
- Responding to the urge to defecate when perceived
- Appropriate use of laxatives:
  - Do not use laxatives, suppositories, or enemas on a regular basis.

- Bulk-forming agents provide insoluble fiber, and are safe for long-term use; it is important to drink at least 6 to 8 glasses of water daily when using these (or any) laxatives.
- Other laxatives such as milk of magnesia, docusate (Colace, DSS), bisacodyl (Dulcolax), cascara, or castor oil should be used only occasionally to relieve constipation.
- Reporting any change in bowel habits such as new or persistent constipation or diarrhea, abdominal pain, black or bloody stools, nausea or anorexia, weakness, or unexplained weight loss to the primary care provider

The Patient with Irritable Bowel Syndrome

Irritable bowel syndrome (IBS), also known as spastic bowel or mucous colitis, is a motility disorder of the lower GI tract. It is a chronic disorder with no identifiable organic cause. IBS is characterized by abdominal pain and bloating with constipation, diarrhea, or both.

Irritable bowel syndrome is common, affecting up to 20% of people in Western civilization. It usually affects young people, with about 50% of patients diagnosed before age 35. There is a higher prevalence of IBS in women than in men (American College of Physicians [ACP], 2007).

Pathophysiology

In IBS, it appears that CNS regulation of the motor and sensory functions of the bowel is altered. Patients with IBS often experience increased motor reactivity of the small bowel and colon in response to stimuli such as food intake, hormonal influences, and physiologic or psychologic stress. IBS is characterized by visceral hypersensitivity and hyperactivity of the GI tract. Hypersecretion of colonic mucus is a common feature of the syndrome.

IBS may develop as a sequela of gastroenteritis, particularly when the infection is caused by *Campylobacter*, *Salmonella*, or *Shigella*.

A lower visceral pain threshold is often found in patients with IBS. Patients may complain of pain, bloating, and distention when intestinal gas levels are normal. Serotonin, a neurotransmitter involved in regulating GI motility, and visceral perception may play a role in IBS. Higher than expected postprandial plasma serotonin levels are noted in some patients with IBS (Fauci et al., 2008).

Psychologic factors such as depression or anxiety have been linked to IBS; however, they have not been identified as causes of the disorder. Recent research does indicate a correlation between emotional, physical, and sexual abuse and IBS.

Manifestations

IBS is characterized by abdominal pain that often is relieved by defecation and a change in bowel habits (see the accompanying Manifestations box). The pain may be either colicky, occurring in spasms, or dull and continuous. Altered patterns of defecation may include the following:

- A change in frequency
- Abnormal stool form (hard or lumpy, loose or watery)
- Altered stool passage (straining, urgency, or a sensation of incomplete evacuation)
- Passage of mucus

The patient may also complain of abdominal bloating and excess gas. Other manifestations include nausea, vomiting, anorexia, fatigue, headache, depression, or anxiety. The abdomen is often tender to palpation, particularly over the sigmoid colon.

Interdisciplinary Care

Irritable bowel syndrome is diagnosed based on the presence of abdominal pain or discomfort at least 3 days per month in the past 3 months that has at least two of the following characteristics: (1) improved with defecation, (2) associated with a change in frequency of elimination; (3) associated with a change in stool form (Fauci et al., 2008). Management is directed toward relieving manifestations and reducing or eliminating precipitating factors. Many patients benefit from cognitive behavioral therapy or psychotherapy (Moynihan, Callahan, Kalsmith, & Moses, 2008).

Diagnosis

The primary purpose of diagnostic testing is to rule out other causes of abdominal pain and altered fecal elimination. The stools may be examined for occult blood, ova and parasites, and white blood cells (WBCs). A sigmoidoscopy, colonoscopy, and/or a small-bowel series (upper GI series with small-bowel follow-through) and barium enema may be performed to visually examine the bowel mucosa, measure intraluminal pressures, and biopsy suspicious lesions. Nursing care for these procedures is outlined in ∞ Chapter 21. Laboratory tests include a complete blood count (CBC) with differential and erythrocyte sedimentation rate to evaluate for anemia from bleeding or a possible tumor. Increased WBCs indicate a bacterial infection.

MANIFESTATIONS of Irritable Bowel Syndrome

- Abdominal pain
  - May be relieved by defecation
  - May be intermittent and colicky or dull and continuous
- Altered bowel elimination
  - Constipation
  - Diarrhea
  - Mucous stools
- Abdominal bloating and flatulence
- Abdominal tenderness, especially over sigmoid colon
- Possible nausea, vomiting

Medications

Although not curative, medications may be prescribed to manage the manifestations of IBS. Bulk-forming laxatives (such as bran, methylcellulose, or psyllium) may help reduce bowel spasm and normalize the number and form of bowel movements. An anticholinergic drug such as dicyclomine (Antispas, Bentyl) or hyoscyamine (Anaspaz) may be ordered to inhibit bowel motility by interfering with parasympathetic stimulation of the gastrointestinal tract. It relieves postprandial abdominal pain when given 30 to 60 minutes before meals. Because of side effects such as dry mouth, blurred vision, and urinary hesitancy, these drugs are used with caution in older adults. In patients with diarrhea, loperamide (Imodium) or diphenoxylate (Lomotil) may be used prophylactically to prevent diarrhea in selected situations.

Antidepressant drugs, including tricyclics and selective serotonin reuptake inhibitors (SSRIs), may help relieve abdominal pain associated with IBS. Although the anticholinergic side effects of the tricyclics (such as desipramine [Norpramin] and imipramine [Tofranil]) may help decrease diarrhea, they have more adverse effects than SSRIs such as sertraline (Zoloft) and fluoxetine (Prozac). Alosetron (Lotronex) is a serotonin receptor antagonist that reduces abdominal pain and diarrhea in patients with IBS. Its use is limited, however, by its association with ischemic colitis.

Nutrition

Many patients with IBS benefit from additional dietary fiber. Adding bran to meals provides added bulk and water content to the stool, reducing the incidence of both loose diarrheal stools and hard, constipated stools. Other dietary changes are specific to individual triggers for IBS manifestations. Some patients may benefit from limiting lactose, fructose, or sorbitol intake (see Table 24–1). When excess gas and flatulence are problems, reducing the intake of gas-forming foods, such as beans, cabbage, apple and grape juices, nuts, and raisins, may be helpful. Caffeinated drinks, such as coffee, tea, and soft drinks, act as gastrointestinal stimulants; limiting intake of these fluids may prove beneficial.

Complementary and Alternative Therapies

Herbal preparations may provide some benefit for patients with IBS. Herbs with an antispasmodic effect, such as anise, chamomile, peppermint, and sage, may be used to reduce the manifestations of IBS. Ginger root can be consumed as a tea or capsule to assist with reduction of gas, bloating, and diarrhea and to improve the functioning of the stomach. Probiotic therapies (such as yogurt with active bacterial cultures) have been shown to benefit patients with IBS, as has hypnosis (Moynihan et al., 2008).

Nursing Care

Patients with IBS rarely require acute care for it as a primary problem. However, nurses frequently interact with these patients in clinics and other community settings.

Assessment

Careful assessment is important to help identify the effects of IBS on the patient. Collect the following assessment data:

- *Health history:* Current manifestations, their onset and duration; current treatment measures; effect of manifestations on

Irritable bowel syndrome is a functional disorder; while the patient's symptoms are real, physical findings often are absent or limited. Consensus groups of physicians practicing in western Europe developed and revised diagnostic criteria for IBS. These criteria include recurrent abdominal pain or discomfort that improves with defecation, a change in the frequency of defecation, and/or a change in the appearance of the stool. Barakzai, Gregory, and Fraser (2007) noted that the prevalence of IBS is lower in Mexican Americans, and wondered if this reflects a cultural bias in the criteria. Using a retrospective study of the medical records of 139 Mexican Americans diagnosed with IBS, they found significant variation in how these patients described their symptoms. While diarrhea, constipation, and abdominal pain frequently were reported, patients also presented with complaints such as dizziness, myalgias, headache, and more vague complaints such as cold bones and cold stomach. Symptoms related by more than half of the patients studied did not meet the current criteria for diagnosing IBS.

IMPLICATIONS FOR NURSING

Culture influences what people perceive, how they interpret it, and what they choose to report as symptoms. As nurses, it is important to remember that culture not only affects what the

patient reports, but also how we hear and interpret what is said. To develop an accurate diagnostic picture, it is important to obtain a complete history, maintain a nonjudgmental attitude about how symptoms are reported, and use a skilled interpreter.

CRITICAL THINKING IN PATIENT CARE

1. In this study, researchers found presenting complaints such as "nervousness" that initially may appear to be vague or unrelated to the ultimate diagnosis. What follow-up questions could you ask when the patient describes such symptoms as "nervousness," or "cold stomach"?
2. When you are talking with your non-native English-speaking patient, she describes a symptom in her native tongue. When you ask her to translate what she said to English, she tells you there is no corresponding English word for what she is describing. How will you proceed?
3. As you are talking with your patient with IBS symptoms, she says, "I might as well just go home and learn to live with this, because nobody seems to believe me, and all of the tests come back normal. I guess I'm just crazy." How will you respond?

---

lifestyle; careful exploration of history of emotional, physical, or sexual abuse. The accompanying nursing research box illustrates the importance of culture in how the patient may relate his or her symptoms.

- *Physical examination:* Apparent general state of health; abdominal shape and contour, bowel sounds, tenderness.

Nursing Diagnoses and Intervention

The primary nursing responsibility to patients with IBS is education; providing referrals and counseling are additional nursing responsibilities. See the previous sections on diarrhea and constipation for selected nursing interventions.

Community-Based Care

Include the following topics in teaching for the patient with IBS:

- The nature of the disorder and the reality of the patient's manifestations

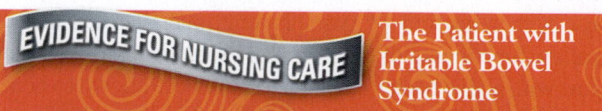

EVIDENCE FOR NURSING CARE   The Patient with Irritable Bowel Syndrome

Selected resources that nurses may find helpful when planning evidence-based nursing care follow.

- National Collaborating Centre for Nursing and Supportive Care. (2008, February). *Irritable bowel syndrome in adults. Diagnosis and management of irritable bowel syndrome in primary care.* London, UK: National Institute for Health and Clinical Excellence (NICE). Retrieved from http://www.guideline.gov/summary/summary.aspx?doc_id=13703
- Dalrymple, J., & Bullock, I. (2008 March). Diagnosis and management of irritable bowel syndrome in adults in primary care: Summary of NICE guidance. *BMJ: British Medical Journal, 336*(7643), 556–558.

- Stress and anxiety reduction techniques, such as meditation, visualization, exercise, "time-out," and progressive relaxation
- Dietary influences that may contribute to IBS and suggested dietary changes, such as additional fiber and water intake
- The use and role of prescribed medications, their adverse effects, and when to contact the physician
- The importance of routine follow-up appointments and of notifying the primary care provider if manifestations change (such as blood in the stool, significant constipation or diarrhea, increasing abdominal pain, or weight loss)

If needed, refer the patient to a counselor or other mental health professional for assistance in dealing with psychologic factors.

The Patient with Fecal Incontinence

Fecal incontinence, the loss of voluntary control of defecation, occurs less frequently than urinary incontinence but is no less distressing to the patient. Multiple factors may contribute to fecal incontinence (Box 24–1). Bowel incontinence is usually considered a symptom, not a disease or disorder. Patients often do not reveal fecal incontinence in discussing health concerns. Little information is available about its incidence and prevalence. Because many of the etiologic factors are more prevalent in the older adult, older patients are more often affected.

Pathophysiology

To understand the pathophysiology of fecal incontinence, it is necessary to understand the normal mechanisms of defecation. The rectum is normally empty. When it is distended by feces entering from the sigmoid colon, the defecation reflex is stimulated. This reflex causes involuntary relaxation of the internal sphincter and stimulates the urge to defecate. When the external

BOX 24–1 Selected Causes of Fecal Incontinence

Neurologic Causes
- Spinal cord injury or disease
- Head injury, stroke, or brain tumor
- Degenerative neurologic disease, such as multiple sclerosis, amyotrophic lateral sclerosis (ALS), dementia
- Diabetic neuropathy

Local Trauma
- Obstetric tears
- Anorectal injury
- Anorectal surgery with sphincter damage

Inflammatory Processes
- Infection
- Radiation

Other Causes
- Diarrhea
- Stool impaction
- Pelvic floor relaxation or loss of sphincter tone
- Tumors

sphincter, which is under both somatic (voluntary) and autonomic (involuntary) control, relaxes, defecation occurs. Adults normally can override the defecation reflex by voluntary contraction of the external sphincter and pelvic floor muscles. The wall of the rectum gradually relaxes, and the urge to defecate subsides.

The most common causes of fecal incontinence are those that interfere with either sensory or motor control of the rectum and anal sphincters. If the external sphincter is paralyzed as a result of spinal cord injury or disease, defecation occurs automatically when the internal sphincter relaxes with the defecation reflex. If sphincter muscles have been damaged or excessive pelvic floor relaxation has occurred, it may not be possible to override the defecation reflex with voluntary control.

Age-related changes in anal sphincter tone and response to rectal distention increase the risk for fecal incontinence in older adults. Resting and maximal anal sphincter pressures are decreased, particularly in older women. In addition, less rectal distention is needed to produce sustained relaxation of the anal sphincter in older females.

Interdisciplinary Care

The diagnosis of fecal incontinence is based on the patient's history. Physical examination of the pelvic floor and anus is performed to evaluate muscle tone and rule out a fecal impaction. Impaired sphincter muscle may be palpable on digital exam. Anorectal manometry or a rectal motility test may be used to evaluate the functional ability of the sphincter muscles. In this test, a small, flexible balloon catheter is introduced into the rectum, and pressures are measured in the rectum and internal and external sphincters. Normally, rectal dilation causes the internal sphincter to relax and the external sphincter to contract. Sigmoidoscopy may be used to examine the rectum and anal canal.

Management of fecal incontinence is directed toward the identified cause. Medications to relieve diarrhea or constipation may be prescribed. A high-fiber diet, ample fluids, and regular exercise are helpful for many patients. Exercises to improve sphincter and pelvic floor muscle tone (Kegel exercises) may be of long-term benefit. ∞ See Chapter 27 for more information about Kegel exercises.

Patients may benefit from using loperamide before meals and prophylactically before running errands or leaving the house. Biofeedback therapy may be used for mentally alert patients with intact sphincter muscles but low muscle tone. With motivation and reinforcement, patients achieve improved sphincter control in response to a stimulus. The goal of biofeedback is to improve sensation, coordination, and strength of the sphincter muscle.

When damage to the sphincter or rectal prolapse (protrusion of rectal mucous membrane through the anus) is the cause of fecal incontinence, surgical repair is the treatment of choice. Surgery may be indicated when conservative measures have not been effective. Permanent colostomy, the creation of an opening from the large bowel on the abdominal wall, is a last choice option for some patients, but it can control fecal output when other measures fail.

✍ Nursing Care

Health Promotion

A bowel training program to establish a regular pattern of elimination often is effective in relieving fecal incontinence. Teach the patient to establish a regular time of day for elimination, usually 15 to 30 minutes after breakfast. A stimulant, such as a cup of coffee, a rectal suppository, or even a phosphate enema, may be given to prompt defecation. Patients with neurologic incontinence may learn to stimulate the anal canal digitally to initiate defecation.

Dietary changes may be useful in managing fecal incontinence. If incontinence occurs only with mild loose or liquid stools, increasing dietary fiber or using a bulking agent to increase stool bulk and solidity may be effective. The majority of the fiber should come from a fiber-rich diet because fiber supplements provide only a limited amount of additional fiber. When incontinence of solid stool occurs, a low-residue diet of foods that are easily digested and absorbed may be prescribed to reduce the frequency of defecation.

Assessment

- *Health history:* Extent, onset, and duration of incontinence; identified contributing factors; history of spinal cord or anorectal injury or surgery; chronic diseases such as diabetes, multiple sclerosis, or other neurologic disorders.
- *Physical examination:* Mental status; general health; examination of perianal tissues; digital rectal examination.

Nursing Diagnoses and Interventions

Bowel Incontinence

Nurses are often responsible for instituting bowel training programs and other measures to manage fecal incontinence.

- Teach caregivers to place the patient on a toilet or commode and provide for privacy at a certain time of day. *Placing the patient in a normal position to defecate at a consistent time of day stimulates the defecation reflex and helps reestablish a pattern of stool evacuation.*
- If necessary, insert a glycerin or bisacodyl (Dulcolax) suppository 15 to 20 minutes before positioning on the toilet or commode. *This helps to stimulate evacuation. Once a regular*

elimination pattern is established, it may be possible to discontinue suppository use.

- Maintain a caring, nonjudgmental manner in providing care. *This promotes a feeling of acceptance when the patient may feel unacceptable.*

> **PRACTICE ALERT**
> Provide room odor control with deodorizer tablets, sprays, or other devices. Controlling odor is important to preserve the patient's self-esteem.

Risk for Impaired Skin Integrity

Good skin care is vital for the patient with fecal incontinence. Stool contains enzymes and other irritating substances that promote skin breakdown when they are not promptly removed. This can lead to pressure ulcers, particularly when a neurologic disorder (such as spinal cord injury, dementia, or stroke) impairs mobility.

- Clean the skin thoroughly with mild soap and water after each bowel movement. *Toilet tissue may be more irritating to the skin and less effective in removing fecal material.*
- Apply a skin barrier cream or ointment after each bowel movement. *These help protect the skin from irritating substances in the feces.*
- If incontinence pads or briefs are used, check frequently for soiling and change when feces is noted. *Although these help protect bedding and clothing from soiling, they can contribute to skin breakdown if they are not checked and changed frequently.*

Community-Based Care

Managing fecal incontinence is a challenging problem for the patient and family caregivers. For the patient with intact cognition, it can be psychologically devastating. The patient may become socially isolated from fear of odor or soiling clothing. Self-esteem may suffer from a sense of lost control over body functions and the inability to provide self-care. It is important to stress that incontinence is never normal (i.e., aging alone is not a cause of incontinence) and often is treatable. Encourage the patient to seek medical evaluation of the problem.

Topics of patient and family education include the following:

- Recommended dietary measures such as consuming a high-fiber diet and ample fluids to maintain soft, formed stool, or a low-residue diet to reduce the number of stools.
- Suggestions for regular exercise to stimulate bowel peristalsis and regular evacuation.
- Use of bulk-forming laxatives, such as psyllium seed (Metamucil), to provide stool bulk and reduce the number of small, liquid stools.
- Prescribed medications (such as loperamide to reduce the number of stools), their appropriate use, and management of adverse effects (such as constipation).
- Bowel training program instructions, including techniques for digital anal stimulation, inserting suppositories, or administering enemas as recommended. For digital anal simulation, teach to insert a lubricated gloved finger through the anal sphincter into the rectum 1.5 to 2 inches while seated on the toilet or commode, then use a circular side-to-side movement to gently stretch the rectal wall until the internal sphincter relaxes.
- The importance of good skin care, particularly if neurologic impairment is present.
- The potential benefits and associated risks of biofeedback and surgical treatment, if recommended.
- Provide referrals for home care or community health services as indicated.

Acute Inflammatory and Infectious Bowel Disorders

The GI tract is particularly vulnerable to inflammation and infection because of its continual exposure to the external environment. Although most pathogens affecting the GI tract are ingested in food or water, infection also may be spread by direct contact, possibly by the respiratory route. Pathogens may also be transmitted sexually through anal intercourse.

Acute disease of the GI tract may be caused by the pathogen itself or by a bacterial or other toxin. Acute inflammatory disorders such as appendicitis and peritonitis result from contamination of damaged or normally sterile tissue by the patient's own endogenous or resident bacteria.

The Patient with Appendicitis

Appendicitis, inflammation of the vermiform appendix, is a common cause of acute abdominal pain. It is the most common reason for emergency abdominal surgery, affecting 10% of the population (McPhee et al., 2008). Appendicitis can occur at any age, but is more common in adolescents and young adults and slightly more common in males than females.

Pathophysiology

The appendix is a tubelike pouch attached to the cecum just below the ileocecal valve. It is usually located in the right iliac region, at an area designated as McBurney's point (Figure 24–1 ■). The function of the appendix is not fully understood, although it may serve as a type of reservoir for beneficial intestinal bacteria.

Obstruction of the proximal lumen of the appendix is apparent in most acutely inflamed appendices. The obstruction is often caused by a *fecalith*, or hard mass of feces. Other obstructive causes include a calculus or stone, a foreign body, inflammation, a tumor, parasites (e.g., pinworms), or edema of lymphoid tissue. Following obstruction, the appendix becomes distended with fluid secreted by its mucosa. Pressure within the lumen of the appendix increases, impairing its blood supply and leading to inflammation, edema, ulceration, and infection. Purulent exudate forms, further distending the appendix. Within 24 to 36 hours, tissue necrosis and gangrene result, leading to perforation if treatment is not initiated. Perforation results in bacterial peritonitis.

Appendicitis can be classified as simple, gangrenous, or perforated, depending on the stage of the process. In simple appendicitis, the appendix is inflamed but intact. When areas of tissue

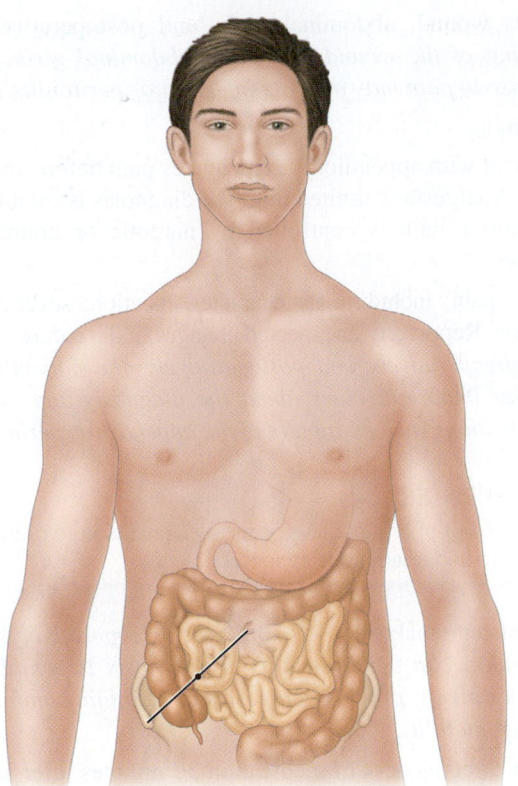

Figure 24–1 ■ McBurney's point, located midway between the umbilicus and the anterior iliac crest in the right lower quadrant. It is the usual site for localized pain and rebound tenderness due to appendicitis.

necrosis and microscopic perforations are present in the appendix, the disorder is called gangrenous appendicitis. A perforated appendix shows evidence of gross perforation and contamination of the peritoneal cavity.

Manifestations

Continuous mild generalized or upper abdominal pain is the initial characteristic manifestation of acute appendicitis. Over the next 4 hours, the pain intensifies and localizes in the right lower quadrant of the abdomen. It is aggravated by moving, walking, or coughing. On palpation, localized and rebound tenderness are noted at McBurney's point. *Rebound tenderness* is demonstrated by relief of pain with direct palpation of McBurney's point followed by pain on release of pressure. Extension or internal rotation of the right hip increases the pain. In addition to pain, a low-grade temperature, anorexia, nausea, and vomiting are often present.

Pain and local tenderness may be less acute in older adults, delaying the diagnosis, and leading to a 15% mortality of perforated appendicitis in the older adult (McPhee et al., 2008). This can present a significant problem; the course of acute appendicitis in older adults is more virulent and complications develop sooner. Pregnant women may develop right lower quadrant, periumbilical, or right subcostal (under the rib cage) pain due to possible displacement of the appendix by the distended uterus.

Complications

Perforation, peritonitis, and abscess are possible complications of acute appendicitis. Perforation is manifested by increased pain and a high fever. It can lead to a small, localized abscess, local

peritonitis, or significant generalized peritonitis. (Peritonitis is discussed in the next section of this chapter.)

A less common disorder is chronic appendicitis, characterized by chronic abdominal pain and recurrent acute attacks at intervals of several months or more. Other conditions, such as inflammatory bowel disease and renal disorders, often cause manifestations attributed to chronic appendicitis.

Interdisciplinary Care

The acutely inflamed appendix can perforate within 24 hours, so rapid diagnosis and treatment are important. Because of this urgency and the low incidence of surgical complications, diagnostic testing and preoperative treatment may be limited. The patient is admitted to the hospital, and intravenous fluids and antibiotics are initiated. Oral food and fluids are withheld until a diagnosis is confirmed. Once the diagnosis is established, an appendectomy is performed.

Diagnosis

Diagnostic and laboratory tests are used to help confirm the diagnosis and rule out other possible causes for the manifestations. Abdominal ultrasound is the most effective test for diagnosing acute appendicitis. Ultrasound examination has reduced the incidence of exploratory surgery and is particularly useful with patients with atypical symptoms, such as older adults. Other diagnostic tests used to accurately diagnose appendicitis include abdominal x-rays, an intravenous pyelogram, a urinalysis, and a pelvic examination. In addition, a WBC count with differential is obtained. With appendicitis, the total white count is elevated (10,000 to 20,000/mm^3), with an increased number of immature WBC (bands).

Medications

Prior to surgery, intravenous fluids are given to restore or maintain vascular volume and prevent electrolyte imbalance. Antibiotic therapy with a third-generation cephalosporin effective against many gram-negative bacteria, such as cefoperazone (Cefobid), cefotaxime (Claforan), ceftazidime (Fortaz), or ceftriaxone (Rocephin), is initiated prior to surgery. The antibiotic is repeated during surgery and continued for at least 48 hours postoperatively. (The nursing implications for cephalosporin antibiotics are discussed in ∞ Chapter 12.) Pain medications are administered as prescribed.

Surgery

The treatment of choice for acute appendicitis is an *appendectomy*, surgical removal of the appendix. Either a laparoscopic approach (insertion of an endoscope to view abdominal contents) or laparotomy (surgical opening of the abdomen) may be used for appendectomy. Laparoscopic appendectomy requires a very small incision through which the laparoscope is inserted. This procedure has several advantages: (1) Direct visualization of the appendix allows definitive diagnosis without laparotomy; (2) postoperative hospitalization is short; (3) postoperative complications are infrequent; and (4) recovery and resumption of normal activities is rapid.

An open appendectomy is performed by laparotomy. A small transverse incision is made at McBurney's point (Figure 24–1); the appendix is isolated and ligated (tied off) to prevent contamination of the site with bowel contents, and then removed. Laparotomy generally is used when the appendix has ruptured. It allows removal of contaminants from the peritoneal cavity by irrigation with sterile normal saline. Occasionally the wound may be left unsutured for periodic irrigation. Recovery is generally uneventful. ∞ Refer to Chapter 4 for discussion of preoperative and postoperative nursing care.

⌀ Nursing Care

A Case Study & Nursing Care Plan for a patient with appendicitis is included on page 667.

Assessment

Because appendicitis can rapidly progress from inflammation to perforation, prompt assessment is vital. Obtain the following assessment data:

- *Health history:* Current manifestations, including onset, duration, progression, and aggravating or relieving factors; most recent food or fluid intake; known medication or other allergies; current medications; history of chronic diseases.
- *Physical examination:* Vital signs including temperature; apparent general health; abdominal shape and contour, bowel sounds, tenderness to light palpation.

Nursing Diagnoses and Interventions

Preoperative nursing care is directed toward preparing the patient physically and psychologically for emergency surgery. Limited time is available for preoperative teaching.

PRACTICE ALERT
Keep the patient with suspected appendicitis NPO, and do not administer laxatives or enemas, which may cause perforation of the appendix. No heat should be applied to the abdomen; this may increase circulation to the appendix and also cause perforation.

Risk for Infection

Preventing complications during the preoperative and postoperative periods is a primary nursing care goal. Perforation and peritonitis are the most likely preoperative complications; postoperative complications include wound infection, abscess, and possible peritonitis.

PRACTICE ALERT
Assess abdominal status frequently, including distention, bowel sounds, and tenderness. Increasing generalized pain, a rigid, boardlike abdomen, and abdominal distention may indicate developing peritonitis.

- Monitor vital signs, including temperature. *Tachycardia and rapid shallow respirations may indicate perforation of the appendix with resulting peritonitis. Fever may develop as well, and the blood pressure may fall if sepsis is present.*
- Maintain intravenous infusion until oral intake is adequate. *Intravenous fluids are given to maintain vascular volume and to provide a route for antibiotic administration.*

- Assess wound, abdominal girth, and postoperative pain. *Swelling of the wound, increased abdominal girth, or an increase in pain may indicate infection or peritonitis.*

Acute Pain

The patient with appendicitis experiences pain before and after surgery. Analgesia is limited until the diagnosis is established. Postoperative pain is controlled by narcotic or nonnarcotic analgesics.

- Assess pain, including its character, location, severity, and duration. Report any unexpected changes in the nature of pain. *Both preoperatively and postoperatively, the patient's pain provides important clues about the diagnosis and possible complications such as rupture of the appendix or peritonitis.*

PRACTICE ALERT
Sudden relief of preoperative pain may signal rupture of the distended and edematous appendix.

- Administer analgesics as ordered. *Preoperatively, pain medication can be given after a diagnosis is established. Postoperatively, provide analgesics to maintain comfort and enhance mobility.*
- Assess effectiveness of medication 30 minutes after administration. Report unrelieved pain. *Pain unrelieved by prescribed analgesic may indicate a complication or the need for further assessment. For example, continued abdominal discomfort and distention may indicate excess intestinal gas that may be better relieved by ambulation.*

Using NANDA, NIC, and NOC

Linkages between a selected NANDA nursing diagnosis, NIC, and NOC for the patient with appendicitis are shown in the chart that follows.

Community-Based Care

Preoperative teaching may be limited by pain and the urgent nature of surgery. Explain why food and fluids are not permitted during this time. If time allows, teach postoperative turning, coughing, deep breathing, and pain management.

NANDA, NIC, AND NOC LINKAGES
The Patient with Appendicitis or Peritonitis

NANDA
> Acute Pain
>
> ⬇
>
> **NIC**
> Analgesic Administration
> Pain Management
> Vital Signs Monitoring
>
> ⬇
>
> **NOC**
> Pain Control
> Comfort Status: Physical
> Vital Signs

Data from NANDA International. (2009). *Nursing diagnoses: Definitions & classification 2009–2011.* Oxford, UK: Wiley-Blackwell; Bulechek, G., Butcher, H., & Dochterman, J. (Eds.). (2008). *Nursing interventions classification (NIC)* (5th ed.). St. Louis, MO: Mosby; and Moorhead, S., Johnson, M., Maas, M., & Swanson, E. (Eds.). (2008). *Nursing outcomes classification (NOC)* (4th ed.). St. Louis, MO: Mosby.

Jamie Lynn is a 19-year-old college student majoring in physical therapy. Ms. Lynn arrives at the emergency department at 1:00 AM complaining of general lower abdominal pain that had started the previous evening. By midnight, the pain was more localized over the right lower quadrant. She also reports nausea and vomiting.

ASSESSMENT

Sue Grady, RN, completes the admission assessment in the emergency department. Ms. Lynn is complaining of nausea and severe abdominal pain, stating, "Walking makes my stomach hurt worse." Physical assessment findings include T 100.2°F (37.8°C), P 84, R 16, and BP 110/70; skin warm to touch; abdomen flat and guarded, with marked tenderness in right lower quadrant. Ms. Lynn's CBC shows WBC 14,000/mm^3; neutrophils 81.1%; lymphocytes 12.5%. The diagnosis of acute appendicitis is made, and Ms. Lynn is transferred to surgery for a laparoscopic appendectomy.

DIAGNOSES

- *Impaired Skin Integrity* related to surgical incision
- *Acute Pain* related to surgical intervention
- *Anxiety* related to situational crisis

EXPECTED OUTCOMES

- Incision will heal without infection or complications
- Will verbalize adequate pain relief
- Will verbalize decreased anxiety
- Will return to preoperative activities

PLANNING AND IMPLEMENTATION

- Assess pain using a pain scale; provide analgesics as needed.
- Teach pain management following discharge.
- Teach abdominal splinting during coughing, turning, or ambulating as needed.
- Teach home care of incision.
- Discuss activity limitations as ordered.
- Instruct to report fever or warmth, redness, or drainage from the incision.

EVALUATION

On discharge the following evening, Ms. Lynn is fully ambulatory. Her appetite has returned, and she is tolerating food and fluids well. Her temperature is normal. The nurse provides Ms. Lynn with written and verbal information on postoperative care following an appendectomy.

CRITICAL THINKING IN THE NURSING PROCESS

1. What is the pathophysiologic basis for Ms. Lynn's elevated WBC?
2. How would Ms. Lynn's postoperative care and teaching differ if she had undergone a laparotomy instead of a laparoscopic appendectomy?
3. Outline a teaching plan to give to patients for home care following an appendectomy.
4. Develop a care plan for Ms. Lynn for the nursing diagnosis *Anxiety* related to a situational crisis.

See Evaluating Your Response in Appendix C.

With uncomplicated appendectomy, the patient often is discharged either the day of surgery or the day following surgery. Postoperative teaching includes the following:

- Wound or incision care, including hand hygiene and dressing change procedures as indicated
- Instructions to report fever, increased abdominal pain, swelling, redness, drainage, bleeding, or warmth of the operative site to the physician
- Activity limitations (e.g., lifting, driving), if any
- Returning to work if appropriate

The Patient with Peritonitis

Peritonitis, inflammation of the peritoneum, is a serious complication of many acute abdominal disorders. It is usually caused by enteric bacteria entering the peritoneal cavity through a perforated ulcer, ruptured appendix, perforated diverticulum (discussed later in this chapter), necrotic bowel, or during abdominal surgery. Pelvic inflammatory disease, gallbladder rupture, abdominal trauma, or peritoneal dialysis can also lead to peritonitis.

Pathophysiology

The peritoneum is a double-layered serous membrane lining the walls (parietal peritoneum) and organs (visceral peritoneum) of the abdominal cavity. There is a potential space between the parietal and visceral layers of the peritoneum that contains a small amount of serous fluid. This space, the peritoneal cavity, normally is sterile.

Peritonitis results from contamination of the normally sterile peritoneal cavity by infection or a chemical irritant. Chemical peritonitis often precedes bacterial peritonitis. Perforation of a peptic ulcer or rupture of the gallbladder releases gastric juices (hydrochloric acid and pepsin) or bile into the peritoneal cavity, causing an acute inflammatory response.

Bacterial peritonitis usually is caused by infection by *Escherichia coli*, *Klebsiella*, *Proteus*, or *Pseudomonas* bacteria, which normally inhabit the bowel. Inflammatory and immune defense mechanisms are activated when bacteria enter the peritoneal space. These defenses can effectively eliminate small numbers of bacteria, but may be overwhelmed by massive or continued contamination. When this occurs, mast cells release histamine and other vasoactive substances, causing local vasodilation and increased capillary permeability. Polymorphonuclear leukocytes (a type of WBC) infiltrate the peritoneum to phagocytize bacteria and foreign matter. Fibrinogen-rich plasma exudate promotes bacterial destruction and forms fibrin clots to seal off and segregate the bacteria. This process helps limit and localize the infection, allowing host defenses to eradicate it. Continued contamination, however, leads to generalized inflammation of the peritoneal cavity. The inflammatory process causes fluid to shift into the peritoneal space (third spacing). Circulating blood volume is depleted, leading to hypovolemia. *Septicemia*, a systemic disease caused by pathogens or their toxins in the blood, may follow.

Manifestations

Manifestations of peritonitis depend on the severity and extent of the infection, as well as the age and general health of the patient. Both local and systemic manifestations are

MANIFESTATIONS of Peritonitis

ABDOMINAL/GASTROINTESTINAL MANIFESTATIONS
- Diffuse or localized pain
- Tenderness with rebound
- Boardlike rigidity
- Diminished or absent bowel sounds
- Distention
- Anorexia, nausea, and vomiting

SYSTEMIC MANIFESTATIONS
- Fever
- Malaise
- Tachycardia
- Tachypnea
- Restlessness
- Confusion or disorientation
- Oliguria

FAST FACTS

Mortality from Peritonitis
- The overall mortality rate associated with peritonitis is about 40%.
- Patients with other medical conditions, older patients, and those with greater bacterial contamination have a higher risk of dying.
- Young people with perforated ulcers or appendicitis, those with less extensive bacterial contamination, and those who receive early surgical intervention have mortality rates of less than 10%.

present (see the accompanying box). The patient often presents with evidence of an *acute abdomen*, an abrupt onset of diffuse, severe abdominal pain. The pain may localize and intensify near the area of infection. Movement may intensify the pain. The entire abdomen is tender, with guarding or rigidity of abdominal muscles. The acute abdomen is often described as boardlike. Rebound tenderness may be present over the area of inflammation. Peritoneal inflammation inhibits peristalsis, resulting in a paralytic ileus. (Paralytic ileus is discussed in a later section of this chapter.) Bowel sounds are markedly diminished or absent, and progressive abdominal distention is noted. Pooling of GI secretions may cause nausea and vomiting. Systemic manifestations of peritonitis include fever, malaise, tachycardia and tachypnea, restlessness, and possible disorientation. The patient may be oliguric (having little urine output) and show signs of dehydration and shock.

The older, chronically debilitated, or immunosuppressed patient may present with few of the classic signs of peritonitis. Increased confusion and restlessness, decreased urinary output, and vague abdominal complaints may be the only manifestations present. These patients are at increased risk for delayed diagnosis, contributing to a higher mortality rate.

Complications

Complications of peritonitis may be life threatening. Abscess formation is common. The very defense mechanisms designed to isolate and localize the infection can protect it from immune responses and systemic antibiotics. Fibrous adhesions in the abdominal cavity are a late complication and may lead to subsequent obstruction.

Without prompt and effective treatment, septicemia and septic shock can develop. Fluid loss into the abdominal cavity may lead to hypovolemic shock. These potentially lethal complications require immediate, aggressive intervention to prevent multiple organ failure and death. Septicemia, shock, and its management are discussed in ∞ Chapter 11.

Interdisciplinary Care

Care of the patient with peritonitis focuses on establishing the diagnosis and identifying and treating its cause as well as the peritonitis. Preventing complications is an important aspect of care.

Diagnosis

Diagnostic tests are performed to establish the diagnosis of peritonitis, rule out other disorders, and help identify the cause. The tests that may be ordered include a WBC count (elevated to approximately $20,000/mm^3$ in peritonitis), blood cultures, abdominal CT scan, liver and renal function studies, serum electrolytes, and a paracentesis (in peritonitis, peritoneal fluid will contain increased protein and WBCs). Increased numbers of immature blood cells are present as the bone marrow releases them in response to the infection.

Medications

Until the infecting organism has been identified, a broad-spectrum antibiotic effective against organisms commonly implicated in peritonitis is prescribed. A beta-lactam antibiotic such as imipenem (Primaxin) or meropenem (Merrem), which has a very broad spectrum of action, may be used. Once culture results have been obtained, antibiotic therapy is modified to the specific organism(s) responsible. Antibiotics that may be ordered include ampicillin (e.g., Omnipen, Polycillin), metronidazole (Flagyl), ciprofloxacin (Cipro), clindamycin (Cleocin), a cephalosporin such as ceftriaxone (Rocephin) or an aminoglycoside antibiotic such as gentamicin (Garamycin) or amikacin (Amikin). Nursing implications for antibiotic therapy are discussed in ∞ Chapter 12. Analgesics are prescribed to promote comfort.

Surgery

If the cause of peritonitis is a perforation, gangrenous bowel, or inflamed appendix, a laparotomy is done to close the perforation or remove the damaged and inflamed tissue. If an abscess is present, it also may be surgically drained or removed.

Peritoneal lavage, washing of the peritoneal cavity with copious amounts of warm isotonic fluid, may be done during surgery. This procedure dilutes residual bacteria and removes gross contaminants, blood, and fibrin clots. In rare instances, peritoneal lavage may be continued for several days following surgery. The solution is infused into the upper portion of the peritoneal cavity and removed via drains in the pelvic cul-de-sac. Careful attention to fluid and electrolyte status and strict aseptic technique are necessary.

Patients who have had laparotomy for peritonitis often return from surgery with either Penrose or closed drain systems such as a Jackson-Pratt drain. In some cases, the incision may be left unsutured. With severe and long-standing peritonitis, the abdomen may be closed temporarily with polypropylene mesh containing a nylon zipper or Velcro to allow repeated exploration of the abdomen and drainage of infectious sites.

Nutrition

Intravenous fluids and electrolyte replacements are administered to maintain vascular volume and fluid and electrolyte balance. Parenteral nutrition is given until adequate oral intake resumes.

Other Treatments

The patient is placed on bed rest in Fowler's position to help localize the infection and promote lung ventilation. Oxygen is often ordered to facilitate cellular metabolism and healing.

INTESTINAL DECOMPRESSION   The inflammatory process of peritonitis often draws large amounts of fluid into the abdominal cavity and the bowel. In addition, peristaltic activity of the bowel is slowed or halted by the inflammation, causing **paralytic ileus** (or *ileus*), impaired propulsion or forward movement of bowel contents. Intestinal decompression is used to relieve abdominal distention, facilitate closure, and minimize postoperative respiratory problems. A nasogastric or long intestinal tube is inserted and connected to continuous drainage (Figure 24–2 ■). If prolonged intestinal decompression is

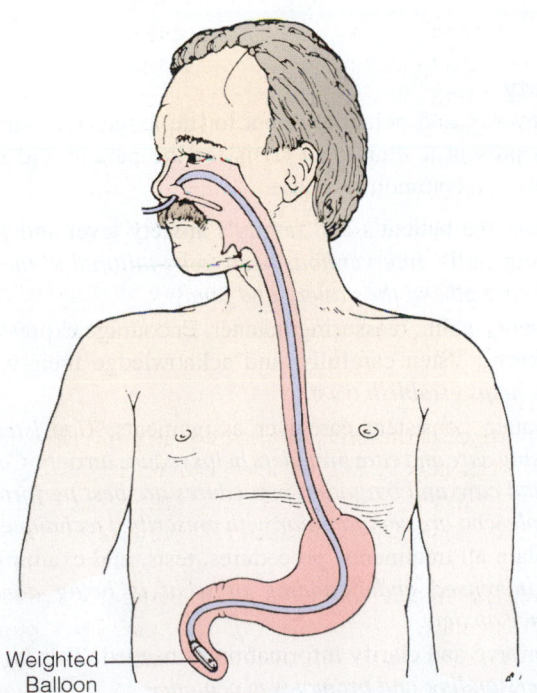

Weighted Balloon

Figure 24–2 ■ The weighted tip or inflated balloon at the end of an intestinal tube is drawn into the intestine by gravity and peristalsis.

anticipated, a jejunostomy may be performed for comfort. Suction is maintained until peristalsis resumes, bowel sounds are present, and the patient is passing flatus. Food and fluids are withheld until intestinal motility has returned and suction is discontinued.

Nursing Care

Peritonitis is a serious illness. Early recognition and treatment are important to minimize the risk of complications.

Assessment

- *Health history:* Pain, its onset, character, severity, location, aggravating and relieving factors; associated symptoms such as anorexia, nausea, vomiting; current and previous history of peptic ulcer disease, gallbladder disease, chronic diseases; current medications.
- *Physical examination:* Vital signs including temperature; level of consciousness; skin color, temperature, warmth, capillary refill and turgor; abdominal shape, contour, bowel sounds, tenderness, tympany, and guarding.

Nursing Diagnoses and Interventions

Patients with peritonitis require intensive nursing and medical care to prevent complications and recover fully. Nursing care priorities include interventions to manage pain, altered fluid balance, altered protection due to infection, and anxiety.

Acute Pain

Abdominal distention and acute inflammation contribute to the pain associated with peritonitis. Surgery further disrupts abdominal muscles and other tissues, causing pain. Effective pain management promotes immune function, healing, mobility, and recovery.

- Assess pain, including its location, severity (using a standard pain scale), and type. Monitor analgesic effectiveness. Report changes to the primary care provider.

> **PRACTICE ALERT**
> Unrelieved pain or a change in the location, severity, or type of pain may indicate spread of infection, abscess formation, or other complications of peritonitis.

- Place in Fowler's or semi-Fowler's position with the knees and feet elevated. *This position reduces stress on abdominal structures and facilitates respirations, promoting comfort.*
- Administer analgesics as ordered on a routine basis or using patient-controlled analgesia (PCA). *Routine analgesic administration maintains a therapeutic blood level and helps maintain comfort, facilitating healing and movement.*
- Teach and assist with adjunctive pain management techniques such as meditation, visualization, massage, and progressive relaxation. *Adjunctive measures augment analgesics and help promote a sense of control over pain.*

Deficient Fluid Volume

In peritonitis, significant amounts of fluid are drawn into the abdominal cavity and bowel, reducing vascular volume and cardiac output. This fluid also may be lost from the body by intestinal suction or through drains placed in the abdomen during surgery. An unsutured incision causes additional significant fluid loss.

■ Maintain accurate intake and output records. Measure urine output every 1 to 2 hours; report output of less than 30 mL/h. Measure gastrointestinal output at least every 4 hours. *Intake and output records provide valuable information about fluid volume status.*

> **PRACTICE ALERT**
> Urine output of less than 30 mL/hr may indicate hypovolemia, decreased cardiac output, and impaired tissue perfusion.

■ Monitor vital signs and hemodynamic parameters such as central venous pressure, cardiac output, and pulmonary artery pressures every hour or as indicated. *These measurements provide important information about fluid and vascular volumes as well as cardiovascular status.*

■ Weigh daily. *Weight is an accurate indicator of fluid status. Rapid weight gains or losses reflect changes in fluid volume.*

■ Assess skin turgor, color, temperature, and mucous membranes at least every 8 hours. *Warm, dry skin with poor turgor and dry, shiny mucous membranes indicate dehydration.*

■ Measure or estimate fluid losses through abdominal drains and on dressings. *Significant amounts of exudative fluid may be lost.*

■ Monitor laboratory values, including hemoglobin and hematocrit, urine specific gravity, serum osmolality and electrolytes, and ABGs. Report changes to the physician. *Laboratory results provide information about fluid and electrolyte status and acid–base balance.*

■ Administer intravenous fluids and electrolytes as ordered. Gastrointestinal drainage may be replaced milliliter for milliliter with a balanced electrolyte solution. *Intravenous fluids are necessary to meet daily fluid intake needs, as well as replace continuing losses of water and electrolytes.*

■ Provide good skin care and frequent oral hygiene. *Fluid deficit increases the risk of skin breakdown and ulceration of mucous membranes.*

Delayed Surgical Recovery

Repeated surgeries, an unsutured incision, and the presence of drains interrupt skin integrity and the body's first line of defense against microorganisms. In addition, immune defenses are stressed by the infection and potential malnutrition. As a result, the risk for impaired healing and further infection is increased.

■ Monitor temperature, pulse rate, and for localized signs of infection such as redness and swelling around incisions and drain sites, increased or purulent drainage, and cloudy or malodorous urine. *Impaired defenses increase the risk for extension of the infection or unrelated infections.*

■ Obtain cultures of purulent drainage from any site. *Early identification of any additional infection allows timely intervention.*

■ Monitor WBC and differential, serum protein, and albumin. *An increased WBC with a higher percentage of immature cells present in the blood is an indicator of infection and normal immune response. Serum albumin and protein levels are indicators of nutritional status as well as immune function.*

■ Practice meticulous hand hygiene and use standard precautions at all times. *Hand hygiene reduces transient bacteria on the skin and remains the most important method of controlling infection. Standard precautions reduce the risk of spreading infection to or from the patient.*

■ Use strict aseptic technique for dressing changes, wound care, and irrigations. *Disruption of the protective barrier of the skin increases the risk of contamination and further infection.*

■ Maintain fluid balance and nutritional status through enteral or parenteral feedings, as indicated. See the following research box for evidence-based recommendations for care of enterally fed patients. *Adequate nutrition and fluid balance are necessary for optimal immune system function.*

> **PRACTICE ALERT**
> An acute infection such as peritonitis causes a stress response with excess energy expenditure and loss of body proteins and cell mass. Glycogen stores are rapidly depleted, and body proteins are used to meet energy needs. Withholding food further complicates this process, leading to rapid development of protein-calorie malnutrition (PCM). PCM impairs the immune response and slows healing.

Anxiety

The severity and potential threat to life associated with peritonitis present a situational crisis for the patient and family. Anxiety is a common response.

■ Assess the patient's and family's anxiety level and present coping skills. *Interventions need to be tailored to the needs and strengths of the patient and family.*

■ Present a calm, reassuring manner. Encourage expression of concerns; listen carefully, and acknowledge their validity. *This helps establish trust.*

■ Maintain consistent caregiver assignments. *Consistency of nursing care and care providers helps reduce anxiety. Complex wound care and irrigation procedures are best performed by people who are very familiar with prescribed techniques.*

■ Explain all treatments, procedures, tests, and examinations. *An increased understanding of what is being done can reduce anxiety.*

■ Reinforce and clarify information as needed. *This improves understanding and promotes acceptance.*

■ Teach and assist with relaxation techniques such as meditation, visualization, and progressive relaxation. *These measures promote positive coping skills and reduce physical manifestations of anxiety.*

MOVING EVIDENCE INTO ACTION | **Enterally Fed, Critically Ill Patient**

A vital component of the treatment and care of critically ill patients (such as those with peritonitis) is providing nutritional support, primarily through enteral feedings. Although this remains the method of choice for this population, and has many advantages, enteral feeding also comes with the risk of bronchopulmonary aspiration as a complication. Aspiration occurs in as many as 40% of patients and up to 50% to 75% of patients who have an endotracheal tube in place. Several methods are currently used to detect aspiration, but not as much information has been published about how to prevent aspiration in enterally fed patients. This study (Sanko, 2004) was conducted to review and synthesize current research in order to make recommendations to improve the quality and safety of administering enteral nutrition to critically ill patients. Recommended prevention techniques included the following:

- Preventing aspiration with feeding tube placement by verifying placement with an x-ray. After verifying the placement, the tube should be securely taped and the external tube length should be measured, noted, and marked on the tube as a reference point for further tube placement checks. If the position of the tube is questioned, the x-ray should be repeated.
- Maintaining the head of the bed at an angle of at least 30 degrees, with 45% being ideal, and stopping feedings 30 to 60 minutes before placing the patient in the supine position.
- Maintaining cuff pressure in patients with artificial airways at 20 to 30 cm H_2O.

Based on published findings, there is not sufficient evidence to support placement of feeding tubes beyond the pylorus or using small-bore tubes to prevent aspiration.

IMPLICATIONS FOR NURSING

Based on this review of the relevant research, it is obvious that more research is needed in this area of care. However, daily assessments of the patient and the feeding tube with multiple methods (including x-ray, external length marking, pH testing, aspirate characteristics, or trypsin/pepsin levels) should be conducted by caregivers who have the knowledge to accurately interpret the results.

CRITICAL THINKING IN PATIENT CARE

1. Aspiration is defined as the inhalation of oropharyngeal or gastric contents into the larynx and lower respiratory tract. The result is usually aspiration pneumonitis or aspiration pneumonia. What assessments would you conduct and monitor to identify these complications?
2. You are on a committee that is evaluating the practice of adding blue dye to feeding solutions in order to better detect aspiration. The literature does not support this method. How and what would you do to convince the committee that this practice should not be continued?
3. What principle supports elevating the head of the bed to prevent aspiration? (Consider gravity and the placement of internal organs with the patient in this position.)

Community-Based Care

Teaching for home care includes the following topics:

- Wound care procedures, including dressing changes or irrigations. Provide verbal and written instructions on how to change dressings or do irrigations as well as where to obtain supplies, and allow opportunities to practice and demonstrate the procedure prior to discharge.
- Prescribed medications, including name and purpose of the drug, potential adverse effects, and their management.
- Manifestations of further infection (redness, heat, swelling, purulent drainage, chills, and fever) and potential complications to be reported to the care provider.
- Prescribed activity restrictions.
- Instructions for a high-calorie, high-protein diet for healing and optimal immune function.

Provide a referral to home health services for assessment, wound care, and further teaching, as needed.

The Patient with Gastroenteritis

Gastroenteritis, or *enteritis*, is an inflammation of the stomach and small intestine. Enteritis may be caused by bacteria, viruses, parasites, or toxins. Upper GI manifestations such as anorexia, nausea, and vomiting are common. Diarrhea of varying intensity and abdominal discomfort are nearly universal features of gastroenteritis.

The infectious organism usually enters the body in contaminated water or food. For this reason, gastroenteritis often is called food poisoning. Viruses commonly cause acute diarrheal illness. Diarrhea due to rotaviruses or the Norwalk virus occurs year-round in both adults and children. These illnesses are generally mild and self-limited, but can have severe consequences in the very young, the very old, or in people with impaired immune function.

Pathophysiology

Bacterial or viral infection of the GI tract produces inflammation, tissue damage, and manifestations by two primary mechanisms:

- *The production of exotoxins.* A number of bacteria produce and excrete an exotoxin that enters the surrounding environment (intestinal lumen), causing damage and inflammation. Exotoxins in the GI tract are often referred to as *enterotoxins*. They impair intestinal absorption and can cause secretion of significant amounts of electrolytes and water into the bowel, resulting in diarrhea and fluid loss. Common bacterial enterotoxins include those produced by *Staphylococcus, Clostridium perfringens, Clostridium botulinum,* some strains of *Escherichia coli, Vibrio cholera,* and *C. difficile.*
- *Invasion and ulceration of the mucosa.* Other bacteria, including some *Shigella, Salmonella,* and *E. coli* species, damage tissue more directly. They invade the intestinal mucosa of the small bowel or colon, producing microscopic ulceration, bleeding, fluid exudate, and water and electrolyte secretion.

In some cases, the mechanism of injury is unclear. It may be a combination of direct and toxic damage. For example, the Norwalk virus damages the mucosa of the jejunum, with fluid and electrolyte secretion.

Manifestations

Although the manifestations of bacterial and viral enteritis vary according to the organism involved, several features are common (see the following Manifestations box). Anorexia, nausea, and vomiting are caused by distention of the upper GI tract by unabsorbed chyme and excess water. Bowel distention, along with irritation of the bowel mucosa and gas production due to fermentation of undigested food, lead to abdominal pain and cramping. Borborygmi, excessively loud and hyperactive bowel sounds, are another result. The abdomen is often distended and tender.

Diarrhea is usually predominant with enteritis. Fluid is secreted into the bowel lumen, and the unabsorbed chyme and electrolytes create an osmotic pull of fluid into the bowel. Motility is stimulated, and stools become watery and frequent. Loss of fluids and electrolytes through diarrhea can lead to the most serious manifestations of enteritis. Fluid volume can be rapidly depleted, leading to dehydration and hypovolemia. Orthostatic hypotension and fever may be noted initially. If fluid loss continues, hypovolemic shock may develop.

Complications

Electrolyte and acid–base imbalances may result from gastroenteritis. Extensive vomiting can lead to metabolic alkalosis due to the loss of hydrochloric acid from the stomach. When diarrhea predominates, metabolic acidosis is more likely. Potassium is lost in either case, leading to hypokalemia. Hyponatremia may develop if fluids are replaced with pure water. Headache, cardiac irregularities, changes in respiratory rate and pattern, malaise and weakness, muscle aching, and signs of neuromuscular irritability are the possible manifestations of these disturbances in homeostasis.

Specific Types of Gastrointestinal Infections

Several gastrointestinal infections produce specific effects that are discussed below and summarized in Table 24–3.

TRAVELER'S DIARRHEA   People traveling to another country frequently develop diarrhea within 2 to 10 days, particularly when there is a significant difference in climate, sanitation standards, or food and drink. Strains of enterotoxin-producing *E. coli*, *Shigella* species, *Salmonella*, and *Campylobacter* are the most frequent causes of traveler's diarrhea (Yates, 2005). Other bacteria and viruses also may cause traveler's diarrhea.

MANIFESTATIONS of Gastroenteritis

GASTROINTESTINAL EFFECTS
- Anorexia, nausea, and vomiting
- Abdominal pain and cramping
- Borborygmi
- Diarrhea

GENERAL EFFECTS
- Malaise, weakness, and muscle aches
- Headache
- Dry skin and mucous membranes
- Poor skin turgor
- Orthostatic hypotension, tachycardia
- Fever

Up to 10 or more loose stools per day and abdominal cramping are common manifestations. Nausea and vomiting are less frequent; fever is rare. Manifestations usually resolve within 2 to 5 days. Complications are rare.

ESCHERICHIA COLI HEMORRHAGIC COLITIS   Most pathologic forms of *E. coli* bacteria cause little more than common traveler's diarrhea. However, some strains, such as serotype 0157:H7, produce a potent enterotoxin in the large intestine after being ingested. This toxin damages bowel mucosa and the endothelial cells of blood vessels in the GI tract. If absorbed, the toxin can damage other blood vessels as well, such as those of the kidney.

Cattle provide the reservoir for *E. coli* 0157:H7. It is usually spread through undercooked beef (hamburger in particular) and unpasteurized milk or apple juice. It may also be spread by direct contact via the fecal–oral route. The onset of hemorrhagic colitis is abrupt, with severe abdominal cramping and watery diarrhea that becomes grossly bloody within 24 hours. Fever may be present.

Hemolytic uremic syndrome and thrombotic thrombocytopenic purpura are significant complications of *E. coli* hemorrhagic colitis, affecting about 5% of people with the disease. Older adults have the highest risk for developing complications.

STAPHYLOCOCCAL FOOD POISONING   Certain foods provide an excellent medium for staphylococcal growth when contaminated and left at room temperature. Examples include meats and fish, dairy products (e.g., custards), and bakery products (e.g., cream-filled pastries). The organism itself does not affect the bowel; the toxin it produces, however, impairs intestinal absorption and acts on receptors in the gut, stimulating the medullary center to produce vomiting.

The onset of staphylococcal food poisoning is abrupt, occurring within 2 to 8 hours after consuming the contaminated food. Nausea and vomiting are severe. Manifestations typically last 3 to 6 hours, and include abdominal cramping, diarrhea, headache, and fever. Complications such as fluid and electrolyte imbalances are rare, but may develop in older adults and people with underlying chronic disease processes.

CHOLERA   *Cholera* is an acute diarrheal illness caused by strains of *Vibrio cholerae*. It is endemic in parts of Asia, the Middle East, and Africa. Cholera is spread by the fecal–oral route through contaminated water or food. The organism produces an enterotoxin, enzymes, and other substances that affect the entire small intestine. Water and electrolytes are secreted into the bowel lumen in response to the toxin. The enzymes and other substances produced by the bacteria may affect mucous protection of bowel endothelium.

Cholera ranges in severity from very mild, with few or no manifestations, to acute and fulminant. Its onset is typically abrupt, with severe, frequent, watery diarrhea. Up to 1 L of stool may be passed in an hour, rapidly depleting fluid volume. Stool is often described as "rice water stool" and is characteristically gray and cloudy, with no fecal odor, blood, or pus. Vomiting may accompany the diarrhea. Other manifestations relate to the loss of fluid and electrolytes: thirst, oliguria, muscle cramps, weakness, and significant signs of dehydration.

TABLE 24–3 Selected Bacterial Infections of the Bowel

DISEASE AND ORGANISM	INCUBATION	PATHOGENESIS	MANIFESTATIONS	MANAGEMENT
Traveler's diarrhea: *Escherichia coli*	24 to 72 hours	Enterotoxin causes hypersecretion of the small intestine.	Abrupt onset of diarrhea; vomiting rare	Prophylactic bismuth subsalicylate; antidiarrheal such as loperamide; 3-day course of norfloxacin, ciprofloxacin, or azithromycin
Hemorrhagic colitis: *E. coli* 0157:H7	1 to 3 days	Enterotoxin causes direct mucosal damage in large intestine; also toxic to vascular endothelial cells.	Severe abdominal cramping, watery diarrhea that becomes grossly bloody; fever; possible complications: hemolytic uremic syndrome and thrombotic thrombocytopenic purpura	Supportive care with fluid replacement and bland diet; may require dialysis or plasmapheresis for complications
Staphylococcal food poisoning	2 to 8 hours	Enterotoxin impairs intestinal absorption and affects vomiting centers in the brain.	Severe nausea and vomiting; abdominal cramping and diarrhea; headache and fever	Fluid and electrolyte replacement as needed
Cholera: *Vibrio cholerae*	1 to 3 days	Enterotoxin affects entire small intestine, causing secretion of water and electrolytes into bowel lumen.	Severe diarrhea with "rice water stool," gray, cloudy, odorless, with no blood or pus; vomiting; thirst, oliguria, muscle cramps, weakness; dehydration and vascular collapse	Oral or intravenous rehydration; possible antimicrobial therapy with tetracycline, doxycycline, or ciprofloxacin, others
Salmonellosis: *Salmonella*	8 to 48 hours	Superficial infection of the GI tract without invasion or production of toxins.	Diarrhea with abdominal cramping, nausea, and vomiting; low-grade fever, chills, weakness	Treatment of symptoms; a third-generation cephalosporin or a fluoroquinolone antibiotic for severe illness
Shigellosis (bacillary dysentery): *Shigella*	1 to 4 days	Local tissue invasion, primarily involving large intestine and distal ileum; endotoxin causes fluid and electrolyte secretion into bowel lumen.	Watery diarrhea with severe abdominal cramping and tenesmus; lethargy	Fluid and electrolyte replacement; correction of acidosis; antibiotic therapy with ciprofloxacin, ceftriaxone, others
Clostridium difficile colitis (*C. difficile*)	1 to 2 weeks	Antibiotic therapy interferes with normal protective bacteria in the colon; *C. difficile* colonizes and releases toxins that cause mucosal inflammation and damage	Diarrhea, abdominal cramps, malaise, fever, anorexia	Cessation of the causative antibiotic; antibiotic therapy with vancomycin or metronidazole (specific for *C. difficile*)

Metabolic acidosis and hypokalemia develop. If untreated, circulatory collapse and acute renal failure may occur.

Recovery from cholera usually occurs spontaneously within 3 to 6 days. With prompt and adequate fluid replacement, mortality is less than 1%.

CLOSTRIDIUM DIFFICILE COLITIS *Clostridium difficile colitis* (*C. difficile* colitis) is associated with antibiotic therapy. Treatment with antibiotics (especially broad-spectrum antibiotics) predisposes to interference with the normal protective bacteria of the colon, leading to colonization by *C. difficile* by the oral–fecal route. Subsequent release of toxins by the bacteria causes mucous damage and inflammation. This is primarily a problem in hospitalized patients, causing diarrhea and abdominal cramping. These manifestations commonly begin within 1 to 2 weeks of antibiotic treatment. It is also being seen in the community in healthy adults. The bacteria can be identified in the stool.

SALMONELLOSIS *Salmonellosis* is food poisoning caused by ingesting raw or improperly cooked foods contaminated with *Salmonella* bacteria. Meat, poultry, eggs, and dairy products commonly are implicated in salmonellosis; recent outbreaks

have been linked to products such as peanuts and alfalfa sprouts. These bacteria cause superficial infection of the GI tract, rarely invading further. They do not produce a toxin.

Manifestations develop 8 to 48 hours after ingesting the bacteria. Diarrhea may be violent with abdominal cramping, nausea, and vomiting. A low-grade fever, chills, and weakness may accompany GI manifestations. The disease usually is self-limited, resolving within 3 to 5 days, although bacteremia may develop.

SHIGELLOSIS (BACILLARY DYSENTERY) *Shigellosis* (or bacillary dysentery) occurs worldwide, and may be endemic or occur in epidemics. Humans are the reservoir for *Shigella* organisms, which are spread directly via the fecal–oral route or indirectly through contaminated food, fomites (inanimate objects), and vectors (such as fleas). The incubation period for shigellosis is 1 to 4 days.

Shigella organisms infect the distal ilium and lower intestine. They invade the tissue, causing inflammation, and they produce an enterotoxin. The result is watery diarrhea containing blood, mucus, and inflammatory exudate. The onset of diarrhea is abrupt, with severe abdominal cramping, and *tenesmus,* a sensation of urgent and continuing need to defecate. Lethargy is common; rarely, neurologic manifestations occur.

In adults, shigellosis is usually mild and self-limiting. Older adults and debilitated patients are at risk for volume depletion and electrolyte imbalances. Secondary infection is another potential complication, as is acute blood loss from mucosal ulcerations.

NOROVIRUS Norovirus-associated gastroenteritis is a highly contagious disease that often occurs in outbreaks within an institution or facility. It is characterized by acute vomiting, watery, nonbloody diarrhea, abdominal cramps, and nausea. Systemic manifestations such as myalgia, malaise, headache, and low-grade fever are common.

Noroviruses are transmitted primarily by the fecal–oral route, either through direct contact or via contaminated food or water. The average incubation period is 12 to 48 hours. The disease tends to be self-limiting, with dehydration its most common complication.

Interdisciplinary Care

The goals of care for gastroenteritis are to manage the manifestations, prevent complications, identify the cause of the infection, and prevent its spread. The history and manifestations provide valuable cues about the cause. Diagnostic testing is used to identify the pathogen and evaluate its effects. In most cases, treatment is supportive, directed toward relieving manifestations, restoring fluid and electrolyte balance, and maintaining function.

Diagnosis

If manifestations are severe or do not resolve within about 48 hours, laboratory testing is used to identify the causative organism and to assess fluid, electrolyte, and acid–base balance. A stool specimen for culture, ova and parasites, and fecal leukocytes usually reveals the infective organism, but may require up to 6 weeks to identify some bacteria. In infections such as botulism, the toxin itself may be isolated in the stool. Contamination of the stool by urine or treatment with antibiotics, bismuth subsalicylate (Pepto-Bismol), or mineral oil may interfere with pathogen growth, altering stool culture results. Use a clean bedpan or collection device to obtain the stool specimen, and instruct the patient to avoid mixing the stool with urine or toilet tissue.

A sigmoidoscopy may be done to differentiate inflammatory bowel disease from infectious processes. It does not replace stool cultures, because the lesions associated with some infectious processes are indistinguishable from those of ulcerative colitis. (Nursing care of the patient having a sigmoidoscopy is discussed in ∞ Chapter 21.)

Serum osmolality and electrolytes and ABGs are done to assess and monitor fluid, electrolyte, and acid–base balance. Common imbalances associated with enteritis and diarrhea are outlined in Table 24–4.

Medications

Acute enteritis usually resolves spontaneously, and no drug treatment is required. If the patient is severely ill and manifestations are prolonged, medications may be prescribed.

Antibiotic therapy specific to the organism may be used to treat bacterial colitis, cholera, salmonellosis, or shigellosis. Ciprofloxacin (Cipro), clarithromycin (Biaxin), erythromycin, amoxicillin/clavulanate (Augmentin), or another antibiotic may be prescribed. Stool culture is obtained prior to starting antibiotics, but treatment may begin before culture results are available. A presumptive diagnosis based on history and presenting manifestations guides the choice of antibiotic.

An antidiarrheal drug may be prescribed to promote comfort and reduce fluid loss. Nursing measures related to antidiarrheal medications are outlined in the Medication Administration box on page 655.

TABLE 24–4 Laboratory Values Associated with Enteritis and Diarrhea

TEST	NORMAL VALUE	CHANGE WITH SIGNIFICANT DIARRHEA
Serum osmolality	280 to 300 mOsm/kg	Increased; levels above 320 mOsm/kg indicate significant dehydration.
Serum potassium	3.5 to 5.3 mEq/L	Decreased due to loss through stool and vomitus; levels below 2.5 mEq/L are critical.
Serum sodium	135 to 145 mEq/L	Decreased due to loss through stool and vomitus; may be significant when fluid losses are replaced with pure water; levels below 120 mEq/L may be critical.
Serum chloride	95 to 105 mEq/L	Increased when sodium loss is greater than chloride loss; decreased with severe diarrhea and with vomiting; possible critical values are below 80 mEq/L or above 115 mEq/L.
Blood gases		
■ pH	Arterial: 7.35 to 7.45	Decreased in metabolic acidosis, a possible result of severe diarrhea; increased in metabolic alkalosis, a possible result of severe vomiting and chloride loss; values below 7.25 or above 7.55 are critical.
■ PCO_2	Arterial: 35 to 45 mmHg	Typically decreased in metabolic acidosis as the body attempts to eliminate excess acid by "blowing off" CO_2; increased with metabolic alkalosis as the body retains CO_2 in an attempt to normalize pH.
■ Bicarbonate	24 to 28 mEq/L	Decreased in metabolic acidosis; increased in metabolic alkalosis.
Hematocrit	Males: 40% to 54%	Increased with dehydration and hypovolemia as a result of concentration of blood cells.
	Females: 36% to 46%	
Urine specific gravity	1.005 to 1.030	Increased with dehydration and hypovolemia as kidneys attempt to conserve fluid.

PRACTICE ALERT
Use of antidiarrheal preparations prolongs the course and increases complication risk in some types of gastroenteritisis, and therefore is contraindicated. Obtain a careful history before recommending these agents to the patient.

Nutrition and Fluids

Replacing lost fluids and electrolytes is vital when vomiting and/or diarrhea are severe or prolonged. In many cases of enteritis, fluid and electrolyte replacement are all that is required until the infection resolves.

Oral rehydration is preferred for replacing physiologic fluids. An oral glucose-electrolyte solution is often well tolerated in sips, even when vomiting is present. Commercial preparations such as Gatorade, All-Sport, and Pedialyte are available. A solution of 5 mL (1 teaspoon) table salt, 5 mL baking soda, 20 mL (4 teaspoons) granulated sugar, and flavoring (such as lemon extract or juice) to 1 L (1 quart) of water also is effective.

Intravenous rehydration may be necessary with severe diarrhea and fluid loss. In some cases, a combination of oral and intravenous fluids may be used to replace lost fluids and maintain vascular volume. Balanced electrolyte solutions, such as glucose in normal saline and Ringer's solution, are used. Lactated Ringer's solution or another alkalinizing solution may be ordered if metabolic acidosis is present.

Gastric Lavage

Gastric lavage and catharsis—in effect, "washing out" the stomach and intestines—may be performed to remove unabsorbed toxin from the GI tract if botulism is suspected. The patient with botulism is closely observed for signs of respiratory distress. Respiratory support with endotracheal intubation or tracheostomy and mechanical ventilation may be required (∞ see Chapter 37).

Plasmapheresis

Plasmapheresis (plasma exchange therapy) may be performed to remove circulating toxins for hemorrhagic colitis caused by *E. coli*. ∞ See Chapter 44 for the nursing care of a patient having this procedure. Potential complications include those associated with intravenous catheters, shifts in fluid balance, and altered blood clotting.

Dialysis

Acute tubular necrosis and renal failure associated with hemorrhagic colitis may necessitate dialysis to remove wastes and prevent severe fluid and electrolyte imbalances and metabolic acidosis. Although acute renal failure often resolves spontaneously and renal function resumes, dialysis can be lifesaving. Either hemodialysis or peritoneal dialysis may be used, generally as a temporary measure. Nursing care related to acute renal failure and dialysis is discussed in ∞ Chapter 28.

∞ Nursing Care

Although *C. difficile* colitis bacterial infections usually are hospital acquired, few patients with acute enteritis require hospitalization. Most are treated in community settings. Assessment,

education, and support of self-care measures are major nursing responsibilities.

Health Promotion

Nurses play a significant role in preventing enteritis as educators, community health providers, and advocates for environmental safety.

Teach the importance of proper food handling and maintaining appropriate temperatures. Raw fruits and vegetables should be thoroughly washed before consuming. Adequate cooking of meat products is vital to prevent disorders such as staphylococcal food poisoning, *E. coli* hemorrhagic colitis, and salmonellosis. Emphasize the importance of not consuming raw meat products, and cooking hamburger, in particular, to the point that no redness is noted in the meat. The highly pathogenic *E. coli* serotype 0157:H7 is present in the gut of infected animals. Meats from the animal may be contaminated with bowel contents. The organism is readily destroyed by heat, so cuts of meat such as steaks or roasts are less likely to cause infection, since the organism is on the outside of the meat. However, the process of grinding hamburger allows *E. coli* to be mixed throughout the meat. Thorough cooking destroys the organism. This pathogen (and others) may be spread through unpasteurized milk. Discuss the dangers of consuming milk that has not been pasteurized and encourage patients to avoid it.

Dairy products, eggs, and egg products left at room temperature provide a good growth medium for bacteria. Discuss the importance of prompt refrigeration of meats and these products to minimize this risk. Many gastrointestinal infections are spread through contaminated water. Encourage travelers to consume only bottled water unless local water supplies are clearly safe. Water purification tablets are available for hikers and campers, and may be used when traveling abroad.

Assessment

- *Health history:* Onset, duration, and severity of manifestations; recent activities such as attending a picnic or potluck, international travel, or camping; other affected members of the household; measures taken to relieve manifestations or replace fluids.
- *Physical examination:* Vital signs including temperature and orthostatic blood pressure; skin color, temperature, moisture, and turgor; peripheral pulses and capillary refill; abdominal shape, contour, bowel sounds, tenderness.

Nursing Diagnoses and Interventions

Diarrhea and fluid volume deficit are priority nursing diagnoses. See the earlier section of this chapter on diarrhea for specific nursing interventions related to these diagnoses. Nausea and vomiting frequently accompany the diarrhea associate with gastroenteritis. Nursing care of the patient experiencing nausea and vomiting is detailed in ∞ Chapter 23.

Community-Based Care

Discuss the following topics with the patient for self-care:

- The importance of good hand hygiene, particularly before handling food and after each bowel movement
- The need to wash clothing and linens contaminated with feces separately in hot water and detergent

- Oral solutions to replace lost fluids and electrolytes
- Appropriate use of antidiarrheal medications if recommended
- Manifestations of complications to report to the healthcare provider

The Patient with a Protozoal Bowel Infection

Parasites live within, on, or at the expense of other organisms. Parasitic intestinal infections are common in developing countries. They include both protozoal and helminthic (parasitic worms) infections. Parasites that infect the bowel usually enter the GI tract through the mouth by the fecal–oral route; some are spread by direct contact or through sexual activity.

Of the protozoal bowel infections, only giardiasis is common in the United States. Amebiasis is found chiefly in the tropics and where sanitation is poor. Cryptosporidiosis, a form of coccidiosis, is an important worldwide cause of sporadic mild diarrhea, traveler's diarrhea, and severe diarrhea in people who are immunocompromised.

Pathophysiology and Manifestations

The most common protozoal infections of the bowel are discussed next and summarized in Table 24–5.

Giardiasis

Giardiasis is a protozoal infection of the upper small intestine caused by *Giardia lamblia*. It is the most common intestinal protozoal pathogen in the United States. Humans and other mammals are the reservoir for *Giardia*. It is spread by the fecal–oral route, usually in contaminated food or water. It is also spread by direct contact. When the cyst form of the organism is ingested, trophozoites emerge in the duodenum and jejunum, attaching themselves to the intestinal mucosa. This leads to superficial invasion, inflammation, and destruction of the mucosa of the small intestine.

Giardiasis may be asymptomatic, although manifestations may develop suddenly or insidiously. Diarrhea is common. It is usually mild, with one or more large, loose stools per day. Diarrhea may be severe, however, with frequent, copious, frothy, malodorous, and greasy stools. Other manifestations include weight loss and weakness; anorexia, nausea, and vomiting; epigastric pain, abdominal cramping and distention, flatulence, and belching. Malabsorption may develop.

Amebiasis

Amebiasis (amebic dysentery) is caused by the protozoon *Entamoeba histolytica*. Several strains of the protozoon have been identified. Humans are the host for this parasite. It usually is transmitted through food or water contaminated by feces and by person-to-person contact. The parasite enters the intestines, where it may live without causing disease, or it may invade the intestinal wall to cause ulceration and inflammation. The cecum, appendix, ascending colon, sigmoid colon, and rectum are most often affected. Ulcers may spread to cause hemorrhage, edema, and mucosal sloughing. The infection may spread via the blood to the liver, lungs, or brain.

Amebiasis is usually asymptomatic. Mild manifestations include abdominal cramps, flatulence, and intermittent diarrhea containing blood and mucus. Severe manifestations of amebic dysentery include frequent watery stools containing blood, mucus, and necrotic tissue; colic, tenesmus, and abdominal tenderness; nausea and vomiting; and fever. The liver may be enlarged and tender to palpation.

Complications are rare, but may include appendicitis, bowel perforation with peritonitis, and fulminating colitis.

TABLE 24–5 Common Protozoal Infections of the Bowel

DISEASE AND ORGANISM	INCUBATION	PATHOGENESIS	MANIFESTATIONS	MANAGEMENT
Giardiasis: *Giardia lamblia*	1 to 3 weeks or more	Trophozoite attaches to mucosa in duodenum and jejunum, causing superficial invasion, inflammation, and tissue destruction.	Diarrhea, mild or severe, daily or intermittent; anorexia, nausea, vomiting; epigastric pain, cramping, distention; flatulence and belching; may be asymptomatic	Metronidazole (Flagyl, others), tinidazole (Tindamax), nitazoxanide (Alinia)
Amebiasis: *Entamoeba histolytica*	2 to 4 weeks	Organisms may reside in large intestine without causing disease or can invade colon wall, causing ulceration; may be carried via blood to liver to produce abscess.	Usually asymptomatic; diarrhea may be mild, with few semiformed mucus-containing stools per day, or severe, with 10 to 20 blood-streaked liquid stools per day; abdominal cramps and flatulence; colic, tenesmus, vomiting, tenderness; fatigue, weight loss; prostration and toxicity	Metronidazole and paromomycin (Humatin) or iodoquinol (Diiodohydroxyquin, Yodoxin); metronidazole or tinidazole for hepatic abscess
Cryptosporidiosis: *Cryptosporidium*	2 to 10 days	Organisms attach to epithelial surface of small bowel (jejunum), causing villous atrophy and mild inflammatory changes; may secrete enterotoxin.	In immunocompetent patients: asymptomatic to profuse, watery diarrhea of sudden onset, abdominal cramping; malaise, fever; anorexia, nausea, vomiting. In immunodeficient patients: profuse watery diarrhea with loss of up to 15 to 20 L/day; severe malabsorption, electrolyte imbalance; weight loss; lymphadenopathy	Self-limiting in immunocompetent patients. For immunodeficient patients: spiramycin, zidovudine (AZT), paromomycin (Humatin), octreotide, eflornithine; fluid and electrolyte replacement; parenteral nutrition as needed

Cryptosporidiosis (Coccidiosis)

Cryptosporidiosis causes sporadic mild diarrhea and traveler's diarrhea in all age groups. In people with impaired immune function, such as those with human immunodeficiency virus (HIV) disease, it causes severe diarrhea, malabsorption, and significant weight loss.

This organism is transmitted by the fecal–oral route. Contaminated water is a frequent source of infection. The organism attaches to epithelium of the small bowel, causing surface damage and inflammation and characteristic watery diarrhea. The disease is self-limited in people with competent immune systems. Watery diarrhea may be accompanied by low-grade fever, nausea, vomiting, abdominal cramps, and general malaise.

Immunocompromised patients develop profuse watery diarrhea with significant fluid and electrolyte losses and severe malabsorption. The organism may be found in the respiratory tract, large intestines, and biliary tract of immunocompromised people. Lymphadenopathy (enlarged lymph nodes) may develop.

Interdisciplinary Care

Management of protozoal bowel infections includes identifying the causative organism and administering medications.

Diagnosis

Diagnostic testing includes a stool examination for ova and parasites, and possibly for their antigens. Many protozoa are shed intermittently rather than continuously; stools are collected sequentially (e.g., every other day for a total of three specimens). These organisms often are fragile, requiring a fresh stool specimen. Serology testing for an immune response to the suspected parasite also may be performed. A sigmoidoscopy may be done to examine the bowel mucosa and collect a stool specimen for examination (in this case, no bowel prep is done prior to the test). When giardiasis is suspected, duodenal aspirate may be stained and examined microscopically for the protozoa. Small bowel biopsy can identify giardiasis or *Cryptosporidium* infection.

MEDICATION ADMINISTRATION   Antiprotozoal Agents

LOCAL (GASTROINTESTINAL) AGENTS

Iodoquinol (Yodoxin, Amebaquin)

Paromomycin (Humatin)

These drugs exert a local amebicidal effect in the intestines and are poorly absorbed when administered orally. Local agents have the advantage of provoking fewer side effects than systemically active agents.

Nursing Responsibilities

- Assess for potential contraindications:
  a. Hypersensitivity to the drug or drug class
  b. Iodoquinol: malnutrition, thyroid disorders; hepatic or renal impairment, optic neuropathy, or hypersensitivity to iodine
  c. Paromomycin: ulcerative bowel lesions; hypersensitivity to aminoglycoside antibiotics, impaired renal function, intestinal obstruction
- Observe for adverse effects: anorexia, nausea, vomiting, abdominal cramping, diarrhea, and increased flatulence; report skin rash, visual disturbances, or changes in blood work to primary care provider.

Health Education for the Patient and Family

- Take as prescribed for the full course of therapy.
- Take with food to reduce gastrointestinal effects.
- Keep follow-up appointments as recommended to evaluate the effects of treatment.
- Report adverse effects to the physician:
  a. Any change in vision
  b. Numbness, tingling, or pain in extremities
  c. Chills, fever, skin rash or boils
  d. A change in urination or character of urine
  e. Diminished hearing or tinnitus
  f. Weight loss, diarrhea, fatty stools
  g. Candidiasis of the mouth or vagina
- Practice good hand hygiene, particularly after using the toilet, to prevent spreading the disease to others.

SYSTEMIC AGENTS

Metronidazole (Flagyl, Satric, Metzol, others)

Furazolidone (Furoxone), albendazole (Albenza)

Patients with symptomatic protozoal infections are generally treated with a systemic antiprotozoal agent. Metronidazole is the most widely used of these antiprotozoal agents and is the drug of choice for treating amebiasis.

Nursing Responsibilities

- Assess for possible contraindications to therapy:
  a. Hypersensitivity to the prescribed agent or related drugs
  b. Liver dysfunction or blood dyscrasias
  c. Concurrent use of alcohol or an MAOI
  d. Pregnancy
- Administer as ordered.
  a. Metronidazole may be given orally after meals or as a continuous or intermittent intravenous infusion.
  b. Administer furazolidone and albendazole orally with meals to minimize gastric distress.
- Observe for possible adverse effects; notify the physician if significant. Gastrointestinal effects are common.
  a. Peripheral neuropathy and CNS effects may occur with metronidazole.
  b. Blood dyscrasias may develop with furazolidone or albendazole; monitor CBC and report abnormal results.
  c. Furazolidone can cause hypoglycemia; carefully monitor blood glucose in diabetic patients.
  d. Report abnormal liver function test results.
- Monitor the character and number of stools; obtain specimens as ordered to evaluate the effectiveness of therapy.

Health Education for the Patient and Family

- Take the drug as prescribed for the full duration of the prescription.
- Taking oral preparations after meals helps minimize gastrointestinal side effects. Notify the physician if nausea and vomiting continue.
- Do not use alcohol while taking these drugs. An antabuse-type response with severe headache, flushing, and vomiting may occur.
- Report adverse effects to the physician, including dizziness and other nervous system changes, sore throats, fatigue, bruising, or infection.
- Candidiasis of the mouth or vagina may occur with metronidazole therapy. Report symptoms to the physician.
- A harmless change in urine color to deep yellow (quinacrine) or rust or brown (metronidazole or chloroquine) may occur while taking these drugs.
- If you are diabetic taking furazolidone, carefully monitor blood glucose levels because hypoglycemia may develop.
- Practice good hand hygiene, particularly after using the toilet, to prevent transmitting the protozoa to others.

Medications

Pharmacologic treatment includes both local and systemic antiparasitic drugs, such as iodoquinol (Amebaquin), paromomycin (Humatin), metronidazole (Flagyl), tinidazole (Tindamax), or nitazoxanide (Alinia). Treatment is usually provided on an outpatient basis. Severe amebic dysentery may require hospitalization for intravenous fluid and electrolyte replacements. Nursing care related to common antiprotozoal drugs is outlined in the Medication Administration box on page 677.

✍ Nursing Care

Nursing assessment, diagnoses, and interventions for the patient with a protozoal GI infection are similar to those indicated for patients with bacterial or viral infections. *Diarrhea* and *Risk for Deficient Fluid Volume* are priority nursing diagnoses. See previous sections of this chapter for specific nursing interventions related to these diagnoses.

Nurses need to teach the public how parasitic diseases are transmitted and how to avoid spreading the infection. Prevention of amebiasis and giardiasis involves the following:

- Provision of safe water supplies
- Appropriate disposal of human feces
- Safe food storage, handling, and preparation
- Adequate hand hygiene after defecating and before handling food

Instruct people living in high-risk areas (e.g., tropical climates, areas with untreated water supplies) to boil, filter, or treat water supplies with iodine to eliminate protozoal contamination. Instruct them to avoid foods that cannot be peeled or cooked. Teach the manifestations of protozoal infections and where to obtain treatment.

Emphasize the importance of keeping toilet areas clean and maintaining good personal hygiene. Advise the patient to avoid rectal contact during sexual activity. Other household members should have stool specimens examined for parasites. Contaminated recreational water (swimming pools, water slides) is increasingly recognized as a potential source of cryptosporidiosis; advise immunocompromised individuals to avoid this exposure.

The Patient with a Helminthic Disorder

Helminths are parasitic worms, capable of causing infectious diseases in humans. Helminths are subclassified as round worms (nematodes), flukes (trematodes), or tapeworms (cestodes).

Pathophysiology

Although all helminths can infect humans, the definitive host and intermediate hosts vary with each organism. In nearly all instances of helminthic disorders, the organism enters the body through the GI tract in contaminated and inadequately cooked foods. Some of these organisms remain in the intestinal tract; others migrate to infect the liver, lungs, or other structures. Table 24–6 summarizes the most common helminths and their effects.

Interdisciplinary Care

The management of helminthic disorders includes diagnostic testing and medications.

Diagnosis

The primary means of diagnosing helminthic disorders is examination of the stool for ova and parasites. Enterobiasis is diagnosed by the presence of the parasite's eggs on the perianal skin or on cellulose tape placed over the anus. A CBC may also be ordered. Anemia may be present, particularly with hookworm disease. *Eosinophilia* (an increased percentage of eosinophils in the blood) is common in helminthic disorders. With trichinosis, serum muscle enzymes such as the creatinine kinase (CK) and aspartate aminotransferase (AST) are typically elevated. Serologic testing for antibodies to the worm may also be performed. Blood, duodenal washings, and cerebrospinal fluid (CSF) may be examined for the presence of the trichinosis larvae. Inflamed muscle may be biopsied.

Medications

Helminthic infections often are treated with a single oral dose or 3-day course of pyrantel pamoate (Antiminth), albendazole (Albenza), or mebendazole (Vermox). Doses may need to be repeated every 2 weeks for patients with heavy infections. These drugs are generally safe, requiring few precautions. Giving the drug after meals minimizes GI side effects. Treatment is followed by a stool culture at 2 weeks to evaluate effectiveness. If necessary, an additional course of the drug is prescribed. Other members of the household are generally also treated.

Most patients with trichinosis recover spontaneously without long-term effects. The intestinal phase of the disease is treated with albendazole, taken twice daily for as long as 60 days, or a 13-day course of mebendazole. Hospitalization may be required during the muscle invasion phase of the disease if the infection is severe. Corticosteroids may be used to reduce the inflammation and manage the manifestations.

✍ Nursing Care

Because many patients with these disorders are asymptomatic, nurses need to be alert for histories that indicate risk and subtle manifestations of the disorder. Use standard precautions to minimize the risk of spreading these infections to other patients. Wear gloves and gowns as necessary to prevent fecal contamination of hands and clothing. On rare occasions, parasites may be present in the sputum or vomitus, so handle these secretions with care. Disinfect toilets, toilet seats, and commodes after use. Teach the patient the importance of hand hygiene after using the toilet and before handling food to prevent reinfection.

Discuss measures to prevent spread of the disease in the household. Emphasize the importance of hygiene measures including changing bedding, daily cleaning of toilets with disinfectant, and hand hygiene.

Many helminthic disorders are acquired by consuming food that has been fecally contaminated or contains larvae of the organism. Explain the importance of not fertilizing food or grain crops with fecal material, particularly human feces. Teach

TABLE 24–6 Selected Helminthic Diseases

	INFECTION	HOST	AREA	PATHOGENESIS	MANIFESTATIONS
Nematode infections	Ascariasis	Humans	Worldwide, cosmopolitan; warm, moist climates	Eggs are ingested in fecally contaminated food and drink; motile larvae migrate to lungs and back to small intestine, where they mature to produce more eggs.	Pulmonary: low-grade fever, cough, blood-tinged sputum, wheezing, dyspnea, substernal chest pain. GI: ulcer-like epigastric pain, vomiting, abdominal distention
	Enterobiasis (pinworm infection)	Humans	Worldwide, cosmopolitan	Infect cecum; eggs deposit on perianal skin, organisms may be transmitted to others or reinfect host by oral ingestion.	Nocturnal perianal and perineal pruritus; insomnia, irritability, restlessness
	Hookworm disease	Humans	Tropics and subtropics	Larvae enter through skin or by ingestion and migrate to lungs, up bronchial tree, and down esophagus to mature in upper small bowel, where they attach and suck blood.	Skin: pruritic dermatitis at site of entry. Pulmonary: dry cough, wheezing, blood-tinged sputum. GI: anorexia, diarrhea, abdominal pain. Systemic: anemia, pallor, cardiac insufficiency
	Trichinosis	Pigs, dogs, cats, rats, many wild animals	Temperate areas where pork is consumed	Larvae are ingested in undercooked meat; adult female burrows into mucosa of small intestine to produce larvae that disseminate via blood and lymphatic system to body tissues and become encysted in striated muscle.	GI: diarrhea, abdominal cramps, malaise. Muscle: fever; muscle pain, tenderness, edema, and spasm. Systemic: periorbital and facial edema, sweating; photophobia and conjunctivitis; manifestations of inflammation in tissues invaded by larvae
Cestode infections	Fasciolopsiasis (intestinal fluke) Tapeworm	Humans; other mammals and fish	Worldwide	Organism is ingested by eating uncooked fish or meat containing embryo cysts, by fecal contamination, or by swallowing infected intermediate hosts, such as arthropods, fleas, or lice; head (scolex) of adult worm attaches in upper small intestine, and eggs form in individual segments.	Large tapeworms: often asymptomatic; infection may cause mild nausea, diarrhea, abdominal pain; anemia, thrombocytopenia, and mild leukopenia. Small tapeworms: may be asymptomatic; diarrhea, abdominal pain, anorexia, vomiting, weight loss, and irritability

patients to cook all meats and fish adequately to destroy possible larvae. In general, pickled or salt-preserved meats and fish are no safer than raw. Smoking, another means of preserving fish and meat, may not achieve temperatures high enough to destroy the organisms. Vegetables grown in soil that may be contaminated with eggs or larvae should be peeled or cooked prior to eating.

Emphasize the importance of safe water supplies. Encourage people traveling to areas in which water supplies are questionable to drink only bottled water or carry purification tablets. Work with patients who have private water systems to protect water from fecal contamination by either humans or animals.

The patient with a helminthic disorder may feel dirty or be ashamed of the disease. Emphasize the prevalence of these disorders, and assure the patient that infection can occur despite good health practices when the eggs or larva of the organism are prevalent.

Chronic Inflammatory Bowel Disorders

The Patient with Inflammatory Bowel Disease

Chronic **inflammatory bowel disease (IBD)** includes two separate but closely related conditions: ulcerative colitis and Crohn's disease. These conditions have a number of similarities.

The etiology of both illnesses is unknown, although current evidence implicates both genetic and environmental factors. IBD occurs more frequently in the United States and northern European nations than it does in southern Europe and countries in the Southern Hemisphere. IBD affects certain ethnic groups more than others, as outlined in the following

Focus on Cultural Diversity box. As many as 1 million Americans have IBD, with that number divided about equally between ulcerative colitis and Crohn's disease (Crohn's & Colitis Foundation of America [CCFA], 2009). It tends to run in families, with 15% to 25% of patients having a close relative with one of the types of IBD (CCFA, 2009). Factors such as an abnormal immune response to microorganisms normally found in the gut are thought to play a role in the development of IBD. Factors such as smoking and oral contraceptive use also affect the risk for IBD.

The peak incidence of IBD is in adolescents and young adults between the ages of 15 and 30 years but it also affects older adults (Fauci et al., 2008). IBD is a chronic and recurrent disease process. Responses to physiologic or psychologic stresses do not cause IBD, but often play a role in exacerbations of the disease.

Despite the similarities, ulcerative colitis and Crohn's disease have distinct differences. Ulcerative colitis primarily affects the large bowel in a continuous pattern, progressing distally to proximally. In Crohn's disease, a patchy pattern of involvement is seen, affecting primarily the small intestine. Ulcerative colitis shows mainly mucosal involvement; in Crohn's disease, the submucosal layers of the bowel are affected. A comparison of ulcerative colitis and Crohn's disease is found in Table 24–7. The Multisystem Effects of Inflammatory Bowel Disease are illustrated on page 682.

Ulcerative Colitis

Ulcerative colitis is a chronic inflammatory bowel disorder that affects the mucosa and submucosa of the colon and rectum. Most people with ulcerative colitis have mild or moderate disease, with six or fewer stools per day. Its onset usually is insidious, with attacks that last 1 to 3 months occurring at intervals of months to years. Typically, only the distal colon is affected, with few systemic manifestations of the disease. Approximately 15% of people with ulcerative colitis develop *fulminant colitis*, with involvement of the entire colon, severe bloody diarrhea, acute abdominal pain, and fever. Patients with fulminant disease are at high risk for complications.

Pathophysiology

The inflammatory process of ulcerative colitis begins at the rectosigmoid area of the anal canal and progresses proximally. In most patients, the disease is confined to the rectum and sigmoid colon. It may progress to involve the entire colon, stopping at the ileocecal junction.

Ulcerative colitis begins with inflammation at the base of the crypts of Lieberkühn in the distal large intestine and rectum. Microscopic, pinpoint mucosal hemorrhages occur, and crypt

TABLE 24–7 Characteristics of Ulcerative Colitis and Crohn's Disease

	CHARACTERISTIC	ULCERATIVE COLITIS	CROHN'S DISEASE
Clinical	Gender	Equal	Equal
	Age at onset	15 to 30 years; secondary peak 60 to 80 years	15 to 30 years; secondary peak 60 to 80 years
	Course of disease	Typically chronic and intermittent	Slowly progressive, relapsing
	Diarrhea	5 to 30 stools per day with blood and mucus	Common, usually less severe than colitis, with no obvious blood or mucus in stool
	Abdominal pain	Cramping in left lower quadrant; relieved by defecation	Cramping or steady right lower quadrant or periumbilical pain; tenderness and mass noted in right lower quadrant
	Nutritional deficit	Common; involves anemia, hypoalbuminemia, and weight loss	Common and significant: involves anemia, weight loss, and multiple vitamin and mineral deficits
	Constitutional manifestations	Fever rare; may have associated arthritic, skin, or other organ involvement, such as erythema nodosum or uveitis	Fever, malaise, fatigue; may have some associated conditions plus urinary complications
Pathologic	Depth of involvement	Mucosa and submucosa	Transmural (entire bowel wall)
	Portion of bowel involved	Typically rectum and sigmoid colon; may extend to involve entire large bowel	Any portion of GI tract; terminal ileum and ascending colon involvement predominates
	Distribution	Continuous from rectum	Patchy; skip lesions
	Appearance of mucosa	Granular, dull, hyperemic, friable; disease uniform in affected bowel; pseudopolyps may be seen	Cobblestone appearance, with areas of normal tissue surrounded by ulceration and fissures
Complications	Acute	Toxic megacolon, perforation, massive hemorrhage	Obstruction, fistulization, abscess formation, malabsorption
	Long term	Colorectal cancer	Colon cancer

abscesses develop (Figure 24–3 ■). These abscesses penetrate the superficial submucosa and spread laterally, leading to necrosis and sloughing of bowel mucosa. Further tissue damage is caused by inflammatory exudates and the release of inflammatory mediators, such as prostaglandins and other cytokines (∞ see Chapter 12 for further discussion of the inflammatory process). The mucosa is red and edematous due to vascular congestion, friable (easily broken), and ulcerated. It bleeds easily, and hemorrhage is common. Edema creates a granular appearance. Pseudopolyps, tonguelike projections of bowel mucosa into the lumen, may develop as the epithelial lining of the bowel regenerates. Chronic inflammation leads to atrophy, narrowing, and shortening of the colon, with loss of its normal haustra.

Manifestations

Diarrhea is the predominant manifestation of ulcerative colitis. Stools contain both blood and mucus. Nocturnal diarrhea may occur. Mild ulcerative colitis is characterized by fewer than 4 stools per day, intermittent rectal bleeding and mucus, and few systemic manifestations. Severe ulcerative colitis can lead to more than 6 to 10 bloody stools per day, extensive colon involvement, anemia, hypovolemia, and malnutrition. Rectal inflammation causes fecal urgency and tenesmus. Left lower quadrant cramping relieved by defecation is common. Other manifestations include fatigue, anorexia, and weakness.

Patients with severe disease may also have systemic manifestations such as arthritis involving one or several joints, skin and mucous membrane lesions, or *uveitis* (inflammation of the uvea, the vascular layer of the eye, which may also involve the sclera and cornea). Some patients develop thromboemboli, with blood vessel obstruction due to clots carried from the site of their formation. The liver and biliary system may be affected by the disease, as may the kidneys, with an increased risk for gallstones, cirrhosis, kidney stones, and ureteral obstruction (Fauci et al., 2008).

Complications

Acute complications of ulcerative colitis include hemorrhage, toxic megacolon, and colon perforation. Massive hemorrhage may occur with severe attacks of the disease. *Toxic megacolon*, a condition characterized by acute motor paralysis and dilation of the colon to greater than 6 cm, may affect part or all of the colon. The transverse segment of the bowel is most often affected. Toxic megacolon may be triggered by the use of laxatives, narcotics, and electrolyte imbalances (Fauci et al., 2008). Manifestations of toxic megacolon include fever, tachycardia, hypotension, dehydration, abdominal tenderness and cramping, and a change in the number of stools per day. Perforation is rare, but the risk of this dangerous complication is increased with toxic megacolon. Perforation leads to peritonitis.

The risk for colorectal cancer is increased in patients with ulcerative colitis. Beginning 8 to 15 years after the diagnosis, annual or biennial colonoscopies with biopsy to detect masses or cell dysplasia are recommended for patients who have extensive ulcerative colitis (Fauci et al., 2008).

Crohn's Disease

Like ulcerative colitis, Crohn's disease, also known as regional enteritis, is a chronic, relapsing inflammatory disorder affecting the gastrointestinal tract. Crohn's disease can affect any portion of the GI tract from the mouth to the anus, but usually affects the terminal ileum and ascending colon. Only the small bowel is involved in nearly 40% of patients with Crohn's disease. The disease is limited to the colon only in 30% of those affected. Both the small and large intestine are involved in the remaining 30% of patients (Porth & Matfin, 2009).

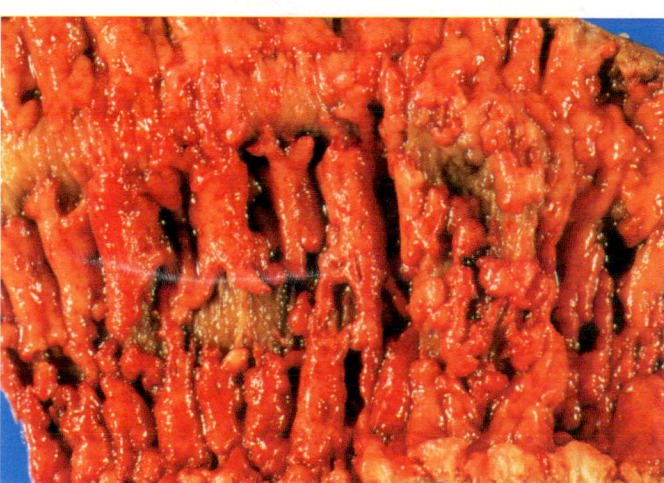

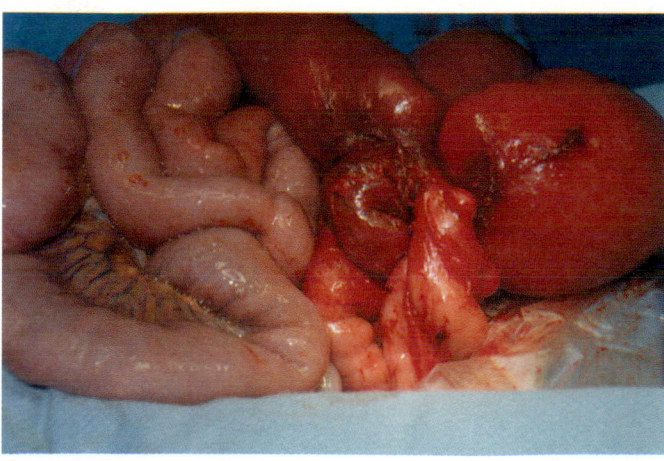

Figure 24–3 ■ *A,* Photomicrograph of the mucosa of the large intestine showing the entrances to the crypts of Lieberkühn. The crypts are the focal points for *B,* ulcerative colitis and *C,* Crohn's disease.

MULTISYSTEM EFFECTS OF
Irritable Bowel Disease

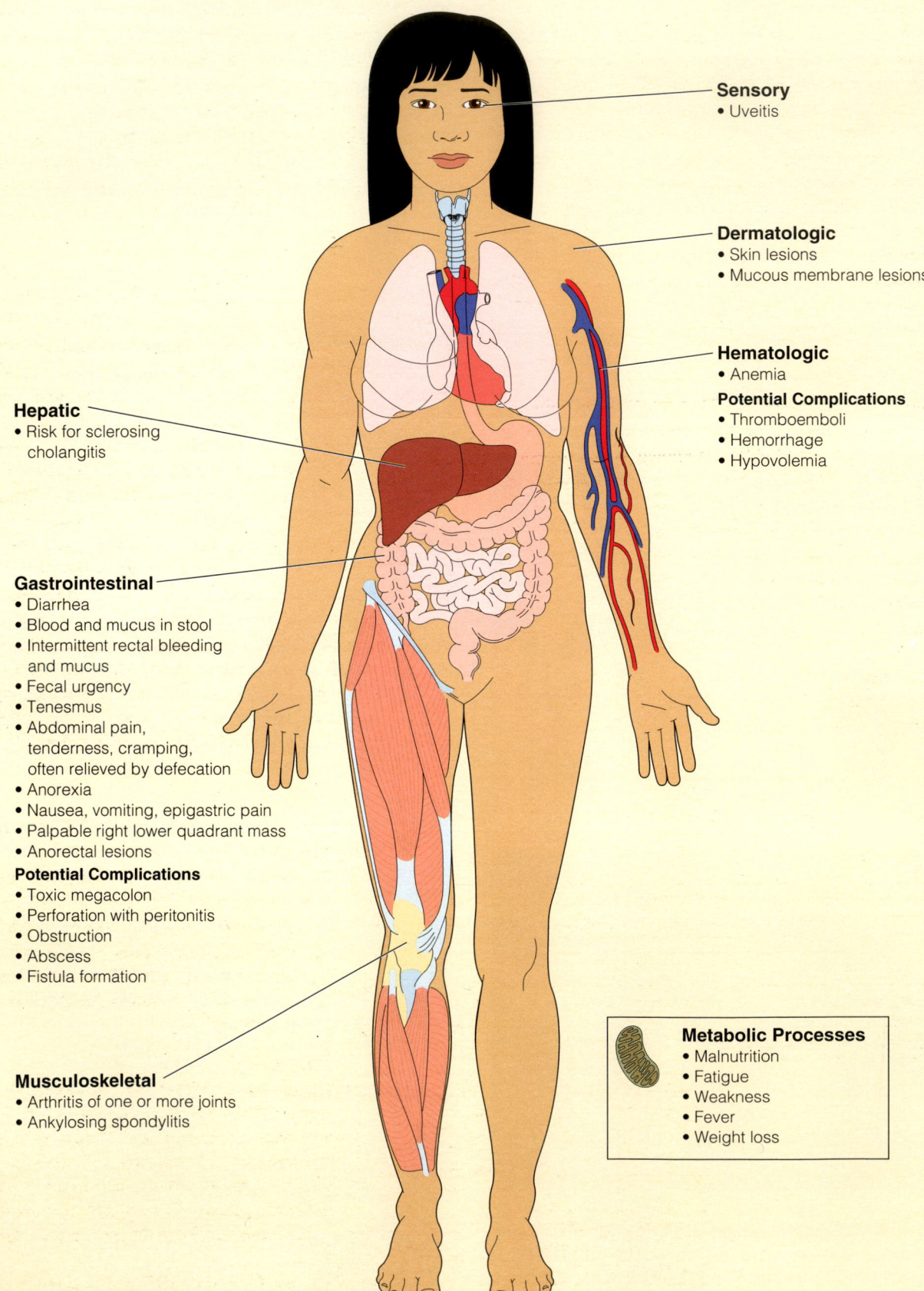

Sensory
- Uveitis

Dermatologic
- Skin lesions
- Mucous membrane lesions

Hematologic
- Anemia

Potential Complications
- Thromboemboli
- Hemorrhage
- Hypovolemia

Hepatic
- Risk for sclerosing cholangitis

Gastrointestinal
- Diarrhea
- Blood and mucus in stool
- Intermittent rectal bleeding and mucus
- Fecal urgency
- Tenesmus
- Abdominal pain, tenderness, cramping, often relieved by defecation
- Anorexia
- Nausea, vomiting, epigastric pain
- Palpable right lower quadrant mass
- Anorectal lesions

Potential Complications
- Toxic megacolon
- Perforation with peritonitis
- Obstruction
- Abscess
- Fistula formation

Musculoskeletal
- Arthritis of one or more joints
- Ankylosing spondylitis

Metabolic Processes
- Malnutrition
- Fatigue
- Weakness
- Fever
- Weight loss

Pathophysiology

Crohn's disease typically begins as a small inflammatory *aphthoid lesion* (shallow ulcers with a white base and elevated margin, similar to a canker sore) of the mucosa and submucosa of the bowel. These initial lesions may regress, or the inflammatory process can progress to involve all layers of the intestinal wall. Deeper ulcerations, granulomatous lesions, and fissures (knife-like clefts that extend deeply into the bowel wall) develop. The inflammatory process involves the entire bowel wall (transmural).

The lumen of the affected bowel assumes a "cobblestone appearance" as fissures and ulcers surround islands of intact mucosa over edematous submucosa. The inflammatory lesions of Crohn's disease are not continuous; rather, they often occur as "skip" lesions with intervening areas of normal-appearing bowel. Some evidence suggests that despite its normal appearance, the entire bowel is affected by this disorder.

As the disease progresses, fibrotic changes in the bowel wall cause it to thicken and lose flexibility, taking on an appearance that has been likened to a rubber hose. The inflammation, edema, and fibrosis can lead to local obstruction, abscess development, and the formation of fistulas between loops of bowel or bowel and other organs (Figure 24–4 ■). Fistulas between loops of bowel are known as enteroenteric fistulas; those that occur between bowel and bladder are known as enterovesical fistulas; and fistulas that occur between bowel and skin are known as enterocutaneous fistulas. Perineal fistulas are relatively common, originating in the ileum.

Depending on the severity and extent of the disease, malabsorption and malnutrition may develop as the ulcers prevent absorption of nutrients. When the jejunum and ileum are affected, the absorption of multiple nutrients may be impaired, including carbohydrates, proteins, fats, vitamins, and folate. Disease in the terminal ileum can lead to vitamin B_{12} malabsorption and bile salt reabsorption. The ulcerations can also lead to protein loss and chronic, slow blood loss with consequent anemia.

Manifestations

Because the GI system involvement in Crohn's disease can be so diverse, manifestations vary among patients. The majority of people with Crohn's disease experience persistent diarrhea. Stools are liquid or semiformed and typically do not contain blood, although blood may be passed if the colon is involved. Abdominal pain and tenderness are also common. The pain may be located in the right lower quadrant and relieved by defecation. A palpable right lower quadrant mass is often present. Systemic manifestations such as fever, fatigue, malaise, weight loss, and anemia are common. Anorectal lesions such as fissures, ulcers, fistulas, and abscesses also are common and may occur years before intestinal disease is apparent. If the stomach and duodenum are involved, nausea, vomiting, and epigastric pain may occur.

Complications

Certain complications of Crohn's disease (e.g., intestinal obstruction, abscess, and fistula) are so common that they are considered part of the disease process. For many patients, the disease initially presents with one of these complications. Intestinal obstruction is a common complication caused by repeated inflammation and scarring of the bowel that leads to fibrosis and stricture. Obstruction of the bowel lumen causes abdominal distention, cramping pain, and borborygmi. Nausea and vomiting may occur.

Fistulas may be asymptomatic, particularly if they occur between loops of small bowel. When fistulization causes an abscess, chills and fever, a tender abdominal mass, and leukocytosis develop. A fistula between the small bowel and colon may exacerbate diarrhea, weight loss, and malnutrition. When the bladder is involved, recurrent urinary tract infections occur.

Perforation of the bowel is uncommon, but can lead to generalized peritonitis. Massive hemorrhage also is an uncommon complication of Crohn's disease. Long-standing Crohn's disease increases the risk of cancer of the small intestine or colon by five to six times. This cancer risk, however, is significantly lower than the risk associated with ulcerative colitis.

Interdisciplinary Care

Interdisciplinary care for inflammatory bowel disease begins by establishing the diagnosis and the extent and severity of the disease. Treatment is supportive, including medications and dietary measures to decrease inflammation, promote intestinal rest and healing, and reduce intestinal motility. Many patients with IBD require surgery at some point to manage the disease or its complications.

Diagnosis

Diagnostic testing is used to establish the diagnosis of IBD, assess the extent of the disease, and evaluate the effects of the disorder. A sigmoidoscopy, colonoscopy, or a barium upper and lower x-ray series is performed to inspect the bowel mucosa for characteristic changes of IBD. (Nursing implications for these diagnostic tests are outlined in ∞ Chapter 21).

Laboratory tests to differentiate IBD and to identify effects and complications of the disease include a stool examination

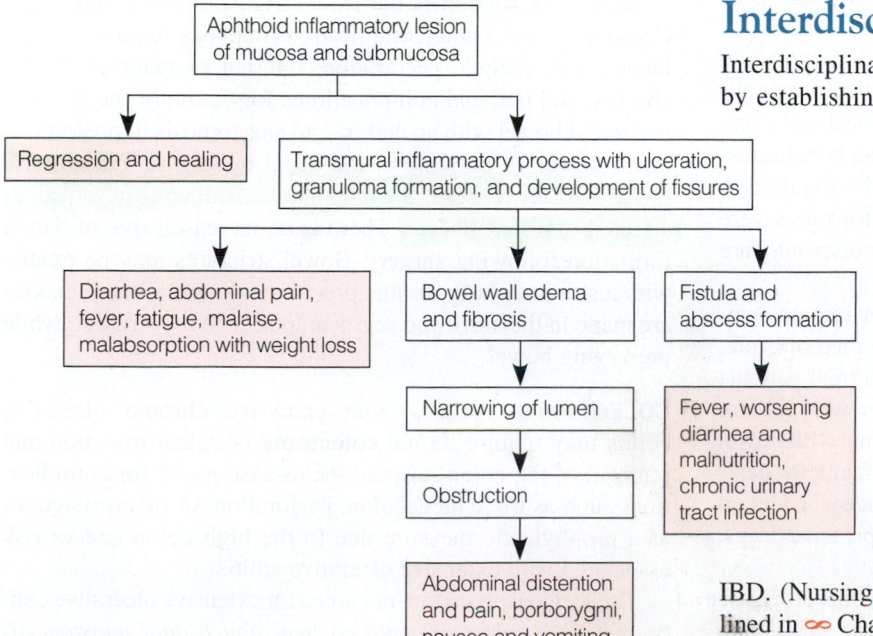

Figure 24–4 ■ The progression of Crohn's disease.

for blood and mucus, and stool cultures to rule out infectious causes of bowel inflammation and diarrhea. CBC with hemoglobin and hematocrit shows anemia from chronic inflammation, blood loss, and malnutrition, and leukocytosis due to inflammation and possible abscess formation. The sedimentation rate and levels of C-reactive protein are typically elevated during periods of acute inflammation. Serum albumin may be decreased because of malabsorption, malnutrition, protein loss through intestinal lesions, and chronic inflammation. Folic acid and serum levels of most vitamins, including A, B complex, C, and the fat-soluble vitamins, often are decreased due to malabsorption. Additional tests for renal and hepatic function may be done if the patient has significant systemic manifestations of the disease.

Medications

The ultimate goal of care is to achieve and maintain remission of the disease and its symptoms. Drug therapy plays a key role in achieving this goal. Locally acting and systemic anti-inflammatory drugs are the primary medications used to manage mild to moderate IBD. Drugs to suppress the immune response may be used to treat patients with severe disease.

Sulfasalazine (Azulfidine) is a sulfonamide antibiotic and anti-inflammatory that is poorly absorbed from the gastrointestinal tract and acts topically on the colonic mucosa to inhibit the inflammatory process. The active anti-inflammatory ingredient in sulfasalazine, 5-aminosalicylic acid (5-ASA), also is available in preparations that do not contain sulfa, such as olsalazine and mesalamine. They have the advantage of causing fewer adverse effects than sulfasalazine. Azo compounds, such as balsalazide and olsalazine, are 5-ASA compounds that are released in the colon and are especially useful to treat ulcerative colitis. Mesalamine (Canasa, Rowasa) is an orally or rectally administered 5-ASA compound that provides topical anti-inflammatory action in the colon of patients with ulcerative colitis. Specific preparations, their method of action, and nursing implications for these medications are outlined in the Medication Administration box on page 685.

For acute exacerbations of IBD, corticosteroids are given to reduce inflammation and induce remission. For ulcerative colitis, the drug may be administered rectally for its local effect and to minimize systemic effects. Hydrocortisone can be administered rectally. Intravenous corticosteroids may be required to treat severe disease; oral preparations are used for less severe manifestations and long-term therapy. Corticosteroids are tapered off once remission has been achieved.

Mercaptopurine (6-MP, Purinethol) and other immunosuppressive agents such as azathioprine (Imuran), methotrexate, and cyclosporine (Sandimmune) can be used to treat patients who have not responded to other treatments or who require chronic steroid therapy. These drugs may allow withdrawal from corticosteroids, maintain remission, and facilitate healing. Long-term therapy may be required to produce a beneficial effect. For more information about immunosuppressive drugs, ∞ see Chapter 13.

Newer treatments for IBD employ other immune response modifiers, such as the monoclonal antibody infliximab (Remicade) to suppress tumor necrosis factor (TNF, an inflammatory mediator substance) in patients who have not responded to standard therapies. Although antibiotic therapy generally is not indicated in IBD, metronidazole (Flagyl) has active anti-inflammatory effects. It may be prescribed to help prevent remission after ileal resection in Crohn's disease. Ciprofloxacin (Cipro) is an alternative to metronidazole.

Antidiarrheal agents, such as loperamide and diphenoxylate, may be given to slow gastrointestinal motility and reduce diarrhea. These drugs are safe for patients with mild, chronic manifestations, but they are not given during acute attacks because they may precipitate toxic dilation of the colon.

Nutrition

Antigens in the diet may stimulate the immune response in the bowel, exacerbating IBD. As a result, dietary management for inflammatory bowel disease is individualized. Some patients benefit from eliminating all milk and milk products from the diet. Increased dietary fiber may help reduce diarrhea and relieve rectal manifestations, but is contraindicated for patients with intestinal strictures caused by repeated inflammation and scarring.

All food may be withheld to promote bowel rest during an acute exacerbation of Crohn's disease. Nutritional status is maintained using enteral or total parenteral nutrition (TPN). ∞ See Chapter 22 for more information about enteral feedings and TPN. TPN carries a higher risk of complications than does enteral nutrition. An elemental diet such as Ensure, which contains all essential nutrients in a residue-free formula, may be prescribed. Elemental diets provide essential nutrients to the small intestine to support cell growth, but are not always palatable.

Surgery

Surgical interventions for IBD differ, depending on the primary disease process and the portion of the bowel affected. Generally, surgery is performed only when necessitated by complications of the disease or failure of conservative treatment measures.

Bowel obstruction is the leading indication for surgery in Crohn's disease. Other complications that may require surgical intervention include perforation, internal or external fistula, abscess, and perianal complications. Resection of the affected portion of bowel with an end-to-end anastomosis to preserve as much bowel as possible is the usual treatment. The disease process tends to recur in other areas following removal of affected bowel segments. There is an increased risk of fistula formation following surgery. Bowel strictures may be treated with a strictureplasty. In this procedure, longitudinal incisions are made in the narrowed segment to relieve the stricture while preserving bowel.

COLECTOMY Patients with extensive chronic ulcerative colitis may require a total colectomy (surgical resection and removal of the colon) to treat the disease itself; for complications such as toxic megacolon, perforation, or hemorrhage; or as a prophylactic measure due to the high colon cancer risk associated with extensive ulcerative colitis.

The surgical procedure of choice for extensive ulcerative colitis is a total colectomy with an ileal pouch-anal anastomosis (IPAA). In this procedure, the entire colon and rectum are

MEDICATION ADMINISTRATION   Inflammatory Bowel Disease

SULFASALAZINE (AZULFIDINE)

Sulfasalazine is an anti-inflammatory drug used for its local effect on the intestinal mucosa in inflammatory bowel disease. The active part of the drug is 5-ASA, which inhibits prostaglandin production in the bowel. Prostaglandin is an important mediator of the inflammatory process; blocking its production reduces inflammation.

Nursing Responsibilities

- Assess for contraindications, including pregnancy or a history of hypersensitivity to sulfonamides or salicylates.
- Assess baseline values for renal function tests (serum creatinine, BUN, urinalysis), liver function tests, and CBC.
- Administer as ordered. Suppositories or retention enemas may be administered at bedtime. Administer oral forms with a full glass of water.
- Have resuscitation equipment available; anaphylactic responses may occur.
- Evaluate for therapeutic response, including reduced number of stools, reduced mucus and blood, and improved stool consistency.
- Monitor for possible adverse responses:
  a. Headache, anorexia, nausea, or vomiting
  b. Skin rash, dermatitis, urticaria, or pruritus
  c. Evidence of blood dyscrasias, such as bleeding, easy bruising, fever
  d. Leukopenia, thrombocytopenia, hemolytic anemia, or agranulocytosis
  e. Changes in urinary output or renal function studies
  f. Evidence of hepatitis or myocarditis

Health Education for the Patient and Family

- Take oral preparations after meals to decrease gastric distress.
- Drink at least 2 quarts of fluid per day to reduce the risk of kidney damage.
- Use sunscreen to prevent burns; this drug increases sensitivity to sun.
- Do not take aspirin, vitamin C, or any other over-the-counter medications containing aspirin or vitamin C without consulting your doctor.
- This medication may interfere with the effectiveness of oral contraceptives; use alternative methods of contraception.
- Notify your doctor if you develop headache, anorexia, nausea, vomiting, skin rash or hives, sore throat or mouth, bleeding gums, joint pain, easy bruising, or fever.

MESALAMINE (ASACOL ROWASA) AND OLSALAZINE (DIPENTUM)

Mesalamine and olsalazine contain the same active ingredient, 5-ASA, as sulfasalazine, but cause fewer adverse effects. Their mechanism of action is the same as that of sulfasalazine. These drugs are available as suppositories, suspension for enema, or oral tablets.

Nursing Responsibilities

- Assess for possible contraindications such as pregnancy, lactation, or hypersensitivity to these drugs or aspirin.
- Administer as ordered. If more than one dose per day is ordered, space doses evenly over the 24-hour period.
- Evaluate for desired effects (as for sulfasalazine) and potential adverse effects.
  a. Nausea, diarrhea, abdominal cramps, or flatulence
  b. CNS effects including headache, dizziness, insomnia, weakness, or fatigue
  c. Rash or itching
  d. Flulike symptoms, general malaise

Health Education for the Patient and Family

- Teach the recommended method of administration, including how to insert rectal suppositories or administer a retention enema.

- Shake suspension forms well prior to using.
- Diarrhea is the most common side effect of these drugs. Notify your doctor if adverse effects occur.

CORTICOSTEROIDS

Methylprednisolone (Medrol, Solu-Medrol)

Prednisolone (Delta-Cortel) Prednisone

Glucocorticoids are hormones produced by the adrenal cortex. These hormones are necessary for the stress response. Cortisol, the main glucocorticoid, has potent anti-inflammatory effects. Corticosteroids are used to treat acute episodes of IBD. Because of their multiple and significant side effects, they are not used to maintain remission.

Nursing Responsibilities

- Assess for conditions that may be adversely affected by corticosteroid drugs: peptic ulcer disease, glaucoma or cataracts, diabetes, or psychiatric disorders.
- Obtain baseline vital signs and weight; monitor both routinely during therapy. Hypertension and weight gain may result from salt and water retention.
- Monitor for edema.
- Administer as ordered. For daily or alternate-day dosing, administer in the morning, when physiologic glucocorticoid levels are highest, to reduce adrenal cortisone suppression.
- Administer oral preparations with food to decrease gastrointestinal side effects. Antacids or histamine H_2-receptor blocking agents, such as cimetidine (Tagamet), may be prescribed during corticosteroid therapy.
- Monitor for desired effects: reduced diarrhea, less blood and mucus in the stool, and less abdominal cramping.
- Monitor for adverse effects:
  a. Increased susceptibility to infection and masking of early signs of infection
  b. Hyperglycemia
  c. Hypokalemia, as manifested by muscle weakness, nausea, vomiting, and cardiac rhythm disturbances
  d. Edema, hypertension, and signs of heart failure
  e. Peptic ulcer formation and possible gastrointestinal hemorrhage (abdominal pain, black or tarry stools, and signs of bleeding)
  f. Changes in mental status, including depression, euphoria, aggression, and behavioral changes
  g. With long-term use, cushingoid effects, such as abnormal fat deposits in the face (moon faces) and trunk (buffalo hump), muscle wasting and thin extremities, thinning of the skin, and osteoporosis

Health Education for the Patient and Family

- Take as prescribed; do not change the dose or time of day. Do not stop the medication abruptly. The dose will be tapered down gradually when the drug is discontinued.
- Notify the physician if adverse or cushingoid effects occur.
- Take with food or at mealtimes to decrease the gastrointestinal effects.
- Monitor weight. If a gain of more than 5 pounds is noted, notify the physician.
- Moderate salt intake and avoid foods and snacks high in sodium, such as processed meats and potato chips. Increase intake of foods high in potassium, such as fruits, vegetables, and lean meats.
- Carry a card or wear a bracelet or tag at all times identifying corticosteroid use.

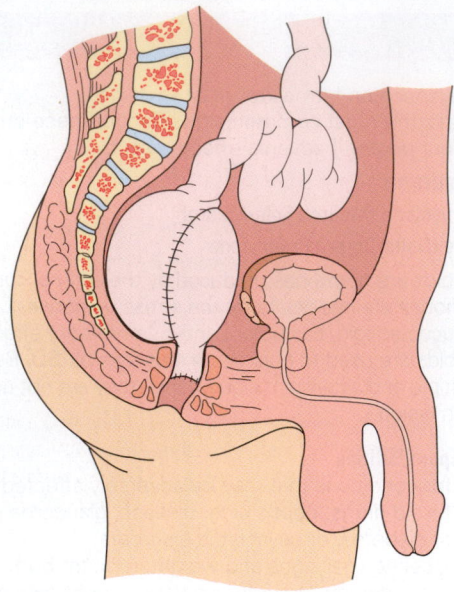

Figure 24–5 ■ Ileal pouch-anal anastomosis (IPAA).

removed; a pouch is formed from the terminal ileum; and the pouch is brought into the pelvis and anastomosed to the anal canal (Figure 24–5 ■). A temporary or loop ileostomy (described in the next section) is generally performed at the same time and is maintained for 2 to 3 months to allow the anal anastomosis to heal. When the healing is complete, the ileostomy is closed, and the patient has six to eight daily bowel movements through the anus. Advanced age, obesity, or other factors may preclude an IPAA. For these patients, a permanent ileostomy or continent ileostomy may be created.

OSTOMY An intestinal ostomy is a surgically created opening between the intestine and the abdominal wall that allows the passage of fecal material. The surface opening is called a **stoma** (Figure 24–6 ■). The precise name of the ostomy depends on the location of the stoma. An **ileostomy** is an ostomy made in the ileum of the small intestine. In an ileostomy, the colon, rectum, and anus are usually completely removed (*total proctocolectomy with permanent ileostomy*). The anal canal is closed, and the end of the terminal ileum is brought to the body surface through the right abdominal wall to form the stoma. A temporary or *loop ileostomy* may be formed to eliminate feces and allow tissue healing for 2 to 3 months following an IPAA. A loop of ileum is brought to the body surface to form a stoma and allow stool drainage into an external pouch. When the ileostomy is no longer necessary, a second surgery is performed to close the stoma and repair the bowel, restoring fecal elimination through the anus.

In a *continent ileostomy* (Figure 24–7 ■), an intra-abdominal reservoir is constructed and a nipple valve formed (the ileum folded back on itself) from the terminal ileum, before it is brought to the surface of the abdominal wall. Stool collects in the internal pouch; the nipple valve prevents it from leaking through the stoma. A catheter is inserted into the pouch to drain the stool.

Nursing care of the patient with an ileostomy is outlined in the following box. Procedure 24–1 on page 688 describes how to apply one- and two-piece drainable ostomy pouches.

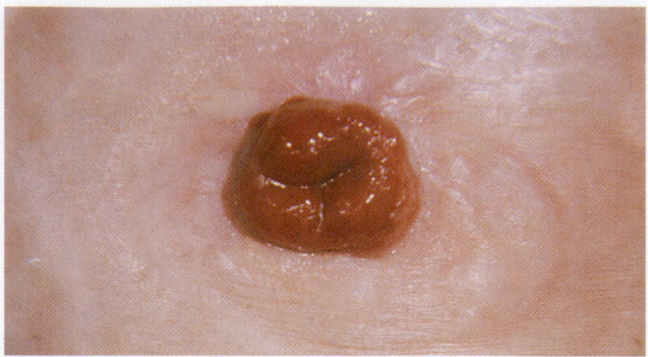

Figure 24–6 ■ A healthy-appearing stoma.
Courtesy of Carol Williams, RN, BS, UC Davis Medical Center.

Complementary and Alternative Therapies

The chronic nature of IBD and adverse effects of many prescribed treatments lead up to 50% of patients with IBD to seek or use complementary and alternative therapies. The most common complementary therapies used by patients with IBD include herbal therapies, nutritional supplements, probiotics, and fish oil (Langmead & Rampton, 2006; Mayo Clinic, 2008). Herbal remedies such as aloe vera gel and curcumin appear to have a beneficial effect, as do Chinese traditional medicine including Jian Pi Ling tablets and Yukui tang tablets. Probiotics, bacteria similar to those normally found in the gut, appear to have a beneficial anti-inflammatory effect in the bowel (Connelly, 2008). Probiotics are available in foods such as yogurt, miso, and soy beverages, as well as in dietary supplements. Results have been mixed in studies of the beneficial effect of fish oil or Omega-3 fatty acid supplements for IBD. Peppermint tea is an excellent tonic for reducing nausea, relieving abdominal pain, and providing a calming effect. Chamomile tea helps to reduce intestinal inflammation (Balch & Stengler, 2004). Anecdotal evidence supports the use of homeopathy to promote comfort in patients with IBD. Acupuncture improves perceived well-being in patients with IBD, but does not appear to effect remission (Langmead & Rampton, 2006). Many complementary and alternative therapies for IBD may interact with prescribed medications; instruct the patient to discuss all potential therapies with the primary care provider. Acupressure, body massage, reflexology, aromatherapy, and stress reduction therapies can also aid in reducing manifestations of IBD.

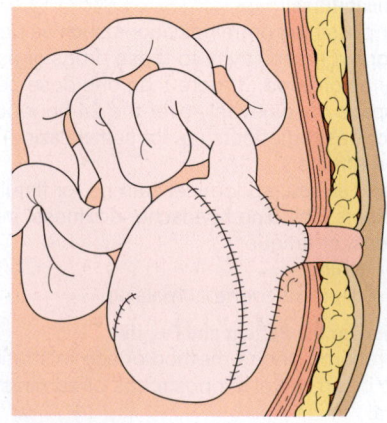

Figure 24–7 ■ Continent (Kock's) ileostomy.

NURSING CARE OF THE PATIENT Having an Ileostomy

PREOPERATIVE CARE

- Provide routine preoperative care and teaching as outlined in ∞ Chapter 4.
- Refer to an enterostomal therapist for marking and teaching about the stoma location, ostomy care, and options for ostomy appliances. *It is important to begin teaching prior to surgery to facilitate learning and acceptance of the ostomy postoperatively.*
- Discuss the availability of a local United Ostomy Association chapter, and provide a referral as necessary or desired. *Local chapters often have members with ostomies who are willing to provide both preoperative and postoperative teaching, listening, and support.*
- Provide preoperative bowel preparation as ordered. *Cathartics, enemas, and preoperative antibiotics are often ordered to reduce the risk of abdominal contamination and infection after surgery.*

POSTOPERATIVE CARE

- Provide routine postoperative care and teaching as outlined in ∞ Chapter 4.
- Apply an ostomy pouch over the stoma. (See Procedure 24–1.) *Stool from an ileostomy is expressed continuously or irregularly, and it is liquid in nature; continuous use of a pouch to collect the drainage is necessary.*
- Assess frequently for bleeding, stoma viability, and function. In the early postoperative period, small amounts of blood in the pouch are expected. A healthy stoma appears pink or red and moist as a result of mucous production (Figure 24–6). It should protrude approximately 2 cm from the abdominal wall. *Frequent assessment is particularly important in the initial postoperative period to ensure stoma health and monitor for possible complications. A dusky, brown, black, or white stoma indicates circulatory compromise. Other possible stoma complications include retraction (indentation or loss of the external portion of the stoma) or prolapse (outward telescoping of the stoma, that is, an abnormally long stoma).*
- As the stoma starts to function, empty the pouch, explaining the procedure to the patient. Initial drainage is dark green, viscid, and usually odorless. Drainage gradually thickens and becomes yellow-brown. Empty the pouch when it is one-third full. Measure drainage, and include it as output on intake and output records. Rinse the pouch and reapply the clamp. *Emptying the pouch when it is no more than one-third full helps prevent the skin seal from breaking as a result of the weight of the pouch. Because of the potential for excess fluid loss through ileostomy drainage, it is important to include it as fluid output.*
- Assess the peristomal skin. Skin around the stoma should remain clean and pink and free of irritation, rashes, inflammation, or excoriation. *Skin complications may arise from appliance irritation or hypersensitivity, excoriation from a leaking appliance, or* Candida albicans, *a yeast infection.*
- Protect peristomal skin from enzymes and bile salts in the ileostomy effluent. Using a skin barrier on the pouch is essential. Change the pouch if leakage occurs or if the patient complains of burning or itching skin. *Enzymes and bile salts normally reabsorbed in the large intestine are irritating to the skin. Excoriation of skin surrounding the stoma impairs the first line of defense against microorganisms and can interfere with the ability to achieve a tight skin seal and prevent pouch leakage.*

- Report the following abnormal assessment findings to the physician:
  a. Allergic or contact dermatitis. *A rash may result from contact with fecal drainage or indicate sensitivity to pouch, paste, tape, or sealant.*
  b. Purulent ulcerated areas surrounding the stoma. *Disruption of the protective barrier of the skin allows bacterial entry.*
  c. A red, bumpy, itchy rash or white-coated area. *This is a manifestation of* Candida albicans, *a yeast infection.*
  d. Bulging around the stoma. *This finding may indicate herniation, caused by loops of intestine protruding through the abdominal wall.*
- Apply protective ointments to the perirectal area of patients with newly functioning ileoanal reservoirs and anastomoses. *This helps protect the skin from the initial stools. As stools thicken and become fewer per day, the patient experiences less perirectal irritation.*

Health Education for the Patient and Family

- While caring for the ostomy, explain procedures to the patient. *Teaching is immediate and ongoing to facilitate acceptance of the ostomy and self-care.*
- Teach to manage the pouch clamp, and to empty, rinse, and perform pouch changes. *Self-care is vital to independence and self-esteem.*
- Instruct how to use an electric razor to shave the peristomal hair if necessary. *An electric razor prevents accidental cutting of the stoma with a razor blade.*
- Teach to check the stoma and peristomal skin with each pouch change. *Ongoing assessment is important for optimal health and function of the stoma and surrounding skin. Stripping of tape or excessively frequent pouch removal may cause mechanical trauma to peristomal skin. Chronic skin irritation by ileostomy effluent may lead to pseudoverracous lesions, or wartlike nodules.*
- Instruct to report abnormal appearance of the stoma or surrounding skin to the physician:
  a. Narrowing of the stoma lumen. *This indicates stenosis and may interfere with fecal elimination.*
  b. Lacerations or cuts in the stoma. *The stoma contains no nerves, so trauma may occur without pain.*
  c. Separation of the stoma from the abdominal surface. *This potential complication may require surgical repair.*
- Emphasize the importance of adequate fluid and salt intake; the risk for dehydration and hyponatremia is increased particularly during hot weather, when fluid is lost through perspiration as well as ileostomy drainage. Water intake should be sufficient to maintain pale urine and an output of at least 1 quart per day. When exercising in hot weather, the patient should consume extra water and salt. High-potassium foods, such as bananas and oranges, may be recommended. *Loss of the reabsorptive surface of the large bowel increases the amount of water and sodium loss in the stool. If the ileostomy is high (more proximal in the ileum), additional potassium losses may also occur.*
- Discuss manifestations of fluid and electrolyte imbalances:
  a. Extreme thirst
  b. Dry skin and oral mucous membrane
  c. Decreased urine output
  d. Weakness, fatigue
  e. Muscle cramps
  f. Abdominal cramps, nausea, vomiting
  g. Shortness of breath
  h. Orthostatic hypotension (feeling faint when suddenly changing positions)

(continued)

| **NURSING CARE OF THE PATIENT** | Having an Ileostomy (continued) |

- Discuss dietary concerns. A low-residue diet is recommended initially (see Table 24–8). Foods that may cause excessive odor or gas are typically avoided as well. *Because food blockage is a potential problem, high-fiber foods are limited, and foods that may cause blockage, such as popcorn, corn, nuts, cucumbers, celery, fresh tomatoes, figs, strawberries, blackberries, and caraway seeds, are avoided. Symptoms of food blockage include abdominal cramping, swelling of the stoma, and absence of ileostomy output for over 4 to 6 hours.*
- Teach self-care measures to relieve food blockage:
  a. Take a warm shower or tub bath. *This can help relax the abdominal muscles.*
  b. Assume a knee–chest position. *The knee–chest position reduces intra-abdominal pressure.*
  c. Drink warm fluids or grape juice if not vomiting. *This provides a mild cathartic effect.*
  d. Massage peristomal area. *Massage may stimulate peristalsis and fecal elimination.*
  e. Remove pouch if the stoma is swollen, and apply a pouch with a larger opening. *If the stoma swells, the pouch may create a mechanical obstruction to output.*
- Notify the physician or enterostomal therapy nurse of the following:
  a. The previous measures fail to relieve the obstruction.
  b. Signs of a partial obstruction persist, including high-volume odorous fluid output, abdominal cramps, nausea, and vomiting.
  c. There is no ileostomy output for 4 to 6 hours.
  d. Signs of fluid and electrolyte imbalance occur, such as weakness, dizziness, lightheadedness, or headache.

Should self-care measures not succeed in breaking up a blockage, ileostomy lavage, as described in Procedure 24–2, may be required.

PROCEDURE 24–1 Changing a One- or Two-Piece Drainable Ostomy Pouch

GATHER SUPPLIES
- Disposable gloves
- One- or two-piece pouch
- Skin barrier paste
- Skin prep
- Clamp
- Pouch deodorant
- Measuring guide
- Adhesive remover
- Skin cleanser
- Washcloths
- Plastic bag

BEFORE THE PROCEDURE
Explain the procedure and provide for privacy.

Follow standard precautions. Don gloves.

PROCEDURE
1. Remove soiled pouch (and the flange if a two-piece pouch) by gently pulling on the pouch or flange and pushing on skin. Use adhesive remover to remove skin barrier paste.
2. Empty pouch, discarding it and the flange (if applicable) in a plastic bag. Save the tail closure clamp. The pouch from a two-piece system may be cleaned out and reused.
3. Cleanse skin and stoma with warm water and skin cleanser or mild soap. Rinse skin and stoma, and pat dry.
4. Note stoma color and peristomal skin condition.
5. If necessary, clip or shave peristomal hair.
6. Use measuring guide or previous pattern to check size of stoma.
   a. Presized pouch: check to verify that size is correct.
   b. Cut-to-fit pouch or flange: Trace the correct size of the stoma onto the back of the flange, and cut the opening to match the pattern. The opening should be no more than 1/8 inch larger than stoma.

7. Apply skin prep to skin covered by a wafer, pouch, or tape. Allow to dry.
8. Remove backings from pouch or flange.
9. Apply a bead of skin barrier paste around the stoma base or around the opening of the pouch or flange. Allow the paste to air-dry for 1 to 2 minutes.
10. Center the pouch or flange over the stoma, and press to adhere.
11. For a two-piece pouch, snap the pouch onto skin barrier flange.
12. Place deodorizing tablets or a few drops of liquid pouch deodorizer (in some cases, antiseptic mouthwash may be used) in the pouch. Apply the clamp.
13. "Picture frame" the pouch with tape to provide extra security.

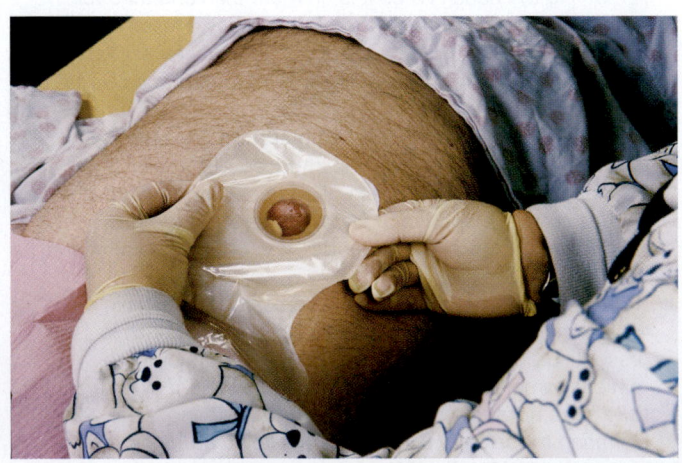

TABLE 24–8 Low-Residue Diet

FOOD GROUP	ALLOWED	AVOID
Beverages	Coffee, teas, juices, carbonated beverages; milk limited to 2 cups per day	Alcohol, prune juice
Breads and cereals	Products made from refined flours (white bread, crackers) or finely milled grains (e.g., corn flakes, crisp rice cereal, puffed wheat)	Whole-grain breads, rolls, or cereal; breads or rolls with seeds, nuts, or bran
Desserts	Gelatins, tapioca, plain custards, or puddings; angel-food or sponge cake; ice cream or frozen desserts without fruit or nuts	Any desserts containing dried fruits, nuts, seeds, or coconut; rich pastries, pies
Fruits	Fruit juices and strained fruits; cooked or canned apples, apricots, cherries, peaches, pears; bananas	All other raw or cooked fruits
Meats and other protein sources	Roasted, baked, or broiled tender or ground beef, veal, pork, lamb, poultry, or fish; smooth peanut butter; cottage, cream, American, or mild cheddar cheeses in small amounts	Tough or spiced meats and those prepared by frying; highly flavored cheeses; nuts
Potatoes, rice, and pasta	Peeled potatoes; white rice; most pasta products	Potato skins, potato chips, or fried potatoes; brown rice; whole-grain pasta products
Sweets	Sugar, honey, jelly, hard candy and gumdrops, plain chocolates	Jam, marmalade; candy made with seeds, nuts, coconut
Vegetables	Vegetable juices and strained vegetables; cooked or canned vegetables	Raw or whole cooked vegetables
Other	Salt, ground seasonings; cream sauce and plain gravy	Chili sauce, horseradish; popcorn, seeds of any kind; whole spices, olives, vinegar

---

PROCEDURE 24–2 Ileostomy Lavage

GATHER SUPPLIES
- Disposable gloves
- Disposable irrigation sleeve
- 60 mL catheter-tipped syringe
- #14 Fr. catheter
- Water-soluble lubricant
- Normal saline for irrigation
- Bedpan
- Clean ostomy pouch

BEFORE THE PROCEDURE

Explain the procedure and provide for privacy.

Follow standard precautions. Don gloves.

PROCEDURE

1. Remove the pouch. Apply disposable irrigation sleeve.
2. Clamp the bottom of the sleeve, or place it into the bedpan.
3. Gently examine stoma digitally to break up any fecal mass proximal to stoma and determine direction of the bowel.

4. Lubricate catheter, and insert into stoma until blockage is reached. If the catheter does not reach the blockage after 8 to 10 cm, notify the physician. This may indicate a more proximal obstruction.
5. Instill 30 to 50 mL normal saline.
6. Remove catheter. Allow stoma to drain.
7. Repeat the procedure until the mass is removed.
8. When the blockage is removed, remove the irrigation sleeve.
9. Clean peristomal skin.
10. Apply pouch and clamp.

AFTER THE PROCEDURE

1. Document the procedure, amount of solution used, consistency of results, and the patient's tolerance of the procedure.
2. Discuss dietary intake to help determine cause of blockage.

Nursing Care

Health Promotion

Although IBD cannot, at this time, be predicted or prevented, effective management may help the patient avoid complications of the disease. Stress the importance of complying with the prescribed treatment regimen and promptly reporting manifestations of exacerbations to the physician.

Assessment

Assessment data related to IBD includes the following subjective and objective data:

- *Health history:* Current manifestations, including onset, duration, severity (number of stools per day, presence of blood or mucus in stool, abdominal pain or cramping, tenesmus); usual diet, ability to maintain weight and nutrition, food intolerances; associated manifestations such as arthralgias, fatigue, malaise; current medications; previous treatment and diagnostic tests.

- *Physical examination:* General appearance; weight; vital signs including orthostatic vitals and temperature; abdominal assessment including shape, contour, bowel sounds, palpation for tenderness and masses, presence of stoma or scars.

Nursing Diagnoses and Interventions

When planning nursing care for the patient with IBD, it is vital to consider the chronic, recurrent nature of the disorder. Teaching is a major aspect of care. Diarrhea and disturbed body image are significant nursing care problems for the patient with IBD. With severe disease, impaired nutrition must be considered a priority problem as well. See the accompanying Case Study & Nursing Care Plan for a patient with ulcerative colitis.

Diarrhea

During an acute exacerbation of IBD, diarrhea can be frequent and painful. The frequency of defecation and associated abdominal pain and cramping may interfere with ADLs and increase the risk for fluid volume deficit and impaired skin integrity.

- Record the frequency, amount, and color of stools using a stool chart. Measure and record liquid stool as output. *The severity of diarrhea is an indicator of the severity of the disease and helps determine the need for fluid replacement.*

> **PRACTICE ALERT**
> Observe stools for obvious blood and test for occult blood as indicated. Report grossly bloody stools (**hematochezia**), which may indicate hemorrhage and necessitate emergency surgery.

- Monitor vital signs every 4 hours. *Tachycardia, tachypnea, and fever may be indicators of fluid volume deficit.*

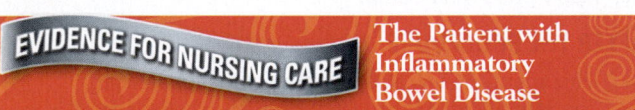

The Patient with Inflammatory Bowel Disease

Selected resources that nurses may find helpful when planning evidence-based nursing care follow.

- Belling, R., McLaren, S., & Woods, L. (2009). Specialist nursing interventions for inflammatory bowel disease. *Cochrane Database of Systemic Reviews, 4.* Art. No.: CD006597. DOI: 10.1002/14651858.CD006597.pub2. Retrieved from http://www.cochrane.org/reviews/en/ab006597.html
- Singh, S., Graff, L. A., & Bernstein, C. N. (2009). Do NSAIDs, antibiotics, infections, or stress trigger flares in IBD? *The American Journal of Gastroenterology, 104,* 1298–1313.
- Smith, G. D., Watson, R., Roger, D., McRorie, E., Hurst, N., Luman, W., & Palmer, K. R. (2002). Impact of a nurse-led counseling service on quality of life in patients with inflammatory bowel disease. *Journal of Advanced Nursing, 38*(2), 152–160. Retrieved from http://www.ncbi.nlm.nih.gov/pubmed

- Weigh daily and record. *Rapid weight loss (over days to a week) usually indicates fluid loss, whereas weight loss over weeks to months may indicate malnutrition.*
- Assess for other indications of fluid deficit: warm, dry skin, poor skin turgor, dry shiny mucous membranes, weakness, lethargy, complaints of thirst. *The extent of fluid loss may not be readily evident with diarrhea, particularly if the patient uses the bathroom without assistance. Systemic manifestations of fluid volume deficit may be the first indicators of the problem.*
- Maintain bowel rest by keeping NPO or limiting oral intake to elemental feedings as indicated. *Bowel rest during an acute exacerbation of IBD promotes healing and reduces diarrhea and other manifestations.*
- Administer prescribed anti-inflammatory and antidiarrheal medications as indicated. *Anti-inflammatory medications reduce the extent of bowel inflammation and diarrhea. Unless contraindicated, antidiarrheal medications help reduce fluid loss and increase comfort.*

> **PRACTICE ALERT**
> When giving antidiarrheal medications to a patient with ulcerative colitis, closely observe for manifestations of toxic megacolon: fever, tachycardia, hypotension, dehydration, abdominal pain and cramping, and an abrupt relief of diarrhea.

- Maintain fluid intake by mouth or intravenously as indicated. *The patient with IBD requires fluid to replace ongoing losses, as well as fluid to meet the usual daily needs of the body. If an elemental diet or total parenteral nutrition is prescribed, additional fluids may be required to meet fluid intake needs.*
- Provide good skin care. *Fluid deficit and tissue dehydration increase the risk for skin excoriations or breakdown.*
- Assess perianal area for irritation or denuded skin from the diarrhea. Use gentle cleansing agents, such as Peri-Wash or Tucks, diaper wipes, or cotton balls saturated with witch hazel. Apply a protective cream, such as zinc oxide–based preparations, to protect skin from the irritating effects of diarrheal stool. *Digestive enzymes in the stool are very corrosive, increasing the risk of skin breakdown where exposed to diarrheal stool.*

Disturbed Body Image

The patient with IBD may experience frustration at not being able to control, or even predict, fecal elimination, particularly when the disease is severe. Diarrhea can interfere with the ability to complete tasks, maintain employment or engage in social activities, and even meet basic needs such as eating, sleeping, and sexual activity. Body image can suffer as a result. Treatment of IBD, be it total colectomy with ileal pouch-anal anastomosis, ileostomy, or chronic corticosteroid therapy, can affect the view of self.

- Accept feelings and perception of self. *Negating or denying the reality of the patient's perception impairs trust.*
- Encourage discussion of physical changes and their consequences as they relate to self-concept. *This demonstrates acceptance and provides an opportunity to express the impact of the disease and its treatment on the patient's life.*

- Encourage discussion about concerns regarding the effect of the disease or treatment on close personal relationships. *This demonstrates understanding and provides an opportunity for the patient to express feelings about the impact of the disease on relationships and significant others.*
- Encourage the patient to make choices and decisions regarding care. *This increases the patient's sense of control over the disease and his or her future.*
- Discuss possible treatment options and their effects openly and honestly. *Open discussion allows more informed decisions.*
- Involve the patient in care, teaching and demonstrating as needed. *This encourages and facilitates independence and decision making.*
- Provide care in an accepting, nonjudgmental manner. *Acceptance of the patient despite potential embarrassment about odors or diarrhea enhances self-esteem.*
- Arrange for interaction with other patients or groups of people with IBD or ostomies. *The patient may feel that no one who has not experienced a similar problem can understand his or her feelings.*
- Teach coping strategies (odor control, dietary modifications, and so on), and support their use. *This facilitates healthy adaptation to the disease.*

Imbalanced Nutrition: Less than Body Requirements

Crohn's disease can significantly alter the bowel's ability to absorb nutrients. In both forms of IBD, blood and protein-rich fluid may be lost in diarrheal stools. With malabsorption and continuing nutrient losses, multiple nutrient deficits can develop, affecting growth and development, healing, muscle mass, bone density, and electrolyte balances.

- Monitor laboratory results, including hemoglobin and hematocrit, serum electrolytes, and total serum protein and albumin levels. *These studies provide an indicator of nutritional status.*
- Provide the prescribed diet: high-kilocalorie, high-protein, low-fat diet with restricted milk and milk products if lactose intolerance is present. *Calories and protein are important to replace lost nutrients. Fat restriction helps reduce diarrhea and nutrient loss, particularly when significant portions of the terminal ileum have been resected.*
- Provide parenteral nutrition as necessary if the patient is unable to absorb enteral nutrients. *Parenteral nutrition can help reverse nutritional deficits and promote weight gain and healing in the patient with acute manifestations.*
- Arrange for dietary consultation. Consider food preferences as allowed. *Providing preferred foods in the prescribed diet increases intake and supports nutritional status.*
- Provide or administer elemental enteral nutrition and supplements as ordered. *Elemental enteral nutritional supplements support healing while providing for bowel rest. They can replace losses and improve nutritional status more rapidly than diet alone.*
- Include family members, the primary food preparer in particular, in teaching and dietary discussions. *Families can reinforce teaching and help the patient maintain required restrictions or kilocalorie intake.*

Using NANDA, NIC, and NOC

Linkages between a selected NANDA nursing diagnosis, NIC, and NOC for the patient with IBD are shown in the chart that follows.

Community-Based Care

IBD is a chronic condition for which the patient provides daily self-management. For this reason, teaching is a vital component of care. Teach the patient and family about the following topics:

- The type of IBD affecting the patient, including the disease process, short- and long-term effects, the relationship of stress to disease exacerbations, and the manifestations of complications
- Prescribed medications, including drug names, desired effects, schedules for tapering the doses if ordered (as with corticosteroids), and possible side effects or adverse reactions and their management
- The recommended diet and the rationale for any specific restrictions
- Use of nutritional supplements such as Ensure to maintain weight and nutritional status
- Indicators of malabsorption and impaired nutrition; recommendations for self-care and when to seek medical intervention
- If discharged with a central catheter and home parenteral nutrition, written and verbal instructions on catheter care, troubleshooting, and parenteral nutrition administration (Have the patient and a family member demonstrate catheter care and parenteral nutrition maintenance.)
- The importance of maintaining a fluid intake of at least 2 to 3 quarts per day, increasing fluid intake during warm weather, exercise, or strenuous work, and when fever is present
- The increased risk for colorectal cancer and importance of regular bowel exams
- Risks and benefits of various treatment options

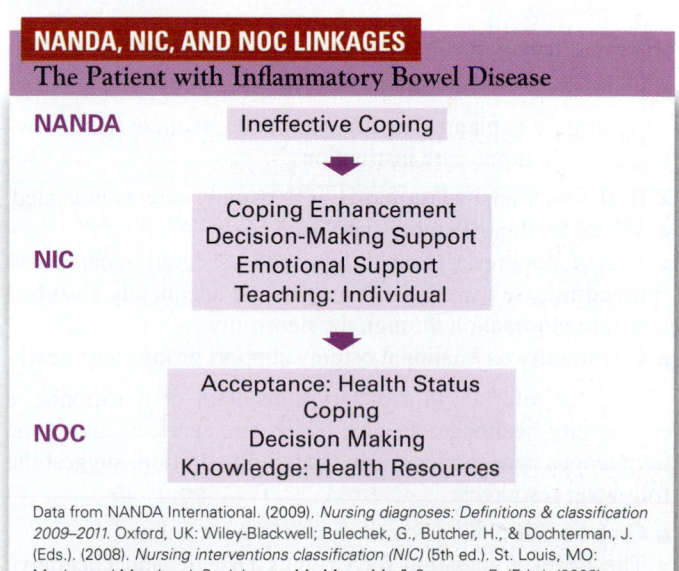

NANDA, NIC, AND NOC LINKAGES
The Patient with Inflammatory Bowel Disease

NANDA — Ineffective Coping

NIC — Coping Enhancement / Decision-Making Support / Emotional Support / Teaching: Individual

NOC — Acceptance: Health Status / Coping / Decision Making / Knowledge: Health Resources

Data from NANDA International. (2009). *Nursing diagnoses: Definitions & classification 2009–2011.* Oxford, UK: Wiley-Blackwell; Bulechek, G., Butcher, H., & Dochterman, J. (Eds.). (2008). *Nursing interventions classification (NIC)* (5th ed.). St. Louis, MO: Mosby; and Moorhead, S., Johnson, M., Maas, M., & Swanson, E. (Eds.). (2008). *Nursing outcomes classification (NOC)* (4th ed.). St. Louis, MO: Mosby.

CASE STUDY & NURSING CARE PLAN   A Patient with Ulcerative Colitis

Cortez Lewis is a 42-year-old real estate agent and mother of three school-age children. She has had ulcerative colitis for 18 years and has been treated with prednisone and sulfasalazine. Over the past 4 months she has been having abdominal pain and cramping and frequent bloody diarrhea stools. During the same period, she has lost 20 lb (9 kg); and has had difficulty maintaining her career. She recently developed several lesions of the lower leg identified as erythema nodosum. A recent colonoscopy revealed extensive involvement of the entire colon. On admission, Mrs. Lewis states, "I'm tired of fighting this disease. I am a prisoner in my home because of the diarrhea." She is admitted for a total proctocolectomy and ileal pouch-anal anastomosis.

ASSESSMENT

Janet Wheeler, RN, completes the admission assessment. Mrs. Lewis now weighs 115 lb (52.2 kg). She complains of abdominal cramping, pain, and frequent bloody diarrhea stools. Several reddened lesions are noted on her lower legs. Physical assessment findings include T 98°F (36.6°C), P 72, R 20, and BP 104/72. Skin cool and pale. Abnormal laboratory findings include hemoglobin 7.3 g/dL (normal 11.7 to 15.7 g/dL); hematocrit 23.3% (normal 35% to 47%); WBC 15,580/mm^3 (normal 3500 to 11,000/mm^3); platelet count 995,000/mm^3 (normal 150,000 to 450,000/mm^3); serum protein 4.6 g/dL (normal 6 to 8 g/dL); serum albumin 2.4 g/dL (normal 3.5 to 5 g/dL). Preparation for surgery is begun.

DIAGNOSES

- *Imbalanced Nutrition: Less than Body Requirements* related to impaired absorption
- *Diarrhea* related to inflammation of bowel
- *Risk for Deficient Fluid Volume* related to abnormal fluid loss
- *Risk for Impaired Tissue Integrity* related to drainage from temporary ileostomy
- *Acute Pain* related to surgical intervention
- *Risk for Sexual Dysfunction* related to temporary ileostomy

EXPECTED OUTCOMES

- Resume prescribed diet within 5 days after surgery.
- Demonstrate normal fecal elimination through the temporary ileostomy.
- Maintain adequate fluid balance.
- Demonstrate appropriate ostomy care prior to discharge.
- Report a tolerable level of discomfort.
- Verbalize feelings about sexuality and acknowledge importance of discussing sexual issues with husband.

PLANNING AND IMPLEMENTATION

- Discuss dietary modifications related to nutritional status and presence of ileostomy. Provide referral to dietitian for diet planning and teaching.
- Teach importance of maintaining a high fluid intake and manifestations of dehydration.
- Teach to empty and change ostomy pouch of choice.
- Teach stoma and peristomal skin assessment with each pouch change.
- Teach food blockage management.
- Refer to local United Ostomy Association.
- Provide list of local medical suppliers for ostomy appliances.

EVALUATION

On discharge, Mrs. Lewis is caring for her ileostomy by demonstrating her ability to empty, rinse, and change the pouch. The enterostomal therapy (ET) nurse has provided written and verbal instructions on ileostomy care. Mrs. Lewis verbalizes her understanding of the recommended diet and the need to limit high-fiber food intake and avoid enteric-coated and timed-release medications. The ET nurse has discussed sexual aspects of having an ileostomy and has given Mrs. Lewis a booklet, "Sex and the Female Ostomate," available through the United Ostomy Association. Mrs. Lewis is looking forward to the planned surgery to close the temporary ileostomy.

CRITICAL THINKING IN THE NURSING PROCESS

1. Why is the patient with an ileostomy at risk for dehydration? How can Mrs. Lewis monitor her fluid status at home?
2. Why were Mrs. Lewis's hemoglobin and hematocrit low on admission? If her hemoglobin had been low but her hematocrit normal on admission, what might be the explanation?
3. Outline a teaching plan that could be given to patients for home care of an ileostomy.
4. Develop a care plan for Mrs. Lewis for the nursing diagnosis *Risk for Impaired Skin Integrity*.

See Evaluating Your Response in Appendix C.

- Importance of informing interdisciplinary care team of complementary and alternative therapy use

If surgery is planned or has been done, include the following topics in home care instructions:

- Ileal pouch-anal anastomosis or ileostomy care as indicated
- Where to obtain ostomy supplies
- Use of nonprescription drugs, such as enteric-coated and timed-release capsules that may not be adequately absorbed before elimination through the ileostomy
- Community and national ostomy support groups (see next)

Provide referrals to a dietary consultant or nutritionist, a community healthcare agency, home care services, and home intravenous care services as indicated. In addition, suggest the following resources:

- Crohn's and Colitis Foundation of America, Inc.
- The Israel Foundation for Crohn's Disease and Ulcerative Colitis
- United Ostomy Association, Inc.

The Patient with Diverticular Disease

Diverticula are small (0.5- to 1.0-cm) outpouchings of the colon that occur in rows (Figure 24–8 ■). Diverticula may occur anywhere in the intestinal tract, excluding the rectum. The vast majority, however, affect the large intestine, with 85% to 95% occurring in the sigmoid colon (Fauci et al., 2008; McPhee, 2008).

FAST FACTS

Diverticular Disease

- People in the United States, Australia, the United Kingdom, and France have high and increasing incidence rates of diverticular disease.
- The incidence of diverticula increases with age, with 5% to 10% of the population older than 45 years of age and almost 80% of those older than 85 years of age experiencing it.
- Most of the people diagnosed with diverticular disease remain asymptomatic.
- Men and women are equally affected.

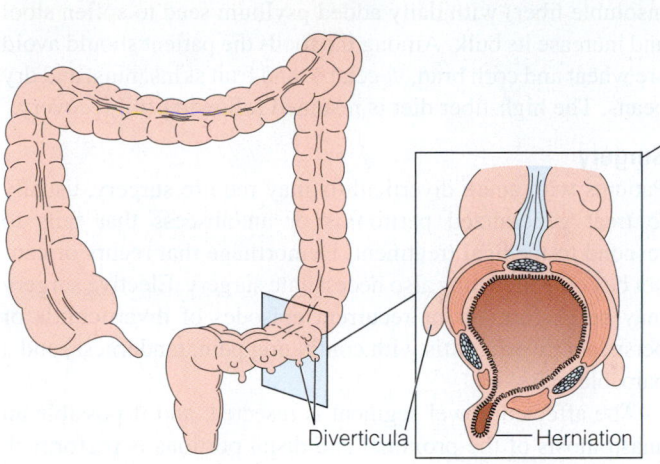

Figure 24–8 ■ Diverticula of the colon.

Cultural factors, diet in particular, are thought to play an important role in the development of diverticula. A diet consisting of highly refined and fiber-deficient foods is believed to be the major factor contributing to the disease. Decreased activity levels and delaying defecation have been suggested as contributing factors. The increasing incidence of diverticula with aging suggests that dietary factors (lack of fiber), a decrease in physical activity, poor bowel habits (neglecting the urge to defecate), and the effects of aging contribute to development of the disease (Porth & Matfin, 2009).

Pathophysiology

Diverticula form when increased pressure within the bowel lumen causes bowel mucosa to herniate through defects in the colon wall. The circular and longitudinal muscles often thicken or hypertrophy in the area affected by diverticula. This narrows the bowel lumen, increasing intraluminal pressure. Deficient dietary fiber and a lack of fecal bulk contribute to muscle hypertrophy and narrowing of the bowel. Contraction of the muscles in response to normal stimuli such as meals may occlude the narrowed lumen, further increasing intraluminal pressure. The high pressure causes mucosa to herniate through the muscle wall, forming a diverticulum. Areas where nutrient blood vessels penetrate the circular muscle layer are the most common sites for diverticula formation.

Diverticulosis

Diverticulosis indicates the presence of diverticula. More than two-thirds of patients with diverticulosis are asymptomatic. When manifestations such as episodic pain (usually left-sided), constipation, and diarrhea occur, they often can be attributed to irritable bowel syndrome (IBS), which commonly accompanies diverticular disease. (IBS is discussed earlier in this chapter.) As the disease progresses, abdominal cramping, narrow stools (decrease in caliber), increased constipation, bleeding in the stools, weakness, and fatigue may develop.

Complications of diverticulosis include hemorrhage and diverticulitis. A diverticulum may bleed, whether it is inflamed or not, possibly due to erosion of an adjacent blood vessel by a fecalith (hard mass) in the diverticulum.

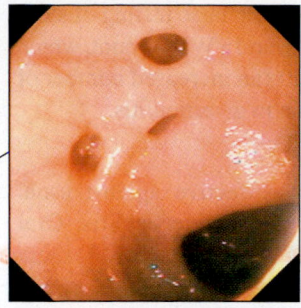

Diverticulitis

Diverticulitis is inflammation in and around the diverticular sac. It typically affects only one diverticulum, usually in the sigmoid colon. Undigested food and bacteria collect in the diverticula, forming a hard mass that impairs the mucosal blood supply, allowing bacterial invasion. Mucosal ischemia leads to perforation. With microscopic perforation, inflammation is localized. Gross perforation of a diverticulum results in more extensive bacterial contamination and can lead to abscess formation or peritonitis.

MANIFESTATIONS Pain is a common manifestation of diverticulitis. It is usually left-sided and may be mild to severe and either steady or cramping. The patient may also experience either constipation or increased frequency of defecation. Depending on the location and severity of the inflammation, nausea, vomiting, and a low-grade fever may occur. On examination, the abdomen may be distended, with tenderness and a palpable mass in the left lower quadrant resulting from the inflammatory response.

The older adult may have less specific manifestations, complaining of vague abdominal pain. A palpable mass and signs of a large bowel obstruction may be present.

COMPLICATIONS Complications associated with diverticulitis (in addition to peritonitis and abscess formation) include bowel obstruction, fistula formation, and hemorrhage. Severe or repeated episodes of diverticulitis may lead to scarring and fibrosis of the bowel wall, further narrowing the bowel lumen. This increases the risk for obstruction of the large bowel. Acutely inflamed tissue may adhere to the small bowel, increasing the potential for small-bowel obstruction as well. Fistulas may form, usually between the sigmoid colon and the bladder. Urinary tract infection is the usual sign of a colovesical fistula. Fistulas may also perforate into the small intestine, ureter, vagina, perineum, or abdominal wall. Bleeding from perforation of a vessel wall can occur with diverticulitis. Although it may be significant, bleeding usually stops spontaneously.

Interdisciplinary Care

Management of diverticular disease varies from no prescribed treatment to surgical resection of affected colon, depending on the severity of the disease and its complications.

Diagnosis

Diagnostic testing is used to identify diverticular disease when the disease is symptomatic or complications develop. In addition to illustrating diverticula, a barium enema and x-rays can reveal segmental spasm and muscular thickening with a narrowed bowel lumen. Flexible sigmoidoscopy or colonoscopy may be done to detect diverticulosis, assess for strictures or bleeding, and rule out tumor as the cause of the patient's manifestations. Abdominal x-ray films may show free abdominal air associated with diverticulitis and perforation. CT scan may be done with or without contrast media to assess inflammation and detect an abscess or fistula.

Flexible Sigmoidoscopy Video

Laboratory tests include hemoccult or guaiac testing of stool to identify the presence of occult blood, and a WBC count, which may show leukocytosis with a left shift (an increased number of immature WBCs) due to inflammation in diverticulitis.

Medications

Systemic broad-spectrum antibiotics effective against usual bowel flora are prescribed to treat acute diverticulitis. Oral antibiotics such as metronidazole (Flagyl) and ciprofloxacin (Cipro) or trimethoprim-sulfamethoxazole (Septra, Bactrim) may be prescribed if manifestations are mild. Rifaximin (Xifaxan) is a poorly absorbed antibiotic that may be used together with fiber to treat uncomplicated diverticular disease. Severe, acute attacks often necessitate hospitalization and treatment with intravenous fluids and antibiotics effective against anaerobic and gram-negative bacteria. Therapy may include a second-generation cephalosporin such as cefoxitin (Mefoxin), or another antibiotic such as piperacillin-tazobactam (Zosyn) or ticarcillin-clavulanate (Timentin). Antibiotics and their nursing implications are discussed in ∞ Chapter 12.

Although a stool softener such as docusate sodium (Colace) may be prescribed, it is important to note that laxatives (which can further increase intraluminal pressure in the colon) are avoided for the patient with diverticular disease.

Nutrition

Dietary modification is central to the management of diverticular disease. It appears that dietary changes can reduce the risk of complications of diverticulosis. A high-fiber diet is recommended; it increases stool bulk, decreases intraluminal pressures, and may reduce spasm (Table 24–9). Bran is a low-cost fiber supplement that can be added to cereal, soups, salads, or other foods. Commercial bulk-forming products, such as psyllium seed (Metamucil) or methylcellulose also may be recommended. These products are discussed in the Medication Administration box on pages 658–659. The patient often is advised to avoid foods with small seeds (such as popcorn, caraway seeds, figs, or berries), which could obstruct diverticula.

Bowel rest is prescribed during an acute episode of diverticulitis. The patient initially may be NPO with intravenous fluids and possibly parenteral nutrition. Feeding is resumed gradually. Initially, a clear liquid diet is prescribed with gradual advancement to a soft, low-roughage diet (i.e., a diet low in insoluble fiber) with daily added psyllium seed to soften stool and increase its bulk. Among the foods the patient should avoid are wheat and corn bran, vegetable and fruit skins, nuts, and dry beans. The high-fiber diet is resumed following full recovery.

Surgery

Patients with acute diverticulitis may require surgery, usually to treat generalized peritonitis or an abscess that fails to respond to medical treatment. Hemorrhage that recurs or cannot be controlled may also necessitate surgery. Elective surgery may be performed for recurrent episodes of diverticulitis or persistent diverticulitis with continuing pain, tenderness, and a palpable mass.

The affected bowel segment is resected, and if possible an anastomosis of the proximal and distal portions is performed. When an acute infection and diverticulitis are present, a two-stage Hartmann procedure is required. A temporary colostomy is created and anastomosis delayed until the inflammation has subsided. A second surgery is performed 2 to 3 months later to reconnect the bowel and close the temporary colostomy.

∞ Nursing Care

Health Promotion

Teaching patients about the benefits of a high-fiber diet is important primary prevention for diverticular disease. Nurses working with groups and individuals in the community should emphasize the importance of a high-fiber diet and its benefits in preventing diverticular disease and other disorders. In facilities such as residential settings, the nurse can work with dietary staff and care providers to increase the amount of fiber in residents' diets, unless this is contraindicated by a preexisting condition.

Assessment

Because most patients with diverticular disease have few or no manifestations, nursing assessment focuses on manifestations of complications.

- *Health history:* Abdominal pain or cramping, chronic constipation or irregular bowel habits; nausea and vomiting; history of diverticular disease or irritable bowel syndrome.
- *Physical examination:* Bowel sounds, presence of abdominal tenderness of masses and location; stool for occult blood.

Nursing Diagnoses and Interventions

Patients with acute diverticulitis are acutely ill and have multiple nursing care needs. The risk of perforation and resulting peritonitis or abscess formation is high. Priority nursing diagnoses include *Acute Pain* and *Anxiety* related to the possibility of a significant complication or possible surgery.

Potential Complication: Perforation

During an acute attack of diverticulitis, inflammation and mucosal ischemia place the patient at risk for perforation and peritonitis. In addition to maintaining bowel rest to reduce the risk of perforation, the nurse monitors for manifestations of perforation and possible sepsis.

- Monitor vital signs including temperature at least every 4 hours. *Tachycardia and tachypnea may be early indications of*

TABLE 24–9	Foods Recommended in a High-Fiber, High-Residue Diet	
FOOD GROUP	**RECOMMENDED FOODS**
Cereals and grains	Wheat or oat bran; cooked cereals, such as oatmeal; dry cereals, such as bran buds or flakes, corn flakes, shredded wheat; whole-grain breads or crackers; brown rice
Fruits	Unpeeled raw apples, peaches, and pears; oranges; blackberries, raspberries, strawberries (may be restricted for the patient with diverticulosis)
Vegetables	Dried beans (navy, kidney, pinto), lima beans; broccoli; peas; corn; squash; raw vegetables, such as carrots, celery, and tomatoes; potatoes (with skins)

increased inflammation and resulting fluid shift. Fever greater than 101°F (38.3°C) may indicate increased inflammation or spread of inflammation. Note, however, that little temperature elevation may occur in the older patient. A change in behavior or increasing lethargy may be subtle indications of infection in the older adult.

- Assess abdomen every 4 to 8 hours or more often as indicated, including measuring abdominal girth, auscultating bowel sounds, and palpating for tenderness. Promptly report significant changes to the physician. *Increasing abdominal distention, a decrease or change in the quality of bowel sounds, and/or increasing tenderness or guarding may indicate spread of the infectious process or peritonitis.*

- Assess for evidence of lower intestinal bleeding by visual examination and guaiac testing of stools for occult blood. *Perforation of a diverticulum may produce either intestinal or intra-abdominal bleeding and require immediate treatment such as surgery.*

- Maintain intravenous fluids, TPN, and accurate intake and output records. *During acute diverticulitis, oral intake is usually prohibited or restricted. Intravenous fluids are given to maintain fluid and electrolyte balance; TPN is used to maintain nutritional status, facilitating healing and recovery.*

Acute Pain

Pain is a common manifestation of acute diverticulitis. It results from inflammation of the bowel and edema of affected tissues. If surgery is required, postoperative pain is managed with narcotic analgesics.

- Ask the patient to rate pain using a 0 to 10 pain scale. Document the level of pain, and note any changes in location or character of pain. *The perception and response to pain is individual and is affected by past experiences, culture, ethnic background, and many other factors. A change in the character or intensity of the pain may indicate a complication such as perforation or abscess formation.*

- Administer prescribed analgesic or maintain PCA as ordered. Assess analgesic effectiveness. Avoid administering morphine. Provide adjunctive medications as ordered, and encourage use of adjunctive techniques, such as relaxation, positioning, and distraction. Notify the physician if pain management is inadequate. *If patient has not obtained adequate pain relief, further assessment and intervention are required.*

- Maintain bowel rest and total body rest (bed rest with limited activity). *Rest helps reduce inflammation and promote healing, increasing comfort.*

- Reintroduce oral foods and fluids slowly, providing a soft, low-fiber diet with bulk-forming agents. *This allows continued healing of the affected bowel while promoting soft, easily expelled stools.*

Anxiety

The patient with acute diverticulitis faces not only hospitalization, but also potential serious complications such as peritonitis and hemorrhage. Surgery and formation of a temporary colostomy may be necessary. Furthermore, episodes of acute diverticulitis are often recurrent, and the patient may fear future problems.

- Assess and document level of anxiety. *Severe anxiety or panic states can interfere with the ability to respond to instructions and assist with care. Low to moderate anxiety levels enhance learning and compliance with prescribed interventions.*

- Demonstrate empathy and awareness of the perceived threat to health. *It is important to recognize and respect the patient's feelings and perceptions as reality.*

- Attend to physical care needs. *This provides reassurance that these needs will be met and relieves concerns about them.*

- Spend as much time as possible with the patient. *Presence of a caring nurse helps relieve fears of abandonment or that help will not be available if needed. It also enhances trust and provides opportunity for expression of fears or concerns.*

- Assess level of understanding about disease and condition. *This allows misperceptions that may contribute to anxiety to be corrected.*

- Encourage supportive family and friends to remain with the patient as much as possible. *This provides a supportive environment for the patient and also distracts from physical concerns.*

- Assist the patient to identify and use appropriate coping mechanisms. *Coping mechanisms provide immediate relief of anxiety while the patient adapts to the situation.*

- Involve the patient and family (as appropriate) in care decisions. *This increases the patient's sense of control over the situation.*

Community-Based Care

The patient with diverticular disease is responsible for self-care. Discuss the following topics for home care:

- Prescribed high-fiber diet and the need to maintain the diet for life to reduce the incidence of complications, including ways to increase dietary fiber

- Complications of diverticular disease and its manifestations

Provide a referral to a dietitian for teaching as indicated. Prior to discharge of the patient with acute diverticulitis, discuss the following:

- Food and fluid limitations, including recommendations for a low-residue diet during the initial period of healing.

- Colostomy management (if a temporary colostomy has been created), including where to obtain supplies and dietary management.

- Planned procedure to reanastomose the colon and revise the colostomy. Refer to community healthcare agencies as indicated.

Malabsorption Syndromes

Malabsorption is a condition in which the intestinal mucosa ineffectively absorbs nutrients—including carbohydrates, proteins, fats, water, electrolytes, minerals, and vitamins—resulting in their excretion in the stool. Many bowel disorders can lead to malabsorption.

Diseases of the small intestine often cause malabsorption. Other medical and/or surgical conditions can result in malabsorption if they affect digestion or the intestinal mucosa. Primary diseases of the small-bowel mucosa, such as sprue, Crohn's disease, and acute infections, can lead to malabsorption.

TABLE 24–10 Selected Causes of Malabsorption

CAUSE	RELATED FACTORS OR CONDITIONS
Impaired absorption	Sprue
	Short bowel syndrome
	Acute enteritis and other bowel infections or infestations
	AIDS-related opportunistic infections and Kaposi's sarcoma
	Celiac disease
	Crohn's disease
	Intestinal ischemia or infarction
	Scleroderma
Impaired digestion	Lactose intolerance
	Gastrectomy
	Chronic pancreatitis, cancer of the pancreas
	Cystic fibrosis
	Biliary obstruction
	Cirrhosis, hepatitis, or liver failure
	Zollinger-Ellison syndrome

It can also result from *maldigestion*, inadequate preparation of chyme for absorption. For example, major gastric resections, pancreatic disorders with impaired pancreatic enzyme secretion, and biliary disorders that affect bile secretion can impair digestion and absorption of chyme. Selected causes of impaired absorption and digestion are listed in Table 24–10.

Regardless of the cause, malabsorption causes common manifestations resulting from impaired absorption of chyme and the nutrients it contains (see Pathophysiology Linkage). Predominant GI manifestations include anorexia; abdominal bloating; diarrhea with loose, bulky, foul-smelling stools; and steatorrhea (fatty stools). Weight loss, weakness, general malaise, muscle cramps, bone pain, abnormal bleeding, and anemia are common systemic manifestations of malabsorption. These manifestations result from malnutrition and fluid loss due to poor absorption.

Three common malabsorption disorders in adults are celiac disease, lactose intolerance, and short bowel syndrome.

The Patient with Celiac Disease

Celiac disease, also known as celiac sprue or nontropical sprue, is a chronic immune-mediated disorder of the small intestine in which the absorption of nutrients, particularly fats, is impaired. It is characterized by sensitivity to the gliadin fraction of gluten, a cereal protein. Gluten is found in wheat, rye, barley, and oats. It is also used as a filler in many prepared foods and in medications.

The cause of celiac disease is unknown; however, genetic and immune factors are known to play a role in its development. Caucasians of European descent are most commonly affected (McPhee et al., 2008). Having a first-degree relative with celiac disease significantly increases the risk. Nearly all people with celiac disease share the HAL-DQ2 allele, although only a small percentage of people with this allele actually have celiac disease (Fauci et al., 2008).

Manifestations of celiac disease often develop in childhood, but may develop at any age. The severity of the disease depends on the extent of mucosal involvement in the intestine and the duration of the disease.

Pathophysiology

Most absorption of nutrients occurs in the small intestine. The mucosa of the small intestine is arranged in microscopic folds, which in turn contain even smaller finger-like projections called villi. The cells of the villi are covered with microscopic hairs, microvilli, projecting from the cell membrane. The folds, villi, and microvilli of the intestinal mucosa provide a huge surface area for nutrient absorption. Cells of the intestines are specialized to absorb different nutrients. Readily digested nutrients are absorbed in the proximal intestine; others are absorbed more distally in the intestines. Nutrients are absorbed by the processes of simple diffusion (water and small lipids), facilitated diffusion (water-soluble vitamins), and active transport (glucose and amino acids). Once absorbed into the cells of the villi, nutrients enter the blood or lymph for systemic distribution.

PATHOPHYSIOLOGY LINKAGE Local and Systemic Manifestations of Malabsorption

CATEGORY	MANIFESTATION	CAUSE
Local (GI)	Diarrhea	Disruption of bowel mucosa impairs absorption of fluid and electrolytes, leading to excess water in the stool
	Abdominal distention	Gas formation from fermentation of undigested carbohydrates
	Steatorrhea	Impaired fat absorption leading to excess fat in feces
Systemic	Weight loss	Carbohydrate, protein, and fat deficit
	Weakness and malaise	Kilocalorie deficit; impaired absorption of micronutrients (vitamins and minerals) leading to nutrient deficiencies, anemia; fluid and electrolyte losses
	Anemia	Vitamin B_{12}, folic acid, and iron deficits impair erythropoiesis
	Bone pain	Calcium and vitamin D deficits lead to bone demineralization
	Muscle cramps, paresthesias	Protein wasting, vitamin B_{12} and electrolyte deficits impair neuromuscular function
	Easy bruising and bleeding	Vitamin K deficit
	Glossitis, cheilosis	Iron, folic acid, and vitamin B_{12} deficits

In celiac disease, it the intestinal mucosa is damaged by an immunologic response. Gliadin acts as an antigen (a substance that induces the formation of antibodies that interact specifically with it), prompting an inappropriate T-cell mediated immune response. People with celiac disease have increased antibodies to other antigens as well. The immune response prompts an inflammatory response in the small bowel, resulting in loss of villi and microvilli. The villi shorten and atrophy, resulting in loss of intestinal folds and absorptive surface. Digestive enzyme production, including disaccharidase and particularly lactase, is reduced as well. The proximal small bowel is affected to the greatest extent, likely due to its greater exposure to dietary gluten.

Manifestations

Manifestations of celiac disease may develop at any age. Local manifestations include abdominal bloating and cramps, diarrhea, and steatorrhea. Systemic manifestations result from the effects of malabsorption and resulting deficiencies. Anemia is common. Patients with celiac disease are often small in stature, and may have delayed maturity. Other signs of nutrient deficiencies include tetany, vitamin deficiencies, muscle wasting, and rickets (impaired bone development). When gluten is removed from the diet, the manifestations resolve.

Gastrointestinal malignancies and intestinal lymphoma are potential complications of celiac disease. Other complications include intestinal ulceration and development of refractory disease, or disease that no longer responds to a gluten-free diet.

Interdisciplinary Care

With any malabsorptive disorder, the initial focus of management is to identify the cause. Once this has been determined, specific therapy can be prescribed.

Diagnosis

Laboratory and diagnostic testing are used to make the differential diagnosis for various causes of malabsorption syndromes and to determine the severity of nutrient deficiencies.

An enteroscopy permits direct examination of intestinal mucosa and collection of a tissue specimen for biopsy. Tissue biopsy is necessary to establish the diagnosis of celiac disease.

Upper GI series with small-bowel follow-through may be done to evaluate the structures of the upper GI tract. With celiac disease, the typical "feathery" pattern of barium in the small bowel is lost, and the barium may precipitate and clump. Nursing implications of diagnostic tests are included in ∞ Chapter 21.

Laboratory tests are used to identify pathophysiologic effects of the disease. Fecal fat is measured to document the presence of steatorrhea. The fat content of stool is increased in many malabsorptive disorders, including celiac disease. Serologic testing for IgA endomysial antibodies and IgG and IgA antigliadin antibodies is used to diagnose celiac disease and evaluate compliance with the prescribed gluten-free diet. Serum levels of protein, albumin, cholesterol, electrolytes, and iron may be ordered to evaluate for nutrient deficiencies. The hemoglobin, hematocrit, and RBC indices are used to evaluate anemia. Prothrombin time is increased in vitamin K deficiency.

Medications

Patients with severe nutritional deficits may require vitamin and mineral supplements, as well as iron and folic acid to correct anemia. Vitamin K may be administered parenterally if the prothrombin time is prolonged. In patients whose disease fails to respond to dietary management, corticosteroids may be ordered to suppress the inflammatory response.

Nutrition

The patient with celiac disease is placed on a gluten-free diet. This treatment is generally successful, as long as the patient avoids gluten totally. Gluten is so widely used in prepared foods that this may be no easy task. Consultation with a dietitian and detailed dietary instructions are necessary. Patients need to become aware of hidden sources of gluten and to analyze dietary labels. Common sources of gluten and foods to be avoided are indicated in Table 24–11.

The prescribed diet is high in calories and protein to correct nutrient deficits. Fat content is restricted to minimize steatorrhea. The diet usually is restricted in lactose as well to compensate for the loss of lactase-containing microvilli. Foods containing lactose may be reintroduced once remission has occurred. Patients with refractory disease may benefit from restriction of other dietary proteins such as soy (Fauci et al., 2008).

TABLE 24–11 Dietary Sources of Gluten

FOOD GROUP	CONTAINS GLUTEN	MAY CONTAIN GLUTEN
Cereals, grains, and grain products	Bread, crackers, cereal, and pasta containing wheat, rye, or barley grain or flour	Seasoned rice and potato mixes
Beverages	Malt, Postum, Ovaltine, beers, and ales	Commercial chocolate milk, cocoa, and other beverage mixes, such as instant tea mix, dietary supplements
Desserts	Cakes, cookies, and pastries made with wheat, rye, or barley flour	Commercial ice cream and sherbet
Meats and other protein sources		Meat loaf, cold cuts and prepared meats, breaded meats; cheese products; soy protein meat substitutes; commercial egg products
Fruits and vegetables		Commercial seasoned vegetable mixes or vegetables with sauce; canned baked beans; commercial pie fillings
Miscellaneous		Commercial salad dressings and mayonnaise; ketchup and prepared mustard; gravy, white sauce; nondairy creamer; syrups; commercial pickles

✍ Nursing Care

Nursing care for the patient with celiac disease focuses on the effects of the disorder on health and nutrition, as well as the patient's ability to manage the disease.

Assessment

- *Health history:* Onset, duration, and severity of manifestations; number and character of stools; previous teaching related to disorder; current treatment and diet.
- *Physical examination:* Vital signs; abdominal shape, contour, bowel sounds; manifestations of malnutrition (e.g., anemia, small stature, muscle wasting, signs of other nutrient deficiencies).

Nursing Diagnoses and Interventions

Diarrhea and malnutrition are significant problems for the patient with celiac disease and the priority foci for nursing intervention.

Diarrhea

Steatorrhea and diarrhea typically occur with celiac disease because fat, water, and other nutrients are poorly absorbed, remaining in the bowel to be eliminated in the stool. Diarrhea can interfere with lifestyle, ADLs, skin integrity, and fluid and electrolyte balance.

- Assess and document the frequency and nature of stools. *Bowel elimination reflects the severity of the disease and efficacy of treatment. With effective treatment, stools become less frequent and more normal in color and appearance.*
- Weigh daily, monitor intake and output, and assess skin turgor and mucous membranes for indications of fluid balance. *Diarrhea increases the risk for hypovolemia and dehydration resulting from excess fluid loss in the stool.*
- Assess and document perianal skin condition. *Frequent defecation can irritate skin and mucous membranes, increasing the risk of breakdown.*
- Encourage a liberal fluid intake. *Oral fluids help replace fluid lost through diarrheal stool.*

Imbalanced Nutrition: Less than Body Requirements

Celiac disease is a chronic condition. With continuing malabsorption, multiple nutrient deficits may occur, resulting in impaired growth and development, impaired healing, muscle wasting, bone disease, and electrolyte imbalances.

- Maintain accurate dietary intake records. *Assessment of dietary intake provides information about compliance with the prescribed diet as well as the adequacy of nutrient intake.*
- Monitor laboratory results, including hemoglobin and hematocrit, serum electrolytes, total serum protein, and albumin levels. *These studies provide information about nutritional status.*
- Arrange for dietary consultation. Provide for food preferences as allowed. *An individualized diet developed to address the patient's food preferences as well as nutrient needs will promote appetite and food intake.*
- Provide the prescribed high-kilocalorie, high-protein, low-fat, gluten-free diet for the patient with celiac sprue. Restrict lactose (dairy product) intake as indicated. *Calories and protein*

are important to replace lost nutrients. Fat restriction helps reduce diarrhea and nutrient loss. Lactose may be restricted during initial treatment, then slowly reintroduced into the diet as the gut heals and its normal structure is restored.

- Provide parenteral nutrition as ordered if the patient is unable to absorb enteral nutrients. *Parenteral nutrition can help reverse nutritional deficits and promote weight gain when manifestations are acute.*
- Encourage nutritional supplements. *Nutritional supplements often are necessary to replace losses and restore nutrient levels to normal more rapidly than diet alone can achieve.*
- Include family members, the primary food preparer in particular, in teaching and dietary discussions. *Families can reinforce teaching and help the patient maintain required restrictions or kilocalorie intake.*

Community-Based Care

The patient with celiac disease has a chronic condition that requires continuing dietary management.

Provide a detailed list of foods that contain gluten and need to be eliminated from the diet, as well as foods that are allowed. Teach the patient and family how to identify gluten-containing commercial products by reading labels and lists of ingredients. Encourage the purchase and use of a gluten-free cookbook. Discuss potential long-term complications of the disorder and manifestations to be reported to the primary care provider.

If corticosteroids have been prescribed, stress the importance of taking the medication as ordered. Emphasize the need to avoid stopping the medication abruptly and to notify all caregivers that a corticosteroid is part of the patient's medication regimen. Instruct to frequently monitor weight. A weight gain of 5 lb (2.3 kg) or more in less than a week usually reflects fluid gain, a possible adverse effect of corticosteroids. Other potential effects include decreased resistance to infection, an impaired inflammatory response, and changes in the metabolism of carbohydrates, proteins, and fats.

The Patient with Lactase Deficiency

For carbohydrates to be absorbed from the small intestine, they first must be broken down into simple sugars, or monosaccharides. Lactose is the primary carbohydrate in milk and milk products. It is a disaccharide, requiring the enzyme lactase for digestion and absorption. Lactase deficiency can lead to *lactose intolerance* and manifestations of malabsorption. Lactase deficiency usually is genetic in origin, but also occurs secondarily to celiac disease, Crohn's disease, and other disorders affecting the mucosa of the small intestine. There is a racial/ethnic component to the disorder, as described in the following Focus on Cultural Diversity box.

Manifestations

Many people with lactase deficiency are asymptomatic. Small to moderate amounts of milk (one to two 8-ounce glasses) may be well tolerated. Manifestations of lactose intolerance include lower abdominal cramping, pain, and diarrhea following milk ingestion. Undigested lactose ferments in the intestine, forming gases that contribute to bloating and flatus. Lactic and fatty acids produced by this fermentation irritate the bowel, leading to increased motility and abdominal cramping. The undigested lactose draws water into the intestine, which contributes to increased motility and diarrhea. The diarrhea associated with lactose intolerance may be explosive.

Interdisciplinary Care

The diagnosis of lactase deficiency usually is based on a history of intolerance to milk and milk products, and a trial of a lactose-free diet. If manifestations resolve when lactose intake is eliminated, the diagnosis of lactase deficiency is confirmed.

Diagnosis

The lactose breath test is a noninvasive test that may be used to diagnose lactase deficiency. Expired hydrogen gas (H_2) is measured following oral administration of 50 g of lactose. If lactose is digested and absorbed normally, then little change occurs in the amount of exhaled H_2 from fasting to postlactose administration. With lactose intolerance, exhaled H_2 increases following lactose administration as the sugar ferments in the bowel.

For the lactose tolerance test, 100 g of lactose solution is orally administered, followed by measurement of blood glucose levels at intervals of 30, 60, and 120 minutes. If lactose is digested and absorbed normally, the blood glucose rises more than 20 mg/dL. The expected blood glucose elevation does not occur in lactase deficiency.

Nutrition

A lactose-free or reduced lactose diet relieves the manifestations of the disorder. Some patients require total elimination of milk and milk products from the diet. Many can tolerate limited amounts of lactose. Milk pretreated with lactase is readily available. Nonprescription lactase enzyme preparations are available to improve milk tolerance. Yogurt containing bacterial lactases may be well tolerated. Calcium supplements are often recommended, particularly for women on a reduced-lactose or lactose-free diet.

∞ Nursing Care

Nursing care for the patient with lactose intolerance focuses on providing education and support. Discuss sources of lactose: Milk, ice cream, and cottage cheese are high in lactose; aged cheese and yogurt contain much smaller amounts. Potential hidden sources of lactose include sherbets, desserts made from milk and milk chocolate, sauces and gravies, and cream soups. Suggest a trial of lactase-treated milk or lactase enzyme supplements. Emphasize the importance of obtaining nutrients

contained in dairy products from other sources. Proteins may be obtained from meats, eggs, legumes, and grains. Other sources of calcium include sardines, oysters, and salmon, as well as plant sources such as beans, cauliflower, rhubarb, and green leafy vegetables.

The Patient with Short Bowel Syndrome

The small bowel may be resected due to tumors, infarction of bowel mucosa, incarcerated hernias, Crohn's disease, trauma, and enteropathy resulting from radiation therapy. Resection of significant portions of the small intestine may result in a condition known as *short bowel syndrome*. The severity of the disorder depends on the total amount of bowel resected, as well as the portions of bowel removed. Removal of the proximal portions, including the duodenum, jejunum, and proximal ileum, and the distal portion of the ileum is associated with more severe malabsorption and manifestations than is resection of midportions of the ileum.

Resection of the small intestine affects the absorption of water, nutrients, vitamins, and minerals. Transit time of ingested foods and fluids is reduced, and digestive processes are impaired. The bowel undergoes an adaptive process in which the remaining villi enlarge and lengthen to increase absorptive surface following resection. For many patients, absorption and bowel function return to preoperative or near-normal levels. Others have continued significant impairment of digestion and absorption, leading to nutrient deficiencies, weight loss, and diarrhea. Short bowel syndrome is associated with an increased risk for kidney stones and gallstones.

Interdisciplinary Care

Management of short bowel syndrome focuses on alleviating manifestations. Patients often simply require frequent, small, high-kilocalorie, high-protein feedings.

Diagnosis

Laboratory and diagnostic studies are used to evaluate nutrient deficiencies. Total serum proteins and albumin are reduced, as are serum levels of folate, iron, vitamins, minerals, and electrolytes. Anemia and a prolonged prothrombin time (indicative of vitamin K deficiency) may develop.

Medications

Multivitamin and mineral supplementation is frequently necessary. Antidiarrheal medications are used to reduce bowel motility, allowing a greater amount of time for nutrient absorption. Some patients are affected by gastric hypersecretion following bowel resection. For these patients, a proton-pump inhibitor such as omeprazole (Prilosec) may be ordered. Patients with severe manifestations of short bowel syndrome may require parenteral nutrition.

∞ Nursing Care

Nursing care for the patient with short bowel syndrome focuses on the problems of potential fluid volume deficit, malnutrition, and diarrhea.

Fluid losses are generally greatest in the initial periods following surgery, warranting the closest attention at that time. Close monitoring of vital signs, intake and output, daily weights, skin turgor, and condition of mucous membranes is vital. It is important to remember that the risk also is high when other abnormal fluid losses occur through, for example, fever, draining wounds, or excess perspiration.

Document nutritional status, including weight, anthropometric measurements, laboratory values, and kilocalorie intake. Provide nutritional supplementation with enteral feedings as needed. Maintain central lines and PN, using aseptic technique.

For diarrhea, document the number and character of stools. Administer antidiarrheal medications as ordered. If the patient is lactose intolerant, limit intake of milk and milk products. Provide good skin care of the perianal region to prevent breakdown from frequent bowel movements. Refer to the discussion of nursing care for the patient with celiac disease for other measures for altered nutrition and diarrhea.

The patient and family affected by this condition require extensive education. Because there is no way to cure or replace the lost bowel at this time, the patient must manage the disorder on a day-to-day basis. Provide instructions about the recommended diet and medication regimen. Emphasize the importance of maintaining an adequate fluid intake, particularly in hot weather or during strenuous exercise. Teach the patient to monitor his or her weight frequently and report changes. Include teaching about possible manifestations of dehydration and nutrient deficiencies that should be reported to the physician. Referring the patient to a dietitian or counselor can help the person cope with what may be a lifelong problem.

Neoplastic Disorders

Cancer remains the second leading cause of death in the United States, preceded only by heart disease. Although cancer may affect any portion of the digestive tract, the large intestine and rectum are the most common sites. Malignant neoplasms of the lower bowel are the second leading cause of death from cancer (after lung cancer), making this a significant healthcare concern.

The Patient with Polyps

A *polyp* is a mass of tissue that arises from the bowel wall and protrudes into the lumen. Polyps may develop in any portion of the bowel, but they occur most often in the sigmoid colon and rectum. They vary considerably in size and may be single or multiple. It is estimated that approximately 30% of people over the age of 50 have polyps. Although most polyps are benign, some have the potential to become malignant. Familial adenomatous polyposis (FAP) is a syndrome with a dominant inheritance pattern that leads to the development of hundreds to thousands of adenomatous polyps. Some of these polyps will inevitably become malignant (Fauci et al., 2008).

Pathophysiology

Polyps are identified by their structure and tissue type. Most polyps are adenomas, benign epithelial tumors that are considered premalignant lesions. Greater than 95% of adenocarcinomas arise from adenomas; however, less than 1% of polyps ever become malignant (Fauci et al., 2008). Of polyps that are removed during colonoscopy, more than 70% are adenomatous (McPhee et al., 2008).

Adenomatous polyps represent disruption of the normal process of cell proliferation to replace epithelial cells lining the intestine. Cells are constantly being reproduced to replace those shed as feces move through the colon. Disruption of the normal process of cell division and maturation can lead to formation of a polyp composed of tightly packed epithelial cells. The cells may appear grossly normal or show signs of dysplasia. Polyps may develop as tubular, villous, or tubulovillous adenomas. Polyps may be named by the way they are attached to the bowel wall as either sessile (raised nodules) or pedunculated (attached by a stalk) (Figure 24–9 ■).

Tubular adenomas (also called pedunculated polyps) are more common than sessile polyps and account for about 65% of benign polyps of the large intestine (Porth & Matfin, 2009).

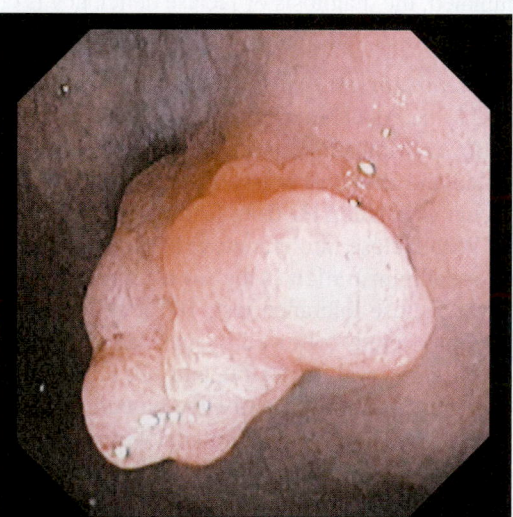

A

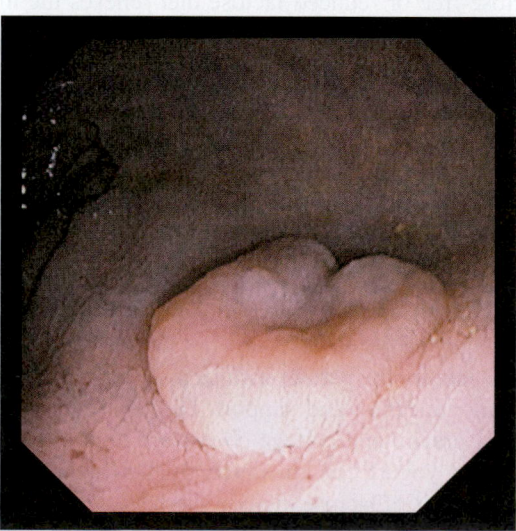

B

Figure 24–9 ■ *A*, Tubular (or pedumculated) and *B*, villous (or sessile) polyps.

A tubular adenoma is a globelike structure attached to the intestinal wall by a thin, stalk-like stem. The incidence of this type of polyp increases with age, although it occurs in all age groups and in both genders. Most are small, 1 cm or less in diameter, although they may be as large as 4 to 5 cm. The malignant potential of these polyps seems to be related to their size. Small adenomas less than 1 cm have a low risk of being malignant, and larger adenomas greater than 1 cm have a much higher risk of harboring malignancy or a high-grade dysplasia.

Villous adenomas (also called sessile polyps) have a broad base and an elevated, cauliflower-like surface (Figure 24–9B). They typically develop in the rectosigmoid colon. This type of polyp is often larger than tubular adenomas, usually more than 5 cm. Villous adenomas are not common, accounting for about 10% of colon polyps. They have a higher malignant potential than tubular adenomas. Some adenomatous polyps contain both tubular epithelium and villi and are known as *tubulovillous adenomas.*

Manifestations

Most polyps are asymptomatic, found coincidentally during routine examination or diagnostic testing. Intermittent painless rectal bleeding, bright or dark red, is the most common presenting complaint. A large polyp may cause abdominal cramping, pain, or manifestations of obstruction. Diarrhea and mucous discharge may be associated with a large villous adenoma.

Interdisciplinary Care

The diagnosis of intestinal polyps is generally based on diagnostic studies such as sigmoidoscopy or colonoscopy. A rectal polyp may be palpable on digital examination, but further studies are necessary to determine its size and type and the extent of colon involvement, and to assess for malignancy. Genetic testing and counseling is offered to patients with or a family history of FAP. First degree relatives of a patient with FAP undergo annual sigmoidoscopy beginning at age 10 years.

Once identified, polyps are removed because of the risk of malignancy. Pedunculated polyps and small villous lesions may be removed during colonoscopy using an electrocautery snare or hot biopsy forceps passed through the scope. This relatively safe procedure has less than a 2% risk of complications such as perforation or hemorrhage. Large villous adenomas are completely excised and examined histologically for evidence of malignancy. In some cases, the colon segment containing the polyp is resected. Patients with FAP usually undergo a total colectomy with ileorectal anastomosis before age 20 years to significantly reduce their risk for developing colon cancer.

Treatment following polypectomy depends on histologic examination of the excised tissue. Because polyps tend to recur, follow-up colonoscopy is recommended in 3 years and then every 5 years if no further polyps are detected. When the polyp is found to be malignant, follow-up care is determined by the tissue type and degree of invasion.

✆ Nursing Care

Health Promotion

The incidence of intestinal polyps increases with age. They affect men and women equally. It is believed that an adenomatous polyp requires more than 5 years of growth to become significant in size and malignant potential. Advise all patients to have a screening for colorectal cancer (with a colonoscopy being the "gold standard" for diagnosis) at age 50 and as recommended thereafter for early detection of polyps (American Cancer Society [ACS], 2008).

Assessment

Polyps are a "silent" disease, with few or no manifestations.

- *Health history:* Rectal bleeding; personal or family history of intestinal polyps or colorectal cancer.

Nursing Diagnoses and Interventions

Nursing care for the patient with polyps focuses on education and assisting the patient through diagnostic testing and polyp removal. Before and after colonoscopy and polypectomy, provide direct care and teaching about the procedure, expected sensations during the procedure, and anticipated postoperative care. Cathartics are prescribed prior to colonoscopy; cleansing enemas may be ordered. Observe for evidence of fluid and electrolyte imbalance during preoperative preparation. If enemas are ordered, use normal saline (not tap water) to reduce the risk of electrolyte imbalances. Following polypectomy, observe closely for possible complications such as hemorrhage.

Community-Based Care

Include the following topics when teaching for home care:

- The significance of polyps and their relationship to colorectal cancer
- The importance of keeping follow-up appointments and undergoing repeat colonoscopy as recommended: at 3 years following polypectomy, then every 5 to 10 years unless additional polyps are found
- Manifestations to report to the physician, such as diarrhea, pain, rectal bleeding, light-headedness, or other indications of possible blood loss

The Patient with Colorectal Cancer

Colorectal cancer (cancer of the colon or rectum) is the third most common cancer diagnosed in the United States. In the United States about 146,970 new cases of colorectal cancer were diagnosed in 2009, and it was expected to cause about 49,920 deaths during that year (ACS, 2009). Earlier diagnosis and improved treatment have improved the survival rate for colorectal cancer. Its incidence, which is nearly equal among men and women, has been declining in the United States for the past 15 years. The incidence of colorectal cancer varies among ethnic groups; see the following Focus on Cultural Diversity box. Colorectal cancer occurs most frequently after age 50. The incidence continues to rise with increasing age. With early diagnosis and treatment, the 5-year survival rate for colorectal cancer is 90%; however, only 39% of colorectal cancers are diagnosed at this early stage.

Although the specific cause of colorectal cancer is unknown, a number of risk factors have been identified (Box 24–2). Genetic factors are linked to the risk for colorectal cancer. Up to 25% of people who develop colorectal cancer have a family history of the disease (Fauci et al., 2008). Persons with familial adenomatous polyposis inevitably will develop colon cancer unless the colon is removed. Hereditary nonpolyposis colorectal cancer (also known as Lynch syndrome) is an autosomal dominant disorder that significantly increases the risk for developing colorectal and other cancers. Tumors associated with Lynch syndrome often affect the ascending colon, and tend to occur at an earlier age. Inflammatory bowel diseases increase the risk of colorectal cancer.

Diet plays a role in the development of colorectal cancer. The disease is prevalent in economically prosperous countries where people consume diets high in calories, meat proteins, and fats. This dietary pattern, common in the United States, is thought to increase the population of anaerobic bacteria in the gut. These anaerobes convert bile acids into carcinogens. Diets high in fruits and vegetables, folic acid, and calcium appear to reduce the risk of colorectal cancer. Cereal fiber, once thought to reduce colorectal cancer risk, does not now appear to play a role either way in its development. Other factors that may reduce the risk of colorectal cancer include regular exercise, taking a daily multivitamin, and the use of aspirin and other NSAIDs.

Pathophysiology

Nearly all colorectal cancers that begin as adenomatous polyps are adenocarcinomas. Most tumors develop in the rectum and sigmoid colon, although any portion of the colon may be affected (Figure 24–10 ■). The tumor typically grows undetected, producing few manifestations. By the time manifestations occur, the disease may have spread into deeper layers of the bowel tissue and adjacent organs. Colorectal cancer spreads by direct extension to involve the entire

BOX 24–2 Risk Factors for Colorectal Cancer

- Age over 50 years
- Polyps of the colon and/or rectum
- Family history of colorectal cancer
- Personal history of colorectal, ovarian, endometrial, or breast cancer
- Inflammatory bowel disease
- Exposure to radiation
- Diet: high animal fat and kilocalorie intake
- Obesity, smoking, and alcohol use

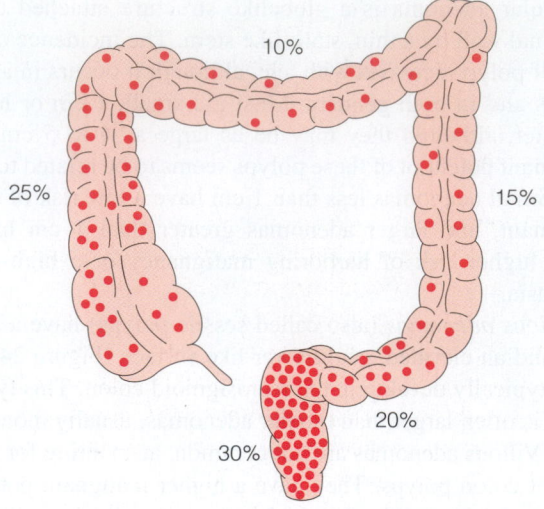

Figure 24–10 ■ The distribution and frequency of cancer of the colon and rectum.

bowel circumference, the submucosa, and outer bowel wall layers. Neighboring structures such as the liver, greater curvature of the stomach, duodenum, small intestine, pancreas, spleen, genitourinary tract, and abdominal wall also may be involved by direct extension. Metastasis to regional lymph nodes is the most common form of tumor spread. This is not always an orderly process; distal nodes may contain cancer cells while regional nodes remain normal. Cancerous cells from the primary tumor may spread by way of the lymphatic system or circulatory system to secondary sites such as the liver, lungs, brain, bones, and kidneys. "Seeding" of the tumor to other areas of the peritoneal cavity can occur when the tumor extends through the serosa or during surgical resection.

Manifestations

Bowel cancer often produces no manifestations until it is advanced. Because it grows slowly, 5 to 15 years of growth may occur before manifestations develop. The manifestations depend on its location, type and extent, and complications. Rectal bleeding is often the initial manifestation that prompts patients to seek medical care. Other common early manifestations include a change in bowel habits, either diarrhea or constipation. Pain, anorexia, and weight loss are characteristic in advanced disease. A palpable abdominal or rectal mass may be present. Occasionally the patient presents with anemia from occult bleeding.

Complications

The primary complications associated with colorectal cancer are (1) bowel obstruction due to narrowing of the bowel lumen by the lesion; (2) perforation of the bowel wall by the tumor, allowing contamination of the peritoneal cavity by bowel contents; and (3) direct extension of the tumor to involve adjacent organs.

Most recurrences of colorectal cancer after tumor removal occur within the first 4 years. The size of the primary tumor does not necessarily relate to long-term survival. The number of involved lymph nodes, penetration of the tumor through the bowel wall, and tumor adherence to adjacent organs are better predictors of the prognosis for the disease.

Interdisciplinary Care

The focus of interdisciplinary care for colorectal cancer is prevention, early detection, and intervention. Colorectal cancer is always treated by surgical resection, with chemotherapy and radiation therapy used as adjuncts.

Prevention

Measures to prevent colon cancer that are considered to be effective and safe include consuming a diet high in fruits and vegetables and low in saturated fat and red meat, regular exercise, maintaining a healthy weight, limiting alcohol consumption, and quitting smoking. Consuming fiber supplements, minerals such as calcium, vitamins, and nonsteroidal anti-inflammatory drugs may help prevent colorectal cancer, but their effect is not yet proven (ACS, 2009). Although considered safe, these measures are the subject of further research to demonstrate conclusive proof of effectiveness.

Screening

The ACS (2008) recommends one of the following testing schedules for the early detection of colorectal cancer, beginning at age 50. These options are acceptable choices for average-risk adults.

- Yearly fecal occult blood test (FOBT) or fecal immuno-chemical test (FIT) or stool DNA test (sDNA).
- Flexible sigmoidoscopy every 5 years, *or*
- double-contrast barium enema every 5 years, *or*
- CT colonography (virtual colonoscopy) every 5 years, *or*
- colonoscopy every 10 years.

Diagnosis

Diagnostic and laboratory tests are used for screening, diagnosis, and monitoring purposes. Diagnostic tests include a sigmoidoscopy or colonoscopy as the primary diagnostic test used to detect and visualize tumors. While flexible sigmoidoscopy can detect 50% to 65% of colorectal cancers, many clinicians recommend colonoscopy. Tissue for biopsy is obtained at the time of endoscopy to confirm cancerous tissue and evaluate cell differentiation (∞ see Chapter 14). Current staging methods primarily use the TNM system, as outlined in Table 24–12. Radiologic examinations may include a chest x-ray to detect tumor metastasis to the lung. Computed tomography (CT) scan, magnetic resonance imaging (MRI), or ultrasonic examination may be used to assess tumor depth and involvement of other organs by direct extension or metastasis.

Laboratory tests used are a fecal occult blood (by guaiac or hemoccult testing) to detect blood in the feces and a CBC to detect anemia resulting from chronic blood loss and tumor growth. Carcinoembryonic antigen (CEA) is a tumor marker that can be detected in the blood of patients with colorectal cancer. CEA levels are used to estimate prognosis, monitor treatment, and detect cancer recurrence.

Surgery

Surgical resection of the tumor, adjacent colon, and regional lymph nodes is the treatment of choice for colorectal cancer. Options for surgical treatment vary from destruction of the tumor by laser photocoagulation performed during endoscopy to abdominoperineal resection with permanent colostomy. When possible, the anal sphincter is preserved and colostomy avoided.

Laser photocoagulation uses a very small, intense beam of light to generate heat in tissues toward which it is directed. The heat generated by the laser beam can be used to destroy small tumors. It is also used for palliative surgery of advanced tumors to remove obstruction. Laser photocoagulation can be performed endoscopically and is useful for patients who cannot tolerate major surgery.

Other surgical treatment options for small, localized tumors include local excision and fulguration. These procedures also may be performed during endoscopy, eliminating the need for abdominal surgery. Local excision may be used to remove a disk of rectum containing a tumor in patients with a small,

TABLE 24–12 The TNM Classification for Colorectal Cancer

STAGE	PRIMARY TUMOR (T)	REGIONAL LYMPH NODES (N)	DISTANT METASTASIS (M)
	TX—Primary tumor cannot be assessed T0—No evidence of primary tumor	NX—Regional lymph nodes cannot be assessed	MX—Presence of distant metastasis cannot be assessed
Stage 0	Tis—Carcinoma *in situ*	N0—No regional lymph node metastasis	M0—No distant metastasis
Stage I	T1—Tumor invades submucosa		
	T2—Tumor invades muscularis propria		
Stage II	T3—Tumor invades through muscularis propria into subserosa or into non peritonealized pericolic or perirectal tissues		
	T4—Tumor perforates visceral peritoneum or directly invades other organs or structures		
Stage III	Any T	N1—Metastasis in one to three pericolic or perirectal lymph nodes	
		N2—Metastasis in four or more pericolic or perirectal lymph nodes	
Stage IV	Any T	Any N	M1—Distant metastasis

well-differentiated, mobile polypoid lesion. *Fulguration* or electrocoagulation is used to reduce the size of some large tumors for patients who are poor surgical risks. This procedure requires general anesthesia and may need to be repeated at intervals.

Most patients with colorectal cancer undergo surgical resection of the colon with anastomosis of remaining bowel as a curative procedure. The distribution of regional lymph nodes determines the extent of resection because these may contain metastatic lesions. Most tumors of the ascending, transverse, descending, and sigmoid colon can be resected.

Tumors of the rectum usually are treated with an abdominoperineal resection in which the sigmoid colon, rectum, and anus are removed through both abdominal and perineal incisions. A permanent sigmoid colostomy is performed to provide for elimination of feces. Nursing care of the patient having bowel surgery is outlined in the accompanying box below.

COLOSTOMY Surgical resection of the bowel may be accompanied by a colostomy for diversion of fecal contents. A **colostomy** is an ostomy made in the colon. It may be created if the bowel is obstructed by the tumor, as a temporary measure to promote healing of anastomoses, or as a permanent means of

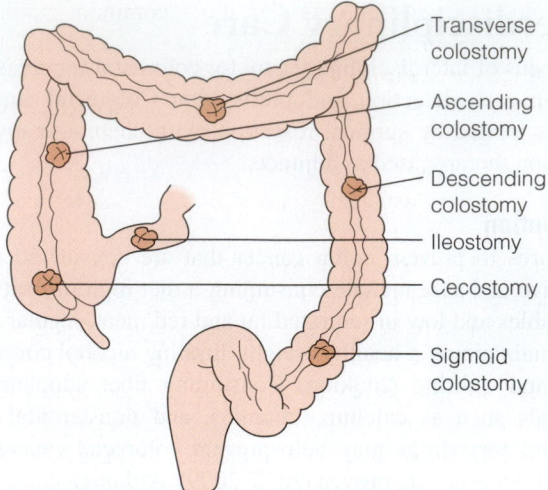

Figure 24–11 ■ Various ostomy levels and sites.

fecal evacuation when the distal colon and rectum are removed. Colostomies take the name of the portion of the colon from which they are formed: ascending colostomy, transverse colostomy, descending colostomy, and sigmoid colostomy (Figure 24–11 ■).

NURSING CARE OF THE PATIENT | **Having Bowel Surgery**

PREOPERATIVE NURSING CARE

- Provide routine preoperative care for the surgical patient as outlined in ∞ Chapter 4.
- Arrange for consultation with ET specialist if appropriate. *The ET nurse is trained to identify and mark an appropriate stoma location, taking into consideration the level of ostomy, skinfolds, and the patient's clothing preferences. Initial ostomy care teaching also is provided by the ET nurse during the preoperative visit.*
- Insert a nasogastric tube if ordered. *Although it is often inserted in the surgical suite just prior to surgery, the nasogastric tube may be placed preoperatively to remove secretions and empty stomach contents.*
- Perform bowel preparation procedures as ordered. *Oral and parenteral antibiotics as well as cathartics and enemas may be prescribed preoperatively to clean the bowel and reduce the risk of peritoneal contamination by bowel contents during surgery.*

POSTOPERATIVE NURSING CARE

- Provide routine care for the surgical patient (∞ Chapter 4).
- Monitor bowel sounds and degree of abdominal distention. *Surgical manipulation of the bowel disrupts peristalsis, resulting in an initial ileus. Bowel sounds and the passage of flatus indicate a return of peristalsis.*
- Assess the position and patency of the nasogastric tube, connecting it to low suction. If the tube becomes clogged, gently irrigate with sterile normal saline. *A nasogastric or gastrostomy tube is used postoperatively to provide gastrointestinal decompression and facilitate healing of the anastomosis. Ensuring its patency is important for comfort and healing.*
- Assess color, amount, and odor of drainage from surgical drains and the colostomy (if present), noting any changes or the presence of clots or bright bleeding. *Initial drainage may be bright red and then become dark and finally clear or*

greenish yellow over the first 2 to 3 days. A change in the color, amount, or odor of the drainage may indicate a complication such as hemorrhage, intestinal obstruction, or infection.

- Alert all personnel caring for the patient with an abdominoperineal resection to avoid rectal temperatures, suppositories, or other rectal procedures. *These procedures could disrupt the anal suture line, causing bleeding, infection, or impaired healing.*
- Maintain intravenous fluids while nasogastric suction is in place. *The patient on nasogastric suction is unable to take oral food and fluids and, moreover, is losing electrolyte-rich fluid through the nasogastric tube. If replacement fluid and electrolytes are not maintained, the patient is at risk for dehydration, sodium, potassium, and chloride imbalance, and metabolic alkalosis.*
- Provide antacids, histamine$_2$ receptor antagonists, and antibiotic therapy as ordered. *These medications may be ordered for the postoperative patient, depending on the procedure performed. Antibiotic therapy is a common measure to prevent infection resulting from contamination of the abdominal cavity with gastric contents.*
- Resume oral food and fluids as ordered. Initial feedings may be clear liquids, progressing to full liquids, and then frequent small feedings of regular foods. Monitor bowel sounds and monitor for abdominal distention frequently during this period. *Oral feedings are reintroduced slowly to minimize abdominal distention and trauma to the suture lines.*
- Begin discharge planning and teaching. Consult with a dietitian for instructions and menu planning; reinforce teaching. Teach about potential postoperative complications such as abdominal abscess, or bowel obstruction, their signs and symptoms, and preventive measures.

A *sigmoid colostomy* is the most common permanent colostomy performed, particularly for cancer of the rectum. It is usually created during an abdominoperineal resection. This procedure involves the removal of the sigmoid colon, rectum, and anus through abdominal and perineal incisions. The anal canal is closed, and a stoma formed from the proximal sigmoid colon. The stoma usually is located on the lower left quadrant of the abdomen.

When a *double-barrel colostomy* is performed, two separate stomas are created (Figure 24–12 ■). The distal colon is not removed, but bypassed. The proximal stoma, which is functional, diverts feces to the abdominal wall. The distal stoma, also called the mucous fistula, expels mucus from the distal colon. It may be pouched or dressed with a 4 × 4 gauge dressing. A double-barrel colostomy may be created for cases of trauma, tumor, or inflammation, and it may be temporary or permanent.

An emergency procedure used to relieve an intestinal obstruction or perforation is called a *transverse loop colostomy*. During this procedure, a loop of the transverse colon is brought out from the abdominal wall and suspended over a plastic rod or bridge, which prevents the loop from slipping back into the abdominal cavity. The loop stoma may be opened at the time of surgery or a few days later at the patient's bedside. The bridge may be removed in 1 to 2 weeks. Transverse loop colostomies are typically temporary.

In a *Hartmann procedure*, a common temporary colostomy procedure, the distal portion of the colon is left in place and is oversewn for closure. A temporary colostomy may be done to allow bowel rest or healing, such as following tumor resection or inflammation of the bowel. It also may be created following traumatic injury to the colon, such as a gunshot wound. Anastomosis of the severed portions of the colon is delayed because bacterial colonization of the colon would prevent proper healing of the anastomosis. About 3 to 6 months following a temporary colostomy, the colostomy is closed and the colon is reconnected. Patients with temporary colostomies require the same care as patients with permanent colostomies. See nursing care for a patient with a colostomy on page 706.

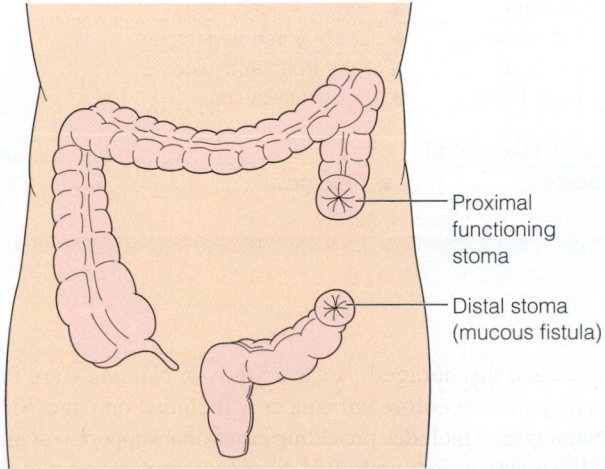

Figure 24–12 ■ A double-barrel colostomy. The proximal stoma is the functioning stoma; the distal stoma expels mucus from the distal colon.

Proximal functioning stoma

Distal stoma (mucous fistula)

Radiation Therapy

Although radiation therapy is not used as a primary treatment for colon cancer, it is used with surgical resection for treating rectal tumors. Small rectal cancers may be treated with intracavitary, external, or implantation radiation. Rectal cancer has a high rate of regional recurrence following complete surgical resection, particularly when the tumor has invaded tissues outside the bowel wall or regional lymph nodes. Pre- or postoperative radiation therapy reduces the recurrence of pelvic tumors, although the effect of radiation therapy on long-term survival is less clear. Radiation therapy is used preoperatively to shrink large rectal tumors enough to permit surgical removal of the tumor.

Chemotherapy

Chemotherapeutic agents, such as intravenous fluorouracil (5-FU) and folinic acid (leucovorin), are also used postoperatively as adjunctive therapy for colorectal cancer. When combined with radiation therapy, chemotherapy reduces the rate of tumor recurrence and prolongs survival for patients with stage II and stage III rectal tumors. The benefit for colon cancers is less clear, but chemotherapy may be used to reduce its spread to the liver and prevent recurrence. Irinotecan (CPT-11) or oxaliplatin may be used in chemotherapy regimens for colorectal cancer. Further discussion about chemotherapy and nursing implications is included in ∞ Chapter 14.

✍ Nursing Care

Health Promotion

Primary prevention of colorectal cancer is a significant nursing care issue. Teach patients the importance of maintaining an optimal weight and staying physically active. Discuss dietary recommendations provided by the ACS for the prevention of colorectal cancer. These recommendations include decreasing the amount of fat, refined sugar, and red meats in the diet while increasing intake of dietary fiber. Foods that contain high amounts of fiber include raw fruits and vegetables, legumes, and whole-grain products.

Stress the importance of regular health examinations, including digital rectal exams. Discuss recommendations for regular hemoccult testing of stool after age 40. Include the importance of seeking medical treatment if blood is noted in or on the stool. Teach patients the warning signs for cancer, including those specific to bowel cancer, such as a change in bowel habits.

Assessment

- *Health history:* Usual bowel patterns and any recent changes; weight loss, fatigue, decreased activity tolerance; presence of blood in the stool; pain with defecation, abdominal discomfort, perineal pain; usual diet; family history of colon cancer, other specific risk factors such as inflammatory bowel disease or colon polyps.
- *Physical examination:* General appearance; weight; abdominal shape, contour; bowel sounds, abdominal tenderness; stool hemoccult or guaiac.

NURSING CARE OF THE PATIENT with a Colostomy

- Assess the location of the stoma and the type of colostomy performed. *Stoma location is an indicator of the section of bowel in which it is located and a predictor of the type of fecal drainage to expect.*
- Assess stoma appearance and surrounding skin condition frequently (see the box on page 687). *Assessment of stoma and skin condition is particularly important in the early postoperative period, when complications are most likely to occur and are most treatable.*
- Position a collection bag or drainable pouch over the stoma. *Initial drainage may contain more mucus and serosanguineous fluid than fecal material. As the bowel starts to resume function, drainage becomes fecal in nature. The consistency of drainage depends on the stoma location in the bowel.*
- If ordered, irrigate the colostomy, instilling water into the colon similar to an enema procedure. *The water stimulates the colon to empty.*
- When a colostomy irrigation is ordered for a patient with a double-barrel or loop colostomy, irrigate the proximal stoma. Digital assessment of the bowel direction from the stoma can assist in determining which is the proximal stoma. *The distal bowel carries no fecal contents and does not need irrigation. It may be irrigated for cleansing just prior to reanastomosis.*
- Empty a drainable pouch or replace the colostomy bag as needed or when it is no more than one-third full. *If the pouch is allowed to overfill, its weight may impair the seal and cause leakage.*
- Provide stomal and skin care for the patient with a colostomy as for the patient with an ileostomy (see the box on page 687). *Good skin and stoma care is important to maintain skin integrity and function as the first line of defense against infection.*
- Use caulking agents, such as Stomahesive or karaya paste, and a skin barrier wafer as needed to maintain a secure ostomy pouch. This may be particularly important for the patient with a loop colostomy. *The main challenge for a patient with a transverse loop colostomy is to maintain a secure ostomy pouch over the plastic bridge.*
- A small needle hole high on the colostomy pouch will allow flatus to escape. This hole may be closed with a Band-Aid and opened only while the patient is in the bathroom for odor control. *Ostomy bags may "balloon" out, disrupting the skin seal, if excess gas collects.*

Health Education for the Patient and Family
- Prior to discharge, provide written, verbal, and psychomotor instruction on colostomy care, pouch management, skin care, and irrigation for the patient. *Whether the colostomy is temporary or permanent, the patient will be responsible for its management. Good understanding of procedures and*

care enhances the ability to provide self-care, as well as self-esteem and control.

- Allow ample time for the patient (and family, if necessary) to practice changing the pouch, either on the patient or a model. *Practice of psychomotor skills improves learning and confidence.*
- If an abdominoperineal resection has been performed, emphasize the importance of using no rectal suppositories, rectal temperatures, or enemas. Suggest that the patient carry medical identification or a Medic-Alert tag or bracelet. *These measures are important to prevent trauma to the tissues when the rectum has been removed.*
- The diet for a patient with a colostomy is individualized and may require no alteration from that consumed preoperatively. Dietary teaching should, however, include information on foods that cause stool odor and gas and foods that thicken and loosen stools. Foods that cause these effects on ostomy output are listed next.

Foods That Increase Stool Odor

■ Asparagus	■ Fish
■ Beans	■ Garlic
■ Cabbage	■ Onions
■ Eggs	■ Some spices

Foods That Increase Intestinal Gas

■ Beer	■ Cucumbers
■ Broccoli	■ Dairy products
■ Brussels sprouts	■ Dried beans
■ Cabbage	■ Peas
■ Carbonated drinks	■ Radishes
■ Cauliflower	■ Spinach
■ Corn	

Foods That Thicken Stools

■ Applesauce	■ Pasta
■ Bananas	■ Pretzels
■ Bread	■ Rice
■ Cheese	■ Tapioca
■ Yogurt	■ Creamy peanut butter

Foods That Loosen Stools

■ Chocolate	■ Highly spiced foods
■ Dried beans	■ Leafy green vegetables
■ Fried foods	■ Raw fruits and juices
■ Greasy foods	■ Raw vegetables

Foods That Color Stools

■ Beets	■ Red gelatin

Nursing Diagnoses and Interventions

In planning and implementing care, consider both physical care needs and emotional response to the diagnosis. Because colorectal cancer is often advanced at the time of diagnosis, the prognosis, even with treatment, may be poor. Denial and anger are common. Extensive abdominal surgery and potentially a colostomy may be necessary, and the effects of chemotherapy and radiation therapy can leave the patient

fatigued and discouraged. A Case Study & Nursing Care Plan for a patient with colorectal cancer is included on page 707.

Nursing care includes providing emotional support, teaching, and direct care before and after diagnostic procedures and surgery and during adjunctive treatments. Priority nursing diagnoses include *Acute Pain, Imbalanced Nutrition,* and *Anticipatory Grieving. Risk for Sexual Dysfunction* should be considered as a priority diagnosis if a colostomy has been created.

- Monitor for adequate pain relief. Use subjective and objective information, including the location, intensity, and character of the pain, as well as nonverbal signs, such as grimacing; muscle tension; apparent dozing; changes in pulse or blood pressure; or rapid, shallow respirations. *The patient may assume that pain is to be expected or tolerated or may fear becoming addicted to analgesic medications. Careful questioning and assessment can provide accurate information about pain status, allowing better control of discomfort.*

- Ask patient to rate pain using a 0 to 10 pain scale. Document the level of pain. *Pain is a subjective experience. Patients perceive and respond to pain differently. Religion and ethnic background may affect the response to pain.*

- Monitor analgesic effectiveness 30 minutes after administration. Monitor for pain relief and adverse effects. *The method*

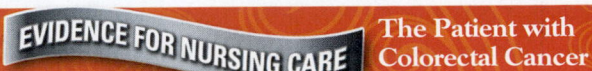

EVIDENCE FOR NURSING CARE — The Patient with Colorectal Cancer

Selected resources that nurses may find helpful when planning evidence-based nursing care follow.

- Daly, J. M., Merchant, M. L., & Levy, B. T. (2009). Colorectal cancer screening. *The American Journal of Nursing, 109*(10), 60–62. doi:10.1097/01.NAJ.0000361496.60341.84
- National Cancer Institute. (2008). *Colon cancer treatment (PDQ®). Health professional version.* Retrieved from www.cancer.gov/cancertopics/pdq/treatment/colon/healthprofessional/

of delivery, dosage, or medication itself may need to be adjusted to provide adequate pain relief.

- Assess the incision for inflammation or swelling; assess drainage catheters and tubes for patency. *Poorly controlled pain or pain that changes may be related to organ distention from an obstructed nasogastric tube, urinary catheter, or wound drain, or may indicate an infection.*

CASE STUDY & NURSING CARE PLAN   A Patient with Colorectal Cancer

William Cunningham is a 65-year-old retired railroad employee, husband, and father of three grown children. For the past 3 months, Mr. Cunningham has noticed small amounts of blood and occasional mucus in his stools. He has a sensation of pressure in the rectum, and notices that his stools are smaller in diameter, about the size of pencil. After palpating a mass on digital examination of the rectum, the physician orders a colonoscopy. A large sessile lesion is found in the rectum and biopsied. The pathology report shows the lesion to be adenocarcinoma. Mr. Cunningham is scheduled for an abdominoperineal resection and sigmoid colostomy.

ASSESSMENT

Madonna Hart, RN, completes the admission assessment. Mr. Cunningham states that his bowel habits have recently changed, but denies pain or other symptoms. Physical assessment findings include T 98.4°F (36.9°C), P 82, R 18, and BP 118/78. He is 70 inches (178 cm) tall and weighs 185 lb (84 kg). Laboratory findings are normal except for the previous pathology report of adenocarcinoma of rectal lesion.

Mr. Cunningham states, "I really don't want a colostomy, but if that is what it takes to get rid of this, I'm ready to get it over with."

DIAGNOSES

- *Acute Pain* related to surgical intervention
- *Risk for Impaired Skin Integrity (Peristomal)* related to fecal drainage and pouch adhesive
- *Risk for Constipation/Diarrhea* related to effects of surgery on bowel function
- *Disturbed Body Image* related to colostomy
- *Risk for Sexual Dysfunction* related to wide rectal incision, radiation therapy, and colostomy

EXPECTED OUTCOMES

- Report pain within an acceptable range that allows ease of movement and ambulation.

- Perform colostomy care using correct technique.
- Demonstrate willingness to discuss changes in sexual function.
- Wear clothing to enhance physical and emotional self-esteem.

PLANNING AND IMPLEMENTATION

- Provide analgesia as ordered, evaluating its effectiveness.
- Discuss foods that cause odor and gas.
- Teach colostomy care.
- Maintain consistent nursing personnel assignment to facilitate trust.
- Refer to the local United Ostomy Association.
- Provide a list of local medical supply companies for ostomy supplies.
- Provide for privacy when teaching and discussing concerns about ostomy.

EVALUATION

On discharge, Mr. Cunningham is able to empty and rinse out his colostomy pouch. He is changing the pouch and caring for surrounding skin appropriately. Ms. Hart has given him verbal and written instructions on colostomy care. He verbalizes understanding of phantom rectal pain, and the importance of avoiding rectal suppositories. He expresses an understanding of the need to avoid heavy lifting, and the importance of follow-up care. Ms. Hart has referred Mr. Cunningham to a home health agency in his community for further questions and follow-up care.

CRITICAL THINKING IN THE NURSING PROCESS

1. What is the cause of phantom rectal pain?
2. Why is it important to discuss dietary concerns with a patient with a colostomy, especially odor- and gas-forming foods?
3. Outline a plan to teach Mr. Cunningham how to irrigate a colostomy.
4. Develop a care plan for Mr. Cunningham for the nursing diagnosis *Disturbed Body Image.*

See Evaluating Your Response in Appendix C.

- Assess the abdomen for distention, tenderness, and bowel sounds. *Intra-abdominal bleeding, peritonitis, or paralytic ileus can cause pain that may be confused with incisional pain.*
- Administer analgesia prior to an activity or procedure. *Adequate pain relief reduces muscle tension, allowing for more comfortable participation in activities.*
- Assist with adjunctive comfort measures, such as positioning, diversional activities, management of environmental stimuli, guided imagery, and teaching relaxation techniques. *These measures enhance the effects of analgesia by reducing muscle tension.*
- Splint incision with a pillow, and teach the patient how to self-splint when coughing and deep breathing *to prevent respiratory complications related to fear of pain.*

Imbalanced Nutrition: Less than Body Requirements

Bowel preparation for diagnostic procedures, surgery, radiation therapy, and chemotherapy place the patient with colorectal cancer at risk for nutritional deficiencies. Fluid and electrolyte replacement is provided following surgery, along with possible PN (∞ see Chapter 22). Adequate kilocalorie and nutrient intake are necessary for healing after surgery. Additionally, if the tumor is advanced, metabolic needs may be increased and the appetite decreased.

- Assess nutritional status, using data such as height and weight, skinfold measurements, body mass index (BMI) calculation (∞ see Chapter 21), and laboratory data including serum albumin level. Refer to dietitian or nutritionist for dietary management. *The patient who is malnourished before beginning aggressive cancer treatment requires more vigorous nutrition management to promote healing.*
- Assess readiness for resumption of oral intake after surgery or procedures using data such as statements of hunger, presence of bowel sounds, passage of flatus, and minimal abdominal distention. *Manipulation of the bowel interrupts peristalsis of the GI tract. It is important to ensure that peristalsis has resumed prior to resumption of oral intake.*
- Monitor and document food and fluid intake. *Documentation helps identify the adequacy of kilocalories and other nutrient intake.*
- Weigh daily. *Weight fluctuation may indicate adequate or inadequate dietary intake.*
- Maintain PN and central intravenous lines as ordered. *Parenteral nutrition prevents tissue catabolism and promotes healing when food intake is disrupted for more than 2 to 3 days.*
- When oral intake resumes, help the patient develop a meal plan that incorporates food preferences and considers the patient's schedule and environment. *Consideration of likes, dislikes, and circumstances in meal planning promotes adequate intake.*

Grieving

When a bowel resection is performed for colorectal cancer, the patient needs to adjust to the loss of a major body part as well as to the diagnosis of cancer. Even when the prognosis for recovery is good, many people perceive cancer as fatal. Supporting the patient and family during the initial stages of grieving can improve physical recovery as well as psychologic coping and eventual adaptation.

- Work to develop a trusting relationship with the patient and family. *This increases the nurse's effectiveness in helping them work through the grieving process.*
- Listen actively, encouraging the patient and family to express their fears and concerns. Assist to identify strengths, past experiences, and support systems:
  - Demonstrate respect for cultural, spiritual, and religious values and beliefs; encourage use of these resources to cope with losses.
  - Encourage discussion of the potential impact of loss on individual family members, family structure, and family function. Assist family members to share concerns with one another.
  - Refer to cancer support groups, social services, or counseling as appropriate.

  These resources can be used throughout the grieving process.

Risk for Sexual Dysfunction

Colorectal cancer and ostomy surgery increase the risk for sexual dysfunction, defined as a change in sexual function so that it becomes unsatisfying, unrewarding, or inadequate (NANDA, 2009). Physical factors that can lead to sexual dysfunction include disruption of nerves and blood vessels that supply the genitals, radiation therapy, chemotherapy, and other medications prescribed after surgery.

Psychologically, an *ostomate* (patient with an ostomy) experiences an altered body image and may develop low self-esteem. The patient may feel undesirable and fear rejection. He or she may be concerned about odors or pouch leakage during sexual activity. This emotional stress can contribute to sexual dysfunction.

- Provide opportunities for the patient and family to express feelings about the cancer diagnosis, ostomy, and effects of other treatments. *Encouraging verbalization of feelings about the diagnosis, ostomy, and treatments provides an opportunity to validate that feelings of anger and depression are normal responses to the diagnosis and change in body function.*
- Provide consistent colostomy care. *An accepting attitude and consistent care that provides a secure appliance and controls odor and leakage instill a sense of confidence in the patient.*
- Encourage expression of sexual concerns. Provide privacy and caregivers who have established trust with the patient and family and are comfortable with discussions about sexual concerns. *Sexuality is a very private concern to most people. The patient and family are not likely to express their concerns openly unless trust has been established.*
- Reassure the patient and significant other that the effect of physical illness and prescribed interventions on sexuality usually is temporary. *The patient and partner may misinterpret an initial decrease in libido as evidence that sexual activity will not be possible or resume following recovery.*
- Refer the patient and partner to social services or a family counselor for further interventions. *Patients are often discharged from acute care settings well before concerns about sexual activity surface. Ongoing counseling provides a continuing resource.*

■ Arrange for a visit from a member of the United Ostomy Association. *People who are living and coping with an ostomy can provide information and support, helping the new ostomate overcome feelings of isolation and rejection.*

Using NANDA, NIC, and NOC

Linkages between a selected NANDA nursing diagnosis, NIC, and NOC for the patient with colorectal cancer are shown in the chart that follows.

Community-Based Care

During the diagnostic and preoperative periods, provide instruction about the following topics:

■ Tests to be performed and preparatory procedures, including dietary restrictions, laxatives, enemas, and food and fluid restrictions just prior to the procedure
■ Recommended postprocedure care and potential adverse effects to report
■ Preoperative care, such as intestinal preparation and food and fluid restrictions

If a colostomy is planned, refer to an enterostomal therapist for stoma placement and initial teaching.

Once treatment has been initiated, include the following topics (as appropriate) in teaching for home care:

■ Pain management
■ Skin care and management of potential adverse effects of radiation therapy and/or chemotherapy (∞ Refer to

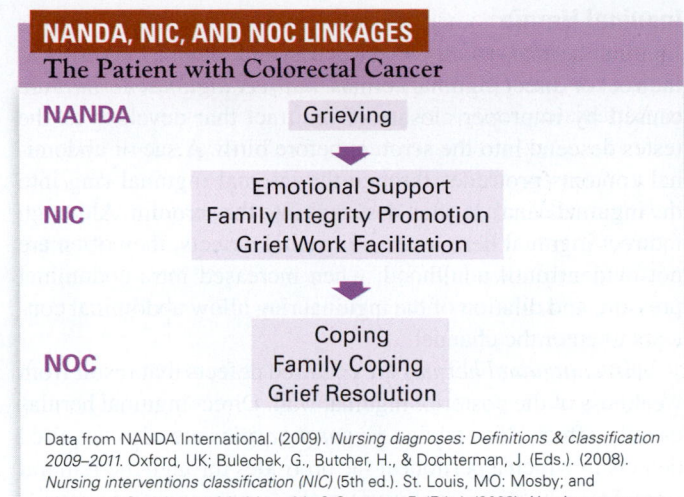

NANDA, NIC, AND NOC LINKAGES
The Patient with Colorectal Cancer

NANDA — Grieving

NIC — Emotional Support / Family Integrity Promotion / Grief Work Facilitation

NOC — Coping / Family Coping / Grief Resolution

Data from NANDA International. (2009). *Nursing diagnoses: Definitions & classification 2009–2011.* Oxford, UK; Bulechek, G., Butcher, H., & Dochterman, J. (Eds.). (2008). *Nursing interventions classification (NIC)* (5th ed.). St. Louis, MO: Mosby; and Moorhead, S., Johnson, M., Maas, M., & Swanson, E. (Eds.). (2008). *Nursing outcomes classification (NOC)* (4th ed.). St. Louis, MO: Mosby.

Chapter 14 for further discussion of teaching needs related to these therapies.)
■ Incision and ostomy care
■ Recommended diet
■ Follow-up appointments and care

If the tumor is inoperable or a cure is not anticipated, provide information about pain and symptom management. Discuss the hospice philosophy and available services. Provide a referral to a local hospice or home health department.

Structural and Obstructive Bowel Disorders

Any portion of the intestines may be affected by a structural or obstructive disorder. Defects in the abdominal wall may allow intra-abdominal contents (such as loops of bowel) to protrude, indirectly affecting bowel function. Likewise, obstructions may result from disease of the bowel itself or from obstruction of the bowel lumen by an external force.

The Patient with a Hernia

A *hernia* is a defect in the abdominal wall that allows abdominal contents to protrude out of the abdominal cavity. Trauma, surgery, and increased intra-abdominal pressure caused by such conditions as pregnancy, obesity, weight lifting, or tumors are risk factors for hernia formation.

Pathophysiology

Hernias are classified by location (Figure 24–13 ■), and may be congenital or acquired. Most hernias occur in the groin (inguinal or femoral hernias). Inguinal hernias often are congenital, caused by improper closure of the tract that develops as the testes descend into the scrotum during fetal development. Groin hernias may be acquired, resulting from weakness of fascia in a region called Hesselbach's area or from dilation of the femoral ring (e.g., during pregnancy and childbirth). Ventral or incisional hernias of the abdominal wall generally are acquired, caused by weakening of normal abdominal wall musculature. Umbilical hernias also are congenital, and usually are

detected in infancy. Hiatal hernias develop in the diaphragm (∞ see Chapter 23).

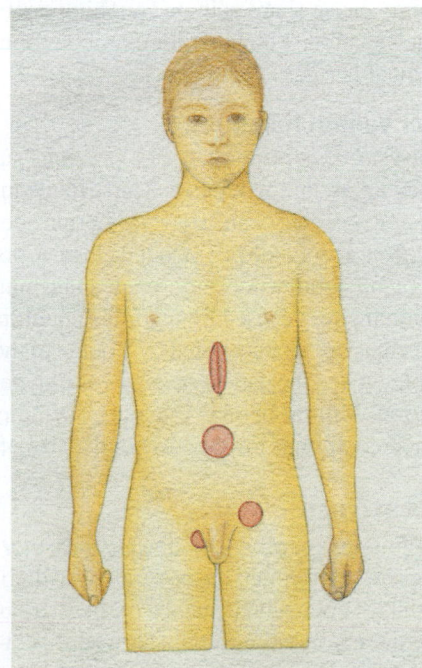

Figure 24–13 ■ An abdominal wall (ventral or incisional) hernia and an inguinal hernia.

Inguinal Hernia

Inguinal hernias usually affect males, and may be classified as indirect or direct inguinal hernias. *Indirect inguinal hernias* are caused by improper closure of the tract that develops as the testes descend into the scrotum before birth. A sac of abdominal contents protrudes through the internal inguinal ring into the inguinal canal. It often descends into the scrotum. Although indirect inguinal hernias are congenital defects, they often are not evident until adulthood, when increased intra-abdominal pressure and dilation of the inguinal ring allow abdominal contents to enter the channel.

Direct inguinal hernias are acquired defects that result from weakness of the posterior inguinal wall. Direct inguinal hernias usually affect older adults. *Femoral hernias* are also acquired defects in which a peritoneal sac protrudes through the femoral ring. These hernias usually affect obese or pregnant women.

Inguinal hernias may produce no symptoms and are discovered during routine physical examination. They may cause a lump, swelling, or bulge in the groin, particularly with lifting or straining. An inguinal hernia may cause sharp pain or a dull ache that radiates into the scrotum. A palpable mass may be present in the groin, although it may be felt only with increased intra-abdominal pressure (as occurs during coughing) and invagination of the scrotum toward the inguinal ring.

Umbilical Hernia

Pregnancy and obesity contribute to the development of umbilical hernias in adults. *Umbilical hernias* may be congenital and evident during infancy, or acquired as the tissue closing the umbilical ring weakens, allowing protrusion of abdominal contents. These hernias are more common in women. Other predisposing factors include multiple pregnancies with prolonged labor, ascites, and large intra-abdominal tumors.

Umbilical hernias tend to enlarge steadily and contain omentum, although they may also contain small or large bowel. The hernia may cause sharp pain on coughing or straining or a dull, aching sensation. Strangulation is a common complication of umbilical hernias.

Incisional or Ventral Hernia

Incisional or *ventral hernias* occur at a previous surgical incision or following abdominal muscle tears. Inadequate healing of the incision or tear can lead to hernia development. Contributing factors include poor wound closure, postoperative infection, age or debility, obesity, inadequate nutrition, and excess incisional stress caused by vigorous coughing.

Ventral hernias are characterized by a bulge at the incisional site, often noted when the patient pulls to a sitting position from a lying position. Ventral hernias often are asymptomatic, and the risk of incarceration is low because of the size of the defect.

Manifestations

Abdominal contents (peritoneum, bowel, and other abdominal organs) can protrude through the abdominal wall to form a sac covered by skin and subcutaneous tissues. In most cases, abdominal contents move into the sac when intra-abdominal pressure increases, then return to the abdominal cavity when pressure returns to normal or when manual pressure is placed on the bulging sac. This is known as a *reducible hernia*.

Complications

The risk for complications is low with a reducible hernia. If the contents of a hernia cannot be returned to the abdominal cavity, it is said to be *incarcerated*. Contents of an incarcerated hernia are trapped, usually by a narrow neck or opening to the hernia. Incarceration increases the risk of complications, including obstruction and strangulation. Obstruction occurs when the lumen of the bowel contained within the hernia becomes occluded, much like the crimping of a hose. A *strangulated hernia* develops when blood supply to bowel and other tissues in the hernia sac is compromised, leading to necrosis. The affected bowel can infarct, leading to perforation with contamination of the peritoneal cavity. Manifestations of a strangulated hernia include severe abdominal pain and distention, nausea, vomiting, tachycardia, and fever.

Interdisciplinary Care

The diagnosis of a hernia is made by a physical examination. The patient is examined in a supine or standing position. A bulge may be seen or felt when the patient coughs or bears down. No laboratory or diagnostic testing is usually required, unless bowel obstruction or strangulation is suspected.

Surgical repair, or *herniorrhaphy*, is the usual treatment of hernia. Surgery is generally well tolerated by people of all ages and carries a much lower risk than the complications of incarceration, obstruction, and strangulation. Emergency surgery is indicated for a hernia that is incarcerated, painful, or tender. In a herniorrhaphy, the abdominal wall defect is closed by suturing or with wire or mesh over the defect. If incarceration has occurred or strangulation is suspected, the abdomen is explored at the time of surgery and any infarcted bowel resected. Heavy lifting and heavy manual labor are restricted for approximately 3 weeks after surgery.

When surgery is contraindicated, the patient may be taught to reduce the hernia by lying down and gently pushing against the mass. A binder or truss may be worn to prevent or control the protrusion. An incarcerated hernia should not be reduced by the patient.

∽ Nursing Care

Assessment

- *Health history:* Manifestations of hernia, such as bulging in the groin or of the abdominal wall when coughing, straining, or moving from lying to standing; pain (abdominal, groin, or scrotal); history of hernia or abdominal surgery.
- *Physical examination:* Observe for bulging of the abdominal wall or around the umbilicus when raising head and shoulders from supine position; wearing gloves, palpate inguinal region for bulges when the patient coughs or bears down (Valsalva maneuver) while standing.

Nursing Diagnoses and Interventions

Herniorrhaphy is generally an uncomplicated procedure, usually performed as same-day surgery. Preoperative assessment and teaching and immediate postoperative care are the primary nursing care needs. Care is similar to that provided for a patient with an appendectomy.

Risk for Ineffective Gastrointestinal Perfusion

When providing care for a patient with a known hernia, the possibility of obstruction and strangulation must be considered throughout nursing assessments. Although nursing interventions may not be able to prevent these complications, rapid identification of the problem allows timely surgical treatment. Prompt treatment may prevent major complications related to infection and peritoneal contamination by bowel contents.

- Assess bowel sounds and abdominal distention at least every 8 hours. *A change in bowel sounds—either cessation of sounds or an onset of hyperactive, high-pitched sounds—may indicate obstruction. With obstruction, abdominal girth may increase.*

> **PRACTICE ALERT**
> Promptly report any acute increase in abdominal, groin, perineal, or scrotal pain. An abrupt increase in the intensity of pain may indicate bowel ischemia due to strangulation.

- Notify primary care provider if the hernia becomes painful or tender. *Pain and tenderness may indicate incarceration and increased risk for strangulation.*
- If signs of possible obstruction or strangulation occur, notify the physician. Place patient in supine position with the hips elevated and knees slightly bent. Withhold all food and fluids (NPO), and begin preparations for surgery. *This position helps relax abdominal muscles and may facilitate reduction of the hernia. Strangulation or obstruction require immediate surgical intervention.*

Community-Based Care

Include the following topics when teaching patients about hernias and home care:

- Rationale for examining the groin and abdomen for bulges
- The nature of hernias, risk factors, and manifestations
- Surgical intervention for hernias
- How to reduce a hernia if necessary
- The importance of seeking immediate medical intervention for signs of strangulation or obstruction
- The need to notify the physician if upper respiratory infection and cough develop preoperatively (forceful coughing is not recommended postoperatively)
- Postoperative pain management and activity restrictions

The Patient with Intestinal Obstruction

Intestinal obstruction is failure of intestinal contents to move through the bowel lumen. Intestinal obstructions may affect either the large or small bowel. The small intestine is more commonly affected; however, bowel obstructions may also occur in the large intestine. Obstruction is the most common reason for small-bowel surgery.

Pathophysiology

Intestinal obstructions may be either mechanical or functional in nature. *Mechanical* obstructions may be caused by (1) problems outside the intestine, such as bands of scar tissue (adhesions) or hernias; (2) problems within the intestine, such as tumors or inflammatory bowel disease; or (3) obstruction of the intestinal lumen. The obstruction may be partial or complete. In some mechanical obstructions, such as a strangulated hernia, blood supply to the affected portion of bowel also is impaired, resulting in necrosis of the affected segment. *Functional* obstruction occurs when peristalsis fails to propel intestinal contents although there is no mechanical obstruction. *Adynamic ileus* (also known as *paralytic ileus* or simply *ileus*) is the most common functional obstruction after abdominal surgery. Obstructions are further classified by the portion of intestine affected.

When the intestine is obstructed, gas and fluid accumulate proximal to and within the obstructed segment, distending the bowel. Swallowed air accounts for most of the gas. Ingested fluid, saliva, gastric juice, and pancreatic secretions contribute to accumulated fluid. Water and sodium are drawn into the bowel lumen, contributing to fluid accumulation, distention, and vascular fluid losses. Distention of the bowel lumen interferes with peristaltic movement, leading to atony and further distention. Significant distention of the bowel lumen compromises blood flow to mucosa, eventually leading to necrosis. Gangrenous bowel may perforate with resulting peritonitis. Rapid bacterial growth in the obstructed bowel can lead to sepsis and death.

Significant bowel distention, vomiting, and third spacing of fluids in the bowel and peritoneal cavity can lead to massive loss of fluids and electrolytes with resulting hypovolemia, hypokalemia, renal insufficiency, and shock.

Small-Bowel Obstruction

Adhesions, or bands of scar tissue, and hernias account for most mechanical small bowel obstructions. In adults, adhesions develop following abdominal surgery or inflammatory processes. Adhesions usually produce a *simple obstruction*, or single blockage in one portion of the intestine (Figure 24–14A ■). The obstruction produced by an incarcerated hernia is a *closed-loop obstruction*, with two different portions of the bowel lumen obstructed (Figure 24–14B).

Tumors, either intrinsic (of the bowel itself) or extrinsic (of another organ but affecting the bowel because of their size), can progressively occlude the bowel lumen and eventually obstruct it (Figure 24–14C). Other, less common causes of bowel obstruction include intussusception (rare in adults) (Figure 24–14D); volvulus, which is the rotation of loops of bowel about a fixed point (Figure 24–14E); foreign bodies; stricture; and inflammatory bowel disease.

Both volvulus and an incarcerated hernia can cause a *strangulated obstruction*. In a strangulated obstruction, not only is the lumen of the bowel obstructed, but the blood supply to the affected portion is also compromised.

In a functional obstruction or adynamic ileus, peristalsis stops due to either neurogenic or muscular impairment. The bowel lumen remains patent, but contents are not propelled forward.

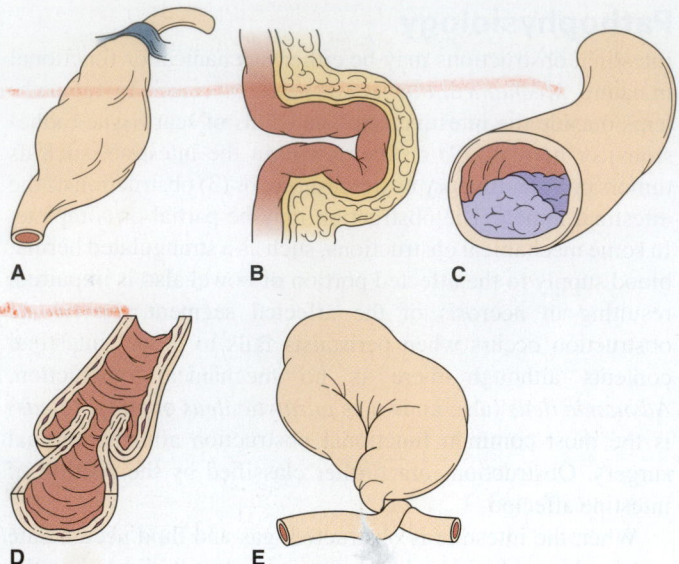

Figure 24–14 ■ Selected causes of mechanical obstruction. *A,* adhesions; *B,* incarcerated hernia; *C,* tumor; *D,* intussusception; and *E,* volvulus.

Temporary ileus commonly follows gastrointestinal surgery. It may result from tissue anoxia or peritoneal irritation due to hemorrhage, peritonitis, or perforation of an organ. Other conditions that can precipitate paralytic ileus include renal colic, spinal cord injuries, uremia, and electrolyte imbalances, hypokalemia in particular. In addition, the effects of some narcotics, anticholinergic drugs, and antidiarrheal medications such as diphenoxylate can produce a functional obstruction.

MANIFESTATIONS   The manifestations of a small-bowel obstruction vary, depending on the type and level of obstruction and how rapidly it develops. Cramping or colicky abdominal pain that may be intermittent or increasing in intensity is

common. Vomiting is common, particularly in high or proximal obstructions, because distention of the lumen stimulates the vomiting center. In a high obstruction, vomitus contains bile and mucus. As bacterial fermentation occurs, vomitus often contains fecal matter, particularly with a low or distal obstruction. Flatus and feces already present in the lower bowel may be expelled early in the obstructive process, but this expulsion ceases as the obstruction continues.

Early in the course of a mechanical obstruction, borborygmi and high-pitched tinkling bowel sounds often are present. Borborygmi may coincide with waves of colicky abdominal pain as the intestine attempts to propel contents past the obstruction. Visible peristaltic waves may be noted in the distended loops of bowel in thin patients. In the later stages, the bowel becomes silent. With a paralytic ileus, bowel sounds are greatly diminished or absent throughout the process. Abdominal distention is minimal with proximal obstructions, but may be pronounced with distal obstruction and paralytic ileus. The abdomen may be tender to palpation as well.

In addition to abdominal and gastrointestinal manifestations, signs of fluid and electrolyte imbalance develop. Hypovolemia can develop rapidly as extracellular fluid is sequestered in the bowel and vomiting occurs. Although early vital signs may be normal, changes are noted as dehydration and hypovolemia develop. The patient becomes tachycardic and tachypneic, and blood pressure falls. Temperature may be elevated. Urine output drops, and signs of hypovolemic shock may be seen. The manifestations of mechanical small bowel obstruction are outlined with their accompanying pathophysiologic processes in the Pathophysiology Linkage box that follows.

COMPLICATIONS   Hypovolemia and hypovolemic shock with multiple organ dysfunction is a significant complication of bowel obstruction and can lead to death. Renal insufficiency from hypovolemia can lead to acute renal failure. Pulmonary

PATHOPHYSIOLOGY LINKAGE   Small Bowel Obstruction

MANIFESTATION	PATHOPHYSIOLOGY
Abdominal pain: intermittent midabdominal, colicky; intensity may initially decrease, then become severe and steady	Peristaltic waves attempt to propel bowel contents past the obstruction. As the bowel becomes increasingly distended, peristalsis is inhibited and pain may decrease in intensity. If unrelieved, distention of bowel lumen impairs mucosal blood supply, leading to ischemia and necrosis. Bowel infarction or perforation may occur, leading to chemical and bacterial peritonitis.
Bowel sounds: initially loud, possibly high-pitched; may correspond with waves of abdominal pain; later infrequent or absent	Initial distention of the bowel proximal to the obstruction stimulates peristalsis as the bowel attempts to propel contents past the obstruction. With further distention and resulting electrolyte imbalances, peristalsis is inhibited and bowel sounds become less frequent to inaudible.
Vomiting	Distention of the bowel stimulates the vomiting center of the brain, which, in turn, stimulates the vomiting reflex.
Abdominal distention	Fluid (saliva, gastric juice, bile, pancreatic secretions) and air are trapped in the bowel proximal to the obstruction.
Hypovolemia, electrolyte imbalance	Normal movement of water and sodium from the bowel lumen to the interstitial and intravascular spaces is initially inhibited. Fluids and electrolytes are lost through vomiting. With continued obstruction and bowel distention, sodium and water move from the vascular system into the bowel lumen, further distending it. Intestinal venous return is inhibited, leading to tissue edema and accumulation of fluid and electrolytes within the peritoneal cavity.

ventilation may be impaired because abdominal distention elevates the diaphragm and interferes with respiratory processes.

Strangulation associated with incarcerated hernia or volvulus impairs the blood supply to the bowel. Gangrene may rapidly result, causing bleeding into the bowel lumen and peritoneal cavity and eventual perforation. With perforation, bacteria and toxins from the strangulated intestine enter the peritoneum and, potentially, the circulation, resulting in peritonitis and possible septic shock. Strangulation greatly increases the risk of mortality.

Large-Bowel Obstruction

Obstruction of the large intestine occurs much less frequently than small-bowel obstruction. Although any portion of the colon may be affected, obstruction usually occurs in the sigmoid segment. Cancer of the bowel is the most common cause; other causes include volvulus, diverticular disease, inflammatory disorders, and fecal impaction.

MANIFESTATIONS Constipation and colicky abdominal pain are usual manifestations of large-bowel obstruction. The pain is often deep and cramping; severe, continuous pain may signal bowel ischemia and possible perforation. Vomiting is a late sign, if it occurs at all. The abdomen is distended, with high-pitched, tinkling bowel sounds with rushes and gurgles. On palpation, localized tenderness or a mass may be noted.

COMPLICATIONS If the ileocecal valve between the small and large intestines is competent, distention proximal to the obstruction is limited to the colon itself. This is known as a *closed-loop obstruction*. It can lead to massive colon dilation as the ileum continues to empty gas and fluid into the colon. Increasing pressure within the obstructed colon impairs circulation to the bowel wall. Gangrene, perforation and peritonitis are potential complications. Massive distention can impair function of the diaphragm, leading to atelectasis. Pressure on the inferior vena cava may impair venous return.

Interdisciplinary Care

The management of a bowel obstruction focuses on relieving the pressure and obstruction, and providing supportive care. The intestine is decompressed, and fluid and electrolyte balance is restored. Surgery may be necessary to relieve a mechanical obstruction or if strangulation is suspected.

Diagnosis

Radiologic studies (x-rays and CT scan) are used to confirm the diagnosis of bowel obstruction. Laboratory testing is used to evaluate for the presence of infection and fluid and electrolyte imbalances.

An abdominal x-ray often shows distended loops of intestine with fluid and gas in a small-bowel obstruction. Free air under the diaphragm indicates a perforation. X-ray or CT scan with contrast media may be required to confirm a mechanical obstruction and assess the completeness of the obstruction. Gastrografin is often used to provide contrast rather than barium when a bowel obstruction is suspected.

Laboratory tests used are WBC, serum amylase, serum osmolality, electrolytes, and arterial blood gases. These tests will show the following results with a bowel obstruction:

- *WBC* often shows mild leukocytosis due to an inflammatory response to changes within the obstructed bowel lumen. With strangulation, leukocytosis is marked.
- *Serum amylase levels* may be elevated, particularly when strangulation is present.
- *Serum osmolality* and *electrolyte levels* are affected by fluid and electrolyte losses from vomiting and fluid sequestering in the bowel lumen. With hypovolemia, the serum osmolality and urine specific gravity increase. Potassium and chloride are lost through vomiting, leading to hypokalemia and hypochloremia.
- ABGs may reveal metabolic alkalosis (pH > 7.45, bicarbonate > 24 mEq/L, PCO_2 > 45 mmHg) with small-bowel obstruction due to loss of hydrochloric acid from the stomach.

Gastrointestinal Decompression

Most partial small-bowel obstructions are successfully treated with gastrointestinal decompression using a nasogastric tube. Functional obstructions respond to treatment with bowel rest and intestinal decompression as well. Current evidence indicates that a standard nasogastric tube is as effective for gastrointestinal decompression as a longer intestinal tube. Collected fluid and gas are removed using low suction until peristalsis resumes or the obstruction is relieved.

Surgery

Surgical intervention is required for complete mechanical obstructions as well as for strangulated or incarcerated obstructions of the small intestine. Patients with incomplete mechanical obstruction may also require surgery if the obstruction persists.

Prior to surgery, a nasogastric tube is inserted to relieve vomiting and abdominal distention and to prevent aspiration of intestinal contents. Fluid and electrolyte balance must be restored before surgery. Isotonic intravenous fluids, such as normal (physiologic) saline, Ringer's solution, or other balanced electrolyte solutions, are used. Additional electrolytes may be added to the solution to correct low levels. It is particularly important to correct hypokalemia prior to surgery. Acid–base imbalances are also addressed, often using intravenous acidifiers or alkalinizing agents. If strangulation has occurred, the patient may require plasma or blood replacement. Intravenous broad-spectrum antibiotics are administered prophylactically (see the section on peritonitis).

Simple mechanical obstruction due to adhesions may be relieved using laparoscopic surgery to remove or lyse the scar tissue. A laparotomy may be performed to allow inspection of the small intestine and removal of infarcted or gangrenous tissue. Obstructing tumors are resected, and foreign bodies are removed. Any bowel that appears to be gangrenous is resected, usually followed by an end-to-end anastomosis of remaining intestine. If a large tumor mass or dense adhesions are found, the area of obstruction may be bypassed by anastomosis of proximal small bowel to small or large intestine distal to the obstruction. Nursing care of the patient having bowel surgery is included in the box on page 704.

Obstructions of the large intestine usually necessitate surgery. The primary goal is to relieve colonic distention and prevent perforation; the secondary goal is to remove the obstructing lesion. In some cases, colonoscopy may be used to relieve the distention. If the patient's condition prohibits major surgery or the obstructing tumor is advanced, laser photocoagulation may be used to enlarge the bowel lumen and a stent inserted to reduce the risk of reobstruction. Removal of the obstructing lesion is the preferred treatment. The proximal and distal bowel segments may be anastomosed, or a permanent colostomy or ileostomy may be required.

Nursing Care

Health Promotion

Teach health promotion activities, such as increasing dietary fiber intake, maintaining a generous fluid intake, and exercising daily to help prevent constipation and possible large-bowel obstruction, particularly in the older adult. Stress the importance of complying with dietary restrictions (such as avoiding popcorn) for patients who experience repeated small-bowel obstructions.

Assessment

Nurses may be instrumental in the early identification of intestinal obstructions in older adults, the homebound patient, or the institutionalized patient. Early identification and intervention significantly reduce morbidity from bowel obstruction.

- *Health history:* Complaints of abdominal pain and bloating, constipation; previous history of bowel obstruction or risk factors such as hernia, inflammatory bowel disease, diverticulosis, or previous abdominal surgery; current medications.
- *Physical examination:* Vital signs including orthostatic blood pressure, temperature; skin color, temperature, texture, and turgor; color and moisture of mucous membranes; abdominal shape, contour, bowel sounds, presence of tenderness or masses on palpation.

Nursing Diagnoses and Interventions

In patients with a suspected or confirmed bowel obstruction, frequent assessment for complications such as fluid and electrolyte imbalance, acid–base imbalances, hypovolemic shock, perforation, and peritonitis is necessary.

Deficient Fluid Volume

Because of the large collection of fluid in the bowel proximal to an obstruction, the accompanying vomiting, and nasogastric suction, the patient with an intestinal obstruction often has a fluid volume deficit. If not corrected promptly, hypovolemic shock, acute renal failure, and multiple organ system dysfunction from poor tissue perfusion may result.

- Monitor vital signs, pulmonary artery pressures, cardiac output (CO), and central venous pressure (CVP) hourly. *A decrease in blood pressure, tachycardia, and tachypnea may indicate hypovolemia. Although invasive, hemodynamic parameters such as pulmonary artery pressures, CO, and CVP allow accurate assessment of fluid volume status.*

- Measure urinary output hourly and nasogastric drainage every 2 to 4 hours. *A urinary output of 30 mL per hour or more usually indicates an adequate glomerular filtration rate (GFR), another indicator of fluid volume. Nasogastric output provides a tool for evaluating fluid replacement needs.*

> **PRACTICE ALERT**
> Promptly report urine output of less than 30 mL per hour. This often indicates hypovolemia and an increased risk for shock and acute renal failure.

- Maintain intravenous fluids and blood volume expanders as ordered. The amount of fluid administered is calculated to meet ongoing fluid needs and replace previous and current losses. *Restoration and maintenance of blood volume are necessary to maintain cardiac output and tissue and organ perfusion.*
- Measure abdominal girth every 4 to 8 hours. Mark the level of measurement on the abdomen. *A reference mark allows consistent, accurate measurements. An increase in abdominal girth indicates increasing intestinal distention.*
- Notify the physician of changes in status. *Changes in vital signs, pain, and signs of increasing distention can indicate the need for immediate surgical intervention.*

Ineffective Gastrointestinal Perfusion

Perfusion of the intestinal wall and mucosa may be impaired by the obstructive process itself (e.g., strangulation or volvulus) or by significant intestinal distention. The goal is to maintain tissue perfusion and promote normal peristalsis and bowel elimination.

- Monitor vital signs hourly. Assess peripheral pulses, skin color, temperature, and capillary refill. *Cardiovascular assessment is vital to detect early signs of hypovolemic shock resulting from sequestering large volumes of fluid in the intestines. Hypovolemia and shock can convert mild bowel ischemia to infarction as the blood supply to the tissue falls.*
- Monitor urine output hourly. Report output of less than 30 mL per hour. *Urine output is a good indicator of the GFR and tissue perfusion. The urine output often falls before vital sign changes are apparent in hypovolemia.*
- Monitor temperature at least every 4 hours. *An elevated temperature may be an early indication of sepsis from bowel perforation as a result of gangrene.*
- Frequently assess pain. *A change in the character of pain or a rapid increase in its intensity may signal bowel infarction or perforation.*
- Maintain NPO status until peristalsis resumes. *Enteral food or fluids may increase distention and bowel ischemia. They also are restricted until the possibility of perforation is eliminated.*

Ineffective Breathing Pattern

Significant abdominal distention from a bowel obstruction can cause the diaphragm to flatten, impairing pulmonary ventilation. Following surgery, splinting of abdominal muscles to avoid pain can lead to shallow respirations. These factors, plus the risk of aspiration of gastrointestinal contents during vomiting, place the patient at high risk for respiratory complications, particularly with a small-bowel obstruction.

- Assess respiratory rate, pattern, and lung sounds at least every 2 to 4 hours. *Tachypnea, shortness of breath, or apparent dyspnea may be early signs of respiratory compromise. Diminished breath sounds, particularly in the bases of the lungs, or crackles indicate poor lung expansion and possible impaired ventilation.*
- Monitor ABG results for possible effects of altered respiratory status. *Tachypnea may lead to respiratory alkalosis as excess carbon dioxide is eliminated. Conversely, impaired chest expansion can lead to respiratory acidosis because of alveolar hypoventilation.*
- Elevate the head of the bed. *Elevating the head of the bed reduces the work of breathing and improves alveolar ventilation by reducing the pressure of abdominal distention on the diaphragm.*
- Provide a pillow or folded bath blanket to use in splinting the abdomen while coughing postoperatively. *Splinting abdominal muscles and incisions improves the ease and effectiveness of coughing postoperatively.*
- Maintain nasogastric or intestinal tube patency. *Maintaining gastrointestinal suction helps reduce abdominal distention and prevent aspiration associated with vomiting.*

- Encourage use of incentive spirometer or other assistive device hourly. *These devices encourage deep breathing, opening distal airways and preventing atelectasis.*
- Contact respiratory therapy as indicated. *The respiratory therapist may suggest or perform additional measures to maintain effective pulmonary ventilation.*
- Provide good oral care at least every 4 hours. *Dehydration and nasogastric suction dry the mucous membranes of the mouth and throat, increasing the risk of bacterial growth. Many respiratory infections result from aspirated organisms.*

Community-Based Care

Include the following topics when teaching the patient with intestinal obstruction in preparation for home care:

- Wound care
- Activity level, return to work, and any other recommended restrictions
- Recommended follow-up care
- Care of temporary colostomy (if appropriate) and planned reanastomosis
- For recurrent obstructions, their cause, early identification of manifestations, and possible preventive measures

Anorectal Disorders

Anorectal lesions include hemorrhoids, a normal condition common to all adults that may become enlarged and painful; anal fissure; anorectal abscess; anorectal fistulas; and pilonidal disease.

The Patient with Hemorrhoids

The anus and anal canal contain two superficial venous plexuses with the hemorrhoidal veins. When pressure on these veins is increased or venous return impeded, they can develop *varices*, or varicosities, becoming weak and distended. This condition is commonly known as *hemorrhoids*, or "piles." When asymptomatic, hemorrhoids are considered to be a normal condition found in all adults.

Pathophysiology and Manifestations

Hemorrhoids develop when venous return from the anal canal is impaired. Straining to defecate increases venous pressure and is the most common cause of distended hemorrhoids. Pregnancy increases intra-abdominal pressure, raising venous pressure, and is another cause of hemorrhoids. Other factors that may contribute to symptomatic hemorrhoids include prolonged sitting, obesity, chronic constipation, and a low-fiber diet.

Hemorrhoids are classed as either internal or external. *Internal* hemorrhoids affect the venous plexus above the mucocutaneous junction of the anus (Figure 24–15 ■). Internal hemorrhoids rarely cause pain, usually presenting with bleeding. Bleeding from internal hemorrhoids is bright red and unmixed with the stool. It can vary in quantity from streaks on toilet tissue to enough to color the water in the

toilet. Recurrent bleeding of internal hemorrhoids may be sufficient to cause anemia. Mucous discharge and a feeling of incomplete evacuation of stool also may be manifestations of internal hemorrhoids.

External hemorrhoids affect the inferior hemorrhoidal plexus below the mucocutaneous junction. Bleeding is rare with external hemorrhoids. Anal irritation, a feeling of pressure, and difficulty cleaning the anal region may be manifestations of external hemorrhoids.

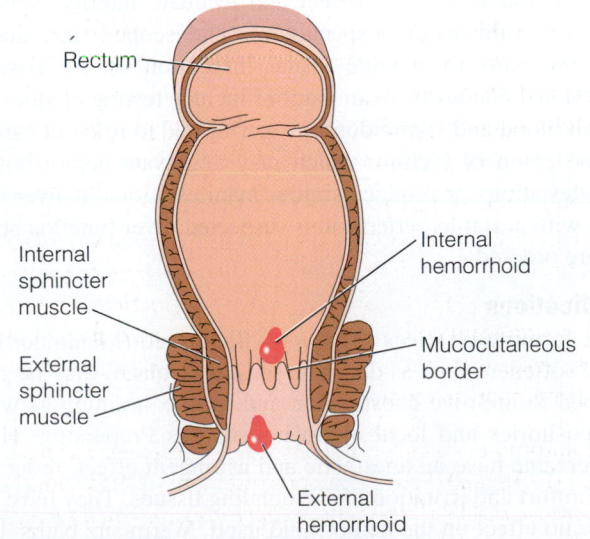

Rectum

Internal sphincter muscle

External sphincter muscle

Internal hemorrhoid

Mucocutaneous border

External hemorrhoid

Figure 24–15 ■ The location of internal and external hemorrhoids.

As they enlarge, hemorrhoids may prolapse or protrude through the anus. Initially, prolapse occurs only with defecation and the hemorrhoids spontaneously regress back into the anal canal. Eventually, the patient may need to manually replace internal hemorrhoids after defecation, or they may become permanently prolapsed, in which case replacement is not possible. Manifestations of permanently prolapsed hemorrhoids include mucous discharge and clothing soilage.

Normal hemorrhoids are not painful. Prolapsed hemorrhoids may become strangulated as a result of congestion and edema, leading to thrombosis. Hemorrhoidal thrombosis causes extreme pain and may lead to infarction of skin and mucosa overlying the hemorrhoid. Internal hemorrhoids associated with portal hypertension in liver disease may bleed profusely if ruptured. (∞ See Chapter 25 for further discussion of portal hypertension.)

A *thrombosed external hemorrhoid* is a thrombosis of the subcutaneous external hemorrhoidal veins of the anal canal, rather than a true hemorrhoid. It appears as a painful bluish hematoma beneath the skin and typically occurs following a sudden increase in venous pressure, for example, heavy lifting, coughing, or straining. Pain is significant at onset but gradually subsides. Spontaneous rupture with bleeding may occur. Thrombosed external hemorrhoids resolve without intervention.

Interdisciplinary Care

Because hemorrhoids are a normal condition, management is conservative unless complications such as permanent prolapse or thrombosis occur.

Diagnosis

Hemorrhoids are diagnosed by the patient's history and by examination of the anorectal area. External hemorrhoids can be seen on visual inspection, especially if thrombosed. The patient is asked to strain (Valsalva's maneuver) during the examination to detect prolapse. Internal hemorrhoids are usually not palpable or tender on digital examination of the rectum. Anoscopic examination is used to detect and evaluate internal hemorrhoids. For this exam, a speculum or endoscope is introduced into the anus to provide visual inspection of the tissues. Additional diagnostic examinations include testing of stool for occult blood and sigmoidoscopy, performed to rule out cancer of the colon or rectum, which may aggravate hemorrhoidal manifestations or produce similar manifestations. If liver disease with portal hypertension is suspected, liver function studies are ordered.

Medications

Bulk-forming laxatives such as psyllium seed (Metamucil) or stool softeners such as docusate sodium (Colace) may be prescribed to improve constipation and reduce straining as well. Suppositories and local ointments such as Preparation H or Nupercaine have an anesthetic and astringent effect, reducing discomfort and irritation of surrounding tissues. They have little or no effect on the hemorrhoid itself. Warm sitz baths, bed rest, and local astringent compresses may be recommended to reduce the swelling of edematous prolapsed hemorrhoids after digital reduction.

Nutrition

Hemorrhoids that are not permanently prolapsed or acutely thrombosed generally are treated conservatively. A high-fiber diet and increased water intake to increase stool bulk, improve its softness, and reduce straining is effective for most patients with internal or external hemorrhoids.

Sclerotherapy

Hemorrhoids that are permanently prolapsed, are thrombosed, or produce significant manifestations may be treated more aggressively. *Sclerotherapy* involves injecting a chemical irritant into tissues surrounding the hemorrhoid to induce inflammation and eventual fibrosis and scarring. It is used to treat recurrent bleeding and early prolapse of internal hemorrhoids. The treatment produces minimal pain. Enlarged or prolapsing hemorrhoids also may be treated with rubber band ligation. A rubber band is placed snugly around the hemorrhoidal plexus and surrounding mucosa, causing the tissue to necrose and slough within 7 to 10 days. Treatment is limited to one hemorrhoidal complex at a time, so repeat treatments may be necessary. Pain should be minimal if the band is placed appropriately; persistent pain following band ligation may signal an infection. Bleeding can occur as the hemorrhoid sloughs. Other procedures used to treat hemorrhoids include cryosurgery, in which hemorrhoids are necrosed by freezing with a cryoprobe; infrared photocoagulation; or electrocoagulation.

Hemorrhoidectomy

Patients with chronic manifestations, permanent prolapse, chronic bleeding and anemia, or painful thrombosed hemorrhoids may be treated surgically with a *hemorrhoidectomy*. In this procedure, hemorrhoids are surgically excised, leaving normal skin and surrounding tissues. This procedure may use conventional techniques or a laser to remove both internal and external hemorrhoids. Few complications are associated with hemorrhoidectomy.

∞ Nursing Care

Primary prevention of symptomatic hemorrhoids involves education of patients of all ages. Stress the importance of maintaining an adequate intake of dietary fiber, a liberal fluid intake, and regular exercise to maintain stool bulk, softness, and regularity. Discuss the need to respond to the urge to defecate rather than postponing defecation. Teach appropriate constipation management, including the use of bulk-forming laxatives.

Most patients with hemorrhoids are treated in community settings where the primary nursing focus is educational. Discuss the appropriate use of over-the-counter preparations and sitz baths for the relief of minor hemorrhoidal manifestations. If necessary, teach patients how to reduce prolapsed hemorrhoids digitally.

Teach manifestations of possible hemorrhoidal complications, such as chronic bleeding, prolapse, and thrombosis. Stress the need to seek medical evaluation if manifestations persist. Discuss the link between manifestations of hemorrhoids and colorectal cancer, and urge the patient to seek medical intervention for persistent, unresolved, or progressive manifestations.

When a hemorrhoidectomy is performed, the patient requires more direct nursing intervention. Postoperative care of

BOX 24–3 Perianal Postoperative Care

Assessment
- Monitor vital signs every 4 hours for 24 hours.
- Inspect rectal dressing every 2 to 3 hours for 24 hours.
- Monitor urinary output.

Pain Control
- Assist to position of comfort, usually side-lying.
- Provide analgesics as prescribed.
- Keep fresh ice packs over the rectal dressing as ordered.
- Assist with sitz bath three to four times per day.
- Provide a flotation pad for use when sitting.

Elimination
- Give stool softeners as prescribed.
- Give an analgesic before the first postoperative bowel movement if possible.
- When tolerated, encourage fluid intake of at least 2000 mL per day.

Patient and Family Teaching
- Take sitz bath after each bowel movement for 1 to 2 weeks after surgery.
- Drink at least 2 quarts of fluid per day.
- Eat adequate dietary fiber, and exercise moderately.
- Take stool softeners as prescribed.
- Report to the physician the following symptoms: rectal bleeding, continued pain on defecation, fever greater than 101°F (38.3°C), purulent rectal drainage.

the patient with perianal surgery is outlined in Box 24–3. Anal packing may be in place for the first 24 hours following the procedure. When removed, observe the patient closely for bleeding. Pain is a common postoperative problem. Although the operative procedure is minor, postoperative discomfort can be significant because the anal region is richly innervated and muscle spasms may occur. In addition to systemic analgesics, sitz baths usually are ordered. These not only help promote relaxation and reduce discomfort but also clean the anal area. Use of a rubber ring or donut device minimizes pressure on the surgical site while the patient sits in the bath.

The patient may remain hospitalized until after the first postoperative bowel movement. Stool softeners, adequate fluids, and analgesia before defecation can reduce anxiety and discomfort. Adequate cleaning following defecation, usually with a sitz bath, is vital.

Whether caring for a patient with hemorrhoids or a hemorrhoidectomy, consider the following nursing diagnoses:

- *Acute* or *Chronic Pain* related to inflamed anal tissues
- *Constipation* related to dietary habits and/or delay of defecation
- *Risk for Infection* related to disruption of anal tissue

The Patient with an Anorectal Lesion

Unlike the rectum, which is relatively insensitive to pain, the anal canal is richly supplied with sensory nerves and highly sensitive to painful stimuli. Lesions of the anorectal area may cause significant pain, particularly with defecation. Infection is a potential complication of anorectal lesions because of contamination by fecal bacteria. The superior boundary of the anal canal (the anorectal juncture or pectinate line) contains 8 to 12 anal crypts where anorectal abscesses or fistulas can form. Lesions of the anorectal area include fissures, abscesses, fistulas, and pilonidal disease.

Anal Fissure

Anal fissures or ulcers occur when the epithelium of the anal canal over the internal sphincter becomes denuded or abraded. Irritating diarrheal stools and tightening of the anal canal with increased sphincter tension are frequent causes of anal fissures. Other factors that may contribute to their development include childbirth trauma, habitual cathartic use, laceration by a foreign body, and anal intercourse. Chronic inflammation and infection of surrounding tissues accompanies an anal fissure.

Patients with anal fissures typically have periods of exacerbation and remission. Because they occur below the mucocutaneous line, anal fissures are painful. The pain occurs with defecation and may be described as tearing, burning, or cutting. Bright red bleeding is noted with a bowel movement. Bleeding is typically minor and noted on toilet tissue. Because of fear of defecation, the patient may develop constipation, which further disrupts normal bowel habits and aggravates manifestations.

The diagnosis of anal fissure is made on gentle digital examination of the anal canal and anoscopy using a small anoscope. Treatment is usually conservative, involving dietary changes to increase fiber intake and stool bulk, increased fluid intake, and use of bulk-forming laxatives. A topical agent such as hydrocortisone cream may be prescribed. Surgical intervention with an internal sphincterotomy, an incision into the internal sphincter to increase its diameter, is considered when the fissure does not heal with medical intervention.

Anorectal Abscess

Invasion of the pararectal spaces by pathogenic bacteria can lead to an *anorectal abscess*. Commonly caused by infection that extends from the anal crypt into a pararectal space, the abscess may appear small but often contains a large amount of pus. Multiple pathogens may be present, including *Escherichia coli*, *Proteus*, streptococci, and staphylococci. Other factors that may contribute to the development of an anorectal abscess include infection of a hair follicle, sebaceous gland, or sweat gland, and abrasions, fissures, or anal trauma. The incidence of anorectal abscess is higher in men.

Pain is the primary manifestation of an anorectal abscess. Sitting or walking may aggravate the pain, but it is unrelated to defecation. External swelling, redness, heat, and tenderness are apparent on examination. With a deeper abscess, swelling may not be visible, but the abscess is palpable on digital examination.

If the abscess either does not drain spontaneously or is not drained surgically, adjacent anatomic spaces will be affected. Systemic sepsis is also a potential complication.

Incision and drainage is the treatment of choice for an anorectal abscess because it rarely resolves with antibiotic therapy alone. This treatment often leads to a persistent fistula, which is surgically closed after the infection has cleared.

Anorectal Fistula

A fistula is a tunnel or tubelike tract with openings at each end. *Anorectal fistulas* have one opening in the anal canal with the other usually found in perianal skin. Most occur spontaneously or as a result of anorectal abscess drainage. Crohn's disease is a predisposing factor to fistula development.

The primary manifestation of an anorectal fistula is intermittent or constant drainage or discharge, which may be purulent. This may be accompanied by local itching, tenderness, and pain associated with defecation.

Digital and anoscopic examination with gentle probing of the fistula tract are used to establish the diagnosis. Although some fistulas may heal spontaneously, the treatment of choice is a fistulotomy. The primary opening of the fistula is removed, and the tract is opened to allow it to heal by secondary intention, from the inside outward. If the sphincter is involved, a two-stage operation may be done to preserve the muscle and prevent fecal incontinence.

Pilonidal Disease

The patient with *pilonidal disease* has an acute abscess or chronic draining sinus in the sacrococcygeal area. Underlying the abscess or sinus is a cyst with granulation tissue, fibrosis, and, often, hair tufts. This disease usually affects young hirsute (hairy) males and is probably due to hair entrapment in deep tissues of the sacrococcygeal area. Some researchers believe that it is a congenital disorder.

The lesion of pilonidal disease is generally asymptomatic unless it becomes acutely infected. Manifestations of acute inflammation accompany infection, including pain, tenderness, redness, heat, and swelling of the affected area. Purulent discharge may be noted from one or more sinuses or openings in the midline.

The preferred treatment option for pilonidal disease is incision and drainage. The sinus tract and underlying cyst are excised and closed by either primary- or secondary-intention healing. The patient may be instructed to remove hair from the area routinely by shaving or using a depilatory to prevent further hair entrapment and recurrence of the problem.

Nursing Care

Patients with anorectal disorders are often treated in the community, and the primary nursing responsibility is education. Teach the importance of maintaining a high-fiber diet and liberal fluid intake to increase stool bulk and softness and thereby decrease discomfort with defecation. Stress the importance of responding to the urge to defecate to prevent constipation.

Following surgical treatment of any of these disorders, teach the patient to keep the perianal region clean and dry. If a dressing is in place, instruct to avoid soiling it with urine or feces during elimination. Following removal of the dressing, teach to clean the area gently with soap and water following a bowel movement. Discuss the use of sitz baths for cleaning and comfort. Suggest taking an analgesic if necessary prior to defecation, but caution that some analgesics may promote constipation. Teach manifestations of infection or other possible complications to report to the physician. If an antibiotic has been prescribed, provide written and verbal instructions about its use, its desired and possible adverse effects, and their management.

CHAPTER HIGHLIGHTS

- Disorders of intestinal motility include diarrhea, constipation, irritable bowel syndrome, and fecal incontinence. Diarrhea is a manifestation of many other bowel disorders, including lactose intolerance, infections, and inflammatory diseases of the bowel. Constipation may be a primary problem (especially for the older adult) or a manifestation of another disorder. Irritable bowel syndrome (IBS) is a functional disorder without any identifiable organic cause. Fecal incontinence is usually considered to be the manifestation of a disorder rather than a disorder itself.
- Appendicitis is an acute inflammation of the vermiform appendix, manifested by abdominal pain that localizes in the right lower quadrant of the abdomen. On palpation, localized and rebound tenderness is present at McBurney's point. It is treated most often with an appendectomy.
- Peritonitis (inflammation of the peritoneum from infection or chemical irritant) is a serious complication of a wide variety of acute abdominal disorders, including perforated ulcer, ruptured appendix, abdominal trauma or surgery, or necrotic bowel. Complications may be life threatening; without prompt and effective treatment, septicemia and septic shock may occur.

- Gastroenteritis, which may result from bacterial or viral infections, parasites, or toxins, is often the result of consuming contaminated water or food. Manifestations include nausea and vomiting, diarrhea, and abdominal discomfort.
- Nurses provide education to help prevent protozoal infections (such as giardiasis, amebiasis, and coccidiosis) and helminthic infestations (roundworms, flukes, or tapeworms). Both types of bowel disorders are treated with medications.
- Chronic inflammatory bowel disease (IBD) includes two separate but closely related conditions: ulcerative colitis and Crohn's disease. Ulcerative colitis affects the mucosa and submucosa of the colon and rectum. Crohn's disease can affect any part of the GI tract, but usually involves the terminal ilium and ascending colon. Diarrhea is common to both disorders. A colectomy (removal of the large colon) may be performed to treat ulcerative colitis; an ileostomy (artificial opening from the abdomen to the ileum) may be performed to treat Crohn's disease.
- Diverticula are saclike projections of mucosa through the muscular layer of the colon. When these sacs become inflamed, the condition is labeled diverticulitis. A diet high in fiber is recommended for self-care.

- Malabsorption syndromes, in which the intestinal mucosa ineffectively absorbs nutrients, may be caused by a wide variety of diseases. However, three common malabsorption disorders in adults are celiac disease, lactase deficiency with resulting lactose intolerance of milk and milk products, and short bowel syndrome (a condition that can develop following resection of the small bowel).

- Malignant tumors of the lower bowel are the second leading cause of death from cancer. The risk of colon cancer may be reduced through health-related screenings and a diet high in fruits, vegetables, folic acid, and calcium. Rectal bleeding is the most common initial manifestation but may not occur until the cancer is well advanced. Surgical treatment is through resection of the bowel, accompanied by a colostomy for diversion of fecal contents.

- A hernia is a defect in the abdominal wall that allows intra-abdominal contents to protrude out of the abdominal cavity. Hernias may follow trauma, surgery, and increased intra-abdominal pressure (as from pregnancy or obesity). Hernias may be congenital or acquired, and may be inguinal, umbilical, incisional, or ventral.

- Intestinal obstructions occur when intestinal contents cannot move through the lumen of the bowel. They may occur in either the large or small intestine, may be partial or complete, and are caused by many factors, ranging from surgical ileus following abdominal surgery to adhesions or tumors.

- Anorectal disorders include hemorrhoids, anorectal lesions (fissures, abscess, and fistula), and pilonidal disease. These disorders are painful and pose a risk for bleeding and infection.

TEST YOURSELF NCLEX-RN® REVIEW

1. A patient presents at the urgent care clinic with complaints of diarrhea for the past week. The nurse should first do which of the following?
   1. Advise the patient to abstain from all food intake until the diarrhea subsides.
   2. Ask the patient to describe the number and character of daily stools.
   3. Question the patient about possible exposure to an enterotoxin or protozoal infection.
   4. Recommend an over-the-counter antidiarrheal preparation such as Pepto-Bismol.

2. Which of the following is of highest priority when caring for a patient admitted with possible appendicitis?
   1. Perform preoperative skin preparation.
   2. Teach postoperative coughing, deep breathing, and exercise.
   3. Withhold all food and fluids.
   4. Insert saline lock for intravenous antibiotic therapy.

3. When teaching a patient with inflammatory bowel disease about prescribed sulfasalazine, the nurse instructs the patient to do which of the following?
   1. Use a sunscreen while taking the drug.
   2. Take the drug on an empty stomach.
   3. Limit fluid intake to 1500 mL per day or less.
   4. Take vitamin C while on the drug.

4. A patient reports frequent large, fatty, foul-smelling stools. The nurse inquires further about which of the following?
   1. possible exposure to enterotoxins in food or water
   2. a history of alternating diarrhea and constipation
   3. known family history of colorectal cancer
   4. the relationship of episodes to particular foods

5. A patient tells the nurse that both his father and grandfather died of colon cancer, and he is worried that he is going to die from "the same horrible disease." Which of the following does the nurse include in her recommendations?
   1. The genetic link is weak in colon cancer, so he should simply follow the usual recommendations for screening.
   2. He should plan for annual digital rectal exams and periodic colonoscopy for early identification of possible tumors.
   3. He should have annual CEA levels drawn to screen for early tumor development.
   4. Significantly increasing his intake of dietary fiber can reduce his risk of developing colon cancer within 5 years.

6. A patient has a nasogastric tube in place to maintain gastric decompression. Which nursing actions are important in monitoring responses to *Deficient Fluid Volume* when caring for this patient? **Select all that apply.**
   1. Low suction is used to decompress the stomach.
   2. Give the patient as much water as he or she wants to drink.
   3. Listen to bowel sounds prior to checking the placement of the NG tube.
   4. Document the amount and color of NG tube drainage every shift.
   5. Keep an accurate record of intake and output every 2 to 4 hours.
   6. Measure abdominal girth every 4 to 8 hours.

7. A patient has developed a paralytic ileus following a recent abdominal surgery. What is the most important nursing consideration when caring for this patient?
   1. Ensure that the patient is able to eat a clear liquid diet.
   2. Maintain the patient on strict bedrest.
   3. Monitor bowel sounds every hour.
   4. Ensure nasogastric tube is functioning.

8. Mrs. Jones has a history of diverticulosis and has been having abdominal pain recently. When educating Mrs. Jones about her diet prior to discharge from the hospital, what type of foods should be excluded from Mrs. Jones's diet?
   1. whole-wheat bread
   2. raspberries
   3. soup
   4. apples

9. Your 85-year-old patient Mr. Allen was admitted with a diagnosis of constipation. Which of the following is important in your discharge education for this patient? **Select all that apply.**
   1. Eat plenty of fresh fruits and vegetables daily.
   2. Take a bisacodyl (Dulcolax) daily.
   3. Drink six to eight glasses of nonalcoholic fluid daily.
   4. Take docusate (Colace) at nighttime only.
   5. Eat whole-wheat bread instead of white bread.
   6. Eat a bran cereal for breakfast.

10. Which of the following nursing interventions are of highest priority when caring for a patient with a small bowel obstruction?
    1. placing the patient in semi-Fowler's position
    2. maintaining nasogastric suction
    3. keeping strict intake and output records
    4. administering prescribed analgesics

See Test Yourself answers in Appendix C.

BIBLIOGRAPHY

American Cancer Society. (2006). *Cancer facts & figures for Hispanics/Latinos 2006–2008.* Atlanta, GA: Author.

American Cancer Society. (2007). *Cancer facts & figures for African Americans 2007–2008.* Atlanta, GA: Author.

American Cancer Society. (2009). *Cancer facts & figures 2009.* Atlanta, GA: Author.

American Cancer Society. (2008). *Colorectal cancer facts & figures 2008-1010.* Atlanta, GA: Author.

American College of Physicians. (2007). In the clinic. Irritable bowel syndrome. *Annals of Internal Medicine, 3 July 2007,* ITC7-1-ITC7-16.

Balch, J. F., & Stengler, M. (2004). *Prescription for natural cures: A self-care guide for treating health problems with natural remedies including diet and nutrition, nutritional supplements, bodywork, and more.* Hoboken, NJ: Wiley & Sons.

Banning, M. (2008). Ageing and the gut. *Nursing Older People, 20*(1), 17–21.

Barakzai, M., Gregory, J., & Fraser, D. (2007). The effect of culture on symptom reporting: Hispanics and irritable bowel syndrome. *Journal of the American Academy of Nurse Practitioners, 19*(2007), 261–267.

Bazensky, I., Shoobridge-Moran, C., & Yoder, L. (2007 February). Colorectal cancer: An overview of the epidemiology, risk factors, symptoms, and screening guidelines. *Medsurg Nursing, 16*(1), 46–51.

Bulechek, G., Butcher, H., & Dochterman, J. (Eds.). (2008). *Nursing interventions classification (NIC)* (5th ed.). St. Louis, MO: Mosby.

Calfee, D. (2008 September). *Clostridium difficile:* A reemerging pathogen. *Geriatrics, 63*(9), 10–14, 21.

Centers for Disease Control and Prevention. (2006). Noroviruses. Retrieved from http://www.cdc.gov/ncidod/dvrd/revb/gastro/norovirus-factsheet.htm

Centers for Disease Control and Prevention. (2009 May 7). Outbreak of *Salmonella* serotype Saintpaul infections associated with eating alfalfa sprouts – United States, 2009. *Morbidity and Mortality Weekly Report, 58*(Early Release May 7, 2009). Retrieved from www.cdc.gov/mmwr

Cokkinides, V., Bandi, P., Siegel, R., Ward E., & Thun, M. (2007). *Cancer prevention & early detection facts & figures 2008.* Atlanta, GA: American Cancer Society.

Connelly, P. (2008 June). *Lactobacillus plantarum–* A literature review of therapeutic benefits. *Journal of the Australian Traditional-Medicine Society, 14*(2), 79–82.

Crohn's & Colitis Foundation of America. (2008). *About ulcerative colitis & procitis.* Retrieved from www.ccfa.org/info/about/ucp

Crohn's & Colitis Foundation of America. (2009). *About Crohn's disease.* Retrieved from http://www.ccfa.org/info/about/crohns

Dalrymple, J., & Bullock, I. (2008 March). Diagnosis and management of irritable bowel syndrome in adults in primary care: Summary of NICE guidance. *BMJ: British Medical Journal, 336*(7643), 556–558.

Dupont, H. (2008). Systematic review: Prevention of travellers' diarrhorea. *Alimentary Pharmacology & Therapeutics, 27,* 741–751.

Fauci, A., Braunwald, E., Kasper, D., Hauser, S., Longo, D., Jameson, J., et al. (2008). *Harrison's principles of internal medicine* (17th ed.). New York, NY: McGraw Hill.

Freeman, L. (2007 May). Responding to small-bowel obstruction. *Nursing 2007, 37*(5), 56hn1–56hn2, 56hn4, 56hn6.

Ginsberg, D., Phillips, S., Wallace, J., & Josephson, K. (2007 June). Evaluating and managing constipation in the elderly. *Urologic Nursing, 27*(3), 191–200.

Guarino, A., Vecchio, A., & Canani, R. (2009 April). Probiotics as prevention and treatment for diarrhea. *Current Opinion in Gastroenterology, 25*(1). Retrieved from www.medscape.com

Heitkemper, M., & Wolff, J. (2007 April). Challenges in chronic constipation. *The Nurse Practitioner, 32*(4), 36–42.

Higgins, R. (2009 February). Abdominal assessment and diagnosis of appendicitis. *Emergency Nurse, 16*(9), 22–24.

Holman, C., Roberts, S., & Nicol, M. (2008 June). Preventing and treating constipation in later life. *Nursing Older People, 20*(5), 22–24.

Kee, J. (2009). *Handbook of laboratory and diagnostic tests with nursing implications* (6th ed.). Upper Saddle River, NJ: Prentice Hall.

Kyle, G. (2009 January). Common bowel problems in older adult care. *Nursing & Residential Care, 11*(1), 22–25.

Kyle, G. (2009 February). Common bowel problems: Constipation risk assessment. *Nursing & Residential Care, 11*(2), 76–79.

Langmead, L., & Rampton, D. (2006). Review article: Complementary and alternative therapies for inflammatory bowel disease. *Alimentary Pharmacology & Therapeutics, 23,* 341–349.

Lindberg, D. (2009 January/February). Hydrogen breath testing in adults. *Gastroenterology Nursing, 32*(1), 19–24.

Managing constipation in the elderly. (2007). *Geriatrics Supplement,* August 2007.

Martin, S. (2008). Against the grain: An overview of celiac disease. *Journal of the American Academy of Nurse Practitioners, 20*(2008), 243–250.

Mayo Clinic. (2008). *Ulcerative colitis.* Retrieved from www.mayoclinic.com/health/ulcerative-colitis/

McPhee, S. Papadakis, M., & Tierney, L., Jr. (2008). *Current medical diagnosis & treatment* (47th ed.). New York, NY: McGraw Hill.

Moorhead, S., Johnson, M., Maas, M., & Swanson, E. (Eds.). (2008). *Nursing outcomes classification (NOC)* (4th ed.). St. Louis, MO: Mosby.

Moynihan, N., Callahan, M., Kalsmith, B., & Moses, P. (2008 February). How do you spell relief for irritable bowel syndrome? C-A-R-E-F-U-L-L-Y. *The Journal of Family Practice, 57*(2), 100–108.

NANDA International. (2009). *Nursing diagnoses: Definitions & classification 2009–2011.* Oxford, UK: Wiley-Blackwell.

National Cancer Institute. (2008). *Colon cancer treatment (PDQ®).* Health professional version. Retrieved from www.cancer.gov/cancertopics/pdq/treatment/colon/healthprofessional/

National Center for Complementary and Alternative Medicine (NCCAM). (2008). *An introduction to probiotics.* Retrieved from http://nccam.nih.gov/health/probiotics

Pontieri-Lewis, V. (2006 August). Basics of ostomy care. *Medsurg Nursing, 15*(4), 199–202.

Porth, C. M., & Matfin, G. (2009). *Pathophysiology: Concepts of altered health states* (8th ed.). Philadelphia, PA: Lippincott.

Rowland, I., Melton, L., Gray, J., Bulpitt, C., Hickson, M., Smith, M., et al. (2008 February). Latest research and thinking into the power of probiotics. *Practice Nurse, 35*(Supplement), 1–4.

Sabol, V., & Carlson, K. (2007 January–March). Diarrhea: Applying research to bedside practice. *AACN Advanced Critical Care, 18*(1), 32–44.

Stahlfeld, K., Hower, J., Homitsky, S., & Madden, J. (2007 June). Is acute appendicitis a surgical emergency? *The American Surgeon, 73,* 626–630.

Thorson, M., Bliss, D., & Savik, K. (2008). Re-examination of risk factors for non-*Clostridium difficile*-associated diarrhea in hospitalized patients. *JAN: Original Research,* 354–364.

Westwood, N., & Travis, S. (2008). Review article: What do patients with inflammatory bowel disease want for their clinical management? *Alimentary Pharmacology & Therapeutics, 27*(Supplement 1), 1–8.

Wilkinson, J., & Ahern, N. (2009). *Prentice Hall nursing diagnosis handbook* (9th ed.). Upper Saddle River, NJ: Prentice Hall.

Willcox, A., & Hayward, M. (2008 July). A guide to travel health. *Emergency Nurse, 16*(4), 30–37.

Wilson, B., Shannon, M., Shields, K., & Stang, C. (2008). *Prentice Hall nurse's drug guide 2008.* Upper Saddle River, NJ: Prentice Hall.

Yantis, M., & Velander, R. (2009 March). Probiotics can thwart antibiotic-associated diarrhea. *Nursing 2009, 39*(3), 58–59.

Yarbo, C., Frogge, M., & Goodman, M. (2005). *Cancer nursing: Principles and practice* (6th ed.). Sudbury, MA: Jones & Bartlett.

Yates, J. (2005). Traveler's diarrhea. *American Family Physician, 71*(11), 2095–2100.

Nursing Care of Patients with Gallbladder, Liver, and Pancreatic Disorders

LEARNING OUTCOMES

1. Describe the pathophysiology of commonly occurring disorders of the gallbladder, liver, and exocrine pancreas.
2. Use knowledge of normal anatomy and physiology to understand the manifestations and effects of biliary, hepatic, and pancreatic disorders.
3. Relate changes in normal assessment data to the pathophysiology and manifestations of gallbladder, liver, and exocrine pancreatic disorders.

CLINICAL COMPETENCIES

1. Assess functional health status of patients with gallbladder, liver, or pancreatic disease.
2. Monitor for, recognize, document, and report expected and unexpected manifestations in patients with gallbladder, liver, or pancreatic disease.
3. Provide appropriate, evidence-based teaching about diagnostic tests and test results for patients with gallbladder, liver, and pancreatic disorders.
4. Integrate appropriate dietary, pharmacologic, and other interdisciplinary measures into nursing care and teaching of the patient with a gallbladder, liver, or pancreatic disorder.
5. Provide safe, patient-centered nursing care for the patient who has surgery of the gallbladder, liver, or pancreas.
6. Integrate psychosocial, cultural, and spiritual considerations into the plan of care for a patient with a gallbladder, liver, or pancreatic disorder.
7. Use evidence-based practice, technology, and information management tools to develop, implement, evaluate, and, as needed, revise the plan of care for patients with disorders of the gallbladder, liver, or pancreas.
8. Provide appropriate patient and family teaching to promote, maintain, and restore functional health status for patients with gallbladder, liver, and pancreatic disorders.

KEY TERMS

ascites, 727
biliary colic, 722
cholecystitis, 722
cholelithiasis, 721
cirrhosis, 736

esophageal varices, 728
hepatitis, 729
jaundice, 728
pancreatitis, 751
paracentesis, 743

portal hypertension, 728
portal systemic encephalopathy, 728
steatorrhea, 753

Gallbladder, liver, and exocrine pancreas disorders may occur as primary disorders, or develop secondarily to other disease processes. The functioning of one organ frequently affects that of another. Duct inflammation or obstruction, and changes in the multiple functions of these organs, can cause significant health effects.

Patients with a gallbladder, liver, or pancreatic disorder may experience pain, metabolic and nutritional disturbances, and altered body image. Nursing care addresses physiologic, emotional, and psychosocial needs of the patient and family.

Gallbladder Disorders

Altered bile flow through the hepatic, cystic, or common bile duct is a common problem and a frequent cause of hospitalization. It often leads to inflammation and other complications. Gallstones are the most common cause of obstructed flow. Tumors and abscesses also can obstruct bile flow.

The Patient with Gallstones

Cholelithiasis is the formation of stones (*calculi* or *gallstones*) within the gallbladder or biliary duct system. Cholelithiasis is a common problem in the United States, affecting more than 10%

of men and 20% of women by age 65 (McPhee et al., 2008). Box 25–1 lists risk factors for gallstones. The incidence of gallstones varies among people of different ethnic backgrounds; see the accompanying Focus on Cultural Diversity box.

Physiology Review

Normally, bile is formed by the liver and stored in the gallbladder. Bile contains bile salts, bilirubin, water, electrolytes, cholesterol, fatty acids, and lecithin. In the gallbladder, some of the water and electrolytes are absorbed, further concentrating

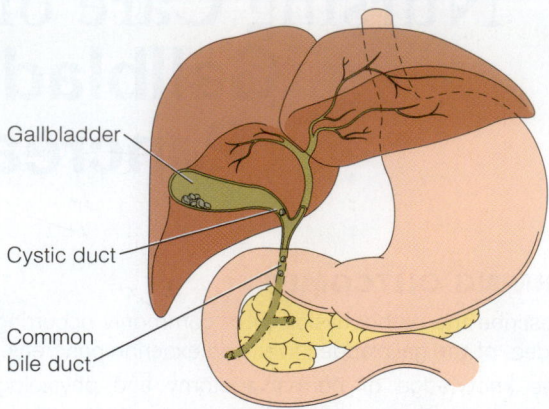

Gallbladder

Cystic duct

Common bile duct

Figure 25–1 ■ Common locations of gallstones.

the bile. Food entering the intestine stimulates the gallbladder to contract and release bile through the common bile duct and sphincter of Oddi into the intestine. The bile salts in bile increase the solubility and absorption of dietary fats.

Pathophysiology and Manifestations

Cholelithiasis

Gallstones form when several factors interact: abnormal bile composition, biliary stasis, and inflammation of the gallbladder. Most gallstones (80%) consist primarily of cholesterol; the rest contain a mixture of bile components. Excess cholesterol in bile is associated with obesity, a high-calorie and high-cholesterol diet, and drugs that lower serum cholesterol levels. When bile is supersaturated with cholesterol, it can precipitate out to form stones. Biliary stasis, or slowed emptying of the gallbladder, contributes to cholelithiasis. Stones do not form when the gallbladder empties completely in response to hormonal stimulation. Slowed or incomplete emptying allows cholesterol to concentrate and increases the risk of stone formation. Finally, inflammation of the gallbladder allows excess water and bile salt reabsorption, increasing the risk for lithiasis.

> **PRACTICE ALERT**
> Certain very-low-calorie diets are associated with a high risk of cholelithiasis. Increased cholesterol concentration in the bile and decreased gallbladder contractions associated with fasting increase the risk of gallstone formation.

Most gallstones are formed in the gallbladder. They then may migrate into the ducts (Figure 25–1 ■), leading to *cholangitis* (duct inflammation). Although some people with cholelithiasis are asymptomatic, many develop manifestations.

> **FOCUS ON CULTURAL DIVERSITY**
> **Gallstones**
>
> Native Americans in both the Northern and Southern Hemispheres, and those of the Pima tribe in particular, have a higher incidence of gallstones than do Caucasians of American or European heritage. This is thought to result from genes that promote efficient calorie use and fat storage—a beneficial trait when the availability of adequate food varies over time. Gallstones composed of cholesterol are less common in African Americans, and Asians have a low incidence of the disease (McPhee et al., 2008).

Early manifestations of gallstones may be vague: epigastric fullness or mild gastric distress after eating a large or fatty meal. Stones that obstruct the cystic duct or common bile duct lead to distention and increased pressure behind the stone. This causes **biliary colic**, a severe, steady pain in the epigastric region or right upper quadrant of the abdomen. The pain may radiate to the back, right scapula, or shoulder. The pain often begins suddenly following a meal, and may last as long as 5 hours. It often is accompanied by nausea and vomiting.

Obstruction of the common bile duct may cause bile reflux into the liver, leading to jaundice, pain, and possible liver damage. If the common duct is obstructed, pancreatic enzymes will be unable to enter the small intestine, and pancreatitis (discussed later in this chapter) becomes a potential complication.

Cholecystitis

Cholecystitis is inflammation of the gallbladder. *Acute cholecystitis* usually follows obstruction of the cystic duct by a stone. The obstruction increases pressure within the gallbladder, leading to ischemia of the gallbladder wall and mucosa. Retained bile causes chemical irritation and bacterial inflammation often follows. The ischemia can lead to necrosis and perforation of the gallbladder wall.

Acute cholecystitis usually begins with an attack of biliary colic. The pain involves the entire right upper quadrant (RUQ), and may radiate to the back, right scapula, or shoulder. Movement or deep breathing may aggravate the pain. The pain usually lasts longer than biliary colic, continuing for 12 to 18 hours. Anorexia, nausea, and vomiting are common. Fever often is present, and may be accompanied by chills. The RUQ is tender to palpation.

Chronic cholecystitis may result from repeated bouts of acute cholecystitis or from persistent irritation of the gallbladder wall by stones. Bacteria may be present in the bile as well. Chronic cholecystitis often is asymptomatic.

Complications of cholecystitis include *empyema*, a collection of infected fluid within the gallbladder; gangrene and perforation with resulting peritonitis or abscess formation; formation of a fistula into an adjacent organ (such as the duodenum, colon, or stomach); or obstruction of the small intestine by a large gallstone (*gallstone ileus*). Table 25–1 compares the manifestations and complications of acute cholelithiasis with those of cholecystitis.

TABLE 25–1 Manifestations and Complications of Cholelithiasis and Cholecystitis

MANIFESTATIONS	CHOLELITHIASIS	CHOLECYSTITIS
Pain	■ Abrupt onset ■ Severe, steady ■ Localized to epigastrium and RUQ of abdomen ■ May radiate to back, right scapula, and shoulder ■ Lasts 30 minutes to 5 hours	■ Abrupt onset ■ Severe, steady ■ Generalized in RUQ of abdomen ■ May radiate to back, right scapula, and shoulder ■ Lasts 12 to 18 hours ■ Aggravated by movement, breathing
Associated symptoms	■ Nausea, vomiting	■ Anorexia, nausea, vomiting ■ RUQ tenderness and guarding ■ Chills and fever
Complications	■ Cholecystitis ■ Common bile duct obstruction with possible jaundice and liver damage ■ Common duct obstruction with pancreatitis	■ Gangrene and perforation with peritonitis ■ Chronic cholecystitis ■ Empyema ■ Fistula formation ■ Gallstone ileus

Interdisciplinary Care

Treatment of the patient with gallstones depends of the acuity of the condition and the patient's overall health status. When gallstones are present but asymptomatic and the patient has a low risk for complications, conservative treatment is indicated. However, when the patient experiences frequent symptoms, has acute cholecystitis, or has very large stones, the gallbladder and stones are usually surgically removed.

Diagnosis

Diagnostic tests are ordered to identify the presence and location of stones, identify possible complications, and help differentiate gallbladder disease from other disorders.

■ *Serum bilirubin* is measured. Elevated direct (conjugated) bilirubin may indicate obstructed bile flow in the biliary duct system (Box 25–2).

■ *Complete blood count (CBC)* may show an elevated WBC count in the presence of inflammation and infection.

■ *Serum amylase* and *lipase* are measured to identify possible pancreatitis related to common duct obstruction.

■ *Ultrasonography of the gallbladder* is a noninvasive exam that can accurately diagnose cholelithiasis with more than 95% accuracy. It also can be used to assess emptying of the gallbladder.

■ *Abdominal x-ray* (flat plate of the abdomen) may show gallstones that have a high calcium content.

■ *Gallbladder scans* (e.g., HIDA, DIDA, or DISIDA scans) use an intravenous radioactive solution that is rapidly extracted from the blood and excreted into the biliary tree to diagnose cystic duct obstruction and acute or chronic cholecystitis.

∞ See Chapter 21 for more information about and the nursing implications of these diagnostic tests.

Medications

Patients who refuse surgery or for whom surgery is inappropriate may be treated with a drug to dissolve the gallstones. Ursodiol (Actigall) and chenodiol (Chenix) reduce the cholesterol content of gallstones, leading to their gradual dissolution. These drugs act by reducing cholesterol production in the liver, thus reducing the cholesterol content of bile. Consequently,

these drugs are most effective in treating stones with high cholesterol content. They are less effective in treating radiopaque stones with high calcium salt content. Ursodiol is generally well-tolerated with few side effects, whereas chenodiol has a high incidence of diarrhea at therapeutic doses. It also is hepatotoxic, so periodic liver function studies are required during therapy.

The primary disadvantages of pharmacologic treatment for gallstones include its cost, long duration (2 years or more), and the high incidence of recurrent stone formation when treatment is discontinued. If infection is suspected, antibiotics may be ordered to cure the infection and reduce associated inflammation and edema. Patients with pruritus (itching) due to severe obstructive jaundice and an accumulation of bile salts on the skin may be given cholestyramine (Questran). This drug binds with bile salts to promote their excretion in the feces. A opioid analgesic such as morphine may be required for pain relief during an acute attack of cholecystitis.

BOX 25–2 Sorting Out Total, Direct, and Indirect Bilirubin Levels

When serum bilirubin levels are drawn, the results usually are reported as the total bilirubin, direct bilirubin, and indirect bilirubin levels. Most bilirubin is formed from hemoglobin, as aging or abnormal RBCs are removed from circulation and destroyed. It is then bound to protein and transported to the liver. This protein-bound bilirubin is called *indirect* or *unconjugated* bilirubin. Once in the liver, bilirubin is separated from the protein and converted to a soluble form, *direct* or *conjugated* bilirubin. Conjugated bilirubin is then excreted in the bile.

■ Total (serum) bilirubin includes both indirect and direct forms. In adults, the normal total bilirubin is 0.1 to 1.2 mg/dL. Total bilirubin levels increase when more is being produced (e.g., RBC hemolysis), or when its metabolism or excretion are impaired (e.g., liver disease or biliary obstruction).

■ Direct (conjugated) bilirubin levels, normally 0.1 to 0.3 mg/dL in adults, rise when its excretion is impaired by obstruction within the liver (e.g., in cirrhosis, hepatitis, exposure to hepatotoxins) or in the biliary system.

■ Indirect (unconjugated) bilirubin levels, normally < 1.0 mg/dL in adults, rise in RBC hemolysis (e.g., sickle cell disease or transfusion reaction).

Treatments

SURGERY *Laparoscopic cholecystectomy* (removal of the gallbladder) is the treatment of choice for symptomatic cholelithiasis or cholecystitis. This minimally invasive procedure has a low risk of complications and generally requires a hospital stay of less than 24 hours. Not all patients are candidates for laparoscopic cholecystectomy, and there is a risk that a laparoscopic cholecystectomy may be converted to a *laparotomy* (surgical opening into the abdomen) during the procedure. See the accompanying box for nursing care for a patient having a laparoscopic cholecystectomy.

When stones are lodged within the ducts, a cholecystectomy with common bile duct exploration may be done. A T-tube (Figure 25–2 ■) is inserted to maintain patency of the duct and promote bile passage while the edema decreases. Excess bile is collected in a drainage bag secured below the surgical site. If it is suspected that a stone has been retained following surgery, a postoperative cholangiogram via the T-tube or direct visualization of the duct with an endoscope may be performed. See the box on page 725 for nursing care for a patient with a T-tube.

Some patients who are poor surgical risks and for whom laparoscopic cholecystectomy is inappropriate may have either a *cholecystostomy* to drain the gallbladder, or a *choledochostomy* to remove stones and position a T-tube in the common bile duct.

NUTRITION Food intake may be eliminated during an acute attack of cholecystitis, and a nasogastric tube inserted to relieve nausea and vomiting. Dietary fat intake may be limited, especially if the patient is obese. If bile flow is obstructed, fat-soluble vitamins (A, D, E, and K) and bile salts may need to be administered.

OTHER THERAPIES In some cases, shock wave lithotripsy may be used with drug therapy to dissolve large gallstones. In *extracorporeal shock wave lithotripsy*, ultrasound is used to align the stones with the source of shock waves and the computerized lithotripter. Positioning is of prime importance throughout the procedure, which usually takes an hour. Mild

NURSING CARE OF THE PATIENT
Having Laparoscopic Cholecystectomy

PREOPERATIVE CARE
- Provide routine preoperative care as ordered (∞ see Chapter 4).
- Assess for manifestations of cholecystitis and other complications of gallstones. *An acutely inflamed gallbladder and ductal system increases surgical complexity and may necessitate open cholecystectomy.*
- Reinforce teaching about the procedure and postoperative expectations, including pain management, deep breathing, and mobilization. *Preoperative teaching reduces anxiety and promotes rapid postoperative recovery.*

POSTOPERATIVE CARE
- Provide routine postoperative recovery care as outlined in ∞ Chapter 4.
- Treat postoperative pain and nausea and vomiting prophylactically and as needed to relieve symptoms. *Postoperative pain is common during the first 24 to 48 hours after surgery. Manipulation of the bowel and insufflation of the abdomen with gas commonly lead to postoperative nausea (Graham, 2008).*
- Assist to chair at bedside as allowed. *Early mobilization promotes lung ventilation and circulation, reducing the potential for postoperative complications.*
- Advance oral intake from ice chips to regular diet as tolerated. *Oral intake can be rapidly resumed due to minimal disruption of the gastrointestinal tract during surgery.*
- Provide and reinforce teaching: pain management, incision care, activity level, postoperative follow-up appointments. *With early discharge, the patient and family assume responsibility for the majority of postoperative care. A clear understanding of this care and expected needs reduces anxiety and the risk of postoperative complications.*
- Initiate follow-up contact 24 to 48 hours after discharge to evaluate adequacy of pain control, incision management, and discharge understanding. *Contact following discharge provides an opportunity to evaluate care and reinforce teaching.*

sedation may be given during the procedure. Nursing care after the procedure includes monitoring for biliary colic, which can result from the gallbladder contracting to remove stone fragments; nausea; and transient hematuria. *Percutaneous cholecystostomy*, ultrasound-guided drainage of the gallbladder, may be done in high-risk patients to postpone or even eliminate the need for surgery.

COMPLEMENTARY THERAPIES The herb goldenseal has been used in treating cholecystitis. One of the active ingredients in goldenseal, berberine, stimulates secretion of bile and bilirubin. It also inhibits the growth of many common pathogens, including those known to infect the gallbladder. A study of the effectiveness of berberine in patients with cholecystitis demonstrated relief of all symptoms. Goldenseal can stimulate the uterus, so it is contraindicated for use during pregnancy and lactation. An herbal formula composed of peppermint and wormwood extracts is believed by some to promote emptying of the gallbladder and increase bile salts, thereby reducing the recurrence and growth of gallstones (Chi, 2008).

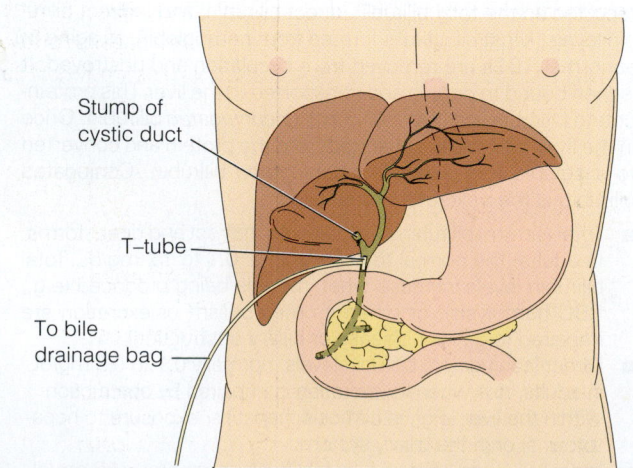

Stump of cystic duct

T–tube

To bile drainage bag

Figure 25–2 ■ T-tube placement in the common bile duct. Bile fluid flows with gravity into a drainage collection device below the level of the common bile duct.

- Ensure that the T-tube is properly connected to a sterile container; keep the tube below the level of the surgical wound. *This position promotes the flow of bile and prevents backflow or seepage of caustic bile onto the skin. The tube itself decreases biliary tree pressure.*
- Monitor drainage from the T-tube for color and consistency; record as output. Normally, the tube may drain up to 500 mL in the first 24 hours after surgery; drainage decreases to less than 200 mL in 2 to 3 days, and is minimal thereafter. Drainage may be blood tinged initially, changing to green-brown. Report excessive drainage immediately (after 48 hours, drainage greater than 500 mL is considered excessive). *Stones or edema and inflammation can obstruct ducts below the tube, requiring treatment.*
- Place in Fowler's position. *This promotes gravity drainage of bile.*
- Assess skin for bile leakage during dressing changes. *Bile irritates the skin; it may be necessary to apply skin protection with karaya or another barrier product.*
- Teach patient how to manage the tube when turning, ambulating, and performing activities of daily living. *Direct pulling or traction on the tube must be avoided.*
- If indicated, teach care of the T-tube, how to clamp it, and signs of infection. *Patients may be discharged home with the tube in place. Reporting early signs of infection facilitates prompt treatment.*

Nursing Care

In addition to the nursing care discussed in this section, a Case Study & Nursing Care Plan for a patient with cholelithiasis is found on page 727.

Health Promotion

Although most risk factors for cholelithiasis cannot be controlled or modified, several can. Modifiable risk factors include obesity, hyperlipidemia, extremely low-calorie diets, and diets high in cholesterol. By contrast, physical activity, a high-fiber and low carbohydrate diet, and consumption of unsaturated fats all appear to have a protective effect, reducing the incidence of gallstones and cholecystitis. Discuss the dangers of "yo-yo" dieting, with cycles of weight loss followed by weight gain, and of extremely low-calorie diets. Encourage patients with high serum cholesterol levels to discuss using cholesterol-lowering drugs with their primary care provider.

Assessment

Assessment data related to cholelithiasis and cholecystitis include the following:

- *Health history:* Current manifestations, including RUQ pain, its character and relationship to meals, duration, and radiation, nausea and vomiting, or other symptoms; duration of symptoms; risk factors or previous history of symptoms; chronic diseases such as diabetes, cirrhosis, or inflammatory bowel disease; current diet; use of oral contraceptives or possibility of pregnancy.

- *Physical assessment:* Current weight; color of skin and sclera; abdominal assessment including light palpation for tenderness; color of urine and stool.
- *Diagnostic tests:* Monitor results of WBC, serum bilirubin, liver enzymes, and pancreatic enzymes (amylase and lipase).

Nursing Diagnoses and Interventions

Priority nursing diagnoses for the patient with cholelithiasis or cholecystitis often include pain related to biliary colic or surgery, imbalanced nutrition related to the effects of altered bile flow and to nausea and anorexia, and risk for infection related to potential rupture of an acutely inflamed gallbladder. Nursing interventions for the patient who has undergone a laparoscopic or open cholecystectomy are similar to those for other patients having abdominal surgery. (∞ See Chapter 4.)

Pain

The pain associated with cholelithiasis can be severe. Sometimes a combination of interventions is indicated.

- Discuss the relationship between fat intake and the pain. Teach ways to reduce fat intake (Box 25–3). *Fat entering the duodenum initiates gallbladder contractions, causing pain when gallstones are present in the ducts.*
- Withhold oral food and fluids during episodes of acute pain. Insert nasogastric tube and connect to low suction if ordered. *Emptying the stomach reduces the amount of chyme entering the duodenum and the stimulus for gallbladder contractions, thus reducing pain.*
- For severe pain, administer morphine, fentanyl, or other narcotic analgesia as ordered. *Recent research indicates that morphine is no more likely to cause spasms of the sphincter of Oddi than meperidine.*
- Place in Fowler's position. *Fowler's position decreases pressure on the inflamed gallbladder.*
- Monitor vital signs, including temperature, at least every 4 hours. *Bacterial infection often is present in acute cholecystitis, and may cause an elevated temperature and respiratory rate.*

Imbalanced Nutrition: Less than Body Requirements

The patient with severe gallbladder disease may develop nutritional imbalances related to anorexia, pain, and nausea following meals, and impaired bile flow that alters absorption of fat and fat-soluble vitamins (A, D, E, and K) from the gut.

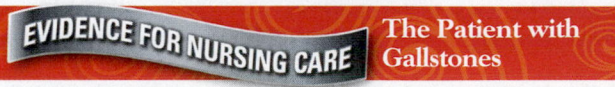

EVIDENCE FOR NURSING CARE   **The Patient with Gallstones**

Selected resources that nurses may find helpful when planning evidence-based nursing care follow.

- Holcomb, S. S. (2008). Acute abdomen: What a pain! *Nursing2008, 38*(9), 34–40.
- Society of American Gastrointestinal and Endoscopic Surgeons (SAGES). (2007, November). *Diagnostic laparoscopy for acute abdominal pain. In: Diagnostic laparoscopy guidelines.* Los Angeles, CA: Society of American Gastrointestinal and Endoscopic Surgeons (SAGES).

BOX 25–3 Examples of High-Fat Foods

- Whole-milk products (e.g., cream, ice cream, cheese)
- Doughnuts, deep-fried
- Avocados
- Sausage, bacon, hot dogs
- Gravies with fat, cream
- Most nuts (e.g., pecans, cashews)
- Corn chips and potato chips
- Butter and cooking oils
- Fried foods (e.g., cheeseburgers, hamburgers, french fries)
- Peanut butter
- Chocolate candies

- Assess nutritional status, including diet history, height and weight, and skinfold measurements (∞ see Chapters 21 and 22). *Even though often obese, patients with gallbladder disease may have an imbalanced diet or may have specific vitamin deficiencies, particularly of the fat-soluble vitamins.*
- Evaluate laboratory results, including serum bilirubin, albumin, glucose, and cholesterol levels. Report abnormal results to the primary care provider. *Elevated serum bilirubin may indicate impaired bilirubin excretion due to obstructed bile flow. A low serum albumin may indicate poor nutritional status. Glucose intolerance and hypercholesterolemia are risk factors for cholelithiasis.*
- Refer to a dietitian or nutritionist for diet counseling to promote healthy weight loss and reduce pain episodes. *A low-carbohydrate, low-fat, higher protein diet reduces symptoms of cholecystitis. While fasting and very-low-calorie diets are contraindicated, a moderate reduction in calorie intake and increased activity levels promote weight loss.*
- Administer vitamin supplements as ordered. *Patients who do not absorb fat well due to obstructed bile flow may require supplements of the fat-soluble vitamins.*

Risk for Infection

An acutely inflamed gallbladder may become necrotic and rupture, releasing its contents into the abdominal cavity. While the resulting infection often remains localized, peritonitis can result from chemical irritation and bacterial contamination of the peritoneal cavity.

PRACTICE ALERT

Rupture of an acutely inflamed gallbladder may be heralded by abrupt but transient pain relief as contents are released from the distended gallbladder into the abdomen. Promptly report this change to the physician.

Following open cholecystectomy (*laparotomy*), the risk for pulmonary infection is significant due to the high abdominal incision.

- Monitor vital signs including temperature every 4 hours. Promptly report vital sign changes or temperature elevation. *Tachycardia, increased respiratory rate, or an elevated temperature may indicate an infectious process.*
- Assess abdomen every 4 hours and as indicated (e.g., when pain level changes abruptly). *Increasing abdominal*

tenderness or a rigid, boardlike abdomen may indicate rupture of the gallbladder with peritonitis.

- Assist to cough and deep breathe or use incentive spirometer every 1 to 2 hours while awake. Splint abdominal incision with a blanket or pillow during coughing. *The high abdominal incision of an open cholecystectomy interferes with effective coughing and deep breathing, increasing the risk of atelectasis and respiratory infections such as pneumonia.*
- Place in Fowler's position and encourage ambulation as allowed. *Fowler's position and ambulating promote lung expansion and airway clearance, reducing the risk of respiratory infections.*
- Administer antibiotics as ordered. *Antibiotics may be given preoperatively to reduce the risk of infection from infected gallbladder contents, and may be continued postoperatively to prevent infection.*

Community-Based Care

Teaching varies, depending on the choice of treatment options for cholelithiasis and cholecystitis. If surgery is not an option, teach about medications that dissolve stones, their use and adverse effects (diarrhea is a common side effect), and maintaining a low-fat and low-carbohydrate diet if indicated. Include an explanation about the role of bile and the function of the gallbladder in terms that the patient and family can understand.

Provide appropriate preoperative teaching for the planned procedure. Discuss the possibility of open cholecystectomy even when a laparoscopic procedure is planned. Teach postoperative self-care measures to manage pain and prevent complications. If the patient will be discharged with a T-tube, provide instructions about its care (see the Nursing Care box on page 725). Discuss manifestations of complications to report to the physician. Stress the importance of follow-up appointments.

Following cholecystectomy, a low-fat diet may be initially recommended. Refer the patient and food preparer to a dietitian to review low-fat foods. (See Box 25–3 for examples of high-fat foods to avoid.) Higher fat foods may be gradually added to the diet as tolerated.

The Patient with Cancer of the Gallbladder

Gallbladder cancer is rare, primarily affecting people over age 65. Women are more likely to develop the disorder. Manifestations of gallbladder cancer include intense pain and a palpable mass in the RUQ of the abdomen. Jaundice and weight loss are common. Gallbladder cancers spread by direct extension to the liver, and metastasize via the blood and lymph system.

At the time of diagnosis, the cancer usually is too advanced to treat surgically. Ninety-five percent of patients with primary cancer of the gallbladder die within 1 year. Radical and extensive surgical interventions may be performed, but the prognosis is poor regardless of treatment. Nursing care is palliative, focusing on maintaining comfort and independence to the extent possible.

CASE STUDY & NURSING CARE PLAN   A Patient with Cholelithiasis

Joyce Red Wing is a 44-year-old married mother of three children. A member of the Chickasaw tribe, she is active in tribal activities and works part time as a cook at a community kitchen. Recently Mrs. Red Wing has noticed a dull pain in her upper abdomen that gets worse after eating fatty foods; nausea and sometimes vomiting accompany the pain. She had a similar pain after the birth of her last child. She is diagnosed with cholelithiasis, and is admitted for a laparoscopic cholecystectomy.

ASSESSMENT

David Corbin, RN, takes Mrs. Red Wing's admission history. It includes intolerance to fatty foods and intermittent "stabbing" abdominal pain that radiates to her back. Her usual diet includes tacos or fried bread and biscuits with gravy for breakfast. She reports "not wanting to eat much of anything lately." She states she has never had surgery before and hopes "everything goes well." Physical assessment includes T 100°F (37.7°C), P 88, R 20, and BP 130/84. She has had a recent 5 lb weight loss, currently weighing 130 lb (59 kg). She is 63 inches (160 cm) tall. Abdominal examination elicits tenderness in the right upper abdominal quadrant. She has no jaundice, chills, or evidence of complications.

DIAGNOSES

- *Imbalanced Nutrition: Less than Body Requirements* related to anorexia and recent weight loss
- *Acute Pain* related to inflamed gallbladder and surgical incisions
- *Risk for Infection* related to potential bacterial contamination of abdominal cavity
- *Anxiety* related to lack of information about perioperative experience

EXPECTED OUTCOMES

- Maintain present weight within 5 lb (2.3 kg) over the next 3 weeks.
- Resume regular diet, decreasing intake of foods high in fat.

- Verbalize adequate pain control after surgery and with activity resumption.
- Remain free of infection.
- Verbalize a decrease in anxiety before surgery.

PLANNING AND IMPLEMENTATION

- Teach about the gallbladder and the function of bile.
- Discuss pre- and postoperative care, including self-care following discharge.
- Promote mobility as soon as allowed after surgery.
- Teach home care of incisions and recognition of signs of infection.
- Review specific high-fat foods to avoid and ways to maintain her weight.
- Provide analgesia as needed postoperatively. Teach appropriate analgesic use after discharge.

EVALUATION

Mrs. Red Wing is discharged the morning after her surgery. She is afebrile, has no signs of infection, and is able to appropriately care for her incisions. She identifies signs of infection and talks about ways to reduce her fat intake while keeping her weight stable. She verbalizes understanding of initial activity restrictions and resumption of normal activities. Mrs. Red Wing states, "It wasn't as bad as I thought it would be at first." She has an appointment to see her surgeon in 1 week.

CRITICAL THINKING IN THE NURSING PROCESS

1. What is the rationale for a low-fat diet with cholelithiasis? Discuss nutritional practices as they relate to the medical problem and Mrs. Red Wing's culture.
2. How would your discharge teaching for Mrs. Red Wing differ if she had had an open cholecystectomy instead of a laparoscopic cholecystectomy?
3. Design a nursing care plan for Mrs. Red Wing for the nursing diagnosis *Fatigue*.

See Evaluating Your Response in Appendix C.

Liver Disorders

The liver is a complex organ with multiple metabolic and regulatory functions. Optimal liver function is essential to health. Because of the significant amount of blood in the liver at all times, it is exposed to the effects of pathogens, drugs, toxins, and possibly malignant cells. As a result, liver cells may become inflamed or damaged, or cancerous tumors may develop.

Physiology Review

The essential functions of the liver include the metabolism of proteins, carbohydrates, and fats. It also is responsible for the metabolism of steroid hormones and most drugs. It synthesizes essential blood proteins, including albumin and clotting factors in particular. The liver detoxifies alcohol and other toxic substances. Ammonia, a toxic by-product of protein metabolism, is converted to urea in the liver for elimination by the kidneys. The liver produces bile, an essential substance for absorbing fats and eliminating bilirubin from the body. Minerals and fat-soluble vitamins are stored in the liver, as is glycogen (stored carbohydrate for energy reserves). The Kupffer cells that line the sinusoids phagocytize foreign cells and damaged blood cells. ∞ See Chapter 21 for more information about the liver.

Common Manifestations of Liver Disorders

Although many different disorders can disrupt liver function, their manifestations relate to three primary effects: disrupted liver cell function, impaired bilirubin conversion and excretion leading to jaundice, and disrupted blood flow through the liver, with resulting portal hypertension.

Hepatocellular Failure

The liver is vital to digestion and metabolism of nutrients; the production of plasma proteins, including those involved in clotting; and the metabolism and excretion of compounds such as bilirubin, steroid hormones, and ammonia, as well as toxins (such as alcohol) and drugs. Impaired function of liver cells has multiple effects, including the following:

- Impaired protein metabolism with decreased production of albumin and clotting factors. Low albumin levels contribute to edema in peripheral tissues and **ascites**, accumulation of fluid in the abdomen (Figure 25–3 ■), as plasma oncotic pressure is reduced. Impaired clotting factor production increases the risk for bleeding.

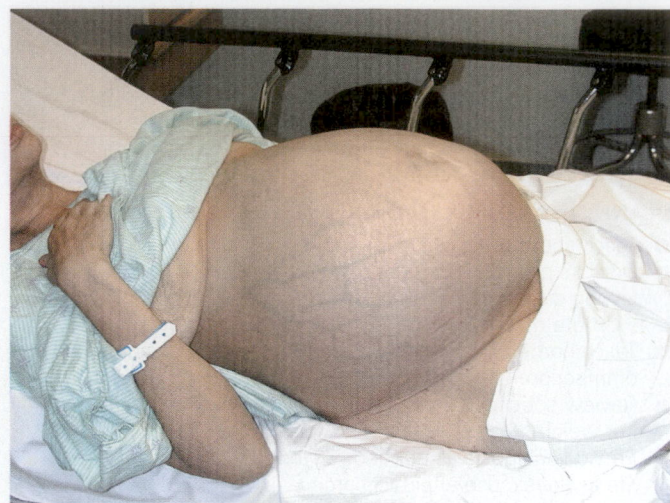

Figure 25–3 ■ In ascites, serous fluid collects in the abdominal cavity, causing uniform distension.

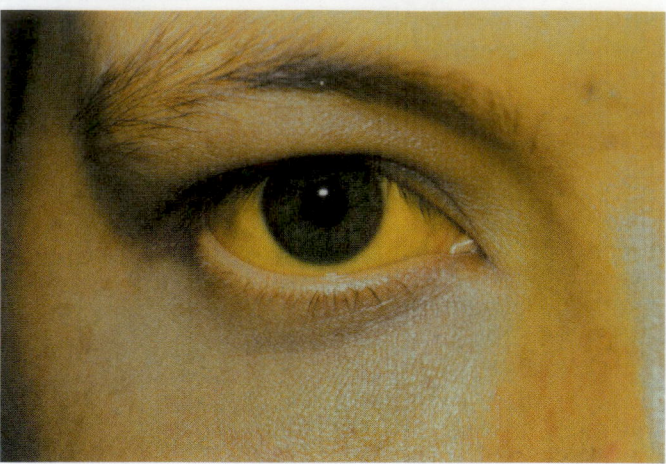

Figure 25–4 ■ Jaundice. Note the yellowing of the white (sclera) of the eye and of the surrounding facial skin.

- Disrupted glucose metabolism and storage with resulting alterations in blood glucose levels (either hyperglycemia or hypoglycemia).
- Reduced bile production that impairs the absorption of lipids and fat-soluble vitamins. Inadequate vitamin K, a fat-soluble vitamin, affects the production of clotting factors, leading to a bleeding tendency.
- Impaired metabolism of steroid hormones (including estrogen and testosterone) leads to feminization in men and irregular menses in women.

Jaundice

Disrupted metabolism and excretion of bilirubin allows it to accumulate in tissues, leading to **jaundice**, yellow staining of tissues (Figure 25–4 ■). Jaundice (also called *icterus*) often is first noticeable in the sclera of the eyes, then the skin.

When RBCs are destroyed (due to cell aging or disease), hemoglobin is released. The hemoglobin molecule breaks up into globin, a protein, and heme, the iron-containing portion of the molecule. In this process, biliverdin, later converted to fat-soluble bilirubin (*unconjugated bilirubin*), is released. The bilirubin binds with albumin to be transported to the liver. In the liver, it is converted to a water-soluble form (*conjugated bilirubin*) to be excreted in the bile. See Box 25–2 for more information about bilirubin metabolism.

Jaundice can result from disruptions at any point in the production and metabolism of bilirubin:

- *Hemolytic jaundice* develops when excess RBC destruction (hemolysis) releases more bilirubin into circulation than the liver is able to process. High blood levels of unconjugated bilirubin are seen.
- *Hepatic jaundice* occurs when impaired liver cell (*hepatocyte*) function disrupts the conversion and excretion of bilirubin. Blood levels of both conjugated and unconjugated bilirubin may be elevated. Stools may appear normal or clay colored, and urine is dark because the conjugated bilirubin is excreted by the kidneys.

- Obstruction of bile flow within the biliary system (the gallbladder and bile ducts) impairs bilirubin excretion, leading to *obstructive jaundice*. Levels of conjugated bilirubin are elevated. Stools are light or clay colored due to lack of bile pigment; and urine is dark because the kidneys excrete bilirubin.

Portal Hypertension

Impaired blood flow through the liver increases pressure in the portal venous system that drains the gastrointestinal tract, the spleen, and surface veins of the abdomen. **Portal hypertension**, increased pressure in the portal system, has several effects when it is prolonged:

- Dilation of veins in the gastrointestinal tract and the abdominal wall. This congestion tends to suppress the appetite and lead to formation of collateral vessels in the distal esophagus, stomach, and rectum. The dilated, congested vessels in the esophagus are known as **esophageal varices**; in the rectum, they lead to the development of hemorrhoids. In advanced liver failure, superficial varices may develop around the umbilicus, a feature known as *caput medusae*.
- Splenomegaly, or enlargement of the spleen.
- Ascites, accumulation of fluid in the peritoneal cavity. Increased hydrostatic pressure in abdominal vessels forces fluid out of the vessels and into the peritoneal cavity. Low serum albumin levels (*hypoalbuminemia*) contribute to fluid accumulation by reducing the osmotic draw of fluid back into vessels.
- **Portal systemic encephalopathy** (or *hepatic encephalopathy*), impaired consciousness and mental status due to the accumulation of toxic waste products in the blood (ammonia in particular) as blood bypasses the congested liver. It appears that factors other than elevated ammonia levels contribute, including toxic fatty acids, altered neurotransmitters, and an imbalance of plasma amino acid ratios. Cerebral edema develops late in the course of liver failure, resulting from both the accumulation of toxins and vascular mechanisms. As cerebral edema

progresses, intracranial pressure increases, cerebral perfusion decreases, and brain cells become hypoxic.

■ *Hepatorenal syndrome* is acute renal failure due to disrupted blood flow to the kidneys. ∞ See Chapter 28 for more information about renal failure.

See the section of this chapter on cirrhosis for more information about the effects and complications associated with portal hypertension.

The Patient with Hepatitis

Hepatitis is inflammation of the liver. It is usually caused by a virus, although it may result from exposure to alcohol, drugs and toxins, or other pathogens. Hepatitis may be acute or chronic in nature. Cirrhosis, discussed in the next section, is a potential consequence of severe hepatocellular damage. Chronic hepatitis also increases the risk for developing liver cancer.

Pathophysiology and Manifestations

The inflammatory process of hepatitis, whether caused by a virus, toxin, or other mechanism, damages hepatic cells and disrupts liver function. Cell-mediated immune responses damage hepatocytes and Kupffer cells, leading to hyperplasia, necrosis, and cellular regeneration. The flow of bile through bile canaliculi and into the biliary system can be impaired by the inflammatory process, leading to jaundice. When the inflammatory process is mild (e.g., hepatitis A), the liver parenchyma is not significantly damaged. The inflammatory processes associated with hepatitis B and hepatitis C, however, can lead to severe liver damage. The metabolism of nutrients, drugs, alcohol, and toxins and the process of bile elimination are disrupted by the inflammation of hepatitis. ∞ See Chapter 21 for more information about the liver, and the preceding section for more information about the effects of disrupted liver function.

Viral Hepatitis

Viral hepatitis is nearly always caused by one of five viruses: hepatitis A virus (HAV), hepatitis B virus (HBV), hepatitis C virus (HCV), the hepatitis B-associated delta virus (HDV), and

hepatitis E virus (HEV). With the exception of HBV, all of the hepatitis viruses are RNA viruses; HBV is a DNA virus. The viruses differ from one another in mode of transmission, incubation period, the severity and type of liver damage they cause, and their ability to become chronic or develop a carrier (asymptomatic) state. The illnesses they cause, however, are clinically very similar. Table 25–2 identifies unique features of the primary hepatitis viruses.

FAST FACTS

In the United States, hepatitis A, hepatitis B, and hepatitis C dominate.

■ Hepatitis A is less common than hepatitis B, with a reported 2,979 acute cases reported in 2007. The rate of hepatitis A infections per 100,000 population has fallen steadily since the introduction of hepatitis A vaccine, to the lowest ever reported rate of 1.0 in 2007.

■ There were 4,519 reported cases of hepatitis B in 2007. The rate of reported hepatitis B infections peaked at 11.5 per 100,000 population in 1985, since then falling to 1.5.

■ In 2007, 849 cases of hepatitis C were reported, for a national rate of 0.3 per 100,000 population.

■ The estimated number of actual new cases of viral hepatitis is significantly higher than the number of reported cases: An estimated 25,000 new cases of hepatitis A, 43,000 new cases of hepatitis B, and 17,000 new cases of hepatitis C are believed to have developed in 2007 (Centers for Disease Control and Prevention [CDC], 2009).

Hepatitis viruses replicate in the liver, indirectly damaging liver cells (hepatocytes). The viruses provoke an immune response that causes inflammation and necrosis of hepatocytes, leading to the clinical presentation of acute disease. Although the extent of damage and the immune response vary among the different hepatitis viruses, the disease itself usually follows a predictable pattern.

No manifestations are present during the incubation period after exposure to the virus. The *prodromal* or *preicteric* (before jaundice) *phase* may begin abruptly or insidiously, with general malaise, anorexia, fatigue, and muscle and body aches.

TABLE 25–2 Comparison of Types of Viral Hepatitis

VIRUS	HEPATITIS A (HAV)	HEPATITIS B (HBV)	HEPATITIS C (HCV)	HEPATITIS D (HDV)	HEPATITIS E (HEV)
Mode of transmission	Fecal–oral	Blood and body fluids; perinatal	Blood and body fluids	Blood and body fluids; perinatal	Fecal–oral
Incubation (in weeks)	2–6	6–24	5–12	3–13	3–6
Onset	Abrupt	Slow	Slow	Abrupt	Abrupt
Carrier state	No	Yes	Yes	Yes	Yes
Possible complications	Rare	Chronic hepatitis Cirrhosis Liver cancer	Chronic hepatitis Cirrhosis Liver cancer	Chronic hepatitis Cirrhosis Fulminant hepatitis	May be severe in pregnant women
Laboratory findings	Anti-HAV antibodies present	Positive HBsAg (HBV surface antigen); anti-HBV antibodies present	Anti-HCV antibodies present	Positive HDVAg (delta antigen) early; anti-HDV antibodies later	Anti-HEV antibodies present

These manifestations often are mistaken for the flu. Nausea, vomiting, diarrhea, or constipation may develop, as well as mild RUQ abdominal pain. Chills and fever may be present.

The *icteric* (jaundiced) *phase* usually begins 5 to 10 days after the onset of symptoms. It is heralded by jaundice of the sclera, skin, and mucous membranes. Inflammation of the liver and bile ducts prevents bilirubin from being excreted into the small intestine. As a result, the serum bilirubin levels are elevated, causing yellowing of the skin and mucous membranes. Pruritus may develop due to deposition of bile salts on the skin. The stools are light brown or clay colored because bile pigment is not excreted through the normal fecal pathway. Instead, the pigment is excreted by the kidneys, causing the urine to turn brown. Whereas patients with acute hepatitis A or B are likely to develop jaundice, many people with hepatitis C do not develop jaundice. As a result, the infection may go undiagnosed for an extended period of time.

During the icteric phase, the initial prodromal manifestations usually diminish even though the serum bilirubin increases. The appetite increases, and the temperature returns to normal. When uncomplicated, spontaneous recovery usually begins within 2 weeks of the onset of jaundice.

The *convalescent phase* follows jaundice and lasts several weeks. During this time, manifestations gradually improve: Serum enzymes decrease, liver pain decreases, and gastrointestinal symptoms and weakness subside. See the accompanying box for the manifestations of each phase of hepatitis.

HEPATITIS A   Hepatitis A, or *infectious hepatitis,* is transmitted by the fecal–oral route via contaminated food, water, shellfish, and direct contact with an infected person. International travel is the primary risk factor for developing hepatitis A; others include close household or sexual contact with an infected partner (CDC, 2009). The virus is in the stool of infected persons up to 2 weeks before symptoms develop. Once jaundice develops, the amount of virus in the stool and the risk of spreading the disease decrease significantly. Although hepatitis A usually has an abrupt onset, it is typically a benign and self-limited disease with few long-term consequences. Symptoms last up to 2 months.

HEPATITIS B   Hepatitis B can cause acute hepatitis, chronic hepatitis, *fulminant* (rapidly progressive) hepatitis, or a carrier state. Less than 5% of adults infected with hepatitis B develop chronic hepatitis (National Institutes of Health [NIH], 2008). In a *carrier state*, the person harbors the active virus and is capable of spreading it to others, even though there are no discernible manifestations of the disease. It is more likely to develop when the virus is acquired at birth from an infected mother (Fauci et al., 2008). This virus is spread through contact with infected blood and body fluids. High-risk groups for hepatitis B include injection drug users, people with multiple sex partners, men who have sex with other men, and people frequently exposed to blood products (such as people on hemodialysis). Healthcare workers are at risk through exposure to blood and needle-stick injuries. Hepatitis B is a risk factor for primary liver cancer, particularly in people who are infected perinatally (Fauci et al., 2008).

In hepatitis B, liver cells are damaged by the immune response to this antigen. Damage may affect only portions or the majority of the liver. The liver shows evidence of injury and scarring, regeneration, and proliferation of inflammatory cells. During the prodromal period, patients with HBV may experience such immune-mediated manifestations as urticaria and other rashes, arthralgias, serum sickness, or glomerulonephritis (Copstead & Banasik, 2010). The disease itself may be asymptomatic.

HEPATITIS C   Hepatitis C, formerly known as non-A, non-B hepatitis, is the primary worldwide cause of chronic hepatitis, cirrhosis, and liver cancer (Porth & Matfin, 2009). It is transmitted through infected blood and body fluids. Injection drug use is the primary risk factor for HCV infection, accounting for nearly half of all new infections (CDC, 2009). Acute hepatitis C usually is asymptomatic; if symptoms do develop, they often are mild and nonspecific. The disease often is recognized long after exposure occurred, when secondary effects of the disease (such as chronic hepatitis or cirrhosis) develop. Only about 15% of acute infections completely resolve; most progress to chronic active hepatitis (Copstead & Banasik, 2010).

> **SAFETY ALERT**
> Nurses frequently care for patients whose hepatitis antigen status is unknown or who have a secondary diagnosis of chronic hepatitis B or C. Exercise Standard Precautions including hand hygiene and personal protective equipment use with all patients to reduce the risk of exposure to these blood borne pathogens.

HEPATITIS DELTA   Hepatitis delta only causes infection in people who also are infected with hepatitis B. It can cause acute or chronic infection, and can increase the severity of HBV infection (Porth & Matfin, 2009). It is transmitted in the same manner as HBV; as the number of people with immunity to HBV has increased, the incidence of hepatitis delta has decreased (Fauci et al., 2008).

HEPATITIS E   Hepatitis E is rare in the United States. It is transmitted by fecal contamination of water supplies in developing areas such as southeast Asia, parts of Africa, and Central

MANIFESTATIONS **of Acute Hepatitis**

PREICTERIC PHASE
- "Flulike" symptoms: malaise, fatigue, fever
- Gastrointestinal: anorexia, nausea, vomiting, diarrhea, constipation
- Muscle aches, polyarthritis
- Mild right upper abdominal pain and tenderness

ICTERIC PHASE
- Jaundice
- Pruritus
- Clay-colored stools
- Brown urine
- Decrease in preicteric phase symptoms (e.g., appetite improves; no fever)

POSTICTERIC/CONVALESCENT PHASE
- Serum bilirubin and enzymes return to normal levels
- Energy level increases
- Pain subsides
- Gastrointestinal: minimal to absent

America. Person-to-person transmission is rare. It primarily affects young adults. It can cause fulminant, fatal hepatitis in pregnant women.

Chronic Hepatitis

Chronic hepatitis is chronic infection of the liver. Although it may cause few symptoms, it is the primary cause of liver damage leading to cirrhosis, liver cancer, and liver transplantation. Three of the known hepatitis viruses cause chronic hepatitis: HBV, HCV, and HDV. Patients with chronic hepatitis may have periods of active liver disease interspersed with periods of inactivity. Liver damage and fibrosis variably progress during periods of disease activity (NIH, 2008). Manifestations of chronic hepatitis include malaise, fatigue, and hepatomegaly. Occasional icteric (jaundiced) periods may occur. Liver enzymes, particularly serum aminotransferase levels, typically are elevated.

In chronic active hepatitis, inflammation extends to involve entire hepatic lobules. Chronic active hepatitis usually leads to cirrhosis and end-stage liver failure.

Fulminant Hepatitis

Fulminant hepatitis is a rapidly progressive disease, with liver failure developing within 2 to 3 weeks after the onset of symptoms. Although uncommon, it is usually related to HBV with concurrent HDV infection.

Toxic Hepatitis

Many substances, including alcohol, certain drugs, and other toxins, can directly damage liver cells. Alcoholic hepatitis can result from chronic alcohol abuse or from an acute toxic reaction to alcohol. Alcoholic hepatitis causes necrosis of hepatocytes and inflammation of the liver parenchyma (functional tissue). Unless alcohol intake is avoided, progression to cirrhosis is common.

Other potential hepatotoxins include acetaminophen, benzene, carbon tetrachloride, halothane, chloroform, and poisonous mushrooms. These substances directly damage liver cells, leading to necrosis. The degree of damage often depends on age and the extent of exposure (dose) to the hepatotoxin. Acetaminophen overdose is the leading cause of acute liver failure.

Autoimmune Hepatitis

Autoimmune hepatitis is a chronic disorder in which a cell-mediated immune response directed against liver cells causes persistent inflammation and necrosis with fibrosis and scarring. Circulating autoantibodies such as antinuclear antibody (ANA) usually are present. Many affected individuals have a personal or family history of other autoimmune disorders, such as rheumatoid arthritis or thyroiditis, suggesting a genetic link to the disorder. Chronic autoimmune hepatitis can ultimately lead to cirrhosis and liver failure.

Interdisciplinary Care

Management of hepatitis focuses on determining its cause, providing appropriate treatment and support, and teaching strategies to prevent further liver damage. Effective management begins with thorough assessment of diagnostic and laboratory data.

Diagnosis

Liver function tests, such as blood levels of bilirubin and enzymes commonly released when liver cells are damaged, are obtained. These include the following:

- *Alanine aminotransferase (ALT)* is an enzyme contained within each liver cell. When liver cells are damaged, ALT is released into the blood. Levels may exceed 1000 U/L or more in acute hepatitis.
- *Aspartate aminotransferase (AST)* is an enzyme found predominantly in heart and liver cells. AST levels rise when liver cells are damaged; with severe damage, blood levels may be 20 to 100 times normal values.
- *Alkaline phosphatase (ALP)* is an enzyme present in liver cells and bone. Serum ALP levels often are elevated in hepatitis, and may remain elevated after ALT and AST levels have returned to normal ranges.
- *Serum bilirubin* levels, including *conjugated* and *unconjugated*, are elevated in viral hepatitis due to impaired bilirubin metabolism and obstruction of the hepatobiliary ducts by inflammation and edema. The bilirubin level decreases as inflammation and edema subside.
- Laboratory tests for viral antigens and their specific antibodies may be done to identify the infecting virus and its state of activity. These tests are summarized in Table 25–2.
- A *liver biopsy* may be done to detect and evaluate chronic hepatitis. (Nursing implications for this test are outlined in ∞ Chapter 21.)

∞ See Chapter 21 for more information about diagnostic tests and their nursing implications.

Medications

PREVENTION Hepatitis A and hepatitis B are preventable diseases. Vaccines are available, as are preparations to prevent the disease following known or suspected exposure.

Vaccines Hepatitis A vaccine provides long-term protection against HAV infection. It is an inactivated whole-virus vaccine available in pediatric and adult formulations. Although more than 95% of adults achieve immunity after one dose of the vaccine, two doses are recommended for full protection. See Table 25–3.

Three doses of hepatitis B vaccine provide immunity to HBV infection in 90% of healthy adults. Because the hepatitis delta virus requires the presence of the hepatitis B virus, hepatitis B vaccine also protects against HDV. Hepatitis B vaccine is a recombinant vaccine. Vaccines produced by different manufacturers may be used interchangeably, although their dosages differ. Older adults are less likely to achieve immunity than younger adults. Patients on hemodialysis and people who are immunocompromised may need larger or more doses of the vaccine to achieve adequate protection. Serologic testing for immunity is recommended on completion of the series for people in these high-risk groups.

A combined hepatitis A and hepatitis B vaccine is available for use. It is recommended for the same high-risk populations as the single vaccines. Three doses are given: the initial dose, followed by doses no sooner than 4 weeks and 6 months later.

TABLE 25–3 CDC Recommendations for Hepatitis Prevention in Adults

DISEASE/STRATEGY	IMMUNIZATION	ADVERSE REACTIONS	POPULATION RECOMMENDATIONS
Hepatitis A			
Prevention	Hepatitis A vaccine (Havrix; VAQTA), 2 doses with at least 6 months between doses Injected IM into deltoid muscle Combined hepatitis A and hepatitis B vaccine (Twinrix), 3 doses (initial dose followed by doses 4 weeks and 6 months later) given IM into deltoid muscle	Pain at injection site	■ Everyone who desires protection from HAV infection ■ International travelers ■ Men who have sex with men ■ Illegal drug users ■ Persons with clotting-factor disorders, chronic liver disease ■ Persons with occupational risk
Postexposure prophylaxis	Standard immune globulin IM into large muscle mass within 2 weeks of exposure Hepatitis A vaccine may be used in healthy people 40 years old and younger	Rare; risk of anaphylaxis in people with IgA deficiency	■ Close contacts of people with known hepatitis A ■ People potentially exposed to hepatitis A at child care center or restaurant with infected food handler
Hepatitis B			
Prevention	Recombinant hepatitis B vaccine (Recombivax HB; Engerix-B), 3 doses (minimum of 16 weeks between dose #1 and #3) given IM into deltoid muscle Combined hepatitis A and hepatitis B vaccine (Twinrix), 3 doses (initial dose followed by doses 4 weeks and 6 months later) given IM into deltoid muscle	Pain at injection site; fatigue, headache	■ Infants and adolescents ■ Adults seeking protection from HBV infection ■ Persons with chronic liver disease ■ Men who have sex with men ■ Prostitutes; heterosexuals with multiple sexual partners ■ People with an STI ■ Injection drug users ■ Long-term male prisoners ■ People on hemodialysis ■ Healthcare workers
Postexposure prophylaxis	Hepatitis B immune globulin (HBIG) given IM into large muscle mass within 24 hours of exposure; concurrent initiation of hepatitis B vaccine series	Infrequent; muscle stiffness, pain	■ Infants born to women with HBV infection ■ Percutaneous or permucosal exposure to HBV when unvaccinated or antibody response is negative or unknown

Source: Centers for Disease Control and Prevention. (2009). *Epidemiology and prevention of vaccine-preventable diseases* (11th ed.). (Atkinson, J., Wolfe, S., Hamborsky, J., & McIntyre, L. Eds.). Washington, DC: Public Health Foundation.

Postexposure Prophylaxis   Postexposure prophylaxis may be recommended for household or sexual contacts of people with HAV or HBV and other people who are known to have been exposed to these viruses. It is not necessary if the exposed person has been vaccinated and is known to be immune.

Hepatitis A prophylaxis is provided by a single dose of immune globulin (IG) given within 2 weeks after exposure. IG is recommended for all people with household or sexual contact with a person known to be infected with hepatitis A. See Table 25–3 for further recommendations.

Hepatitis B postexposure prophylaxis is indicated for people exposed to the hepatitis B virus. Hepatitis B immune globulin (HBIG) is given to provide for short-term immunity. HBV vaccine may be given concurrently. Candidates for postexposure prophylaxis include those with known or suspected percutaneous or permucosal contact with infected blood, sexual partners of patients with acute HBV or who are HBV carriers, and household contacts of patients with acute HBV infection (National Immunization Program, 2005).

DISEASE TREATMENT   Nearly all people with acute viral hepatitis recover fully without pharmacologic treatment. Severe cases of acute hepatitis B may be treated with an antiretroviral drug such as lamivudine (Epiver, Heptovir), adefovir (Hepsera), entecavir (Baraclude), tenofovir (Viread) or telbivudine (Tyzeka). Treatment is not indicated for mild to moderate cases (Fauci et al., 2008). Acute hepatitis C generally is treated with interferon alpha, an antiviral agent, to reduce the risk of chronic hepatitis C. While single drug treatment with interferon α is common, a long-acting interferon (peginterferon or Pegasys) may be combined with the antiviral drug ribavirin (Rebetol, Virazole). Combination therapy with peginterferon and ribavirin is the treatment of choice for chronic hepatitis C. See the accompanying Medication Administration feature for nursing responsibilities related to interferons and antiviral drugs.

Interferon α interferes with viral replication, reducing the viral load. It is given by intramuscular or subcutaneous injection. Virtually all patients treated with interferon develop a

INTERFERON ALPHA

Conventional interferons

Interferon alfa-2a (Roferon-A)

Interferon alfa-2b (Intron A)

Interferon alfacon-1 (Infergen)

Long-acting interferons:

Peginterferon alfa-2a (Pegasys)

Peginterferon alfa-2b (PEG-Intron)

Human interferons have antiviral, immunosuppressive, and antineoplastic activity. Interferon alpha interferes with viral replication by blocking the virus from entering host cells, inhibiting syntheses of viral RNA and proteins, and viral release from host cells. Conventional interferons have a short half-life and must be administered several times weekly; long-acting preparations can be given once weekly. Long-acting preparations have a higher incidence of adverse effects, however.

Nursing Responsibilities

- Administer by subcutaneous injection. Do not use if solution is discolored or contains visible particulates.
- Monitor for manifestations of hypersensitivity (e.g., angioedema or bronchoconstriction); immediately notify physician and administer emergency treatment as needed to maintain cardiorespiratory status.
- Monitor CBC, platelet count, and renal and liver function studies. Frequently assess mental status. Withhold the drug and notify the physician of significant changes in lab values, manifestations of neuropsychiatric effects, severe abdominal pain, or changes in vision.

Patient Education

- This drug may cause flulike symptoms with fever, fatigue, body aches, headache, and chills. These symptoms tend to diminish over time with continued use of the drug. If approved by your physician, acetaminophen may be used to promote comfort.
- Notify your doctor immediately if you become severely depressed or develop thoughts of suicide, have severe chest pain or difficulty breathing, notice unusual bleeding or

bruising or have bloody diarrhea, notice a change in your vision, develop severe stomach or lower back pain, or notice a new or worsening skin condition.

- Keep all appointments for lab tests and follow-up visits to your doctor.
- Women: Use a reliable means of birth control and notify your physician immediately if you become pregnant.

ANTIRETROVIRAL DRUGS (NUCLEOSIDE/NUCLEOTIDE ANALOGS)

Lamivudine (Epiver-HBV)

Adefovir (Hepsera)

Entecavir (Baraclude)

Tenofovir (Viread)

Telbivudine (Tyzeka)

The nucleoside/nucleotide analog antiretroviral drugs were originally developed for treating HIV infection and now also are approved for HBV treatment, although the recommended doses differ for these two uses. These drugs inhibit synthesis of viral DNA. Therapy with antiretroviral drugs may be prolonged as relapse is common when the drug is stopped. Viral resistance to the drug also is a concern.

Nursing Responsibilities

- Administer PO as ordered.
- Monitor baseline and periodic renal and liver function tests, CBC with differential, blood chemistries, and serum electrolytes. Notify the physician of significant changes.
- Lactic acidosis is a risk with these drugs; monitor for manifestations such as hyperventilation, lethargy, and ABG values indicative of metabolic acidosis. Withhold the drug and notify the physician if manifestations of lactic acidosis develop.

Patient Teaching

- Take the drug as prescribed.
- Notify your doctor if you develop severe abdominal pain, nausea, vomiting or anorexia, or if you become jaundiced.
- Symptoms of recurrent hepatitis B may develop after you stop taking this drug; notify your physician if this occurs.

flulike syndrome with fever, fatigue, muscle aches, headache, and chills. Acetaminophen helps alleviate some of these adverse effects, which tend to decrease over time. Depression also is a common adverse effect of this drug. Instruct patients to contact their physician if suicidal thoughts or manifestations of depression develop. Ribavirin has two major adverse effects: hemolytic anemia and birth defects. Blood counts are obtained before and during treatment to detect early signs of hemolytic anemia. Because of the risk for birth defects, this drug is contraindicated for use during pregnancy, and two reliable methods of birth control must be used by women taking the drug and female sexual partners of men taking the drug.

In addition to interferon α or peginterferon, options for treating chronic hepatitis B include antiviral drugs such as lamivudine or adefovir. Using an antiviral drug in combination with an interferon reduces liver inflammation and fibrosis. Although side effects are minimal, patients may become resistant to the beneficial effects of these drugs. Entecavir is the most potent of the HBV antivirals and may be used as an alternate to lamivudine or adefovir. Treatment of acute hepatitis also includes as-needed bed rest, adequate nutrition as tolerated, and avoidance of strenuous activity, alcohol, and agents that

are toxic to the liver. In most cases, clinical recovery takes 3 to 16 weeks.

Complementary Therapies

Milk thistle, with its active ingredient silymarin, has been used by herbalists to treat liver disease for over 2000 years. Clinical studies have demonstrated that treatment with silymarin promotes quality of life and reduces symptoms in patients with hepatitis C. It also is beneficial for patients who have liver damage due to toxins, cirrhosis, and alcoholic liver disease. Silymarin is a powerful antioxidant that also promotes liver cell growth; it has not been shown, however, to decrease viral activity or reduce liver inflammation (National Center for Complementary and Alternative Medicine, 2008).

Herbalists also may use licorice root to treat hepatitis. It has both antiviral and anti-inflammatory effects. Long-term use of licorice root, however, can lead to hypertension and affect fluid and electrolyte balance.

Herbal preparations also may be used to relieve the adverse effects of interferon alpha. Ginger can help relieve nausea, and St. John's wort is used for the depression associated with interferon alpha.

Nursing Care

Health Promotion

Nurses play an instrumental role in preventing the spread of hepatitis. Stress the importance of hygiene measures such as hand hygiene after toileting and before all food handling. Discuss the dangers of injection drug use and, with drug users, of sharing needles or other equipment. Encourage all sexually active patients to use safer sexual practices such as abstinence, mutual monogamy, and barrier protection (such as male or female condoms).

Discuss recommendations for hepatitis A and hepatitis B vaccine with people in high or moderate risk groups for these infections. Ensure that nurses and other healthcare workers at risk for exposure to blood and body fluids are effectively vaccinated against hepatitis A and B. Encourage all people with known or probable exposure to HAV or HBV to obtain postexposure prophylaxis. See the accompanying nursing research feature for a study of healthcare workers' attitudes toward infected peers.

Assessment

Collect assessment data related to hepatitis, such as the following:

- *Health history:* Current manifestations, including anorexia, nausea, vomiting, abdominal discomfort, changes in bowel elimination or color of stools; muscle or joint pain, fatigue; changes in color of skin or sclera; duration of symptoms; known exposure to hepatitis; high-risk behaviors such as injection drug use or multiple sexual partners; previous history of liver disorders; current medications, prescription and over the counter.
- *Physical assessment:* Vital signs including temperature; color of sclera and mucous membranes; skin color and condition; abdominal contour and tenderness; color of stool and urine.
- *Diagnostic tests:* Serum bilirubin, liver function tests, serologic antibody–antigen levels.

Nursing Diagnoses and Interventions

Patients with acute or chronic hepatitis usually are treated in community settings; rarely is hospitalization required. Nursing care focuses on preventing spread of the infection to others and promoting the patient's comfort and ability to provide self-care.

Risk for Infection (Transmission)

An important goal when caring for patients with acute viral hepatitis is preventing spread of the infection.

- Use standard precautions. Practice meticulous hand hygiene. *The hepatitis viruses are spread by direct contact with feces or blood and body fluids. Standard precautions and good hand hygiene protect both healthcare workers and other patients from exposure to the virus.*
- For patients with HAV or HEV, use standard precautions and contact isolation if fecal incontinence is present. *The fecal–oral route is the primary mode of transmission of these viruses. Other hepatitis viruses are transmitted through blood and other body fluids.*
- Encourage prophylactic treatment of all members of household and intimate sexual contacts. *Prophylactic treatment of people in close contact with the patient decreases their risk of contacting the disease or, if already infected, the severity of the disease.*

SAFETY ALERT

If the patient diagnosed with hepatitis A is employed as a food handler or child care worker, contact the local health department to report possible exposure of patrons. Maintain confidentiality. Prophylactic treatment of people who have possibly been exposed to the virus can prevent a local epidemic of the disease.

MOVING EVIDENCE INTO ACTION   Applying Evidence to Practice

Although the number of healthcare workers infected with blood borne pathogens such as HBV and HCV is small, those instances in which the infection has been transmitted to patients by the infected worker have received widespread publicity. Calls for testing of all healthcare workers or for restricting the practice of infected workers have been raised.

Kagan, Ovadia, and Kaneti (2008) studied nurses' and physicians' knowledge, attitudes, and opinions regarding disclosure and practice restrictions of healthcare workers infected with a blood borne pathogen. Although a correlation was found between knowledge about blood borne pathogens and attitudes toward infected healthcare workers, this study did not find a correlation between knowledge and opinions about disclosure of infection status or practice restrictions. There was, however, a correlation noted between attitudes toward infected workers and opinions regarding disclosure and oractuce restrictions.

IMPLICATIONS FOR NURSING

Of the major blood borne pathogens, HBV is associated with a significantly higher risk of transmission to and from healthcare workers than are HCV or HIV. Interestingly, participants in this study were more likely to have a positive attitude toward

healthcare workers infected with HBV and less likely to endorse self-disclosure and practice restrictions. Nurses need appropriate information and knowledge in order to accurately respond to patient's questions and concerns about blood borne pathogens.

CRITICAL THINKING IN PATIENT CARE

1. In this study, participants reported a more positive attitude toward healthcare workers infected with HBV than those infected with HCV or HIV. What factors do you think may have contributed toward this difference in attitudes?
2. Do you believe that nurses infected with a blood borne pathogen should disclose their status to patients for whom they provide care? Why or why not? Should a physician with HBV or HCV restrict his or her practice? If so, in what ways?
3. A coworker you know to be infected with HBV tells you that she is considering a position in a hemodialysis clinic. You know that patients undergoing hemodialysis fall within a high risk group for contracting hepatitis B. How will you respond to your coworker? What additional knowledge or information do you need to develop your response?

Source: Kagan, H., Ovadia, K., & Kaneti, T. (2008). Physicians' and nurses' vies on infected health care workers. *Nursing Ethics, 15*(5), 573–585.

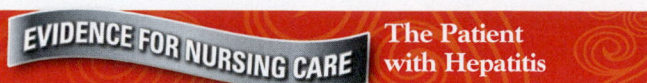

EVIDENCE FOR NURSING CARE — The Patient with Hepatitis

Selected resources that nurses may find helpful when planning evidence-based nursing care follow.

- Davenport, A. & Myers, F. (2009). How to protect yourself after body fluid exposure. *Nursing2009, 39*(5), 22–28.
- National Institutes of Health. (2008 October). NIH Consensus Development Conference statement on management of hepatitis B. *NIH Consensus and State-of-the-Science Statement, 25*(2), 1–29.

Fatigue

Fatigue and possible weakness are common in acute hepatitis. Although bed rest is rarely indicated, adequate rest periods and limitation of activities may be necessary. Many patients with acute hepatitis may be unable to resume normal activity levels for 4 or more weeks.

- Encourage planned rest periods throughout the day. *Adequate rest is necessary for optimal immune function.*
- Assist to identify essential activities and those that can be deferred or delegated to others. *Identifying essential and nonessential activities promotes the patient's sense of control.*
- Suggest using level of fatigue to determine activity level, with gradual resumption of activities as fatigue and sense of well-being improves. *Fatigue associated with activity is an indicator of appropriate and inappropriate activity levels. As recovery progresses, increasing activity levels are tolerated with less fatigue.*

Imbalanced Nutrition: Less than Body Requirements

Adequate nutrition is important for immune function and healing in patients with acute or chronic hepatitis.

- Help plan a diet of appealing foods that provides a high-kilocalorie intake of approximately 16 carbohydrate kilocalories per kilogram of ideal body weight. *Sufficient energy is required for healing; adequate carbohydrate intake can spare protein.*
- Encourage planning food intake according to symptoms of the disease. Discuss eating smaller meals and using between-meal snacks to maintain nutrient and calorie intake. *Patients with acute hepatitis often are more anorexic and nauseated in the afternoon and evening; planning the majority of calorie intake in the morning helps maintain adequate intake. Limiting fat intake and the size of meals may reduce the incidence of nausea.*
- Instruct to avoid alcohol intake and diet drinks. *Alcohol avoidance is vital to prevent further liver damage and promote healing. Diet drinks (e.g., diet sodas or juice drinks) provide few calories when an increased calorie intake is needed for healing.*
- Encourage use of nutritional supplements such as Ensure or instant breakfast drinks to maintain calorie and nutrient intake. *Nutritional supplement drinks are an additional source of concentrated calories and nutrients.*

Disturbed Body Image

Jaundice and associated rashes and itching can affect the patient's body image. Nursing measures to prevent skin breakdown and address body image are discussed in the following section on cirrhosis.

Using NANDA, NIC, and NOC

Linkages between a selected NANDA nursing diagnosis, NIC, and NOC for the patient with viral hepatitis are shown in the chart that follows.

Community-Based Care

Provide discharge teaching to patients and their families for home care. Include the following topics:

- Recommended prophylactic treatment
- Infection control measures such as frequent hand hygiene; not sharing eating utensils; avoiding food handling or preparation activities by the patient with hepatitis A; abstaining from sexual relations during acute infection; and using barrier protection if a carrier or for chronic infection
- Managing fatigue and limited activity
- Managing pruritus and maintaining skin integrity: use warm, not hot water when bathing; use mild or no soap; limit duration of baths and showers; pat dry, do not rub, apply an alcohol-free lotion soon after bathing to retain skin moisture; wear loose cotton garments that allow moisture to evaporate from skin; reduce room temperature, especially at night, to prevent overheating; keep fingernails short, and wear cotton mittens or gloves as needed to prevent scratching during sleep
- Promoting nutrient intake
- Avoiding hepatic toxins such as alcohol, acetaminophen, and selected other drugs; encourage to alert all care providers to presence of infection
- Recommended follow-up

If chronic hepatitis B or C is being treated with medications, teach how to administer the drug, its dosing schedule, precautions, and management of adverse effects. Stress the importance of keeping follow-up appointments, including recommended laboratory testing.

NANDA, NIC, AND NOC LINKAGES
The Patient with Viral Hepatitis

NANDA	Imbalanced Nutrition: Less than Body Requirements
NIC	Energy Management / Nutrition Management
NOC	Energy Conservation / Nutritional Status: Nutrient Intake

Data from NANDA International. (2009). *Nursing diagnoses: Definitions & classification 2009–2011* Oxford, UK: Wiley-Blackwell; Bulechek, G., Butcher, H., & Dochterman, J. (Eds.). (2008). *Nursing interventions classification (NIC)* (5th ed.). St. Louis, MO: Mosby; and Moorhead, S., Johnson, M., Maas, M., & Swanson, E. (Eds.). (2008). *Nursing outcomes classification (NOC)* (4th ed.). St. Louis, MO: Mosby.

The Patient with Cirrhosis

Cirrhosis is characterized by fibrosis of liver tissue leading to decreased mass, impaired liver function, and altered blood flow. Cirrhosis was previously thought to be an irreversible condition; now, however, it is recognized that fibrosis may be reversed when the underlying cause is eliminated (Fauci et al., 2008).

FAST FACTS

- Cirrhosis is the 12th leading cause of death in the United States overall.
- In adults ages 25 to 64 years, however, cirrhosis/chronic liver disease is the 7th leading cause of death.
- Overall, the death rate due to cirrhosis and chronic liver disease in men is more than twice that of women (National Center for Health Statistics [NCHS], 2009).

Alcoholic cirrhosis is the most common type of cirrhosis in the United States. Chronic hepatitis B or C also are leading causes of cirrhosis, particularly in people who consume alcohol excessively. Other causes include prolonged obstruction of the biliary (bile drainage) system; long-term, severe right heart failure, and uncommon liver disorders. The incidence and mortality attributable to cirrhosis and chronic liver disease vary significantly among populations. See the accompanying Focus on Cultural Diversity box.

Pathophysiology

In cirrhosis, functional liver tissue is gradually destroyed and replaced by fibrous scar tissue. As hepatocytes and liver lobules are destroyed, the metabolic functions of the liver are lost. Structurally abnormal nodules encircled by connective tissue develop. This fibrous connective tissue forms constrictive bands that disrupt blood and bile flow within liver lobules. Blood no longer flows freely through the liver to the inferior vena cava. This restricted blood flow leads to portal hypertension, increased pressure in the portal venous system.

Alcoholic Cirrhosis

Alcoholic or Laënnec's cirrhosis is the end result of alcoholic liver disease. Its development is directly related to alcohol consumption: total amount of alcohol consumed, number of years

FOCUS ON CULTURAL DIVERSITY
Cirrhosis

- Although cirrhosis/chronic liver disease is the 12th leading cause of death overall in the United States, it is the 6th leading cause of death for people of Native American (including Alaska Natives) and Hispanic (or Latino) origin.
- Native American men have the highest incidence and mortality rate from cirrhosis and chronic liver disease, followed by Native American women, Hispanic men, and women of Hispanic or Latino origin (NCHS, 2009).
- At this time, there is no clear explanation for these differences. Contributory factors may include the following:
  - Socioeconomic factors that lead to greater stress and alcohol consumption among certain populations
  - Patterns of alcohol consumption (e.g., consuming alcohol without food calories)
  - Variations in alcohol metabolism among populations
  - As yet unidentified immunologic or genetic factors

of excessive alcohol consumption, and blood alcohol levels. Women develop cirrhosis at lower overall levels of alcohol use than men. This may relate to the effects of estrogen and less effective metabolism of alcohol in women, resulting in higher blood alcohol levels.

Alcohol causes metabolic changes in the liver: Triglyceride and fatty acid synthesis increases, and the formation and release of lipoproteins decrease, leading to fatty infiltration of hepatocytes (fatty liver). At this stage, abstinence from alcohol can allow the liver to heal. With continued alcohol abuse, the disease progresses. Inflammatory cells infiltrate the liver (alcoholic hepatitis), causing necrosis, fibrosis, and destruction of functional liver tissue. In the final stage of alcoholic cirrhosis, regenerative nodules form, and the liver shrinks and develops a nodular appearance. Malnutrition commonly accompanies alcoholic cirrhosis. See Pathophysiology Linkage: Cirrhosis, and Pathophysiology Illustrated: Cirrhosis and Portal Hypertension on the following pages.

Posthepatic Cirrhosis

Advanced progressive liver disease resulting from chronic hepatitis B or C, autoimmune hepatitis, or from nonalcoholic fatty liver disease is known as posthepatic or postnecrotic cirrhosis. Chronic viral hepatitis is the leading cause of posthepatic cirrhosis in the United States. About 25% of persons with chronic hepatitis B or C will eventually develop cirrhosis. The immune response is responsible for producing liver damage and fibrosis in chronic and autoimmune hepatitis. The liver is shrunken and nodular, with extensive liver cell loss and fibrosis. The obesity epidemic is seen as a major factor contributing to an increased incidence of cirrhosis due to nonalcoholic fatty liver disease.

Biliary Cirrhosis

When bile flow is obstructed within the liver or in the biliary system, retained bile damages and destroys liver cells close to the interlobular bile ducts. This leads to inflammation, fibrosis, and formation of regenerative nodules. Within the liver, bile ducts are narrowed or obstructed, leading to elevated bilirubin levels and progressive liver failure.

Manifestations and Complications

Early in the course of cirrhosis, few manifestations may be present. The liver usually is enlarged and may be tender. A dull, aching pain in the epigastric area or RUQ may be present. Other early signs include weight loss, weakness, and anorexia. Bowel function is disrupted with diarrhea or constipation.

As the disease progresses, manifestations related to liver cell failure and portal hypertension develop. Impaired metabolism causes such manifestations as bleeding, ascites, gynecomastia (breast enlargement) in men and infertility in women, jaundice, and neurologic changes. Portal hypertension accounts from such manifestations as ascites, peripheral edema, anemia, and low WBC and platelet counts. See Multisystem Effects of Cirrhosis on page 738.

Portal Hypertension

Increased pressure in the portal system causes blood to be rerouted to adjoining lower pressure vessels. This *shunting* of blood involves collateral vessels. Affected veins, which become

PATHOPHYSIOLOGY LINKAGE Cirrhosis

MANIFESTATIONS	UNDERLYING PATHOPHYSIOLOGY
Edema, ascites	■ Impaired hepatocyte function impairs plasma protein synthesis (hypoalbuminemia) ■ Disrupted hormone balance due to loss of metabolic and detoxification functions ■ Metabolism of aldosterone is impaired, leading to salt and water retention; disrupted renal blood flow contributes to fluid retention ■ Increased hydrostatic pressure in portal venous system
Bleeding, bruising	■ Decreased clotting factor synthesis related to impaired hepatocyte function ■ Increased platelet destruction by enlarged spleen ■ Impaired vitamin K absorption and storage
Esophageal varices, hemorrhoids	■ Increased pressure in portal venous system with development of weak, thin-walled vessels, particularly in the lower esophagus, rectum, and abdominal wall
Gastritis, anorexia, diarrhea	■ Engorged veins in gastrointestinal system disrupt normal appetite mechanisms ■ Alcohol ingestion ■ Impaired bile synthesis and fat absorption
Abdominal wall vein distention (caput medusae)	■ Portal hypertension
Jaundice	■ Impaired bilirubin metabolism due to disrupted hepatocyte function ■ Bile excretion is impaired by fibrosis and obstruction of biliary channels
Malnutrition, muscle wasting	■ Impaired nutrient metabolism ■ Impaired fat absorption ■ Impaired hormone metabolism
Anemia, leukopenia, increased risk for infection	■ Bleeding ■ Increased blood cell destruction by spleen
Asterixis, encephalopathy	■ Accumulated metabolic toxins ■ Impaired ammonia metabolism and excretion
Gynecomastia, infertility, impotence	■ Altered sex hormone metabolism

engorged and congested, are located in the esophagus, rectum, and abdomen. Portal hypertension increases the hydrostatic pressure in vessels of the portal system. Increased hydrostatic pressure in the capillaries pushes fluid out, contributing to ascites formation.

Splenomegaly

The spleen enlarges (splenomegaly) because portal hypertension causes blood to be shunted into the splenic vein. Splenomegaly increases the rate at which red and white blood cells and platelets are removed from circulation and destroyed. This increased blood cell destruction leads to anemia, leukopenia, and thrombocytopenia.

Ascites

Ascites is the accumulation of plasma-rich fluid in the abdominal cavity. Although portal hypertension is the primary cause of ascites, decreased serum proteins and increased aldosterone also contribute to the fluid accumulation. *Hypoalbuminemia*, low serum albumin, decreases the colloidal osmotic pressure of plasma. This pressure normally holds fluid in the intravascular compartment; when plasma colloidal osmotic pressure decreases, fluid escapes into extravascular compartments. *Hyperaldosteronism*, an increase in aldosterone levels, causes sodium and water retention, contributing to ascites and generalized edema.

Esophageal Varices

Esophageal varices are enlarged, thin-walled veins that form in the submucosa of the esophagus. These collateral vessels form when blood is shunted from the portal system due to portal hypertension. The thin-walled varices may rupture, causing massive hemorrhage; even eating high-roughage foods can precipitate bleeding. Thrombocytopenia, platelet deficiency, and impaired production of clotting factors by the liver contribute to the risk for hemorrhage.

Portal Systemic Encephalopathy

Portal systemic encephalopathy (*hepatic encephalopathy*) results from accumulation of neurotoxins in the blood and cerebral edema. Ammonia, a by-product of protein metabolism, contributes to hepatic encephalopathy. Ammonium ion is produced as proteins and amino acids are broken down by bacteria in the intestinal tract. Normally, the ammonia produced is then converted by the liver to urea before entering the general circulation. As functional liver tissue is destroyed, ammonia can no longer be converted to urea, and it accumulates in the blood. Other nervous system depressants, such as narcotics and tranquilizers, also can contribute to hepatic encephalopathy. Box 25–4 lists selected precipitating factors for hepatic encephalopathy. Accumulation of other metabolic toxins are thought to contribute as well.

PATHOPHYSIOLOGY ILLUSTRATED
Cirrhosis and Portal Hypertension

Normal liver

The liver contains multiple lobules made up of plates of hepatocytes, the functional cells of the liver, surrounded by small capillaries called sinusoids. These sinusoids receive a mixture of venous and arterial blood from branches of the portal vein and hepatic artery. Blood from the sinusoids drains into the central vein of the lobule. Hepatocytes produce bile, which drains outward to bile ducts.

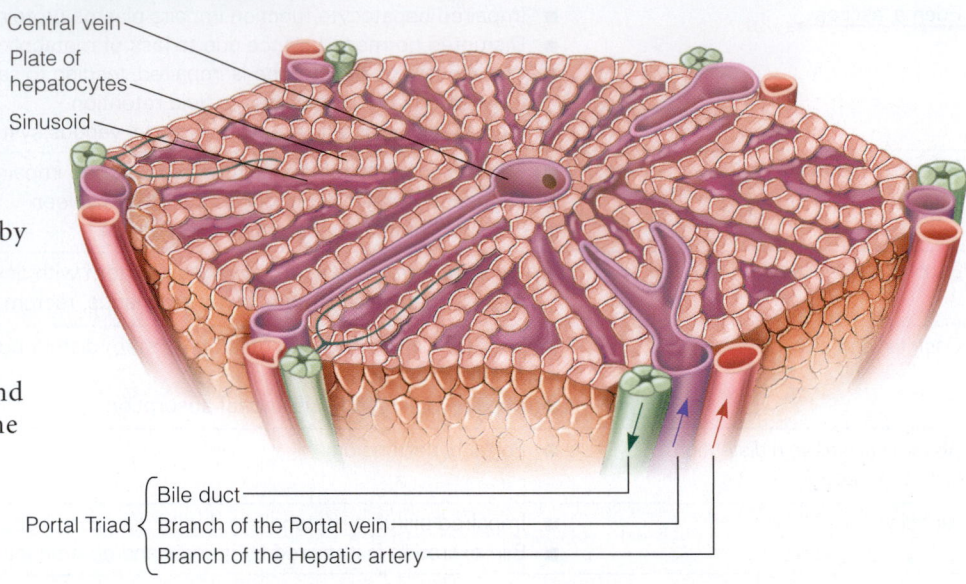

Central vein
Plate of hepatocytes
Sinusoid

Portal Triad {
Bile duct
Branch of the Portal vein
Branch of the Hepatic artery

Fatty liver

Ingested alcohol is primarily metabolized in the liver. Acetaldehyde, formed when alcohol is metabolized, damages hepatocytes and impairs the oxidation of fatty acids. As a result, fat accumulates within hepatocytes and liver lobules. Other alcohol metabolism byproducts, including oxygen free radicals, promote inflammation and may stimulate autoantibody production.

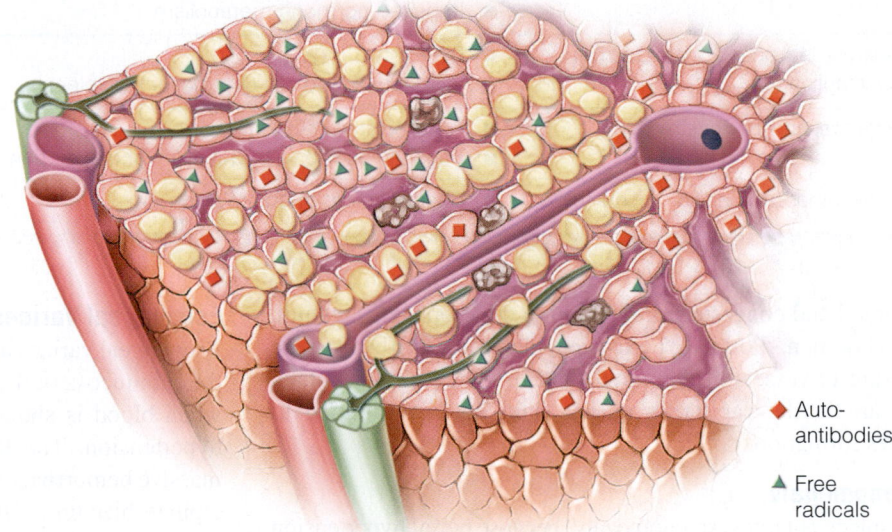

♦ Auto-antibodies

▲ Free radicals

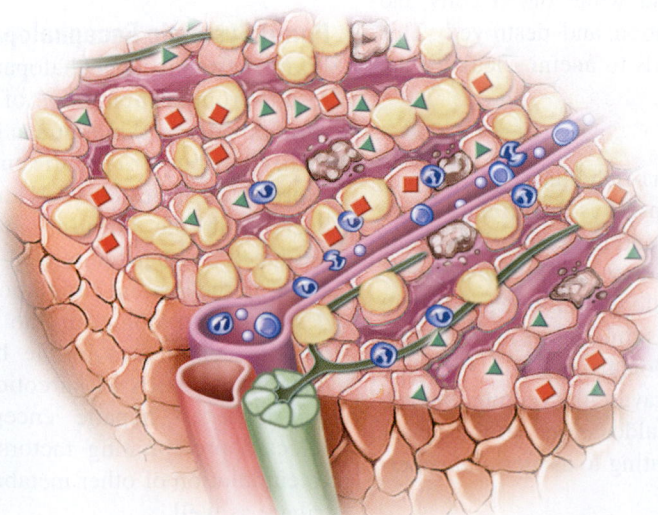

Alcoholic hepatitis

With continued alcohol intake, liver cells degenerate and spotty cellular necrosis occurs. Inflammatory cells such as polymorphonuclear leukocytes and lymphocytes infiltrate the lobule.

Alcoholic cirrhosis

Cellular necrosis and inflammation transform some liver cells into fibroblasts that produce and deposit collagen. Weblike bands of connective tissue develop around the portal triads and central vein, eventually connecting with one another. Small islands of liver cells continue to regenerate, forming nodules. Hepatocyte destruction outpaces regeneration. As a result of cell loss, fibrosis and scarring, the liver shrinks and becomes hard and nodular.

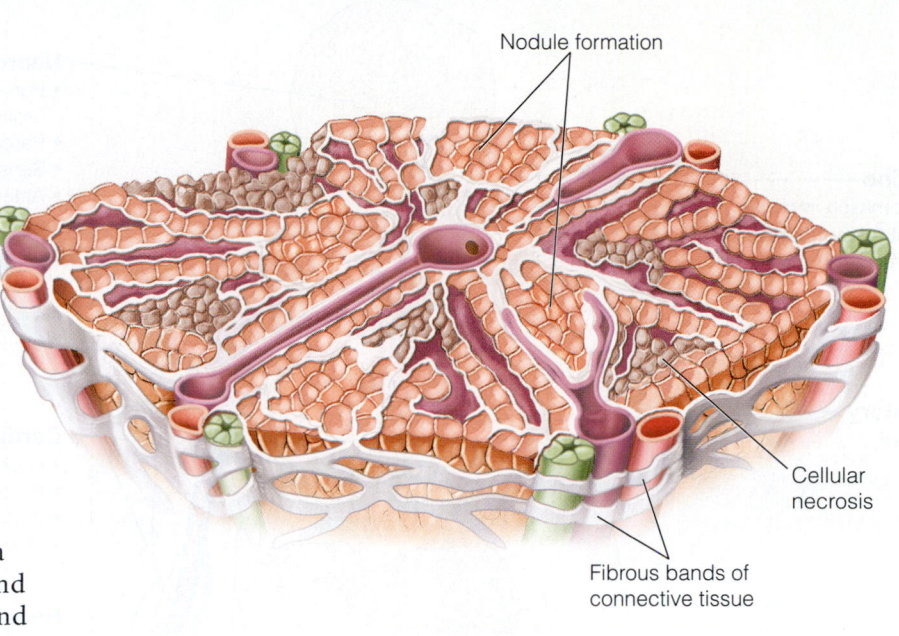

Nodule formation

Cellular necrosis

Fibrous bands of connective tissue

Portal hypertension

Bands of fibrotic scar tissue obstruct the sinusoids and blood flow from the portal vein to the hepatic vein. Pressure in the portal venous system, which drains the gastrointestinal tract, pancreas, and spleen, increases. This increased pressure opens collateral vessels in the esophagus, anterior abdominal wall, and rectum, allowing blood to bypass the obstructed portal vessels. Prolonged portal hypertension leads to the development of (1) varices (fragile, distended veins) in the lower esophagus, stomach, and rectum; (2) splenomegaly (an enlarged spleen); (3) ascites (accumulation of fluid in the abdomen); and (4) portal systemic encephalopathy (disrupted CNS function with altered consciousness).

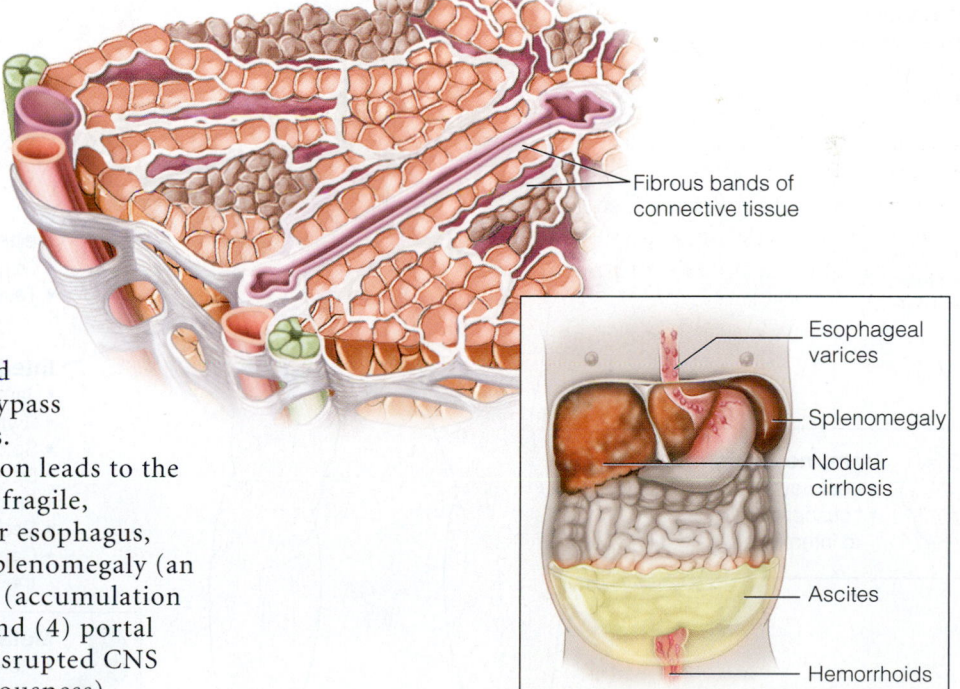

Fibrous bands of connective tissue

Esophageal varices

Splenomegaly

Nodular cirrhosis

Ascites

Hemorrhoids

MULTISYSTEM EFFECTS OF
Cirrhosis

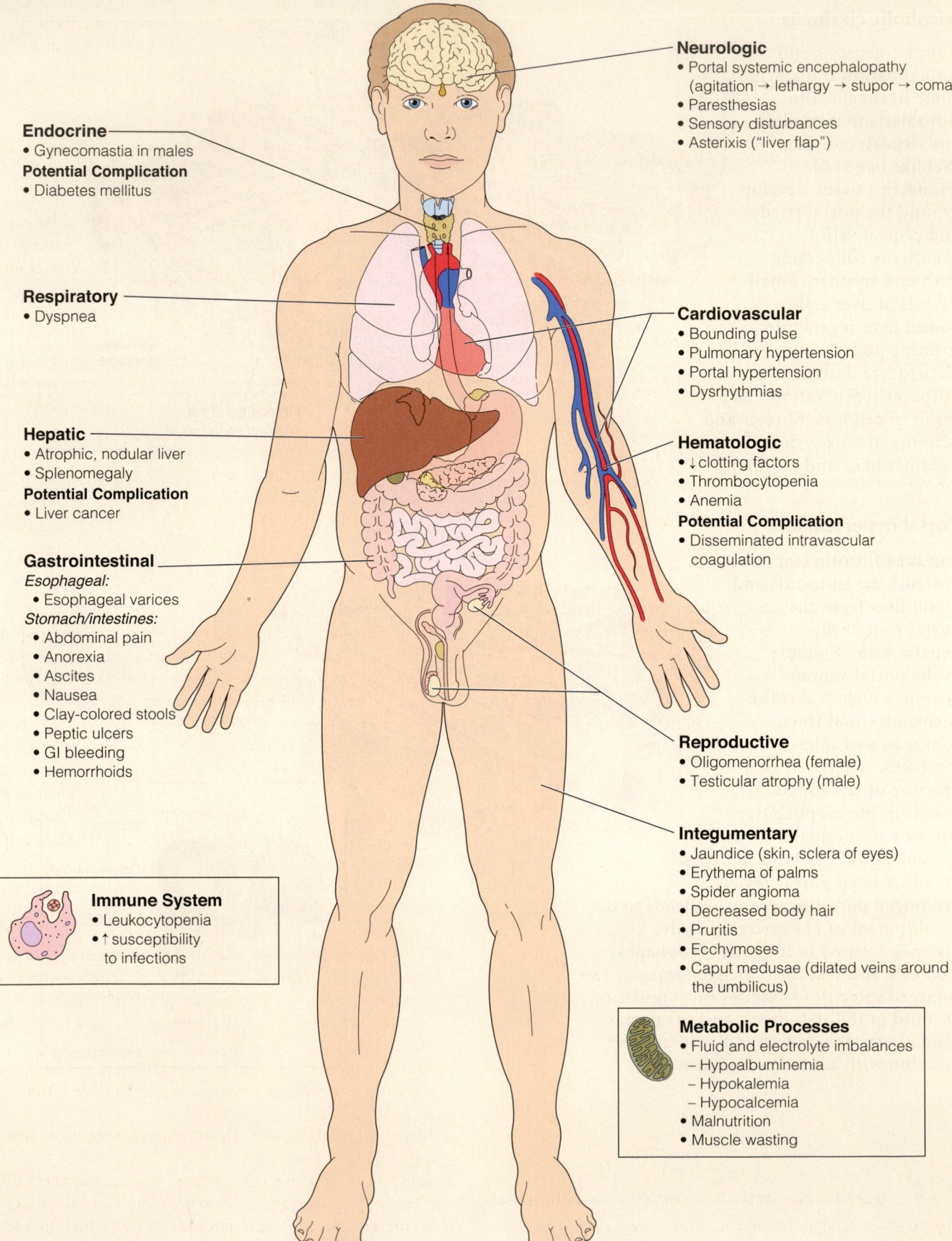

Neurologic
- Portal systemic encephalopathy (agitation → lethargy → stupor → coma)
- Paresthesias
- Sensory disturbances
- Asterixis ("liver flap")

Endocrine
- Gynecomastia in males

Potential Complication
- Diabetes mellitus

Respiratory
- Dyspnea

Cardiovascular
- Bounding pulse
- Pulmonary hypertension
- Portal hypertension
- Dysrhythmias

Hepatic
- Atrophic, nodular liver
- Splenomegaly

Potential Complication
- Liver cancer

Hematologic
- ↓ clotting factors
- Thrombocytopenia
- Anemia

Potential Complication
- Disseminated intravascular coagulation

Gastrointestinal
Esophageal:
- Esophageal varices

Stomach/intestines:
- Abdominal pain
- Anorexia
- Ascites
- Nausea
- Clay-colored stools
- Peptic ulcers
- GI bleeding
- Hemorrhoids

Reproductive
- Oligomenorrhea (female)
- Testicular atrophy (male)

Integumentary
- Jaundice (skin, sclera of eyes)
- Erythema of palms
- Spider angioma
- Decreased body hair
- Pruritis
- Ecchymoses
- Caput medusae (dilated veins around the umbilicus)

Immune System
- Leukocytopenia
- ↑ susceptibility to infections

Metabolic Processes
- Fluid and electrolyte imbalances
  – Hypoalbuminemia
  – Hypokalemia
  – Hypocalcemia
- Malnutrition
- Muscle wasting

BOX 25–4 Factors Precipitating Portal Systemic Encephalopathy

- High serum ammonia level
- Constipation
- Blood transfusions
- Gastrointestinal bleeding
- Medications: sedatives, tranquilizers, narcotic analgesics, anesthetics
- Hypoxia
- Severe infection
- Surgery

Asterixis (liver flap), a muscle tremor that interferes with the ability to maintain a fixed position of the extremities and causes involuntary jerking movements, is an early sign of portal systemic encephalopathy. Asterixis primarily affects the upper extremities, but also may affect the tongue and feet. Asterixis is elicited by instructing the patient to extend the arms and dorsiflex the wrists. If present, asterixis causes a downward flapping of the hands (Figure 25–5 ■). Changes in personality and mentation develop; agitation, restlessness, impaired judgment, and slurred speech also are early manifestations of hepatic encephalopathy. As it progresses, confusion, disorientation, and incoherence develop. Cerebral edema that leads to increased intracranial pressure and cerebral hypoxia is the leading cause of death in people with portal systemic encephalopathy and liver failure.

Hepatorenal Syndrome

Although the cause is unclear, renal failure with azotemia (excess nitrogenous waste products in the blood), sodium retention, oliguria, and hypotension may develop in patients with advanced cirrhosis and ascites. Hepatorenal syndrome appears to be the result of imbalanced blood flow, leading to constriction of vessels leading to and within the kidneys. The syndrome may be precipitated by gastrointestinal bleeding, aggressive diuretic therapy, or by an unknown cause.

Spontaneous Bacterial Peritonitis

Patients with cirrhosis and ascites may develop bacterial peritonitis, even in the absence of known contamination of the

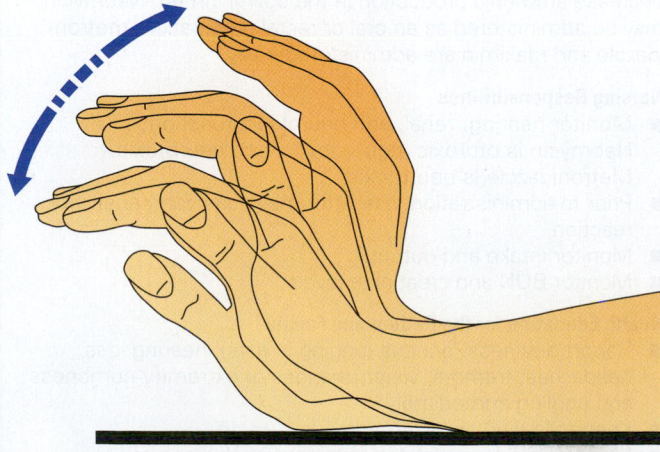

Figure 25–5 ■ Asterixis. Note the downward tremor of the hand on dorsiflexion of the wrist.

peritoneal cavity or other specific risk factors (e.g., paracentesis). The inflammatory response to peritonitis worsens ascites by increasing the permeability of capillaries in the mesentery. The manifestations of spontaneous bacterial peritonitis may be subtle, with increased abdominal discomfort or pain, fever, increasing ascites, worsening encephalopathy, and an overall decline in condition.

Interdisciplinary Care

Care for the patient with cirrhosis is holistic, addressing physiologic, psychosocial, and spiritual needs. The importance of including the family in the plan of care cannot be overemphasized, particularly if alcohol abuse is identified as the cause. Alcohol abstinence is critical: Fewer than 50% of patients who have experienced complications of cirrhosis and who continue to drink will survive for 5 years. The prognosis improves with abstinence, and liver transplant may be a treatment option in abstinent patients (Fauci et al., 2008).

Treatment of cirrhosis is supportive, directed at slowing the progression to liver failure and reducing complications. Treatment includes medications to help regulate protein metabolism, maintenance of fluid and electrolyte balance, and supportive therapies, including treatment of underlying problems, such as malnutrition, anemia, bleeding, encephalopathy, renal failure, and infections.

Diagnosis

Studies to confirm the diagnosis of cirrhosis and identify its cause and effects are performed. Diagnostic tests may include the following:

- *Liver function studies* include *ALT*, *AST*, and *ALP*. All may be elevated in cirrhosis, but usually not as severely as in acute hepatitis. Elevations in these enzymes may not correlate well with the extent of liver damage in cirrhosis.
- *CBC with platelets* is done. A low RBC count, hemoglobin, and hematocrit demonstrate anemia related to bone marrow suppression, increased RBC destruction, bleeding, and deficiencies of folic acid and vitamin B_{12}. Platelets are low, related to increased destruction by the spleen. Leukopenia (low WBC count) also relates to splenomegaly.
- *Coagulation studies* show a prolonged prothrombin time due to impaired production of coagulation proteins and lack of vitamin K.
- *Serum electrolytes* are measured. Hyponatremia is common, due to hemodilution. Hypokalemia, hypophosphatemia, and hypomagnesemia also are frequently seen, related to malnutrition and altered renal excretion of these electrolytes.
- *Bilirubin* levels are usually elevated in severe cirrhosis, including both direct (conjugated) and indirect (unconjugated) bilirubin.
- *Serum albumin* levels show hypoalbuminemia due to impaired liver production.
- *Serum ammonia* levels are elevated because the liver fails to effectively convert ammonia to urea for renal excretion.
- *Serum glucose* and *cholesterol* levels frequently are abnormal in patients with cirrhosis.

■ *Abdominal ultrasound* is performed to evaluate liver size, detect ascites, and identify liver nodules. Ultrasound may be used in conjunction with *Doppler studies* to evaluate blood flow through the liver and spleen.

■ *Esophagoscopy* (upper endoscopy) may be done to determine the presence of esophageal varices.

■ *Liver biopsy* is not always necessary to diagnose cirrhosis, but may be done to distinguish cirrhosis from other forms of liver disease. See page 575 for nursing implications for a patient having a liver biopsy. Figure 21–8 shows the site and position for liver biopsy. Biopsy may be deferred if the bleeding time is prolonged (such as a prothrombin time [PT] greater than 3 seconds over the control).

∞ See Chapter 21 for more information about and the nursing implications of the aforementioned diagnostic tests.

Medications

Medications are used to treat the complications and effects of cirrhosis; they do not reverse or slow the process of cirrhosis itself. Known hepatotoxic drugs and alcohol are avoided, as are drugs metabolized by the liver (e.g., barbiturates, sedatives, hypnotics, and acetaminophen). Several groups of drugs are commonly prescribed. See the Medication Administration box for nursing responsibilities and patient teaching for commonly used drugs in patients with cirrhosis.

■ Diuretics reduce fluid retention and ascites. Spironolactone (Aldactone) is frequently the drug of first choice because it addresses one of the causes of ascites—increased aldosterone levels. If additional diuresis is necessary, a loop diuretic such as furosemide (Lasix) may be added to the regimen.

■ Medications to reduce the nitrogenous load and lower serum ammonia levels are added when manifestations of hepatic encephalopathy develop. Commonly administered medications are lactulose and antibiotics such as neomycin, metronidazole, or rifaximin. Lactulose reduces the number of ammonia-forming organisms in the bowel and increases the acidity of colon contents, converting ammonia into ammonium ion. Ammonium ion is not absorbable, and is excreted in the feces. Neomycin sulfate is a locally acting antibiotic that also reduces the number of ammonia-forming bacteria in the bowel. Because it is toxic to the kidneys and auditory system, it is alternated with metronidazole. Metronidazole is a systemic antibiotic effective against common Gram-negative bacteria that inhabit the bowel. Peripheral neuropathy is a

---

MEDICATION ADMINISTRATION   **The Patient with Cirrhosis**

DIURETICS

Spironolactone (Aldactone)

Furosemide (Lasix)

Spironolactone is a potassium-sparing diuretic that competes with aldosterone. It reduces ascites by increasing renal excretion of fluid and decreasing aldosterone levels. Furosemide is a loop diuretic that promotes the excretion of potassium. Drugs may be given in combination if serum potassium level permits.

Nursing Responsibilities

■ Monitor ECG, serum potassium, BUN, creatinine levels, and hydration status.
■ Weigh daily.
■ Carefully monitor intake and output.
■ Monitor for signs of hyperkalemia if taking spironolactone alone: bradycardia; widening QRS, spiking T waves, or ST segment depression on ECG; diarrhea; and muscle twitching.
■ Assess for hyponatremia: confusion, lethargy, apprehension.

Health Education for the Patient and Family

■ Maintain diet and fluid restrictions as prescribed.
■ Report increases in weight or edema.
■ Immediately report signs of hyponatremia, hyperkalemia, or hypokalemia (∞ see Chapter 10).
■ Expect increased urinary output; take medications in morning hours to avoid nocturia.

LAXATIVES

Lactulose (Cephulac, Chronulac)

Lactulose is a disaccharide laxative that is not absorbed by the gastrointestinal tract. It reduces the number of ammonia-producing bacteria and lowers the pH in the colon. The lower pH (increased acidity) converts ammonia to ammonium ion, a nonabsorbable form that is excreted in the feces. Lactulose also pulls water into the bowel lumen, increasing the number of daily stools.

Nursing Responsibilities

■ Assess bowel sounds and abdominal girth.
■ Maintain accurate stool chart.
■ Adjust dose to achieve two to four soft stools per day.
■ Monitor electrolytes and hydration.

Health Education for the Patient and Family

■ Drink adequate fluids.
■ Report diarrhea; if present, decrease dose. You should have an average of two to four stools per day.
■ This drug may cause nausea. Continue taking the drug; taking it with crackers or a soft drink may reduce nausea.

ANTI-INFECTIVE AGENTS

Neomycin sulfate (Neo Tabs)

Metronidazole (Flagyl)

Rifaximin (Xifaxan)

These antibiotics act in the gut to reduce intestinal bacteria and decrease ammonia production in the bowel lumen. Neomycin may be administered as an oral or rectal preparation; metronidazole and rifaximin are administered orally.

Nursing Responsibilities

■ Monitor hearing, renal, and neurologic functions. Neomycin is ototoxic, nephrotoxic, and neurotoxic. Metronidazole is neurotoxic.
■ Prior to administration, check for previous hypersensitivity reaction.
■ Monitor intake and output.
■ Monitor BUN and creatinine levels.

Health Education for the Patient and Family

■ Report dizziness, tinnitus (ringing in ears), hearing loss, headaches, tremors, vision changes or extremity numbness and tingling immediately.
■ Keep follow-up appointments.
■ Maintain fluids; avoid dehydration. (Teach signs of dehydration.)

potential toxic effect of metronidazole. Rifaximin, a poorly absorbed antibiotic, acts locally within the bowel and has few adverse or toxic effects.

■ A beta-blocker such as nadolol (Corgard) or propranolol (Inderal) may be given to reduce portal hypertension and prevent bleeding of esophageal varices.

■ Ferrous sulfate and folic acid are given as indicated to treat anemia. Vitamin K may be ordered to reduce the risk of bleeding. When bleeding is acute, packed RBCs, fresh frozen plasma, or platelets may be administered to restore blood components and promote hemostasis.

■ Antacids are prescribed as indicated. A drug regimen to treat *H. pylori* infection may also be effective (∞ see Chapter 23).

■ Oxazepam (Serax), a benzodiazepine antianxiety/sedative drug, is not metabolized by the liver, and may be used to treat acute agitation.

Nutrition and Fluid Management

Dietary support is an essential part of care for the patient with cirrhosis. Dietary needs change as hepatic function fluctuates.

■ Sodium intake is restricted to under 2 g/day, and fluids are restricted as necessary to reduce ascites and generalized edema. Fluids are often limited to 1500 mL/day. Fluid needs are calculated based on response to diuretic therapy, urine output, and serum electrolyte values.

■ Unless serum ammonia levels are high, a palatable diet with adequate calories and protein is recommended. Although dietary protein restriction has previously been recommended for patients with cirrhosis and hepatic encephalopathy, it is now recognized that the effects of protein-calorie malnutrition are more damaging than protein consumption (Fauci et al., 2008; Wolf, 2008). Vegetable proteins may be recommended along with restricted red meat consumption. Parenteral nutrition is used as needed to maintain nutritional status when food intake is limited.

■ Vitamin and mineral supplements are ordered based on laboratory values. Deficiencies in the B-complex vitamins, particularly thiamin, folate, and B_{12}, and the fat-soluble vitamins A, D, and E are common. These vitamins may need to be administered in a water-soluble form. Patients with alcohol-induced cirrhosis are at high risk for magnesium deficiency, which needs to be replaced.

Complication Management

ASCITES **Paracentesis**, aspiration of fluid from the peritoneal cavity, may be a diagnostic or a therapeutic procedure. It may be done therapeutically to relieve severe ascites that does not respond to diuretic therapy. The goal of paracentesis is to relieve respiratory distress caused by excess fluid in the abdomen. Ascites fluid may be withdrawn in moderate amounts of 500 mL to 1 L daily to reduce the risk of fluid and electrolyte imbalances. Large-volume paracentesis, withdrawal of 4 to 6 L of fluid at one time, may be used. Albumin is often administered intravenously during large-volume paracentesis to maintain intravascular volume as the pressure of the ascites fluid in the abdomen is relieved. Nursing care for the patient undergoing paracentesis are listed in the accompanying box. Figure 25–6 ■ shows insertion sites and patient positioning during paracentesis.

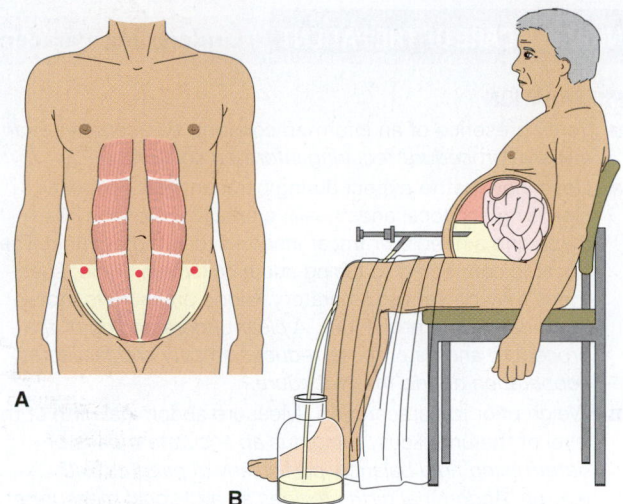

Figure 25–6 ■ Sites and position for paracentesis. *A,* Potential sites of needle or trocar insertion to avoid abdominal organ damage. *B,* The patient sits comfortably; in this position, the intestines float back and away from the insertion site.

ESOPHAGEAL VARICES Primary care for esophageal varices involves screening with endoscopy. When varices are identified, beta blocker therapy may be initiated to lower portal venous pressure or endoscopic variceal ligation or sclerotherapy may be performed. In *variceal ligation* or *banding,* small rubber bands are placed on varices to occlude blood flow. *Endoscopic sclerosis* involves injecting a sclerosing agent directly into the varices to induce inflammation and clotting. ∞ See Chapter 21 for the nursing implications of endoscopy.

Bleeding esophageal varices are life threatening and require intensive care management. Restoration of hemodynamic stability is the first priority. A central line is inserted and central venous and pulmonary artery pressures are monitored (∞ see Chapter 31). Blood is given to restore blood volume, and fresh frozen plasma may be administered to restore clotting factors. Somatostatin or octreotide, drugs that constrict blood vessels in the gut, are given intravenously to reduce blood flow in the portal venous system.

When the blood pressure and cardiac output have stabilized, upper endoscopy is performed to evaluate and treat the varices. A large nasogastric tube is inserted prior to endoscopy, and gastric lavage (irrigation of the stomach with large quantities of normal saline) is performed to improve visualization. During endoscopy, the varices may be banded or sclerosed to reduce the risk of recurrent bleeding. *Balloon tamponade* of bleeding varices may be used if bleeding cannot be controlled through vasoconstriction or if endoscopy is unavailable or contraindicated by the patient's condition. A multiple-lumen nasogastric (NG) tube (such as a Sengstaken-Blakemore tube or a Minnesota tube) is inserted, and the gastric and esophageal balloons are inflated to apply direct pressure on the bleeding varices (Figure 25–7 ■). Tension is applied to the tube to further compress the varices. Balloon tamponade carries a number of risks, including aspiration,

---

NURSING CARE OF THE PATIENT **Undergoing Paracentesis**

PREPARATION

- Verify presence of an informed consent. *Paracentesis is an invasive procedure requiring informed consent.*
- Describe what to expect during paracentesis: Following cleansing and local anesthesia, a small incision may be made and a needle or trocar inserted to withdraw fluid. The trocar is connected to tubing and a collection bottle; specimens may be sent to laboratory. Blood pressure is monitored during the procedure. *A clear understanding of the procedure and its purpose reduces anxiety and facilitates cooperation during the procedure.*
- Weigh prior to paracentesis. Measure abdominal girth at the level of the umbilicus. *Weight is an accurate means of determining fluid balance, particularly in patients with edema. Abdominal girth provides an additional measure of the effectiveness of paracentesis.*
- Assess vital signs for baseline. *Fluid shifts during and after paracentesis can affect cardiovascular stability. Baseline vital signs provide a reference for subsequent measurements.*
- Have patient void immediately prior to the test. *The bladder must be empty prior to paracentesis to reduce the risk for bladder puncture.*

- Position seated, either on the side of the bed or in a chair, with feet supported. *The sitting position allows ascites fluid to collect in the lower abdomen, facilitating its removal.*

AFTER THE PROCEDURE

- A small dressing is placed over the puncture site after the needle is withdrawn. There may be some fluid leakage from the site. *Depending on the size of the trocar inserted and the amount of remaining ascites fluid, the insertion puncture may not immediately seal, allowing fluid to escape.*
- Monitor vital signs every 15 minutes for 1 hour, every 30 minutes for 1 hour, then every 4 hours. Measure abdominal girth and obtain weight. *Removal of large amounts of fluid from the abdominal cavity can cause significant fluid shifts with resulting vascular instability. Weight and abdominal girth measurements provide information about fluid balance.*
- Salt-poor albumin may be given after the procedure to replace lost protein. *Removing ascites fluid reduces pressure within the peritoneal cavity. In the patient with hypoalbuminemia and portal hypertension, a significant amount of vascular fluid can escape as a result, leading to hypovolemia. Albumin is given to increase plasma oncotic pressure, helping retain fluid within the vascular system.*

---

airway obstruction, and tissue ischemia and necrosis. An endotracheal tube is inserted prior to nasogastric intubation to support the airway and reduce the risk of aspiration. This short-term measure is used only until more definitive treatment can be done. Without definitive treatment, rebleeding is common when balloon tamponade is discontinued.

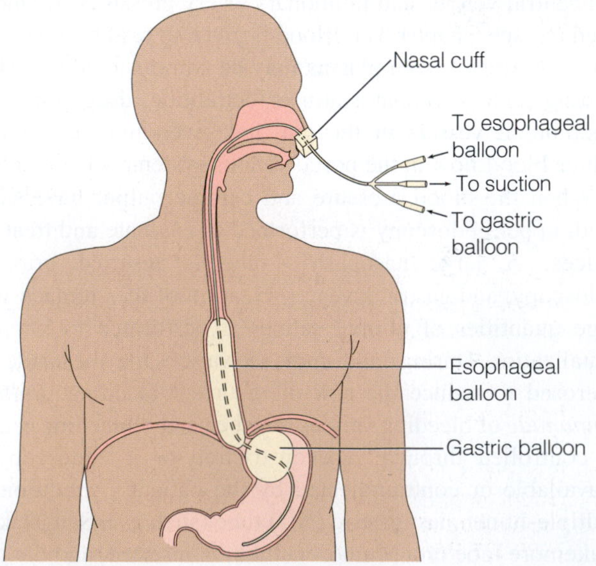

Figure 25–7 ■ Triple-lumen nasogastric tube (Sengstaken-Blakemore) used to control bleeding esophageal varices.

SAFETY ALERT

When caring for a patient with a multiple-lumen NG tube, always deflate the esophageal balloon before the gastric balloon. This practice prevents the balloon from becoming misplaced and occluding the airway. Always keep an appropriate syringe at the bedside to deflate the esophageal balloon should the patient develop respiratory distress.

PORTAL HYPERTENSION *Transjugular intrahepatic portosystemic shunt (TIPS)* may be used as an emergency measure to relieve portal hypertension and its complications of esophageal varices and ascites. A channel is created through the liver tissue using a needle inserted transcutaneously (Figure 25–8 ■). An expandable metal stent is inserted into this channel to allow blood to flow directly from the portal vein into the hepatic vein, bypassing the cirrhotic liver. The shunt relieves pressure in esophageal varices and allows better control of fluid retention with diuretic therapy. Stenosis and occlusion of the shunt are frequent complications. TIPS also increases the risk of developing hepatic encephalopathy (due to decreased perfusion of the liver and impaired ammonia metabolism) and may reduce long-term survival. It generally is used as a short-term measure until liver transplant is performed.

Surgery

Liver transplantation is indicated for some patients with irreversible, progressive cirrhosis. A decline in functional status, increasing bilirubin levels, falling albumin levels, and increasing problems with complications that respond poorly to treatment

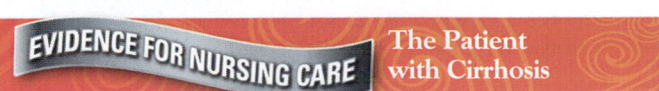

Figure 25–8 ■ Transjugular intrahepatic portosystemic shunt (TIPS). *A,* Guided by angiography, a balloon catheter inserted via the jugular vein is advanced to the hepatic veins and through the substance of the liver to create a portacaval (portal vein-to-vena cava) channel. *B,* A metal stent is positioned into the channel, and expanded by inflating the balloon. *C,* The stent remains in place after the catheter is removed, creating a shunt for blood to flow directly from the portal vein into the hepatic vein.

are indications for liver transplantation. Malignancy, active alcohol or drug abuse, and poor surgical risk are contraindications for the surgery. See the box for nursing care of the patient undergoing a liver transplant.

Nursing Care

In addition to the nursing care discussed in this section, a Case Study & Nursing Care Plan for a patient with alcoholic cirrhosis is found on page 748.

Health Promotion

For most patients, high-risk behaviors are the risk factors for cirrhosis. With all patients (including children and young adults), stress the relationship between alcohol and drug abuse and liver disorders. While many patients tolerate alcohol use in moderation with no adverse effects on the liver, excess alcohol use is the leading cause of cirrhosis. Injection drug use also is a significant risk factor, increasing the risk for contracting blood-borne hepatitis (B, C, or D). These types of viral hepatitis can lead to chronic hepatitis and, ultimately, to cirrhosis. Provide information and referral as appropriate for hepatitis B immunization. Discuss abstinence or safer sex practices as another measure to prevent viral hepatitis and potential liver damage.

Assessment

Assessment data related to cirrhosis include the following:

- *Health history:*   Current manifestations, including abdominal pain or discomfort, recent weight loss, weakness, and anorexia; altered bowel elimination; excess bleeding or bruising; abdominal distention; jaundice, pruritus; altered libido or impotence; duration of symptoms; history of liver or gallbladder disease; pattern and extent of alcohol or injection drug use; use of other prescription and nonprescription drugs.
- *Physical assessment:*   Vital signs; mental status; color and condition of skin and mucous membranes; peripheral pulses and presence of peripheral edema; abdominal assessment including appearance, shape and contour, bowel sounds, abdominal girth, percussion for liver borders, and palpation for tenderness and liver size.

Nursing Diagnoses and Interventions

Nursing care of the patient with cirrhosis presents many challenges because liver function affects all body systems. The nurse is responsible for coordinating care among care providers. Many nursing diagnoses may apply. The diagnoses discussed in this section focus on problems with fluid and electrolyte balance, disturbed thought processes, risk for bleeding, skin integrity, and nutrition.

Excess Fluid Volume

Cirrhosis affects water and salt regulation due to portal hypertension, hypoalbuminemia, and hyperaldosteronism. Signs of fluid volume overload and portal hypertension may develop: ascites, peripheral edema, internal hemorrhoids and varices, and prominent abdominal wall veins. Careful monitoring is necessary, because treatment measures can lead to further fluid and electrolyte imbalances.

EVIDENCE FOR NURSING CARE   **The Patient with Cirrhosis**

Selected resources that nurses may find helpful when planning evidence-based nursing care follow.

- Garcia-Tsao, G., & Bosch, J. (2010). Management of varices and variceal hemorrhage in cirrhosis. *New England Journal of Medicine, 362*(9), 823–832.
- Les, I., Doval, E., Flavià, M., Jacas, C., Cárdenas, G., Esteban, R., et al. (2010). Quality of life in cirrhosis is related to potentially treatable factors. *European Journal of Gastroenterology & Hepatology, 22*(2), 221–227.
- O'Shea, R., Dasarathy, S., McCullough, A., (2010, January). Alcoholic liver disease. *Hepatology, 51*(1), 307–28. Retrieved from http://www.guideline.gov/summary/summary.aspx?ss=15&doc_id=15477&nbr=007577&string=cirrhosis
- Runyon, B., & AASLD Practice Guidelines Committee. (2009, June). Management of adult patients with ascites due to cirrhosis: An update. *Hepatology, 49*(6), 2087-107. Retrieved from http://www.guideline.gov/summary/summary.aspx?ss=15&doc_id=14887&nbr=007373&string=cirrhosis

NURSING CARE OF THE PATIENT | Undergoing Liver Transplantation

PREOPERATIVE CARE

- Obtain a complete nursing history and physical examination. *A complete preoperative nursing assessment provides baseline data for comparison after surgery.*
- Provide routine preoperative care as ordered (∞ see Chapter 4). *Preoperative care is similar to that provided for other patients undergoing major surgery.*
- Discuss preoperative and postoperative expectations with the patient and family. Introduce to the intensive care unit, and discuss anticipated drainage tubes and supportive measures in the immediate postoperative period. Provide information about visiting policies and family accommodations (if available). *Preoperative teaching helps relieve anxiety in the patient and family members. Patients return from surgery to an intensive care or specialized care unit. Restrictions on the number of visitors and the time they may spend with the patient are common.*
- Once a donor liver is located, check for evidence of infection; if no infection is present, begin preoperative antibiotics as ordered. *An acute or chronic infection may contraindicate liver transplantation as drugs given postoperatively to suppress rejection of the transplanted organ also impair the ability to fight infection.*

POSTOPERATIVE CARE

- Provide routine postoperative care as outlined in ∞ Chapter 4.
- Maintain airway and ventilatory support until awake and alert. *Until the new liver clears the anesthesia, the patient requires measures to support respirations and ventilation.*
- Monitor temperature and implement rewarming measures (such as warming blankets, heating lamps, and head covers) as indicated. *The patient often is hypothermic after liver transplant, necessitating careful rewarming while maintaining hemodynamic stability.*
- Frequently monitor hemodynamic pressures, including arterial blood pressure, central venous pressure, and pulmonary artery pressures. *Postoperative fluid volume status may be difficult to determine without careful pressure measurements. The rate and type of fluids administered are determined by hemodynamic status.*

- Monitor urine output hourly; maintain careful intake and output records. Weigh daily. *Urine output and weight provide additional information about fluid volume status. In addition, renal function may be altered after liver transplant; acute renal failure is a significant risk.* ∞ *See Chapter 28 for more information about acute renal failure and its management.*
- Monitor for signs of active bleeding, including excess drainage, increasing abdominal girth, bloody nasogastric drainage, black tarry stools, tachypnea, tachycardia, diminished peripheral pulses, or pallor. Report immediately. *Altered coagulation in the early postoperative period increases the risk for bleeding. Blood products to replace volume and clotting factors may be necessary.*
- Monitor serum electrolytes and laboratory values related to blood coagulation, liver function, and renal function. Report abnormal results or significant changes immediately. *Electrolyte imbalances are common postoperatively. Altered liver or renal function tests may indicate rejection of the transplanted liver or acute renal failure. Other early signs of transplant rejection include fever, a drop in bile output, or a change in bile color and viscosity.*
- Monitor neurologic status. *With good function of the transplanted organ, mental status should clear within days of the transplant.*
- Provide discharge teaching:
  a. Teach how to reduce risk of infection, and signs of infection to report.
  b. Instruct how to recognize and report signs of organ rejection.
  c. Discuss all medications, including their purpose, schedule, adverse effects, and potential long-term effects. Stress the importance of complying with all prescribed medications and postoperative precautions for the remainder of the patient's life.
  d. Discuss possible changes in body image and psychologic responses to receiving a transplanted organ. Refer to a counselor or support group as indicated.
  e. Refer for home health services for continued assessment and teaching.
  f. Stress importance of continued follow-up with transplant team and primary care provider.

- Weigh daily. Assess for jugular vein distention, measure abdominal girth daily, and check for peripheral edema. Monitor intake and output. *Careful assessment is important to detect fluid shifts.*
- Assess urine specific gravity. *Specific gravity measures the concentration of urine, an indicator of hydration.*

PRACTICE ALERT
Monitor the patient with cirrhosis for signs of impaired renal function, such as oliguria, a fixed specific gravity of about 1.012, central edema (around the eyes and of the face), and increasing serum creatinine and BUN levels. Such signs may indicate hepatorenal syndrome or acute renal failure from another cause.

- Provide a low-sodium diet (500 to 2000 mg/day) and restrict fluids as ordered. *Excess sodium leads to water retention, and can increase fluid volume, ascites, and portal hypertension.*

Risk for Acute Confusion

Accumulated nitrogenous waste products and other metabolites affect mental status and thought processes. Effects of portal systemic encephalopathy can range from mild confusion to agitation to coma.

- Assess neurologic status, including level of consciousness and mental status. Observe for signs of early encephalopathy: changes in handwriting, speech, and asterixis. *Early identification of evidence of encephalopathy allows prompt intervention—subtle changes in neurologic functioning are important!*

PRACTICE ALERT
Closely monitor patients who have experienced gastrointestinal bleeding for signs of portal systemic encephalopathy. Blood in the intestinal tract is digested as a protein, increasing serum ammonia levels and the risk for portal systemic encephalopathy.

- Avoid factors that may precipitate portal systemic encephalopathy. Avoid hepatotoxic medications and CNS depressant drugs. *Cautious use of medications and close monitoring can eliminate iatrogenic causes of encephalopathy.*

- If possible, plan for consistent nursing care assignments. *Consistent care providers facilitate early identification of subtle neurologic changes indicative of portal systemic encephalopathy.*

- Administer medications or enemas as ordered to reduce nitrogenous products. Monitor bowel function and provide measures to promote regular elimination and prevent constipation. *Oral or rectally administered (per enema) medications are ordered to reduce intestinal bacteria and the ammonia they produce. Regular bowel elimination promotes protein and ammonia elimination in the feces.*

- Orient to surroundings, person, and place; provide simple explanations and reassurance. *Modification of verbal interactions to level of understanding and mental status may reduce anxiety and agitation.*

Risk for Bleeding
Impaired coagulation, esophageal varices, and possible acute gastritis place the patient with cirrhosis at significant risk for hemorrhage. Clotting is altered by vitamin K deficiency; impaired manufacture of coagulation Factors II, VII, IX, and X; and increased platelet destruction due to splenomegaly.

- Monitor vital signs; report tachycardia or hypotension. *Increased pulse and decreasing blood pressure may indicate hypovolemia due to hemorrhage.*

- Institute bleeding precautions (Box 25–6). *Preventive measures can decrease the risk for active bleeding.*

- Monitor coagulation studies and platelet count. Report abnormal results. *Coagulation studies help determine the risk for bleeding and the need for treatment.*

- Carefully monitor the patient who has had bleeding esophageal varices for evidence of rebleeding: hematemesis, hematochezia (bright blood in the stool) or tarry stools, signs of hypovolemia or shock. *Rebleeding is common following variceal hemorrhage, especially within the first week.*

> **PRACTICE ALERT**
> Carefully monitor the respiratory status of the patient with a Sengstaken-Blakemore or Minnesota tube. Displacement of the tube can obstruct the airway unless an endotracheal tube is in place. The esophageal balloon prevents the patient from swallowing oral secretions, increasing the risk for aspiration. Keep the head of the bed elevated to 45 degrees to reduce the risk of aspiration and promote gas exchange.

Impaired Skin Integrity
Severe jaundice with bile salt deposits on the skin may cause pruritus. Scratching related to the pruritus damages the skin and impairs its integrity. Malnutrition, particularly protein deficiency, and edema also increase the risk for tissue breakdown and impaired skin integrity.

> **BOX 25–5 Bleeding Precautions**
> - Prevent constipation.
> - Avoid rectal temperatures or enemas.
> - Avoid injections; if needed, use small-gauge needle and apply gentle pressure.
> - Monitor platelet count, PT, and aPPT.
> - Assess for ecchymotic areas and areas of purpura.
> - Apply pressure to bleeding sites. After venipuncture, apply direct pressure for at least 5 minutes.
> - Use only a soft toothbrush.
> - Avoid blowing nose.
> - Assess oral cavity for bleeding gums.

- Use warm water rather than hot water when bathing. *Hot water increases pruritus.*

- Use measures to prevent dry skin: Apply an emollient or lubricant as needed to keep skin moist, avoid soap or preparations with alcohol, and do not rub the skin. *Dry skin contributes to pruritus.*

- If indicated, apply mittens to the hands to prevent scratching. *Patients with encephalopathy may not understand the need to refrain from scratching.*

- Institute measures to prevent skin and tissue breakdown: Turn at least every 2 hours, use an alternating pressure mattress, and frequently assess skin condition. *Frequent position changes relieve pressure and promote circulation and tissue oxygenation.*

- Administer prescribed antihistamine (to relieve pruritus) cautiously. *Decreased liver function increases the risk for altered drug responses.*

Imbalanced Nutrition: Less than Body Requirements
The patient with cirrhosis is at risk for malnutrition for a number of reasons: possible chronic alcohol use, anorexia, impaired vitamin and mineral absorption, and impaired protein metabolism. In addition, salt restrictions may make the diet less palatable and appealing to the patient.

- Weigh daily. Instruct to weigh at least weekly at home. *Weight is a good indicator of both nutritional status and fluid balance. Short-term weight fluctuations tend to reflect fluid balance, while longer term changes in weight are more reflective of nutritional status.*

- Provide small meals with between-meal snacks. *A small meal is more appealing for an anorexic patient. Between-meal snacks help maintain adequate calorie and nutrient intake.*

- Unless protein is restricted due to impending portal systemic encephalopathy, promote protein and nutrient intake by providing nutritional supplements such as Ensure or instant breakfasts. *The sodium and protein content of all meals and snacks must be calculated when maintaining restrictions of these nutrients.*

- Arrange for consultation with a dietitian for diet planning while hospitalized and at home. *The dietitian can provide detailed instructions, sample menus, and suggestions for improving the palatability of the diet and promoting intake.*

CASE STUDY & NURSING CARE PLAN   A Patient with Alcoholic Cirrhosis

Richard Wright is a 48-year-old divorced father of two teenagers. Mr. Wright has been admitted to the community hospital with ascites and malnutrition. He has had three previous hospital stays for cirrhosis, the most recent being 6 months ago.

ASSESSMENT

Mr. Wright is lethargic but responds appropriately to verbal stimuli. He complains of "spitting up blood the past week or so" and says, "I'm just not hungry." He has lost 20 lb (9 kg) since his previous admission. He is jaundiced and has petechiae and ecchymoses on his arms and legs. Liz Mowdi, Mr. Wright's nurse, notes pitting pretibial edema. Abdominal assessment reveals a tight, protuberant abdomen with caput medusae. The liver margin is not palpable; the spleen is enlarged. Vital signs are T 100°F (37.7°C), P 110, R 25, and BP 110/70.

Abnormal laboratory results include WBC 3700/mm^3 (normal 4300 to 10,800/mm^3); RBC 4.0 million/mm^3 (normal 4.6 to 5.9 million/mm^3); platelets 75,000/mm^3 (normal 150,000 to 350,000/mm^3); serum ammonia 105 μm/dL (normal 35 to 65 μm/dL); total bilirubin 4.9 mcg/dL (normal 0.1 to 1.0 mcg/dL); and serum sodium 150 mEq/L (normal 135 to 145 mEq/L). Potassium, hemoglobin, hematocrit, total protein, and albumin levels are markedly decreased. Hepatic enzymes are elevated. Blood urea nitrogen and creatinine levels are marginally elevated. Oxygen saturation (O$_2$ sat) is 88% (normal range: 96% to 100%) per pulse oximetry.

Endoscopy shows bleeding from gastric ulcer, and the diagnosis of alcoholic cirrhosis with gastritis is made. Mr. Wright is started on Aldactone, 25 mg PO q8h; Riopan, 30 mL 2 h p.c. and hs; lactulose, 30 mL qh until onset of diarrhea, then 15 mL tid; and 800 mg sodium diet; fluid restriction of 1500 mL/day.

DIAGNOSES

- *Impaired Gas Exchange* related to pressure of ascites fluid on the diaphragm as manifested by tachypnea and decreased oxygen saturation
- *Excess Fluid Volume* related to electrolyte imbalance and hypoalbuminemia as manifested by ascites and peripheral edema
- *Imbalanced Nutrition: Less than Body Requirements* related to anorexia and possible alcohol abuse as manifested by weight loss and low serum protein levels
- *Risk for Acute Confusion* related to effects of high ammonia levels as manifested by lethargy
- *Risk for Bleeding* related to impaired platelet formation and portal hypertension

EXPECTED OUTCOMES

- Respiratory rate and O$_2$ sats will be within normal limits.
- Abdominal girth will decrease by 1 to 2 cm per day; peripheral edema will decrease.
- Will gain 1 lb (0.45 kg) per week without evidence of increased fluid retention. Serum albumin levels will return to normal range.
- Will be alert and oriented; serum ammonia levels are within normal range.
- Will demonstrate no further evidence of active bleeding.
- Will verbalize willingness to join a community support group.

PLANNING AND IMPLEMENTATION

- Weigh daily.
- Provide high-calorie, low-salt, low-protein diet with between-meal snacks.
- Maintain stool chart.
- Assign same nurses to care as much as possible to facilitate evaluation of mental status. Promptly report changes in status or laboratory values.
- Measure abdominal girth every 8 hours, marking level of measurement.
- Institute bleeding precautions.
- Elevate head of bed; assist to chair with legs elevated tid as tolerated.
- Include significant others in care and teaching; refer to community agencies for discharge follow-up.

EVALUATION

A week after admission, Mr. Wright's ascites has decreased and no further active bleeding is noted. His serum protein levels have increased, and his laboratory values are improving. No further bruising is noted during hospitalization. Although he shows a 5-lb weight loss as excess water is eliminated, he is consuming 100% of his diet. His serum ammonia levels have returned to normal. On discharge, O$_2$ sat is 96%; respirations are 18. Lactulose will be continued on discharge.

Ms. Mowdi provides both written and verbal information about the medication and cirrhosis, including measures to prevent complications. Mr. Wright and his children express interest in Alcoholics Anonymous and Al-Anon and are referred to those agencies. Prior to discharge, follow-up appointments are made with a psychiatric social worker and a primary caregiver.

CRITICAL THINKING IN THE NURSING PROCESS

1. Describe the relationship between portal hypertension, liver dysfunction, and ascites.
2. Outline a 1-day menu for a low-protein, low-sodium, high-calorie diet.
3. What is the pathophysiologic basis for portal systemic encephalopathy? What are the nursing responsibilities related to lactulose and neomycin?
4. Design a nursing care plan for Mr. Wright for the diagnosis *Ineffective Coping*.

See Evaluating Your Response in Appendix C.

Using NANDA, NIC, and NOC

Linkages between a selected NANDA nursing diagnosis, NIC, and NOC for the patient with cirrhosis are shown in the chart that follows.

Community-Based Care

Cirrhosis is a chronic, progressive disease. As such, the patient and family assume major roles in managing the disease and its manifestations and in preventing complications. Teaching topics for home care include the following:

- The absolute necessity of avoiding alcohol and other hepatotoxic drugs. Suggest inpatient or community-based alcohol treatment programs and Alcoholics Anonymous as indicated.
- Diet and fluid intake restrictions and recommendations. Include suggestions to promote nutritional intake and increase the flavor of food when sodium is restricted.
- Prescribed medications, their timing, intended and adverse effects, and manifestations to report to the primary care provider.
- Bleeding precautions (see Box 25–5).

NANDA, NIC, AND NOC LINKAGES
The Patient with Cirrhosis

NANDA → Ineffective Protection

↓

NIC → Environmental Management: Safety
Self-Responsibility Facilitation
Bleeding Precautions
Skin Surveillance

↓

NOC → Neurologic Status
Health Promoting Behavior
Blood Coagulation
Tissue Integrity:
Skin and Mucous Membranes

Data from NANDA International. (2009). *Nursing diagnoses: Definitions & classification 2009–2011.* Oxford, UK: Wiley-Blackwell; Bulechek, G., Butcher, H., & Dochterman, J. (Eds.). (2008). *Nursing interventions classification (NIC)* (5th ed.). St. Louis, MO: Mosby; and Moorhead, S., Johnson, M., Maas, M., & Swanson, E. (Eds.). (2008). *Nursing outcomes classification (NOC)* (4th ed.). St. Louis, MO: Mosby.

- Manifestations of potential complications to be reported to the primary care provider. Stress the importance of promptly reporting evidence of gastrointestinal bleeding for prompt intervention for potential hemorrhage.
- Skin care techniques to reduce pruritus and the risk of damage.
- Ways to manage fatigue and conserve energy.

Provide referrals for home health services, dietary consultation, social services, and counseling as needed by the patient and family. Suggest local support groups where available. If appropriate, suggest hospice services for the patient with end-stage liver disease.

The Patient with Cancer of the Liver

Primary liver cancer is uncommon in the United States, accounting for only 0.5% to 2% of all cancers (American Cancer Society [ACS], 2009). It is, however, a common malignancy worldwide. Hepatocellular carcinoma is common in parts of Asia and Africa, where the incidence is as high as 500 cases per 100,000 people. This higher incidence is linked to chronic hepatitis B or C infection. The incidence of primary liver cancer in men is nearly double that in women. The incidence of liver cancer is higher in Hispanics than it is in Black and non-Hispanic Whites; Blacks have a higher incidence than Whites (ACS, 2006; ACS 2007). The prognosis for primary liver cancer is poor, in part because the disease often is advanced at the time of diagnosis. Metastasis to the liver from primary tumors of the lung, breast, and gastrointestinal tract are relatively common.

Pathophysiology

About 80% to 90% of primary hepatic cancers arise from the liver's parenchymal cells (hepatocellular carcinoma); the remainder form in the bile ducts (cholangiocarcinoma). Regardless of the origin, the progress of the disease is similar.

BOX 25–6 **Suspected Causes of Primary Liver Cancer**

- Chronic hepatitis C infection
- Chronic hepatitis B infection
- Cirrhosis, regardless of type
- Aflatoxin (a toxin produced by *Aspergillus* molds) exposure
- Chronic ethanol consumption
- Nonalcoholic fatty liver (steatohepatitis or NASH)

Several etiologic factors have been identified (Box 25–6). Most primary liver cancer in the United States is related to alcoholic cirrhosis, HBV, or HCV.

The underlying pathophysiology of primary liver cancer is damage to hepatocellular DNA. This damage may be caused by integration of HBV or HCV into the DNA or by repeated cycles of cell necrosis and regeneration that facilitate DNA mutations. HBV and aflatoxins damage a specific tumor suppressor gene, p53. Tumors may be limited to one specific area, may occur as nodules throughout the liver, or may develop as surface infiltrates. The tumor interferes with normal hepatic function, leading to biliary obstruction and jaundice, portal hypertension, and metabolic disruptions (hypoalbuminemia, hypoglycemia, and bleeding disorders). It also may secrete bile products and produce hormones (paraneoplastic syndrome) that may lead to polycythemia, hypoglycemia, and hypercalcemia. Tumors usually grow rapidly and metastasize early.

Manifestations

Initial manifestations of liver cancer develop insidiously and often are masked by the presence of cirrhosis or chronic hepatitis. Weakness, anorexia, weight loss, fatigue, and malaise are common early manifestations. Abdominal pain and a palpable mass in the right upper quadrant are common presenting symptoms. See the following box for manifestations of primary liver cancer. Ascites and jaundice may be present at diagnosis. Signs of liver failure with portal hypertension, splenomegaly, and altered metabolism develop as the tumor progresses.

Interdisciplinary Care

Ultrasound of the liver is used as a screening tool for liver cancer. CT scan with contrast and MRI are used to determine tumor size and extent. A liver biopsy is done to confirm the diagnosis and identify the tumor type or origin. See the box on page 575 for the nursing implications of liver biopsy. Serum alpha-fetoprotein (AFP) levels, normally low in nonpregnant adults, rise in most patients with hepatocellular cancer.

MANIFESTATIONS of Primary Liver Cancer

- Malaise
- Anorexia
- Lethargy
- Weight loss
- Fever of unknown origin
- Jaundice
- Feeling of abdominal fullness
- Painful right upper quadrant mass
- Manifestations of liver failure

Small, localized tumors may be surgically resected, or destroyed using radiofrequency ablation or injection of an agent such as ethanol directly into the tumor. Most tumors, however, have spread extensively or have distant metastasis at the time of diagnosis, so this is frequently not an option. Additionally, patients with underlying liver disease such as cirrhosis may not tolerate loss of additional functional liver tissue. Liver transplantation may be done for stage I or II tumors (no apparent lymph node involvement or distant metastasis). Liver transplantation is limited as a treatment option by the availability of donor organs.

Radiation therapy may be used to shrink the tumor, decreasing pressure on surrounding organs and reducing pain. Chemotherapy may be used as primary treatment for advanced tumors. Direct continuous hepatic arterial infusion with an implanted pump has shown promise in prolonging survival rates. ∞ See Chapter 14 for nursing care for patients receiving radiation therapy or chemotherapy.

Nursing Care

Encourage patients with risk factors for primary liver cancer to avoid alcohol and other substances that may further damage the liver. Urge them to discuss regular screening for liver tumors (such as serum AFP levels) with their primary care physician.

Both the patient and the family need extensive nursing support. Controlling pain is a priority. Because of the poor prognosis, early referral for hospice services may be appropriate.

Nursing diagnoses, interventions, and teaching for the patient with liver cancer are similar to those for patients with cirrhosis (see pages 745–749).

The Patient with Liver Trauma

Blunt or penetrating trauma to the abdomen can damage the liver. Liver trauma is frequently seen in combination with injuries to other abdominal organs. Motor vehicle crashes, stab or gunshot wounds, and iatrogenic sources such as liver biopsy are among the causes of these injuries.

Pathophysiology and Manifestations

Liver trauma generally causes bleeding due to the vascularity of the organ. Liver injury may cause a surface hematoma, hematoma within the liver parenchyma, laceration of liver tissue, or disruption of vessels leading to or from the liver. Severe bleeding can rapidly disrupt hemodynamic stability and lead to shock.

> **PRACTICE ALERT**
> Bleeding due to liver trauma may not be immediately apparent. Instruct the patient with apparent or potential liver trauma to immediately report light-headedness, rapid heart rate, shortness of breath, thirst, or increasing abdominal pain.

Interdisciplinary Care

Diagnostic peritoneal lavage is often used along with CT scan to diagnose liver trauma. The procedure is performed by making a small abdominal incision into the peritoneum (after the bladder has been emptied), and inserting a small catheter into the peritoneal cavity. If blood is immediately detected, the patient is taken directly to surgery for abdominal exploration. If frank bleeding is not apparent, a liter of isotonic fluid is instilled into the abdomen, then drained and sent for laboratory analysis.

Intravenous fluids, fresh frozen plasma, platelets, and other clotting factors are administered to restore blood volume and promote hemostasis. Hemodynamic status is closely monitored; continued instability may indicate a need for surgical intervention to control hemorrhage. Postoperative nursing care focuses on preventing pulmonary complications, such as atelectasis, and detecting and preventing infection.

Nursing Care

Nursing care of the patient with liver trauma focuses on fluid management and other supportive care related to shock. Keeping family members informed is an important aspect of care, especially during the period of patient instability. Diagnoses include the following:

- *Deficient Fluid Volume* related to hemorrhage
- *Risk for Infection* related to wound or abdominal contamination
- *Risk for Bleeding* related to impaired coagulation

The Patient with Liver Abscess

Liver abscesses usually are bacterial or amoebic (protozoal) in origin. Bacterial abscesses may follow trauma or surgical procedures, including biopsy. Multiple or single abscesses occur most commonly in the right lobe. Amoebic abscesses most frequently occur following infestation of the liver by *Entamoeba histolytica*. Amoebic infestation is associated with poor hygiene, unsafe sexual practices, or travel in areas where drinking water is contaminated.

Pathophysiology and Manifestations

Following bacterial or amoebic invasion of the liver, healthy tissue is destroyed, leaving an area of necrosis, inflammatory exudate, and blood. This damaged region becomes walled off from the healthy liver tissue. Pyogenic (bacterial) liver abscess may be caused by cholangitis, or distant or intra-abdominal infections, such as peritonitis or diverticulitis. *Escherichia coli* is the most frequently identified causative organism. The onset of pyogenic abscess is usually sudden, causing acute symptoms such as fever, malaise, vomiting, hyperbilirubinemia, and pain in the right upper abdomen.

The infection pathway for amoebic hepatic abscesses usually is the portal venous circulation from the right colon. Generally, the onset of amoebic abscess is insidious.

Interdisciplinary Care

Hepatic abscess is diagnosed through biopsy, hepatic aspirate, blood and fecal cultures, and CT scan and ultrasound studies. Therapy is based on identifying the causative organism through laboratory cultures. Pyogenic abscesses are treated with antibiotics to which the causative organism is sensitive.

Pharmacologic agents used for amebic hepatic abscess are the same as those used for intestinal amebic infestation (∞ see Chapter 24); combination therapy is commonly used. Two commonly used drugs for treating amebic liver abscesses are metronidazole (Flagyl) and iodoquinol (Diquinol). Both medications can cause gastrointestinal symptoms. Bone marrow suppression is a risk with metronidazole.

If the abscess does not respond to antibiotic therapy, percutaneous aspiration or surgical drainage may be done. In these procedures, a *percutaneous closed-catheter drain* is placed in the abscess to promote drainage of purulent material.

∞ Nursing Care

A major aspect of nursing care is prevention; teaching patients to avoid contaminated water and foods is especially important. Nursing interventions include teaching hikers to treat water and food handlers to wash hands thoroughly.

Patients who have a liver abscess require supportive care to prevent dehydration from the accompanying fever, nausea, vomiting, and anorexia. Careful monitoring of fluid and electrolyte status is indicated, as are comfort measures for abdominal pain. Possible nursing diagnoses include the following:

- *Risk for Deficient Fluid Volume* related to effects of prolonged fever and vomiting
- *Readiness for Enhanced Knowledge* related to transmission of amebic abscess
- *Activity Intolerance* related to pain and weakness

Exocrine Pancreas Disorders

The pancreas is both an exocrine and an endocrine gland. It is made up of two basic cell types, each having different functions. The exocrine cells produce enzymes that empty through ducts into the small intestine, whereas the endocrine cells produce hormones that enter the bloodstream directly. Disorders of the exocrine pancreas affect the secretion and glandular control of digestive enzymes, whereas disorders of the endocrine pancreas affect the production of hormones necessary for normal carbohydrate, protein, and fat metabolism. Disorders of the exocrine pancreas are discussed in this section of the chapter; diabetes mellitus, a disorder of the endocrine pancreas, is discussed in ∞ Chapter 20.

The Patient with Pancreatitis

Pancreatitis, or inflammation of the pancreas, is characterized by the release of pancreatic enzymes into the tissue of the pancreas itself, leading to hemorrhage and necrosis. Pancreatitis may be either acute or chronic. About 5000 new cases of acute pancreatitis are diagnosed every year in the United States. It is a serious disease, with a mortality rate of approximately 10% (Fauci et al., 2008). Hospitalizations for acute pancreatitis have increased over the past 15 years. Additionally, the incidence of hospitalization for acute pancreatitis is higher in Blacks than it is in Whites (Fagenholz et al., 2007). Alcoholism and gallstones are the primary risk factors for acute pancreatitis, however, the etiology of about 30% of cases is unclear.

The incidence of chronic pancreatitis is less clear because many people with chronic pancreatitis do not have classic manifestations of the disease. Patients with chronic pancreatitis may have long-term effects of the disease, with chronic changes in enzyme and hormone production.

Physiology Review

Knowledge of the normal structure and functions of the exocrine pancreas is important to understand how inflammation affects it and the patient. The exocrine pancreas consists of lobules of acinar cells. The acinar cells secrete digestive enzymes and fluids (pancreatic juices) into ducts that empty into the main pancreatic duct (the duct of Wirsung). The pancreatic duct joins the common bile duct and empties into the

duodenum through the ampulla of Vater (in some people the main pancreatic duct empties directly into the duodenum). The epithelial lining of the pancreatic ducts secretes water and bicarbonate to modify the composition of the pancreatic secretions. Pancreatic enzymes are secreted primarily in an inactive form and are activated in the intestine, a modification that prevents digestion of pancreatic tissue by its own enzymes (Porth & Matfin, 2009). The pancreatic enzymes, with related functions, are as follows:

- Proteolytic enzymes, including trypsin, chymotrypsin, carboxypolypeptidase, ribonuclease, and deoxyribonuclease, which break down dietary proteins
- Pancreatic amylase, which breaks down starch
- Lipase, which breaks down fats into glycerol and fatty acids

Pathophysiology

Acute Pancreatitis

Acute pancreatitis is an inflammatory disorder that involves self-destruction of the pancreas by its own enzymes through autodigestion. The milder form of acute pancreatitis, *interstitial edematous pancreatitis*, leads to inflammation and edema of pancreatic tissue. It often is self-limiting. The more severe form, *necrotizing pancreatitis*, is characterized by inflammation, hemorrhage, and ultimately necrosis of pancreatic tissue.

Acute pancreatitis is more common in middle adults; its incidence is higher in men than in women. Gallstones are the leading cause of acute pancreatitis, with alcohol being the second leading cause (Fauci et al., 2008). Some patients recover completely, others experience recurring attacks, and still others develop chronic pancreatitis. The mortality and symptoms depend on the severity and type of pancreatitis, as well as the patient's age and general health. Organ failure (respiratory failure in particular) is the leading cause of death in acute pancreatitis (Fauci et al., 2008).

Although the exact cause of pancreatitis is not known, the following factors may activate pancreatic enzymes within the pancreas, leading to autodigestion, inflammation, edema, and/or necrosis.

- Gallstones may obstruct the pancreatic duct or cause bile reflux, activating pancreatic enzymes in the pancreatic duct system.

■ Alcohol causes duodenal edema, and may increase pressure and spasm in the sphincter of Oddi, obstructing pancreatic outflow. It also stimulates pancreatic enzyme production, thus raising pressure within the pancreas.

Other factors associated with acute pancreatitis include tissue ischemia or anoxia, trauma or surgery, pancreatic tumors, third-trimester pregnancy, infectious agents (viral, bacterial, or parasitic), elevated calcium levels, and hyperlipidemia. Some medications have been linked with this disorder, including thiazide diuretics, estrogen, steroids, salicylates, and NSAIDs.

Regardless of the precipitating factor, the pathophysiologic process begins with the release of activated pancreatic enzymes into pancreatic tissue. Activated proteolytic enzymes, trypsin in particular, digest pancreatic tissue and activate other enzymes such as phospholipase A, which digests cell membrane phospholipids, and elastase, which digests the elastic tissue of blood vessel walls. This leads to proteolysis, edema, vascular damage and hemorrhage, and necrosis of parenchymal cells. Cellular damage and necrosis release activated enzymes and vasoactive substances that produce vasodilation, increase vascular permeability, and cause edema. A large volume of fluid may shift from circulating blood into the retroperitoneal space, the peripancreatic spaces, and the abdominal cavity.

MANIFESTATIONS Acute pancreatitis develops suddenly, typically with an abrupt onset of continuous severe epigastric and abdominal pain. This pain commonly radiates to the back and is relieved somewhat by sitting up and leaning forward. The pain often is initiated by a fatty meal or excessive alcohol intake.

Other manifestations include nausea and vomiting; abdominal distention and rigidity; decreased bowel sounds; tachycardia; hypotension; elevated temperature; and cold, clammy skin. Within 24 hours, mild jaundice may appear. Retroperitoneal bleeding may occur 3 to 6 days after the onset of acute pancreatitis; signs of bleeding include bruising in the flanks (Turner's sign) or around the umbilicus (Cullen's sign). See the accompanying Manifestations box below.

COMPLICATIONS Systemic complications of acute pancreatitis include intravascular volume depletion with shock, acute tubular necrosis and renal failure (∞ see Chapter 28 for more information about acute renal failure), and acute respiratory distress syndrome (ARDS). Hypovolemic shock and acute renal failure usually develop within 24 hours after the onset of acute pancreatitis. Manifestations of ARDS may be seen 3 to 7 days after its onset, particularly in patients who have experienced severe volume depletion. ∞ See Chapter 38 for more information about ARDS.

Localized complications include pancreatic necrosis, abscess, pseudocysts, and pancreatic ascites. Pancreatic necrosis causes an inflammatory mass that may be infected. It may lead to shock and multiple organ failure. A pancreatic abscess may form late in the course of the disease (6 or more weeks after its onset), causing an epigastric mass and tenderness (McPhee et al., 2008). Pancreatic pseudocysts, encapsulated collections of fluid, may develop both within the pancreas itself and in the abdominal cavity (Figure 25–9 ■). They may impinge on other structures, or may rupture, causing generalized peritonitis. Rupture of a pseudocyst or of the pancreatic duct can lead to pancreatic ascites. Pancreatic ascites is recognized by gradually increasing abdominal girth and persistent elevation of the serum amylase level without abdominal pain.

Chronic Pancreatitis

Chronic pancreatitis is characterized by chronic inflammation, fibrosis, and gradual destruction of functional pancreatic tissue. In contrast to acute pancreatitis, which is reversible, chronic pancreatitis is an irreversible process that eventually leads to pancreatic insufficiency. Alcoholism is the primary risk factor for chronic pancreatitis in the United States. Malnutrition is a major worldwide risk factor. About 10% to 20% of chronic pancreatitis is idiopathic, with no identified cause. A genetic mutation on a gene associated with cystic fibrosis may play a role in these cases. Children or young adults with cystic fibrosis may develop chronic pancreatitis as well.

MANIFESTATIONS of Acute and Chronic Pancreatitis

ACUTE PANCREATITIS
- Abrupt onset of severe epigastric and left upper quadrant pain, may radiate to back
- Nausea, vomiting; fever
- Decreased bowel sounds; abdominal distention and rigidity
- Tachycardia, hypotension; cold, clammy skin
- Possible jaundice
- Positive Turner's sign (flank ecchymosis) or Cullen's sign (periumbilical ecchymosis)

CHRONIC PANCREATITIS
- Recurrent epigastric and LUQ pain, radiates to back
- Anorexia, nausea and vomiting, weight loss
- Flatulence, constipation
- Steatorrhea

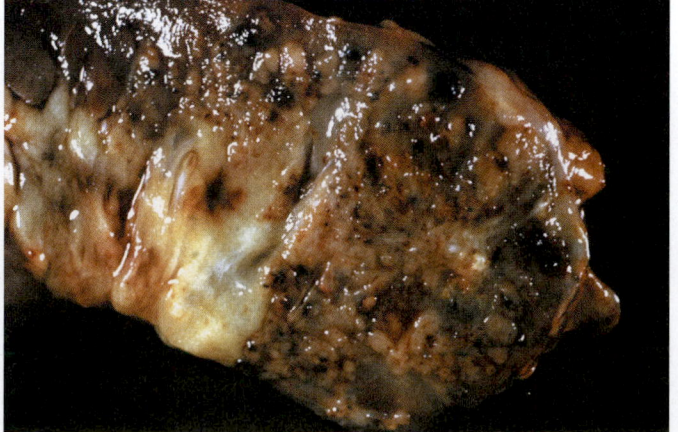

Figure 25–9 ■ Acute pancreatitis. Gross clinical specimen of a pancreas affected by acute pancreatitis. Pseudocyst, a pus-filled bleb seen as the yellow area (lower left center), is a potential complication of acute pancreatitis.

In chronic pancreatitis related to alcoholism, pancreatic secretions have an increased concentration of insoluble proteins. These proteins calcify, forming plugs that block pancreatic ducts and the flow of pancreatic juices. This blockage leads to inflammation and fibrosis of pancreatic tissue. In other cases, a stricture or stone may block pancreatic outflow, causing chronic obstructive pancreatitis. In chronic pancreatitis, recurrent episodes of inflammation eventually lead to fibrotic changes in the parenchyma of the pancreas, with loss of exocrine function. This leads to malabsorption from pancreatic insufficiency. If endocrine function is disrupted as well, clinical diabetes mellitus may develop.

MANIFESTATIONS Chronic pancreatitis typically causes recurrent episodes of epigastric and left upper abdominal pain that radiates to the back. This pain may last for days to weeks. As the disease progresses, the interval between episodes of pain becomes shorter. Other manifestations include anorexia, nausea and vomiting, weight loss, flatulence, constipation, and **steatorrhea** (fatty, frothy, foul-smelling stools caused by a decrease in pancreatic enzyme secretion).

COMPLICATIONS Complications of chronic pancreatitis include malabsorption, malnutrition, and possible peptic ulcer disease. Pancreatic pseudocyst or abscess may form, or stricture of the common bile duct may develop. Diabetes mellitus may develop, and there is an increased risk for pancreatic cancer. Opioid addiction related to frequent, severe pain episodes is common.

Interdisciplinary Care

Acute pancreatitis often is a mild, self-limiting disease. Treatment focuses on reducing pancreatic secretions and providing supportive care. Treatment to eliminate the causative factor is begun after the acute inflammatory process resolves. Severe necrotizing pancreatitis may require intensive care management. Treatment for chronic pancreatitis often focuses on managing pain and treating malabsorption and malnutrition.

Diagnosis

The laboratory tests that may be ordered when pancreatitis is suspected are summarized in Table 25–4. Diagnostic studies include the following:

- *Ultrasonography* can identify gallstones, a pancreatic mass, or pseudocyst.
- *Endoscopic ultrasonography* can detect changes indicative of chronic pancreatitis in the pancreatic duct and parenchyma.
- *Contrast-enhanced CT scan* may be ordered to identify pancreatic enlargement, ductal calcifications, fluid collections in or around the pancreas, and perfusion deficits in areas of necrosis.
- *Magnetic resonance cholangiopancreatography (MRCP)* is a noninvasive test that allows visualization of the bile and pancreatic ducts.
- *Endoscopic retrograde cholangiopancreatography (ERCP)* may be performed to diagnose chronic pancreatitis and to differentiate inflammation and fibrosis from carcinoma.
- *Percutaneous fine-needle aspiration biopsy* may be performed to differentiate chronic pancreatitis from cancer of the pancreas; the cells that are aspirated are examined for malignancy.

More information about these tests and their nursing implications can be found in ∞ Chapter 21.

Medications

The treatment of acute pancreatitis is largely supportive. Opioid analgesics such as morphine sulfate or hydromorphone (Dilaudid) are used as needed to control pain. Prophylactic antibiotics are prescribed for patients with severe or necrotizing pancreatitis to prevent infection.

Patients with chronic pancreatitis may also require analgesics, but are closely monitored to prevent drug dependence. Pancreatic enzyme supplements are given to manage abdominal pain and reduce steatorrhea (see the Medication Administration box on page 754). Patients with chronic pancreatitis may need to remain on pancreatic enzyme supplements for life. H_2 blockers such as cimetidine (Tagamet) and ranitidine (Zantac), and proton-pump inhibitors such as omeprazole

TABLE 25–4 Laboratory Tests in Exocrine Pancreatic Disorders

TEST	NORMAL VALUE	SIGNIFICANCE
Serum amylase	30 to 170 units/L	Rises within 2 to 12 hours of onset of acute pancreatitis to two to three times normal. Returns to normal in 3 to 4 days.
Serum lipase	14 to 280 units/L	Levels rise in acute pancreatitis; remain elevated for 7 to 14 days.
Urine amylase	4 to 37 units/L/2h	Urine amylase levels rise in acute pancreatitis.
Serum glucose	70 to 110 mg/dL	May be transient elevation in acute pancreatitis.
Serum bilirubin	0.1 to 1.2 mg/dL	Compression of the common duct may increase bilirubin levels in acute pancreatitis.
Serum alkaline phosphatase (ALP)	42 to 136 units/L	Compression of the common duct may increase levels in acute pancreatitis.
Serum calcium	9 to 11 mg/dL or 4.5 to 5.5 mEq/L	Hypocalcemia develops in up to 25% of patients with acute pancreatitis.
White blood cells	4500/mm³ to 10,000/mm³	Leukocytosis indicates inflammation and is usually present in acute pancreatitis.

MEDICATION ADMINISTRATION — The Patient with Chronic Pancreatitis

PANCREATIC ENZYME REPLACEMENT
Pancrelipase (Lipancreatin)

Pancrelipase enhances the digestion of starches and fats in the gastrointestinal tract by supplying an exogenous source of the enzymes protease, amylase, and lipase. The drug promotes nutrition and decreases the number of bowel movements.

Nursing Responsibilities
- Assess for allergy to pork protein.
- Monitor frequency and consistency of stools.
- Weigh every other day. Record weights.

- Give with meals; if not enteric coated, H_2 antagonists or antacids may be given concurrently to prevent destruction of the enzymes by hydrochloric acid.
- Monitor for side effects: rash, hives, respiratory difficulty, hematuria, hyperuricemia, or joint pain.

Health Education for the Patient and Family
- Take with meals or snacks.
- If medicine is enteric coated, do not crush, chew, or mix with alkaline foods (e.g., milk, ice cream).
- Be sure to follow prescribed diet.
- Continue taking this drug until or unless advised by physician that it is no longer necessary.

(Prilosec) may be given to neutralize or decrease gastric secretions. Octreotide (Sandostatin), a synthetic hormone, suppresses pancreatic enzyme secretion and may also be used to relieve pain in chronic pancreatitis.

Treatments

NUTRITION Oral food and fluids generally are withheld during acute episodes of pancreatitis to reduce pancreatic secretions and promote rest of the organ. A nasogastric tube may be inserted and connected to suction. Intravenous fluids are administered to maintain vascular volume, and total parenteral nutrition (TPN) is initiated. Oral food and fluids are begun once the serum amylase levels have returned to normal, bowel sounds are present, and pain disappears. A low-fat diet is ordered, and alcohol intake is strictly prohibited.

SURGERY If the pancreatitis is the result of a gallstone lodged in the sphincter of Oddi, an *endoscopic transduodenal sphincterotomy* may be performed to remove the stone. When cholelithiasis is identified as a causative factor, a cholecystectomy is performed once the acute pancreatitis has resolved. Surgical procedures to promote drainage of pancreatic enzymes into the duodenum or resection of all or part of the pancreas may be done to provide pain relief in patients with chronic pancreatitis. Large pancreatic pseudocysts may be drained endoscopically or surgically.

COMPLEMENTARY THERAPIES Several complementary therapies may be used in conjunction with traditional treatments for patients with acute or chronic pancreatitis. Fasting or use of low-salt, low-fat vegetarian diets may reduce episodes of recurrent pain. Qigong, a system of gentle exercise, meditation, and controlled breathing, is believed to balance the flow of qi (a vital life force) through the body. Qigong lowers the metabolic rate, and may reduce the stimulation of pancreatic enzyme secretion. Magnetic field therapy also may be employed for patients with pancreatitis. All complementary therapies should be prescribed by a trained and competent practitioner.

Nursing Care

In addition to the nursing care discussed in this section, a Case Study & Nursing Care Plan for a patient with acute pancreatitis is found on page 755.

Health Promotion

Teach patients who abuse alcohol about the risk for developing pancreatitis. Advise abstinence to reduce this risk, and refer to an alcohol treatment program or Alcoholics Anonymous.

Assessment

Assessment data related to acute or chronic pancreatitis include the following:

- *Health history:* Current manifestations; abdominal pain (location, nature, onset and duration, identified precipitating factors); anorexia, nausea, or vomiting; flatulence, diarrhea, constipation, or stool changes; recent weight loss; history of previous episodes or gallstones; alcohol use (extent and duration); current medications.
- *Physical assessment:* Vital signs including orthostatic vitals and peripheral pulses; temperature; skin temperature and color, presence of any flank or periumbilical ecchymoses; abdominal assessment including bowel sounds, presence of distention, tenderness, or guarding.

Nursing Diagnoses and Interventions

Nursing care for the patient with acute pancreatitis focuses on managing pain, nutrition, and maintaining fluid balance.

Acute Pain

Obstruction of pancreatic ducts and inflammation, edema, and swelling of the pancreas caused by pancreatic autodigestion cause severe epigastric, left upper abdominal, or midscapular back pain. The pain often is accompanied by nausea and vomiting, abdominal tenderness, and muscle guarding.

- Using a standard pain scale (∞ see Chapter 9), assess pain, including location, radiation, duration, and character. Note nonverbal cues of pain: restlessness or remaining rigidly still; tense facial features; clenched fists; rapid, shallow respirations; tachycardia; and diaphoresis. Administer analgesics on a regular schedule. *Pain assessment before and after analgesic administration measures its effectiveness. Administering analgesics on a regular schedule prevents pain from becoming established, severe, and difficult to control. Unrelieved pain has negative consequences; for example, pain, anxiety, and restlessness may increase pancreatic enzyme secretion.*

CASE STUDY & NURSING CARE PLAN   A Patient with Acute Pancreatitis

Rose Schliefer is a 59-year-old wife, mother of three, and grandmother of four. She has been hospitalized for the past 6 weeks for acute hemorrhagic pancreatitis and pseudocyst. The pancreatitis was caused by gallstones. Mrs. Schliefer spent 3 weeks in intensive care, and then underwent surgery to remove the gallstones and to insert drains into the pseudocyst. Prior to discharge, she had progressed to a soft, high-carbohydrate, low-fat diet; had all drains removed; and was able to walk in the hall. Mrs. Schliefer was referred to a community health agency in her home town for continued follow-up.

ASSESSMENT

Lee Quinn, the community health nurse, assesses Mrs. Schliefer at home after discharge. Mrs. Schliefer is thin and appears anxious and tired. She states that she lost 30 lb (13.6 kg) in the hospital and now weighs only 102 lb (46 kg). She is 66 inches (168 cm) tall. Her vital signs are within normal limits. Mrs. Schliefer has a well-healed upper abdominal scar and two small wounds (from drains) on each side of her abdomen. The wounds are closed but still have scabs. Her skin is cool and dry, and turgor is poor. She is alert and oriented and responds appropriately to questions. Blood glucose levels are normal. Mrs. Schliefer states that her main problems are lack of energy and lack of appetite for the low-fat diet that has been ordered. Mrs. Schliefer's husband and daughters express concern about their ability to provide care. Although they have been taught all about the disease and how to provide care, they still are not sure they know exactly what should be done now that Mrs. Schliefer is at home.

DIAGNOSES

- *Fatigue* related to decreased metabolic energy production
- *Imbalanced Nutrition: Less than Body Requirements* related to prolonged hospitalization, dietary restrictions, and impaired digestion
- *Bathing Self-Care Deficit* (Level II: requires help of another person, supervision, and teaching) related to decreased strength and endurance
- *Risk for Caregiver Role Strain* related to inexperience with caregiving tasks

EXPECTED OUTCOMES

- Set priorities for daily and weekly activities, and incorporate a rest period into daily activity.
- Gain 1 to 2 lbs per week.
- Bathe and maintain personal hygiene without assistance.
- Family members will verbalize comfort with providing necessary care.

PLANNING AND IMPLEMENTATION

- Explain causes of fatigue. Review effects of pancreatitis, surgery, and acute illness on energy levels.

- Develop activity goals, incorporating small, incremental steps toward achieving goals. Mrs. Schliefer indicates that she wants to cook a meal for the whole family. To reach this goal, she will do the following:
  a. Schedule the meal when her energy level is highest.
  b. List actions necessary to prepare the meal and delegate difficult tasks to family members.
  c. Ask daughters to reorganize the kitchen to avoid unnecessary steps.
  d. Plan the meal no sooner than the third week after being home.
- Instruct her to do the following:
  a. Rest in bed each day from 1:00 PM to 3:00 PM.
  b. Eat six small meals a day with family members or friends.
  c. Sit and rest quietly for 15 minutes before eating.
- Discuss dietary restrictions and how to adapt them to usual diet.
- Advise to use shower chair and develop self-care goals for bathing and hygiene in small steps. Add self-care tasks gradually as tolerated.
- Discuss division of responsibilities for physical care, home maintenance, and medical care with family members.
- Encourage family discussion of concerns about future; acknowledge family strengths.

EVALUATION

One month after discharge, Mrs. Schliefer and her family have established new routines based on her energy levels. Mrs. Schliefer now fixes lunch because she feels best during midday. She and her husband share this time together without interruption. Mrs. Schliefer still rests during the day but can now provide self-care. She has gained only 2 lb, but states that she is getting used to the new diet and that "things are even starting to taste good without butter." She also says that sitting quietly before meals is helpful and that she prefers eating six small meals a day. Mr. and Mrs. Schliefer and their daughters agree that their initial worries about Mrs. Schliefer's care have been resolved; now they all know what they must do, and the future looks much brighter.

CRITICAL THINKING IN THE NURSING PROCESS

1. Your patient with acute pancreatitis is also an alcoholic. Describe assessments that indicate the beginnings of withdrawal.
2. Discuss the pathophysiologic basis of hypovolemic shock in acute necrotic pancreatitis.
3. Outline a teaching plan that includes specific foods to omit and to include in a high-carbohydrate, low-protein, low-fat diet.
4. Develop a plan of care for the nursing diagnosis *Impaired Home Maintenance*.

See Evaluating Your Response in Appendix C.

PRACTICE ALERT

Regularly assess respiratory status (at least every 4 to 8 hours), including respiratory rate, depth, and pattern; breath sounds; oxygen saturation; and arterial blood gas results. Report tachypnea, adventitious or absent breath sounds, oxygen saturation levels below 92%, $PaO_2 < 70$ mmHg or $PaCO_2 > 45$ mmHg. Severe abdominal pain causes shallow respirations and hypoventilation, and suppresses cough effectiveness, which can lead to pooling of secretions, atelectasis, and pneumonia.

- Maintain NPO status and nasogastric tube patency as ordered. *Gastric secretions stimulate hormones that stimulate pancreatic secretion, aggravating pain. Eliminating oral intake and maintaining gastric suction reduce gastric secretions. Nasogastric suction also decreases nausea, vomiting, and intestinal distention.*
- Maintain bed rest in a calm, quiet environment. Encourage use of nonpharmacologic pain management techniques such as meditation and guided imagery. *Decreasing physical movement and mental stimulation decreases metabolic rate,*

gastrointestinal secretion, pancreatic secretions, and resulting pain. Adjunctive pain relief measures enhance the effectiveness of analgesics (∞ see Chapter 9).

- Assist to a comfortable position, such as a side-lying position with knees flexed and head elevated 45 degrees. *Sitting up, leaning forward, or lying in a fetal position tends to decrease pain caused by stretching of the peritoneum by edema and swelling.*

- Remind family and visitors to avoid bringing food into the patient's room. *The sight or smell of food may stimulate secretory activity of the pancreas through the cephalic phase of digestion.*

Imbalanced Nutrition: Less than Body Requirements

The effects of pancreatitis and its treatment may result in malnutrition. Inflammation increases metabolic demand and frequently causes nausea, vomiting, and diarrhea. At a time of increased metabolic demand, NPO status and gastric suction further decrease available nutrients. In the patient with chronic pancreatitis, loss of digestive enzymes affects the digestion and use of nutrients.

- Monitor laboratory values: serum albumin, serum transferrin, hemoglobin, and hematocrit. *Serum albumin, serum transferrin (which transports iron in the blood), hemoglobin, and hematocrit levels are decreased in malnutrition. Decreased pancreatic enzymes affect protein catabolism and absorption; decreased transferrin affects iron absorption and transport, thereby decreasing hematocrit and hemoglobin levels.*

- Weigh daily or every other day. *Short-term weight changes (over hours to days) accurately reflect fluid balance, whereas weight changes over days to weeks reflect nutritional status.*

- Maintain stool chart; note frequency, color, odor, and consistency of stools. *Protein and fat metabolism are impaired in pancreatitis; undigested fats are excreted in the stool. Steatorrhea indicates impaired digestion and, possibly, an increase in the severity of pancreatitis.*

- Monitor bowel sounds. *The return of bowel sounds indicates return of peristalsis; nasogastric suction usually is discontinued within 24 to 48 hours thereafter.*

- Administer prescribed intravenous fluids and/or TPN. *Intravenous fluids are given to maintain hydration. TPN is used to provide fluids, electrolytes, and kilocalories when fasting is prolonged (more than 2 to 3 days).*

- Provide oral and nasal care every 1 to 2 hours. *Fasting and nasogastric suction increase the risk for mucous membrane irritation and breakdown.*

- When oral intake resumes, offer small, frequent feedings. Provide oral hygiene before and after meals. *Oral hygiene decreases oral microorganisms that can cause foul odor and taste, decreasing appetite. Small, frequent feedings reduce pancreatic enzyme secretion and are more easily digested and absorbed.*

Risk for Deficient Fluid Volume

Acute pancreatitis can lead to a fluid shift from the intravascular space into the abdominal cavity (third spacing). Third spacing of fluid may cause hypovolemic shock, affecting cardiovascular function, respiratory function, renal function, and mental status.

- Assess cardiovascular status every 4 hours or as indicated, including vital signs, cardiac rhythm, hemodynamic parameters (central venous and pulmonary artery pressures); peripheral pulses and capillary refill; and skin color, temperature, moisture, and turgor. *These measurements are indicative of fluid volume status and are used to monitor response to treatment. Stable values are as follows: heart rate less than 100; blood pressure within 10 mmHg of baseline; central venous pressure 0 to 8 mmHg; pulmonary wedge pressure 8 to 12 mmHg; cardiac output approximately 5 L/min; and skin warm, dry, with good turgor and color. (∞ See Chapter 11 for a full discussion of hypovolemic shock.)*

- Monitor renal function. Obtain hourly urine output; report if less than 30 mL per hour. Weigh daily. *Urine output of less than 30 mL per hour indicates decreased renal perfusion or acute renal failure, a major complication of acute pancreatitis. Weight changes are an effective indicator of fluid volume status.*

- Monitor neurologic function, including mental status, level of consciousness, and behavior. *Hypotension and hypoxemia may decrease cerebral perfusion, causing changes in mental status, decreased level of consciousness, and changes in behavior. In addition, alcohol withdrawal is a risk in the patient with acute pancreatitis.*

Using NANDA, NIC, and NOC

Linkages between a selected NANDA nursing diagnosis, NIC, and NOC for the patient with pancreatitis are shown in the chart that follows.

Community-Based Care

The patient with pancreatitis is often acutely ill and, along with family members, needs information about both hospital procedures and self-care at home following discharge. During the acute stage, keep explanations brief and simple.

Prior to discharge, teach the patient and family about the disease and how to prevent further attacks of inflammation. Include the following topics as appropriate:

- Alcohol can cause stones to form, blocking pancreatic ducts and the outflow of pancreatic juice. Continued alcohol intake is likely to cause further inflammation and destruction of the pancreas. Avoid alcohol entirely.

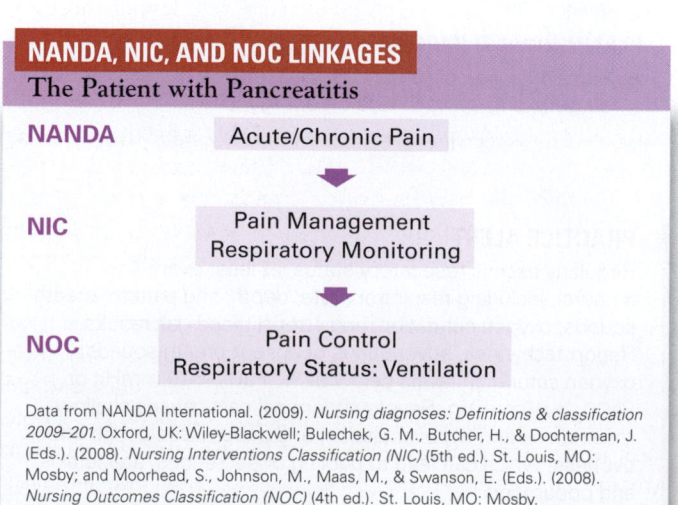

NANDA, NIC, AND NOC LINKAGES

The Patient with Pancreatitis

NANDA	Acute/Chronic Pain
NIC	Pain Management Respiratory Monitoring
NOC	Pain Control Respiratory Status: Ventilation

Data from NANDA International. (2009). *Nursing diagnoses: Definitions & classification 2009–201.* Oxford, UK: Wiley-Blackwell; Bulechek, G. M., Butcher, H., & Dochterman, J. (Eds.). (2008). *Nursing Interventions Classification (NIC)* (5th ed.). St. Louis, MO: Mosby; and Moorhead, S., Johnson, M., Maas, M., & Swanson, E. (Eds.). (2008). *Nursing Outcomes Classification (NOC)* (4th ed.). St. Louis, MO: Mosby.

- Smoking and stress stimulate the pancreas and should be avoided.
- If pancreatic function has been severely impaired, discuss appropriate use of pancreatic enzymes, including timing, dose, potential side effects, and monitoring of effectiveness.
- A low-fat diet is recommended. Provide a list of high-fat foods to avoid. Crash dieting and binge eating also should be avoided as they may sometimes precipitate attacks. Spicy foods, coffee, tea, or colas, and gas-forming foods stimulate gastric and pancreatic secretions and may precipitate pain. Avoid them if this occurs.
- Report symptoms of infection (fever of 102°F [38.8°C] or more, pain, rapid pulse, malaise) because a pancreatic abscess can develop after initial recovery.

Refer to a dietitian or nutritionist for diet teaching as needed. If appropriate, refer to community agencies, such as Alcoholics Anonymous, or to an alcohol treatment program. Provide referrals to community or home health agencies as needed for continued monitoring and teaching at home.

The Patient with Pancreatic Cancer

Cancer of the pancreas accounts for approximately 3% of all cancers. It is, however, one of the most lethal cancers: The 5-year survival rate is only about 5%. An estimated 42,470 new cases occurred in the United States in 2009, with approximately 35,240 deaths from cancer of the pancreas occurring the same year (American Cancer Society, 2009). The incidence of pancreatic cancer increases after age 50. The incidence is higher in Blacks than in Whites.

FAST FACTS

Identified risk factors for pancreatic cancer include:
- Cigarette smoking—the incidence is twice as high in smokers as in nonsmokers
- Chronic pancreatitis
- Diabetes mellitus
- Cirrhosis
- Obesity, high-fat diet; possibly red meat consumption
- Genetic predisposition

In contrast to acute and chronic pancreatitis, alcohol abuse and gallstones are not identified risk factors for pancreatic cancer.

Pathophysiology and Manifestations

Most cancers of the pancreas occur in the exocrine pancreas, are adenocarcinomas, and are fatal within 1 to 3 years after diagnosis.

Cancer of the pancreas often causes few symptoms until advanced. Early manifestations are nonspecific, including anorexia, nausea, weight loss, flatulence, and dull epigastric pain. The pain increases in severity as the tumor grows. Other manifestations depend on the location of the tumor. Cancer of the head of the pancreas, which is the most common site, often obstructs bile flow through the common bile duct and the ampulla of Vater, resulting in jaundice, clay-colored stools, dark urine, and pruritus. Cancer of the body of the pancreas presses on the celiac ganglion, causing pain that increases when the person eats or lies supine. Cancer of the tail of the pancreas often causes no symptoms until it has metastasized. Other late manifestations include a palpable abdominal mass and ascites. Because the manifestations are nonspecific, up to 85% of patients with cancer of the pancreas do not seek health care until the cancer becomes too far advanced for a cure.

Interdisciplinary Care

Early cancers of the head of the pancreas may be resectable. A pancreatoduodenectomy (commonly called Whipple's procedure) is performed to remove the head of the pancreas, the entire duodenum, the distal third of the stomach, a portion of the jejunum, and the lower half of the common bile duct. The common bile duct is then sutured to the end of the jejunum, and the remaining pancreas and stomach are sutured to the side of the jejunum (Figure 25–10 ■). Radiation and chemotherapy are often used in addition to surgery.

Postoperative nursing care of the patient undergoing Whipple's procedure is outlined on page 758. Immediate postoperative care is often provided in the intensive care unit.

The patient with pancreatic cancer has multiple problems requiring nursing care. ∞ Chapter 14 provides a discussion of care of the patient with cancer; the nursing diagnoses and interventions discussed for the patient with pancreatitis are also appropriate for the patient with pancreatic cancer.

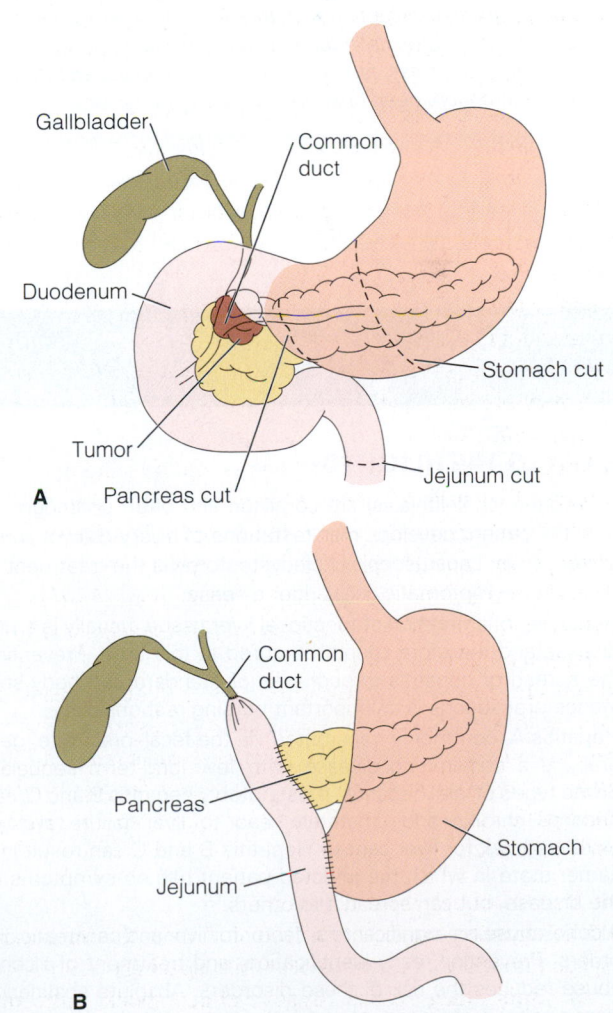

Figure 25–10 ■ Pancreatoduodenectomy (Whipple's procedure): *A*, areas of resection; *B*, appearance following resection.

NURSING CARE OF THE PATIENT   Undergoing Whipple's Procedure

PREOPERATIVE CARE

- Provide routine preoperative nursing care as outlined in ∞ Chapter 4.
- Clarify teaching and learning as needed. Provide psychologic support for patient and family. *The patient and family faced with a diagnosis of pancreatic cancer may require reinforcement of teaching as anxiety, fear, and possible denial can interfere with learning.*

POSTOPERATIVE CARE

- Provide postoperative care as outlined in ∞ Chapter 4.
- Maintain in semi-Fowler's position. *Semi-Fowler's position facilitates lung expansion and reduces stress on the anastomosis and suture line.*
- Maintain low gastrointestinal suction. If drainage is not adequate, obtain an order to irrigate, using minimal pressure. Do not reposition nasogastric tube. *Pressure within the operative area from retained secretions increases intraluminal pressure and places stress on the suture line. Forceful irrigations and repositioning of the nasogastric tube may disrupt the suture line.*
- Maintain pain control using analgesics as prescribed (PCA, infusion, or given on a regular basis). Assess effectiveness of pain management. *Doses higher than normal may be required if narcotic analgesics have been used prior to surgery to manage pain. Increased pain may indicate complications such as disruption of suture line, leakage from anastomosis, or peritonitis. Adequate pain management increases resistance to stress, facilitates healing, and increases the ability to cough, deep breathe, and change position.*

- Assist with coughing, deep breathing, and changing position every 1 to 2 hours. Splint incision during coughing and deep breathing. *The location of the incision makes coughing and deep breathing more painful. The prolonged surgical procedure, anesthesia, location of incision, and immobility increase the risk of retained secretions, atelectasis, and pneumonia. Changing position facilitates drainage of secretions; effective coughing and deep breathing remove secretions and open distal alveoli.*
- Monitor for complications:
  a. Take vital signs every 2 to 4 hours or as indicated; immediately report changes (such as elevated temperature; hypotension; weak, thready pulse; increased or difficult respirations).
  b. Assess skin color, temperature, moisture, and turgor.
  c. Measure urinary output, gastrointestinal output, and drainage from any other tubes; monitor amount and type of wound drainage.
  d. Assess level of consciousness.
  e. Assess abdomen, including contour, bowel sounds, tenderness. Report increasing abdominal pain or signs of acute abdomen (rigid, board-like abdomen).
  f. Monitor results of laboratory tests, especially arterial blood gases, hemoglobin, and hematocrit.
  The major complications following Whipple's procedure are hemorrhage, bile leak, hypovolemic shock, and hepatorenal failure. The assessments listed provide information about the patient's status and alert the nurse to abnormal findings that signal the onset of these complications.

CHAPTER HIGHLIGHTS

- Gallstones (cholelithiasis) are common and often unrecognized until the patient develops manifestations of biliary colic or acute cholecystitis. Laparoscopic cholecystectomy is the treatment of choice for symptomatic gallbladder disease.
- Hepatitis, inflammation of functional liver tissue, usually is a viral disease and therefore cannot be cured at this time. Preventing the spread of hepatitis through use of standard and body substance precautions is an important nursing responsibility.
- Hepatitis A, commonly transmitted via the fecal–oral route, generally is a self-limiting disease with few long-term sequelae. Some types of viral hepatitis, most notably hepatitis B and C, can become chronic and ultimately lead to liver failure and an increased risk for liver cancer. Hepatitis B and C can result in a carrier state in which the infected patient has no symptoms of the disease, but can spread it to others.
- Alcohol abuse is a significant risk factor for liver and pancreatic disorders. Prevention, early identification, and treatment of alcohol abuse reduces the risk of these disorders. Absolute abstinence from alcohol is an important part of the treatment plan for patients with liver and pancreatic disorders.

- Cirrhosis leads to portal hypertension and liver failure, which, in turn, account for most of the manifestations and complications of the disorder. Complications such as ascites, splenomegaly, esophageal varices, and portal systemic encephalopathy affect multiple body systems and significantly contribute to mortality and morbidity associated with cirrhosis.
- Bleeding from esophageal varices may be massive, resulting in a medical emergency and requiring prompt control to maintain cardiac output.
- Acute pancreatitis often develops as a complication of gallstones. Acute pancreatitis often resolves with no long term consequences. Chronic pancreatitis is more frequently related to alcohol abuse and can lead to continuing pain and digestive disruptions.
- All of the accessory organs of digestion (the gallbladder, liver, and pancreas) can be a primary site of malignancy. Cancer of the gallbladder is uncommon; hepatocellular and pancreatic cancer are more common and their incidence is increasing. These cancers often are advanced when diagnosed, reducing treatment options and the chance for cure.

TEST YOURSELF NCLEX-RN® REVIEW

1. When assessing the patient admitted for a laparoscopic cholecystectomy, the nurse would expect to find which of the following?
   1. a history of right upper quadrant pain
   2. obvious jaundice of the sclera and skin
   3. complaints of recurrent heartburn and acid reflux
   4. complaints of chills, fever, nausea, and vomiting

2. Which of the following does the nurse include in her teaching for a patient with acute cholecystitis? **Select all that apply.**
   1. Avoid consumption of foods high in fat such as gravies and peanut butter.
   2. Limit your intake to dry crackers and clear liquids during episodes of acute pain.
   3. A low-carbohydrate diet such as the Atkins diet is recommended for weight loss.
   4. Call your doctor if you develop severe abdominal pain and a temperature.
   5. Surgery for gallstones is optional; they pose little risk when fat intake is minimal.

3. During an outbreak of hepatitis A traced to a food handler at a local restaurant, the nurse teaches staff at the restaurant that the most cost-effective means of protecting customers from further outbreaks is to do which of the following?
   1. insist that all food handlers be immunized against hepatitis A
   2. test all new employees for hepatitis A antigen
   3. wash hands thoroughly before handling food and after using the bathroom
   4. use gloves for handling food if any cuts or scrapes are on hands

4. The nurse would evaluate teaching as effective when a patient with chronic hepatitis C states which of the following?
   1. "I will reduce my alcohol intake and use only acetaminophen for pain relief."
   2. "I understand that I must return to the doctor every year for a follow-up liver biopsy."
   3. "Even though no treatment is available for this disease, I plan to live a long life."
   4. "I will avoid donating blood and will use barrier protection during sex."

5. When evaluating for people possibly exposed to hepatitis A by a recently diagnosed patient, the nurse inquires about which of the following?
   1. sexual partners within the past 6 months
   2. close household contacts within the past 4 weeks
   3. food preparation activities since the development of jaundice
   4. immunization status of the patient

6. A patient hospitalized with cirrhosis, ascites, and mild hepatic encephalopathy suddenly vomits 200 mL of bright red blood. Which of the following should the nurse do first?
   1. Insert a nasogastric tube.
   2. Place in Fowler's position.
   3. Contact the physician.
   4. Check stool for occult blood.

7. The nurse caring for a patient scheduled for an abdominal paracentesis instructs the patient to do which of the following?
   1. avoid eating or drinking fluid for 6 hours prior to the procedure
   2. scrub the abdomen with antiseptic soap before the procedure
   3. empty the bladder before the procedure
   4. report excess flatus following the procedure to the physician

8. A patient hospitalized with severe ascites due to cirrhosis develops a fever and confusion. The nurse should do which of the following?
   1. auscultate bowel sounds and palpate for abdominal tenderness
   2. inquire about headache and check for nuchal rigidity
   3. observe for neck vein distention and auscultate lung sounds
   4. measure abdominal girth and percuss for shifting dullness

9. A 54-year-old woman admitted with acute pancreatitis says, "I don't understand how I got this disease. I thought alcoholics got pancreatitis—I never drink." Which of the following is the most appropriate response by the nurse?
   1. "Was there a time in your life that you did drink heavily?"
   2. "It also is prevalent in smokers; do you smoke cigarettes?"
   3. "Gallstones also are a risk factor. We'll evaluate for them."
   4. "Intravenous drug use is a risk factor. Do you use drugs by injection?"

10. The nurse caring for a patient returning to the unit following Whipple's procedure identifies which of the following as of highest priority in the plan of care?
    1. referral to a smoking cessation program
    2. frequent turning, coughing, and deep breathing exercises
    3. early mobilization including ambulation as tolerated
    4. maintaining patency of the nasogastric tube

See Test Yourself answers in Appendix C.

BIBLIOGRAPHY

American Cancer Society. (2009). *Cancer facts and figures 2009*. Atlanta, GA: Author.

American Cancer Society. (2007). *Cancer facts & figures for African Americans 2007–2008*. Atlanta, GA: Author.

American Cancer Society. (2006). *Cancer facts & figures for Hispanics/Latinos 2006–2008*. Atlanta, GA: Author.

American College of Physicians. (2008). In the clinic. Hepatitis C. *Annals of Internal Medicine, 3 June 2008,* ITC1-ITC16.

Baltimore, J., & Davidson, J. (2007 March). Caring for a patient with acute cholecystitis. *Nursing2007, 37*(3), 64hn1-64hn2, 64hn4.

Belogia, E., Costa, J., Gareen I., Grem, J., Inadomi, J., Kern, E., et al. (2009). National Institutes of Health Consensus Development Conference Statement: Management of hepatitis B. *Annals of Internal Medicine 2009, 150,* 104–110.

Brenner, Z., & Krenzer, M. (2010, January). Understanding acute pancreatitis. *Nursing, 40*(1), 32-37.

Bulechek, G., Butcher, H., & Dochterman, J. (2008). *Nursing interventions classification (NIC)* (5th ed.). St. Louis, MO: Mosby.

Cainelli, F. (2008). Hepatitis C virus infection in the elderly: Epidemiology, natural history and management. *Drugs Aging 2008, 25*(1), 9–18.

Centers for Disease Control and Prevention. (2009). *Epidemiology and prevention of vaccine-preventable diseases* (11th ed.). (Atkinson, W., Wolfe, S., Hamborski, J., & McIntyre, L., Eds.). Washington, DC: Public Health Foundation.

Centers for Disease Control and Prevention. (2009 May 22). Surveillance for acute viral hepatitis – United States, 2007. *MMWR 2009, 58*(SS-3).

Chi, T. (2008 April). Efficacy of an herbal extract formula on gallbladder conditions. *Nutritional Perspectives: Journal of the Council on Nutrition of the American Chiropractic Association, 31*(2), 4–5, 7–9.

Chronic pancreatitis. (2007 December 1). *American Family Physician, 76*(11), 1679–1688.

Copstead, L. C., & Banasick, J. L. (2010). *Pathophysiology* (4th ed.). St. Louis, MO: Saunders.

Diestag, J. (2008 October 2). Hepatitis B virus infection. *New England Journal of Medicine, 359*(14), 1486–1500.

DiPiro, J., Talbert, R., Yee, G., Matzke, G., Wells, B., & Posey, L. (2008). *Pharmacotherapy: A pathophysiologic approach* (7th ed.). New York, NY: McGraw Hill.

Elwood, D. (2008 December). Cholecystitis. *Surgical Clinics of North America, 88*(6), 1241–1252.

Fagenholz, P., Castillo, C., Harris, N., Pelletier, A., & Camargo, C., Jr. (2007 July). Increasing United States hospital admissions for acute pancreatitis, 1988–2003. *Annals of Epidemiology, 17*(7), 491–197.

Fauci, A., Kasper, D., Braunwald, E., Hauser, S., Longo, D., Jameson, J., et al. (Eds.). (2008). *Harrison's principles of internal medicine* (17th ed.). New York, NY: McGraw-Hill.

Fontaine, K. L. (2005). *Complementary & alternative therapies for nursing* (2nd ed.). Upper Saddle River, NJ: Prentice Hall Health.

Goenka, N., Subramanian, S., Weston, P., & Vora, J. (2007 July–August). Nonalcoholic fatty liver disease: More than 'just a bit of fatty liver.' *Practical Diabetes International, 24*(6), 305–308.

Graham, L. (2009 October 22). Care of patients undergoing laparoscopic cholecystectomy. *Nursing Standard, 23*(7), 41–48.

Lambou-Gianoukos, S., & Heller, S. (2008 December). Lithogenesis and bile metabolism. *Surgical Clinics of North America, 88*(6), 1175–1194.

Lehne, R. (2007). *Pharmacology for nursing care* (6th ed.). St. Louis, MO: Saunders.

Maheshwari, A., Ray, S., & Thuluvath, P. (2008 July 26). Acute hepatitis C. *Lancet, 372*(9635), 321–332.

Marchiondo, K. (2010, January). Acute Pancreatitis. *MEDSURG Nursing, 19*(1), 54-55.

McCance, K. L., & Huether, S. E. (2006). *Pathophysiology: The biologic basis for disease in adults & children* (5th ed.). St. Louis, MO: Mosby.

McPhee, S., Papadakis, M., & Tierney, L. (2008). *Current medical diagnosis & treatment* (47th ed.). New York, NY: Lange Medical Books/McGraw-Hill.

Moorhead, S., Johnson, M., Maas, M., & Swanson, E. (2008). *Nursing outcomes classification (NOC)* (4th ed.). St. Louis, MO: Mosby.

Nair, R., Lawler, L., & Miller, M. (2007 December 1). Chronic pancreatitis. *American Family Physician, 76*(11), 1679–1688.

NANDA International. (2009). *Nursing diagnoses: Definitions & classification 2009–2011.* Oxford, UK: Wiley-Blackwell.

National Center for Complementary and Alternative Medicine, National Institutes of Health. (2008). *Get the facts. CAM and hepatitis C: A focus on herbal supplements.* (NCCAM Pub. No. D422). Retrieved from www.nccam.nih.gov

National Center for Complementary and Alternative Medicine, National Institutes of Health. (2008). *Herbs at a glance. Milk thistle.* Retrieved from www.nccam.nih.gov

National Center for Health Statistics. (2009 April). Deaths: Final data for 2006. *National Vital Statistics Reports, 57*(14).

National Center for Health Statistics. (2009). *Health, United States, 2008, with chartbook.* Hyattsville, MD: Author.

National Institute of Diabetes and Digestive and Kidney Diseases. (2007 Winter). NIDDK explores causes, treatment, and research challenges for acute liver failure. *Digestive Diseases News,* Winter 2007, 1–2, 6.

National Institutes of Health. (2008 October). NIH Consensus Development Conference statement on management of hepatitis B. *NIH Consensus and State-of-the-Science Statement, 25*(2), 1–29.

Poll, R. (2009). Improving awareness of the hepatitis C virus. *Practice Nursing, 20*(3), 131–132.

Porth, C., & Matfin, G. (2009). *Pathophysiology: Concepts of altered health states* (8th ed.). Philadelphia: Lippincott.

Riehl, M. (2007 April). Help your patient cope with pancreatic cancer. *Nursing2007, 37*(4). 54–57.

Ross, S. (2008 September). Milk thistle (silybum marianum): An ancient botanical medicine for modern times. *Holistic Nursing Practice, 22*(5), 299–300.

Rothrock, J. (2007). *Alexander's care of the patient in surgery* (13th ed.). St. Louis, MO: Mosby.

Rustgi, V. (2007). The epidemiology of hepatitis C infection in the United States. *Journal of Gastroenterology 2007, 42,* 513–521.

Sanders, G., & Kingsnorth, A. (2007 August 11). Gallstones. *BMJ: British Medical Journal, 335*(7614), 295–299. See, A., & Irvine, L. (2010). Modern management of acute biliary pancreatitis in pregnancy. *Journal of Obstetrics & Gynaecology, 30*(4), 410–411.

Sun, V., & Sarna, L. (2008 October). Symptom management in hepatocellular carcinoma. *Clinical Journal of Oncology Nursing, 12*(5), 759–766.

Ward, J. (1008 May). Editorial. Time for renewed commitment to viral hepatitis prevention. *American Journal of Public Health, 98*(5), 779–780.

Wilkinson, J., & Ahern, N. (2009). *Nursing diagnosis handbook* (9th ed.). Upper Saddle River, NJ: Prentice Hall Health.

Wolf, D. (2008 August). Encephalopathy, hepatic. *eMedicine Gastroenterology,* August 14, 2008. Retrieved from http://emedicine.medscape.com

Building Clinical Competence
Responses to Altered Gastrointestinal Function

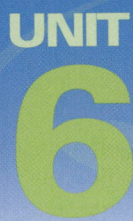

Functional Health Pattern: Nutritional-Metabolic

Think about patients with altered gastrointestinal function for whom you have cared in your clinical experiences.

- What were their major medical diagnoses?

- What kinds of manifestations did each of these patients have? Were these signs and symptoms similar or very different?

- How did the patients' manifestations and eating behaviors affect their nutritional status? Were they on a prescribed diet? Did they use dietary supplements? Did they have difficulty chewing or swallowing? Were they gaining or losing weight?

- How did the patients' health status affect their elimination patterns? Had the bowel routine changed recently? If so, how? Did they use laxatives? If so, how often and what type? Did they use any medications that affect bowel movements? Had they had a colonoscopy or other diagnostic tests of the rectum or colon? Did they have an ostomy?

Responses to altered gastrointestinal function commonly affect the nutritional-metabolic and the elimination health patterns. The Nutritional-Metabolic Health Pattern describes the pattern of food and fluid consumption in relation to metabolic need. Nutritional and gastrointestinal disorders affect nutritional status in two primary ways:

- Lack of proper nutrients (e.g., poor eating habits, anorexia or nausea, impaired GI absorption) can lead to nutritional disorders such as malnutrition, reduced energy, and impaired tissue repair and healing.

- Excess intake of nutrients can result in nutritional disorders such as obesity, alcoholic cirrhosis, or cholelithiasis.

The Elimination Health Pattern describes patterns of excretory function, including bowel function and the patient's perception of what is "normal." Bowel elimination can be affected by food and fluid intake, GI disorders, medications, and indirect factors such as perception, psychologic status, and exercise patterns. Bowel disorders affect the elimination pattern in two primary ways:

- Interfering with formation of a formed fecal mass, leading to diarrhea.

- Interfering with bowel transit and defecation, resulting in constipation.

The purposes of the gastrointestinal system are to intake food, break the food into molecules of nutrients, absorb these nutrients into the blood, and finally to excrete solid waste. The nutrients promote growth, maintenance, and repair damaged tissue of the body. Categories of nutrients include proteins, carbohydrates, fats, vitamins, and minerals. Manifestations such as the following affect nutrient intake:

- **Nausea** (*unpleasant, wave-like sensations in the stomach; feelings of urge or need to vomit*)

- **Heartburn** (*backflow of gastric contents into esophagus causes high acidity of stomach contents in esophagus resulting in pain and irritation of mucosa lining the esophagus*)

- **Pain** (*swollen tissue, inflammatory changes cause tissue damage, which stimulates pain receptors that transmit pain impulses to the brain*)

Bowel elimination is the end process of digestion. Nutrients are absorbed during digestion and indigestible materials are eliminated from the body through the gastrointestinal tract. Bowel disorders interrupt normal patterns of elimination, leading to manifestations such as the following:

- **Diarrhea** (*mucosal inflammation causes plasma, serum protein, blood, and mucus to increase fluidity and bulk of stool, which results in increased rate of propulsion of loose, watery stool*)

- **Constipation** (*decreased motility, denial of urge to defecate, or decreased fluid intake causes hard, dry stool, which results in difficulty passing stool*)

- **Flatus** (*excessive amount of air or gas in the intestines causes distention of the intestines with mild to moderate pain, which results in passage of excessive air or gas*)

Priority nursing diagnoses within the Nutritional-Metabolic Health Pattern that may be appropriate for patients with gastrointestinal disorders follow:

- *Imbalanced Nutrition: Less than Body Requirements* as evidenced by decreased food intake, weight loss, dry and brittle hair, weakness

- *Deficient Fluid Volume* as evidenced by dry mucous membranes, poor skin turgor, thirst, increased body temperature

- *Impaired Skin Integrity* as evidenced by disruption of skin surface, pain, itching

- *Impaired Tissue Integrity* as evidenced by poor wound healing

Nursing diagnoses from other health patterns often are of high priority for patients with gastrointestinal disorders include the following:

- *Acute Pain* (Cognitive-Perceptual Health Pattern)

- *Nausea* (Cognitive-Perceptual Health Pattern)

- *Fatigue* (Activity-Exercise Health Pattern)

Priority nursing diagnoses within the Elimination Health Pattern that may be appropriate for patients with bowel disorders include the following:

- *Bowel Incontinence* as evidenced by urgency, inability to delay defecation, or fecal staining of clothing.

- *Diarrhea* as evidenced by frequent, large or watery stools, abdominal cramping, and hyperactive bowel sounds.

- *Constipation* as evidenced by difficulty defecating, hard and dry stool, distended abdomen, or excessive flatus.

- *Risk for Impaired Liver Function* as evidenced by excess alcohol intake, exposure to viral hepatitis, or presence of gallstones.

Nursing diagnoses from other functional health patterns may be of high priority for patients with bowel elimination disorders follow:

- *Acute Pain* (Cognitive-Perceptual Health Pattern)

- *Anxiety* (Self-Perception-Self-Concept Health Pattern)

- *Imbalanced Nutrition: Less than Body Requirements* (Nutritional-Metabolic Health Pattern)

CLINICAL SCENARIO

Directions: *Read the following clinical scenario and answer the questions that follow. To complete this exercise successfully you will not only use knowledge of the content in this unit, but also principles related to setting priorities and maintaining patient safety.*

You have been assigned to work with the following four patients for the 0700 shift on a medical-surgical unit. Significant data obtained during report is as follows:

- Thomas Jones, aged 56, was admitted with cirrhosis of the liver. He transferred to your unit yesterday after a 3-day stay in ICU for treatment of esophageal varices. Significant history includes daily alcohol consumption (6 to 12-pack of beer or a pint of liquor daily for several years) and history of smoking (2 packs per day for the past 30 years). Current vital signs are T100°F, P 96, R 28, BP 150/90. He complains of abdominal tenderness and dyspnea. Treatment for the bleeding problems has been successful but he appears anxious and irritable.

- Tonya Cooper, aged 21, was admitted yesterday with dehydration, weakness, and fainting. Upon assessment her weight is 90 lbs (40.9 kg) and height is 5'5". Her vital signs are T 97° F, P 70, R 26, BP 90/56 mm Hg with orthostatic BP of 70/48 mm Hg. She has a history of bouts of anorexia nervosa and laxative use for 3 years. She has an IV infusing with 0.9% NaCl with added KCL. She is to be monitored for food intake and watched for one hour after meals. She is ringing her call light to get up to the bathroom.

- Paul Bruner, age 86, was admitted the previous evening with sharp abdominal pain. During the admission assessment, a mass was palpated in his abdomen. His vital signs on admission were temperature 100.4°F, pulse 88, respirations 26, and blood pressure 150/86. He is scheduled for surgery at 10:30 and needs two enemas prior to surgery.

- Grace Freeman is a 36-year-old who had a temporary colostomy placed five days ago due to an abdominal injury from a motor vehicle accident. Vital signs at 0400 were temperature 98.6°F, pulse 78, respirations 14, and blood pressure 112/78. She put on her call light for assistance as her colostomy bag is full and she needs help emptying it.

Question

1. What life style changes did your patients need to make in order to improve their nutritional status? How did you help them identify these changes? How did your assist each patient to meet their elimination needs?

Questions

Priority Setting

1. In what order would you visit these patients after report? What is the rationale for your choice?
   A. _____
   B. _____
   C. _____
   D. _____

Health Promotion

1. Besides nutrition teaching, what other health promotion topics should be discussed with each patient?
   A. _____
   B. _____
   C. _____
   D. _____

2. Teaching appropriate constipation management includes which actions? **Select all that apply.**
   A. Decrease dietary fiber.
   B. Increase fluid intake.
   C. Increase exercise activity.
   D. Use bulk-forming laxatives.
   E. Use enemas daily.

3. When teaching the importance of early detection of malignant tumors, the nurse should include which of the following as the most common initial clinical manifestation of malignant tumors of the lower bowel?
   A. rectal bleeding
   B. diarrhea
   C. rectal pain
   D. constipation

Nursing Process

1. What priority nursing diagnoses would you choose for each of the patients presented previously? Explain the rationale for your choices.

	Nursing Diagnosis	Rationale
Thomas Jones		
Tonya Cooper		
Paul Bruner		
Grace Freeman		

2. When Mr. Jones was admitted to the emergency department, which laboratory studies would you expect to draw? **Select all that apply.**
   A. AST
   B. troponins
   C. ALK
   D. Complete blood cell count
   E. LDH
   F. ADH

3. To prepare Mr. Jones for an esophagoscopy, the nurse institutes which the following interventions?
   A. Explains that it is not a painful procedure but he will be medicated for pain
   B. Keeps the patient NPO for 12 hours prior to the procedure
   C. Inserts a large nasogastric tube and irrigates the stomach to improve visualization
   D. Positions the patient in a supine position with the head slightly hyperextended

4. Write a discharge teaching plan for Mrs. Freeman regarding how to take care of the colostomy at home.

Communication

1. In planning discharge for Ms. Cooper, the family and patient participate in teaching and diet counseling sessions. Which is the priority item for the family and Ms. Cooper to follow after discharge?
   A. Monitor weight regularly to determine further weight loss.
   B. Use rewards for food and caloric intake rather than for weight gain.
   C. Gradually increase the amount of food taken at meals.
   D. Attend support groups for people with eating disorders.

2. If Ms. Cooper says to you, "I don't know why everyone is so concerned about what I do with my life." How will you respond?

3. While giving Mr. Bruner an enema he states, "I'm not sure I need this surgery. If I have cancer I might as well die. It's my daughter who thinks I should do this." How should the nurse respond?

Delegation

1. For each patient, what assessment data and nursing interventions can be delegated to a nursing assistant?

2. What instruction will you give the nursing assistant assisting Ms. Cooper with her meals?

Content-Specific Questions

1. While performing a venipuncture on a patient with hepatitis B, a nurse receives a needle stick. What steps should be taken to provide safety for the nurse?

2. Patients with celiac disease are placed on a gluten-free diet. The patient understands dietary instructions when the patient chooses which meal?
   A. Corned beef sandwich on rye bread
   B. Tossed green salad with oatmeal raisin cookie
   C. Eggs and bacon with whole wheat toast
   D. Tomato soup with cornbread

3. Patients with severe diarrhea may develop metabolic acidosis. Which arterial blood gases indicate metabolic acidosis?
   A. pH 7.45, PCO2 40 mmHg, Bicarbonate 25 mEq/L
   B. pH 7.28, PCO2 30 mmHg, Bicarbonate 19 mEq/L
   C. pH 7.55, PCO2 50 mmHg, Bicarbonate 30 mEq/L
   D. pH 7.33, PCO2 36 mmHg, Bicarbonate 24 mEq/L

4. To prepare a patient for a colonoscopy, the nurse teaches the patient to implement which interventions?
   A. Maintain a liquid diet for 4 days prior to the procedure.
   B. Remain NPO for 4 hours prior to the procedure.
   C. Administer bowel preparation the evening before the procedure.
   D. Administer a cleansing enema the evening before the procedure.

5. When assessing a patient with large bowel obstruction, which clinical manifestations are noted on assessment?
   A. tachycardia and diarrhea
   B. colicky abdominal pain and constipation
   C. severe abdominal cramping and vomiting
   D. dull bowel sounds and nausea

CASE STUDY: Joseph Brown

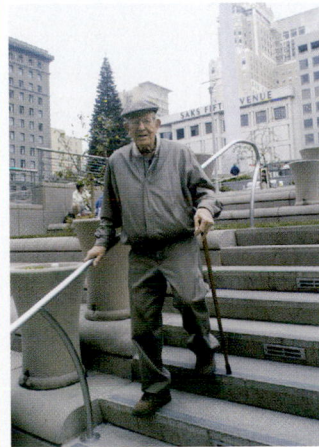

Joseph Brown, aged 82, has a history of hypertension and angina pectoris for which he takes furosemide, atenolol, and Nitrostat. His son brings him to the hospital after finding him weak, confused, and in need of good hygiene. Mr. Brown feels that he cooked some outdated food that made him ill. He states he has had nausea, vomiting, and diarrhea for the past 2 days. He also states he has not been able to take his medications for the past 2 days and feels that his heart is beating too fast.

Admission assessment shows temperature 101.6°F, pulse 102, respirations 20, and blood pressure 130/70. His height is 5'10" and he weighs 150 lbs. He states that his usual weight is 165 lbs. His skin color is pale. His abdomen is distended, tender to palpation, and has hyperactive bowel sounds. He complains of nausea and a sore rectum from bouts of diarrhea. He appears tired and listless.

Mr. Brown is diagnosed with acute gastroenteritis. In acute gastroenteritis, bacterial or viral infection damages GI mucosa directly or produces exotoxins that inflame and damage the GI mucosa. Intestinal absorption is impaired and water and electrolytes are secreted into the bowel, leading to diarrhea and fluid loss. Manifestations of acute gastroenteritis are nausea, vomiting, anorexia, diarrhea, and abdominal pain. Complications include dehydration, fluid and electrolyte imbalances, acid–base imbalance, and possible hypovolemic shock. Due to Mr. Brown's nausea, diarrhea, and weight loss, the nursing diagnosis of *Imbalanced Nutrition: Less than Body Requirements* is a priority for nursing care.

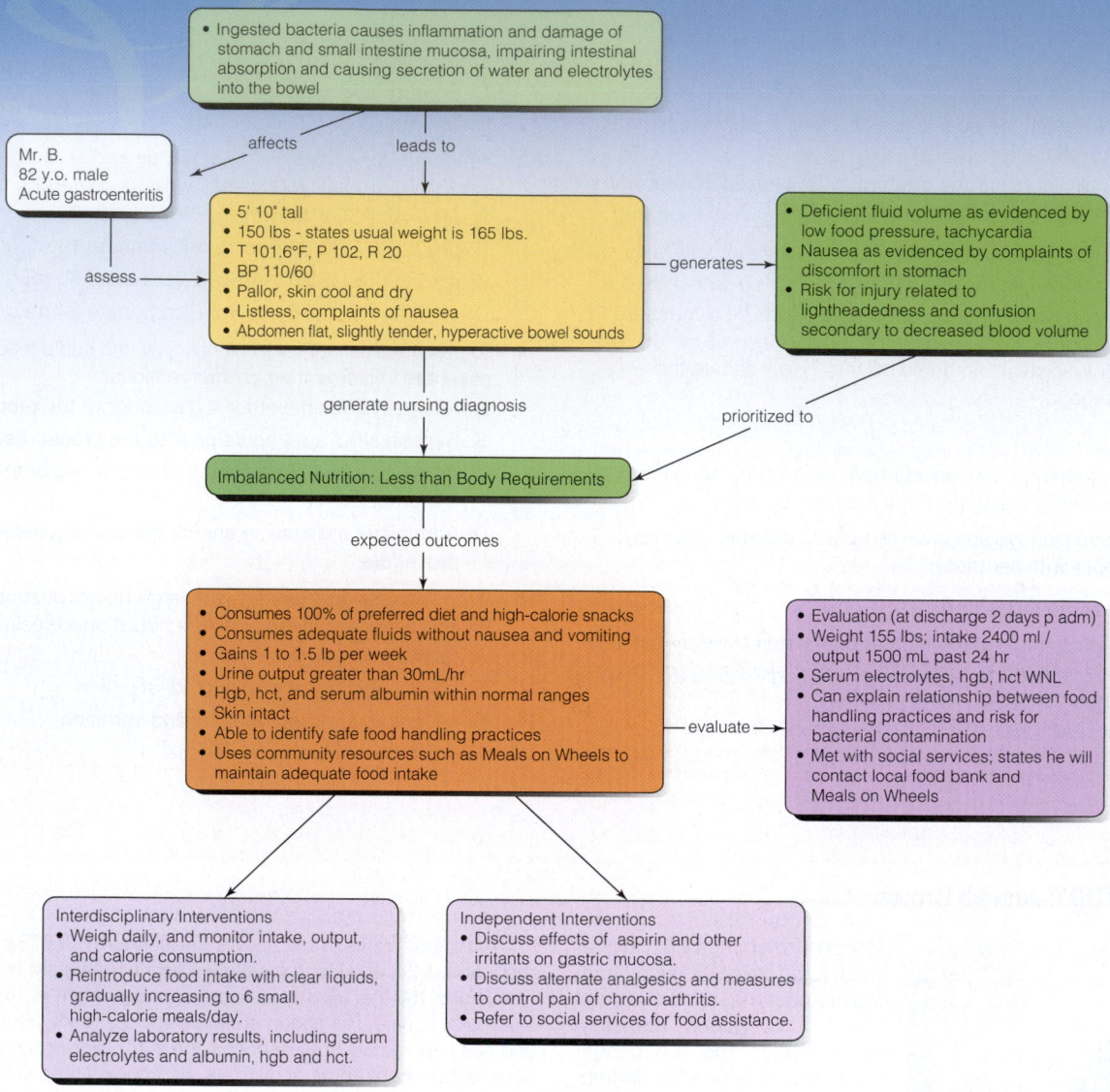

- Ingested bacteria causes inflammation and damage of stomach and small intestine mucosa, impairing intestinal absorption and causing secretion of water and electrolytes into the bowel

Mr. B.
82 y.o. male
Acute gastroenteritis

affects   leads to

assess

- 5' 10" tall
- 150 lbs - states usual weight is 165 lbs.
- T 101.6°F, P 102, R 20
- BP 110/60
- Pallor, skin cool and dry
- Listless, complaints of nausea
- Abdomen flat, slightly tender, hyperactive bowel sounds

generates

- Deficient fluid volume as evidenced by low food pressure, tachycardia
- Nausea as evidenced by complaints of discomfort in stomach
- Risk for injury related to lightheadedness and confusion secondary to decreased blood volume

generate nursing diagnosis

prioritized to

Imbalanced Nutrition: Less than Body Requirements

expected outcomes

- Consumes 100% of preferred diet and high-calorie snacks
- Consumes adequate fluids without nausea and vomiting
- Gains 1 to 1.5 lb per week
- Urine output greater than 30mL/hr
- Hgb, hct, and serum albumin within normal ranges
- Skin intact
- Able to identify safe food handling practices
- Uses community resources such as Meals on Wheels to maintain adequate food intake

evaluate

- Evaluation (at discharge 2 days p adm)
- Weight 155 lbs; intake 2400 ml / output 1500 mL past 24 hr
- Serum electrolytes, hgb, hct WNL
- Can explain relationship between food handling practices and risk for bacterial contamination
- Met with social services; states he will contact local food bank and Meals on Wheels

Interdisciplinary Interventions
- Weigh daily, and monitor intake, output, and calorie consumption.
- Reintroduce food intake with clear liquids, gradually increasing to 6 small, high-calorie meals/day.
- Analyze laboratory results, including serum electrolytes and albumin, hgb and hct.

Independent Interventions
- Discuss effects of aspirin and other irritants on gastric mucosa.
- Discuss alternate analgesics and measures to control pain of chronic arthritis.
- Refer to social services for food assistance.

Activity:

1. After reviewing the case study and concept map, do you agree that *Imbalanced Nutrition: Less than Body Requirements* is the highest priority nursing diagnosis for this patient? Why or why not?

2. Go to the Pearson Nursing Student Resources for this book at www.nursing.pearsonhighered.com to write a concept map using the nursing diagnosis *Deficient Fluid Volume.*

See answers and hints in Appendix C.

Elimination Pattern PART III

UNIT 7
Responses to Altered Urinary
Elimination 767

Functional Health Patterns with Related Nursing Diagnoses

HEALTH PERCEPTION HEALTH MANAGEMENT

- Perceived health status
- Perceived health management
- Health care behaviors: health promotion and illness prevention activities, medical treatments, follow-up care

VALUE-BELIEF

- Values, goals, or beliefs (including spirituality) that guide choices or decisions
- Perceived conflicts in values, beliefs, or expectations that are health related

COPING-STRESS-TOLERANCE

- Capacity to resist challenges to self-integrity
- Methods of handling stress
- Support systems
- Perceived ability to control and manage situations

NUTRITIONAL-METABOLIC

- Daily consumption of food and fluids
- Favorite foods
- Use of dietary supplements
- Skin lesions and ability to heal
- Condition of the integument
- Weight, height, temperature

PART III

Elimination (Urinary) Patterns: Examples of related NANDA Nursing Diagnoses

- Deficient Fluid Volume
- Excess Fluid Volume
- Functional Urinary Incontinence
- Impaired Urinary Elimination
- Overflow Urinary Incontinence
- Reflex urinary Incontinence
- Stress Urinary Incontinence
- Risk for Electrolyte Imbalance
- Risk for Imbalance Fluid Volume
- Risk for Ineffective Renal Perfusion
- Urinary Retention

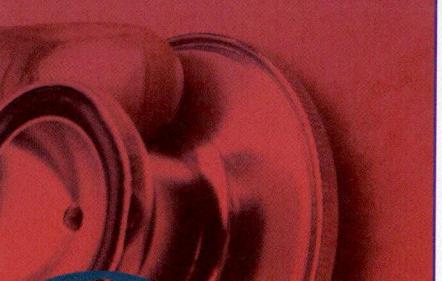

SEXUALITY-REPRODUCTIVE

- Satisfaction with sexuality or sexual relationships
- Reproductive pattern
- Female menstrual and perimeno-pausal history

ELIMINATION

- Patterns of bowel and urinary excretion
- Perceived regularity or irregularity of elimination
- Use of laxatives or routines
- Changes in time, modes, quality or quantity of excretions
- Use of devices for control

ROLE-RELATIONSHIP

- Perception of major roles, relationships, and responsibilities in current life situation
- Satisfaction with or disturbances in roles and relationships

ACTIVITY-EXERCISE

- Patterns of personally relevant exercise, activity, leisure, and recreation
- ADLs which require energy expenditure
- Factors that interfere with the desired pattern (e.g., illness or injury)

SELF-PERCEPTION– SELF-CONCEPT

- Attitudes about self
- Perceived abilities, worth, self-image, emotions
- Body posture and movement, eye contact, voice and speech patterns

SLEEP-REST

- Patterns of sleep and rest/relaxation in a 24-hr period
- Perceptions of quality and quantity of sleep and rest
- Use of sleep aids and routines

COGNITIVE-PERCEPTUAL

- Adequacy of vision, hearing, taste, touch, smell
- Pain perception and management
- Language, judgment, memory, decisions

Responses to Altered Urinary Elimination

7

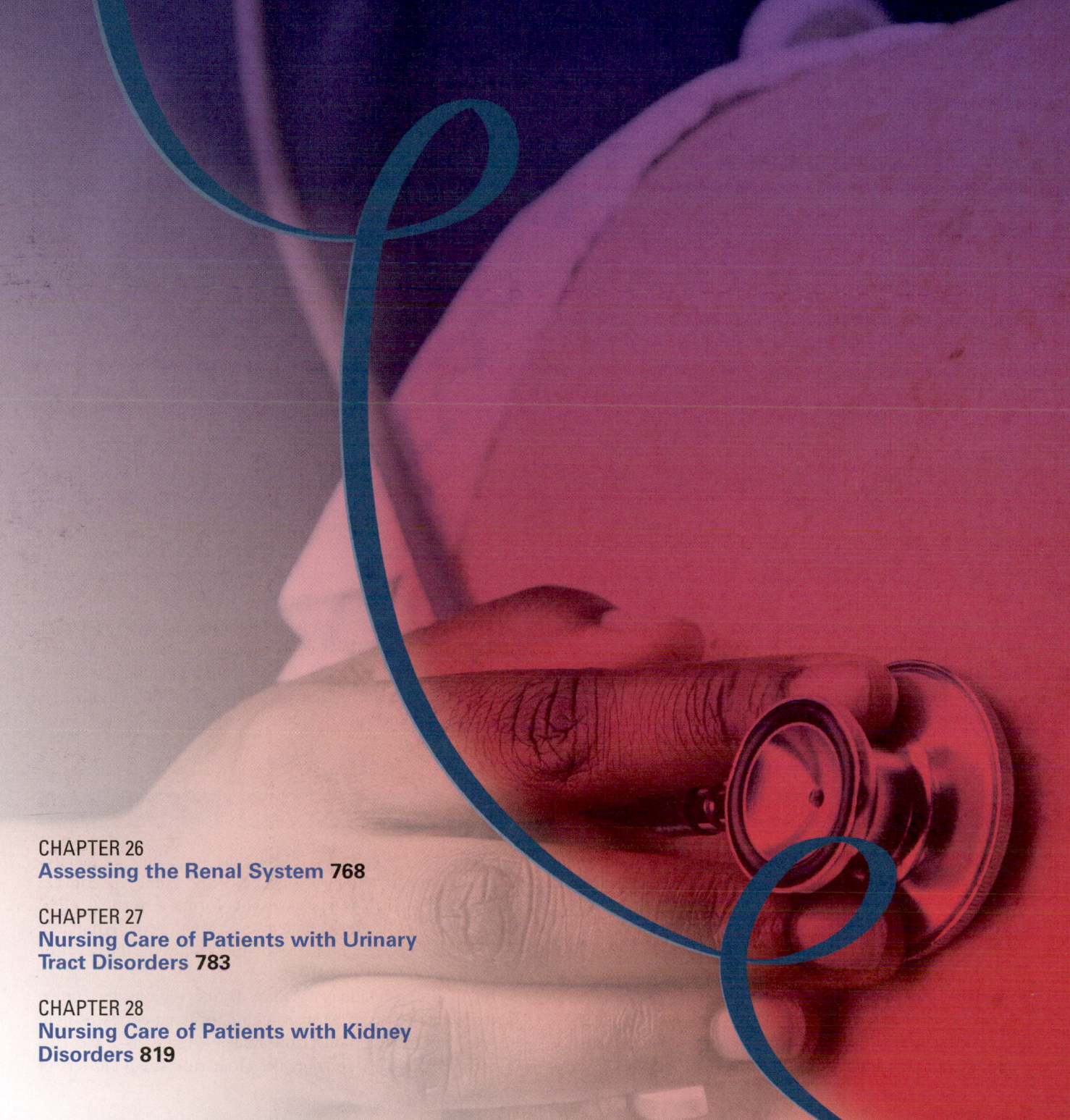

CHAPTER 26   Assessing the **Renal System**

LEARNING OUTCOMES

1. Describe the anatomy, physiology, and functions of the renal system.
2. Identify specific topics for consideration during a health history interview of the patient with health problems involving the renal system.
3. Describe techniques used to assess the integrity and function of the renal system.
4. Give examples of genetic disorders of the renal system.
5. Describe normal variations in assessment findings for the older adult.
6. Identify abnormal findings that may indicate alterations in urinary elimination.

CLINICAL COMPETENCIES

1. Conduct and document a health history for patients who have or are at risk for alterations in renal function.
2. Conduct and document a physical assessment of the renal system.
3. Monitor the results of diagnostic tests and report abnormal findings.

EQUIPMENT NEEDED

- Urine specimen cup
- Disposable gloves
- Stethoscope

KEY TERMS

dysuria, *777*	micturition, *773*	urea, *772*
hematuria, *771*	nocturia, *779*	

The functions of the renal system (also called the urinary system) are to regulate body fluids, to filter metabolic wastes from the bloodstream, to reabsorb needed substances and water into the bloodstream, and to eliminate metabolic wastes and water as urine. Disorders of the renal system affect the whole body, and may result in alterations in fluid and electrolyte balance, cardiovascular function, and nutritional status. In turn, healthy renal system function depends on the health of other body systems, especially the circulatory, endocrine, and nervous systems.

Anatomy, Physiology, and Functions of the Renal System

The organs of the renal system are the paired kidneys, the paired ureters, the urinary bladder, and the urethra (Figure 26–1 ■). Each structure is essential to the total functioning of the renal system.

The Kidneys

The two kidneys are located outside the peritoneal cavity and on either side of the vertebral column at the levels of T_{12} through L_3. These highly vascular, bean-shaped organs are approximately 4.5 inches (11.4 cm) long and 2.5 inches (6.4 cm) wide. The lateral surface of the kidney is convex; the medial surface is concave and forms a vertical cleft, the hilum. The ureter, renal artery, renal vein, lymphatic vessels, and nerves enter or exit the kidney at the level of the hilum.

Internally, each kidney has three distinct regions: the cortex, medulla, and pelvis. The outer region, or renal cortex, is light in color and has a granular appearance (Figure 26–2 ■). This region of the kidney contains the glomeruli, small clusters of

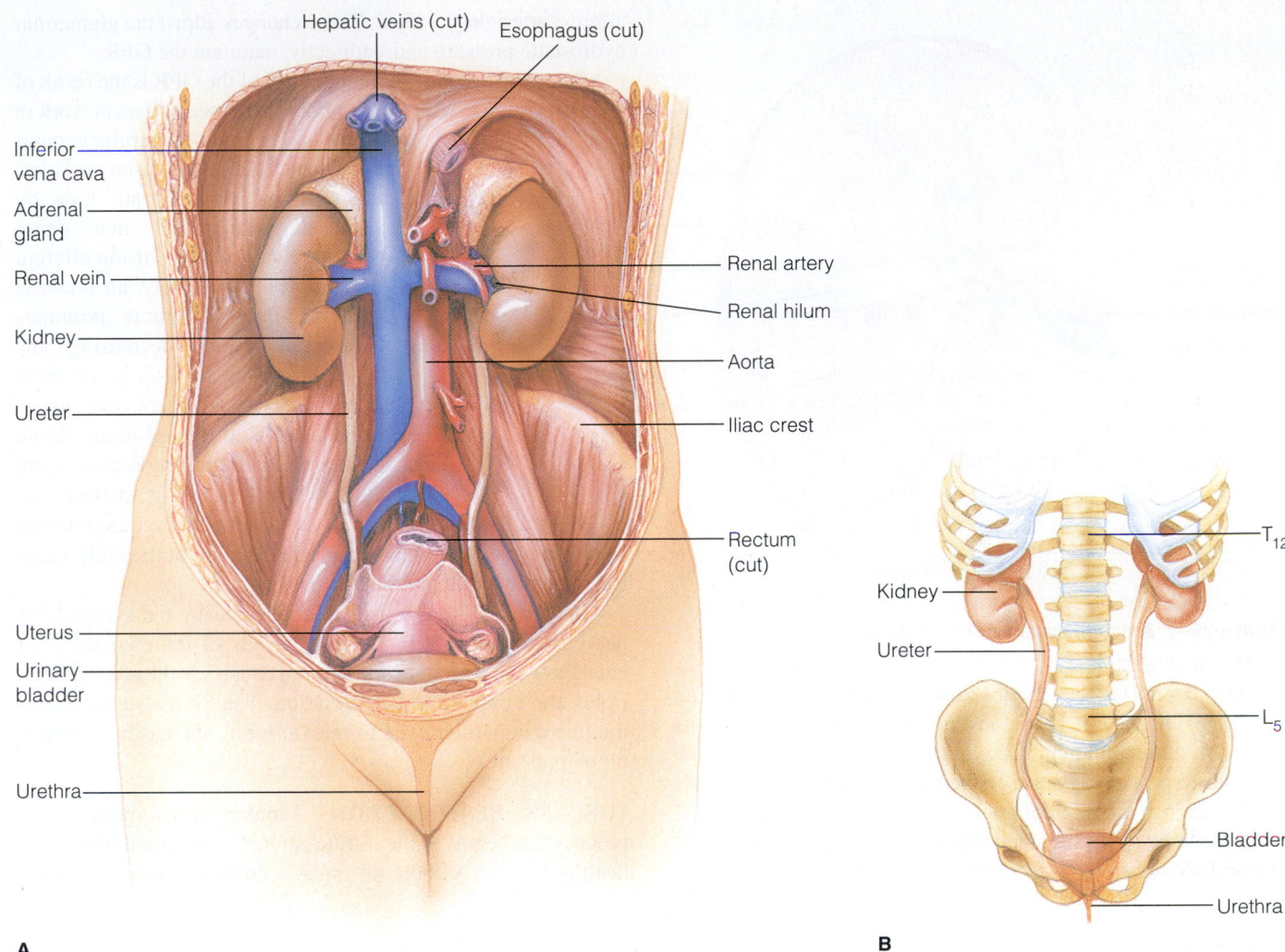

Figure 26–1 ■ The renal system. *A,* Anterior view of the renal system in a female. *B,* The kidneys are shown in relation to the vertebrae and ribs.

capillaries. The glomeruli bring blood to and carry waste products from the nephrons, the functional units of the kidney.

The renal medulla, just below the cortex, contains cone-shaped tissue masses called renal pyramids, formed almost entirely of bundles of collecting tubules. The collecting tubules that make up the pyramids channel urine into the innermost region, the renal pelvis. The renal pelvis is continuous with the ureter as it leaves the hilum. Branches of the pelvis, the calyces, extend toward the medulla and serve to collect urine and empty it into the pelvis. From the pelvis, urine is channeled through the ureter and into the bladder for storage. The walls of the calyces, the renal pelvis, and the ureter contain smooth muscle that moves urine along by peristalsis.

Formation of Urine

Each kidney contains approximately 1 million nephrons, which process the blood to make urine (Figure 26–3 ■). Each nephron contains a tuft of capillaries called the glomerulus, which is completely surrounded by the glomerular capsule (or Bowman's space). The complex structures of the kidneys process about 180 L (47 gal) of blood-derived fluid each day. Of this amount, only 1% is excreted as urine; the rest is returned to

the circulation. (Normal and abnormal findings of urine on laboratory analysis are listed in Table 26–1.) Urine formation is accomplished entirely by the nephron through three processes: glomerular filtration, tubular reabsorption, and tubular secretion (Figure 26–4 ■).

GLOMERULAR FILTRATION   Glomerular filtration is a passive process in which hydrostatic pressure forces fluid and solutes through a membrane. The amount of fluid filtered from the blood into the capsule per minute is called the glomerular filtration rate (GFR). Three factors influence this rate: the total surface area available for filtration, the permeability of the filtration membrane, and the net filtration pressure.

Net filtration pressure is responsible for the formation of filtrate and is determined by two forces: hydrostatic pressure (push) and osmotic pressure (pull). The glomerular hydrostatic pressure pushes water and solutes across the membrane. This pressure is opposed by the osmotic pressure in the glomerulus (primarily the colloid osmotic pressure of plasma proteins in the glomerular blood) and the capsular hydrostatic pressure exerted by fluids within the glomerular capsule. The difference between these forces determines the net filtration pressure, which is directly proportional to the GFR.

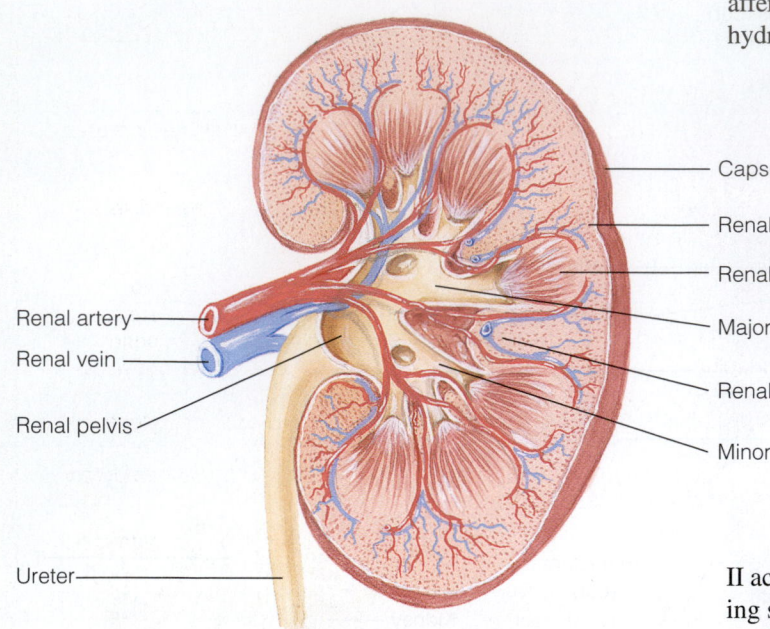

Figure 26–2 ■ Internal anatomy of the kidney.

The normal GFR in both kidneys is 120 to 125 mL/min in adults. This rate is held constant under normal conditions by renal autoregulation. The myogenic mechanism, which responds to pressure changes in the renal blood vessels, controls the diameter of the afferent arterioles to achieve autoregulation. An increase in systemic blood pressure causes the renal vessels to constrict, whereas a decrease in blood pressure causes the

afferent arterioles to dilate. These changes adjust the glomerular hydrostatic pressure and, indirectly, maintain the GFR.

Another control of the GFR is the result of the renin–angiotensin mechanism at work in the kidneys. The juxtaglomerular apparatus, located in the distal tubules, responds to slow filtrate flow by releasing chemicals that cause intense vasodilation of the afferent arterioles. Conversely, an increase in the flow of filtrate promotes vasoconstriction, decreasing the GFR. A sustained drop in systemic blood pressure triggers the juxtaglomerular cells to release renin. Renin acts on a plasma globulin, angiotensinogen, to release angiotensin I, which is in turn converted to angiotensin II. As a vasoconstrictor, angiotensin II activates vascular smooth muscle throughout the body, causing systemic blood pressure to rise.

Glomerular filtration is also controlled by the sympathetic nervous system (SNS). During periods of extreme stress or emergency, SNS system stimulation constricts the afferent arterioles and inhibits filtrate formation. The SNS also stimulates the juxtaglomerular cells to release renin, increasing systemic blood pressure.

TUBULAR REABSORPTION   Tubular reabsorption is a process that begins as the filtrate enters the proximal tubules. In healthy kidneys, almost all organic nutrients such as glucose

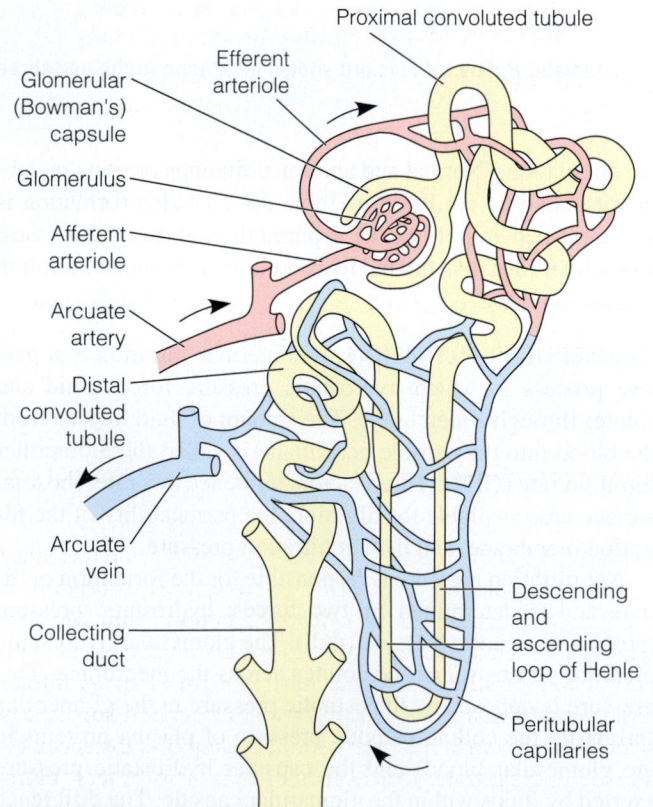

Figure 26–3 ■ The structure of a nephron, showing the glomerulus within the glomerular capsule.

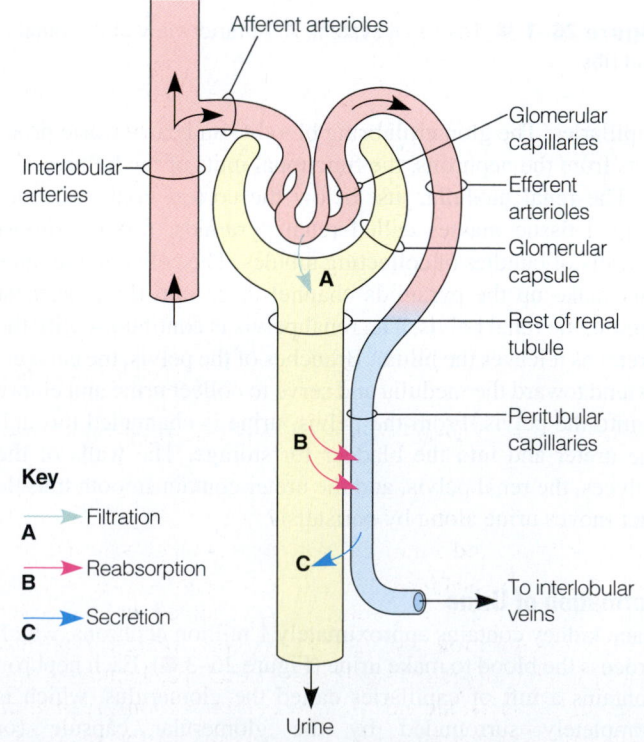

Figure 26–4 ■ Schematic view of the three major mechanisms by which the kidneys adjust to the composition of plasma: *A,* glomerular filtration; *B,* tubular reabsorption; and *C,* tubular secretion.

TABLE 26–1 Normal Results and Abnormal Findings: Urinalysis

CHARACTERISTIC OR COMPONENT	NORMAL RESULTS	ABNORMAL FINDING WITH POSSIBLE CAUSE
Color	Light straw to amber yellow	■ Red, dark, smoky color may be the result of blood in the urine (**hematuria** or menstrual blood). ■ Cloudy urine occurs from infection (pyuria) ■ Colorless urine indicates very dilute urine, such as in overhydration, kidney disease, alcohol ingestion, or diabetes insipidus. ■ Very dark yellow urine indicates dehydration and/or fever. ■ Red or red brown urine may be caused by sulfisoxazole-phenazopyridine (Azo Gantrisin), phenytoin (Dilantin), cascara, chlorpromazine (Thorazine), docusate calcium, and phenolphthalein (Doxidan); and by carrots, rhubarb, and food coloring. ■ Orange urine is caused by fever, urobilin, phenazopyridine (Pyridium), amidopyrine, nitrofurantoin, sulfonamides, carrots, beets, and food coloring. ■ Blue or green urine is caused by *Pseudomonas*, amitriptyline (Elavil), methylene blue, methocarbamol (Robaxin), and yeast concentrate. ■ Brown or black urine is caused by Lysol poisoning, melanin, bilirubin, methemoglobin, porphyrin, cascara, and injectable iron.
Appearance	Clear	■ Hazy or cloudy urine indicates bacteria, pus, RBCs, WBCs, phosphates, prostatic fluid spermatozoa, or urates. ■ Milky urine is the result of fats or pyuria. ■ Yellow foam results from bilirubin, bile, or severe cirrhosis of the liver. ■ A dark yellow to brownish color is seen with deficient fluid volume.
Odor	Aromatic	■ Ammonia smell increases as urine stands outside the body. ■ Urinary tract infection (UTI) causes a foul or unpleasant odor, depending on the causative organism. ■ Asparagus causes a distinctive odor. ■ Mousy odors result from phenylketonuria. ■ Sweet or fruity odors occur in starvation and diabetic ketoacidosis.
pH	4.5–8.0	■ < 4.5: metabolic acidosis, respiratory acidosis, diet high in meat protein, ammonium chloride, and mandelic acid ■ > 8.0: bacteriuria, UTI, antibiotics (neomycin, kanamycin), sulfonamides, sodium bicarbonate, acetazolamide (Diamox), potassium citrate
Specific gravity	1.005–1.030	■ < 1.005: diabetes insipidus, overhydration, renal disease, severe potassium deficit ■ > 1.030: dehydration, fever, diabetes mellitus, vomiting, diarrhea, contrast media
Protein	2–8 mg/dL	■ > 8 mg/dL: proteinuria, exercise, fever, stress, acute infection, kidney disease, lupus erythematosus, leukemia, multiple myeloma, cardiac disease, toxemia of pregnancy, septicemia, lead, mercury, neomycin, barbiturates, sulfonamides
Glucose	Negative	■ > 15 mg/dL or + 4: diabetes mellitus, stroke, Cushing's syndrome, anesthesia, glucose infusions, severe stress, infections, ascorbic acid, aspirin, cephalosporins, and epinephrine
Ketones	Negative	■ + 1 to 3: ketoacidosis, starvation, high-protein diet
RBCs	Rare	■ > 2 per low-power field: kidney trauma, kidney diseases, renal calculi, cystitis, excess aspirin, anticoagulants, sulfonamides, menstrual contamination
WBCs	3–4	■ > 4 per low-power field: UTI, fever, strenuous exercise, kidney diseases
Casts	Occasional hyaline	■ Fever, kidney diseases, heart failure

and amino acids are reabsorbed. However, the tubules constantly regulate and adjust the rate and degree of water and ion reabsorption in response to hormonal signals. Reabsorption may be active or passive. Substances reclaimed through active tubular reabsorption are usually moving against electrical and/or chemical gradients. These substances, including glucose, amino acids, lactate, vitamins, and most ions, require an ATP-dependent carrier to be transported into the interstitial space. In passive tubular reabsorption, which includes diffusion and osmosis, substances move along their gradient without expenditure of energy.

TUBULAR SECRETION The final process in urine formation is tubular secretion, which is essentially reabsorption in reverse. Substances such as hydrogen and potassium ions, creatinine, ammonia, and organic acids move from the blood of the peritubular capillaries into the tubules themselves as filtrate. Thus, urine consists of both filtered and secreted substances. Tubular secretion is important for disposing of substances not already in the filtrate, such as medications. This process eliminates undesirable substances that have been reabsorbed by passive processes and rids the body of excessive potassium ions. It is also a vital force in the regulation of blood pH.

Maintaining Normal Composition and Volume of Urine

Maintaining the normal composition and volume of urine involves a countercurrent exchange system. In this system, fluid flows in opposite directions through the parallel tubes of the loop of Henle and the vasa recta, tiny capillaries that run along the loop of Henle. Fluid is exchanged across these parallel membranes in response to a concentration gradient (Figure 26–5 ■). When the filtrate enters the proximal convoluted tubule, its osmolality (at 300 mOsm/kg) is essentially the same as that of the plasma and the interstitial fluid of the renal cortex.

Urine is composed, by volume, of about 95% water and 5% solutes. The largest component of urine by weight is **urea** (a nitrogenous waste product formed in the liver from the breakdown of amino acids). Other solutes normally excreted in the urine include sodium, potassium, phosphate, sulfate, creatinine, uric acid, calcium, magnesium, and bicarbonate.

Clearing Waste Products

The kidneys excrete water-soluble waste products and other chemicals or substances from the body. This process is called renal plasma clearance, which refers to the ability of the kidneys to clear (cleanse) a given amount of plasma of a particular substance in a given time (usually 1 minute). The kidneys clear 25 to 30 g of urea each day. They also clear creatinine (an end product of creatine phosphate, found in skeletal muscle), uric acid (a metabolite of nucleic acid metabolism), and ammonia as well as bacterial toxins and water-soluble drugs.

Renal Hormones

Hormones either activated or synthesized by the kidneys include the active form of vitamin D, erythropoietin, and natriuretic hormone.

Vitamin D is necessary for the absorption of calcium and phosphate by the small intestine. In an inactive form, vitamin D enters the body either by dietary intake or through the action of ultraviolet rays on cholesterol in the skin. Activation occurs in two steps, the first in the liver and the second in the kidneys. The renal step is stimulated by parathyroid hormone, which in turn responds to a decreased plasma calcium level. Erythropoietin stimulates the bone marrow to produce red blood cells in response to tissue hypoxia. The stimulus for the production of erythropoietin by the kidneys is decreased oxygen delivery to kidney cells. The right atria of the heart releases natriuretic hormone in response to increased volume and

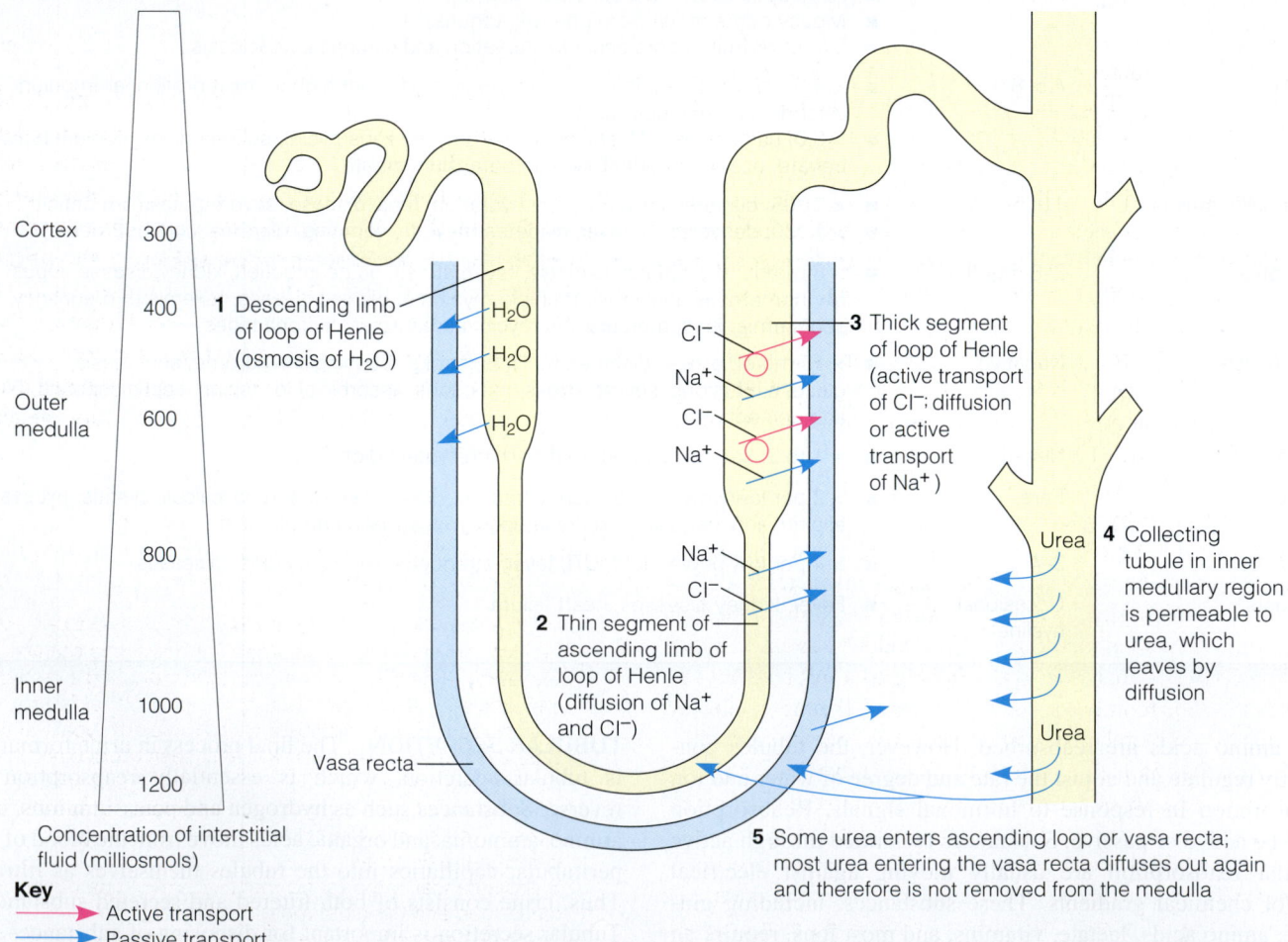

Figure 26–5 ■ The countercurrent exchange system is responsible for establishing and maintaining an osmotic gradient necessary to the composition, volume, and pH of urine.

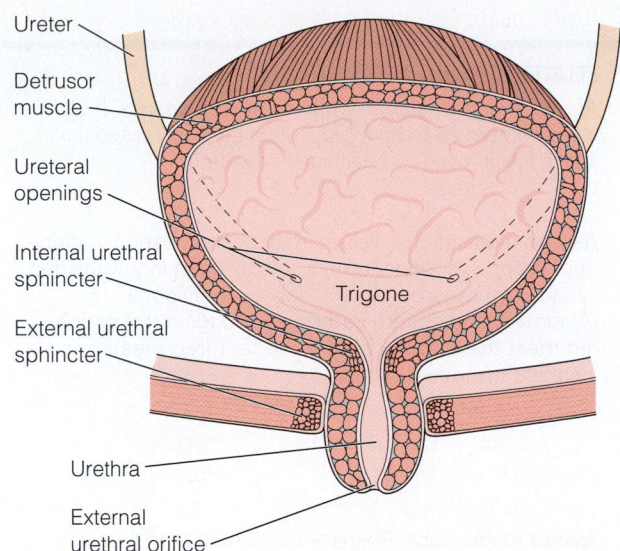

Ureter

Detrusor muscle

Ureteral openings

Internal urethral sphincter

Trigone

External urethral sphincter

Urethra

External urethral orifice

Figure 26–6 ■ Internal view of the urinary bladder and trigone.

stretch, as occurs in increased extracellular volume. This hormone inhibits ADH secretion, so that the collecting tubules are less porous and a large amount of dilute urine is produced.

The Ureters, Urinary Bladder, and Urethra

The ureters are bilateral tubes approximately 10 to 12 inches (26 to 30 cm) long. They transport urine from the kidney to the bladder through peristaltic waves originating in the renal pelvis. The wall of the ureter has three layers: an inner epithelial mucosa, a middle layer of smooth muscle, and an outer layer of fibrous connective tissue. The urinary bladder is posterior to the symphysis pubis and serves as a storage site for urine. In males, the bladder lies immediately in front of the rectum; in females, the bladder lies in front of the vagina and the uterus. Openings for the ureters and the urethra are inside the bladder: The trigone is the smooth triangular portion of the base of the bladder outlined by the openings for the ureters and urinary bladder. (See Figure 26–6 ■.)

The size of the bladder varies with the amount of urine it contains. In healthy adults, the bladder holds about 300 to 500 mL of urine before internal pressure rises and signals the need to empty the bladder through **micturition** (also called urination or voiding). However, the bladder can hold more than twice that amount if necessary. The bladder has an internal urethral sphincter that relaxes in response to a full bladder and signals the need to urinate. A second external urethral sphincter is formed by skeletal muscle and is under voluntary control.

The urethra is a thin-walled muscular tube that channels urine to the outside of the body. It extends from the base of the bladder to the external urinary meatus. In females, the urethra is approximately 1.5 inches (3 to 5 cm) long, and the urinary meatus is anterior to the vaginal orifice. In males, the urethra is approximately 8 inches (20 cm) long and serves as a channel for semen as well as urine. The prostate gland encircles the urethra at the base of the bladder in males. The male urinary meatus is located at the end of the glans penis.

Assessing Renal System Function

Renal system function is assessed by findings from diagnostic tests, a health assessment interview to collect subjective data, and a physical assessment to collect objective data.

Diagnostic Tests

The results of diagnostic tests of renal system function are used to support the diagnosis of a specific disease, to provide information to identify or modify the appropriate medication or therapy used to treat the disease, and to help nurses monitor the patient's responses to treatment and nursing care interventions. Diagnostic tests to assess the structures and functions of the renal system are described in the box. More information is included in the discussion of specific disorders in ∞ Chapters 27 and 28.

Regardless of the type of diagnostic test, the nurse is responsible for explaining the procedure and any special preparation needed, assessing for medication use that may affect the outcome of the tests, ensuring the consent form is signed (if necessary), supporting the patient during the examination as necessary, documenting the procedures as appropriate, and monitoring the results of the tests. The nurse is also responsible for postprocedure care and patient teaching for self-care at home.

Genetic Considerations

When conducting a health assessment interview and physical assessment, it is important for the nurse to consider genetic influences on adult health. During the health assessment interview, ask about family members with health problems affecting kidney function, or of family members diagnosed with polycystic disease or diabetes mellitus. During the physical assessment, assess for any manifestations that might indicate a genetic disorder (see Genetic Considerations). If data are found to indicate genetic risk factors or alterations, ask about genetic testing and refer for appropriate genetic counseling and evaluation. ∞ Chapter 8 provides further information about genetics in medical-surgical nursing.

GENETIC CONSIDERATIONS
Examples of Renal System Disorders

- Adult polycystic kidney disease (APKD) is linked to a familial chromosome 16 disorder. The disease is characterized by large cysts in one or both kidneys and a gradual loss of kidney tissue with resultant chronic renal failure.
- Chronic renal failure may be a complication of type 1 and type 2 diabetes mellitus (DM), but is seen more often in patients with type 1 DM. Type 1 and type 2 DM are classified as multifactorial inheritance disorders because both genetic and environmental factors are necessary for onset of the disorder.
- Bladder cancer is the fourth most common type of cancer in men and the ninth most common cancer in women. Genetic factors related to chromosome 9 are interrelated with risk factors such as smoking and exposure to industrial chemicals to cause bladder cancer.

DIAGNOSTIC TESTS of the Renal System

NAME OF TEST	PURPOSE & DESCRIPTION	RELATED NURSING INTERVENTIONS
Blood urea nitrogen (BUN)	This blood test measures urea. Increased levels may result from dehydration, vomiting, diarrhea, digested blood, or prerenal/renal failure. Normal values: 5–25 mg/dL	Assess hydration status, which may affect results. If BUN is elevated from 26 to 35 mg/dL, encourage increased fluid intake (if approved by healthcare provider).
Creatinine (serum)	This blood test is used to diagnose kidney dysfunction. Creatinine is a by-product of the breakdown of muscle and is excreted by the kidneys. When 50% or more nephrons are destroyed, serum creatinine levels rise. Normal BUN/creatine ratio is 10:1. Values are not affected by hydration status. Normal value: Serum: 0.5–1.5 mg/dL. (Older adults and women may have decreased values due to decreased muscle mass.)	Assess medications; values may be increased by antibiotics (cephalosporins, amphotericin B, aminoglycosides, kanamycin) ascorbic acid, L-dopa, methyldopa (Aldomet), and lithium carbonate. Suggest not eating red meat the evening before the test (red meats can increase the value).
Creatinine clearance	A 24-hour urine test to identify renal dysfunction and to monitor renal function. Normal value: 85–135/min Women and older adults may have slightly lower values.	Assess medications: Phenacetin, steroids, and thiazides may decrease creatinine clearance; ascorbic acid, steroids, L-dopa, methyldopa (Aldomet), and cefoxitin may increase creatinine clearance. Levels of creatinine are elevated in hypothyroidism, hypertension, pregnancy, and exercise. Ask the patient to void and discard first voiding. Instruct patient, family, and staff (if hospitalized) to save all urine for a clearly designated 24-hour period, maintaining the specimen in the container on ice or in the refrigerator.
Cystatin C	This blood test may be used as an alternative to creatinine and creatinine clearance to screen for and monitor kidney dysfunction in people suspected of having kidney diseases. Cystatin C is a cysteine proteinase inhibitor that is filtered by the kidneys; increased concentrations in the blood indicate kidney dysfunction. Results of the test are not affected by muscle mass, gender, age or race.	No special preparation is required.
CT scan of kidneys	The CT scan allows evaluation of kidney size, tumors, abscesses, suprarenal masses, and obstructions. A contrast dye may be administered orally or injected IV, allowing increased visualization of the density of renal tissue and masses in comparison to an ultrasound.	Assess the patient for allergies to iodine, x-ray contrast dye, and seafood. Assess medications: Oral hypoglycemic agents are contraindicated for use with iodinated contrast. Ensure that serum creatinine and BUN levels are available. Tell the patient to remain NPO for 4 hours prior to the test, and that laxatives or enemas may be ordered to remove gas or fecal material from the bowel. Posttest, monitor for and tell the patient to report allergic reactions to the dye (rash, itching, headache, vomiting), and to increase fluid intake to help excrete the dye.
Cystometrogram (CMG) (voiding cystogram)	This test is conducted to evaluate bladder capacity and neuromuscular functions of the bladder, urethral pressures, and causes of bladder dysfunction. A measured quantity of fluid is instilled into the bladder, and the filling capacity and voiding pressures are measured. Normal value: Urine stream strong and uninterrupted, normal filling pattern and sensation of fullness; bladder capacity: 300–600 mL; urge to void: >150 mL; fullness felt: 300 mL.	Tell patient that the bladder will be filled and during filling he or she will be asked to describe the first urge to void, and the sensation of being unable to delay urination any longer.

DIAGNOSTIC TESTS of the Renal System (continued)

NAME OF TEST	PURPOSE & DESCRIPTION	RELATED NURSING INTERVENTIONS
Cystoscopy (cystogram), cystography	Direct visualization of the bladder wall and urethra is accomplished by using a cystoscope. During the procedure small renal calculi can be removed from the ureter, bladder, or urethra, and tissue biopsy can be done. It also permits determination of the cause of hematuria or UTI. A stent may be inserted during the procedure to facilitate urinary drainage past an obstruction. A retrograde pyelogram may be done during the cystoscopy. By instilling a contrast dye into the bladder (cystography), neurogenic bladder, fistulas, tumors, or ruptures can be identified. The test may be done with either local or general anesthesia.	Assess history of cystitis or prostatitis (these disorders could result in sepsis after the procedure), hypersensitivity to anesthetics, and urinary patterns (amount, color, odor). Take and record vital signs. Following the procedure, assess for complications (hemorrhage, bladder perforation, urinary retention) and report gross hematuria (blood in the urine). Apply heat to the lower abdomen or assist with sitz bath if ordered to relieve pain and muscle spasms. Tell the patient to avoid alcoholic drinks for 2 days, to increase fluid intake, and that a slight burning sensation with voiding may occur for a day or two. Instruct the patient to immediately notify the physician if the urine remains bloody for more than three voidings after the procedure, or if bright bleeding, low urine output, abdominal or flank pain, chills, or fever develops.
GFR, estimated GFR (eGFR)	A measured GFR is considered the most accurate means of detecting changes in kidney function. Because the GFR is a complicated measurement to obtain, an eGFR can be used. The eGFR is calculated based on the serum creatinine, age, gender, and (in some instances) racial origin. The National Kidney Foundation recommends that the eGFR be calculated automatically every time a creatinine test is done. Normal Value: 90–120 mL/min	No special preparation is necessary.
Intravenous pyelogram (IVP), retrograde pyelogram	An IVP is a radiologic examination done to visualize the entire renal tract to identify abnormal size, shape, and function of the kidneys or to detect renal calculi (stones), tumors, or cysts. A radiopaque substance is injected IV and a series of x-rays taken. A retrograde pyelogram is a radiologic examination done to evaluate the structures of the ureters and kidney pelvis. It may be performed alone or in conjunction with a cystoscopy.	Schedule IVP prior to any ordered barium test or gallbladder studies using contrast material. Ask about allergy to seafood, iodine, or radiologic contrast dye. Notify physician or radiologist if allergies are known. Assess medications: Oral hypoglycemic agents are contraindicated for use with iodinated contrast. Assess renal and fluid status, including serum osmolality, creatinine, and blood urea nitrogen (BUN) levels. Notify the physician of any abnormal values. Instruct the patient to complete ordered pretest bowel preparation, including prescribed laxative or cathartic the evening before the test, and an enema or suppository the morning of the test. Tell the patient not to eat food for 8 to 12 hours prior to the test; clear liquids are allowed. Take and record vital signs. Instruct the patient to contact the healthcare provider for any delayed reactions to the dye (breathing difficulty, rash, itching, rapid heart beat).
MRI of the kidneys	An MRI is used to visualize the kidneys by assessing computer-generated films of radiofrequency waves and changes in magnetic fields.	Inform patient of need to lie still during the examination. Assess for any metallic implants (such as pacemakers, clips on brain aneurysms, body piercings, tattoos, shrapnel). If present, notify imaging physician. Remove transdermal medication patches (both OTC and prescribed) unless otherwise ordered (FDA, 2009). Replace the patch following the procedure. Tell the patient to inform the staff about the patch when making the appointment and when completing the admission information. Ask if patient is pregnant; if so the test is not performed. Ask about claustrophobia; if this is a problem request the patient to ask for a relaxing medication to take prior to the MRI.
Portable ultrasonic bladder scan	This test is used to obtain information about residual urine. Warmed ultrasound gel is applied over the lower abdomen, and the ultrasound probe is placed just above the pubic bone. The scanner shows an outline of the bladder and displays the amount of urine in the bladder in milliliters. Obtain several readings and use the largest (the most accurate). Print the information, place it on the patient's chart, and document the residual urine amount.	No special preparation is needed, but the test is usually not used for pregnant women. Report a residual amount more than 100 mL.

(continued)

DIAGNOSTIC TESTS of the Renal System (continued)

NAME OF TEST	PURPOSE & DESCRIPTION	RELATED NURSING INTERVENTIONS
Renal arteriogram or angiogram	This radiologic test is done to visualize renal blood vessels to detect renal artery stenosis, renal thrombosis or embolism, tumors, cysts, or aneurysm; to determine the causative factor for hypertension; and to evaluate renal circulation. A contrast medium is injected into the femoral artery.	Assess for allergy to iodine, seafood, or other contrast dye from other x-ray procedures. Assess medications: Oral hypoglycemic agents are contraindicated for use with iodinated contrast; anticoagulants should be discontinued. Instruct the patient to take a laxative or cleansing enema the night before the test (if ordered) and to remain NPO for 8 to 12 hours prior to the test. Take and record vital signs. Ask the patient to void and remove dentures and jewelry before the test. After the test, monitor for bleeding from the femoral artery, restrict activity for a day, assess peripheral pulses, and monitor urine output. Instruct the patient to contact the healthcare provider for any delayed reactions to the dye (such as breathing difficulty, rash, itching, rapid heart beat, decreased urine output).
Renal biopsy	A renal biopsy is performed to determine the cause of renal disease, to rule out cancer metastasis to the kidney, or if rejection is occurring with a kidney transplant. It is performed by using a cystoscope, excising a wedge of kidney tissue, or through the skin with a biopsy needle (percutaneous route).	If a general anesthetic is used, ask the patient not to eat or drink fluids for 8 to 12 hours before the biopsy. Take and record vital signs. Note hemoglobin and hematocrit values and report abnormal findings. After the biopsy, if the percutaneous route was used, apply pressure to the site for about 20 minutes to prevent bleeding. Assess bowel sounds if surgical interventions were used. Tell the patient to increase oral fluid intake and to report decreased urination or burning on urination.
Renal scan	This test is done to evaluate kidney blood flow, location, size, and shape; and to assess kidney perfusion and urine production. Radioactive isotopes are injected IV and radiation detector probes are placed over the kidneys to monitor activity in the kidneys. Radioisotope distribution in the kidneys is scanned and graphed. Nonfunctioning tissue, such as in tumors and cysts, appears as cold spots.	Ask patient to drink several glasses of water prior to the test. Obtain weight and have patient void. After the procedure, increase fluid intake.
Renal ultrasound	This noninvasive test is conducted to detect renal or perirenal masses, identify obstructions, and diagnose renal cysts and solid masses. It is done by applying a conductive gel to the skin and placing a small external ultrasound probe on the patient's skin. Sound waves are recorded on a computer as they are reflected off tissues.	No special preparation is needed.
Residual urine (postvoiding residual urine)	A residual urine test is conducted to measure the amount of urine left in the bladder after voiding. **Normal value:** < 50 mL	Ask the patient to void in a collection device and measure the amount. Immediately after voiding, catheterize using sterile technique and a straight catheter. Drain bladder completely. Document time, amount voided, amount obtained on catheterization, color, clarity, odor, and any other significant data. Report amount of residual urine if it is more than 100 mL.
Urinalysis (UA)	An examination of the constituents of a sample of urine in order to establish a baseline, to provide data for diagnosis, or to monitor results of treatment. Normal findings and abnormal findings with causes are outlined in Table 26–1.	Provide a clean specimen cup for a sample of urine. An early morning specimen is preferred. Note on the laboratory slip if the patient is menstruating (some menstrual blood may be present in the urine sample if so). Assess medications, fluid status, and foods that might affect urinalysis results. Tell the patient to refrigerate the specimen until it can be taken for analysis.

DIAGNOSTIC TESTS of the Renal System (continued)

NAME OF TEST	PURPOSE & DESCRIPTION	RELATED NURSING INTERVENTIONS
Urine culture (midstream, clean-catch)	A culture of a urine sample is conducted to identify the causative organism of a UTI. Normal value: <10,000 organisms/mL (urine is sterile but urethra contains bacteria and a few WBCs) Values of >100,000 organisms/mL indicate UTI	Provide a sterile container for the urine sample. Ask women to separate labia with one hand and clean labia with other hand, using sterile cotton sponges saturated with a cleansing solution, and wiping three times front to back. Ask men to retract the foreskin and cleanse glans with three cotton sponges saturated with a cleansing solution, using a circular motion. After cleaning, tell patient to begin voiding and then collect specimen in the container (initial voiding will contain urethral contaminants). If patient is unable to void, it may be necessary to obtain a specimen by urinary catheterization. Ask the patient to wait to take antibiotics or sulfonamides until after the specimen is taken and to refrigerate the specimen until it can be taken for testing. If the patient is taking antibiotics, it should be listed on the laboratory slip.
Uroflowmetry	This test measures the volume of urine voided per second.	Ask the patient to increase fluid intake and refrain from voiding for several hours before the test to ensure a full bladder and a strong urge to void during testing. Tell the patient he or she will be asked to urinate into a funnel.

Health Assessment Interview

A health assessment interview to determine problems with renal structure and function may be conducted during a health screening, may focus on a chief complaint (such as burning on urination or difficulty starting the stream when urinating), or may be part of a total health assessment. As with alterations in bowel function, patients with problems with renal system function may be embarrassed to talk about renal elimination patterns. It is often helpful to discuss less personal information first.

Assess the patient's current urinary status. Focus questions on changes in patterns of urination, changes in the urine, and pain. Assess changes in patterns of urination by asking the patient the following questions: How many times a day do you urinate? Do you feel that you empty your bladder each time? How many times do you get up at night to urinate? Do you experience a very strong desire to urinate and feel that you just cannot wait? Have you noticed that you urinate small amounts of dark, strong-smelling urine?

Changes in the urine that should be explored include the presence of blood or a cloudy appearance of the urine. If the patient has noticed blood, explore the use of medications (such as anticoagulants or dye-containing drugs) or bleeding problems. Cloudy, foul-smelling urine often indicates infection (pyuria); ask the patient about temperature elevations, chills, and general malaise. Cloudy urine in men may result from retrograde ejaculation (when semen is discharged into the bladder instead of from the penis) during intercourse.

If the patient reports pain (**dysuria**), explore its location, duration, and intensity. Kidney pain is experienced in the back and the costovertebral angle (the angle between the lower ribs and adjacent vertebrae) and may spread toward the umbilicus. Renal colic (pain in response to renal calculi moving through the ureter) is severe, sharp, stabbing, and excruciating; often it is felt in the flank, bladder, urethra, testes, or ovaries. Bladder and urethral pain is usually dull and continuous but may be experienced as spasms. The patient with a distended bladder experiences constant pain increased by any pressure over the bladder.

Information about surgeries or other treatment of previous renal problems is essential to the health history, as is a family history of altered structure or function. A family history of renal problems may be the first clue to abnormalities in the patient's renal function. Explore information regarding family occurrence of end-stage renal disease, renal calculi, and frequent infections as well as related problems such as hypertension and diabetes mellitus.

Questions about lifestyle, diet, and work history should explore cigarette smoking and/or exposure to toxic industrial or environmental chemicals (to identify risks for cancer), usual fluid intake, type of fluid intake, and self-care measures to replace fluids lost during work or physical activity in hot temperatures.

Interview questions categorized by functional health patterns are listed in the box on page 778.

Physical Assessment

The structure and function of the renal system is assessed by examination of the skin, abdomen, kidneys, bladder, and urinary meatus. Guidelines for abdominal assessment are outlined in ∞ Chapter 21. Normal age-related findings for the older adult are summarized in the Nursing Care of the Older Adult box on page 779.

Physical assessment of the renal system may be performed as part of a total health assessment, as part of an abdominal assessment, or as part of the back examination (for the kidneys). The techniques of inspection, auscultation, palpation, and percussion are used.

PRACTICE ALERT
Auscultate immediately after inspection because percussion or palpation may increase bowel motility and interfere with sound transmission during auscultation.

Before beginning the assessment, ask the patient to provide a clean-catch urine specimen (if ordered) and give the patient a specimen cup. Assess the specimen for color, odor, and clarity before you send it to the laboratory.

FUNCTIONAL HEALTH PATTERN INTERVIEW   Renal System

Functional Health Pattern	Interview Questions and Leading Statements
Health Perception-Health Management	■ Have you ever had a bladder or kidney disease, injury, or surgery? Describe. ■ If so, how was the problem treated? ■ Describe your usual intake of fluids for a 24-hour period. What type of fluids do you drink? ■ Have you ever smoked? If so, how many cigarettes per day? ■ Describe the problem you are having with your kidneys or bladder. ■ Are you taking medications for this or any other health problem? If so, what do you take and how often? ■ *For women:* Describe how you care for yourself when you urinate (for example, direction of wiping with tissue). ■ If you have a surgical diversion of urine, describe how you care for yourself (what skin and appliance care do you do, how often do you empty the bag?). ■ Do you wear or have you ever worn an external catheter, indwelling catheter, or incontinence briefs? Explain. ■ Have you ever done self-catheterization? If so, why and how often?
Nutritional-Metabolic	■ How much coffee, tea, or alcohol do you drink in a 24-hour period? ■ Have you ever limited your fluid intake? Explain. ■ Do you limit the amount of salt you eat? Explain. ■ Do you have swelling in your ankles? If so, what do you do?
Elimination	■ How many times a day do you urinate? Has there been a change in your usual pattern of urination? ■ Do you experience a sudden urge to urinate? ■ Has there been a change in your urine, such as a change in amount, color, or odor? Have you ever noticed blood in your urine or on the tissue after you wipe? ■ Is it difficult for you to begin or end your flow of urine? ■ Have you ever had problems controlling your urine when you laugh, sneeze, or cough? ■ Do you have any discharge from your urethra? Explain.
Activity-Exercise	■ Do your urinary problems interfere with your activities of daily living? Explain. ■ Describe your usual energy level. Has there been a change? Explain. ■ Have you ever been taught to do Kegel exercises to help you control your urination? If so, how often do you practice these?
Sleep-Rest	■ Does a problem with urination interfere with your ability to sleep and rest? Explain. ■ Has there been a change in the number of times you wake up at night to urinate? Explain.
Cognitive-Perceptual	■ Do you have any pain or burning when you urinate? ■ Have you experienced any tenderness or pain over the lower sides of your back or severe pain that spreads over your lower abdomen? If so, describe its location, intensity, aggravating factors, and duration.
Self-Perception-Self-Concept	■ How does having this condition make you feel about yourself?
Role-Relationships	■ How does having this condition affect your relationships with others?
Sexuality-Reproductive	■ Has this condition interfered with your usual sexual activity?
Coping-Stress-Tolerance	■ Has having this condition created stress for you? ■ Have you experienced any kind of stress that makes this condition worse? Explain. ■ Describe what you do when you feel stressed.
Value-Belief	■ Describe how specific relationships or activities help you cope with this problem. ■ Describe specific cultural beliefs or practices that affect how you care for and feel about this problem. ■ Is there anything interfering with your spiritual beliefs, needs or practices during your illness? What can I or another caregiver do to help you with your spiritual needs? ■ Are there any specific treatments that you would not use to treat this condition?

At the beginning of the assessment, the patient may be sitting or lying supine. Prior to the examination, collect all necessary equipment and explain the techniques to the patient to decrease anxiety. Because the examination involves exposure of the genital area, give the patient a gown and drape the patient appropriately to minimize exposure.

Guidelines for percussion and palpation of the kidneys are outlined in Box 26–1.

NURSING CARE OF THE OLDER ADULT **Age-Related Renal System Changes**

AGE-RELATED CHANGE	SIGNIFICANCE
Kidneys: ↓ size of renal cortex and number of nephrons, ↓ growth of renal tissue, ↑ risk of atherosclerosis, all of which may result in atrophy of the kidneys.	■ Decreased renal blood flow. ■ Decreased GFR by about 50% between ages 20 and 90.
Renal tubules: ↓ function, with less effective exchange of substances, water and sodium conservation and suppression of ADH secretion in presence of hypoosmolality.	■ Risk of hyponatremia and **nocturia** (voiding more often at night). ■ Effects of medications may be altered (with decreased filtration). ■ Decreased reabsorption of glucose may result in 1+ proteinuria and glycosuria, which are not of major clinical significance.
Bladder: ■ Muscles weaken and bladder capacity decreases. ■ More difficult to empty bladder. ■ Delayed micturition reflex.	■ Urinary retention is more common. ■ Urinary frequency, urgency, and nocturia are more common with aging. ■ Larger amounts of residual urine present after voiding. ■ Some stress incontinence may occur, especially in women who have had several children. ■ Urinary incontinence is *not* a normal outcome of aging.

BOX 26–1 Guidelines for Physical Assessment of the Kidneys

Percussion of the Kidneys

Percussion of the kidneys helps assess pain or tenderness. Assist the patient to a sitting position, and stand behind the patient. For indirect percussion, place the palm of your nondominant hand over the costovertebral angle (see Figure *A*). Strike this area with the ulnar surface of your dominant hand, curled into a fist (see Figure *B*). For direct percussion, also strike the area over the costovertebral angle with the ulnar surface of your dominant hand, curled into a fist. Repeat the technique for the other kidney. You should do percussion of the kidneys with only enough force so the patient feels a gentle thud. Percussion is usually done at the end of the assessment.

Palpation of the Kidneys

Although the technique of palpation of the kidneys is outlined here, this technique is best performed by an advanced practitioner, because it involves deep palpation. In addition, the kidneys are difficult to palpate.

Assist the patient to the supine position and stand at the right side of the patient. To palpate the left kidney, reach across the patient and place your left hand under the patient's left flank with your palm upward. Elevate the left flank with your fingers, displacing the kidney upward. Ask the patient to take a deep breath and use the palmer surface of your right hand to palpate the kidney (Figure *C*). Repeat the technique for the right kidney.

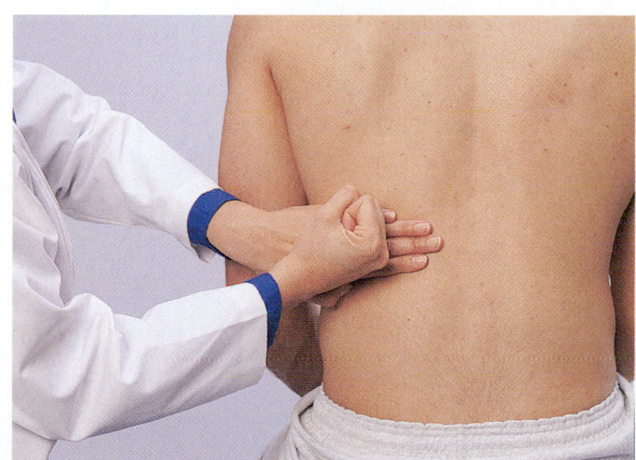
B

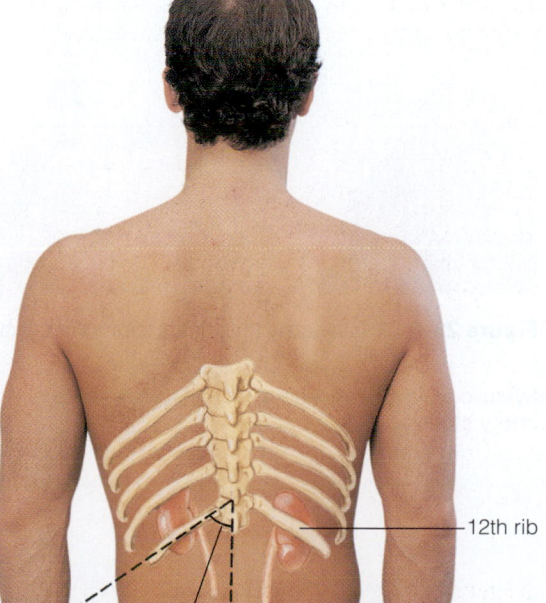
A
Costovertebral angle — 12th rib

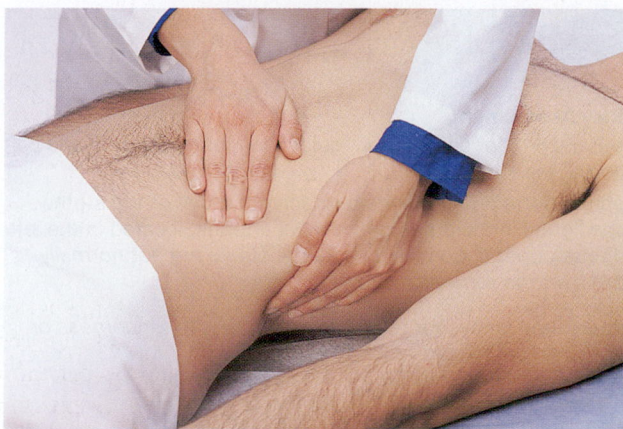
C

Renal Assessments

Technique/Normal Findings	Abnormal Findings

Skin Assessment

Inspect the skin and mucous membranes, noting color, turgor, and excretions. *The color of skin and mucous membranes should be even and appropriate to the age and race of the patient; skin should be dry with no visible excretions.*

- Pallor of the skin and mucous membranes may indicate kidney disease with resultant anemia.
- Decreased turgor of the skin may indicate dehydration.
- Edema (generalized or in the lower extremities) may indicate fluid volume excess. (Changes in skin turgor may indicate renal insufficiency with either excess fluid loss or retention.)
- An accumulation of uric acid crystals, called uremic frost, may be seen on the skin of the patient with late-stage renal failure.

Abdominal Assessment

Inspect the abdomen, noting size, symmetry, masses or lumps, swelling, distention, glistening, or skin tightness.

The abdomen should be slightly concave, symmetric, and without distention or masses.

- Enlargements or asymmetry may indicate a hernia or superficial mass.
- If the urinary bladder is distended, it rises above the symphysis pubis as a rounded mass.
- Distention, glistening, or skin tightness may be associated with fluid retention.
- Ascites is an accumulation of fluid in the peritoneal cavity.

Urinary Meatus Assessment

This technique is not part of a routine assessment, but it is an important component in patients with health problems of the renal system.

For the male patient: With the patient in a sitting or standing position, compress the tip of the glans penis with the gloved hand to open the urinary meatus (Figure 26–7 ■).

For the female patient: With the patient in the dorsal lithotomy position, spread the labia with your gloved hand to expose the urinary meatus.

The urinary meatus should be midline and free of redness, lesions, or discharge.

- Increased redness, swelling, or discharge from the urinary meatus may indicate infection or sexually transmitted infection.
- Ulceration of the urinary meatus may indicate a sexually transmitted infection.
- Hypospadias is displacement of the urinary meatus to the ventral surface of the penis.
- Epispadias is displacement of the urinary meatus to the dorsal surface of the penis.

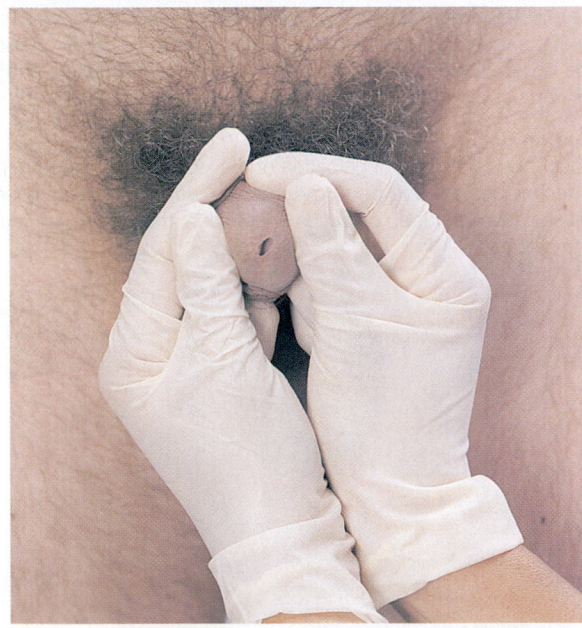

Figure 26–7 ■ Inspecting the urinary meatus of the male.

Kidney Assessment

See Box 26–1 for assessment guidelines for percussion and palpation of the kidneys.

Auscultate the renal arteries by placing the bell of the stethoscope lightly in the areas of the renal arteries, located in the left and right upper abdominal quadrants. *Bruits are not normally heard over the renal arteries.*

Percuss the kidneys for tenderness or pain. *No tenderness or pain should be elicited.*

- Systolic bruits ("whooshing" sounds) may indicate renal artery stenosis.

- Tenderness and pain on percussion of the costovertebral angle suggest glomerulonephritis or glomerulonephrosis.

Technique/Normal Findings	Abnormal Findings
Palpate the kidneys. The lower pole of the right kidney may be palpable with deep palpation; the remaining right kidney and the left kidney are normally not palpable. *If palpable, they should be nontender, bilaterally of appropriate size and density, and without palpable masses.*	■ A mass or lump may indicate a tumor or cyst. ■ Tenderness or pain on palpation may suggest an inflammatory process. ■ A soft kidney that feels spongy may indicate chronic renal disease. ■ Bilaterally enlarged kidneys may suggest polycystic kidney disease. ■ Unequal kidney size may indicate hydronephrosis.
Bladder Assessment Percuss the bladder for tone and position. *The bladder should be midline without dullness.*	■ A dull percussion tone over the bladder of a patient who has just urinated may indicate urinary retention. ■ A distended bladder may be palpated at any point from the symphysis pubis to the umbilicus and is felt as a firm, rounded organ. It indicates urinary retention.

SAMPLE DOCUMENTATION
Assessment of Renal System Function

Home visit made to 66-year-old woman with end-stage chronic kidney failure. Skin pale and oral mucous membranes dry. 4+ edema in ankles and feet. Eyelids swollen. Skin tight and shiny over abdomen and bilateral lower extremities. Abdomen distended and tender on light palpation; further palpation deferred. Urinary bladder not palpable. Urine output for past 24 hours is 15 mL.

TEST YOURSELF NCLEX-RN® REVIEW

1. A nurse is assessing the renal system of an older woman. Which statement by the woman would indicate a health problem?
   1. "I sometimes have to get up at night to urinate."
   2. "When I have to urinate, I really feel an urge to go."
   3. "My doctor told me I have a slight amount of protein in my urine."
   4. "I leak urine all the time."
2. A patient has been vomiting for 4 hours. What hormone is increased as a result?
   1. thyroxine
   2. renin
   3. aldosterone
   4. ADH
3. What diagnostic test can be used to determine GFR as well as glomerular damage?
   1. routine urinalysis
   2. renal scan
   3. creatinine clearance
   4. renal biopsy
4. What gland encircles the male urethra at the base of the bladder?
   1. spleen
   2. pancreas
   3. prostate
   4. adrenal
5. During a health history interview, a patient tells the nurse that she has to get up to void several times a night. This finding is documented as which of the following?
   1. polyuria
   2. nocturia
   3. dysuria
   4. hematuria
6. What question would the nurse ask a patient prior to an IVP?
   1. "Are you allergic to shellfish?"
   2. "Do you have burning on urination?"
   3. "Have you ever had kidney stones?"
   4. "Why are you having this test?"
7. Before beginning the physical assessment of the renal system, the nurse should ask the patient to do which of the following?
   1. empty the bladder
   2. take several deep breaths
   3. provide a urine specimen
   4. drink several glasses of water
8. Following surgery, a patient has not voided for 12 hours. What assessment should the nurse make?
   1. Palpate for bladder distention.
   2. Auscultate for bowel sounds.
   3. Inspect for edema of the urethra.
   4. Percuss for gastric tympany.

9. Which renal system disorder is believed to be the result of genetic and environmental factors?
1. hematuria
2. incontinence
3. kidney infection
4. bladder cancer

10. What assessment would the nurse use to assess hydration status of a patient?
1. auscultation of renal arteries
2. palpation for skin turgor
3. percussion for dullness over bladder
4. palpation of both kidneys

See Test Yourself answers in Appendix C.

Pearson Nursing Student Resources

Find additional review materials at
nursing.pearsonhighered.com

Prepare for success with additional NCLEX®-style practice questions, interactive assignments and activities, Web links, animations and videos, and more!

BIBLIOGRAPHY

Armstrong, J., & Mitchell, E. (2008). Comprehensive nursing assessment in the care of older people. *Nursing Older People, (20)*1, 36–40.

Bently, J. (2007). History taking in the Australian outback: Haematuria. *British Journal of Nursing, 16*(4), 231.

Bickley, L., & Szilagyi, P. (2005). *Bates' guide to physical examination and history taking* (9th ed.). Philadelphia: Lippincott.

Dowling-Castronovo, A. (2004). Try this: Best practices in nursing care to older adults from the Hartford Institute for Geriatric Nursing. Urinary incontinence assessment. *Dermatology Nursing, 16*(1), 97–98.

Eliopoulos, C. (2006). *Gerontological nursing* (6th ed.). Philadelphia: Lippincott Williams & Wilkins.

Flasar, C. (2008). What is urine specific gravity? *Nursing, 38*(7), 14.

Holcomb, S. S. (2008a). Acute abdomen: What a pain! *Nursing, 38*(9), 34–40.

Holcomb, S. S. (2008b). Third spacing: When body fluid shifts. *Nursing, 37*(8), 50–53.

Ind, D. (2006). Fluid assessment. *Renal Society of Australian Journal, 2*(3), 51–52.

Johnson, V. (2007). Voiding dysfunction. *Urologic Nursing, 27*(1), 84.

Kee, J. (2009). *Prentice Hall handbook of laboratory & diagnostic tests with nursing implications.* (6th ed.). Upper Saddle River, NJ: Pearson Prentice Hall.

Naish, W., & Haliam, M. (2007). Urinary tract infection: Diagnosis and management. *Nursing Standard, 21*(23), 50–59, 60.

National Institute of Health. (2008). *Genes and Disease: Glands and Hormones.* Available http://www.ncbi.nlm.nih.gov/books/bookres.fegi/gnd/pdf.html

Nursing guidelines for assessment and management of urinary retention in hospitalized older adults. (2007). *Australian Nursing Journal, 15*(2), 22–23.

Palmer, M. (2004). Physiologic and psychologic age-related changes that affect urologic patients. *Urologic Nursing, 24*(4), 247–252, 257.

Perform abdominal assessment, or risk missing life-threatening trauma injury: Don't allow "invisible" injuries to escape detection in your ED. (2004). *ED Nursing, 7*(7), 73–75.

Porth, C. (2007). Essentials of *pathophysiology: Concepts of altered health states* (2nd ed.). Philadelphia: Lippincott. Williams & Wilkins.

Weber, J., & Kelley, J. (2009). *Health assessment in nursing* (4th ed.). Philadelphia: Lippincott Williams & Wilkins.

Wilson, L. A. (2005). Urinalysis. *Nursing Standard, 19*(35), 51–54.

LEARNING OUTCOMES

1. Identify populations at risk for common urinary tract disorders and behaviors that increase the risk.
2. Explain the pathophysiology of common urinary tract disorders.
3. Describe the manifestations of urinary tract disorders, relating manifestations to the pathophysiology of the disorder.
4. Discuss the nursing implications of medications and treatments prescribed for patients with urinary tract disorders.
5. Describe invasive and surgical procedures used in treating urinary tract disorders.

CLINICAL COMPETENCIES

1. Assess the functional health status of patients with urinary tract disorders, using data to determine priority nursing diagnoses and select individualized nursing interventions.
2. Identify, report, and document abnormal or unexpected assessments, monitoring patient status.
3. Use evidence-based research to plan and implement nursing care for patients with urinary tract disorders.
4. Integrate the interdisciplinary plan of care into care for patients with urinary tract disorders.
5. Knowledgeably and safely administer prescribed medications and treatments for patients with urinary tract disorders.
6. Provide effective nursing care for patients undergoing invasive procedures or surgery of the urinary tract.
7. Plan and provide appropriate teaching for prevention of and self-care of urinary tract disorders.
8. Evaluate patient responses, revising plan of care as needed to promote, maintain, or restore functional health of patients with urinary tract disorders.

KEY TERMS

cystectomy, 802
cystitis, 785
dysuria, 785
hematuria, 785
hydronephrosis, 794
lithiasis, 792

lithotripsy, 795
neurogenic bladder, 807
nocturia, 785
pyelonephritis, 785
renal colic, 794
ureteral stent, 787

ureteroplasty, 787
urgency, 785
urinary calculi, 792
urinary diversion, 802
urinary incontinence (UI), 809

The urinary system includes the kidneys, ureters, urinary bladder, and urethra. This organ system can be affected by a variety of disorders, including congenital malformations, infections, obstructions, trauma, tumors, and neurologic conditions. Any portion of the system—from the kidney through the urethra—can be affected with serious or even life-threatening consequences unless the problem is appropriately diagnosed and treated. Kidney disorders can affect urine production and waste elimination directly, and are discussed in the next chapter. Disorders of the urinary drainage system (the kidney pelvis, ureters, bladder, and urethra) may obstruct urine flow or spread to the kidneys, affecting urine production and elimination. The anatomy and physiology and nursing assessment related to the urinary tract is presented in ∞ Chapter 26.

When caring for patients with urinary tract disorders, it is important to consider the patient's modesty in voiding, possible difficulty in discussing the genitals, embarrassment about being exposed for examination and testing, and fear of changes in body image or function. These psychosocial issues may interfere with the patient's willingness to seek help, discuss treatment, and learn about preventive measures.

Nursing interventions for patients with urinary tract disorders are directed toward primary prevention, early detection, and management of the disorder through health teaching and nursing care.

The Patient with a Urinary Tract Infection

Bacterial infections of the urinary tract are a common reason for seeking health services, second only to upper respiratory infections. Community acquired urinary tract infections (UTIs) are common in young women, and unusual in men under the age of 50.

Risk Factors for UTI

Patients can be predisposed to UTI by a variety of factors (Box 27–1). Some risk factors cannot be changed (e.g., aging and the short urethra of the female). In women, sexual activity increases the risk for UTI, thought to result from bacteria introduced into the bladder via the urethra during sexual intercourse. Use of spermicidal compounds with a diaphragm, cervical cap, or condom alters the normal bacterial flora of the vagina and perineal tissues and further increases the risk for UTI. Some females lack a normally protective mucosal enzyme and have decreased levels of cervicovaginal antibodies to enterobacteria, further increasing their risk. Prostatic hypertrophy and bacterial prostatitis are risk factors among males. Circumcision appears to have a protective effect. Unprotected anal intercourse also is a risk factor. Congenital or acquired factors contributing to the risk of infection include urinary tract obstruction by tumors or calculi, structural abnormalities such as strictures, impaired bladder innervation, bowel incontinence, and chronic diseases such as diabetes mellitus. Pregnancy increases the risk of UTI and asymptomatic bacteriuria due to hormonal effects, physical compression by the expanding uterus, and pregnancy-related changes in the bladder mucosa (Rahn, 2008).

Instrumentation of the urinary tract (e.g., catheterization or cystoscopy) is a major risk factor for UTI. Even when performed under strict aseptic conditions, catheterization can result in bladder infection. The placement of the catheter prevents the flushing action of voiding, and bacteria may ascend to the bladder either through the catheter lumen or via exudate between the urethral mucosa and the catheter.

Older patients have an increased incidence of UTI. The greatest degree of increase is seen in men, as the ratio of female-to-male UTI in older adults changes from 50:1 to less than 5:1. An increased risk of urinary stasis, chronic disease states (such as diabetes mellitus), and an impaired immune response contribute to the higher incidence of UTI in the older adult. In men, the prostate typically enlarges with aging, potentially resulting in urinary retention as the urethra narrows. Prostatic secretions are lessened, diminishing their protective, antibacterial effect. In older women, loss of tissue elasticity and weakening of perineal muscles often contribute to the development of a cystocele or rectocele. Resulting changes in bladder and urethral position increase the risk of incomplete bladder emptying.

Physiology Review

The urinary tract is normally sterile above the urethra. Adequate urine volume, a free flow from the kidneys through the urinary meatus, and complete bladder emptying are the most important mechanisms maintaining sterility. Pathogens that enter and contaminate the distal urethra are washed out during voiding. Other defenses for maintaining sterile urine include its normal acidity and bacteriostatic properties of the bladder and urethral cells. The peristaltic activity of the ureters and a competent vesicoureteral junction help maintain sterility of the upper urinary tract. As the ureter enters the bladder, its distal portion tunnels between the mucosa and muscle layers of the bladder wall (Figure 27–1 ■). During voiding, increased *intravesicular* (within the bladder) pressure compresses the ureter, preventing *reflux*, or backflow of urine toward the kidneys. In males, a long urethra and the antibacterial effect of zinc in prostatic fluid also help prevent contamination of this normally sterile environment.

BOX 27–1 **Risk Factors for UTI**

Female
- Short, straight urethra
- Proximity of urinary meatus to vagina and anus
- Sexual intercourse
- Use of diaphragm and spermicidal compounds for birth control
- Pregnancy

Male
- Being uncircumcised
- Prostatic hypertrophy

Both
- Aging
- Urinary tract obstruction
- Neurogenic bladder dysfunction
- Vesicoureteral reflux
- Genetic factors
- Catheterization
- Anal intercourse

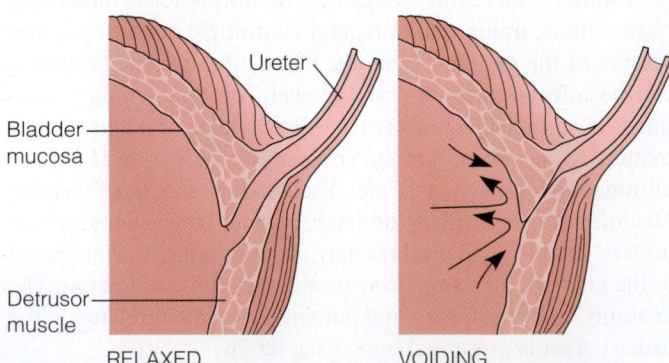

Figure 27–1 ■ A competent vesicoureteral junction. Note how increased intravesicular pressure during voiding occludes the distal portion of the ureter, preventing reflux.

Pathophysiology and Manifestations

Pathogens usually enter the urinary tract by ascending from the mucous membranes of the perineal area into the lower urinary tract. Bacteria that have colonized the urethra, vagina, or perineal tissues are the usual source of infection (Porth & Matfin, 2009). From the bladder, bacteria may continue to ascend the urinary tract, eventually infecting the *parenchyma* (functional tissue) of the kidneys. Hematogenous spread of infection to the urinary tract is rare. Infections introduced in this manner are usually associated with previous damage or scarring of the urinary tract. Bacteria introduced into the urinary tract may cause asymptomatic bacteriuria or an inflammatory response with manifestations of UTI. Asymptomatic bacteriuria is commonly found in pregnant women, the elderly, and patients with diabetes mellitus or who have an indwelling urinary catheter (Lin & Fajardo, 2008).

UTIs can be categorized in several ways. Anatomically, they may affect the lower or the upper urinary tract. Lower urinary tract infections include *urethritis*, inflammation of the urethra; *prostatitis*, inflammation of the prostate gland (discussed in ∞ Chapter 48); and **cystitis**, inflammation of the urinary bladder. The most common upper urinary tract infection is **pyelonephritis**, inflammation of the kidney and renal pelvis. The infection may involve superficial tissues such as the bladder mucosa, or may invade other tissues such as prostate or renal tissues. Epidemiologically, UTIs are identified as community acquired or catheter associated.

Cystitis

Cystitis, inflammation of the urinary bladder, is the most common UTI. The infection tends to remain superficial, involving the bladder mucosa. The mucosa becomes hyperemic (red) and may hemorrhage (Figure 27–2 ■), and the inflammatory response causes pus to form. This process causes the classic manifestations associated with cystitis. Typical presenting symptoms of cystitis include **dysuria** (painful or difficult urination), urinary frequency and **urgency** (a sudden, compelling need to urinate), and **nocturia** (voiding two or more times at night). In addition, the urine may have a foul odor and appear cloudy (*pyuria*) or bloody (**hematuria**) because of mucus, excess white cells in the urine, and bleeding of the inflamed bladder wall. Suprapubic pain and tenderness also may be present. See the following box for manifestations of cystitis.

Cystitis in adult females usually results from colonization of the bladder by bacteria normally found in the lower gastrointestinal tract. These bacteria gain entry by ascending the short, straight female urethra. In addition to the risk factors listed on page 784, personal hygiene practices and voluntary urinary retention can contribute to the risk for UTI in women.

Older patients may not experience the classic symptoms of cystitis. Instead, they often present with nonspecific manifestations such as nocturia, incontinence, confusion, behavior change, lethargy, anorexia, or "just not feeling right." Fever may be present; however, hypothermia also may develop in an older adult.

Although the bacteriostatic effect of prostatic fluid and a longer urethra provide an effective barrier to bladder infection for adult males, in elderly men an enlarged prostate can impede urine flow, leading to incomplete bladder emptying and urinary stasis. Bacteria are not completely flushed with voiding, allowing colonization of the bladder.

Cystitis is usually uncomplicated and readily responds to treatment. When left untreated, the infection can ascend to involve the kidneys. Severe or prolonged infection may lead to sloughing of bladder mucosa and ulcer formation. Chronic cystitis can lead to bladder stones (discussed later in this chapter).

Catheter-Associated UTI

At least 10% to 15% of hospitalized patients with indwelling urinary catheters develop bacteriuria. The longer the catheter remains in place, the greater the risk for infection. Bacteria, including *E. coli*, *Proteus*, *Pseudomonas*, and *Klebsiella*, reach the bladder by either migrating through the column of urine within the catheter or by moving up the mucous sheath of the urethra outside the catheter. Bacteria enter the catheter system at the connection between the catheter and drainage system or through the emptying tube of the drainage bag. Colonization of perineal skin by bowel flora is a common source of infection in catheterized women. Causative organisms associated with catheter-associated UTI are more likely to demonstrate antibiotic resistance than those found in community-acquired UTI (Fauci et al., 2008).

Catheter-associated UTIs often are asymptomatic. Gram-negative bacteremia is the most significant complication associated with these UTIs. Most catheter-associated UTIs resolve quickly when the catheter is removed and a short course of antibiotic is administered. Intermittent catheterization carries a lower risk of infection than does an indwelling catheter, and is preferred for patients who are unable to empty their bladder by voiding.

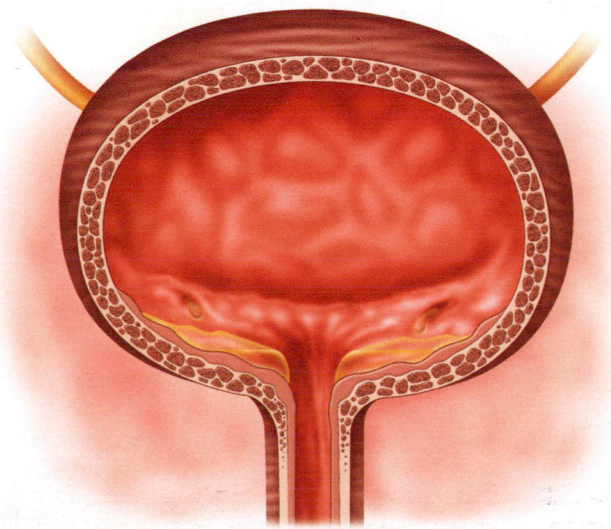

Figure 27–2 ■ Appearance of the bladder wall affected by cystitis.

MANIFESTATIONS of Cystitis

- Dysuria
- Pyuria
- Frequency
- Hematuria
- Urgency
- Suprapubic discomfort
- Nocturia

Pyelonephritis

Pyelonephritis is inflammation of the renal pelvis and parenchyma, the functional kidney tissue. *Acute pyelonephritis* is a bacterial infection of the kidney; *chronic pyelonephritis* is associated with nonbacterial infections and inflammatory processes that may be metabolic, chemical, or immunologic in origin.

ACUTE PYELONEPHRITIS Acute pyelonephritis usually results from an infection that ascends to the kidney from the lower urinary tract. Asymptomatic bacteriuria or cystitis can lead to acute pyelonephritis. Risk factors include pregnancy (because of slowed ureteral peristalsis), urinary tract obstruction, and congenital malformation. Urinary tract trauma, scarring, calculi (stones), kidney disorders such as polycystic or hypertensive kidney disease, and chronic diseases such as diabetes may also contribute to pyelonephritis. *Vesicoureteral reflux*, a condition in which urine moves from the bladder back toward the kidney, is a common risk factor in children who develop pyelonephritis and is also seen in adults when bladder outflow is obstructed.

The infection spreads from the renal pelvis to the renal cortex. The pelvis, calyces, and medulla of the kidney are primarily affected, with white blood cell (WBC) infiltration and inflammation. The kidney becomes grossly edematous. Localized abscesses may develop on the cortical surface of the kidney. As with cystitis, *E. coli* is the organism responsible for 85% of the cases of acute pyelonephritis. Other organisms commonly found include *Proteus* and *Klebsiella*, bacteria that normally inhabit the intestinal tract.

The onset of acute pyelonephritis is typically rapid, with chills and fever, malaise, vomiting, flank pain, costovertebral tenderness, urinary frequency, and dysuria (see the following Manifestations box). Symptoms of cystitis also may be present. The older adult may present with a change in behavior, acute confusion, incontinence, or a general deterioration in condition.

CHRONIC PYELONEPHRITIS Chronic pyelonephritis involves chronic inflammation and scarring of the tubules and interstitial tissues of the kidney. It is a common cause of chronic kidney disease. It may develop as a result of UTIs or other conditions that damage the kidneys, such as hypertension or vascular conditions, severe vesicoureteral reflux, or obstruction of the urinary tract.

The patient with chronic pyelonephritis may be asymptomatic or have mild manifestations such as urinary frequency, dysuria, and flank pain. Hypertension can develop as kidney tissue is destroyed.

MANIFESTATIONS of Acute Pyelonephritis

URINARY	SYSTEMIC
▪ Urinary frequency	▪ Vomiting
▪ Dysuria	▪ Diarrhea
▪ Pyuria	▪ Acute fever
▪ Hematuria	▪ Shaking chills
▪ Flank pain	▪ Malaise
▪ Costovertebral tenderness	

Interdisciplinary Care

Treatment of UTI focuses on eliminating the causative organism, preventing relapse or reinfection, and identifying and correcting any contributing factors. Drug treatment with antibiotics and urinary anti-infectives is commonly used. In some cases, surgery may be indicated to correct contributing factors.

Diagnosis

Laboratory testing for UTI includes the following:

- *Urinalysis* to assess for pyuria, bacteria, and blood cells in the urine. A bacteria count greater than 100,000 (10^5) per milliliter is indicative of infection. Rapid tests for bacteria in the urine include using a *nitrite dipstick* (which turns pink in the presence of bacteria) and the *leukocyte esterase test*, an indirect method of detecting bacteria by identifying lysed or intact WBCs in the urine.

  Urine should be collected via suprapubic aspiration or by midstream clean-catch specimen; if necessary, straight catheterization or "mini-cath," with strict aseptic technique, may be used. Catheterization is avoided if possible to reduce the risk of further infection. ∞ See Chapter 26 for nursing care related to collecting a urinalysis specimen.

- *Gram stain of the urine* may be done to identify the infecting organism by shape and characteristic (gram-positive or gram-negative).

- *Urine culture and sensitivity* tests may be ordered to identify the infecting organism and the most effective antibiotic. Culture requires 24 to 72 hours, so treatment to eliminate the most common organisms often is initiated without culture.

SAFETY ALERT

Obtain urine specimens from a patient with an indwelling urinary catheter by briefly (15 minutes or less) clamping the proximal drainage tubing, then withdrawing urine directly from the port using sterile technique. Sterile technique is necessary to reduce the risk of catheter-associated UTI.

- *WBC with differential* may be done to detect typical changes associated with infection, such as *leukocytosis* (elevated WBC) and increased numbers of neutrophils.

In men and in adult women with recurrent infections or persistent bacteriuria, additional diagnostic testing may be ordered to evaluate for structural abnormalities and other contributing factors:

- *Intravenous pyelography (IVP)* is used to evaluate for structural or functional abnormalities, such as vesicoureteral reflux, of the kidneys, ureters, and bladder.

- *Voiding cystourethrography* may be ordered to detect structural or functional abnormalities of the bladder and urethral strictures. This test has a lower risk of allergic response to the contrast dye than IVP.

- *Cystoscopy* may be used to diagnose conditions such as prostatic hypertrophy, urethral strictures, bladder calculi, tumors, polyps or diverticula, and congenital abnormalities. A tissue biopsy may be obtained during the procedure, and other interventions performed (e.g., stone removal or stricture dilation).

■ *Manual pelvic* or *prostate examinations* are done to assess for structural changes of the genitourinary tract, such as prostatic enlargement, cystocele, or rectocele.

Nursing implications for these diagnostic procedures are presented in ∞ Chapter 26.

Medications

Most acute uncomplicated infections of the lower urinary tract can be treated with a short course of antibiotic therapy. Upper urinary tract infections, in contrast, usually require longer treatment to eradicate the infecting organism and prevent recurrence.

Short-course therapy (a 3-day course of treatment) reduces treatment cost, increases compliance, and has a lower rate of side effects. Oral trimethoprim-sulfamethoxazole (TMP-SMX), SMX, TMP, or a quinolone antibiotic such as ciprofloxacin (Cipro), norfloxacin (Noroxin), or levofloxacin (Levaquin, Quixin) may be ordered.

Men and women with pyelonephritis, urinary tract abnormalities or stones, or a history of previous infections with antibiotic-resistant infections require a 7- to 10-day course of a fluoroquinolone antibiotic such as ciprofloxacin, levofloxacin, or an alternate antibiotic. The patient with severe illness may need hospitalization and intravenous antibiotic therapy. Imipenem-cilastatin (Primaxin), or an antibiotic combination such as IV ampicillin and gentamicin or ceftriaxone (Rocephin) may be prescribed for severe illness or sepsis associated with UTI. ∞ See Chapter 12 for the nursing implications for antibiotic therapy.

The outcome of treatment for UTI is determined by follow-up urinalysis and culture. *Cure*, as evidenced by no pathogens present in the urine, is the desired outcome. Treatment *failure* occurs when therapy fails to eradicate bacteria in the urine. *Recurrent infection* occurs when a persistent source of infection causes repeated infection after initial cure. *Reinfection* is the development of a new infection with a different pathogen following successful UTI treatment.

> **PRACTICE ALERT**
> Follow-up urine culture is scheduled 10 days to 2 weeks following completion of antibiotic therapy for UTI to ensure that bacteria have been eradicated from the urinary tract.

Patients who experience frequent symptomatic UTIs may be treated with prophylactic antibiotic therapy with a drug such as TMP-SMZ, TMP, or nitrofurantoin (Furadantin, Macrodantin, Macrobid). TMP and nitrofurantoin do not achieve effective plasma concentrations at recommended doses, but do reach effective concentrations in the urine. Nitrofurantoin also may be used to treat UTI in pregnant women. Nursing implications for these urinary anti-infectives and for phenazopyridine (Pyridium), a urinary analgesic, are outlined in the following Medication Administration box.

Antibiotics and urinary anti-infectives are not generally recommended to treat asymptomatic bacteriuria except in pregnant women. The preferred treatment for catheter-associated UTI is removal of the indwelling catheter followed by a 10- to 14-day course of antibiotic therapy to eliminate the infection.

Surgery

Surgery may be indicated for recurrent UTI if diagnostic testing indicates calculi, structural anomalies, or strictures that contribute to the risk of infection. Table 27–1 lists major causes of urinary tract obstruction that may contribute to UTI.

Stones, or *calculi*, in the renal pelvis or in the bladder are an irritant and provide a matrix for bacterial colonization. Treatment may include surgical removal of a large calculus from the renal pelvis or cystoscopic removal of bladder calculi. *Percutaneous ultrasonic pyelolithotomy* or *extracorporeal shock wave lithotripsy* (described in the next section of this chapter) may be used instead of surgery to crush and remove stones. (See the Diagnostic Tests box on pages 774–777 for nursing care related to cystoscopy.)

Ureteroplasty, surgical repair of a ureter, may be indicated for structural abnormality or stricture of a ureter. This may be combined with a ureteral reimplantation if vesicoureteral reflux is present. The patient returns from these surgeries with an indwelling urinary catheter (Foley or suprapubic) and a **ureteral stent** (a thin catheter inserted into the ureter to provide for urine flow and ureteral support), which remains in place for 3 to 5 days. Care of the patient with a ureteral stent is outlined in the box on page 789.

COMPLEMENTARY THERAPIES Complementary therapies such as aromatherapy or herbal preparations may be used in conjunction with antibiotics to treat UTI. Research supports the use of cranberry products to prevent UTI in women with recurrent symptomatic infections. Blueberry juice also is commonly used to prevent and treat UTI. Adding bergamot, sandalwood, lavender, or juniper oil to bath water helps relieve the discomfort of UTI. Herbal supplements such as saw palmetto have a urinary antiseptic effect, and may be beneficial in treating or preventing UTI. Consult a qualified herbologist for recommended doses and appropriate use.

TABLE 27–1 Major Causes of Urinary Tract Obstruction by Location

LOCATION	OBSTRUCTIVE PROCESS
Kidney pelvis	Calculi (stones)
	Polycystic kidney disease
	Infection and scarring
Ureters	Calculi
	Scarring and stricture
	Congenital defects or strictures
	External processes such as pregnancy, tumors, lymph node enlargement
Bladder	Neurogenic bladder
	Tumors
	Calculi and other foreign bodies
Urethra	Benign prostatic hypertrophy
	Tumors
	Scarring and stricture
	Trauma

MEDICATION ADMINISTRATION   Urinary Anti-Infectives and Analgesics

URINARY ANTI-INFECTIVES

Nitrofurantoin (Furadantin, Macrodantin, Macrobid)

Trimethoprim (Proloprim, Trimpex)

Urinary anti-infectives are usually used prophylactically to prevent recurrence of UTI in patients with frequent symptomatic infections. Nitrofurantoin also may be used to treat UTI in pregnant women.

Nursing Responsibilities

- Ensure adequate fluid intake (1500 to 2000 mL/day) to maintain a urine output of at least 1500 mL of urine per 24 hours. Do not overhydrate.
- Administer with meals to minimize GI side effects, such as nausea, gastric upset, and abdominal cramping.
- Trimethoprim is contraindicated for use in patients with renal or hepatic impairment; nitrofurantoin is contraindicated for patients with impaired renal function. Report abnormal laboratory values such as elevated creatinine or BUN, bilirubin, alanine aminotransferase (ALT), aspartate aminotransferase (AST), and lactic dehydrogenase (LDH).
- Use with caution in older or chronically ill patients. Monitor closely for adverse effects.
- Do not administer trimethoprim to pregnant women because of possible adverse effects on the fetus.
- Monitor the patient taking nitrofurantoin for an acute or chronic pulmonary reaction with manifestations of dyspnea, cough, chills, fever, and chest pain. Discontinue the drug and notify the physician.
- Nitrofurantoin may cause peripheral neuropathy, especially in older patients and adult diabetics. Notify the physician if symptoms develop.
- Nitrofurantoin oral suspension may stain the teeth; have the patient rinse the mouth thoroughly after administering.
- Monitor for signs of phenytoin toxicity (sedation, ataxia, and increased blood levels) if trimethoprim is given concurrently. Phenytoin doses may need to be reduced.

Health Education for the Patient and Family

- These drugs are used along with hygiene practices to prevent recurrent UTI. Take as directed, even when no symptoms are present.
- Drink six to eight glasses of water or fluid per day while taking these drugs.
- Take the drug with meals or food to reduce gastric effects; however, avoid milk products because they may interfere with absorption.

- Trimethoprim should not be taken during pregnancy. Contact your physician before attempting to become pregnant.
- Contact your doctor if you develop any of the following: chest pain, difficulty breathing, cough, chills, and fever; numbness and tingling or weakness of the extremities; rash or pruritus (itching).
- If you are taking an oral suspension of nitrofurantoin, rinse your mouth thoroughly after each dose to avoid staining the teeth.
- Nitrofurantoin turns the urine brown. This is not harmful and subsides when the drug is discontinued.
- If you are taking trimethoprim along with phenytoin (Dilantin) or a related anticonvulsant, contact your doctor if you become sedated or begin to stagger.

URINARY ANALGESIC

Phenazopyridine (Pyridium)

Phenazopyridine is a urinary tract analgesic that may be used for symptomatic relief of the pain, burning, frequency, and urgency associated with UTI during the first 24 to 48 hours of therapy. Its use is somewhat controversial because it does not treat the infection and may delay effective treatment in the patient with recurrent UTI who saves a dose or two "for the next time."

Nursing Responsibilities

- Monitor renal function (urine output, weight, serum creatinine, and BUN) during treatment; report changes.
- Stop the drug and contact the physician if sclera or skin become yellow tinged. This may indicate reduced excretion and toxicity.

Health Education for the Patient and Family

- Take with meals to minimize gastric upset.
- Consume 2 to 3 quarts of fluid daily while taking this drug.
- If you are a diabetic, check your blood sugars regularly while taking this drug.
- This drug turns urine orange or red. Protect your clothing from staining.
- Contact lenses may become stained if worn while taking this drug.
- Promptly contact your doctor if symptoms of UTI recur; do not take phenazopyridine before you seek medical treatment.
- If you develop itching or notice a yellow tinge to your skin or eyes, stop taking the drug and notify the physician.

∂ Nursing Care

Health Promotion

Teach measures to prevent UTI to all patients, particularly to young, sexually active women. Encourage patients to maintain a generous fluid intake of 2.0 to 2.5 quarts per day, increasing intake during hot weather or strenuous activity. Discuss the need to avoid voluntary urinary retention, emptying the bladder every 3 to 4 hours. Instruct women to cleanse the perineal area from front to back after voiding and defecating. Teach to void before and after sexual intercourse to flush out bacteria introduced into the urethra and bladder. Teach measures to maintain the integrity of perineal tissues: Avoid bubble baths, feminine hygiene sprays, and vaginal douches; wear cotton briefs, avoid synthetic materials; if postmenopausal, use hormone replacement therapy or estrogen cream. Unless contraindicated, suggest measures to

maintain acid urine: Drink two glasses of low-sugar cranberry juice daily; take ascorbic acid (vitamin C), and avoid excess intake of milk and milk products, other fruit juices, and sodium bicarbonate (baking soda).

Assessment

Focused assessment data for the patient with a UTI includes the following:

- *Health history:* Current symptoms, including frequency, urgency, burning on urination, voidings per night; color, clarity, and odor of urine; other manifestations such as lower abdominal, back, or flank pain; nausea or vomiting; fever; duration of symptoms and any treatment attempted; history of previous UTIs and their frequency; possibility of pregnancy and type of birth control used; chronic diseases such as diabetes; current medications and any known allergies.

NURSING CARE OF THE PATIENT with a Ureteral Stent

Ureteral stents are used to maintain patency and promote healing of the ureters (see the following figure). A stent may be temporary, used during and after a surgical procedure, or it may be used for longer periods in patients with ureteral obstruction due to tumors, strictures, or other causes.

Stents may be positioned during surgery or cystoscopy. They are made of a nontoxic material such as silicone or polyurethane, with side drainage holes placed along the length of the stent. Stents are radiopaque for easy radiographic identification. One or both ends of the stent may be pigtail or J shaped to prevent migration.

- Label all drainage tubes including stents for easy identification. Attach each catheter and stent to a separate closed drainage system. *Careful labeling allows close monitoring of output from all sources and reservoirs. Separate drainage systems minimize the risk of infection.*
- If the stent has been brought to the surface, secure it and maintain its position. *The stent is usually placed in the renal pelvis. It is important to secure it well to prevent trauma to the kidney, inadvertent removal of the stent, and ureter obstruction.*
- Monitor urine output, including color, consistency, and odor. Monitor for signs of infection or bleeding: fever, tachycardia, pain, hematuria, and cloudy or malodorous urine. *The stent facilitates urine flow but may become obstructed because of bleeding, calculi, or sediment. Obstruction may result in hydronephrosis and kidney damage. The stent itself is a foreign body in the urinary tract and can increase the risk of UTI.*
- Maintain fluid intake, encouraging fluids that acidify urine, such as low-sugar apple, cranberry, and blueberry juice.

The stent can precipitate calculus formation as well as UTI. Increasing fluid intake and acidifying the urine help prevent these complications.

- For an indwelling stent, stress the need for regular follow-up to monitor for and prevent complications such as UTI and calculi. *The patient with an indwelling stent may tend to forget that the stent is in place and become lax in compliance with follow-up and preventive measures.*

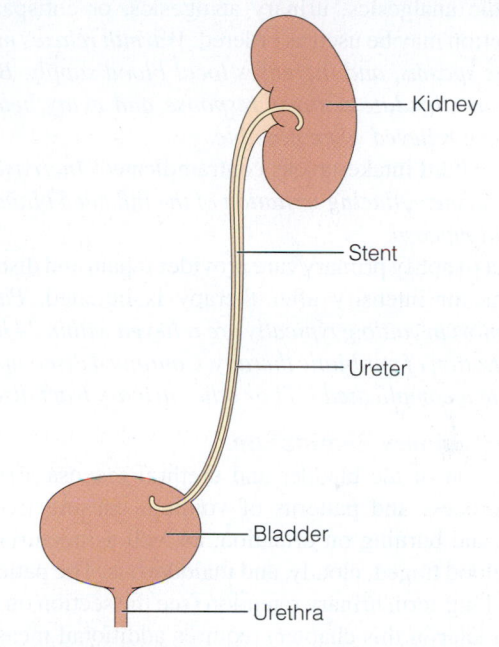

- Kidney
- Stent
- Ureter
- Bladder
- Urethra

- *Physical examination:* General health; vital signs including temperature; abdominal shape, contour, tenderness to palpation (especially suprapubic); percuss for costovertebral tenderness (see Box 26–1).

∞ See Chapter 26 for complete nursing assessment of the urinary system.

Nursing Diagnoses and Interventions

The patient's general health, abilities for self-care, and risk factors that may contribute to UTI are considered when planning and implementing nursing care for the patient with a UTI. Priority nursing diagnoses focus on comfort, urinary elimination, and teaching/learning needs. A Case Study & Nursing Care Plan for the patient with cystitis can be found on page 792.

Acute Pain

Pain is a common manifestation of both lower and upper UTI. Urinary tract pain is caused primarily by distention and increased pressure within the tract. The severity of the pain is related to the rate at which inflammation and distention develop, not their degree.

In cystitis, inflammation causes a sensation of fullness; dull, constant suprapubic pain; and possibly low back pain. The inflamed bladder wall and urethra cause dysuria, pain, and burning on urination. Bladder spasms may develop, causing periodic severe, stabbing discomfort. Pain associated with pyelonephritis is often steady and dull, localized to the outer abdomen or flank region. Urologic disorders rarely cause central abdominal pain.

- Assess pain: timing, quality, intensity, location, duration, and aggravating and alleviating factors. *A change in the nature, location, or intensity of the pain could indicate an extension of the infection or a related but separate problem.*

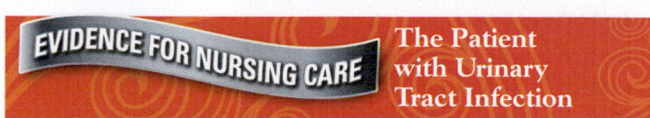

EVIDENCE FOR NURSING CARE — The Patient with Urinary Tract Infection

Selected resources that nurses may find helpful when planning evidence-based nursing care follow.

- American College of Obstetricians and Gynecologists (ACOG). (2008 March). *Treatment of urinary tract infections in nonpregnant women.* Washington, DC: Author.
- Gotelli, J., Merryman, P., Carr, C., McElveen, L., Epperson, C., & Bynum, D. (2008 December). A quality improvement project to reduce the complications associated with indwelling urinary catheters. *Urologic Nursing, 28*(6), 465–467, 473.
- Lin, K., & Fajardo, K. (2008 July 1). Clinical guidelines. Screening for asymptomatic bacteriuria in adults: Evidence for the U. S. Preventive Services Task Force reaffirmation recommendation statement. *Annals of Internal Medicine, 149*(1), W-20–W-24.
- Robinson, S., Allen, L., Barnes, M., Berry, T., Foster, T., Friedrich, L., et al. (2007 June). Development of an evidence-based protocol for reduction of indwelling urinary catheter usage. *MEDSURG Nursing, 16*(3), 157–161.

- Teach or provide comfort measures such as warm sitz baths, warm packs or heating pads, and balanced rest and activity. Systemic analgesics, urinary analgesics, or antispasmodic medication may be used as ordered. *Warmth relaxes muscles, relieves spasms, and increases local blood supply. Because pain can stimulate a stress response and delay healing, it should be relieved when possible.*
- Increase fluid intake unless contraindicated. *Increased fluid dilutes urine, reducing irritation of the inflamed bladder and urethral mucosa.*
- Instruct to notify primary care provider if pain and discomfort continue or intensify after therapy is initiated. *Pain and discomfort in voiding typically are relieved within 24 hours of the initiation of antibiotic therapy. Continued discomfort may indicate a complicated UTI or other urinary tract disorder.*

Impaired Urinary Elimination
Inflammation of the bladder and urethral mucosa affects the normal process and patterns of voiding, causing frequency, urgency, and burning on urination, as well as nocturia. Urine may be blood tinged, cloudy, and malodorous. The patient with short- or long-term urinary retention (see the section on urinary retention later in this chapter) requires additional measures to assess for and prevent UTI.

- Monitor (or instruct the patient to monitor) color, clarity, and odor of urine. *Urine should return to clear yellow within 48 hours, unless drug therapy causes a change in the color of urine. If clarity does not return, further investigation may be necessary.*

- Instruct to avoid caffeinated drinks, including coffee, tea, and cola; citrus juices; drinks containing artificial sweeteners; and alcoholic beverages. *Caffeine, citrus juices, and artificial sweeteners irritate bladder mucosa and the detrusor muscle, and can increase urgency and bladder spasms.*
- Use strict aseptic technique and a closed urinary drainage system when inserting a straight or indwelling urinary catheter. Insert indwelling catheters to the full recommended length (4 or more inches in women and to the bifurcation in men) before inflating the balloon. *Bacteria colonizing the perineal tissues or on the nurse's hands can be introduced into the bladder during catheterization. Aseptic technique reduces this risk. Inflation of the balloon while in the urethra damages urethral tissues and can cause significant discomfort for the patient.*

- When possible, use intermittent straight catheterization to relieve urinary retention. Remove indwelling urinary catheters as soon as possible. *Using intermittent straight catheterization allows the bladder to fill and completely empty in a more normal manner, maintaining physiologic function. The risk of infection associated with an indwelling catheter is about 3% to 5% per day of catheterization (Fauci et al., 2008). See the accompanying box for evidence-based practice for reducing the risk of catheter-associated UTI.*
- Maintain the closed urinary drainage system, and use aseptic technique when emptying the catheter drainage bag. Maintain gravity flow, preventing reflux of urine into the bladder from the drainage system. *Bacteria can enter the drainage system when its integrity is interrupted (e.g., disconnecting the catheter from the drainage system) or during emptying of the drainage bag. These bacteria can ascend the column of urine to the bladder, causing UTI.*
- Provide perineal care on a regular basis and following defecation. Use antiseptic preparations only as ordered. *Regular cleansing of perineal tissues reduces the risk of colonization by bowel or other bacteria. While antiseptic solutions may be ordered for catheter care, they can dry perineal tissues and reduce normal flora, increasing the risk of colonization by pathogens, and should not routinely be used.*

Readiness for Enhanced Self Health Maintenance
The patient with a urinary tract infection is at an increased risk for future UTI and needs to understand the disease process, risk factors, measures to prevent recurrent infection, diagnostic procedures, and home care. In addition, once the manifestations of UTI are relieved, motivation to continue the treatment plan declines. Failure to complete the full course of therapy and recommended follow-up can lead to continued bacteriuria and recurrent infections.

- Teach how to obtain a midstream clean-catch urine specimen. *Cleansing of the urinary meatus and perineal area reduces contamination of the specimen by external cells and bacteria. Ninety percent of urethral bacteria are cleared in the first 10 mL of voided urine; a midstream specimen is representative of urine in the bladder.*
- Assess knowledge about the disease process, risk factors, and preventive measures. *The patient may have little understanding of UTI, its causes, and contributing factors.*
- Discuss the prescribed treatment plan and the importance of taking all prescribed antibiotics.

MOVING EVIDENCE INTO ACTION   **Reducing Catheter-Associated Complications**

Insertion of an indwelling (retention) catheter is a commonly performed procedure in hospitals, with up to 25% of patients having an indwelling catheter at some time during hospitalization. Furthermore, catheters often remain in place when there is no clear indication for their continued use. Indwelling catheters are not only associated with an increased risk for UTI, but also often affect the patient's comfort and mobility as well. Nurses on an older adult acute care unit determined that approximately 24% of the patients were catheterized at any one time (Gotelli et al., 2008). Of these, more than half had no clear indication for catheterization. Using a nurse-driven protocol, the need for catheterization was assessed using specific criteria (e.g., aggressive diuretic or fluid therapy, accurate monitoring of intake and output, management of urinary incontinence with stage 3 pressure ulcers), and the catheter removed when criteria were no longer met. As a result, the prevalence of catheterization dropped from 24% at any given time to just over 16%.

IMPLICATIONS FOR NURSING
Although a physician's order is required for inserting an indwelling catheter, nurses often are in the best position to evaluate the need for continued catheterization as the patient progresses. This study demonstrated the effectiveness of (1) providing

nurses with clear criteria for assessing the need for catheterization, and (2) empowering nurses to remove an indwelling catheter and implement a bladder retraining program when criteria are no longer met. These nursing actions can have a positive impact on patient outcomes, reducing the risk for catheter-associated infection and other complications.

CRITICAL THINKING IN PATIENT CARE
1. This summary notes several of the criteria used to determine the continued need for an indwelling urinary catheter. What other criteria would you consider in determining the appropriateness of continued catheterization? Provide justification for the criteria you identify.
2. An indwelling urinary catheter has been called a "one-point restraint." Identify why this is the case, and discuss potential noninfectious complications of urinary catheterization.
3. Patients who have had a urinary catheter in place for an extended period may require a bladder retraining program. Develop such a program for an older adult in an acute care or post-acute care setting.

Source: Gotelli, J., Merryman, P., Carr, C., McElveen, L., Epperson, C., & Bynum, D. (2008 December). A quality improvement project to reduce the complications associated with indwelling urinary catheters. *Urologic Nursing, 28* (6), 465–467, 473.

- Help the patient develop a plan for taking medications, such as taking them with meals (unless contraindicated) or setting out all doses for the day in the morning. *Missed doses of antibiotic can result in subtherapeutic blood levels and reduced effectiveness. Taking medication in association with a regular daily activity such as meals helps patients remember doses.*
- Instruct to keep appointments for follow-up and urine culture. *Follow-up urine culture, often scheduled 7 to 14 days after completion of antibiotic therapy, is vital to ensure complete eradication of bacteria and prevent relapse or recurrence.*
- Teach measures to prevent future UTI (see the preceding Health Promotion section). *Keeping urine dilute and acidic and voiding regularly flush bacteria out of the bladder and urethra. The proximity of the female urethral meatus to the vagina and anus increases the risk of bacterial contamination, especially during intercourse. Bubble baths, feminine hygiene sprays, synthetic fibers, and douches may dry and irritate perineal tissues, promoting bacterial growth.*

Using NANDA, NIC, and NOC
Linkages between a selected NANDA nursing diagnosis, NIC, and NOC for the patient with a urinary tract infection are shown in the chart that follows.

Community-Based Care
Because both upper and lower urinary tract infections are usually managed in the community, teaching is the most important nursing intervention. Provide instruction on the following topics:
- Risk factors for UTI and how to minimize or eliminate these factors through increased fluid intake, regular elimination, and personal hygiene measures
- Early manifestations of UTI and the importance of seeking medical intervention promptly
- Maintaining optimal immune system function by attending to physical and psychosocial stressors, such as lack

of adequate rest, poor nutrition, and high levels of emotional stress
- The importance of completing the prescribed treatment and keeping follow-up appointments
- Minimizing the risk of UTI when an indwelling urinary catheter is necessary:
  - Use alternatives to an indwelling catheter when possible. For urinary incontinence, try scheduled toileting, incontinence pads or diapers, and external catheters if possible. For urinary retention, teach the patient or a family member to perform straight catheterization every 3 to 4 hours using clean technique.
  - Teach care measures such as perineal care, managing and emptying the collection chamber, maintaining a closed system, and bladder irrigation or flushing if ordered when an indwelling catheter is necessary.

NANDA, NIC, AND NOC LINKAGES
The Patient with Urinary Tract Infection

NANDA	Impaired Urinary Elimination

NIC	Pain Management Teaching: Prescribed Medication Teaching: Individual

NOC	Comfort Status: Physical Infection Severity Knowledge: Treatment Regimen

Data from NANDA International. (2009). *Nursing diagnoses: Definitions and classification 2009–2011*. Oxford, UK: Wiley-Blackwell; Bulechek, G., Butcher, H., & Dochterman, J. (Eds.). (2008). *Nursing interventions classification (NIC)* (5th ed.). St. Louis, MO: Mosby; and Moorhead, S., Johnson, M., Maas, M., & Swanson, E. (Eds.). (2008). *Nursing outcomes classification (NOC)* (4th ed.). St. Louis, MO: Mosby.

Miija Waisanen is a 25-year-old second-year nursing student. She was recently married, and she and her husband live in an apartment near the college she attends. Mrs. Waisanen has never been pregnant, and she is using a diaphragm for birth control. She presents at the local urgent care clinic complaining of low back pain, frequency, urgency, and burning on urination that began the day before.

ASSESSMENT

Patrice Ramiros, RN, admits Mrs. Waisanen to the clinic. Mrs. Waisanen denies having had similar symptoms in the past or ever having been diagnosed with a UTI. She describes her pain as a constant, dull ache that does not change with movement. She feels the need to urinate almost constantly, but experiences difficulty in starting her stream, and burning pain and cramping when voiding. She reports getting up four times the night before to urinate. She denies painful intercourse and states that her last menstrual period began only 2 weeks ago. Physical examination reveals: BP 112/68; P 90 and regular, afebrile. Suprapubic tenderness noted but no flank or costovertebral angle tenderness. Clean-catch urine specimen shows hematuria, multiple WBCs, and a bacteria count greater than 10^5 per milliliter.

The nurse practitioner prescribes trimethoprim-sulfamethoxazole (TMP-SMZ) 160 mg/800 mg PO bid for 3 days, and aspirin or acetaminophen 650 mg PO every 4 hours as needed for pain. Mrs. Waisanen is instructed to return to the clinic in 7 days for a follow-up urine culture, or sooner if her symptoms do not improve.

DIAGNOSES

- *Acute Pain* related to infection and inflammatory process in the urinary tract
- *Impaired Urinary Elimination* related to inflammation as evidenced by frequency, urgency, nocturia, and dysuria
- *Readiness for Enhanced Self Health Management* related to risk factors for and treatment of UTI

EXPECTED OUTCOMES

- Report relief of low back pain and burning on urination.
- Regain a normal voiding pattern without frequency, urgency, nocturia, and abnormal urine characteristics.

- Verbalize understanding of the disease process, related risk factors, follow-up instructions, and symptoms of recurrence indicating the need for medical attention.

PLANNING AND IMPLEMENTATION

- Teach comfort measures: warm sitz baths, a heating pad on low heat applied to her lower back or abdomen, rest, increased fluid intake, avoiding caffeinated beverages, and aspirin or acetaminophen as ordered.
- Advise to refrain from sexual intercourse until infection and inflammation have cleared to avoid further irritation of inflamed tissues.
- Discuss the possible relationship between using a diaphragm for birth control and UTI in women.
- Discuss dietary and hygiene practices to prevent UTI, symptoms indicating the need for further intervention, and the risks of undertreatment.

EVALUATION

Six months later, Mrs. Waisanen rotates through the urgent care clinic for her community-based nursing experience. Ms. Ramiros asks how she is doing. Mrs. Waisanen reports that her symptoms and urine cleared within about a day after starting the antibiotic and she has had no further problems. She has seen her women's healthcare nurse practitioner to change her birth control to oral contraceptives, increased her intake of fluid and vitamin C, and no longer puts off urinating until she "has time to go!"

CRITICAL THINKING IN THE NURSING PROCESS

1. What physiologic and psychosocial factors put Mrs. Waisanen at risk for developing a UTI?
2. Compare and contrast the benefits and drawbacks to short-course therapy versus conventional therapy for UTI.
3. Develop a care plan for Mrs. Waisanen for the nursing diagnosis *Ineffective Health Maintenance.*

See Evaluating Your Response in Appendix C.

The Patient with Urinary Calculi

Urinary calculi, stones in the urinary tract, are the most common cause of upper urinary tract obstruction (Porth & Matfin, 2009). The term **lithiasis** means "stone formation." When the stones form in the kidney, it is known as *nephrolithiasis*; when they form elsewhere in the urinary tract (for example, the bladder), it is called *urolithiasis*. Stones may form and obstruct the urinary tract at any point (Figure 27–3 ■). In the United States and other industrialized countries, renal or kidney stones are the most common.

Incidence and Risk Factors

Urolithiasis is common, accounting for approximately 2 million doctor visits and 166,000 hospital stays annually (NKUDIC, 2009). In the United States, the incidence varies by region, with the highest frequency in southern and midwestern states. Males are affected more often than females. Calculi are more common among Whites than Blacks. Most people affected are in young or middle adulthood.

Although the majority of stones are idiopathic (having no demonstrable cause), a number of risk factors have been identified. The greatest risk factor for stone formation is a prior personal or family history of urinary calculi. A genetic predisposition toward the accumulation of certain mineral substances in the urine or a congenital lack of protective factors may explain the familial link. Other identified risk factors include dehydration with resultant increased urine concentration, immobility, and excess dietary intake of calcium, oxalate, or proteins. Gout, hyperparathyroidism, and urinary stasis or repeated infections also contribute to calculus formation.

Physiology Review

Normally, a balance exists in the kidneys between the need to conserve water and to eliminate poorly soluble materials such as calcium salts. This balance is affected by factors such as diet, environmental temperature, and activity. Protective inorganic and organic substances in the urine, such as pyrophosphate, citrate, and glycoproteins, normally inhibit stone formation.

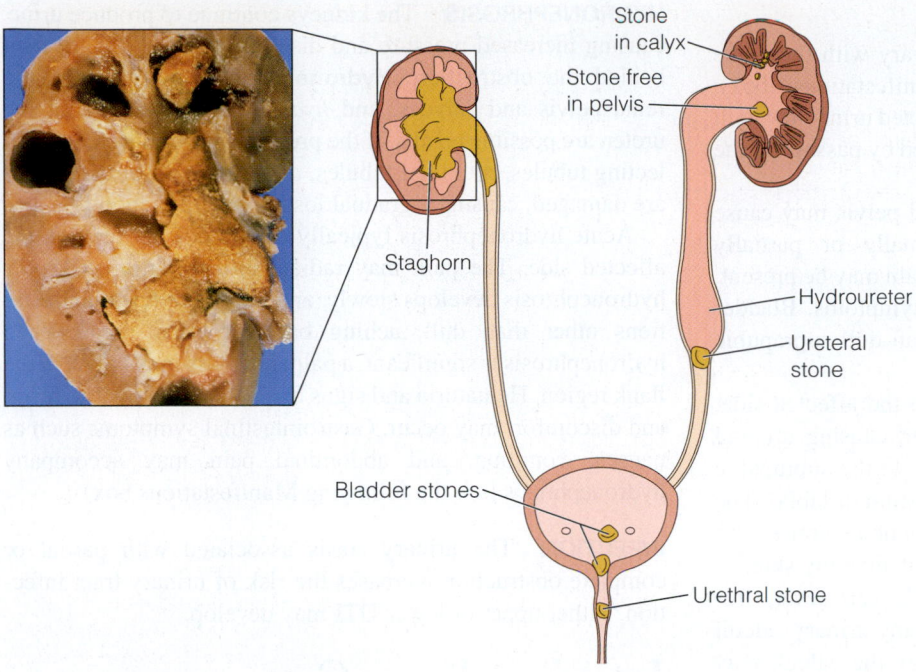

Figure 27–3 ■ Development and location of calculi within the urinary tract.

Source: Dr. E. Walker/Photo Researchers, Inc.

Pathophysiology

Three factors contribute to urolithiasis: supersaturation, nucleation, and lack of inhibitory substances in the urine.

When the concentration of an insoluble salt in the urine is very high, that is, when the urine is supersaturated, crystals may form. Usually, these crystals disperse and are eliminated because the bonds holding them together are weak. However, a nucleus of crystals may develop stable bonds to form a stone. More often, crystals form around an organic matrix or mucoprotein nucleus to become a stone. The stimulus required to initiate crystallization in supersaturated urine may be minimal. Ingesting a meal high in insoluble salt, or decreased fluid intake as occurs

during sleep, allows the concentration to increase to the point where precipitation occurs and stones are formed and grow. When fluid intake is adequate, no stone growth occurs. The acidity or alkalinity of the urine and the presence or absence of calculus-inhibiting compounds also affect lithiasis.

Most (70% to 80%) kidney stones are *calcium stones*, composed of calcium oxalate and/or calcium phosphate. These stones are generally associated with high concentrations of calcium in the blood or urine. *Uric acid stones* develop when the urine concentration of uric acid is high. They are more common in men, and may be associated with gout. Genetic factors contribute to the development of uric acid stones and calcium stones. *Struvite* (magnesium-ammonium phosphate) *stones* are associated with UTI caused by urease-producing bacteria such as *Proteus*. These stones can grow to become very large, filling the renal pelvis and calyces. They often are called *staghorn stones* because of their shape (see Figure 27–3 ■). *Cystine stones* are rare, and are associated with a genetic defect. The types of renal calculi, contributing factors, and recommended dietary modifications are listed in Table 27–2.

> **MEMORY CUE**
> - Most urinary stones form in the renal pelvis and are composed primarily of calcium salts.
> - Men are more frequently affected by urinary stones than women.
> - Loss of calcium from the bones (e.g., due to immobility) and dehydration are major risk factors for urinary stones.

TABLE 27–2 Risk Factors and Interventions for Renal Calculi

STONE TYPE AND INCIDENCE	RISK FACTORS	MANAGEMENT
Calcium phosphate and/or oxalate 70%–80%	Hypercalciuria and hypercalcemia: hyperparathyroidism, immobility, bone disease, vitamin D intoxication, multiple myeloma, renal tubular acidosis, prolonged steroid intake Alkaline urine Dehydration Inflammatory bowel disease	Pharmacology: Thiazide diuretics, phosphates Dietary: Limit foods high in sodium and protein, increase foods that acidify urine Other: Increase hydration, exercise
Struvite 15%–20%	UTIs, especially *Proteus* infections	Pharmacology: Antibiotic therapy for UTI Other: Surgical intervention or lithotripsy to remove stone
Uric acid 5%–10%	Gout, increased purine intake, acid urine	Pharmacology: Potassium citrate, allopurinol Dietary: Low purine diet Other: Increase hydration
Cystine (uncommon)	Genetic defect, acid urine	Pharmacology: Penicillamine, sodium bicarbonate Dietary: Sodium restriction Other: Increase hydration

Manifestations

The symptoms caused by urinary calculi vary with their size and location (see the following Manifestations box). Manifestations develop as a result of obstructed urine flow with resulting distention, and tissue trauma caused by passage of the rough-edged, crystalline stone.

Calculi affecting the kidney calyces and pelvis may cause few symptoms. If the stone has gradually or partially obstructed urinary flow, dull, aching flank pain may be present, but renal calculi often are silent, without symptoms. Bladder calculi may cause few symptoms other than dull suprapubic pain with exercise or after voiding.

Renal colic, acute, severe flank pain on the affected side, develops when a stone obstructs the ureter, causing ureteral spasm. The pain of renal colic may radiate to the suprapubic region, groin, and external genitals (the scrotum or labia). The severity of the pain often causes a sympathetic response with associated nausea, vomiting, pallor, and cool, clammy skin.

Manifestations of UTI, including chills and fever, frequency, urgency, and dysuria, may accompany urinary calculi at any level. Trauma to the urinary tract by the calculi may cause gross or microscopic hematuria. Gross hematuria is often the only sign of bladder stones.

Complications

Urinary stones may obstruct urine flow at any point of the urinary tract, leading to complications such as hydronephrosis and urinary stasis with subsequent infection.

Obstruction

Stones can obstruct the urinary tract at any point from the calyces of the kidney to the distal urethra, impeding the outflow of urine. If the obstruction develops slowly, there may be few or no symptoms, whereas sudden obstruction (e.g., blockage of a ureter by a passing stone) may cause severe manifestations. Urinary tract obstruction can ultimately lead to renal failure. The degree of obstruction, its location, and the duration of impaired urine flow determine the effect on renal function.

HYDRONEPHROSIS The kidneys continue to produce urine, causing increased pressure and distention of the urinary tract behind the obstruction. **Hydronephrosis**, distention of the renal pelvis and calyces, and *hydroureter*, distention of the ureter, are possible results. If the pressure is unrelieved, the collecting tubules, proximal tubules, and glomeruli of the kidney are damaged, causing a gradual loss of renal function.

Acute hydronephrosis typically causes colicky pain on the affected side. The pain may radiate into the groin. Chronic hydronephrosis develops slowly, and may have few manifestations other than dull, aching back or flank pain. When hydronephrosis is significant, a palpable mass may be felt in the flank region. Hematuria and signs of UTI such as pyuria, fever, and discomfort may occur. Gastrointestinal symptoms such as nausea, vomiting, and abdominal pain may accompany hydronephrosis (see the following Manifestations box).

INFECTION The urinary stasis associated with partial or complete obstruction increases the risk of urinary tract infection. Either upper or lower UTI may develop.

Interdisciplinary Care

Management of urinary calculi focuses on relieving acute symptoms, destroying or removing stones, and preventing further stone formation. Asymptomatic stones (those not causing pain, infection, or obstruction) are treated conservatively.

Diagnosis

Laboratory and diagnostic tests that may be ordered when urinary calculi are suspected include the following:

- *Urinalysis* to assess for hematuria and the presence of WBCs and crystal fragments. The urine pH is helpful in identifying the type of stone.
- *Chemical analysis* of any stones passed in the urine determines the type of stone and suggests measures to prevent further stone formation. Retrieving stones or teaching the patient to do so is a nursing responsibility. All urine is strained and may be saved. Any visible stones or sediment are sent for analysis.
- *Urine calcium*, *uric acid*, and *oxalate* levels measure the amount of these substances excreted over a 24-hour period, and may be assessed to help identify possible causes of lithiasis. Elevated calcium levels occur in hyperparathyroidism, Cushing's syndrome, and osteoporosis, all of which may contribute to lithiasis. Uric acid levels may be elevated in

---

MANIFESTATIONS of Urinary Calculi

KIDNEY STONES
- Often asymptomatic
- Dull, aching flank pain
- Microscopic hematuria
- Manifestations of UTI

URETERAL STONES
- Renal colic
  - Acute, severe flank pain on affected side
  - Often radiates to suprapubic region, groin, and external genitals
- Nausea, vomiting, pallor, and cool, clammy skin

BLADDER STONES
- May be asymptomatic
- Dull suprapubic pain, possibly associated with exercise or voiding
- Gross or microscopic hematuria
- Manifestations of UTI

MANIFESTATIONS of Acute and Chronic Hydronephrosis

ACUTE
- Acute, colicky pain; may radiate into groin
- Hematuria, pyuria
- Fever
- Nausea, vomiting, abdominal pain

CHRONIC
- Dull, aching flank pain
- Hematuria, pyuria
- Fever
- Palpable flank mass

patients with gout and those at risk for forming uric acid calculi. Urine oxalate excretion may help to differentiate calcium oxalate from calcium phosphate stones.

- *Serum calcium, phosphorus,* and *uric acid* levels may be obtained to help identify factors contributing to calculus formation.
- *KUB* (kidneys, ureters, and bladder) x-ray of the lower abdomen may show calculi as opacities in the kidneys, ureters, and bladder.
- *Renal ultrasonography* uses reflected sound waves to detect stones and evaluate the kidneys for possible hydronephrosis.
- *Spiral computed tomography (CT) scan* of the kidney, with or without contrast medium, shows calculi, ureteral obstruction, and other renal disorders.
- *Cystoscopy* is used to visualize and possibly remove calculi from the urinary bladder and distal ureters.

Nursing implications and care for patients undergoing these tests and procedures is outlined in ∞ Chapter 26.

Medications

An acute episode of renal colic is treated with analgesia, medications to promote stone passage, and hydration. A narcotic analgesic such as morphine sulfate is given, often intravenously, to relieve pain and reduce ureteral spasm. Indomethacin, a nonsteroidal anti-inflammatory drug (NSAID), given as a suppository, may reduce the amount of narcotic analgesia required for acute renal colic. An oral alpha-adrenergic blocker such as tamsulosin (Flomax) or a calcium-channel blocker such as nifedipine (Adalat CC, Procardia) is prescribed to relax ureteral muscle and promote passage of the stone (Stevermer & Ewigman, 2008). Oral or intravenous fluids reduce the risk of further stone formation and promote urine output.

After analysis of the calculus, various medications may be ordered to inhibit or prevent further lithiasis. A thiazide diuretic, frequently prescribed for calcium calculi, acts to reduce urinary calcium excretion and is very effective in preventing further stones. Potassium citrate alkalinizes urine (raises the pH) and is often prescribed to prevent stones that tend to form in acidic urine (uric acid, cystine, and some forms of calcium stones). See Table 27–2 for other preparations related to types of stones. Nursing responsibilities focus on teaching the patient about the prescribed medication, its importance in preventing further stone formation, and potential adverse effects.

Nutrition and Fluid Management

Diet modifications may be prescribed to change the character of the urine and prevent further lithiasis.

Increased fluid intake of 2.5 to 3.0 L per day is recommended, regardless of stone composition. A fluid intake to ensure the production of approximately 2.0 to 2.5 L of urine a day prevents the stone-forming salts from becoming concentrated enough to precipitate. Fluid intake should be spaced throughout the day and evening. Some authorities recommend that patients drink one to two glasses of water at night to prevent concentration of urine during sleep.

Recommended dietary changes may include reduced intake of the primary substance forming the calculi. For calcium stones, however, restricting dietary calcium may actually increase the risk of stone formation while promoting bone loss. A low-sodium restricted-protein diet has been shown to be more effective in preventing the recurrence of calcium stones. Dietary sodium also is restricted in patients who form cystine stones (Fauci et al., 2008).

The patient with uric acid stones requires a diet low in purines. Organ meats, sardines, and other high-purine foods are eliminated from the diet. Foods with moderate levels of purines, such as red and white meats and some seafood, may be limited.

In addition to limiting certain foods, the diet may be modified to maintain a urinary pH that does not promote lithiasis. Uric acid and cystine stones tend to form in acid urine. Foods that tend to alkalinize the urine may be recommended. Because alkaline urine promotes formation of calcium stones and urinary tract infections, the diet may be modified to lower the pH of the urine. Foods that affect urinary pH and foods high in various stone components are summarized in Table 27–3.

Treatment

Treatment of existing calculi depends on the location of the stone, the extent of obstruction, renal function, the presence or absence of UTI, and the patient's general state of health. In general, the stone is removed if it is causing severe obstruction, infection, unrelieved pain, or serious bleeding.

Lithotripsy, using sound or shock waves to crush a stone, is the preferred treatment for urinary calculi. Several techniques are available. *Extracorporeal shock wave lithotripsy (ESWL)* is a noninvasive technique for fragmenting kidney stones using shock waves generated outside the body. Acoustic shock waves are aimed under fluoroscopic guidance at the stone (Figure 27–4 ■). These shock waves travel through soft tissue without causing damage, but shatter the stone as its greater density stops their progress. Repeated shock waves pulverize the stone into fragments small enough to be eliminated in the urine. The procedure may require 30 minutes to 2 hours to complete. Intravenous sedation generally is adequate to maintain comfort during the procedure. See the box on page 796 for nursing care of the patient undergoing a lithotripsy procedure.

TABLE 27–3 Teaching Patients with Urolithiasis: Possible Food and Fluid Modifications

Foods high in oxalate	Asparagus, beer and colas, beets, cabbage, celery, chocolate and cocoa, fruits, green beans, nuts, tea, tomatoes
Purine-rich foods	Goose, organ meats, sardines and herring, venison; moderate in beef, chicken, crab, pork, salmon, veal
Acidifying foods	Cheese, cranberries, eggs, grapes, meat and poultry, plums and prunes, tomatoes, whole grains
Alkalinizing foods	Green vegetables, fruit (except as noted above), legumes, milk and milk products, rhubarb

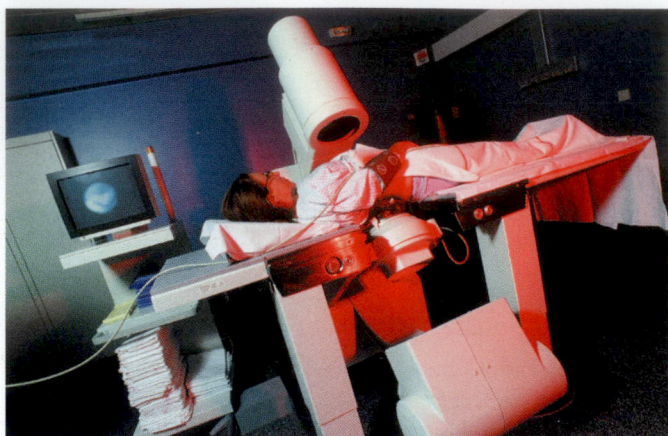

Figure 27–4 ■ Extracorporeal shock-wave lithotripsy. Acoustic shock waves generated by the shock wave generator travel through soft tissue to shatter the urinary stone into fragments, which are then eliminated in the urine.

Source: Photo Researchers, Inc.

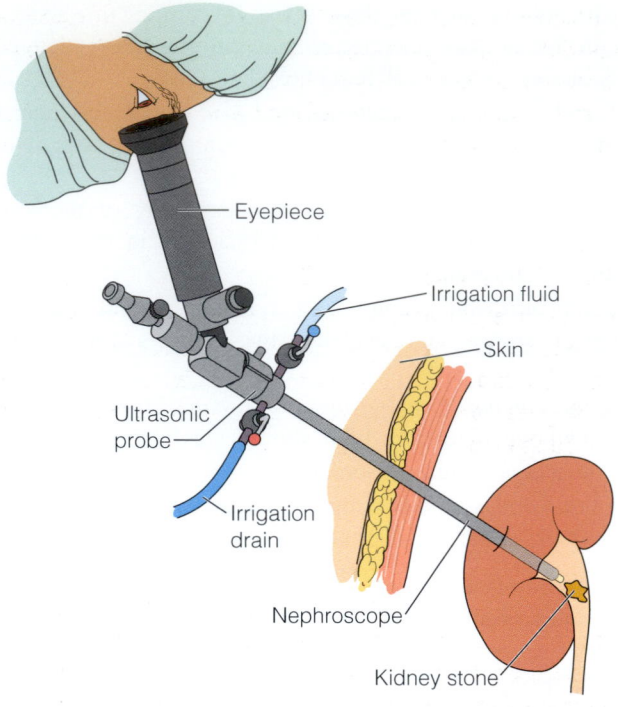

Figure 27–5 ■ Percutaneous ultrasonic lithotripsy. A nephroscope is inserted into the renal pelvis, and ultrasonic waves are used to fragment the stone. The fragments then are removed through the nephroscope.

Lithotripsy also may be performed using a percutaneous ultrasonic or laser technique. *Percutaneous nephrolithotomy* uses a nephroscope inserted into the kidney pelvis through a small flank incision (Figure 27–5 ■). The stone is fragmented using a small ultrasonic transducer or laser, and the fragments are removed through the nephroscope. In a *ureteroscopy* procedure, laser beams are used to disintegrate the stone, without damaging soft tissue. A ureteroscope (passed up the ureter from the bladder during cystoscopy) is used to guide the laser probe into direct contact with the stone.

A double J stent may be inserted into the affected ureter to maintain its patency following ESWL or other lithotripsy procedures. (See the box on page 789 for nursing care of the patient with a ureteral stent.)

On rare occasions, surgical intervention is necessary to remove a calculus in the renal pelvis or ureter. *Ureterolithotomy* is incision in the affected ureter to remove a calculus. *Pyelolithotomy* is incision into and removal of a stone from the kidney pelvis. A staghorn calculus that invades the calyces and renal parenchyma may require a *nephrolithotomy* for removal. ∞ See Chapter 4 for care of the surgical patient.

NURSING CARE OF THE PATIENT   Having Lithotripsy

PREOPERATIVE CARE

- Assess knowledge and understanding of the procedure, providing information as needed. *Anxiety is reduced, and recovery is enhanced and hastened when the patient is fully prepared for surgery.*
- Follow directions from the radiology department, physician, or anesthetist for withholding food and fluids and for bowel preparation prior to surgery. *Conscious sedation, general anesthesia, or spinal anesthesia may be required, depending on the procedure. Fecal material in the bowel may impede fluoroscopic visualization of the kidney and stone.*

POSTOPERATIVE CARE

- In the initial period, monitor vital signs frequently. *The kidney is highly vascular; therefore, hemorrhage and resulting shock are potential complications of lithotripsy. Bleeding may be internal or retroperitoneal and difficult to detect.*
- Monitor amount, color, and clarity of urine output. *Urine is often bright red initially, but bleeding should diminish within 48 to 72 hours. Cloudy urine may indicate the presence of an infection.*

- Maintain placement and patency of urinary catheters. Anchor ureteral catheters or nephrostomy tubes securely. Irrigate gently if ordered. *A kinked or plugged catheter may result in hydroureter, hydronephrosis, and kidney damage. Decreased urinary output and flank pain are possible symptoms of obstructed urine flow. Excessive force in irrigation may cause trauma and bleeding.*
- Prepare for discharge by teaching care of the indwelling catheter, urine-collection device, and incision site (if present). Teach signs and symptoms to report: urine leakage from incision for more than 4 days, symptoms of infection, pain, bright hematuria. *Many patients are discharged with dressings and catheters in place. The patient and family need necessary information to provide self-care.*
- Teach measures to reduce the risk of further lithiasis. *Many patients have repeated episodes of lithiasis and renal colic. Prevention of stone formation is important to preserve renal function.*

Bladder stones may be removed using an instrument passed through a cystoscope to crush the stones. The remaining stone fragments are then irrigated out of the bladder using an acid solution to counteract the alkalinity that precipitated stone formation.

∽ Nursing Care

Nursing care for the patient with urolithiasis is directed at providing for comfort during acute renal colic, assisting with diagnostic procedures, ensuring adequate urinary output, and teaching the patient information necessary to prevent future stone formation.

Health Promotion

Discuss the importance of maintaining an adequate fluid intake with all patients. Stress the need to increase fluid intake during warm weather and strenuous exercise or physical labor. Discuss the relationship between weight-bearing activity and retention of calcium in the bones. Encourage all patients to remain as physically active as possible to prevent bone resorption (loss) and possible hypercalciuria.

Instruct patients with known gout to maintain a generous fluid intake so as to produce at least 2 L of urine every day. Discuss the risk of lithiasis with patients who have frequent UTIs, and teach measures to reduce the incidence of UTI and the risk for lithiasis.

Assessment

Obtain subjective and objective assessment data specific to urolithiasis:

- *Health history:* Complaints of flank, back, or abdominal pain, radiation, characteristics and timing, aggravating or relieving factors; other symptoms such as nausea and vomiting; possible contributing factors such as dehydration; previous or family history of kidney stones; current or previous treatment measures.

- *Physical examination:* General appearance including position, vital signs; skin color, temperature, moisture, turgor; abdominal, flank, or costovertebral tenderness; amount, color, and characteristics of urine (presence of hematuria, bacteria, pyuria, pH).

Nursing Diagnoses and Interventions

See the Case Study & Nursing Care Plan on page 799 for additional nursing diagnoses and interventions.

Acute Pain

Pain is the primary outward manifestation of urolithiasis, particularly when a stone lodges within a ureter, causing acute obstruction and distention. Invasive and noninvasive procedures to remove or crush stones also may be painful. Patients undergoing surgery also experience incisional pain.

- Assess pain using a standard pain scale and its characteristics. Administer analgesia as ordered and monitor its effectiveness. *The intensity, type of pain, and its responsiveness to analgesia provide valuable clues as to its cause. Regular administration of prescribed analgesics controls pain more effectively than waiting until pain becomes intolerable. Administering an ordered NSAID on a routine schedule may significantly reduce the need for narcotic analgesia in patients with renal colic.*

- Unless contraindicated, encourage fluid intake and ambulation in the patient with renal colic. *Increased fluids and ambulation increase urinary output, facilitating movement of the calculus through the ureter and decreasing pain.*

- Use nonpharmacologic measures such as positioning, moist heat, relaxation techniques, guided imagery, and diversion as adjunctive therapy for pain relief. *Adjunctive pain relief measures can enhance the effectiveness of analgesics and other prescribed treatment.*

- If surgery has been performed, monitor urinary output, catheters, incision, and wound drainage. *Pain may be a symptom of proximal distention due to a blocked catheter. Infection or hematoma at the surgical site can significantly increase perceived pain.*

Impaired Urinary Elimination

Obstruction of the urinary tract is the primary problem associated with urolithiasis. Obstruction can ultimately lead to stasis, infection, or irreversible renal damage.

- Monitor amount and character of urine output. If catheterized, measure output hourly. Document any hematuria, dysuria, frequency, urgency, and pyuria. Strain all urine for stones, saving any recovered stones for laboratory analysis. *The amount of urine output helps determine possible urinary*

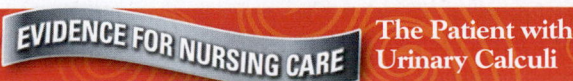

EVIDENCE FOR NURSING CARE — The Patient with Urinary Calculi

Selected resources that nurses may find helpful when planning evidence-based nursing care follow.

- Baumgarten, D. A., Francis, I. R., Bluth, E. I., Bush, Jr., W. H., Casalino, D. D., Curry, N. S., et al. (2007). ACR Appropriateness Criteria® acute onset flank pain, suspicion of stone disease. *National Guideline Clearinghouse.* Retrieved from http://www.guideline.gov/summary/summary.aspx?doc_id=11563&nbr=005991&string=urinary+AND+calculi

- Tiselius, H., Alken, P., Buck C, Gallucci, M., Knoll, T., Sarica, K., et al. (2008 March). *Guidelines on urolithiasis.* Arnhem, The Netherlands: European Association of Urology (EAU. Retrieved from http://www.guideline.gov/summary/summary.aspx?ss=15&doc_id=12528&nbr=006452&string=urolithiasis

tract obstruction and adequacy of hydration. Hematuria, gross or microscopic, is often associated with calculi and with procedures used to remove stones, such as cystoscopy or lithotripsy. A change in the amount of hematuria may indicate stone passage or a complication. Dysuria, frequency, urgency, and cloudy urine are symptoms of UTI, often associated with urolithiasis. Antibiotic therapy may be required. Analysis of stones recovered from the urine can direct measures to prevent further lithiasis.

> ### PRACTICE ALERT
> A stone that completely obstructs the ureter can lead to hydronephrosis and kidney damage on the affected side. Report symptoms of hydronephrosis such as dull flank pain or aching and changes in renal function studies (BUN and serum creatinine). Because the other kidney continues to function, urine output may not fall significantly with obstruction of one ureter. A drop in eGFR or rising BUN and serum creatinine levels may be early signs of renal failure.

■ Maintain patency and integrity of all catheter systems. Secure catheters well, label as indicated, and use sterile technique for all ordered irrigations or other procedures. *A kinked or plugged catheter, particularly a ureteral catheter or nephrostomy tube, may damage the urinary system. Labeling catheters can prevent mistakes, such as inappropriate irrigation or clamping. Any catheter increases the risk of infection; aseptic technique in all procedures reduces this risk.*

Readiness for Enhanced Knowledge
The patient with urolithiasis has multiple learning needs. These include information about the disease and its possible consequences, any diagnostic or therapeutic procedures performed, and strategies to prevent future lithiasis.

■ Assess understanding and previous learning. *Relating information to previously learned material enhances retention and understanding.*
■ Present all material in a manner appropriate to knowledge base, developmental and educational level, and current needs. *Learning is an active process that requires the patient's participation. Tailoring teaching to the individual increases involvement.*
■ Teach about all diagnostic and treatment procedures. *Knowing what to expect reduces anxiety, enhances compliance, and hastens recovery.*
■ If the patient will be managed in the community, teach to
  ■ collect and strain all urine, saving any stones.
  ■ report stone passage to the physician and bring the stone in for analysis.
  ■ report any changes in the amount or character of urine output to physician.
    When pain can be managed with oral analgesics, urinary stones are managed in the community. The patient needs to know how and why to collect the calculus and indicators of complications, such as reduced urine output and cloudy or bloody urine.

■ Teach measures to prevent further urolithiasis:
  ■ Increase fluid intake to 2500 to 3500 mL per day.
  ■ Follow recommended dietary guidelines.
  ■ Maintain activity level to prevent urinary stasis and bone resorption.
  ■ Take medications as prescribed.
The risk of recurrent lithiasis is approximately 50%; however, this risk can be reduced by measures to prevent conditions favoring stone formation.

■ Teach about the relationship between urinary calculi and UTI, emphasizing preventive measures and the importance of prompt treatment. *Urinary tract infection promotes urolithiasis and thus requires prompt treatment to reduce this risk.*

Using NANDA, NIC, and NOC
Linkages between a selected NANDA nursing diagnosis, NIC, and NOC for the patient with urinary calculi are shown in the chart that follows.

Community-Based Care
The patient with urinary calculi needs to know how to manage existing stones and what to do to reduce the risk of future stone formation. Discuss the following topics to prepare the patient and family for home care:

■ Importance of maintaining a fluid intake adequate to produce 2.0 to 2.5 quarts of urine per day
■ Prescribed medications, their management, and potential adverse effects
■ Dietary recommendations
■ Prevention, recognition, and management of UTI
■ Any further diagnostic or treatment measures planned

When the patient is to be discharged with dressings, a nephrostomy tube, or a catheter, teach the patient and family about the following:

■ How to change dressings, maintaining aseptic technique
■ Assessment of the wound and skin for healing and possible complications such as infection or skin breakdown

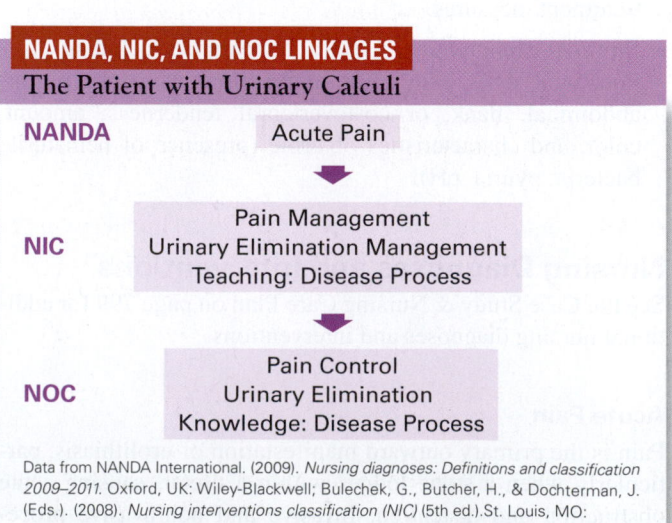

NANDA, NIC, AND NOC LINKAGES
The Patient with Urinary Calculi

NANDA — Acute Pain

NIC — Pain Management / Urinary Elimination Management / Teaching: Disease Process

NOC — Pain Control / Urinary Elimination / Knowledge: Disease Process

Data from NANDA International. (2009). *Nursing diagnoses: Definitions and classification 2009–2011.* Oxford, UK: Wiley-Blackwell; Bulechek, G., Butcher, H., & Dochterman, J. (Eds.). (2008). *Nursing interventions classification (NIC)* (5th ed.).St. Louis, MO: Mosby; and Moorhead, S., Johnson, M., Maas, M., & Swanson, E. (Eds.). (2008). *Nursing outcomes classification (NOC)* (4th ed.). St. Louis, MO: Mosby.

CASE STUDY & NURSING CARE PLAN   A Patient with Urinary Calculi

Richard Leton, aged 44, owns a small business. He is admitted to the medical unit from the emergency department (ED) after awakening at 4:00 AM with severe right-sided pain. His CBC is normal, and urinalysis reveals microscopic hematuria, but no protein or bacteria. A renal ultrasound shows a 4- to 5-mm stone partially obstructing the right ureter.

Stephen Phillips, Mr. Leton's admitting nurse, notes that he is pale, diaphoretic, and very anxious. He complains of nausea and asks for an emesis basin. Mr. Leton received 4 mg of intravenous morphine sulphate and 20 mg nifedipine PO shortly after admission to the ED, approximately 2.5 hours ago. He denies pain at this time, but says, "I'm scared to death that it'll come back—I couldn't even move, it hurt so bad."

ASSESSMENT

Mr. Leton's history reveals no previous episodes of renal calculi. He felt well until the pain awakened him during the night. He admits that he has been working under a deadline to complete a construction project and that he probably has not been drinking enough fluids "considering how hot it's been." Physical assessment findings include T 100.4°F (38.0°C) PO, P 98, R 24, and BP 160/86. Color is pale to ashen, skin cool and moist. Abdomen firm with moderate tenderness in the right upper outer quadrant. The ED physician orders an IV of 5% dextrose in 1/2 normal saline at 200 mL/h until nausea relieved, then PO fluids of at least 3000 mL/24 h; nifedipine 20 mg PO every 8 hours; morphine sulfate (MS) 2 to 10 mg IV prn severe pain; indomethacin (Indocin) 50 mg per rectal suppository q8h; promethazine (Phenergan) 25 mg PO or per suppository q6h prn nausea; activity to tolerance; and strain all urine, sending recovered stones for analysis.

DIAGNOSES

- *Anxiety* related to anticipation of recurrent severe pain
- *Risk for Imbalanced Nutrition: Less than Body Requirements* related to nausea
- *Acute Pain* related to partial obstruction of right ureter by calculus
- *Impaired Urinary Elimination* related to partial obstruction of ureter by calculus
- *Readiness for Enhanced Knowledge* about disease process, contributing factors, and management

EXPECTED OUTCOMES

- Demonstrate reduced anxiety by relaxed facial expression, vital signs within his normal range, and ability to rest when not disturbed.
- Consume at least 50% of diet and 100% of ordered fluids without nausea or vomiting.

- Request analgesia as needed at onset of pain; report effective pain relief.
- Maintain urine output of 2500 mL/24 h with no signs of infection or obstruction (such as increased pain, dysuria, pyuria, or hematuria).
- Relate an understanding of the process of urolithiasis and contributing factors.
- Verbalize dietary and fluid intake, and other measures to reduce risk of future stone formation.

PLANNING AND IMPLEMENTATION

- Reassure that measures to prevent further episodes of renal colic are being implemented, and that medication is available to relieve pain promptly.
- Assess the effectiveness of analgesia and its adverse effects, especially nausea.
- Maintain IV as ordered until oral fluid intake exceeds 200 mL of fluid per hour while awake.
- Measure and strain all urine. Assess urine for color, clarity, and odor.
- Teach about urolithiasis and its risk factors, especially as they relate to Mr. Leton.
- Teach the importance of maintaining a high fluid intake, especially when working outdoors in hot weather, recommended dietary modifications and their rationale, ordered medications and their effects, how to identify and prevent UTI, and symptoms that should be reported to the physician.

EVALUATION

Mr. Leton passed the obstructing stone the evening after admission and is discharged the following day. On discharge, he denies pain or nausea, his urine is clear and pale yellow, and urinalysis is normal. Laboratory analysis shows that the calculus was calcium oxalate. Mr. Leton is able to state the importance of continuing a high fluid intake. He verbalizes that he will reduce his intake of sodium, modify his protein intake, and that he will increase his intake of foods to acidify his urine. He is able to list foods to include in his diet. He states, "You'd better believe I'll follow my diet, drink my water, and make sure I don't get an infection. I hope to never feel pain like that again!"

CRITICAL THINKING IN THE NURSING PROCESS

1. What factors contributed to the onset and timing of Mr. Leton's ureteral colic?
2. What is the rationale for administering indomethacin, an NSAID, to a patient with ureteral colic?
3. Why did Mr. Phillips include a nursing intervention to assess for a relationship between Mr. Leton's nausea, his pain, and the ordered analgesic agent?

See Evaluating Your Response in Appendix C.

- How to manage drainage systems and maintain their patency
- Emptying drainage bags and assessing urine output
- When to contact the physician and recommendations for follow-up care

The Patient with a Urinary Tract Tumor

A malignancy can develop in any part of the urinary tract; however, 90% develop in the bladder, about 8% develop in the renal pelvis, and only 2% develop in the ureter or urethra (Fauci et al., 2008). When diagnosed early, the 5-year survival rate for bladder cancer is 93% (American Cancer Society [ACS], 2009).

Incidence and Risk Factors

An estimated 70,980 new cases of bladder cancer were diagnosed in the United States in 2009, and 14,330 people died as a result of the disease. The incidence of bladder cancer is nearly four times higher in men than it is in women, and about twice as high in White men as it is in Black men (ACS, 2009). Most people who develop bladder cancer are over age 60.

Two major factors are implicated in the development of bladder cancer: the presence of carcinogens in the urine and chronic inflammation or infection of bladder mucosa. Cigarette smoking is the primary risk factor for bladder cancer. The risk in smokers is twice that of nonsmokers (ACS, 2009). The chemicals and dyes used in the plastics, rubber, and cable industries; substances in the work environment of textile workers, leather finishers, spray painters, and petroleum workers; and high levels of arsenic in drinking water also are associated with a higher risk. Additional risk factors for bladder cancer include residence in an urban area, chronic UTIs, and bladder calculi. The parasite *Schistosoma haematobium*, endemic to Egypt and the Sudan, also increases the risk for bladder cancer (Porth & Matfin, 2009). The risk for bladder cancer appears to be reduced by increasing the intake of fluids and vegetables (ACS, 2009).

> **FAST FACTS**
> The major risk factors for bladder cancer are the following:
> - Male gender, aged > 60, residence in urban area
> - Cigarette smoking
> - Occupational exposure to dyes or solvents
> - Chronic UTI or bladder calculi

Pathophysiology

Most urinary tract malignancies arise from epithelial tissue. Transitional epithelium lines the entire tract from the renal pelvis through the urethra. Carcinogenic breakdown products of certain chemicals and from cigarette smoke are excreted in the urine and stored in the bladder, possibly causing a local influence on abnormal cell development. Squamous cell carcinoma of the urinary tract occurs less frequently than transitional epithelial cell tumors.

Urinary tract tumors begin as nonspecific cellular alterations that develop into either flat or papillary lesions. These lesions may be either superficial or invasive. Most bladder tumors are papillary lesions (*papillomas*), a polyp-like structure attached by a stalk to the bladder mucosa (Figure 27–6 ■). Papillomas are generally superficial, noninvasive tumors that bleed easily and frequently recur (Fauci et al., 2008). They rarely progress to become invasive, and the prognosis for recovery is good.

Carcinoma *in situ* (CIS), which occurs less frequently, is a poorly differentiated flat tumor that invades directly and is associated with a poorer prognosis. These tumors often initially present as superficial lesions, later progressing to

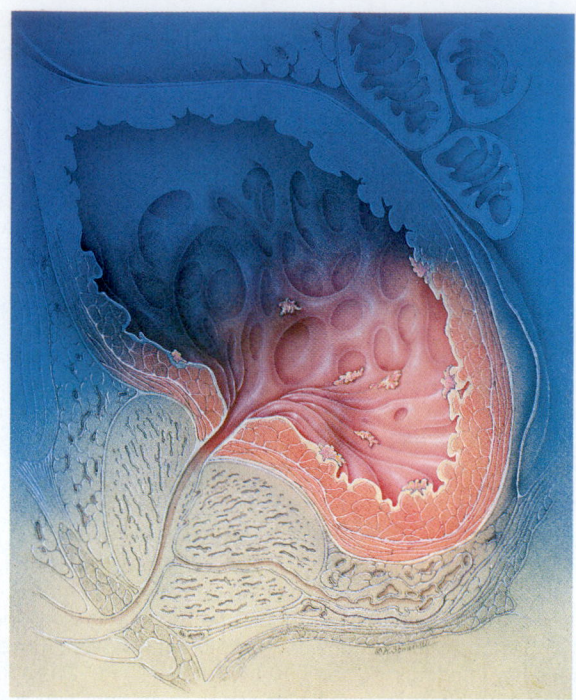

Figure 27–6 ■ Papillary transitional cell carcinoma of the urinary bladder.

Source: Custom Medical Stock Photo, Inc.

become invasive (Figure 27–7 ■). Grade I tumors are highly differentiated and rarely progress to become invasive, whereas grade III tumors are poorly differentiated and usually progress (Fauci et al., 2008). The tumor, node, metastasis (TNM) system, outlined in Table 27–4, is used to stage bladder tumors. ∞ See Chapter 14 for more information about tumor grading and staging. When metastasis occurs, the pelvic lymph nodes, lungs, bones, and liver are most commonly involved.

Manifestations

Painless hematuria is the presenting sign in 75% of urinary tract tumors. Hematuria may be gross or microscopic and is often intermittent, causing delay in seeking treatment. Inflammation surrounding the tumor occasionally causes manifestations of a UTI, including frequency, urgency, and dysuria. Ureteral tumors may cause colicky pain from obstruction.

TABLE 27–4 Bladder Tumor Staging

DEPTH OF INVOLVEMENT	STAGE	TNM (TUMOR, NODE, METASTASIS) STAGE	TUMOR INVOLVEMENT
Superficial	Cis	T_a	Limited to the bladder mucosa
	I	T_1	Involvement of the bladder mucosa and submucosal layers
Invasive	II	T_2	Invasion of superficial muscle of bladder wall
		T_{3a}	Deep muscle invasion
	III	T_{3b}	Involvement of perivesicular fat
	IV	$T_{3-4}N_+$	Regional (pelvic) lymph node involvement
		$T_{3-4}M_1$	Metastasis to distant lymph nodes or organs

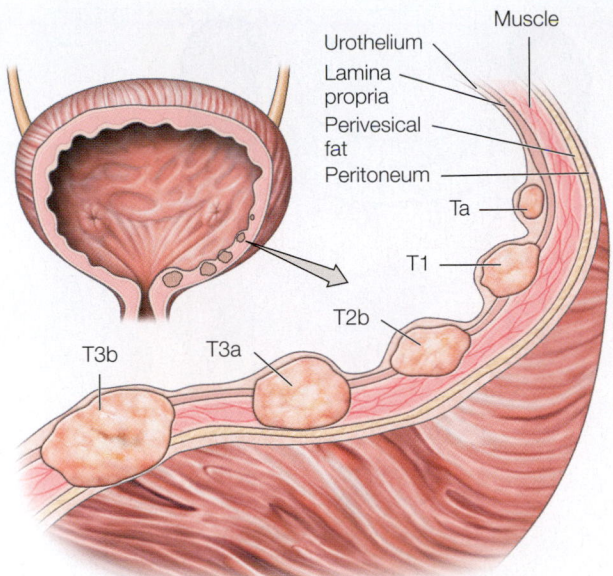

Figure 27–7 ■ Stages of bladder tumor development and invasiveness, beginning at the 3 o'clock position of the bladder and continuing in a clockwise manner.

Tumors of the urinary tract typically cause few outward signs and may not be discovered until obstructed urine flow causes flank pain or renal failure.

PRACTICE ALERT
Intermittent painless hematuria is the most common presenting symptom of bladder cancer. Instruct all patients with painless hematuria to contact their physician for follow-up testing.

Interdisciplinary Care

Treatment of the patient with a tumor of the urinary tract focuses on removing or destroying the cancerous tissue, preventing further invasion or metastasis, and maintaining renal and urinary function.

Diagnosis

When a urinary tract tumor is suspected, the following diagnostic tests may be ordered:

- *Urinalysis* is done to evaluate for hematuria. Gross or microscopic hematuria is often the first indicator of a neoplasm in the urinary tract.
- *Urine cytology*, microscopic examination of cells in the urine, is performed to identify abnormal cells (tumor or

pretumor cells). Periodic urine cytology is recommended for patients at high risk for bladder cancer or its recurrence due to carcinogen exposure.

- *Ultrasound of the bladder* is a noninvasive test to detect bladder tumors. *Intravenous pyelography* may reveal a rigid deformity of the bladder wall, obstruction of urine flow at the point of the tumor, or bladder filling or emptying defects.
- *Cystoscopy* and *ureteroscopy* allow direct visualization, assessment, and biopsy of lesions of the urethra, bladder, or ureters to provide definitive diagnosis of urinary tract tumors.
- *CT scan* or *MRI* is primarily used to evaluate tumor invasion or metastasis.

∞ See Chapter 26 for nursing care related to these diagnostic tests.

Medications

Immunologic or chemotherapeutic agents administered by intravesical instillation (into the bladder) may be used either as the primary treatment for bladder cancer when multiple early lesions are present or to prevent recurrence following endoscopic tumor removal. Bacille Calmette-Guérin (BCG; BCGLive, TheraCys) is a suspension of attenuated *Mycobacterium bovis* used to treat CIS and recurrent bladder tumors. Instillation into the bladder causes a local inflammatory reaction that eliminates or reduces superficial tumors. Systemic mycobacterial infection is a rare complication of intravesical BCG therapy that may require antituberculin treatment. Other chemotherapeutic agents also may be administered intravesically, including thiotepa, mitomycin C, and interferon. Bladder irritation, frequency, dysuria, and contact dermatitis are possible adverse reactions to intravesical chemotherapy. Suppression of bone marrow function also can occur as a result of intravesical treatment.

Radiation Therapy

Radiation therapy primarily is used as palliative treatment for inoperable tumors and patients who cannot tolerate surgery. Radiation therapy may also be used in combination with systemic chemotherapy to improve local and distant relapse rates (∞ see Chapter 14).

Surgery

A number of surgical procedures, ranging from simple resection of noninvasive tumors to removal of the bladder and surrounding structures, are used to treat urinary tract tumors. Indications for each procedure and specific nursing implications are outlined in Table 27–5.

TABLE 27–5 Surgical Procedures to Treat Bladder Tumors

PROCEDURE	INDICATIONS	NURSING IMPLICATIONS
Transurethral resection of bladder tumor	Diagnose and treat superficial bladder tumors; control bleeding	Maintain continuous bladder irrigation postoperatively; monitor for excessive bleeding; ensure catheter patency. Increase fluids to 2500–3000 mL/day. Give stool softeners to prevent straining.
Partial cystectomy	Resect solitary, isolated tumor at stage T_2 or T_3 not involving trigone	Maintain patency of urethral and/or suprapubic catheter to make sure suture lines are free of pressure; monitor for excess bleeding.
Complete or radical cystectomy	Remove large, invasive tumors; involvement of trigone	Permanent urinary diversion is required. Maintain patency and position of stents; urethral catheter may be in place to drain pelvic cavity.

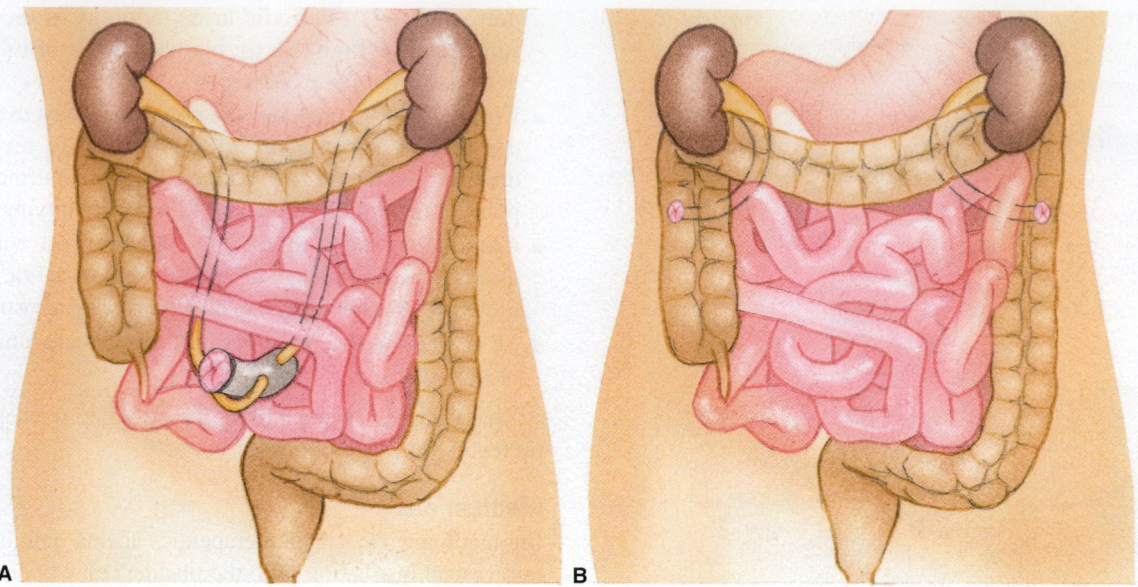

Figure 27–8 ■ Common urinary diversion procedures. *A,* Ileal conduit. A segment of ileum is separated from the small intestine and formed into a tubular pouch with the open end brought to the skin surface to form a stoma. The ureters are connected to the pouch. *B,* Bilateral cutaneous urostomy. The ureters are brought to the surface of the abdomen to form individual stomas.

Transurethral tumor resection may be performed by excision, *fulguration* (destruction of tissue using electric sparks generated by high-frequency current), or *laser photocoagulation* (use of light energy to destroy abnormal tissue). Laser surgery carries the lowest risk of bleeding and perforation of the bladder wall. Following cystoscopic tumor resection, patients are followed at 3-month intervals for tumor recurrence. Recurrences may develop anywhere in the urinary tract, including the renal pelvis, ureter, or urethra.

Cystectomy, surgical removal of the bladder, is necessary to treat invasive cancers. Partial cystectomy may be done to remove a solitary lesion; however, radical cystectomy is the standard treatment for invasive tumors. The bladder and adjacent muscles and tissues are removed. In men, the prostate and seminal vessels are also removed, resulting in impotence. In women, a total hysterectomy and bilateral salpingo-oophorectomy (removal of the uterus, fallopian tubes, and ovaries) accompanies the procedure, causing sterility. At the time of surgery, a **urinary diversion** is created to provide for urine collection and drainage. An *ileal conduit* (Figure 27–8A ■), or a *bilateral cutaneous urostomy* (Figure 27–8B), or a *continent urinary diversion* is created to collect and drain urine. Table 27–6 describes the most frequently used urinary diversion techniques.

Surgical procedures to remove tumors involving other portions of the urinary tract vary according to the site and stage of the tumor. When the distal ureter is involved, the tumor may be resected and the ureter implanted into the opposite ureter to provide for drainage. A proximal ureteral tumor necessitates removal of the ureter and kidney on the affected side.

TABLE 27–6 Urinary Diversion Procedures

PROCEDURE	DESCRIPTION	NURSING CONSIDERATIONS
Ileal conduit	Portion of ileum is isolated from small intestine, leaving vascular, lymphatic, and neural connections intact; ileum is formed into pouch with open end brought to surface to form a stoma; ureters are inserted into pouch.	Most common urinary diversion. Continuous urine drainage necessitates appliance. Postoperative edema may interfere with urine output. Risk of infection is less than for cutaneous ureterostomy, but potential for reflux is high. Good skin care vital because of constant contact with urine.
Cutaneous urostomy	Each ureter is brought to the surface of the abdomen to form a stoma.	Continuous urine drainage requires dual appliances. Risk of infection is high due to direct route from the skin to the kidneys. Good skin care is vital because of constant contact with urine.
Continent urinary reservoir	A portion of the stomach, colon, or small intestine is used to form a reservoir to which the ureters are attached. Nipple valves are formed to prevent reflux. A nipple valve and stoma may be formed or the pouch may be attached to the urethral stump, avoiding creation of a stoma.	Drainage collection device not necessary. Patient must be able and motivated to manage self-catheterization. Reservoir may absorb urea and electrolytes, resulting in imbalances. Significant portion of bowel is required to form pouch and stoma.

See the box on page 804 for nursing care of the patient undergoing tumor resection and a urinary diversion.

∞ Nursing Care

The patient who undergoes treatment for a tumor of the urinary tract has many nursing care needs because of alterations in the functional health patterns of elimination, health perception-health management, cognitive-perceptual, self-perception-self-concept, role-relationships, and coping-stress-tolerance.

Health Promotion

Encourage all patients not to smoke. Provide referral to smoking cessation programs or clinics for patients who wish to quit smoking. Encourage patients at high risk for developing bladder cancer (see page 800) to have periodic examinations, including urinalysis and possible urine cytology.

Assessment

Nursing assessment related to urinary tract cancer includes both subjective and objective information:

- *Health history:* Risk factors; history of hematuria or manifestations of UTI (dysuria, frequency, urgency, pyuria); lower abdominal discomfort or flank pain.
- *Physical examination:* General health; abdominal tenderness; urine for analysis.

Nursing Diagnoses and Interventions

Maintaining urinary output is the priority nursing care focus for the patient with a bladder tumor. For additional potential nursing diagnoses and interventions for the patient with a bladder tumor, see the Case Study & Nursing Care Plan that follows.

Impaired Urinary Elimination

Whether the patient has undergone transurethral resection of a bladder tumor or radical cystectomy with urinary diversion, urinary elimination is altered at least temporarily.

- Monitor urine output from all catheters, stents, and tubes for amount, color, and clarity hourly for the first 24 hours postoperatively, then every 4 to 8 hours. *Decreased urine output may indicate impaired catheter or drainage system patency. Prompt intervention is necessary to prevent hydronephrosis. A change in color or clarity may indicate a complication such as hemorrhage or infection.*

PRACTICE ALERT
Promptly report urine output of less than 30 mL per hour, which may indicate low vascular volume or renal insufficiency. Prompt intervention is vital to restore cardiac output and prevent acute renal failure.

- Label all catheters, stents, and their drainage containers. Maintain separate closed gravity drainage systems for each. *Clear identification of each tube can prevent errors in irrigating and calculating outputs. Separate closed systems minimize the risk and extent of potential bacterial contamination and resultant infection.*

PRACTICE ALERT
Use aseptic techniques and strictly follow guidelines for irrigating catheters. Catheters placed in the kidney pelvis are irrigated using gentle pressure and small amounts of fluid (10 to 15 mL) to avoid damaging renal tissues.

- Secure ureteral catheters and stents with tape; prevent kinking or occlusion; and maintain gravity flow by keeping drainage bag below level of kidneys. *Impaired urine flow can lead to urinary retention and distention of the bladder, a newly created reservoir, or the renal pelvis (hydronephrosis).*
- Encourage fluid intake of 3000 mL per day. *Increased fluid intake maintains a high urinary output, reducing the risk of infection. Dilute urine is less irritating to the skin surrounding the stoma site. Electrolyte reabsorption from reservoirs may increase risk of calculi; high fluid intake and urine output reduce this risk.*

PRACTICE ALERT
Monitor urine output closely for first 24 hours after stents or ureteral catheters are removed. Edema or stricture of ureters may impede output, leading to hydronephrosis and kidney damage.

- Encourage activity to tolerance. *Ambulation promotes drainage of urine from reservoirs and helps prevent calcium loss from bones, which could precipitate calculus formation.*

Risk for Impaired Skin Integrity

The skin surrounding the stoma site of an ileal conduit is at risk for irritation and breakdown. Because urine is acidic and contains high concentrations of electrolytes, it has a corrosive

BOX 27–2 Urinary Stoma Care

- Gather all supplies: a clean, disposable pouch; liquid skin barrier or barrier ring; 4-by-4 gauze squares; stoma guide; adhesive solvent; clean gloves; and a clean washcloth.
- Assess knowledge, learning needs, and ability and willingness to assist with procedure. Explain the procedure as needed.
- Use standard precautions.
- Remove old pouch, pulling gently away from skin. Warm water or adhesive solvent may be used to loosen the seal if necessary.
- Assess stoma. Normally the stoma is bright red and appears moist. Report a dark purple, black, or very pale stoma to the physician. Slight bleeding with cleansing is normal, especially in the immediate postoperative period.
- Prevent urine flow during cleaning by placing a rolled gauze square or tampon over the stoma opening.
- Cleanse skin around the stoma with soap and water, rinse, and pat or air dry.
- Use the stoma guide to determine correct size for the bag opening and/or protective ring seal. Trim the bag or seal as needed.
- Apply skin barrier; allow to dry.
- Apply the bag with an opening no more than 1 to 2 mm wider than outside of stoma. Allow no wrinkles or creases where the bag contacts the skin.
- Connect bag to the urine-collection device. Dispose of old pouch, used supplies, and gloves appropriately. Wash hands.
- Chart procedure, including stoma appearance and response of the patient.

NURSING CARE OF THE PATIENT   Having a Cystectomy and Urinary Diversion

PREOPERATIVE CARE

■ Provide routine preoperative care as outlined in ∞ Chapter 4.

■ Assess knowledge of the proposed surgery and its long-term implications, clarifying misunderstandings and discussing concerns. *Patients having surgery for cancer of the urinary tract are trying to cope with the diagnosis of cancer and may not fully understand the surgery and its potential effects. Open discussion can facilitate postoperative recovery and adjustment.*

■ Begin teaching about postoperative tubes and drains, self-care of stoma, and control of drainage and odor. *Postoperative physiologic and psychologic stressors may interfere with learning. A basic understanding of what to expect in the way of tubes, drains, and procedures reduces stress in the immediate postoperative period. Preoperative teaching can enhance recall and postoperative learning.*

■ Assist in identifying stoma site, avoiding folds of skin, bones, scar tissue, and the waistline or belt area. Be sure to consider the patient's occupation and style of clothing. The site should be visible to the patient and accessible for manipulation. *Stoma placement is a vital component of adjustment and self-care. Care is taken to place the stoma away from areas of constant irritation by clothing or movement. It should be located so that the patient can cover and disguise the collecting device, maintain the seal to prevent leakage, and effectively cleanse and maintain the site.*

■ Perform bowel-preparation activities as ordered. *Bowel preparation is done to prevent fecal contamination of the peritoneal cavity and to decompress the bowel during surgery.*

POSTOPERATIVE CARE

■ Provide routine postoperative care (∞ see Chapter 4).

■ Monitor intake and output carefully, assessing urine output every hour for the first 24 hours, then every 4 hours or as ordered. Call the physician if urine output is less than 30 mL per hour. *Tissue edema and bleeding may interfere with urinary output from stoma, catheters, or drains. Maintenance of urine outflow is vital to prevent hydronephrosis and possible*

renal damage. A urine output of at least 30 mL per hour is necessary for effective renal function.

■ Assess color and consistency of urine. Expect pink or bright red urine fading to pink and then clearing by the third postoperative day. Urine may be cloudy due to mucus production by bowel mucosa. *Bright red blood in the urine from a urinary diversion may indicate hemorrhage, necessitating further surgery. Excessive cloudiness or malodorous urine may indicate infection.*

■ Assess size, color, and condition of the stoma and surrounding skin every 2 hours for the first 24 hours, then every 4 hours for 48 to 72 hours. Expect the stoma to appear bright red and slightly edematous initially. Slight bleeding during cleansing is normal. *Compromised circulation causes the stoma to appear pale, gray, or cyanotic or blanch when touched. Other complications, such as infection or impaired healing, may be evidenced by a change in the appearance of the stoma or incision.*

■ Irrigate the ileal diversion catheter with 30 to 60 mL of normal saline every 4 hours or as ordered. *Mucus produced by the bowel wall may accumulate in the newly devised reservoir or obstruct catheters.*

■ Monitor serum electrolyte values, acid–base balance, and renal function tests such as BUN and serum creatinine. *Reabsorption of electrolytes from reservoirs created by portions of bowel may result in electrolyte imbalance and metabolic acidosis. Optimal renal function is necessary to maintain a normal state of homeostasis.*

■ Teach the patient and family about stoma and urinary diversion care, including odor management, skin care, increased fluid intake, pouch application and leakage prevention, self-catheterization for patients with continent reservoirs, and signs of infection and other complications. *The ability to provide self-care is a significant factor in the adjustment to a changed body image. Teaching family members facilitates acceptance and adjustment. The family also needs this knowledge in case illness or disability interferes with the self-care capacity.*

effect on skin. In addition, adhesives and sealants used to prevent pouch leakage may irritate the skin.

■ Assess peristomal skin for redness, excoriation, or signs of breakdown. Assess for urine leakage from catheters, stents, or drains. Keep the skin clean and dry. Change wet dressings. *Intact skin is the first line of defense against infection. Impaired skin integrity may lead to local or systemic infection and impaired healing.*

■ Ensure gravity drainage of urine collection device or empty bag every 2 hours. *Overfilling of the collection bag may damage the seal, allowing leakage and contact of urine with skin.*

■ Change urine collection appliance as needed, removing any mucus from stoma. See Box 27–2 for care of a urinary drainage stoma. *Meticulous care and protection of skin surrounding stoma can maintain integrity and prevent breakdown.*

Disturbed Body Image

A radical cystectomy and urinary diversion affect the patient's body image. In most cases, an abdominal stoma is created, requiring either a drainage appliance or regular catheterization

of the stoma to drain urine. Removal of the prostate and seminal vesicles or the uterus and ovaries leaves the patient sterile. If radiation or chemotherapy is planned as adjunctive therapy, the patient may experience hair loss, stomatitis, nausea and vomiting, or other disturbing side effects of therapy.

■ Use therapeutic communication techniques, actively listening and responding to the patient's and family's concerns. *Patients must know their feelings and concerns are respected and valued. Denial, anger, guilt, bargaining, or depression are common during grieving and normal for a patient undergoing a significant change in body image.*

■ Recognize and accept behaviors that indicate use of coping mechanisms, encouraging adaptive mechanisms. *The patient may initially use defensive coping mechanisms such as denial, minimization, and dissociation from the immediate situation to reduce anxiety and maintain psychologic integrity. Adaptive mechanisms include learning as much as possible about the surgery and its effects, practicing procedures, setting realistic goals, and rehearsing various alternative outcomes.*

CASE STUDY & NURSING CARE PLAN   A Patient with a Bladder Tumor

Ben Hussain is a 61-year-old automobile salesman. He is married and has five children, all of whom are grown and living away from home. One week ago, Mr. Hussain became alarmed when his urine became bright red. Even though he had no other symptoms, he called his physician. The physician ordered a urinalysis and urine cytology, revealing gross hematuria and poorly differentiated abnormal cells. Cystoscopy and tissue biopsy confirm a stage C tumor involving the bladder trigone. Mr. Hussain is admitted for a radical cystectomy and continent urinary diversion.

ASSESSMENT

Mr. Hussain's admission history, obtained by Tara Mills, RN, his primary nurse, indicates that he has lost 10 to 15 pounds during the last few months. He smoked two to three packs of cigarettes per day for 40 years, but cut back to a pack a day about a year ago. He says he could not quit smoking entirely. He drinks five to six cups of coffee daily and consumes a moderate amount of alcohol, averaging three to four drinks a day. Mr. Hussain says that he is "a little nervous about surgery and what they're going to find." Ms. Mills notes that he fidgets and talks rapidly throughout their interview. He also expresses concern about how he will handle the pain after surgery, because he had never been hospitalized before his cystoscopy. Physical assessment findings include T 98.2°F (36.7°C) PO, P 84, R 18, and BP 154/86. Examinations of the skin, neuromuscular, and cardiac systems are within normal limits. Scattered expiratory crackles are noted on auscultation of lung fields. Bowel sounds are very active; Mr. Hussain explains that he began taking his bowel-preparation laxative the day before admission. Slight tenderness is noted in the suprapubic region. Mr. Hussain's urine is clear and bright pink. CBC and chemistry screening results are within normal limits. Surgery is planned for 9:00 AM the following day.

DIAGNOSES

- *Anxiety* related to undetermined extent of disease and fear of pain
- *Readiness for Enhanced Knowledge* related to care and management of continent urinary diversion
- *Impaired Urinary Elimination* related to cystectomy and urinary diversion
- *Risk for Impaired Gas Exchange* related to smoking history and effects of anesthesia

EXPECTED OUTCOMES

- Verbalize decreased feelings of anxiety.
- Demonstrate appropriate postoperative pain relief through subjective reports of pain severity and objective findings.
- Be able to care for urinary diversion and surrounding skin prior to discharge.
- Demonstrate self-catheterization of stoma using appropriate technique prior to discharge.

- Maintain normal urine output with acceptable color and clarity and no signs of infection.
- Maintain adequate gas exchange as evidenced by good skin color, O_2 saturation greater than 95%, and clear lung sounds on auscultation.

PLANNING AND IMPLEMENTATION

- Spend as much time as possible with Mr. Hussain and his family preoperatively, answering questions fully and encouraging expression of fears.
- Provide written and verbal explanations when feasible.
- Administer analgesia on a regular basis for the first 48 to 72 hours. Monitor for objective signs of unrelieved pain.
- Explain all procedures related to stoma and diversion care as they are being performed.
- Encourage Mr. Hussain to look at stoma and touch it when ready.
- Teach stoma and skin care, as well as self-catheterization, emphasizing measures to prevent skin irritation and urinary tract infection.
- Monitor urine output, color, clarity, and consistency every hour for first 24 hours, then every 4 hours for 24 hours, then every 8 hours. Report output of less than 30 mL per hour, bright bleeding, excessively cloudy or malodorous urine.
- Assist with use of incentive spirometer every hour while awake. Ambulate as soon as possible. Assess lung sounds every 4 hours, reporting increased crackles or diminished breath sounds.
- Refer Mr. and Mrs. Hussain to local stoma group on discharge.

EVALUATION

On discharge, Mr. Hussain has performed self-catheterization and stoma and skin care several times. His wife also is able to catheterize the stoma and demonstrate skin care. His urine is pale yellow and slightly cloudy. Mr. Hussain is ambulating independently and using oxycodone (Percocet) twice a day for pain relief. His lungs are clear, and he is very proud of having "survived" 7 days without a cigarette. He says, "Now I'm going to shoot for 7 weeks, then 7 months, then 7 years without a smoke!" A home health referral is made to continue teaching Mr. Hussain to care for his diversion and appliance.

CRITICAL THINKING IN THE NURSING PROCESS

1. How does cigarette smoking contribute to the increased risk of urinary tract tumors?
2. Suppose Mr. Hussain had become confused, disoriented, and tremorous and had begun to experience visual hallucinations 2 to 3 days postoperatively. What would you suspect the cause to be? What would be the appropriate response?
3. Develop a care plan for Mr. Hussain for the nursing diagnosis *Risk for Sexual Dysfunction*.

See Evaluating Your Response in Appendix C.

- Encourage looking at, touching, and caring for the stoma and appliance as soon as possible. Allow the patient to proceed gradually, providing support and encouragement. *Accepting the stoma as part of the self is vital to adapting to the changed body image and is indicated by a willingness to provide self-care.*
- Discuss concerns about returning to usual activities, perceived relationship changes, and resumption of sexual relations. Provide referral to support group or provide for contact with someone who has successfully adjusted to a urinary

diversion. *Patients and families may be reluctant to discuss topics of concern. An atmosphere of openness and acceptance facilitates expression of concerns and anxieties related to the changed body image.*

Risk for Infection

Diagnostic instrumentation procedures, surgical manipulation, and disruption of normal urinary tract defense mechanisms increase the risk of ascending urinary tract infection. When an ileal conduit or artificial bladder is created using bowel tissue, the normal bacteriostatic activity of bladder mucosa is lost. In addition, the peristaltic action of the ureters may be disrupted, and the vesicoureteral junction no longer prevents urine reflux. Adjunctive chemotherapy or radiation treatments may impair normal immune function and further increase the risk of infection.

- Maintain separate closed drainage systems, keeping drainage bags lower than the kidney, and prevent loops or kinks in drainage tubing, which impede urine flow. *Although urine is sterile when it leaves the kidney, bacteria grow rapidly in urine. Prevention of urine reflux is essential to preventing UTI.*
- Monitor for signs of infection: elevated temperature, cloudy or foul-smelling urine, hematuria, general malaise, back or abdominal pain, and nausea and vomiting. *Infection undermines the healing process. Early detection and treatment help prevent long-term consequences such as chronic pyelonephritis.*

> **PRACTICE ALERT**
> Impaired immune function (due to aging or the effects of chemotherapy) and urine cloudiness (related to the effects of urine on ileal mucosa) can mask usual signs of UTI such as fever and altered urine clarity. Be alert for more generalized manifestations such as increased fatigue and malaise.

- Teach signs and symptoms of infection and self-care measures to prevent UTI. *The patient with a cystectomy and ileal diversion, urostomy, or continent reservoir is at risk of UTI for life because of impaired urinary defense mechanisms. Using clean or aseptic technique in providing care, increasing fluid intake, and using measures to acidify urine minimize this risk to a certain degree but do not eliminate it.*

Community-Based Care

The need for individual and family teaching for the patient who has had surgery to treat a urinary tract tumor is significant. For many patients, surgery means a lifelong change in urinary elimination. Even the patient who has undergone transurethral excision of bladder tumors requires follow-up cystoscopy on a regular basis and needs to be alert for signs of tumor recurrence.

The patient who has had a urinary diversion needs teaching about care of the stoma and surrounding skin, prevention of urine reflux and infection, signs and symptoms of UTI and renal calculi, and, in some cases, self-catheterization using clean technique.

The Patient with Urinary Retention

Urinary retention, incomplete emptying of the bladder, can lead to overdistention of the bladder, poor detrusor muscle contractility, and inability to urinate. If the problem persists, hydroureter and hydronephrosis can result.

Physiology Review

Normally, bladder emptying is controlled by the interaction of muscle tone and the autonomic nervous system. The sympathetic nervous system (SNS) relaxes the detrusor muscle, allowing the bladder to fill with urine. The internal sphincter, a

continuation of the detrusor muscle, remains closed during filling. Pressures within the bladder remain low during filling, in contrast to high sphincter and urethral pressures. Voluntary muscles of the external sphincter and pelvic floor help maintain these high pressures. When the bladder contains 150 to 300 mL of urine, signals from stretch receptors in the bladder wall are transmitted to the spinal cord and cerebral cortex. Reflexive bladder emptying can be consciously inhibited. During *micturition* (bladder emptying), parasympathetic stimulation causes the detrusor muscle of the bladder fundus to contract, opening the internal sphincter. The external sphincter then relaxes, allowing urine to flow out.

Pathophysiology

Either mechanical obstruction of the bladder outlet or a functional problem can cause urinary retention. *Benign prostatic hypertrophy (BPH) is a common cause;* difficulty initiating and maintaining urine flow is often the presenting complaint in men with BPH. Fecal impaction may be a contributing factor in urinary retention, particularly in older adults or immobile patients. Acute inflammation associated with infection or trauma of the bladder, urethra, or perineal tissues may also interfere with micturition. Scarring due to repeated UTI can lead to urethral stricture and a mechanical obstruction. Bladder calculi may also obstruct the urethral opening from the bladder.

Surgery, particularly abdominal or pelvic surgery, may disrupt detrusor muscle function, leading to urine retention. Drugs also may interfere with its function. Anticholinergic medications such as atropine, glycopyrrolate (Robinul), propantheline bromide (Pro-Banthine), scopolamine hydrochloride (Transderm-Scop), and others can lead to acute urinary retention and bladder distention. Many other drug groups have anticholinergic side effects and may cause urinary retention. Among these are anti-anxiety agents such as diazepam (Valium), antidepressant and tricyclic drugs such as imipramine (Tofranil), antiparkinsonian drugs, antipsychotic agents, and some sedative/hypnotic drugs. In addition, antihistamines common in over-the-counter cough, cold, allergy, and sleep-promoting drugs have anticholinergic effects and may interfere with bladder emptying. Diphenhydramine (Benadryl) is an example of a nonprescription antihistamine.

Voluntary urinary retention (particularly common among nurses!) may lead to overfilling of the bladder and a loss of detrusor muscle tone.

Manifestations

The patient with urinary retention is unable to empty the bladder completely. Overflow voiding or incontinence may occur, with 25 to 50 mL of urine eliminated at frequent intervals. Assessment reveals a firm, distended bladder that may be displaced to one side of midline. Percussion of the lower abdomen reveals a dull tone, reflective of fluid in the bladder.

Severe urinary retention with resulting bladder distention impairs the ability of the vesicoureteral junction to prevent backflow of urine into the ureters (see Figure 27–1 on page 784). Reflux of urine from the distended bladder distends the ureters (hydroureter) and kidneys (hydronephrosis).

Hydronephrosis impairs renal function, and acute renal failure can result. ∞ See Chapter 28 for more information about acute renal failure.

Interdisciplinary Care

Urinary retention is confirmed using a bladder scan or by inserting a urinary catheter (if possible) and measuring the urine output. Use of a bladder scan is preferred to reduce the risk of UTI.

An indwelling urinary catheter or intermittent straight catheterization can prevent urinary retention and overdistention of the bladder. Cholinergic medications such as bethanechol chloride (Urecholine), which promote detrusor muscle contraction and bladder emptying, may be used. A medication with no anticholinergic side effects may be substituted when urinary retention is related to drug therapy.

Mechanical obstructions are treated by removing or repairing the obstruction when possible. Resection of the prostate gland may be done for urinary retention related to BPH. Bladder calculi are removed, and measures to prevent their formation are instituted.

♋ Nursing Care

Health promotion measures to prevent urinary retention include monitoring urine output in at-risk patients and evaluating drug regimens for medications known to interfere with detrusor muscle function. Pay particular attention to elimination when these drugs are ordered for (or used by) a patient with BPH or other mechanical obstruction of urine flow.

Impaired Urinary Elimination

Nursing measures to promote urination include placing the patient in normal voiding position and providing for privacy. Additional measures include running water, placing the patient's hands in warm water, pouring warm water over the perineum, or taking a warm sitz bath.

In acute urinary retention, catheterization may be necessary to relieve bladder distention and prevent hydronephrosis. Use a relatively small catheter (16 Fr. for a man, 14 Fr. for a woman). A coudé-tipped catheter is passed more easily in the older man with an enlarged prostate. Using 2% lidocaine gel (10 mL injected into the male urethra or 6 mL injected into the female urethra) reduces discomfort during catheterization and the risk of catheter-associated infection and promotes pelvic muscle relaxation (Bardsley, 2005). Carefully observe the patient as the distended bladder drains.

> **PRACTICE ALERT**
> Some patients may experience a vasovagal response, becoming pale, sweaty, and hypotensive if the bladder is rapidly drained. Draining urine in 500-mL increments and clamping the catheter for 5 to 10 minutes between increments may prevent this response. Hematuria also may occur with rapid bladder decompression. Promptly notify the physician if hematuria develops.

Home care for the patient with urinary retention varies, depending on the cause. Some patients may be taught intermittent self-catheterization. Instruct all patients who have experienced urinary retention to avoid over-the-counter drugs that affect micturition, especially those with an anticholinergic effect (allergy and cold medications, many nonprescription sleep aids). Other home care measures include double-voiding (urinate, remain on the toilet for 2 to 5 minutes, then urinate again), scheduled voiding, or, when other measures fail, an indwelling catheter. When an indwelling catheter is necessary, teach the patient and family to use clean technique when changing from overnight bag to leg bag, and to promptly report signs of UTI to the primary care provider.

The Patient with Neurogenic Bladder

The neurologic connections influencing bladder filling, the perception of fullness and the need to void, and bladder emptying are complex. Disruption of the central or peripheral nervous systems may interfere with normal mechanisms, causing **neurogenic bladder**.

Pathophysiology

As noted in the physiology section on urinary retention, bladder filling and emptying are controlled by the central nervous system (CNS). This neurologic control can be disrupted at any level: the cerebral cortex (voluntary impulses), the micturition center of the midbrain, the spinal cord tracts, or the peripheral nerves of the bladder itself.

Spastic Bladder Dysfunction

A simple reflex arc exists between the bladder and the spinal cord at levels S_2 through S_4. The stimulus of more than 400 mL of urine in the bladder causes reflex contraction of the detrusor muscle and bladder emptying unless voluntary control (cerebral input) is used to suppress it. Disruption of CNS transmission above the sacral spinal cord segment typically leads to *spastic neurogenic bladder*. Both sensory and voluntary control of urination are interrupted partially or totally, while the sacral reflex arc remains intact. The stimuli generated by bladder filling cause frequent spontaneous detrusor muscle contraction and involuntary bladder emptying. Spinal cord injury above the sacral segment is the most common cause of a spastic bladder. Other causes include stroke, multiple sclerosis, and other CNS lesions.

Flaccid Bladder Dysfunction

Damage to the sacral spinal cord at the level of the reflex arc, the cauda equina, or the sacral nerve roots causes loss of detrusor muscle tone and a *flaccid neurogenic bladder*. The perception of bladder fullness is lost, and the bladder becomes overdistended, with weak and ineffective detrusor muscle contractions. Flaccid neurogenic bladder is seen with myelomeningocele and during the spinal shock phase of a spinal cord injury above the sacral region. During the spinal shock phase, all reflex activity below the level of spinal cord injury is suppressed.

Peripheral neuropathies may also cause bladder atony and overfilling. Either sensory or motor pathways (or both) may be disrupted, leading to incomplete bladder emptying and large residual volumes after voiding. Diabetes mellitus is the most common cause of peripheral bladder neuropathy. Other causes include multiple sclerosis, chronic alcoholism, and prolonged overdistention of the bladder.

Interdisciplinary Care

Management of neurogenic bladder focuses on maintaining continence and avoiding complications associated with overfilling or incomplete emptying of the bladder. Because self-care is the goal, teaching is a primary intervention for the healthcare team.

Diagnosis

The following diagnostic tests may be ordered for the patient with a neurogenic bladder:

- *Urine culture* to detect possible UTI related to impaired bladder function.
- *Urinalysis* and *eGFR, serum creatinine* and *BUN* to evaluate renal function. See Table 28–2 on page 826 for normal BUN and creatinine levels. Ascending infection or hydronephrosis

resulting from bladder overfilling and vesicoureteral reflux can damage the kidneys. Impaired renal function may lead to blood cells or protein in the urine, and elevated BUN and creatinine levels.

- *Postvoid bladder scan* to measure residual urine. Amounts greater than 50 mL may indicate ineffective detrusor muscle contractions, common in neurogenic bladder.
- *Cystometrography* to evaluate bladder filling and the detrusor muscle tone and function. See page 774 for nursing care of the patient undergoing cystometrography.

Medications

Medications may be prescribed to increase or decrease the contractility of the detrusor muscle, to increase or decrease the tone of the internal sphincter, or to relax the external urethral sphincter.

Bethanechol, a cholinergic drug, stimulates detrusor muscle contraction in flaccid neurogenic bladder. It is generally used to manage short-term urinary retention (e.g., following surgery or childbirth). It may be used in combination with bladder-training techniques to promote complete emptying of a neurogenic

---

MEDICATION ADMINISTRATION   The Patient with Neurogenic Bladder

ANTICHOLINERGIC DRUGS TO TREAT SPASTIC BLADDER

Darifenacin (Enablex)
Oxybutynin (Ditropan, Ditropan XL)
Solifenacin succinate (VESIcare)
Trospium (Sanctura)
Tolterodine (Detrol, Detrol LA)
Propantheline bromide (Pro-Banthine)
Flavoxate hydrochloride (Urispas)

Anticholinergic drugs inhibit the response to acetylcholine, relaxing the detrusor muscle and increasing internal sphincter tone. The combination of detrusor relaxation and internal sphincter contraction increases the bladder capacity of patients with spastic or hyperreflexive neurogenic bladder. Of these medications, darifenacin, solifenacin succinate, and tolterodine have the most specific effects on the detrusor muscle with fewer anticholinergic side effects.

Nursing Responsibilities

- Assess for contraindications, such as glaucoma, gastrointestinal or urinary tract obstruction, severe ulcerative colitis or toxic megacolon, unstable cardiovascular status, or myasthenia gravis.
- Observe for the desired effect of increased bladder capacity with decreased incontinence and spasm.
- Monitor for possible interaction with other drugs such as narcotic analgesics, antidysrhythmic medications, antihistamines, antidepressants, or psychoactive drugs.
- Monitor heart rate and blood pressure, especially when given to patients with known cardiovascular disease.
- Assess for adverse effects such as urinary hesitancy or retention, dysrhythmias, mental status changes, and gastrointestinal disturbances.

Health Education for the Patient and Family

- Take the drug as ordered. Some of these drugs (e.g., trospium) need to be taken on an empty stomach for optimal absorption, others may be taken irrespective of food intake.
- Promptly report eye pain, rapid heart beat, difficulty breathing, rash or hives, or changes in mental function to your primary care provider.

- These drugs may cause drowsiness or blurred vision. Use caution when driving, operating machinery, or performing other tasks requiring mental acuity.
- Hard candies help relieve dry mouth associated with these drugs.
- Do not use alcohol or nonprescription antihistamines while taking these drugs.

CHOLINERGIC DRUGS TO STIMULATE MICTURITION

Bethanechol chloride (Urecholine)

Bethanechol stimulates the parasympathetic nervous system, increasing detrusor muscle tone and producing a contraction strong enough to initiate micturition. It is used primarily to treat acute postoperative and postpartum urinary retention.

Nursing Responsibilities

- Assess for contraindications, including hypersensitivity, hyperthyroidism, peptic ulcer disease, asthma, significant bradycardia or hypotension, coronary heart disease, epilepsy, and parkinsonism.
- Do not give to patients who have had recent gastrointestinal or bladder surgery or those with possible gastrointestinal or urinary tract obstruction.
- Give oral forms on an empty stomach to reduce the risk of nausea and vomiting.
- Administer parenteral bethanechol subcutaneously. Keep atropine, the antidote for bethanechol overdose or toxicity, available.
- Observe for desired effect within 30 to 60 minutes after oral administration, 5 to 15 minutes after injection.
- Assess for adverse effects such as malaise, headache, abdominal cramping, nausea, hypotension with reflex tachycardia, wheezing, and dyspnea.

Health Education for the Patient and Family

- Take the medication 1 hour before or 2 hours after meals.
- Use caution when rising from a recumbent or sitting position; you may feel dizzy or light-headed.

bladder. Anticholinesterase drugs such as neostigmine (Prostigmin) and pyridostigmine (Mestinon) also may be used to increase detrusor muscle tone.

Anticholinergic drugs (parasympathetic blockers) relax the detrusor muscle and contract the internal sphincter, increasing bladder capacity in patients with spastic bladder dysfunction. Oxybutynin (Ditropan), tolterodine (Detrol), darifenacin (Enablex), solifenacin succinate (VESIcare), and trospium (Sanctura) inhibit the muscarinic effects of acetylcholine on smooth muscle, reducing detrusor muscle spasticity and promoting bladder filling. Other anticholinergic drugs also may be used, including propantheline (Pro-Banthine) or flavoxate (Urispas). Dry mouth, blurred vision, and constipation are potential adverse effects of anticholinergic medications. See the Medication Administration box for drugs used to modify detrusor muscle activity on the previous page.

Nutrition
Dietary measures to reduce the risk for UTI and urinary calculi may be suggested for the patient with neurogenic bladder. A moderate to high fluid intake and a diet that acidifies the urine are helpful. Cranberry juice is recommended to maintain urine acidity. See Table 27–3 for additional foods to include or avoid in the diet to help prevent UTI and urolithiasis. The timing of fluid intake may be regulated to promote continence.

Bladder Retraining
Patients with spastic neurogenic bladder may use measures to stimulate reflex voiding, allowing scheduled toileting. Techniques include using trigger points, for example, stroking or pinching the abdomen, inner thigh, or glans penis. Pulling pubic hairs, tapping the suprapubic region, or inserting a gloved finger into the rectum and gently stretching the anal sphincter can also stimulate urination.

The *Credé's method* (applying pressure to the suprapubic region with the fingers of one or both hands), manual pressure on the abdomen, and the Valsalva maneuver (bearing down while holding one's breath) promote bladder emptying for the patient with a spastic or flaccid bladder.

> **PRACTICE ALERT**
> Increasing lower abdominal and bladder pressure with the Credé's method can stimulate autonomic dysreflexia in some patients with spinal cord injuries. Autonomic dysreflexia is a medical emergency in which the blood pressure rises rapidly due to SNS stimulation.

∞ See Chapter 44 for a discussion of autonomic dysreflexia.

The patient with a flaccid bladder may require catheterization to completely empty the bladder. An indwelling catheter may be used initially, but intermittent catheterization is preferred. Clean intermittent self-catheterization is performed every 3 to 4 hours to prevent overdistention of the bladder (see Procedure 43–1).

Surgery
Surgery may be required when urination cannot be effectively managed using more conservative measures. *Rhizotomy*, or destruction of the nerve supply to the detrusor muscle or the external sphincter, may be used for patients with hyperreflexia

or spasticity. Urinary diversion is another surgical technique used when conservative management fails. Implantation of an artificial sphincter may be useful for some patients with neurogenic bladder. See Table 27–6 for urinary diversion techniques and page 802 for nursing care of the patient undergoing a urinary diversion.

Nursing Care
Nursing care of the patient with a neurogenic bladder is directed toward promoting urinary drainage and continence, preventing complications, and teaching the patient and family self-care techniques.

Assessment
Nursing assessment for neurogenic bladder includes obtaining a complete nursing history, focusing on information related to CNS or spinal cord injury or disease, as well as disorders that affect the peripheral nervous system (e.g., diabetes). Ask about measures used to stimulate or control urination. Inspect and palpate the lower abdomen and suprapubic region for tenderness or bladder distention. Percuss the suprapubic region for a dull percussion tone indicative of a full bladder. Dullness up to the level of the umbilicus indicates at least 500 mL of urine in the bladder (Gray, 2000). Assess urine for color, clarity, and odor. Collect a specimen for analysis as indicated.

Nursing Diagnoses and Interventions
Although each patient has individual nursing care needs, examples of nursing diagnoses appropriate for the patient with a neurogenic bladder include the following:

- *Impaired Urinary Elimination* related to impaired bladder innervation
- *Toileting Self-Care Deficit* related to neurologic injury
- *Risk for Impaired Skin Integrity* related to urinary incontinence
- *Risk for Infection* related to impaired urination reflex

Community-Based Care
Include the following in teaching for the patient with neurogenic bladder and family members:

- Measures to stimulate reflex voiding and promote bladder emptying
- Use of prescribed medications, including desired and adverse effects, and interactions with other drugs
- Manifestations of UTI or urolithiasis, and measures to reduce the risk of these complications

The Patient with Urinary Incontinence
The most common manifestation of impaired bladder control is **urinary incontinence (UI)**, or involuntary urination. UI can have a significant impact on patients, leading to physical problems such as skin breakdown, infection, and rashes. Psychosocial consequences include embarrassment, isolation and withdrawal, feelings of worthlessness and helplessness, and depression.

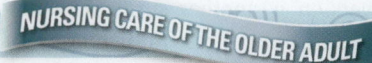

NURSING CARE OF THE OLDER ADULT   **Minimizing the Risk for UTI and UI**

Older adults have a higher incidence of two common urinary tract disorders: UTI and UI.

URINARY TRACT INFECTION

Aging affects normal protective mechanisms to prevent UTI. The pH of urine increases with aging, allowing bacteria to grow and multiply more readily. Glucosuria, more common in older adults due to the higher incidence of diabetes, facilitates bacterial growth. Incomplete bladder emptying and urinary retention are more common due to problems such as prostatic hypertrophy in men, bladder prolapse in women, and neurogenic bladder in both sexes. Changes in vaginal pH in women and decreased prostatic secretions in men may also contribute to an increased incidence of UTI.

While many UTIs in older adults are asymptomatic and self-limited, infections can lead to bacteremia, sepsis, and shock. Manifestations of UTI in the elderly include dysuria, urgency, frequency, incontinence, occasional hematuria, and confusion. Symptoms such as fever, chills, and flank pain and tenderness may be absent. Dementia may make diagnosis more difficult.

URINARY INCONTINENCE

UI, the involuntary loss of urine, is a common problem in older adults. While incontinence should never be considered a *normal* consequence of aging, age-related changes contribute to its development. Bladder capacity tends to decline with age and involuntary bladder muscle contractions are more common. Fluid ingested during the day tends to be excreted later in the day and into the night. In women, decreased estrogen levels and pelvic muscle relaxation decrease bladder outlet and urethral resistance pressures. Decreased estrogen also causes atrophic vaginitis and urethritis, with manifestations of dysuria and urgency. In men, the prostate enlarges with aging. Other risk factors for UI in older adults include impaired mobility and chronic degenerative diseases, impaired cognition, medications, low fluid intake, diabetes, and stroke.

Assessing for Home Care

Assessment for urinary problems in the older adult focuses on risk factors, the extent and manifestations of the disorder, and contributing factors. Using clear language, ask about problems with urine loss, its frequency, and any contributing factors. Inquire about frequency, urgency, and burning on urination. Identify current medications and the time of day each is taken. Assess patterns of fluid intake and output. Assess the abdomen for evidence of bladder distention or tenderness. Perform a mental status examination if indicated.

Assess the home environment (whether in the community or a residential living facility) for possible barriers to urinary elimination:

- Inadequate lighting, particularly at night
- Narrow doorways that may interfere with access to the toilet
- Inadequate toilet facilities
- The need for mobility aids such as safety bars, a raised toilet seat, or a bedside commode

Teaching for Home Care

Discuss the following points to help prevent UTI and UI in the older adult:

- Maintain a generous fluid intake. Reduce or eliminate fluid intake after the evening meal to reduce nocturia.
- Wear comfortable clothing that is easy to remove for toileting.
- Maintain good hygiene, but do not bathe more often than necessary; frequent bathing and feminine hygiene sprays or douches may dry perineal tissues, increasing the risk of UTI or UI.
- Perform pelvic muscle exercises (Kegel exercises) several times a day to increase perineal muscle tone.
- Reduce consumption of caffeine-containing beverages (coffee, tea, colas), citrus juices, and artificially sweetened beverages containing NutraSweet.
- Use behavioral techniques such as scheduled toileting, habit training, and bladder training to reduce the frequency of incontinence. *Scheduled toileting* is toileting at regular intervals (e.g., every 2 to 4 hours). *Habit training* is toileting the patient on a schedule that corresponds with the normal pattern. *Bladder training* gradually increases the bladder capacity by increasing the intervals between voidings and resisting the urge to void.
- See your primary care provider regularly for a pelvic or prostate exam.
- For women, discuss possible benefits and risks of hormone replacement therapy, physical therapy, or surgery to treat incontinence.
- Report a change in urine color, odor, or clarity, or symptoms such as burning, frequency, or urgency to your primary care provider.

Resources for Home Care

- National Association for Continence website

Incidence and Prevalence

Up to 25 million people in the United States have some degree of urinary incontinence. The estimated cost of managing UI is $14.2 billion yearly (Bradway et al., 2008). UI is especially common among older patients (see the box above). UI often leads to institutionalization; in long-term care, foster care, and homebound populations, the incidence is more than 50% (National Association for Continence, 2009; NKUDIC, 2009). The actual prevalence of urinary incontinence is nearly impossible to determine. Embarrassment and the availability of products to protect clothing and prevent detection contribute to patients' not seeking evaluation of and treatment for incontinence.

FAST FACTS

- UI is especially common among older patients. Although the prevalence of urinary incontinence increases in older adults, it is *not* a normal consequence of aging and it *can* be treated.
- An estimated 38% or more of women aged 60 and older experience UI.
- Among men aged 60 and older, the prevalence is about 17%.
- Annual healthcare costs associated with UI exceed $463 million; when the amount spent on commercial products to manage UI is included, spending likely exceeds $14 billion annually.

Pathophysiology

Urinary continence requires input from the CNS, a bladder able to expand and contract and sphincters that can maintain a urethral pressure higher than that in the bladder. Intact cognition, mobility, motivation, and manual dexterity also are necessary to maintain continence. Mechanically, incontinence results when the pressure within the urinary bladder exceeds urethral resistance, allowing urine to escape. Any condition causing higher than normal bladder pressures or reduced urethral resistance can potentially result in incontinence. Relaxation of the pelvic musculature, disruption of cerebral and nervous system control, and disturbances of the bladder and its musculature are common contributing factors.

Incontinence may be an acute, self-limited disorder, or it may be chronic. The causes may be congenital or acquired, reversible or irreversible. Congenital disorders associated with incontinence include *epispadias* (absence of the upper wall of the urethra), and *meningomyelocele* (a neural tube defect in which a portion of the spinal cord and its surrounding meninges protrude through the vertebral column). CNS or spinal cord trauma, stroke, and chronic neurologic disorders such as multiple sclerosis and Parkinson's disease are examples of acquired, irreversible causes of incontinence. Reversible causes include acute confusion, medications such as diuretics or sedatives, prostatic enlargement, vaginal and urethral atrophy, UTI, and fecal impaction.

Incontinence is commonly categorized as stress incontinence, urge incontinence (also known as overactive bladder), overflow incontinence, and functional incontinence. Table 27–7 summarizes each type with its physiologic cause and associated factors. *Mixed incontinence*, with elements of both stress and urge incontinence, is common. *Total incontinence* is loss of all voluntary control over urination, with urine loss occurring without stimulus and in all positions.

Incontinence is associated with an increased risk for falls, fractures, pressure ulcers, urinary tract infection, and depression. It contributes to the stress of caregivers, and often is a factor in institutionalizing the patient.

Interdisciplinary Care

UI management is directed at identifying and correcting the cause if possible. If the underlying disorder cannot be corrected, techniques to manage urine output can often be taught.

Evaluation for incontinence begins with a complete history, including specific questions about lower urinary tract symptoms and the duration, frequency, volume, and associated circumstances of urine loss. A voiding diary (Figure 27–9 ■) is often used to collect detailed information. The history also includes information about chronic or acute illnesses, previous surgeries, and current medication use, both prescription and over the counter.

Physical assessment includes abdominal, rectal, and pelvic assessment as well as evaluation of mental and neurologic status, mobility, and dexterity. Findings often associated with incontinence in women include weak abdominal and pelvic muscle tone, cystocele or urethrocele, and atrophic vaginitis. In men, an enlarged prostate gland is the physical finding most commonly associated with incontinence.

See the Moving Evidence into Action feature on page 813 for evidence-based practice for diagnosing lower urinary tract symptoms in women.

TABLE 27–7 Types of Urinary Incontinence

	DESCRIPTION	PATHOPHYSIOLOGY	CONTRIBUTING FACTORS
Stress	Loss of urine associated with increased intra-abdominal pressure during sneezing, coughing, lifting. Quantity of urine lost is usually small.	Relaxation of pelvic musculature and weakness of urethra and surrounding muscles and tissues leads to decreased urethral resistance.	■ Multiple pregnancies ■ Decreased estrogen levels ■ Short urethra, change in angle between bladder and urethra ■ Abdominal wall weakness ■ Prostate surgery ■ Increased intra-abdominal pressure due to tumor, ascites, obesity
Urge	Involuntary loss of urine associated with a strong urge to void	Hypertonic or overactive detrusor muscle leads to increased pressure within bladder and inability to inhibit voiding.	■ Neurologic disorders such as stroke, Parkinson's disease, multiple sclerosis; peripheral nervous system disorders ■ Detrusor muscle overactivity associated with bladder outlet obstruction, aging, or disorders such as diabetes
Overflow	Inability to empty bladder, resulting in overdistention and frequent loss of small amounts of urine	Outlet obstruction or lack of normal detrusor activity leads to overfilling of bladder and increased pressure.	■ Spinal cord injuries below S_2 ■ Diabetic neuropathy ■ Prostatic hypertrophy ■ Fecal impaction ■ Drugs, especially those with anticholinergic effect
Functional	Incontinence resulting from physical, environmental, or psychosocial causes	Ability to respond to the need to urinate is impaired.	■ Confusion or dementia ■ Physical disability or impaired mobility ■ Therapy or sedation ■ Depression ■ Regression

Your Daily Voiding Diary   Date _____

This diary will help you and your healthcare team identify factors causing bladder control problems. Choose a 24-hour period when you can record your fluid intake (type and amount), urine output and episodes of urine leakage, any strong urge to void just prior to leaking, and your activity when leak episodes occur. The line below illustrates how to use your diary.

Time 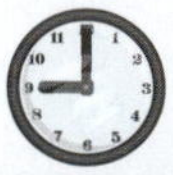	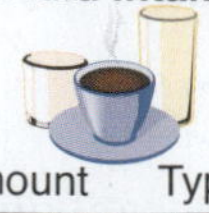 Fluid Intake		Urine Output 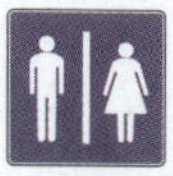			Leaks 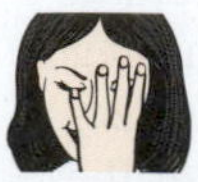			Urge		Activity
	Amount	Type							Yes	No	
7 am	2 cups	coffee	sm	(med)	lg	(sm)	med	lg	Yes		walking
			sm	med	lg	sm	med	lg			
			sm	med	lg	sm	med	lg			
			sm	med	lg	sm	med	lg			
			sm	med	lg	sm	med	lg			
			sm	med	lg	sm	med	lg			
			sm	med	lg	sm	med	lg			
			sm	med	lg	sm	med	lg			
			sm	med	lg	sm	med	lg			
			sm	med	lg	sm	med	lg			
			sm	med	lg	sm	med	lg			
			sm	med	lg	sm	med	lg			
			sm	med	lg	sm	med	lg			
			sm	med	lg	sm	med	lg			
			sm	med	lg	sm	med	lg			
			sm	med	lg	sm	med	lg			
			sm	med	lg	sm	med	lg			
			sm	med	lg	sm	med	lg			

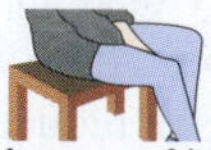

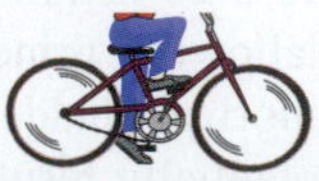

I used___pads today.   I used___diapers today.

Questions to ask my health care team: _____

_____

_____

Figure 27–9 ■ A sample voiding diary.

Source: Adapted from *Your Daily Bladder Diary*, National Kidney and Urologic Diseases Information Center, National Institute of Diabetes and Digestive and Kidney Disease (NIDDK), National Institutes of Health.

Diagnosis

With an appropriate history and physical examination, diagnostic testing rarely is required. Certain tests may, however, be done to rule out UTI or to guide treatment.

- *Urinalysis* and *urine culture* using a clean-catch specimen are done to rule out infection and other acute causes of incontinence.
- *Postvoiding residual (PVR) volume* is measured to determine how completely the bladder empties with voiding. Less than 50 mL PVR is expected; when 100 mL or more is obtained, further testing is indicated.
- *Cystometrography* is used to assess neuromuscular function of the bladder by evaluating detrusor muscle function, pressure within the bladder, and the filling pattern of the bladder.
- *Uroflowmetry* is a noninvasive test used to evaluate voiding patterns.
- *Cystoscopy* or *ultrasonography* may be ordered to identify structural disorders contributing to incontinence, such as an enlarged prostate or a tumor.

Nursing implications for the specialized studies for urinary incontinence are outlined in ∞ Chapter 26.

Medications

Both stress and urge incontinence may improve with drug treatment.

Drugs that contract the smooth muscles of the bladder neck may reduce episodes of mild stress incontinence. Duloxetine (Cymbalta), a drug that inhibits the uptake of both norepinephrine and serotonin, is the drug of choice for treating stress UI that is not fully controlled with nonpharmacologic treatment (e.g., teaching, pelvic muscle exercise). In clinical trials, this drug reduced the frequency of UI and the number of voidings per day, particularly when combined with pelvic floor muscle training. Adverse effects such as nausea, headache, insomnia and constipation are common with duloxetine, limiting its usefulness for many patients (DiPiro et al., 2008).

When incontinence is associated with postmenopausal atrophic vaginitis, estrogen therapy may be effective. Both systemic estrogens and local creams are used.

Patients with urge incontinence may be treated with preparations that increase bladder capacity. Anticholinergic drugs inhibit muscarinic receptors of the parasympathetic nervous system, reducing detrusor muscle contractions. A number of drugs have been approved to treat urge UI, including oxybutynin (Ditropan

MOVING EVIDENCE INTO ACTION — Lower Urinary Tract Symptoms in Women

The underdiagnosis and inadequate treatment of UI is a commonly recognized problem; less well recognized is the extent to which women experience lower urinary tract symptoms (LUTS) with or without accompanying UI. LUTS include storage symptoms (e.g., frequency, urgency, and nocturia), voiding symptoms (slow stream, hesitancy, straining, and terminal dribble), and postmicturition symptoms (incomplete bladder emptying, postvoiding dribble). Various studies have indicated that up to 67% of women over age 18 years experience LUTS; the prevalence increases with aging. Many women are reluctant to seek treatment for LUTS; when they do, primary care providers often do not offer appropriate treatment information.

IMPLICATIONS FOR NURSING

Asking specific questions about LUTS can facilitate identification of symptoms affecting the patient's qualify of life. Accurate assessment and diagnosis is vital to planning and implementing appropriate care and achieving the desired outcomes of continence and quality of life. Successful treatment promotes self-esteem and provides positive reinforcement for continuing planned strategies.

CRITICAL THINKING IN PATIENT CARE

1. Identify at least five questions you should ask a patient to determine the presence of LUTS. How will you follow up to identify the potential effect of LUTS on the patient's quality of life (consider activities of daily living [ADLs], employment, social interactions, intimate relationships)?
2. Identify patient teaching for a woman who experiences frequency, urgency, nocturia and postvoid dribbling but who only occasionally loses urine.
3. What nursing care measures and patient teaching will you provide for the patient with stress incontinence that may not be appropriate or necessary for the patient with urge incontinence? For the patient with urge incontinence but not stress incontinence?
4. Develop a nursing care and teaching plan using the nursing diagnosis *Readiness for Enhanced Urinary Elimination*.

Source: Bradway, C., Coyne, K., Irwin, D., & Kopp, Z. (2008). Lower urinary tract symptoms in women–A common but neglected problem. *Journal of the American Academy of Nurse Practitioners, 20*(2008), 311–318.

---

and the extended release form, Ditropan XL), tolterodine (Detrol and its longer acting form, Detrol LA), trospium (Sanctura), darifenacin (Enablex), and solifenacin (VESIcare). These drugs can be taken once or twice a day, and have fewer side effects than less specific anticholinergic drugs. These drugs are contraindicated for the patient with acute glaucoma. Urinary retention is a potential side effect that must be considered when these drugs are used (see the Medication Administration box on page 808). Studies about the use and effectiveness of botulinum toxin A to control detrusor muscle overactivity are currently underway in the United States and Europe. Botulinum toxin A is injected directly into the muscle; its effects last for a period of 3 to 9 months, necessitating repeated injections (DiPiro et al., 2008).

Surgery

Surgery may be used to treat stress incontinence associated with cystocele or urethrocele and overflow incontinence associated with an enlarged prostate gland.

Suspension of the bladder neck, a technique that brings the angle between the bladder and urethra closer to normal, is effective in treating stress incontinence associated with urethrocele in 80% to 95% of patients. A laparoscopic, vaginal, or abdominal approach may be used to perform this surgery. Care of the patient with a bladder neck suspension is outlined in the accompanying box.

Prostatectomy, using either the transurethral or suprapubic approach, is indicated for the patient who is experiencing overflow incontinence as a result of an enlarged prostate gland and urethral obstruction. Care of the patient with a prostatectomy is outlined in ∞ Chapter 49.

Other surgical procedures of potential benefit in the treatment of incontinence include implantation of an artificial sphincter, formation of a urethral sling to elevate and compress the urethra, and augmentation of the bladder with bowel segments to increase bladder capacity.

NURSING CARE OF THE PATIENT
Having a Bladder Neck Suspension

PREOPERATIVE CARE
- Provide routine preoperative care and teaching as outlined in ∞ Chapter 4.
- Discuss the need to avoid straining and the Valsalva maneuver postoperatively. Suggest measures such as increasing fluid and fiber intake and using a stool softener to prevent postoperative constipation. *Straining and increased abdominal pressure during the Valsalva maneuver may place excessive stress on suture lines and interfere with healing.*

POSTOPERATIVE CARE
- Provide routine postoperative care as outlined in ∞ Chapter 4.
- Monitor urine output, including quantity, color, and clarity. Expect urine to be pink initially, gradually clearing. *Bright red urine, excessive vaginal drainage, or incisional bleeding may indicate hemorrhage. Instrumentation of the urinary tract increases the potential for UTI; cloudy urine may be an early sign.*
- Maintain stability and patency of suprapubic and/or urethral catheters. Secure catheters in position. *Maintaining bladder decompression eliminates pressure on suture lines. Preventing movement or pulling on catheters reduces the risk for resultant pressure on surgical incisions.*
- Carefully monitor urine output after catheter removal. *Difficulty voiding is common following catheter removal. Early intervention to prevent bladder distention is important to prevent pressure on suture lines.*
- If the urethral or suprapubic catheter will remain in place on discharge, teach proper care to the patient and family members as needed. *Appropriate self-care and early recognition of problems reduce the risk for significant complications.*

Complementary Therapies

Biofeedback and relaxation techniques may help reduce episodes of UI. Biofeedback uses electronic monitors to teach conscious control over physiologic responses of which the individual is not normally aware. Developing awareness of perceptible information allows the patient to gain voluntary control over urination. Biofeedback is widely used to manage urinary incontinence.

⌘ Nursing Care

Health Promotion

Although UI rarely causes serious physical effects, it frequently has significant psychosocial effects, and can lead to lowered self-esteem, social isolation, and even institutionalization. Get the word out—inform all patients that UI is not a normal consequence of aging and that treatments are available. To reduce the incidence of UI, teach all women to perform pelvic floor muscle (Kegel) exercises (Box 27–3) to improve perineal muscle tone. Advise women to seek advice from their women's healthcare or primary care practitioner about using topical hormone therapy during menopause to maintain perineal tissue integrity. Advise older men to have routine prostate examinations to prevent urethral obstruction and overflow incontinence. Pelvic floor muscle exercises also may benefit men who experience UI following prostatectomy, but evidence supporting this is limited.

Assessment

Nursing assessment for the patient with UI includes both subjective and objective data:

- *Health history:* Voiding diary; frequency of incontinent episodes, amount of urine loss and activities associated with incontinence; methods used to deal with incontinence; use of Kegel exercises or medications; any chronic diseases, related surgeries, etc.; effects of incontinence on usual activities, including social activities.

BOX 27–3 Pelvic Floor Muscle (Kegel) Exercises

- Identify the pelvic muscles with these techniques:
  - Stop the flow of urine during voiding and hold for a few seconds.
  - Tighten the muscles at the vaginal entrance around a gloved finger or tampon.
  - Tighten the muscles around the anus as though resisting defecation.
- Perform exercises by tightening pelvic muscles, holding for 10 seconds, and relaxing for 10 to 15 seconds. Continue the sequence (tighten, hold, relax) for 10 repetitions.
- Keep abdominal muscles and breathing relaxed while performing exercises.
- Initially, exercises should be performed twice per day, working up to four times a day.
- Encourage exercising at a specific time each day or in conjunction with another daily activity (such as bathing or watching the news). Establish a routine because these exercises should be continued for life.
- Assistive devices, such as vaginal cones and biofeedback, may be useful for patients who have difficulty identifying appropriate muscle groups.

- *Physical examination:* Physical and mental status, including any physical limitations or impaired cognition; inspect, palpate, and percuss abdomen for bladder distention; inspect perineal tissues for redness, irritation, or tissue breakdown; observe for bulging of bladder into vagina when bearing down; assess pelvic muscle tone as indicated.

Nursing Diagnoses and Interventions

In planning nursing care, consider the patient's mental status, mobility, and motivation. Behavioral techniques can be effective, but require long-term commitment and the physical and mental capability to use them.

Nursing care and modification of routines can restore continence fully or partially even in the institutionalized patient. Scheduled toileting, bladder training, and prompted voiding combined with positive reinforcement such as praise can reduce the need for diapers, incontinence pads, and indwelling catheters.

See the Case Study & Nursing Care Plan on page 816 for additional nursing diagnoses and interventions for the patient with urinary incontinence.

Readiness for Enhanced Urinary Elimination

Exercises to strengthen pelvic floor muscles, dietary modifications, and bladder training programs often are effective to restore and maintain continence.

- Instruct to keep a voiding diary, recording the time and amount of all fluid intake and urinary output, status at the time of voiding (dry or wet) and on arising from sleep, and activities. *Voiding diaries provide valuable information for identifying the type of incontinence and possible measures to reduce or eliminate incontinent episodes.*
- Teach pelvic floor muscle exercises (see Box 27–3). Instruct to consciously tighten pelvic muscles when the need to void is perceived and to relax the abdomen while walking to the bathroom. *Improved pelvic muscle strength helps retain urine and prevent stress incontinence by increasing urethral pressure. Exercises also decrease abnormal detrusor muscle contractions, decreasing pressure within the bladder.*

PRACTICE ALERT
Do not advise patients who have difficulty emptying the bladder completely to stop urine flow while voiding to identify pelvic floor muscles. Repeated interruption of micturition can interfere with complete bladder emptying and increase the risk for UTI.

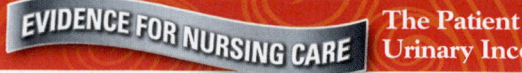
EVIDENCE FOR NURSING CARE — The Patient with Urinary Incontinence

Selected resources that nurses may find helpful when planning evidence-based nursing care follow.

- Dowling-Castronovo, A., & Bradway, C. (2008). Urinary Incontinence. *Nursing Standard of Practice Protocol: Urinary incontinence (UI) in older adults admitted to acute care.* Hartford Institute for Geriatric Nursing, New York University College of Nursing.

- Using the patient's voiding diary, suggest dietary and fluid intake modifications to reduce stress and urge incontinence. Include limiting caffeine, alcohol, citrus juice, and artificial sweetener consumption; limiting fluid intake to no less than 1.5 to 2.0 L per day; and limiting evening fluid intake. *Caffeine, alcohol, and citrus juices are bladder irritants and tend to promote detrusor instability, increasing the risk of urge incontinence. Artificial sweeteners may also irritate the bladder. Fluid intake of 1.5 to 2.0 L per day is adequate to maintain health for most patients; excess fluid may increase stress incontinence if bathroom facilities are not readily available.*

> **PRACTICE ALERT**
> Limiting total fluid intake to less than 1.5 to 2.0 L per day is not recommended for patients with UI. Inadequate fluid increases urine concentration, leading to bladder wall irritation and possibly increasing problems of urge incontinence.

Toileting Self-Care Deficit

Functional incontinence may be the predominant problem in an institutionalized older adult. Limited mobility, impaired vision, dementia, lack of access to facilities and privacy, and tight staffing patterns increase the risk for incontinence in previously continent residents. The primary problem in functional incontinence is an outside factor that interferes with the ability to respond normally to the urge to void. An immobilized patient may wet the bed if a call light is not within reach; a patient with Alzheimer's disease may perceive the urge to void but be unable to interpret its meaning or respond by seeking a bathroom. For these patients, self-care deficit in toileting is a primary problem.

- Assess physical and mental abilities and limitations, usual voiding pattern, and ability to assist with toileting. *A thorough assessment allows planned interventions to address specific needs and promote independence.*
- Provide assistive devices as needed to facilitate independence, such as raised toilet seats, grab bars, a bedside commode, or night-lights. *Fostering independence in toileting bolsters self-concept and maintains a positive body image.*
- Plan a toileting schedule based on the patient's normal elimination patterns to achieve approximately 300 mL of urine output with each voiding. *Allowing the bladder to fill to a point at which the urge to void is experienced and then emptying it completely helps maintain normal bladder capacity and bacteriostatic functions.*
- Position for ease of voiding—sitting for females, standing for males—and provide privacy. *Normal positioning, usual toileting facilities, and privacy enhance the ability to void on schedule and empty the bladder completely.*
- Adjust fluid intake so that the majority of fluids are consumed during times of the day when the patient is most able to remain continent. Unless fluids are restricted, maintain a fluid intake of at least 1.5 to 2.0 L per day. *An adequate fluid intake is vital to promote hydration and urinary function. Overly concentrated urine can irritate the bladder, increasing incontinence.*
- Assist with clothing that is easily removed (e.g., elastic-waist pants or loose dresses). Velcro and zipper fasteners may be easier to use than snaps and buttons. *Clothing that is difficult to remove can increase the risk of incontinence in the patient with mobility problems or impaired dexterity.*

Impaired Social Interaction

Urinary incontinence increases the risk for social isolation due to embarrassment, fear of not having ready access to a bathroom, body odor, or other factors. Social isolation, in turn, can increase problems of incontinence, because normal cues and relationships are lost, and the need to remain dry is less strongly felt.

- Assess reasons for and extent of social isolation. Verify the degree of social isolation with the patient or significant other. *Do not assume that social isolation is only related to urinary incontinence. Other problems frequently associated with aging (such as a hearing deficit) may be primary or contributing factors.*
- Refer patient for urologic examination and incontinence evaluation. *Patients who assume that urinary incontinence is a normal part of the aging process may not be aware of treatment options.*
- Explore alternative coping strategies with patient, significant other, staff, and other healthcare team members. *Protective pads or shields, good perineal hygiene, scheduled voiding, and clothing that does not interfere with toileting can enhance continence.*

Using NANDA, NIC, and NOC

Linkages between a selected NANDA nursing diagnosis, NIC, and NOC for the patient with urinary incontinence are shown in the chart that follows.

Community-Based Care

Because UI is a contributing factor in the institutionalization of many older people, patient and family teaching can have a significant impact on maintaining independence and residence in the community. Address possible causes of incontinence and appropriate treatment measures. Refer for urologic examination if not already completed. Discuss fluid intake management, perineal care, and products for clothing protection.

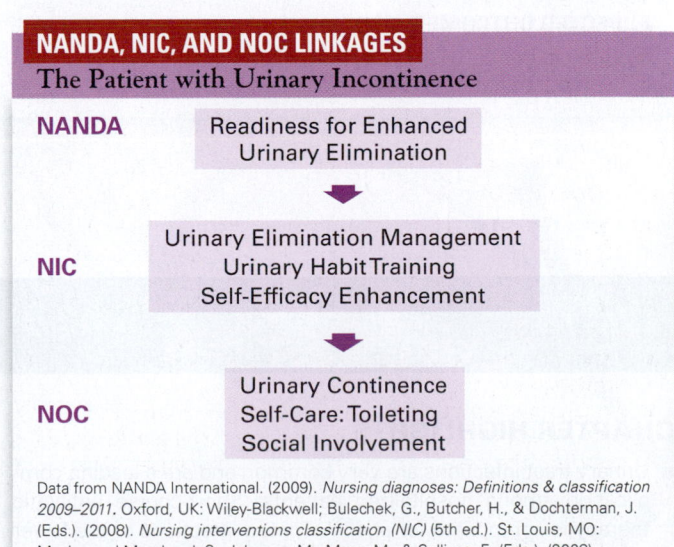

NANDA, NIC, AND NOC LINKAGES
The Patient with Urinary Incontinence

NANDA
Readiness for Enhanced Urinary Elimination

NIC
Urinary Elimination Management
Urinary Habit Training
Self-Efficacy Enhancement

NOC
Urinary Continence
Self-Care: Toileting
Social Involvement

Data from NANDA International. (2009). *Nursing diagnoses: Definitions & classification 2009–2011.* Oxford, UK: Wiley-Blackwell; Bulechek, G., Butcher, H., & Dochterman, J. (Eds.). (2008). *Nursing interventions classification (NIC)* (5th ed.). St. Louis, MO: Mosby; and Moorhead, S., Johnson, M., Maas, M., & Sullivan, E. (Eds.). (2008). *Nursing outcomes classification (NOC)* (4th ed.).St. Louis, MO: Mosby.

CASE STUDY & NURSING CARE PLAN   A Patient with Urinary Incontinence

Anna Giovanni, a 76-year-old retired teacher, has been widowed for 10 years and lives alone. Mrs. Giovanni's eldest daughter expresses concern that her mother seems increasingly reluctant to leave her apartment to visit friends and family. She reports a strong odor of urine throughout her mother's apartment and that her mother's bed is often wet. She expresses worry about needing to place her mother in a nursing home if she cannot continue to live independently.

ASSESSMENT

Jane Oberle, RN, a nurse practitioner, examines Mrs. Giovanni who admits that she has problems with urine leakage when laughing and coughing, and a strong urge to void on hearing the sound of running water. At night, her urge to void is so strong that she often cannot reach the bathroom in time. Mrs. Giovanni denies a history of UTIs, neurologic disorders, or difficulty with her bowels. She had a hysterectomy at age 52 and was on hormone replacement therapy for about 10 years afterward. She is taking digoxin 0.125 mg daily, furosemide 40 mg twice daily, and potassium chloride 20 mEq three times daily for mild heart failure.

Physical assessment reveals a moderate cystourethrocele and atrophy of vaginal and vulvar tissues. Moderate perineal dermatitis is noted. Pelvic floor strength is weak. Urinalysis is within normal limits, and postvoiding residual urine is 5 mL.

Analysis of Mrs. Giovanni's voiding diary shows moderate consumption of tea and juices throughout the day, with nine daytime voidings and four night voidings with an average volume of about 250 mL per void. She notices urine leakage most often in the late afternoon and at night. Ms. Oberle identifies a diagnosis of stress incontinence with an urgency component and decides to try a conservative approach before referring Mrs. Giovanni for further testing and possible cystourethrocele repair. She prescribes estrogen cream, tolterodine (Detrol), and a barrier cream to treat Mrs. Giovanni's vulvitis.

DIAGNOSES

- *Stress Urinary Incontinence* related to weak pelvic floor musculature and tissue atrophy
- *Urge Urinary Incontinence* related to excess intake of caffeine and citrus juices
- *Impaired Skin Integrity* related to constant contact of urine with perineal tissues
- *Ineffective Coping* related to inability to control urine leakage

EXPECTED OUTCOMES

- Remain dry between voidings and at night.
- Demonstrate improved perineal muscle strength.
- Regain and maintain perineal skin integrity.
- Return to her previous level of social activity.

PLANNING AND IMPLEMENTATION

- Teach how to identify pelvic floor muscles and how to perform Kegel exercises.
- Suggest drinking decaffeinated tea and noncitrus fruit juices (grape, apple, and cranberry).
- Encourage to minimize fluid intake after evening meal.
- Change afternoon dose of furosemide from 9:00 PM to 3:00 PM.
- Instruct to void by the clock, gradually increasing intervals from every 45 to 60 minutes to every 2 to 2.5 hours. Advise to maintain shorter voiding intervals for 2 to 3 hours after furosemide doses.
- Teach to cleanse perineal area, wiping front to back, after each voiding or incident of urine leakage.
- Introduce commercial products available for clothing and furniture protection, encouraging experimentation to identify the most helpful product(s).
- Provide a commode for bedside at night and adequate lighting to prevent injury.
- Schedule follow-up visits and evaluations to reinforce teaching.

EVALUATION

Three months after her initial visit, Mrs. Giovanni states that she is doing very well, experiencing only occasional leakage of small amounts of urine, primarily when sneezing, coughing, or laughing. She finds a minipad adequate for protection and is often able to remain dry all day. She has had no further problems with enuresis since changing her evening furosemide dose to late afternoon and limiting her fluids after dinner. She can make it to the bathroom and no longer needs the bedside commode. Her perineal tissue is intact, and she demonstrates improved muscle strength. Her daughter says her mother is beginning to resume her normal social activities, and that she is no longer worried about her mother's ability to care for herself independently.

CRITICAL THINKING IN THE NURSING PROCESS

1. What factors in Mrs. Giovanni's past medical history and current medication regimen contributed to her nighttime incontinence?
2. What is the rationale for including an intervention to teach Mrs. Giovanni about perineal cleansing as part of her care plan?
3. Develop a care plan for Mrs. Giovanni for the nursing diagnosis *Situational Low Self-Esteem* related to urinary incontinence.

See Evaluating Your Response in Appendix C.

CHAPTER HIGHLIGHTS

- Urinary tract infections are very common and are a leading complication among hospitalized patients. Short-course antibiotic therapy is appropriate for uncomplicated infections of the lower urinary tract that are not associated with the presence of an indwelling urinary catheter.
- Teach patients about perineal hygiene and the importance of maintaining adequate fluid intake as measures to help prevent UTI.
- Urinary stones (most commonly kidney stones in the United States) can obstruct the urinary tract at any level, and cause significant pain as they move from the kidney through the ureter.

Instruct patients who have had a kidney stone to maintain a generous fluid intake, particularly during exercise and warm weather, to reduce the risk of further stone formation.

- The risk for bladder cancer is greater among men than women, and cigarette smoking is the most significant risk factor for bladder cancer. Most tumors can be resected transurethrally if diagnosed early, before spreading to deeper layers of the bladder wall, the lymph nodes, and adjacent tissue.

- When resection of the urinary bladder is necessary, a urinary diversion is created to collect urine. A collection appliance must be worn constantly on an ileal conduit; when a continent urinary diversion is created, the pouch is emptied by intermittent catheterization of the stoma.

- Urinary retention may occur as a result of some medications, neurologic damage or disease, or obstruction (e.g., an enlarged prostate gland). If the underlying condition cannot be treated, medications or intermittent catheterization are used to promote bladder emptying.

- Older adults in particular are at risk for urinary incontinence, a treatable condition. A health history, voiding diary, and diagnostic testing are used to establish the type of urinary incontinence and direct treatments such as surgery, pelvic floor muscle exercises, medications, and scheduled toileting.

TEST YOURSELF NCLEX-RN® REVIEW

1. A 23-year-old woman presents to the urgency clinic with symptoms of a UTI. The nursing history reveals that the patient was treated 3 months previously for a UTI. What additional question should the nurse ask?
   1. "Did you complete your antibiotic prescription for your first UTI?"
   2. "What form of birth control are you using?"
   3. "Does your partner have similar symptoms?"
   4. "How much fluid do you drink each day?"

2. A 58-year-old woman presents at her primary care provider's office with symptoms of frequency, urgency, nocturia, dysuria, and cloudy, rust-colored urine for the third time in the past 2 years. The nurse should plan to include which of the following in her teaching for this patient? **Select all that apply.**
   1. return to the office in 10 days for follow-up culture
   2. preprocedure instruction for an IVP
   3. the potential benefits of estrogen vaginal cream
   4. recommendations for perineal cleansing
   5. recommendations for screening cystoscopy

3. Recognizing the risk for urolithiasis in the immobilized patient, the nurse appropriately plans to do which of the following?
   1. Administer a calcium supplement.
   2. Regularly monitor urine pH.
   3. Maintain an indwelling urinary catheter.
   4. Increase fluid intake to 3000 mL per day.

4. A patient admitted with possible kidney stones develops sudden complaints of acute crampy pain on the left side that radiates into the groin. He is nauseated, and vomits clear fluid. On voiding, his urine is pink. The most appropriate response by the nurse is which of the following?
   1. Obtain a bladder scan to assess for residual urine.
   2. Administer the prescribed narcotic analgesic.
   3. Notify the physician.
   4. Strain all urine.

5. The nurse teaching a group of community members about wellness and disease prevention includes which of the following as a measure to reduce the risk for bladder cancer?
   1. Do not start smoking; if you smoke, stop.
   2. Avoid using hair dyes and pesticides in the home.
   3. Limit your intake of coffee and other caffeinated beverages.
   4. Empty your bladder every 2 hours.

6. At a local health fair, a man remarks to the nurse that his urine occasionally appears pink. He wonders if this is anything to be concerned about. How should the nurse respond?
   1. Instruct the man to notify his physician if he develops pain or difficulty voiding.
   2. Advise the man to make an appointment to see his physician.
   3. Instruct the man to track the relationship between urine color and his activities.
   4. Tell the man to increase his fluid intake to 2 1/2 to 3 quarts per day.

7. The nurse evaluates her teaching as effective when the patient with a newly created continent ileal diversion is able to do which of the following?
   1. Demonstrate care for the collection device.
   2. State the importance of promptly reporting cloudy urine to the physician.
   3. Demonstrate self-catheterization of the stoma.
   4. Identify factors contributing to his risk for bladder cancer.

8. The nurse identifies which of the following as a high-priority goal for a patient with stress incontinence?
   1. can identify products for protecting clothing and furniture
   2. states chronic and benign nature of the disorder
   3. performs pelvic floor muscle exercises as taught at least twice a day
   4. limits intake of beverages containing artificial sweeteners

9. A patient tells the nurse that she has difficulty getting to the bathroom in time to prevent urine leaks once she feels the need to void. What teaching should the nurse provide?
   1. Limit intake of caffeine-containing beverages, particularly in the evening.
   2. Establish a voiding schedule, emptying her bladder at least every 2 hours.
   3. Discuss potential benefits of bladder suspension surgery with her physician.
   4. Wear clothing that is easily removed for toileting.

10. The nurse caring for a patient in the spinal shock phase following spinal cord injury appropriately plans to do which of the following?
    1. Insert a Foley catheter to accurately measure output.
    2. Stimulate voiding using Credé's method.
    3. Assess for urinary retention following each voiding.
    4. Catheterize with straight catheter every 3 to 4 hours.

See Test Yourself answers in Appendix C.

BIBLIOGRAPHY

American Cancer Society. (2009). *Cancer facts and figures 2009.* Atlanta: Author.

American College of Obstetricians and Gynecologists (ACOG). (2008 March). Treatment of urinary tract infections in nonpregnant women. Washington, DC: Author.

Barclay, L. (2008 March 17). New guidelines for management of urinary tract infection in nonpregnant women. *Medscape Medical News.* Retrieved from www.medscape.com

Bardsley, A. (2005). Use of lubricant gels in urinary catheterization. *Nursing Standard, 20*(8), 41–46.

Bishop, T. (2008 June 6). Urinalysis (urine testing) can provide valuable information about a patient's condition, allowing the detection of systemic disease and infection. *Practice Nurse 2008, 35*(12), 18–20.

Bradway, C., Coyne, K., & Kopp, Z. (2008). Lower urinary tract symptoms in women–A common but neglected problem. *Journal of the American Academy of Nurse Practitioners, 20*(2008), 311–318.

Bulechek, G., Butche, H., & Dochterman, J. (Eds.). (2008). *Nursing interventions classification (NIC)* (5th ed.). St. Louis, MO: Mosby.

Copstead, L. & Banasik, J. (2010). *Pathophysiology* (4th ed.). St. Louis, MO: Elsevier/Saunders.

Davis, C. (2008 April). The cost of containment. *Nursing Older People, 20*(3), 24–26.

DiPiro, J., Talbert, R., Yee, G., Matzke, G., Wells, B., & Posey, L. M. (2008). *Pharmacotherapy: A pathophysiologic approach* (7th ed.). New York, NY: McGraw-Hill.

Dowling-Castronovo, A., & Bradway, C. (2008). Urinary Incontinence. Nursing Standard of Practice Protocol: Urinary incontinence (UI) in older adults admitted to acute care. Hartford Institute for Geriatric Nursing, New York University College of Nursing.

Dowling-Castronovo, A., & Specht, J. (2009 February). Assessment of transient urinary incontinence in older adults. *American Journal of Nursing, 109*(2), 62–71.

Fauci, A., Kasper, D., Braunwald, E., Hauser, S., Longo, D., Jameson, J., et al. (Eds.). (2008). *Harrison's principles of internal medicine* (17th ed.). New York, NY: McGraw-Hill.

Fontaine, K. L. (2005). *Complementary & alternative therapies for nursing practice* (2nd ed.). Upper Saddle River, NJ: Prentice Hall.

Gotelli, J., Merryman, P., Carr, C., McElveen, L., Epperson, C., & Bynum, D. (2008 December). A quality improvement project to reduce the complications associated with indwelling urinary catheters. *Urologic Nursing, 28*(6), 465–467, 473.

Katz, A. (2009 March). When worlds collide: Urinary incontinence and female sexuality. *American Journal of Nursing, 109*(3), 59–63.

Kee, J. (2009). *Handbook of laboratory and diagnostic tests with nursing implications* (6th ed.). Upper Saddle River, NJ: Pearson Prentice Hall.

Lajiness, M. (2008 October). Common antibiotics for the treatment of urinary tract infections. *Urologic Nursing, 28*(5), 387–389.

Lin, K., & Fajardo, K. (2008 July 1). Clinical guidelines. Screening for asymptomatic bacteriuria in adults: Evidence for the U. S. Preventive Services Task Force reaffirmation recommendation statement. *Annals of Internal Medicine, 149*(1), W-20–W-24.

McPhee, S., Papadakis, M., & Tierney, L., Jr. (Eds.). (2008). *Current medical diagnosis & treatment* (47th ed.). New York, NY: McGraw Hill.

Moorhead, S., Johnson, M., Maas, M., & Swanson, E. (Eds.). (2008). *Nursing outcomes classification (NOC)* (4th ed.). St. Louis, MO: Mosby.

NANDA International. (2009). *Nursing diagnoses definitions and classification 2009–2011.* Oxford, UK: Wiley-Blackwell.

National Kidney and Urologic Diseases Information Clearinghouse. (2009). *Kidney and urologic diseases statistics for the United States.* Retrieved from www.kidney.niddk.nih.gov

National Kidney Foundation. (2008). *The problem of kidney and urologic disease.* Retrieved from www.kidney.org

Nursing guidelines for assessment and management of urinary retention in hospitalized older adults. (2007 August). *Australian Nursing Journal, 15*(2), 22–23.

Paige, N., & Nagami, G. (2009 February). The top 10 things nephrologists wish every primary care physician knew. *Mayo Clinic Proceedings, 84*(2), 180–186.

Palmer, M. (2008). Urinary incontinence quality improvement in nursing homes: Where have we been? Where are we going? *Urologic Nursing, 28*(6), 439–444.

Palmer, M., & Newman, D. (2007 March). Bladder matters: Urinary incontinence and estrogen. *American Journal of Nursing, 107*(3), 35–36, 38.

Pickett, S. (2008 October 17). The basics. Urinary tract infection. *GP: General Practitioner, October 2007,* 37, 39.

Porth, C., & Matfin, G. (2009). *Pathophysiology: Concepts of altered health states* (8th ed.). Philadelphia: Lippincott.

Rahn, D. (2008 October). Urinary tract infections: Contemporary management. *Urologic Nursing, 28*(5), 333–341.

Research backs cranberries for preventing urinary tract infections in women. (2008 April). *Harvard Women's Health Watch.* Retrieved from www.health.harvard.edu

Richards, S. (2008 June 6). Urinary tract infection. *Practice Nurse, 35*(11), 16–18.

Robinson, S., Allen, L., Barnes, M., Berry, T., Foster, T., Friedrich, L., et al. (2007 June). Development of an evidence-based protocol for reduction of indwelling urinary catheter usage. *MEDSURG Nursing, 16*(3), 157–161.

Rosh, A. (2009 April 5). Suprapubic aspiration. Retrieved from www.emedicine.medscape.com

Rothrock, J. C. (2007). *Alexander's care of the patient in surgery* (13th ed.). St. Louis, MO: Mosby.

Spencer, J. W., & Jacobs, J. J. (2003). *Complementary and alternative medicine: An evidence-based approach* (2nd ed.). St. Louis, MO: Mosby.

Stevemer, J., & Ewigman, B. (2008 April). Drugs help pass more ureteral stones. *The Journal of Family Practice, 57*(4), 224–227.

Stokowski, L. (2009). Preventing catheter-associated urinary tract infections. *Medscape Nurses 2009.* Retrieved from www.medscape.com

Wilkinson, J., & Ahern, N. (2009). *Nursing diagnosis handbook* (9th ed.). Upper Saddle River, NJ: Prentice Hall.

Wilson, B., Shannon, M., Shields, K., & Stang, C. (2008). *Nurse's drug guide.* Upper Saddle River, NJ: Prentice Hall.

Nursing Care of Patients with Kidney Disorders

LEARNING OUTCOMES

1. Describe the pathophysiology of common kidney disorders, relating pathophysiology to normal functions and manifestations of the disorder.
2. Discuss risk factors for kidney disorders and nursing measures to reduce these risks.
3. Explain diagnostic studies used to identify disorders of the kidneys and their effects.
4. Discuss the effects and nursing implications for medications and treatments used for patients with kidney disorders.
5. Compare and contrast renal replacement therapies, including dialysis and kidney transplant, to manage acute and chronic renal failure.

CLINICAL COMPETENCIES

1. Assess the functional health status of patients with kidney disorders.
2. Recognize, monitor, document, and report unexpected or abnormal manifestations in patients with kidney disorders.
3. Provide safe and effective nursing care for patients undergoing renal replacement therapies, surgery involving the kidneys, or renal transplant.
4. Using assessed data and current standards of practice, determine priority nursing diagnoses and interventions for patients with renal disorders.
5. Plan and implement evidence-based nursing care for patients with renal disorders using research and best practices.
6. Collaborate and coordinate with the patient and other members of the interdisciplinary team to prioritize and implement care.
7. Provide teaching appropriate to the patient and situation for patients with kidney disorders.
8. Evaluate patient responses to care, revising the plan of care as needed to promote, maintain, or restore functional health status for patients with renal disorders.

KEY TERMS

acute renal failure, *836*
acute tubular necrosis, *837*
azotemia, *822*
chronic kidney disease (CKD), *848*
dialysis, *840*
glomerular filtration rate, *820*

glomerulonephritis, *822*
hematuria, *821*
hemodialysis, *840*
nephrectomy, *832*
nephrotic syndrome, *824*
oliguria, *822*

peritoneal dialysis, *840*
proteinuria, *821*
renal failure, *835*
ultrafiltration, *840*
uremia, *849*

The internal environment of the body normally remains in a relatively constant or *homeostatic* state. The kidneys help maintain homeostasis by regulating the composition and volume of extracellular fluid. They excrete excess water and solutes and also can conserve water and solutes when deficits occur. In addition, the kidneys help regulate acid–base balance and they excrete metabolic wastes. Regulation of blood pressure is also a key function of the kidneys.

Both primary kidney disorders (such as glomerulonephritis) and systemic diseases (such as diabetes mellitus) can affect renal function. In the United States, more than 23 million people (about 13% of adults) have chronic kidney disease (National Kidney and Urologic Diseases Information Clearinghouse [NKUDIC], 2009). Every year, approximately 1 in every 1000 people in the United States develops end-stage renal disease (ESRD), the final phase of chronic renal disease in which little or no kidney function remains. Chronic renal disease accounted for more than 87,500 deaths in 2006, and is a major cause of lost work time and wages (NKUDIC, 2009). Ironically, the increased prevalence of chronic renal disease in recent years is partially related to the success of dialysis and transplantation.

Age-Related Changes in Kidney Function

Glomeruli in the renal cortex (∞ see Chapter 26 for a review of normal kidney structure and function) are lost with aging, reducing kidney mass. Because of the large functional reserve of the kidneys, however, renal function remains adequate unless additional stressors affect the renal system. The **glomerular filtration rate (GFR)**, the amount of filtrate made by the kidneys per minute, declines due to age-related factors affecting the renovascular system (such as arteriosclerosis, decreased renal vascularity, and decreased cardiac output). By age 80, the GFR may be less than half of what it was at age 30.

Age-related changes in renal function have significant implications. The kidneys are less able to concentrate urine and compensate for increased or decreased salt intake. When combined with diminished effectiveness of antidiuretic hormone (ADH) and a reduced thirst response, both common in aging, this decreased ability to concentrate urine increases the risk for dehydration. Potassium excretion may be decreased because of lower aldosterone levels. As a result, fluid and electrolyte imbalances are more common and potentially critical in the older patient.

Decreased GFR in the older adult also reduces the clearance of drugs excreted through the kidneys. This reduced clearance prolongs the half-life of drugs and may necessitate lower drug

doses and longer dosing intervals. Common medications affected by decreased GFR include the following:

- Cardiac drugs: digoxin, procainamide
- Antibiotics: aminoglycosides, tetracyclines, cephalosporins
- Histamine H_2 antagonists: cimetidine
- Antidiabetic agents: chlorpropamide.

When caring for older adults, it is especially important to monitor drugs that are toxic to the renal tubules. Radiologic dyes and aminoglycoside, tetracycline, and the cephalosporin antibiotics are part of this group.

Age-related changes in renal function and related nursing implications are summarized in Table 28–1.

The Patient with Polycystic Kidney Disease

Polycystic kidney disease, a hereditary disease characterized by formation of fluid-filled cysts and massive kidney enlargement, affects both children and adults. This disease has two forms: The autosomal dominant form primarily affects adults; the autosomal recessive form is present at birth (Porth & Matfin, 2009). Autosomal recessive polycystic kidney disease is rare. It usually is diagnosed prenatally or in infancy. Renal failure generally develops during childhood, necessitating kidney transplant or dialysis. Autosomal dominant polycystic kidney disease (ADPKD) is relatively common, affecting 1 in every 400 to 1000 people and accounting for approximately 4.5% of patients with ESRD in the United States (Fauci et al., 2008; NKUDIC, 2009). See the genetics box that follows. This section focuses on autosomal dominant polycystic kidney disease, the more common form of the disorder.

Pathophysiology

Renal cysts are fluid-filled sacs affecting the nephron, the functional unit of the kidneys. The cysts, which arise from tubular epithelial cells, may range in size from microscopic to several centimeters in diameter and affect the renal cortex and medulla of both kidneys. Cysts may detach from the tubule, continuing to enlarge by active fluid secretion. As the cysts enlarge and multiply, the kidneys also enlarge. Although only a small percentage of nephrons are involved, the cysts compress adjacent

---

TABLE 28–1 Nursing Implications of Age-Related Changes in Kidney Function

FUNCTIONAL CHANGE	EFFECT	IMPLICATIONS
Decreased GFR	Decreased clearance of drugs excreted primarily through the kidneys increases drug half-life and blood levels, and risk of drug toxicity	Monitor carefully for signs of toxicity, especially when administering digoxin, aminoglycoside antibiotics, tetracycline, vancomycin, chlorpropamide, procainamide, cimetidine, and cephalosporin antibiotics.
Decreased number of functional nephrons; lower levels of aldosterone; increased resistance to ADH	Decreased ability to conserve water and sodium; impaired potassium excretion; and decreased hydrogen ion excretion, resulting in reduced ability to compensate for acidosis	Monitor for dehydration and hyponatremia; maintain fluid intake of 1500 to 2500 mL/day unless contraindicated; monitor for hyperkalemia, especially if taking a potassium-sparing diuretic, heparin, angiotensin-converting enzyme (ACE) inhibitor, beta-blocker, or NSAID; increased risk for acidosis.
Reduced numbers of functional nephrons	Decreased renal reserve with increased risk of failure	Avoid giving nephrotoxic drugs if possible; monitor urine output and blood chemistries for early signs of renal failure.

renal parenchyma. Renal blood vessels and nephrons are compressed and obstructed, leading to tissue ischemia. This activates the renin-angiotensin system within the kidney. Functional tissue is destroyed, with compression, ischemia, and accumulation of inflammatory mediators likely playing a role (Figure 28–1 ■).

People affected by polycystic kidney disease often develop cysts elsewhere in the body, including the liver, spleen, pancreas, lungs, and reproductive organs. Up to 40% of people with ADPKD develop liver cysts, which may bleed or become infected. Diverticular disease of the colon is common, and may lead to perforation of the bowel (Fauci et al., 2008). About 25% of people with polycystic kidney disease have cardiac valve abnormalities, including mitral valve prolapse ("floppy" mitral valves) and aortic valve insufficiency. The risk of subarachnoid or cerebral hemorrhage from a ruptured cerebral aneurysm is significantly increased in patients with ADPKD.

Manifestations

Polycystic kidney disease is slowly progressive. Symptoms usually develop by age 40 to 50. Common manifestations include flank pain, microscopic or gross **hematuria** (blood in the urine), **proteinuria** (proteins in the urine), and *polyuria* and

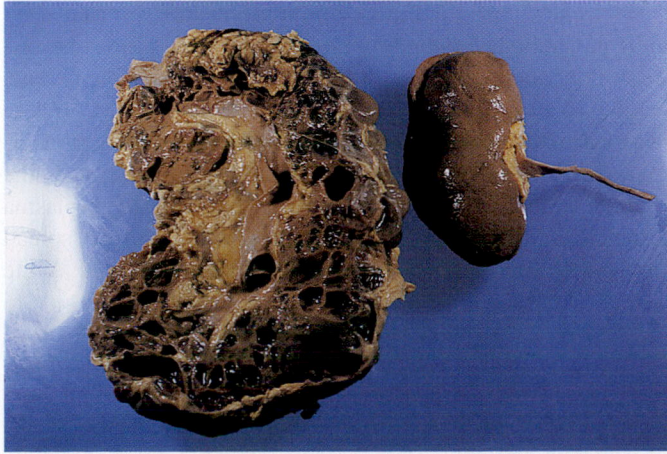

Figure 28–1 ■ A polycystic kidney. The functional tissue of the kidneys is gradually destroyed and replaced with fluid-filled cysts.

Source: A. Glauberman/Photo Researchers, Inc.

nocturia, as the concentrating ability of the kidney is impaired. Urinary tract infection and renal calculi are common, as cysts interfere with normal urine drainage. Most patients develop hypertension from disruption of renal vessels. The kidneys become palpable, enlarged, and knobby. Symptoms of renal insufficiency and chronic renal failure typically develop by age 60 to 70. The progression to ESRD tends to occur more rapidly in Blacks and in men.

Interdisciplinary Care

Diagnostic tests used to determine the extent of polycystic kidney disease include the following:

- *Renal ultrasonography* is the diagnostic procedure of choice for polycystic kidney disease.
- *Computed tomography (CT) scan* of the kidney may be used to detect cystic disease at an earlier stage when there is a positive family history.
- *Genetic testing* for ADPKD type 1 and type 2 is available, and is particularly important when a family member is being considered as a potential kidney donor.

∞ See Chapter 26 for the nursing implications of these tests.

Management of adult polycystic kidney disease is largely supportive. Care is taken to avoid further renal damage by nephrotoxic substances, UTI, obstruction, or hypertension. A fluid intake of 2000 to 2500 mL per day is encouraged to help prevent UTI and lithiasis. Hypertension associated with polycystic disease is generally controlled using a multidrug regimen that includes an angiotensin-converting enzyme (ACE) inhibitor or angiotensin receptor blocker (ARB) (∞ see Chapter 32). Ultimately, dialysis or renal transplantation is required. Patients with polycystic kidney disease are typically good candidates for transplantation because of the absence of associated systemic disease, but may still experience effects of the extrarenal elements of the disease.

∞ Nursing Care

For those with adult polycystic kidney disease, an autosomal dominant disorder, discuss genetic counseling and screening of family members for evidence of the disease. Consider the following nursing diagnoses when planning care for the patient with polycystic kidney disease:

- *Excess Fluid Volume* related to impaired renal function
- *Grieving* related to potential loss of kidney function
- *Readiness for Enhanced Knowledge* regarding measures to help preserve kidney function
- *Risk for Ineffective Coping* related to potential genetic transmission of the disorder to offspring.

Teach the patient with polycystic kidney disease about the disease, its genetic nature, and usual course. Discuss measures to maintain optimal renal function. Instruct to maintain a fluid intake of at least 2500 mL per day. Include additional information about preventing UTI (such as hygiene measures) and early manifestations of UTI. Stress the importance of seeking treatment to prevent further kidney damage. Advise to avoid drugs that are potentially toxic to the kidneys and to check with the primary care provider before taking any new drug. Discuss the potential benefits of genetic counseling with the patient and family.

The Patient with a Glomerular Disorder

Disorders and diseases involving the glomerulus are the leading cause of chronic kidney disease in the United States. They are the underlying disease process for more than half of those people needing dialysis and result in a significant number of deaths per year (NKUDIC, 2009).

Glomerular disorders may be either primary, involving mainly the kidney, or secondary to a multisystem disease or hereditary condition. Primary glomerular disease is often immunologic or idiopathic in origin. Diabetes mellitus, undiagnosed or inadequately treated hypertension, systemic lupus erythematosus (SLE), and Goodpasture's syndrome are frequently implicated in secondary glomerular disorders.

FAST FACTS

- Glomerular disorders and diseases are the leading cause of chronic kidney disease in the United States.
- Hematuria, proteinuria, and hypertension often are early manifestations of glomerular disorders.
- Acute poststreptococcal glomerulonephritis (also called acute proliferative glomerulonephritis) is the most common primary glomerular disorder.
- Diabetes mellitus, hypertension, and SLE are common causes of secondary glomerulonephritis.

Physiology Review

The glomerulus is a tuft of capillaries surrounded by a thin, double-walled capsule (Bowman's capsule) (see Figure 26–3). About 20% of the resting cardiac output flows through the glomeruli of the kidneys, forming approximately 180 L of plasma ultrafiltrate. More than 99% of this filtrate is reabsorbed in the renal tubules. The rate of glomerular filtration is controlled by opposing forces: The pressure and amount of blood flowing through the glomeruli promote filtration, and the pressure in Bowman's capsule and colloid osmotic (*oncotic*) pressure of the blood oppose it. The total surface area of glomerular capillaries also affects the GFR. The glomerular capillary membrane has three layers: the capillary endothelial layer, the basement membrane, and the capsule epithelial layer. Water and the smallest solutes (such as electrolytes) pass freely across this membrane, whereas larger molecules (such as plasma proteins) are retained in the blood.

Pathophysiology

Glomerular disease affects both the structure and function of the glomerulus, disrupting glomerular filtration. The capillary membrane becomes more permeable to plasma proteins and blood cells. This increased permeability in the glomerulus causes the manifestations common to glomerular disorders: hematuria, proteinuria, and edema. The GFR falls, leading to **azotemia** (increased blood levels of nitrogenous waste products) and hypertension. Glomerular involvement may be diffuse (involving all glomeruli) or focal (involving some glomeruli while others remain essentially normal).

Both hematuria and proteinuria are caused by glomerular capillary membrane damage, which allows blood cells and proteins to escape from the blood into the glomerular filtrate. Hematuria may be either gross or microscopic. Proteinuria is considered to be the most important indicator of glomerular injury, because it increases progressively with increased glomerular damage. Loss of plasma proteins leads to *hypoalbuminemia* (low serum albumin levels), which in turn reduces the plasma oncotic pressure (osmotic pressure created by plasma proteins), leading to edema.

As plasma proteins are lost, the forces opposing filtration diminish, and the amount of filtrate increases. The increased flow of filtrate stimulates the renin–angiotensin–aldosterone mechanism (∞ see Chapter 26), producing vasoconstriction and a resulting fall in GFR. Increased aldosterone production causes salt and water retention, which further contribute to edema. As the GFR falls, filtration and elimination of nitrogenous wastes, including urea, decrease, causing azotemia. **Oliguria**, urine output of less than 400 mL in 24 hours, may result from the decreased GFR. Hypertension results from fluid retention and disruption of the renin–angiotensin system, a key regulator of blood pressure.

The major primary glomerular disorders include acute glomerulonephritis, rapidly progressive glomerulonephritis, nephrotic syndrome, and chronic glomerulonephritis. Diabetic nephropathy and lupus nephritis are the most common secondary forms of glomerular disease.

Acute Postinfectious Glomerulonephritis

Glomerulonephritis is inflammation of the glomerular capillary membrane. Acute glomerulonephritis can result from systemic diseases or primary glomerular diseases, but acute postinfectious glomerulonephritis (also known as acute post-streptococcal glomerulonephritis) is the most common form. Infection of the pharynx or skin with group A beta-hemolytic streptococcus is the usual initiating event for this disorder. Staphylococcal or viral infections, such as hepatitis B, mumps, or varicella (chickenpox), can lead to a similar postinfectious acute glomerulonephritis. This primarily childhood disease also can affect adults.

In acute postinfectious glomerulonephritis, circulating antigen–antibody immune complexes formed during the primary infection become trapped in the glomerular membrane, leading to an inflammatory response. The complement system is activated, and vasoactive substances and inflammatory mediators are released. Endothelial cells proliferate, and the glomerular membrane swells and becomes permeable to plasma proteins and blood cells. Renal involvement is diffuse, spread throughout the kidneys. See Pathophysiology Illustrated: Acute Glomerulonephritis on page 823.

MANIFESTATIONS AND COMPLICATIONS Acute postinfectious glomerulonephritis is characterized by an abrupt onset of hematuria, proteinuria, salt and water retention, and evidence of azotemia occurring 10 to 14 days after the initial infection. The urine often appears brown or cola-colored. Salt and water retention increase extracellular fluid volume, leading to hypertension and edema. The edema is primarily noted in the face, particularly around the eyes (*periorbital* edema). Dependent

PATHOPHYSIOLOGY ILLUSTRATED

Acute Postinfectious Glomerulonephritis

Infection from group A beta-hemolytic Streptococcus causes an immune response that causes inflammation and damage to the glomeruli. Protein and red blood cells are allowed to pass through the glomeruli. Blood flow to the glomeruli is reduced due to obstruction with damaged cells and renal insufficiency results, leading to the retention of sodium, water, and waste.

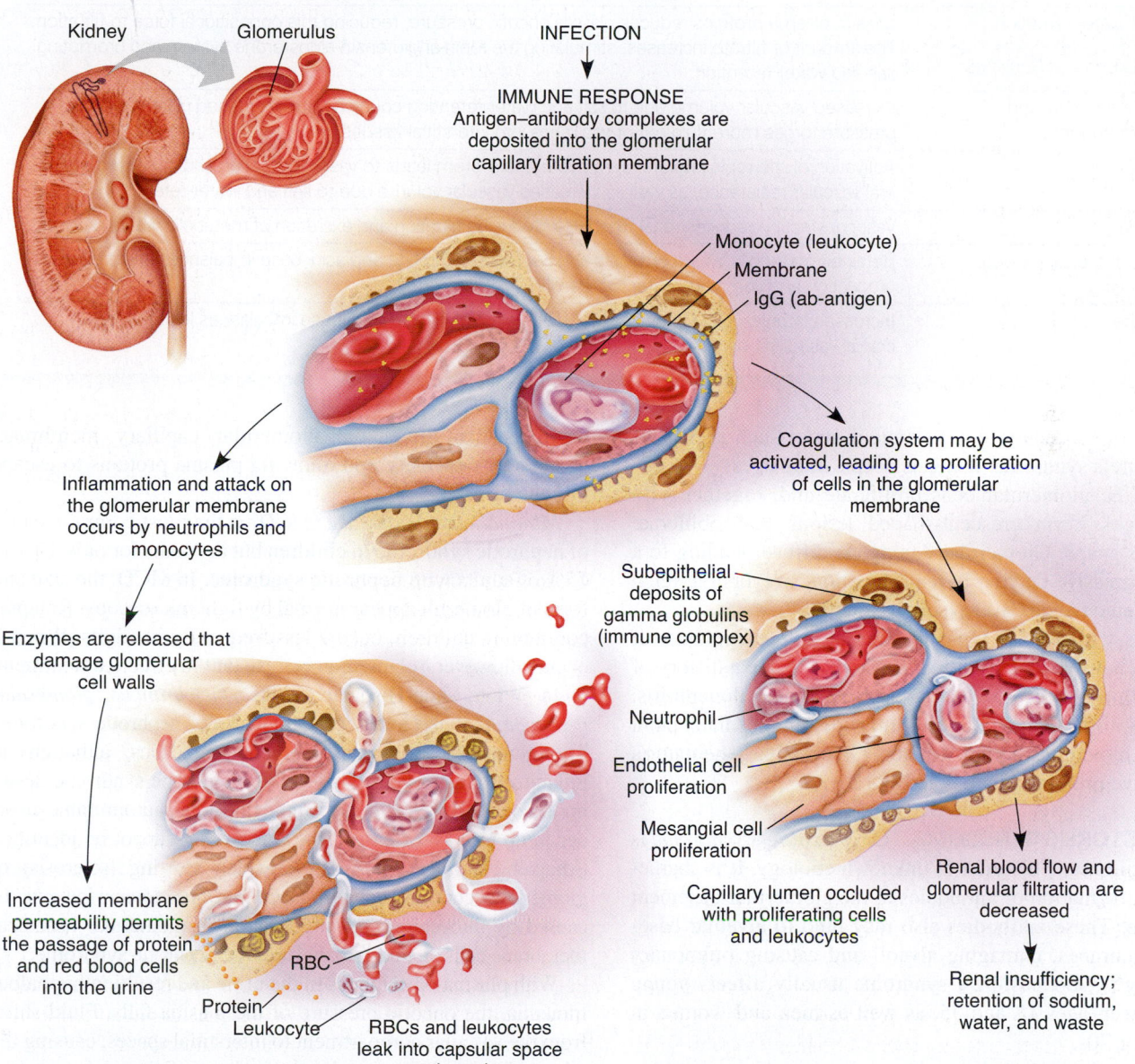

Kidney   Glomerulus

INFECTION

IMMUNE RESPONSE
Antigen–antibody complexes are deposited into the glomerular capillary filtration membrane

Monocyte (leukocyte)
Membrane
IgG (ab-antigen)

Inflammation and attack on the glomerular membrane occurs by neutrophils and monocytes

Coagulation system may be activated, leading to a proliferation of cells in the glomerular membrane

Enzymes are released that damage glomerular cell walls

Subepithelial deposits of gamma globulins (immune complex)

Neutrophil

Endothelial cell proliferation

Mesangial cell proliferation

Increased membrane permeability permits the passage of protein and red blood cells into the urine

RBC

Protein

Leukocyte

RBCs and leukocytes leak into capsular space causing edema

Capillary lumen occluded with proliferating cells and leukocytes

Renal blood flow and glomerular filtration are decreased

Renal insufficiency; retention of sodium, water, and waste

edema, affecting the hands and upper extremities in particular, may also be noted. Other manifestations may include fatigue, anorexia, nausea and vomiting, and headache (see the Pathophysiology Linkages table on page 824).

The older adult may have less apparent symptoms. Nausea, malaise, arthralgias, and proteinuria are common manifestations; hypertension and edema are seen less often. Pulmonary infiltrates may occur early in the disorder, often due to worsening of a preexisting condition such as heart failure.

The prognosis for adults with acute glomerulonephritis is less favorable than it is for children. The symptoms may resolve spontaneously within 10 to 14 days. Full recovery is usual in children, whereas 60% or more affected adults recover completely. The remainder have persistent symptoms, and some have permanent kidney damage (Porth & Matfin, 2009).

Rapidly Progressive Glomerulonephritis

Rapidly progressive glomerulonephritis (RPGN), which also may be known as crescentic glomerulonephritis, is characterized by manifestations of severe glomerular injury without a specific, identifiable cause. This type of glomerulonephritis often progresses to renal failure within months. It may be idiopathic

PATHOPHYSIOLOGY LINKAGE   Acute Glomerulonephritis

MANIFESTATION	RELATED PATHOPHYSIOLOGY
Hematuria, cola-colored urine	Disruption of the glomerular capillary membrane allows red blood cells to escape from the vascular system into Bowman's capsule, ultimately being excreted in the urine
Proteinuria	Plasma proteins cross the damaged glomerular capillary membrane, becoming part of the filtrate and excreted urine
Salt and water retention	Loss of plasma proteins reduces plasma oncotic pressure, reducing this oppositional force to filtration. The amount of filtrate increases, stimulating the renin-angiotensin-aldosterone system and prompting salt and water retention.
Edema, periorbital and facial, dependent	Increased vascular volume due to salt and water retention coupled with decreased plasma oncotic pressure forces more fluid out of capillaries into interstitial tissues.
Hypertension	Activation of the renin-angiotensin-aldosterone system leads to vasoconstriction and increased peripheral vascular resistance, as well as increased vascular volume due to salt and water retention.
Azotemia	Vasoconstriction reduces renal blood flow, reducing filtration and excretion of metabolic waste products.
Fatigue, anorexia, nausea, and vomiting	Retained metabolic waste products and fluid and electrolyte and acid–base imbalances affect energy production and vomiting centers in the CNS.
Headache	Increased intravascular volume and fluid and electrolyte and acid–base imbalances lead to intracranial vasodilation.

(primary), or secondary to a systemic disorder such as SLE or Goodpasture's syndrome. It affects people of all ages.

In RPGN, glomerular cells proliferate and, together with macrophages, form crescent-shaped lesions that obliterate Bowman's space. Glomerular damage is diffuse, leading to a rapid, progressive decline in renal function. Irreversible renal failure often develops over weeks to months.

Patients with RPGN typically present with complaints of weakness, nausea, and vomiting. Some may relate a history of a flulike illness preceding the onset of the glomerulonephritis. Other symptoms include oliguria and abdominal or flank pain. Moderate hypertension may develop. On urinalysis, hematuria and massive proteinuria are noted.

GOODPASTURE'S SYNDROME   *Goodpasture's syndrome* is a rare autoimmune disorder of unknown etiology. It is characterized by formation of antibodies to the glomerular basement membrane. These antibodies also may bind to alveolar basement membranes, damaging alveoli and causing pulmonary hemorrhage. Goodpasture's syndrome usually affects young men between ages 18 and 35, as well as men and women in their 60s or 70s.

Although the glomeruli may be nearly normal in appearance and function in Goodpasture's syndrome, extensive cell proliferation and crescent formation characteristic of rapidly progressive glomerulonephritis are more common. Renal manifestations include hematuria, proteinuria, and edema. Rapid progression to renal failure may occur. Alveolar membrane damage can lead to mild or life-threatening pulmonary hemorrhage. Cough, shortness of breath, and hemoptysis (bloody sputum) are early respiratory manifestations.

Nephrotic Syndrome

Nephrotic syndrome is a group of clinical findings as opposed to a specific disorder. It is characterized by massive proteinuria, hypoalbuminemia, hyperlipidemia, and edema. A number of disorders can affect the glomerular capillary membrane, changing its porosity and allowing plasma proteins to escape into the urine.

Minimal change disease (MCD) is the most common cause of nephrotic syndrome in children but accounts for only 10% to 15% of adults with nephrotic syndrome. In MCD, the size and form of glomeruli appear normal by light microscopy. Relapse, common in children, occurs less frequently in adults. When it occurs, however, relapse can be resistant to effective treatment.

In White, non-Hispanic adults, *membranous glomerulonephropathy* is the most common cause of nephrotic syndrome. The glomerular basement membrane thickens, although no inflammation is present. This form of nephrotic syndrome develops secondarily to malignancy, infection, or an autoimmune disorder in up to 30% of cases. The cause often cannot be identified (idiopathic). *Focal sclerosis*, in which scarring (sclerosis) of glomeruli occurs, and *membranoproliferative glomerulonephritis*, caused by thickening and proliferation of glomerular basement membrane cells, are additional forms of nephrotic syndrome.

With plasma protein loss in the urine and resulting hypoalbuminemia, the oncotic pressure of the plasma falls. Fluid shifts from the vascular compartment to interstitial spaces, causing the edema characteristic of nephrotic syndrome. Salt and water retention, possibly due to activation of the renin–angiotensin system, contribute to the edema. Edema may be severe, affecting the face and periorbital area as well as dependent tissues (Figure 28–2 ■).

Loss of plasma proteins stimulates the liver to increase albumin production and lipoprotein synthesis. As a result, serum triglyceride and low-density lipoprotein (LDL) levels increase, as do urine lipids (*lipiduria*). Hyperlipidemia increases the risk for atherosclerosis in patients with nephrotic syndrome.

Thromboemboli (mobilized blood clots) are a relatively common complication of nephrotic syndrome. Loss of clotting and anticlotting factors along with plasma proteins are thought to disrupt the coagulation system, increasing the risk for renal venous thrombosis, deep venous thrombosis, and pulmonary

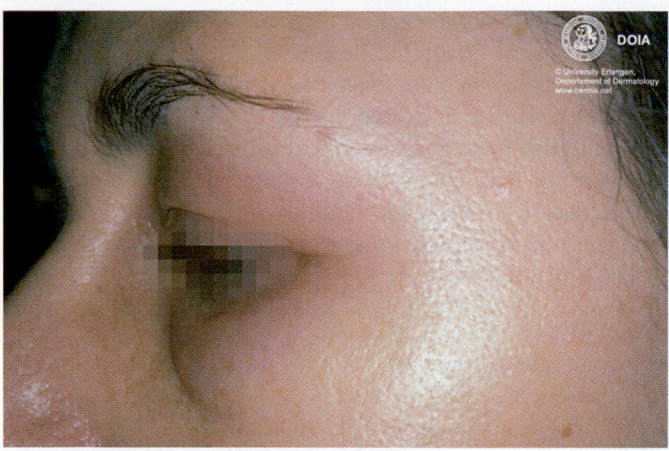

Figure 28–2 ■ Severe edema characteristic of nephrotic syndrome.

embolism. Renal venous thrombosis can cause flank or groin pain on one or both sides, gross hematuria, and a reduced GFR.

Nephrotic syndrome usually resolves without long-term effects in children. The prognosis for adults is less optimistic because the syndrome often occurs secondarily to another disorder. Many adults do not recover completely, experiencing persistent proteinuria and potentially, progressive renal impairment.

Chronic Glomerulonephritis

Chronic glomerulonephritis is typically the result of progressive glomerular disorders such as RPGN, lupus nephritis, or diabetic nephropathy. In many cases, however, no previous glomerular disease has been identified.

Slow, progressive destruction of the glomeruli and a gradual decline in renal function are characteristic of chronic glomerulonephritis. The kidneys decrease in size symmetrically, and their surfaces become granular or roughened. Eventually, entire nephrons are lost.

Symptoms develop insidiously, and the disease is often not recognized until signs of renal failure develop. Chronic glomerulonephritis may also be diagnosed when hypertension and impaired renal function are found coincidentally during a routine physical examination or treatment for an unrelated disorder. Viral or bacterial infectious diseases can exacerbate the disorder, prompting its diagnosis.

The course of chronic glomerulonephritis varies, with years to decades between the diagnosis and the development of end-stage renal failure.

Diabetic Nephropathy

Diabetic nephropathy, kidney disease common in the later stages of diabetes mellitus (DM), is the leading cause of chronic kidney disease in North America. About 40% of patients with diabetes develop nephropathy; because type 2 diabetes is more prevalent, it accounts for a higher portion of patients with chronic kidney disease. Diabetes-associated kidney lesions are more common in Blacks, Native Americans, and Pacific Islanders (Fauci et al., 2008).

Initial evidence of microproteinuria indicating renal damage is typically seen within 5 to 10 years after the onset of diabetes. Overt proteinuria and nephropathy generally develop within another 5 to 10 years of the onset of microproteinuria.

The characteristic lesion of diabetic nephropathy is glomerulosclerosis and thickening of the glomerular basement membrane. As the disease progresses, the glomerular capillary lumen narrows, reducing the surface area for glomerular filtration. Arteriosclerosis, a common feature of long-term diabetes and hypertension, contributes to the disease, as do nephritis and tubular lesions. Pyelonephritis, inflammation of the kidney, is also implicated in the development of diabetic nephropathy. A further discussion of diabetic nephropathy is found in ∞ Chapter 20.

Lupus Nephritis

Systemic lupus erythematosus (SLE) is an inflammatory autoimmune disorder affecting the connective tissue of the body. Most patients with SLE develop kidney abnormalities related to their disease; many develop manifestations of nephritis (Fauci et al., 2008). Circulating immune complexes deposited in the glomerulus as well as those that form within the glomerular capillary wall trigger an inflammatory response leading to glomerular injury in SLE. Manifestations of lupus nephritis range from microscopic hematuria to massive proteinuria. Its progression may be slow and chronic or *fulminant*, with a sudden onset and the rapid development of renal failure. End-stage kidney disease eventually develops in about 20% of patients with lupus nephritis. Improved management of the underlying disease, immunotherapy, dialysis, and renal transplantation have significantly improved the prognosis in recent years.

Interdisciplinary Care

Management of all types of glomerulonephritis, acute and chronic, primary and secondary, focuses on identifying the underlying disease process and preserving kidney function. In most glomerular disorders, there is no specific treatment to achieve a cure. Treatment goals are to maintain renal function, prevent complications, and support the healing process.

Diagnosis

Laboratory and diagnostic testing are valuable to identify the cause of glomerulonephritis and evaluate kidney function.

The following studies may be ordered to help identify the underlying cause or etiology:

- *Throat or skin cultures* detect infection by group A beta-hemolytic streptococci. Although poststreptococcal glomerulonephritis typically follows the acute infection by 1 to 2 weeks, treatment to eradicate any remaining organisms is initiated to minimize antibody production.
- *Antistreptolysin O (ASO) titer* and other tests detect streptococcal *exoenzymes* (bacterial enzymes that stimulate the immune response in acute poststreptococcal glomerulonephritis). Other titers such as antistreptokinase (ASK) or anti-deoxyribonuclease B (ADNAase B) may be obtained as well.
- *Erythrocyte sedimentation rate (ESR)* may be elevated in acute poststreptococcal glomerulonephritis and in lupus nephritis.
- *KUB* (kidney, ureter, bladder) *abdominal x-ray* may show enlarged kidneys in acute glomerulonephritis, whereas bilateral small kidneys are typical of late chronic glomerulonephritis.

■ *Kidney scan* demonstrates delayed uptake and excretion of the radioactive material in glomerular diseases.

■ *Biopsy* is the most reliable diagnostic procedure for glomerular disorders. Biopsy helps determine the type of glomerulonephritis, the prognosis, and appropriate treatment.

∞ See Chapter 26 for the nursing implications of diagnostic tests used to evaluate glomerular disorders.

The following studies are used to evaluate kidney function:

■ *Blood urea nitrogen (BUN)* is measured. Urea is eliminated from the body by filtration in the glomerulus; minimal amounts are reabsorbed in the renal tubules. Glomerular diseases interfere with filtration and elimination of urea nitrogen, causing blood levels to rise. Normal BUN values are listed in Table 28–2. Levels up to 50 mg/dL or 17.7 mmol/L indicate mild azotemia, and levels higher than 100 mg/dL or 35.7 mmol/L indicate severe renal impairment.

■ *Serum creatinine* is a good indicator of kidney function. Levels greater than 4 mg/dL indicate serious renal impairment.

■ *Urine creatinine* levels decrease when renal function is impaired because it is not effectively eliminated from the body.

■ *eGFR (estimated GFR)* is a calculated value used to evaluate renal function. Four variables are used to calculate the eGFR: serum creatinine, age in years, gender, and race (African American or other). Values of 60 mL/min/1.73 m^2 or higher are within the normal range for adults (20 years old and above), and may simply be reported as > 60 mL/min/1.73 m^2.

■ *Creatinine clearance* may be used to evaluate the GFR. The *clearance*, or amount of blood cleared of creatinine in 1 minute, depends on the amount and pressure of blood being filtered and the filtering ability of the glomeruli. Disorders such as glomerulonephritis affect glomerular filtration, decreasing the creatinine clearance.

■ *Serum electrolytes* are evaluated because impaired kidney function alters their excretion.

■ *Urinalysis* often shows red blood cells (RBCs) and proteins in the urine of patients with a glomerular disorder. These substances, normally too large to enter glomerular filtrate, escape due to increased porosity of glomerular capillaries in glomerular disorders.

Medications

Although no drugs are available to cure glomerular disorders, medications are used to treat underlying disorders, reduce inflammation, and manage the symptoms.

Antibiotics are prescribed for the patient with poststreptococcal glomerulonephritis to eradicate any remaining bacteria, removing the stimulus for antibody production. Nephrotoxic antibiotics, such as the aminoglycoside antibiotics, streptomycin, and some cephalosporins, are avoided.

Aggressive immunosuppressive therapy is used to treat acute inflammatory processes such as rapidly progressive glomerulonephritis, Goodpasture's syndrome, and exacerbations of SLE. When begun early, immunosuppressive therapy significantly reduces the risk of end-stage renal disease and renal failure. Prednisone, a glucocorticoid, is prescribed in relatively large doses of 1 mg per kilogram of body weight per day (e.g., a 160-pound man would receive 70 to 75 mg per day). Other immunosuppressive agents such as cyclophosphamide (Cytoxan) or azathioprine (Imuran) are prescribed in conjunction with corticosteroids. Corticosteroid use in poststreptococcal glomerulonephritis may actually worsen the condition, so it is avoided.

TABLE 28–2 Changes in Laboratory Values Associated with Kidney Disease

TEST	NORMAL VALUE	VALUE IN RENAL DISEASE
Blood urea nitrogen (BUN)	5–25 mg/dL Slightly higher in older adults	25–50 mg/dL or higher
BUN/Creatinine ratio	10:1 (BUN:creatinine) to 20:1	Decreased ratio in acute tubular necrosis; increased in glomerular disease, azotemia
Creatinine, serum	0.5–1.5 mg/dL Slightly lower in females, older adults	Elevated; levels > 4 mg/dL indicate severe impairment of renal function
Creatinine clearance	85–135 mL/min Slightly lower in females Values decline in older adults	Reduced renal reserve: 32.5–85.0 mL/min Renal insufficiency: 6.5–32.5 mL/min Renal failure: < 6.5 mL/min
eGFR	≥ 60 mL/min/1.73 m^2	Decreased in renal impairment
Serum albumin	3.5–5 g/dL; lower in older adults	Decreased in nephrotic syndrome
Serum electrolytes	Potassium: 3.5–5.3 mEq/L	Increased in renal insufficiency
	Sodium: 135–145 mEq/L	Decreased in nephrotic syndrome
	Calcium: 4.5–5.5 mEq/L or 9–11 mg/dL	Decreased in renal failure
	Phosphorus: 2.5–4.5 mg/dL	Increased in renal failure
Red blood cell count	Female: 4.0–5.0 million/mm^3	Decreased in chronic kidney disease
	Male: 4.6–6.0 million/mm^3	
Urine creatinine	1 – 2 g/24 hours	Decreased in disorders of impaired renal function
Urine protein	25–150 mg/24 hours	Increased in disorders of impaired renal function
Urine red blood cells	< 2/HPF; no RBC casts	Present in glomerular disorders

Oral glucocorticoids such as prednisone also are used in high doses to induce remission of nephrotic syndrome. When glucocorticoids alone are ineffective, other immunosuppressive agents such as cyclophosphamide or chlorambucil (Leukeran) may be used to induce or maintain remission. ∞ See Chapter 13 for more information about corticosteroids and other immunosuppressive drugs.

ACE inhibitors or angiotensin-receptor blockers (ARBs) may be ordered to reduce protein loss associated with nephrotic syndrome and slow the progression of renal failure. They have a protective effect on the kidney in patients with diabetic nephropathy.

Antihypertensives are prescribed to maintain the blood pressure within normal levels. Blood pressure management is important because systemic and renal hypertension are associated with a poorer prognosis in patients with glomerular disorders.

Treatments

Restricted activity may be recommended during the acute phase of poststreptococcal glomerulonephritis. When the edema of nephrotic syndrome is significant or the patient is hypertensive, sodium intake may be restricted to 1 to 2 g per day. Dietary protein may be restricted if azotemia is present. When proteins are restricted, those included in the diet should be complete or high-value proteins. Complete proteins supply the essential amino acids required for growth and tissue maintenance. Complete and incomplete proteins are compared in Table 28–3.

Plasma exchange therapy (also called *plasmapheresis*), a procedure to remove damaging antibodies from the plasma, is used in conjunction with immunosuppressive therapy to treat RPGN and Goodpasture's syndrome. Plasma and glomerular-damaging antibodies are removed using a blood cell separator. The RBCs are then returned to the patient along with albumin or human plasma to replace the plasma removed. This procedure is usually done in a series of treatments. It is not without risk, and informed consent is required. Potential complications of plasma exchange therapy include those associated with intravenous catheters, fluid volume shifts, and altered coagulation.

Renal failure resulting from a glomerular disorder may necessitate dialysis to restore fluid and electrolyte balance and remove waste products from the body. Dialysis procedures and related nursing care are explained in the acute renal failure section later in this chapter.

Nursing Care

Health Promotion

Discuss the importance of effectively treating streptococcal infections in all age groups to help reduce the risk for acute glomerulonephritis. Stress the importance of completing the full course of antibiotic therapy to eradicate the infecting bacteria. Teach patients with diabetes mellitus and SLE about potential renal effects of their disease. Discuss measures to reduce the risk of associated nephritis, such as effectively managing the disease, treating hypertension, and avoiding drugs and substances that are potentially toxic to the kidneys.

Assessment

∞ Review Chapter 26 for complete assessment of the renal and urinary systems. Focused assessment data related to glomerular disorders include the following:

■ *Health history:* Complaints of facial or peripheral edema or weight gain, fatigue, nausea and vomiting, headache, general malaise, abdominal or flank pain; cough or shortness of breath; changes in amount, color, or character of urine (e.g., frothy urine); history of skin or pharyngeal streptococcal infection, diabetes, SLE, or kidney disease; current medications.
■ *Physical examination:* General appearance; vital signs; weight; presence of periorbital, facial, or peripheral edema; inspect skin for lesions, infection; inspect throat, obtain culture as indicated; obtain urine specimen for color, character, odor.

Nursing Diagnoses and Interventions

Nursing care is supportive and educational. Monitoring renal function and fluid volume status are key components of care, as is protecting the patient from infection. Both manifestations of glomerular disorders and their treatment can interfere with a patient's ability to maintain usual roles and responsibilities. For additional potential nursing diagnoses and interventions, see the Case Study & Nursing Care Plan on page 829.

Excess Fluid Volume

Excess fluid volume and resulting edema are common manifestations of glomerular disorders. When proteins are lost in the urine, the oncotic pressure of plasma falls, and fluid shifts into the interstitial spaces. The body responds to this fluid shift by

TABLE 28–3 Complete and Incomplete Protein Sources

	COMPLETE PROTEINS	INCOMPLETE PROTEINS
Definition	Provide all essential amino acids needed for growth and tissue maintenance	Lack one or more essential amino acids or contain inadequate proportions
Examples	Milk, eggs, cheese, meats, poultry, fish, and soy	Vegetables, breads, cereals and grains, legumes, seeds, and nuts

EVIDENCE FOR NURSING CARE — The Patient with Glomerulonephritis

Selected resources that nurses may find helpful when planning evidence-based nursing care follow.

■ Nguyen, T., & Toto, R. (2008). Slowing chronic kidney disease progression: results of prospective clinical trials in adults. *Pediatric Nephrology, 23*(9), 1409–1422.
■ Singapore Ministry of Health. (2007 March). *Glomerulonephritis.* Singapore: Singapore Ministry of Health. Retrieved from http://www.guideline.gov/summary/summary.aspx?doc_id=10845&nbr=005660&string=glomerulonephritis

retaining sodium and water to maintain intravascular volume, leading to excess fluid volume.

- Monitor vital signs, including blood pressure, apical pulse, respirations, and breath sounds, at least every 4 hours. Report significant changes. *Excess fluid increases the cardiac workload and the blood pressure. Tachycardia may result. Associated electrolyte imbalances can cause dysrhythmias. Increased pulmonary vascular pressure can lead to pulmonary edema, tachypnea, dyspnea, and crackles (rales) in the lungs.*
- Record intake and output every 4 to 8 hours, or more frequently as indicated. *Accurate intake and output records help determine fluid volume status.*

PRACTICE ALERT
Weigh daily, using consistent technique (time of day, scale, and clothing). Accurate daily weights are the best indicator of approximate fluid balance.

- Monitor serum electrolytes, hemoglobin and hematocrit, BUN, and creatinine. *Glomerular disorders affect fluid balance and may alter electrolyte balance as well, potentially leading to complications such as cardiac dysrhythmias (∞ see Chapter 10). Increased intravascular volume can result in low hemoglobin and hematocrit values. BUN and creatinine provide information about renal function.*
- Maintain fluid restriction as ordered. Offer ice chips (in limited and measured amounts) and frequent mouth care to relieve thirst. With the patient, develop a fluid intake schedule. *Fluids may be restricted to reduce fluid overload, edema, and hypertension. Ice chips and frequent mouth care moisten mucous membranes and help relieve thirst while maintaining oral tissue integrity. Including the patient in planning fluid intake promotes a sense of control and understanding of the treatment regimen.*

PRACTICE ALERT
Carefully monitor and regulate intravenous infusions; include fluid used to dilute IV medications as intake. Significant "hidden" fluid intake can occur with intravenous medication administration.

- Arrange dietary consultation regarding sodium or protein restricted diets. *Including the patient and dietitian in planning allows individualization of the diet to patient preferences. The glomerular disorder may reduce appetite; considering food preferences can help maintain adequate nutrition.*
- Monitor for desired and adverse effects of prescribed medications. *Diuretic therapy helps reduce excess fluid volume; however, glomerular disorders can affect the patient's response to treatment. In addition, diuretics can exacerbate the electrolyte imbalances and muscle weakness often associated with glomerular disorders.*
- Provide frequent position changes and good skin care. *Perfusion may be altered by tissue edema, increasing the risk of breakdown.*

Fatigue

Fatigue is a common manifestation of glomerular disorders. Anemia, loss of plasma proteins, headache, anorexia, and nausea compound this fatigue. The ability to maintain usual physical and mental activities may be impaired.

- Document energy level. *As glomerular function improves, fatigue begins to resolve, and energy increases.*
- Schedule activities and procedures to provide adequate rest and energy conservation. Prevent unnecessary fatigue. *Adequate rest and energy conservation reduce fatigue and improve the patient's ability to tolerate and cope with required treatments and activities.*
- Assist with ADLs as needed. *The goal is to conserve limited energy reserves.*
- Discuss the relationship between fatigue and the disease process with patient and family. *Understanding the nature of the disease and associated fatigue helps the patient and family cope with reduced energy and comply with prescribed rest.*
- Reduce energy demands with frequent, small meals and short periods of activity. Limit the number of visitors and visit length. *Small, frequent meals reduce the energy needed for eating and digestion. Limiting visitors and visit length helps conserve energy. In addition, nurses can assist the fatigued patient who may be reluctant to ask visitors to leave.*

Risk for Infection

The effects of both the glomerular disorder and treatment with anti-inflammatory and cytotoxic drugs can depress the immune system, increasing the risk for infection. The anti-inflammatory effect of corticosteroids may also mask early manifestations of infection.

PRACTICE ALERT
Monitor vital signs, temperature, and mental status every 4 hours. An elevated temperature may indicate infection; anti-inflammatory drugs may moderate this response, however. Tachycardia, increasing lethargy, or confusion may be the initial signs of infection.

- Assess frequently for other signs of infection such as purulent wound drainage, productive cough, adventitious breath sounds, and red or inflamed lesions. Monitor for manifestations of UTI, such as dysuria, frequency and urgency, and cloudy, foul-smelling urine. *Early identification and treatment of infection is important to prevent systemic complications in the susceptible patient.*
- Monitor CBC, focusing on the WBC and differential. *An elevated WBC and increased numbers of immature WBCs in the blood (left shift) may be early indicators of infection.*
- Use good hand hygiene technique. Protect from cross-infection by providing a private room and restricting ill visitors. *Patients with decreased resistance to infection need increased protection.*
- Avoid or minimize invasive procedures. *Maintaining the protective skin barrier is especially important for the patient with altered immune status.*

CASE STUDY & NURSING CARE PLAN A Patient with Acute Glomerulonephritis

Jung-Lin Chang is a 23-year-old graduate student in biology. He presents at the university health center with brown and foamy urine. The physician there admits him to the infirmary and orders a throat culture, ASO titer, CBC, BUN, serum creatinine, and urinalysis.

ASSESSMENT
Connie King, the nurse admitting Mr. Chang, notes that his history is essentially negative for past kidney or urinary problems. He relates having had a "pretty bad" sore throat a couple of weeks before admission. However, it was during midterms, so he took a few antibiotics he had from a previous bout of strep throat, increased his fluids, and did not see a doctor. The sore throat resolved, and he felt well until noticing the change in his urine. He admits that his eyes seemed a little puffy, but he thought this was due to lack of sleep and fatigue. He has eaten little the past 2 days, but was not alarmed because his food intake is irregular most of the time.

Physical assessment findings include T 98.8°F (37.1°C) PO, P 98, R 18, and BP 136/90. Weight 165 pounds (75 kg), up from his normal of 160 (72.5 kg). Moderate periorbital edema and edema of hands and fingers noted.

Throat culture is negative, but the ASO titer is high. CBC essentially normal. BUN 42 mg/dL, serum creatinine 2.1 mg/dL. Urinalysis reveals the presence of protein, red blood cells, and RBC casts. A subsequent 24-hour urine protein analysis shows 1025 mg of protein (normal 30 to 150 mg/24 hours).

The physician diagnoses acute poststreptococcal glomerulonephritis and places Mr. Chang on bed rest with bathroom privileges. He orders fluid restriction (1200 mL/day) and a restricted sodium and protein diet.

DIAGNOSES
- *Excess Fluid Volume* related to plasma protein deficit and sodium and water retention
- *Risk for Imbalanced Nutrition: Less than Body Requirements* related to anorexia
- *Anxiety* related to prescribed activity restriction
- *Readiness for Enhanced Self-Health Management* related to glomerulonephritis and treatment

EXPECTED OUTCOMES
- Maintain blood pressure within normal limits.
- Return to usual weight with no evidence of edema.
- Consume adequate calories following prescribed dietary limitations.
- Verbalize reduced anxiety regarding ability to continue studies.
- Demonstrate an understanding of acute glomerulonephritis and prescribed treatment regimen.

PLANNING AND IMPLEMENTATION
- Vital signs every 4 hours; notify physician of significant changes.
- Weigh daily; intake and output every 8 hours.
- Schedule fluids allowing 650 mL on day shift, 450 mL on evening shift, and 100 mL on night shift.
- Arrange dietary consultation to plan a diet that includes preferred foods as allowed.
- Provide small meals with high-carbohydrate between-meal snacks.
- Encourage Mr. Chang to talk about his condition and its potential effects.
- Assist with problem solving and exploring options for maintaining studies.
- Enlist friends and family to listen and provide support.
- Teach Mr. Chang and his family about acute glomerulonephritis and prescribed treatment.
- Instruct in appropriate antibiotic use.

EVALUATION
Mr. Chang is released from the infirmary after 4 days. He decides to return to his parents' home for the 6 to 12 weeks of convalescence prescribed by his doctor. Mr. Chang's renal function gradually returns to normal with no further azotemia and minimal proteinuria after 4 months. He verbalizes understanding of the relationship between the strep throat, his inappropriate use of antibiotics, and the glomerulonephritis. He says, "I may not always remember to take every pill on time in the future, but I sure won't save them for the next time again!"

CRITICAL THINKING IN THE NURSING PROCESS
1. How did Mr. Chang's use of "a few" previously prescribed antibiotics to treat his sore throat affect his risk for developing poststreptococcal glomerulonephritis?
2. What additional risk factors did Mr. Chang have for developing glomerulonephritis?
3. The initial manifestations of acute poststreptococcal glomerulonephritis and rapidly progressive glomerulonephritis are very similar. What diagnostic test would the physician use to make the differential diagnosis? Develop a plan of care for a patient undergoing this examination.

See Evaluating Your Response in Appendix C.

- If catheterization is required, use sterile intermittent straight catheterization or maintain a closed drainage system for an indwelling catheter. Prevent urine reflux from the drainage system to the bladder or the bladder to the kidneys by ensuring a patent, gravity flow system. *The urinary tract is a frequent entry point for infection, particularly in the hospitalized or institutionalized patient. Maintaining strict asepsis during catheterization is vital. Intermittent catheterization is associated with a lower risk of UTI than an indwelling catheter.*
- Provide a nutritionally sound diet with complete proteins. *A well-balanced, nutritionally sound diet is important to maintain nutritional status and support immune function.*

- Teach measures to prevent infection. *Care often is provided in the home, requiring the patient and family to use appropriate infection control measures.*

Ineffective Role Performance
The manifestations and treatment of glomerular disorders can affect the ability to maintain usual roles and activities. Fatigue and muscle weakness may limit physical and social activities. Activity limitations may be ordered to minimize the degree of proteinuria. If azotemia is present, malaise, nausea, and mental status changes can interfere with role function. Facial and periorbital edema affect the patient's self-esteem and may lead to isolation.

- Establish a strong therapeutic relationship. *It is important to gain the patient's trust and confidence.*
- Encourage self-care and participation in decision making. *Increased autonomy helps restore self-confidence and reduce powerlessness.*
- Provide time for verbalization of thoughts and feelings; listen actively, acknowledging and accepting fears and concerns. *Adequate time and active listening encourage expression of concerns and the effect of the disease or treatments on daily life. This helps the patient deal with the illness, its treatment, and associated losses.*
- Support coping skills, helping the patient identify personal strengths. *This support helps the patient gain confidence.*
- When possible, enlist the support of family, other patients, and friends. *These people can provide physical, psychologic, emotional, and social support.*
- Discuss the effect of the disease and treatments on roles and relationships, helping identify potential changes in roles, relationships, and lifestyle. Help the patient and family develop a plan for alternative behaviors and relationships, encouraging the patient to maintain usual roles to the extent possible. *Developing a plan helps reduce the strain of role changes and maintain a sense of dignity and control.*
- Provide accurate and optimistic information about the disorder and its short- and long-term effects. *The patient and family need accurate information to plan for the future.*
- Evaluate the need for additional support and social services for the patient and family. Provide referrals as indicated. *Depending on patient and family strengths, the severity of the disorder, and its treatment and prognosis, ongoing social support services may be necessary to facilitate coping and adaptation.*

Using NANDA, NIC, and NOC

Linkages between a selected NANDA nursing diagnosis, NIC, and NOC for the patient with glomerular disorder are shown in the chart that follows.

NANDA, NIC, AND NOC LINKAGES

The Patient with a Glomerular Disorder

NANDA

Fatigue

↓

NIC

Energy Management
Coping Enhancement
Nutrition Management

↓

NOC

Energy Conservation
Coping
Nutritional Status: Energy

Data from NANDA International. (2009). *Nursing Diagnoses: Definitions and Classification 2009–2011.* Oxford, UK: Wiley-Blackwell; Bulechek, G., Butcher, H., and Dochterman, J. (Eds.). (2008). *Nursing interventions classification (NIC)* (5th ed.). St. Louis, MO: Mosby; and Moorhead, S., Johnson, M., Maas, M., and Swanson, E. (Eds.). (2008). *Nursing outcomes classification (NOC)* (4th ed.). St. Louis, MO: Mosby.

Community-Based Care

Glomerular disorders may be self-limited or progressive. In either case, the course is lengthy, ranging from months to years. Self-management is essential. Provide instructions for the patient and family, including the following topics:

- Information about the disease and the prognosis
- Prescribed treatment, including activity and diet restrictions; the use and potential effects, both beneficial and adverse, of all medications
- Risks, manifestations, prevention, and management of complications such as edema and infection
- Signs, symptoms, and implications of improving or declining renal function
- Measures to prevent further kidney damage, such as nephrotoxic drugs to avoid
- Community resources, such as home care providers and support groups.

The Patient with a Vascular Kidney Disorder

Renal function is dependent on an adequate supply of blood. Blood supports renal cell metabolism and is vital to kidney function, the nephron in particular. The kidney can regulate fluid, electrolyte, and acid–base balance and serve as a major organ of excretion only when its blood supply is sufficient. Vascular disorders such as hypertension and atherosclerosis, therefore, can have a significant impact on renal function.

Hypertension

Hypertension, sustained elevation of the systemic blood pressure, can result from or cause kidney disease.

Prolonged hypertension damages the walls of arterioles and accelerates the process of atherosclerosis. This damage primarily affects the heart, brain, kidneys, eyes, and major blood vessels. In the kidney, arteriosclerotic lesions develop in the *afferent* (leading into) and *efferent* (going out of) arterioles and the glomerular capillaries. The glomerular filtration rate declines and tubular function is affected, resulting in proteinuria and microscopic hematuria. Uncontrolled or poorly controlled hypertension is the second leading cause of chronic kidney disease in the United States, accounting for nearly one-fourth of current cases (NKUDIC, 2009).

Malignant hypertension is a rapidly progressive form of hypertension that can develop in patients with untreated primary hypertension. The diastolic pressure is in excess of 120 mmHg and may be as high as 150 to 170 mmHg. Malignant hypertension affects less than 1% of hypertensive patients; it is more common in African Americans than in people of European ancestry. Untreated, malignant hypertension causes a rapid decline in renal function due to vessel changes, renal ischemia, and infarction.

Approximately 5% to 10% of hypertensive patients have *secondary hypertension*, which is actually a manifestation of an underlying disease. Renal vascular disease and diseases of the renal parenchyma, such as diabetic nephropathy, are commonly associated with secondary hypertension.

Management of hypertension to maintain the blood pressure within an optimal range is vital to prevent kidney damage. When hypertension is secondary to kidney disease, adequate blood pressure control can slow the decline in renal function. Hypertension and its management is discussed in depth in ∞ Chapter 32.

Renal Artery Stenosis

Renal artery stenosis (RAS) causes about 5% of all cases of hypertension (Fauci et al., 2008). It can affect one or both kidneys.

Renal artery stenosis is most often caused by atherosclerosis, particularly in older adults. The lumen of the renal artery is gradually occluded by plaque, affecting blood flow to the kidney. One or both kidneys may be affected. Atherosclerotic renovascular disease is more commonly found in people with evidence of coronary heart disease or peripheral vascular disease. Detailed discussion about the pathophysiology of atherosclerosis can be found in ∞ Chapter 30. In younger women, RAS is usually due to fibromuscular dysplasia, structural abnormalities of the arterial wall.

Renal artery stenosis stimulates the renin-angiotensin system as well as the sympathetic nervous system. Hypertension develops, along with flushing and significant blood pressure variations. Most patients have evidence of chronic kidney disease and significant cardiovascular risk by the time RAS is diagnosed. An epigastric bruit (murmur) and other manifestations of vascular insufficiency may also be present.

Doppler ultrasonography is used to screen for RAS. The affected kidney appears small and atrophied on renal ultrasound. Magnetic resonance angiography (MRA) and renal angiography with contrast allow visualization of renal blood vessels and are used to diagnose RAS

Conservative therapy is used for most patients with RAS. ACE inhibitors or angiotensin-receptor blockers (ARBs) are used along with diuretics and other antihypertensive drugs to control blood pressure. In some cases, percutaneous transluminal angioplasty is performed to dilate the affected vessel and position a stent to maintain patency. In this procedure, a balloon-tipped catheter is inserted via the femoral artery and aorta to dilate the renal artery. While this procedure is often effective, particularly in fibromuscular dysplasia, it is not without risk, including loss of renal function (Fauci et al., 2008).

Nursing care of the patient with RAS focuses on collaborating with the interdisciplinary team to achieve target blood pressures, monitoring renal function, implementing measures to preserve remaining renal function (e.g., ensuring adequate hydration, preventing urinary tract infection, and avoiding nephrotoxic medications), and teaching the patient and family about the prescribed treatment.

Renal Artery Occlusion

Renal arteries can be occluded by either a primary process affecting the renal vessels or by emboli, clots, or other foreign material. Risk factors for acute renal artery thrombosis (formation of a blood clot in the renal artery) include severe abdominal trauma, vessel trauma from surgery or angiography, aortic or renal artery aneurysms, and severe aortic or renal artery atherosclerosis. Emboli from the left side of the heart can travel via the aorta to occlude the renal artery. Emboli may form as a result of a trial fibrillation (irregular and uncoordinated electrical activity of the atria), following myocardial infarction, as vegetative growths on heart valves associated with bacterial endocarditis, or from fatty plaque in the aorta.

Renal arterial occlusion may be asymptomatic when the occlusion develops slowly and the affected vessels are small. Acute occlusion leading to ischemia and infarction typically causes sudden, severe localized flank pain, nausea and vomiting, fever, and hypertension. Hematuria and oliguria may occur. In the older patient, the new onset of hypertension or worsening of previously controlled hypertension may signal renal artery thrombosis.

Laboratory studies reveal leukocytosis (elevated WBC), and elevated renal enzyme levels, including aspartate transaminase (AST) and lactic dehydrogenase (LDH). These enzymes, normally present in renal cells, are released into the circulation when cells necrose and die. With bilateral arterial occlusion and infarction, renal function deteriorates rapidly, leading to acute renal failure (Fauci et al., 2008).

Surgery to restore blood flow to the affected kidney may be indicated for acute occlusion. Management usually is more conservative, using anticoagulant therapy, intrarenal fibrinolysis, hypertension control, and supportive treatment.

Renal Vein Occlusion

A thrombus (clot) formed in a renal vein can occlude the vessel. The cause of the thrombus often is unclear. In adults, renal venous thrombosis usually occurs with nephrotic syndrome. Other predisposing factors include pregnancy, oral contraceptive use, and certain malignancies.

Gradual or acute deterioration of renal function may be the only manifestation of renal vein occlusion. If the thrombus breaks loose, it can become a pulmonary embolism. The definitive diagnosis is made by visualizing the thrombus through renal venography.

Fibrinolytic drugs such as streptokinase or tissue plasminogen activator (tPA) may be given to dissolve or break up the thrombus. Anticoagulant therapy also is used to prevent further clotting and pulmonary emboli. Renal function often improves with treatment.

The Patient with Kidney Trauma

The kidneys are relatively well-protected by the rib cage, back muscles, and abdominal contents, but trauma due to blunt force or penetrating injury may inflict damage. Many renal injuries heal uneventfully, but prompt diagnosis and immediate treatment can be lifesaving in the event of major damage.

Pathophysiology and Manifestations

Blunt force is the most common cause of kidney injury. Falls, motor vehicle crashes, and sports injuries can damage the kidney. Damage may occur from a direct blow, as a result of rapid acceleration/deceleration injury, or a combination. The injury may be minor, causing a contusion or small hematoma, or more serious, resulting in laceration or other damage. The kidney may fragment or "shatter," causing significant blood loss and urine extravasation. Tearing of the renal artery or vein may cause rapid hemorrhage, with shock and possible death.

Gunshot wounds, knife wounds, impalement injuries, and fractured ribs can penetrate the kidney. Minor penetrating injuries may lacerate the capsule or renal cortex. Major injuries include laceration or destruction of renal parenchyma or the vascular supply. Renal artery, renal vein, and renal pelvis lacerations are critical injuries.

The primary manifestations of kidney trauma are hematuria (gross or microscopic), flank or abdominal pain, and oliguria or anuria. There may be localized swelling, tenderness, or ecchymoses in the flank region. Retroperitoneal bleeding from the kidney may cause Turner's sign, a bluish discoloration of the flank. Signs of shock may be present, including hypotension, tachycardia, tachypnea, cool and pale skin, and an altered level of consciousness.

Interdisciplinary Care

Hemoglobin and hematocrit levels fall in significant renal injury with hemorrhage. Hematuria is typically noted on urinalysis. AST levels rise within 12 hours of significant renal trauma. Renal ultrasonography is used to diagnose bleeding and kidney damage. A CT scan with contrast may be performed to visualize renal structures and establish a definitive diagnosis.

Treatment of minor kidney injuries is generally conservative, including bed rest and observation. In these injuries, bleeding is typically minor and self-limiting. With major or critical trauma, immediate treatment focuses on controlling hemorrhage and treating or preventing shock. Surgery may be required to stop the bleeding. Major lacerations may require surgical repair, partial nephrectomy, or total **nephrectomy** (removal) of the damaged kidney.

Nursing Care

Nursing care for the patient who has experienced renal trauma focuses on timely and accurate assessment and appropriate intervention to preserve life and prevent complications. Obtain a urine specimen for analysis when kidney trauma is suspected. Monitor level of consciousness, vital signs, skin color and temperature, and urine output for possible signs of shock. ∞ See Chapter 11 for additional nursing care measures for the patient who has had a traumatic injury or who develops shock.

The Patient with a Renal Tumor

Renal tumors may be either benign or malignant, primary or metastatic. Benign renal tumors are infrequent and are often found only on autopsy. Primary renal malignancies account for about 2% of adult cancers and approximately 12,980 deaths per year (American Cancer Society, 2009). Most primary renal tumors arise from renal cells; a primary tumor also may develop in the renal pelvis, although less frequently. Metastatic lesions to the kidney are associated with lung and breast cancer, melanoma, and malignant lymphoma.

Males are affected by renal cancer more than females by a 2:1 ratio. The highest incidence is seen in people over the age of 55 years. Smoking and obesity are risk factors; chronic irritation associated with renal calculi may also contribute. Some

---

MANIFESTATIONS of Renal Tumors

- Microscopic or gross hematuria
- Flank pain
- Palpable abdominal mass
- Fever
- Fatigue
- Weight loss
- Anemia or polycythemia

---

renal cancers are associated with genetic factors. Patients with ESRD also may develop renal cancer.

Pathophysiology and Manifestations

Most (90% to 95%) primary renal tumors are renal cell carcinomas (Fauci et al., 2008; Porth & Matfin, 2009). These tumors arise from tubular epithelium and can occur anywhere in the kidney. The tumor, which can range in size up to several centimeters, has clearly defined margins and contains areas of ischemia, necrosis, and hemorrhage. Renal tumors tend to invade the renal vein, and often have metastasized when first identified. Metastases tend to occur in the lungs, bone, lymph nodes, liver, and brain.

Renal tumors are often silent, with few manifestations. The classic triad of symptoms, gross hematuria, flank pain, and a palpable abdominal mass, is seen in only about 10% of people with renal cell carcinoma. Hematuria, often microscopic, is the most consistent symptom. Systemic manifestations include fever without infection, fatigue, and weight loss. See the Manifestations box on this page.

The tumor may produce hormones or hormone-like substances, including parathyroid hormone, prostaglandins, prolactin, renin, gonadotropins, and glucocorticoids. These substances produce *paraneoplastic syndromes*, with additional manifestations such as hypercalcemia, hypertension, and hyperglycemia. The progression of renal cell carcinomas varies from prolonged periods of stable disease to very aggressive. Table 28–4 outlines the staging and prognosis for renal cell cancers.

Interdisciplinary Care

Hematuria is often the only initial manifestation of renal cancer; its presence indicates a need for further diagnostic studies, including the following:

- *Renal ultrasonography* to detect renal masses and differentiate cystic kidney disease from renal carcinoma
- *CT scan* to of the abdomen determine tumor density, local extension of the tumor, and regional lymph node or vascular involvement (Figure 28–3 ■)
- *Chest x-ray, bone scan, MRI,* and *liver function studies* to identify potential metastases

Radical nephrectomy is the treatment of choice for stage I or II kidney tumors. In a radical nephrectomy, the adrenal gland, upper ureter, fat and fascia surrounding the kidney, as well as the entire kidney, are removed. Regional lymph nodes may also be resected. Although nephrectomy can be done using a laparoscopic approach, laparotomy primarily is used for radical nephrectomy. See the Nursing Care box for care of the patient having a nephrectomy.

TABLE 28–4 Renal Cell Cancer Staging

STAGE	EXTENT OF TUMOR	PROGNOSIS
I	Confined to the kidney capsule	> 90% 5-year survival
II	Invasion through the capsule but confined to local fascia	85% 5-year survival
III	Regional lymph node, ipsilateral renal vein, or inferior vena cava involvement	60% 5-year survival
IV	Locally invasive or distant metastases	10% or less 5-year survival

Source: Adapted from Fauci, A. et al. (Eds.). (2008). *Harrison's principles of internal medicine* (17th ed.). New York: McGraw-Hill.

No chemotherapy drug consistently causes tumor regression in patients with advanced renal carcinoma. Drugs that inhibit the growth of new blood vessels (called angiogenesis inhibitors or antiangiogenesis agents) are used as first-line treatment for advanced renal cancer. Interleukin 2 has lead to prolonged remission in a small proportion of patients, and may be used (DiPiro et al., 2008; Fauci et al., 2008).

ℰℴ Nursing Care

Nursing Diagnoses and Interventions

Nursing care for the patient with renal cancer focuses on needs related to the cancer diagnosis and to the surgical intervention. Postoperative pain may be significant and the risk for respiratory complications is high. The remaining kidney must be protected from damage to preserve renal function. Psychologically, the patient may grieve the loss of a major organ and the diagnosis of cancer.

Acute Pain

The size and location of the incision used for a radical nephrectomy (Figure 28–4 ■) make pain management a challenge. Intercostal blocks, patient-controlled analgesia (PCA), or routine analgesic administration can effectively relieve the discomfort. Nursing care focuses on assessing pain relief, providing supportive measures to enhance analgesia, and ensuring that pain or the fear of pain does not lead to respiratory complications.

- Assess frequently for adequate pain relief. Use a standard pain scale and nonverbal signs such as grimacing, tense body position, apparent dozing, elevated pulse, change of blood pressure, or rapid, shallow respirations. Notify the physician of inadequate pain relief. *The patient may assume that pain is to be expected or may fear becoming addicted to analgesics. Careful questioning and assessment allow effective pain management. Responses to analgesics are individual, and the prescribed dose may need to be adjusted.*
- Assess the incision for inflammation or swelling and drainage catheters and tubes for patency. *An obstructed catheter can lead to hydronephrosis, hematoma, or abscess, increasing incisional pain.*

> **PRACTICE ALERT**
> Assess for abdominal distention, tenderness, and bowel sounds. Intra-abdominal bleeding, peritonitis, or paralytic ileus can cause pain that may be confused with incisional pain.

- Use adjunctive pain relief measures such as positioning, diversional activities, management of environmental stimuli, guided imagery, and relaxation techniques. *These can enhance the effects of analgesia.*

Ineffective Breathing Pattern

The location of the incision combined with the respiratory depressant effects of narcotic analgesics increases the risk for respiratory complications in the patient who has had a nephrectomy.

- Position to promote respiratory excursion, using semi-Fowler's position and side-lying positions as allowed and tolerated. *Lung expansion is improved in semi-Fowler's and Fowler's positions.*

> **PRACTICE ALERT**
> Assess respiratory status frequently, including rate and depth, cough, breath sounds, oxygen saturation, and temperature. Pneumothorax on the operative side is common. Early identification and intervention can prevent major respiratory complications.

- Change position frequently, ambulate as soon as possible. *These measures promote lung expansion and the movement of mucus out of airways.*

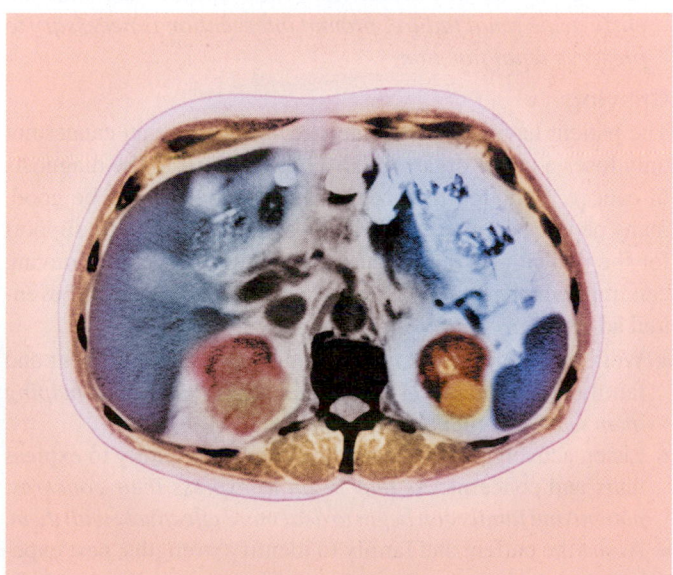

Figure 28–3 ■ A tumor of the right kidney is seen in the lower left of this color CT scan of the abdomen. The front of the body is at top in this view; the two kidneys (dark red) are seen either side of the spine (black, lower center). The tumor distorts the shape of the right kidney. The well-defined orange mass in the left kidney is a cyst.

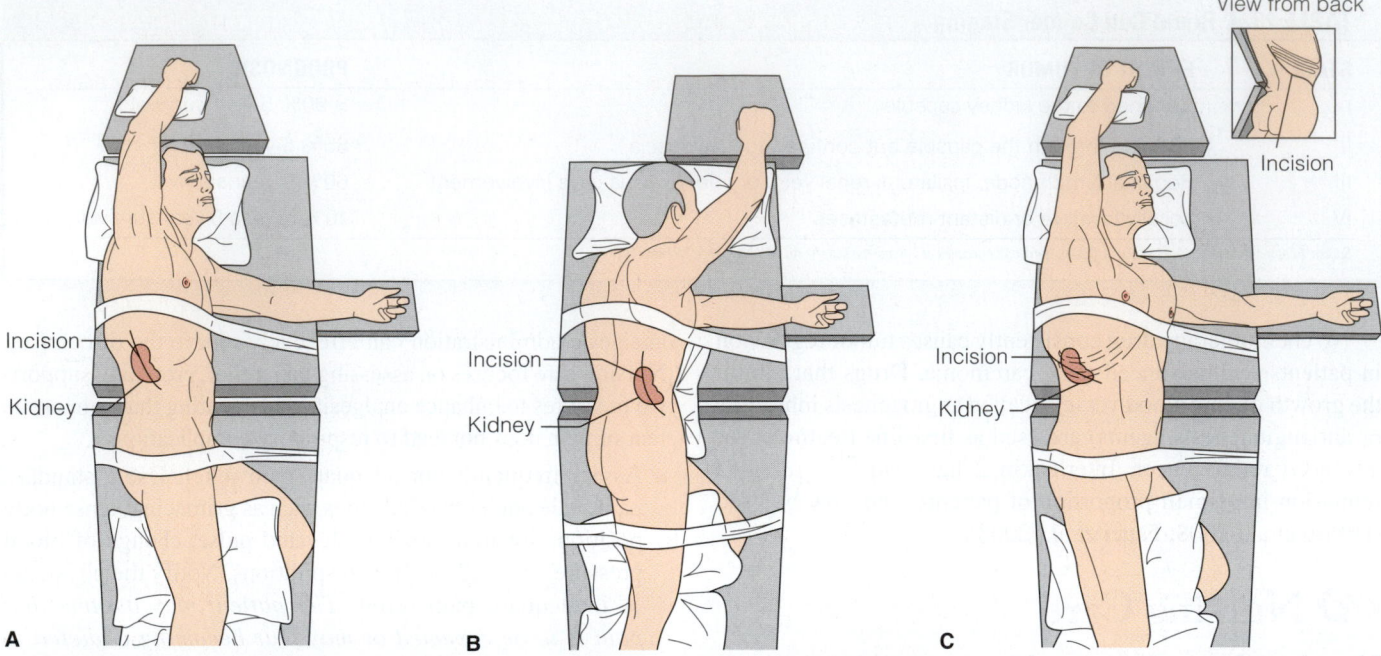

Figure 28–4 ■ Incisions used for kidney surgery: *A*, flank; *B*, lumbar; and *C*, thoracoabdominal.

■ Encourage frequent (every 1 to 2 hours) deep breathing, spirometer use, and coughing. Assist to splint the incision. *These measures promote alveolar ventilation, gas exchange, and airway clearance.*

Risk for Impaired Urinary Elimination

Surgery involving the urinary tract increases the risk for altered renal function and urine elimination. In addition, removal of one kidney dictates extra caution to maintain renal circulation, a sterile urinary tract, and free urine flow.

■ Monitor vital signs, CVP, and urine output every 1 to 2 hours initially, then every 4 hours. *Hypovolemia due to hemorrhage, diuresis, or fluid sequestering (third spacing) reduces blood flow to the kidney and increases the risk of renal ischemia with possible acute tubular necrosis and acute renal failure.*

■ Frequently assess the amount and nature of drainage on surgical dressings and from drainage tubes, stents, and catheters. Measure and record output from each drain or catheter separately. *Frequent and accurate assessment of drainage helps to identify excess bleeding, abnormal fluid loss, infection, or other potential surgical complications.*

> **PRACTICE ALERT**
> Prevent kinking, twisting, or tension on drains and tubes. Do not clamp. Irrigate carefully and only with a physician's order. Notify the physician immediately if any tube becomes dislodged. It is vital to maintain the patency of drains, particularly any affecting the remaining kidney, to prevent the excess pressure of hydronephrosis.

■ Maintain fluid intake with intravenous fluids until oral intake is resumed. Encourage an intake of 2000 to 2500 mL per day as soon as the patient tolerates oral liquids. *A liberal fluid intake prevents dehydration, helps to dilute any nephrotoxic substances, and promotes good urinary output.*

■ Use strict aseptic technique in caring for all urinary catheters, tubes, stents, drains, and incisions. *Asepsis is vital to prevent infection and possible compromise of the remaining kidney.*

■ Following catheter removal, assess frequently for urinary retention. Notify the physician if the patient is unable to void within 4 to 6 hours or if manifestations of retention (distended bladder, discomfort, urinary dribbling) develop. *Maintenance of urine output is vital to prevent stasis and possible complications such as infection and hydronephrosis.*

■ Monitor laboratory results, including urinalysis, BUN, serum creatinine, and serum electrolytes. Report abnormal findings to the physician. *Abnormal values may indicate early acute renal failure; prompt intervention is necessary to preserve renal function.*

Grieving

The patient having a radical nephrectomy for renal cancer not only loses a major organ but also has to adjust to the diagnosis of cancer. Although the prognosis for recovery may be good, many people perceive cancer as always fatal. Providing support for the patient and family during the initial stages of grieving can improve physical recovery, psychologic coping, and eventual adaptation.

■ Work to develop a trusting relationship with the patient and family. *Trust increases the nurse's effectiveness in helping them work through the process of grieving.*

■ Listen actively, encouraging the patient and family to express fears and concerns. *As they begin to express their concerns, patient and family can begin to deal more effectively with them.*

■ Assist the patient and family to identify strengths, past experiences, and support systems. *These resources can be employed in working through the grieving process.*

■ Demonstrate respect for cultural, spiritual, and religious values and beliefs; encourage use of these resources to cope with losses. *Value and belief systems can provide a structure and form for dealing with the grieving process.*

NURSING CARE OF THE PATIENT   Having A Nephrectomy

PREOPERATIVE CARE

- Provide routine preoperative care as outlined in ∞ Chapter 4.
- Report abnormal laboratory values to the surgeon. *Bacteriuria, blood coagulation abnormalities, or other significant abnormal values may affect surgery and postoperative care.*
- Discuss operative and postoperative expectations as indicated, including the location of the incision (Figure 28–4) and anticipated tubes, stents, and drains. *Preoperative teaching about postoperative expectations reduces anxiety for the patient and family during the early postoperative period.*

POSTOPERATIVE CARE

- Provide routine postoperative care as described in ∞ Chapter 4.
- Frequently assess urine color, amount, and character, noting any hematuria, pyuria, or sediment. Promptly report oliguria or anuria, as well as changes in urine color or clarity. *Preserving function of the remaining kidney is critical; frequent assessment allows early intervention for potential problems.*
- Note the placement, status, and drainage from ureteral catheters, stents, nephrostomy tubes, or drains. Label each clearly. Maintain gravity drainage; irrigate only as ordered. *Maintaining drainage tube patency is vital to prevent potential hydronephrosis. Bright bleeding o+r unexpected drainage may indicate a surgical complication.*
- Support the grieving process and adjustment to the loss of a kidney. *Loss of a major organ leads to a body image change and grief response. When renal cancer is the underlying diagnosis, the patient may also grieve the loss of health and potential loss of life.*

- Provide the following home care instructions for the patient and family:
  a. The importance of protecting the remaining kidney by preventing UTI, renal calculi, and trauma. ∞ See Chapter 27 for measures to prevent UTI and calculi. *Damage to the remaining kidney by UTI, renal calculi, or trauma can lead to renal failure.*
  b. Maintain a fluid intake of 2000 to 2500 mL per day. *This important measure helps prevent dehydration and maintain good urine flow.*
  c. Gradually increase exercise to tolerance, avoiding heavy lifting for a year after surgery. Participation in contact sports is not recommended to reduce the risk of injury to the remaining kidney. *Lifting is avoided to allow full tissue healing. Trauma to the remaining kidney could seriously jeopardize renal function.*
  d. Care of the incision and any remaining drainage tubes, catheters, or stents. *This routine postoperative instruction is vital to prepare the patient for self-care and prevent complications.*
  e. Report signs and symptoms to the physician, including manifestations of UTI (dysuria, frequency, urgency, nocturia, cloudy, malodorous urine) or systemic infection (fever, general malaise, fatigue), redness, swelling, pain, or drainage from the incision or any catheter or drain tube site. *Prompt treatment of postoperative infection is vital to allow continued healing and prevent compromise of the remaining kidney.*

- Encourage discussion of the potential impact of loss on the patient and the family structure and function. Assist family members to share concerns with one another. *Sharing of fears and concerns among family members promotes involvement and support of the entire family unit so that the individual is not left to cope alone.*
- Refer to cancer support groups, social services, or counseling as appropriate. *Support groups and counseling services provide additional resources for coping.*

Community-Based Care

If renal cancer was detected at an early stage and cure is anticipated, teaching for home care focuses on protecting the remaining kidney. Include the following measures to prevent infection, renal calculi, hydronephrosis, and trauma:

- Maintain a fluid intake of 2000 to 2500 mL per day, increasing the amount during hot weather or strenuous exercise.
- Urinate when the urge is perceived, and before and after sexual intercourse.
- Properly clean the perineal area.
- Watch for manifestations of UTI and understand the importance of early and appropriate evaluation and intervention.
- If the patient is an older adult male, he should watch for manifestations of prostatic hypertrophy, a major cause of urinary tract obstruction. Stress the importance of routine screening examinations.
- Avoid contact sports such as football or hockey; use measures to prevent motor vehicle accidents and falls, which could damage the kidney.

Renal Failure

Renal failure is a condition in which the kidneys are unable to remove accumulated metabolites from the blood, leading to altered fluid, electrolyte, and acid–base balance. The cause may be a primary kidney disorder, or renal failure may occur secondary to a systemic disease or other urologic defects. Renal failure may be either acute or chronic. Acute renal failure has an abrupt onset and with prompt intervention is often reversible. Chronic kidney disease (CKD) which may culminate in renal failure, develops slowly and insidiously, often producing few symptoms until the kidneys are severely damaged and unable to meet the excretory needs of the body. Acute renal failure and the final stages of chronic kidney disease are characterized by azotemia, increased levels of nitrogenous wastes in the blood.

Acute Renal Failure Video

Renal failure is common and costly. In 2006, more than 110,800 new patients began receiving treatment for end-stage renal disease (ESRD). Annually, more than 354,700 patients with ESRD undergo dialysis, about 18,000 have kidney transplants, and another 77,650 are awaiting kidney transplants. The annual cost of ESRD treatment (in 2006 dollars) is $33.6 billion. The cost is also measured in lives and lifestyle. The 5-year survival rate for patients undergoing dialysis is about 33% (NKUDIC, 2009). Although many patients report satisfaction with their quality of life, often patients on dialysis are unable to work, and the family structure may disintegrate under the strain of treatment.

The Patient with Acute Renal Failure

Acute renal failure (ARF) is a rapid decline in renal function (over hours to days) with azotemia and fluid and electrolyte imbalances. The most common causes of acute renal failure are ischemia and nephrotoxins. The kidney is particularly vulnerable to both because of the amount of blood that passes through it. A fall in blood pressure or volume can cause ischemia of kidney tissues. Nephrotoxins in the blood damage renal tissue directly.

Incidence and Risk Factors

Approximately 5% to 7% of all hospitalized patients develop ARF; the incidence jumps to as much as 30% in critical and special care units (Fauci et al., 2008). The mortality rate for ARF in seriously ill patients is up to 60%. This high death rate is probably more related to the populations affected by ARF— older patients and the critically ill—than to the disorder itself (Porth & Matfin, 2009).

Major trauma or surgery, infection, hemorrhage, severe heart failure, severe liver disease, and lower urinary tract obstruction are risk factors for ARF. Drugs and radiologic contrast media that are toxic to the kidney (*nephrotoxic*) also increase the risk for ARF. Older adults develop ARF more frequently due to their higher incidence of serious illness, hypotension, major surgeries, diagnostic procedures, and treatment with nephrotoxic drugs. The older adult also may have some degree of preexisting renal insufficiency associated with aging.

Physiology Review

The functional unit of the kidneys, the nephron (see Figure 26–3), produces urine through three processes: glomerular filtration, tubular reabsorption, and tubular secretion. In the

glomerulus, a filtrate of water and small solutes is formed. The solute concentration of this filtrate is equal to that of plasma, with the exception of large molecules such as plasma proteins and blood cells. The GFR, the amount of filtrate formed per minute, is affected by blood volume and pressure, the autonomic nervous system, and other factors. From the glomerulus, the filtrate flows into the *tubules*, where its composition is changed by the processes of *tubular reabsorption* and *tubular secretion*. Most water and many filtered solutes such as electrolytes and glucose are reabsorbed. Metabolic waste products such as urea, hydrogen ion, ammonia, and some creatinine are secreted into the tubule for elimination. By the time urine exits the collecting duct into the renal pelvis, 99% of the filtrate has been reabsorbed.

Pathophysiology

The causes and pathophysiology of acute renal failure are commonly categorized as prerenal, intrinsic, and postrenal ARF. Prerenal ARF is the most common, accounting for about 55% of the total. In *prerenal ARF*, hypoperfusion and ischemia lead to acute renal failure without directly affecting the integrity of kidney tissues. *Intrinsic* (or *intrarenal*) *ARF*, due to direct damage to functional kidney tissue, is responsible for another 40%. Urinary tract obstruction with resulting kidney damage is the precipitating factor for *postrenal ARF*, the least common form (~5%). Table 28–5 summarizes the causes of acute renal failure.

Prerenal ARF

Prerenal ARF results from conditions that affect renal blood flow and perfusion. Any disorder that significantly decreases vascular volume, cardiac output, or systemic vascular resistance can affect renal blood flow. The kidneys normally receive 20% to 25% of the cardiac output to maintain the GFR. A drop in renal blood flow to less than 20% of normal causes the GFR to fall. As the filtration of substances by the glomeruli is reduced, less reabsorption of substances in the tubule is required. As a result, kidney cells require less energy and oxygen, and their metabolism slows. Prerenal ARF is rapidly reversed when blood flow is restored, and the renal parenchyma remains undamaged. Continued ischemia can lead to tubular cell necrosis and significant nephron damage. Intrinsic ARF due to ischemic injury may result. See Pathophysiology Illustrated: Acute Renal Failure on page 838.

Postrenal ARF

Obstructive causes of acute renal failure are classified as postrenal. Any condition that prevents urine excretion can lead to postrenal ARF. Benign prostatic hypertrophy is the most

TABLE 28–5 Causes of Acute Renal Failure

	CAUSE	EXAMPLES
Prerenal	Hypovolemia	Hemorrhage, dehydration, excess fluid loss from GI tract, burns, wounds
	Low cardiac output	Heart failure, cardiogenic shock
	Altered vascular resistance	Sepsis, anaphylaxis, vasoactive drugs
Intrarenal	Glomerular/microvascular injury	Glomerulonephritis, DIC, vasculitis, hypertension, toxemia of pregnancy, hemolytic uremic syndrome
	Acute tubular necrosis	Ischemia due to conditions associated with prerenal failure; toxins such as drugs, heavy metals; hemolysis, rhabdomyolysis (muscle cell breakdown)
	Interstitial nephritis	Acute pyelonephritis, toxins, metabolic imbalances, idiopathic
Postrenal	Ureteral obstruction	Calculi, cancer, external compression
	Urethral obstruction	Prostatic enlargement, calculi, cancer, stricture, blood clot

common precipitating factor. Others include renal or urinary tract calculi and tumors. ∞ See Chapter 27 for further discussion of urinary tract obstruction.

Intrinsic (Intrarenal) ARF

Intrinsic or intrarenal failure is characterized by acute damage to the renal parenchyma and nephrons. Intrarenal causes include diseases of the kidney itself and acute tubular necrosis, the most common intrarenal cause of ARF.

In acute glomerulonephritis, glomerular inflammation can reduce renal blood flow and cause ARF. Vascular disorders affecting the kidney, such as vasculitis (inflammation of the blood vessels), malignant hypertension, and arterial or venous occlusion, can damage nephrons sufficiently to result in acute renal failure.

ACUTE TUBULAR NECROSIS Nephrons are especially susceptible to injury from ischemia or exposure to nephrotoxins. **Acute tubular necrosis (ATN)**, destruction of tubular epithelial cells, causes an abrupt and progressive decline of renal function. Prolonged ischemia is the primary cause of ATN. When ischemia and nephrotoxin exposure occur concurrently, the risk for ATN and tubular dysfunction is especially high. Risk factors for ischemic ATN include major surgery, severe hypovolemia, sepsis, trauma, and burns. The impact of ischemia resulting from vasodilation and fluid loss in sepsis, trauma, and burns often is compounded by toxins released by bacteria or from damaged tissue.

Ischemia lasting more than 2 hours causes severe and irreversible damage to kidney tubules with patchy cellular necrosis and sloughing. The GFR is significantly reduced as a result of (1) ischemia, (2) activation of the renin–angiotensin system, and (3) tubular obstruction by cellular debris, which raises the pressure in the glomerular capsule.

Common nephrotoxins associated with ATN include the aminoglycoside antibiotics and radiologic contrast media. Many other drugs (e.g., NSAIDs and some chemotherapy drugs), heavy metals such as mercury and gold, and some common chemicals such as ethylene glycol (antifreeze) are also potentially toxic to the renal tubule. The risk for ATN is higher when nephrotoxic drugs are given to older patients or patients with preexisting renal insufficiency, and when used in combination with other nephrotoxins. Dehydration increases the risk by increasing the toxin concentration in nephrons.

Nephrotoxins destroy tubular cells by both direct and indirect effects. As tubular cells are damaged and lost through necrosis and sloughing, the tubule becomes more permeable. This increased permeability results in filtrate reabsorption, further reducing the ability of the nephron to eliminate wastes.

Rhabdomyolysis caused by release of excess myoglobin from injured skeletal muscles can cause ATN. Myoglobin is a protein that acts as the oxygen reservoir for muscle fibers, much as hemoglobin does for the blood. Muscle trauma, strenuous exercise, hyperthermia or hypothermia, drug overdose, infection, and other factors can precipitate rhabdomyolysis. The myoglobin clogs renal tubules causing ischemic injury, and contains an iron pigment that directly damages the tubules. *Hemolysis*, red blood cell destruction, releases hemoglobin into the circulation with much the same effect as rhabdomyolysis.

Course and Manifestations

The course of acute renal failure due to ATN typically includes three phases: initiation, maintenance, and recovery.

Initiation Phase

The initiation phase may last hours to days. It begins with the initiating event (e.g., hemorrhage) and ends when tubular injury occurs. If ARF is recognized and the initiating event is effectively treated during this phase, the prognosis is good. The initiation phase of ARF has few symptoms; in fact, it is often identified only when manifestations of the maintenance phase develop.

Maintenance Phase

The maintenance phase of ARF is characterized by a significant fall in GFR and tubular necrosis. Oliguria may develop, although many patients continue to produce normal or near-normal amounts of urine (nonoliguric ARF). Even though urine may be produced, the kidney cannot efficiently eliminate metabolic wastes, water, electrolytes, and acids from the body during the maintenance phase of ARF. Azotemia, fluid retention, electrolyte imbalances, and metabolic acidosis develop. These abnormalities are more severe in the oliguric patient than in the nonoliguric one, leading to a poorer prognosis with oliguria.

PATHOPHYSIOLOGY ILLUSTRATED
Acute Renal Failure

The initial kidney injury is usually associated with an acute condition such as sepsis, trauma, and hypotension, or the result of treatment for an acute condition with a nephrotoxic medication. Injury to the kidney can occur because of glomerular injury, vasoconstriction of capillaries, or tubular injury. All consequences of injury lead to decreased glomerular filtration and oliguria.

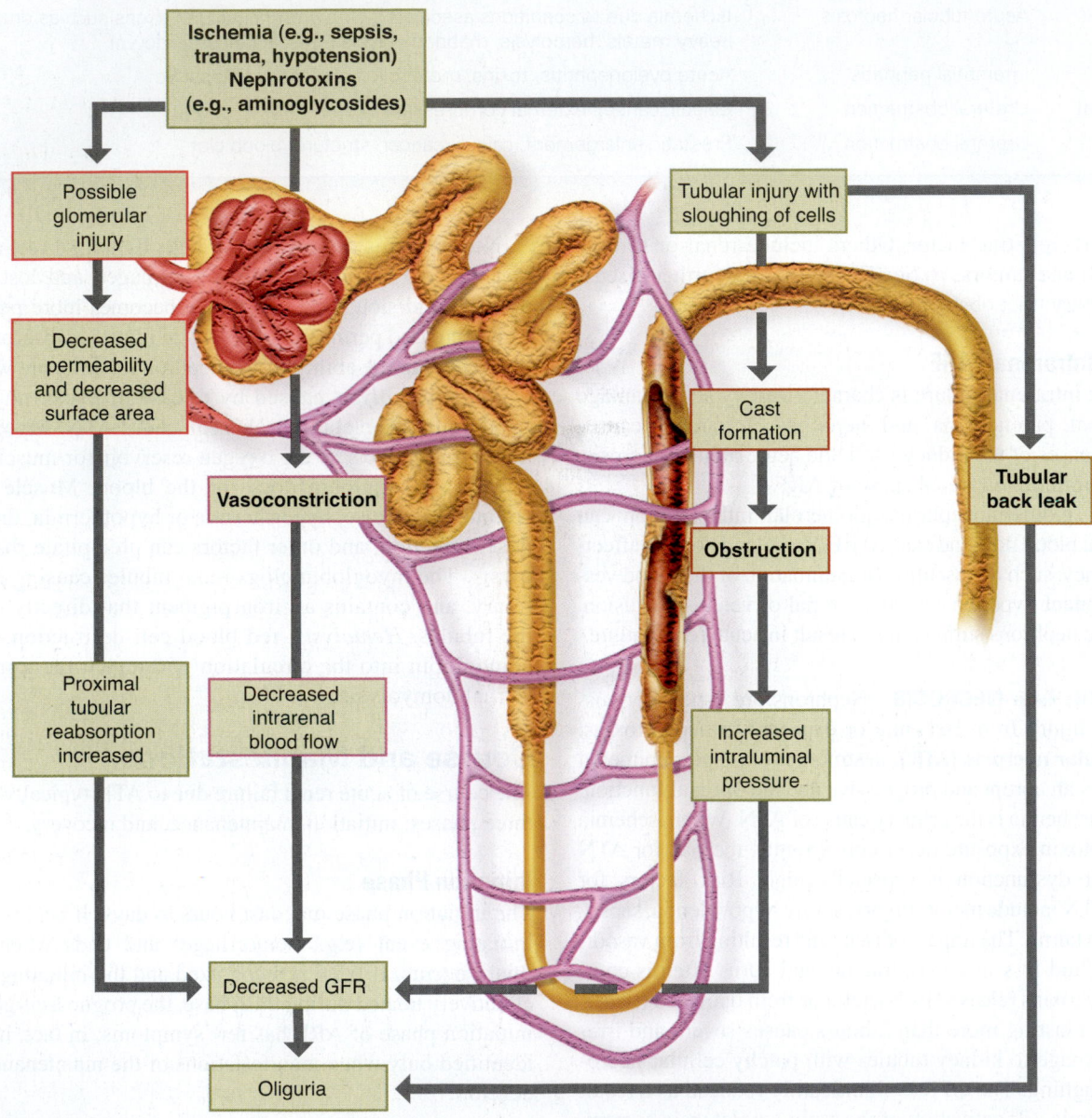

During the maintenance phase, salt and water retention cause edema, increasing the risk for heart failure and pulmonary edema. Impaired potassium excretion leads to hyperkalemia. When the serum potassium level is greater than 6.0 to 6.5 mEq/L, manifestations of its effect on neuromuscular function develop. These include muscle weakness, nausea and diarrhea, electrocardiographic changes, and possible cardiac arrest. Other electrolyte imbalances include hyperphosphatemia and hypocalcemia. Metabolic acidosis results from impaired hydrogen ion elimination by the kidneys.

Erythropoietin secretion by the kidneys is suppressed in ARF, causing anemia to develop after several days. Immune function may be impaired, increasing the risk for infection. Other manifestations of the maintenance phase include the following:

- Edema and hypertension due to salt and water retention
- Confusion, disorientation, agitation or lethargy, hyperreflexia, and possible seizures or coma due to azotemia and electrolyte and acid–base imbalances
- Anorexia, nausea, vomiting, and decreased or absent bowel sounds

- Uremic syndrome if ARF is prolonged (see the section on chronic kidney disease that follows)

Recovery Phase

The recovery phase of ARF is characterized by a process of tubule cell repair and regeneration and gradual return of the GFR to normal or pre-ARF levels. Diuresis may occur as the nephrons and GFR recover, and retained salt, water, and solutes are excreted. Serum creatinine, BUN, potassium, and phosphate levels remain high and may continue to rise in spite of increasing urine output. Renal function improves rapidly during the first 5 to 25 days of the recovery phase, and continues to improve for up to 1 year.

Interdisciplinary Care

Preventing acute renal failure is a goal in caring for all patients, especially those in high-risk groups. Maintaining an adequate vascular volume, cardiac output, and blood pressure is vital to preserve kidney perfusion. Nephrotoxic drugs are avoided whenever possible. When a nephrotoxic drug or substance must be used, the risk of ARF can be reduced by using the minimum effective dose, maintaining hydration, and eliminating other known nephrotoxins from the medication regimen.

Treatment goals for acute renal failure are to (1) identify and correct the underlying cause, (2) prevent additional kidney damage, (3) restore the urine output and kidney function, and (4) compensate for renal impairment until kidney function is restored. Fluid and electrolyte balance is a key component in managing ARF.

The patient's history and physical assessment can provide clues about the initiating event for ARF. Impaired perfusion for as few as 30 minutes may cause significant renal ischemia.

Diagnosis

Diagnostic tests are used to identify the cause of acute renal failure and monitor its effects on homeostasis:

- *Urinalysis* often shows the following abnormal findings in acute renal failure:
  a. A fixed specific gravity of 1.010 (equal to the specific gravity of plasma) because the tubules are unable to concentrate the filtrate
  b. Proteinuria if glomerular damage is the cause of ARF
  c. The presence of RBCs (due to glomerular dysfunction), WBCs (related to inflammation), and renal tubular epithelial cells (indicating ATN)
  d. Cell casts, which are protein and cellular debris molded in the shape of the tubular lumen. In ARF, red and white blood cells and renal tubular epithelial casts may be present. Brownish pigmented casts and positive tests for occult blood indicate hemoglobinuria or myoglobinuria.
- *Serum creatinine, BUN, BUN/creatinine ratio*, and *eGFR* are used to evaluate renal function. In ARF, serum creatinine levels increase rapidly, within 24 to 48 hours of the onset. The BUN/creatinine ratio is reduced, and the eGFR falls in ARF. Creatinine levels generally peak within 5 to 10 days. Creatinine and BUN levels tend to increase more slowly when urine output is maintained. The onset of recovery is marked by a halt in the rise of the serum creatinine and BUN.

- *Serum electrolytes* are monitored to evaluate the fluid and electrolyte status. The serum potassium rises at a moderate rate and is often used to indicate the need for dialysis. Hyponatremia is common, due to the water excess associated with ARF.
- *Arterial blood gases* often show a metabolic acidosis due to the kidneys' inability to adequately eliminate metabolic wastes and hydrogen ions (∞ see Chapter 10).
- *CBC* shows reduced RBCs, moderate anemia, and a low hematocrit. ARF affects erythropoietin secretion and RBC production. Iron and folate absorption may also be impaired, further contributing to anemia.

Laboratory findings associated with kidney disease are summarized in Table 28–2.

- *Renal ultrasonography* is used to identify obstructive causes of renal failure, and to differentiate acute renal failure from end-stage chronic kidney disease. In ARF, the kidneys may be enlarged, whereas they typically appear small and shrunken in chronic kidney disease.
- *CT scan* or *MRI* also may be done to evaluate kidney size and identify possible obstructions.
- *Renal biopsy* may be necessary to differentiate between acute and chronic renal failure.

∞ See Chapter 26 for nursing implications of tests used to identify causes of renal failure.

Medications

The primary focus in drug management for acute renal failure is to restore and maintain renal perfusion and to eliminate drugs that are nephrotoxic from the treatment regimen.

Intravenous fluids and blood volume expanders are given as needed to restore renal perfusion. Dopamine (Intropin), administered in low doses by intravenous infusion, increases renal blood flow. Dopamine is a sympathetic neurotransmitter that improves cardiac output and dilates blood vessels of the mesentery and kidneys when given in low therapeutic doses. Atrial natriuretic peptide (ANP) also may increase the GFR by selectively dilating the afferent arterioles and constricting efferent arterioles (Cheung et al., 2008).

If restoration of renal blood flow does not improve urinary output, a loop diuretic such as furosemide (Lasix) or an osmotic diuretic such as mannitol may be given with intravenous fluids. The purpose is twofold. First, if nephrotoxins are present, the combination of fluids and potent diuretics may, in effect, "wash out" the nephrons, reducing toxin concentration. Second, establishing urine output may prevent oliguria, and reduce the degree of azotemia and fluid and electrolyte imbalances. In some cases, a combination of a loop diuretic and a thiazide diuretic may be used to reestablish urine output and manage salt and water retention associated with ARF.

Aggressive hypertension management limits renal injury when ARF is associated with disorders such as toxemia and pregnancy-induced hypertension. ACE inhibitors, ARBs, or other antihypertensive medications are used to control arterial pressures.

All drugs that are either directly nephrotoxic or that may interfere with renal perfusion (such as potent vasoconstrictors) are discontinued. NSAIDs, nephrotoxic antibiotics such as the aminoglycosides, and other potentially harmful drugs (e.g., contrast media) are avoided throughout the course of acute renal failure.

The patient in acute renal failure has an increased risk of gastrointestinal bleeding, probably related to the stress response and impaired platelet function. Regular doses of antacids, histamine H_2-receptor antagonists (e.g., famotidine or ranitidine), or a proton-pump inhibitor such as omeprazole (Prilosec), are often ordered to prevent GI hemorrhage.

Hyperkalemia may require active intervention as well as restricted potassium intake. Serum levels of greater than 6.5mEq/L are treated to prevent cardiac effects of hyperkalemia. With significant hyperkalemia, calcium chloride, bicarbonate, and insulin and glucose may be given intravenously to reduce serum potassium levels by moving potassium into the cells. A potassium-binding exchange resin such as sodium polystyrene sulfonate (Kayexalate, SPS Suspension) may be given orally or by enema. This agent removes potassium from the body by exchanging sodium for potassium, primarily in the large intestine. When given orally, it is often combined with sorbitol to prevent constipation. Rectally, it is instilled as a retention enema, allowed to remain in the bowel for approximately 30 to 60 minutes, and then irrigated out using a tap-water enema.

Aluminum hydroxide (AlternaGEL, Amphojel, Nephrox), an antacid, is used to control hyperphosphatemia in renal failure. It binds with phosphates in the GI tract, which are then excreted in the feces.

Because many drugs are eliminated from the body by the kidney, drug dosages may need to be adjusted. Doses within the usual range can lead to potentially toxic blood levels, because their elimination is slowed and half-life prolonged. Nursing implications for medications commonly prescribed for the patient in ARF are summarized in the Medication Administration box.

Fluid Management

Once vascular volume and renal perfusion are restored, fluid intake is usually restricted. The allowed daily fluid intake is calculated by allowing 500 mL for insensible losses (respiration, perspiration, bowel losses) and adding the amount excreted as urine (or lost in vomitus) during the previous 24 hours. For example, if a patient with ARF excretes 325 mL of urine in 24 hours, the patient is allowed a fluid intake (including oral and intravenous fluids) of 825 mL for the next 24 hours. Fluid balance is carefully monitored, using accurate weight measurements and the serum sodium as the primary indicators. Hemodynamic monitoring may be initiated to aid in fluid management of the critically ill patient. ∞ See Chapter 31 for more information about hemodynamic monitoring.

Nutrition

Renal insufficiency and the underlying disease process increase the rate of *catabolism* (the breakdown of body proteins) and decrease the rate of *anabolism* (body tissue repair). The patient with ARF needs adequate nutrients and calories to prevent catabolism. Proteins may be limited to 0.6 g per kilogram of body weight per day to minimize the degree of azotemia. Dietary proteins should be of high biologic value (rich in essential amino acids). Carbohydrates are increased to maintain adequate calorie intake and provide a protein-sparing effect.

Parenteral nutrition providing amino acids, concentrated carbohydrates, and fats may be instituted when the patient cannot consume an adequate diet (e.g., due to nausea, vomiting, or underlying critical illness). The disadvantages of parenteral nutrition in the patient with ARF are the high volume of fluid required and the risk for infection through the venous line.

Renal Replacement Therapy

Manifestations of *uremia*, organ dysfunction due to accumulated metabolic wastes, severe fluid overload, hyperkalemia, or metabolic acidosis in a patient with renal failure, indicate a need to replace renal function. **Dialysis** is the diffusion of solute molecules across a semipermeable membrane from an area of higher solute concentration to one of lower concentration. It is used to remove excess fluid and metabolic waste products in renal failure. Early use of dialysis can reduce the rate of complications. Dialysis may also be used to rapidly remove nephrotoxins in acute tubular necrosis. While dialysis compensates for lost renal elimination functions, it does not replace lost erythropoietin production. Anemia is a continuing problem for the patient receiving dialysis.

In dialysis, blood is separated from a dialysis solution (*dialysate*) by a semipermeable membrane. Either **hemodialysis**, a procedure in which blood passes through a semipermeable membrane filter outside the body, or **peritoneal dialysis**, which uses the peritoneum surrounding the abdominal cavity as the dialyzing membrane, may be used for the patient with ARF.

Hemofiltration is closely related to dialysis. It may be used in critically ill patients unable to tolerate dialysis procedures. Hemofiltration may be combined with hemodialysis in a procedure called *hemodiafiltration*.

INTERMITTENT HEMODIALYSIS Hemodialysis uses the principles of diffusion and ultrafiltration to remove electrolytes, waste products, and excess water from the body. Blood is taken from the patient via a vascular access and pumped to the dialyzer (Figure 28–5 ■). The porous membranes of the dialyzer unit allow small molecules such as water, glucose, and electrolytes to pass through, but block larger molecules such as serum proteins and blood cells. The dialysate, a solution of approximately the same composition and temperature as normal extracellular fluid, passes along the other side of the membrane. Small solute molecules move freely across the membrane by diffusion. The direction of movement for any substance is determined by the concentrations of that substance in the blood and the dialysate. Electrolytes and waste products such as urea and creatinine diffuse from the blood into the dialysate. If it is necessary to add something to the blood, such as calcium to replace depleted stores, it can be added to the dialysate to diffuse into the blood. Excess water is removed by creating a higher hydrostatic pressure of the blood moving through the dialyzer than of the dialysate, which flows in the opposite direction. This process is known as **ultrafiltration**.

Initially, patients with ARF typically undergo hemodialysis for 3 to 4 hours daily, then three to four sessions per week as indicated. Hemodialysis is not used if the patient is hemodynamically

MEDICATION ADMINISTRATION The Patient with Acute Renal Failure

LOOP DIURETICS
Bumetanide (Bumex)

Ethacrynic acid (Edecrin)

Furosemide (Lasix)

Torsemide (Demadex)

The loop diuretics, named for their primary site of action in the loop of Henle, are highly effective diuretics used in early ARF to reestablish urine flow and convert oliguric renal failure to nonoliguric renal failure. Loop diuretics may be given with intravenous dopamine to promote renal blood flow. In ATN due to a nephrotoxin, loop diuretics are used to clear the toxin from the nephrons more rapidly. Loop diuretics cause potassium wasting, which is generally not a concern in ARF because renal failure impairs normal potassium elimination.

Nursing Responsibilities
- Assess weight and vital signs for baseline data.
- Monitor intake and output, daily weight (or more frequently as ordered), vital signs, skin turgor, and other indicators of fluid volume status frequently.
- Assess for orthostatic hypotension because these potent diuretics can lead to hypovolemia.
- Monitor laboratory results, especially serum electrolyte, glucose, BUN, and creatinine levels.
- Administer by mouth or, if ordered, by intravenous injection or infusion:
  a. Furosemide injection at a rate of no more than 20 mg per minute; continuous infusion at 10 to 20 mg/hr
  b. Ethacrynic acid 50 mg diluted with 50 mL of normal saline at a rate of no more than 10 mg per minute
  c. Bumetanide undiluted over at least 1 minute or diluted in lactated Ringer's solution, normal saline, or 5% dextrose in water for infusion
  d. Torsemide undiluted over at least 2 minutes
- Assess response. Urine output typically increases within 10 minutes after intravenous administration.
- Monitor hearing and for complaints such as tinnitus. High doses of loop diuretics increase the risk of ototoxicity, especially with ethacrynic acid. These effects may be reversible if detected early and the drug is discontinued.
- Avoid administering concurrently with other ototoxic agents, such as aminoglycoside antibiotics and cisplatin.

Health Education for the Patient and Family
- Unless contraindicated, maintain a fluid intake of 2 to 3 quarts per day.
- Rise slowly from lying or sitting positions, because a fall in blood pressure may cause light-headedness.
- Take in the morning and, if ordered twice a day, late afternoon to avoid sleep disturbance.
- Take with food or milk to prevent gastric distress.
- NSAIDs interfere with the effectiveness of loop diuretics and should be avoided.

OSMOTIC DIURETICS
Mannitol (Osmitrol, Isotol)

Urea (Ureaphil)

The osmotic diuretics act by increasing the osmotic draw in the blood and urine. In the blood, the effect is to pull extracellular water into the vascular system, increasing the GFR. These substances are then freely filtered in the glomerulus and increase the osmotic draw of the urine, inhibiting water reabsorption. The effect is to increase urine volume and flow. In addition, osmotic diuretics dilute waste products in the urine, decreasing the risk of renal damage due to excess concentrations.

Nursing Responsibilities
- Assess urine output. Osmotic diuretics are used in early renal failure to maintain urine output but are contraindicated in anuria. A test dose may be administered; urine output of 30 mL per hour following the test dose shows an adequate response.
- Do not give these diuretics to patients who have heart failure or who are severely dehydrated. They increase vascular volume and may worsen heart failure. These drugs are not effective unless extracellular volume is adequate.
- Administer mannitol intravenously, diluting before use if indicated. Check solution for crystallization. Dissolve crystals by warming the solution slightly. Infuse 15% to 25% mannitol solutions through a filter over 30 to 90 minutes.
- Administer urea intravenously, diluting in 100 mL of 5% or 10% dextrose in water for every 30 g of urea. Administer no faster than 4 mL per minute through a filter.
- Monitor vital signs, breath sounds, and urinary output.
- Discontinue the drug if signs of heart failure or pulmonary edema develop or if renal function continues to decline.

Health Education for the Patient and Family
- Report shortness of breath, headache, chest pain, or dizziness immediately.

ELECTROLYTES AND ELECTROLYTE MODIFIERS
Calcium chloride

Calcium gluconate

Sodium bicarbonate

Sodium polystyrene sulfonate (Kayexalate)

Calcium chloride or gluconate and sodium bicarbonate are administered intravenously in the initial management of hyperkalemia. Calcium is also administered to correct hypocalcemia and reduce hyperphosphatemia. (Calcium and phosphate have a reciprocal relationship in the body: as the level of one rises, the level of the other falls.) Sodium bicarbonate helps correct acidosis and move potassium back into the intracellular space. Sodium polystyrene sulfonate is not used to replace an electrolyte, but to remove excess potassium from the body by exchanging sodium for potassium in the large intestine.

Nursing Responsibilities
- Assess serum electrolyte levels prior to and during therapy. Report rapid shifts or adverse responses to the physician.
- Administer as appropriate:
  a. Intravenous calcium chloride at less than 1 mL per minute; intravenous calcium gluconate at 0.5 mL per minute. Inject into a large vein through a small-bore needle; avoid infiltration because extravasation of intravenous solution will cause tissue necrosis.
  b. Intravenous sodium bicarbonate infusion over 4 to 8 hours; oral tablets as prescribed.
  c. Sodium polystyrene sulfonate as an oral solution mixed with sorbitol to prevent constipation, or as a retention enema mixed with warm water. Leave in the bowel for 30 to 60 minutes, irrigate using a small tap-water enema.
- Monitor for adverse reactions, such as dysrhythmias, electrolyte imbalances, and metabolic alkalosis.

Health Education for the Patient and Family
- Intravenous calcium may make you light-headed; remain in bed for at least 30 minutes after administration.
- Chew sodium bicarbonate tablets and follow with 8 ounces of water. Do not take with milk.
- Retain the sodium polystyrene sulfonate enema as long as possible.

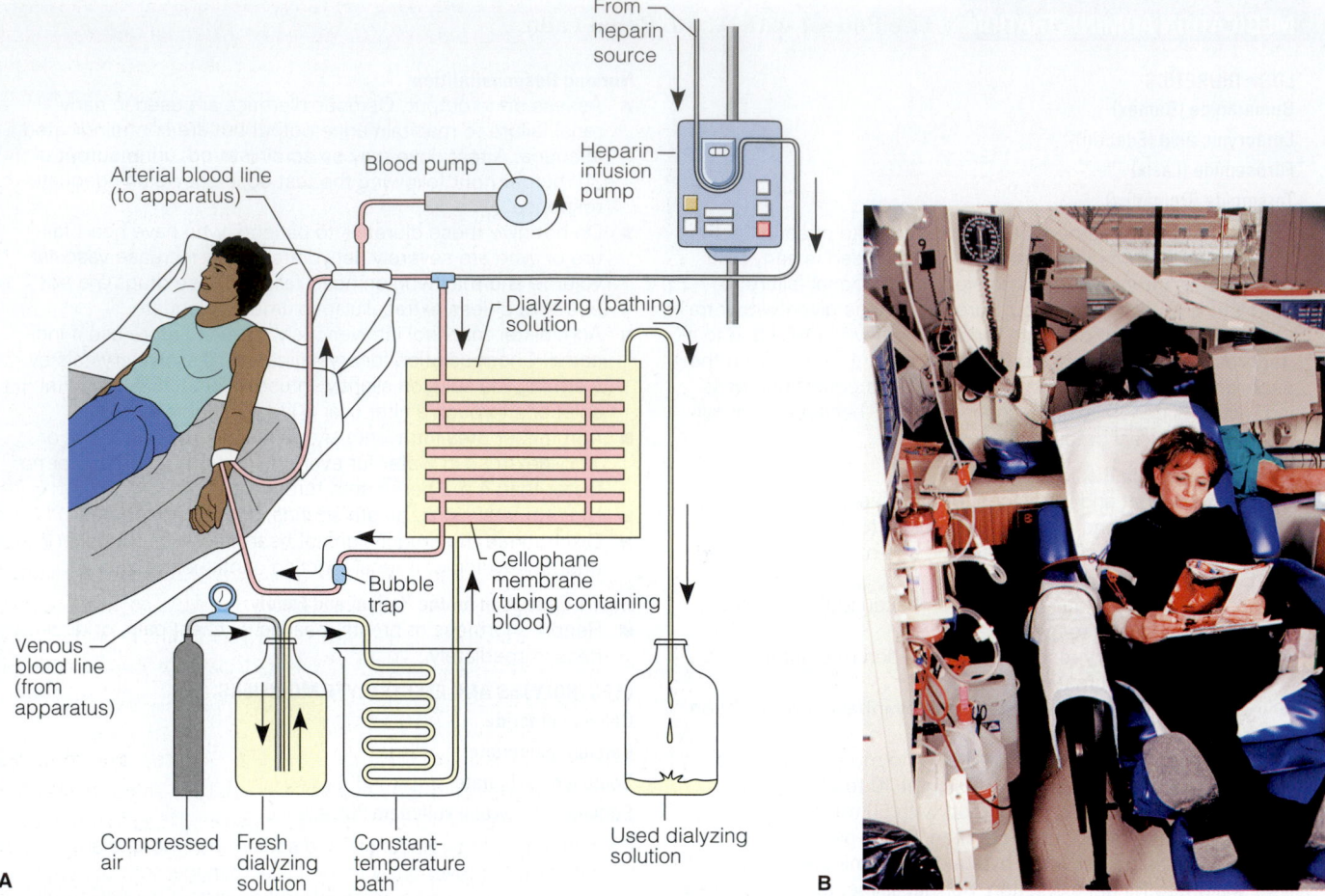

Figure 28–5 ■ *A*, The components of a hemodialysis system. *B*, A woman receiving kidney dialysis.

unstable (e.g., with hypotension or low cardiac output). Following are complications associated with hemodialysis:

■ Hypotension, the most frequent complication during hemodialysis, is related to changes in serum osmolality, rapid removal of fluid from the vascular compartment, vasodilation, and other factors.

■ Bleeding is related to altered platelet function associated with uremia and the use of heparin during dialysis.

■ Infection (local or systemic) is related to WBC damage and immune system suppression. *Staphylococcus aureus* septicemia is commonly associated with contamination of the vascular access site. Patients on chronic hemodialysis have higher rates of hepatitis B, hepatitis C, cytomegalovirus, and HIV infection than the general population.

See the box on page 844 for nursing care of the patient undergoing hemodialysis.

CONTINUOUS RENAL REPLACEMENT THERAPY   Patients with acute renal failure may be unable to tolerate hemodialysis and rapid fluid removal if their cardiovascular status is unstable (e.g., due to trauma, major surgery, heart failure). *Continuous renal replacement therapy* (also called *sustained renal replacement therapy*) is a hemofiltration procedure that allows more gradual fluid and solute removal. In CRRT, blood is continuously circulated through a highly porous hemofilter for a period of 8 to 12 or more hours (Figure 28–6 ■). A large central catheter usually is used to provide venous access.

Excess water and solutes such as electrolytes, urea, creatinine, uric acid, and glucose drain into a collection device. Fluid is replaced with normal saline or a balanced electrolyte solution as needed during CRRT. This slower process helps maintain hemodynamic stability and avoid complications associated with rapid changes in ECF composition. The most common CRRT techniques are outlined in Table 28–6.

CRRT is typically performed in an intensive care unit or specialized nephrology unit. A double-lumen venous catheter is used for most types of CRRT. Strict aseptic technique is vital in caring for vascular access sites to reduce the risk of infection.

VASCULAR ACCESS   Acute or temporary vascular access for hemodialysis or CRRT usually is gained by inserting a double-lumen catheter into the subclavian, jugular, or femoral vein. The double-lumen catheter has a central partition separating the blood withdrawal side of the catheter from the return side. Blood is drawn into the catheter through small openings in the proximal portion of the catheter, and returned to the circulation through an opening in the distal end of the catheter to avoid withdrawing the blood that has just been dialyzed.

For longer term vascular access, an *arteriovenous (AV) fistula* (Figure 28–7 ■) is created. In preparation for fistula formation, the nondominant arm is not used for venipuncture or blood pressure measurement during renal failure. The fistula is created by surgical anastomosis of an artery and vein, usually the radial artery and cephalic vein. It takes about a month

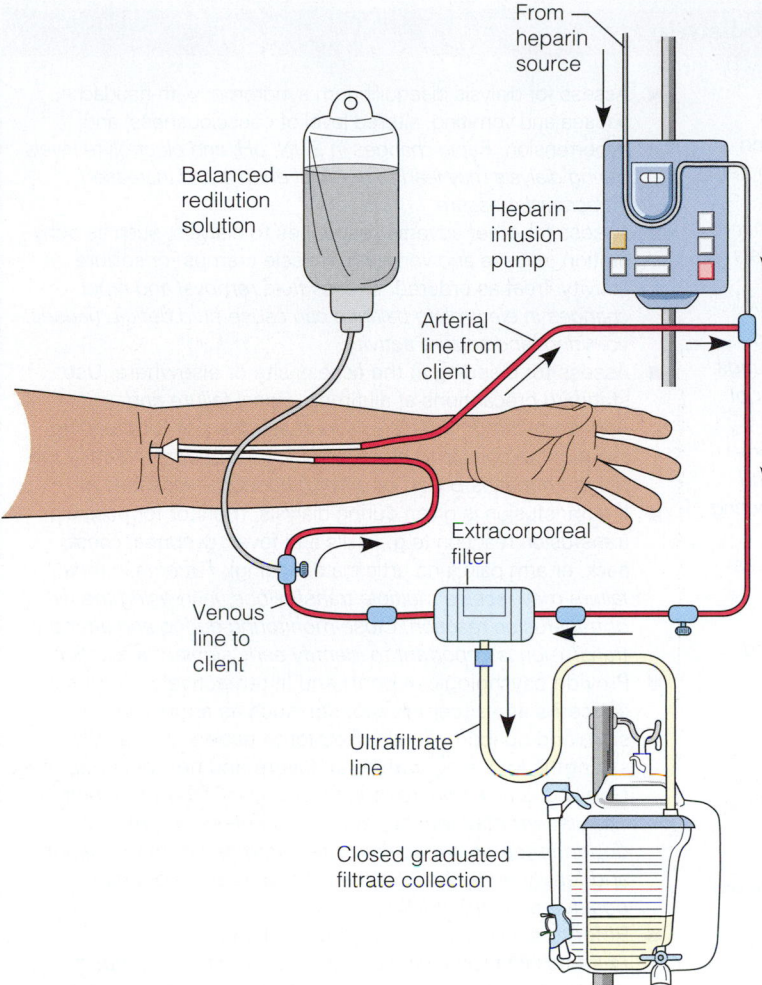

Balanced redilution solution

From heparin source

Heparin infusion pump

Arterial line from client

Extracorporeal filter

Venous line to client

Ultrafiltrate line

Closed graduated filtrate collection

Figure 28–6 ■ Continuous venovenous hemofiltration (CVVH).

for the fistula to mature so that it can be used for taking and replacing blood during dialysis. A functional AV fistula has a palpable pulsation and a bruit on auscultation. Venipunctures and blood pressures are avoided on the arm with the fistula.

In chronic renal failure, an *arteriovenous graft* is most often used for vascular access. The graft, a tube made of Gor-Tex, is surgically implanted and connects the artery and the vein. Blood flows through the graft from the artery to the vein. Occasionally, an *external AV shunt* connecting a peripheral artery with a peripheral vein is used for vascular access.

The rate of complications and mortality associated with catheter access is higher than with AV fistulas or grafts. Ideally, an AV fistula or graft is created as soon as the potential need for

long-term renal replacement therapies is identified. Localized AV fistula, graft, or shunt problems can occur, however. Infection and clotting or thrombosis are the most common shunt problems. Aneurysms may also develop. Both infection and thrombosis can lead to systemic complications such as septicemia and embolization. These local complications may cause the fistula or graft to fail, necessitating development of a new site. The psychologic impact of AV fistula or graft failure is significant, often causing depression and low self-esteem.

PERITONEAL DIALYSIS   In peritoneal dialysis, the highly vascular peritoneal membrane serves as the dialyzing surface (Figure 28–8 ■). Warmed sterile dialysate is instilled into the peritoneal cavity through a catheter inserted into the peritoneal cavity. Metabolic waste products and excess electrolytes diffuse into the dialysate while it remains in the abdomen. Water movement is controlled using dextrose as an osmotic agent to draw it into the dialysate. The fluid is then drained by gravity out of the peritoneal cavity into a sterile bag. This process of dialysate infusion, dwell time of the solution in the abdomen, and drainage is repeated at prescribed intervals.

Because excess fluid and solutes are removed more gradually in peritoneal dialysis, it poses less risk for the unstable patient; however, this slower rate of metabolite removal can be a disadvantage in ARF. Peritoneal dialysis increases the risk for developing peritonitis. It is contraindicated for patients who have had recent abdominal surgery, significant lung disease, or peritonitis. See the box on page 845 for nursing care of the patient having peritoneal dialysis.

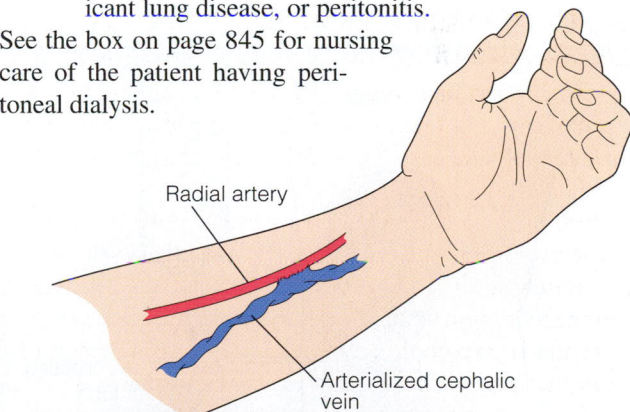

Radial artery

Arterialized cephalic vein

Figure 28–7 ■ An arteriovenous fistula.

TABLE 28–6 Continuous Renal Replacement Therapies		
TYPE	**INDICATIONS**	**DESCRIPTION**
Continuous venovenous hemofiltration (CVVH)	Remove fluid and some solutes	Venous blood circulates through a hemofilter, replacement fluid is added, and blood returned to patient; ultrafiltrate collects in a drainage bag.
Continuous venovenous hemodiafiltration (CVVHDF)	Remove fluid and waste products	Venous blood circulates through a hemofilter surrounded by dialysate, replacement fluid is added, and blood then is returned to patient; ultrafiltrate collects in a drainage bag.
Continuous venovenous hemodialysis (CVVHD)	Remove fluid and waste products	Venous blood circulates through a hemofilter surrounded by dialysate, and then returns to patient through double-lumen venous catheter; ultrafiltrate collects in a drainage bag.

Dialysis Nurse Video

NURSING CARE OF THE PATIENT   Undergoing Hemodialysis

PREDIALYSIS CARE

■ Assess vital signs, including orthostatic blood pressures (lying, sitting, and standing), apical pulse, respirations, and lung sounds. *These data provide baseline information to help evaluate the effects of hemodialysis. Hypertension may indicate excess fluid volume. The patient who is hypotensive may not tolerate rapid fluid volume changes during dialysis. Abnormal heart sounds (e.g., a gallop or murmur) and changes in heart rate or rhythm may indicate excess fluid volume or electrolyte imbalance. Fluid overload may also cause dyspnea, tachypnea, and rales or crackles in the lungs.*

■ Record weight. *Weight changes are an effective indicator of fluid volume.*

■ Assess vascular access site for a palpable pulsation or vibration and an audible bruit and for inflammation. *Infection and thrombus formation are the most common problems affecting the access site in hemodialysis patients.*

■ Alert all personnel to avoid using the extremity with the vascular access site (or the nondominant arm, if long-term access has not been established) for blood pressures or venipuncture. *These procedures may damage vessels and lead to failure of the arteriovenous fistula.*

POSTDIALYSIS CARE

■ Assess and document vital signs, weight, and vascular access site condition. *Rapid fluid and solute removal during dialysis may lead to orthostatic hypotension, cardiopulmonary changes, and weight loss.*

■ Monitor BUN, serum creatinine, serum electrolyte, and hematocrit levels between dialysis treatments. *These values help determine the effectiveness of the treatment, the need for fluid and diet restrictions, and the timing of future dialysis sessions. The anemia associated with renal failure does not improve with dialysis, and iron and folate supplements or periodic blood transfusions may be needed.*

■ Assess for dialysis disequilibrium syndrome, with headache, nausea and vomiting, altered level of consciousness; and hypertension. *Rapid changes in BUN, pH, and electrolyte levels during dialysis may lead to cerebral edema and increased intracranial pressure.*

■ Assess for other adverse responses to dialysis, such as dehydration, nausea and vomiting, muscle cramps, or seizure activity. Treat as ordered. *Excess fluid removal and rapid changes in electrolyte balance can cause fluid deficit, nausea, vomiting, and seizure activity.*

■ Assess for bleeding at the access site or elsewhere. Use standard precautions at all times. *Renal failure and heparinization during dialysis increase the risk for bleeding. Frequent exposure to blood and blood products increase the risk for hepatitis B or C or other bloodborne diseases.*

■ If a transfusion is given during dialysis, monitor for possible transfusion reaction (e.g., chills and fever; dyspnea; chest, back, or arm pain; and urticaria or itching). *Patients in renal failure may receive multiple transfusions, increasing the risk of transfusion reaction. Close monitoring during and after the transfusion is important to identify early signs of a reaction.*

■ Provide psychologic support and listen actively. Address concerns and accept responses such as anger, depression, and noncompliance. Reinforce patient and family strengths in coping with renal failure and hemodialysis. *Grieving is a normal response to loss of organ function. The patient may feel hopeless or helpless and resent dependence on a machine. The nurse can help the patient and family work through these responses and focus on positive aspects of living.*

■ Refer to social services and counseling as indicated. *Patients with renal failure may need additional support services to help them adapt to and live with their disease.*

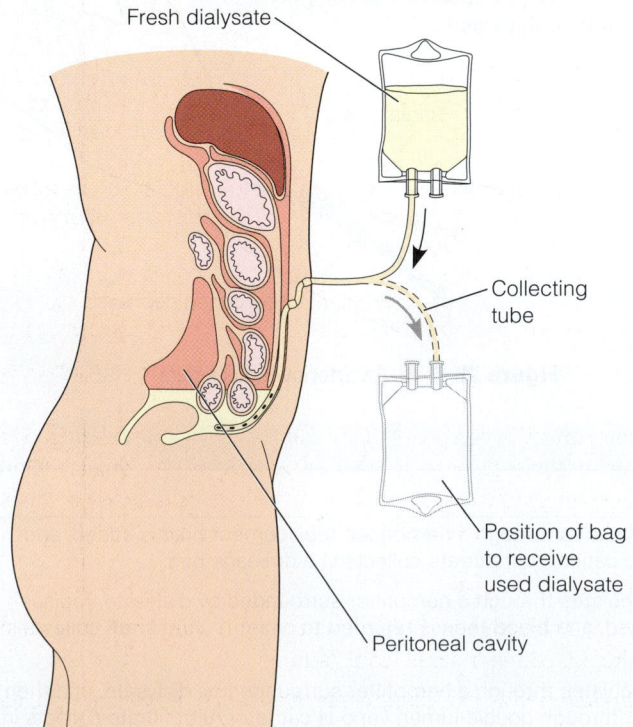

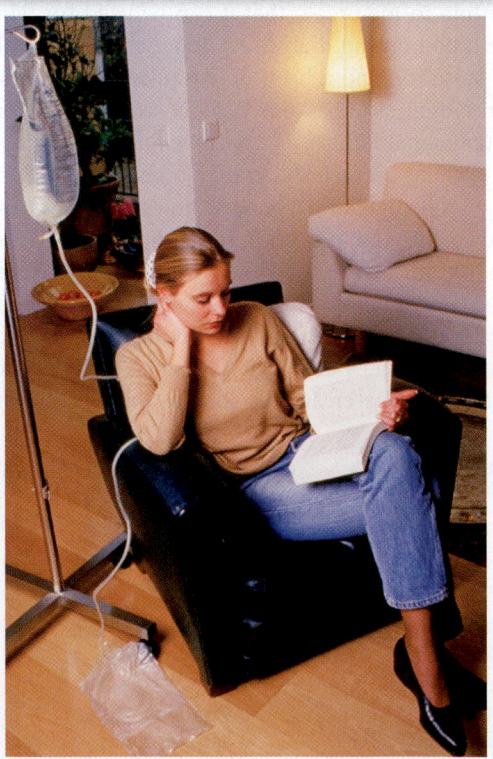

A   B

Figure 28–8 ■ *A,* The components of peritoneal dialysis. *B,* A woman receiving peritoneal dialysis at home.

Fresh dialysate

Collecting tube

Position of bag to receive used dialysate

Peritoneal cavity

PREDIALYSIS CARE

- Document vital signs including temperature, orthostatic blood pressures (lying, sitting, and standing), apical pulse, respirations, and lung sounds. *These baseline data help assess fluid volume status and tolerance of the dialysis procedure. Hypertension, abnormal heart or lung sounds, or dyspnea may indicate excess fluid volume. Poor respiratory function may affect the ability to tolerate peritoneal dialysis. Temperature measurement is vital, because infection is the most common complication of peritoneal dialysis.*

- Weigh daily or between dialysis runs as indicated. *Weight is an accurate indicator of fluid volume status.*

- Note BUN, serum electrolyte, creatinine, pH, and hematocrit levels prior to peritoneal dialysis and periodically during the procedure. *These values are used to assess the efficacy of treatment.*

- Measure and record abdominal girth. *Increasing abdominal girth may indicate retained dialysate, excess fluid volume, or early peritonitis.*

- Maintain fluid and dietary restrictions as ordered. *Fluid and diet restrictions help reduce hypervolemia and control azotemia.*

- Have the patient empty the bladder prior to catheter insertion. *Emptying the bladder reduces the risk of inadvertent puncture.*

- Warm the prescribed dialysate solution to body temperature (98.6°F or 37°C) using a warm water bath or heating pad on low setting. *Dialysate is warmed to prevent hypothermia.*

- Explain all procedures and expected sensations. *Knowledge helps reduce anxiety and elicit cooperation.*

INTRADIALYSIS CARE

- Use strict aseptic technique during the dialysis procedure and when caring for the peritoneal catheter. *Peritonitis is a common complication of peritoneal dialysis; sterile technique reduces the risk.*

- Add prescribed medications to the dialysate; prime the tubing with solution and connect it to the peritoneal catheter, taping connections securely and avoiding kinks. *This allows dialysate to flow freely into the abdominal cavity and prevents leaking or contamination.*

- Instill dialysate into the abdominal cavity over a period of approximately 10 minutes. Clamp tubing and allow the dialysate to remain in the abdomen for the prescribed dwell time. Keep drainage tubing clamped at all times during instillation and dwell time. *Dialysate should flow freely into the abdomen if the peritoneal catheter is patent. Dialysis, the exchange of solutes and water between the blood and*

dialysate, occurs across the peritoneal membrane during the dwell time.

- During instillation and dwell time, observe closely for signs of respiratory distress, such as dyspnea, tachypnea, or crackles. Place in Fowler's or semi-Fowler's position and slow the rate of instillation slightly to relieve respiratory distress if it develops. *Respiratory compromise may result from rapid dialysate instillation or overfilling of the abdomen or from a diaphragmatic defect that allows fluid to enter the thoracic cavity.*

- After prescribed dwell time, open drainage tubing clamps and allow dialysate to drain by gravity into a sterile container. Note the clarity, color, and odor of returned dialysate. *Blood or feces in the dialysate may indicate organ or bowel perforation; cloudy or malodorous dialysate may indicate an infection.*

- Accurately record amount and type of dialysate instilled (including any added medications), dwell time, and the amount and character of the drainage. *When more dialysate drains than has been instilled, excess fluid has been lost (output). If less dialysate is returned than has been instilled, a fluid gain has occurred (intake).*

- Monitor BUN, serum electrolyte, and creatinine levels. *These values are used to assess the effectiveness of dialysis.*

- Troubleshoot for possible problems during dialysis:
  a. Slow dialysate instillation. Increase the height of the container and reposition the patient. Check tubing and catheter for kinks. Check abdominal dressing for wetness, indicating leakage around the catheter. *Slow dialysate flow may be related to a partially obstructed tube or catheter.*
  b. Excess dwell time. *Prolonged dwell time may lead to water depletion or hyperglycemia.*
  c. Poor dialysate drainage. Lower the drainage container, reposition, check for tubing kinks. Check abdominal dressing. *Tubing or catheter obstruction can also interfere with dialysate drainage.*

POSTDIALYSIS CARE

- Assess vital signs, including temperature. *Comparison of pre- and postdialysis vital signs helps identify beneficial and adverse effects of the procedure.*

- Time meals to correspond with dialysis outflow. *Scheduling meals while the abdomen is empty of dialysate enhances intake and reduces nausea.*

- Teach the patient and family about the procedure. *The patient may elect to use peritoneal dialysis at home to manage end-stage renal disease and prevent uremia.*

Nursing Care

Health Promotion

Acute renal failure often can be prevented by measures that maintain fluid volume and cardiac output and reduce the risk of exposure to nephrotoxins. Carefully monitor critically ill, postoperative, and other at-risk patients for early signs of hypovolemia (low urine output; altered mental status; changes in vital signs, skin color, or temperature). Promptly report a fall in urine output to less than 30 mL per hour and other evidence of decreased cardiac output. Maintain intravenous fluids as ordered. Alert the physician if

the patient is receiving more than one nephrotoxic drug or if a nephrotoxic drug is ordered for a dehydrated patient. Closely observe patients receiving blood or blood cells for early signs of transfusion reaction and intervene appropriately.

Assessment

Both subjective and objective data are useful when assessing the patient with acute renal failure:

- *Health history:* Complaints of anorexia, nausea, weight gain, or edema; recent exposure to a nephrotoxin such as an aminoglycoside antibiotic or radiologic procedure using an injected contrast medium; previous transfusion reaction; chronic diseases such as diabetes, heart failure, or kidney disease.

- *Physical examination:* Vital signs including temperature; urine output (amount, color, clarity, specific gravity, presence of blood cells or protein); weight; skin color, peripheral pulses; presence of edema (periorbital or dependent); lung sounds, heart sounds, and bowel tones.

Nursing Diagnoses and Interventions

The patient with acute renal failure has numerous nursing care needs related not only to the renal failure but also to the underlying condition that precipitated it. Priority nursing care needs relate to fluid volume alterations, appetite and nutrition, and teaching/learning. For additional nursing diagnoses and interventions see the Case Study & Nursing Care Plan on page 847.

Excess Fluid Volume

In acute renal failure, the kidneys often cannot excrete adequate urine to maintain a normal extracellular fluid balance. Fluid retention is greater in oliguric renal failure than in non-oliguric failure. Rapid weight gain and edema indicate fluid retention. In addition, heart failure and pulmonary edema may develop. In the older adult or severely debilitated patient, fluid retention can present a significant management problem.

- Maintain hourly intake and output records. *Accurate intake and output records help guide therapy, especially fluid restrictions.*
- Weigh daily or more frequently, as ordered. Use standard technique (same scale, clothing, or coverings) to ensure accuracy. *Rapid weight changes are an accurate indicator of fluid volume status, particularly in the oliguric patient.*
- Assess vital signs at least every 4 hours. *Hypertension, tachycardia, and tachypnea may indicate excess fluid volume.*

> **PRACTICE ALERT**
> Frequently assess breath and heart sounds, neck veins for distention, and back and extremities for edema. Report abnormal findings. Adventitious breath sounds (crackles), abnormal heart sounds such as an S_3 or S_4 gallop, distended neck veins, and peripheral edema may indicate hypervolemia, heart failure, or pulmonary edema.

- If not contraindicated, place in semi-Fowler's position *to enhance cardiac and respiratory function.*
- Report abnormal serum electrolyte values and manifestations of electrolyte imbalance. The patient with ARF is at particular risk for the following electrolyte imbalances:
  a. *Hyperkalemia* due to impaired potassium excretion. Manifestations include irritability, nausea, diarrhea, abdominal cramping, cardiac dysrhythmias, and ECG changes.
  b. *Hyponatremia* due to water retention. Manifestations include nausea, vomiting, and headache, with possible central nervous system (CNS) manifestations of lethargy, confusion, seizures, and coma.
  c. *Hyperphosphatemia* due to decreased phosphate excretion. Manifestations include hyperreflexia, paresthesias, and possible tetany.
  ARF impairs electrolyte and water excretion, causing multiple electrolyte imbalances.

EVIDENCE FOR NURSING CARE   **The Patient with Acute Renal Failure**

Selected resources that nurses may find helpful when planning evidence-based nursing care follow.

- Papanicolaou, N., Francis, I. R., Casalino, D. D., Arellano, R. S., Baumgarten, D. A., Curry, N. S., et al. (2008). ACR Appropriateness Criteria® renal failure.. Reston, VA: American College of Radiology (ACR). Retrieved from http://www.guideline.gov/summary/summary.aspx?doc_id=13685&nbr=007019&string=acute+AND+renal+AND+failure
- Patel, S. S., & Holley, J. L. (2008). Withholding and withdrawing dialysis in the intensive care unit: Benefits derived from consulting the *Renal Physicians Association/American Society of Nephrology Clinical Practice Guideline*, shared decision-making in the appropriate initiation of and withdrawal from dialysis. *Clinical Journal of the American Society of Nephrology, 3*, 587–93.
- Rauen, C. A., Makic, M. B. F., & Bridges, E. (2009). Evidence-based practice habits: Transforming research into bedside practice. *Critical Care Nurse, 29*(2), 46–59.

- Restrict fluids as ordered. Provide frequent mouth care and encourage using hard candies to decrease thirst. If ice chips are allowed, include the water content (approximately one-half of the total volume) as intake. *Fluids are restricted to minimize fluid retention and complications of fluid volume excess.*
- Administer medications with meals. *Giving oral medications with meals minimizes ingestion of excess fluids.*
- Turn frequently and provide good skin care. *Edema decreases tissue perfusion and increases the risk of skin breakdown, especially in the older or debilitated patient.*

Imbalanced Nutrition: Less than Body Requirements

Anorexia and nausea associated with renal failure often interfere with food intake and nutrition. In addition, the disease process leading to ARF may contribute to increased nutritional needs for healing and decreased food intake.

- Monitor and record food intake, including the amount and type of food consumed. *A detailed intake record helps guide decisions about nutritional status and necessary supplements.*
- Weigh daily. *Weight changes over time (days to weeks) reflect nutritional status, while rapid weight changes are more reflective of fluid volume status. In ARF, weight may remain stable or increase due to fluid retention even though tissue mass is being lost.*
- Arrange for dietary consultation to plan meals within prescribed limitations that consider the patient's food preferences. *Diets restricted in protein, salt, and potassium can be unpalatable; intake and appetite improve when preferred foods are included as allowed.*
- Engage the patient in planning daily menus. *Participation in meal planning increases the patient's sense of control and autonomy.*
- Allow family members to prepare meals within dietary restrictions. Encourage family members to eat with the patient. *Familiar foods and social interaction encourage eating and increase enjoyment of meals.*
- Provide frequent, small meals or between-meal snacks. *These measures promote food intake in the fatigued or anorectic patient.*

Judy Devak is driving home late one evening when she loses control of her car trying to avoid hitting a deer in the road. Her car strikes a tree and rolls into a deep ditch beside the road, out of sight of passing cars. The wreck is not discovered until 2 hours later. On arrival at the accident scene, the paramedics find Ms. Devak hypotensive: BP 90/60, P 120, and R 24. She is alert and in severe pain with a fractured right femur. After immobilizing Ms. Devak's neck and back and extricating her from the car, they apply a traction splint to her leg and transport her to the local hospital.

ASSESSMENT

Katie Leaper, RN, obtains a nursing history on Ms. Devak's admission to the intensive care unit. Ms. Devak indicates that she has been healthy, having experienced only minor illnesses and chickenpox as a child. She has never been hospitalized, and knows of no allergies to medications. Ms. Devak is not currently taking prescription or nonprescription drugs. Physical assessment findings include T 97.4°F (36.3°C) PO, P 100, R 18, and BP 124/68. Skin pale, cool, and dry, with multiple scrapes, minor abrasions, and bruises on face and extremities. A linear bruise is noted on her chest and abdomen from the seat belt. Lung sounds clear, heart tones normal, and abdomen tender but soft to palpation. Right leg alignment maintained with skeletal traction. One unit of whole blood was infused prior to ICU admission; a second unit is currently infusing. An indwelling urinary catheter and a nasogastric tube are in place.

During the first few hours after admission, Ms. Leaper notes that Ms. Devak's hourly output has dropped from 55 mL to 45 to 28 mL of clear yellow urine. The physician orders a 500-mL intravenous fluid challenge, STAT urinalysis, BUN, and serum creatinine. The fluid challenge elicits only a slight increase in urine output. Urinalysis results show a specific gravity of 1.010 and the presence of WBCs, red and white cell casts, and tubular epithelial cells in the sediment. Ms. Devak's BUN is 28 mg/dL; her serum creatinine is 1.5 mg/dL. The physician diagnoses probable acute renal failure and orders a nephrology consultation. In addition, the physician orders aluminum hydroxide, 10 mL every 2 hours per nasogastric tube, and ranitidine 50 mg intravenously every 8 hours.

DIAGNOSES

- *Acute Pain* related to injuries sustained in accident
- *Anxiety* related to being in the intensive care unit
- *Risk for Excess Fluid Volume* related to impaired renal function
- *Impaired Physical Mobility* related to skeletal traction
- *Ineffective Protection* related to injuries and invasive procedures

EXPECTED OUTCOMES

- Report adequate pain control.
- Verbalize reduced anxiety.

- Maintain stable weight and vital signs within normal range.
- Maintain skin integrity.
- Use the trapeze appropriately to adjust position in bed while maintaining body alignment.
- Remain free of infection, bleeding, or respiratory distress.

PLANNING AND IMPLEMENTATION

- Maintain PCA.
- Assess frequently for pain control and response to analgesia.
- Encourage expression of thoughts, feelings, and fears about condition and placement in ICU.
- Document vital signs and heart and lung sounds at least every 4 hours.
- Weigh every 12 hours.
- Document hourly intake and output.
- Restrict fluids as ordered, including diluent for all intravenous medications as intake.
- Assist with mouth care every 3 to 4 hours; allow frequent rinsing of mouth and ice chips as allowed.
- Assist with position changes at least every 2 hours; teach use of the overhead trapeze.
- Monitor frequently for signs of infection, bleeding, or respiratory distress.

EVALUATION

After just over 3 days of oliguria, Ms. Devak's urine output increases. By the end of the fourth day she is excreting 60 to 80 mL/h of urine. Although her BUN, serum creatinine, and potassium levels remain high, they never reach a critical point, and dialysis is not required. She is transferred from the ICU on the fifth day after admission. When Ms. Devak is able to begin eating, she is placed on a low-potassium diet, restricted to 50 g of protein. Her renal function gradually improves. By discharge, results of her renal function studies, including BUN and serum creatinine, are nearly normal. Ms. Devak verbalizes an understanding of the need to avoid nephrotoxins such as NSAIDs until allowed by her physician.

CRITICAL THINKING IN THE NURSING PROCESS

1. What was the most likely specific precipitating factor for Ms. Devak's acute renal failure? Did anything else contribute to her risk?
2. Why did the physician prescribe aluminum hydroxide and ranitidine? Consider both the acute renal failure and Ms. Devak's placement in the intensive care unit.
3. Ms. Devak is at risk for respiratory distress related to potential fluid volume excess. How does her fractured femur further contribute to risk for respiratory distress?
4. Develop a care plan for Ms. Devak for the nursing diagnosis of *Deficient Diversional Activity*.

See Evaluating Your Response in Appendix C.

- Administer antiemetics as ordered and provide mouth care prior to meals. *Nausea and a metallic taste in the mouth, common manifestations of uremia, can decrease food intake.*
- Administer parenteral nutrition as ordered if the patient is unable to eat or tolerate enteral nutrition. *Preventing or slowing tissue catabolism is important for the patient with ARF.*

Readiness for Enhanced Knowledge

The patient with ARF has multiple learning needs. These include information about ARF, diagnostic and laboratory studies, management strategies, and implications for the recovery period.

- Assess anxiety level and ability to comprehend instruction. Tailor information and presentation to developmental level and physical, mental, and emotional status. *The patient with ARF may be critically ill or have uremic effects that hinder learning. During the initial stages of ARF it may be necessary to limit information to immediate concerns.*

- Assess knowledge and understanding. *To enhance understanding and retention, relate information presented to previous learning.*
- Teach about diagnostic tests and therapeutic procedures. *Teaching reduces anxiety and improves understanding and cooperation.*
- Discuss dietary and fluid restrictions. *These measures may be continued after discharge.*
- If the patient is discharged prior to the recovery phase of ARF, teach the signs and symptoms of complications, such as fluid volume excess or deficit, heart failure, and electrolyte imbalances. *As kidney function returns, urine output increases, but the concentrating ability of the nephrons and electrolyte excretion remain impaired. This impaired function increases the risk of excess fluid loss, possible dehydration, orthostatic hypotension, and electrolyte imbalance.*
- Teach how to monitor weight, blood pressure, and pulse. *These are important means of assessing fluid status.*
- Instruct to avoid nephrotoxic drugs and chemicals for up to 1 year following an episode of ARF. *During recovery, nephrons are vulnerable to damage by nephrotoxins such as NSAIDs, some antibiotics, radiologic contrast media, and heavy metals. Because alcohol can increase the nephrotoxicity of some materials, discourage alcohol ingestion.*

Using NANDA, NIC, and NOC

Linkages between a selected NANDA nursing diagnosis, NIC, and NOC for the patient with acute renal failure are shown in the chart that follows.

Community-Based Care

Often the patient is critically ill when ARF develops. Critical illness and the resulting state of patient and family crisis can impair learning and retention of information. Include family members in teaching during the initial stages to promote understanding of what is happening and the reasons for specific treatment measures. Inclusion of the family reduces their anxiety, and provides a valuable resource for reinforcing patient teaching about care after discharge.

NANDA, NIC, AND NOC LINKAGES
The Patient with Acute Renal Failure

NANDA — Excess Fluid Volume

NIC — Hemodynamic Regulation / Fluid/Electrolyte Management

NOC — Cardiopulmonary Status / Electrolyte and Acid/Base Balance / Fluid Balance

Data from NANDA International. (2009). *Nursing diagnoses: Definitions & classification 2009–2011.* Oxford, UK: Wiley-Blackwell; Bulechek, G., Butcher, H., & Dochterman, J. (Eds.). (2008). *Nursing interventions classification (NIC)* (5th ed.). St. Louis, MO: Mosby; and Moorhead, S., Johnson, M., Maas, M., & Swanson, E. (Eds.). (2008). *Nursing outcomes classification (NOC)* (4th ed.). St. Louis, MO: Mosby.

Patient teaching needs for home care include the following:
- Avoiding exposure to nephrotoxins, particularly those in over-the-counter products
- Preventing infection and other major stressors that can slow healing
- Monitoring weight, blood pressure, and pulse
- Manifestations of relapse
- Continuing dietary restrictions
- Knowing when to contact the physician

The Patient with Chronic Kidney Disease

Although the kidneys usually recover from acute injury, many chronic conditions can lead to progressive renal tissue destruction and loss of function. Nephron units are lost and renal mass decreases, with progressive deterioration of glomerular filtration, tubular secretion, and reabsorption. This process may progress slowly for many years without being recognized. **Chronic kidney disease (CKD)** is defined by the presence of kidney damage for three or more months and the level of kidney function (National Kidney Foundation [NKF], 2002). Eventually, the kidneys are unable to excrete metabolic wastes and regulate fluid and electrolyte balance adequately, a condition known as kidney failure or end-stage renal disease (ESRD), the final stage of CKD.

The incidence of ESRD is increasing, particularly in older adults. In 2006, more than 110,000 people started treatment for ESRD for a total of about 503,000 people undergoing ESRD treatment (NKUDIC, 2009). See the box on page 849 for nursing care of the older adult with CKD.

FAST FACTS
- The incidence of CKD and ESRD is significantly higher in people aged 65 and older.
- African Americans have the highest incidence of ESRD, followed by Native Americans, Asian/Pacific Islanders, and European Americans.
- People of Hispanic origin have a higher incidence of CKD and ESRD than non-Hispanics.
- Men are more likely to be affected by CKD and ESRD than women.
- Diabetes mellitus is the leading cause of CKD, followed by hypertension, glomerulonephritis, and cystic kidney disease (USRDS, 2008).

Conditions causing CKD typically involve diffuse, bilateral disease of the kidneys with progressive destruction and scarring of the entire nephron. As indicated in Figure 28–9 ■, diabetes is the leading cause of ESRD in all population groups in the United States. Hypertension closely follows diabetes as a major cause of ESRD; in many patients, these disorders coexist (USRDS, 2008).

Pathophysiology

The pathophysiology of CKD varies, depending on the underlying disease process. Table 28–7 outlines common pathologic processes leading to nephron destruction, CKD, and kidney

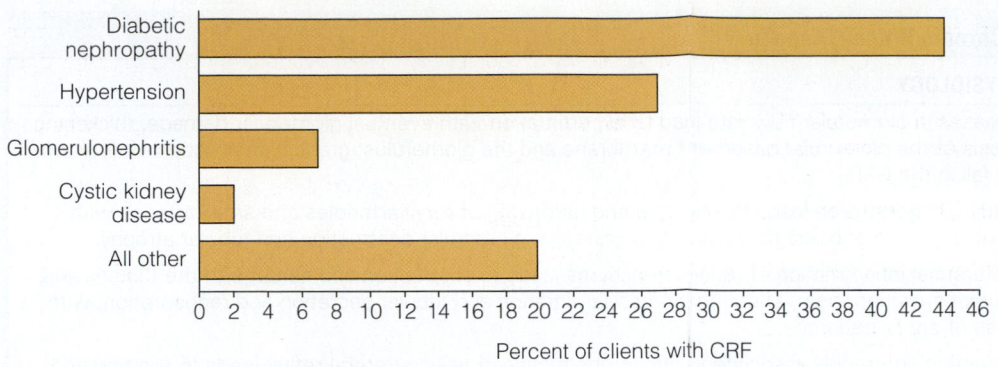

Figure 28–9 ■ The most common causes of chronic renal failure (USRDS, 2008).

failure. Regardless of the initiating cause, glomerulosclerosis and interstitial inflammation and fibrosis are characteristic of CKD and contribute to declining renal function (Copstead & Banasik, 2010). Entire nephron units are gradually destroyed. In the early stages, as nephrons are lost, remaining functional nephrons hypertrophy. Glomerular capillary flow and pressure increase in these nephrons, and more solute particles are filtered to compensate for lost renal mass. This increased demand predisposes the remaining nephrons to glomerular sclerosis (scarring), resulting in their eventual destruction. Proteinuria resulting from glomerular damage is thought to contribute to tubular injury This process of continued loss of nephron function may continue even after the initial disease process has resolved (Fauci et al., 2008).

The course of CKD is variable, progressing over a period of months to many years. In the early stage, often called *decreased renal reserve*, unaffected nephrons compensate for the lost

nephrons. The GFR is slightly decreased, and the patient is asymptomatic with normal BUN and serum creatinine levels. As the disease progresses and the GFR falls further, hypertension and some manifestations of *renal insufficiency* may be seen. Any further insult to the kidneys at this stage (such as infection, dehydration, exposure to nephrotoxins, or urinary tract obstruction) can further reduce function and precipitate the onset of *renal failure* or overt uremia. The serum creatinine and BUN levels rise sharply, the patient becomes oliguric, and manifestations of uremia are seen. In ESRD, the final stage of CKD, the GFR is less than 10% of normal and renal replacement therapy is necessary to sustain life. Table 28–8 summarizes the stages of chronic kidney disease.

Manifestations and Complications

Chronic kidney disease often is not identified until its final, uremic stage is reached. **Uremia**, which literally means "urine in the blood," refers to the syndrome or group of symptoms associated with ESRD. In uremia, fluid and electrolyte balance is altered, the regulatory and endocrine functions of the kidney are impaired, and accumulated metabolic waste products affect essentially every other organ system.

Early manifestations of uremia include nausea, apathy, weakness, and fatigue, symptoms that often are dismissed as a

NURSING CARE OF THE OLDER ADULT   Chronic Kidney Disease

Structural and functional changes occur in the aging kidney. Structurally, the number of nephrons decreases. The GFR declines, resulting in decreased renal clearance of drugs. Urine-concentrating ability decreases, and the kidney is less able to conserve sodium. Renal compensation for acid–base imbalances takes longer. Despite these changes, the kidney retains its ability to regulate fluid and electrolyte homeostasis remarkably well unless additional stresses are added. Any additional stressors such as hypotension, exposure to nephrotoxic drugs, or an inflammatory process such as glomerulonephritis may precipitate renal failure in the older adult.

The manifestations of chronic kidney disease often are missed in aging patients (e.g., edema may be attributed to heart failure or high blood pressure to preexisting hypertension). Serum creatinine levels may rise slowly. Because older adults have less muscle mass, they produce less creatinine, a by-product of muscle cell metabolism. Likewise, the BUN may remain within normal limits.

The same measures are used to treat ESRD in older adults as in younger people. Hemodialysis, peritoneal dialysis, and renal transplantation are appropriate if necessary. Treatment options (including conservative treatment or no treatment) and their potential benefits and ramifications should be clearly explained.

Assessing for Home Care

A number of factors should be considered in assessing the older adult's ability to manage treatment such as dialysis at home:

- Does the patient have reasonable access to a dialysis center or outpatient unit? Is transportation available?
- Would home hemodialysis be appropriate? Is a caregiver available to be trained to manage dialysis? Does the patient's home have appropriate electrical and plumbing fixtures?
- Would continuous ambulatory peritoneal dialysis be appropriate? Does the patient have the manual dexterity, will, and cognitive ability to manage dialysis infusions? If not, would intermittent peritoneal dialysis using a dialyzing machine be more appropriate?
- Are family members or other support persons available to provide assistance to the patient as needed?

Resources for Home Care

The following resources may be useful for patients with kidney disease:

- American Association of Kidney Patients
  800-749-2257
  813-636-8100
- American Kidney Fund
  800-638-8289
  866-300-2800 (Spanish help line)
- National Kidney Foundation
  800-622-9010

TABLE 28–7 Pathophysiology of Chronic Kidney Disease

CAUSE	PATHOPHYSIOLOGY
Diabetic nephropathy	Initial increases in glomerular flow rate lead to hyperfiltration with eventual glomerular damage, thickening and sclerosis of the glomerular basement membrane and the glomerulus; gradual destruction of nephrons leads to a fall in the GFR.
Hypertensive nephrosclerosis	Long-standing hypertension leads to sclerosis and narrowing of renal arterioles and small arteries with subsequent reduction of blood flow leading to ischemia, glomerular destruction and tubular atrophy.
Chronic glomerulonephritis	Chronic interstitial inflammation of renal parenchyma leads to obstruction and damage to the tubules and capillaries that surround them, affecting glomerular filtration and tubular secretion and reabsorption, with gradual loss of entire nephrons.
Chronic pyelonephritis	Chronic infection commonly associated with an obstructive or vesicoureteral reflux leads to scarring and deformity of renal calyces and pelvis, resulting in intrarenal reflux and nephropathy.
Polycystic kidney disease	Multiple bilateral cysts compress renal tissue impairing renal perfusion and leading ischemia, renal vascular remodeling, and release of inflammatory mediators, which damage and destroy normal kidney tissue.
Systemic lupus erythematosus	Immune complexes form in capillary basement membrane leading to inflammation and sclerosis with focal, local, or diffuse glomerulonephritis.

viral infection or influenza. As the condition progresses, frequent vomiting, increasing weakness, lethargy, and confusion develop. The Multisystem Effects of Uremia are illustrated on page 852.

Fluid and Electrolyte Effects

Loss of functional kidney tissue impairs its ability to regulate fluid, electrolyte, and acid–base balance. In the early stages of CKD, impaired filtration and reabsorption lead to proteinuria, hematuria, and decreased urine-concentrating ability. Salt and water are poorly conserved, and risk for dehydration increases. Polyuria, nocturia, and a fixed specific gravity of 1.008 to 1.012 are common. As the GFR decreases and renal function deteriorates further, sodium and water retention are common, necessitating salt and water restrictions.

Hyperkalemia develops as renal failure progresses. Manifestations of hyperkalemia, such as muscle weakness, paresthesias, and ECG changes, are not usually seen until the GFR is less than 5 mL/min. Phosphate excretion is also impaired,

leading to hyperphosphatemia and hypocalcemia. Reduced calcium absorption due to impaired vitamin D activation also contributes to hypocalcemia. Hypermagnesemia develops with advancing renal failure; magnesium-containing antacids are avoided for this reason.

As renal failure advances, hydrogen ion excretion and buffer production are impaired, leading to metabolic acidosis. Respiratory rate and depth increase (Kussmaul's respirations) to compensate for metabolic acidosis. Although metabolic acidosis is often asymptomatic, other possible manifestations include general malaise, weakness, headache, nausea and vomiting, and abdominal pain (∞ see Chapter 10).

Cardiovascular Effects

Cardiovascular disease is a common cause of death in ESRD, and results from accelerated atherosclerosis. Hypertension, hyperlipidemia, and glucose intolerance all contribute to the process. Cerebral and peripheral vascular manifestations of atherosclerosis are also seen.

TABLE 28–8 Stages of Chronic Kidney Disease

STAGE	GLOMERULAR FILTRATION RATE	DESCRIPTION & MANIFESTATIONS
Stage 1	> 90 mL/min/1.73 m²	Kidney damage with normal or increased GFR
		Asymptomatic; normal BUN and creatinine
Stage 2	60–89 mL/min/1.73 m²	Mildly decreased GFR
		Asymptomatic, possible hypertension; blood work generally within normal limits
Stage 3	30–59 mL/min/1.73 m²	Moderate GFR decrease
		Hypertension; possible anemia and fatigue, anorexia, possible malnutrition, bone pain; slight elevation of BUN and serum creatinine
Stage 4	15–29 mL/min/1.73 m²	Severely decreased GFR
		Hypertension, anemia, malnutrition, altered bone metabolism; edema, metabolic acidosis, hypercalcemia; possible uremia; azotemia with increasing BUN and serum creatinine levels
Stage 5	< 15 mL/min/1.73 m²	End-stage renal disease
		Kidney failure with azotemia and overt uremia

Adapted from National Kidney Foundation. (2002). K/DOQI Clinical practice guidelines for chronic kidney disease: Evaluation, classification and stratification. *American Journal of Kidney Disease, 39*, S1–S266, Retrieved from www.kdoqi.org.

Systemic hypertension is a common manifestation of CKD. Hypertension results from excess fluid volume, increased renin–angiotensin activity, increased peripheral vascular resistance, and decreased prostaglandins. Increased extracellular fluid volume also can lead to edema and heart failure. Pulmonary edema may result from heart failure and increased permeability of the alveolar capillary membrane.

Retained metabolic toxins can irritate the pericardial sac, causing an inflammatory response and signs of pericarditis. *Cardiac tamponade*, a potential complication of pericarditis, occurs when inflammatory fluid in the pericardial sac interferes with ventricular filling and cardiac output. Once a common complication of uremia, pericarditis is less common when dialysis is initiated early.

Hematologic Effects

Anemia is common in CKD, caused by multiple factors. The kidneys produce erythropoietin, a hormone that controls RBC production. In renal failure, erythropoietin production declines. Retained metabolic toxins further suppress RBC production and contribute to a shortened RBC life span. Nutritional deficiencies (iron and folate) and increased risk for blood loss from the GI tract also contribute to anemia.

Anemia contributes to manifestations such as fatigue, weakness, depression, and impaired cognition. It also affects cardiovascular function, and may be a major contributing factor to coronary heart disease and heart failure associated with ESRD.

Renal failure impairs platelet function, increasing the risk of bleeding disorders such as epistaxis and GI bleeding. The mechanism of impaired platelet function associated with renal failure is poorly understood.

Immune System Effects

Uremia increases the risk for infection. High levels of urea and retained metabolic wastes impair all aspects of inflammation and immune function. The WBC declines, humoral and cell-mediated immunity are impaired, and phagocyte function is defective. Both the acute inflammatory response and delayed hypersensitivity responses are affected (Porth & Matfin, 2009). Fever is suppressed, often delaying the diagnosis of infection.

Gastrointestinal Effects

Anorexia, nausea, and vomiting are the most common early symptoms of uremia. Hiccups also are commonly experienced. Gastroenteritis is frequent. Ulcerations may affect any level of the GI tract and contribute to an increased risk of GI bleeding. Peptic ulcer disease is particularly common in uremic patients. *Uremic fetor*, a urine-like breath odor often associated with a metallic taste in the mouth, may develop. Uremic fetor can further contribute to anorexia.

Neurologic Effects

Uremia alters both central and peripheral nervous system function. CNS manifestations occur early and include changes in mentation, difficulty concentrating, fatigue, and insomnia. Psychotic symptoms, seizures, and coma are associated with advanced uremic encephalopathy.

Peripheral neuropathy is also common in advanced uremia. Both the sensory and motor tracts are involved. The lower limbs are initially affected. "Restless leg syndrome," sensations of crawling or creeping, prickling, or itching of the lower legs with frequent leg movement, increases during rest. Paresthesias and sensory loss typically occur in a "stocking-glove" pattern. As uremia progresses, motor function is also impaired, causing muscle weakness, decreased deep tendon reflexes, and gait disturbances.

Musculoskeletal Effects

Hyperphosphatemia and hypocalcemia associated with uremia stimulate parathyroid hormone secretion. Parathyroid hormone causes increased calcium resorption from bone. In addition, osteoblast (bone-forming) and osteoclast (bone-destructing) cell activity is affected. This bone resorption and remodeling, combined with decreased vitamin D synthesis and decreased calcium absorption from the GI tract, lead to *renal osteodystrophy*, also known as renal rickets. Osteodystrophy is characterized by *osteomalacia*, softening of the bones, and *osteoporosis*, decreased bone mass. Bone cysts may develop. Manifestations of osteodystrophy include bone tenderness, pain, and muscle weakness. The patient is at increased risk for spontaneous fractures.

Endocrine and Metabolic Effects

Accumulated waste products of protein metabolism are a primary factor involved in the effects and manifestations of uremia. Serum creatinine and BUN levels are significantly elevated. Uric acid levels are increased, contributing to an increased risk of gout.

Tissues become resistant to the effects of insulin in uremia, leading to glucose intolerance. High blood triglyceride levels and lower than normal high-density lipoprotein (HDL) levels contribute to the accelerated atherosclerotic process.

Reproductive function is affected. Pregnancies are rarely carried to term, and menstrual irregularities are common. Reduced testosterone levels, low sperm counts, and impotence affect the male patient with ESRD.

Dermatologic Effects

Anemia and retained pigmented metabolites cause pallor and a yellowish hue to the skin in uremia. Dry skin with poor turgor, a result of dehydration and sweat gland atrophy, is common. Bruising and excoriations are frequently seen. Metabolic wastes not eliminated by the kidneys may be deposited in the skin, contributing to itching or pruritus. In advanced uremia, high levels of urea in the sweat may result in *uremic frost*, crystallized deposits of urea on the skin.

Interdisciplinary Care

Early management of CKD focuses on eliminating or controlling factors that may cause additional kidney damage and further decrease renal function. Included are measures to slow the progression of the disease to ESRD. Additional treatment goals include the following:

- Maintain nutritional status while minimizing the accumulation of toxic waste products and manifestations of uremia.
- Identify and treat complications of CKD.
- Prepare for renal replacement therapies such as dialysis or renal transplant.

MULTISYSTEM EFFECTS OF
Uremia

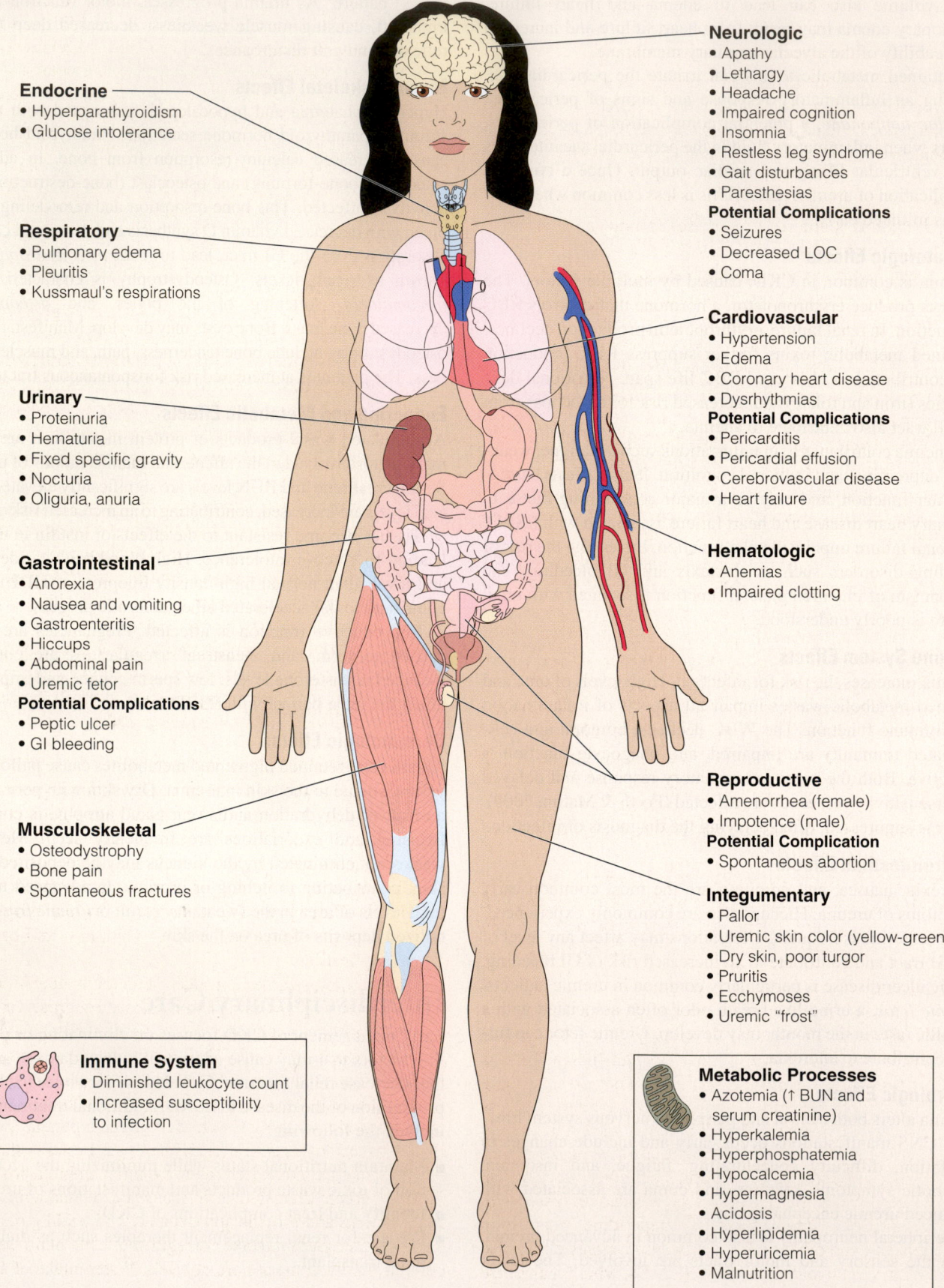

Endocrine
- Hyperparathyroidism
- Glucose intolerance

Respiratory
- Pulmonary edema
- Pleuritis
- Kussmaul's respirations

Urinary
- Proteinuria
- Hematuria
- Fixed specific gravity
- Nocturia
- Oliguria, anuria

Gastrointestinal
- Anorexia
- Nausea and vomiting
- Gastroenteritis
- Hiccups
- Abdominal pain
- Uremic fetor

Potential Complications
- Peptic ulcer
- GI bleeding

Musculoskeletal
- Osteodystrophy
- Bone pain
- Spontaneous fractures

Immune System
- Diminished leukocyte count
- Increased susceptibility to infection

Neurologic
- Apathy
- Lethargy
- Headache
- Impaired cognition
- Insomnia
- Restless leg syndrome
- Gait disturbances
- Paresthesias

Potential Complications
- Seizures
- Decreased LOC
- Coma

Cardiovascular
- Hypertension
- Edema
- Coronary heart disease
- Dysrhythmias

Potential Complications
- Pericarditis
- Pericardial effusion
- Cerebrovascular disease
- Heart failure

Hematologic
- Anemias
- Impaired clotting

Reproductive
- Amenorrhea (female)
- Impotence (male)

Potential Complication
- Spontaneous abortion

Integumentary
- Pallor
- Uremic skin color (yellow-green)
- Dry skin, poor turgor
- Pruritis
- Ecchymoses
- Uremic "frost"

Metabolic Processes
- Azotemia (↑ BUN and serum creatinine)
- Hyperkalemia
- Hyperphosphatemia
- Hypocalcemia
- Hypermagnesia
- Acidosis
- Hyperlipidemia
- Hyperuricemia
- Malnutrition

Diagnosis

Diagnostic testing is used both to identify CKD and to monitor kidney function. A number of tests may be performed to determine the underlying renal disorder. Once the diagnosis is established, renal function is monitored primarily through blood levels of metabolic wastes and electrolytes. ∞ See Chapter 26 for the nursing implications of selected tests.

- *Urinalysis* is done to measure urine specific gravity and detect abnormal urine components. In CKD, the specific gravity may be fixed at approximately 1.010 due to impaired tubular secretion, reabsorption, and urine concentrating ability. Abnormal proteins, blood cells, and cellular casts may also be noted in the urine.
- *Urine culture* is ordered to identify any urinary tract infection that may hasten the progress of CKD.
- *BUN* and *serum creatinine* are obtained to evaluate kidney function and assess the progress of renal failure. A BUN of 20 to 50 mg/dL signals mild azotemia; levels greater than 100 mg/dL indicate severe renal impairment. Uremic symptoms are seen when the BUN is around 200 mg/dL or higher. Serum creatinine levels of greater than 4 mg/dL indicate serious renal impairment.
- *eGFR* is used to evaluate the GFR and stage of chronic kidney disease. The eGFR is a calculated value determined using a formula that includes the serum creatinine, patient's age, gender, and race (African American or non-African American).
- *Serum electrolytes* are monitored throughout the course of CKD. The serum sodium may be within normal limits or low because of water retention. Potassium levels are elevated but usually remain below 6.5 mEq/L. Serum phosphate is elevated, and the calcium level is decreased. Metabolic acidosis is identified by a low pH, low CO_2, and low bicarbonate levels.
- *CBC* reveals moderately severe anemia with a hematocrit of 20% to 30% and a low hemoglobin. The number of RBCs and platelets is reduced.
- *Renal ultrasonography* is done to evaluate kidney size. In CRF, kidney size decreases as nephrons are destroyed and kidney mass is reduced.
- *Kidney biopsy* may be done to identify the underlying disease process if this is unclear. It is also used to differentiate acute from chronic failure. Kidney biopsy may be performed in surgery or done percutaneously using needle biopsy.

Medications

Chronic kidney disease affects both the pharmacokinetic and pharmacodynamic effects of drug therapy. Most medications are excreted primarily by the kidney. The half-life and plasma levels of many drugs increase in chronic kidney disease. Drug absorption may be decreased when phosphate-binding agents are administered concurrently. Proteinuria can significantly reduce plasma protein levels, leading to manifestations of toxicity when highly protein-bound drugs are given. In addition, any potentially nephrotoxic agent is avoided or used with extreme caution. Drugs such as meperidine, metformin (Glucophage), and other oral hypoglycemic agents eliminated by the kidney are avoided entirely. NSAIDs, which may cause a further decline in kidney function, also are avoided (Fauci et al., 2008).

Angiotensin-converting enzyme (ACE) inhibitors and angiotensin receptor blockers (ARBs) have been shown to slow the progression of CKD, and often are used for this purpose. Diuretics such as furosemide or other loop diuretics may be prescribed to reduce extracellular fluid volume and edema. Diuretic therapy also can reduce hypertension and cause potassium wasting, lowering serum potassium levels. Other antihypertensive agents are used to maintain the blood pressure within normal levels, slow the progress of renal failure, and prevent complications of coronary heart disease and cerebral vascular disease. ACE inhibitors are preferred, although any class of antihypertensive agent may be prescribed (∞ see Chapter 32).

Other drugs may be used to manage electrolyte imbalances and acidosis. Sodium bicarbonate or calcium carbonate may be used to correct mild acidosis. Oral phosphorus binding agents such as calcium carbonate or calcium acetate are given to lower serum phosphate levels and normalize serum calcium levels. Aluminum hydroxide may be used in acute treatment of hyperphosphatemia. Its use is limited to short term by complications such as encephalopathy and osteodystrophy associated with long-term administration of aluminum-containing preparations (McPhee et al., 2008). Vitamin D supplements may be given to improve calcium absorption.

If the serum potassium rises to dangerously high levels, a combination of bicarbonate, insulin, and glucose may be given intravenously to promote potassium movement into the cells. Sodium polystyrene sulfonate (Kayexalate), a potassium-ion exchange resin, can be given either orally or rectally (as an enema).

Folic acid and iron supplements are given to combat anemia associated with chronic renal failure. A multiple vitamin preparation is also often prescribed, because anorexia, nausea, and dietary restrictions may limit nutrient intake.

Nutrition and Fluid Management

Maintaining adequate nutrition and preventing protein-calorie malnutrition is the focus of nutritional management during early stages of CKD. As renal function declines, the elimination of water, solutes, and metabolic wastes is impaired. Accumulation of these wastes in the body leads to uremic symptoms. Dietary modifications can slow the progress of nephron destruction, reduce uremic symptoms, and help prevent complications.

Unlike carbohydrates and fats, the body is unable to store excess proteins. Unused dietary proteins are degraded into urea and other nitrogenous wastes, which are then eliminated by the kidneys. Protein-rich foods also contain inorganic ions such as hydrogen ion, phosphate, and sulfites that are eliminated by the kidneys. A daily protein intake of 0.6 g/kg of body weight, or approximately 40 g/day for an average male patient, provides the amino acids necessary for tissue repair. Proteins should be of high biologic value, rich in the essential amino acids (NKF, 2002). Carbohydrate intake is increased to maintain energy requirements and provide approximately 35 kcal/kg per day.

Water and sodium intake are regulated to maintain the extracellular fluid volume at normal levels. Water intake of 1 to 2 L per day is generally recommended to maintain water balance. Sodium is restricted to 2 g per day initially. More stringent water and sodium restrictions may be necessary as renal failure progresses. The patient is instructed to monitor weight daily and report any weight gain in excess of 5 pounds over a 2-day period.

In stages 4 and 5, potassium and phosphorous intake are also restricted. Potassium intake is limited to less than 60 to 70 mEq/day (normal intake is about 100 mEq/day) (McPhee et al., 2008). The patient is cautioned to avoid using salt substitutes, which typically contain high levels of potassium chloride. Foods high in phosphorus include eggs, dairy products, and meat.

Renal Replacement Therapies

When pharmacologic and dietary management strategies are no longer effective to maintain fluid and electrolyte balance and prevent uremia, dialysis or kidney transplantation is considered.

A number of considerations affect the choice of long-term treatment. Hemodialysis and peritoneal dialysis each have advantages and disadvantages. Establishing vascular access for hemodialysis may take several months. Planning ahead to develop the access before dialysis is necessary can ease the transition to dialysis. Established access is not a consideration for peritoneal dialysis. The peritoneal catheter can be placed and treatment initiated as soon as it is indicated. When dialysis treatments will be performed at home, initiating instruction before it is required can result in more effective learning. If a family member will serve as a dialysis helper, training begins prior to the onset of uremia.

If transplantation is considered, tissue typing and identification of potential living related donors can be done prior to the onset of ESRD. To make an informed decision, both the patient and the potential donor need to understand the risks, benefits, and options available. If the decision for transplant is made early, dialysis can potentially be avoided. The patient's age, concurrent health problems, donor availability, and personal preference influence the choice of renal replacement therapy.

DIALYSIS   Approximately 65% of all people being treated for ESRD in the United States are receiving dialysis at an average maintenance cost of about $66,000 per year (USRDS, 2008). For the patient who is not a candidate for renal transplantation or who has had a transplant failure, dialysis is life sustaining.

The most common therapies for ESRD in the United States are hemodialysis performed in a dialysis center, followed by kidney transplant and peritoneal dialysis (USRDS, 2008). Both hemodialysis and peritoneal dialysis can be done in the home, but few patients use home hemodialysis. Of the two, peritoneal dialysis is typically the choice for at-home treatment. Because the morbidity and mortality for each are comparable, factors such as the desire and ability to manage home care, employment, and availability of a dialysis center become the primary factors influencing the choice of hemodialysis or peritoneal dialysis.

Patients on long-term dialysis have a higher risk for complications and death than the general population. Many have other severe diseases along with ESRD. Infection and cardiovascular disease are common causes of illness and death. The 1-year

survival rate for patients receiving dialysis is nearly 79%; long-term survival, however, falls to 33% at 5 years and about 10% at 10 years (NKUDIC, 2009).

The decision to initiate dialysis is not easy. Like insulin therapy for the diabetic, dialysis manages the symptoms of ESRD but does not cure it. Dialysis is a constant factor of life, requiring thinking and planning ahead at all times. Patients on dialysis may not be able to maintain a job. Families often fall apart with the day-to-day stress. Even with dialysis, the patient may have constant flulike symptoms, never feeling truly well. Patients on hemodialysis may feel powerless because of their dependence on others for treatment. On the other hand, home peritoneal dialysis places a continuing burden on the patient to maintain treatment. In the end, the patient may choose to discontinue treatment, preferring death over continued dialysis.

Hemodialysis for ESRD typically is done three times a week for a total of 9 to 12 hours. The amount of dialysis needed (or dialysis dose) is individually determined by factors such as body size and residual renal function, dietary intake, and concurrent illness. Hypotension and muscle cramps are common complications during hemodialysis treatments. Infection and vascular access problems are common long-term complications of hemodialysis. Cardiovascular disease is the leading cause of death for patients receiving hemodialysis. The death rate from cardiovascular disease is higher in patients on hemodialysis than those on peritoneal dialysis or who have had a kidney transplant for reasons that are unclear (Fauci et al., 2008). See the previous section on ARF and the box on page 844 for more information about hemodialysis and related nursing care.

Peritoneal dialysis is currently used by approximately 5% of people who require long-term dialysis in the United States. In Canada and Europe, 35% to 45% of patients with ESRD are treated with peritoneal dialysis. In third world countries, peritoneal dialysis is used to treat the majority of patients with ESRD.

Continuous ambulatory peritoneal dialysis (CAPD) is the most common form of peritoneal dialysis used. Dialysate (2 L) is instilled into the peritoneal cavity, and the catheter is sealed. The patient can then continue normal daily activities, emptying the peritoneal cavity and replacing the dialysate every 4 to 6 hours. No special equipment is needed. A variation of CAPD is continuous cyclic peritoneal dialysis (CCPD), which uses a delivery device during nighttime hours and a continuous dwell during the day. CAPD can be performed anywhere, and CCPD allows for home treatment at night, leaving the patient free during the day.

Peritoneal dialysis has several advantages over hemodialysis. Heparinization and vascular complications associated with an AV fistula are avoided. The clearance of metabolic wastes is slower but more continuous, avoiding rapid fluctuations in extracellular fluid composition and associated symptoms. More liberal intake of fluids and nutrients is often allowed for the patient on CAPD. While glucose absorbed from dialysate can increase blood glucose levels in the diabetic, regular insulin can be added to the infusion to manage hyperglycemia. The patient on peritoneal dialysis is better able to self-manage the treatment regimen, reducing feelings of helplessness.

The major disadvantages of peritoneal dialysis include less effective metabolite elimination and risk of infection (peritonitis). Peritoneal dialysis may not be effective for large patients with no residual kidney function. Serum triglyceride levels increase with peritoneal dialysis. Finally, the presence of an indwelling peritoneal catheter may cause a body image disturbance. See the previous section of this chapter and the box on page 845 for more information about dialysis and nursing care for the patient undergoing peritoneal dialysis.

KIDNEY TRANSPLANT Kidney transplant has become the treatment of choice for many patients with ESRD. Kidneys are the solid organ most commonly transplanted, and to date kidney transplantation is the most successful of transplantation procedures. The first kidney transplant was performed in 1954; the donor and recipient were identical twins. Kidney transplant as a treatment for ESRD is limited primarily by availability of organs. In 2006, more than 18,000 people received a kidney transplant; however, there currently are more than 85,000 awaiting a transplant (OPTN: Organ Procurement and Transplantation Network, 2009).

Kidney transplant improves both survival and quality of life for the patient with ESRD. The patient on dialysis has a 64.3% probability of surviving after 2 years of dialysis; the transplant

---

NURSING CARE OF THE PATIENT Having a Kidney Transplant

PREOPERATIVE CARE

■ Provide routine preoperative care as outlined in ∞ Chapter 4.

■ Assess knowledge and feelings about the procedure, answering questions and clarifying information as needed. Listen and address concerns about surgery, the source of the donor organ, and possible complications. *Addressing concerns and reducing preoperative anxiety improve postoperative recovery.*

■ Continue dialysis as ordered. *Continued renal replacement therapy is necessary to manage fluid and electrolyte balance and prevent uremia prior to surgery.*

■ Administer immunosuppressive drugs as ordered before surgery. *Immunosuppression is initiated before transplantation to prevent immediate graft rejection.*

POSTOPERATIVE CARE

■ Provide routine postoperative care as outlined in ∞ Chapter 4.

■ Maintain urinary catheter patency and a closed system. *Catheter patency is vital to keep the bladder decompressed and prevent pressure on suture lines. A closed drainage system minimizes the risk for urinary tract infection.*

■ Measure urine output every 30 to 60 minutes initially. *Careful assessment of urine output helps determine fluid balance and transplant function. Acute tubular necrosis is a common early complication, usually due to tissue ischemia during the period between removal of the kidney from the donor and transplantation. Oliguria is an early sign.*

■ Monitor vital signs and hemodynamic pressures closely. *Diuresis may occur immediately, resulting in hypovolemia, low cardiac output, and impaired perfusion of the transplanted kidney.*

■ Maintain fluid replacement, generally calculated to replace urine output over the previous 30 or 60 minutes, milliliter for milliliter. *Fluid replacement is vital to maintain vascular volume and tissue perfusion.*

■ Administer diuretics as ordered. *Loop and/or osmotic diuretics such as furosemide or mannitol may be used to promote postoperative diuresis.*

■ Remove the catheter within 2 to 3 days or as ordered. Encourage to void every 1 to 2 hours and assess frequently for signs of urinary retention following catheter removal. *The bladder may have atrophied prior to surgery, reducing its capacity. Urinary retention places stress on suture lines and increases the risk of infection.*

■ Monitor serum electrolytes and renal function tests. *These tests are used to monitor graft function and fluid and electrolyte status. Electrolyte imbalances may develop as the transplanted kidney begins to function and diuresis occurs. Elevated serum creatinine and BUN levels may be early signs of rejection or graft failure.*

■ Monitor for possible complications:
  a. *Hemorrhage* from an arterial or venous anastomosis can be either acute or insidious. Indicators include swelling at the operative site, increased abdominal girth, and signs of shock, including changes in vital signs and level of consciousness. *Hemorrhage is a surgical emergency, requiring prompt recognition and treatment to preserve the graft.*
  b. *Ureteral anastomosis failure* causes urine leakage into the peritoneal cavity. It may be marked by decreased urine output with abdominal swelling and tenderness. *Failure of the ureteral anastomosis requires surgical intervention.*
  c. *Renal artery thrombosis* is characterized by an abrupt onset of hypertension and reduced GFR. *Renal artery thrombosis can result in transplant failure.*
  d. *Infection* due to immunosuppression is an immediate and continuing risk. The inflammatory response is blunted, and infection may not significantly elevate the temperature. Monitor for signs such as change in level of consciousness, cloudy or malodorous urine, or purulent drainage from the incision. *Prevention and prompt treatment of infections are particularly important in the immunosuppressed patient.*

■ Include the following in predischarge teaching for the patient and family:
  a. The use and effects of prescribed medications, including antihypertensive medications, immunosuppressive agents, prophylactic antibiotics, and others as ordered.
  b. Monitoring vital signs (including temperature) and weight.
  c. Manifestations of organ rejection, such as swelling and tenderness over the graft site, fever, joint aching, weight gain, and decreased urinary output. Stress the importance of promptly reporting signs and symptoms to the physician.
  d. Ordered or recommended dietary restrictions such as restricted carbohydrate and sodium intake, and increased protein intake.
  e. Measures to prevent infection, such as avoiding crowds and obviously ill individuals.
  The patient and family will manage care after discharge, and therefore need a good understanding of what to expect, how to monitor graft status, and measures to reduce the adverse effects of medications.

■ Provide psychologic support, address concerns, and provide information as needed. *The patient knows that transplant success is not guaranteed. In addition, the patient has often been managing a chronic disease independently and is used to having a degree of control. Providing information and allowing the patient to retain control relieves anxiety and improves recovery.*

BOX 28–1 How Deceased Donor Kidneys Are Allocated for Transplant

The scarcity of organs for transplant raises questions about how deceased donor kidneys are allocated—who receives a kidney and who does not. Past inequities in the allocation process (e.g., more men than women, more Caucasians than people of other ethnicities, more rich than poor, and more young than old) led to the development of the United Network for Organ Sharing (UNOS) in 1986. UNOS has policies for organ distribution, including kidneys, hearts, livers, and other transplanted organs.

UNOS maintains national, regional, and local lists of patients awaiting transplants. When an organ becomes available, donor information is entered into the UNOS computer. The computer then runs a match program, generating a list of patients ranked by criteria such as blood and tissue type, organ size, and medical urgency of the patient. Factors such as time on the waiting list and distance between the donor and the transplant center also are considered. A candidate with a perfect match (six HLAs in common) and compatible blood type gets priority for the kidney, regardless of region or geographic area. Otherwise, the list of patients in the local area is checked first, then the regional list of patients awaiting transplant. If no match is found in the region, the organ becomes available to patients nationwide.

The UNOS allocation system, standardized fees, and Medicare coverage for transplantation have done much to ensure equitable access to available kidneys. Still, controversy exists. Patients with resources for travel may register in several different regions for an organ. Up to 10% of patients receiving a transplant in any center may be foreign nationals competing with U.S. citizens for scarce organ resources. A transplant center can accept or reject a candidate for transplant who has lost a kidney because of noncompliance.

As long as the demand for kidneys exceeds the supply of donor organs, it is likely that controversy will exist regarding their allocation. Nurses can help by identifying potential donors and contacting the transplant coordinator. In addition, nurses can inform the public about organ donation and the allocation system, and encourage donation.

recipient has a greater than 91.7% probability of survival after 2 years. At 5 years, the difference is even greater: 33.1% for dialysis compared with more than 80.2% for transplant (NKU-DIC, 2008). The transplant patient is no longer tethered to a dialysis catheter, machine, or center. Dietary and fluid restrictions are reduced, and the body image is more "whole."

Most transplanted kidneys are obtained from deceased donors; however, transplants from living donors are increasing. In 2009, of transplanted kidneys, 45% came from living donors, most of whom were related to the recipient (OPTN, 2009). With both deceased and living donor transplants, a close match between blood and tissue type is desired. Human leukocyte antigens (HLAs) are compared between the donor and recipient; six antigens in common is considered to be a "perfect" match. The success of well-matched living-donor transplants is better than for deceased donor organ transplants, with a 1-year graft survival of 95.1% compared to 89% for deceased donor transplants (OPTN, 2009). Close tissue matching probably accounts for the better outcome with living donors. People with normal kidneys who are in good physical health may donate a kidney. Predonation counseling is vital: Nephrectomy is major surgery and involves a risk that trauma or disease may damage the remaining kidney in the future. If the transplant fails, the psychologic impact on the donor can be significant. Nursing care of the patient having a nephrectomy is summarized in the box on page 835.

Ideally, deceased donor kidneys are obtained from people who meet the criteria for brain death, are less than 65 years old, and are free of systemic disease, malignancy, or infection, including HIV and hepatitis B or C. Expanded deceased donor criteria may allow donation of a kidney from a deceased donor who is older than 65 years or who has cardiovascular disease (hypertension or stroke) or an elevated serum creatinine (UNOS, 2008). Kidneys are removed after brain death has been determined, and are preserved by hypothermia or a technique called continuous hypothermic pulsatile perfusion. A kidney preserved by hypothermia is transplanted within 24 to 48 hours. Continuous pulsatile perfusion allows up to 3 days before transplantation. The system used to allocate deceased donor kidneys for transplantation is outlined in Box 28–1.

The donor kidney is placed in the lower abdominal cavity of the recipient, and the renal artery, vein, and ureter are anastomosed (Figure 28–10 ■). The renal artery of the donor kidney is connected to the hypogastric artery, and the renal vein to the iliac vein. The ureter is connected to one of the recipient's ureters or directly to the bladder, using a tunnel technique to prevent reflux. Nursing care for the patient having a kidney transplant is outlined in the box on page 855.

Unless the donor and recipient are identical twins, the grafted organ stimulates an immune response to reject the transplanted organ. Immunosuppressive drugs minimize this response. Azathioprine or mycophenolate mofetil are commonly used, often in combination with prednisone, a corticosteroid. Cyclosporine, a potent immunosuppressive, also may be used. These drugs suppress a portion of the immune system and

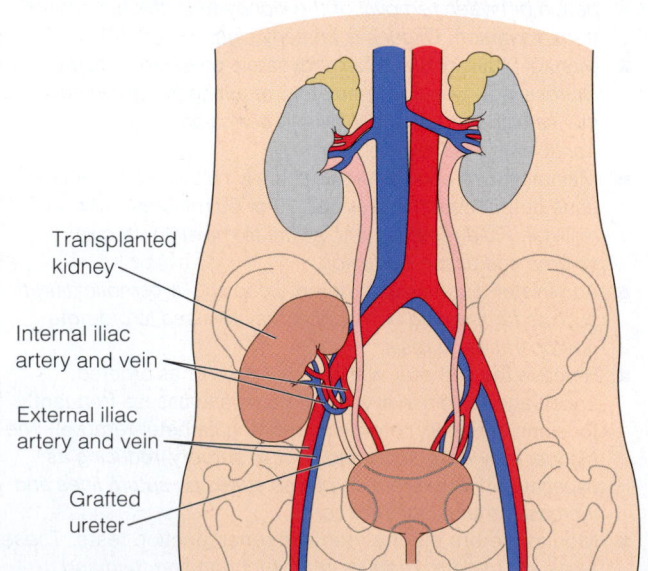

Transplanted kidney

Internal iliac artery and vein

External iliac artery and vein

Grafted ureter

Figure 28–10 ■ Placement of a transplanted kidney in the iliac fossa with anastomosis to the hypogastric artery, iliac vein, and bladder.

the inflammatory response, increasing the risk for infections and cancers with long-term therapy. The nursing implications of immunosuppressive therapy are outlined in ∞ Chapter 13.

Glucocorticoids such as prednisone and methylprednisolone are used for both maintenance of immunosuppression and to treat acute rejection episodes. Side effects of long-term corticosteroid use include impaired wound healing, emotional disturbances, osteoporosis, and cushingoid effects on glucose, protein, and fat metabolism.

Azathioprine inhibits both cellular and humoral immunity. Because this drug is rapidly metabolized by the liver, the dose may not need to be altered in the presence of renal failure. Bone marrow suppression, abnormalities of liver function, and alopecia are the primary significant adverse effects for azathioprine. The action of mycophenolate mofetil is similar to that of azathioprine. Its advantages are minimal bone marrow suppression and increased potency in preventing or reversing rejection of the transplanted organ (Fauci et al., 2008).

Cyclosporine primarily affects cellular immunity, the helper T cells in particular. Among its many adverse effects, which include hepatotoxicity and hirsutism, nephrotoxicity is a primary concern for the kidney transplant patient.

Even with immunosuppressive therapy, the transplanted kidney can be rejected at any time. Either acute or chronic rejection may develop. *Acute rejection* develops within months of the transplant. It is caused by a cellular immune response with T-lymphocyte proliferation (Porth & Matfin, 2009). Few manifestations may be apparent other than a rise in serum creatinine and possible oliguria. Methylprednisolone, a glucocorticoid, and OKT3 monoclonal antibody (∞ see Chapter 13) are used to manage acute rejection episodes. OKT3 can cause severe systemic reactions, including chills, fever, hypotension, headache, and possible pulmonary edema (Fauci et al., 2008). *Chronic rejection*, which may develop months to years following the transplant, is a major cause of graft loss. Both humoral and cellular immune responses are involved in chronic rejection. It does not respond to increased immunosuppression. The presenting manifestations of chronic rejection—progressive azotemia, proteinuria, and hypertension—are those of progressive renal failure.

Hypertension is a possible complication of kidney transplant, resulting from graft rejection, renal artery stenosis, or renal vasoconstriction. Patients may develop glomerular lesions and manifestations of nephrosis. Hypertension and altered blood lipids (increased LDLs and decreased HDLs) increase the risk of death from myocardial infarction and stroke following transplant (Fauci et al., 2008).

Long-term immunosuppression has adverse effects as well. Infection is a continuing threat. Bacterial and viral infections may develop, as well as fungal infections of the blood, lungs, and CNS. Tumors are also common, with carcinoma *in situ* of the cervix, lymphomas, and skin cancers most prevalent. The risk of congenital anomalies is increased in infants whose mothers have undergone immunosuppressive therapy. Corticosteroid use may lead to bone problems, gastrointestinal disorders such as peptic ulcer disease, and cataract formation.

✐ Nursing Care

Health Promotion

Measures to reduce the risk of CKD focus on preventing kidney disease and appropriately managing diabetes and hypertension. Promote early and effective treatment of all infections, particularly skin and pharyngeal infections caused by streptococcal bacteria. Discuss measures to reduce the risk for urinary tract infections, and stress the importance of prompt treatment to eradicate the infecting organism. Discuss the relationship between diabetes, hypertension, and kidney disease. Emphasize that maintaining blood glucose levels and the blood pressure within the recommended ranges reduces the risk of adverse effects on the kidneys. Ensure that all patients with less than optimal renal function are well-hydrated, particularly when a nephrotoxic drug is prescribed or anticipated. Finally, encourage the patient with ESRD to investigate options for early transplantation to avoid long-term dialysis.

Assessment

Both subjective and objective data are used to assess the patient with CKD:

- *Health history:* Complaints of anorexia, nausea, weight gain, or edema; current treatment (if any), including type and frequency of dialysis or previous kidney transplant; chronic diseases such as diabetes, heart failure, or kidney disease.
- *Physical examination:* Mental status; vital signs including temperature, heart and lung sounds, and peripheral pulses; urine output (if any); weight; skin color, moisture, condition; presence of edema (periorbital or dependent); bowel tones; presence and location of an AV fistula, shunt, graft, or peritoneal catheter.

See the box on page 859 for assessment of the older adult with ESRD.

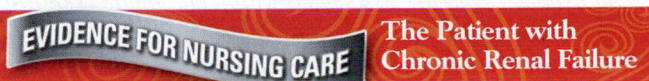

EVIDENCE FOR NURSING CARE — The Patient with Chronic Renal Failure

Selected resources that nurses may find helpful when planning evidence-based nursing care follow.

- Lin, Y-F., Wu, V-C., Ko, W-J, Chen, Y-S., Chen, Y-M., Li, W-Y. et al. (2009). Residual urine output and postoperative mortality in maintenance hemodialysis patients. *American Journal of Critical Care*, 18(5), 446–55.

- Michigan Quality Improvement Consortium. (2008 November). *Diagnosis and management of adults with chronic kidney disease.* Southfield, MI: Michigan Quality Improvement Consortium. Retrieved from http://www.guideline.gov/summary/summary.aspx?ss=15&doc_id=13824&nbr=&string=

- National Collaborating Centre for Chronic Conditions. (2008 September). *Chronic kidney disease. Early identification and management of chronic kidney disease in adults in primary and secondary care.* London, UK: National Institute for Health and Clinical Excellence (NICE). Retrieved from http://www.guideline.gov/summary/summary.aspx?ss=15&doc_id=14330&nbr=&string=

Nursing Diagnoses and Interventions

Whether the patient with ESRD is facing long-term dialysis or renal transplantation, a number of nursing care needs can be identified. This section focuses on nursing care related to impaired renal function, nutritional deficits due to dietary restrictions and nausea, increased risk for infection, and changes in body image. Also see the Case Study & Nursing Care Plan on page 860 for additional potential nursing diagnoses and interventions for the patient with chronic kidney disease.

Risk for Ineffective Renal Perfusion

Capillaries are an integral part of the nephron. As nephrons are destroyed, kidney perfusion progressively declines. As renal perfusion and nephron function fall, the kidney is less able to maintain fluid and electrolyte balance and eliminate waste products from the body.

- Monitor intake and output, vital signs including orthostatic blood pressures, and weight. *These provide important data to identify changes in fluid volume.*

> **PRACTICE ALERT**
> Weight changes are a more accurate indicator of fluid volume status in the oliguric or anuric patient than intake and output measurements.

- Restrict fluids as ordered. *As renal function declines, the ability to eliminate excess fluid is impaired.*
- Monitor respiratory status, including lung sounds, every 4 to 8 hours. *Fluid volume overload may lead to heart failure and possible pulmonary edema.*
- Monitor BUN, serum creatinine, eGFR, pH, electrolytes, and CBC. Report significant changes. *As renal function declines, the GFR falls and progressive azotemia with increasing BUN and serum creatinine is seen. Metabolic acidosis develops as the kidney is unable to eliminate hydrogen ions and conserve bicarbonate. Hyponatremia, hyperkalemia, hyperphosphatemia, and hypocalcemia are associated with renal failure. The RBC count, hemoglobin, and hematocrit decline due to deficient erythropoietin to stimulate cell production in the bone marrow. An acute fall in hemoglobin and hematocrit may indicate GI bleeding, a risk in patients with ESRD.*
- Report manifestations of electrolyte imbalances, such as cardiac dysrhythmias and other ECG changes, muscle tremors and possible tetany, and Kussmaul's respirations. *Manifestations of electrolyte imbalance may indicate the need for intervention.*
- Administer medications to treat electrolyte imbalances as ordered. *Medications may be prescribed to help maintain electrolyte and acid–base balance and prevent adverse effects of imbalances.*

> **SAFETY ALERT**
> Monitor carefully for desired and adverse effects of all medications. Impaired renal function affects drug elimination and increases the risk for toxic effects.

- Administer antihypertensive medications as ordered. *Hypertension management is an important factor in slowing the progression of CKD.*

- Time activities and procedures to allow rest periods. *The anemia associated with CKD may cause significant fatigue and activity intolerance.*

Imbalanced Nutrition: Less than Body Requirements

Anorexia, nausea, and vomiting are common manifestations of CKD and uremia. The patient often has a metallic taste and bad breath, which also diminish appetite. A diet restricted in protein and sodium will compound these problems. Food intake may be insufficient to meet metabolic needs. Catabolism, the breakdown of body proteins to meet energy needs, exacerbates azotemia and uremia.

- Monitor food and nutrient intake as well as episodes of vomiting. *Careful monitoring helps determine the adequacy of intake.*
- Weigh daily before breakfast. *This provides the most accurate measurement. Remember that a gain of 2 pounds or more over a 24-hour period is more likely to reflect fluid retention than a gain in body mass.*
- Administer antiemetic agents 30 to 60 minutes before eating. *Antiemetics reduce nausea and the risk of vomiting with food intake.*
- Assist with mouth care prior to meals and at bedtime. *Mouth care improves taste, stimulates the appetite, and maintains the integrity of oral mucous membranes.*
- Serve small meals and provide between-meal snacks. *Small meals are less likely to prompt nausea and help improve food intake.*
- Arrange for a dietary consultation. Provide preferred foods to the extent possible, and involve the patient in planning daily menus. Encourage family members to bring food as dietary restrictions allow. *Providing preferred foods within restrictions promotes intake.*
- Monitor nutritional status by tracking weight, laboratory values such as serum albumin and BUN, and anthropometric measurements (∞ see Chapters 21 and 22). *Indicators of impaired nutrition develop gradually and may be subtle. Careful assessment is important.*
- Administer parenteral nutrition as prescribed. Routinely monitor blood glucose levels, and use strict aseptic technique when handling the solution and venous access site. *Parenteral nutrition may be necessary to prevent catabolism and increasing azotemia. Hyperglycemia and infection are risks associated with parenteral nutrition (∞ see Chapter 22). Immune system suppression associated with renal failure further increases the risk for infection.*

Risk for Infection

Chronic kidney disease affects the immune system and leukocyte function, increasing susceptibility to infection. Invasive devices required for hemodialysis or peritoneal dialysis add to this risk. The patient who has had a kidney transplant remains on immunosuppressive therapy for life, further depressing the immune system and increasing the risk for infection.

- Use standard precautions and good hand hygiene technique at all times. *Hand hygiene is a primary means of preventing the transfer of organisms. Patients who are on hemodialysis or who have had multiple blood transfusions to treat anemia have an increased risk for hepatitis B, hepatitis C, and HIV infection.*

CASE STUDY & NURSING CARE PLAN   A Patient with End-Stage Renal Disease

Walter Cohen, 45 years old, is the print shop manager at a local community college. He has been a type 1 diabetic since the age of 20, and was diagnosed with diabetic nephropathy 10 years ago. Despite blood pressure control with antihypertensive medications and frequent blood glucose monitoring with insulin coverage, he developed overt proteinuria 5 years ago and has now progressed to end-stage renal disease. He enters the nephrology unit for temporary hemodialysis to relieve uremic symptoms. While there, a CAPD catheter will be inserted. Mr. Cohen's desire to continue working is the primary factor in his choice of CAPD over hemodialysis.

ASSESSMENT

Richard Gonzalez, Mr. Cohen's care manager, obtains a nursing assessment. Mr. Cohen states that his diabetes has always been difficult to control. He has had numerous hypoglycemic episodes and has been hospitalized "four or five times" for ketoacidosis. Recently he has developed symptoms of peripheral neuropathy and increasing retinopathy. He attributed his lack of appetite, nausea, vomiting, and fatigue over the past month to "a touch of the flu." His weight remained stable, so he did not worry about not eating much.

Physical assessment findings include T 97.8°F (36.5°C) PO, P 96, R 20, and BP 178/100. Skin cool and dry, with minor excoriations on forearms and lower legs. Breath odor fetid. Scattered fine rales noted in bilateral lung bases. Soft S_3 gallop noted at cardiac apex. Bilateral pitting edema of lower extremities to just below the knees; fingers and hands also edematous. Abdominal assessment essentially normal, with hypoactive bowel sounds. Urinalysis shows a specific gravity of 1.011, gross proteinuria, and multiple cell casts. CBC results: RBC 2.9 million/mm³; hemoglobin 9.4 g/dL; hematocrit 28%. Blood chemistry abnormalities include BUN 198 mg/dL; creatinine 18.5 mg/dL; sodium 125 mEq/L; potassium 5.7 mEq/L; calcium 7.1 mg/dL; phosphate 6.8 mg/dL. A temporary jugular venous catheter will be placed for hemodialysis the next day, followed by peritoneal catheter insertion later in the week.

DIAGNOSES

- *Excess Fluid Volume* related to failure of kidneys to eliminate excess body fluid
- *Imbalanced Nutrition: Less than Body Requirements* related to effects of uremia
- *Impaired Skin Integrity* of lower extremities related to dry skin and itching
- *Risk for Infection* related to invasive catheters and impaired immune function

EXPECTED OUTCOMES

- Adhere to the prescribed fluid restriction of 750 mL per day.
- Demonstrate reduced extracellular fluid volume by weight loss, decreased peripheral edema, clear lung sounds, and normal heart sounds.
- Consume and retain 100% of prescribed diet, including snacks.
- Demonstrate healing of lower extremity skin lesions.

- Remain free of infection.
- Demonstrate appropriate peritoneal catheter care and CAPD.

PLANNING AND IMPLEMENTATION

- Space fluids, allowing 400 mL from 0700 to 1500, 200 mL from 1500 to 2300, and 100 mL from 2300 to 0700.
- Provide mouth care at least every 4 hours and before every meal.
- Keep sugarless hard candy and ice chips at the bedside; include ice consumed as fluid intake.
- Weigh daily before breakfast; monitor vital signs, and heart and lung sounds, every 4 hours.
- Document intake and output every 4 hours.
- Arrange dietary consultation for menu planning.
- Administer prescribed antiemetic 1 hour before meals.
- Monitor food intake, noting percentage and types of food consumed.
- Clean lesions on lower extremities every 8 hours and assess healing.
- Teach CAPD procedure and peritoneal catheter care.
- Assist to identify strengths and needs in health regimen management.

EVALUATION

Mr. Cohen was hospitalized for 2 weeks, undergoing four hemodialysis sessions to reduce uremic symptoms. An arteriovenous fistula has been created in his left arm in case he should need hemodialysis in the future. He begins peritoneal dialysis the second week, and by discharge he is able to manage the catheter care and dialysis runs with the help of his wife. His heart and lung sounds are normal, and he has minimal peripheral edema on discharge. The excoriations on his legs have healed. His temperature is normal, and no evidence of infection is noted. Mr. Cohen remains anorectic and slightly nauseated, but is eating most of his prescribed diet and snacks. He has lost 10 pounds with excess fluid removal by dialysis, but his weight remains stable during the second week. Mr. Cohen and his wife have been introduced to another patient who has been on CAPD for several years and promises to help them with problem solving.

CRITICAL THINKING IN THE NURSING PROCESS

1. How does diabetes mellitus damage the kidneys and lead to CKD? Why is this more significant for a patient with type 1 diabetes than for someone with type 2 diabetes (∞ see Chapter 20)?
2. Why do high levels of urea in the blood often cause changes in cognition and mental status? What manifestations of encephalopathy would you expect to see?
3. How might Mr. Cohen's insulin dosage and diet need to be changed with the institution of peritoneal dialysis? Why?
4. Develop a care plan for the nursing diagnosis *Disturbed Body Image.*

See Evaluating Your Response in Appendix C.

SAFETY ALERT

Use strict aseptic technique when managing ports, catheters, and incisions, to reduce the risk of introducing infectious organisms when immune responses are impaired.

- Monitor temperature and vital signs at least every 4 hours. *A low-grade fever or increased pulse rate may indicate an infection in the immunosuppressed patient.*

- Monitor WBC count and differential. *Increased WBCs may indicate a bacterial infection; decreased WBCs may indicate viral infection. A shift in the differential showing more immature WBCs (bands) in circulation is another indicator of infection.*
- Culture urine, peritoneal dialysis fluid, and other drainage as indicated. *Culture is done to verify the presence of pathogens.*

MOVING EVIDENCE INTO ACTION — Patients with Early Chronic Kidney Disease

In a study of patients with early CKD, nurse researchers in Canada looked at patients' perceptions of health, kidney disease, and the supports these patients needed to manage their disease (Costantini et al., 2008). The study included 14 patients between ages 19 and 69.

The researchers identified that these patients went through a process they termed "renegotiating life with chronic kidney disease." Soon after the initial diagnosis, patients engaged in a discovery process, searching for evidence of the disease (when the patient often was free of symptoms) and coming to realize the life-long nature of their disease. Discovery both required disease-specific information and prompted realization of the need for additional information on self-care and managing the disease. Researchers identified this as the process of learning to live with kidney disease and assuming increasing responsibility for managing the disease.

IMPLICATIONS FOR NURSING

Patients with any chronic disease, including CKD need information and support to become effective self-health managers. While the disease may have a common name, each individual has unique needs—the information and support desired by a 19-year-old with CKD may be very different than that for a 69-year-old. Treating all patients with ESRD holistically, respecting their individual and unique characteristics and experience, is vital to promote acceptance and autonomy. Listen carefully, responding to each person's concerns. Discuss the effects of the disease and its treatment on the patient's life, marital and family relationships, and socialization. Suggest strategies to manage prescribed medications, diet and fluid restrictions, and day-to-day symptoms. Whenever appropriate, provide information about treatment options, allowing the patient to determine the preferred alternative.

CRITICAL THINKING IN PATIENT CARE

1. Identify assessment tools and data you could use to evaluate the knowledge and learning readiness of a patient with early CKD.
2. What interventions can you, as the nurse, implement to promote autonomy and acceptance in the patient with CKD? How might these interventions differ for young, middle, and older adults?
3. Develop a teaching plan for a 19-year-old single woman newly diagnosed with CKD and a teaching plan for a 69-year-old married man with newly identified CKD.

PRACTICE ALERT
Monitor clarity of dialysate return. Dialysate should return clear in the patient undergoing peritoneal dialysis. Cloudy dialysate may indicate peritonitis, the most common complication of peritoneal dialysis, and should be reported and cultured.

- Provide good respiratory hygiene including position changes, coughing, and deep breathing. *These measures improve clearance of respiratory secretions, reducing the risk for infection.*
- Restrict visits from obviously ill people. Teach the patient and family about the risk for infection and measures to reduce the spread of infection. *The patient's resistance to infection is impaired, necessitating extra caution in preventing unnecessary exposures.*

Disturbed Body Image

Chronic disease and impaired kidney function can affect the patient's body image. Hemodialysis requires an arteriovenous fistula or shunt; a permanent peritoneal catheter is required for peritoneal dialysis. While kidney transplant can restore an image of wholeness, a visible scar remains and the organ may be perceived as "foreign."

- Involve the patient in care, including meal planning, dialysis, and catheter, port, or incision care to the extent possible. *Involvement improves acceptance and stimulates discussion about the effect of the disease and treatment measures on the patient's life.*
- Encourage expression of feelings and concerns, accepting perceptions and feelings without criticism. *Self-expression enhances the patient's self-worth and acceptance.*
- Include the patient in decision making and encourage self-care. *Increased autonomy enhances the patient's sense of control, independence, and self-worth.*
- Support positive gains, but do not support denial. *The patient may have difficulty accepting the renal failure, but adaptation to the loss is important.*

- Help the patient develop and achieve realistic goals. *Realistic goals allow the patient to see progress.*
- Provide positive reinforcement and feedback. *These measures support growth and adaptation.*
- Reinforce effective coping strategies. *Reinforcement helps the patient develop positive versus negative strategies for coping.*
- Facilitate contact with a support group or other community members affected by renal failure. *The patient benefits by providing and receiving support in a group of people going through similar circumstances.*
- Refer for mental health counseling as indicated or desired. *Counseling can help the patient develop effective coping and adaptation strategies.*

Using NANDA, NIC, and NOC

Linkages between a selected NANDA nursing diagnosis, NIC, and NOC for the patient with chronic kidney disease are shown in the chart that follows.

Community-Based Care

Chronic renal failure and ESRD are long-term processes that require patient management. No matter what treatment option is chosen (hemodialysis, peritoneal dialysis, or renal transplantation), day-to-day management falls to the patient and family. See the accompanying Nursing Research box. Teaching for home care includes the following topics:

- Nature of chronic kidney disease and renal failure, including expected progression and effects
- Monitoring weight, vital signs, and temperature
- Prescribed medications, including purpose, intended effect, and potential adverse effects and their management
- Prescribed dietary and fluid restrictions (Involve the patient, a dietitian, and the family member usually responsible for cooking. Include strategies to manage nausea and relieve thirst within allowed fluid limits.)

- How to assess and protect a fistula or shunt for hemodialysis (or the extremity to be used if one is anticipated)
- Peritoneal catheter care and the procedure for peritoneal dialysis as indicated (Include a family member or significant other, in case the patient is unable to perform the procedure independently at some time.)
- Following kidney transplant, prescribed medications, adverse effects and their management, infection prevention, graft protection, and manifestations of organ rejection

Refer to a dietitian for diet planning and counseling. If home hemodialysis is planned, refer the designated dialysis helper for formal training. Both the National Kidney Foundation and the American Association of Kidney Patients may be able to provide support and educational materials for the patient with ESRD (see the box on page 859). Local and state chapters of these organizations can provide additional support.

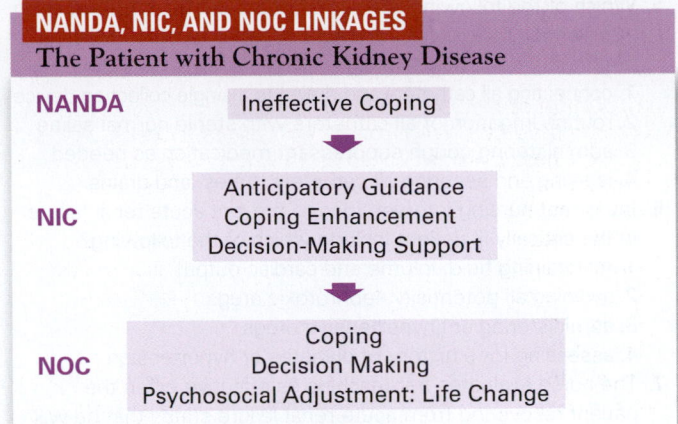

NANDA, NIC, AND NOC LINKAGES
The Patient with Chronic Kidney Disease

NANDA — Ineffective Coping

NIC — Anticipatory Guidance / Coping Enhancement / Decision-Making Support

NOC — Coping / Decision Making / Psychosocial Adjustment: Life Change

Data from NANDA International. (2009). *Nursing diagnoses: Definitions and classification 2009–2011.* Oxford, UK: Wiley-Blackwell; Bulechek, G., Butcher, H., and Dochterman, J. (Eds.). (2008). *Nursing interventions classification (NIC)* (5th ed.). St. Louis, MO: Mosby; and Moorhead, S., Johnson, M., Maas, M., and Swanson, E. (Eds.). (2008). *Nursing outcomes classification (NOC)* (4th ed.). St. Louis, MO: Mosby.

CHAPTER HIGHLIGHTS

- Congenital and acquired disorders of the kidneys can profoundly affect urinary elimination and ultimately all body systems.
- Glomerulonephritis, inflammation of the glomerulus of the kidney, leads to loss of proteins and blood cells in the urine, a decrease in the glomerular filtration rate, and severe edema.
- The renal and cardiovascular systems are closely interrelated. Vascular disorders, such as hypertension, renal artery stenosis, or obstruction of the renal artery or vein, can have serious consequences in terms of renal function.
- Renal cell malignancies, while uncommon, often are not evident until the cancer is advanced and has metastasized to other sites.

- Acute renal failure is a frequent complication of critical illnesses, typically occurring in people with no prior history of kidney disorders. Ischemic and nephrotoxic damage to the kidney are the most common precipitating factors for ARF.
- Chronic kidney disease can be the result of numerous systemic and kidney disorders, such as diabetes mellitus, hypertension, systemic lupus erythematosus, and chronic glomerulonephritis.
- When the kidneys fail, renal replacement therapies are necessary to eliminate metabolic waste products and sustain life. Dialysis and kidney transplant are the primary renal replacement therapies used.

TEST YOURSELF NCLEX-RN® REVIEW

1. The physician orders digoxin 0.125 mg three times per week for an 82-year-old patient with heart failure. Which of the following is an appropriate response by the nurse?
   1. Question the order because older patients may require larger doses due to protein loss in the urine.
   2. Administer the drug as ordered, monitoring the patient for manifestations of toxicity.
   3. Assess the patient's eGFR before administering the drug at this dose.
   4. Use 0.25-mg digoxin tablets, cutting the tablet in half to save money for the patient.

2. A patient newly diagnosed with polycystic kidney disease asks if there is anything his children need to know about their risk for getting the disorder. How should the nurse respond?
   1. Because the condition was just diagnosed, there is no risk of passing the condition on to his children.
   2. When his children prepare to marry, they and their potential partners should undergo genetic testing to determine if their children will be at risk.
   3. The adult form of this disorder is transmitted as a dominant gene; each child has a 50% risk of having inherited the defective gene.
   4. His children would have developed symptoms of the disorder *in utero* or shortly after birth if they had inherited the defective gene.

3. In obtaining a nursing history from a 22-year-old patient admitted with a diagnosis of acute glomerulonephritis, the nurse specifically asks the patient about a recent history of which of the following?
   1. urinary tract infection
   2. strep throat
   3. x-ray using contrast media
   4. illicit drug use

4. The nurse evaluates his teaching for a patient with acute glomerulonephritis as effective when the patient does which of the following?
   1. chooses soy or animal proteins for allowed grams of protein in diet
   2. states the need to remain on bed rest until his urine returns to clear yellow
   3. demonstrates care for the vascular shunt or peritoneal catheter
   4. limits fluid intake to less than 1500 mL per day

5. Which of the following is an appropriate postoperative nursing intervention for the patient who has had a partial or total nephrectomy?
   1. connecting all catheters and drains to a single collection device
   2. routine irrigation of all catheters with sterile normal saline
   3. administering cough suppressant medication as needed
   4. labeling and securing all catheters, tubes, and drains

6. Important nursing interventions to prevent acute renal failure in the critically ill patient include which of the following?
   1. maintaining fluid volume and cardiac output
   2. avoiding all potentially nephrotoxic drugs
   3. administering antihypertensive drugs
   4. assessing for a history of diabetes or hypertension

7. The nurse evaluates her teaching as effective when the patient recovering from acute renal failure states that he will do which of the following?
   1. Limit his fluid intake to 1500 mL or less per day.
   2. Consume only vegetable proteins.
   3. Avoid taking drugs that may be nephrotoxic.
   4. Self-catheterize for residual urine at least once a week.

8. The nurse caring for a patient preparing to undergo hemodialysis includes which of the following in the plan of care? **Select all that apply.**
   1. Obtain weight and orthostatic vital signs.
   2. Assess blood pressure of extremity where fistula has been created.
   3. Monitor serum creatinine, BUN, and hematocrit levels.
   4. Determine urine specific gravity and pH.
   5. Restrict fluid and protein intake.

9. An appropriate goal of nursing care for a patient with end-stage renal disease is the patient will be able to do which of the following?
   1. Identify a live-in caregiver.
   2. State the advantages and disadvantages of types of renal replacement therapies.
   3. Demonstrate the ability to independently perform hemodialysis in the home.
   4. Relate the hospice philosophy and identify indicators of the need for hospice care.

10. Following a kidney transplant, the nurse notes that the patient's urine is cloudy. How should the nurse respond?
    1. Record the finding.
    2. Increase the intravenous flow rate.
    3. Irrigate the urinary catheter.
    4. Notify the physician.

Pearson Nursing Student Resources

Find additional review materials at
nursing.pearsonhighered.com
Prepare for success with additional NCLEX®-style practice questions, interactive assignments and activities, Web links, animations and videos, and more!

BIBLIOGRAPHY

American Cancer Society. (2009). *Cancer facts and figures 2009.* Atlanta, GA: Author.

Barone, C. P., Martin-Watson, A. L., & Barone, G. W. (2004). The postoperative care of the adult renal transplant recipient. *Medsurg Nursing, 13*(5), 286–302.

Brown, D., & Martindale, A. (2008). Urinary tract trauma – diagnosis and management. *Trauma, 10,* 5–11.

Bulechek, G., Butcher, H., & Dochterman, J. (Eds.). (2008). *Nursing interventions classification (NIC)* (5th ed.). St. Louis, MO: Mosby.

Cheung, C., Ponnusamy, A., & Anderton, J. (2008). Management of acute renal failure in the elderly patient: A clinician's guide. *Drugs & Aging, 25*(6), 455–476.

Copstead, L. C., & Banasik, J. L. (2010). *Pathophysiology* (4th ed.). St. Louis, MO: Elsevier/Saunders.

Costantini, L., Beanlands, H., McCay, E., Cattran, D., Hladunewich, M., & Francis, D. (2008, March–April). The self-management experience of people with mild to moderate chronic kidney disease. *Nephrology Nursing Journal, 35*(2), 147–155.

DiPiro, J., Talbert, R., Yee, G., Matzke, G., Wells, B., & Posey, L. (2008). *Pharmacotherapy: A pathophysiologic approach* (7th ed.). New York, NY: McGraw Hill.

Fauci, A., Kasper, D., Braunwald, E., Hauser, S., Longo, D., Jameson, J., et al. (Eds.). (2008). *Harrison's principles of internal medicine* (17th ed.). New York: McGraw-Hill.

Kendrick, M. (2008 September 24). What's the point of measuring eGFR? *Pulse, 24 September 2008.* Available at www.pulsetoday.co.uk.

Kinzner, C., & Hain, D. (2007 November–December). Understanding the eGFR. *Nephrology Nursing Journal, 34*(6), 655–657.

Kohtz, C., & Thompson, M. (2007 September). Preventing contrast medium-induced nephropathy. *American Journal of Nursing, 107*(9), 40–49.

Lu, D., McCarthy, A., Lanning, L., Delaney, C., & Porter, C. (2007 May–June). A descriptive study of individuals with membranoproliferative glomerulonephritis. *Nephrology Nursing Journal, 34*(3), 295–302.

Marshall, M., Golper, T., Shaver, M., Alam, M., & Chatoth, D. (2001). Sustained low-efficiency dialysis for critically ill patients requiring renal replacement therapy. *Kidney International, 60,* 777–785.

McCance, K. L., & Huether, S. E. (2010). *Pathophysiology: The biologic basis for disease in adults & children* (6th ed.). St. Louis, MO: Mosby.

McPhee, S., Papadakis, M., & Tierney, L., Jr. (Eds.). (2008). *Current medical diagnosis & treatment* (47th ed.). New York: McGraw-Hill.

Menezes, F., Wey, S., Peres, C., Medina-Pestana, J., & Camargo, L. (2008 August). Risk factors for surgical site infection in kidney transplant recipients. *Infection Control & Hospital Epidemiology, 29*(8), 771–773.

Moorhead, S., Johnson, M., Maas, M., & Swanson, E. (Eds.). (2008). *Nursing outcomes classification (NOC)* (4th ed.) St. Louis, MO: Mosby.

NANDA International. (2009). *Nursing diagnoses: Definitions and classification 2009–2011.* Oxford, UK: Wiley-Blackwell.

National Kidney Disease Education Program. (2008). Health professionals. Chronic kidney disease (CKD) information. Retrieved from www.nkdep.nih.gov.

National Kidney and Urologic Diseases Information Clearinghouse. (2009). *Kidney and urologic disease statistics for the United States* (NIH Publication No. 09-3895). Retrieved from http://www.niddk.nih.gov/kudiseases/kidney/pubs/kustats

National Kidney Foundation. (2002). K/DOQI Clinical practice guidelines for chronic kidney disease: Evaluation, classification and stratification. *American Journal of Kidney Disease, 39*(supplement 1), S1-S266. Retrieved from www.kdoqi.org

National Kidney Foundation. (2009). The problem of kidney and urologic disease. Retrieved from www.kidney.org

Olson, D. (2007 March). Arranging live organ donation over the internet. *American Journal of Nursing, 107*(3), 69–72.

Organ Procurement and Transplantation Network. (2009

August). Donors recovered in the U.S. by donor type. Retrieved from http://optn.transplant.hrsa.gov/

Organ Procurement and Transplantation Network. (2009 August). Kidney Kaplan-Meyer graft survival rates for transplants performed 1997–2004. Retrieved from http://optn.transplant.hrsa.gov/

Peiffer, K. (2007 March). Brain death and organ procurement. *American Journal of Nursing, 107*(3), 58–67.

Phillips, A. (2009 January-February). Autosomal dominant polycystic kidney disease: A case study. *Nephrology Nursing Journal, 36*(1), 41–47.

Porth, C., & Matfin, G. (2009). *Pathophysiology: Concepts of altered health states* (8th ed.). Philadelphia: Lippincott.

Racial differences in trends of end-stage renal disease by primary diagnosis – United States, 1994–2004. (2007 March 23). *MMWR: Morbidity & Mortality Weekly Report, 56*(11), 253–256.

Russell, S. (2008 February). Responding to 2 threats to the kidney. *Nursing, 38*(2), 36–40.

Spencer, J. W., & Jacobs, J. J. (2003). *Complementary and alternative medicine: An evidence-based approach* (2nd ed.). St. Louis, MO: Mosby.

Sque, M., Long, T., Payne, S., & Allardyce, D. (2007). Why relatives do not donate organs for transplants: 'Sacrifice' or 'gift of life'? *Journal of Advanced Nursing, 61*(2), 134–144.

United Network for Organ Sharing: Policies. (2008–2009). Retrieved from www.unos.org

U.S. Renal Data System. (2008). *USRDS 2008 Annual data report: Atlas of chronic kidney disease and end-stage renal disease in the United States.* Bethesda, MD: National Institutes of Health, National Institute of Diabetes and Digestive and Kidney Diseases.

Wilkinson, J., & Ahern, N. (2009). *Nursing diagnosis handbook* (9th ed.). Upper Saddle River, NJ: Prentice Hall.

Functional Health Pattern: Elimination

Think about patients with altered urinary elimination for whom you have cared.

- What were their major medical diagnoses? Was the urinary elimination problem their primary diagnosis or a secondary one? Was it present on admission of the patients to the healthcare system or did it develop during the course of care?

- What kinds of manifestations did each of these patients have? Were these manifestations similar or different?

- Which health care behaviors affected the patients' elimination status? What was their amount and type of fluid intake? Did they take any medications?

- The Elimination Health Pattern includes patterns of urinary elimination, including urine formation, flow, and micturition. It is affected by disorders of the kidneys, ureters, urinary bladder, and urethra. The urinary system regulates body fluids, filters metabolic wastes from the bloodstream, reabsorbs essential substances and water back into the bloodstream, and eliminates metabolic wastes and water as urine.

- Kidney disorders affect the production of urine, elimination of waste products from the body, and regulatory processes such as fluid and electrolyte and acid–base balance, blood pressure, and RBC formation. Disorders of the urinary tract (kidneys, ureters, urinary bladder, and urethra) can interfere with the flow and excretion of urine produced in the kidneys.

Alterations in the structure and function of the urinary system may cause either local or systemic manifestations such as the following:

- **Dysuria** (*inflamed urinary tract tissue causes the release of inflammatory chemicals, which causes irritation of nociceptors and leads to pain*)

- **Hematuria** (*inflamed or damaged urinary tract tissue leads to increased capillary permeability, which causes RBCs to be released into the urine*)

- **Proteinuria** (*damage to glomerulus allows large protein molecules to enter filtrate; protein is detectable in the urine*)

- **Hypertension** (*impaired water and electrolyte excretion, disruption of the renin-angiotensin-aldosterone system cause hypervolemia and increased peripheral vascular resistance, which results in increased blood pressure*)

Priority nursing diagnoses within the elimination functional health pattern that may be appropriate for patients with urinary disorders include the following:

- *Impaired Urinary Elimination*
- *Urinary Incontinence (Stress, Urge, Total)*
- *Urinary Retention*

Nursing diagnoses from other functional health patterns that often are of high priority for the patient with a urinary elimination disorder include the following:

- *Ineffective Health Maintenance* (Health Perception-Health Management Pattern)

- *Acute Pain* (Cognitive-Perceptual Pattern)
- *Excess Fluid Volume* (Nutritional-Metabolic Pattern)

Question

1. When the patient has difficulty starting the urinary stream, what can the nurse do to assist with voiding?

Questions

Refer to the Clinical Scenario on the next page to answer the following questions.

Priority Setting

1. In what order would you visit these patients after report?
   A. _____
   B. _____
   C. _____
   D. _____

Health Promotion

1. In order to prevent urinary tract infection, what should Agnes Smith be taught?

2. In order to prevent further kidney stones, what should Joseph Rouse be taught about his diet?

3. In order to prevent further kidney damage, what should Angela Baldwin be taught about her diet?

Nursing Process

1. What priority nursing diagnoses would you choose for each of the patients presented? What is the rationale for your choice?

	Nursing Diagnosis	Rationale
Phillip Jones		
Agnes Smith		
Joseph Rouse		
Angela Baldwin		

2. Philip Jones is complaining of inability to void. A bladder scan indicates that there is 800 mL of urine in the bladder. Which interventions does the nurse perform?
   A. Insert a urinary catheter and completely drain the bladder at once.
   B. Insert a urinary catheter and drain urine in 500 mL increments.
   C. Ambulate Mr. Jones to the bathroom to try to void and run water in the sink.
   D. Give Mr. Jones a glass of water to drink to encourage voiding.

Directions: *Read the following clinical scenario and answer the questions that follow. To complete this exercise successfully you will not only use knowledge of the content in this unit, but also principles related to setting priorities and maintaining patient safety.*

You have been assigned to work with the following four patients for the 0700 shift on a renal medical-surgical unit. Significant data obtained during report is as follows:

- Phillip Jones is a 45-year-old who was admitted two days ago after a fall from a deer hunting stand. He experienced a bruised right kidney and numerous ecchymotic areas to the right side from the fall. His vital signs are temperature 99°F, pulse 98, respirations 28, and blood pressure 110/68. He is complaining of abdominal pain and difficulty urinating.

- Agnes Smith is an 84-year-old who was admitted 2 hours ago with complaints of urinary incontinence, anorexia, confusion

and lethargy. Her vital signs on admission were temperature 97°F, pulse 88, respirations 20, and blood pressure 148/90. The physician ordered trimethoprim-sulfamethoxazole (Bactrim) to be started as soon as possible.

- Joseph Rouse is a 45-year-old who is to undergo surgery for removal of uric acid stones after having a failed lithotripsy. His vital signs are temperature 99.6°F, pulse 94, respirations 24, blood pressure 112/68. His skin is pale, cool and clammy. He is complaining of nausea, severe left-sided flank pain with spasms, and lightheadedness.

- Angela Baldwin is a 34-year-old who has a medical history of systemic lupus erythematosus. She was admitted with complaints of left flank pain and generalized edema. Urinalysis results indicate hematuria and proteinuria. Vital signs are temperature 100°F, pulse 88, respirations 26, and blood pressure 144/90. She is admitted for aggressive immunosuppressive therapy.

3. Which nursing actions are instituted for Philip Jones following kidney trauma?
   A. Monitor level of consciousness and urine output.
   B. Monitor vital signs for hypotension and bradycardia.
   C. Observe for hypertension and check urine for hematuria.
   D. Observe urine for oliguria and proteinuria.

4. After Joseph Rouse returned from surgery, the nurse needs to report which urinary output?
   A. 20 mL per hour
   B. 40 mL per hour
   C. 300 mL per 8 hours
   D. 400 mL per 8 hours

Communication

1. The physician ordered trimethoprim-sulfamethoxazole (Bactrim) for Agnes Smith's uncomplicated cystitis. Mrs. Smith understands the length of antibiotic therapy when she verbalizes which statement?
   A. "I should be able to return home after three days of antibiotics."
   B. "I can be discharged after five days of antibiotics."
   C. "I need to stay in the hospital for one week to finish the antibiotics."
   D. "I can stay in the hospital for five days of antibiotics and take five days of antibiotics at home."

2. If Angela Baldwin asks, "Are these urinary problems I am having an indication that the lupus is getting worse?" How will you respond?

Delegation

1. What data collection and interventions can be delegated to a nursing assistant for each patient?
   A. _____
   B. _____

C. _____
D. _____

Content-Specific Questions

1. The physician orders phenazopyridine (Pyridium) for relief of pain and burning with cystitis. What should the nurse teach the patient about the use of this medication?
   A. Take the medication with antacids to prevent stomach upset.
   B. Drink less fluid to allow the drug to concentrate in the bladder.
   C. The drug turns the urine and other body secretions orange or red.
   D. Stop taking the drug if nausea and diarrhea occur.

2. The patient diagnosed with uric acid stones is ordered to follow a diet low in purines. Which is the meal plan lowest in purines?
   A. liver with onions and potatoes
   B. chicken sandwich with French fries
   C. spaghetti with ground beef meat sauce
   D. macaroni and cheese with stewed tomatoes

3. When assessing a patient with glomerulonephritis, which manifestations are indicative of an early disease process?
   A. pyuria, leukocytosis, and hyperthermia
   B. hematuria, proteinuria, and hypertension
   C. dysuria, hyperglycemia, and hypertension
   D. oliguria, flank pain, and hypotension

4. Which are risk factors of urinary tract infections? **Select all that apply.**
   A. Circumcision in males
   B. decreased cervicovaginal antibodies
   C. sexual intercourse in women
   D. short urethra in men
   E. aging in men
   F. urinary catheterization

5. Which is the most accurate indicator of fluid volume status in the oliguric or aneuric patient?
   A. intake and output
   B. weight changes
   C. restrict fluids
   D. BUN and creatinine levels

6. The most reliable diagnostic procedure to determine glomerular disorders is which diagnostic test?
   A. kidney scan
   B. antistreptolysin O titer
   C. kidney biopsy
   D. blood urea nitrogen

CASE STUDY: Amos Jenkins

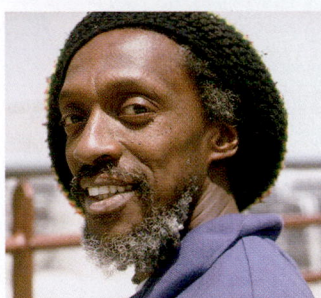

Amos Jenkins is a 45-year-old Black male who has been a truck driver for the past 20 years. He is admitted to the hospital with complaints of nausea for one week, weakness, fatigue, loss of appetite, and feeling very depressed. He has a past medical history of type 1 diabetes mellitus, hypertension, and diabetic neuropathy. Upon admission, his vital signs are temperature 98.7°F, pulse 96, respirations 20, and blood pressure 170/100. He has bilateral pitting edema to lower extremities. His fingers and hands are also edematous. He complains of dry and itching skin. His urine is collected for a urinalysis and blood work is drawn and sent to the laboratory. Results returned with a specific gravity of 1.011, gross hematuria, BUN 198 mg/dL, and creatinine 18.5 mg/dL.

Based on his past medical history and current findings, a medical diagnosis of chronic kidney disease is determined. In CKD, entire nephron units are gradually destroyed. In the early stages remaining functional nephrons hypertrophy. Glomerular capillary flow and pressure increase in the nephrons to compensate for lost renal mass. Increased demand on the remaining nephrons leads to glomerular sclerosis or scarring with eventual nephron destruction. As the disease progresses, renal insufficiency develops, with eventual renal failure. The manifestations of CKD are nausea, apathy, weakness, fatigue, proteinuria, hematuria, polyuria, nocturia, and pale and dry skin. As the disease progresses, manifestations uremia develop, including vomiting, increasing weakness, paresthesias, lethargy, confusion, headache, abdominal pain, urine-like breath odor, and uremic frost. Complications of chronic renal failure are fluid and electrolyte imbalance, acid–base imbalance, hypertension, hyperlipidemia, glucose intolerance, pulmonary edema, anemia, bleeding disorders, osteodystrophy, sexual impotence, psychotic symptoms, seizures, and coma.

Based on Mr. Jenkins's assessment and past medical history, the nursing diagnosis of *Impaired Urinary Elimination* is appropriate for planning nursing interventions.

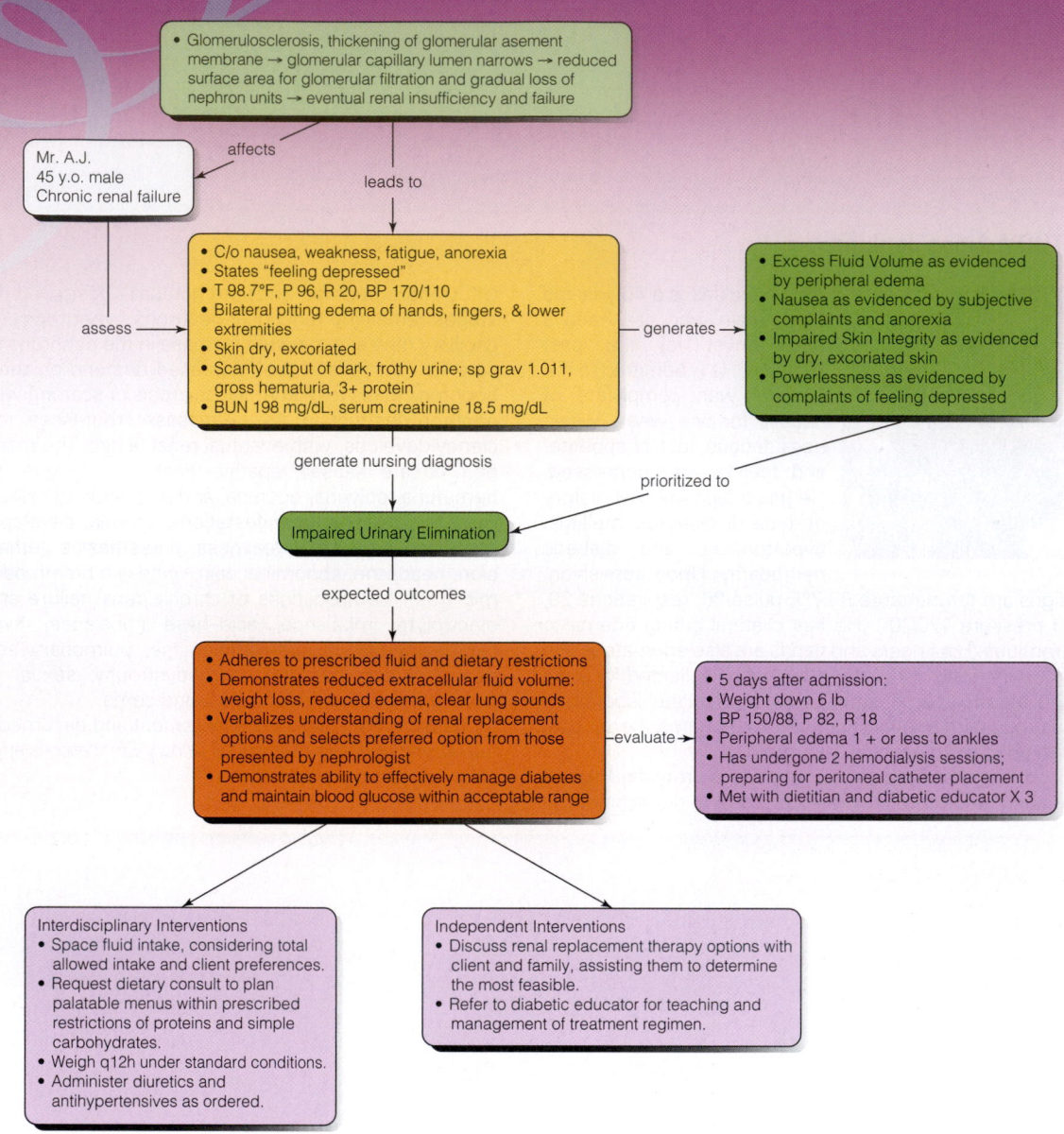

- Glomerulosclerosis, thickening of glomerular asement membrane → glomerular capillary lumen narrows → reduced surface area for glomerular filtration and gradual loss of nephron units → eventual renal insufficiency and failure

Mr. A.J.
45 y.o. male
Chronic renal failure

affects

leads to

assess

- C/o nausea, weakness, fatigue, anorexia
- States "feeling depressed"
- T 98.7°F, P 96, R 20, BP 170/110
- Bilateral pitting edema of hands, fingers, & lower extremities
- Skin dry, excoriated
- Scanty output of dark, frothy urine; sp grav 1.011, gross hematuria, 3+ protein
- BUN 198 mg/dL, serum creatinine 18.5 mg/dL

generates

- Excess Fluid Volume as evidenced by peripheral edema
- Nausea as evidenced by subjective complaints and anorexia
- Impaired Skin Integrity as evidenced by dry, excoriated skin
- Powerlessness as evidenced by complaints of feeling depressed

generate nursing diagnosis

prioritized to

Impaired Urinary Elimination

expected outcomes

- Adheres to prescribed fluid and dietary restrictions
- Demonstrates reduced extracellular fluid volume: weight loss, reduced edema, clear lung sounds
- Verbalizes understanding of renal replacement options and selects preferred option from those presented by nephrologist
- Demonstrates ability to effectively manage diabetes and maintain blood glucose within acceptable range

evaluate

- 5 days after admission:
- Weight down 6 lb
- BP 150/88, P 82, R 18
- Peripheral edema 1 + or less to ankles
- Has undergone 2 hemodialysis sessions; preparing for peritoneal catheter placement
- Met with dietitian and diabetic educator X 3

Interdisciplinary Interventions
- Space fluid intake, considering total allowed intake and client preferences.
- Request dietary consult to plan palatable menus within prescribed restrictions of proteins and simple carbohydrates.
- Weigh q12h under standard conditions.
- Administer diuretics and antihypertensives as ordered.

Independent Interventions
- Discuss renal replacement therapy options with client and family, assisting them to determine the most feasible.
- Refer to diabetic educator for teaching and management of treatment regimen.

Activity:

1. After reviewing the concept map, is there anything you would change to make it more understandable?

2. Go to the Pearson Nursing Student Resources for this book at www.nursing.pearsonhighered.com to write a concept map addressing the nursing diagnosis *Readiness for Enhanced Knowledge* related to planned peritoneal dialysis.

   See answers and hints in Appendix C.

Appendix A: Standard Precautions

Standard precautions are designed to reduce the risk of transmission of microorganisms from both recognized and unrecognized sources of infection. They are the primary strategies for preventing nosocomial infections within institutions, and are important to protect healthcare workers as well. Standard precautions apply to (1) blood; (2) all body fluids, secretions, and excretions except sweat, regardless of whether or not they contain visible blood; (3) nonintact skin; and (4) mucous membranes. Standard precautions are applied to all patients receiving care in any healthcare setting, regardless of their diagnosis or presumed infection status. Although these precautions are specifically designed for healthcare settings, they also may be implemented in providing home care or in other community-based care settings.

Hand Hygiene

- Avoid unnecessary touching of surfaces in the patient-care area.
- Perform hand hygiene (a) after touching blood, body fluids, secretions, excretions, and contaminated items, whether or not gloves are worn; (b) immediately after removing gloves, even if gloves appear to be intact; (c) between contacts with patients; and (d) when otherwise indicated to prevent transfer of organisms to other patients. You may need to wash your hands between tasks and procedures on the same patient to prevent cross-contaminating different body sites.
- Use soap and warm water for hand hygiene when hands are visibly dirty or contaminated with blood, other body fluids, or material containing body proteins.
- If hands are not visibly soiled, use an alcohol-based hand rub for routinely decontaminating hands in all other situations.

Personal Protective Equipment

Gloves

- Wear clean, nonsterile gloves when touching blood, body fluids, secretions, excretions, and contaminated items.
- Put on clean gloves just before touching mucous membranes and nonintact skin.
- Change your gloves between tasks and procedures on the same patient after contacting material that may contain a high concentration of microorganisms.
- Wear gloves for all invasive procedures such as performing venipuncture or other vascular or surgical procedures.
- Wear gloves if you have cuts, scratches, or other breaks in the skin.
- Remove gloves promptly after use, before touching noncontaminated items and surfaces, and before going to another patient; perform hand hygiene immediately after removing gloves.

Mask, Eye Protection, Face Shield

Wear a mask and eye protection or a face shield to protect mucous membranes of your eyes, nose, and mouth during procedures and patient-care activities that are likely to generate splashes or sprays of blood, body fluids, secretions, or excretions (including suctioning of the respiratory tract or endotracheal intubation). Wear a surgical mask when assisting with lumbar puncture or when material is injected into the spinal canal or subdural space.

Gown

Wear a gown (clean, disposable) to protect your skin and prevent soiling of clothing during procedures and patient-care activities that are likely to generate splashes or sprays of blood, body fluids, secretions, or excretions. Remove soiled gowns promptly, washing your hands immediately after gown removal.

Respiratory Hygiene/Cough Etiquette

Implement measures to control respiratory secretions of patients (and people accompanying them) with manifestations of a respiratory infection on entry into the healthcare setting:

- Post signs alerting patients to cover their mouths/noses when coughing or sneezing, use and dispose of tissues, and perform hand hygiene after contacting respiratory secretions.
- Provide tissues and no-touch receptacles (e.g., a waste container with a foot pedal) for tissue disposal.
- Provide instructions and resources (e.g., alcohol-based hand rub dispensers) for hand hygiene in or near patient waiting areas.
- As appropriate, offer masks to coughing patients, and encourage them to sit at least 3 feet away from other patients in the waiting area.

Environmental Control

Follow hospital procedures for routine care, cleaning, and disinfecting environmental surfaces, beds, bed rails, bedside equipment, and other frequently touched surfaces.

Equipment

Handle used patient-care equipment that is soiled with blood, body fluids, secretions, and excretions in a way that prevents exposing your skin and mucous membranes, contaminating your clothing, and transferring microorganisms to other patients or environments. Ensure that reusable equipment is cleaned and appropriately reprocessed before using for the care of another patient.

Linen

Handle and transport linens soiled with blood, body fluids, secretions, and excretions in a manner that prevents exposing your skin and mucous membranes, contaminating your clothing, and transferring microorganisms to other patients and environments. Place soiled linen in leakage-resistant bags at the location where it is used.

Occupational Health and Bloodborne Pathogens

- Take care to prevent injuries when using needles, scalpels, and other sharps; when handling sharp instruments after procedures; when cleaning used instruments; and when disposing of used needles.
- Never recap used needles, manipulate them using both hands, or handle them in a manner that directs the point of a needle toward any part of your body. If it is necessary to protect the needle prior to disposal, use a one-handed "scoop" technique or mechanical device to hold the needle sheath.
- Do not remove used needles from disposable syringes by hand; do not bend, break, or otherwise manipulate used needles by hand.
- Place used disposable syringes and needles, scalpel blades, and other sharp items in appropriate puncture-resistant containers located as close as practical to the area in which the items were used.
- Place reusable syringes and needles in a puncture-resistant container for transport to the reprocessing area.
- Use mouthpieces, resuscitation bags, or other ventilation devices as an alternative to mouth-to-mouth resuscitation methods whenever possible.

Safe Injection Practices

When using needles, cannulas that replace needles, and intravenous delivery systems do the following:

- Use aseptic technique to avoid contaminating sterile equipment.

- Needles, cannulas, and syringes are single-use items; never use the same syringe, needle, or cannula for more than one patient (even if used to enter or connect to a patient's IV fluid or administration set).
- Use intravenous fluid infusion and administration sets for one patient only and appropriately discard after using.
- Use single-dose vials of parenteral medications whenever possible; do not use the same single-dose vial for more than one patient or combine left-over contents with that from another vial.
- Use a sterile syringe and needle or cannula to access multiple-dose vials if necessary to use; do not store the vial in the patient-care area and discard if sterility is compromised or questionable.

Patient Placement

Place patients who contaminate the environment or who do not (or are not expected to) assist in maintaining appropriate hygiene or environmental control (e.g., an ambulatory, confused patient with fecal incontinence) in a private room.

Source: Centers for Disease Control and Prevention. (2007). *Standard Precautions. Excerpt from Guideline for Isolation Precautions: Preventing Transmission of Infectious Agents in Healthcare Settings 2007.* Atlanta: Public Health Service, U.S. Department of Health and Human Services, Centers for Disease Control and Prevention. Retrieved from www.cdc.gov/ncidod/dhqp/gl_isolation_standard.html#

Appendix B: 2009–2011 NANDA-Approved Nursing Diagnoses

Activity Intolerance
Activity Intolerance, Risk for
Activity Planning, Ineffective
Airway Clearance, Ineffective
Anxiety
Anxiety, Death
Aspiration, Risk for
Attachment, Risk for Impaired
Autonomic Dysreflexia
Autonomic Dysreflexia, Risk for
Bleeding, Risk for
Blood Glucose Level, Risk for Unstable
Body Image, Disturbed
Body Temperature: Imbalanced, Risk for
Bowel Incontinence
Breastfeeding, Effective
Breastfeeding, Ineffective
Breastfeeding, Interrupted
Breathing Pattern, Ineffective
Cardiac Output, Decreased
Caregiver Role Strain
Caregiver Role Strain, Risk for
Childbearing Process, Readiness for
    Enhanced
Comfort, Impaired
Comfort, Readiness for Enhanced
Communication, Impaired Verbal
Communication, Readiness for Enhanced
Confusion, Acute
Confusion, Acute, Risk for
Confusion, Chronic
Constipation
Constipation, Perceived
Constipation, Risk for
Contamination
Contamination, Risk for
Coping: Community, Ineffective
Coping: Community, Readiness for
    Enhanced
Coping, Defensive
Coping: Family, Compromised
Coping: Family, Disabled
Coping: Family, Readiness for Enhanced
Coping, Ineffective
Coping, Readiness for Enhanced
Decisional Conflict
Decision Making, Readiness for Enhanced
Denial, Ineffective
Dentition, Impaired
Development: Delayed, Risk for
Diarrhea
Disuse Syndrome, Risk for
Diversional Activity, Deficient
Electrolyte Imbalance, Risk for

Energy Field, Disturbed
Environmental Interpretation Syndrome,
    Impaired
Failure to Thrive, Adult
Falls, Risk for
Family Processes, Dysfunctional
Family Processes, Interrupted
Family Processes, Readiness for Enhanced
Fatigue
Fear
Fluid Balance, Readiness for Enhanced
Fluid Volume, Deficient
Fluid Volume, Deficient, Risk for
Fluid Volume, Excess
Fluid Volume, Imbalanced, Risk for
Gas Exchange, Impaired
Gastrointestinal Motility, Dysfunctional
Gastrointestinal Motility, Dysfunctional,
    Risk for
Grieving
Grieving, Complicated
Grieving, Risk for Complicated
Growth, Disproportionate, Risk for
Growth and Development, Delayed
Health Behavior, Risk-Prone
Health Maintenance, Ineffective
Health Management, Ineffective Self
Health Management, Readiness for
    Enhanced Self
Health-Seeking Behaviors (Specify)
Home Maintenance, Impaired
Hope, Readiness for Enhanced
Hopelessness
Human Dignity, Risk for Compromised
Hyperthermia
Hypothermia
Immunization Status, Readiness for
    Enhanced
Infant Behavior, Disorganized
Infant Behavior, Disorganized, Risk for
Infant Behavior, Organized, Readiness for
    Enhanced
Infant Feeding Pattern, Ineffective
Infection, Risk for
Injury, Risk for
Insomnia
Intracranial Adaptive Capacity, Decreased
Jaundice, Neonatal
Knowledge, Deficient
Knowledge, Readiness for Enhanced
Latex Allergy Response
Latex Allergy Response, Risk for
Liver Function, Impaired, Risk for
Loneliness, Risk for
Maternal/Fetal Dyad, Risk for Disturbed

Memory, Impaired
Mobility: Bed, Impaired
Mobility: Physical, Impaired
Mobility: Wheelchair, Impaired
Moral Distress
Nausea
Neglect, Self
Neglect, Unilateral
Neurovascular Dysfunction: Peripheral,
    Risk for
Noncompliance (Specify)
Nutrition, Imbalanced: Less than Body
    Requirements
Nutrition, Imbalanced: More than Body
    Requirements
Nutrition, Imbalanced: More than Body
    Requirements, Risk for
Nutrition, Readiness for Enhanced
Oral Mucous Membrane, Impaired
Pain, Acute
Pain, Chronic
Parenting, Impaired
Parenting, Readiness for Enhanced
Parenting, Risk for Impaired
Perfusion, Decreased Cardiac Tissue,
    Risk for
Perfusion, Ineffective Cerebral Tissue,
    Risk for
Perfusion, Ineffective Gastrointestinal,
    Risk for
Perfusion, Ineffective Peripheral Tissue
Perfusion, Ineffective Renal, Risk for
Perioperative Positioning Injury, Risk for
Personal Identity, Disturbed
Poisoning, Risk for
Post-Trauma Syndrome
Post-Trauma Syndrome, Risk for
Power, Readiness for Enhanced
Powerlessness
Powerlessness, Risk for
Protection, Ineffective
Rape-Trauma Syndrome
Relationship, Readiness for Enhanced
Religiosity, Impaired
Religiosity, Readiness for Enhanced
Religiosity, Risk for Impaired
Relocation Stress Syndrome
Relocation Stress Syndrome, Risk for
Resilience, Impaired Individual
Resilience, Risk for Compromised
Resilience, Readiness for Enhanced
Role Conflict, Parental
Role Performance, Ineffective
Sedentary Lifestyle
Self-Care, Readiness for Enhanced

Self-Care Deficit: Bathing
Self-Care Deficit: Dressing
Self-Care Deficit: Feeding
Self-Care Deficit: Toileting
Self-Concept, Readiness for Enhanced
Self-Esteem, Chronic Low
Self-Esteem, Situational Low
Self-Esteem, Risk for Situational Low
Self-Mutilation
Self-Mutilation, Risk for
Sensory Perception, Disturbed (Specify: Auditory, Gustatory, Kinesthetic, Olfactory, Tactile, Visual)
Sexual Dysfunction
Sexuality Pattern, Ineffective
Shock, Risk for
Skin Integrity, Impaired
Skin Integrity, Risk for Impaired
Sleep, Readiness for Enhanced
Sleep Deprivation

Sleep Pattern, Disturbed
Social Interaction, Impaired
Social Isolation
Sorrow, Chronic
Spiritual Distress
Spiritual Distress, Risk for
Spiritual Well-Being, Readiness for Enhanced
Spontaneous Ventilation, Impaired
Stress Overload
Sudden Infant Death Syndrome, Risk for
Suffocation, Risk for
Suicide, Risk for
Surgical Recovery, Delayed
Swallowing, Impaired
Therapeutic Regimen Management: Ineffective Family
Thermoregulation, Ineffective
Tissue Integrity, Impaired
Transfer Ability, Impaired

Trauma, Risk for
Trauma, Vascular, Risk for
Urinary Elimination, Impaired
Urinary Elimination, Readiness for Enhanced
Urinary Incontinence, Functional
Urinary Incontinence, Overflow
Urinary Incontinence, Reflex
Urinary Incontinence, Stress
Urinary Incontinence, Urge
Urinary Retention
Weaning Response, Dysfunctional
Violence: Other-Directed, Risk for
Violence: Self-Directed, Risk for
Walking, Impaired
Wandering

Source: NANDA International. (2009). *Nursing diagnoses: Definitions and classification 2009–2011.* Oxford, UK: Wiley-Blackwell. Used with permission.

Appendix C: Test Yourself, End of Unit, and Evaluate Your Response Answers

Test Yourself Answers

Chapter 1: Medical-Surgical Nursing in the Twenty-first Century

1. **Answer: 2 Rationale:** This is done in order to standardize the different healthcare professions nationally and develop guidelines of practice.
2. **Answer: 4 Rationale:** Critical thinking is needed in order to perform nursing assessments, prioritize patient care, evaluate treatment and education needs, and address any potential safety issues.
3. **Answer: 1 Rationale:** The patient is an integral part of developing a care plan. It is very important to include the patient in order to establish individualized goals to best meet the needs of the patient. Nurses develop a partnership with the patient when initiating the plan of care.
4. **Answer: 2, 1, 5, 4, 3 Rationale:** Assessment is the first step to determine the needs of the patient. Based on this information, individualized goals and outcomes can be established. Next, the planning stage determines what is necessary to meet the expected outcomes. These expected outcomes should be short-term and realistic, and should be adjusted as necessary. Implementation follows, which is when the plan is put into action. The final step is evaluation. The plan is evaluated to determine the degree of success of the individualized goals and outcomes. The outcomes may be met, partially met, or not met. This is the time when it may be necessary to change the plan and outcomes in order to best meet the patient's needs. The patient should be involved in each step of the nursing process.
5. **Answer: 3 Rationale:** Although there are many layers of care involved in nursing, the foundation for all aspects of nursing is the knowledge base. Without a strong knowledge base, nurses would not be able to develop clinical competency or practice, or provide holistic care.
6. **Answer: 4 Rationale:** The educator role is the most important function for nurses when developing and providing health information to patients.
7. **Answer: 1 Rationale:** Situations involving a difference of opinion between patients and healthcare providers may arise. The nurse plays an integral part in these situations by assisting and supporting the patient's decision making through advocacy.
8. **Answer: 2 Rationale:** When a nurse is responsible for assignments and determining appropriate work activities for other members of the nursing team, this is a leadership or manager role. This role can be formal or informal.
9. **Answer: 2 Rationale:** Critical pathways are developed to address general standards of care and outcomes for a specific patient population. This often helps to simplify the nursing process, but the nurse still must individualize the plan for the patient.
10. **Answer: 3 Rationale:** The nurse is ultimately responsible for the vital signs performed by unlicensed personnel. If there is any question regarding the readings, it is the nurse's responsibility to evaluate the results, repeat anything in question, and inform the provider as necessary.

Chapter 2: Health and Illness in Adults

1. **Answer: 4 Rationale:** Many patients have underlying disease processes, and daily medications are necessary to assist in maintaining good health. Thus, the definition of wellness is actively practicing healthy behaviors, rather than the absence of disease or illness.
2. **Answer: 1, 2, 4, 5 Rationale:** Genetic makeup can predispose patients for many different chronic illnesses or diseases. Cognitive abilities can affect the understanding, or lack of understanding, a patient has regarding how to maintain wellness. Age can affect health as many chronic illnesses become more problematic with age. Age can also affect cognitive abilities and affect other senses necessary to maintain wellness, such as hearing, sight, smell, and taste. Race can also be a factor of health, as many chronic illnesses are more prevalent in particular races and can also be more difficult to manage, such as hypertension in the Black population.
3. **Answer: 2 Rationale:** Sickle cell disease is an autosomal recessive disease that is primarily found in patients of African descent.
4. **Answer: 1 Rationale:** Practicing safer sex is the only choice with a focus on prevention.
5. **Answer: 2 Rationale:** Assuming the sick role is when you take on the responsibility of calling to explain your illness and you do not go to class as a result.
6. **Answer: 4 Rationale:** A congenital illness is a disorder that a person is born with, often as a result of a physiological imperfection.
7. **Answer: 2 Rationale:** The most important factor when referring to a chronic illness is that it lasts for a lifetime. Although manifestations may wax and wane, and remissions may occur, the underlying disease still exists.
8. **Answer: 1 Rationale:** Although Mr. Jones is at risk for multiple illnesses, the system at greatest risk is the cardiovascular system. He has many risk factors for cardiovascular disease including age, overweight, smoking, and sedentary lifestyle.
9. **Answer: 2 Rationale:** Accident prevention in the home is a very important topic to present to senior citizens. This population is at greatest risk for falls and injury in the home due to sensory problems including vision loss, unsteady gait, loss of sensation to hot and cold, and loss of sense of smell and taste to identify spoiled food.
10. **Answer: 3, 4 Rationale:** Recognizing that dying is a part of living is part of adjusting to aging and recognizing the bodily changes that occur as a result of aging. Coping with loss is part of the grieving process that the widowed spouse must endure as the result of death of a loved one.

Chapter 3: Community and Home-Based Care of Adults

1. **Answer: 3 Rationale:** The focus of community-based nursing care is to provide direct care to individuals and their families with acute or chronic health problems.
2. **Answer: 1 Rationale:** Access to healthcare services may be more challenging for rural residents due to transportation issues. Urban residents often have easier access to public transportation to obtain healthcare services.

3. **Answer: 1 Rationale:** Assessment questions related to transportation, financial, personal, physical, and emotional assistance can help the nurse determine the person's social support system.

4. **Answer: 4 Rationale:** Respite care provides assistance to full-time caregivers and helps relieve some of the stress associated with this huge responsibility.

5. **Answer: 1, 3, 4, 5 Rationale:** All four of these individuals can potentially benefit from home-care services.

6. **Answer: 4 Rationale:** The role of advocate occurs when the nurse explores, informs, supports, and affirms the choices of a patient. These activities include advanced directives, living wills, and durable power of attorney for health care.

7. **Answer: 1, 3, 4 Rationale:** Overloaded extension cords, several throw rugs, cluttered floor space, and expired medications are all environmental threats to safety.

8. **Answer: 2 Rationale:** It is important to determine the priorities of needs from the patient and family perspective before establishing a plan of rehabilitative care.

9. **Answer: 2 Rationale:** Health teaching about the importance of effective hand hygiene, the use of gloves, proper handling of linens, disposal of wastes, and the practice of standard precautions can help to control infection in the home.

10. **Answer: 4 Rationale:** Only interventions identified on the treatment plan are covered by private insurance, Medicare, or Medicaid; therefore, treatment plans are a requirement for reimbursement.

Unit 1 Building Clinical Competence: Dimensions of Medical-Surgical Nursing
Functional Health Pattern: Health Perception-Health Management

Functional Health Patterns
Hint: Ask patients to tell you how they feel and why they think they feel this way.

Priority Setting
1.
   A. The distance and travel time between patients.
   B. The estimated time for each visit.
   C. Tom Smith needs IV antibiotics at 0930.
   Rationale: An absolute plan cannot be addressed without knowing more about the setting. Because all patients are relatively stable, who is seen first is not critical. The nurse should plan a route that would allow adequate time for each visit. Mr. Smith's visit will take at least 90 minutes because IV vancomycin takes a minimum of 60 minutes to infuse. Thirty minutes will be allowed for set up and clean up of the infusion. The dressing can be changed while the antibiotic is infusing. The route should be planned to avoid back-tracking (if possible) to be most efficient and cost effective.

Health Promotion
1. An important part of primary prevention is to provide patient teaching related to his or her primary diagnosis. What primary prevention interventions will you talk to each patient about? The following are examples of answers to this question. Other answers are also possible.
   A. Cora Swank: Ms. Swank should have instruction in adequate fiber and fluids in her diet and daily activity. *Rationale: These primary prevention interventions will help with bowel function as well as regaining strength following surgery, facilitating healing and maintaining optimum health.*

   B. Tom Smith: Mr. Smith should be encouraged to wear appropriate safety equipment during high-risk activities such as riding motorcycles. Appropriate safety equipment includes helmet, gloves, long sleeves, long pants, and boots. *Rationale: Proper use of safety equipment can prevent head injury and decrease the chance of soft tissue damage during an accident.*

   C. Marguerite Garcia: Mrs. Garcia should be encouraged to talk with family members or friends daily. If she fails to contact these people daily, they should be responsible to physically check on her to be sure she is OK. *Rationale: Elderly patients living alone are at risk for falls and injury. A responsible person(s) should be in contact with them daily. Should the elderly patient fail to make contact, someone must physically check on the patient's well-being.*

   D. Sebastian Huian: Mr. Huian should be encouraged to stop smoking and provided with information about local stop-smoking programs. *Rationale: Evidence shows smoking contributes to hypertension and stroke. By stopping smoking Mr. Huian can lower his risk for further strokes. His left-sided weakness could also pose a fire risk if he should drop the lit cigarette.*

2. C. *Rationale: Tertiary level of prevention includes providing training to a patient to become productive to society within the limitation of the patient's abilities. Primary level of prevention is developing a healthy lifestyle to prevent illness, such as maintaining a balanced diet and stopping smoking. Secondary level of prevention is screening for and treating illnesses.*

Nursing Process
1.
   A. Cora Swank: Assess abdominal incision for healing. Assess skin around the ostomy, and the intactness of the ostomy appliance. Assess the amount, color, and consistency of stool. Assess pain control. *Rationale: Ms. Swank is a postoperative patient and it is important to assess the amount of healing.*

   B. Tom Smith: Assess the leg wound for healing, amount and type of drainage, and intactness of wound dressing. Assess pain management. Assess condition of the IV site and the patency of the IV needle. *Rationale: It is important for the nurse to evaluate the effectiveness of treatment by assessing the condition of the wound. The patency and condition of an IV must be determined before administration of any medication. Infection and slow healing of injuries can result in chronic pain, which must be evaluated.*

   C. Marguerite Garcia: Besides obtaining a blood pressure and blood glucose, assess heart and lung sounds. Assess the feet and lower legs for the condition of the skin, normal sensation, pulses, and the presence of swelling. *Rationale: Hypertension and congestive heart failure can cause irregular pulse, moist lung sounds, and swelling and decreased circulation in the feet. Diabetes can cause peripheral nerve damage.*

   D. Sebastian Huian: Assess vital signs, a neurological status including the degree of left-sided weakness, and Sebastian's functional abilities for self-care. *Because Mr. Huian was just discharged from rehabilitation and this is the first time the home health nurse is responsible for his care, it is important to obtain a baseline of his neurological and functional status.*

2. Each patient could have more than one nursing diagnosis. The following is not all-inclusive.

	Nursing Diagnosis	Rationale
Cora Swank	*Actue Pain* related to recent surgery *Risk for Impaired Skin Integrity* related to recent surgery and colostomy	*Patient is 10 days post-op. While pain should be less, mild to moderate analgesics may be required.* *Skin irritation can occur at operative site and around the colostomy appliance.*
Tom Smith	*Acute Pain* related to left leg injury and infection *Impaired Skin Integrity* related to wound infection	*Even though the leg injury was some time ago, healing has not taken place. In this situation acute pain can become chronic in nature.* *There is an obviously infected wound.*
Marguerite Garcia	*Risk for Knowledge Deficit* related to hypertension and type II diabetes *Risk for Noncompliance* of self-administration of medication	*The scenario implies that Mrs. Garcia may not be taking her medication as prescribed. It is important for the nurse to assess her and determine the need for information or other interventions.*
Sebastian Huian	*Risk for Self-Care Deficit*: bathing/ hygiene, dressing/grooming, feeding, toileting	*Because of Mr. Huian's recent CVA and discharge from rehabilitation, he is at risk for self-care deficit in the home environment.*

3. A, C, E. *Rationale: The patient is more likely to follow the plan of care when the nurse has established an atmosphere of trust and has rapport with the patient. To develop a plan of care, the nurse needs to assess the environment to determine the patient's safety needs and to obtain the patient's input into the goals to be accomplished.*

4. Ask Mrs. Garcia to plan a menu for a week and then determine if she has selected low sodium foods. *Rationale: The best way to determine a patient's understanding of teaching is to have him or her repeat the information or demonstrate his or her knowledge.*

Communication

1. Report your assessment findings and the plan for home care that was established with the patient and family. *Rationale: It is important to communicate assessment findings and plan of care to provide a baseline for evaluating patient progress.*

Delegation

1. A home health aid can take Mrs. Garcia's blood pressure, blood glucose, and observe Mrs. Garcia taking her medication. If Mrs. Garcia takes her medication when the home health aid is not present, the aid can report the medication is or is not in the medication container. *Rationale: Home health aids can be taught to take all vital signs and obtain capillary blood glucose values. In most cases, home health aids can remind patients to take their medication and can assist them in opening containers. Home health aids cannot evaluate the effectiveness of medication.*

Nursing Ethics

1. The nurse should explain that dating the patient is not allowed. *Rationale: It is not ethical to date a patient or to give him or her the impression that a personal relationship will occur in the future. Once the nurse–patient relationship is no longer established, and the nurse does not have a professional responsibility to provide nursing care, a personal relationship could be established.*

Concept Map

Hint: A concept map is one way to visualize the relationships between nursing diagnosis. Be creative in diagramming these relationships. It will be helpful to review Meeting Health Needs of Adults in Chapter 2 as you develop your concept map for Risk-Prone Health Behavior.

Chapter 4: Nursing Care of Patients Having Surgery

1. **Answer: 2 Rationale:** The nurse's primary responsibility to informed consent is serving as a witness to the patient signature on the consent form.
2. **Answer: 2 Rationale:** When patients are discharged soon after surgery, they need increased information about complications so they will recognize abnormal manifestations as early as possible and report these to the healthcare provider.
3. **Answer: 3 Rationale:** Nonsteroidal anti-inflammatory drugs (NSAIDs) potentiate analgesia and reduce inflammation caused from surgery.
4. **Answer: 4 Rationale:** Creatinine levels specifically reflect renal clearance. When creatinine is increased above normal levels, renal impairment needs to be considered.
5. **Answer: 3 Rationale:** Redness or swelling in the calf may be a manifestation of DVT in the circulatory system distal to the surgery.
6. **Answer: 3 Rationale:** All orders must be cancelled when the patient is admitted to surgery and must be re-ordered following surgery.
7. **Answer: 4 Rationale:** Anesthetic agents cause paralysis and block sympathetic nervous system control. This blocks manifestations of hypoglycemia and could prevent recognition of the condition.
8. **Answer: 3 Rationale:** Administering analgesics on a regular schedule in the immediate postoperative period enhances pain control.
9. **Answer: 4 Rationale:** Remaining in a fixed position for a long period of time impairs circulation, which increases the risk of pressure ulcers; joint stiffness develops from lack of flexion so that pain occurs when the joint is flexed.
10. **Answer: 4 Rationale:** Hypothermia is associated with bleeding from the surgical site and increases cardiac ischemia, which in turn increases the risk of cardiac mortality.

Chapter 5: Nursing Care of Patients Experiencing Loss, Grief, and Death

1. **Answer: 3 Rationale:** Only the person experiencing loss can evaluate his or her experiences. This is highly individualized and cannot be judged by others.
2. **Answer: 1 Rationale:** Anger is a common response to the diagnosis of a terminal illness.
3. **Answer: 2 Rationale:** A strong support system of friends and family is extremely important in helping one through the grieving process and to cope with loss.
4. **Answer: 1 Rationale:** Culture dictates the rituals of mourning, providing a pathway to express the loss.

5. **Answer: 2 Rationale:** A living will expresses the exact wishes of a patient regarding expectations for medical care. It addresses what the patient is willing to or not willing to endure to sustain life.

6. **Answer: 3 Rationale:** Hospice care, representing a model of care rather than a location for care, is for patients suffering from terminal illnesses.

7. **Answer: 4 Rationale:** The nurse would respect the patient's wishes and withhold pain medications.

8. **Answer: 1 Rationale:** It is thought that the sense of hearing is the last sense to go before death occurs.

9. **Answer: 3 Rationale:** It is important to continue to manage pain at all times of life, especially in end-of-life care.

10. **Answer: 2 Rationale:** The open-ended statement of acknowledging to the woman "This must be a difficult time for you" provides an opportunity for her to express her feelings as she recognizes the nurse's willingness to listen.

Chapter 6: Nursing Care of Patients with Problems of Substance Abuse

1. **Answer: 2 Rationale:** A blood alcohol level (BAL) greater than 0.08% is considered legal intoxication in most states.

2. **Answer: 1 Rationale:** Open-ended questions about drug or alcohol use should be asked in a nonthreatening, nonjudgmental, matter-of-fact manner (for example, beginning with how, what, and andandand and when).

3. **Answer: 4 Rationale:** Thiamine replacement is typically ordered for patients with chronic alcoholism, which can lead to thiamine deficiency and neurological impairments.

4. **Answer: 3 Rationale:** All CNS depressants (including alcohol, benzodiazepines, and barbiturates) have a potentially dangerous progress of withdrawal. Severe withdrawal or delirium tremens is a medical emergency.

5. **Answer: 3 Rationale:** Disulfiram is a form of aversion therapy that prevents the breakdown of alcohol, causing physical illness if taken while drinking alcohol.

6. **Answer: 3 Rationale:** Patients who receive care from an impaired nurse may complain of ineffective pain control and may report they did not receive medications while that nurse was on duty.

7. **Answer: 2 Rationale:** The smoking rates for women have steadily increased and it is now the leading known cause of preventable death and disease among women.

8. **Answer: 4 Rationale:** It is recommended that patients wear a medic alert bracelet while on naltrexone (ReVia).

9. **Answer: 1 Rationale:** A realistic goal for substance abusers is the identification of healthy coping mechanisms, relaxation, and stress reduction techniques to decrease the risks of substance abuse.

10. **Answer: 3 Rationale:** *Ineffective Denial* is the best choice. Patients need assistance to recognize and change maladaptive behaviors related to substance abuse.

Chapter 7: Nursing Care of Patients Experiencing Disasters

1. **Answer: 3 Rationale:** Although emergencies can typically be handled by available emergency services, disasters involve multiple services and agencies working together.

2. **Answer: 3 Rationale:** Nurses are an integral part in assisting with disasters. However, they do not serve in a leadership role in the command center. Their role is in assisting with triage and in meeting the emergency healthcare needs of those injured or involved in the disaster.

3. **Answer: 4 Rationale:** Reverse triage is necessary when there are limited resources to care for multiple people injured in a disaster. This is so the majority of people can be helped with the resources currently available.

4. **Answer: 3 Rationale:** It is important to recognize that a patient whose primary language is not English may not read in his or her primary language. This can create a significant problem when providing health education. It is important to have someone translate all information to the patient and have the patient explain what has been taught in order to ensure proper understanding of the information.

5. **Answer: 3 Rationale:** PPE should lessen the likelihood of occupational injury and/or illness, but proper precautions also must be taken to ensure safety. This can be as simple as proper hand hygiene after removing gloves, or following isolation guidelines.

6. **Answer: 2 Rationale:** Decontamination cannot begin in the hot zone as this is the area of greatest contamination. It is important to decontaminate the area outside of the hot zone to prevent its spread.

7. **Answer: 1 Rationale:** A dirty bomb is a bomb that carries a radiological signature and can cause contamination and radiation poisoning.

8. **Answer: 2 Rationale:** Radiation sickness is the direct result of exposure to ionizing radiation, which causes cellular mutation. This condition must be treated rapidly or death may result as the cells continue to mutate and die.

9. **Answer: 3 Rationale:** Older adults have individual needs. Some may be more independent than others regarding the degree of support needed in emergencies, whereas others may require multiple resources and support in an evacuation.

10. **Answer: 4 Rationale:** Nurses often are so involved in caring for others they tend to neglect themselves. In disaster situations, nurses may also suffer from loss while caring for others. As a result the nurse may feel overwhelmed and be as traumatized as those for whom he or she is caring.

Unit 2 Building Clinical Competence: Alterations in Patterns of Health

Functional Health Pattern: Health Perception-Health Management

Functional Health Patterns
Hint: There are many ways we increase the patient's comfort without realizing we are doing so.

Priority Setting
1.
   A. John Linzer should be seen first. Even with a DNR order, Mr. Linzer and his family need support during the dying process. If death is not imminent, the nurse may be able to leave the room after providing reassurance and instruction.
   B. Peter Black should be seen second. Numbness in the legs can be a sign of an undetected nerve injury that must be assessed and diagnosed rapidly to prevent permanent damage.
   C. Paul Goetz should be seen third. He is exhibiting signs of alcohol withdrawal and needs assessment and medication to alleviate the symptoms. A sitter should be designated to stay with Mr. Goetz to ensure his safety.
   D. Mary Black should be seen last. Her condition is the most stable and surgery is not scheduled for several hours.

Health Promotion
1. To facilitate healing of a fracture, Mrs. Black should have increased calories, protein, calcium, and vitamin D.
2. C. *Rationale: This meal plan contains the necessary nutrients with the fewest empty calories.*

Nursing Process

1.

    A. Peter Black: A complete neurological assessment is needed with emphasis on the lower extremities. All abrasions and lacerations should be assessed for bleeding and signs of infection.

    B. Mary Black: Assess the left ankle for pain and bruising. All abrasions and ecchymotic areas should be assessed for bleeding.

    C. John Linzer: Assess for signs of impending death, including level of consciousness, mottling, and respiratory pattern.

    D. Paul Goetz: Assess for continued signs of alcohol withdrawal including combativeness, orientation, hallucinations, diaphoresis, and nausea.

2.

	Nursing Diagnosis	Rationale
Peter Black	*Risk for Neurovascular Dysfunction* related to injury	*Mr. Black's most urgent problem is recent numbness in his legs.*
Mary Black	*Anxiety* related to hospitalization of children and upcoming surgery	*Mrs. Black's physical status is stable. She is requesting to see her children before surgery.*
John Linzer	*Death Anxiety* related to terminal illness	*Even when the patient and family have had time to prepare for death, anxiety is common in the final hours.*
Paul Goetz	*Disturbed Sensory Perception (Visual)* related to alcohol withdrawal	*Mr. Goetz is seeing spiders and exhibiting other symptoms of alcohol withdrawal.*

3.

    A. Administer pain medications as ordered. *Rationale: Maintaining comfort is a high priority for all patients.*

    B. Turn every 1 to 2 hours. *Rationale: Repositioning adds comfort to the bed-fast patient.*

    C. Provide hygiene, oral care every 1 hour, peri-care following each incontinence, and bed bath daily. *Rationale: Often the patient breathes through the mouth in the last stage of life. Hygiene care is essential to comfort.*

    D. Provide oral liquids as tolerates. *Rationale: As long as swallowing is intact, oral fluids prevent dehydration and add comfort.*

    E. Establish therapeutic communication. Encourage patient to share feelings with family members. *Rationale: The dying patient may need to communicate final wishes, thoughts, and feelings with friends and family.*

4. D. *Rationale: Use a nonjudgmental approach to develop a trusting nurse–patient relationship to be able to spend time with the patient to discuss his feelings, fears, and anxieties.*

5. Ativan (lorazepam) is a benzodiazepine anxiolytic agent that produces calmness. Mr. Goetz should be evaluated for a decrease in anxiety, agitation, and hallucinations.

6. B. *Rationale: Frequent coughing helps to remove anesthetic agents from the lungs to prevent pneumonia.*

Communication

1. Report the results of your neuro assessment including time symptoms began, the location of the numbness, and any other abnormal findings.

2. Give a brief report to the pediatric nurse regarding Mr. and Mrs. Black's condition, the change in Mr. Black's neurological status, and Mrs. Black's upcoming surgery. *Rationale: The pediatric nurse needs information about both Mr. and Mrs. Black's condition in order to be supportive of the Black children. Other family members may be needed to make decisions regarding the children's health care if the parents are unable to make informed decisions because of their own health status.*

Delegation

1.

    A. Peter Black: Obtaining vital signs and performing basic ADLs can be delegated to the nursing assistant. Mr. Black should not get out of bed; therefore, a urinal should be provided. Until specifically ordered by the physician, he should be kept NPO, so frequent oral care may be necessary.

    B. Mary Black: Besides obtaining vital signs, the nursing assistant can assist with elimination. Mrs. Black's ankle needs to remain immobile, so she will need assistance with transferring to the commode or a wheelchair if she is allowed to visit her children on the pediatric unit.

    C. John Linzer: Vital signs and physical care including hygiene, turning, and positioning can be delegated.

    D. Paul Goetz: Safety is an important factor for Mr. Goetz. A nursing assistant can be delegated to be a sitter in the room at all times. The nursing assistant can also obtain vital signs and assist with ADLs.

Nursing Ethics

1. Paul Goetz asks you to bring him some beer. He says, "You can smuggle it in and no one will know." How will you respond? "No, Paul, I cannot bring you a beer. I know you feel you need alcohol. Even though I cannot provide it for you, I can give you the prescribed medication that will help you get through the detoxification. I can also be sure the counselor sees you as soon as possible." *Rationale: It is not ethical to provide alcohol to the chemically dependent patient. However, in order to maintain a therapeutic relationship, the nurse should offer prescribed medication and psychological support.*

2. D. *Rationale: Nurses must first know how to take care of themselves in a disaster in order to be able to assist others.*

Concept Map

Hint: Changing the shapes of the boxes or adding color can further demonstrate the interconnectedness of the concepts. For the second part of this activity, you may find it helpful to review Chapter 5 and Box 1-5.

Chapter 8: Genetic Implications of Adult Health Nursing

1. Answer: 2 Rationale: In an autosomal dominant condition, you only need one of the genotypes to have the condition. An autosomal dominant condition is not a sex-linked disease and is not found on the x or y chromosomes.

2. Answer: 1, 3 Rationale: Fabry disease is an x-linked genetic disorder. Since the male provides the y chromosome to a male offspring, the male cannot pass on this disease to male offspring. The female can pass this disorder on. Also, which grandmother (maternal or fraternal) is not stated, and if the grandmother was not affected, she could be a carrier since her brother had the disease.

3. Answer: 4 Rationale: It is a nurse's responsibility to explain what is involved in genetic testing. It is not the nurse's responsibility to discuss potential outcomes, as this is the responsibility of the genetic counselor.

4. Answer: 4 Rationale: Mitochondrial mutations are only passed from the mother. This is because mitochondria are primarily found in ova and not sperm. This is considered a matrilineal pattern of inheritance. An affected female will pass the condition on to her children; however, an affected male will not.

5. **Answer: 2 Rationale:** Performing a family history assessment helps the nurse know what is important to focus on regarding health promotion and maintenance when planning prophylactic screening and treatment.

6. **Answer: 2 Rationale:** Retention of information decreases during times of high stress, such as being diagnosed with a genetic disorder.

7. **Answer: 1, 2, 4 Rationale:** Most genetic specialists will complete chromosomal studies and provide information about the condition; this information will in turn facilitate decision making.

8. **Answer: 1, 2, 4 Rationale:** Minor physical anomalies are simply visual. However, an atrial-septal health defect is a functional defect, which can impair activity and cause severe complications as the patient gets older.

9. **Answer: 3 Rationale:** A family history for mutation of the MLH/MSH2 gene greatly increases the risk for colon cancer.

10. **Answer: 4 Rationale:** GINA is a federal law designed to protect consumers from discrimination by employers and health insurance companies based on genetic information.

Chapter 9: Nursing Care of Patients in Pain

1. **Answer: 2 Rationale:** Chronic pain is defined as pain that has persisted for 6 or more months. Low back pain is the most common cause of chronic pain.

2. **Answer: 4 Rationale:** Initial or "fast" pain is sharp and well-defined as the stimulus is transmitted along myelinated A delta fibers to the thalamus and cerebral cortex. The smaller unmyelinated C fibers transmit the stimulus more slowly, producing a second or "slow" pain, which is less well-localized, dull, and throbbing.

3. **Answer: 1, 2, 5 Rationale:** NSAIDs are more effective when taken on a scheduled basis rather than PRN. These drugs, when effective (particularly for musculoskeletal pain), can cause gastrointestinal bleeding and hypertension, necessitating regular follow-up.

4. **Answer: 1 Rationale:** Transdermal patches of opioid are slowly absorbed, reaching a therapeutic level 12 to 72 hours after application. The drug can accumulate in the body tissues, leading to a toxic level accompanied by manifestations such as sleepiness or respiratory difficulty.

5. **Answer: 3 Rationale:** The quality of the pain is assessed through descriptive statements such as sharp, burning, stabbing, dull, etc.

6. **Answer: 3 Rationale:** Pain is objective; the patient provides the most accurate information about its intensity.

7. **Answer: 2 Rationale:** Constipation is a common side effect of opioids narcotics, especially when used on a regular basis.

8. **Answer: 1 Rationale:** Research has shown that patients with moderate cognitive impairment can use a pain scale to indicate the intensity of pain. The faces pain scale may be more accurate and effective in the cognitively impaired adult.

9. **Answer: 3 Rationale:** The combination of glucosamine and chondroitin has been shown to reduce pain in patients with moderate to severe knee pain.

10. **Answer: 1 Rationale:** Rigorous physical activity such as running prompts the release of endorphins (natural opioids-like substances). Endorphins bind with opioids receptors in the CNS, inhibiting the transmission of pain signals.

Chapter 10: Nursing Care of Patients with Altered Fluid, Electrolyte, and Acid–Base Balance

1. **Answer: 1 Rationale:** Ringer's solution is an isotonic, balanced electrolyte solution that can expand plasma volume and help restore electrolyte balance.

2. **Answer: 4 Rationale:** In fluid volume deficit, there is less volume in the vascular system, which decreases venous return and cardiac output, leading to manifestations of dizziness, orthostatic hypotension, and flat neck veins. The heart rate increases and the blood pressure falls.

3. **Answer: 1, 3, 4 Rationale:** Frequent neurological checks are necessary as hypernatremia draws water out of brain cells, causing them to shrink. As the brain shrinks, tension is placed on cerebral vessels, which may cause them to tear and bleed. Hypernatremia affects mental status and brain function (including orientation to time, place, and person), as can rapid correction of hypernatremia. Fluid replacement is the primary treatment for hypernatremia. Maintaining intravenous access is necessary for administration of fluids and possible emergency medications.

4. **Answer: 2 Rationale:** Hypokalemia affects nerve impulse transmission, including the transmission of cardiac impulses. The patient may develop ECG changes and atrial or ventricular dysrhythmias.

5. **Answer: 4 Rationale:** Calcium should be taken with a full glass of water to allow maximum absorption.

6. **Answer: 1 Rationale:** A positive Chvostek's sign indicates increased neuromuscular excitability, commonly associated with both hypomagnesemia and hypocalcemia. Additional manifestations of hypomagnesemia include confusion, hallucinations, and possible psychoses. Administration of magnesium sulfate helps restore magnesium balance and neuromuscular function.

7. **Answer: 1 Rationale:** The pH is indicative of acidosis (less than 7.35), and the bicarbonate level is low (less than 22 mEq/L), indicating bicarbonate deficit as cause of the acidosis. In addition, the $PaCO_2$ is low (less than 35 mmHg), indicating respiratory compensation for the excess acid.

8. **Answer: 1, 3, 5 Rationale:** The slow respiratory rate leads to inadequate alveolar ventilation. As a result, carbon dioxide is not effectively eliminated from the blood, causing it to accumulate. This increases carbonic acid levels, leading to respiratory acidosis, as indicated by the low pH and high $PaCO_2$. Excess carbon dioxide causes vasodilation, leading to warm, flushed skin, particularly in acute respiratory acidosis.

9. **Answer: 2 Rationale:** Gastric suctioning removes highly acidic gastric secretions, increasing the risk of metabolic alkalosis.

10. **Answer: 3 Rationale:** The patient is demonstrating classic manifestations of respiratory alkalosis, a potential complication of mechanical ventilation when the rate or volume of ventilations are too high. Arterial blood gases provide the data necessary to confirm and treat this problem.

Chapter 11: Nursing Care of Patients Experiencing Trauma and Shock

1. **Answer: 4 Rationale:** Although all of the choices can be sources of injury or death in adults of all ages, motor vehicle crashes remain the leading cause of injury.

2. **Answer: 1 Rationale:** Airway obstruction is the first and foremost risk to assess for, as this represents the ABCs of life support: A = airway, B = breathing, C = circulation. A patent airway must be the number one priority for survival.

3. **Answer: 2 Rationale:** Assessing airway patency is the first step in the ABCs of life support in any setting.

4. **Answer: 3 Rationale:** The priority assessment, regardless of setting, is airway patency.

5. **Answer: 2 Rationale:** The endotoxins released from bacteria in septic shock stimulate the release of vasoactive proteins causing peripheral vasodilation and decreased peripheral resistance.

6. **Answer: 1 Rationale:** Direct pressure to the wound is the best method to manage uncontrolled bleeding.

7. **Answer: 1 Rationale:** Trauma is defined as injury to human tissues from the transfer of energy.

8. **Answer: 3 Rationale:** A transfusion reaction is a risk from a blood transfusion.

9. **Answer: 2 Rationale:** Widespread vasodilation can cause distributive shock as the blood pressure drops dangerously due to the very low peripheral vascular resistance.

10. **Answer: 1 Rationale:** Ultimately there is a systemic imbalance between oxygen supply and demand.

Chapter 12: Nursing Care of Patients with Infections

1. **Answer: 3 Rationale:** Acquired passive immunity is the result of a gamma globulin infusion following exposure to hepatitis A. This type of immunity is short-lived and usually lasts only about 4 weeks.

2. **Answer: 3 Rationale:** If a culture and sensitivity is ordered, obtain it before beginning treatment so the anti-infective medication does not alter the ability to identify the causative organisms.

3. **Answer: 4 Rationale:** Although the exact mechanism of action is unknown, aspirin inhibits prostaglandin synthesis.

4. **Answer: 1 Rationale:** Increased banded neutrophils is a response to bacterial infection. This is called a "shift to the left."

5. **Answer: 2 Rationale:** Contact precautions, wearing gloves and gowns for direct contact.

6. **Answer: 1 Rationale:** The T cells of the immune system adapt to kill intracellular organisms.

7. **Answer: 1 Rationale:** Thrombocytosis is best explained as increased platelets.

8. **Answer: 4 Rationale:** When there is a nursing diagnosis of *Risk for Infection*, it can pertain to the patient, caregivers, or other patients. It addresses the possibility that the patient cannot fight infection, the staff is potentially at risk for developing an infection from the infected patient, or the other patients are at risk for becoming infected from the infected patient.

9. **Answer: 4 Rationale:** When administering antibiotics, the nurse must be aware of potential hypersensitivity reactions. It is important to monitor for any hypersensitivities in addition to providing education about the infection, antibiotic, and any potential side effects of treatment.

10. **Answer: 3 Rationale:** Wearing gloves, gowns, and goggles when coming in contact with contaminated body fluids is considered to be a standard procedure.

Chapter 13: Nursing Care of Patients with Altered Immunity

1. **Answer: 4 Rationale:** Anaphylaxis is the most severe form of type 1 IgE reactions. When an allergen is introduced for which there is circulating IgE specific to the allergen a cascade leading to anaphylaxis is initiated.

2. **Answer: 1 Rationale:** This type of rejection episode is the most common and most treatable.

3. **Answer: 3 Rationale:** These manifestations are indicative of a respiratory infection caused by PCP.

4. **Answer: 4 Rationale:** When a patient tests positive for HIV, this means that antibodies to the AIDS virus are present in the blood. HIV does not equal AIDS.

5. **Answer: 2 Rationale:** As Retrovir can cause bone marrow suppression, leukopenia can be an adverse reaction of Retrovir.

6. **Answer: 2 Rationale:** Of all of the choices available, the allergen prick testing has the lowest risk of anaphylaxis because there is the smallest amount of allergen entering the bloodstream.

7. **Answer: 2 Rationale:** When hypersensitivity is suspected it is important to avoid any further exposure to the potential cause. The best way to do this is by replacing all tubing and attaching a new line primed with NS.

8. **Answer: 2 Rationale:** Protease inhibitors and nucleoside analogs are associated with serious metabolic problems such as diabetes mellitus.

9. **Answer: 4 Rationale:** The priority when initiating or changing HIV drug therapy regimens is the patient's willingness to adhere to the drug regimen. Since the side effects can be difficult and challenging to overcome, many patients are not willing to continue with their therapy.

10. **Answer: 4 Rationale:** Antithymocyte globulin (ATC) is used to induce immunosuppression immediately following a transplant. Its purpose is to bind with the peripheral lymphocytes and mononuclear cells to remove them from circulation and prevent them from being able to reject the new organ.

Chapter 14: Nursing Care of Patients with Cancer

1. **Answer: 3 Rationale:** Metastasis occurs when cells from a primary tumor site travel through the lymphatic system or bloodstream to find a secondary target.

2. **Answer: 1 Rationale:** Encouraging the patient to express his feelings about the cancer diagnosis is the most valuable and powerful intervention that could be offered.

3. **Answer: 3 Rationale:** It is important not to rub or scratch the treated skin areas, as this can cause irritation to the surface of the skin as well as breaks in the skin. Rubbing may also wipe off the ink markings, which are important landmarks to ensure that the radiation treatments are directed to the correct location.

4. **Answer: 2 Rationale:** Providing an antiemetic prior to chemotherapy is an excellent preventative treatment to prevent nausea and vomiting following chemotherapy.

5. **Answer: 3 Rationale:** Although all of these choices can be a result of chemotherapy, the one that is directly affected with bone marrow suppression is a low platelet count of 50,000.

6. **Answer: 3 Rationale:** Chemotherapy is not cell type specific. It simply targets cells that are rapidly dividing, which can be both cancer cells and healthy cells. It is important to understand that the destruction of normal cells can cause other manifestations such as mucositis, hair loss, and bone marrow suppression.

7. **Answer: 1 Rationale:** External radiation therapy is when the radiation is initiated outside of the body, directed towards the patient, and is set to deliver to a certain depth for a specified period of time. This exposure is meant to destroy the cancer cells the radiation comes into direct contact with.

8. **Answer: 2 Rationale:** Tumor lysis syndrome can cause high levels of uric acid. Patients are often treated with allopurinol to help excrete the uric acid in the urine.

9. **Answer: 3 Rationale:** The S phase is when DNA replication occurs. This is when the cell is beginning mitosis and the chromosomes multiply from 23 to 46. They then migrate toward each axis in preparation for division of the cell.

10. **Answer: 1 Rationale:** Oncogenes, genes that stimulate cell growth, require something to activate them in order to cause this reaction.

Unit 3 Building Clinical Competence: Pathophysiology and Patterns of Health

Functional Health Pattern: Health Perception-Health Management

Functional Health Patterns

Hint: There are many nonpharmacologic or complementary therapies the nurse can initiate without a physician's order.

Priority Setting

A. Allen Barber should be seen second. *Rationale: Post-op pain of 8/10 on day 4 is very unusual and could indicate beginning dehiscence.*

B. Tamra Sanders should be seen first. *Rationale: Severe chest pain and shortness of breath could indicate life-threatening change in conditions.*

C. Mia Windham should be seen third. *Rationale: Bloody diarrhea can lead to severe dehydration, hemorrhage, and shock, but there is no indication that Ms. Windham is in immediate danger.*

D. Harry Anderson should be seen fourth. *Rationale: Harry's confusion can result in his calling for help. While he should be checked on to determine his safety, a CAN could be assigned to stay with him.*

Health Promotion

1. B. *Rationale: A high-protein and high-kilocalorie diet provides necessary nutrients to meet metabolic and tissue healing needs. High fiber can increase intestinal motility and cause diarrhea, further increasing weight loss. High vitamins can cause vitamin overdose.*

2. Allen Barber should be taught to manage his diabetes to maintain blood glucose levels within normal ranges. *Rationale: Wound healing is facilitated by normal glucose levels.*

Nursing Process

1.

A. Allen Barber: Pain scale, direct visualization of surgical wound, and abdominal sounds. *Rationale: It appears the surgical wound is infected, which delays healing. This wound infection could result in intestinal complications and wound dehiscence.*

B. Tamra Sanders: Heart and lung sounds, oxygen saturation. Rationale: Sickle cells can obstruct circulation to any organ. Ms. Sanders's symptoms could indicate a blockage in circulation to the heart or lungs or both, which could be life–threatening.

C. Mia Windham: Abdominal sounds, further incidence of bloody diarrhea, skin condition on hands and feet, location and description of rash. *Rationale: Ms. Windham must be assessed for worsening signs of tissue rejection.*

D. Harry Anderson: Neuro assessment including pupils, clearness of speech, strength in arms and legs, and changes in levels of confusion. Observe for signs of seizure activity. *Rationale: HIV/AIDS affects the nervous system. The nurse must observe for signs of worsening of Harry's condition.*

2.

	Nursing Diagnosis	Rationale
Allen Barber	*High Risk for Impaired Skin Integrity as evidenced by worsening inflammation at surgical site*	*Worsening inflammation indicates an infectious process that can result in wound dehiscence.*
Tamra Sanders	*Impaired Gas Exchange as evidenced by chest pain and shortness of breath*	*Maintaining breathing and circulation is always the highest priority.*
Mia Windham	*Ineffective Management of Therapeutic Regimen as evidenced by signs of tissues rejection*	*Ms. Windham received a bone marrow transplant in treatment of leukemia. It appears her body is rejecting the transplanted tissue.*
Harry Anderson	*Altered Health Maintenance as evidenced by increased confusion and risk for seizure activity*	*As AIDS progresses, Mr. Anderson will have increased difficulty in maintaining his health status.*

3. Tamra Sanders should be placed in semi-fowlers to high fowlers position. *Rationale: Sitting in an upright position causes the abdominal contents to move away from the diaphragm and eases inhalation.*

4. B. *Rationale: Use saline for wound cleansing. Soap and harsh cleansers like povidone-iodine or hydrogen peroxide cause drying and tissue damage.*

5. A. *Rational: Diarrhea increases bicarbonate loss, resulting in metabolic acidosis.*

6. A. *Rationale: White blood cell count indicates extent of inflammatory process, erythrocyte sedimentation rate detects inflammation, and C-reactive protein indicates presence of inflammatory process.*

Communication

1. The doctor must be told about the amount of bloody diarrhea Ms. Windham has had in the last 24 hours, the amount of pain she is experiencing, any change in the rash on her extremities, and any new symptoms. *Rationale: The doctor must be kept up-to-date on Ms. Windham's symptoms of tissue rejection.*

2. C. *Rationale: A child born to carrier parents has a 25% chance of inheriting sickle cell anemia.*

3. Determine Ms. Sanders's level of cognitive development and communicate with her in developmentally appropriate terms. *Rationale: People with Down's syndrome have a wide variety of cognitive abilities. It is important communicate in developmentally appropriate terms, not age appropriate terms.*

Delegation

1.

A. Allen Barber: Delegate vital signs, obtaining blood glucose levels and assistance with ADLs including hygiene, elimination, and ambulation. Rationale: Obtaining vital signs and BG values can be safely delegated to a trained nursing assistant. A 4-day postoperative patient should be able to provide much of his own care, but would need some assistance that could be provided by unlicensed personnel.

B. Tamra Sanders: Delegate vital signs, ADLs, and a sitter. Rationale: Ms. Sanders may need a sitter due to Down's syndrome and chest pain with shortness of breath. While the nursing assistant cannot assess changes in her condition, he or she can summon help and initiate CPR if necessary.

C. Mia Windham: Delegate vital signs, ADLs, and I&O. Rationale: The nursing assistant is able to record intake and output and notify the RN of further bloody diarrhea.

D. Harry Anderson: Delegate vital signs, ADLs, and sitter. Rationale: Due to Mr. Anderson's confusion and risk of seizure activity, a sitter may be necessary to maintain patient safety.

Related Questions

1. D. *Rationale: Supine position with legs elevated increases venous return. Trendelenburg causes abdominal organs to press against the diaphragm, compromising respirations.*

2. D. *Rationale: Notify the physician if WBCs fall below 4000 and platelets fall below 75,000 prior to administering any cytotoxic agents due to being at risk for developing infections.*

3. D. *Rationale: A severe anaphylactic reaction may be treated with 1:100,000 concentration of epinephrine intravenously.*

4. Flushed face, burning sensation along a vein, dyspnea, hypotension, lumbar pain, fever. *Rationale: Clumping of RBCs blocks blood vessels, decreasing circulation to vital organs. Hemolysis of RBCs causes a release of hemoglobin into blood that can block renal circulation.*

5. A, D, E. *Rationale: Maintain a diet low in fat and high in fiber as well as increasing vegetables and fruits in the diet. Increase intake of vitamins E, C, and beta-carotene and omega-3 oils. Limit charcoal grilled meats.*

Concept Map

Hint: Providing care to enable the patient to manage his or her health needs involves providing verbal as well as written information. The patient must be able to verbalize understanding of the information. For the second part of this activity, consider the factors underlying Mr. Blount's breathing pattern in developing your concept map.

Chapter 15: Assessing the Integumentary System

1. **Answer: 2 Rationale:** The layer that has the most glands and hair follicles located in it is the dermis.

2. **Answer: 3 Rationale:** Melanin is the pigment found in skin that is responsible for tanning.

3. **Answer: 1, 2 Rationale:** Inspection is the first assessment technique to check the skin surface. The next assessment step is to palpate any areas of the skin that appear abnormal in order to get a better understanding of depth and size of any lesions.

4. **Answer: 1 Rationale:** Erythema often occurs as a result of increased body temperature. This occurs when the capillaries in the skin dilate to release some of the heat caused from the increased body temperature.

5. **Answer: 3 Rationale:** Often new soap can cause skin irritation and itching. It is important to determine if there is anything that has changed to cause this irritation. This is the easiest variable to assess.

6. **Answer: 1 Rationale:** A decreased skin turgor is a sign of dehydration.

7. **Answer: 4 Rationale:** Edema begins in the distal extremities. The best place to assess for this is the ankle/foot area.

8. **Answer: 4 Rationale:** Lichenification is a condition in which the skin cells multiply, causing what appears to be thickened and calloused skin. The skin often has a rough and leathery appearance to it.

9. **Answer: 4 Rationale:** Angiomas are a common finding in older patients.

10. **Answer: 3 Rationale:** Head lice deposit and attach small white eggs to the hair shaft.

11. **Answer: 4 Rationale:** A family history increases the risk for skin cancer.

Chapter 16: Nursing Care of Patients with Integumentary Disorders

1. **Answer: 3 Rationale:** The best way to help moisturize the skin is to apply a moisturizing agent after bathing.

2. **Answer: 1 Rationale:** Nevi are the skin lesions that can become malignant and need to be monitored for any change.

3. **Answer: 4 Rationale:** Psoriasis causes abnormal growth and division of epidermal cells, causing keratosis. The use of ultraviolet light therapy helps to slow down this cellular division, which decreases the lesions and keratosis associated with psoriasis.

4. **Answer: 2 Rationale:** Actinic keratosis is a premalignant skin lesion, with the risk of developing into a malignancy.

5. **Answer: 4 Rationale:** A linear pattern of painful vesicles indicates shingles, a varicella infection. The virus remains along a nerve from a previous infection with chickenpox.

6. **Answer: 2 Rationale:** Anyone can have lice. Major infestations often occur in areas where many people are in close proximity, especially in the public school setting.

7. **Answer: 1 Rationale:** People with fair skin, blond hair, and freckles are at increased risk for nonmelanoma skin cancers.

8. **Answer: 1 Rationale:** A change in the color or size of a nevus is cause for concern when evaluating for the possibility of melanoma.

9. **Answer: 2 Rationale:** Skin tears may occur as a result of the shearing force of pulling a patient up in bed. Prevention includes lifting, rather than pulling the patient up in bed.

10. **Answer: 3 Rationale:** Dermabrasion is a skin treatment that helps to reduce the appearance of acne scarring and other skin imperfections.

Chapter 17: Nursing Care of Patients with Burns

1. **Answer: 3 Rationale:** In the emergent phase of burn management, it is important to monitor electrolyte levels frequently. Initially the patient is at risk for fluid and electrolyte imbalances, especially for decreased serum potassium levels. This can cause an increased risk for arrhythmias.

2. **Answer: 4 Rationale:** A full thickness burn is not painful, as the nerves have also been affected from the burn. In this situation, pain is not a good sign. It tells the nurse that the depth of the burn goes beyond the nerves. Superficial partial thickness, and deep partial thickness burns will still be very painful to the patient, as the nerves remain intact or exposed.

3. **Answer: 4 Rationale:** The larger the surface area of the burn and the deeper the burn, the more at risk the patient is for burn shock. A high-voltage electrical accident will cause a deeper burn and since this scenario explains that > 50% of the body is affected, this places the patient at the highest risk.

4. **Answer: 2 Rationale:** Silvadene cream can cause neutropenia. It is important for the nurse to monitor the patient's WBC count daily to assess for any changes, which could indicate neutropenia. Although this is the most important intervention, it is also important to keep the patient as comfortable as possible. Premedicating is definitely not a bad idea, as burn dressing changes can be very painful and the Silvadene will help debride the burn.

5. **Answer: 2 Rationale:** The Parkland Formula uses lactated Ringer's solution, administered at 4 mL $\times$ kg $\times$ % TBSA burn, with 50% of the total volume infused in the first 8 hours, and the remaining 50% over the next 16 hours. This would be 4 $\times$ 70 $\times$ 50% = 14,000 $\times$ 50% = 7000.

6. **Answer: 1 Rationale:** Urine output is the most sensitive indicator of fluid resuscitation success. A decrease in urine output is seen in dehydration and a recovery from dehydration is seen with an increase in urine output.

7. **Answer: 4 Rationale:** A decreased left radial pulse is cause for alarm in this type and location of burn. This can be the first symptom seen in compartment syndrome and is a surgical emergency.

8. **Answer: 2 Rationale:** The "rule of nines" is a method of quickly estimating the percentage of TBSA affected by a burn injury. It is most useful in emergency situations but is not accurate for estimating TBSA in adults who are short, obese, or very thin. Anterior trunk = 18%, perineum = 1%, left arm = 9%. These are added together to equal 28%.

9. **Answer: 1, 3, 5, 6 Rationale:** Teaching injury prevention is a very important job in nursing. Burns are a common injury in the home. It is important to help older adults understand ways to help prevent burns. Wearing close-fitting clothing when cooking can help prevent shirtsleeves or scarves from catching on fire. The water temperature of the water heater should not be set above 120°F. This can help prevent burns from water scalding. Installing antiscald devices can also help prevent water burns. As older adults often have decreased olfactory senses, having a neighbor routinely check for the odor of gas can help prevent fires.

10. **Answer: 3 Rationale:** A 15% carbon monoxide level would cause only mild manifestations of dizziness at this stage. Later stages with higher levels will cause the remaining manifestations of the skin color change, drowsiness, and hypotension.

Unit 4 Building Clinical Competence: Responses to Altered Integumentary Structure and Function

Functional Health Pattern: Nutritional-Metabolic

Functional Health Patterns
Hint: Besides contacting the dietitian, the nurse can encourage intake of food and fluids by providing small frequent amounts of the patient's choice of food and drink.

Priority Setting
1.
   A. Mrs. Carter should be seen first. *Rationale: She may need pain medications and should not have to wait for pain relief.*
   B. Mr. Johnson should be seen second. *Rationale: It is important to have him ready for surgery on time at 0800. The nursing assistant can obtain vital signs and help him with urinary elimination while you are seeing Mrs. Carter.*
   C. Mr. Jenkins should be seen third. *Rationale: If new lesions are appearing, they should be assessed and documented, but this is not urgent.*
   D. Mr. Ugandi should be seen last. *Rationale: Discharge is anticipated and teaching should begin as soon as possible, but the other patients' needs are higher priority at this time.*

Health Promotion
1. A. *Rationale: Foods high in protein, such as eggs, milk, and meat, are required for tissue growth and maintenance. Foods high in iron, such as meat, poultry, and eggs, are required for increased red blood cell production and preventing anemia.*
2. D. *Rationale: A cool environment will decrease itching, and light cotton clothing will decrease pain from material rubbing on lesions.*

Nursing Process
1.

	Nursing Diagnosis	Rationale
Mr. Johnson	*Anxiety* related to upcoming surgery	*Even though Mr. Johnson has had previous surgeries and should know what to expect, each surgery carries risks that cause anxiety.*
Mrs. Carter	*Pain* in R. leg related to cellulitis	Because of the number of pain receptors in the skin, cellulitis is very painful.
Mr. Jenkins	*Hopelessness*	Mr. Jenkins is concerned that new lesions are forming, which is out of his control.
Mr. Ugandi	*Knowledge Deficit* related to home care of Toxic Epidermal Necrolysis	Mr. Ugandi has a chronic, progressive disease (AIDS) and is being discharged to continue healing from Toxic Epidermal Necrolysis. He needs instruction in self-care within any limitations of AIDS.

2. 18%. *Rationale: Arms are 4.5% each, and anterior trunk is 9% for a total burn area of 18%.*
3. A. *Rationale: Clinical manifestations of infection of the dermis and subcutaneous tissue are redness, swelling, and pain.*
4. C. *Rationale: Hypersensitivity reactions to mafenide acetate include pruritus, edema, facial edema, and urticaria.*

Communication
1. "Mr. Jenkins, I know this is very difficult for you and sometimes you might feel that dying would be better than the burning pain you are experiencing. I'm sorry, but because there is no cure for herpes zoster, the sores can come back. There are some medications you can take that decrease the chance of them recurring. I'll have your doctor talk with you about them. Is there anything else you want to talk about? *Rationale: Honest, direct answers to questions are preferred. At age 86, Mr. Jenkins may be telling you that he is feeling hopeless and may give up. It is important to keep communication lines open.*

Delegation
1. What data collection and interventions can be delegated to a nursing assistant for each patient?
   A. Mr. Johnson: Vital signs, assistance with elimination, transfer to stretcher/transport to surgery, preparing room for his return from surgery.
   B. Mrs. Carter: Vital signs, hygiene, nutrition, turning/activity.
   C. Mrs. Jenkins: Vital signs, hygiene, nutrition, turning/activity. Remind the nursing assistant of contact precautions to prevent spread of infection.
   D. Mr. Ugandi: Vital signs, hygiene, nutrition, turning/activity. Remind the nursing assistant of standard precautions to prevent spread of infection.

Content-Specific Questions
1. A, C, D. E. *Rationale: Burn injuries cause the body to increase energy expenditure and to utilize nutrients for healing.*
2. D. *Rationale: Burns destroy the protective layer of the skin; therefore, due to losses through an open wound, fluid and electrolyte imbalances occur.*
3. B. *Rationale: A quadriplegic is unable to reposition him- or herself without assistance, which places the patient at high risk for pressure ulcers.*
4. A, C, E. *Rationale: These preventative measures are ways to prevent overexposure to the UVA rays of the sun that cause sunburns.*
5. B. *Rationale: Morphine causes respiratory depression. Respiratory rate below 12 is depressed and may require intervention.*

Concept Map

Hint: The differences in distribution of fat and fluid between male and female patients can be significant. Electric burns cause tissue destruction at the point of entry and point of exit as well as internal tissue between those points. The concept map must reflect this tissue damage and related nursing diagnoses.

Chapter 18: Assessing the Endocrine System

1. **Answer: 2 Rationale:** ADH (antidiuretic hormone) causes the distal tubules of the kidneys to reabsorb water, which would decrease the urine output.
2. **Answer: 3 Rationale:** A low calcium level may be tested by the Trousseau's sign. A positive test causes the fingers and hand to contract on the arm where a blood pressure cuff is inflated.
3. **Answer: 1 Rationale:** Excessive amounts of glucocorticoids cause manifestations of immunosuppression with depression of the inflammatory response and inhibition of the effectiveness of the immune system.
4. **Answer: 3 Rationale:** When assessing the endocrine system, it is important to look for manifestations of diabetes. One of the first manifestations is polydipsia, which is increased thirst.
5. **Answer: 2 Rationale:** The thyroid gland is assessed for the size and consistency to assess for goiters, enlargement, or nodules.
6. **Answer: 2 Rationale:** Assess for Chvostek's sign by tapping a finger in front of the ear, at the angle of the jaw. A positive sign causes facial grimacing with repeated contractions of the facial muscle.
7. **Answer: 4 Rationale:** A TSH (thyroid-stimulating hormone) level is the most accurate indicator of thyroid function.
8. **Answer: 3 Rationale:** Thyroid nodules are a normal finding in the older adult.
9. **Answer: 2 Rationale:** Rough, dry skin is often found in patients with hypothyroidism.
10. **Answer: 4 Rationale:** Increased deep tendon reflexes are seen in hyperthyroidism.

Chapter 19: Nursing Care of Patients with Endocrine Disorders

1. **Answer: 1 Rationale:** A self-generated antibody attaches to TSH receptors in the thyroid and results in increased TH production.
2. **Answer: 3 Rationale:** The thyroid gland takes up iodine in any form (including radioactive iodine) and concentrates it within the gland, decreasing the number of cells that produce TH.
3. **Answer: 3 Rationale:** This is a compensatory but ineffective effort to produce more TH by enlarging the gland itself.
4. **Answer: 4 Rationale:** Cushing's syndrome is the result of excessive cortisone; in this case a side effect of cortisone administration.
5. **Answer: 2 Rationale:** Patients with Addison's disease are often stressed by infection or trauma; additional doses of steroids may be needed to prevent crisis. Therefore, patients are urged to carry injectable cortisone and a syringe at all times.
6. **Answer: 2 Rationale:** As blood volume expands, neurons become edematous and irritability occurs.
7. **Answer: 2 Rationale:** Patients with this disorder are at risk for pathological fractures of the bones because of the decreased density of the bone.
8. **Answer: 3 Rationale:** Increased serum calcium decreases neuromuscular excitability, which decreases bowel motility.
9. **Answer: 4 Rationale:** Patients with Addison's disease have decreased cortisone but compensatory mechanisms increase ACTH, which causes skin to appear deeply suntanned or bronzed.
10. **Answer: 1 Rationale:** With a sudden stoppage of steroids, the adrenal cortex cannot recuperate rapidly enough to increase production because it has been suppressed with exogenous steroids.

Chapter 20: Nursing Care of Patients with Diabetes Mellitus

1. **Answer: 1 Rationale:** Ninety-five percent of patients diagnosed with type 1 DM have genetic markers indicating increased susceptibility for the development of type 1 DM.
2. **Answer: 3 Rationale:** A deficit of insulin increases the liver's production of ketone bodies and increased release of free fatty acids. Bicarbonate production is decreased and acid buffering is impaired, resulting in metabolic acidosis.
3. **Answer: 4 Rationale:** Caloric need decreases with aging; unless dietary intake also decreases (and exercise increases), weight gain ensues. Obesity is a risk factor for the development of type 2 DM.
4. **Answer: 3 Rationale:** Changes in sensation, such as numbness or tingling, support this diagnosis.
5. **Answer: 3 Rationale:** Visual inspection of the feet each day is important in preventing more serious complications.
6. **Answer: 3 Rationale:** Since it is clear, Lantus (glargine) could be confused with regular insulin. Regular insulin is short acting in 4 to 6 hours and Lantus is long acting in 24 to 28 hours.
7. **Answer: 3 Rationale:** Only regular insulin can safely be administered intravenously for diabetic ketoacidosis.
8. **Answer: 3 Rationale:** Levels of Hgb A1C greater than 6.5% demonstrate elevated or erratic glucose control over time and support a diagnosis of DM.
9. **Answer: 3 Rationale:** No intermediate- or long-acting insulin is given the day of surgery since dietary intake postoperatively is uncertain. IV glucose (5%) and regular insulin in equally divided doses will compensate for the increase in serum glucose until the patient is eating and drinking normally.
10. **Answer: 4 Rationale:** Insulin is absorbed more rapidly when injected subcutaneously in the abdomen.

Unit 5 Building Clinical Competence: Responses to Altered Endocrine Function

Functional Health Pattern: Nutritional-Metabolic

Functional Health Patterns

Hint: Many endocrine disorders affect metabolism and therefore the patient's need for nutrients. The patient's nutritional intake may be more than or less than body requirements.

Priority Setting

1.
   A. Mrs. Rant should be seen first. *Rationale: Relieving pain is a high priority, especially when the patient's blood pressure is elevated.*
   B. Mr. Blew should be seen second. *Rationale: The effectiveness of admission treatment of his extremely high blood glucose should be determined.*
   C. Mr. Rite should be seen third. *Rationale: While he has been stable, he is exhibiting signs of increased intracranial pressure and must be assessed.*
   D. Mrs. Fox can be seen last. *Rationale: Her vital signs are stable and she is waiting for labs to be drawn.*

Health Promotion

1. Teach Mr. Blew to provide foot care including inspecting his feet daily using a mirror, wearing well-fitting shoes/slippers at all times, caring for his nails, and reporting sores or red skin to his healthcare provider. He should be taught to monitor is blood glucose.

2. A. *Rationale: Hyperparathyroidism is excess in serum calcium levels. Increased fluids and decreased calcium and vitamin A & D supplements are the appropriate treatment.*

Nursing Process
1.

	Nursing Diagnosis	Rationale
Mr. Blew	*Knowledge Deficit* related to self-care of diabetes mellitus, including signs of hyperglycemia, hypoglycemia, and treatment	*A patient with severe hyperglycemia has many nursing diagnoses, the priority is to teach symptoms of worsening condition so the patient can report appropriately to the nurse.*
Mrs. Rant	*Pain* related to renal calculi	*Passing renal calculi causes severe flank pain.*
Mrs. Fox	*Potential for Self-Care Deficit* related to age and depressed condition on admission	*Ability to care for self must be evaluated prior to discharge.*
Mr. Rite	*Risk for Impaired Thought Processes* including cognitive, voluntary, and involuntary control	*The patient is exhibiting signs on increased intracranial pressure, which can rapidly become worse and threaten his life.*

2. B. *Rationale: Signs and symptoms of hypoglycemia are tachycardia, hypotension, and shakiness.*
3. C. *Rationale: Three to six days after a closed head injury, the patient may develop diabetes insipidus due to increased intracranial pressure.*
4. B. *Rationale: The patient must take a pulse prior to taking the medication; a pulse > 100 must be reported to the doctor.*
5. A, B, E, F. *Rationale: Laboratory tests used to monitor diabetes management are fasting blood glucose levels, glycosylated hemoglobin, abnormal electrolyte levels indicating DKA or HHS, and cholesterol levels to monitor for increased risk of cardiovascular impairments.*

Communication
1. C. *Rationale: Fast-acting carbohydrates, such as juice or milk may be administered to raise the blood glucose level.*
2. "I don't know at this time if that will be necessary. We will be assessing Mrs. Fox's ability to care for herself. We will also get information from the doctor. I will have the discharge coordinator contact you to discuss these issues." *Rationale: It is important that elderly patients be given time to improve following a major health event. An evaluation of their ability to care for themselves is necessary as a part of discharge planning.*

Delegation
1. The nurse can delegate the following tasks to a nursing assistant. *Rationale: All tasks must be within the legal scope of practice for the nursing assistant and the facility policy.*
A. Mr. Blew: vital signs, blood glucose
B. Mrs. Rant: vital signs, strain all urine for stones
C. Mrs. Fox: vital signs, assisting with ADLs with instruction for patient to be as independent as possible
D. Mr. Rite: vital signs

Related Questions
1. A. *Rationale: Clinical manifestations of hyperthyroidism are increased perspiration (diaphoresis), diarrhea from increased gastrointestinal motility, and weight loss with increased appetite.*

2. D. *Rationale: Hemorrhage or edema may compress the trachea causing respiratory distress.*
3. A. *Rationale: Classic clinical manifestations of metabolic syndrome are hypertension, abdominal obesity, and blood glucose > 110 mg/dL.*
4. A. *Rationale: Electrolyte imbalances with untreated Cushing's syndrome are hypernatremia, hypokalemia, and hyperglycemia.*

Concept Map
Hint: More details can add to understanding and consistent care. Review information in Chapter 20 regarding type 2 diabetes and the long-term complications of diabetes to assist in developing your concept map for Mr. Gregg's risk for neurovascular dysfunction.

Chapter 21: Assessing the Gastrointestinal System
1. Answer: 2 Rationale: Proteins derived from animal foods (meats, fish, poultry, cheese, eggs, yogurt, and milk) are complete.
2. Answer: 2 Rationale: Vitamin K is an essential element for blood clotting and, without sufficient levels, bleeding can occur.
3. Answer: 4 Rationale: An elevated amylase indicates that the pancreatic enzymes, released during acute pancreatic inflammation, are digesting their own tissues.
4. Answer: 1 Rationale: The condition of the patient's teeth, possible difficulty for her to chew comfortably, and her dry mouth because of decreased production of saliva in the older adult may cause a nutritional deficit because she will tend to eat food that is easier to chew and swallow.
5. Answer: 4 Rationale: In patient with ascites of the liver of more than 500 mL, a method of determining fluid presence is palpating dullness in the abdomen in the supine position and then on the right side. The presence of dullness moving in these two positions indicates ascites with shifting dullness pattern.
6. Answer: 3 Rationale: Internal hemorrhoids occur with impaired venous return during evacuation of stool or increased abdominal pressure in pregnancy causing distension of veins of the anus.
7. Answer: 4 Rationale: A patient with an ostomy should have questions answered about the consistency of the stool. This information may indicate location of the opening within the intestinal tract and demonstrate how the bowel is functioning.
8. Answer: 4 Rationale: A stool specimen will supply the opportunity to directly exam the feces and detect presence of intestinal parasites.
9. Answer: 2 Rationale: Polyps have been documented as increased risk factors for developing cancer; therefore, removal is indicated to prevent neoplastic cell development.
10. Answer: 4 Rationale: Colon cancer is often an inherited disorder; knowledge of family history is important.

Chapter 22: Nursing Care of Patients with Nutritional Disorders
1. Answer: 3 Rationale: The lack of regular exercise in daily life means less expenditure of energy; therefore, nutrients are stored as fat. Research has shown that adopted children's weight is related to their biological parents. "Fast foods" are a contributing factor.
2. Answer: 2 Rationale: This response informs the patient of the calorie–pound relationship and involves the patient in the planning strategies to improve and maintain weight loss.
3. Answer: 1 Rationale: Recent weight loss is the most prevalent finding in protein-calorie malnutrition. Skinfold thickness is decreased and the patient demonstrates lethargy and drowsiness.

4. **Answer: 3 Rationale:** Small-bore feeding tubes displace easily. Accurate placement is evaluated by aspirating contents and checking the pH. In the stomach the pH is < 4.

5. **Answer: 4 Rationale:** An identified contributing factor to anorexia is family pressure. Family therapy commonly is an important part of the interdisciplinary treatment plan.

6. **Answer: 2 Rationale:** A BMI greater than 25 and central obesity as indicated by a waist–hip ratio of 1 or greater are associated with a higher risk for hypertension, elevated lipid levels, heart disease, and stroke. These conditions have the greatest effect on health over time.

7. **Answer: 4, 5 Rationale:** Because this drug causes dry mouth and potential for constipation, fluids are important to maintain function. The drug is intended to be taken along with a restricted calorie diet for weight loss.

8. **Answer: 1, 2, 4, 5 Rationale:** There are many contributing factors that influence nutrition in the home-bound older adult such as inability to shop for nutritional foods, and the ability to afford and to prepare nutritional food. There are also psychosocial issues of depression and loneliness since eating is a social affair; this could well influence the amount and proportion of caloric intake. Arranging for food to be brought to the patient and for the patient to be transported to a senior center for a meal may solve the weight loss issue and no further interventions may be necessary. Referral to the primary care provider is necessary.

9. **Answer: 4 Rationale:** Beginning oral intake of nutrients as soon as possible after surgery is the best way to prevent malnutrition.

10. **Answer: 1 Rationale:** One of the postoperative complications with gastric bypass surgery is an anastomotic leak causing peritonitis. These manifestations could be related to this condition and the surgeon needs to be notified.

Chapter 23: Nursing Care of Patients with Upper Gastrointestinal Disorders

1. **Answer: 4 Rationale:** The use of tobacco and drinking alcohol are the two primary risk factors for oral cancers.

2. **Answer: 2, 5 Rationale:** Placing the head of the bed on blocks and avoiding lying down for at least 3 hours after eating will help prevent backflow of gastric content into the esophagus by decreasing the pressure on the lower esophageal sphincter.

3. **Answer: 1 Rationale:** The most common contributing factor to acute stress gastritis is the interruption of the integrity of the gastric lining by gastric irritants such as aspirin and/or NSAIDs. A period of gastric rest, followed by a slow progression to regular dietary intake is advised.

4. **Answer: 4 Rationale:** A peptic ulcer is an interruption of the integrity of the gastric lining; perforation is the most lethal complication of this process. It produces inflammation, infection, and possibly shock.

5. **Answer: 3 Rationale:** Frequent small meals with solid foods or liquids, not both, are effective in controlling the hyperosmolar problem of dumping syndrome.

6. **Answer: 2 Rationale:** Bright bleeding from the mouth could indicate perforation of the esophageal wall or vessel rupture by invasion of a tumor.

7. **Answer: 1 Rationale:** These manifestations indicate a possible hypersensitivity response to the antibiotics. Anaphylaxis could occur, so this is an emergency situation.

8. **Answer: 3 Rationale:** The discomfort of stomatitis is aggravated by eating; viscous lidocaine to reduce mouth pain is important to promote nutrition.

9. **Answer: 3 Rationale:** Maintaining patency of the nasogastric tube following gastric surgery is vital to prevent pressure gastric distension and pressure on the suture line. Irrigating gently with NS, if ordered, is the appropriate action. If unable to open tube, notify surgeon.

10. **Answer: 3, 4, 5 Rationale:** Severe pain may be a manifestation of perforation of the ulcer. Oral food and fluids are withheld to prevent vomiting and prepare for possible surgery. The patient is placed in Fowler's position to localize drainage to the pelvic area, and the physician is notified to ensure prompt diagnosis and treatment.

Chapter 24: Nursing Care of Patients with Bowel Disorders

1. **Answer: 2 Rationale:** The nurse should first assess the number, frequency, and water content of stools to support the diagnosis of diarrhea and estimate fluid and electrolyte loss.

2. **Answer: 3 Rationale:** Appendectomy, often performed on an emergency basis, is the usual treatment for appendicitis. Withholding food and fluids are the most appropriate measures in preparing the patient for surgery.

3. **Answer: 1 Rationale:** Sulfasalazine makes the patient susceptible to sunburn so a sunscreen should be used while outside.

4. **Answer: 4 Rationale:** Steatorrhea is a manifestation of malabsorption, and may relate to celiac disease. Exposure to foods containing gluten may trigger manifestations such as these.

5. **Answer: 2 Rationale:** The recommendation for patient health with this familial history of cancer is to monitor for polyps and tumors early through annual digital examinations and periodic colonoscopy. Research has proven a direct genetic link of polyps and cancer development (20%).

6. **Answer: 4, 5, 6 Rationale:** The documentation and frequent measuring of nasogastric output will help maintain vascular volume with replacement of fluids, and the color will indicate if drainage is normal. Measuring abdominal girth will assist in determining if increased intestinal distension is occurring.

7. **Answer: 4 Rationale:** It is most important to maintain the patency of the nasogastric tube to remove gastric secretions and air that may apply pressure to the anastomosis site and cause failure of the suture line. Keeping the stomach decompressed is important to prevent vomiting that could also cause damage to the anastomosis site.

8. **Answer: 2 Rationale:** Raspberry seeds can cause obstruction to the diverticular opening and set up the environment to initiate diverticulitis.

9. **Answer: 1, 3, 5, 6 Rationale:** Fresh fruits and vegetables, whole wheat bread, and bran cereal supply roughage and fiber in the diet that can assist in the evacuation of fecal material and lessen the possibility of developing diverticulum, the incidence of which is high in this age group. Adequate liquid is important to prevent hard, formed stools that are difficult to pass. Taking daily laxatives can decrease the normal bowel reflexes. Colace can be administered safely either in the morning or at nighttime.

10. **Answer: 2 Rationale:** Gastrointestinal decompression removes gastric juices, reducing the amount of accumulated fluid and gas proximal to the obstruction and the risk for bowel ischemia and necrosis.

Chapter 25: Nursing Care of Patients with Gallbladder, Liver, and Pancreatic Disorders

1. **Answer: 1 Rationale:** Right upper quadrant pain following ingestion of a fatty meal is the typical manifestation experienced by patients with cholelithiasis. Chills, fever, nausea, and vomiting may indicate an infection and contraindicate surgery at this time.

2. **Answer: 1, 4 Rationale:** Acute cholecystitis usually develops from a stone obstructing the cystic duct, preventing release of bile from the gallbladder. High fatty foods like gravies and peanut butter stimulate contraction of the obstructed gallbladder,

causing pain. The patient should be instructed to call the physician if severe abdominal pain and a fever are experienced

3. **Answer: 3 Rationale:** Hepatitis A is transmitted by oral-fecal route from an infected person handling food, water, or fish, or through direct contact without washing hands before handling food or after using the bathroom.

4. **Answer: 4 Rationale:** Hepatitis C is transmitted through contact with blood or body fluids.

5. **Answer: 2 Rationale:** The hepatitis A virus can be transmitted before manifestations of the disease (including jaundice) develop; therefore, it is important to identify people who have had direct contact with the newly diagnosed patient.

6. **Answer: 2 Rationale:** Maintaining a patent airway is of highest priority. Placing the patient in Fowler's position may prevent aspiration of blood and should be the primary action.

7. **Answer: 3 Rationale:** It is important to empty the bladder prior to the paracentesis to make sure the bladder is not punctured during the procedure.

8. **Answer: 1 Rationale:** The nurse should assess bowel sounds and palpate for tenderness since spontaneous bacterial infection can develop with ascites, producing fever and worsening encephalopathy.

9. **Answer: 3 Rationale:** In women, the most common contributing factor to development of acute pancreatitis is a gallstone obstructing the duct.

10. **Answer: 4 Rationale:** Maintaining a patent nasogastric tube is vital to prevent accumulation of gastric secretions and pressure on the anastomoses created in Whipple's procedure.

Unit 6 Building Clinical Competence: Responses to Altered Gastrointestinal Function

Functional Health Pattern: Nutritional-Metabolic

Functional Health Patterns

Hint: Even small suggestions to change life style can have a big impact on the patient's health status. Identify what communication you used to answer these questions.

Priority Setting

1.
   A. Thomas Jones should be seen first. *Rationale: Mr. Jones is becoming anxious and irritable, which are signs of DTs from alcohol withdrawal. He needs to be evaluated and treated.*
   B. Paul Bruner should be assessed second. *Rationale: Mr. Bruner is scheduled for surgery and enemas must be given with time to expel the fluid. Assessment must be done before the enemas are given.*
   C. Tonya Cooper should be seed third. *Rationale: Ms. Cooper needs assistance to use the bedpan. Her orthostatic blood pressure is too low for it to be safe to get her out of bed.*
   D. Grace Freeman should be assessed fourth. *Rationale: While the colostomy bag needs to be changed, it is not harmful to leave it for a few minutes. Changing the bag is an optimal time for patient teaching, which will take some time.*

Health Promotion

1.
   A. Thomas Jones: Discuss alcohol treatment, stop-smoking programs, and ways to prevent injury and infection.
   B. Tonya Cooper: Discuss the need for increased fluids and prevention of falls that might occur due to weakness and fainting.

   C. Paul Bruner: Discuss the need for progressive activity to prevent pneumonia and DVT; following surgery he will need a balanced diet, high in protein, to promote healing.
   D. Grace Freeman: Discuss the need for daily activity to promote bowel elimination.

2. B, C, D. *Rationale: Liquids soften the stool, exercise increases gastric motility, and bulk-forming laxatives create bulk and draw water into the intestines, which soften the stool, preventing constipation.*

3. A. *Rationale: The most common initial clinical manifestation is rectal bleeding due to impaired integrity of the rectal tissue.*

Nursing Process

1. A, C, D, E. *Rationale: On admission a baseline for the extent of blood loss and life impairment must be determined.*

2.

	Nursing Diagnosis	Rationale
Thomas Jones	*High Risk for Noncompliance: medical management of cirrhosis*	*Patients with advanced cirrhosis and alcoholism find it difficult to change long-standing behavior.*
Tonya Cooper	*Fluid Volume Deficit*	*Ms. Cooper has such severe fluid volume deficit that she has developed orthostatic hypotension.*
Paul Bruner	*Reactive Depression related to abdominal mass and upcoming surgery*	*At 86 years of age, many people lack the mental energy to overcome major medical issues and become depressed.*
Grace Freeman	*Impaired Skin Integrity*	*The colostomy has altered the integrity of the skin. The application of the bag can also further impair the skin.*

3. C. *Rationale: Blood in the stomach can prevent locating the source of the bleeding. Flushing the stomach with cold saline can slow bleeding as well as rinse the blood from the stomach.*

4. The teaching plan should include types of appliances, how to remove and apply the appliance, how to remove flatus from the appliance, skin inspection, and skin care. Also include contact information for professional support and local ostomy support groups.

Communication

1. B. *Rationale: Rewarding good behavior helps to develop a positive self-concept. Monitoring daily food intake provides data of balanced nutrients where weight gain does not.*

2. "We are concerned for you because your blood pressure is so low you can go into shock and die. It is your life, but we care about you and don't want you hurting yourself." *Rationale: The nurse must be honest with the patient and express concern and caring for the patient's welfare.*

3. The nurse should respond with, "I understand your concerns. Have you discussed your feelings with your daughter and the doctor? I can have them come and talk with you before the surgery if you would like." *Rationale: The nurse must respond to the patient's wishes. It is important to facilitate communication between Mr. Bruner, his daughter, and the surgeon.*

Delegation

1. For each patient, vital signs and assisting with ADLs can be delegated. The nursing assistant may need to stay with Mr. Jones or Ms. Cooper to prevent them from hurting themselves. The nursing assistant can help get Ms. Green ready for surgery but cannot administer medication.

2. Tell the nursing assistant assisting Ms. Cooper with her meals to stay with her and prevent her from stimulating vomiting for at least one hour after she eats.

Content-Specific Questions

1. The nurse will need to complete an incident report form and be seen by the hospital infection control department. Blood should be drawn to establish a baseline in case the nurse becomes Hepatitis B positive. Facility policy should be followed.

2. D. *Rationale: Gluten is found in wheat, rye, barley, and oats. Patients on a gluten-free diet can have corn.*

3. B. *Rationale: In metabolic acidosis, pH is decreased below 7.35, pCO2 is decreased below 35 mmHg, and Bicarbonate is decreased below 22 mmEq/L.*

4. C. *Rationale: Instruct the patient to administer a bowel preparation the evening before to cleanse the intestines prior to the procedure.*

5. B. *Rationale: The usual clinical manifestations of large bowel obstruction are constipation and colicky abdominal pain.*

Concept Map

Hint: In identifying the priority nursing diagnosis, look at the circumstances and time frame of the patient's illness and weight loss. You may find it helpful to review Chapter 10 as you consider this question and develop a concept map for the nursing diagnosis of *Deficient Fluid Volume*.

Chapter 26: Assessing the Renal System

1. **Answer: 4 Rationale:** Leakage of urine is not a normal manifestation in women of any age.

2. **Answer: 4 Rationale:** ADH is increased to limit the excretion of water in the urine to maintain fluid balance.

3. **Answer: 3 Rationale:** Creatinine clearance is a test that determines the filtering ability of the glomeruli and the blood circulation to them. If the clearance is decreased, the glomeruli are damaged or the circulation is slowed.

4. **Answer: 3 Rationale:** The prostate surrounds the male urethra at the base of the bladder.

5. **Answer: 2 Rationale:** Nocturia is defined as two or more voidings during the night.

6. **Answer: 1 Rationale:** The contrast media used in IVPs cause some adverse reactions in patients that are allergic to iodine or products containing iodine. Shellfish contain iodine.

7. **Answer: 3 Rationale:** Collecting a urine specimen allows the examiner to assess the urine for color, odor, and clarity before the exam.

8. **Answer: 1 Rationale:** Anesthetic agents used during surgery may cause problems with initiating voiding. Palpation will determine if the bladder is distended.

9. **Answer: 4 Rationale:** Bladder cancer is believed to result from genetic and environmental factors.

10. **Answer: 2 Rationale:** Skin turgor is the best assessment technique to determine hydration of patients.

Chapter 27: Nursing Care of Patients with Urinary Tract Disorders

1. **Answer: 2 Rationale:** The form of birth control, especially for those using a diaphragm and spermicidal gel, can alter the vaginal flora and increase the risk of UTIs. The reoccurrence time factor of the UTI is too long to be a failure to complete antibiotic treatment the first time.

2. **Answer: 1, 3, 4 Rationale:** The nurse needs to inform the patient that a urine culture in 10 days is done to ensure antibiotic therapy was effective. In a perimenopausal woman vaginal cream may maintain tissue integrity to prevent bacterial colonization of perineal tissues; instructions on cleansing may prevent further infections.

3. **Answer: 4 Rationale:** Increasing fluid intake to 3000 mL per day will produce enough urine to prevent stone-forming salts from concentrating sufficiently to precipitate.

4. **Answer: 3 Rationale:** These are manifestations of renal colic and possible ureteral obstruction. Prompt diagnosis and treatment is vital to prevent hydroureter and hydronephrosis should the ureter be completely obstructed.

5. **Answer: 1 Rationale:** Bladder cancer is two times more prevalent in smokers than nonsmokers.

6. **Answer: 2 Rationale:** Painless hematuria is the usual presenting manifestation of bladder cancers and should be evaluated quickly for best outcome.

7. **Answer: 3 Rationale:** The patient with a newly created continent ileal diversion will have to demonstrate self-catheterization since this is the only way to empty the continent ileal diversion. There is no collection device in this surgical procedure.

8. **Answer: 3 Rationale:** Stress incontinence should not be viewed as a normal result of aging, but as a treatable problem. Pelvic floor muscle exercises strengthen perineal muscles, increasing urinary sphincter control, and will reduce the incidence of incontinence.

9. **Answer: 1 Rationale:** Inability to retain urine long enough to reach the toilet following perception of the need to urinate is characteristic of urge incontinence. Caffeine and artificial sweeteners are bladder irritants, causing instability of the detrusor muscle and aggravating manifestations. Restricting intake of fluids containing these substances in the evening reduces nocturia.

10. **Answer: 4 Rationale:** Catheterizing the patient every 3 to 4 hours with a straight catheter prevents overdistension of the bladder and the increased risk for infection associated with an indwelling catheter.

Chapter 28: Nursing Care of Patients with Kidney Disorders

1. **Answer: 2 Rationale:** The GFR tends to decrease with aging, decreasing drug excretion and increasing the risk for toxicity. Administering smaller doses less frequently reduces the risk, but the patient needs continued monitoring for manifestations of digoxin toxicity.

2. **Answer: 3 Rationale:** The adult form of polycystic kidney disease (PKD) is transmitted in an autosomal dominant pattern. Each child has a 50% chance of inheriting the disease.

3. **Answer: 2 Rationale:** The most common cause of acute glomerulonephritis is an abnormal immune response to beta-hemolytic streptococcus A infection, usually strep throat.

4. **Answer: 1 Rationale:** Soy or animal proteins are complete proteins necessary for growth and tissue maintenance. Complete proteins are preferred when total protein intake is restricted, as in acute glomerulonephritis.

5. **Answer: 4 Rationale:** Postoperatively, it is important to monitor separately all drainage device volumes to determine function of each catheter or drain and prevent hydronephrosis.

6. **Answer: 1 Rationale:** Ischemia is the most common cause of acute renal failure (ARF); therefore, maintaining fluid volume, cardiac output, and renal output are the highest priority nursing interventions to prevent renal failure.

7. **Answer: 3 Rationale:** Nephrotoxic drugs, including over-the-counter products, can produce further damage to the kidney cells and should be avoided.

8. **Answer: 1, 3 Rationale:** Weight and orthostatic vital signs are indicators of fluid volume status and electrolyte balance. Laboratory tests are monitored to evaluate the effects of treatment.

9. **Answer: 2 Rationale:** The patient's ability to state advantages and disadvantages of renal replacement therapies indicates understanding of treatment options and the ability to make informed decisions on treatment. Patients may be able to live independently or with the assistance of a part-time caregiver.

10. **Answer: 4 Rationale:** Cloudy urine could be a manifestation of an infection. Prompt treatment is vital to preserve integrity of the transplanted organ in an immunosuppressed patient.

Unit 7 Building Clinical Competence: Responses to Altered Urinary Elimination

Functional Health Pattern: Elimination

Functional Health Patterns
Hint: Be creative in identifying possible interventions.

Priority Setting
1.
   A. Joseph Rouse should be seen first. *Rationale: He has severe pain; tachycardia; and cool, pale, clammy skin following surgery. These can indicate early shock and must be evaluated and reported to the primary care provider.*
   B. Philip Jones should be seen second. *Rationale: Abdominal pain associated with being unable to void could indicate internal bleeding or blockage of the urinary system. These issues must be evaluated and reported to the primary care provider.*
   C. Agnes Smith can be seen third. *Rationale: While Mrs. Smith seems to be stable, if she is confused she may not be able to summon help if needed.*
   D. Angela Baldwin can be seen last. *Rationale: Nephritis can become life threatening and her health status must be evaluated; however, she is able to summon help if needed.*

Health Promotion
1. Agnes Smith should be taught to drink plenty of fluids and to provide perineal care several times daily.
2. Joseph Rouse should be taught to drink adequate fluids and to limit foods high in calcium and oxalate.
3. Angela Baldwin should be taught to limit fluids, and to follow the sodium and protein restrictions prescribed by the primary care provider.

Nursing Process
1.

	Nursing Diagnosis	Rationale
Phillip Jones	*Urinary Retention* related to kidney trauma	*Swelling from trauma can cause urinary retention.*
Agnes Smith	*Urinary Incontinence* related to urinary infection	*Patients with UTI can develop urge incontinence. The incontinent patient is also more at risk for UTI.*
Joseph Rouse	*Pain* related to kidney surgery	*Severe pain can be a sign of postoperative complication of internal bleeding.*

Angela Baldwin	*Fluid Volume Excess* related to nephritis associated with SLE	*Without normal kidney function, fluid volume excess develops, putting stress on the heart and other internal organs.*

2. B. *Rationale: Draining urine in 500 mL increments may prevent a vasovagal response from draining the bladder too rapidly.*
3. A. *Rationale: With kidney trauma, the nursing actions are to monitor for level of consciousness, vital signs, skin color and temperature, and urine output for possible signs of shock. Signs of shock, such as hypotension, tachycardia, tachypnea, cool and pale skin, and altered level of consciousness may be present.*
4. A. *Rationale: Urine output of less than 30 mL is a sign of decreased renal and cardiac output. It needs to be reported to the physician promptly.*

Communication
1. A. *Rationale: Three-day medications therapy with trimethoprim-sulfamethoxazole (Bactrim) is the recommended treatment for uncomplicated cystitis.*
2. The nurse should respond, "It seems that the urinary complications you are having are associated with the lupus. Let's ask the doctor to discuss this with you when she comes in this morning." *Rationale: By acknowledging that the urinary symptoms might be associated with the lupus the nurse shows honesty. Because the nurse cannot diagnose medical problems, referring the patient to the primary care provider is appropriate.*

Delegation
1. For each patient, the nursing assistant can obtain vital signs, record intake and output, and provide ADLs.

Content-Specific Questions
1. C. *Rationale: Pyridium turns the urine and other body secretions a red or orange.*
2. D. *Rationale: Foods high in purines are organ meats and those moderate in purines are beef, chicken, pork. The patient on a low-purine diet needs to decrease eating these types of foods.*
3. B. *Rationale: Hematuria, proteinuria, and hypertension are the classic early manifestations of glomerulonephritis.*
4. B, C, F. *Rationale: Decreased cervicovaginal antibodies, sexual intercourse, short urethra, and aging in women are risk factors for urinary tract infections. Circumcision is a protective mechanism in men. Any patient is at risk when urinary catheter is inserted.*
5. B. *Rationale: Weight changes are a more accurate indicator of fluid volume status than intake and output, restricting fluids, and monitoring labs for BUS and creatinine.*
6. C. *Rationale: The most reliable diagnostic procedure for glomerular disorders is kidney biopsy. It determines the type of glomerulonephritis, the prognosis, and appropriate treatment.*

Concept Map
Hint: Note that in the evaluation section of the concept map provided, Mr. Jenkins has undergone hemodialysis and is preparing for placement of a peritoneal dialysis catheter. Review the section on renal replacement therapies for nursing care and patient teaching related to peritoneal dialysis.

Chapter 29: Assessing the Cardiovascular and Lymphatic Systems
1. **Answer: 3 Rationale:** Hemorrhage would decrease the total volume of blood and venous return, which would decrease stroke volume and likewise cardiac output.

2. **Answer: 3 Rationale:** Since pain is subjective, a numerical rating scale assesses what is the patient's perception of pain intensity.

3. **Answer: 1 Rationale:** This is the location of the apex of the heart and can be assessed at left midclavicular, fifth intercostal space on most patients.

4. **Answer: 2 Rationale:** Bradycardia is defined as a pulse rate < 60 beats per minute.

5. **Answer: 3 Rationale:** Fatigue would indicate that the body's tissues are not receiving adequate oxygenation. O_2 is carried by the hemoglobin molecule on the RBC; if RBC numbers are very low there are insufficient numbers to carry adequate oxygen to meet demands.

6. **Answer: 2 Rationale:** Platelet plug formation is the first step in clotting. If the count is low, fewer platelets are available for clotting; therefore, with tissue injury, platelets are not available and bruising occurs.

7. **Answer: 1 Rationale:** The thickness of the blood will affect the ability of the blood to flow through the vessels, thus increasing the peripheral vascular resistance (PVR).

8. **Answer: 2 Rationale:** Auscultating with the bell of the stethoscope will identify soft sounds such as the carotid arteries and identify any bruits.

9. **Answer: 3 Rationale:** A murmuring or blowing sound is the definition of a bruit.

10. **Answer: 4 Rationale:** Notify the physician immediately; these manifestations indicate a severe decrease in perfusion to the leg, and cells are dying from lack of blood flow.

Chapter 30: Nursing Care of Patients with Coronary Heart Disease

1. **Answer: 3 Rationale:** Stopping smoking decreases the risk of coronary heart disease by 50%.

2. **Answer: 1 Rationale:** These manifestations could indicate myopathy, a serious potential complication of statin drugs that needs to be reported promptly.

3. **Answer: 2 Rationale:** Stable angina is predictable and it is associated with increased activity and relieved by rest and nitrates.

4. **Answer: 4 Rationale:** Reestablishing coronary blood flow and cardiac tissue perfusion within 20 to 45 minutes is imperative to minimize damage to the myocardium.

5. **Answer: 2 Rationale:** The cardiac catheter used to insert the stent is usually inserted via the femoral artery, a large, high-pressure vessel. The leg is maintained in extension for a prescribed period after the procedure to reduce the risk of bleeding, hematoma formation, or clot formation at the insertion site.

6. **Answer: 4 Rationale:** Relieving pain in AMI decreases sympathetic nervous system stimulation and cardiac work. Pain relief is of highest priority, although the other goals also are appropriate for the patient with AMI.

7. **Answer: 1 Rationale:** Fibrinolytic therapy, administered to restore myocardial perfusion, disrupts the clotting cascade and can lead to potentially serious bleeding. Establishing bleeding precautions is vital to preserve physiologic integrity.

8. **Answer: 3 Rationale:** A CK of 320 U/L, four times the normal level, is indicative of muscle tissue damage; in the patient with acute chest pain it often indicates acute myocardial infarction.

9. **Answer: 2 Rationale:** Mobitz type II AV block often is associated with a large anterior MI and a high mortality rate. Pacemaker therapy may be necessary to maintain effective ventricular contractions and cardiac output.

10. **Answer: 1 Rationale:** Sinus bradycardia may be well-tolerated in some patients. Assessment is important before treating. However, if decreased mental status and hypotension is present, intervention is necessary.

Chapter 31: Nursing Care of Patients with Cardiac Disorders

1. **Answer: 1 Rationale:** Normal ejection fraction is 60%; an ejection fraction of 25% indicates severe impairment of ventricular function.

2. **Answer: 3 Rationale:** Interdisciplinary treatment goals for the patient with heart failure are to reduce the cardiac workload and improve pump effectiveness. Loss of excess fluid, as indicated by weight loss, reduces cardiac work. The drop in heart rate and reduced pulmonary vascular congestion are indicative of improved cardiac pump.

3. **Answer: 2, 4, 5 Rationale:** In left ventricular failure, the cardiac output falls and pressure in the pulmonary vascular system increases. This leads to fatigue, increasing dyspnea, and crackles in the lung bases.

4. **Answer: 4 Rationale:** Calibrating and leveling the system during each shift ensures accuracy and consistency of measurements.

5. **Answer: 2 Rationale:** Morphine is given intravenously to relieve anxiety; it also is a venous vasodilator, reducing venous return and cardiac work.

6. **Answer: 1 Rationale:** A pericardial friction rub, a grating sound, is a characteristic sign of pericarditis so it is expected, but should be documented in the patient's record.

7. **Answer: 4 Rationale:** Effective treatment for acute infective endocarditis requires long-term intravenous antibiotic therapy to eliminate the infecting organisms.

8. **Answer: 3 Rationale:** The murmur of mitral valve stenosis would be heard during diastole (when blood is flowing through the stenotic valve from the atrium to the ventricle) at the apex of the heart.

9. **Answer: 2 Rationale:** Anticoagulant therapy to prevent clot formation is necessary following insertion of a mechanical valve.

10. **Answer: 1 Rationale:** In hypertrophic cardiomyopathy, manifestations may not develop until the demand for oxygen increases, such as with athletes during activity, causing sudden death due to a ventricular dysrhythmia. This type of cardiomyopathy is not a filling problem but rather an obstruction to ejection of blood to the body to meet oxygen demand.

Chapter 32: Nursing Care of Patients with Vascular and Lymphatic Disorders

1. **Answer: 3 Rationale:** Hypertension generally is asymptomatic.

2. **Answer: 1 Rationale:** While lasagna made with whole-grain pasta, low-fat cheese, and vegetables or lean meats would be allowed, this answer demonstrates the need for additional teaching.

3. **Answer: 2, 4 Rationale:** First-dose hypotension and orthostatic hypotension are potential adverse effects of this drug, as is persistent cough.

4. **Answer: 1 Rationale:** These manifestations indicate a possible arterial occlusion. This is an emergency; immediate intervention is necessary to preserve the extremity.

5. **Answer: 4 Rationale:** Endovascular approach on an 86-year-old patient would mean less surgical risk and faster recovery.

6. **Answer: 4 Rationale:** Patients with peripheral atherosclerosis may have paresthesias and decreased hair on the affected extremity.

7. **Answer: 2, 3, 1, 4, 5 Rationale:** First, smoking cessation, because nicotine causes vasoconstriction, further decreasing blood flow; next, daily skin inspections looking for breaks in integrity to prevent infections; third, maintaining feet by regular cleansing, cotton socks, and protecting feet by wearing shoes; fourth, regular daily exercise to develop collateral circulation; and fifth, weight loss if necessary to keep patient mobile.

8. **Answer: 2 Rationale:** Anticoagulant therapy will be continued after discharge; understanding the importance of follow-up care and monitoring for adverse effects is vital.
9. **Answer: 1 Rationale:** Elevating the legs and wearing elastic stockings may relieve the discomfort associated with varicose veins.
10. **Answer: 3 Rationale:** Careful skin and foot care is a high priority to prevent skin breakdown and potential infection.

Chapter 33: Nursing Care of Patients with Hematologic Disorders

1. **Answer: 3 Rationale:** Red blood cells and the hemoglobin they contain carry oxygen to the tissues; in anemia, the oxygen-carrying capacity of blood is reduced, leading to exertional dyspnea.
2. **Answer: 1 Rationale:** During gastric resection, intrinsic factor production may decrease, leading to vitamin B_{12} deficiency anemia with associated neurologic deficits such as numbness and tingling of extremities.
3. **Answer: 2 Rationale:** Prior to bone marrow transplant, chemotherapy or total body irradiation is used to destroy leukemic cells in the bone marrow. Normal blood cells also are destroyed, causing significant risk for infection and bleeding.
4. **Answer: 1, 3, 5 Rationale:** AML causes both neutropenia and thrombocytopenia, with resulting increased risk for infection and bleeding. A private room and oral hygiene help reduce infection risk, and a soft, bland diet reduces trauma to oral mucosal membranes.
5. **Answer: 1 Rationale:** The correct response is open-ended and allows the patient to state more specifically what he is concerned about.
6. **Answer: 3 Rationale:** Multiple-drug chemotherapy regimes are effective at different phases of the cell cycle, allowing lower doses of individual drugs to decrease adverse effects and produce more effective tumor destruction.
7. **Answer: 4 Rationale:** A new onset of severe pain may signal a pathological fracture and needs to be reported.
8. **Answer: 2 Rationale:** A platelet count of 60,000/mm³ is significantly low (normal 150,000–450,000/mm³), increasing the risk of bleeding and bruising with minor trauma.
9. **Answer: 1 Rationale:** The most common form of classic hemophilia is transmitted as an x-linked recessive disorder passed from mother to son; therefore, the daughter may be a carrier.
10. **Answer: 4 Rationale:** A platelet infusion replaces those platelets used in the abnormal clotting process of DIC.

Unit 8 Clinical Competencies: Responses to Altered Cardiac Function
Functional Health Pattern: Activity-Exercise Patterns

Functional Health Patterns
Hint: Think about the timing of ADLs and other necessary treatments. Think about safety measures while the patient is in the hospital as well as at home.

Priority Setting
1.
   A. Scott Jacoby should be seen first. *Rationale: Mr. Jacoby needs to be ready for the bone marrow biopsy this morning. The degree of his mental abilities is unclear. The patient with Down's syndrome often needs simple instruction and reassurance.*
   B. Arnold Markus should be seen second. *Rationale: Mr. Markus has started having isolated PVCs and crackles in the lower lobes of the lungs. These signs can indicate a worsening of the CHF, which needs to be evaluated.*
   C. Theresa Cartwright can be seen third. *Rationale: Mrs. Cartwright can summon help if needed. Treatment has been initiated, but the Heparin IV must be monitored.*
   D. Betty Williams should be seen last. *Rationale: Mrs. Williams's vital signs and heart rhythm are stable.*

Health Promotion
1. Mr. Markus should be taught to eat a low-sodium diet to help prevent water retention. He should avoid obviously salty foods, limit the use of salt during cooking, and refrain from adding salt at the table.
2. Mrs. Williams should be taught to manage her type 2 diabetes, to stop smoking, and to control her hypertension. She should be given the resources (professional resources and support groups) she needs. She should be encouraged to eat a healthy diet and engage in exercise as recommended by her healthcare provider.
3. The nurse should discuss dietary restriction because of anticoagulant therapy. Not massaging or deeply rubbing the legs, wearing anti-embolitic stockings, and taking care to prevent trauma should also be discussed.

Nursing Process
1.

	Nursing Diagnosis	Rationale
Betty Williams	*Risk for Activity Intolerance* related to MI	*A weakened heart may not be able to sustain a high level of activity. Mrs. Williams should increase activity gradually.*
Arnold Markus	*Decreased Cardiac Output*	*Mr. Markus's heart is weak and unable to pump effectively.*
Theresa Cartwright	*Anxiety* related to unexpected hospitalization and uncertainty about the seriousness of her illness	*Mrs. Cartwright is a mother of young children who need her at home.*
Scott Jacoby	*High Risk for Infection* related to upper respiratory infection and possible pathology of the bone marrow	*Mr. Jacoby currently has an infection and has symptoms of bone marrow pathology (possible leukemia). This puts him at greater risk for further infection.*

2. C. *Rationale: While fluid in the lungs will alter lung sounds, oxygen saturation levels indicate the ability of the lungs to function and the heart to circulate the blood.*
3. D. *Rationale: A PVC falling on the T wave of the previous beat can cause the life-threatening dysrhythmia ventricular fibrillation.*
4. A. *Rationale: Assessment should be completed before initiating interventions. A full symptom assessment should be completed before administering the prescribed nitroglycerine tablet.*
5. B. *Rationale: Fever and burning on urination would indicate a urinary tract infection. Mr. Jacoby is at risk for infection, so these symptoms are significant.*

6. B, F. *Rationale: Prothrombin time (PT) and International Normalized Ration (INR) are monitored to determine the dosage levels of warfarin therapy.*

Communication

1. C. *Rationale: Mrs. Cartwright needs to continue to take birth control pills to prevent pregnancy, as Coumadin is a teratogenic drug.*

2. You should explain that her heart has been weakened by the heart attack, but with time it can heal and strengthen. It will be important for her to follow the doctor's instructions.

Delegation

1.

A. Mrs. Williams: The nursing assistant can obtain vital signs and assist with a bed bath unless the doctor has ordered a warm shower. Mrs. Williams will also need blood glucose values obtained.

B. Mr. Markus: The nursing assistant can obtain vital signs and assist with a warm shower and ambulation.

C. Mrs. Cartwright: The nursing assistant can obtain vital signs. Since Mrs. Cartwright will be on bedrest, she will need assistance with all ADLs.

D. Mr. Jacoby: The nursing assistant can obtain vital signs, assist with ADLs, and assist with preparation for bone marrow biopsy. The nursing assistant may accompany the patient to the procedure if support is needed.

Related Questions

1. C. *Rationale: The patient with a mitral valve replacement will be prescribed long-term anticoagulant therapy. Patients with a history of duodenal ulcer are at increased risk of intestinal bleeding and must be monitored closely.*

2. B. *Rationale: Venous stasis impairs delivery of nutrients and oxygen to peripheral tissues.*

3. C. *Rationale: Keep fingers and toes warm to prevent spasms of the small arteries in the digits.*

4. B. *Rationale: Cardizem may cause bradycardia. Notify the physician if the heart rate is less than 60 beats per minute.*

5. D. *Rationale: Use enough direct pressure to control bleeding. Pressure on the femoral artery or a tourniquet will occlude the blood vessels and decrease tissue perfusion, and should only be used as a last resort to save a life.*

Concept Map

Hint: Review Unit 7 to determine the impact of chronic kidney disease on hypertension. The concept map for Unit 8 (this one) would reflect both disorders.

Chapter 34: Assessing the Respiratory System

1. Answer: 4 Rationale: The apex or top of the lungs is located just below the clavicle.

2. Answer: 3 Rationale: A family history of lung cancer is a risk factor for developing lung cancer.

3. Answer: 4 Rationale: Bronchovesicular breath sounds are normal; the nurse would take and record the vital signs as usual.

4. Answer: 1 Rationale: As the body temperature rises the bond between oxygen and hemoglobin decreases so less oxygen binds and unloading is enhanced.

5. Answer: 2 Rationale: Thoracentesis is the removal of fluid around the lung.

6. Answer: 3 Rationale: Information about illness management is important in identifying health problems.

7. Answer: 2 Rationale: Wheezes are continuous musical sounds heard in the chest.

8. Answer: 4 Rationale: If the patient had a lung removed, breath sounds would be absent from that side because without air movement no sound would be generated.

9. Answer: 3 Rationale: While auscultating the lungs, the patient should take slow deep breaths to allow adequate time for air to go into and out of the lungs. Breathing through the mouth amplifies the sound, making it easier to hear.

10. Answer: 2 Rationale: Decreased diaphragmatic movement on the left side should be documented; it is an expected outcome with pneumothorax on the left since air movement and diaphragm movement would be decreased.

Chapter 35: Nursing Care of Patients with Upper Respiratory Disorders

1. Answer: 4 Rationale: Over-the-counter nasal spray is the best choice to relieve URI manifestations in the patient with hypertension, since its effects are local, not systemic. The duration of use is limited to prevent rebound.

2. Answer: 2 Rationale: Yearly influenza vaccinations are the most effective way of preventing flu and pneumonia in this group.

3. Answer: 1 Rationale: Completion of the antibiotic medication is the most important in order to cure the bacterial infection and prevent reoccurrence.

4. Answer: 3 Rationale: Posterior nasal packing obstructs the nares and may compromise oxygenation. Oxygenation has the highest priority.

5. Answer: 4 Rationale: Fracture of other facial bones may accompany nasal fracture, damaging the dura and causing spinal fluid leak. A positive glucose indicates the presence of spinal fluid.

6. Answer: 3, 5, 6 Rationale: The manifestations of sleep apnea include daytime sleepiness, elevated BP, and complaints of morning headache.

7. Answer: 1 Rationale: Persistent voice hoarseness may be the first sign of a laryngeal tumor, necessitating follow-up diagnostic testing.

8. Answer: 3 Rationale: With stage I laryngeal cancer, radiation can cure the cancer, and preserve the voice. This cancer does metastasize to other areas.

9. Answer: 4, 5, 2, 1, 3 Rationale: Maintaining airway patency is of highest priority. The head may need additional support because of the removal of neck muscles. Frequent, small meals help meet metabolic needs; swallowing may be difficult and the effort may produce fatigue. Regaining speech will require practice and assistance from a speech therapist. Loss of the voice will result in grieving; encouraging expression of feelings can facilitate gradual acceptance of the loss.

10. Answer: 2 Rationale: When providing tracheostomy care, the nurse secures clean ties before removing soiled ones to prevent accidental dislodgement of the tube.

Chapter 36: Nursing Care of Patients with Ventilation Disorders

1. Answer: 4 Rationale: Unless oxygenation is compromised by the inflammatory process, the sputum specimen is obtained first.

2. Answer: 1, 4, 5, 2, 3 Rationale: Overall gray skin color and bluish tinge to lips indicate hypoxemia; supplemental oxygen is highest priority. Second, raise the head of the bed to promote chest expansion and alveolar ventilation. Assessment of oxygen saturation and breath sounds provide important information to be provided to the physician.

3. Answer: 3 Rationale: A 9 mm induration is a positive result in a patient with HIV disease.

4. **Answer: 2 Rationale:** When teaching a patient who is taking INH, the nurse needs to include information on adverse effects such as numbness and tingling of extremities to the doctor.

5. **Answer: 3 Rationale:** Smoking cessation is important with the diagnosis of lung cancer to prevent further damage from the chemicals in the cigarettes.

6. **Answer: 3, 4 Rationale:** Chest tube drainage that is red, free-flowing, and exceeds 70mL/hour indicates hemorrhage and must be reported. Vital signs and level of consciousness are measured to evaluate cardiac output and hemodynamic stability.

7. **Answer: 1 Rationale:** The patient having a thoracentesis needs to sit upright, leaning forward during the procedure to spread the rib cage for easier placement of the needle.

8. **Answer: 4 Rationale:** A patient with a fractured rib would be urged to use a small pillow to splint the area when coughing to reduce the movement of rib cage and pain.

9. **Answer: 2 Rationale:** A respiratory rate of 36 indicates respiratory distress, and is of greatest concern.

10. **Answer: 1 Rationale:** Tension pneumothorax displaces structures in the mediastinum, including the great vessels. Cardiac output may be severely compromised, resulting in inadequate oxygen delivery and nutrients to cells and tissues.

Chapter 37: Nursing Care of Patients with Gas Exchange Disorders

1. **Answer: 2 Rationale:** Ineffective airway clearance is the highest priority because it impairs alveolar ventilation and the exchange of oxygen and carbon dioxide at the capillaries, decreasing the blood and tissue oxygen levels.

2. **Answer: 1 Rationale:** The physician needs to be informed because this indicates increasing fatigue and impending respiratory failure.

3. **Answer: 3 Rationale:** The patient should be taught to use the anti-inflammatory drug as needed to treat acute episodes of wheezing.

4. **Answer: 1 Rationale:** Development of a barrel chest due to air trapping is an expected finding in COPD.

5. **Answer: 3 Rationale:** During an acute exacerbation of COPD, keeping the SaO_2 above 90% is an appropriate goal.

6. **Answer: 4 Rationale:** In some patients with COPD, decreased arterial oxygen concentrations drive respirations. Administered O_2 may decrease the drive to breathe; however, many patients with COPD require supplemental oxygen.

7. **Answer: 1, 2, 4, 5 Rationale:** Thick, tenacious, milky white sputum and fever indicate possible infection. Difficulty coughing up mucus and increased shortness of breath and fatigue indicate potential early manifestations of respiratory failure.

8. **Answer: 2 Rationale:** These manifestations may indicate pulmonary embolism. Oxygen is administered to support gas exchange and tissue oxygenation.

9. **Answer: 1 Rationale:** Restlessness and tachypnea are early signs of respiratory failure caused by hypoxemia and stimulation of the respiratory center.

10. **Answer: 4 Rationale:** Patent airways are necessary to maintain effective alveolar ventilation and gas exchange.

Unit 9 Building Clinical Competence: Responses to Altered Respiratory Function
Functional Health Pattern: Activity-Exercise Patterns

Functional Health Patterns
Hint: **To facilitate breathing the nurse must not only think about positioning, but also how to maintain a patent airway and facilitate oxygen/carbon dioxide exchange.**

Priority Setting
1.
   A. James Mohr should be seen first. *Rationale: Mr. Mohr has been coughing, and because of the tracheostomy he may be unable to clear his airway. Immediate suctioning is needed to open the airway.*
   B. Maggie Sawyer should be seen second. *Rationale: Ms. Sawyer could be having a pulmonary embolism, which can be life-threatening.*
   C. Jack Holt should be seen third. *Rationale: Mr. Holt's vital signs are elevated and he is experiencing pain with breathing. He may need medication for pain.*
   D. Amy Campbell should be seen last. *Rationale: While Ms. Campbell is wheezing, her vital signs and oxygen saturation level appear the most stable.*

Health Promotion
1. Patients with COPD need high-calorie, high-protein diets without excessive carbohydrates, which can increase levels of carbon dioxide, adding stress to the lungs.
2. Allow family members or significant others to remain with the patient while maintaining a quiet environment. Assist with guided imagery, relaxation techniques, and gentle massage, and administer medication as needed.

Nursing Process
1.

	Nursing Diagnosis	Rationale
Jack Holt	*Pain in Chest* related to breathing difficulty and frequent cough	*Chest pain caused by frequent coughing can diminish coughing effort, which results in mucus remaining in lungs.*
Maggie Sawyer	*Impaired Gas Exchange* as evidenced by sudden onset of difficulty breathing, chest pain, coughing, restlessness, and a feeling that she is going to die	*Ms. Sawyer's history of deep vein thrombosis can result in pulmonary embolism (PE). PE blocks blood to the alveoli, resulting in impaired gas exchange.*
James Mohr	*Ineffective Airway Clearance* related to trauma and tracheostomy	*A tracheostomy tube irritates the trachea, causing increased mucus and cough. The tube can become obstructed with mucus.*
Amy Campbell	*Ineffective Airway Clearance* as evidenced by wheezing	*Bronchospasm that occurs during an asthma attack obstructs the air flow into and out of the lungs.*

2. C. *Rationale: Wearing a mask is standard precaution for a patient with a droplet infection.*
3. B. *Rationale: The patient is positioned with the area to be drained above the trachea or mainstem bronchus. Head down allows gravity to facilitate drainage of secretions.*
4. D. *Rationale: Stretching the legs and walking every 1 to 2 hours when traveling will reduce the risk of pulmonary embolism. Hose that bind around the knee and use of pillows can contribute to deep vein thrombus formation and subsequently pulmonary embolism.*

5. C. *Rationale: Showering and bathing are allowed as long as the tracheostomy is protected from the flow of water.*

6. B. *Rationale: Short-acting bronchodilators are used first to dilate the bronchi quickly (albuterol), followed by longer-acting bronchodilators (atrovent), and lastly preventative medications (cromolyn).*

Communication

1. "Chronic asthma is a life-long disease, but with treatment it can be controlled. Most patients lead a very productive life."

Delegation

1. What data collection and interventions can be delegated to a nursing assistant for each patient?

A. Jack Holt: The nursing assistant can obtain vital signs and oxygen saturation, and assist with ADLs. Frequent oral care, disposing of contaminated tissues, and supplying clean ones is needed.

B. Maggie Sawyer: The nursing assistant can obtain vital signs and oxygen saturation, assist with ADLs, assist with set up of oxygen, and stay with the patient in case further assistance is needed.

C. James Mohr: The nursing assistant can obtain vital signs and oxygen saturation, and assist with ADLs. He or she should call the RN immediately if the patient coughs productively and indicates the airway is becoming blocked.

D. Amy Campbell: The nursing assistant can obtain vital signs and oxygen saturation, and assist with ADLs. He or she should notify the RN immediately if the patient develops severe respiratory distress. Adjusting the oxygen is not a nursing assistant function.

Content-Specific Questions

1. A. *Rationale: Arterial blood gases are drawn to evaluate gas exchange and hypoxemia. Carboxyhemoglobin levels determine carbon monoxide poisoning. Electrolytes are drawn if water aspiration is a possibility.*

2. A. *Rationale: A pH of less than 7.35 indicates acidosis. A pCO_2 greater than 45 mmHG indicates a respiratory problem. These results indicate respiratory acidosis.*

3. B. *Rationale: Corticosteroids have to be weaned off due to adrenal atrophy caused by taking them.*

4. D. *Rationale: Early signs of pulmonary tuberculosis are fatigue, weight loss, anorexia, low-grade afternoon fever, night sweats, and a dry cough. Purulent and/or blood-tinged sputum are later manifestations.*

5. A, C, E. *Rationale: Age-related changes in the older adults are decreased elastic recoil of lungs, loss of skeletal muscle strength, less elastic and more fibrotic alveoli, increases in residual volume, and decreased effectiveness of coughing.*

Concept Map

Hint: As you plan interventions to address Mrs. Hamer's nutritional status, consider the impact of her chronic lung disease on her oxygenation needs, nutrition/fluid needs, and ADLs.

Chapter 38: Assessing the Musculoskeletal System

1. **Answer: 3 Rationale:** Long bones have two broad ends that are called epiphyses.

2. **Answer: 1 Rationale:** *Abduction* is the term for moving an extremity away from the midline of the body.

3. **Answer: 1 Rationale:** Patients with gout have increased serum uric acid and if medication for treating gout is effective the serum level of uric acid should be decreased.

4. **Answer: 4 Rationale:** Women in their 60s are usually post-menopausal, and are at risk for decreased bone density as well as for fractures due to osteoporosis.

5. **Answer: 3 Rationale:** With decreased bone mass and decreased calcium absorption, the bones become brittle and at risk for fractures.

6. **Answer: 2 Rationale:** When assessing facial muscle strength the nurse would ask the patient to stick out his or her tongue.

7. **Answer: 4 Rationale:** Crepitation is a grating sound as the joint moves.

8. **Answer: 3 Rationale:** The ballottement test is used to assess for fluid in the knee joint.

9. **Answer: 2 Rationale:** Scoliosis is the term used to describe a lateral curve in the spine.

10. **Answer: 1 Rationale:** Pain and limited mobility are the most common manifestations of musculoskeletal disorders.

Chapter 39: Nursing Care of Patients with Musculoskeletal Trauma

1. **Answer: 2 Rationale:** Ice used on a sprained ankle immediately after injury will cause vasoconstriction of the blood vessels to decrease edema and pain.

2. **Answer: 3 Rationale:** A compound fracture means bone has broken the skin, which is the first line of defense against bacterial invasion.

3. **Answer: 3 Rationale:** Pale, cold fingers of an older woman with a cast could indicate decreased circulation to the hand.

4. **Answer: 4 Rationale:** Calcium deposits in the fracture site allow callus to begin to form as healing occurs.

5. **Answer: 2 Rationale:** Cyanosis and lack of sensation in the toes indicates decreased circulation and pressure on nerves; if this is not relieved soon permanent damage could occur.

6. **Answer: 2 Rationale:** Patients with deep vein thrombosis of the lower extremity require careful monitoring of the respiratory system for complications of emboli.

7. **Answer: 2 Rationale:** Patients who have suffered musculoskeletal injuries have soft tissue damage, muscle spasm, and swelling causing acute pain.

8. **Answer: 1 Rationale:** During the first 24 hours after amputation the remaining extremity is elevated above the level of the heart to promote venous return and decrease swelling.

9. **Answer: 4 Rationale:** Phantom limb pain is experienced by a majority of amputees, especially in the early postoperative period.

10. **Answer: 4 Rationale:** The amputated finger should be wrapped in a clean cloth, put in a plastic bag, and placed on ice (although not directly on ice, which could cause tissue frostbite) to preserve tissue. This will preserve the amputated finger so that it can be surgically reattached.

Chapter 40: Nursing Care of Patients with Musculoskeletal Disorders

1. **Answer: 2 Rationale:** *Risk for Falls* is the most significant nursing diagnosis in terms of long-term disability because falls may cause fractures in the patient with osteoporosis.

2. **Answer: 4 Rationale:** Most patients with osteoarthritis use NSAIDs for control of discomfort from disease.

3. **Answer: 2 Rationale:** Patients with gout have increased serum levels of uric acid.

4. **Answer: 3 Rationale:** In patients with osteoporosis and osteomalacia, fractures are a potential complication because of lack of calcium intake and vitamin D intake.

5. **Answer: 1 Rationale:** Being overweight by 30 pounds is indicative of an increased risk for osteoarthritis, especially in the joints of the legs.

6. **Answer: 3 Rationale:** By monitoring vital signs, hemoglobin, and hematocrit, the nurse can determine early if the fluid volume is deficient (caused by excessive bleeding), or if blood supply to an extremity is compromised.

7. **Answer: 1 Rationale:** Fever and weight loss are found in patients with rheumatoid arthritis.

8. **Answer: 3 Rationale:** In the nursing diagnosis *Ineffective Protection*, the most important intervention for the patient with SLE would be to practice careful hand hygiene, as SLE patients are at risk for opportunistic and severe infection.

9. **Answer: 4 Rationale:** Most cases of Lyme disease occur when an infected tick remains embedded for at least 24 hours.

10. **Answer: 2 Rationale:** Septic arthritis is a medical emergency; if not diagnosed quickly and treatment begun, destruction of the affected joint may occur.

Unit 10 Building Clinical Competence: Responses to Altered Musculoskeletal Function
Functional Health Pattern: Activity-Exercise Patterns

Functional Health Patterns
Hint: Because protecting the patient from falling is a top priority, the nurse uses many basic techniques to protect the patient when ambulating, but also turning, positioning, and transferring.

Priority Setting
1.
  A. Joyce Stevens should be seen first. *Rationale: Petechiae, difficulty breathing, and confusion can be signs of life-threatening pulmonary embolism that must be evaluated immediately.*
  B. Jesse Drummond should be seen second. *Rationale: While phantom pain is common following an amputation, Mr. Drummond had a bilateral amputation, which increases his anxiety and pain. The nurse needs to assess the stumps to determine if complications are also adding to the pain level.*
  C. José Rivera should be seen third. *Rationale: Mr. Rivera may need pain medication. The upcoming surgery may be causing anxiety, which increases pain.*
  D. Kim Wong should be seen last. *Rationale: Her vital signs do not indicate immediate concern, and results from the blood tests are needed to determine the cause of the symptoms.*

Health Promotion
1. Ms. Stevens should be taught to eat a diet high in protein to promote healing and high in calcium to strengthen bones. If she is prescribed anticoagulant medication, she may need to limit her intake of food high in vitamin K.
2. Yes. He needs high protein to heal and high calcium to strengthen his weakened bones.

Nursing Process
1.

	Nursing Diagnosis	Rationale
Jesse Drummond	*Impaired Physical Mobility* related to bilateral amputation	*Mr. Drummond had both legs amputated. He will be wheelchair bound unless he is able to get prosthetic legs.*
Joyce Stevens	*Ineffective Breathing Pattern*	*Ms. Stevens is exhibiting signs of pulmonary embolism, a life-threatening complication.*
José Rivera	*Altered Tissue Perfusion* related to surgery, gun shot wound, and osteomyelitis	*The circulation to the tissue of the upper leg was damaged by the gun shot. Subsequent infection impairs circulation further.*
Kim Wong	*Altered Tissue Perfusion*	*The symptoms of swollen joints, pain, and cyanotic digits indicates lack of circulation.*

2. B. *Rationale: Pushing the stump against soft and then harder surfaces will help toughen the skin.*
3. A. *Rationale: Anti-DNA antibodies are a specific indicator of systemic lupus erythematosus. Patients also have anemia, leukopenia, thrombocytopenia, and elevated eosinophil sedimentation rate.*
4. A. *Rationale: Place the patient in a private room and use standard precautions with good hand hygiene to prevent spread of the infection.*

Communication
1. "Mr. Drummond, I am sorry your legs hurt. What you are describe is called phantom pain and is very common immediately after amputation. Generally the pain eases as healing occurs. I will get you some medication. When your doctor gets here, I will have him talk with you more about your pain."
2. "Ms. Wong, I know it is hard for you to wait for the results of your tests, but until we have them, the doctor cannot determine if you have lupus or not. Once a diagnosis is made the options for treatment can be discussed with you. I will have the doctor talk with you as soon as possible."

Delegation
1.
  A. Jesse Drummond: The nursing assistant can obtain vital signs and help with all ADLs.
  B. Joyce Stevens: The nursing assistant can obtain vital signs, help with all ADLs, and help with the hip exerciser as directed and supervised by the RN.
  C. José Rivera: The nursing assistant can obtain vital signs, help transfer the patient to surgery, and set up the post-op room for his return.
  D. Kim Wong: The nursing assistant can obtain vital signs and help with all ADLs.

Content-Specific Questions
1. D. *Rationale: The patient with an above-the-knee amputation should not sit for prolonged periods of time, as prolonged sitting can lead to hip contracture.*
2. B. *Rationale: Meats, seafood, beans, spinach, asparagus are high-purine foods.*
3. D. *Rationale: Patients with autoimmune diseases are at increased risk of coronary heart disease such as myocardial infarction.*
4. C. *Rationale: The most toxic effects of NSAIDS are gastric irritation, ulceration, and bleeding.*
5. A, C, D, E, G. *Rationale: The 5 Ps of a neurovascular assessment are pain, pulses, pallor, paresis, and paresthesia.*

6. A. *Rationale: Smoking reduces bone density in menopausal women, making them at risk for osteoporosis.*
7. C. *Rationale: All answers are correct but the most important is to follow a regimen of rest, ice, compression, and elevation for 24 to 48 hours to reduce swelling and pain.*

Concept Map

Hint: Are there other Independent Interventions that can help this patient with impaired physical mobility? Which other identified nursing diagnosis would you identify as of highest priority during the first 48 hours after admission? Five days after the accident?

Chapter 41: Assessing the Nervous System

1. **Answer: 4 Rationale:** The blood-brain barrier controls the environment within by allowing oxygen, carbon dioxide, lipids, glucose, and water into the capillaries but preventing entry of urea, creatinine, toxins, proteins, and antibiotics.
2. **Answer: 3 Rationale:** The lower motor neurons maintain muscle tone and reflexes; any damage could result in loss of reflexes.
3. **Answer: 3 Rationale:** Cerebrospinal fluid (CSF) cushions the brain tissue and spinal cord, protects them from trauma, provides nourishment to the brain, and removes waste products.
4. **Answer: 1 Rationale:** The posterior spinal roots contain cells that discriminate fine touch sensations such as dull and sharp; therefore, damage to these roots would mean the patient would be unable to detect dull or sharp sensation.
5. **Answer: 1 Rationale:** The sympathetic division of the ANS has the purpose of preparing the body to handle stressful events, such as a near auto crash, by increasing heart rate, force of contraction, vasodilation of coronary arteries, and increased mental alertness.
6. **Answer: 2 Rationale:** Auscultation is not used in assessing the neurologic system.
7. **Answer: 1 Rationale:** A cotton ball and a safety pin would be used to assess sensations of light, dull, and sharp on the face.
8. **Answer: 4 Rationale:** In patients who are unconscious the corneal reflex is absent, so when the cornea is touched with a wisp of cotton, the patient does not blink.
9. **Answer: 3 Rationale:** A tongue depressor is used on the posterior section of the tongue to illicit a gag reflex, testing cranial nerve IX.
10. **Answer: 2 Rationale:** In decorticate posturing the upper arms are close to the body; the elbows, wrists, and fingers are flexed; and the legs are extended with internal rotation.

Chapter 42: Nursing Care of Patients with Intracranial Disorders

1. **Answer: 4 Rationale:** Normally the RAS and cerebral hemispheres control respirations with a regular pattern; however, when they are damaged, the lower brainstem responds to changes in $PaCO_2$, resulting in irregular respiratory patterns.
2. **Answer: 2 Rationale:** The unconscious patient with impaired gag or swallowing reflexes would be at risk for aspiration since saliva and any fluids taken by mouth could not be swallowed normally.
3. **Answer: 2 Rationale:** Osmotic diuretics increase the osmolality of blood by excreting water and leaving solutes; as a result, the water in the brain would is drawn into the vascular space.
4. **Answer: 3 Rationale:** Motor responses to a direct stimuli such as "squeeze my hand" are the best way to identify changes in mental status.
5. **Answer: 1, 2, 3 Rationale:** A patient with an altered LOC would probably have blood glucose to check for hypoglycemia, electrolytes to check for metabolic disturbances (especially sodium), and toxicology to test for drug or alcohol toxicity.

6. **Answer: 3 Rationale:** Serum osmolality would assess water and solute balance in the blood, indicating the hydration status of the patient.
7. **Answer: 2 Rationale:** Numbness and tingling in the corner of the patient's mouth that disappears within minutes or hours is a manifestation of temporary occlusion of the middle cerebral artery.
8. **Answer: 1 Rationale:** Hypertension is the greatest risk factor for a stroke because sustained systolic and diastolic pressure damage cerebral blood vessels.
9. **Answer: 3 Rationale:** The motor pathways of the nervous system cross at the medulla and spinal cord, meaning damage to the left cerebral vessel will demonstrate neurologic deficits on the right side, an effect called contralateral.
10. **Answer: 4 Rationale:** Tissue plasminogen activator is given within the first 3 hours of the ischemic stroke to cause fibrinolysis of the clot.

Chapter 43: Nursing Care of Patients with Spinal Cord Disorders and CNS Infections

1. **Answer: 3 Rationale:** SCI at the C1-C4 level produces respiratory paralysis and the patient will be unable to breathe on his or her own, so a ventilator will be necessary to maintain respiratory function.
2. **Answer: 1, 2, 4 Rationale:** Corticosteroids will be used to decrease cord edema. Vasopressors will be used to treat bradycardia or hypotension from spinal shock. Analgesics will be used to control pain.
3. **Answer: 1 Rationale:** In a patient with spinal cord injury no impulses are transmitted between the brain and spinal cord and the cord does not function at all, producing spinal shock that may last from minutes to weeks or months.
4. **Answer: 2 Rationale:** Autonomic dysreflexia can be caused by kinked catheter tubing that allows the bladder to become full, triggering massive vasoconstriction below the injury site and producing the manifestations of this process. The other answers will not cause autonomic dysreflexia.
5. **Answer: 1, 3, 5 Rationale:** In teaching prevention of back injuries the nurse would incorporate principles of proper body mechanics, which are spread feet apart, use large leg muscles, and work as close to the object as possible. Bending from the waist to lift rather than sometimes rolling or pushing will contribute to back injuries.
6. **Answer: 2 Rationale:** Monitor for signs of nerve root compression by assessing hand grips and arm strength, ability to move the fingers, and ability to detect touch.
7. **Answer: 1 Rationale:** The patient with a spinal cord tumor (regardless of type) requires nursing interventions to provide management of acute pain.
8. **Answer: 3 Rationale:** Young adults living in close proximity (such as college students living in a dormitory) are at a greater risk of contracting bacterial meningitis.
9. **Answer: 3 Rationale:** Mosquito control with repellants, insecticides, and protective clothing; destruction of the insect larvae and elimination of breeding places, such as pools of stagnant water; and community mosquito control programs can help prevent meningitis and encephalitis.
10. **Answer: 2 Rationale:** Tetanus is completely preventable by active immunization.

Chapter 44: Nursing Care of Patients with Neurologic Disorders

1. **Answer: 1, 2 Rationale:** Dementia is a general term used to describe the outcome of the death of neurons, and the cognitive and behavioral manifestations of AD.

2. **Answer: 3 Rationale:** Memory deficits are usually the first indication of AD. They are subtle and may not be noticed by friends and family until the patient exhibits unsafe behaviors.

3. **Answer: 1 Rationale:** *Fatigue* affects all patients with MS regardless of type or severity.

4. **Answer: 3 Rationale:** Interferons are used to reduce exacerbations in patients with multiple sclerosis and enhance immune function.

5. **Answer: 4 Rationale:** When teaching a young adult with MS it is important to stress avoidance of extremes of heat and cold since maintaining a constant body temperature will decrease exacerbations of manifestations, and heat slows down transmission of nerve impulses.

6. **Answer: 2 Rationale:** Parkinson's disease manifestations appear when the brain cells no longer produce enough dopamine to inhibit acetylcholine; this results in uncoordinated motor movement.

7. **Answer: 3 Rationale:** With the gait changes, balance problems, and possible orthostatic hypotension, patients with PD are at increased risk for falls. This safety issue needs to be addressed with the caregivers.

8. **Answer: 4 Rationale:** Antiglutamate is the drug classification used to treat ALS because it prevents the release of glutamic acid and protects against toxicity of neurons.

9. **Answer: 3 Rationale:** When teaching patients about Bell's palsy, the nurse needs to tell the patient that one side of the face will not move normally since the affected nerve supplies the muscles that produce expression on one side of the face.

10. **Answer: 1 Rationale:** Riluzole (Rilutek) is administered without food at the same time each day.

Unit 11 Building Clinical Competence: Responses to Altered Neurologic Function
Functional Health Pattern: Cognitive-Perceptual

Functional Health Patterns
Hint: Because neurological disorders can affect many aspects of the patient's ability to function independently, there are numerous things the nurse must assist with to maintain patient safety.

Priority Setting
1.
   A. Cesar Phillips should be seen first. *Rationale: BP 170/110 before medication 1.5 hours ago. The effectiveness of this treatment must be evaluated.*
   B. Louie Hernandez should be seen second. *Rationale: Mr. Hernandez may have swallowing difficulty and therefore may have difficulty keeping his airway clear. Aphasia may prevent him from summoning help if needed. Frequent observation is needed.*
   C. Tonya Walton should be seen second. *Rationale: The increasing head pain can indicate complications after neurosurgery and must be evaluated.*
   D. Jane Thomas should be seen last. *Rationale: Ms. Thomas is the most stable and has no urgent needs.*

Health Promotion
1. Ms. Thomas should be taught not to lift or move anything over 10 pounds until her surgeon approves. Once healing is complete, she must lift by using her legs, not her back. *Rationale: Lifting can traumatize the incision and prevent adequate healing. Using the back to lift heavy objects can cause further injury to lumbar discs.*
2. Both Mr. Hernandez and Mr. Phillips have been smokers for a long time. They should be informed that smoking increases blood pressure, which can lead to stroke. They should be provided with information on local stop-smoking programs. *Rationale: Research shows that smoking increases the risk of hypertension, strokes, and heart disease. Many stop-smoking programs are effective.*

Nursing Process
1. B. *Rationale: Heart sounds and pain assessment are part of a beginning-of-shift baseline assessment. Because Mr. Hernandez may be having difficulty swallowing, assessing fluid balance is important.*
2. C. *Rationale: The previous nurse gave Ms. Walton Tylenol ES for a headache of 6 on a scale of 1 to 10. You should evaluate the effectiveness of this medication by determining the current pain level on the same 1 to 10 scale.*
3. D. *Rationale: Mr. Phillips was given an antihypertensive medication 1.5 hours ago. Because his blood pressure was 170/110 when the medication was given, a blood pressure of 145/90 would indicate that the medication was effective.*
4. A, B, D, E. *Rationale: All of these are topics that should be discussed before discharge. There is no indication that Ms. Thomas is overweight.*
5. A, D, E. *Rationale: White blood cell count would indicate the presence of infection. Hematocrit and hemoglobin would indicate fluid balance and hemostasis. These are priorities after any surgery.*
6. B. *Rationale: Increased headache that is not controlled with medication indicates increased intracranial pressure and must be reported to the physician.*

Communication
1. Explain to Mrs. Phillips that the MRI indicated that a stroke has caused her husband's symptoms. Acknowledge that strokes are more common in older people, but that Mr. Phillips is at risk because of his uncontrolled hypertension and smoking. *Rationale: Mrs. Phillips is grieving the loss of her husband's function and needs accurate information and reassurance.*
2. Explain that it is too early to determine how much permanent neurologic deficits Mr. Hernandez will have. Explain that Mr. Hernandez's rehabilitation will be evaluated frequently and plans will be discussed with her at that time. *Rationale: Over time, rehabilitation can be effective in restoring neurologic function. The amount of permanent neurologic deficit cannot be determined until this time.*

Delegation
1.
   A. Mr. Hernandez: The nursing assistant can obtain vital signs and assist with ADLs. Instruct him or her not to provide oral intake until swallowing evaluation is obtained.
   B. Ms. Thomas: The nursing assistant can obtain vital signs and assist with ADLs. Remind the him or her to assist the patient to log roll to prevent twisting of the lumbar spine.
   C. Mr. Phillips: The nursing assistant can obtain vital sings and assist with ADLs. Mr. Phillips should remain in bed and will need assistance to turn every 2 hours.
   D. Ms. Walton: The nursing assistant can obtain vital signs and assist with ADLs. Ms. Walton should remain in bed, and will need assistance turning every 2 hours.

Content-Specific Questions
1. The disciplines the nurse should include in a discharge planning meeting would be Medicine, Physical Therapy, Occupational Therapy, Speech Therapy, Dietitian, and Social Work. The patient and/or a family member should also be included. These disciplines can provide valuable input for planning rehabilitation services.

2. Yes, with the exception that speech therapy would not be necessary because the patient with cervical injury can still speak. Respiratory therapy would be a valuable addition because the patient may experience respiratory distress and have difficulty clearing the airway.

Concept Map

Hint: **When planning care for the patient with impaired swallowing, consider not only independent nursing interventions, but also patient, family, and caregiver teaching as well as appropriate referrals.**

Chapter 45: Assessing the Eye and Ear

1. **Answer: 2 Rationale:** When the cornea is touched the patient will blink as a mechanism to protect it from foreign objects.
2. **Answer: 4 Rationale:** Presbyopia develops in older adults as the lens of the eye looses its ability to adjust, requiring the patient to hold papers farther away in order to focus and read.
3. **Answer: 2 Rationale:** Tuning forks are used to assess if hearing loss is conductive or sensorineural.
4. **Answer: 1 Rationale:** As the light enters the lens, the rays bend and are focused on a single point on the retina; this focusing is called accommodation.
5. **Answer: 4 Rationale:** Patients having a test of refraction will have the pupil dilated to examine the internal eye structures.
6. **Answer: 3 Rationale:** Receptors within the inner ear maintain equilibrium by responding to changes in head position in order to coordinate body movements and balance.
7. **Answer: 1 Rationale:** The Snellen eye chart measures the patient's ability to read letters at a standard distance of twenty feet. The patient reads the smallest line possible, and the numbers on the side indicate visual acuity, for example, 20/20, 20/30.
8. **Answer: 1 Rationale:** The examiner can whisper a word 1 or 2 feet behind the patient, asking the patient to repeat the word; this may provide a rough estimate of hearing acuity.
9. **Answer: 2 Rationale:** The vestibular structures maintain balance. As the person ages this function may decrease and the patient may be at risk for falling.
10. **Answer: 4 Rationale:** The examiner must have a normal visual field when assessing the visual field of a patient because the examiner's field becomes the standard or norm. If the examiner does not have normal visual field then the results of this part of the exam will be inaccurate.

Chapter 46: Nursing Care of Patients with Eye and Ear Disorders

1. **Answer: 4 Rationale:** The highest priority for residents with moderate to severe hearing or vision impairment is safety.
2. **Answer: 2 Rationale:** In teaching a patient with newly diagnosed glaucoma, the nurse emphasizes the importance of taking eye drops as prescribed on a continuing basis to control intraocular pressure and prevent vision loss.
3. **Answer: 3 Rationale:** Timolol is a beta adrenergic blocker that can decrease myocardial contractility and impair cardiac function in the patient with heart failure.
4. **Answer: 4 Rationale:** The highest priority for a patient with repeated attacks of vertigo and tinnitus is maintenance of safety. Sitting when an attack occurs reduces the risk of injury from falling.
5. **Answer: 1 Rationale:** Following eye surgery, patients are placed in semi-Fowler's or Fowler's position to reduce intraocular pressure and edema.

6. **Answer: 3 Rationale:** Immediate referral to an ophthalmologist is necessary because the manifestations suggest a detached retina. Immediate treatment is necessary to optimize sight restoration.
7. **Answer: 1, 2, 3, 4, 5 Rationale:** All the assessments should be included because each provides information about infection and possible location in the ear.
8. **Answer: 4 Rationale:** Aging is a risk factor for cerumen impaction because there is less and it is harder and drier. The nurse should inspect the ear canal for patency.
9. **Answer: 1 Rationale:** One-on-one social interactions in a quiet environment facilitate effective communication for the patient with a severe hearing deficit.
10. **Answer: 2 Rationale:** Cataract removal is elective surgery, generally performed only when visual impairment interferes with activities of daily living.

Unit 12 Building Clinical Competence: Responses to Altered Visual and Auditory Function
Functional Health Pattern: Cognitive-Perceptual Pattern

Functional Health Patterns

Hint: **When the patient cannot see clearly, the nurse must be diligent to maintain a safe environment including helping others to be aware of safety measures. The nurse can use a variety of communication techniques when working with hearing impaired patients. If written communication is used, the nurse must be sure the patient can read and write.**

Priority Setting
1.
A. Kenneth Koch should be seen first. *Rationale: Mr. Koch is having severe pain and needs to be assessed and medicated.*
B. Georgia Stanley should be seen second. *Rationale: Ms. Stanley is scheduled for x-rays and an MRI. She must be assessed before she leaves her room.*
C. Andrew Hardy should be seen third. *Rationale: Mr. Hardy's blood glucose was 600 on admission and must be reevaluated do determine the effectiveness of treatment.*
D. Gladys Harvey should be seen last. *Rationale: Ms. Harvey is experiencing routine post-op recovery and is stable.*

Health Promotion
1. Teach Ms. Stanley to avoid sudden head movements and position changes, to take prescribed medications, and to lie down in a quiet darkened room when feeling an impending attack. Discuss with her methods to maintain safety if an attack occurs when she is driving a car or using other mechanical equipment.
2. Teach Mr. Hardy to control his diabetes and make appropriate referrals for diabetic education. Teach him to take his prescribed antihypertensive medication, to be seen by an ophthalmologist annually, and to report black spots, floaters, cobwebs, or eye pain immediately.
3. D. *Rationale: Loud noises above 85 decibels may cause hearing loss.*

Nursing Process
1.

	Nursing Diagnosis	Rationale
Andrew Hardy	*Altered Nutrition: More than Body Requirements*	*Mr. Hardy had a blood glucose of 600. Lowering the blood glucose level is the highest priority for him.*

Gladys Harvey	*Sensory-Perceptual Alterations: Input Deficit* related to eye surgery	*Ms. Harvey's vision is decreased due to R eye patch from surgery.*
Georgia Stanley	*High Risk for Injury* related to vertigo	*Ms. Stanley has been experiencing vertigo that has resulted in falling.*
Kenneth Koch	*Pain* related to ear surgery	*Mr. Koch is experiencing pain at 9 on a scale of 1 to 10.*

2. D. *Rationale: Laser photocoagulation is the treatment for both forms of diabetic retinopathy. This treatment seals the leaking microaneurysms, and proliferating vessels are destroyed to reduce further damage.*

3. B. *Rationale: After eye surgery, place the patient in semi-Fowler's or Fowler's position on the unaffected side.*

4. C. *Rationale: Grilled chicken with lettuce and tomato are low in sodium. Ketchup, cheese, and potato chips are high in sodium.*

5. A, B, F. *Rationale: Diagnostic studies for Ménière's disease are caloric testing, Rinne and Weber tests, and glycerol test. These studies test impaired vestibular function and hearing.*

6. B. *Rationale: Coughing or sneezing increases intraocular pressure and may lead to postoperative complications. Avoid lifting more than 5 pounds. Lie on the unaffected side. Maintain eye patch to prevent injury to the eye.*

Communication

1. B, D, E, F. *Rationale: To improve communication with a patient with hearing loss, speak in a normal tone while facing the patient, and use short sentences and pauses to increase comprehension. Speak at a normal rate and avoid over articulating to make lip-reading easier. Reduce environmental noises to decrease distractions.*

Delegation

1.
   A. Andrew Hardy: The nursing assistant can obtain vital signs and blood glucose by finger stick, and assist with ambulating to maintain safety.
   B. Gladys Harvey: The nursing assistant can obtain vital signs and assist with ADLs as needed, including ambulation to maintain safety.
   C. Georgia Stanley: The nursing assistant can obtain vital signs, assist with ADLs, assist with ambulation to maintain safety, and prepare the room for the patient's return from radiology.
   D. Kenneth Koch: The nursing assistant can obtain vital signs and assist with ADLs as needed, including ambulation to maintain safety.

Content-Specific Questions

1. A. *Rationale: Hyphema is bleeding into the anterior chamber of the eye. Assessment of hyphema includes eye pain, decreased visual acuity, and seeing a reddish tint.*

2. A. *Rationale: Gentamicin may damage the eighth cranial nerve, resulting in hearing loss.*

3. C. *Rationale: The correct way to administer ear drops is to have the patient lie on the unaffected side, pull the pinna up and back, instill the ear drops, and have the patient remain on the side for approximately 5 minutes.*

Concept Map

Hint: Are there more detailed Independent Interventions that you can identify for this patient? Review Chapter 20 as you develop your second concept map addressing this patient's risk for visual impairment. How do your nursing diagnosis and planned interventions compare between the two concept maps?

Chapter 47: Assessing the Male and Female Reproductive Systems

1. **Answer: 3 Rationale:** The obese male may have enlarged breasts, called gynecomastia.
2. **Answer: 4 Rationale:** In the female, the clitoris is an erectile organ similar to the penis in the male.
3. **Answer: 2 Rationale:** The explanation should begin by explaining that the prostate gland surrounds the urethra.
4. **Answer: 1 Rationale:** PSA is the diagnostic test used to diagnose and monitor prostate cancer.
5. **Answer: 1 Rationale:** Testicular self-examination is one method of providing health management.
6. **Answer: 3 Rationale:** Following menopause the estrogen level drops and cholesterol increases, putting the woman at risk for cardiovascular disease.
7. **Answer: 1 Rationale:** When women of reproductive age become pregnant, menstruation normally stops until after delivery.
8. **Answer: 4 Rationale:** Pap smears are used to detect cervical cancers and precancerous lesions of the cervix.
9. **Answer: 3 Rationale:** Palpation is used to detect any lumps or changes in breast tissues.
10. **Answer: 2 Rationale:** Vaginal bleeding after menopause is not normal and should be reported to the healthcare provider.

Chapter 48: Nursing Care of Men with Reproductive System and Breast Disorders

1. **Answer: 4 Rationale:** This is stated in an appropriate way to allow the patient to feel free to ask any questions about his sexual concerns.
2. **Answer: 2 Rationale:** In a health teaching session with young men, the nurse should tell them about retracting the foreskin while showering, and cleaning regularly to decrease the presence of collection of secretions under the foreskin, which has been shown to increase the risk of penile cancer.
3. **Answer: 1 Rationale:** Sexually active men who have gonorrhea are especially susceptible to inflammation or infection of the epididymis.
4. **Answer: 2 Rationale:** Testicular cancer commonly occurs between the ages of 15 and 40.
5. **Answer: 3 Rationale:** Men with chronic prostatitis should increase their fluid intake to 3L/day and void often to decrease the irritation when voiding.
6. **Answer: 2, 4 Rationale:** In digital rectal examination for BPH, the prostate is asymmetrical and enlarged, while in prostate cancer the exam shows nodules and a fixed position. PSA is specific to the prostate and is released by both benign and malignant cells; however, in BPH the amounts of the free form of PSA and complex PSA would be different.
7. **Answer: 2 Rationale:** As the prostate enlarges around the urethra it begins to obstruct the outflow of urine from the bladder during urination, causing problems with urinary retention, frequency, and urgency.
8. **Answer: 3 Rationale:** The nurse needs to notify the surgeon because dark red fluid with obvious clots and painful bladder spasms could indicate that the patient may be hemorrhaging postoperatively.
9. **Answer: 1 Rationale:** Prostate cancer is the most common type of malignancy in American men.
10. **Answer: 4 Rationale:** Some studies have shown an increase in prostate cancer in men with diets high in red meats and fats. Informing the community of this relationship could help men change their dietary habits to decrease the risk of prostate cancer.

Chapter 49: Nursing Care of Women with Reproductive System and Breast Disorders

1. **Answer: 1 Rationale:** The nurse acknowledging the problem stated by the patient gives credence for the patient, but because the nurse is uncomfortable addressing the issue herself, she refers the patient to the physician.
2. **Answer: 2, 3, 4 Rationale:** Osteoporosis, cardiovascular disease, and fractures are all related to estrogen deprivation.
3. **Answer: 1200 Rationale:** This level can be achieved through diet and supplements if necessary.
4. **Answer: 1 Rationale:** Kegel exercises strengthen perineal muscle tone and minimize stress incontinence.
5. **Answer: 2 Rationale:** A health-promotion seminar for reducing the risk of cervical cancer should contain information about safe sex methods that reduce the incidence of genital infections from HPV, which is the most important risk factor.
6. **Answer: 4 Rationale:** For a woman with PMS, the nurse would recommend a decrease in sodium intake to help minimize the fluid retention due to the increased production of aldosterone, which results in sodium retention and edema.
7. **Answer: 2 Rationale:** Endometrial implantations tend to atrophy and disappear after menopause since ovarian hormones no longer stimulate them.
8. **Answer: 1, 3, 4 Rationale:** A teaching plan for home care of a woman following an abdominal hysterectomy should include no lifting to decrease chances of hemorrhage, reporting temperature > 100°F since this may be a sign of infection, and taking regular rest periods since she may be tired for several days postoperatively.
9. **Answer: 4 Rationale:** Risk factors for breast cancer are doubled for the 64-year-old with a positive family history.
10. **Answer: 3 Rationale:** *Grieving* is an appropriate nursing diagnosis since she is losing a portion of her body.

Chapter 50: Nursing Care of Patients with Sexually Transmitted Infections

1. **Answer: 2 Rationale:** Women and infants are disproportionately affected by STIs because women may not experience manifestations of the disease and pass the infection on to the infant through vaginal birth.
2. **Answer: 1 Rationale:** STIs must be treated by treating both partners to prevent reinfection from one to the other, since manifestations are not always demonstrated when the infection is present.
3. **Answer: 1, 4, 5 Rationale:** Topics of information when teaching a male to prevent an STI should include using a new condom with each sex act, careful handling to prevent damage to condom, and withdrawal from the vagina when the penis is erect, holding the condom against the base of the penis to prevent contamination of the penis.
4. **Answer: 4 Rationale:** Blisters and ulcers appear on the penis of a patient infected with genital herpes.
5. **Answer: 1 Rationale:** Genital warts are caused by a viral infection (not yeast).
6. **Answer: 4 Rationale:** Women with HPV genital infection should be advised to have a pelvic exam and Pap smear every year since this infection causes an increased risk in developing cervical cancer, and the annual exams would identify the cancer early.
7. **Answer: 2 Rationale:** Itching is the most common manifestation experienced by a woman with a vaginal infection.
8. **Answer: 3 Rationale:** When teaching a woman with an STI experiencing severe genital discomfort, a simple recommendation is to wear cotton underwear because it absorbs moisture and allows airflow better than other materials.
9. **Answer: 1 Rationale:** The male urethra and female cervix are initially affected by the gonorrheal organism.
10. **Answer: 3 Rationale:** Syphilis is a systemic infection that is caused by a spirochete that can affect a developing fetus.

Unit 13 Building Clinical Competence: Responses to Altered Reproductive Function
Functional Health Pattern: Sexuality-Reproductive Pattern

Functional Health Patterns
Hint: Think about your nonverbal communication techniques that can put the patient at ease and increase the patient's comfort.

Priority Setting
1. In what order would you visit these patients after report?
   A. Wendy Torrell should be seen first. *Rationale: Ms. Torrell has had major abdominal bleeding and is at risk for impaired tissue perfusion.*
   B. Tara Morris should be seen second. *Rationale: She has an elevated temperature and a significant infection that must be assessed. Her IV antibiotics need to be administered on time.*
   C. Barney Green should be seen third. *Rationale: Because Mr. Green is a postoperative patient, he is at risk for bleeding and infection. His output needs to be assessed because the Foley catheter was removed.*
   D. Regina Perkins should be seen last. *Rationale: Ms. Perkins is stable and is ready for discharge. By assessing her last, the nurse can provide discharge teaching at the same time.*

Health Promotion
1. Ms. Torrell should be encouraged to eat foods high in iron and folic acid, including dark green vegetables and deep yellow fruits and vegetables. She should take prescribed iron supplements and eat high-fiber foods to maintain normal bowel function.
2. Ms. Morris should be instructed to abstain from sexual intercourse until the infection has cleared. She should be instructed to use condoms unless she is in a monogamous relationship.

Nursing Process
1.

	Nursing Diagnosis	Rationale
Wendy Torrell	*Fluid Volume Deficit* related to blood loss	*Ms. Torrell lost enough blood to require replacement of 2 units of whole blood.*
Barney Green	*Altered Urinary Elimination Patterns* related to TURP	*Mr. Green is dribbling urine after the catheter is removed.*
Tara Morris	*Infection of Reproductive Organs* as evidenced by purulent vaginal drainage, pain, and fever	*Infection must be resolved to prevent damage to the reproductive organs.*
Regina Perkins	*Knowledge Deficit* related to postoperative care	*Ms. Perkins is recovering normally and is ready for discharge instruction.*

2. B. *Rationale: For Ms. Torrell the abdominal binder is used to control intra-abdominal bleeding. Abdominal binders can be used to support the abdominal muscles especially in obese patients, but there is no indication that these were the purpose in Ms. Torrell's case.*

3. C. *Rationale: Absorption of isotonic irrigating fluids during and after surgery may cause a hypervolemic and hyponatremic state.*

4. A. *Rationale: All are correct. The most important is to take all medications for the prescribed amount of doses to completely cure the infection.*

5. A. *Rationale: Beef and eggs are high in heme iron. Brown rice is high in nonheme iron. Heme iron foods promote absorption of nonheme iron foods when eaten together. Broccoli, asparagus, kidney beans, and green, leafy vegetables are high in folic acid.*

Communication

1. Some reproductive infections can cause scar tissue of the fallopian tubes. There would be a possibility of having difficulty becoming pregnant or developing a tubal pregnancy if that occurs. The doctor or healthcare provider can provide more information in her specific case.

2. Dribbling urine after the Foley catheter is removed following a TURP is common. Usually the dribbling stops once complete healing occurs. It is too early to determine if dribbling will be permanent.

Delegation

1.

A. Wendy Torrell: The nursing assistant can obtain vital signs, empty the Foley catheter every hour, and provide ADLs. He or she should be instructed not to get Ms. Torrell out of bed and to keep her NPO until it is determined surgery will not be necessary.

B. Barney Green: The nursing assistant can obtain vital signs and assist with ADLs. Mr. Green may need assistance with ambulation.

C. Tara Morris: The nursing assistant can obtain vital signs and assist with ADLs. He or she should be instructed to obtain a temperature every 2 hours until it is within normal limits for 24 hours.

D. Regina Perkins: The nursing assistant can obtain vital signs and offer breakfast prior to discharge. He or she can assist with packing belongings and can take Ms. Perkins to her car in a wheelchair once the discharge process is complete.

Content-Specific Questions

1. D. *Rationale: The priority nursing diagnosis with endometriosis is* Anxiety *related to risk for loss of reproductive function due to increased risk of infertility.*

2. B. *Rationale: Cialis is incompatible with many medications, such as nitrates, alpha blockers, antibiotics, and antifungals.*

3. A, C, F. *Rationale: VDRL and RPR blood tests measure syphilis antibody production. FTA-ABS is an antibody test used for symptomatic patients who test negative to VDRL.*

4. B. *Rationale: To prevent radiation damage to others, avoid close contact with pregnant women, infants, and children. Other factors related to radiation therapy are to sleep alone for the first week, eat less red meat, and use condoms for sexual contact.*

5. D. *Rationale: Vaginal bleeding after intercourse or between menstrual periods may be the first symptom of cervical cancer. Other answers are later symptoms of cervical cancer.*

6. C. *Rationale: Condoms provide the best protection of birth control when being treated for gonorrhea.*

Concept Map

Hint: **As you prioritize identified nursing diagnoses and interventions, think about the other physical problems the patient has or might have and the psychological issues with which she must cope. Reviewing Chapter 14 will be helpful in developing your second concept map for this patient.**

Evaluate Your Response: Cues for Critical Thinking Questions

Chapter 4: Nursing Care of Patients Having Surgery
A Patient Having Surgery

1. Safety concerns include ambulating and not tripping over scatter rugs or clutter. See the information in Chapter 3 on safety in the home.

2. Medications used to prevent an occurrence such as infection are called prophylactic medications. Her risks for infection are from the surgical wound and microvascular circulation in bone. Teach her to take the complete course of antibiotics prescribed and about the possible side effects of the antibiotic. Encourage her to notify the physician if side effects or adverse events occur.

3. When blood stops flowing, it clots. Her immobility is a concern and puts her at risk for thrombosis and emboli. She has a risk for bleeding secondary to the anticoagulant and should inform healthcare providers such as dentists that she is taking the anticoagulant.

4. Consider the risk for osteoporosis in addition to the degenerative changes Mrs. Overbeck experienced. She will need calcium sources and vitamin D.

Chapter 5: Nursing Care of Patients Experiencing Loss, Grief, and Death
A Patient Experiencing Loss and Grief

1. Review the physical manifestations of grief described in the chapter and compare and contrast those with the ones verbalized by Mrs. Rogers.

2. Consider the benefits of including Mrs. Rogers's daughter in a meeting of the staff. What type of questions would be most useful in making the daughter feel a part of the plan of care? Why would a statement such as "Why don't you do more for your mother" be inappropriate?

3. Consider the losses Mrs. Rogers has experienced. Review the material in the chapter on responses to loss. Think about the reasons you would not say, "Oh, you have a lot to live for." Think of two or three questions or statements that would help you assess the reason why Mrs. Rogers said this to you.

Chapter 6: Nursing Care of Patients with Problems of Substance Abuse
A Patient Having Withdrawal from Alcohol

1. Consider the interactions of prescribed or over-the-counter medications with alcohol. What if the patient has not taken prescribed medications because of chronic alcoholism?

2. Review the effects of Antabuse. Make a list of possible interactions and side effects.

3. *Imbalanced Nutrition: Less than Body Requirements* is an appropriate nursing diagnosis when a patient does not have sufficient nutritional intake to meet metabolic needs. What in Mr. Russell's history and physical assessment supports this diagnosis? What nutritional information should you provide?

Chapter 7: Nursing Care of Patients Experiencing Disasters

A Patient with Injuries from a Natural Disaster

1. Consider how Mr. Jones put himself at risk for infection (see Chapter 12). How could Mr. Jones have avoided exacerbating his skin lesions?
2. Since Mr. Jones has a history of elevated blood pressure that has not been consistently treated or monitored, cardiac status should be evaluated. Which tests are indicated? Also, could his decreased sensation and poor healing be related to cardiac impairment? Mr. Jones also has identifying data in his history and physical to suggest diabetes. Identify this data and tests that would be indicated.
3. Review risk factors for and causes and manifestations of infection in Chapter 12. Identify the factors that contributed to Mr. Jones's fever.
4. Consider Mr. Jones's environmental and personal situations. What information do you have about Mr. Jones that indicates a lack of interest in health maintenance? Are there signs of a change in outlook?

Chapter 9: Nursing Care of Patients in Pain

A Patient Experiencing Chronic Pain

1. Review the factors that affect an individual's response to pain. What have you observed in your own family and friends, as well as patients for whom you have cared?
2. Reflect on the benefits and disadvantages of each alternative. Make your decision based on knowledge about pain and about medications for pain.
3. What factors in Ms. Akers's illness and treatment increase her risk for constipation? What would you include in the plan specific to fluid intake and diet?

Chapter 10: Nursing Care of Patients with Altered Fluid, Electrolyte, and Acid–Base Balance

A Patient with Hypokalemia

1. Review the physiologic effects of potassium, especially its intracellular and neuromuscular effects.
2. Review the potential sites and causes of excess potassium loss.
3. Think about the effects of diuretics on potassium balance and the effects of hypokalemia on digitalis therapy. What is the primary indication for digitalis therapy and how does this contribute to the interaction of these three factors?
4. Review the section in Chapter 24 on the causes and management of constipation.

A Patient with Hyperkalemia

1. Review the causes and manifestations of hyperkalemia.
2. What are the potential effects of hyperkalemia on cardiac conduction? At what level of hyperkalemia are these likely to be seen?
3. Review collaborative treatment measures to rapidly reduce potassium levels. Why would these be used with a K1 of 8.5?
4. Think about the effects of anxiety on learning as you develop a plan to provide teaching to avoid future episodes of hyperkalemia. As you develop your plan, remember the potential long-term effects of chronic renal failure.

A Patient with Acute Respiratory Acidosis

1. Review normal gas exchange across the alveolar-capillary membrane and the processes that drive this exchange. Then review the role that carbon dioxide plays as a potential acid.
2. Describe the effect of acidosis on cerebral neurons. What manifestations of mental impairment may result?

3. Consider risk factors for choking such as alcohol consumption, taking large bites of food, or inadequate chewing.

Chapter 11: Nursing Care of Patients Experiencing Trauma and Shock

A Patient with Multiple Injuries

1. The definition of *Deficient Fluid Volume* is decreased intravascular, interstitial, and/or intracellular fluid. Which of Mrs. Souza's vital signs would support this definition? What other assessments could you make that would further support this diagnosis?
2. Consider the physiology of cellular metabolism. How long do brain cells live without oxygen? What happens if circulation is improved but the airway is blocked?
3. What can cause restlessness? Consider comfort, elimination, oxygenation, emotional status, and immobility.
4. List the multiple possibilities for entry of pathogens into the human body. Would age and physical condition increase the risk? What about transmission from healthcare personnel?

A Patient with Septic Shock

1. Review the pharmacologic effects of vasopressors. Consider the pathologic basis for septic shock and how these medications may be effective.
2. Review the content on respiratory acidosis in Chapter 10. What do these findings tell you? What is present in Ms. Huang's physical status that would cause these manifestations?
3. Review the content about colloidal intravenous solutions in this chapter. What would you expect these solutions to do when they are administered? How does this correlate to cardiac output? How do you assess increased circulatory volume?

Chapter 12: Nursing Care of Patients with Infections

A Patient with Acquired Immunity

1. Review the adult immunizations listed in this chapter. Consider the geographical area in which the patient lives. For example, patients living in areas at risk for Lyme disease should check with their physician about the new Lyme disease vaccine.
2. Review the concept of acquired immunity and the discussion of immunization in this chapter. What affect could nonimmunized persons have on their family and community?
3. Identify possible systemic and local reactions associated with immunizations. List manifestations that the patient should report to the primary caregiver.

Chapter 13: Nursing Care of Patients with Altered Immunity

A Patient with HIV Infection

1. Considering Ms. Lu's age, how effective is her immune system? How could lifestyle factors affect immune status?
2. At this stage of Ms. Lu's diagnosis, would you expect the physician to order a viral load test? Why or why not?
3. To what community resources could you refer Ms. Lu and her fiancé regarding their desire to have a child?

Chapter 14: Nursing Care of Patients with Cancer

A Patient with Cancer

1. Review content on altered nutrition in Chapter 22 and the content in this chapter on the nursing diagnosis *Imbalanced Nutrition: Less than Body Requirements*. Make a list of diagnostic tests for malnutrition with normal values.
2. Consider the type of cancers Mr. Casey has been diagnosed as having. Where in the body do these malignancies commonly metastasize? What would cause the pain?

3. Review a pharmacology book for medications that increase appetite and make a list of those appropriate to Mr. Casey.
4. Review the content in Chapter 11 on septic shock and outline manifestations. Develop a plan of care for Mr. Casey that is structured by priority of nursing diagnoses.

Chapter 16: Nursing Care of Patients with Integumentary Disorders

A Patient with Herpes Zoster

1. Consider environmental, economic, and language barriers. What agencies in your own city or state exist to provide help? What can you do other than make referrals? If you do make a referral, to whom would it be?
2. Review skin assessment guidelines in Chapter 15. How would you determine that the lesions had not improved? What manifestations would indicate secondary infection of the lesions? What would you do next if the lesions are still very painful and have not improved?
3. *Ineffective Role Performance* is defined as patterns of behavior and self-expression that do not match environmental context, norms, and expectations. Related factors include inadequate or inappropriate linkage with the healthcare system and poverty. Based on this information, what interventions would you use? How would you evaluate the effectiveness of your interventions?

A Patient with Malignant Melanoma

1. List reasons why people do not seek health care. Do you believe nurses can effect change? If so, what community activities would be most effective?
2. Consider attitudes toward the possibility of future illnesses. How would this affect your plan? What do you believe would be most effective in teaching this age group?
3. Think about what you know about taking prescribed antibiotics as well as the side effects of antibiotic therapy. What would you suggest that Mr. Sanders do?
4. *Powerlessness* is the perception that one's own actions will not significantly affect an outcome. Is this a common response to the diagnosis of cancer? Consider types of communications and interventions that would allow greater decision making for Mr. Sanders.

Chapter 17: Nursing Care of Patients with Burns

A Patient with a Major Burn

1. Review the effects of the major burn wound on the renal and gastrointestinal systems. What assessments would indicate effective fluid resuscitation?
2. What type of burns did Mr. Howard have on his arms? Consider the effect of compression on the peripheral vascular system. What assessments would you make to identify this complication?
3. Consider the type of pain the patient has. What do you think might happen if the narcotics were given by other routes, such as oral or intramuscular?
4. Review the effects of a major burn. Consider the damage to cell wall integrity and capillary beds. What effect does the shift of proteins and sodium have on intravascular volume?

Chapter 19: Nursing Care of Patients with Endocrine Disorders

A Patient with Graves' Disease

1. What effect does increased TH have on metabolism and cardiac rate and stroke volume? How does this effect compare to that of sympathetic stimulation?

2. Consider the effect of elevating any body part, such as elevating your leg above heart level for a sprained ankle. How does this affect venous return?
3. You will need to consider Mrs. Manuel from both a medical and a surgical perspective. How would you teach her to care for her incision? With removal of most of the thyroid gland, what manifestations would you be sure she knew about? What should she do if these occur?

A Patient with Hypothyroidism

1. Make a list of changes in body systems that occur with aging and with decreased TH levels. How would you determine what assessment findings were abnormal?
2. Consider the effects of the following factors: weakness, fatigue, problems with memory. What would you recommend she do in her home to increase her safety?
3. Prepare a list of manifestations of hyperthyroidism. Be sure they are in terms a patient would understand.

A Patient with Cushing's Syndrome

1. Review Ms. Domico's lab results and compare them to normal results. What altered the findings in her case?
2. How many ways can you think of to assess fluid balance? Consider weight, I&O, and skin. What other assessments provide information?
3. How does fatigue differ from "just being tired"? Would increasing hours of sleep be an intervention you would include? Why or why not?

A Patient with Addison's Disease

1. Review the functions of the hormones of the adrenal cortex in Chapter 18. Consider the effects of stress, and formulate your response with rationale.
2. Review content on fluid imbalance in Chapter 10. Make a list of assessments you might make that would indicate severe dehydration. What is the pathophysiology of fluid loss in the patient with Addison's disease?
3. Review content on sodium and potassium in Chapter 10 and make a list of foods you would suggest Mr. Sardoff eat.

Chapter 20: Nursing Care of Patients with Diabetes Mellitus

A Patient with Type 1 DM

1. How do the increased urinary output and increased osmolarity of the blood plasma affect the fluid status of the body? What is the response of the body to decreased intravascular volume?
2. Consider the effects of nicotine on blood vessels. How would these effects, when combined with the pathologic effects of long-standing hyperglycemia, affect blood vessel walls?
3. Review the information about chronic illness in Chapter 2. Powerlessness is a perceived lack of control over a situation and/or one's ability to significantly affect an outcome. What types of statements by a patient would help you make this nursing diagnosis?
4. Compare and contrast the developmental needs and tasks of the young adult and the older adult (see Chapter 2). Consider the teaching materials that might have to be adapted to physical changes in the older adult.

Chapter 22: Nursing Care of Patients with Nutritional Disorders

A Patient with Obesity

1. Review the physiology of cholesterol formation in the body and the factors that affect this process.

2. Consider developmental stages and teaching strategies for adult learners.

3. Think about individual factors, family and support group influences, and cultural factors that may affect recommended weight loss and exercise strategies.

A Patient with Malnutrition

1. Review the physiology of albumin and cholesterol formation in the body.

2. Review Mrs. Chow's diet and compare it to the food pyramid or recommendations for food intake to formulate your response.

3. Consider cultural influences and the patient's preferred foods as you plan a diet that is high in calories and protein.

Chapter 23: Nursing Care of Patients with Upper Gastrointestinal Disorders

A Patient with Oral Cancer

1. Review the major risk factors for oral cancer and identify the populations most likely to have these risk factors.

2. Work with your classmates to plan (and implement) an education program, considering the developmental/teaching needs of this group of young people.

3. Think about the possible causes for Mr. Chavez's refusal to talk (remember that assessment is the first step of the nursing process). How will you identify factors contributing to his behavior?

A Patient with Peptic Ulcer Disease

1. Review the physiology of the gastric mucosal barrier and the pathogenesis of peptic ulcer disease, and the effect of *H. pylori* infection on these processes.

2. Review physiologic responses to stress in your physiology or nursing fundamentals text; compare and apply this information with the physiology of the gastric mucosal barrier and the pathophysiology of ulcer development.

3. Consider Mr. O'Donnell's occupation and schedule, as well as the prescribed medications and when each should be taken.

4. Using journal and text resources as well as your classmates, identify as many stress reduction techniques as possible. Then sort your list into those that could be used while working, and identify ways to effectively teach each technique.

A Patient with Gastric Cancer

1. Review the healing process and the normal physiology of the stomach as you formulate your answer to this question.

2. Consider the surgery, immediate postoperative care, and what the patient and family should expect in developing your teaching plan.

3. Review Chapter 14 and nursing care related to chemotherapy.

4. Again, review Chapter 14 for nursing care measures for patients with cancer; also review Chapter 22 for strategies to prevent and manage malnutrition.

Chapter 24: Nursing Care of Patients with Bowel Disorders

A Patient with Acute Appendicitis

1. Review the acute inflammatory response to an infectious process and the role WBCs play in the immune response.

2. Review Chapter 4. Consider factors such as incision size, abdominal muscle disruption, and manipulation of the bowel in developing your response.

3. Consider points such as pain management, resumption of activities, incision care, and potential complications in developing your teaching plan. Consider the patient's education and developmental stage as well.

4. Review the effects of anxiety on recovery and learning. Identify nursing measures to reduce situational anxiety.

A Patient with Ulcerative Colitis

1. Review normal functions of the small and large intestine. Review the usual location of an ileostomy. Review fluid volume deficit in Chapter 10 for manifestations and assessment data.

2. Think about the effect of chronic blood loss and review the effect of malnutrition on the hemoglobin and hematocrit.

3. Review the home care section of inflammatory bowel disease for teaching points to include.

4. Review nursing care for the patient with diarrhea, as well as the procedure for ileostomy care.

A Patient with Colorectal Cancer

1. Review peripheral innervation and impulse transmission in your anatomy and physiology textbook; think about how nerves in the rectal region are disrupted in an abdominoperineal resection. Also review the phantom pain phenomenon in Chapter 9.

2. Compare elimination through a colostomy with "normal" bowel elimination through the anus. How do they differ in terms of the passage of flatus?

3. Review Procedure 24–1. Also review the procedure for administering an enema in your fundamentals or skills textbook.

4. Review this nursing diagnosis in your nursing diagnosis or nursing care planning handbook; be sure to individualize your plan to Mr. Cunningham's situation and needs.

Chapter 25: Nursing Care of Patients with Gallbladder, Liver, and Pancreatic Disorders

A Patient with Cholelithiasis

1. Review the composition of gallstones, as well as the physiology of gallbladder function and bile. Research and discuss dietary practices of the Chickasaw tribe (or of Native Americans).

2. Review Chapter 4 for care related to a laparotomy (incision into the abdomen).

3. As you develop your plan, consider Mrs. Red Wing's culture, job, and family obligations.

A Patient with Alcoholic Cirrhosis

1. Review the anatomy and physiology of the liver and its circulation, as well as the pathophysiology of cirrhosis and its complications.

2. Consult your nutrition textbook as needed for foods that are high in calories but low in protein and sodium. When planning for limited protein intake, be sure to include high-quality proteins and limit intake of lower-quality proteins such as legumes.

3. Review the pathophysiology of hepatic encephalopathy to develop your responses to this question.

4. Review therapeutic communication skills; consult your nursing diagnosis and care planning text book as you develop this care plan.

A Patient with Acute Pancreatitis

1. Review Chapter 6 for assessment data indicative of alcohol withdrawal.

2. Review both the pathophysiology of acute pancreatitis and the acute inflammatory process.

3. Consult your nutrition textbook or the American Dietetic Association website.

4. Consult your nursing care planning textbook to develop this care plan.

Chapter 27: Nursing Care of Patients with Urinary Tract Disorders

A Patient with Cystitis

1. Consider risk factors for UTI as well as factors affecting Mrs. Waisanen's immune function.
2. Consider the indications for short-course antibiotic therapy and the indications for conventional therapy. Think about factors such as cost, compliance, and the risk for adverse effects, as well as how antibiotics work to eradicate bacteria.
3. Identify why *Ineffective Health Maintenance* may be an appropriate nursing diagnosis for Mrs. Waisanen and the individual factors contributing to this diagnosis as you plan care.

A Patient with Urinary Calculi

1. Review the risk factors for urinary lithiasis.
2/3. Using the medications section of interdisciplinary care for the patient with urinary calculi in this chapter and your pharmacology textbook or drug handbook, review analgesia for the patient with renal colic and the intended and adverse effects of the drugs given to Mr. Leton.

A Patient with a Bladder Tumor

1. Review the risk factors for urinary tract tumors, looking for commonalities and considering the physiology of the bladder and urine formation and elimination.
2. Remembering that patients rarely present with one isolated health problem, review Mr. Hussain's health history for possible contributing factors to these manifestations. Then review Chapter 6 for nursing care of the patient with substance abuse. Why might Mr. Hussain experience alcohol withdrawal after 2 to 3 days of hospitalization?
3. Considering the surgery performed and its potential effects on physical function and body image, use your nursing care planning book or guide to identify possible interventions and outcomes for this nursing diagnosis.

A Patient with Urinary Incontinence

1. Consider the effects of menopause and estrogen deficiency on genital tissues, as well as the desired and possible adverse effects of Mrs. Giovanni's medications.
2. Consider not only Mrs. Giovanni's nursing diagnosis of *Impaired Skin Integrity*, but also her risk factors for urinary tract infection.
3. Identify factors that may contribute to situational low self-esteem in Mrs. Giovanni and nursing interventions to address this diagnosis.

Chapter 28: Nursing Care of Patients with Kidney Disorders

A Patient with Acute Glomerulonephritis

1. Review Chapter 12 and the use of antibiotics to treat infection.
2. Review Mr. Chang's history and the risk factors for acute glomerulonephritis.
3. Review the diagnostic tests used to differentiate different forms of glomerulonephritis.

A Patient with Acute Renal Failure

1. Of the categories of causative factors for acute renal failure (prerenal, intrarenal, postrenal), review the two most common and compare Ms. Devak's history and physical examination findings with these categories.
2. Consider the effects of renal failure and the stress response on other body systems. You may want to review peptic ulcer disease and stress gastritis in Chapter 23.
3. Consider both the phases of acute renal failure and their physiologic effects, as well as potential complications of a fractured femur.

4. When planning nursing care related to *Deficient Diversional Activity*, consider Ms. Devak's developmental stage, usual state of health, and mechanisms currently being used to maintain femur alignment.

A Patient with End-Stage Renal Disease

1. Review the usual onset, pathophysiology, and long-term effects of type 1 and type 2 diabetes (Chapter 20).
2. Consider the effects of urea and ammonia (both neurologic toxins) on brain function.
3. Consider the physiology of dialysis, the composition of dialysis solutions (dialysate), as well as potential planned and unplanned effects of peritoneal dialysis.
4. As you develop your response, think about not only the mechanism by which peritoneal dialysis is delivered, but also possible effects of the peritoneal dialysis cycle on body image.

Chapter 30: Nursing Care of Patients with Coronary Heart Disease

A Patient with Coronary Artery Bypass Surgery

1. Identify Mr. Clements's modifiable risk factors as you develop your plan. What barriers might need to be overcome to implement strategies to reduce his risk factors?
2. What strategies can you use to overcome denial without creating hostility or impairing the patient–nurse relationship?
3. Consider traditional family roles as well as those roles that are unique to these individuals. Identify measures you can use to enlist the spouse's support.
4. Think about therapeutic communications as you formulate your response. Will your age or gender potentially affect your ability to respond effectively to these concerns? Would referral to another healthcare provider be appropriate?

A Patient with Acute Myocardial Infarction

1. Review immediate treatment measures for MI. Are other means available for reestablishing coronary artery perfusion? If you are in a rural area without immediate access to a cardiac catheterization lab, how will this affect your response?
2. Review the section of this chapter on dysrhythmias and their treatment. Research protocols for treating frequent PVCs in the post-MI patient at your clinical facility.
3. Review the goals of cardiac rehabilitation and Mrs. Williams's individual risk factors as you develop your teaching plan.
4. Consider the value of using a therapeutic response to Mrs. Williams's statement concerning smoking. Also consider the risks associated with cigarette smoke. How can you respond without supporting Mrs. Williams's desire to smoke and without precipitating anger or resistance? Review Chapter 6.

A Patient with Supraventricular Tachycardia

1. Review the effects of sympathetic and parasympathetic nervous system stimulation on cardiac function.
2. Review the section on supraventricular tachycardias, as well as the antidysrhythmic medications for other treatment options.
3. Use your pharmacology textbook as you develop your teaching plan.

Chapter 31: Nursing Care of Patients with Cardiac Disorders

A Patient with Heart Failure

1. Review the prescribed medications and their interactions. Do not forget to consider Mr. Jackson's age in assessing his risk for toxicity and interactions.
2. Review therapeutic communications skills and the use of open-ended statements to evaluate the underlying message of Mr. Jackson's statement.

3. Review exercise recommendations for the patient with heart failure as well as cardiac rehabilitation principles (Chapter 30).
4. Review the rationale for aspirin therapy in the patient with CHD and its effects on platelets and clotting as you formulate your response.
5. Review Chapter 42 for causes of stroke and the section of Chapter 30 on atrial fibrillation.

A Patient with Mitral Valve Prolapse
1. Review the pathophysiology and manifestations of MVP, as well as the general treatment measures for valve disorders.
2. Think about the effects of progressive conditioning on cardiac function.
3. Consider the anxiety associated with heart conditions and with a potentially progressive disorder that could affect childbearing and other life activities, as well as ultimately necessitate surgery.
4. Review the manifestations of MVP and of mitral regurgitation.

Chapter 32: Nursing Care of Patients with Vascular and Lymphatic Disorders

A Patient with Hypertension
1. Review Mrs. Spezia's assessment data and the risk factors for primary hypertension.
2. Review the pathophysiology of primary hypertension and of obesity (Chapter 22), as well as the relationship between hypertension and coronary heart disease.
3. Think about resources that are available in your community for homeless people. Talk to community health and social service agencies to identify additional resources.
4. Correlate Mrs. Spezia's assessment data, the pathophysiology of hypertension, and the long-term effects of stress.
5. Use your nursing care planning and nursing diagnosis textbooks to help develop your care plan.

A Patient with Peripheral Vascular Disease
1. Review treatments for peripheral atherosclerosis, as well as lifestyle measures for preventing and treating atherosclerosis and coronary heart disease (Chapter 30).
2. Compare the pathophysiology of peripheral atherosclerosis, intermittent claudication, and coronary heart disease (Chapter 30) to identify similarities and differences.
3. Review the actions of beta blockers and their role in angina prophylaxis.
4. Use your nursing care planning and nutrition textbooks to help develop your care plan.

A Patient with Deep Vein Thrombosis
1. Review the pathophysiologic processes of venous thrombosis and inflammation.
2. Think about questions you could ask for further information as well as potential resources for Mrs. Hipps.
3. Consider assessment data to evaluate Mrs. Hipps's limitations and resources, as well as community resources to help meet her needs.
4. Use your nursing diagnosis and care planning textbooks to develop your plan of care.

Chapter 33: Nursing Care of Patients with Hematologic Disorders

A Patient with Folic Acid Deficiency Anemia
1. Consider the effects of Mrs. Matthews's rapid weight loss on fluid balance, as well as the effects of tissue hypoxia on cardiac output.

2. Refer to this chapter and your nutrition text. Be sure to consider Mrs. Matthews's age in designing your menu.
3. Consider factors such as Mrs. Matthews's recent dietary history, the folic acid content of foods, and other pertinent factors in the history and physical assessment.
4. In addition to general factors to consider for the older adult (don't forget transportation among other factors), also consider the possible effect of Mrs. Matthews's recent loss and the grieving process.

A Patient with Acute Myelocytic Leukemia
1. Review the physiology of white blood cells, and the immune and inflammatory responses.
2. Think about the risks created by hospitalization in terms of exposure to infection and invasive procedures.
3. Think about the effect of inability to perform self-care on self-esteem, self-confidence, and perception of power and control.
4. Use information provided in the nursing care and home care sections of this chapter as well as in Chapter 12.
5. Use your nursing care planning and fundamentals texts to develop your care plan.

A Patient with Hodgkin's Disease
1. Review Chapter 14 and the effects of chemotherapy and radiation on cancerous cells. Think about the advantages of combining these two therapies in terms of short- and long-term desired and adverse effects.
2. Consider the primary and potential risks for infection in community settings as you design your teaching plan. What teaching strategies will you use for a young adult with Mr. Quito's education and experience?
3. Review theories of development and the developmental tasks for the young adult.
4. Use your nursing fundamentals and nursing care planning texts for reference in developing your care plan.

A Patient with Hemophilia
1. Review the pathophysiology of hemophilia and its effect on the clotting process.
2. Consider both the ABCs and Maslow's hierarchy of needs as you respond to this question.
3. Think about the genetic transmission of hemophilia. How might Mr. Cruise's hemophilia affect any children that he has? Grandchildren?
4. Review your nursing fundamentals book, nursing skills book, and intravenous therapy text to develop your teaching plan. Also consider previous learning and developmental levels.
5. What evidence supports his as an appropriate nursing diagnosis for Mr. Cruise?

Chapter 35: Nursing Care of Patients with Upper Respiratory Disorders

A Patient with Peritonsillar Abscess
1/2. Review the manifestations of upper respiratory infections and management of these disorders.
3. Think about the primary uses of the nose, mouth, and pharynx as you consider nursing diagnoses related to upper respiratory disorders.

A Patient with Nasal Trauma
1. Consider other measures to restore the patient's sense of control over the situation. Consider the potentially traumatic effects of suction on the mucous membranes as well as possible infection control risks.

2. Review the implications and potential dangers of CSF leakage to help you develop your care plan.

3. Think about the benefits and drawbacks of immediate and delayed rhinoplasty.

A Patient with Total Laryngectomy

1. Review the options for speech rehabilitation. If available, practice using a speech generator. Practice esophageal speech.

2. Use your nursing care planning and nursing diagnoses handbook to develop your care plan. Consider Mr. Tom's age, occupation, and marital status in your plan of care.

3. Review Chapter 4 for surgical nursing care interventions, as well as your nursing fundamentals textbook for wound care strategies.

4. Consider measures to promote airway clearance and ventilation of all lung fields.

Chapter 36: Nursing Care of Patients with Ventilation Disorders

A Patient with Pneumonia

1. Review Mrs. O'Neal's assessment data and compare her history with identified risk factors for pneumonia.

2. Review normal immune and inflammatory responses and the role of white blood cells in these processes.

3. Review Chapter 11 and altered immune responses for the physiology and effects of anaphylactic shock.

4. Use your nursing care planning and nursing diagnosis textbooks to help develop your care plan.

A Patient with Tuberculosis

1. Consider available resources for mentally ill patients, as well as community and public health resources. Consider measures to ensure compliance with the prescribed treatment.

2. Contact your local public health department, the discharge planner for your unit, or the social services department in your clinical facility to help identify available resources.

3. Use the nursing care section under Pneumonia, and your nursing diagnosis or care planning handbook as you develop your care plan.

A Patient with Lung Cancer

1. Review Chapter 14 and use your pharmacology text to research the effects of these drugs and the rationale for combination chemotherapy.

2. Use Chapter 14 and your pharmacology text to identify probable side effects of this treatment regimen. Then use your nursing care planning book to identify appropriate nursing diagnoses and interventions.

3. Review the pathophysiology and collaborative care sections for lung cancer to develop your response to this question.

Chapter 37: Nursing Care of Patients with Gas Exchange Disorders

A Patient with COPD

1. Review the processes by which cigarette smoke inflicts damage on lung tissue. Use your pediatric and pathophysiology texts for additional information.

2. Review the physiology of the respiratory drive, as well as the effects of chronic elevated carbon dioxide levels in the blood.

3. Review the manifestations of COPD and its complications as well as the section of this chapter on respiratory failure.

4. Use your nursing diagnosis handbook to help identify appropriate goals and interventions for this nursing diagnosis.

A Patient with ARDS

1. As you respond to this question, consider additional treatment measures for ARDS and respiratory failure. Also consider the potential long-term consequences and complications of intubation and mechanical ventilation. Discuss strategies for communicating with Ms. Adamson's family and supporting coping and decision making by Ms. Adamson and her family in an instance such as this.

2. Think about the precipitating factors for ARDS and the factors that may precipitate respiratory failure in a patient with COPD. Consider the probable overall respiratory and general health status of the individual affected by each of these conditions.

3. Review the precipitating factors for ARDS and discuss strategies to prevent them.

4. Use your nursing care planning book to identify appropriate goals and nursing interventions for this nursing diagnosis.

Chapter 39: Nursing Care of Patients with Musculoskeletal Trauma

A Patient with a Hip Fracture

1. Consider Mrs. Carbolito's age and the fact that she is postmenopausal. What effect does estrogen have on bone health? What might have increased her risk for falls?

2. Review the principles of traction application. What purpose does it serve prior to surgery? What words could you use that she would understand? Think about the effects of trauma, pain, and suddenly finding oneself in a strange environment on listening and understanding verbal communications.

3. List how each of these manifestations would affect skin integrity, food intake, and bone healing.

A Patient with a Below-the-Knee Amputation

1. Design a sequential plan for Mr. Rocke's self-care of the stump. Consider his readiness to learn and the complexity of the care. Is there a risk in letting him assume total responsibility from the beginning? Why or why not?

2. List the factors used to describe Mr. Rocke. How do these affect his ability or willingness to follow up with medical care? What community agencies are available where you live or go to school that would be good sources of assistance and support for Mr. Rocke?

3. Review the information about exercise. How would Mr. Rocke's choice not to do exercises affect his ability to use a prosthesis to walk?

Chapter 40: Nursing Care of Patients with Musculoskeletal Disorders

A Patient with Osteoporosis

1. Review the effects of nicotine and caffeine on blood circulation to bones. What effect does alcohol play in bone loss?

2. Review foods that increase blood cholesterol levels. What is considered a normal cholesterol level? You may need to read content in Chapter 31. Knowing the patient needs calcium, what type of dairy products would you recommend?

3. List activities for the patient who is not able to be ambulatory. How many of the activities on your list would help prevent osteoporosis?

4. *Risk for Trauma* is defined as an increased risk for accidental tissue injury, such as a fracture. What interventions would you teach Mrs. Bauer to reduce this risk?

A Patient with Osteoarthritis

1. Review information about serum creatinine and BUN in a laboratory studies textbook or on the web. What medications are Mr. Cerulli taking that may be affecting these findings? Consider what teaching is necessary related to these findings.
2. What assessments are significant for confusion? If necessary, review content related to confusion. Review Mr. Cerulli's history in the case study and determine factors that may have contributed to his risk for confusion before, during, and after surgery.
3. *Acute Confusion* is defined as an abrupt onset of a cluster of global, transient changes and disturbances in attention, cognition, psychomotor activity, level of consciousness, and/or sleep–wake cycle. What assessments could you make to support this diagnosis for Mr. Cerulli? What interventions might you design for this diagnosis?

A Patient with Rheumatoid Arthritis

1. Think about the role differences in a 42-year-old woman and a 72-year-old woman. On the other hand, consider the effects of a chronic illness that may have been present for 30 years. Would your plan differ? Why or why not?
2. List the possible disabilities that may be caused by rheumatoid arthritis. How do you believe these would affect Mrs. James? What agencies in your community are available for support of people with this type of illness? Where would you go for literature to give Mrs. James?
3. *Ineffective Role Performance* is defined as behaviors and expressions that do not match norms or expectations. Do you believe this is an appropriate nursing diagnosis for Mrs. James? Why or why not? What interventions could be implemented for this diagnosis?

Chapter 42: Nursing Care of Patients with Intracranial Disorders

A Patient with a Seizure Disorder

1. List the teaching topics you would include for Ms. Carlson. Consider how her needs (e.g., for safety) would differ if she lived alone.
2. Describe statements you could use to help Ms. Carlson understand not only the dangers but also the legal issues involved. What if Ms. Carlson does not recognize these concerns?
3. What type of questions could you ask Ms. Carlson to determine why she feels this way? Would you personally find it embarrassing? How can you facilitate Ms. Carlson's understanding for this recommendation?

A Patient with a Stroke

1. What subjective manifestations does the patient with hypertension have? (Review content in Chapter 32.)
2. Consider referral to community resources as a volunteer tutor for adult literacy, gardening, and/or woodworking. Tutoring college students is another option.
3. Use statements that will encourage Mr. Boren to talk about his arm and how he feels about being unable to use it.

A Patient with a Subdural Hematoma

1. Review the manifestations of the types of intracranial hematomas. What assessments are specific to a subdural hematoma? Why is it important to know this?
2. What are some other interventions that might be used? How could family help? What if no family members are available?
3. *Acute Confusion* is a sudden onset of changes in attention, cognition, psychomotor activity, level of consciousness, and/or

sleep–wake cycle. What would you determine as priority nursing diagnoses and interventions for Mr. Lee?

A Patient with a Brain Tumor

1. Review content in the chapter on increased intracranial pressure and intracranial surgery. List collaborative and nursing interventions to decrease increased intracranial pressure.
2. What do these manifestations indicate? What would be your priority assessment? Who would you notify?
3. Practice the use of therapeutic communications and what response you would make.
4. Consider the reasons Ms. Lange feels powerless. What nursing interventions might decrease this feeling?

Chapter 43: Nursing Care of Patients with Spinal Cord Disorders and CNS Infections

A Patient with an SCI

1. What are the developmental tasks of a 19-year-old? How does the inability to meet these tasks affect emotional responses?
2. Think about questions that explore Mr. Valdez's fears in relation to sexuality. Practice questions and statements with friends until you are not embarrassed to ask them.
3. Consider how your own values and beliefs may differ from those of a patient.
4. What baseline assessments and information are necessary before developing a plan for urinary elimination needs? Why would self-catheterization be an option? What are the risks of long-term Foley catheterization?

A Patient with Bacterial Meningitis

1. List the environmental stimuli in the hospital setting. How could these be decreased? What effect do these stimuli have on cognition and behavior that is altered by an intracranial infection?
2. Think about how you would feel if Mr. Cook tried to hit you. How would you respond to him? To whom would you report this?
3. Why would Mr. Cook have pain? How would pain be manifested during the initial treatment period? Is it important to consider the respiratory effects of narcotics for him? Defend your answer.

Chapter 44: Nursing Care of Patients with Neurologic Disorders

A Patient with Alzheimer's Disease

1. Think about what information you would need and how you would collect it. Consider such factors as the age of family members, educational level of family members, and stage of the patient's AD. What else would you need to know?
2. Review the suggested activities in this section of the chapter. What others can you think of or have you seen used successfully? Osteoarthritis often results in joint stiffness and pain as well as problems with mobility. Would this affect your interventions? If so, how could they be adapted?
3. Consider the type of foods that might be prepared, the timing of meals, and interventions that might be used to decrease agitation before or during meals.

A Patient with Multiple Sclerosis

1. Outline a typical day's activities for Mr. McMurphy that would provide a balance between activity and rest. What assessments would you make to evaluate the effectiveness of this plan?
2. Consider how respiratory infections are spread. Why is Mr. McMurphy at increased risk?
3. The definition of *Risk for Injury* is that one is at risk as a result of environmental conditions interacting with the person's adaptive

and defensive resources. What factors in this patient's history and physical status would support this diagnosis? What interventions would you include in the care plan and why?

A Patient with Parkinson's Disease

1. Consider the adaptations that might be made to clothing and shoes. What adaptive devices might be useful?

2. What information would you need to know before you develop your interventions? Include that from Mr. Avneil and what might be available in the community and the long-term care facility.

3. *Chronic Sorrow* is a recurring pattern of sadness in response to continual loss. Consider the type of communications you would need to use with Mr. Avneil to identify his degree of sorrow. What other assessment might provide cues to support this diagnosis (think about eating and sleeping)? How might an activity such as reminiscence help?

Chapter 46: Nursing Care of Patients with Eye and Ear Disorders

A Patient with Glaucoma and Cataracts

1. What is the pathophysiology of glaucoma? How does a cataract affect glaucoma?

2. Consider the effects of corticosteroids on glaucoma. If Mrs. Rainey is to administer several medications at home, identify specific teaching guidelines for her.

3. Would you request a referral for home health visits? Why or why not? Think about the effect of transferring her for a brief admission to an assisted-living facility.

Chapter 48: Nursing Care of Men with Reproductive System and Breast Disorders

A Man with Prostate Cancer

1. Why would Mr. Turner be at risk for altered skin integrity? Outline the interventions you would include on his teaching plan that would promote skin integrity as he cares for himself at home.

2. Noncompliance is defined as behaviors that do not coincide with the therapeutic plan agreed upon by the person and the healthcare professional. Do you think Mr. Turner fully understood his treatment and agreed with his follow-up care? What could be done in the preoperative phase of Mr. Turner's care to better ensure his understanding and desire to have continued medical care?

3. What assessments indicate that Mr. Turner does or does not have bladder distention? Would you report this? If so, to whom?

Chapter 49: Nursing Care of Women with Reproductive System and Breast Disorders

A Woman with Endometriosis

1. What is the relationship between Mrs. Hall's manifestations and a decreased RBC count? Review the information in Chapter 32 and list assessments you would make to identify anemia.

2. List nonthreatening questions you would use to begin the discussion. How might it help to ask these questions at the beginning of the interview? Then list questions that you might use to collect data about the couple's sexual history. Would you be embarrassed to ask them? If so, how might this in turn affect their responses?

3. *Situational Low Self-Esteem* is the state in which a person develops a negative perception of self-worth in response to a current situation. What information in Mrs. Hall's history might provide data to support this nursing diagnosis?

A Woman with Cervical Cancer

1. Consider developmental needs and how they differ by age.

2. Review the effects of radiation, discussed in Chapter 14.

3. Does fatigue differ from "feeling tired"? Can the fatigue from radiation be decreased? If so, how?

A Woman with Breast Cancer

1. Review the information in the chapter on the genetic factors that pose a risk for developing breast cancer. How could you explain this in terms understandable by Mrs. Clemments and her daughters?

2. List the different types of mastectomies. Consider the implications of the differences, and how this would affect your nursing care.

3. Review the information on chemotherapy in Chapter 14. List the types of chemotherapy and its common side effects. Consider the classifications of medications that are used to treat these side effects.

4. What factors in the treatment of Mrs. Clemments's treatment might disrupt the amount and quality of her sleep? What interventions might be used to improve her sleep pattern?

Chapter 50: Nursing Care of Patients with Sexually Transmitted Infections

A Patient with Gonorrhea

1. What manifestations does Ms. Cirit have that are typical of the disease? Would you make other assessments? If so, what are they?

2. Review the discussion of HIV in Chapter 13. Do you believe it is true that infection with gonorrhea may increase the risk of HIV? If so, how would you explain this to Ms. Cirit?

3. *Impaired Social Interaction* is a state of aloneness or rejection experienced by an individual that is perceived as negative. What assessments of Ms. Cirit might support this diagnosis? What interventions and expected outcomes would you develop?

A Patient with Syphilis

1. Describe the assessments you would expect to find in a man with early syphilis.

2. Consider topics such as number of sex partners, patterns of sexual activity, and use of safe sex practices. What other topics should be explored? How can you ask these questions without being embarrassed or embarrassing the patient?

3. List possible statements you might make. Do you believe this is a nursing responsibility? If you do not feel comfortable with this topic, what could you do?

GLOSSARY

Abrasion Partial-thickness denudation of an area of integument, generally resulting from falls or scrapes.

Absence seizure (petit mal seizure) A type of generalized seizure characterized by a sudden brief cessation of all motor activity accompanied by a blank stare and unresponsiveness.

Accommodation The ability of the eye to adjust to variations in distance.

Achalasia Absence of peristalsis of the esophagus and high gastroesophageal sphincter pressure resulting in dilation and loss of tone in the esophagus.

Acidosis The condition in which the hydrogen ion concentration increases above normal (reflected in a pH below 7.35).

Acids A substance that releases hydrogen ions in solution.

Acne Disorder of the pilosebaceous (hair and sebaceous gland) structure, resulting in eruption of papules or pustules.

Acoustic neuroma or schwannoma Benign tumor of cranial nerve VIII.

Acquired immune deficiency syndrome (AIDS) A specific group of diseases or conditions that are indicative of severe immunosuppression related to infection with the human immunodeficiency virus.

Acquired immunity Immunity developed after exposure to a pathogen. See *Active immunity.*

Acromegaly Meaning literally "enlarged extremities," this is a condition resulting from excessive growth hormone secretion during adulthood.

Actinic keratosis Also called senile or solar keratosis, this is an epidermal skin lesion directly related to chronic sun exposure and photodamage.

Active immunity Production of antibodies or development of immune lymphocytes against specific antigens.

Active transport Movement of molecules across cell membranes and epithelial membranes against a concentration gradient; requires energy.

Acute coronary syndrome (ACS) A condition of unstable cardiac ischemia; includes unstable angina and acute myocardial ischemia with or without significant myocardial tissue injury.

Acute gastritis A benign, self-limiting disorder associated with ingestion of gastric irritants such as aspirin, alcohol, caffeine, or foods contaminated with certain bacteria.

Acute illness An illness that occurs rapidly, lasts for a relatively short time, and is self-limiting.

Acute lymphoblastic leukemia (ALL) Abnormal proliferation of lymphoblasts in the bone marrow, lymph nodes, and spleen; the most common type of leukemia in children and young adults.

Acute myeloblastic leukemia (AML) Uncontrolled proliferation of myeloblasts (granulocyte precursors) and hyperplasia of bone marrow and the spleen; the most common acute leukemia in adults.

Acute myocardial infarction (AMI) Necrosis (death) of myocardial cells.

Acute pain Pain of sudden onset that is usually self-limited and localized; it lasts for less than 6 months and has an identifiable cause, such as trauma, surgery, or inflammation.

Acute renal failure Abrupt onset of renal failure, often reversible.

Acute respiratory distress syndrome (ARDS) Noncardiac pulmonary edema and progressive refractory hypoxemia.

Acute tubular necrosis (ATN) A syndrome of abrupt and progressive decline in tubular and glomerular function.

Adaptive immune response A specific and systemic immune initiated by and directed against particular antigens.

Adaptive immunity Long-lasting and specific response of the lymphocytes to antigens.

Addiction A primary, chronic neurobiologic disease characterized by compulsive use of a substance despite negative consequences, such as health threats or legal problems.

Addisonian crisis A life-threatening response to acute adrenal insufficiency. Triggers include surgery, acute systemic illness, trauma, or abrupt withdrawal of long-term corticosteroid therapy.

Advance directive Also called a *living will*, this is a document in which a patient formally states preferences for health care in the event that he or she later becomes mentally incapacitated, and names a person who has durable power of attorney to serve as a substitute decision maker to implement the patient's stated preferences.

Aesthetic surgery See *Cosmetic surgery.*

Afterload The force the ventricles must overcome to eject their blood volume; the pressure in the arterial system ahead of the ventricles.

Agnosia The inability to recognize one or more subjects that were previously familiar; agnosia may be visual, tactile, or auditory.

Agranulocytosis Severe neutropenia, with less than 200 cells/µm.

Alcohol Alcohol and other CNS depressants act on other neurotransmitters in the brain such as gamma-aminobutyric acid (GABA). GABA is the most prevalent inhibitory neurotransmitter in the brain and has a major role in decreasing neuronal excitability. Alcohol creates an additive effect with GABA, further inhibiting arousal and depressing the autonomic nervous system.

Alcoholic cirrhosis (Laënnec's cirrhosis) The end result of alcoholic liver disease.

Alkalis Alkalis are bases that accept hydrogen ions in solution.

Alkalosis The condition where the hydrogen ion concentration decreases below normal (reflected in a pH above 7.45).

Alleles Different forms of a gene or DNA occupying the same place on a pair of chromosomes; an allele for each gene is inherited from each parent.

Allergy A hypersensitivity response to environmental or exogenous antigens.

Allografts Grafts between members of the same species but who have different genotypes and HLA antigens. See also *Homograft.*

Alopecia Loss of hair; baldness.

Alzheimer's disease (AD) A form of dementia characterized by progressive, irreversible deterioration of the general intellectual functioning.

Amenorrhea Absence of menstruation.

Amphetamine Central nervous system stimulant that causes arousal and an elevation of mood with a sense of increased strength, mental capacity, self-confidence, and a decreased need for food and sleep.

Amputation Partial or total removal of a body part.

Amyotrophic lateral sclerosis (ALS) Progressive, degenerative neurologic disease characterized by weakness and wasting of the involved muscles, without any accompanying sensory or cognitive changes; also called *Lou Gehrig's disease.*

Analgesic A medication that reduces or eliminates the perception of pain.

Anaphylactic shock Shock resulting from a widespread hypersensitivity reaction (called *anaphylaxis*). The pathophysiology in this type of shock includes vasodilation, pooling of blood in the periphery, and hypovolemia with altered cellular metabolism.

Anaphylaxis An acute systemic type I hypersensitivity reaction that occurs in response to an injected antigen.

Anaplasia The regression of a cell to an immature or undifferentiated cell type.

Anasarca Severe, generalized edema.

Androgens Hormones synthesized in the testes, ovaries, and adrenal cortex that promote expression of male sex characteristics.

Anemia An abnormally low number of circulating RBCs, hemoglobin concentration, or both.

Anergy Inability to react to specific antigens.

Anesthesia State produced by medications given intravenously, intraspinally, subcutaneously, or by inhalation to create temporary partial or total loss of sensation and consciousness in a patient for invasive procedures such as surgery or painful diagnostic tests.

Aneurysm Abnormal dilation of a blood vessel, commonly at a site of a weakness or tear in the vessel wall.

Angina pectoris (angina) Chest pain resulting from reduced coronary blood flow that causes a temporary imbalance between myocardial blood supply and demand.

Angioma (hemangioma) Benign vascular tumor.

Anion gap The difference between the sum of two measured anions, chloride and bicarbonate, and the principal measured cation, sodium.

Ankylosing spondylitis A chronic inflammatory arthritis that primarily affects the axial skeleton, leading to pain and progressive stiffening and fusion of the spine.

Anorexia Loss of appetite.

Anorexia nervosa An eating disorder characterized by a body weight less than 85% of expected for age and height, and an intense fear of gaining weight.

Anorgasmia Absence of orgasm.

Anosmia Inability to smell.

Anthropometric measurements Measurement of height, weight, triceps skin folds, and midarm circumference.

Antibodies Immunoglobulin molecules that bind with an antigen to inactivate it.

Antibody-mediated (humoral) immune response Activation of B cells to produce antibodies to respond to antigens such as bacteria, bacterial toxins, and free viruses.

Anticipatory grieving A combination of intellectual and emotional responses and behaviors by which people adjust their self-concept in the face of a potential loss.

Antigen A substance capable of evoking a specific immune response; usually a protein which the body recognizes as foreign, causing an immune response to be stimulated.

Antigenic substances Agents such as microorganisms, cells and tissues from other humans or animals, and some inorganic substances that stimulate an immune response.

Aortic valve The semilunar valve between the left ventricle of the heart and the aorta. It prevents blood from flowing backward into the ventricle.

Aortitis Inflammation of the aorta, usually the aortic arch.

Aphasia Defective or absent language function.

Apical impulse A normal, palpable pulsation (thrust) in the area of the midclavicular line in the left fifth intercostal space. It can be seen on inspection in about half of the adult population.

Aplastic anemia A condition manifested by failure of the bone marrow to produce all three types of blood cells.

Apnea Cessation of breathing lasting from a few seconds to a few minutes.

Appendectomy Surgical removal of the appendix.

Appendicitis Inflammation of the vermiform appendix.

Apraxia The inability to carry out a motor pattern (such as drawing a figure) even when strength and coordination are adequate.

Areflexia Lack of normal reflexes.

Arterial blood gas (ABG) A laboratory test used to evaluate acid–base balance and gas exchange.

Arteriovenous (AV) malformation A congenital intracranial lesion, formed by a tangled collection of dilated arteries and veins, that allows blood to flow directly from the arterial into the venous system, bypassing the normal capillary network.

Arthralgia Joint pain.

Arthritis Joint inflammation.

Arthroplasty The reconstruction or replacement of a joint.

Ascites Excess fluid in the peritoneal cavity.

Asphyxiation Oxygen deprivation.

Asthma Chronic inflammatory disorder of the airways that is characterized by recurrent episodes of wheezing, breathlessness, chest tightness, and coughing.

Astigmatism A condition that develops with abnormal curvature of the cornea or eyeball, causing the image to focus at multiple points on the retina.

Ataxia Uncoordinated, irregular gait and muscle movement; weakness.

Atelectasis Collapse of lung tissue following obstruction of the bronchus or bronchioles.

Atherosclerosis A form of arteriosclerosis in which deposits of fat and fibrin obstruct and harden the arteries.

Atopic dermatitis (eczema) Common inflammatory skin disorder of unknown cause.

Atrial kick Delivery of an additional bolus of blood to the ventricles resulting from atrial systole; occurs just prior to ventricular systole.

Atrial natriuretic peptide (ANP) A hormone released by atrial muscle cells in response to distention from fluid overload.

Aura Sensation preceding generalized seizure activity; may be a vague sense of uneasiness or an abnormal sensation.

Auscultatory gap A temporary disappearance of sound between the systolic and diastolic BP.

Autografting Transplanting of the patient's own tissue; the most successful type of tissue transplant.

Autoimmune disorder Failure of immune system to recognize itself, resulting in normal host tissue being targeted by immune defenses.

Autonomic dysreflexia Exaggerated sympathetic response that occurs in patients with spinal cord injuries at or above the T_6 level.

Autosome A single chromosome from any one of the 22 pairs of chromosomes not involved in sex determination (X or Y); humans have 22 pairs of autosomes.

Azotemia Increased blood levels of nitrogenous waste products.

B lymphocytes (B cells) Bursa-equivalent lymphocytes responsible for synthesizing antibodies in response to specific antigens.

Bacterial vaginosis Nonspecific vaginitis.

Bactericidal Capable of killing organisms without immune system intervention.

Bacteriostatic Inhibits growth of microorganisms, leaving the destruction to the host's immune system.

Bacteriuria Bacteria in the urine.

Balanced suspension traction Traction in which several forces of pull work in unison to raise and support the patient's injured extremity off the bed and maintain its alignment.

Balloon tamponade The application of pressure to stop esophageal bleeding using an inflatable balloon.

Bariatrics The healthcare science that focuses on patients who are extremely obese.

Basal cell carcinoma Epithelial tumor that is believed to originate either from the basal layer of the epidermis or from cells in the surrounding dermal structures. These tumors are characterized by an impaired ability of the basal cells of the epidermis to mature into keratinocytes, with mitotic division beyond the basal layer.

Basal metabolic rate (BMR) Test to measure the energy used when the body is at rest; rarely used due to the availability of more accurate thyroid tests.

Base excess (BE) A calculated value also known as buffer base capacity. Base excess reflects the degree of acid–base imbalance by indicating the status of the body's total buffering capacity.

Bases (or alkalis) Substances that accept hydrogen ions in solution.

Bell's palsy (facial paralysis) Disorder of the facial nerve (seventh cranial nerve), characterized by unilateral paralysis of the facial muscles.

Benign prostatic hyperplasia (BPH) Enlargement of the prostate gland.

Bereavement The time of mourning experienced after a loss.

Bile A greenish, watery solution containing bile salts, cholesterol, bilirubin, electrolytes, water, and phospholipids.

Biliary colic A severe, steady pain in the epigastric region or upper right quadrant of the abdomen caused by obstruction and increased pressure in the bile duct.

Binge-eating disorder A nutritional disorder characterized by recurrent episodes of binge eating—eating an excessive amount of food during a defined period of time and a sense of loss of control over eating during binge episodes.

Biofeedback An electronic method of measuring autonomic physiologic responses, such as brain waves, muscle contraction, and skin temperature, and then "feeding" this information back to the patient.

Biological markers Stable segments of DNA important for the construction of chromosome maps.

Bioterrorism Use of an etiologic agent (disease) to cause harm or kill a population, food, and/or livestock.

Biotherapy Treatment that modifies the biologic processes that result in malignant cells, primarily through enhancing the person's own immune responses.

Bivalving Process of splitting a cast down both sides to alleviate pressure on the injured extremity.

Blood clot See *Thrombus*.

Blood flow The volume of blood transported in a vessel, in an organ, or throughout the entire circulation over a given period of time.

Blood pressure The tension or pressure exerted by blood against arterial walls.

Blunt trauma The type of trauma that occurs when there is no communication from the damaged tissues to the outside environment.

Body mass index (BMI) Used to identify excess adipose tissue, BMI is calculated by dividing the weight (in kilograms) by the height (in meters squared, m^2).

Bone marrow transplant (BMT) Infusion of bone marrow cells to restore bone marrow function after chemotherapy or radiation. Allogeneic BMT uses donor bone marrow cells from a donor; autologous BMT uses the patient's own bone marrow.

Borborygmus The presence of excessive loud and hyperactive bowel sounds.

Botulism A severe, life-threatening form of food poisoning caused by *Clostridium botulinum*.

Brachytherapy A type of radiation therapy in which the source of radiation is placed directly into or adjacent to the tumor, a technique that delivers a high dose to the tumor and a lower dose to normal tissue.

Bradycardia A heart rate of less than 60 beats per minute.

Bradykinesia Slowed movements due to muscle rigidity.

Bradypnea Abnormally low respiratory rate.

Brain abscess Infection with a collection of purulent material within the brain tissue.

Brain death The cessation of cerebral blood flow with global brain infarction and permanent loss of all brain function.

Brain death criteria Clinical signs used to determine whether a comatose patient is brain dead.

Breakthrough pain Pain that exceeds baseline chronic or persistent pain, with or without baseline analgesia.

Bronchiectasis Permanent abnormal dilation of one or more large bronchi and destruction of bronchial walls, usually accompanied by infection.

Bronchitis Inflammation of the bronchi (airways).

Bruit An adventitious sound heard during auscultation; of venous or arterial origin.

Buffer A substance that prevents major changes in pH by removing or releasing hydrogen ions.

Bulimia nervosa An eating disorder characterized by recurring episodes of binge eating followed by purge behaviors such as self-induced vomiting, use of laxatives or diuretics, fasting, or excessive exercise.

Burn An injury resulting from exposure to heat, chemicals, radiation, or electric current.

Burn shock Hypovolemic shock resulting from the shift of a massive amount of fluid from the intracellular and intravascular compartments into the interstitium following burn injury.

Bursitis Inflammation of the bursa.

Cachexia The wasted physical appearance characteristic of cancer and other chronic illnesses. It is characterized by rapid depletion of the body's protein, particularly in skeletal muscle, with less rapid loss of fat.

Caffeine A methylxanthine stimulant that increases the heart rate and acts as a diuretic.

Calculi Presence of abnormal concentration or stones in the body occur in the gallbladder, kidneys, ureters, bladder, or urethra.

Cancer A family of complex diseases with manifestations that vary according to body system and type of tumor cells involved; marked by uncontrolled growth and the spread of abnormal cells.

Candidiasis Infection of mucous membranes caused by *Candida albicans*, a yeast-like fungus.

Cannabis sativa Cannabis sativa is the source of marijuana.

Carbuncle A group of infected hair follicles.

Carcinogen Cancer-causing agent.

Carcinogenesis The production or origin of cancer.

Carcinoma A tumor arising from epithelial tissue.

Cardiac arrest Sudden failure of the heart to pump.

Cardiac cycle The contraction and relaxation of the heart during one heartbeat.

Cardiac index (CI) Cardiac output adjusted for body size.

Cardiac output (CO) The amount of blood pumped by the ventricles into the pulmonary and systemic circulations in 1 minute.

Cardiac rehabilitation A long-term program of medical evaluation, exercise, risk factor modification, education, and counseling designed to limit the physical and psychologic effects of cardiac illness and improve the patient's quality of life.

Cardiac reserve The ability of the heart to respond to the body's changing need for cardiac output.

Cardiac tamponade Compression of the heart due to pericardial effusion, trauma, cardiac rupture, or hemorrhage.

Cardiogenic shock Shock that occurs when the heart's pumping ability is compromised to the point that it cannot maintain cardiac output and adequate tissue perfusion.

Cardiomegaly Enlargement of the heart.

Cardiomyopathy Primary abnormality of the heart muscle that affects its structural or functional characteristics.

Cardiovascular disease (CVD) Generic term for disorders of the heart and blood vessels.

Carpal spasm Decreased calcium levels cause the patient's hand and fingers to contract in response to occlusion of the blood supply by a blood pressure cuff (Trousseau's sign).

Carpal tunnel syndrome Compression of the median nerve as a result of inflammation and swelling of the synovial lining of the tendon sheaths.

Carrier Any individual who carries a single copy of an altered gene or mutation for a recessive condition on one chromosome of a chromosome pair and an unaltered form of that gene on the other chromosome. A carrier generally is not affected by the gene alteration; on the average, each person in the general population is a carrier of five or six gene mutations for recessive disorders.

Carriers (related to infections) Harbor the pathogen without showing evidence of clinical disease.

Catabolism Biochemical process involving the breakdown of complex structures into simpler forms.

Cataract Opacification (clouding) of the lens of the eye.

Celiac disease (celiac sprue, nontropical sprue) Chronic hereditary disorder characterized by sensitivity to the gliadin fraction of gluten, a cereal protein.

Cell cycle The four phases that occur during growth and development of a cell.

Cell-mediated (cellular) immune response Direct or indirect inactivation of antigen by lymphocytes.

Cellulitis A localized infection of the dermis and subcutaneous tissue.

Central pain Related to a lesion in the brain that may spontaneously produce high-frequency bursts of impulses that are perceived as pain.

Central nervous system depressants Central nervous system depressants, including barbiturates, benzodiazepines, paraldehyde, meprobamate, and chloral hydrate, are subject to abuse.

Central obesity See *Upper body obesity.*

Cerebral concussion Transient, temporary, neurogenic dysfunction caused by mechanical force to the brain.

Cerebral contusion Bruise on the surface of the brain.

Cerebral edema An increase in the volume of brain tissue due to abnormal accumulation of fluid in brain cells.

Cerumen Earwax.

Chalazion Granulomatous cyst or nodule of the lid.

Chancre Hard, syphilitic primary ulcer.

Cheilosis Cracks at corners of the mouth seen in vitamin B-complex deficiencies, especially riboflavin.

Chemotherapy Cancer treatment involving the use of cytotoxic medications to decrease tumor size, adjunctive to surgery or radiation therapy, or to prevent or treat suspected metastases.

Chlamydia A group of syndromes caused by *Chlamydia trachomatis*, a bacterium that behaves like a virus spreading within a host cell; spread by sexual contact and to the neonate by passage through the birth canal of an infected mother.

Cholecystectomy Removal of the gallbladder.

Cholecystitis Inflammation of the gallbladder, usually associated with stones in the cystic or common bile duct.

Cholelithiasis Formation of stones (calculi) within the gallbladder or biliary duct system.

Cholera Acute diarrheal illness caused by certain strains of *Vibrio cholerae.*

Chorea Jerky, rapid, involuntary movements.

Chromosome Genetic material carried by each cell; found in the cell nucleus.

Chronic bronchitis Excessive secretion of bronchial mucus characterized by a productive cough lasting 3 or more months in 2 consecutive years.

Chronic gastritis Disorders characterized by progressive and irreversible changes in the gastric mucosa.

Chronic illness A condition that requires continuing management over a long period—years or even decades.

Chronic hepatitis Chronic infection of the liver; the primary cause of liver damage leading to cirrhosis, liver cancer, and liver transplantation.

Chronic kidney disease (CKD) The presence of kidney damage for three or more months with loss of nephron units and decreased renal mass leading to progressive deterioration of glomerular filtration, tubular secretion, and reabsorption.

Chronic lymphocytic leukemia (CLL) Proliferation and accumulation of small, abnormal, mature lymphocytes in the bone marrow, peripheral blood, and body tissues; least common type of the major leukemias.

Chronic myelogenous leukemia (CML) Abnormal proliferation of all bone marrow elements, usually associated with a chromosome abnormality (the Philadelphia chromosome).

Chronic obstructive pulmonary disease (COPD) Chronic air flow obstruction due to chronic bronchitis and/or emphysema.

Chronic otitis media Condition involving permanent perforation of the tympanic membrane, with or without recurrent pus formation and often accompanied by changes in the mucosa and bony structures (ossicles) of the middle ear.

Chronic pain Prolonged pain, usually lasting longer than 6 months; pain that persists after the condition causing it has resolved; may be malignant or nonmalignant in origin

Chronic sorrow A cyclical, recurring, and potentially progressive pattern of pervasive sadness experienced in response to continual loss, throughout the trajectory of an illness or disability.

Chronic stump pain The result of neuroma formation, causing severe burning pain.

Chronic venous insufficiency A chronic disorder of inadequate venous return.

Chvostek's sign Contraction of the lateral facial muscles in response to tapping the face in front of the ear; caused by decreased blood calcium levels.

Chyme Thick, fluid mixture of food and gastric juices formed in the stomach during the digestive process.

Circulating nurse A registered nurse who coordinates and manages a wide range of activities before, during, and after surgical procedures.

Cirrhosis A progressive, irreversible disorder, eventually leading to liver failure; the end stage of chronic liver disease.

Closed fracture (simple fracture) Break in continuity of bone with skin still intact.

Clubbing Enlargement and blunting of the terminal portion of the fingers; associated with chronic hypoxemia.

Cluster headache A severe, unilateral vascular headache that occurs in groups, or clusters and is characterized by exacerbations and remissions; predominantly experienced by men ages 20 to 40.

Coagulation The process of creating a fibrin meshwork that cements blood components together to form an insoluble clot.

Cocaine A highly addictive stimulant/euphoric drug extracted from the leaves of the coca plant.

Code of ethics An established and agreed-on group of principles of conduct that provide a frame of reference for nursing behaviors that are congruent with professional values.

Cold sore See *Herpes simplex.*

Cold zone Considered the "safe zone" during a disaster, it is adjacent to the warm zone and is the area where a more in-depth triage of victims would occur; survivors may find shelter in this area, and command and control vehicles would be found here as well as the emergency transport vehicles.

Colectomy Surgical removal of the colon.

Collateral channels Connections between small arteries.

Collateral vessels Accessory pathways connected to the smaller arteries in the coronary system.

Colorectal cancer Malignant tumor arising from the epithelial tissues of the colon or rectum.

Colostomy Ostomy made in the colon.

Comedones Noninflammatory acne lesions.

Community-based care Centers on individual and family healthcare needs. The nurse practicing community-based care provides direct services to individuals to manage acute or chronic health problems and to promote self-care. The care is provided in the local community, is culturally competent, and is family centered.

Compartment A space enclosed by a fibrous membrane or fascia.

Compartment syndrome Condition in which excess pressure constricts the structures within a compartment and reduces circulation to muscles and nerves.

Complex regional pain syndrome Extremity pain that is severe, diffuse, and burning, and accompanied by vasomotor changes that affect skin color and temperature.

Concussion Brain injury resulting from a violent jar, shake, or impact with an object.

Conjunctivitis Inflammation of the conjunctiva.

Consanguinity Related by having a common ancestor; close blood relationship.

Conscious sedation Anesthesia that provides analgesia and amnesia, but in which the patient remains conscious. Patients are able to breathe independently and are cardiovascularly stable.

Consciousness A condition in which a person is aware of self and environment and is able to respond appropriately to stimuli; full consciousness requires both normal arousal and full cognition.

Constipation The infrequent (two or fewer bowel movements weekly) or difficult passage of stools.

Contact dermatitis Type of dermatitis caused by a hypersensitivity response or chemical irritation.

Continuous renal replacement therapy (CRRT) A form of hemodialysis in which blood is continuously circulated through a highly porous hemofilter from artery to vein or vein to vein.

Contractility The inherent capability of the cardiac muscle fibers to shorten.

Contracting The negotiation of a cooperative working agreement between the nurse and patient that is continuously renegotiated.

Contractures Permanent shortening of connective tissues.

Contralateral deficit Manifestations of a stroke on the side of the body opposite the side of the brain that is damaged.

Contusion Superficial tissue injury resulting from blunt trauma, such as a kick or blow from an object, that causes the breakage of small blood vessels and bleeding into the surrounding tissue.

Conventional weapons Weapons such as bombs and guns that are used more frequently than nonconventional terrorist weapons.

Convergence Moving the eyes inward toward the nose to see an object close to the face.

Co-occurring disorders Concurrent diagnosis of a substance-use disorder and a psychiatric disorder. One disorder can precede and cause the other, such as the relationship between alcoholism and depression.

Cor pulmonale Condition of right ventricular hypertrophy and failure that results from long-standing pulmonary hypertension.

Core competencies Standards that a profession agrees are essential for a person to be deemed competent in his or her field.

Corneal reflex Closure of eyelids (blinking) due to corneal irritation.

Corneal ulcer Local necrosis of the cornea, may be caused by infection, exposure trauma, or the misuse of contact lenses.

Coronary heart disease (CHD) Heart disease caused by impaired blood flow to the myocardium.

Coryza (rhinorrhea) Profuse nasal discharge.

Cosmetic surgery (aesthetic surgery) One of two fields within plastic surgery. Cosmetic surgery enhances the attractiveness of normal features.

Crackles Discontinuous lung sounds heard by auscultation; can be fine or coarse. Produced by air passing over airway secretions or the opening of collapsed airways.

Crepitation A grating sound heard on movement of a joint.

Creutzfeldt-Jakob disease (CJD, spongiform encephalopathy) Rare, progressive neurologic disease that causes brain degeneration without inflammation.

Critical pathway A healthcare plan designed to provide care with a multidisciplinary, managed action focus; developed for specific diagnoses, usually those that are high volume, high risk, and high cost.

Critical thinking Self-directed thinking that is focused on what to believe or do in a specific situation.

CRNA Certified registered nurse anesthetist; a nurse certified in anesthesia administration.

Crohn's disease (regional enteritis) Chronic, relapsing inflammatory disorder affecting the gastrointestinal tract.

Crossing over A process that occurs during meiosis in which homologous maternal and paternal chromosomes break and exchange corresponding sections of DNA and then rejoin; this process can cause an exchange of alleles between chromosomes and provides human diversity.

Cryosurgery The destruction of tissue by cold or freezing with agents such as fluorocarbon sprays, carbon dioxide snow, nitrous oxide, and liquid nitrogen.

Curettage The removal of lesions with a curette, a semisharp cutting instrument.

Curling's ulcers Acute ulcerations of the stomach or duodenum that form following a burn injury.

Cushing's ulcers Stress ulcers occurring as sequelae of head injury or central nervous system surgery.

Cutaneous melanoma See *Malignant melanoma*.

Cyanosis A bluish discoloration of the skin and mucous membranes due to oxygen deficiency.

Cystectomy Complete surgical removal of the urinary bladder and adjacent muscles and tissues.

Cystic fibrosis (CF) Inherited disorder of the exocrine glands that results in the secretion of abnormal amounts of mucus.

Cystitis Inflammation of the urinary bladder.

Cysts Benign closed sacs in or under the skin surface that are lined with epithelium and contain fluid or a semisolid material.

Cytokines Hormone-like polypeptides produced primarily by monocytes, macrophages, and T cells. Cytokines act as messengers of the immune system, facilitating communication between the cells to adjust or vary the inflammatory reaction or to initiate immune cell proliferation and differentiation.

Dawn phenomenon A rise in blood glucose between 4 AM and 8 AM that is not a response to hypoglycemia.

Death Irreversible cessation of circulatory and respiratory functions or irreversible cessation of all functions of the entire brain, including the brainstem.

Death anxiety Worry or fear related to death or dying.

Debridement Process of removing dead tissue from a wound.

Decerebrate posturing Abnormal posture with the neck extended; the jaw clenched; arms pronated, extended, and close to the sides; legs extended; and feet plantar flexed. Results from lesions of the midbrain, pons, or diencephalons.

Decorticate posturing Abnormal posture with the upper arms close to the sides; the elbows, wrists, and fingers flexed; the legs extended and internally rotated; and the feet plantar flexed. Results from lesions of the corticospinal tracts.

Deep venous thrombosis (DVT) Blood clot (thrombus) formation and inflammation within a deep vein, usually in the pelvis or lower extremities; a common complication of hospitalization, surgery, and immobilization.

Deformation Alteration of the spinal cord and soft tissues caused by abnormal movements from acceleration and deceleration forces.

Dehiscence An unintended separation of wound margins due to incomplete healing.

Dehydration Loss of water.

Delayed healing Healing that occurs at a slower rate than expected.

Delegation To effectively assign appropriate work activities to other members of the healthcare team. When the nurse delegates nursing care activities to another person, that person is authorized to act in the place of the nurse, while the nurse retains the accountability for the activities performed.

Delirium tremens (DT) A medical emergency usually occurring 3 to 5 days following alcohol withdrawal and lasting 2 to 3 days; characterized by paranoia, disorientation, delusions, visual hallucinations, elevated vital signs, vomiting, diarrhea, and diaphoresis.

Dementia A global impairment of cognitive function that usually is progressive and may be permanent; interferes with normal social and occupational activities.

Demyelination Destruction or removal of the myelin sheaths of nerves.

Depolarization The rapid inflow of sodium ions, causing an electrical change in which the inside of a cell becomes positive in relation to the outside.

Dermatitis Acute or chronic inflammation of the skin characterized by erythema and pain or pruritus.

Dermatome Area of skin innervated by cutaneous branches of a single spinal nerve.

Dermatophytes Fungi that cause superficial skin infections.

Dermatophytoses Superficial fungal infection of the skin; also called *ringworm*.

Diabetes insipidus A deficit of ADH causes excretion of large amounts of dilute urine, in some instances as much as 12 L/day. The patient has extreme thirst and drinks large volumes of water. If unable to replace the water loss, the patient becomes dehydrated and hypernatremic. Even though hyperosmolality is present, the urine is dilute and has a low specific gravity.

Diabetes mellitus (DM) Group of chronic disorders of the endocrine pancreas, all categorized under a broad diagnostic label. The condition is characterized by inappropriate hyperglycemia caused by a relative or absolute deficiency of insulin or by a cellular resistance to the action of insulin.

Diabetic ketoacidosis (DKA) A form of metabolic acidosis induced by stress in a person with type 1 diabetes.

Diabetic nephropathy A disease of the kidneys characterized by the presence of albumin in the urine, hypertension, edema, and progressive renal insufficiency.

Diabetic neuropathies Disorders of the peripheral nerves and the autonomic nervous system manifesting one or more of the following: sensory and motor impairment, muscle weakness and pain, cranial nerve disorders, impaired vasomotor function, impaired gastrointestinal function, and impaired genitourinary function.

Diabetic retinopathy The collective name for the changes in the retina that occur in the person with diabetes. The retinal capillary structure undergoes alterations in blood flow, leading to retinal ischemia and a breakdown in the blood retinal barrier.

Dialysate Dialysis solution.

Dialysis The diffusion of solute molecules across a semipermeable membrane from an area of higher concentration to one of lower concentration.

Diaphoresis Copious production of sweat.

Diarrhea An increase in the frequency, volume, and fluid content of the stool.

Diastolic blood pressure The minimum pressure maintained by elastic arterial walls during diastole (cardiac relaxation) to maintain blood flow through capillary beds; averages 80 mmHg in a healthy adult.

Differentiation A process occurring over many cell cycles that allows cells to specialize in certain tasks.

Diffuse brain injury (DBI) A brain injury from a high-speed acceleration–deceleration accident with widespread disruption of axons in the white matter.

Diffuse esophageal spasm Nonperistaltic contraction of esophageal smooth muscle.

Diffusion The process by which solute molecules move from an area of high solute concentration to an area of low solute concentration to become evenly distributed.

Dilemma A choice between two unpleasant, ethically troubling alternatives.

Diplopia Unilateral or bilateral double vision.

Disability The degree of observable and measurable impairment.

Disaster Event that requires extraordinary efforts beyond those needed to respond to everyday emergencies.

Disease Literally meaning "without ease," this term describes alterations in structure and function of the body or mind. Diseases may have mechanical, biologic, or normative causes.

Dislocation Separation of contact between two bones of a joint.

Dissection (aortic) A life-threatening emergency caused by a tear in the intima of the aorta with hemorrhage into the media.

Disseminated intravascular coagulation (DIC) A disruption of hemostasis characterized by widespread intravascular clotting and bleeding; a syndrome that develops as a complication of many other disorders.

Distributive shock Also called *vasogenic shock*, this includes several types of shock that result from widespread vasodilation and decreased peripheral resistance.

Diverticula Saclike projections of mucosa through the muscular layer of the colon.

Diverticulitis Inflammation in and around the diverticular sac; typically affects only one diverticulum, usually in the sigmoid colon.

Diverticulosis Indicates the presence of diverticula.

Dominant A characteristic or gene that is apparent even when the relevant gene is present in only one copy; a person with a dominant gene usually expresses that gene trait.

Do-not-resuscitate (DNR or "no-code") order Usually written by the physician for the patient who has a terminal illness or is near death, this order is usually based on the wishes of the patient and family that no cardiopulmonary resuscitation be performed for respiratory or cardiac arrest.

Dual diagnosis The coexistence of substance abuse/dependence and a psychiatric disorder in one individual (used interchangeably with *dual disorder* and *co-occurring disorders*).

Dual disorder See *Dual diagnosis*.

Dumping syndrome Complication of partial gastrectomy characterized by nausea, weakness, sweating, palpitation, syncope, sensation of warmth, and occasionally diarrhea.

Duodenal ulcers Peptic ulcer disease affecting the duodenum.

Durable power of attorney A document that can delegate the authority to make health, financial, and/or legal decisions on a person's behalf. It must be in writing and must state that the designated person is authorized to make healthcare decisions.

Dwarfism A condition characterized by short stature; insufficient pituitary growth hormone is one cause.

Dysarthria Difficulty speaking.

Dysfunctional uterine bleeding (DUB) Vaginal bleeding that is usually painless but abnormal in amount, duration, or time of occurrence.

Dysmenorrhea Pain associated with menstruation.

Dyspareunia Painful intercourse.

Dysphagia Difficulty swallowing.

Dysphonia Change in the tone of voice.

Dysplasia The loss of DNA control over differentiation occurring in response to adverse conditions.

Dyspnea Difficult or labored breathing.

Dysrhythmia Abnormal heart rate or rhythm.

Dysuria Painful urination.

Ecchymosis A flat, irregularly shaped lesion (bruise) of varying size with no pulsation; caused by blood collecting under skin.

Ectopic beats Impulses originating outside normal conduction pathways of the heart.

Edema Accumulation of fluid in the body's tissues; an excess accumulation of fluid in the interstitial space.

Ejection fraction (EF) The percentage of total blood remaining in the ventricle at the end of diastole (relaxation); normal is 50% to 70%.

Electrical bone stimulation Application of electrical current at the fracture site to treat fractures that are not healing appropriately. The electrical stress increases the migration of osteoblasts and osteoclasts to the fracture site. Mineral deposition increases, promoting bone healing.

Electrocardiography The graphic recording of the heart's electrical activity detected and recorded through electrodes placed on the surface of the body.

Electrolytes Substances that dissociate in solution to form charged particles called ions.

Electrosurgery The destruction or removal of tissue with high-frequency alternating current.

Embolic CVA Cerebrovascular accident occurring when a blood clot or clump of matter traveling through the cerebral blood vessels becomes lodged in a vessel too narrow to permit further movement.

Embolism Sudden obstruction of a blood vessel by a clot or debris.

Emergency Encompasses an unforeseen combination of circumstances calling for immediate action for a range of victims from one to many.

Emphysema Destruction of the walls of the alveoli, with resulting enlargement of abnormal air spaces.

Empyema Accumulation of purulent exudate in the pleural cavity.

Encephalitis An acute inflammation of the parenchyma of the brain or spinal cord.

End of life The final days or weeks of life when death is imminent.

Endocarditis Inflammation of the endocardium.

Endometriosis A condition in which multiple, small implants of endometrial tissue develop throughout the pelvic cavity.

Endoscopy Inspection of organs or cavities of the body using an endoscope.

Endotoxins Found in the cell wall of gram-negative bacteria, endotoxins are released only when the cell is disrupted. They act as activators of many human regulatory systems, producing fever, inflammation, and potentially clotting, bleeding, or hypotension when released in large quantities.

End-stage renal disease The final stage of chronic renal failure in which the kidneys are unable to excrete metabolic wastes and regulate fluid and electrolyte balance adequately; characterized by a glomerular filtration rate of less than 5% of normal.

Enophthalmos Sunken appearance of the eyes.

Enteral nutrition Administration of liquid nutritional formulas to meet calorie and protein needs in patients unable to consume adequate food; also called *tube feeding*.

Enucleation Surgical removal of an eye.

Epicondylitis (tennis elbow, golfer's elbow) Inflammation of the tendon at its point of origin into the bone.

Epididymitis Infection or inflammation of the epididymis.

Epidural hematoma (extradural hematoma) A collection of blood between the dura and the skull.

Epilepsy A disorder characterized by chronic seizure activity.

Epistaxis Nosebleed.

Equianalgesia/Equianalgesic Approximate equivalent doses of opioid analgesics as compared to morphine sulfate.

Erectile dysfunction Inability to attain and maintain an erection sufficient to permit satisfactory sexual intercourse.

Erosive gastritis See *Stress-induced (erosive gastritis)*.

Erysipelas Infection of the skin most often caused by group A *streptococci*.

Erythema A reddening of the skin.

Erythropoiesis Red blood cell production.

Eschar Hard, leathery crust that covers a burn wound and harbors necrotic tissue.

Escharotomy Surgical removal of eschar from the torso or extremity to prevent circumferential constriction.

Esophageal varices Enlarged, thin-walled veins that form in the submucosa of the esophagus.

Esophagojejunostomy Removal of the entire stomach with anastomosis of the distal esophagus to the jejunum.

Estrogen Hormone produced by the ovaries.

Ethics Principles of conduct. Ethical behavior is concerned with moral duty, values, obligations, and the distinction between right and wrong.

Euthanasia From the Greek for painless, easy, gentle, or good death, now commonly used to signify a killing prompted by a humanitarian motive.

Euthyroid Term describing normal thyroid hormone function.

Evisceration Protrusion of body contents through a surgical wound.

Exacerbation A period during chronic illness in which symptoms reappear.

Exfoliative dermatitis Inflammatory skin disorder characterized by excessive peeling or shedding of skin.

Exophthalmos Protrusion of the eyeballs.

Exotoxins Soluble proteins secreted into surrounding tissue by the microorganism. Exotoxins are highly poisonous, causing cell death or dysfunction.

External otitis Inflammation of the ear canal.

Extracapsular fractures Fractures of the trochanteric region.

Extracorporeal shock-wave lithotripsy (ESWL, transcutaneous shock-wave lithotripsy) Noninvasive technique for fragmenting kidney stones using shock waves generated outside the body.

Faith community nursing Also known as parish nursing, this is a nontraditional, community-based way of providing health promotion and health restoration nursing interventions to specific groups of people.

Family Two or more persons joined by emotional closeness and shared bonds and who identify themselves as being part of a family.

Fasciculations Involuntary twitching.

Fasciectomy (fascial excision) Process of excising the wound to the level of fascia.

Fat embolism syndrome (FES) Characterized by neurologic dysfunction, pulmonary insufficiency, and a petechial rash on the chest, axilla, and upper arms due to fat globules lodged in the pulmonary vascular bed or peripheral circulation.

Fecal impaction A rock-hard or putty-like mass of feces in the rectum.

Fecal incontinence Loss of voluntary control of defecation.

Fecalith A hard mass of feces.

Fibrocystic changes (FCC) Physiologic nodularity and breast tenderness that increases and decreases with the menstrual cycle.

Fibroid tumors (uterine leiomyoma) Solid benign tumors originating from smooth muscle of the uterus.

Fibromyalgia (fibrositis) A common rheumatic syndrome characterized by musculoskeletal pain, stiffness, and tenderness.

Filtration The process by which water and dissolved substances (solutes) move from an area of higher hydrostatic pressure to an area of lower hydrostatic pressure.

Fistula Abnormal opening or passage between two organs or spaces that are normally separated or an abnormal passage to the outside of the body.

Flaccidity Decreased muscle tone in disease or trauma of the lower motor neurons.

Flail chest Free-floating segment of the chest wall, resulting from two or more consecutive ribs fractured in multiple places.

Flap A piece of tissue whose free end is moved from a donor site to a recipient site while maintaining a continuous blood supply through its connection at the base or pedicle.

Flatus Gas in the digestive tract.

Fluid resuscitation Replacement of the extensive fluid and electrolyte losses associated with major burn injuries.

Fluid volume deficit (FVD) A decrease in intravascular, interstitial, and/or intracellular fluid in the body.

Fluid volume excess (FVE) Excess extracellular fluid resulting from retention of both water and sodium in the body.

Folic acid deficiency anemia An anemia resulting from folic acid deficiency, a necessary nutrient for DNA synthesis and RBC maturation.

Folliculitis Bacterial infection of the hair follicle, most commonly caused by *Staphylococcus aureus*.

Fracture A break in a bone usually due to trauma.

Freestanding outpatient surgical facilities Surgical units independent of a hospital with or without financial connections to a hospital or healthcare organization.

Friction rub The sound heard when two dry surfaces are rubbed together.

Frostbite An injury of the skin from freezing.

Full-thickness burn A burn that involves all layers of the skin, including the epidermis, dermis, and epidermal appendages.

Fulminant hepatitis Hepatitis with a rapid and severe onset and course.

Furuncle Often called a boil, but also an inflammation of the hair follicle.

Fusiform excision The removal of a full thickness of the epidermis and dermis, usually with a thin layer of subcutaneous tissue.

Galactorrhea Lactation not associated with pregnancy or nursing.

Gastric lavage Irrigation of the stomach with large quantities of normal saline.

Gastric mucosal barrier A protective barrier consisting of lipids, bicarbonate ions, and mucous gel that protects the stomach lining from the damaging effects of gastric juices.

Gastric outlet obstruction Obstruction of the pyloric region of the stomach and duodenum that impairs gastric outflow; a potential complication of peptic ulcer disease.

Gastric ulcers Ulcers of the stomach lining, usually in the lesser curvature and antrum; more common in older adults.

Gastritis Inflammation of the stomach lining.

Gastroduodenostomy (Billroth I) Excision of the pylorus of the stomach with the anastomosis of the upper stomach to the duodenum; commonly used partial gastrectomy procedure.

Gastroenteritis Inflammation of the gastrointestinal tract; not a specific disease, but a group of syndromes or a collection of related manifestations.

Gastroesophageal reflux Backward flow of gastric contents into the esophagus.

Gastroesophageal reflux disease (GERD) The reflux of acidic gastric contents into the lower esophagus.

Gastrojejunostomy (Billroth II) Subtotal excision of the stomach with closure of the duodenum and side-to-side anastomosis of the jejunum to the stomach; commonly used partial gastrectomy procedure.

Gastroparesis Slowed gastrointestinal motility, which causes early satiety.

Gene A sequence of DNA on a chromosome that represents a fundamental unit of heredity; occupies a specific spot on a chromosome (gene locus).

Gene expression When the protein product of a gene is visible (for example, through the presence of a body structure or identifiable through biochemical tests such as insulin or phenylalanine levels).

General anesthesia Deep sedation, which includes analgesia and muscle paralysis. This type of anesthesia requires respiratory maintenance without the aid of the patient's respiratory musculature.

Genital herpes (herpes simplex genitalis) An infection of the external genitalia caused by herpes simplex genitalis; transmitted by vaginal, anal, or oral–genital contact.

Genital warts (condyloma acuminatum, venereal warts) A sexually transmitted condition caused by the human papilloma virus.

Genotype The genes and the variations therein that a person inherits from his or her parents.

Germ cells Cells that give rise to a sperm or egg.

Gigantism Gigantism occurs when GH hypersecretion begins before puberty and the closure of the epiphyseal plates. The person becomes abnormally tall, often exceeding 7 ft (213 cm) in height, but body proportions are relatively normal.

Gingivitis Inflammation of the gums, characterized by redness and bleeding.

Gland Tissue that produces secretions or synthesizes hormones.

Glaucoma Condition characterized by increased intraocular pressure of the eye and a gradual loss of vision.

Glomerular filtration rate (GFR) The rate at which plasma is filtered through the glomeruli of the kidney.

Glomerulonephritis Inflammation of the capillary loops of the glomeruli.

Glossitis Inflammation of the tongue.

Glucocorticoid A group of hormones secreted by the adrenal cortex; they regulate carbohydrate levels in the body.

Gluconeogenesis Formation of glucose from fats and proteins.

Glucose-6-phosphate dehydrogenase (G6PD) anemia Anemia due to a hereditary defect in RBC metabolism.

Glucosuria Excessive glucose in urine.

Glycogenolysis Breakdown of liver glycogen to glucose.

Goiter An enlarged thyroid gland. Enlargement results from both inadequate and excessive synthesis of thyroid hormones.

Gonorrhea (GC, clap) An infection caused by *Neisseria gonorrhoeae* that is transmitted by direct sexual contact or during delivery of a neonate by an infected mother.

Gout A metabolic disorder characterized by hyperuricemia and acute inflammatoryarthritis triggered by urate crystallization within joints and deposits of insoluble urates in connective tissues of the body.

Grief The emotional response to loss and its accompanying changes.

Grieving The internal process the person uses to work through the response to loss.

Guillain-Barré syndrome (GBS) Acute demyelinating disorder of the peripheral nervous system characterized by progressive, usually rapid muscle weakness and paralysis.

Gynecomastia Breast enlargement in men.

Hallucinogens Drugs that produce hallucinations.

Hallux valgus (bunion) The enlargement and lateral displacement of the first metatarsal.

Hammertoe (claw toe) The dorsiflexion of the first phalanx with accompanying plantar flexion of the second and third phalanges.

Handicap The total adjustment to disability that limits functioning at a normal level.

Hazardous materials Substances that pose a potential risk to life, health, or property if they are released because of their chemical, biologic, or physical nature.

Health "A state of complete physical, mental, and social well-being, and not merely the absence of disease or infirmity" (WHO, 1974, p. 1).

Healthcare surrogate An individual selected to make medical decisions when a person is no longer able to make them for his- or herself.

Health–illness continuum A visual representation of health as a dynamic process, with high-level wellness at one extreme of the continuum and death at the opposite extreme.

Heart block A block in the normal conduction pathways.

Heart failure Inability of the heart to pump adequate blood to meet the metabolic demands of the body.

Heave An excessive thrust.

Hemangioma See *Angioma*.

Hemarthrosis The collection of blood in a joint.

Hematemesis Blood in the vomit.

Hematochezia Blood in the stool.

Hematoma A contusion with a large amount of bleeding.

Hematopoiesis Blood cell formation.

Hematuria Blood in the urine.

Hemianopia Loss of half of the visual field of one or both eyes.

Hemiparesis Weakness of one side of the body.

Hemiplegia Paralysis in one-half of the body vertically.

Hemodialysis A procedure in which electrolytes, waste products, and excess water are removed from the body by diffusion and ultra-filtration as blood passes by an artificial semipermeable membrane outside the body.

Hemodynamics Study of the forces involved in blood circulation.

Hemoglobin The oxygen-carrying protein within RBCs; composed of the heme molecule and globin, a protein molecule.

Hemolysis The process of RBC destruction.

Hemolytic anemia Premature destruction (lysis) of RBCs.

Hemophilia A group of hereditary clotting factor disorders that lead to persistent and potentially severe bleeding.

Hemophilia A (classic hemophilia) The most common type of hemophilia, caused by clotting factor VIII deficiency.

Hemophilia B (Christmas disease) Hemophilia caused by factor IX deficiency.

Hemoptysis Bloody sputum.

Hemorrhage Rapid or excessive bleeding.

Hemorrhagic CVA (intracranial hemorrhage) Cerebrovascular accident occurring when a cerebral blood vessel ruptures.

Hemorrhoids (piles) Clusters of dilated veins in swollen anal tissue.

Hemostasis Control of bleeding.

Hemothorax Blood in the pleural space.

Hepatic encephalopathy Altered consciousness, mentation, and motor function affecting cirrhotic patients.

Hepatitis Inflammation of the liver, usually caused by a virus; may be acute or chronic.

Hepatorenal syndrome Renal failure accompanied by azotemia, sodium retention, oliguria, and hypotension in patients with cirrhosis and ascites.

Hernia A defect in the abdominal wall that allows abdominal contents to protrude out of the abdominal cavity.

Herniated intervertebral disk Rupture of the cartilage surrounding the intervertebral disk with protrusion of the nucleus pulposus.

Herpes simplex (fever blister, cold sore) Acute viral infections of the skin and mucous membranes caused by two types of herpesvirus: HSV I and HSV II.

Herpes zoster (shingles) Viral infection of a nerve supplying a dermatome section of the skin caused by varicella zoster, the same herpesvirus that causes chickenpox.

Heterograft (xenograft) Skin obtained from an animal, usually a pig.

Heterozygous Nonidentical copies of a particular gene (different alleles) on the paired chromosomes.

Hiatal hernia Protrusion of part of the stomach through the esophageal hiatus of the diaphragm into the mediastinal cavity.

Hirsutism Increased growth of coarse hair, usually on the face and trunk.

Histocompatibility The ability of cells and tissues to survive transplantation without immunologic interference by the recipient.

Holistic health care Care in which all aspects of a person (physical, psychosocial, cultural, spiritual, and intellectual) are considered as essential components of individualized care.

Home care Services for patients who are in need of treatment or support to function effectively in the home environment.

Homeostasis The body's tendency to maintain a state of physiologic balance in the presence of constantly changing conditions.

Homograft (allograft) Human tissue (skin, cornea, organs) used in skin graft or tissue transplant.

Homologous Chromosomes that are members of the same pair and normally have the same number and arrangement of genes; usually one copy is from the mother and the other copy is from the father.

Homonymous hemianopia Impaired vision or blindness in one side of both eyes.

Homozygous Identical copies of a particular gene (same alleles) on both paired chromosomes.

Hordeolum (sty) Staphylococcal abscess that may occur on either the external or internal margin of the lid.

Hormone Chemical messengers secreted via body fluids that have specific targets where they increase or inhibit organ functions.

Hospice (hospice care) A special component of home care, designed to provide medical, nursing, social, psychologic, and spiritual care for terminally ill patients and their families. Hospice care relies on a philosophy of relieving pain and suffering and allowing the patient to die with dignity in a comfortable environment.

Hot zone The site of a disaster where a weapon was released or where contamination occurred.

Human genome The total amount of the DNA (genes) in an individual's cells.

Human immunodeficiency virus (HIV) Virus responsible for AIDS.

Huntington's disease Progressive, degenerative, inherited neurologic disease characterized by increasing dementia and chorea; also called *chorea*.

Hydrocele Fluid-filled mass within the scrotum.

Hydrocephalus An abnormal accumulation of cerebrospinal fluid within the cerebral ventricles.

Hydronephrosis Distention of the kidney pelvis and calyces with urine behind an obstruction.

Hydroureter Distention of the ureter with urine.

Hypercapnia Increased blood levels of carbon dioxide.

Hyperglycemia Elevated blood glucose levels, which causes osmotic diuresis and, if chronic, damages blood vessel epithelium and renal glomeruli.

Hyperopia (farsightedness) A condition in which the eyeball is short, causing the image to focus behind the retina.

Hyperosmolar hyperglycemic state (HHS) A condition of very high blood glucose with adequate insulin to prevent ketosis, a complication of type 2 DM.

Hyperparathyroidism A disorder that results from an increase in the secretion of parathyroid hormone (PTH), which regulates normal serum levels of calcium.

Hyperplasia An increase in the number or density of normal cells.

Hypersensitivity Exaggerated response of the immune system to an antigen.

Hypertension Excess pressure in the arterial portion of systemic circulation.

Hyperthyroidism A disorder caused by excessive production and delivery of thyroid hormone to the tissues.

Hypertrophic scar Overgrowth of dermal tissue that remains within the boundaries of the wound.

Hypervolemia Excess intravascular fluid.

Hyphema Bleeding into the anterior chamber of the eye, possibly as the result of blunt eye trauma.

Hypoglycemia Low blood glucose levels.

Hypoparathyroidism A disorder that results from abnormally low PTH levels. The most common cause is damage to or inadvertent removal of all of the parathyroid glands during thyroidectomy. The lack of circulating PTH causes hypocalcemia and an elevated blood phosphate level.

Hypothyroidism A disorder that results when the thyroid gland produces an insufficient amount of TH.

Hypovolemia Decreased circulating blood volume.

Hypovolemic shock Shock caused by a decrease in intravascular volume of 15% or more. This form of shock is caused by the loss of whole blood, blood plasma, or extracellular fluid.

Hypoxemia Decreased oxygen concentration in the blood, measured by PaO_2.

Hypoxia Insufficient supply of oxygen to the tissues.

Ichthyosis An inherited dermatologic condition in which the skin is dry, fissured, and hyperkeratotic; the surface of the skin has the appearance of fish scales.

Ileostomy An ostomy made in the ileum of the small intestine.

Illness The response a person has to a disease; integrates the patient's perception, as well as the pathophysiologic alterations and the psychologic effects of those alterations.

Immunity The protection of the body from disease.

Immunocompetent Possessing an immune system that can identify antigens and effectively destroy or remove them.

Immunocompromised Possessing an immune response that has been weakened by a disease or an immunosuppressive agent.

Immunoglobulin (Ig) A protein that functions as an antibody.

Immunosuppression Inability of the immune system to respond to an antigen. Occurs in response to disease or medications; may be intentional to prevent rejection of transplants or a side effect of some medications.

Impairment A disturbance in structure or function resulting from physiologic or psychologic abnormalities.

Impetigo Infection of the skin caused by either *Staphylococcus aureus* or beta-hemolytic streptococci.

Impotence Inability to achieve or maintain an erection.

Incidental pain A type of breakthrough pain that is predictable because it is associated with movement such as turning or coughing.

Increased intracranial pressure (IICP, intracranial hypertension) Sustained elevated pressure (10 mmHg or higher) within the cranial cavity.

Independent nursing care Care provided by nurses within the scope of their practice without the direction or supervision of a physician.

Infection Colonization by and multiplication of an organism within a host. The host can be any organism capable of supporting the nutritional and physical growth requirements of the microorganism, for example, humans.

Inflammation A complex, nonspecific, adaptive response to injury that brings fluid, dissolved substances, and blood cells into the interstitial tissues where the invasion or damage has occurred.

Inflammatory bowel disease (IBD) Chronic inflammation of the bowel common to a group of conditions that includes Crohn's disease and ulcerative colitis.

Influenza Highly contagious viral respiratory disease characterized by coryza, fever, cough, and constitutional manifestations such as headache and malaise.

Informed consent Disclosure of risks associated with the intended procedure or operation to the patient. The language of the document varies according to statutory and common law of each state.

Inhalants Inhaled solvents categorized into three types: anesthetics, volatile nitrites, and organic solvents.

Innate adaptive immunity Specific and nonspecific responses that prevent or limit the entry of invaders into the body, thereby limiting the extent of tissue damage and reducing the workload of the adaptive immune system.

Insulin A hormone that facilitates entry of glucose into fat and muscle cells for energy.

Insulin reaction Hypoglycemia in patients with type 1 diabetes mellitus.

Interdisciplinary care Care provided by members of the healthcare team in addition to medical professionals. Usually includes team members who address psychosocial and spiritual issues as well as physical care.

Intermittent claudication Cramping, aching ischemic pain in the calves, thighs, and buttocks that occurs with a predictable level of activity and is relieved by rest.

Intracerebral hematomas A collection of blood in the brain tissue, most often located in the frontal or temporal lobes.

Intracranial aneurysm Saccular outpouching of a cerebral artery that occurs at the site of a weakness in the vessel wall.

Intracranial hypertension See *Increased intracranial pressure*.

Intracranial pressure (ICP) The pressure within the cranial cavity, usually measured as the pressure within the lateral ventricles.

Intraductal papilloma A tiny wartlike growth on the inside of the peripheral mammary duct that causes discharge from the nipple.

Intraoperative phase The time during surgery, from beginning to end.

Iron deficiency anemia The most common type of anemia; results from inadequate iron for optimal RBC formation.

Irritable bowel syndrome (IBS) A motility disorder of the gastrointestinal tract characterized by alternating periods of constipation and diarrhea.

Ischemia Deficient blood flow to tissue resulting in reduced oxygen delivery.

Ischemic Deprived of oxygen.

Islets of Langerhans Hormone-producing cells (alpha cells, beta cells, and delta cells) scattered through the pancreas.

Isograft Tissue transplant where the donor and recipient are identical twins.

Jaundice Yellow-to-orange color visible in the skin and mucous membranes; most often the result of a hepatic disorder.

Joint arthroplasty Reconstruction or replacement of a joint.

Kaposi's sarcoma (KS) A vascular malignancy (a tumor of the endothelial cells lining small blood vessels) that presents as vascular macules, papules, or violet lesions affecting the skin and viscera. It is often the presenting symptom of AIDS.

Keloid Elevated, irregularly shaped, progressively enlarging scar arising from excessive amounts of collagen in the stratum corneum during scar formation in connective tissue repair.

Keratitis Inflammation of the cornea.

Keratin Keratin is a fibrous, water-repellent protein that gives the epidermis its tough, protective quality.

Keratosis Any skin condition in which there is a benign overgrowth and thickening of the cornified epithelium.

Ketoacidosis A condition of very high blood glucose and insufficient insulin that results in accumulation of ketones and fatty acids in the blood; a form of metabolic acidosis.

Ketonuria The presence of ketones in the urine.

Ketosis An accumulation of ketone bodies produced during the oxidation of fatty acids.

Kindling Long-term changes in brain neurotransmission that occur after repeated detoxifications.

Kinesthesia The ability to perceive movement and sense of position.

Korotkoff's sounds Sounds heard during auscultation of blood pressure.

Korsakoff's psychosis Secondary dementia caused by thiamine (B_1) deficiency that may be associated with chronic alcoholism; characterized by progressive cognitive deterioration, confabulation, peripheral neuropathy, and myopathy.

Kussmaul's respirations Deep, rapid respirations associated with compensatory mechanisms.

Kwashiorkor (protein energy malnutrition, PEM) Chronic protein deficiency with adequate calories to meet body needs.

Kyphosis Exaggerated thoracic curvature of the spine, common in older adults.

Labyrinthectomy Surgical removal of the labyrinth.

Labyrinthitis Inflammation of the inner ear.

Laceration Open wound that results from sharp cutting or tearing. Injuries to the integument are at risk for contamination from dirt, debris, or foreign objects.

Lacunar strokes Thrombotic stroke of smaller cerebral blood vessels in deeper parts of the brain or brain stem.

Laminectomy Removal of the lamina of the vertebrae.

Laparoscopic cholecystectomy Removal of the gallbladder using an endoscope.

Laryngectomy Removal of the larynx.

Laryngitis Inflammation of the larynx.

Leiomyoma See *Fibroid tumor*.

Leukemia A group of chronic malignant disorders of white blood cells and WBC precursors; characterized by replacement of bone marrow by malignant immature WBCs, abnormal immature circulating WBCs, and infiltration of malignant cells into other tissues.

Leukocytes Also called white blood cells, these are the primary cells involved in both nonspecific and specific immune system responses. These cells isolate the infecting organism or injury, destroy pathogens, and promote healing.

Leukocytosis An increase in the number of leukocytes in the blood (above 10,/mm^3), usually caused by infection.

Leukopenia Abnormal decrease of circulating leukocytes, usually below 5/mm^3; occurs when bone marrow activity is suppressed or when leukocyte destruction increases.

Leukoplakia Formation of white patches or spots on the mucous membranes or tongue; these lesions may become malignant.

Libido Sexual desire.

Lichen planus Benign inflammatory disorder of the mucous membranes and skin.

Lift A more sustained thrust than normal.

Lipoatrophy Atrophy of subcutaneous tissue.

Liposuction A method of changing the contours of the body by aspirating fat from the subcutaneous layer of tissue.

Lithiasis Stone formation.

Lithotripsy Crushing of renal calculi.

Living will A document that provides written directions about life-prolonging procedures to provide instructions when a person can no longer communicate in a life-threatening situation.

Lobectomy Surgical removal of a single lobe of lung.

Locked-in syndrome Patient is alert and fully aware of the environment, but is unable to communicate through speech or movement as a result of blocked efferent pathways to the brain.

Lordosis Increased lumbar curve.

Loss Loss may be defined as an actual or potential situation in which a valued object, person, body part, or emotion that was formerly present is lost or changed and can no longer be seen, felt, heard, known, or experienced. A loss may be temporary or permanent, complete or partial, objectively verifiable or perceived, physical or symbolic.

Lower body obesity (peripheral obesity) A waist-to-hip ratio of less than 0.8 in an obese individual.

Lung abscess Localized area of lung destruction or necrosis and pus formation.

Lung compliance Distensibility of the lungs.

Lyme disease An inflammatory disorder caused by a spirochete, *Borrelia burgdorferi*, which is transmitted primarily by ticks.

Lymphadenopathy The enlargement of lymph nodes (over 1 cm) with or without tenderness. It may be caused by inflammation, infection, or malignancy of the nodes or the regions drained by the nodes.

Lymphangitis Inflammation of a lymphatic vessel.

Lymphedema Edema of an extremity due to accumulated lymph; may be primary or secondary, resulting from inflammation, obstruction, or removal of lymphatic vessels.

Lymphocytes Lymphocytes account for 20% to 40% of circulating leukocytes. Lymphocytes are the principal effector and regulator cells of specific immune responses.

Lymphoid tissues Connective tissues containing lymphocytes; include tissues of the bone marrow, thymus, lymph nodes, and spleen.

Lymphoma Malignancy of lymphoid tissue.

Macrophages Monocytes mature into macrophages after settling into tissue. Macrophages are large phagocytes. They are important in the body's defense against chronic infections.

Macular degeneration Destructive changes in the macula due to injury or gradual failure of the outer pigmented layer of the retina (the retinal layer adjacent to the choroid), which removes cellular waste products and keeps the retina attached to the choroid.

Malabsorption A condition in which nutrients are ineffectively absorbed by the intestinal mucosa, resulting in their excretion in the stool.

Malignant hypertension A hypertensive emergency, marked by a diastolic pressure greater than 120 mmHg.

Malignant melanoma (cutaneous melanoma) Skin cancer that arises from melanocytes.

Malignant pain Pain associated with a life-threatening illness such as cancer but not limited to cancer pain.

Malnutrition Inadequate nutrient intake to meet body needs; may include deficiency of major nutrients (calories, carbohydrates, proteins, and fats) or micronutrients such as vitamins and minerals.

Manifestations Signs and symptoms of a disease or condition caused by alterations in structure or function.

Man-made disasters Either accidental or intentional, they are complex emergencies, technological disasters, material shortages, and other disasters not caused by natural hazards.

Marasmus (protein energy undernutrition) Insufficient protein and calorie intake to meet metabolic needs.

Mass casualty incidents Situations in which 100 or more casualties are involved, significantly overwhelming available emergency medical services, facilities, and resources.

Mastoidectomy Surgical removal of infected mastoid air cells.

Mastoiditis Bacterial infection of the mastoid process.

Maturity-onset diabetes of the young (MODY) Diabetes in young obese adults.

Mean arterial pressure (MAP) The average pressure in the arterial circulation throughout the cardiac cycle; the product of cardiac output and systemic vascular resistance (SVR).

Medical-surgical nursing The health promotion, health care, and illness care of adults, based on knowledge derived from the arts and sciences and shaped by knowledge (the science) of nursing.

Meiosis The reduction of division of the cell occurring only in the sex cells of the testes and ovaries when the amount of genetic material is reduced in half (23 chromosomes).

Melanin Skin pigment that forms a protective shield to protect keratinocytes and nerve endings in the dermis from the damaging effects of ultraviolet light.

Melena Black, tarry stool that contains old, digested blood.

Ménière's disease Chronic disorder of unknown cause characterized by recurrent attacks of vertigo with tinnitus and a progressive unilateral hearing loss.

Meningitis Inflammation of the meninges of the brain and spinal cord.

Menopause Permanent cessation of menses.

Menorrhagia Excessive or prolonged menstruation.

Menstrual cycle Cyclic buildup of the uterine lining, ovulation, and sloughing of the lining occurring approximately every 28 days in nonpregnant females of childbearing age.

Menstruation Periodic shedding of the uterine lining in a woman of childbearing age who is not pregnant.

Metabolism Consisting of the breakdown of complex structures into simpler forms to produce energy (catabolism) and the combination of simpler molecules to produce and maintain more complex structures necessary to living organisms (anabolism).

Metaplasia A change in the normal pattern of differentiation such that dividing cells differentiate into cell types not normally found in that location in the body.

Metastasis Secondary tumor; the process by which spreading of malignant neoplasms occurs; the transfer of disease from one organ or part to another not directly connected with it.

Methcillin-resistant *Staphylococcus aureus* (MRSA) A strain of antibiotic-resistant *S. aureus* that colonizes the skin and nares.

Metrorrhagia Bleeding between menstrual periods; may be caused by hormonal imbalances, pelvic inflammatory disease, cervical or uterine polyps, uterine fibroids, or cervical or uterine cancer.

Microalbuminuria Protein in the urine.

Micturition Releasing urine from the urinary bladder (voiding).

Mild concussion Brain trauma resulting in a brief loss of consciousness that lasts from seconds to hours.

Minor trauma Injury to a single part or system of the body, usually treated in the hospital or emergency department.

Mitigation The action taken to prevent or reduce the harmful effects of a disaster on human health or property, it involves future-oriented activities to prevent subsequent disasters or to minimize their effects.

Mitosis The process of making new cells by cell division. Cell division through mitosis results in two cells called *daughter cells* that are genetically identical to the original cell, or *mother cell*, and to each other.

Mitral valve (bicuspid valve) Valve between the left atrium and ventricle in the heart; prevents blood from flowing backwards into the atrium.

Monosomic (monosomy) When one member of the chromosome pair is missing, for example, Turner syndrome (45, XO).

Morbid obesity Weight greater than 100% over ideal body weight.

Morton's neuroma A tumor-like mass formed within the neurovascular bundle of the intermetatarsal spaces.

Mosaicism A chromosome variation or abnormality that occurs after fertilization during mitosis at an early cell stage so not all cells are affected with the variation; for example, a child who is mosaic for Down syndrome will have some cells with two copies of chromosome 21 and some that have an extra chromosome 21.

Mourning The actions or expressions of the bereaved, including the symbols, clothing, and ceremonies that make up the outward manifestations of grief.

Multifactorial Health conditions determined by multiple factors, including genetic and environmental factors, each having an additive effect.

Multiple casualty incidents Incidents in which more than 2 but fewer than 100 persons are injured.

Multiple myeloma A malignancy in which plasma cells multiply uncontrollably and infiltrate the bone marrow, lymph nodes, spleen, and other tissues.

Multiple sclerosis (MS) A chronic demyelating autoimmune disease of the central nervous system.

Multiple trauma Most often the result of a motor vehicle crash, this type of trauma requires immediate intervention specifically focused on ensuring survival.

Murmur Sound made by turbulent blood flow through the heart.

Muscular dystrophy (MD) A group of inherited muscle diseases that cause progressive muscle degeneration and wasting.

Myasthenia gravis Chronic, progressive neuromuscular disorder characterized by fatigue and severe weakness of skeletal muscles.

Myelodysplastic syndrome A group of blood disorders characterized by abnormal-appearing bone marrow and cytopenia (low numbers of circulating blood cells). MDS is not a single disease; at least five variations of the disorder have been identified.

Myocarditis Inflammatory disorder of the heart muscle.

Myopia (nearsightedness) A condition in which the eyeball is elongated, causing the image to focus in front of the retina instead of on it.

Myringotomy Incision of the tympanic membrane.

Myxedema Systemic condition that develops from inadequate levels of thyroid hormone (hypothyroidism).

Myxedema coma A life-threatening complication of long-standing, untreated hypothyroidism, characterized by severe metabolic disorders (hyponatremia, hypoglycemia, lactic acidosis), hypothermia, cardiovascular collapse, impaired cognition, and coma.

Natural disasters Disasters caused by acts of nature or emerging diseases; some are unexpected and some are predictable through advanced meteorological technologies.

Natural killer cells (NK cells, null cells) Large, granular lymphocytes (found in the spleen, lymph nodes, bone marrow, and blood) that provide immune surveillance and resistance to infection, and play an important role in the destruction of early malignant cells.

Nausea An unpleasant sensation of sickness or queasiness; may or may not be followed by vomiting.

Necrosis Tissue cell death.

Neglect syndrome (unilateral neglect) A disorder of attention. In this syndrome, the person cannot integrate and use perceptions from the affected side of the body or from the environment on the affected side and, hence, ignores that part.

Neoplasm A mass of new tissue (a collection of cells) that grows independently of its surrounding structures and has no physiologic purpose.

Nephrectomy Removal of the kidney.

Nephrotic syndrome A condition marked by massive proteinuria, hypoalbuminemia, hyperlipidemia, and edema.

Neuralgia Nerve pain.

Neurogenic bladder Dysfunctional urinary bladder due to lesion of central or peripheral nervous system.

Neurogenic shock Shock resulting from an imbalance between parasympathetic and sympathetic stimulation of vascular smooth muscle. If parasympathetic overstimulation or sympathetic understimulation persists, sustained vasodilation occurs, and blood pools in the venous and capillary beds.

Neuropathic pain Pain resulting from abnormal impulse processing by the peripheral and central nervous systems following injury to the peripheral nerves.

Neuropathy Damage to peripheral nerves causing hyper- or hyposensation and leading to neuropathic pain and injury.

Neutropenia A decrease in circulating neutrophils.

Nevi (moles) Flat or raised macules or papules with rounded, well-defined borders.

Nicotine Nicotine, a stimulant, is found in tobacco and enters the system via the lungs (cigarettes and cigars) and oral mucous membranes (chewing tobacco as well as smoking).

Nociceptive pain Pain caused by stimulation of peripheral or visceral pain receptors.

Nociceptors Sensory nerve fibers that conduct pain impulses from the periphery to the central nervous system.

Nocturia Voiding two or more times at night.

Node Elements of the immune system connected by lymphatics. Upregulates immune function; does not synthesize hormones.

Nonconventional terrorist weapons Chemical, biological, and nuclear weapons of terrorism; used less frequently than conventional terrorist weapons.

Non-Hodgkin's lymphoma (NHL) Lymphoid tissue malignancies that do not contain Reed–Sternberg cells.

Nonunion A state that exists when the ends of a fracture fail to heal together.

Normal sinus rhythm (NSR) Normal heart rhythm, in which impulses originate in the sinus node and travel through normal conduction pathways without delay.

Nosocomial Pertaining to or occurring in a hospital.

Nosocomial infection Infection contracted during residence in a hospital or extended care facility.

Nuclear terrorism Use of a nuclear device to cause mass murder and devastation.

Nursing process The series of critical thinking activities nurses use as they provide care to patients; this logical approach to care ensures that patients receive comprehensive and effective care.

Nutrients Substances found in food that are used by the body to promote growth, maintenance, and repair.

Nutrition The process by which the body ingests, absorbs, transports, uses, and eliminates food.

Nystagmus Rapid involuntary eye movements.

Obesity An excess of body fat (adipose tissue).

Obstructive shock Shock caused by an obstruction in the heart or great vessels that either impedes venous return or prevents effective cardiac pumping action.

Occult blood/bleeding Blood or bleeding that is hidden or not readily apparent.

Office-based surgical suites A setting for many elective surgeries, although increasing malpractice insurance premiums have influenced their decline.

Oligomenorrhea Scant menses.

Oliguria Urine output of less than 400 mL in 24 hours.

Oncogene Gene capable of triggering cancerous characteristics.

Oncologic emergencies In caring for patients with cancer, nurses may encounter a number of emergency situations in which their role may be pivotal to the patient's survival. Most of these emergencies require astute observations, accurate judgments, and rapid action once the problem has been identified.

Oncology The study of cancer.

Onycholysis The separation of the distal nail plate from the nail bed.

Onychomycosis A fungal or dermatophyte infection of the nail plate.

Opiates Analgesics derived from the opium plant; produce analgesia by binding to opioid receptors within and outside the CNS; the most potent analgesics available, and the treatment of choice for acute moderate-to-severe pain. Examples include morphine, codeine, and fentanyl (Durgesic, Actiq). Also called narcotic analgesics.

Orchitis Infection or inflammation of the testicle.

Orthopnea Difficulty breathing when supine.

Orthostatic hypotension A decrease in systolic blood pressure of more than 10 to 15 mmHg and a drop in diastolic blood pressure on standing.

Osmosis The process by which water moves across a selectively permeable membrane from an area of lower solute concentration to an area of higher solute concentration.

Ossification The process of bone formation.

Osteitis deformans See *Paget's disease of bone*.

Osteoarthritis (OA) (degenerative joint disease) The most commonly occurring of all forms of arthritis. This disease is characterized by loss of articular cartilage in articulating joints and hypertrophy of the bones at the articular margins.

Osteomalacia (adult rickets) Metabolic bone disorder characterized by inadequate mineralization of bone matrix.

Osteomyelitis Infection within the bone that can lead to tissue death and necrosis.

Osteophytes Bony outgrowths often called "joint mice."

Osteoporosis Literally defined as "porous bones," a metabolic bone disorder characterized by loss of bone mass, increased bone fragility, and an increased risk of fractures.

Osteotomy An incision into or transection of the bone.

Ostomy General term for an operation in which an artificial opening is created.

Otitis media Inflammation or infection of the middle ear.

Otorrhea Leakage of cerebrospinal fluid through the ear.

Otosclerosis Abnormal bone formation in the osseous labyrinth of the temporal bone causing the footplate of the stapes to become fixed or immobile in the oval window. The result is a conductive hearing loss.

Ovarian cycle The female cycle that occurs from puberty until menopause in which the production of ova occur.

Oxyhemoglobin The combined form of hemoglobin and oxygen; found in arterial blood, it carries oxygen to body tissues.

Pacemaker A pulse generator used to provide an electrical stimulus to the heart when the heart fails to generate or conduct its own at a rate that maintains the cardiac output.

PaCO$_2$ Partial pressure of carbon dioxide in arterial blood.

Paget's disease of bone (osteitis deformans) A skeletal disorder that results from excessive osteoclastic activity. Paget's disease is characterized by bone deformity, especially of the long bones of the lower limbs, the pelvis, the lumbar vertebrae, and the skull.

Pain A subjective response to both physical and psychologic stressors.

Pain threshold The point at which a stimulus elicits a pain response.

Pain tolerance The amount of pain a person can endure before responding to it.

Palliative care An area of care that has evolved out of the hospice experience, but exists outside of hospice programs and is not restricted to the end of life. Palliative care is focused on the relief of physical, mental, and spiritual distress for individuals who have an incurable illness and is used earlier in the disease experience than hospice care. The goal of palliative care is to prevent and relieve suffering by early assessment and treatment of pain and other physical, psychosocial, and spiritual needs to improve the patient's quality of life.

Pallor Lack of color; paleness of skin.

Pancreatitis Inflammation of the pancreas.

Pannus Granulation tissue that forms in joints affected by rheumatoid arthritis and leads to the formation of scar tissue that immobilizes the joint.

PaO$_2$ Partial pressure of oxygen in arterial blood.

Papilledema Swelling of the optic nerve.

Paracentesis Aspiration of fluid from the peritoneal cavity.

Paralytic ileus Impaired propulsion or forward movement of bowel contents.

Paraplegia Paralysis of the lower portion of the body, sometimes involving the lower trunk.

Parasites Organisms that live within, on, or at the expense of the patient.

Parenteral nutrition (PN or TPN) Intravenous administration of carbohydrates (high concentrations of dextrose), protein (amino acids), electrolytes, vitamins, minerals, and fat emulsions.

Paresthesia An abnormal sensation of the skin, such as numbness, burning, or pricking.

Parish nursing A nontraditional, community-based way of providing health promotion and health restoration nursing interventions to a spiritual community.

Parkinson's disease (PD) Progressive, degenerative neurologic disease characterized by nonintentional tremor, bradykinesia, and muscle rigidity.

Paronychia An infection of the cuticle of the fingernails or toenails.

Paroxysmal Abrupt onset and termination.

Paroxysmal nocturnal dyspnea (PND) Attacks of acute shortness of breath that occur at night, waking up the patient.

Partial gastrectomy Removal of a portion of the stomach, usually the distal half to two-thirds.

Partial seizures Seizures that involve a restricted part of one cerebral hemisphere; may be simple partial (without loss of consciousness) or complex partial (with loss of consciousness).

Partial-thickness burn Burn that involves the entire dermis and the papillae of the dermis (superficial partial-thickness burn) or extends into the hair follicles (deep partial-thickness burn).

Passive immunity Temporary protection—provided by antibodies produced by other people or animals—against disease-producing antigens. Protection is gradually lost when these acquired antibodies are used up either by natural degradation or by combining with the antigen.

Pathogens Virulent organisms rarely found in the absence of disease.

Patient The person with whom and for whom nursing care is designed and implemented.

Patient-controlled analgesia (PCA) A pump with a control mechanism that allows the patient to self-manage pain.

Pediculosis capitis An infestation with head lice.

Pediculosis corporis An infestation with body lice.

Pediculosis pubis An infestation with pubic lice (often called "crabs").

Pelvic inflammatory disease (PID) A term used to describe infection of the pelvic organs.

Pemphigus vulgaris Chronic disorder of the skin and oral mucous membranes characterized by vesicle (blister) formation.

Penetrance The percentage or likelihood that an individual who has inherited a gene mutation will actually express the disease signs and symptoms in his or her lifetime.

Penicillin-resistant *Streptococcus pneumoniae* **(PRSP)** Infection transmitted by droplets from the respiratory tract; requires transmission-based droplet precautions.

Peptic ulcer/peptic ulcer disease (PUD) A break in the mucous lining of the gastrointestinal tract where it comes in contact with gastric juice; may affect any area of the gastrointestinal tract exposed to acid-pepsin secretions, including the esophagus, stomach, or duodenum.

Pericarditis Inflammation of the pericardium.

Perioperative nursing A specialized area of nursing practice that incorporates the three phases of the surgical experience: preoperative, intraoperative, and postoperative.

Peripheral vascular disease (PVD) Impaired blood supply to peripheral tissues, particularly the lower extremities.

Peripheral vascular resistance (PVR) The opposing forces or impedance to blood flow as the arterial channels become more and more distant from the heart.

Peristalsis Alternating waves of contraction and relaxation of involuntary muscles.

Peritoneal dialysis Procedure in which electrolytes, waste products, and excess water are removed from the body by diffusion using the peritoneum surrounding the abdominal cavity as the dialyzing membrane.

Peritonitis Inflammation of the peritoneum.

Pernicious anemia Anemia resulting from failure to absorb dietary vitamin B_{12} due to lack of intrinsic factor.

Persistent vegetative state (PVS) Condition of complete unawareness of self and the environment.

Personal protective equipment (PPE) Equipment used for the protection of personnel including gloves, masks, goggles, gowns, and biologic disposal bags (red bags); may also include hoods, helmets, head gear, and impermeable suits.

Pertussis (whooping cough) A highly contagious acute upper respiratory infection caused by the bacterium *Bordetella pertussis*.

Phagocytosis A process by which a foreign agent or target cell is engulfed, destroyed, and digested. Neutrophils and macrophages, known as phagocytes, are the primary cells involved in phagocytosis.

Phantom limb pain A confusing pain syndrome that occurs following surgical or traumatic amputation of a limb. The patient experiences pain in the missing body part even though there is complete mental awareness that the limb is gone.

Pharyngitis Acute inflammation of the pharynx.

Phenotype The expression of a person's entire physical, biochemical, and physiologic makeup, as determined by the individual's genotype and environmental factors.

Phimosis Constriction of the foreskin so that it cannot be retracted over the glans penis.

Plasmapheresis (plasma exchange) Removal of the plasma component from whole blood.

Plastic surgery The alteration, replacement, or restoration of visible portions of the body, performed to correct a structural or cosmetic defect.

Platelets (thrombocytes) Cell fragments that have no nucleus and cannot replicate.

Pleural effusion Collection of excess fluid in the pleural space.

Pleuritis Inflammation of the pleura.

Pneumonectomy Removal of an entire lung.

Pneumonia Inflammation of the lung parenchyma (the respiratory bronchioles and alveoli).

Pneumothorax Results when air enters the pleural space due to blunt and penetrating injuries to the chest.

Polycystic kidney disease A hereditary disease characterized by cyst formation and massive kidney enlargement.

Polycythemia (erythrocytosis) Excess RBCs characterized by a hematocrit higher than 55%.

Polydipsia Excessive thirst.

Polymorphisms The DNA sequences that are natural variations in a gene usually having no adverse effects on the individual.

Polymyositis A systemic connective-tissue disorder characterized by inflammation of connective tissue and muscle fibers leading to muscle weakness and atrophy.

Polyp Mass of tissue that arises from the bowel wall and protrudes into the lumen.

Polyphagia Excessive eating.

Polysubstance abuse The simultaneous use of many substances.

Polyuria Excessive output of urine.

Portal hypertension Elevated pressure in the portal venous system that causes rerouting of blood to adjoining lower pressure vessels.

Portal systemic (hepatic) encephalopathy Impaired consciousness and mental status due to the accumulation of toxic waste products in the blood (ammonia in particular) as blood bypasses the congested liver.

Postconcussion syndrome Persistent headache, dizziness, irritability, insomnia, impaired memory and concentration, and learning problems following a concussion; may last for several weeks or up to 1 year.

Postoperative phase Period when a procedure or surgery has been completed and the patient is recovering from the stress associated with the surgery.

Postpoliomyelitis syndrome A complication of a previous infection by the poliomyelitis virus.

Preload The amount of cardiac muscle fiber tension or stretch that exists at end diastole, just before ventricular contraction.

Premature ejaculation A common ejaculatory disorder in which semen is ejaculated before completion of sexual intercourse.

Premenstrual syndrome (PMS) Complex of symptoms characterized by irritability, depression, edema, and breast tenderness preceding the monthly menses.

Preoperative phase Time when preparation of the patient for surgery is conducted and completed.

Preparedness Actions that address preparations for and actions in dealing with the consequences of a disaster.

Presbycusis Age-related loss of the ability to hear high-frequency sounds, may occur because of cochlear hair cell degeneration or loss of auditory neurons in the organ of Corti.

Presbyopia Impaired near vision resulting from a loss of elasticity of the lens of the eye.

Pressure ulcer Ischemic lesion of the skin and underlying tissue caused by external pressure that impairs the flow of blood and lymph.

Priapism Sustained, painful erection that lasts at least 4 hours and is not associated with sexual arousal.

Primary hypertension (idiopathic, essential) A persistently elevated systemic blood pressure.

Primary polycythemia (polycythemia vera) A neoplastic stem cell disorder characterized by overproduction of red blood cells and, to a lesser extent, white blood cells and platelets.

Professional boundaries The borders between the vulnerability of the patient and the power of the nurse.

Progesterone Hormone produced by the ovary; works with estrogen to control the menstrual cycle.

Proptosis Forward displacement of the eye.

Prostatitis Inflammation of the prostate gland.

Protein-calorie malnutrition (PCM) Deficient protein and calories to meet metabolic needs.

Proteinuria Abnormal proteins in the urine.

Proto-oncogenes Normal genes that promote cell growth and repair.

Pruritus Subjective itching sensation producing an urge to scratch.

Psoriasis Chronic, noninfectious skin disorder that is characterized by raised, reddened, round circumscribed plaques covered by silvery white scales.

Psychogenic pain Pain that is experienced in the absence of any diagnosed physiologic cause or event.

Psychostimulants Psychostimulants such as cocaine and amphetamines have a high potential for abuse. Euphoria is the main subjective effect associated with cocaine and amphetamines, leading to addiction.

Ptosis Drooping of the eyelid.

Pulmonary edema An abnormal accumulation of fluid in the interstitial tissue and alveoli of the lung.

Pulmonary embolism Sudden occlusion of blood flow in a portion of the pulmonary vascular system, causing a ventilation-perfusion imbalance and impaired gas exchange.

Pulmonary hypertension Condition in which the pulmonary arterial pressure is elevated to an abnormal level.

Pulmonic valve The semilunar valve between the right ventricle and the pulmonary artery.

Pulse Rhythmic pressure wave that can be felt over an artery.

Pulse deficit Condition in which the radial pulse is less than the apical pulse, indicating weak, inefficient left ventricular contractions.

Pulse pressure The difference between the systolic and diastolic blood pressure.

Puncture wound Wound that occurs when a sharp or blunt object penetrates the integument.

Pupillary light reflex Reflex in which the pupil contracts in response to a bright light.

Pyelonephritis Upper urinary tract inflammation affecting the kidney and renal pelvis.

Pyoderma Purulent bacterial infection of skin.

Pyuria Pus in the urine.

Quadriplegia See *Tetraplegia*.

Quality assurance The process of ensuring quality control activities that evaluate, monitor, or regulate the standard of services provided to the consumer.

Rabies Viral (rhabdovirus) infection of the central nervous system transmitted by infected saliva that enters the human body through a bite or an open wound.

Radiation sickness One of the results of DNA mutation inside cells exposed to ionizing radiation.

Radiation therapy Therapy that uses radiation to kill a tumor, to reduce its size, to decrease pain, or to relieve obstruction.

Radiculopathy A condition in which one or more nerves, especially nerve roots, do not function normally.

Radiological dispersion bomb Also called a "dirty bomb," it consists of a conventional explosive such as trinitrotoluene (TNT) packed with radioactive waste by-products from nuclear reactors that discharges deadly radioactive particles into the environment.

Raynaud's disease/phenomenon Disorders characterized by episodes of intense vasospasm in the small arteries and arterioles of the fingers and possibly the toes.

Reactive arthritis (Reiter's syndrome) An acute, nonpurulent inflammatory arthritis that complicates a bacterial infection of the genitourinary or gastrointestinal tracts.

Rebound tenderness Pain that occurs with withdrawal or release of pressure applied during abdominal palpation.

Recessive A characteristic that is apparent only when two copies of the gene encoding it are present, one from the mother and one from the father.

Reconstruction The recovery aspect of disaster response; during this period restoration, reconstitution, and mitigation take place.

Recovery The fifth of 5 stages of disaster. Activities include rebuilding and returning to some semblance of "normalcy" but also includes mitigation activities or planning to prevent subsequent disasters or to minimize the effects of future disasters.

Red blood cell (RBCs, erythrocytes) Blood cells shaped like a biconcave disk that contain hemoglobin required for oxygen transport to body tissues; the most common type of blood cell.

Referral source A person recommending home care services and supplying the agency with details about the patient's needs. The source may be a physician, nurse, social worker, therapist, or discharge planner.

Referred pain Pain that is perceived in an area distant from the site of the stimuli.

Reflex sympathetic dystrophy A group of poorly understood posttraumatic conditions involving persistent pain, hyperesthesias, swelling, changes in skin color and texture, changes in temperature, and decreased motion.

Reflux, urinary Backflow of urine toward the kidneys.

Refraction The bending of light rays as they pass from one medium to another medium of different optical density.

Refractory period A period in which myocardial cells are resistant to stimulation.

Regional anesthesia Anesthesia that desensitizes the area to be operated but does not involve the full central nervous system or cause sedation.

Regurgitation (valvular) Backflow of blood through an incompletely closed valve into the area it just left.

Rehabilitation The process of learning to live to one's maximum potential with a chronic impairment and its resultant functional disability.

Reiter's syndrome See *Reactive arthritis*.

Remission A period in which symptoms are not experienced even though the disease is still clinically present.

Renal artery stenosis Narrowing of the renal artery.

Renal colic Acute, severe, intermittent pain in the flank and upper outer abdominal quadrant generally associated with acute obstruction of a ureter and resulting ureteral spasm.

Renal failure A condition in which the kidneys are unable to remove accumulated metabolites from the blood, resulting in altered fluid, electrolyte, and acid–base balance.

Renal impairment (decreased renal reserve) A glomerular filtration rate of approximately 50% of normal with normal BUN and serum creatinine levels.

Renal insufficiency A glomerular filtration rate of 20% to 50% of normal with azotemia and some manifestations of renal failure.

Renal transplant The surgical insertion of a functioning kidney.

Renin–angiotensin mechanism An intrinsic system that responds to renal perfusion; a fall in renal blood flow (e.g. due to low BP or cardiac output) stimulates renin release, ultimately leading to vasoconstriction and sodium and water retention and increased BP and cardiac output.

Repolarization Restoration of the resting cell membrane potential following generation of an action potential.

Respiratory failure Inability of lungs to oxygenate the blood and remove carbon dioxide adequately to meet the body's needs, even at rest.

Respite care Short-term or intermittent home care, often using volunteers. These services exist to give the primary caregiver some relief from the burden of full-time care.

Response Occurs in the emergency stage of disaster response, after the impact of the disaster event has occurred, the community has been rapidly assessed for damage, and the types and extent of injuries suffered as well as the immediate needs of the community have been determined.

Reticular activating system (RAS) A system of reticular neurons within the reticular formation that passes steady streams of impulses through thalamic relays in order to stimulate the cerebral cortex into wakefulness.

Retinal detachment Separation of the retina or sensory portion of the eye from the choroid.

Retinitis pigmentosa Hereditary degenerative disease characterized by retinal atrophy and loss of retinal function progressing from the periphery to the central region of the retina.

Retractions A pulling in of the tissue of the precordium; a slight retraction just medial to the midclavicular line at the area of the apical impulse is normal and is more likely to be visible in thin patients.

Retrograde ejaculation Seminal fluid discharged into the bladder.

Reverse triage Working from the principle of the greatest good for the greatest number, reverse triage is an "upside-down triage" used in mass casualty events in which the victims who are most severely injured, requiring extensive resources with little chance of surviving, are treated last.

Rheumatic disorders Inflammatory diseases of connective tissues that affect joints, the muscles, and bones.

Rheumatic fever A systemic inflammatory disease caused by an abnormal immune response to pharyngeal infection by group A beta-hemolytic streptococci.

Rheumatic heart disease (RHD) Slowly progressive valvular deformity following acute or repeated attacks of rheumatic fever; characterized by rigid and deformed valve leaflets, fused valve commissures, and fibrosis of chordae tendineae.

Rheumatoid arthritis A chronic systemic autoimmune disease that causes inflammation of connective tissue, primarily in the joints.

Rhinitis Inflammation of the nasal cavities.

Rhinoplasty Surgical reconstruction of the nose.

Rhinorrhea Leakage of cerebrospinal fluid through the nose.

Ruptured disk See *Herniated intervertebral disk*.

Salmonellosis A form of food poisoning caused by ingestion of foods contaminated with one or more varieties of *Salmonella* bacteria.

Sarcoidosis Systemic disease characterized by granulomas in the lungs, lymph nodes, liver, eyes, skin, and other organs.

Sarcoma A tumor arising from supportive tissues.

Scabies Parasitic infestation caused by the mite *Sarcoptes scabiei*.

Sciatica Pain over the sciatic nerve.

Scleroderma (systemic sclerosis) Hardening of the skin, a chronic condition characterized by the formation of excess fibrous connective tissue and diffuse fibrosis of the skin and internal organs.

Sclerotherapy The removal of benign skin lesions with a sclerosing agent that causes inflammation with fibrosis of tissue.

Scoliosis A lateral curvature of the spine.

Scrub person Prepares the sterile field, surgical supplies, and equipment for surgical procedures; also assists surgeon and physician assistant by passing instruments, suctioning blood, and maintaining the sterile field.

Seborrheic dermatitis Common and chronic inflammatory disorder of the skin that involves the scalp, eyebrows, eyelids, ear canals, nasolabial folds, axillae, and trunk. The cause is unknown.

Sebum Sebaceous glands are found all over the body except on the palms and soles. These glands secrete an oily substance called sebum, which softens and lubricates the skin and hair and also decreases water loss from the skin in low humidity. Sebum also protects the body from infection by killing bacteria.

Secondary hypertension Elevated blood pressure resulting from an identifiable underlying process.

Seizure An episode of excessive and abnormal discharge of electrical activity within the central nervous system.

Semen Fluid containing sperm secreted by the male reproductive system glands.

Seminoma A tumor from seminal or germ tissue.

Septic arthritis The type of arthritis that develops when a joint space is invaded by a pathogen.

Septic shock One part of a progressive syndrome called systemic inflammatory response syndrome (SIRS). Beginning with an infection, SIRS progresses to bacteremia, then sepsis, then septic shock, and finally multiple organ failure syndrome.

Seroconversion Antibody response to a disease or vaccine.

Serum bicarbonate The serum bicarbonate (HCO_3^-) reflects the renal regulation of acid–base balance. It is often called the metabolic component of arterial blood gases. The normal HCO_3^- value is 22 to 26 mEq/L.

Severe acute respiratory syndrome (SARS) Lower respiratory illness of unknown etiology; spread by close person-to-person contact.

Sex chromosomes The chromosomes X or Y that indicate gender.

Sexually transmitted infection (STI, sexually transmitted disease, venereal disease) Any infection transmitted by sexual contact, including vaginal, oral, and anal intercourse.

Shigellosis (bacillary dysentery) An acute bowel infection caused by microorganisms of the *Shigella* genus.

Shingles See *Herpes zoster*.

Shock A clinical syndrome characterized by a systemic imbalance between oxygen supply and demand. This imbalance results in a state of inadequate blood flow to the peripheral tissues, causing life-threatening cellular dysfunction, hypotension, and oliguria.

Sickle cell anemia A hereditary, chronic hemolytic anemia characterized by episodes of sickling, during which RBCs become abnormally crescent shaped.

Sickle cell crisis Severe episodes of fever and intense pain that are the hallmark of sickle cell anemia.

Sinusitis Inflammation of the mucous membranes of one or more of the sinuses.

Sjögren's syndrome An autoimmune disorder that causes inflammation and dysfunction of exocrine glands throughout the body.

Skeletal traction Application of a pulling force through placement of pins into the bone.

Skin graft Surgical method of detaching skin from a donor site and placing it in a recipient site, where it develops a new blood supply from the base of the wound.

Skin tags Soft papules on a pedicle.

Skin traction Traction in which the cradle-like sleeve placed around the extremity exerts its pulling force through the patient's skin.

Sleep apnea Absence of airflow through the upper airways for 10 or more seconds.

Somatic cell Any cell in the body that is not a sex cell (ova and sperm).

Somatic pain Pain arising from nerve receptors originating in the skin or close to the surface of the body.

Somogyi phenomenon A morning rise in blood glucose to hyperglycemic levels following an episode of nocturnal hypoglycemia and a counterregulatory hormone response.

Spasticity Increased muscle tone in diseases involving the corticospinal motor tract.

Spermatocele A mobile, usually painless mass containing dead spermatozoa that forms in the epididymis.

Spinal cord injury (SCI) Injury to spinal cord, usually due to trauma.

Spinal cord tumors Benign or malignant, primary or metastatic tumor of the spinal cord.

Spinal shock Temporary loss of reflex function below the level of injury to the spinal cord.

Splenomegaly Enlargement of the spleen.

Sprain Tearing or stretching of a ligament that results from a twisting motion.

Sprue A chronic primary disorder of the small intestine in which the absorption of nutrients, particularly fats, is impaired.

Squamous cell carcinoma Malignant tumor of the squamous epithelium of the skin or mucous membranes.

Standard A statement or criterion that can be used by a profession and by the general public to measure quality of practice.

Starvation Inadequate dietary intake; the condition of being without food for long periods of time.

Status asthmaticus Severe, prolonged asthma that does not respond to routine treatment. Without aggressive therapy, status asthmaticus can lead to respiratory failure with hypoxemia, hypercapnia, and acidosis.

Status epilepticus Continuous seizure activity with only very short periods of calm occurring between intense and persistent seizures.

Steatorrhea Greasy, frothy, yellow stools resulting from excess fat in the feces.

Stem cell transplant (SCT) Infusion of donor stem cells to replace the recipient's blood cell lines (WBCs, RBCs, and platelets).

Stem cells (hemocytoblasts) Bone marrow precursor cells for all blood cells.

Stenosis Condition where valve leaflets fuse together and are unable to open or close fully.

Stoma Surface opening.

Stomatitis Inflammation of the oral mucosa.

Straight traction A pulling force applied in a straight line to the injured body part resting on the bed.

Strain Stretching or tearing of muscle fibers that results in bleeding into the tissues.

Stress incontinence Loss of usually less than 50 mL of urine occurring with increased abdominal pressure.

Stress-induced (erosive) gastritis Inflammation and superficial erosions of the gastric mucosa that may occur as a complication of other life-threatening conditions such as shock, severe trauma, major surgery, sepsis, burns, or head injury.

Striae A line above or below tissue that differs in color and texture from surrounding tissue.

Stridor High-pitched, harsh inspiratory sound indicative of upper airway obstruction.

Stroke (brain attack, cerebrovascular accident, CVA) A condition in which neurologic deficits occur as a result of decreased blood flow to a focal (localized) area of brain tissue from a blood clot, an embolus, or a cerebral vessel rupture.

Stroke volume (SV) The amount of blood pumped into the aorta with each contraction of the left ventricle.

Subdural hematoma A localized mass of blood that collects between the dura mater and the arachnoid mater.

Subluxation Partial separation (or dislocation) of the bones of a joint.

Substance abuse The use of any chemical in a fashion inconsistent with medical or culturally defined social norms despite physical, psychologic, or social adverse effects.

Substance dependence A severe condition occurring when the use of a chemical substance is no longer under an individual's control for at least 3 months. Continued use of the substance usually persists despite adverse effects on the person's physical condition, psychologic health, and interpersonal relationships (used interchangeably with addiction).

Sudden cardiac death (SCD) Unexpected death occurring within 1 hour of the onset of cardiovascular symptoms.

Sundowning A behavioral change in Alzheimer's disease characterized by increased agitation, time disorientation, and wandering during afternoon and evening hours.

Superficial burn Burn involving only the epidermal layer of the skin; most often results from damage from sunburn, ultraviolet light, minor flash injury (from a sudden ignition or explosion), or mild radiation burn associated with cancer treatment.

Surfactant A lipoprotein produced by the alveolar cells; interferes with adhesion of water molecules, reducing surface tension and helping to expand lungs.

Surge capacity The healthcare system's ability to rapidly expand beyond normal services to meet the increased demand for qualified personnel, medical care, and public health in the event of a large-scale disaster.

Surgery An invasive medical procedure performed to diagnose or treat illness, injury, or deformity. Although surgery is a medical treatment, the nurse assumes an active role in caring for the patient before, during, and after surgery.

Surgical debridement The process of excising a wound to the level of fascia (fascial excision) or sequentially removing thin slices of a burn wound to the level of viable tissue (sequential excision).

Surveillance Collecting and analyzing data to establish a baseline and determine a point at which there is a change or trend in the health of the population.

Syndrome of inappropriate ADH secretion (SIADH) A disorder characterized by high levels of ADH in the absence of serum hypoosmolality. Manifestations of SIADH occur as a result of water retention, hyponatremia, and serum hypo-osmolality. Blood volume expands, but the plasma is diluted.

Synovitis Inflammation of the synovial membrane lining the articular capsule of a joint.

Syphilis A sexually transmitted infection caused by a spirochete that may invade almost any body tissue or organ. It enters the body through a break in the skin or mucous membranes, and can be transferred to the fetus through the placental circulation.

Systemic lupus erythematosus (SLE) A chronic, inflammatory immune complex connective tissue disease.

Systemic sclerosis (scleroderma) Hardening of the skin; a chronic disease characterized by the formation of excess fibrous connective tissue and diffuse fibrosis of the skin and internal organs.

Systole A phase during which the ventricles contract and eject blood into the pulmonary and systemic circuits.

Systolic blood pressure The arterial pressure wave produced by ventricular contraction (systole); averages 120 mmHg in healthy adults.

T lymphocytes (T cells) Type of lymphocyte that matures in the thymus gland.

Tachycardia A heart rate exceeding 100 beats per minute.

Tachypnea Abnormally rapid respiratory rate.

Tendonitis Inflammation of a tendon.

Tension headache Poorly localized headache characterized by ill-defined bilateral head aching, tightness, pressure, or a viselike feeling.

Tension pneumothorax A condition in which an injury to the chest allows air to enter but not escape the pleural cavity.

Terrorism Defined by the U.S. Department of Defense as the "calculated use of violence or the threat of violence to inculcate fear; intended to coerce or to intimidate governments or societies in the pursuit of goals that are generally political, religious or ideological."

Testicular torsion Twisting of the testes and spermatic cord.

Testosterone Male hormone produced in the testes.

Tetanus Disorder of the nervous system caused by a neurotoxin elaborated by *Clostridium tetani*.

Tetany Tonic muscular spasms.

Tetraplegia (formerly called quadriplegia) Injury to cervical segments of the cord thus impairing function of the arms, trunk, legs, and pelvic organs.

Thalassemia An inherited disorder of hemoglobin synthesis in which either the alpha or beta chains of the hemoglobin molecule are missing or defective.

Third spacing The accumulation and sequestration of trapped extracellular fluid in an actual or potential body space as a result of disease or injury.

Thoracentesis Invasive procedure in which fluid (or occasionally air) is removed from the pleural space with a needle.

Thoracotomy Incision of the chest wall to gain access to the lung for surgery.

Thrill Palpable vibration over the precordium or an artery.

Thromboangiitis obliterans (Buerger's disease) An occlusive vascular disease involving inflammation, spasm, and clot formation in small- and medium-sized peripheral arteries.

Thrombocytopenia A platelet count of less than 100, per milliliter of blood.

Thromboembolus A thrombus that breaks loose from the vessel wall.

Thrombophlebitis See *Venous thrombosis*.

Thrombotic cerebrovascular accident Cerebrovascular accident caused by occlusion of a vessel by a thrombus (a blood clot) on the interior wall of an artery.

Thrombus A blood clot that adheres to a vessel wall.

Thrust A visible pulsation.

Thyroid storm or crisis An extreme state of hyperthyroidism that is rare today because of improved diagnosis and treatment methods. Those affected are usually people with untreated hyperthyroidism (most often Graves' disease) and people with hyperthyroidism who have experienced a stressor, such as an infection, trauma, untreated diabetic ketoacidosis, or manipulation of the thyroid gland during surgery. Thyroid crisis is a life-threatening condition.

Thyroidectomy Surgical removal of the thyroid gland.

Thyroiditis Inflammation of the thyroid gland.

Thyrotoxicosis Another term for hyperthyroidism.

Tidal volume (TV) The amount of air (approximately 500 mL) moved in and out of the lungs with each normal, quiet breath.

Tinea capitis A fungal infection of the scalp.

Tinea corporis A fungal infection of the body.

Tinea pedis A fungal infection of the toenails and feet.

Tinnitus Perception of sound such as ringing, buzzing, or roaring in the ears.

Titrate To increase or decrease the dose in small increments.

Tolerance A cumulative state in which a particular dose of a chemical elicits a smaller response than before. With increased tolerance, the individual needs higher and higher doses to obtain the desired effect.

Tonic-clonic seizures Alternating contraction (tonic phase) and relaxation (clonic phase) of muscles during seizure activity.

Tonsillitis Acute inflammation of the palatine tonsils.

Tophi Small white nodules in subcutaneous tissue composed of urate deposits resulting from gout.

Total colectomy Surgical removal of the entire colon.

Total gastrectomy Removal of the entire stomach.

Total hip arthroplasty (THA) Replacement of both the femoral head and the acetabulum.

Total parenteral nutrition (TPN) Intravenous administration of carbohydrates (high concentrations of dextrose), protein (amino acids), electrolytes, vitamins, minerals, and fat emulsions.

Toxic epidermal necrolysis (TEN) Rare, life-threatening disease in which the epidermis peels off the dermis in sheets, leaving large areas of denuded skin.

Toxic megacolon A condition characterized by acute motor paralysis and dilation of the colon.

Traction The application of a straightening or pulling force to return or maintain the fractured bones in normal anatomic position.

Transcutaneous electrical nerve stimulation (TENS) A unit that consists of a low-voltage transmitter connected by wires to electrodes that are placed by the patient as directed by the physical therapist. The patient experiences a gentle tapping or vibrating sensation over the electrodes. The patient can adjust the voltage to achieve maximum pain relief.

Transdermal Medication absorbed through the skin without injection.

Transfusion An infusion of blood or blood components.

Transient ischemic attack (TIA) Brief period of localized cerebral ischemia that causes neurologic deficits lasting for less than 24 hours.

Transjugular intrahepatic portosystemic shunt (TIPS) Used to relieve portal hypertension and its complications of esophageal varices and ascites. A channel is created through the liver tissue using a needle inserted transcutaneously; an expandable metal stent is inserted into this channel to allow blood to flow directly from the portal vein into the hepatic vein, bypassing the cirrhotic liver. The shunt relieves pressure in esophageal varices and allows better control of fluid retention with diuretic therapy. Generally it is used as a short-term measure until liver transplant is performed.

Translocation The joining of a part of or a whole chromosome to another separate chromosome.

Trauma The injury to human tissues and organs resulting from the transfer of energy from the environment.

Traumatic brain injury (TBI) A traumatic insult to the brain capable of causing physical, intellectual, emotional, social, and vocational changes.

Tremors Rhythmic movement.

Triage Means "sorting." Triage is a continuous process in which patient priorities are reassigned as needed treatments, time, and the condition of the patients change.

Tricuspid valve The valve between the right atrium and right ventricle of the heart; prevents blood from flowing backwards into the atrium.

Trigeminal neuralgia (tic douloureux) A chronic disease of the trigeminal cranial nerve (cranial nerve V) that causes severe facial pain.

Triglycerides Molecules of glycerol with fatty acids used to transport and store fats in body tissues.

Trisomy 21 Possessing three chromosomes instead of the usual two as in trisomy 21 or Down syndrome where an additional copy of chromosome 21 is present.

Trousseau's sign Contraction of the hand and fingers (carpal spasm) in response to occlusion of the blood supply by a blood pressure cuff; caused by decreased blood calcium levels.

Tuberculosis (TB) Chronic, recurrent infectious disease caused by *Mycobacterium tuberculosis*; usually affects the lungs, although any organ can be affected.

Tumor marker A protein molecule detectable in serum or other body fluids. This marker is used as a biochemical indicator of the presence of a malignancy.

Tympanoplasty Surgical reconstruction of the middle ear.

Type 1 diabetes One of two types of diabetes characterized by the destruction of beta cells, usually leading to absolute insulin deficiency.

Type 2 diabetes One of two types of diabetes, the characteristics of which may range from predominantly insulin resistance with relative insulin deficiency to a predominantly secretory defect with insulin resistance. There is no immune destruction of beta cells.

Ulcer A lesion of the skin or mucous membranes.

Ulcerative colitis Chronic inflammatory bowel disorder of the mucosa and submucosa of the colon and rectum.

Ultrafiltration Removal of excess body water using a hydrostatic pressure gradient.

Uniform Anatomical Gift Act Legislation that requires people to be informed about their options related to organ donation.

Unilateral neglect State in which a patient is unaware of and inattentive to one side of the body.

Upper body obesity (central obesity) Excess intra-abdominal fat characterized by a waist-to-hip ratio greater than 1 in men and 0.8 in women.

Urea An end product of protein metabolism, eliminated in the urine.

Uremia Literally "urine in the blood"; the syndrome or group of symptoms associated with end-stage renal failure.

Ureteral stent Thin catheter inserted into the ureter to provide for urine flow and ureteral support.

Ureteroplasty Surgical repair of a ureter.

Urgency A sudden, compelling need to urinate.

Urinary calculi Calculi or "stones" in the urinary tract.

Urinary diversion Procedure to provide for urine collection and drainage following cystectomy. The most common urinary diversion is the ileal conduit.

Urinary drainage system The ureters, urinary bladder, and urethra.

Urinary incontinence (UI) Involuntary urination.

Urinary retention Incomplete emptying of the bladder.

Urolithiasis Development of stones within the urinary tract.

Urticaria Hives.

Vaccine Suspensions of whole or fractionated bacteria or viruses that have been treated to make them nonpathogenic.

Valsalva's maneuver Closing the glottis and contracting the diaphragm and abdominal muscles to increase intra-abdominal pressure.

Valvular heart disease Interference of blood flow to, within, and from the heart.

Vancomycin intermediate-resistant *Staphylococcus aureus* (VISA) A form of *S. aureus* with intermediate resistance to vancomycin.

Varicocele Dilation of the pampiniform venous complex of the spermatic cord.

Varicose veins Irregular, tortuous veins with incompetent valves.

Vasectomy Sterilization procedure in which a portion of the spermatic cord is removed.

Vasoconstriction Smooth muscle contraction that narrows the vessel lumen.

Vasodilation Smooth muscle relaxation that expands the vessel lumen.

Vasogenic shock See *Neurogenic shock*.

Venous thrombosis (thrombophlebitis) Blood clot (thrombus) formation on the wall of a vein, accompanied by inflammation of the vein wall and obstructed venous blood flow.

Vertigo Sensation of whirling or rotation.

Very low calorie diet (VLCD) A protein-sparing modified fast (400 to 800 kcal/day or less) under close medical supervision that may be used to treat significant obesity.

Vesicoureteral reflux Condition in which urine moves from the bladder back toward the kidney.

Visceral pain Pain arising from body organs. It is dull and poorly localized because of the low number of nociceptors.

Vital capacity The sum of TV (tidal volume) + IRV (inspiratory reserve volume) + ERV (expiratory reserve volume); approximately 4500 mL in healthy patients.

Vitamin B_{12} deficiency anemia Anemia due to inadequate vitamin B_{12} consumption or impaired absorption.

Vitiligo Abnormal patchy loss of melanin from the skin.

Volatile acids Acids eliminated from the body as a gas.

Volkmann's contracture A common complication of elbow fractures; can result from unresolved compartment syndrome. Arterial blood flow decreases, leading to ischemia, degeneration, and contracture of the muscle.

Vomiting The forceful expulsion of the contents of the upper GI tract resulting from contraction of muscles in the gut and abdominal wall.

Von Willebrand's disease The most common hereditary bleeding disorder, caused by a deficit of or defective von Willebrand factor.

Warm zone Adjacent to the hot zone of a disaster, the area where decontamination of victims or triage and emergency treatment takes place; also called the control zone.

Warts (verrucae) Lesions of the skin caused by the human papillomavirus.

Weaning Process of removing the patient from ventilator support and reestablishing spontaneous, independent respirations.

Weber test A test of hearing; a vibrating tuning fork is placed on the midline of the top of the head and the patient is asked to describe where the sound is heard. Normally, sound is heard equally in both ears.

Wellness An integrated method of functioning oriented toward maximizing an individual's potential within the environment.

Wernicke's encephalopathy Caused by thiamine (B_1) deficiency and characterized by nystagmus, ptosis, ataxia, confusion, coma, and possible death. Thiamine deficiency is common in chronic alcoholism.

Wheezes Continuous, musical sounds caused by narrowing of the lumen in a respiratory passage.

White blood cell (WBCs, leukocytes) The blood cells that contribute to the body's defense against microorganisms.

Wild-type gene The most common type of gene; designated as normal.

Withdrawal Cessation of use of a substance to which an individual has become addicted.

Withdrawal symptoms Constellation of signs and symptoms that occurs in physically dependent individuals when they discontinue drug use.

Xenograft A transplant from an animal species to a human.

Xeroderma A chronic skin condition characterized by dry, rough skin.

Xerosis Dry skin.

Xerostomia Excessive dryness of the mucous membranes due to chemotherapy or radiation.

X-linked Any gene found on the X chromosome, or traits determined by such genes; also refers to the specific mode of inheritance of such genes. One altered gene on an X chromosome in a male can produce disease, such as hemophilia.

X-linked dominant Rare conditions with differential gender outcomes from an altered gene on the X chromosome. For example, if a male is affected, the condition is severe and often lethal. A family history of multiple male miscarriages may be a sign of an X-linked dominant condition.

X-linked recessive The result of an altered gene on the X chromosome. All males with this alteration will express the consequences due to only having one X chromosome. Females may not express the consequence if they have a second normal X chromosome.

Zollinger–Ellison syndrome Peptic ulcer disease caused by a gastrinoma, or gastrin-secreting tumor of the pancreas, stomach, or intestines.

INDEX

Page numbers followed by *f* indicate figures and those followed by *t* indicate tables, boxes, or special features.

acute arterial occlusion, 1048
aneurysm, 1037, 1038*t*
appendicitis, 665–66
benign prostatic hyperplasia, 1662–64, 1662*f*
bone tumors, 1387
brain tumors, 1471, 1471*f*
burns, 460, 462
  autografting, 462
  escharotomy, 460, 460*f*
  surgical debridement, 460
cancer, 358–60
  biopsy, 359*t*
  endoscopy, 359*t*
  lapasoscopy, 359*t*
cardiomyopathy, 1014
central nervous system infection, 1501
cervical cancer, 1695
colorectal cancer, 703–5
COPD, 1244
corneal disorders, 1582–83, 1582*f*
Cushing's syndrome (hypercortisolism), 509
cystic fibrosis, 1251
cysts, 1691
diabetes mellitus, 539
diverticular disease, 694
dysfunctional uterine bleeding, 1685–87
endocarditis, 994
endometrial cancer, 1698
endometriosis, 1693
epilepsy, 1445–46
erectile dysfunction, 1652
eye disorders, 1585*t*, 1603, 1603*t*
gallstones, 724
GERD, 624
glaucoma, 1594
hearing loss, 1616, 1617*f*
hyperparathyroidism, 506
hyperthyroidism, 497
hypothyroidism, 502
increased intracranial pressure, 1440
inflammatory bowel disease
  colectomy, 684, 686
  ostomy, 686
inner ear disorders, 1612
intestinal obstruction, 713–14
kidneys, 834*f*
laryngeal cancer, 1166–67
lung cancer, 1221, 1222*t*
macular degeneration, 1599
melanoma, 430
multiple sclerosis, 1519
neurogenic bladder, 809
nonmelanoma skin cancer, 426
obesity, 594–95
obstructive sleep apnea, 1163
pancreatitis, 754
Parkinson's disease, 1530
pelvic inflammatory disease, 1733
peptic ulcer disease, 638
pericarditis, 999
peritonitis, 668–69
pneumothorax, 1210
pressure ulcer, 437
prostate cancer, 1668–69, 1669*t*
pulmonary embolism, 1258
seizures, 1445–46
skin cancer
  Mohs' surgery, 426
sinusitis, 1148
spinal cord injuries, 1484
spinal cord tumors, 1497
spinal deformity, 1393
stomach cancer, 645–46
testicular cancer, 1658
thrombocytopenia, 1107
trigeminal neuralgia, 1546
urinary incontinence, 813

urinary tract infection, 787
urinary tract tumor
  cystectomy, 801*t*
  partial cystectomy, 801*t*
  transurethral resection of bladder tumor, 801*t*, 802
  urinary diversion, 802, 802*f*, 802*t*
valvular heart disease, 1007–8
varicose veins, 1060
venous thrombosis, 1052, 1054
Surgical assistant, 67
Surgical Care Improve Project (SCIP), 56
Surgical cholangiogram, 574*t*
Surgical debridement, 460
Surgical scrub, 69
Surgical site infections (SSIs), 60*t*, 61, 294
Suspensory ligament, 1559*f*
Sutures, removal, 79
SV. *See* Stroke volume (SV)
SVR. *See* Systemic vascular resistance (SVR)
Swan-neck deformity, 1364, 1365*f*
Sweat glands, 390*t*, 392
Sweeteners, 537
Symmetrel. *See* Amantadine
Sympathectomy, 174, 174*f*
Sympathetic nervous system, 253, 806, 876, 1019
Sympatholytics, 1026*t*
Sympathomimetics, 954–55
Symptoms, in acute illness, 22
Synaral. *See* Fluoxetine
Synarthrosis joints, 1290*t*
Synchronized cardioversion, 955–56, 957*t*
Synchronized intermittent mandatory ventilation (SIMV), 1266
Syndrome of inappropriate ADH secretion (SIADH), 516–17, 1219
Synovial joints, 1292, 1293*f*, 1293*t*
Synovitis, 1300*t*
Synthetic amylin hormone, 535*t*
Syphilis
  Case Study & Nursing Care Plan, 1731*t*
  interdisciplinary care
    diagnosis, 1729–30
    medications, 1730
  latent or tertiary, 1729
  manifestations, 1729, 1730*t*
  nursing care
    anxiety, 1731–32
    assessment, 1730
    community-based care, 1732
    nursing diagnoses and interventions, 1731
    risk for injury, 1731
    situational low self-esteem, 1732
  pathophysiology, 1729
  primary, 1729, 1729*f*
  secondary, 1729
Syphilis screening tests, 1631*t*
Systemic circulation, 872, 873*f*, 1255
  arteries, 877*f*
  veins, 878*f*
Systemic inflammatory response syndrome (SIRS), 259
Systemic lupus erythematosus (SLE), 315, 850*t*
  fast facts, 1374
  interdisciplinary care
    diagnosis, 1377
    medications, 1377, 1378*t*
    treatments, 1377
  manifestations, 1375*f*, 1375–77, 1376*f*, 1377*t*
  nursing care
    community-based care, 1379
    diagnoses and interventions, 1378–79
  pathophysiology, 1375

Systemic sclerosis
  fast facts, 1389
  interdisciplinary care
    diagnosis, 1389
    medications, 1389–90
    physical therapy, 1390
  manifestations, 1389*f*, 1389
  nursing care
    community-based care, 1390
    interventions, 1390
  pathophysiology, 1389
Systemic vascular resistance (SVR), 253
Systole, 873, 874*f*
Systolic blood pressure, 1019
Systolic heart failure, 974

T

Tachypnea, 1135*t*, 1146
Tacrine hydrochloride, 1513*t*
Tacrolimus, 320*t*
Tachydysrhythmias, 946
Tadalafil, 1652
Tagamet. *See* Cimetidine
Talwin. *See* Pentazocine
Tamiflu. *See* Oseltamivir
Tamofen. *See* Tamoxifen
Tamoxifen, 361, 1342, 1708, 1709*t*
Tamsulosin, 795, 1662
Tangier disease, 569*t*
Tapeworm, 679*t*
Target cells, 1074
Tar preparations, 408
Tasmar. *See* Tolcapone
Tavist. *See* Clesmastine
Taxol. *See* Paclitaxel
T cells, 270*t*, 272–73
T-cell suppressors, 320*t*
Team nursing, 14
Teeth, age-related changes, 576*t*
Tegretol. *See* Carbamazepine
Telangiectases, 396*t*, 407
Telbivudine, 732
Telemetry, 954
Teletherapy, 365
Temporal lobe, 1409*f*, 1410*t*
TEN. *See* Toxic epidermal necrolysis (TEN)
Tendonitis, 1300*t*
Tendons, 1290, 1292–93
Tennis elbow, 1308
Tenofovir, 732
TENS. *See* Transcutaneous electrical nerve stimulation (TENS)
Tensilon. *See* Edrophonium chloride
Tension pneumothorax, 241, 1207, 1208*f*, 1209
Teratoma, 1657
Terazosin, 1662
Terminal weaning, 1269
Terrorism
  bioterrorism, 126, 126*t*
  definition, 125
  nuclear/radiologic, 126–27
  weapons used in, 125
Tertiary intention, 78, 78*f*
Testes, 1630, 1632*t*
  disorders
    cancer. *See* Testicular cancer
    orchitis, 1656–57
    torsion, 1657
  self-examination, 1658*t*

Special Features